SAUNDERS DICTIONARIES AND VOCABULARY AIDS

Dorland's Illustrated Medical Dictionary

Dorland's Pocket Medical Dictionary

Chabner: The Language of Medicine

Cole: The Doctor's Shorthand

Jablonski: Illustrated Dictionary of Eponymic Syndromes and Diseases

Leader & Leader: Dictionary of Comparative Pathology and Experimental Biology

Miller-Keane: Encyclopedia and Dictionary of Medicine, Nursing, and Allied Health

Sloane: The Medical Word Book – A Spelling and Vocabulary Guide to Medical Transcription

Sloane: The Legal Speller

Encyclopedia and Dictionary of Medicine, Nursing, and Allied Health

Second Edition

by the late BENJAMIN F. MILLER, M.D.
and
CLAIRE BRACKMAN KEANE, R.N., B.S., M.Ed.

with 139 illustrations, including 16 color plates; 36 tables; 12 appendices

W. B. SAUNDERS COMPANY • Philadelphia • London • Toronto

W. B. Saunders Company: West Washington Square
Philadelphia, PA 19105

1 St. Anne's Road
Eastbourne, East Sussex BN21 3UN, England

1 Goldthorne Avenue
Toronto, Ontario M8Z 5T9, Canada

Encyclopedia and Dictionary of Medicine, Nursing, and Allied Health ISBN 0-7216-6357-5

Last digit is the print number: 9 8 7 6 5 4 3 2 1

PUBLISHER'S FOREWORD
TO THE FIRST EDITION

Behind every encyclopedia/dictionary lie immense labor, high purpose and great hope. Whether that labor has been well done, purpose fulfilled and hope justified is a determination to be made only by the reader. As Johnson so bluntly put it in the Preface to his *Dictionary of the English Language,* "The value of a work must be estimated by its use; it is not enough that a dictionary delights the critic, unless at the same time, it instructs the learner."

Therefore as the reader considers the pages to follow and whether their millions of individual letters have been well put together, he should know what philosophy has animated this work and what use has been foreseen for it.

Its philosophy can be simply put. Especially in a time of expanding details of knowledge, the first requirement for teaching, learning and communication by scientists and professional persons is the existence of an agreed-upon vocabulary of terms. Indeed the first and vital step in learning any discipline is mastery and understanding of its language. It is the intent of this *Encyclopedia and Dictionary of Medicine and Nursing* to provide precisely such an authoritative vocabulary for students and learners of all ages and degrees in the nursing and paramedical sciences.

Although a dictionary must have authority, it may not pretend to dictate. The language of science has not descended to us in a state of uniformity and perfection. Words are like their authors; when they are not gaining strength, they are generally losing it.

In fine, the purpose of an encyclopedia/dictionary is to afford a body of knowledge built upon usage – not upon fixed canons of philology. The skill of such a work lies in its understanding of usage, its reasoned selection of terms, its accuracy and usefulness of definition and its rational adjudication of conflict in terminology. These characters in the work have had their achievement through a variety of means.

The Authors: Creation of this reference source has involved the special knowledge and assistance of many people; but the carrying out of its essential concepts has been the responsibility of its two authors, Benjamin F. Miller, M.D., and Claire Brackman Keane, R.N.

Dr. Miller's sudden death occurred after he had completed work on this manuscript of the Encyclopedia/Dictionary but before he could see it brought to print. He would have relished seeing the printed work, for Dr. Miller was, above all, a bookish man. He felt that "a good book is the best of friends, the same today and forever."

His professional life was given to clinical investigation to which he made significant contribution as Director of the May Institute and whose findings he applied dynamically to the practice of internal medicine, especially the management of cardiovascular disease. At the same time he somehow found time for both the reading and writing of books. His experience as Editor-in-Chief of the *Modern Medical Encyclopedia* honed to a sharp edge his innate capacity to present complex matters in concise and readily understandable form. The Golden Press has graciously allowed adaptation of some of the entries of his *Encyclopedia* for use in the present work.

Dr. Miller was fortunate above all in his coauthor, Claire Brackman Keane, who brought to the work long and thoughtful experience in nursing education, nursing service and textbook authorship. To her critical mind every word was a new and unavoidable challenge. To selection and definition she brought a capacious memory and a sharp sense of what constitutes relevance and usefulness of detail.

The Consultants: Accuracy of the work has demanded not only contemporaneity of content but provision of altogether new definitions keeping pace with the great advances in the sciences which comprise the mosaic of medicine, such as the swift-moving disciplines of genetics, neuroscience, molecular biology, pharmacology, biochemistry and microbiology. Here both authors and publisher have been fortunate in being able to consult with the foremost authors of basic-science texts in English. It is a pleasure to record that the response to calls for counsel and specific advices was always prompt and helpful. To his writers of books in all areas of medicine, nursing and their supporting sciences the publisher owes a debt of gratitude that cannot be repaid but is reflected in the authority of the work here presented.

The Sources: These have been many and varied; but the authors have freely called upon two splendid lexicons for help—the current editions of *Dorland's Illustrated Medical Dictionary* and *Dorland's Pocket Medical Dictionary.* Occasionally entries from these two dictionaries have been sharpened or simplified or revised, in these instances the dictionaries providing a sure entry point for such elaboration and modification.

In one area the authors alone have been responsible for the framing of suitable entries. These are the encyclopedic terms. Their purpose has been to provide a full picture of the nature of disease and disease process, and of the principles of nursing management. Tables too are an important part of the useful encyclopedic character of the work, and their formulations have been checked and rechecked against original sources to secure an error-free compendium of specific data.

Illustrations: The drawing of fresh figures for the work has been under the supervision of Grant Lashbrook, Art Director of the Saunders Company; and the 16 anatomic plates in color represent a distillation of morphologic knowledge useful to both the beginning student and the experienced nurse and physician.

Typography: The alphabet is an extraordinarily ancient and ingenious device for communication and storage of information, and even the present-day forms of its letters derive from Roman and Arabic sources. Hence it is appropriate that typography (an expression of the alphabet) be traditional and conservative. Design of this book has been in the hands of Lorraine Battista, who has given just care to its openness, legibility and attractiveness. Such a small device as beginning each subentry on a new line consults not economy but the convenience of the reader and pleasantness of the page.

Comparative Brevity: Partly by concision of expression, partly by tough-minded selection and partly by ignoring useless accretions of the past this Encyclopedia/Dictionary has been kept modest in size. It is not, in the Duke of Gloucester's phrase, "another damned, thick, square book," but rather an inviting book in large format whose consultation will be rewarding and may justify the hopes with which its preparation was attended.

Finally, the use of this book of words will be assisted by appreciation of the essential fact that words are not things-in-themselves—they are rather *signs* of things, whose validity and use rest upon convention, the purpose of lexicography being the codification and clarification of these conventions. Again we may quote Johnson: "I am not yet so lost in lexicography as to forget that *words are the daughters of earth, and that things are the sons of heaven.* Language is only the instrument of science, and words are but the signs of ideas: I wish, however, that the instrument might be less apt to decay and that signs might be permanent, like the things which they denote."

W. B. SAUNDERS COMPANY

PREFACE
TO THE SECOND EDITION

The second edition of the Encyclopedia and Dictionary includes the allied health sciences in its title to reflect the concept of patient care as a shared responsibility of all members of the health care team. Territorial boundaries that delineate the area of function and expertise of each discipline are becoming increasingly more blurred. Team leadership is no longer the prerogative of any one discipline, but rather the function of the person or group best suited to meet the needs of a particular patient at a particular time and in a particular health care setting. This requires a commitment to values that transcend personal and professional goals. It further demands a knowledge and appreciation of the contribution each team member can make toward achieving the goal of quality health care.

In this second edition the supportive, preventive, and therapeutic aspects of patient care are presented under the heading *Patient Care* in recognition of the concept of patient-centered care. Decisions regarding new entries and the reorganization and updating of those that appeared in the first edition were based on the belief that a published work intended to serve an expanding community of health care professionals and paraprofessionals should strive to seek and emphasize commonalities in knowledge and skills needed in the delivery of health care.

Further, it has been assumed that a primary objective of all members of the health care team is assisting clients in health maintenance and disease prevention, and that the achievement of that objective in no small way depends on the cooperative efforts of an informed client. Therefore patient education has been stressed throughout the second edition. The Appendix contains a new listing of sources for patient education materials as well as an updated list of agencies and organizations concerned with the promotion of health and management of disease.

Also new in the Appendix are a compilation of laboratory reference values and a tabulation of the Recommended Dietary Allowances of the Food and Nutrition Board.

It is not possible to identify by name all of the persons who have shared in the preparation of the second edition. I am particularly grateful to those readers who expressed their thoughts and made known their suggestions for improvement of the first edition. For suggestions regarding the inclusion of additional material in the allied health sciences, I am especially indebted to Drs. Lucille Daniels, Catherine Worthingham, Stanley S. Raphael, and Irwin Ziment. A very special note of thanks must go to Nancy Raley, who conscientiously typed the manuscript with astounding skill and accuracy. Robert E. Wright, former Nursing Editor of the W. B. Saunders Co., and Helen Dietz, Senior Nursing Editor, provided continuous support and direction. It was

Mr. Wright who first approached me about co-editing the Encyclopedia/Dictionary with Dr. Benjamin Miller, and I am profoundly grateful to him for that opportunity. John Friel, Dictionary Editor, and his Associate Editor, Kitty McCullough, have fulfilled their editorial responsibilities far beyond the call of duty. To each of these and to all who have brought this second edition to fruition I wish to extend a sincere "Thank you."

CLAIRE B. KEANE
Athens, Georgia

CONTENTS

NOTES
ON THE USE OF THIS BOOK

Cross References

Words set in SMALL CAPITALS denote cross references. They are used liberally, and the reader is well advised to turn to the term so noted, because he will find important additional information there. For example, within the definition for *rejection* there is a cross reference to TRANSPLANTATION, because the problem of rejection is discussed fully in the encyclopedic definition for *transplantation.* In the *pregnancy* definition a cross reference to ABORTION shows the reader that a fuller discussion of that subject is given at *abortion.*

Compound Terms

Terms composed of a noun modified by a descriptive or eponymic designation are defined under the adjective or eponym when logic dictates. Thus, the definition for *plastic surgery* appears at *plastic,* not at *surgery. Parkinson's disease* is defined at *Parkinson's,* not at *disease. Boric acid* is defined at *boric,* not at *acid.*

In certain cases, when the logical placement of the full definition seems less clear-cut, a summary definition is given as a subentry under the noun entry, and a cross reference directs the reader to the complete definition at the modifying term. This is done, for example, in the *balance* entry, where the subentry for *acid-base balance* gives a one-sentence definition and a cross reference to the main definition in the A's. *Bell's palsy* is treated similarly, with the full definition at *Bell's* and a short definition and cross reference at *palsy.*

It is hoped that this system will save the reader time and effort by giving the full information where he is most likely to look for it.

Sequence of Entries

Entries are alphabetized according to the sequence of their letters, regardless of space or hyphens that may occur between them. Thus sequences such as

heart	carbon
heartbeat	carbonate
heart block	carbon dioxide
heartburn	carbonemia
heart failure	carbonic acid
heart-lung machine	carbonize
heart murmur	carbon monoxide

appear in that order. An exception to this occurs in eponymous terms: only the proper name is considered in such instances. That is, the apostrophe s ('s) is ignored, as is the second word of the eponym. Thus *Kline test* precedes *Klinefelter's syndrome, Leydig cells* precedes *leydigarche, Parkinson's disease* precedes *parkinsonian,* and so on.

Pronunciation

The pronunciation of words is indicated by a simple phonetic respelling in parentheses. Diacritical markings to distinguish vowel sounds are used only when necessary.

An unmarked vowel ending a syllable is long (ba′be).

An unmarked vowel in a syllable ending with a consonant is short (ab-dukt′).

A long vowel in a syllable that must end with a consonant is indicated by a macron (be-hāv′yer).

A short vowel that constitutes or ends a syllable is marked with a breve (ĕ-de′mah; ab′stĭ-nens).

The syllable *ah* is used for the sound of *a* in open, unaccented syllables (ah-bor′shun).

The primary accent in a word is indicated by a bold face, single accent. The secondary accent is indicated by a light face, double accent.

Abbreviations

Abbreviations used in the text of the definitions are few and fairly obvious. They include

adj. (adjective)	It. (Italian)
Fr. (French)	L. (Latin)
Ger. (German)	pl. (plural)
Gr. (Greek)	

In elaboration of entries that are themselves abbreviations, the words "abbreviation for" have been omitted.

COMBINING FORMS
IN MEDICAL TERMINOLOGY*

The following is a list of combining forms encountered frequently in the vocabulary of medicine. A dash or dashes are appended to indicate whether the form usually precedes (as *ante-*) or follows (as *-agra*) the other elements of the compound or usually appears between the other elements (as *-em-*). Following each combining form, the first item of information is the Greek or Latin word, or both a Greek and a Latin word, from which it is derived. Those words that are not printed in Greek characters are Latin. Information necessary to an understanding of the form appears next in parentheses. Then the meaning or meanings of the word are given, followed where appropriate by reference to a synonymous combining form. Finally, an example is given to illustrate the use of the combining form in a compound English derivative.

a-	ἀ- (*n* is added before words beginning with a vowel) negative prefix. Cf. in-[3]. *a*metria
ab-	*ab* away from. Cf. apo-. *ab*ducent
abdomin-	*abdomen, abdominis*. *abdomin*oscopy
ac-	See ad-. *ac*cretion
acet-	*acetum* vinegar. *acet*ometer
acid-	*acidus* sour. *acid*uric
acou-	ἀκούω hear. *acou*esthesia. (Also spelled acu-)
acr-	ἄκρον extremity, peak. *acro*megaly
act-	*ago, actus* do, drive, act. re*act*ion
actin-	ἀκτίς, ἀκτῖνος ray, radius. Cf. radi-. *actin*ogenesis
acu-	See acou-. osteo*acu*sis
ad-	*ad* (*d* changes to *c, f, g, p, s,* or *t* before words beginning with those consonants) to. *ad*renal
aden-	ἀδήν gland. Cf. gland-. *aden*oma
adip-	*adeps, adipis* fat. Cf. lip- and stear-. *adip*ocellular
aer-	ἀήρ air. an*aer*obiosis
aesthe-	See esthe-. *aesthe*sioneurosis
af-	See ad-. *af*ferent
ag-	See ad-. *ag*glutinant
-agogue	ἀγωγός leading, inducing. galact*agogue*
-agra	ἄγρα catching, seizure. pod*agra*
alb-	*albus* white. Cf. leuk-. *albo*cinereous
alg-	ἄλγος pain. neur*alg*ia
all-	ἄλλος other, different. *all*ergy
alve-	*alveus* trough, channel, cavity. *alve*olar
amph-	See amphi-. *amph*eclexis
amphi-	ἀμφί (*i* is dropped before words beginning with a vowel) both, doubly. *amphi*celous
amyl-	ἄμυλον starch. *amyl*osynthesis
an-[1]	See ana-. *an*agogic
an-[2]	See a-. *an*omalous
ana-	ἀνά (final *a* is dropped before words beginning with a vowel) up, positive. *ana*phoresis
ancyl-	See ankyl-. *ancyl*ostomiasis
andr-	ἀνήρ, ἀνδρός man. gyn*andr*oid
angi-	ἀγγεῖον vessel. Cf. vas-. *angi*emphraxis
ankyl-	ἀγκύλος crooked, looped. *ankyl*odactylia. (Also spelled ancyl-)
ant-	See anti-. *ant*ophthalmic
ante-	*ante* before. *ante*flexion
anti-	ἀντί (*i* is dropped before words beginning with a vowel) against, counter. Cf. contra-. *anti*pyogenic
antr-	ἄντρον cavern. *antr*odynia
ap-[1]	See apo-. *ap*heter
ap-[2]	See ad-. *ap*pend
-aph-	ἅπτω, ἀφ- touch. dys*aph*ia. (See also hapt-)
apo-	ἀπό (*o* is dropped before words beginning with a vowel) away from, detached. Cf. ab-. *apo*physis
arachn-	ἀράχνη spider. *arachn*odactyly
arch-	ἀρχή beginning, origin. *arch*enteron

*Compiled by Lloyd W. Daly, A.M., Ph.D., Litt, D., Allen Memorial Professor of Greek, University of Pennsylvania.

arter(i)-	ἀρτηρία elevator (?), artery. *arterio*sclerosis, peri*arter*itis
arthr-	ἄρθρον joint. Cf. articul-. syn*arthr*osis
articul-	*articulus* joint. Cf. arthr-. dis*articul*ation
as-	See ad-. *as*similation
at-	See ad-. *at*trition
aur-	*auris* ear. Cf. ot-. *aur*inasal
aux-	αὔξω increase. enter*auxe*
ax-	ἄξων or *axis* axis. *ax*ofugal
axon-	ἄξων axis. *axon*ometer
ba-	βαίνω, βα- go, walk, stand. hypno*ba*tia
bacill-	*bacillus* small staff, rod. Cf. bacter-. actino*bacill*osis
bacter-	βακτήριον small staff, rod. Cf. bacill-. *bacter*iophage
ball-	βάλλω, βολ- throw. *ball*istics. (See also bol-)
bar-	βάρος weight. pedo*bar*ometer
bi-[1]	βίος life. Cf. vit-. aero*bi*c
bi-[2]	*bi-* two (see also di-[1]). *bi*lobate
bil-	*bilis* bile. Cf. chol-. *bil*iary
blast-	βλαστός bud, child, a growing thing in its early stages. Cf. germ-. *blast*oma, zygoto*blast*.
blep-	βλέπω look, see. hemia*blep*sia
blephar-	βλέφαρον (from βλέπω; see blep-) eyelid. Cf. cili-. *blephar*oncus
bol-	See ball-. em*bol*ism
brachi-	βραχίων arm. *brachi*ocephalic
brachy-	βραχύς short. *brachy*cephalic
brady-	βραδύς slow. *brady*cardia
brom-	βρῶμος stench. podo*brom*idrosis
bronch-	βρόγχος windpipe. *bronch*oscopy
bry-	βρύω be full of life. em*bry*onic
bucc-	*bucca* cheek. disto*bucc*al
cac-	κακός bad, abnormal. Cf. mal-. *cac*odontia, arthro*cace*. (See also dys-)
calc-[1]	*calx, calcis* stone (cf. lith-), limestone, lime. *calc*ipexy
calc-[2]	*calx, calcis* heel. *calc*aneotibial
calor-	*calor* heat. Cf. therm-. *calor*imeter
cancr-	*cancer, cancri* crab, cancer. Cf. carcin-. *cancr*ology. (Also spelled chancr-)
capit-	*caput, capitis* head. Cf. cephal-. de*capit*ator
caps-	*capsa* (from *capio;* see cept-) container. en*caps*ulation
carbo(n)-	*carbo, carbonis* coal, charcoal. *carbo*hydrate, *carbon*uria
carcin-	καρκίνος crab, cancer. Cf. cancr-. *carcin*oma
cardi-	καρδία heart. lipo*cardi*ac
cary-	See kary-. *cary*okinesis
cat-	See cata-. *cat*hode
cata-	κατά (final *a* is dropped before words beginning with a vowel) down, negative. *cata*batic
caud-	*cauda* tail. *caud*ad
cav-	*cavus* hollow. Cf. coel-. con*cave*
cec-	*caecus* blind. Cf. typhl-. *cec*opexy
cel-[1]	See coel-. amphi*cel*ous
cel-[2]	See -cele. *cel*ectome
-cele	κήλη tumor, hernia. gastro*cele*
cell-	*cella* room, cell. Cf. cyt-. *cell*iferous
cen-	κοινός common. *cen*esthesia
cent-	*centum* hundred. Cf. hect-. Indicates fraction in metric system. [This exemplifies the custom in the metric system of identifying fractions of units by stems from the Latin, as centimeter, decimeter, millimeter, and multiples of units by the similar stems from the Greek, as hectometer, decameter, and kilometer.] *cent*imeter, *centi*pede
cente-	κεντέω puncture. Cf. punct-. entero*cente*sis
centr-	κέντρον or *cenrum* point, center. neuro*centr*al
cephal-	κεφαλή head. Cf. capit-. en*cephal*itis
cept-	*capio, -cipientis, -ceptus* take, receive. re*cept*or
cer-	κηρός or *cera* wax. *cer*oplasty, *cer*omel
cerat-	See kerat-. a*cerat*osis
cerebr-	*cerebrum*. *cerebr*ospinal
cervic-	*cervix, cervicis* neck. Cf. trachel-. *cervic*itis
chancr-	See cancr-. *chancr*iform
cheil-	χεῖλος lip. Cf. labi-. *cheil*oschisis
cheir-	χείρ hand. Cf. man-. macro*cheir*ia. (Also spelled chir-)
chir-	See cheir-. *chir*omegaly
chlor-	χλωρός green. a*chlor*opsia
chol-	χολή bile. Cf. bil-. hepato*chol*angeitis
chondr-	χόνδρος cartilage. *chondr*omalacia
chord-	χορδή string, cord. peri*chord*al
chori-	χόριον protective fetal membrane. endo*chori*on
chro-	χρώς color. poly*chro*matic
chron-	χρόνος time. syn*chron*ous
chy-	χέω, χυ- pour. ec*chy*mosis
-cid(e)	*caedo, -cisus* cut, kill. infanti*cide*, germi*cid*al
cili-	*cilium* eyelid. Cf. blephar-. super*cili*ary
cine-	See kine-. auto*cine*sis
-cipient	See cept-. in*cipient*
circum-	*circum* around. Cf. peri-. *circum*ferential
-cis-	*caedo, -cisus* cut, kill. ex*cis*ion
clas-	κλάω, κλασ- break. cranio*clas*t
clin-	κλίνω bend, incline, make lie down. *clin*ometer
clus-	*claudo, -clusus* shut. Maloc*clus*ion
co-	See con-. *co*hesion
cocc-	κόκκος seed, pill. gono*cocc*us
coel-	κοῖλος hollow. Cf. cav-. *coel*enteron. (Also spelled cel-)
col-[1]	See colon-. *col*ic
col-[2]	See con-. *col*lapse

colon- κόλον lower intestine. *colon*ic
colp- κόλπος hollow, vagina. Cf. sin-. endo*colp*itis
com- See con-. *com*masculation
con- *con-* (becomes co- before vowels or *h;* col- before *l;* com- before *b, m,* or *p;* cor- before *r*) with, together. Cf. syn-. *con*traction
contra- *contra* against, counter. Cf. anti-. *contra*indication
copr- κόπρος dung. Cf. sterco-. *copr*oma
cor-[1] κόρη doll, little image, pupil. iso*cor*ia
cor-[2] See con-. *cor*rugator
corpor- *corpus, corporis* body. Cf. somat-. intra*corpor*al
cortic- *cortex, corticis* bark, rind. *cortic*osterone
cost- *costa* rib. Cf. pleur-. inter*cost*al
crani- κρανίον or *cranium* skull. peri*crani*um
creat- κρέας, κρεατ- meat, flesh. *creat*orrhea
-crescent *cresco, crescentis, cretus* grow. ex*crescent*
cret-[1] *cerno, cretus* distinguish, separate off. Cf. crin-. dis*crete*
cret-[2] See -crescent. ac*cret*ion
crin- κρίνω distinguish, separate off. Cf. cret-[1]. endo*crin*ology
crur- *crus, cruris* shin, leg. brachio*crur*al
cry- κρύος cold. *cry*esthesia
crypt- κρύπτω hide, conceal. *crypt*orchism
cult- *colo, cultus* tend, cultivate. *cult*ure
cune- *cuneus* wedge. Cf. sphen-. *cune*iform
cut- *cutis* skin. Cf. derm(at)-. sub*cut*aneous
cyan- κύανος blue. antho*cyan*in
cycl- κύκλος circle, cycle. *cycl*ophoria
cyst- κύστις bladder. Cf. vesic-. nephro*cyst*itis
cyt- κύτος cell. Cf. cell-. plasmo*cyt*oma
dacry- δάκρυ tear. *dacry*ocyst
dactyl- δάκτυλος finger, toe. Cf. digit-. hexa*dactyl*ism
de- *de* down from. *de*composition
dec-[1] δέκα ten. Indicates multiple in metric system. Cf. dec-[2]. *dec*agram
dec-[2] *decem* ten. Indicates fraction in metric system. Cf. dec-[1]. *dec*ipara, *dec*imeter
dendr- δένδρον tree. neuro*dendr*ite
dent- *dens, dentis* tooth. Cf. odont-. inter*dent*al
derm(at)- δέρμα, δέρματος skin. Cf. cut-. endo*derm*, *dermat*itis
desm- δεσμός band, ligament. syn*desm*opexy
dextr- *dexter, dextr-* right-hand. ambi*dextr*ous
di-[1] *di-* two. *di*morphic. (See also bi-[2])
di-[2] See dia-. *di*uresis.
di-[3] See dis-. *di*vergent.
dia- διά (*a* is dropped before words beginning with a vowel) through, apart. Cf. per-. *dia*gnosis
didym- δίδυμος twin. Cf. gemin-. epi*didym*al
digit- *digitus* finger, toe. Cf. dactyl-. *digit*igrade
diplo- διπλόος double. *diplo*myelia
dis- *dis-* (*s* may be dropped before a word beginning with a consonant) apart, away from. *dis*location
disc- δίσκος or *discus* disk. *disc*oplacenta
dors- *dorsum* back. ventro*dors*al
drom- δρόμος course. hemo*drom*ometer
-ducent See duct-. ad*ducent*
duct- *duco, ducentis, ductus* lead, conduct. ovi*duct*
dur- *durus* hard. Cf. scler-. in*dura*tion
dynam(i)- δύναμις power. *dynam*oneure, neuro*dynamic*
dys- δυσ- bad, improper. Cf. mal-. *dys*trophic. (See also cac-)
e- *e* out from. Cf. ec- and ex-. *e*mission
ec- ἐκ out of. Cf. e- *ec*centric
-ech- ἔχω have, hold, be. syn*ech*otomy
ect- ἐκτός outside. Cf. extra-. *ect*oplasm
ede- οἰδέω swell. *ede*matous
ef- See ex-. *ef*florescent
-elc- ἕλκος sore, ulcer. enter*elc*osis. (See also *helc-*)
electr- ἤλεκτρον amber. *electr*otherapy
em- See en-. *em*bolism, *em*pathy, *em*phlysis
-em- αἷμα blood. an*em*ia. (See also hem(at)-)
en- ἐν (*n* changes to *m* before *b, p,* or *ph*) in, on. Cf. in-[2]. *en*celitis
end- ἔνδον inside. Cf. intra-. *end*angium.
enter- ἔντερον intestine. dys*enter*y
ep- See epi-. *ep*axial
epi- ἐπί (*i* is dropped before words beginning with a vowel) upon, after, in addition. *epi*glottis
erg- ἔργον work, deed. en*erg*y
erythr- ἐρυθρός red. Cf. rub(r)-. *erythr*ochromia
eso- ἔσω inside. Cf. intra-. *eso*phylactic
esthe- αἰσθάνομαι, αἰσθη- perceive, feel. Cf. sens-. an*esthe*sia
eu- εὖ good, normal. *eu*pepsia
ex- ἐξ or *ex* out of. Cf. e-. *ex*cretion
exo- ἔξω outside. Cf. extra-. *exo*pathic
extra- *extra* outside of, beyond. Cf. ect- and exo-. *extra*cellular
faci- *facies* face. Cf. prosop-. brachio*faci*olingual

-facient *facio, facientis, factus, -fectus* make. Cf. poie-. cale*facient*
-fact- See facient-. arte*fact*
fasci- *fascia* band. *fascio*rrhaphy
febr- *febris* fever. Cf. pyr-. *febr*icide
-fect- See -facient. de*fect*ive
-ferent *fero, ferentis, latus* bear, carry. Cf. phor-. ef*ferent*
ferr- *ferrum* iron. *ferro*protein
fibr- *fibra* fibre. Cf. in-[1]. chondro*fibr*oma
fil- *filum* thread. *fil*iform
fiss- *findo, fissus* split. Cf. schis-. *fiss*ion
flagell- *flagellum* whip. *flagell*ation
flav- *flavus* yellow. Cf. xanth-. ribo*flav*in
-flect- *flecto, flexus* bend, divert. de*flect*ion
-flex- See -flect-. re*flex*ometer
flu- *fluo, fluxus* flow. Cf. rhe-. *flu*id
flux- See flu-. af*flux*ion
for- *foris* door, opening. per*for*ated
-form *forma* shape. Cf. -oid. ossi*form*
fract- *frango, fractus* break. re*fract*ive
front- *frons, frontis* forehead, front. naso*front*al
-fug(e) *fugio* flee, avoid. vermi*fuge*, centri*fug*al
funct- *fungor, functus* perform, serve, function. mal*funct*ion
fund- *fundo, fusus* pour. in*fund*ibulum
fus- See fund-. dif*fus*ible
galact- γάλα, γάλακτος milk. Cf. lact-. dys*galact*ia
gam- γάμος marriage, reproductive union. a*gam*ont
gangli- γάγγλιον swelling, plexus. neuro*gangli*itis
gastr- γαστήρ, γαστρός stomach. cholangio*gastr*ostomy
gelat- *gelo, gelatus* freeze, congeal. *gelat*in
gemin- *geminus* twin, double. Cf. didym-. quadri*gemin*al
gen- γίγνομαι, γεν-, γον- become, be produced, originate, or γεννάω produce, originate. cyto*gen*ic
germ- *germen, germinis* bud, a growing thing in its early stages. Cf. blast-. *germ*inal, ovi*germ*
gest- *gero, gerentis, gestus* bear, carry. con*gest*ion
gland- *glans, glandis* acorn. Cf. aden-. intra*gland*ular
-glia γλία glue. neuro*glia*
gloss- γλῶσσα tongue. Cf. lingu-. tricho*gloss*ia
glott- γλῶττα tongue, language. *glott*ic
gluc- See glyc(y)-. *gluc*ophenetidin
glutin- *gluten, glutinis* glue. ag*glutin*ation
glyc(y)- γλυκύς sweet. *glyc*emia, *glycyr*rhizin. (Also spelled gluc-)
gnath- γνάθος jaw. ortho*gnath*ous
gno- γιγνώσκω, γνω- know, discern. dia*gno*sis
gon- See gen-. amphi*gony*
grad- *gradior* walk, take steps. retro*grade*
-gram γράφω, γραφ- + -μα scratch, write, record. cardio*gram*
gran- *granum* grain, particle. lipo*gran*uloma
graph- γράφω scratch, write, record. histo*graphy*
grav- *gravis* heavy. multi*grav*ida
gyn(ec)- γυνή, γυναικός woman, wife. andro*gyny*, *gynec*ologic
gyr- γῦρος ring, circle. *gyro*spasm
haem(at)- See hem(at)-. *haem*orrhagia, *haemat*oxylon
hapt- ἅπτω touch. *hapt*ometer
hect- ἑκτ- hundred. Cf. cent-. Indicates multiple in metric system. *hect*ometer
helc- ἕλκος sore, ulcer. *helc*osis
hem(at)- αἷμα, αἵματος blood. Cf. sanguin-. *hem*angioma, *hemato*cyturia. (See also -em-)
hemi- ἡμι- half. Cf. semi-. *hemi*ageusia
hen- εἷς, ἑνός one. Cf. un-. *hen*ogenesis
hepat- ἧπαρ, ἥπατος liver. gastro*hepat*ic
hept(a)- ἑπτά seven. Cf. sept-[2]. *hept*atomic, *hepta*valent
hered- *heres, heredis* heir. *hered*oimmunity
hex-[1] ἕξ six. Cf. sex-. *hex*yl-. An *a* is added in some combinations.
hex-[2] ἔχω, ἐχ- (added to σ becomes ἑξ-) have, hold, be. ca*chexy*
hexa- See hex-[1]. *hexa*chromic
hidr- ἱδρώς sweat. hyper*hidr*osis
hist- ἱστός web, tissue. *hist*odialysis
hod- ὁδός road, path. *hod*oneuromere. (See also od- and -ode[1])
hom- ὁμός common, same. *homo*morphic
horm- ὁρμή impetus, impulse. *horm*one
hydat- ὕδωρ, ὕδατος water. *hydat*ism
hydr- ὕδωρ, ὑδρ- water. Cf. lymph-. achlor*hydr*ia
hyp- See hypo-. *hyp*axial
hyper- ὑπέρ above, beyond, extreme. Cf. super-. *hyper*trophy
hypn- ὕπνος sleep. *hypn*otic
hypo- ὑπό (*o* is dropped before words beginning with a vowel) under, below. Cf. sub-. *hypo*metabolism
hyster- ὑστέρα womb. colpo*hyster*opexy
iatr- ἰατρός physician. ped*iatr*ics
idi- ἴδιος peculiar, separate, distinct. *idi*osyncrasy
il- See in-[2, 3]. *il*linition (in, on), *il*legible (negative prefix)
ile- See ili- [ile- is commonly used to refer to the portion of the

intestines known as the ileum]. *ile*ostomy
ili- *ilium* (*ileum*) lower abdomen, intestines [ili- is commonly used to refer to the flaring part of the hip bone known as the ilium]. *ili*osacral
im- See in-[2,3]. *im*mersion (in, on), *im*perforation (negative prefix)
in-[1] ἶς, ἰνός fiber. Cf. fibr-. *in*osteatoma
in-[2] *in* (*n* changes to *l*, *m*, or *r* before words beginning with those consonants) in, on. Cf. en-. *in*sertion
in-[3] *in-* (*n* changes to *l*, *m*, or *r* before words beginning with those consonants) negative prefix. Cf. a-. *in*valid
infra- *infra* beneath. *infra*orbital
insul- *insula* island. *insul*in
inter- *inter* among, between. *inter*carpal
intra- *intra* inside. Cf. end- and eso-. *intra*venous
ir- See in-[2,3]. *ir*radiation (in, on), *ir*reducible (negative prefix)
irid- ἶρις, ἴριδος rainbow, colored circle. kerato*irid*ocyclitis
is- ἴσος equal. *is*otope
ischi- ἰσχίον hip, haunch. *ischi*opubic
jact- *iacio*, *iactus* throw. *jact*itation
ject- *iacio*, *-iectus* throw. in*ject*ion
jejun- *ieiunus* hungry, not partaking of food. gastro*jejun*ostomy
jug- *iugum* yoke. con*jug*ation
junct- *iungo*, *iunctus* yoke, join. con*junct*iva
kary- κάρυον nut, kernel, nucleus. Cf. nucle-. mega*kary*ocyte. (Also spelled cary-)
kerat- κέρας, κέρατος horn. *kerat*olysis. (Also spelled cerat-)
kil- χίλιοι one thousand. Cf. mill-. Indicates multiple in metric system. *kil*ogram
kine- κινέω move. *kine*matograph. (Also spelled cine-)
labi- *labium* lip. Cf. cheil-. gingivo*labi*al
lact- *lac*, *lactis* milk. Cf. galact-. gluco*lact*one
lal- λαλέω talk, babble. glosso*lal*ia
lapar- λαπάρα flank. *lapar*otomy
laryng- λάρυγξ, λάρυγγος windpipe. *laryng*endoscope
lat- *fero*, *latus* bear, carry. See -ferent. trans*lat*ion
later- *latus*, *lateris* side. ventro*later*al
lent- *lens*, *lentis* lentil. Cf. phac-. *lent*iconus
lep- λαμβάνω, ληπ- take, seize. cata*lep*tic
leuc- See leuk-. *leuc*inuria
leuk- λευκός white. Cf. alb-. *leuk*orrhea. (Also spelled leuc-)
lien- *lien* spleen. Cf. splen-. *lien*ocele
lig- *ligo* tie, bind. *lig*ate
lingu- *lingua* tongue. Cf. gloss-. sub*lingu*al
lip- λίπος fat. Cf. adip-. glyco*lip*in
lith- λίθος stone. Cf. calc-[1]. nephro*lith*otomy
loc- *locus* place. Cf. top-. *loc*omotion
log- λέγω, λογ- speak, give an account. *log*orrhea, embry*ology*
lumb- *lumbus* loin. dorso*lumb*ar
lute- *luteus* yellow. Cf xanth-. *lute*oma
ly- λύω loose, dissolve. Cf. solut-. kerato*lys*is
lymph- *lympha* water. Cf. hydr-. *lymph*adenosis
macr- μακρός long, large. *macr*omyeloblast
mal- *malus* bad, abnormal. Cf. cac- and dys-. *mal*function
malac- μαλακός soft. osteo*malac*ia
mamm- *mamma* breast. Cf. mast-. sub*mamm*ary
man- *manus* hand. Cf. cheir-. *man*iphalanx
mani- μανία mental aberration. *mani*graphy, klepto*mania*
mast- μαστός breast. Cf. mamm-. hyper*mast*ia
medi- *medius* middle. Cf. mes-. *medi*frontal
mega- μέγας great, large. Also indicates multiple (1,000,000) in metric system. *mega*colon, *mega*dyne. (See also megal-)
megal- μέγας, μεγάλου great, large. acro*megal*y
mel- μέλος limb, member. sym*mel*ia
melan- μέλας, μέλανος black. hippo*melan*in
men- μήν month. dys*men*orrhea
mening- μῆνιγξ, μήνιγγος membrane. encephalo*mening*itis
ment- *mens*, *mentis* mind. Cf. phren-, psych- and thym-. de*ment*ia
mer- μέρος part. poly*mer*ic
mes- μέσος middle. Cf. medi-. *mes*oderm
met See meta-. *met*allergy
meta- μετά (*a* is dropped before words beginning with a vowel) after, beyond, accompanying. *meta*carpal
metr-[1] μέτρον measure. stereo*metr*y
metr-[2] μήτρα womb. endo*metr*itis
micr- μικρός small. photo*micr*ograph
mill- *mille* one thousand. Cf. kil-. Indicates fraction in metric system. *milli*gram, *milli*pede
miss- See -mittent. intro*miss*ion
-mittent *mitto*, *mittentis*, *missus* send. inter*mittent*

mne-	μιμνήσκω, μνη- remember. pseudo*mne*sia
mon-	μόνος only, sole. *mono*plegia
morph-	μορφή form, shape. poly*morph*onuclear
mot-	*moveo, motus* move. vaso*mot*or
my-	μῦς, μυός muscle. inoleio*my*oma
-myces	μύκης, μύκητος fungus. myelo*myces*
myc(et)-	See -myces. asco*mycet*es, strepto*myc*in
myel-	μυελός marrow. polio*myel*itis
myx-	μύξα mucus. *myx*edema
narc-	νάρκη numbness. topo*narc*osis
nas-	*nasus* nose. Cf. rhin-. palato*nas*al
ne-	νέος new, young. *ne*ocyte
necr-	νεκρός corpse. *necr*ocytosis
nephr-	νεφρός kidney. Cf. ren-. para*nephr*ic
neur-	νεῦρον nerve. esthesio*neure*
nod-	*nodus* knot. *nod*osity
nom-	νόμος (from νέμω deal out, distribute) law, custom. tax*onomy*
non-	*nona* nine. *non*acosane
nos-	νόσος disease. *nos*ology
nucle-	*nucleus* (from *nux, nucis* nut) kernel. Cf. kary-. *nucle*ide
nutri-	*nutrio* nourish. mal*nutri*tion
ob-	*ob* (*b* changes to *c* before words beginning with that consonant) against, toward, etc. *ob*tuse
oc-	See ob-. *oc*clude.
ocul-	*oculus* eye. Cf. ophthalm-. *ocul*omotor
-od-	See -ode[1]. peri*od*ic
-ode[1]	ὁδός road, path. cath*ode*. (See also hod-)
-ode[2]	See -oid. nemat*ode*
odont-	ὀδούς, ὀδόντος tooth. Cf. dent-. orth*odont*ia
-odyn-	ὀδύνη pain, distress. gastr*odyn*ia
-oid	εἶδος form. Cf. -form. hy*oid*
-ol	See ole-. cholester*ol*
ole-	*oleum* oil. *ole*oresin
olig-	ὀλίγος few, small. *olig*ospermia
omphal-	ὀμφαλός navel. peri*omphal*ic
onc-	ὄγκος bulk, mass. hemat*onc*ometry
onych-	ὄνυξ, ὄνυχος claw, nail. an*onych*ia
oo-	ᾠόν egg. Cf. ov-. peri*oo*thecitis
op-	ὁράω, ὀπ- see. erythr*op*sia
ophthalm-	ὀφθαλμός eye. Cf. ocul-. ex*ophthalm*ic
or-	*os, oris* mouth. Cf. stom(at)-. intra*or*al
orb-	*orbis* circle. sub*orb*ital
orchi-	ὄρχις testicle. Cf. test-. *orchi*opathy
organ-	ὄργανον implement, instrument. *organ*oleptic
orth-	ὀρθός straight, right, normal. *orth*opedics
oss-	*os, ossis* bone. Cf. ost(e)-. *oss*iphone
ost(e)-	ὀστέον bone. Cf. oss-. en*ost*osis, *oste*anaphysis
ot-	οὖς, ὠτός ear. Cf. aur-. par*ot*id
ov-	*ovum* egg. Cf. oo-. syn*ov*ia
oxy-	ὀξύς sharp. *oxy*cephalic
pachy(n)-	παχύνω thicken. *pachy*derma, myo*pachyn*sis
pag-	πήγνυμι, παγ- fix, make fast. thoraco*pag*us
par-[1]	*pario* bear, give birth to. primi*par*ous
par-[2]	See para-. *par*epigastric
para-	παρά (final α is dropped before words beginning with a vowel) beside, beyond. *para*mastoid
part-	*pario, partus* bear, give birth to. *part*urition
path-	πάθος that which one undergoes, sickness. psycho*path*ic
pec-	πήγνυμι, πηγ- (πηκ- before τ) fix, make fast. sym*pec*tothiene. (See also pex-)
ped-	παῖς, παιδός child. ortho*ped*ic
pell-	*pellis* skin, hide. *pell*agra
-pellent	*pello, pellentis, pulsus* drive. re*pellent*
pen-	πένομαι need, lack. erythrocyto*pen*ia
pend-	*pendeo* hang down. ap*pend*ix
pent(a)-	πέντε five. Cf. quinque-. *pent*ose, *penta*ploid
peps-	πέπτω, πεψ- (before σ) digest brady*peps*ia
pept-	πέπτω digest. dys*pept*ic
per-	*per* through. Cf. dia-. *per*nasal
peri-	περί around. Cf. circum-. *peri*phery
pet-	*peto* seek, tend toward. centri*pet*al
pex-	πήγνυμι, πηγ- (added to σ becomes πηξ-) fix, make fast. hepato*pex*y
pha-	φημί, φα- say, speak. dys*pha*sia
phac-	φακός lentil, lens. Cf. lent-. *phac*osclerosis. (Also spelled phak-)
phag-	φαγεῖν eat. lipo*phag*ic
phak-	See phac-. *phak*itis
phan-	See phen-. dia*phan*oscopy
pharmac-	φάρμακον drug. *pharmac*ognosy
pharyng-	φάρυγξ, φαρυγγ- throat. glosso*pharyng*eal
phen-	φαίνω, φαν- show, be seen. phos*phene*
pher-	φέρω, φορ- bear, support. peri*pher*y
phil-	φιλέω like, have affinity for. eosino*phil*ia
phleb-	φλέψ, φλεβός vein. peri*phleb*itis
phleg-	φλέγω, φλογ- burn, inflame. adeno*phleg*mon
phlog-	See phleg-. anti*phlog*istic
phob-	φόβος fear, dread. claustro*phob*ia
phon-	φωνή sound. echo*phon*y

phor-	See pher-. Cf. -ferent. exo*phor*ia
phos-	See phot-. *phos*phorus
phot-	φῶς, φωτός light. *phot*erythrous
phrag-	φράσσω, φραγ- fence, wall off, stop up. Cf. sept-[1]. dia*phrag*m
phrax-	φράσσω, φραγ- (added to σ becomes φραξ-) fence, wall off, stop up. em*phrax*is
phren-	φρήν mind, midriff. Cf. ment-. meta*phren*ia, meta*phren*on
phthi-	φθίνω decay, waste away. ophthalmo*phthi*sis
phy-	φύω beget, bring forth, produce, be by nature. noso*phy*te
phyl-	φῦλον tribe, kind. *phyl*ogeny
-phyll	φύλλον leaf. xantho*phyll*
phylac-	φύλαξ guard. pro*phylac*tic
phys(a)-	φυσάω blow, inflate. *phys*ocele, *physa*lis
physe-	φυσάω, φυση- blow, inflate. em*physe*ma
pil-	*pilus* hair. e*pil*ation
pituit-	*pituita* phlegm, rheum. *pituit*ous
placent-	*placenta* (from πλακοῦς) cake. extra*placent*al
plas-	πλάσσω mold, shape. cine*plas*ty
platy-	πλατύς broad, flat. *platy*rrhine
pleg-	πλήσσω, πληγ- strike. di*pleg*ia
plet-	*pleo, -pletus* fill. de*plet*ion
pleur-	πλευρά rib, side. Cf. cost-. peri*pleur*al
plex-	πλήσσω, πληγ- (added to σ becomes πληξ-) strike. apo*plex*y
plic-	*plico* fold. com*plic*ation
pne-	πνοιά breathing. traumato*pne*a
pneum(at)-	πνεῦμα, πνεύματος breath, air. *pneum*odynamics, *pneumato*thorax
pneumo(n)-	πνεύμων lung. Cf. pulmo(n)-. *pneumo*centesis, *pneumon*otomy
pod-	πούς, ποδός foot. *pod*iatry
poie-	ποιέω make, produce. Cf. -facient. sarco*poie*tic
pol-	πόλος axis of a sphere. peri*pol*ar
poly-	πολύς much, many. *poly*spermia
pont-	*pons, pontis* bridge. *ponto*cerebellar
por-[1]	πόρος passage. myelo*por*e
por-[2]	πῶρος callus. *por*ocele
posit-	*pono, positus* put, place. re*posit*or
post-	*post* after, behind in time or place. *post*natal, *post*oral
pre-	*prae* before in time or place. *pre*natal, *pre*vesical
press-	*premo, pressus* press. *press*oreceptive
pro-	πρό or *pro* before in time or place. *pro*gamous, *pro*cheilon, *pro*lapse
proct-	πρωκτός anus. entero*proct*ia
prosop-	πρόσωπον face. Cf. faci-. di*prosop*us
pseud-	ψευδής false. *pseud*oparaplegia
psych-	ψυχή soul, mind. Cf. ment-. *psych*osomatic
pto-	πίπτω, πτω- fall. nephro*pto*sis
pub-	*pubes* & *puber, puberis* adult. ischio*pub*ic. (See also puber-)
puber-	*puber* adult. *puber*ty
pulmo(n)-	*pulmo, pulmonis* lung. Cf. pneumo(n)-. *pulmo*lith, cardio*pulmon*ary
puls-	*pello, pellentis, pulsus* drive. pro*puls*ion
punct-	*pungo, punctus* prick, pierce. Cf. cente-. *punct*iform
pur-	*pus, puris* pus. Cf. py-. sup*pur*ation
py-	πύον pus. Cf. pur-. nephro*py*osis
pyel-	πύελος trough, basin, pelvis. nephro*pyel*itis
pyl-	πύλη door, orifice. *pyl*ephlebitis
pyr-	πῦρ fire. Cf. febr-. galacto*pyr*a
quadr-	*quadr-* four. Cf. tetra-. *quadr*igeminal
quinque-	*quinque* five. Cf. pent(a)-. *quinque*cuspid
rachi-	ῥαχίς spine. Cf. spin-. encephalo*rachi*dian
radi-	*radius* ray. Cf. actin-. ir*radi*ation
re-	*re-* back, again. *re*traction
ren-	*renes* kidneys. Cf. nephr-. ad*ren*al
ret-	*rete* net. *ret*othelium
retro-	*retro* backwards. *retro*deviation
rhag-	ῥήγνυμι, ῥαγ- break, burst. hemor*rhag*ic
rhaph-	ῥαφή suture. gastror*rhaphy*
rhe-	ῥέω flow. Cf. flu-. diar*rhe*al
rhex-	ῥήγνυμι, ῥηγ- (added to σ becomes ῥηξ-) break, burst. metror*rhex*is
rhin-	ῥίς, ῥινός nose. Cf. nas-. basi*rhin*al
rot-	*rota* wheel. *rot*ator
rub(r)-	*ruber, rubri* red. Cf. erythr-. bili*rub*in, *rubr*ospinal
salping-	σάλπιγξ, σάλπιγγος tube, trumpet. *salping*itis
sanguin-	*sanguis, sanguinis* blood. Cf. hem(at)-. *sanguin*eous
sarc-	σάρξ, σαρκός flesh. *sarc*oma
schis-	σχίζω, σχιδ- (before τ or added to σ becomes σχισ-) split. Cf. fiss-. *schis*torachis, rachi*schis*is
scler-	σκληρός hard. Cf. dur-. *scler*osis
scop-	σκοπέω look at, observe. endo*scop*e
sect-	*seco, sectus* cut. Cf. tom-. *sect*ile
semi-	*semi-* half. Cf. hemi-. *semi*flexion
sens-	*sentio, sensus* perceive, feel. Cf. esthe-. *sens*ory

sep- σήπω rot, decay. *seps*is

sept-[1] *saepio, saeptus* fence, wall off, stop up. Cf. phrag-. naso*sept*al

sept-[2] *septem* seven. Cf. hept(a)-. *sept*an

ser- *serum* whey, watery substance. *ser*osynovitis

sex- *sex* six. Cf. hex-[1]. *sex*digitate

sial- σίαλον saliva. poly*sial*ia

sin- *sinus* hollow, fold. Cf. colp-. *sin*obronchitis

sit- σῖτος food. para*sit*ic

solut- *solvo, solventis, solutus* loose, dissolve, set free. Cf. ly-. dis*solut*ion

-solvent See solut-. dis*solvent*

somat- σῶμα, σώματος body. Cf. corpor-. psycho*somat*ic

-some See somat-. dictyo*some*

spas- σπάω, σπασ- draw, pull. *spas*m, *spas*tic

spectr- *spectrum* appearance, what is seen. micro*spectr*oscope

sperm(at)- σπέρμα, σπέρματος seed. *sperm*acrasia, *spermat*ozoon

spers- *spargo, -spersus* scatter. dis*pers*ion

sphen- σφήν wedge. Cf. cune-. *sphen*oid

spher- σφαῖρα ball. hemi*sphere*

sphygm- σφυγμός pulsation. *sphygmo*manometer

spin- *spina* spine. Cf. rachi-. cerebro*spin*al

spirat- *spiro, spiratus* breathe. in*spirat*ory

splanchn- σπλάγχνα entrails, viscera. neuro*splanchn*ic

splen- σπλήν spleen. Cf. lien-. *splen*omegaly

spor- σπόρος seed. *spor*ophyte, zygo*spore*

squam- *squama* scale. de*squam*ation

sta- ἵστημι, στα- make stand, stop. genesi*sta*sis

stal- στέλλω, σταλ- send. peri*stal*sis. (See also stol-)

staphyl- σταφυλή bunch of grapes, uvula. *staphyl*ococcus, *staphyl*ectomy

stear- στέαρ, στέατος fat. Cf. adip-. *stear*odermia

steat- See stear-. *steat*opygous

sten- στενός narrow, compressed. *sten*ocardia

ster- στερεός solid. chole*ster*ol

sterc- *stercus* dung. Cf. copr-. *sterco*porphyrin

sthen- σθένος strength. a*sthen*ia

stol- στέλλω, στολ- send. dia*stol*e

stom(at)- στόμα, στόματος mouth, orifice. Cf. or-. ana*stom*osis, *stomato*gastric

strep(h)- στρέφω, στρεπ- (before τ) twist. Cf. tors-. *streph*osymbolia, *strep*tomycin. (See also stroph-)

strict- *stringo, stringentis, strictus* draw tight, compress, cause pain. con*strict*ion

-stringent See strict-. a*stringent*

stroph- στρέφω, στροφ- twist. ana*stroph*ic. (See also strep(h)-)

struct- *struo, structus* pile up (against). ob*struct*ion

sub- *sub* (*b* changes to *f* or *p* before words beginning with those consonants) under, below. Cf. hypo-. *sub*lumbar

suf- See sub-. *suf*fusion

sup- See sub-. *sup*pository

super- *super* above, beyond, extreme. Cf. hyper-. *super*motility

sy- See syn-. *sy*stole

syl- See syn-. *syl*lepsiology

sym- See syn-. *sym*biosis, *sym*metry, *sym*pathetic, *sym*physis

syn- σύν (*n* disappears before *s*, changes to *l* before *l*, and changes to *m* before *b*, *m*, *p*, and *ph*) with, together. Cf. con-. myo*syn*izesis

ta- See ton-. ec*ta*sis

tac- τάσσω, ταγ- (τακ- before τ) order, arrange. a*tac*tic

tact- *tango, tactus* touch. con*tact*

tax- τάσσω, ταγ- (added to σ becomes ταξ-) order, arrange. a*tax*ia

tect See teg-. pro*tect*ive

teg- *tego, tectus* cover. in*teg*ument

tel- τέλος end. *tel*osynapsis

tele- τῆλε at a distance. *tele*ceptor

tempor- *tempus, temporis* time, timely or fatal spot, temple. *tempo*romalar

ten(ont)- τένων, τένοντος (from τείνω stretch) tight stretched band. *ten*odynia, *ten*onitis, *tenon*tagra

tens- *tendo, tensus* stretch. Cf. ton-. ex*tens*or

test- *testis* testicle. Cf. orchi-. *tes*titis

tetra- τετρα- four. Cf. quadr-. *tetra*genous

the- τίθημι, θη- put, place. syn*the*sis

thec- θήκη repository, case. *theco*stegnosis

thel- θηλή teat, nipple. *thel*erethism

therap- θεραπεία treatment. hydro*therapy*

therm- θέρμη heat. Cf. calor-. dia*therm*y

thi- θεῖον sulfur. *thi*ogenic

thorac- θώραξ, θώρακος chest. *thoraco*plasty

thromb- θρόμβος lump, clot. *thrombo*penia

thym- θυμός spirit. Cf. ment-. dys*thym*ia

thyr- θυρεός shield (shaped like a door θύρα). *thyr*oid

tme-	τέμνω, τμη- cut. axono*tme*sis
toc-	τόκος childbirth. dys*toc*ia
tom-	τέμνω, τομ- cut. Cf. sect-. appendec*tom*y
ton-	τείνω, τον- stretch, put under tension. Cf. tens-. peri*tone*um
top-	τόπος place. Cf. loc-. *top*esthesia
tors-	*torqueo, torsus* twist. Cf. strep-. ex*tors*ion
tox-	τοξικόν (from τόξον bow) arrow poison, poison. *tox*emia
trache-	τραχεῖα windpipe. *trache*otomy
trachel-	τράχηλος neck. Cf. cervic-. *trachel*opexy
tract-	*traho, tractus* draw, drag. pro*tract*ion
traumat-	τραῦμα, τραύματος wound. *traumat*ic
tri-	τρεῖς, τρία or *tri-* three. *tri*gonid
trich-	θρίξ, τριχός hair. *trich*oid
trip-	τρίβω rub. en*trip*sis
trop-	τρέπω, τροπ- turn, react. sito*trop*ism
troph-	τρέφω, τροφ- nurture. a*trophy*
tuber-	*tuber* swelling, node. *tuber*cle
typ-	τύπος (from τύπτω strike) type. a*typ*ical
typh-	τῦφος fog, stupor. adeno*typh*us
typhl-	τυφλός blind. Cf. cec-. *typhl*ectasis
un-	*unus* one. Cf. hen-. *un*ioval
ur-	οὖρον urine. poly*ur*ia
vacc-	*vacca* cow. *vacc*ine
vagin-	*vagina* sheath. in*vagin*ated
vas-	*vas* vessel. Cf. angi-. *vas*cular
vers-	See vert-. in*vers*ion
vert-	*verto, versus* turn. di*vert*iculum
vesic-	*vesica* bladder. Cf. cyst-. *vesico*vaginal
vit-	*vita* life. Cf. bi-^{1}. de*vit*alize
vuls-	*vello, vulsus* pull, twitch. con*vuls*ion
xanth-	ξανθός yellow, blond. Cf. flav- and lute-. *xanth*ophyll
-yl-	ὕλη substance. cacod*yl*
zo-	ζωή life, ζῷον animal. micro*zo*aria
zyg-	ζυγόν yoke, union. *zyg*odactyly
zym-	ζύμη ferment. en*zym*e

A

A angstrom; mass number.

A. accommodation; ampere; anode (anodal); anterior; axial.

a [L.] *arte'ria* (artery); atto-.

a- word element [L.], *without; not.*

Å angstrom.

$\mathbf{A_2}$ aortic second sound (see HEART SOUNDS).

A.A. achievement age; Alcoholics Anonymous.

$\overline{\overline{aa}}$ [L. pl.] *arte'riae* (arteries).

aa [Gr.] *an'a* (of each), in prescriptions.

A.A.A.S. American Association for the Advancement of Science.

A.A.I.N. American Association of Industrial Nurses.

A.A.P. American Association of Pathologists.

A.A.P.B. American Association of Pathologists and Bacteriologists.

A.A.P.M.R. American Academy of Physical Medicine and Rehabilitation.

ab [L.] preposition, *from.*

ab- word element [L.], *from; off; away from.*

abacterial (a″bak-te′re-al) free from bacteria.

abarognosis (ah-bar″og-no′sis) loss of sense of weight.

abarthrosis (ab″ar-thro′sis) abarticulation.

abarticular (ab″ar-tik′u-ler) not affecting a joint; at a distance from a joint.

abarticulation (ab″ar-tik″u-la′shun) 1. synovial joint. 2. a dislocation.

abasia (ah-ba′ze-ah) inability to walk. adj., **aba′sic, abat′ic.**

a.-asta′sia, astasia-abasia.

a. atac′tica, abasia with uncertain movements, due to a defect of coordination.

choreic a., abasia due to chorea of the limbs.

paralytic a., abasia due to paralysis.

paroxysmal trepidant a., spastic a., abasia due to spastic stiffening of the legs on attempting to stand.

trembling a., a. trep′idans, abasia due to trembling of the legs.

abatement (ah-bāt′ment) decrease in severity of a pain or symptom.

abdomen (ab-do′men) the portion of the body between the thorax and the pelvis. adj., **abdom′inal.** Within this part of the body is the abdominal cavity, which is separated from the chest area by the diaphragm. The cavity, which is lined with a membrane known as the peritoneum, contains the stomach, large and small intestines, liver, spleen, pancreas, kidneys, appendix, gallbladder, urinary bladder, and other structures.

acute a., surgical a., an acute intra-abdominal condition of abrupt onset, usually associated with pain due to inflammation, perforation, obstruction, infarction or rupture of abdominal organs, and usually requiring emergency surgical intervention.

abdomin(o)- word element, *abdomen.*

abdominocentesis (ab-dom″ĭ-no-sen-te′sis) paracentesis of the abdomen (see also abdominal PARACENTESIS).

abdominocystic (ab-dom″ĭ-no-sis′tik) pertaining to the abdomen and gallbladder.

abdominohysterectomy (ab-dom″ĭ-no-his″tĕ-rek′to-me) hysterectomy through an abdominal incision.

abdominohysterotomy (ab-dom″ĭ-no-his″tĕ-rot′o-me) hysterotomy through an abdominal incision.

abdominoscopy (ab-dom″ĭ-nos′ko-pe) examination of the abdomen.

abdominovaginal (ab-dom″ĭ-no-vaj′ĭ-nal) pertaining to the abdomen and vagina.

abduce (ab-dūs′) to abduct, or draw away.

abducens (ab-du′senz) [L.] drawing away.

a. nerve, the sixth cranial nerve; it arises from the pons and supplies the lateral rectus muscle of the eyeball, allowing for motion. Paralysis of the nerve causes diplopia (double vision).

abducent (ab-du′sent) abducting.

abduct (ab-dukt′) to draw away from an axis or the median plane.

abduction (ab-duk′shun) the act of abducting; the state of being abducted.

abductor (ab-duk′tor) that which abducts.

Abernethy's sarcoma (ab′er-ne″thēz) a malignant fatty tumor occurring mainly on the trunk.

aberratio (ab″er-a′she-o) [L.] aberration.

aberration (ab″er-a′shun) 1. deviation from the normal or usual. 2. imperfect refraction or focalization of a lens.

chromatic a., unequal refraction by a lens of light rays of different lengths passing through it, producing a blurred image and a display of colors.

dioptric a., spherical a., inability of a spherical lens to bring all rays of light to a single focus.

abetalipoproteinemia (a-ba″tah-lip″o-pro″te-in-e′me-ah) a hereditary syndrome marked by a lack of β-lipoproteins in the blood and by acanthocytosis, hypocholesterolemia, progressive ataxic neuropathy, atypical retinitis pigmentosa involving the macula, and malabsorption.

abionergy (ab″e-on′er-je) abiotrophy.

abiosis (ab″e-o′sis) absence or deficiency of life. adj., **abiot′ic.**

abiotrophy (ab″e-ot′ro-fe) progressive loss of vitality of certain tissues or organs leading to disorders or loss of function; applied especially to degenerative hereditary diseases of late onset, e.g., Huntington's chorea. adj., **abiotroph′ic.**

abirritant (ab-ir′ĭ-tant) 1. diminishing irritation; soothing. 2. an agent that relieves irritation.

abirritation (ab-ir″ĭ-ta′shun) diminished irritability; atony.

ablactation (ab″lak-ta′shun) weaning.

ablate (ab-lāt′) to remove, especially by cutting.

ablatio (ab-la′she-o) [L.] detachment.

a. ret′inae, detachment of the retina.

ablation (ab-la′shun) 1. separation or detachment;

extirpation; eradication. 2. removal, especially by cutting.

ablepharia (a″blef-a′re-ah) congenital reduction or absence of the eyelids. adj., **ableph′arous.**

ablepharon (a-blef′ah-ron) ablepharia.

ablepsia (a-blep′se-ah) blindness.

abluent (ab′lu-ent) 1. detergent; cleansing. 2. a cleansing agent.

abnerval (ab-ner′val) passing from a nerve through a muscle; said of electric currents.

abnormality (ab″nor-mal′ĭ-te) 1. the state of being unlike the usual condition. 2. a malformation.

aborad (ab-o′rad) away from the mouth.

aboral (ab-o′ral) opposite to, or remote from, the mouth.

abort (ah-bort′) to arrest prematurely a disease or developmental process; to expel the products of conception before the fetus is viable.

abortifacient (ah-bor″tĭ-fa′shent) 1. causing abortion. 2. an agent that induces abortion.

abortion (ah-bor′shun) termination of pregnancy before the fetus is viable. In the medical sense, the terms abortion and miscarriage both refer to the termination of pregnancy before the fetus is capable of survival outside the uterus. In general language, however, abortion most often refers to deliberate interruption of pregnancy, whereas miscarriage connotes a spontaneous or natural loss of the fetus. Because of this distinction made by the average lay person, care should be exercised in the use of the word abortion when speaking of a spontaneous loss of the fetus.

It is rare for a fetus to survive if it weighs less than 1000 gm., or if the pregnancy is terminated before 20 weeks of gestation. These factors are, however, difficult to determine with a high degree of accuracy while the fetus is still *in utero;* survival of the fetus delivered near the end of the second trimester often depends to a great extent on the availability of personnel and equipment capable of supporting life until the infant develops sufficiently.

Viability of the fetus outside the uterus is frequently used as the determining factor in deciding the legality and morality of induced abortion. Whether this is a valid criterion is essentially based on whether one believes that the fetus is human from the moment of conception or that it achieves humanity at some point during physical development. Those who oppose abortion on moral grounds believe that the fetus is human or potentially human and that destruction of the fetal body is tantamount to murder.

The liberalization of abortion laws has resulted in a dramatic increase in the number of abortions performed in physicians' offices, clinics, and hospitals. While this has diminished the occurrence of septic abortions performed at the hands of unscrupulous abortionists and has improved the possibility of safe and uneventful physical recovery from an induced abortion, the issue remains highly controversial and charged with emotion. Members of the health team who may be involved in the performance of abortion procedures often must resolve a personal dilemma and carefully examine their attitudes and beliefs about the deliberate termination of pregnancy. If conflicts and doubts are not resolved, there is a strong possibility that those who participate in abortions will have difficulty remaining nonjudgmental in their dealings with clients. Many women who choose to have an abortion are themselves anxious and confused about the physical and psychological outcomes of the procedure. Pre- and post-abortion counseling are recommended.

The patient should know that other alternatives are available and that an abortion after 20 weeks is inadvisable for medical and other reasons. Preabortion counseling in the psychological, religious, and legal aspects of abortion should be readily available, with immediate referral to the proper resources when indicated. Although delay in carrying out the procedure may increase the risk of complications, no patient should be encouraged to go through with an abortion until she has had time and sufficient counseling to reach a rational decision. During post-abortion counseling there should be a discussion of various methods of contraception. The client will need information on the advantages and disadvantages of each method, her responsibilities in preventing future unwanted pregnancies, and available help in initiating and following through on a program of effective CONTRACEPTION.

PATIENT CARE. The type of care required and the complications to be avoided in abortion will depend on the stage of pregnancy at the time of termination and whether the abortion is spontaneous, is induced under sterile conditions, or is performed by an unskilled abortionist or the patient herself.

In general the two major difficulties associated with abortion are hemorrhage and infection. Perforation of the uterine wall can occur if curettage is employed as a procedure for the removal of the uterine contents, particularly if the abortion is done by someone other than a gynecologist. Another condition that may arise as a result of improper curettage is retention of fragments of the fetal-placental tissue. Unless these fragments are removed and the uterine cavity thoroughly emptied, there is danger of hemorrhage and infection. Hemorrhage is most likely to occur during or immediately after loss of the fetus. Patients who are being treated on an outpatient basis should be instructed to report severe cramps or bleeding beyond the expected spotting. The number of perineal pads used during a given period of time can help determine the amount of blood loss. Other signs of excessive bleeding are restlessness, extreme thirst, and pallor.

Elevation of body temperature usually indicates infection, as does the presence of a foul-smelling vaginal discharge and pelvic pain. As soon as the diagnosis of a uterine infection has been established, the patient is started on a regimen of antibiotic therapy, rest, and measures to facilitate the body's healing processes.

Intravenous fluids and blood transfusions may be needed to replace blood and body fluids. Since acute renal failure is a common complication of postabortion sepsis, it is important to keep an accurate record of fluid intake and output on these patients. Peculiar characteristics as well as the amount of urine should be recorded.

Cervical dilation accompanies all types of abortion and therefore requires perineal care as long as there is vaginal discharge. To further insure against infection via the dilated cervix, the patient should be instructed not to douche, have sexual intercourse, or use tampons for six weeks after the abortion.

The psychological aspects of patient care are varied and complex. If the abortion is induced there may or may not be emotional repercussions. In general most specialists agree that the patient who was emotionally stable and free from psychological problems prior to the abortion will be able to return to her normal routine within a month. This is not to say that abortion does not leave emotional scars in most cases. Religious backround, moral attitudes, and social and cultural mores have some effect on one's ability to accept or reject the deliberate termination of pregnancy.

American literature on emotional response to abortion suggests that serious psychiatric complications occur in slightly less than 10 percent. It is suggested that there is a high risk of psychiatric illness when the patient has ambivalent feelings about the termination of pregnancy, is coerced by her family or physician, has the feeling that the decision was not her own, is having the abortion for medical reasons, or has had a pre-existing psychiatric illness.

The nurse who strongly objects to abortion is legally and morally free to choose not to participate in the procedure itself and is advised to avoid situations in which she has responsibility for the care of patients who have chosen abortion as a means of ending an unwanted pregnancy.

In cases of spontaneous or habitual abortion, patient care is directed toward emotional support of the patient and acceptance of her feelings of bitterness, grief, guilt, relief, and other emotions associated with the loss of the fetus. The patient should be able to express her feelings in an open, nonjudgmental, and nonthreatening environment.

TECHNIQUES OF INDUCED ABORTION. The technique chosen to terminate pregnancy depends on the stage of pregnancy at the time the abortion is done and the policies of the physician and institution.

Menstrual Extraction. This is a form of suctioning in which a flexible cannula is inserted through an undilated cervix for the purpose of removing the fertilized ovum and endometrium. The cannula is attached to a syringe, which is used to aspirate the uterine contents and induce the onset of the "missed period." There is some objection to the use of this technique; it is not always effective and a second procedure may be required.

Suction Curettage. This is the procedure of choice in pregnancies up to 12 weeks, the optimum time being 8 to 10 weeks, by which time pregnancy has been definitely established and the cervix has softened and is more easily dilated. The procedure involves dilation of the cervix followed by vacuum suctioning of the uterus and is performed under local anesthesia, usually in a physician's office or outpatient clinic. Some physicians follow the dilation and suctioning with gentle scraping of the uterine wall to assure removal of all fragments of the fetal body, placenta, and amniotic sac. A common, though not frequent complication is infection related to pre-existing vaginitis and pelvic inflammatory disease.

Vacuum curettage using a laminaria tent is sometimes done when the pregnancy is too far advanced for manual dilation of the cervix, but not mature enough for more complex surgical procedures. This usually encompasses the period between the 12th and 16th week of pregnancy when manual dilation is likely to produce tearing of the cervix. *Laminaria* is a genus of seaweed whose dried stems expand when exposed to moisture. Sterilized cylinders of the stems are inserted into the cervix 18 to 24 hours prior to vacuum curettage, for the purpose of gradually dilating the cervix. The day after insertion the patient is admitted to the hospital and given an oxytocic agent to stimulate uterine contractions. Vacuum suctioning and curettage are then done to remove the conceptus.

Intra-amniotic Injection. The injection of a hypertonic saline solution or prostaglandin via a needle and catheter inserted directly into the amniotic sac is the most frequently used procedure for termination of pregnancy in the second trimester. The patient is hospitalized for this procedure, because she goes into labor and therefore requires continuous care during labor, delivery, and the postpartal period.

When the saline, or "salting out," procedure is done, there is considerable risk of accidental intravenous injection of the saline, which may cause renal and cardiac difficulties, hypernatremia, and cerebral convulsions. After insertion of the needle through the abdominal and uterine wall, approximately 200 ml. of amniotic fluid are withdrawn and replaced with 20 percent saline solution. Contractions usually begin about 12 hours after injection of the saline, and abortion commonly occurs within 36 hours. A continuous oxytocin drip may be administered to hasten delivery. Subsequent curettage may be required to assure complete removal of residual tissue. In some cases abortion does not occur after the first injection, and a second injection of saline is needed.

Prostaglandin injections have the advantage of not requiring aspiration of amniotic fluid, nor is administration of oxytocin necessary. The physician injects 8 ml. (40 mg.) of prostaglandin into the amniotic sac; within 30 minutes contractions begin and abortion takes place within 20 hours. In most cases the fetus is delivered in the patient's bed.

Hysterotomy. This procedure is similar to a cesarean section and carries a higher morbidity than does intra-amniotic injection. It is recommended only for rare cases in which an injection procedure is contraindicated.

complete a., complete expulsion of all the products of conception.

criminal a., termination of pregnancy by illegal interference. In spite of the discovery of antibiotics and improved medical techniques, the mortality from criminal abortions is tragically high because most of these patients wait until too late to seek medical attention. The high rate of maternal deaths from criminal abortion can also be attributed to the drastic and often incredibly unsanitary measures used to terminate the pregnancy. The most frequent complications are severe hemorrhage, sepsis, renal failure, and septic shock.

early a., abortion within the first 12 weeks of pregnancy.

habitual a., spontaneous abortion occurring in three or more successive pregnancies.

incomplete a., abortion in which parts of the products of conception are retained in the uterus.

induced a., abortion brought on intentionally by medication or instrumentation.

inevitable a., abortion in which termination cannot be prevented.

missed a., retention of a dead embryo for more than 8 weeks.

septic a., abortion in which uterine infection is spread to the systemic circulation.

spontaneous a., abortion occurring naturally. It has been estimated that 10 to 12 per cent of all pregnancies end in spontaneous abortion. Habitual aborters are uncommon, but they account for the high percentage of abortions of this type. The woman who has repeated abortions should have a comprehensive examination to determine the cause of this disorder. Hormonal imbalances, especially those involving the progestational hormones, and emotion and psychologic disturbances frequently play an important role in spontaneous abortion. Early prenatal care, under the supervision of an obstetrician, may prevent spontaneous termination of pregnancy.

When spontaneous abortion does occur, the patient should notify her physician at once in order to prevent serious complications that may develop. Any material such as clots or bits of tissue should be saved for laboratory examination. Hemorrhage, shock, and infection are the most frequent hazards of spontaneous abortion. Treatment usually consists of DILATION AND CURETTAGE to remove tissues that may be retained in the uterus. If the abortion is complete, the attending physician may consider a surgical procedure unnecessary. In any event the patient should consult her physician at the first sign of bleeding or cramping during pregnancy.

therapeutic a., abortion induced legally by a qualified physician for medical or other reasons.

threatened a., a condition in which there are signs of premature expulsion of the products of conception.

abortionist (ah-bor′shun-ist) one who performs criminal abortions.

abortive (ah-bor′tiv) 1. incompletely developed. 2. abortifacient.

abortus (ah-bor′tus) a dead or nonviable fetus (weighing less than 17 ounces, or 500 gm., at birth).

abrachia (ah-bra′ke-ah) congenital absence of the arms.

abrachiocephalia (ah-bra″ke-o-sĕ-fa′le-ah) a developmental anomaly with absence of the head and arms.

abrasion (ah-bra′zhun) a wound caused by rubbing or scraping the skin or mucous membrane. A "skinned knee" and a "floor burn" are common examples. To treat the injury, the wound should be washed, a mild antiseptic such as hydrogen peroxide applied, and the wound covered with sterile gauze.

abrasive (ah-bra′siv) 1. causing abrasion. 2. an agent that produces abrasion.

abreaction (ab″re-ak′shun) the release of tension and anxiety associated with the emotional reliving of past, especially repressed, events (catharsis).

abreuography (ab″roo-og′rah-fe) photofluorography.

abruptio (ah-brup′she-o) [L.] separation.

a. placen′tae, premature separation of a normally situated placenta (see also PLACENTA).

abscess (ab′ses) a localized collection of pus in a cavity formed by the disintegration of tissue. Abscesses are usually caused by specific microorganisms that invade the tissues, often by way of small wounds or breaks in the skin. An abscess is a natural defense mechanism in which the body attempts to localize an infection and "wall off" the microorganisms so that they cannot spread throughout the body. As the microorganisms destroy the tissue, an increased supply of blood is rushed to the area. The cells, bacteria, and dead tissue accumulate in a clump of cream-colored liquid, which is the pus. The accumulating pus and the adjacent swollen, inflamed tissues press against the nerves, causing pain. The concentration of blood in the area causes redness. The abscess sometimes "comes to a head" (localizes) by itself and breaks through the skin or other tissues, allowing the pus to drain. Local applications of heat may be used to facilitate localization and drainage.

A skin abscess, no matter how small, should never be squeezed since pressure against the inflamed tissues is likely to spread the infection. Small abscesses frequently drain and heal themselves; larger abscesses and internal abscesses should always be treated by a physician, who may find it necessary to incise the abscess to allow for drainage of the exudate. Sulfonamide drugs and some of the antibiotics often help combat the infection.

alveolar a., a localized suppurative inflammation of tissues about the apex of the root of a tooth.

amebic a., an abscess cavity of the liver resulting from liquefaction necrosis due to entrance of *Entamoeba histolytica* into the portal circulation in amebiasis; amebic abscesses may also affect the lungs, brain, and spleen.

Bezold's a., a subperiosteal abscess of the temporal bone.

Brodie's a., a circumscribed abscess in bone, caused by hematogenous infection, that becomes a chronic nidus of infection.

cold a., one of slow development and with little inflammation, usually tuberculous.

diffuse a., a collection of pus not enclosed by a capsule.

miliary a., one composed of numerous small collections of pus.

milk a., abscess of the breast occurring during lactation.

perianal a., one beneath the skin of the anus and the anal canal.

peritonsillar a., a localized accumulation of pus in the peritonsillar tissue subsequent to suppurative inflammation of the tonsil; called also quinsy.

phlegmonous a., one associated with acute inflammation of the subcutaneous connective tissue.

primary a., one formed at the seat of the infection.

stitch a., one developed about a stitch or suture.

thecal a., one in the sheath of a tendon.

wandering a., one that burrows into tissues and finally points at a distance from the site of origin.

abscissa (ab-sis′ah) the horizontal line in a graph along which are plotted the units of one of the factors considered in the study, as time in a time-temperature study. The other line is called the ordinate.

abscission (ab-sish′un) removal of a part or growth by cutting.

abscopal (ab-sko′p′l) pertaining to the effect that irradiation of a tissue has on a nonirradiated tissue.

absent-mindedness (ab′sent-mīnd″ed-nes) preoccupation to the extent of being unaware of one's immediate surroundings.

absorb (ab-sorb′) to attract and incorporate other material, as through a membrane.

absorbance (ab-sor′bans) in radiology, a measure of the ability of a medium to absorb radiation, expressed as the logarithm of the quotient of the intensity of the radiation entering the medium divided by that leaving it.

absorbefacient (ab-sor″bĕ-fa′shent) 1. causing absorption. 2. an agent that promotes absorption.

absorbent (ab-sorb′ent) 1. able to take in, or suck up and incorporate. 2. a tissue structure involved in absorption. 3. a substance that absorbs or promotes absorption.

absorption (ab-sorp′shun) 1. the act of taking up or in by specific chemical or molecular action; especially the passage of liquids or other substances through a surface of the body into body fluids and tissues, as in the absorption of the end products of DIGESTION into the villi that line the intestine. 2. in psychology, devotion of thought to one object or activity only. 3. in radiology, uptake of energy by matter with which the radiation interacts.

chemical a., any process by which one substance in liquid or solid form penetrates the surface of another substance.

a. coefficient, a measure of the reduction of radiant energy resulting from its passage through a substance. See also COEFFICIENT OF ABSORPTION.

digestive a., the passage of the end products of DIGESTION from the gastrointestinal tract into the blood and lymphatic vessels and the cells of tissues. Absorption of this kind can take place either by diffusion or by active transport.

radiation a., the dissipation of radiant energy as it passes through matter. This phenomenon is of particular importance in diagnostic and therapeutic radiology, which depends on the interaction between ionizing radiations and matter. As radiation passes through matter, it is absorbed by an amount dependent on the atomic and molecular structure and thickness of the substance, and the energy of the primary photons. If radiations pass through a medium of living or nonliving material without absorption (loss of energy), no biologic or photographic effects can occur. In true absorption the photons of radiation waves give up or transfer all of their energy to electrons within the atoms of the matter through which they are passing.

absorptive (ab-sorp′tiv) having the power of absorption; involving absorption.

abstinence (ab′stĭ-nens) a refraining from the use or indulgence in food, stimulants, or coitus.

a. syndrome, withdrawal symptoms.

abstraction (ab-strak′shun) 1. the mental process of forming abstract ideas. 2. the withdrawal of any ingredient from a compound. 3. malocclusion in which the occlusal plane is farther from the eye-ear plane, causing lengthening of the face.

abulia (ah-bu′le-ah) loss or deficiency of will power, initiative, or drive. adj., **abu′lic.**

abutment (ah-but′ment) the anchorage tooth for a bridge.

Ac chemical symbol, *actinium.*

a.c. [L.] *an′te ci′bum* (before meals).

acacia (ah-ka′shah) the dried gummy exudate from stems and branches of species of *Acacia,* prepared as a mucilage or syrup. It is used as a suspending agent for drugs in pharmaceutical preparations, as an emollient and demulcent and, in solution, as in an intravenous infusion in shock.

acalcicosis (ah-kal″sĭ-ko′sis) a condition due to deficiency of calcium in the diet.

acalculia (a″kal-ku′le-ah) inability to do mathematical calculations.

acampsia (a-kamp′se-ah) rigidity of a part or limb.

acanth(o)- word element [Gr.], *sharp spine; thorn.*

acantha (ah-kan′tha) 1. the spine. 2. a spinous process of a vertebra.

acanthesthesia (ah-kan″thes-the′ze-ah) a sensation of a sharp point pricking the body.

acanthion (ah-kan′the-on) a point at the base of the anterior nasal spine.

Acanthocephala (ah-kan″tho-sef′ah-lah) a phylum of elongate, mostly cylindrical organisms (thorny-headed worms) parasitic in the intestines of all classes of vertebrates.

acanthocephaliasis (ah-kan″tho-sef″ah-li′ah-sis) infection with worms of the phylum Acanthocephala.

acanthocephalous (ah-kan″tho-sef″ah-lus) pertaining to or caused by worms of the phylum Acanthocephala.

Acanthocephalus (ah-kan″tho-sef′ah-lus) a genus of parasitic worms (phylum Acanthocephala).

Acanthocheilonema (ah-kan″tho-ki″lo-ne′mah) a genus of long, threadlike worms.

A. per′stans, *Dipetalonema perstans.*

acanthocyte (ah-kan′tho-sīt) an erythrocyte with protoplasmic projections giving it a thorny appearance; seen in abetalipoproteinemia.

acanthocytosis (ah-kan″tho-si-to′sis) the presence in the blood of acanthocytes, characteristically seen in abetalipoproteinemia.

acantholysis (ah″kan-thol′ĭ-sis) loss of cohesion between the cells of the prickle cell layer of the skin and between it and the layer above. adj., **acantholyt′ic.**

a. bullo′sa, epidermolysis bullosa.

acanthoma (ak″an-tho′mah) a tumor in the prickle cell layer of the skin.

acanthosis (ak″an-tho′sis) diffuse hypertrophy or thickening of the prickle cell layer of the skin. adj., **acanthot′ic.**

a. ni′gricans, diffuse acanthosis with gray or black pigmentation, chiefly in body folds, occurring in an adult form, often associated with an internal carcinoma (called *malignant acanthosis nigricans*) and in a benign, nevoid form, more or less generalized. A benign form associated with obesity, which is sometimes due to endocrine disturbance, is called *pseudoacanthosis nigricans.*

acanthrocyte (ah-kan′thro-sīt) acanthocyte.

acapnia (ah-kap′ne-ah) decrease of carbon dioxide in the blood. adj., **acap′nic.**

acarbia (ah-kar′be-ah) decrease of bicarbonate in the blood.

acardia (ah-kar′de-ah) a developmental anomaly with absence of the heart.

acardiacus (ah″kar-di′ah-kus) [L.] having no heart.

acardius (ah-kar′de-us) an imperfectly formed twin fetus without a heart and invariably lacking other body parts.

acariasis (ak″ah-ri′ah-sis) infestation with mites.

acaricide (ah-kar′ĭ-sīd) an agent that destroys mites.

acarid (ak′ah-rid) a tick or a mite of the order Acarina.

Acarina (ak″ah-ri′nah) an order of arthropods (class Arachnoidea), including mites and ticks.

acarinosis (ah-kar″ĭ-no′sis) any disease caused by mites; acariasis.

acarodermatitis (ak″ah-ro-der″mah-ti′tis) skin inflammation due to bites of parasitic mites (acarids).

a. urticarioi′des, grain itch.

acarologist (ak″ah-rol′o-jist) a specialist in acarology.

acarology (ak″ah-rol′o-je) the scientific study of mites and ticks.

acarophobia (ak″ah-ro-fo′be-ah) morbid dread or delusion of infestation by mites.

Acarus (ak′ah-rus) a genus of small mites.

A. folliculo′rum, *Demodex folliculorum.*

A. scab′iei, *Sarcoptes scabiei.*

A. si′ro, a mite that causes vanillism in vanilla pod handlers.

acaryote (ah-kār′e-ōt) 1. non-nucleated. 2. a non-nucleated cell.

acatalasemia (a″kat-ah-la-se′me-ah) acatalasia.

acatalasia (a″kat-ah-la′ze-ah) a rare hereditary disease seen mostly in the Japanese, marked by congenital absence of catalase; it may be associated with recurrent infections of oral structures.

acatamathesia (ah-kat″ah-mah-the′ze-ah) 1. loss or impairment of the power to understand speech. 2. impairment of any one of the perceptive faculties, due to a central lesion.

acataphasia (ah-kat″ah-fa′ze-ah) a speech disorder, with inability to express one's thoughts in a connected manner, due to a central lesion.

acathexia (ak″ah-thek′se-ah) inability to retain bodily secretions. adj. **acathec′tic.**

A.C.C. American College of Cardiology.

accelerator (ak-sel′er-a″tor) [L.] an agent or apparatus that increases the rate at which something occurs or progresses.

a. globulin, clotting factor V.

serum prothrombin conversion a. (SPCA), clotting factor VII.

serum thrombotic a., a factor in serum that has procoagulant properties and the ability to induce blood CLOTTING.

acceptor (ak-sep′tor) a substance that unites with another substance.

hydrogen a., the molecule accepting hydrogen in an oxidation-reduction reaction.

accessory (ak-ses′o-re) supplementary or affording aid to another similar and generally more important thing.

a. nerve, the eleventh cranial nerve; it originates in the medulla oblongata and provides motion for the sternocleidomastoid and trapezius muscles of the neck. Called also spinal accessory nerve.

accident prone (ak′sĭ-dent prōn′) specially susceptible to accidents owing to psychological factors.

accipiter (ak-sip′ĭ-ter) a facial bandage with tails like the claws of a hawk.

acclimation (ak-lĭ-ma′shun) the process of becoming accustomed to a new environment.

accommodation (ah-kom″o-da′shun) adjustment, especially adjustment of the eye for seeing objects at various distances. This is accomplished by the ciliary muscle, which controls the LENS of the eye, allowing it to flatten or thicken as is needed for distant or near vision.

absolute a., the accommodation of either eye separately.

amplitude of a., the total amount of accommodative power of the eye; the difference in refractive power of the eye when adjusted for near and for far vision. The amplitude diminishes as age increases because elasticity of the lens is decreased. Called also range of accommodation.

histologic a., changes in morphology and function of cells following changed conditions.

negative a., adjustment of the eye for long distances by relaxation of the ciliary muscle.

positive a., adjustment of the eye for short distances by contraction of the ciliary muscle.

a. reflex, the coordinated changes that occur when the eye adapts itself for near vision; they are constriction of the pupil, convergence of the eyes, and increased convexity of the lens.

accouchement (ah-ko͞osh-maw′) [Fr.] childbirth; delivery; labor.

a. forcé, rapid forcible delivery by one of several methods; originally, rapid dilatation of the cervix with the hands, followed by version and extraction of the fetus.

accretion (ah-kre′shun) 1. growth by addition of material. 2. accumulation. 3. adherence of parts normally separated.

Ace bandage (ās) trademark for a bandage of woven elastic material.

aceclidine (as-sek′lĭ-dēn) a cholinergic agent.

acedapsone (as″ĕ-dap′sōn) a dapsone derivative having antimalarial and leprostatic activities.

acellular (a-sel′u-lar) not cellular in structure.

acelomate (ah-se′lo-māt) having no coelom or body cavity.

acenocoumarol (ah-se″no-koo′mah-rol) a compound used as an anticoagulant.

acentric (a-sen′tric) 1. not central; not located in the center. 2. lacking a centromere, so that the chromosome will not survive cell divisions.

acephalobrachia (ah-sef″ah-lo-bra′ke-ah) congenital absence of the head and arms.

acephalocardia (ah-sef″ah-lo-kar′de-ah) congenital absence of the head and heart.

acephalocardius (ah-sef″ah-lo-kar′de-us) a monster without a head or heart.

acephalochiria (ah-sef″ah-lo-ki′re-ah) congenital absence of the head and hands.

acephalocyst (ah-sef′ah-lo-sist″) a true hydatid cyst that fails to produce brood capsules.

acephalogaster (ah-sef″ah-lo-gas′ter) a fetus without a head or stomach.

acephalogastria (ah-sef″ah-lo-gas′tre-ah) congenital absence of the head, chest, and stomach.

acephalopodia (ah-sef″ah-lo-po′de-ah) congenital absence of the head and feet.

acephalopodius (ah-sef″ah-lo-po′de-us) a fetus without a head or feet.

acephalorachia (ah-sef″ah-lo-ra′ke-ah) congenital absence of the head and vertebral column.

acephalostomia (ah-sef″ah-lo-sto′me-ah) congenital absence of the head, with the mouth aperture on the upper aspect of the body.

acephalothoracia (ah-sef″ah-lo-tho-ra′se-ah) congenital absence of the head and thorax.

acephalous (ah-sef′ah-lus) headless.

acephalus (ah-sef′ah-lus) a headless fetus.

acerin (ah′ser-in) an extract from the dried fruit of the Norway maple, *Acer plantanoides,* effective against *Escherichia coli* and the vaccinia virus.

acervuline (ah-ser′vu-līn) aggregated; heaped up; said of certain glands.

acervulus (ah-ser′vu-lus), pl. *acer′vuli* [L.] sandy matter in or about the pineal body and other parts of the brain.

acetabular (as″ĕ-tab′u-lar) pertaining to the acetabulum.

acetabulectomy (as″ĕ-tab″u-lek′to-me) excision of the acetabulum.

acetabuloplasty (as″ĕ-tab′u-lo-plas′te) plastic repair of the acetabulum.

acetabulum (as″ĕ-tab′u-lum) the cup-shaped cavity on the lateral surface of the hip bone, receiving the head of the femur.

sunken a., Otto pelvis.

acetal (as′ĕ-tal) an organic compound formed by a combination of an aldehyde with an alcohol.

acetaldehyde (as″et-al′de-hīd) a colorless volatile liquid, CH_3CHO, found in freshly distilled spirits, that is irritating to mucous membranes and has a general narcotic action. It is also an intermediate in the metabolism of alcohol.

acetaminophen (as″et-am′ĭ-no-fen″) a compound used as an analgesic and antipyretic.

acetanilid (as″ĕ-tan′ĭ-lid) a white powder, slightly soluble in water, used as an analgesic and antipyretic, particularly in combination with other drugs in various proprietary preparations such as headache remedies. Habituation may occur and the drug is little used because its continued use may lead to methemoglobinemia.

acetarsol, acetarsone (as″et-ar′sol; as″et-ar′sōn) an arsenical used in the treatment of amebic dysentery and trichomonas vaginalis.

acetate (as′ĕ-tāt) a salt of acetic acid.

acetazolamide (as″et-ah-zol′ah-mīd) a diuretic of the carbonic anhydrase inhibitor type, useful in the treatment of cardiac edema. It is also used to reduce intraocular pressure in the treatment of glaucoma. Side effects of the drug are minor but an electrolyte imbalance with potassium depletion may occur.

Acetest (ah′sĕ-test) trademark for reagent tablets containing sodium nitroprusside, aminoacetic acid, disodium phosphate, and lactose. A drop of urine is placed on a tablet on a sheet of white paper; if significant quantities of acetone are present the tablet changes from a purple tint (1+), to lavender (2+), to moderate purple (3+), or to deep purple (4+).

acetic (ah-se′tik, ah-set′ik) pertaining to vinegar or its acid; sour.

a. acid, a short-chain, saturated fatty acid, the characteristic component of vinegar. It has the odor of vinegar and a sharp acid taste. A 36.5 per cent solution of acetic acid is used topically as a caustic and rubefacient. A dilute acetic acid solution (6 per cent) may be used as an antidote to alkali. Glacial acetic acid is a 99.4 per cent solution.

acetimeter (as″ĕ-tim′ĕ-ter) an instrument for measuring the acetic acid in a fluid.

acetoacetic acid (ah-se″to-ah-se′tik) one of the KETONE BODIES formed in the body in metabolism of certain substances, particularly in the liver in the combustion of fats. It is present in the body in increased amounts in abnormal conditions such as DIABETES MELLITUS and starvation.

Acetobacter (ah-se″to-bak′ter) a genus of bacteria important in completion of the carbon cycle and in production of vinegar.

acetohexamide (as″ĕ-to-heks′ah-mīd) an oral hypoglycemic.

acetone (as′ĕ-tōn) a compound, $CH_3 \cdot CO \cdot CH_3$, with solvent properties and characteristic odor, obtained by fermentation or produced synthetically; it is a by-product of acetoacetic acid. Acetone is one of the KETONE BODIES produced in abnormal amounts in DIABETES MELLITUS. (See also KETOSIS.)

a. bodies, acetone, acetoacetic acid, and beta-oxybutyric acid, being intermediates in fat metabolism. Also called KETONE BODIES.

acetonemia (as″ĕ-to-ne′me-ah) ketonemia.

acetonitrile (as″ĕ-to-ni′tril) methyl cyanide, CH_3-CN, a colorless acid.

acetonuria (as″ĕ-to-nu′re-ah) ketonuria.

acetophenazine (as″ĕ-to-fen′ah-zēn) a compound used as a tranquilizer.

acetophenetidin (as″ĕ-to-fĕ-net′ĭ-din) phenacetin.

acetrizoate sodium (as″ĕ-tri′zo-āt so′de-um) the sodium salt of acetrizoic acid, used as a contrast medium.

acetyl (as′ĕ-til) the monovalent radical, CH_3CO, a combining form of acetic acid.

a. peroxide, a powerful oxidizing agent.

a. sulfisoxazole, a sulfanilamide used as an anti-infective.

acetylaniline (as″ĕ-til-an′ĭ-lin) acetanilid.

acetylation (ah-set″ĭ-la′shun) introduction of an acetyl radical into an organic molecule.

acetyl-beta-methylcholine (as″ĕ-til-ba″tah-meth″il-ko′lēn) methacholine.

acetylcarbromal (as″ĕ-til-kar-bro′mal) a sedative drug used primarily to relieve tension and anxiety and as a daytime sedative.

acetylcholine (as″ĕ-til-ko′lēn) a reversible acetic acid ester of choline, normally present in many parts of the body and having important physiologic functions, such as the transmission of nerve impulses; used as a parasympathomimetic agent.

acetylcholinesterase (as″ĕ-til-ko″lin-es′ter-ās) an enzyme present in nervous tissue, muscle, and red cells that catalyzes the hydrolysis of acetylcholine to choline and acetic acid; called also true CHOLINESTERASE. Abbreviated AChE.

acetylcysteine (as″ĕ-til-sis′te-in) a mucolytic agent used to reduce the viscosity of secretions of the respiratory tract.

acetyldigitoxin (as″ĕ-til-dij″ĭ-tok′sin) an oral digitalis preparation derived from lanatoside, used to improve function of the failing heart. It provides a more rapid curve of action than digitoxin and is less completely absorbed, but is not actually less toxic.

acetylene (ah-set′ĭ-lēn) 1. a colorless, combustible gas with a garlic-like odor. 2. the type of a class of unsaturated (triple-bonded) organic compounds.

acetylphenylhydrazine (as″ĕ-til-fen″il-hi′drah-zēn) an erythrocyte depressant which has been used in the treatment of polycythemia.

acetylsalicylic acid (ah-sēt′il-sal-ĭ-sil′ik) aspirin, a commonly used analgesic, antipyretic, and antirheumatic drug. It is available in pure form or in combination with a variety of drugs.

A.C.G. American College of Gastroenterology.

AcG accelerator globulin (clotting factor V).

ACh acetylcholine.

achalasia (ak″ah-la′ze-ah) failure to relax of the smooth muscle fibers of the gastrointestinal tract at any junction of one part with another; especially failure of the lower esophagus to relax with swallowing, due to degeneration of ganglion cells in the wall of the organ.

The cause of achalasia is unknown, but anxiety and emotional tension seem to aggravate the condition and precipitate attacks. As the condition progresses there is dilatation of the esophagus (megaesophagus) above the constriction and absence of peristalsis in the area.

SYMPTOMS. The patient complains of a feeling of fullness in the sternal region; vomiting frequently occurs, and there may be aspiration of the esophageal contents into the respiratory passages. As a result of this aspiration the patient may develop pneumonia or atelectasis.

Diagnosis is confirmed by x-ray studies using barium and by visual examination of the area by esophagoscope.

TREATMENT. Conservative treatment of mild cases consists of advising the patient to eat a bland diet that is low in bulk. Very large meals should be avoided and all foods should be eaten slowly with frequent drinking of fluids during the meal. To reduce the possibility of aspiration of esophageal contents during sleep, the patient is instructed to sleep with his head and shoulders elevated.

For severe constriction surgical relief may be necessary. The incision, which includes the lower esophagus and upper stomach wall, is made down to but not through the intestinal mucosa. This allows for stretching of the mucosa to accommodate food passing through. Approach is made through an incision into the chest; thus, preoperative care and postoperative care are the same as for elective chest surgery (see also THORACIC SURGERY).

AChE acetylcholinesterase.

ache (āk) 1. continuous pain, as opposed to sharp pangs or twinges. An ache can be either dull and constant, as in some types of backache, or throbbing, as in some types of headache and toothache. 2. to suffer such pain.

acheilia (ah-ki′le-ah) a developmental anomaly with absence of the lips. adj., **achei′lous.**

acheiria (ah-ki′re-ah) 1. a developmental anomaly with absence of the hands. 2. a sensation of loss of the hands, seen in hysteria.

acheiropodia (ah-ki″ro-po′de-ah) a developmental anomaly characterized by absence of both hands and feet.

Achilles tendon (ah-kil′ēz) the strong tendon at the back of the heel that connects the calf muscles (triceps surae muscle) to the heel bone. The name is derived from the legend of the Greek hero Achilles, who was vulnerable only in one heel. Tapping the Achilles tendon normally produces the Achilles REFLEX, or ankle jerk. Failure or exaggeration of this reflex indicates disease or injury to the nerves of the leg muscles or of a part of the spinal cord.

achillobursitis (ah-kil″o-bur-si′tis) inflammation of the bursae about the Achilles tendon.

achillodynia (ah-kil″o-din′e-ah) pain in the Achilles tendon or its bursa.

achillorrhaphy (ak″il-lor′ah-fe) suturing of the Achilles tendon.

achillotenotomy (ah-kil″o-ten-ot′o-me) surgical division of the Achilles tendon.

achlorhydria (a″klōr-hi′dre-ah) absence of hydrochloric acid from gastric juice; associated with PERNICIOUS ANEMIA, stomach cancer, and pellagra. adj., **achlorhy′dric.**

achloropsia (a″klo-rop′se-ah) inability to distinguish green colors.

acholia (a-ko′le-ah) lack or absence of bile secretion. adj., **acho′lic.**

acholuria (ak″o-lu′re-ah) absence of bile pigments from the urine.

achondrogenesis (a-kon″dro-jen′ĕ-sis) a hereditary disorder characterized by hypoplasia of bone, resulting in markedly shortened limbs; the head and trunk are normal.

achondroplasia (a-kon″dro-pla′ze-ah) a disorder of cartilage formation in the fetus, leading to a type of DWARFISM. adj., **achondroplas′tic.**

Achorion (ah-ko′re-on) *Trichophyton.*

achrestic (ah-kres′tik) caused not by absence of a necessary substance, but by inability to utilize such a substance.

achromasia (ak″ro-ma′se-ah) 1. lack of normal skin pigmentation. 2. the inability of tissues or cells to be stained.

achromat, achromate (ak′ro-mat″; ah-kro′māt) a person who is totally color blind.

achromatic (ak″ro-mat′ik) 1. producing no discoloration, or staining with difficulty. 2. pertaining to achromatin. 3. refracting light without decomposing it into its component colors. 4. pertaining to complete lack of color vision.

achromatin (ah-kro′mah-tin) the faintly staining groundwork of a cell nucleus.

achromatism (ah-kro′mah-tizm) 1. the quality or the condition of being achromatic. 2. achromatopia.

achromatolysis (ah-kro″mah-tol′ĭ-sis) disorganization of cell achromatin.

achromatophil (ak″ro-mat′o-fil, a″kro-mat′o-fil) 1. not easily stainable. 2. an organism or tissue that does not stain easily.

achromatopia (ah″kro-mah-to′pe-ah) defective visual perception of colors. adj., **achromatop′ic.**

achromatosis (ah-kro″mah-to′sis) 1. deficiency of pigmentation in the tissues. 2. lack of staining power in a cell or tissue.

achromatous (a-kro′mah-tus) colorless.

achromaturia (a-kro″mah-tu′re-ah) colorless state of the urine.

achromia (a-kro′me-ah) absence of normal color; specifically, a condition of erythrocytes in which their centers are paler than normal (central achromia). adj., **achro′mic.**

achromocyte (ah-kro′mo-sīt) a red cell artifact that stains more faintly than intact red cells.

achromophil (ah-kro′mo-fil) achromatophil.

Achromycin (ak″ro-mi′sin) trademark for preparations of tetracycline hydrochloride, a broad-spectrum antibiotic.

achylia (a-ki′le-ah) absence of hydrochloric acid and enzymes in the gastric secretions.

achylous (a-ki′lus) deficient in chyle.

achymia (a-ki′me-ah) deficiency of chyme.

acicular (ah-sik′u-lar) needle-shaped.

acid (as′id) 1. sour. 2. a substance that yields hydrogen ions in solution and from which hydrogen may be displaced by a metal to form a salt. All acids react with bases to form salts and water (neutralization). Other properties of acids include a sour taste and the ability to cause certain dyes to undergo a color change. A common example of this is the ability of acids to change litmus paper from blue to red.

Acids play a vital role in the chemical processes that are a normal part of the functions of the cells and tissues of the body. A stable balance between acids and bases in the body is essential to life. (See also ACID-BASE BALANCE.) For the various acids, see under the specific name, such as acetic acid.

amino a., any one of a class of organic compounds containing the amino and the carboxyl group, occurring naturally in plant and animal tissues and forming the chief constituents of protein. (See also AMINO ACID.)

bile a's, organic compounds—glycocholic acid and taurocholic acid—formed in the liver and secreted in the bile.

a. burn, injury to tissues caused by an acid, such as sulfuric acid or nitric acid. Emergency first aid for an acid burn of the skin includes (1) immediate and thorough washing of the burn with water; (2) calling a physician; and (3) continued bathing of the burn in water until the physician arrives. (See also BURN.)

fatty a., any monobasic aliphatic acid containing only carbon, hydrogen, and oxygen. (See also FATTY ACID.)

inorganic a., an acid containing no carbon atoms.

keto a's, compounds containing the groups CO (carbonyl) and COOH (carboxyl).

nucleic a's, substances that constitute the prosthetic groups of the nucleoproteins and contain phosphoric acid, sugars, and purine and pyrimidine bases. See also NUCLEIC ACIDS.

organic a., an acid containing the carboxyl group, COOH.

a. phosphatase, a phosphatase that is active in an acid environment.

acidaminuria (as″id-am″ĭ-nu′re-ah) excess of amino acid in the urine.

acid-ash diet a special diet prescribed for the purpose of lowering the urinary pH so that alkaline salts will remain in solution. The diet may be given to aid in the elimination of fluid in certain kinds of edema, in the treatment of some types of urinary tract infection, and to inhibit the formation of alkaline urinary calculi. Meat, fish, eggs, and cereals are emphasized, with little fruit and vegetables and no milk or cheese.

acid-base balance a state of equilibrium between acidity and alkalinity of the body fluids; also called hydrogen ion (H^+) balance because, by definition, an acid is a substance capable of giving up a hydrogen ion during a chemical exchange, and a base is a substance that can accept it. The positively charged hydrogen ion (H^+) is the active constituent of all acids.

Most of the body's metabolic processes produce acids as their end products, but a somewhat alkaline body fluid is required as a medium for vital cellular activities. Therefore chemical exchanges of hydrogen ions must take place continuously in order to maintain a state of equilibrium. An optimal pH (hydrogen ion concentration) between 7.35 and 7.45 must be maintained; otherwise, the enzyme systems and other biochemical and metabolic activities will not function normally.

Although the body can tolerate and compensate for slight deviations in acidity and alkalinity, if the pH drops below 7.30, the potentially serious condition of ACIDOSIS exists. If the pH goes higher than 7.50, the patient is in a state of ALKALOSIS. In either case the disturbance of the acid-base balance is considered serious, even though there are control mechanisms by which the body can compensate for an upward or downward change in the pH. Shifts in the pH of body fluids are controlled by three major regulatory systems which may be classified as *chemical* (the buffer systems), *biologic* (blood and cellular activity), and *physiologic* (the lungs and kidneys).

CHEMICAL CONTROLS. The chemical buffer systems are dependent on the capability of certain substances to either combine with or release hydrogen ions. In the plasma and the intracellular and interstitial fluids there are three major buffer systems that regulate hydrogen ion activity: the carbonic acid–bicarbonate system, the protein buffer system, and the phosphate buffer system.

Of these three, the *carbonic acid–bicarbonate system* is the most important in fluids outside the cell. It is the most extensive and is the first to react to an acid-base imbalance. Carbonic acid and bicarbonate are both derived from water and carbon dioxide and therefore exist in large quantities in the body. Carbonic acid is, however, weakly ionized and needs to coexist with its salt in order to effectively remove excess hydrogen or hydroxyl ions from the extracellular fluids. Hence it is actually the *carbonic acid and sodium bicarbonate* buffer system that works to maintain normal levels of hydrogen ion concentrations in the extracellular fluids. It is important to remember that these two chemical components must be in the ratio of 1:20; that is, for every one part of carbonic acid (H_2CO_3) there must be twenty parts of sodium bicarbonate ($NaHCO_3$). It is not the absolute amount of each component that is crucial in the control of acid-base balance, but the ratio of the one substance to the other. The carbonic acid–bicarbonate buffer system is capable of either accepting or releasing hydrogen ions without forcing the pH to dangerous levels.

The *protein buffer system* is especially remarkable because proteins are powerful buffers that can function as either acid or base, depending on the state of the body fluids. This system is active in the plasma and in intracellular and extracellular fluids.

The *phosphate buffer system* operates in much the same way as the carbonic acid–bicarbonate system but is more active within the cell than in extracellular fluids.

Although the chemical buffer systems react almost instantaneously to a change in the pH of the body fluids, they cannot provide sustained regulation of the pH because they are absorbed rapidly and cannot be replaced immediately. The hydrogen ions that are not handled by the chemical buffer

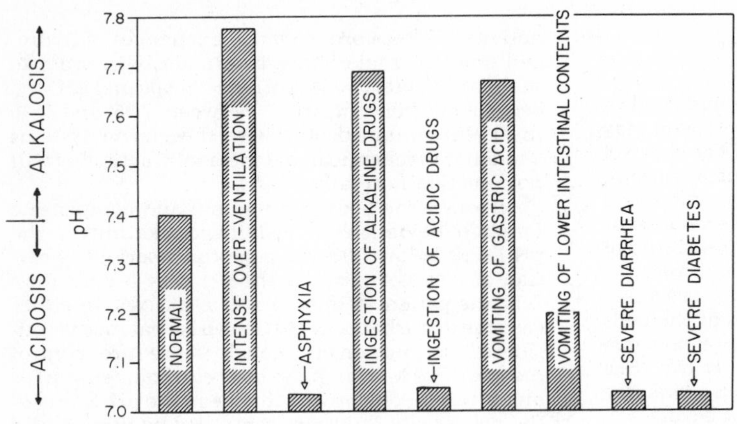

pH of the body fluids in various acid-base disorders. (From Guyton, A. C.: Function of the Human Body. 4th ed. Philadelphia, W. B. Saunders Co., 1974.)

systems become the responsibility of other regulatory controls which respond less rapidly but are not less important.

BIOLOGIC REGULATORS. This type of control is concerned with the shifting of excess acid or alkali in and out of the cell. As an excess ions cross over the cell membrane they must do so in combination with ions of the opposite charge, or in exchange for ions of the same charge. Sodium and potassium are the two cations most often exchanged for the positively charged hydrogen ion.

The hemoglobin-oxyhemoglobin system is another regulatory control. As chloride leaves the oxygenated blood cells and enters the plasma, the bicarbonate moves from the plasma and crosses over into the cellular fluid. This reciprocal exchange between bicarbonate and chloride is a continuous process.

PHYSIOLOGIC REGULATORS. The lungs begin to compensate for an acid-base imbalance within minutes of its onset. They do this by regulating the retention or the excretion of carbon dioxide. If acidosis is present, respiratory activity is increased so that CO_2 is blown off before it unites with the water in the blood to form carbonic acid. If alkalosis is present, respiratory activity is automatically decreased, CO_2 is retained, and carbonic acid is produced to neutralize the excess alkali.

The kidneys act as regulators by reabsorbing bicarbonate when it is needed to control excess acidity and by excreting it when there is a deficit of acid in the body. The kidneys also facilitate the excretion of excess hydrogen ions in combination with phosphate ions (in the form of phosphoric acid), or in combination with ammonia (excreted in the form of ammonium).

Imbalances of the acid-base ratio are discussed under ACIDOSIS and ALKALOSIS. Diagnosis and monitoring of either of these conditions are greatly enhanced by periodic determination of the pH and by BLOOD GAS ANALYSIS.

acidemia (as″ĭ-de′me-ah) abnormal acidity of the blood.

acid-fast (as′id-fast) not readily decolorized by acids after staining; said of bacteria, especially *Mycobacterium tuberculosis.*

acidic (ah-sid′ik) of or pertaining to an acid; acid-forming.

acidifier (ah-sid′ĭ-fi″er) an agent that causes acidity; a substance used to increase gastric acidity.

acidity (ah-sid′ĭ-te) 1. the quality of being acid; the power to unite with positively charges ions or with basic substances. 2. excess acid quality, as of the gastric juice.

acidophilic (as″ĭ-do-fil′ik) 1. easily stained with acid dyes. 2. growing best on acid media.

acidophilism (as″ĭ-dof′ĭ-lizm) the state produced by acidophilic adenoma of the pituitary gland, resulting in ACROMEGALY.

acidosis (as″ĭ-do′sis) a pathologic condition resulting from accumulation of acid or depletion of the alkaline reserve (bicarbonate content) in the blood and body tissues, and characterized by increase in hydrogen ion concentration (decrease in pH). adj., **acidot′ic.** The optimal ACID-BASE BALANCE is maintained by chemical buffers, biologic activities of the cells, and effective functioning of the lungs and kidneys. The opposite of acidosis is ALKALOSIS.

It is rare that acidosis occurs in the absence of some underlying disease process but in cases of mild acidosis the symptoms may be overlooked. The more obvious signs of severe acidosis are muscle twitching, involuntary movement, cardiac arrhythmias, disorientation, and coma.

In general, treatment consists of intravenous or oral administration of sodium bicarbonate or sodium lactate solutions and correction of the underlying cause of the imbalance. Many cases of severe acidosis can be prevented by careful monitoring of the patient whose primary illness predisposes him to increased levels of acidity or decreased bicarbonate levels. Such care includes effective teaching of self-care to the diabetic so that the disease remains under control. Patients receiving intravenous therapy, especially those having a fluid deficit, and those with biliary or intestinal intubation should be watched closely for early signs of acidosis. Others predisposed to acidosis are patients with shock, hyperthyroidism, advanced circulatory failure, or liver disease. Respiratory acidosis can develop in any patient suffering from a respiratory disorder capable of causing alveolar hypoventilation, or from chemical or physical trauma to the medullary respiratory centers.

compensated a., a condition in which the compensatory mechanisms have returned the pH toward normal.

diabetic a., a metabolic acidosis produced by accumulation of ketones in uncontrolled diabetes mellitus.

hypercapnic a., respiratory acidosis.

hyperchloremic a., renal tubular acidosis.

metabolic a., acidosis resulting from accumulation in the blood of keto acids (derived from fat metabolism) at the expense of bicarbonate, thus diminishing the body's ability to neutralize acids. This type of acidosis can occur when there is an acid gain, as in diabetic ketoacidosis, lactic acidosis, poisoning, and failure of the renal tubules to reabsorb bicarbonate. It can also result from bicarbonate loss due to diarrhea or a gastrointestinal fistula.

The symptoms of metabolic acidosis include weakness, malaise, and headache. As the acid level goes up these symptoms progress to stupor, unconsciousness, coma, and death. The breath of the patient may have a fruity odor owing to the presence of acetone, and he may experience vomiting and diarrhea. Loss of fluids can deplete his fluid content and aggravate the acidosis. Hyperventilation may occur as a result of stimulation of the hypothalamus. BLOOD GAS ANALYSIS will reveal a lowered pH and an elevated Pa_{CO_2}.

TREATMENT AND PATIENT CARE. Treatment of metabolic acidosis is primarily concerned with control of the underlying causes. Diabetic ketoacidosis may be corrected by the administration of insulin and fluids. In acute renal failure the patient requires DIALYSIS, and in chronic uremic acidosis the condition is controlled by restricting sodium intake and buffering with bicarbonate.

The patient's vital signs should be checked frequently to assess the progress of compensation. A rising pulse rate may indicate respiratory compensation, a drop in blood pressure frequently occurs as a result of hypovolemia in the diabetic-acidotic patient, and cardiac arrhythmias can be caused by increased calcium levels in the blood.

A careful recording of intake and output provides a means of determining the kidneys' ability to regulate the ACID-BASE BALANCE. Safety measures to avoid injury during involuntary muscular contractions should be carried out. (See also CONVULSIONS.) Mouth care using an alkaline mouthwash such as baking soda reduces the discomfort from mouth acids. Nursing measures to relieve discomfort from vomiting and to avoid the hazards of aspiration of vomitus are required. Education of the patient and his family in the prevention of acute episodes of metabolic acidosis is of primary importance.

renal tubular a., a metabolic acidosis resulting from impairment of the reabsorption of bicarbonate by the renal tubules, the urine being alkaline.

respiratory a., acidosis resulting from ventilatory failure and subsequent retention of carbon dioxide. *Acute* respiratory acidosis occurs when there is a relatively sudden malfunction of respiratory activities, as in upper airway obstruction, acute infections and inflammation of the lung and bronchial tissues, and pulmonary edema. In acute respiratory acidosis the compensatory chemical buffer systems are of limited benefit in restoring the ACID-BASE BALANCE because they depend on normal blood circulation and tissue perfusion for optimal effect. The physiologic regulators, the lungs and kidneys, are of little help because the lungs are malfunctioning and the kidneys require more time to compensate than the acute condition permits.

Chronic respiratory acidosis results from gradual and irreversible loss of ventilatory function, as in COPD. Although the patient in this condition does have an increased retention of CO_2, there is time for the kidneys to compensate by retaining bicarbonate and thereby maintaining a pH within tolerable limits. If, however, the patient develops even a minor respiratory infection, he is subject to a rapidly developing state of acute acidosis because his lungs cannot be depended upon to remove more than a minimal amount of CO_2.

TREATMENT AND PATIENT CARE. The initial treatment for respiratory acidosis is to establish an airway immediately and maintain adequate ventilation and hydration. Acute cases may require ENDOTRACHEAL INTUBATION or TRACHEOSTOMY. INTERMITTENT POSITIVE PRESSURE BREATHING (IPPB) is used to avoid CO_2 narcosis. Beyond a certain point the respiratory center may cease responding to the higher CO_2 levels and breathing will stop abruptly. Drugs which further depress the respiratory center (narcotics, hypnotics, and tranquilizers) must be avoided. Patients in the acute stage must be watched for cessation of breathing and cardiac arrest. CARDIOPULMONARY RESUSCITATION may be required to revive the patient.

It is recommended that oxygen be administered at a rate of no more than 1 to 2 liters per minute because of the danger of removing the hypoxic stimulus to breathing. The rate of oxygen flow should be closely correlated with blood gas studies.

Measures which facilitate breathing are essential to patient care during respiratory acidosis. Frequent turning, coughing, and deep breathing exercises to encourage oxygen–carbon dioxide exchange are beneficial, as is SUCTIONING when needed to remove secretions obstructing the airway. POSTURAL DRAINAGE, unless contraindicated by the patient's condition, may be effective in promoting adequate ventilation.

starvation a., a metabolic acidosis due to accumulation of ketones following a severe caloric deficit.

acid-proof (as′id-pro͞of) acid-fast.

acidulous (ah-sid′u-lus) moderately sour.

acidum (as′ĭ-dum) [L.] acid.

aciduria (as″ĭ-du′re-ah) the excretion of acid in the urine. See also specific forms, such as aminoaciduria, orotic aciduria, etc.

aciduric (as″ĭ-du′rik) capable of growing in extremely acid media.

acinar (as′ĭ-nar) pertaining to or affecting an acinus or acini.

acinetic (as″ĭ-net′ik) akinetic.

aciniform (ah-sin′ĭ-form) grapelike.

acinitis (as″ĭ-ni′tis) inflammation of the acini of a gland.

acinose, acinous (as′ĭ-nōs), (as′ĭ-nus) made up of acini.

acinus (as′ĭ-nus), pl. *ac′ini* [L.] any of the smallest lobules of a compound gland.

acladiosis (ah-klad″e-o′sis) an ulcerative skin disease caused by the fungus *Acladium castellani.*

Acladium (ah-kla′de-um) a genus of fungus sometimes infecting man.

aclasia, aclasis (ah-kla′ze-ah; ak′lah-sis) pathologic continuity of structure, as in chondrodystrophy.

diaphyseal a., hereditary multiple exostoses.

acleistocardia (ah-klīs″to-kar′de-ah) an open state of the foramen ovale of the fetal heart.

acme (ak′me) the critical stage or crisis of a disease.

acne (ak′ne) a disorder of the skin with eruption of papules or pustules; more particularly, acne vulgaris.

a. congloba'ta, conglobate a., severe acne with many comedones, marked by suppuration, cysts, sinuses, and scarring.

cystic a., acne with the formation of cysts enclosing a mixture of keratin and sebum in varying proportions.

a. indura'ta, a progression of papular acne, with deep-seated and destructive lesions that may produce severe scarring.

keloid a., keloid folliculitis.

a. necrot'ica, acne varioliformis.

a. necrot'ica milia'ris, a rare and chronic form of folliculitis of the scalp, occurring principally in adults, with formation of tiny superficial pustules which are destroyed by scratching (see also ACNE VARIOLIFORMIS).

a. neonato'rum, a condition found in newborn infants with oily skins, characterized by comedones, papules, and pustules on nose, cheeks, and forehead.

a. papulo'sa, acne vulgaris with the formation of papules.

a. rosa'cea, rosacea.

tropical a., a severe and extensive form of acne occurring in hot, humid climates, with nodular, cystic, and pustular lesions chiefly on the back, buttocks, and thighs; conglobate abscesses frequently form, especially on the back.

a. variolifor'mis, a rare condition with reddish-brown, papulopustular umbilicated lesions, usually on the brow and scalp; probably a deep variant of acne necrotica miliaris.

a. vulga'ris, chronic acne, usually occurring in adolescence, with comedones (blackheads), papules, nodules, and pustules on the face, neck, and upper part of the trunk.

At the beginning stages of adulthood, there is an increase in hormonal activity and glandular secretion, including increased production of sebum from the sebaceous glands in the skin. In girls this may be more pronounced at the time of the menstrual period. Certain foods also cause an increase in the activity of the sebaceous glands, the worst offenders being chocolate, nuts, sharp cheeses, and fatty foods. If a hair follicle opening on the surface of the skin is small or is clogged by dirt or heavy cosmetics, the fatty material made by the sebaceous glands accumulates, and a "bump" appears under the skin, or a whitehead or blackhead (comedo) shows on the surface. The dark color of blackheads is caused not by dirt but by the discoloring effect of air on the fatty material in the clogged follicle. If this substance becomes infected, as it often does, a pimple results. The temptation to squeeze the unsightly pimple should be resisted. A squeeze can break the membrane around the pimple and spread the infection to the surrounding tissue. The result is more pimples, scars, and pits.

This story is all too familiar to young people. It is not enough to be reminded that "you'll grow out of it," although this is generally true. Acne does tend to disappear with maturity. If the adolescent is excessively troubled with this condition, the scars may be mental as well as physical.

TREATMENT. The first step is to discover and eliminate any food that encourages acne. The skin must be kept clean, particularly in the areas where acne is most apt to appear, such as the face, chest, and back. With plain soap, fairly hot water, and a clean washcloth, the skin is washed, but not scrubbed so hard as to cause injury, and then rinsed with cold water. Sometimes the physician may recommend an antibacterial soap. Towels should be changed at least daily. Hair should be shampooed frequently, and hairbrush, comb, and powder puff should be kept scrupulously clean. All creams and greasy lotions should be avoided, and the follicles should not be plugged with heavy makeup or "pore-closing" beauty aids.

Blackheads are removed with a comedo extractor after the skin has been soaked in warm sudsy water to loosen them. Extractors can be purchased at most drugstores, and should be used instead of fingers. If the blackhead comes out easily, the spot should be touched with rubbing alcohol (70 per cent). If it does not, it should be left alone for a while.

Severe cases of acne require more intensive and complicated treatment, which only a physician can provide. Some cases require therapy by a dermatologist.

When acne has left permanent, disfiguring scars, there are medical techniques that can remove or improve the blemishes. One method is planing with a rotary, high-speed brush. This removes the outer layer of pitted skin, leaving the growing layer and the layers containing the glands and hair follicles. New epithelium grows from the layers underneath; it is rosy at first and gradually becomes normal in color. The technique has also been used successfully in removing some types of disfigurations resulting from accidents. This so-called "sand-paper surgery" or dermabrasion is recommended only for selected cases of acne. It must be performed by a qualified specialist.

acnegenic (ak″ne-jen′ik) producing acne.

acneiform (ak-ne′ĭ-form) resembling acne.

acoelomate (a-se′lo-māt) 1. without a coelom or body cavity. 2. an acoelomate animal.

aconite (ak′o-nīt) dried tuberous root of *Aconitum napellus;* a counterirritant and local anesthetic.

aconitine (ah-kon′ĭ-tin) an alkaloid that is the active principle of aconite.

acorea (ah″ko-re′ah) absence of the pupil.

acoria (ah-ko′re-ah) insatiable appetite.

acouesthesia (ah-koo″es-the′ze-ah) acoustic sensibility.

acoumeter (ah-koo′mĕ-ter) an instrument for measuring the accuracy or acuteness of the hearing.

acoustic (ah-koos′tik) relating to sound or hearing.

acoustics (ah-koos′tiks) the science of sound and hearing.

acoustogram (ah-koos′to-gram) the graphic tracing of the curves of sounds produced by motion of a joint.

A.C.P. American College of Pathologists; American College of Physicians.

acquired (ah-kwīrd′) incurred as a result of factors acting from or originating outside the organism; not inherited.

A.C.R. American College of Radiology.

acragnosis (ak″rag-no′sis) acroagnosis.

acral (a′kral) affecting the extremities.

acrania (a-kra′ne-ah) partial or complete absence of the cranium. adj., **acra′nial.**

acranius (a-kra′ne-us) a monster in which the cranium is absent or rudimentary.

acridine (ak′rĭ-dēn) a crystalline alkaloid from anthracene, the basis of certain dyes.

acriflavine (ak″rĭ-fla′vin) an antiseptic dye used for topical application; average strength is 1:1000 to 1:8000 solution.

acrisorcin (ak″rĭ-sor′sin) a topical antifungal used in the treatment of tinea versicolor.

acritical (a-krit′ĭ-kal) having no crisis.

acro- word element [Gr.], *extreme; top; extremity.*

acroagnosis (ak″ro-ag-no′sis) lack of sensory recognition of a limb.

acroanesthesia (ak″ro-an″es-the′ze-ah) anesthesia of the extremities.

acrobrachycephaly (ak″ro-brak″e-sef′ah-le) abnormal height of the skull, with shortness of its anteroposterior dimension.

acrocentric (ak″ro-sen′trik) having the centromere toward one end of the replicating chromosome.

acrocephalia (ak″ro-sĕ-fa′le-ah) oxycephaly.

acrocephalic (ak″ro-sĕ-fal′ik) oxycephalic.

acrocephalosyndactyly (ak″ro-sef″ah-lo-sin-dak′tĭ-le) oxycephaly associated with webbing of the fingers or toes.

acrocephaly (ak″ro-sef′ah-le) oxycephaly.

acrochordon (ak″ro-kor′don) a pedunculated skin tag occurring principally on the neck, upper chest, and axillae in women of middle age or older.

acrocinesis (ak″ro-si-ne′sis) acrokinesia.

acrocyanosis (ak″ro-si″ah-no′sis) persistent cyanosis of the fingers and hands or the toes and feet, with mottled blue or red discoloration, coldness, and profuse sweating of the digits.

acrodermatitis (ak″ro-der″mah-ti′tis) inflammation of the skin of the hands or feet.

chronic atropic a., a. chron′ica atroph′icans, chronic inflammation of the skin of the extremities, leading to atrophy of the cutis.

a. contin′ua, continuous a., chronic inflammation of the skin of the extremities, in some cases becoming generalized.

enteropathic a., a. enteropath′ica, a hereditary disorder of infancy, with a vesiculopustulous dermatitis preferentially located periorificially and on the head, elbows, knees, hands, and feet, associated with gastrointestinal disturbances, chiefly manifested by diarrhea, and total alopecia.

a. per′stans, acrodermatitis continua.

acrodermatosis (ak″ro-der″mah-to′sis) any disease of the skin of the hands and feet.

acrodynia (ak″ro-din′e-ah) a disease of infancy and early childhood marked by pain and swelling in, and pink coloration of, the fingers and toes and by listlessness, irritability, failure to thrive, profuse perspiration, and sometimes scarlet coloration of the cheeks and tip of the nose. It is due to absorption of mercury. Called also erythredema polyneuropathy and pink disease.

acroesthesia (ak″ro-es-the′ze-ah) 1. exaggerated sensitiveness. 2. pain in the extremities.

acrognosis (ak″rog-no′sis) sensory recognition of the limbs.

acrohypothermy (ak″ro-hi′po-ther″me) abnormal coldness of the hands and feet.

acrokeratosis verruciformis (ak″ro-ker″ah-to′sis ver-roo″sĭ-for′mis) a hereditary dermatosis characterized by the presence of numerous flat wartlike papules on the dorsal aspect of the hand, foot, elbow, and knee.

acrokinesia (ak″ro-ki-ne′se-ah) abnormal motility or movement of the extremities.

acrolein (ak-ro′le-in) a volatile liquid from the decomposition of glycerin.

acromegaly (ak″ro-meg′ah-le) abnormal enlargement of the extremities of the skeleton—nose, jaws, hands, and feet—resulting from hypersecretion of the growth hormone of the PITUITARY GLAND. The condition is relatively rare and occurs in adults. In children overproduction of growth hormone stimulates growth of long bones and results in GIGANTISM, in which the child grows to exaggerated heights. With adults, however, growth of the long bones has already stopped, so that the bones most affected are those of the face, the jaw, and the hands and feet.

Overproduction of growth hormone is most often due to a tumor of the pituitary, and in such cases the condition is treated by surgical removal of the tumor or radiotherapy, or a combination of the two.

acromelalgia (ak″ro-mel-al′je-ah) erythromelalgia.

acromicria (ak″ro-mi′kre-ah) abnormal smallness of the extremities of the skeleton—nose, jaws, hands, and feet.

acromio- word element [Gr.], *acromion.*

acromioclavicular joint (ah-kro″me-o-klah-vik′u-lar) the point at which the clavicle joins with the acromion.

acromiohumeral (ah-kro″me-o-hu′mer-al) pertaining to the acromion and humerus.

acromion (ah-kro′me-on) the lateral extension of the spine of the scapula, forming the highest point of the shoulder. adj., **acro′mial.**

acromionectomy (ah-kro″me-on-ek′to-me) resection of the acromion.

acromiothoracic (ah-kro″me-o-tho-ras′ik) pertaining to the acromion and thorax.

acromphalus (ah-krom′fah-lus) 1. bulging of the navel; sometimes a sign of umbilical hernia. 2. the center of the navel.

acroneurosis (ak″ro-nu-ro′sis) any neuropathy of the extremities.

acropachy (ak′ro-pak″e) clubbing of the fingers.

acropachyderma (ak″ro-pak″e-der′mah) thickening of the skin over the face, scalp, and extremities, clubbing of the extremities, and deformities of the long bones.

acroparalysis (ak″ro-pah-ral′ĭ-sis) paralysis of the extremities.

acroparesthesia (ak″ro-par″es-the′ze-ah) an abnormal sensation, such as tingling, numbness, pins and needles, in the digits.

acropathy (ak-rop′ah-the) any disease of the extremities.

acrophobia (ak″ro-fo′be-ah) morbid fear of heights.

acroposthitis (ak″ro-pos-thi′tis) inflammation of the prepuce.

acroscleroderma (ak″ro-skle″ro-der′mah) acrosclerosis.

acrosclerosis (ak″ro-sklĕ-ro′sis) a combination of Raynaud's disease and scleroderma of the distal parts of the extremities, especially of the digits, and of the neck and face, particularly the nose.

acrotism (ak'ro-tizm) absence or imperceptibility of the pulse. adj., **acrot'ic.**

A.C.S. American Cancer Society; American Chemical Society; American College of Surgeons.

ACTH adrenocorticotropic hormone, a hormone produced by the anterior lobe of the PITUITARY GLAND that stimulates the cortex of the ADRENAL GLAND to secrete its hormones, including corticosterone. If production of ACTH falls below normal, the adrenal cortex decreases in size, and production of the cortical hormones declines. Called also adrenocorticotropin and corticotropin.

ACTH is prescribed to stimulate the adrenal glands in the treatment of some allergies, including asthma, and it has anti-inflammatory properties that sometimes help in the treatment of rheumatoid arthritis. It has been used experimentally in a large number of disorders.

Actidil (ak'tĭ-dil) trademark for preparations of triprolidine, an antihistamine.

actin (ak'tin) a muscle protein localized in the I band of myofibrils; acting along with myosin particles, it is responsible for the contraction and relaxation of muscle.

acting out (ak'ting owt) the behavioral expression of hidden emotional conflicts, such as hostile feelings, in various kinds of neurotic behavior, as a defense pattern analogous to somatic conversion.

actinic (ak-tin'ik) producing chemical action; said of rays of light beyond the violet end of the spectrum.

actinism (ak'tĭ-nizm) the chemical property of light rays.

actinium (ak-tin'e-um) a chemical element, atomic number 89, atomic weight 227, symbol Ac. (See table of ELEMENTS.)

actino- word element [Gr.], *ray; radiation.*

actinobacillosis (ak"tĭ-no-bas"ĭ-lo'sis) an actinomycosis-like disease of domestic animals caused by *Actinobacillus ligniere'sii,* in which the bacilli form radiating structures in the tissues; sometimes seen in man.

Actinobacillus (ak"tĭ-no-bah-sil'us) a genus of gram-negative bacteria capable of infecting cattle and other domestic animals, but rarely man.

A. ligniere'sii, the causative agent of actinobacillosis.

A. mall'ei, *Pseudomonas mallei.*

actinochemistry (ak"tĭ-no-kem'is-tre) the chemistry of radiant energy.

actinodermatitis (ak"tĭ-no-der"mah-ti'tis) dermatitis from exposure to x-rays.

actinogen (ak-tin'o-jen) any radioactive substance.

actinogenesis (ak"tĭ-no-jen'ĕ-sis) the formation or production of actinic rays.

actinogenic (ak"tĭ-no-jen'ik) producing rays, especially actinic rays.

actinology (ak"tĭ-nol'o-je) 1. the study of radiant energy. 2. the science of the chemical effects of light.

actinolyte (ak-tin'o-līt) an apparatus for concentrating the rays of electric light in phototherapy.

Actinomadura (ak"tĭ-no-mad'u-rah) a genus of actinomycetes including *A. madu'rae,* the cause of maduromycosis in which the granules in the discharged pus are white, and *A. pelletier'ii,* the cause of maduromycosis in which the granules are red.

actinometer (ak"tĭ-nom'ĕ-ter) an instrument for measuring the penetrating power of radiant energy.

Actinomyces (ak"tĭ-no-mi'sēz) a genus of actinomycetes.

A. bo'vis, a gram-positive microorganism causing actinomycosis in cattle.

A. israe'li, the microorganism causing actinomycosis in humans.

actinomyces (ak"tĭ-no-mi'sēz) an organism of the genus *Actinomyces.* adj., **actinomycet'ic.**

actinomycete (ak"tĭ-no-mi'sēt) a moldlike bacterium (order Actinomycetales) occurring as elongated, frequently filamentous cells, with a branching tendency. adj., **actinomycet'ic.**

actinomycin (ak"tĭ-no-mi'sin) a family of antibiotics from various species of *Streptomyces,* which are active against bacteria and fungi; it includes the antineoplastic agents cactinomycin (actinomycin C) and dactinomycin (actinomycin D).

actinomycoma (ak"tĭ-no-mi-ko'mah) a tumor-like reactive lesion due to *Actinomyces.*

actinomycosis (ak"tĭ-no-mi-ko'sis) an infection involving the deeper tissues of the skin and mucous membranes and caused by *Actinomyces.* The head and neck are most often involved, the lesions beginning as painless, tumor-like masses around the jaw and neck. Later these masses break down and begin to suppurate with discharge of the exudate through a network of sinuses extending through the skin. Intraperitoneal abscesses and lung abscesses may also occur. The source of infection is unknown, although the mouth is thought to be the portal of entry because the organisms are often found in decayed teeth and in the tonsillar crypts of persons who are otherwise normal.

The infection progresses slowly, without remission, and without at first seeming to affect the general health of the patient. If it is not treated successfully the condition may eventually be fatal.

Treatment is usually with sulfonamide drugs or penicillin. X-ray therapy may be employed for local lesions and in some cases corticosteroids may help eliminate the infection.

actinon (ak'tĭ-non) a radioactive isotope of radon, symbol An.

actinotherapy (ak"tĭ-no-ther'ah-pe) treatment of disease by rays of light, especially ultraviolet rays.

action (ak'shun) the accomplishment of an effect, whether mechanical or chemical, or the effect so produced.

cumulative a., the sudden and markedly increased action of a drug after administration of several doses.

reflex a., an involuntary response to a stimulus conveyed to the nervous system and reflected to the periphery, passing below the level of consciousness (see also REFLEX).

activated resin self-curing resin.

activator (ak'tĭ-va"tor) a substance that makes another substance active or that renders an inactive enzyme capable of exerting its proper effect.

plasminogen a., a substance that activates plasminogen and converts it into plasmin.

tissue a., fibrinokinase.

active transport (ak'tiv trans'port) the movement of ions or molecules across the cell membranes and epithelial layers, usually against a concentration gradient, resulting directly from the expenditure of metabolic energy. For example, under normal circumstances more potassium ions are present within the cell and more sodium ions extracellularly. The process of maintaining these normal differences in electrolytic composition between the intracellular fluids is active transport. The process differs from simple diffusion or osmosis in that it requires the expenditure of metabolic energy.

activity (ak-tiv′ĭ-te) the quality or process of exerting energy or of accomplishing an effect.

displacement a., irrelevant activity produced by an excess of one of two conflicting drives in a person.

enzyme a., the catalytic effect exerted by an enzyme, expressed as units per milligram of enzyme (*specific* activity) or molecules of substrate transformed per minute per molecule of enzyme (*molecular* activity).

optical a., the ability of a chemical compound to rotate the plane of polarization of plane-polarized light.

actomyosin (ak″to-mi′o-sin) the system of actin filaments and myosin particles constituting muscle fibers and responsible for the contraction and relaxation of muscle.

acuity (ah-ku′ĭ-te) acuteness or clearness.

acumeter (ah-koo′mĕ-ter) acoumeter.

acuminate (ah-ku′mĭ-nāt) sharp-pointed.

acupressure (ak′u-presh″er) compression of a blood vessel by inserted needles.

acupuncture (ak′u-pungk″chur) the Chinese practice of inserting needles into specific points along the "meridians" of the body to relieve the discomfort associated with painful disorders, to induce surgical anesthesia, and for preventive and therapeutic purposes.

In general, acupuncture is employed to treat functional disorders rather than organic diseases that bring about severe tissue changes. It may be employed in combination with other therapies in the treatment of degenerative diseases. Acupuncture as a form of anesthesia is considered by traditional Chinese practitioners to be a minor part of acupuncture practice.

Advocates of acupuncture base the practice on the concept of a vital energy flow or life force (*c′hi*) which circulates through the body along meridians similar to the blood, lymphatic, and neural circuits. It is believed that there are two energy flows and that these forces are in everything in the universe. *Yang*, the positive principle, tends to stimulate and to contract; *yin*, the negative principle, tends to sedate and to expand. Health depends upon the equilibrium of yang and yin, first in the body and secondly in the universe.

The therapeutic objective of acupuncture is to rectify an imbalance in the energy flow. This is accomplished by the insertion of needles at specific points along the meridians. The needles are inserted in the skin to varying depths according to the point of insertion and the condition being treated. They may be left in place for varying lengths of time and are vibrated manually or electrically.

Traditionally an Oriental practice, acupuncture is a subject of increasing interest among physicians from the Western countries.

acus (a′kus) a needle or needle-like process.

acute (ah-kūt) 1. sharp. 2. having severe symptoms and a short course.

acyanotic (ah-si″ah-not′ik) not characterized or accompanied by cyanosis.

acyesis (ah″si-e′sis) 1. sterility in a woman. 2. absence of pregnancy.

acyl (as′il) an organic radical derived from an organic acid by removal of the hydroxyl group.

Acylanid (as″il-an′id) trademark for acetyldigitoxin, a digitalis preparation derived from lanatoside.

acylation (as″ĭ-la′shun) introduction of an acyl radical into the molecules of a compound.

acystia (a-sis′te-ah) congenital absence of the bladder.

acystinervia (a-sis″tĭ-ner′ve-ah) paralysis of the bladder.

A.D. [L.] *au′ris dex′tra* (right ear).

ad [L.] preposition, *to.*

A.D.A. American Dental Association; American Diabetes Association; American Dietetics Association.

adactylia, adactyly (a″dak-til′e-ah; a-dak′tĭ-le) congenital absence of the fingers or toes. adj., **adac′tylous.**

Adam's apple a subcutaneous prominence at the front of the throat produced by the thyroid cartilage of the LARYNX.

adamantine (ad″ah-man′tin) pertaining to the enamel of the teeth.

adamantinoma (ad″ah-man″tĭ-no′mah) ameloblastoma.

adamantoblast (ad″ah-man′to-blast) ameloblast.

adamantoblastoma, adamantoma (ad″ah-man″to-blas-to′mah; ad″ah-man-to′mah) ameloblastoma.

Adams' disease (ad′amz) Adams-Stokes disease.

Adams-Stokes disease (ad′amz stōks) a condition characterized by sudden attacks of unconsciusness, with or without convulsions, which frequently accompanies heart block; called also Stokes-Adams disease.

adaptation (ad″ap-ta′shun) adjustment, especially of the pupil to light, or of an organism to environmental conditions.

color a., 1. changes in visual perception of color with prolonged stimulation. 2. adjustment of vision to degree of brightness or color tone of illumination.

dark a., adaptation of the eye to vision in the dark or in reduced illumination.

light a., adaptation of the eye to vision in the sunlight or in bright illumination (photopia), with reduction in the concentration of the photosensitive pigments of the eye.

adaptometer (ad″ap-tom′ĕ-ter) an instrument for measuring the time required for retinal adaptation, i.e., for regeneration of the visual purple; used in detecting night blindness, vitamin A deficiency, and retinitis pigmentosa.

color a., an instrument to demonstrate adaptation of the eye to color or light.

addict (ad′ikt) a person exhibiting addiction.

addiction (ah-dik′shun) physiologic or psychologic dependence on some agent (e.g., alcohol, drug), with a tendency to increase its use (see also DRUG ADDICTION).

Addis count (ad′is) the determination of the number of red blood cells, white blood cells, epithelial cells, casts, and the protein content in an aliquot of a 12-hour urine specimen, used in the diagnosis and management of kidney disease.

Addison's disease (ad'ĭ-sunz) a disease caused by the underfunctioning of the ADRENAL GLANDS, named for Thomas Addison, the 19th-century English physician who first identified it. Addison's disease is comparatively rare, and although it is known to be due to a failure of the adrenal glands, the cause of this failure is not always certain. Tuberculosis of the adrenals accounts for less than half the cases, and idiopathic atrophy of the glands for most of the rest.

A major symptom of the disease is generalized weakness which results from muscle fatigue and inability to maintain a stable level of glucose for energy. The deficit of cortisol produces muscle weakness and trembling, and mental changes manifested as anxiety, depression, and other mood disorders. Gastrointestinal symptoms include nausea, vomiting, and diarrhea. Fluid loss due to electrolyte imbalance brings about loss of weight, hypotension, and dizziness. Pigmentation of the skin and membranes of the mouth occur as the high brain centers, in an effort to stimulate the adrenals, also stimulate pigment cells in the skin.

Medications used for treatment of Addison's disease include a wide range of MINERALCORTICOIDS and GLUCOCORTICOIDS. With proper administration of these hormones and an adequate intake of sodium chloride, patients with Addison's disease have a good chance of remaining healthy.

An important aspect of patient care is education of the patient and his family in regard to the symptoms of inadequate and excess steroid replacement, and the need to report these symptoms so that dosage can be adjusted. It is recommended that the patient wear a medical identification tag stating that he has the disease and is receiving steroid therapy.

addisonian crisis (ad"ĭ-so'ne-an) symptoms of fatigue, nausea and vomiting, weight loss, hypotension, and collapse accompanying an acute attack of Addison's disease.

addisonism (ad'ĭ-sun-izm") symptoms seen in pulmonary tuberculosis, consisting of debility and pigmentation, resembling Addison's disease.

additive (ad'ĭ-tiv) 1. characterized by addition. (See also under EFFECT.) 2. a substance added to another to improve its appearance, increase its nutritive value, etc.

adduct (ah-dukt') to draw toward a center or median line.

adduction (ah-duk'shun) the act of adducting; the state of being adducted.

adductor (ah-duk'tor) that which adducts.

adenalgia (ad"ĕ-nal'je-ah) pain in a gland.

adenase (ad'ĕ-nās) a deaminizing enzyme of the spleen, liver, and pancreas that converts adenine into hypoxanthine and ammonia.

adenasthenia (ad"en-as-the'ne-ah) deficient glandular activity.

adendritic (ah"den-drit'ik) without dendrites.

adenectomy (ad"ĕ-nek'to-me) excision of a gland.

adenectopia (ad"ĕ-nek-to'pe-ah) displacement of a gland.

adeniform (ah-den'ĭ-form) gland-shaped.

adenine (ad'ĕ-nīn) a purine present in nucleoproteins of cells of plants and animals. Adenine and guanine are essential components of NUCLEIC ACIDS. The end product of the metabolism of adenine in man is URIC ACID.

adenitis (ad"ĕ-ni'tis) inflammation of a gland.

adenization (ad"ĕ-nĭ-za'shun) assumption by other tissue of an abnormal glandlike appearance.

adeno- word element [Gr.], *gland.*

adenoacanthoma (ad"ĕ-no-ak"an-tho'mah) adenocarcinoma in which some of the cells exhibit squamous differentiation.

adenoameloblastoma (ad"ĕ-no-ah-mel"o-blas-to'mah) an odontogenic tumor with formation of ductlike structures in place of or in addition to a typical ameloblastic pattern.

adenoblast (ad'ĕ-no-blast") an embryonic forerunner of gland tissue.

adenocarcinoma (ad"ĕ-no-kar"sĭ-no'mah) carcinoma derived from glandular tissue or in which the tumor cells form recognizable glandular structures. **alveolar c.**, adenocarcinoma composed of cells arranged in the form of alveoli.

adenocele (ad'ĕ-no-sēl") a cystic adenomatous tumor.

adenocellulitis (ad"ĕ-no-sel"u-li'tis) inflammation of a gland and the cellular tissue around it.

adenochondroma (ad"ĕ-no-kon-dro'mah) a tumor containing both glandular and cartilaginous elements.

adenocystoma (ad"ĕ-no-sis-to'mah) adenoma in which there is cyst formation.

adenocyte (ad'ĕ-no-sīt") a mature secretory cell of a gland.

adenodynia (ad"ĕ-no-din'e-ah) pain in a gland.

adenoepithelioma (ad"ĕ-no-ep"ĭ-the"le-o'mah) a tumor composed of glandular and epithelial elements.

adenogenous (ad"ĕ-noj'ĕ-nus) orginating from glandular tissue.

adenohypophysis (ad"ĕ-no-hi-pof'ĭ-sis) the anterior or glandular portion of the hypophysis cerebri (see also PITUITARY GLAND). adj., **adenohypophys'eal.**

adenoid (ad'ĕ-noid) 1. resembling a gland. 2. in the plural, hypertrophy of the glandular tissue that normally exists in the nasopharynx of children and is known as the pharyngeal tonsil. Enlargement of this tissue may cause obstruction of the outlet from the nose so that the child breathes chiefly through

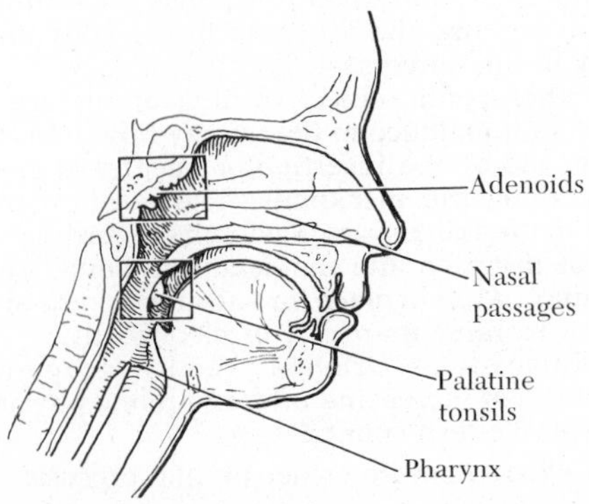

Adenoids.

the mouth, or the eustachian tube may be blocked, with pain in the ear or a sense of pressure resulting. It also may prepare the way for infections of the middle ear and occasionally interferes with hearing.

Prolonged obstruction by enlarged adenoids produces a typical "adenoid facies." The child appears to be dull and apathetic, and has some degree of nutritional deficiency and hearing loss, and some delay in growth and development.

Surgical excision of the enlarged tissue is called adenoidectomy.

adenoidectomy (ad″ĕ-noi-dek′to-me) surgical excision of the adenoids. The operation is usually performed in conjunction with tonsillectomy since both the adenoids and palatine tonsils tend to become enlarged after repeated infections of the throat. The preoperative and postoperative care in adenoidectomy is similar to that in TONSILLECTOMY and is described under that heading.

adenoiditis (ad″ĕ-noi-di′tis) inflammation of the adenoids.

adenolipoma (ad″ĕ-no-lĭ-po′mah) a tumor composed of both glandular and fatty tissue elements.

adenolipomatosis (ad″ĕ-no-lip″o-mah-to′sis) the formation of numerous adenolipomas in the neck, axilla, and groin.

adenology (ad″ĕ-nol′o-je) the sum of knowledge regarding glands.

adenolymphitis (ad″ĕ-no-lim-fi′tis) lymphadenitis; inflammation of lymph nodes.

adenolymphoma (ad″ĕ-no-lim-fo′mah) a cystic salivary-gland tumor containing epithelial and lymphoid tissue, affecting almost exclusively the parotid gland.

adenoma (ad″ĕ-no′mah) a benign epithelial tumor in which the cells form recognizable glandular structures or in which the cells are derived from glandular epithelium.

acidophilic a., a tumor arising from the acidophilic cells of the anterior lobe of the pituitary gland; called also eosinophilic adenoma. Such tumors produce ACROMEGALY and GIGANTISM.

basophilic a., a tumor arising from the basophilic cells of the anterior lobe of the pituitary gland.

chromophobe a., a tumor arising from the chromophobe cells of the anterior lobe of the pituitary gland.

a. des′truens, adenocarcinoma.

eosinophilic a., acidophilic adenoma.

Hürthle cell a., see under H.

sebaceous a., hypertrophy or benign hyperplasia of a sebaceous gland.

a. seba′ceum, nevoid hyperplasia of sebaceous glands, forming multiple yellow papules or nodules on the face.

villous a., a large soft papillary polyp on the mucosa of the large intestine.

adenomalacia (ad″ĕ-no-mah-la′she-ah) undue softness of a gland.

adenomatosis (ad″ĕ-no″mah-to′sis) the formation of numerous adenomatous growths.

adenomatous (ad″ĕ-no′mah-tus) pertaining to adenoma or to nodular hyperplasia of a gland.

adenomere (ad′ĕ-no-mēr″) the blind terminal portion of the glandular cavity of a developing gland, being the functional portion of the organ.

adenomyofibroma (ad″ĕ-no-mi″o-fi-bro′mah) a fibroma containing both glandular and muscular elements.

adenomyoma (ad″ĕ-no-mi-o′mah) a tumor made up of endometrium and muscle tissue, found in the uterus, or more frequently in the uterine ligaments.

adenomyomatosis (ad″ĕ-no-mi″o-mah-to′sis) the presence of multiple adenomyomas.

adenomyometritis (ad″ĕ-no-mi″o-mĕ-tri′tis) adenomyosis of the uterus.

adenomyosarcoma (ad″ĕ-no-mi″o-sar-ko′mah) adenosarcoma containing striated muscle.

adenomyosis (ad″ĕ-no-mi-o′sis) invasion of the muscular wall of an organ (e.g., uterus) by glandular tissue.

adenopathy (ad″ĕ-nop′ah-the) enlargement of glands, especially of the lymph nodes.

adenopharyngitis (ad″ĕ-no-far″in-ji′tis) inflammation of the adenoids and pharynx, usually involving the tonsils.

adenosarcoma (ad″ĕ-no-sar-ko′mah) adenoma blended with sarcoma.

adenosclerosis (ad″ĕ-no-sklĕ-ro′sis) hardening of a gland.

adenosine (ah-den′o-sēn) a structural subunit of ribonucleic acid (RNA) composed of a pentose sugar (D-ribose) and adenine. It also functions as a coenzyme in the metabolic functions of the cell, particularly in biochemical processes during which energy is released from nutrients to promote vital cellular functions.

Adenosine, in combination with three phosphate radicals, forms the nucleotide ATP (*adenosine triphosphate*). The last two phosphate radicals are joined to the rest of the molecule by a "high-energy" bond, so called because each bond contains about 7000 calories of energy per mole of ATP. This high-energy bond is very labile and can split instantly whenever energy is needed to promote cellular functions.

When the energy is released as the high-energy bond is broken, the ATP loses one phosphate radical and ADP (*adenosine diphosphate*) is formed. Energy derived from the breakdown of cellular nutrients is then used to unite phosphoric acid to ADP to form ATP again. These reactions are cyclic, occurring over and over again to energize vital functions of the cell.

a. 3′:5′-cyclic phosphate, cyclic AMP; a cyclic nucleotide participating in the activities of many hormones, including catecholamines, ACTH, and vasopressin. Because this compound is formed from ATP by the action of adenyl cyclase, which in turn is stimulated by the interaction of the aforementioned hormones with the plasma membrane of target cells, it has been called the "second messenger" in the mechanism of hormone action.

a. diphosphate, a compound containing adenosine and two phosphoric acid radicals, formed by the hydrolysis of adenosine triphosphate (ATP), with release of one high-energy bond; abbreviated ADP.

a. monophosphate, adenylic acid; the compound formed after the loss of the second phosphate radical from ATP; abbreviated AMP. Cyclic AMP is adenosine 3′:5′-cyclic phosphate.

a. triphosphatase, ATPase; an enzyme that catalyzes the splitting of adenosine triphosphate, releasing the terminal phosphate group and forming adenosine diphosphate; the energy released is used in the cell's biological activities.

a. triphosphate, a compound composed of adenosine and three phosphate radicals; abbreviated ATP. This intermediary compound has the ability to enter into many reactions, some of them with nutrients to extract energy from them and some within the cells to provide energy for their operation (see ADENOSINE). ATP is present in the cytoplasm and nucleoplasm of all cells. It is used to promote three major types of cellular activities: (1) the transport of glucose and other substances across the cell membrane; (2) the synthesis of proteins and a host of other chemical compounds throughout the cell; and (3) the performance of mechanical work, as in muscle cells.

adenosis (ad″ĕ-no′sis) 1. any disease of a gland. 2. abnormal development of a gland.

adenotome (ad′ĕ-no-tōm) an instrument for excising glands.

adenotomy (ad″ĕ-not′o-me) 1. anatomy, incision, or dissection of glands. 2. incision of adenoids.

adenotonsillectomy (ad″ĕ-no-ton″sĭ-lek′to-me) removal of the tonsils and adenoids.

adenovirus (ad″ĕ-no-vi′rus) any of a large group of viruses causing disease of the upper respiratory tract and conjunctiva, and also present in latent infections in normal persons; many induce malignancy in certain species.

adenylic acid (ad″ĕ-nil′ik) adenosine monophosphate; a component of nucleic acid, consisting of adenine, ribose, and phosphoric acid.

adermia (ah-der′me-ah) congenital defect or absence of the skin.

ADH antidiuretic hormone.

adhesion (ad-he′zhun) union of two surfaces that are normally separate; also, any fibrous band that connects them. Surgery within the abdomen sometimes results in adhesions from scar tissue. As an organ heals, fibrous scar tissue forms around the incision. This scar tissue may cling to the surface of adjoining organs, causing them to kink. Adhesions are usually painless and cause no difficulties, although occasionally they produce obstruction or malfunction by distorting the organ. They can also occur following peritonitis and other inflammatory conditions. They may occur in the pleura, in the pericardium, and around the pelvic organs, in addition to the abdomen. Surgery is sometimes recommended to relieve adhesions.

adhesiotomy (ad-he″ze-ot′o-me) surgical division of adhesions.

adhesive (ad-he′siv) pertaining to, characterized by, or causing close adherence of adjoining surfaces. 2. a substance that causes close adherence of adjoining surfaces.

a. tape, a strip of fabric or other material evenly coated on one side with a pressure-sensitive adhesive material.

adiadochokinesia (ah-di″ah-do″ko-ki-ne′ze-ah) inability to perform fine, rapidly repeated, coordinated movements.

adiaphoria (ah-di″ah-fo′re-ah) nonresponse to stimuli as a result of previous similar stimuli.

Adie's pupil (a′dēz) a pupil that responds to accommodation and convergence in a slow, delayed fashion, as in Adie's syndrome. Called also tonic pupil.

Adie's syndrome (a′dēz) a syndrome consisting of a pathologic pupil reaction (pupillotonia), the most important element of which is a myotonic condition on accommodation; the pupil on the affected side contracts to near vision more slowly than does the pupil on the opposite side, and it also dilates more slowly. The affected pupil does not usually react to light (direct or indirect), but it may do so in an abnormal fashion. Certain tendon reflexes are absent or diminished, but there are no motor or sensory disturbances, nor are there demonstrable changes indicative of disease of the nervous system.

adip(o)- word element [L.], *fat.*

adipectomy (ad″ĭ-pek′to-me) excision of adipose tissue.

adiphenine (ad″ĭfen′ēn) an antispasmodic used as the hydrochloride salt.

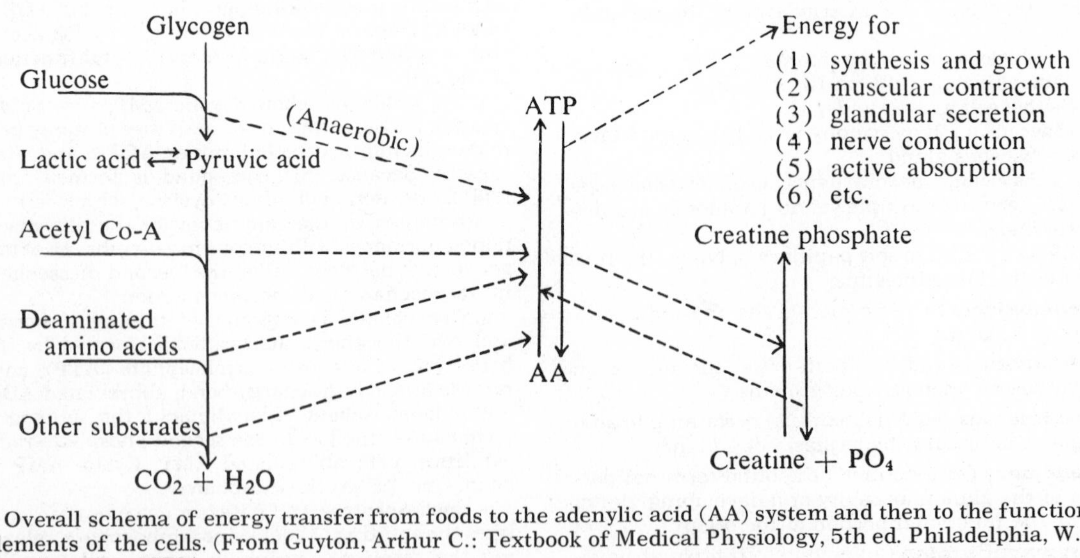

Overall schema of energy transfer from foods to the adenylic acid (AA) system and then to the functional elements of the cells. (From Guyton, Arthur C.: Textbook of Medical Physiology, 5th ed. Philadelphia, W. B. Saunders Co., 1976.)

adipic (ah-dip′ik) pertaining to fat.

adipocele (ad′ĭ-po-sēl″) a hernia containing fat.

adipocellular (ad″ĭ-po-sel′u-lar) composed of fat and connective tissue.

adipofibroma (ad″ĭo-po-fi-bro′mah) a fibrous tumor with fatty elements.

adipogenic, adipogenous (ad″ĭ-po-jen′ik; ad″ĭ-poj′ĕ-nus) producing fat.

adipokinesis (ad″ĭ-po-ki-ne′sis) the mobilization of fat in the body.

adipokinin (ad″ĭ-po-ki′nin) a factor from the anterior pituitary that accelerates mobilization of stored fat.

adipolysis (ad″ĭ-pol′ĭ-sis) the digestion of fats. adj. **adipolyt′ic.**

adiponecrosis (ad″ĭ-po-nĕ-kro′sis) necrosis of fatty tissue.

a. neonato′rum, a. subcuta′nea, induration of subcutaneous fat, thought to be caused by obstetric trauma, in newborn infants.

adipopexis (ad″ĭ-po-pek′sis) the fixation or storing of fat.

adipose (ad′ĭ-pōs) fatty.

adiposis (ad″ĭ-po′sis) a condition marked by deposits or degeneration of fatty tissue.

a. cerebra′lis, fatness from cerebral pituitary disease.

a. doloro′sa, a painful condition due to pressure on nerves caused by fatty deposits.

a. hepat′ica, fatty degeneration of liver.

a. tubero′sa simplex, adiposis dolorosa in which the fatty degeneration occurs in nodular masses.

adiposity (ad″ĭ-pos′ĭ-te) obesity.

adiposogenital dystrophy (ad″ĭ-po-so-jen′ĭ-tal dis′tro-fe) abnormal distribution of fat (obesity) accompanied by underdevelopment of the genitalia. The condition is caused by damage to certain parts of the HYPOTHALAMUS, with a decrease in the secretion of gonadotropic hormones from the anterior lobe of the PITUITARY GLAND. Treatment depends on the primary cause of the condition, usually a tumor or infection involving the hypothalamus. Called also adiposogenital syndrome and Fröhlich's syndrome.

adiposuria (ad″ĭ-po-su′re-ah) the occurrence of fat in the urine.

adipsia (a-dip′se-ah) absence of thirst; abnormal avoidance of drinking.

aditus (ad′ĭ-tus), pl. *ad′itus* [L.] an entrance or opening; used in anatomic nomenclature for various passages in the body.

adjuvant (ad′joo-vant) 1. assisting or aiding. 2. a substance that aids another, such as an auxiliary remedy.

adnerval, adneural (ad-ner′val), (ad-nu′ral) toward a nerve.

adnexa (ad-nek′sah) [L., pl.] appendages; accessory organs, as of the eye (*adenx′a oc′uli*) or uterus (*adnex′a u′teri*). adj., **adnex′al.**

adolescence (ad″o-les′ens) the period between the onset of PUBERTY and the cessation of physical growth. adj., **adoles′cent.** During adolescence, boys and girls undergo the extensive physical changes of puberty; these changes sometimes create emotional difficulties. The adolescent has two main problems: he must adjust himself to the changes in his body; and he must also adjust himself socially—that is, he must learn to live independently, and to be responsible for himself.

Adolescents are usually extremely sensitive about their appearance. They should never be ridiculed on account of it, and great care should be taken to avoid causing them embarrassment. For example, nicknames like "Chubby" and "Skinny," which imply some physical peculiarity, should be avoided as far as possible, however affectionately intended. Adolescents may be particularly sensitive about their weight. They often go through a temporary stage of being overweight or underweight, and it is usually a matter of time before the situation rights itself. Good nutrition is very important at this stage. Adolescence is a period of exceptionally rapid growth and strenuous exercise, and young people's bodies need especially good and complete diets if they are to develop properly. Their food must be rich in protein to make new muscle and body tissue, minerals for the growth of bones, vitamins for good general health, and enough supplementary carbohydrates and fat to provide energy. For more detailed information about the value of different foods, see NUTRITION.

Many adolescents are susceptible to ACNE, BOILS, and other skin complaints; this is mainly because the level of new hormones pouring into the blood is not yet stabilized, and the normal lubricating oil produced by the sebaceous glands in the skin thickens and forms plugs in the hair follicles. Bacteria find a ready home in these fatty plugs, and the follicular pores become infected, with the formation of pimples and boils.

adoral (ad-o′ral) 1. situated near the mouth. 2. directed toward the mouth.

ADP adenosine diphosphate.

adren(o)- (ah-dre′no) word element [L.], *adrenal glands.*

adrenal (ah-dre′nal) 1. near the kidney. 2. of or produced by the adrenal glands. 3. an adrenal gland.

a. gland, a small endocrine gland that rests on top of each kidney; called also suprarenal gland. Like other endocrine glands, the two adrenals secrete hormones into the blood, which carries them to various parts of the body where they can exert their effects. Each adrenal gland is actually a gland within a gland: the outer shell, or cortex, and the inner core, or medulla.

CORTEX. The adrenal cortex plays a vital role in the chemistry of the body. Its hormones, known as corticosteroids, are divided into three groups: GLUCOCORTICOIDS (cortisol [or hydrocortisone], cortisone, and corticosterone), MINERALOCORTICOIDS (aldosterone and desoxycorticosterone, and also corticosterone), and androgens. Progesterone and estrogen are also present in the adrenal secretion in small amounts.

The glucocorticoids help control the metabolism of protein, fat, and carbohydrate. The mineralocorticoids influence the concentration of sodium and potassium in body fluids, exerting an important role in fluid and electrolyte balance. If both adrenal cortices are removed or cease to function, the patient cannot live long unless he receives supportive adrenocortical hormones.

Like other endocrine glands, the cortex is under the control of the PITUITARY GLAND. The pituitary exercises its control by way of its adrenocorticotropic hormone, familiarly known as ACTH, which stimulates the cortex to secrete its hormones.

Diseases of the adrenal cortex are serious but rare. They cause the cortex to overproduce or underproduce its hormones. Two of the commonest of these rare diseases are ADDISON'S DISEASE (underproduction of hormones) and CUSHING'S SYNDROME (overproduction of hormones).

MEDULLA. The two hormones produced by the adrenal medulla are epinephrine (Adrenalin) and norepinephrine (noradrenalin). Their secretion is controlled by the HYPOTHALAMUS. The actions of these two hormones are similar and they are referred to as "sympathomimetic" agents because they mimic the actions of the sympathetic nervous system. They affect automatic responses of the body such as cardiac activity, gastrointestinal motility, dilatation of the pupil of the eye, and various metabolic activities. Epinephrine affects the conversion of glycogen in the liver into glucose, greatly increases the metabolic rate, and increases the cardiac output. Norepinephrine causes vascular constriction, thereby raising the arterial pressure. In general, it can be said that these hormones have almost exactly the same effects as direct sympathetic stimulation except that the hormonal effects are more prolonged.

Hyperfunction of the adrenal medulla is usually due to a tumor (PHEOCHROMOCYTOMA) and the chief symptom is hypertension.

a. insufficiency, hypofunction of the adrenal gland, particularly the cortex, leading to symptoms of weakness and loss of sodium, chloride, and water. See also ADDISON'S DISEASE.

a. rest tumor, masculinovoblastoma.

adrenalectomy (ah-dre″nah-lek′to-me) surgical excision of an adrenal gland. This procedure is indicated when a disorder of the adrenal gland, such as CUSHING'S SYNDROME or PHEOCHROMOCYTOMA, causes an overproduction of adrenal hormones. In some instances of severe Cushing's syndrome, total bilateral adrenalectomy is performed. Adrenalectomy also has been advocated for therapy of some cases of metastatic breast cancer.

Adrenalin (ah-dren′ah-lin) trademark for epinephrine, an adrenergic agent.

adrenergic (ad″ren-er′jik) activated or transmitted by epinephrine; said of nerve fibers that liberate sympathin at a synapse when a nerve impulse passes, i.e., the sympathetic fibers.

a. agent, a substance that duplicates most of the effects of stimulation of the sympathetic nervous system.

a.-blocking agent, a drug that blocks the secretion of epinephrine and norepinephrine at the post-ganglionic nerve endings of the sympathetic nervous system. By blocking these adrenergic substances, which cause constriction of blood vessels and increased cardiac output, adrenergic-blocking agents produce a dilatation of the blood vessels and a decrease in cardiac output. They are classified as antihypertensive drugs. Guanethidine sulfate and methyldopa are examples of adrenergic-blocking agents. During therapy with these drugs, patients should avoid strenuous exercise, which is likely to produce a sudden drop in the blood pressure. Another difficulty to be expected with these drugs is postural hypotension.

a. receptors, postulated sites on effector organs innervated by postganglionic adrenergic fibers of the sympathetic nervous system, classified as α-adrenergic and β-adrenergic receptors according to their reaction to norepinephrine and epinephrine respectively, and to certain blocking and stimulating agents.

adrenocortical (ah-dre″no-kor′tĭ-kal) pertaining to or arising from the cortex of the adrenal gland.

a. hormone, one of the steroids produced by the adrenal cortex (see also CORTICOSTEROID).

adrenocorticomimetic (ah-dre″no-kor″tĭ-ko-mi-met′ik) having effects similar to those of hormones of the adrenal cortex.

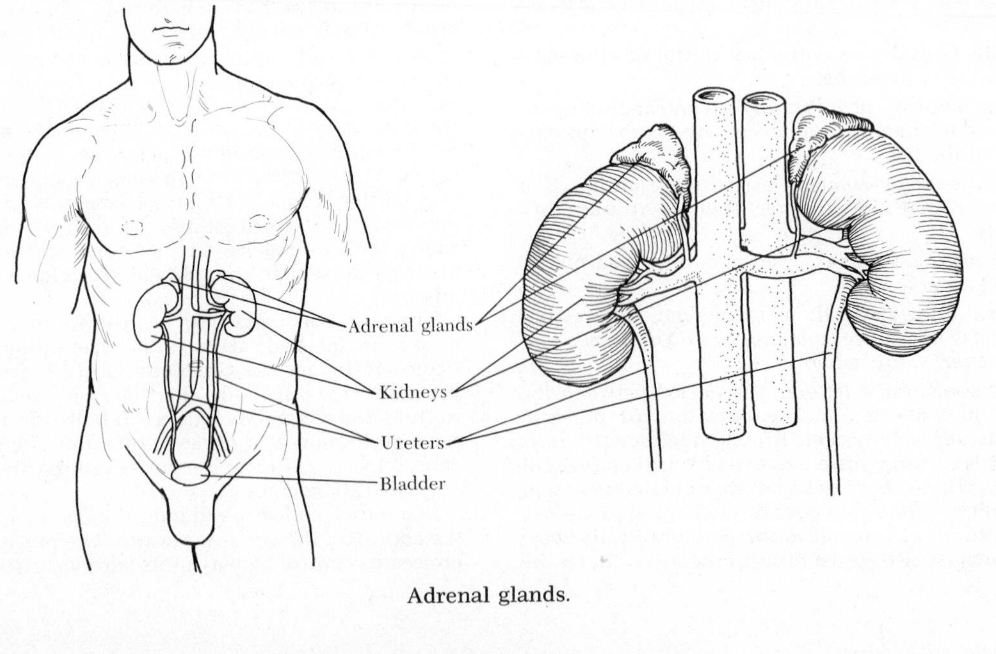

Adrenal glands.

adrenocorticotrophic (ah-dre″no-kor″tĭ-ko-trof′ik) adrenocorticotropic; corticotropic.

adrenocorticotrophin (ah-dre″no-kor″tĭ-ko-trof′in) adrenocorticotropic hormone, or CORTICOTROPIN (see also ACTH).

adrenocorticotropic (ah-dre″no-kor″tĭ-ko-trōp′ik) having a stimulating effect on the adrenal cortex; corticotropic.

a. hormone, ACTH, a hormone secreted by the anterior PITUITARY GLAND that has a stimulaing effect on the ADRENAL CORTEX (see also CORTICOTROPIN).

adrenocorticotropin (ah-dre″no-kor″tĭ-ko-tro′pin) adrenocorticotropic hormone (ACTH), or CORTICOTROPIN.

adrenogenital syndrome (ah-dre″no-jen′ĭ-tal) a group of symptoms associated with alterations of the sex characters and due to abnormally increased production of androgens by the adrenal glands. The term most commonly applies to the development of masculine traits in the female or premature puberty in male children. The condition may be congenital, in which case it is due to an inherited defect of the adrenal gland, or acquired, developing as a result of a tumor or hyperplasia of the adrenals.

SYMPTOMS. Females with the congenital form may be reared as boys because of masculinization of the external genitalia. Males may show sexual prococity, with development of the reproductive organs, appearance of pubic hair, and excessive body growth in early childhood. In acquired adrenogenital syndrome there is appearance of masculine secondary sex characters in the female, and precocious puberty in the male.

TREATMENT. When an adrenal tumor is the underlying cause of the disorder, it is removed surgically. Other treatment consists of administration of corticoids such as cortisone and prednisone. Estrogen therapy is successful in some cases.

adrenolytic (ah-dre″no-lit′ik) antagonizing the action of epinephrine or of the adrenal gland.

adrenomegaly (ah-dre″no-meg′ah-le) abnormal enlargement of the adrenal gland.

adrenopathy (ad″ren-op′ah-the) any disease of the adrenal glands.

Adriamycin (a″dre-ah-mi′sin) trademark for a preparation of doxorubicin, an antineoplastic antibiotic.

adsorb (ad-sorb′) to attract and retain other material on the surface.

adsorbent (ad-sorb′ent) 1. pertaining to or characterized by adsorption. 2. a substance that attracts other materials or particles to its surface.

gastrointestinal a., a substance, usually a powder, taken to adsorb gases, toxins, and bacteria in the stomach and intestines. Examples include activated charcoal and kaolin.

adsorption (ad-sorp′shun) the action of a substance in attracting and holding other materials or particles on its surface.

adtorsion (ad-tor′shun) a turning inward of both eyes.

adult (ah-dult′) having attained full growth or maturity, or an organism that has done so.

adulteration (ah-dul″ter-a′shun) addition of an impure, cheap, or unnecessary ingredient to cheat, cheapen, or falsify a preparation.

advancement (ad-vans′ment) detachment of a portion of tissue, especially muscle, and reattachment at an advanced point, as is done with an eye muscle for correction of strabismus.

capsular a., attachment of Tenon's capsule in front of its normal position.

adventitia (ad″ven-tish′e-ah) the outer coat of an organ or structure, especially the outer coat of an artery.

adventitious (ad″ven-tish′us) not normal to a part.

adynamia (ad″dĭ-na′me-ah) lack of normal or vital powers. adj. **adynam′ic.**

aec- for words beginning thus, see those beginning, *ec-*.

Aedes (a-e′dēz) a genus of mosquitoes, including approximately 600 species.

A. aegyp′ti, the mosquito that transmits the causative organisms of yellow fever and dengue.

aeg- for words beginning thus, see those beginning *eg-*.

aeration (a″er-a′shun) 1. the exchange of carbon dioxide for oxygen by the blood in the lungs. 2. the charging of a liquid with air or gas.

aeriform (ār′ĭ-form, a-er′ĭ-form) resembling air; gaseous.

aero- (a′er-o) word element [Gr.], *air; gas.*

Aerobacter (a″er-o-bak′ter) a genus of bacteria that includes two species, *A. aero′genes* and *A. cloa′cae.*

aerobe (a′er-ōb) a microorganism that lives and grows in the presence of free oxygen. adj. **aero′bic.**

facultative a., one that can live in the presence of oxygen, but does not require it.

obligate a., one that cannot live without oxygen.

aerobiology (a″er-o-bi-ol′o-je) the study of the distribution of living organisms (microorganisms) by the air.

aerobiosis (a″er-o-bi-o′sis) life requiring free oxygen.

aerocele (a′er-o-sēl) a tumor formed by air filling an adventitious pouch, such as laryngocele and tracheocele.

epidural a., a collection of air between the dura mater and the wall of the vertebral column.

aerodermectasia (a″er-o-der″mek-ta′ze-ah) subcutaneous or surgical emphysema.

aerodontalgia (a″er-o-don-tal′je-ah) pain in the teeth due to lowered atmospheric pressure at high altitudes.

aerodynamics (a″er-o-di-nam′iks) the science of air or gases in motion.

aeroembolism (a″er-o-em′bo-lizm) obstruction of a blood vessel by air or gas.

aerogen (a′er-o-jen″) a gas-producing bacillus.

aerogenesis (a″er-o-jen′ĕ-sis) formation or production of gas.

aerohydrotherapy (a″er-o-hi″dro-ther′ah-pe) therapeutic use of air and water.

aeropathy (a″er-op′ah-the) bends (decompression sickness).

aerophagia (a″er-o-fa′je-ah) habitual swallowing of air.

aerophilic, aerophilous (a″er-o-fil′ik; a″er-of′ĭ-lus) requiring air for proper growth.

aeroplethysmograph (a″er-o-plĕ-thiz′mo-graf) an apparatus for graphically recording respiratory volumes.

aerosinusitis (a″er-o-si″nŭ-si′tis) barosinusitis.

aerosol (a′er-o-sol″) a colloid system in which solid or liquid particles are suspended in a gas, especially a suspension of a drug or other substance to be dispensed in a cloud or mist.

Aerosol therapy is a major component of RESPIRATORY THERAPY in the treatment of bronchopulmonary disease. The major purpose of aerosol therapy is the delivery of medications or humidity or both to the mucosa of the respiratory tract and pulmonary alveoli.

Agents delivered by aerosol therapy may act in a number of ways: (1) to relieve spasm of the bronchial muscles and reduce edema of the mucous membranes, (2) to render bronchial secretions more liquid so that they are more easily removed, (3) to humidify the respiratory tract, and (4) to administer antibiotics locally by depositing them in the respiratory tract.

Physical and chemical substances used as medical aerosols include drugs that act as BRONCHODILATORS and DECONGESTANTS, e.g., epinephrine, ephedrine, isoproterenol, atropine, and the steroids. Wetting agents administered as aerosols to render the bronchial secretions more liquid include tyloxapol (Alevaire), sodium ethasulfate (Tergemist), and acetylcysteine (Mucomyst). The selection of one or more antibiotics to be given as aerosol therapy is determined by the patient's specific condition and the preference of the attending physician. Most standard antibiotic drugs are available in aerosol form.

In general, the respiratory therapist is concerned with factors that affect how deeply aerosol particles can penetrate into the bronchial tract and the locations at which these particles are deposited on the bronchial mucosa and alveolar tissues. Depth of penetration is affected by particle size. Particles as large as 100 microns and as small as 5 microns are trapped in the nose. Those which are 5 to 2 microns in size are deposited somewhere in the respiratory tract proximal to the alveoli. Deposition in the alveoli is 90% to 100% for particles 2 to 1 micron in size.

Because aerosol particles are so small, they present the phenomenon of brownian movement as they are bombarded by the molecules of the gas in which they are carried. The velocity with which these particles move about directly affects their diffusion and deposition onto nearby surfaces. Thus the type of aerosol generator used in aerosol therapy is of primary importance.

Another factor affecting penetration and deposition of aerosol particles that should be of concern to respiratory therapists and other members of the health team who are teaching patients the techniques of effective aerosol therapy is that of ventilatory pattern. The ideal pattern of breathing for optimum delivery of aerosol particles is that of slow, moderate deep breathing with breath holding at the end of each inspiration.

a. clearance, removal of particles that have been deposited in the respiratory tissues. Clearance may occur by ciliary transport, by phagocytosis, by encapsulation and immobilization in a deposit of fibrous tissue (in which case the particles remain in the body), and by dissolving in tissue fluid and subsequently diffusing into the general circulation where the particles are metabolized.

a. deposition, the depositing of aerosol particles onto a nearby surface, especially deposition or retention of the particles within the respiratory system. Closely related to aerosol penetration and affected by the same factors.

a. penetration, the maximum distance aerosol particles can be carried into the respiratory tract by inhaled air. Depth of penetration increases as particle size decreases. Factors affecting where aerosol particles will be deposited and how deeply they can penetrate are: gravity, kinetic activity of gas molecules, inertial impaction, physical nature of the particle, and the ventilatory pattern.

Aerosporin (a″er-o-spōr′in) trademark for a preparation of polymyxin B sulfate.

aerotitis (a″er-o-ti′tis) barotitis.

aerotonometer (a″er-o-to-nom′ĕ-ter) a device used in measuring the tension of the blood gases.

aes- for words beginning thus, see those beginning *es-*.

Æsculapius (es″cu-la′pe-us) the god of healing in Roman mythology. The staff of Æsculapius, a rod or staff with a snake entwined around it, is a symbol of medicine and is the official insignia of the American Medical Association (see also CADUCEUS).

aet- for words beginning thus, see those beginning *et-*.

afebrile (a-feb′ril) without fever.

affect (af′ekt) emotional tone or feeling.

affection (ah-fek′shun) a morbid condition or diseased state.

affective (ah-fek′tiv) pertaining to emotional tone or feeling.

a. psychosis, a severely disabling disorder of mood or emotional feeling, with profound effect upon thought and behavior. The disorder is characterized by changes in mood from manic to depressive, or the patient may exhibit the manic or the depressive reaction only, or variants of the two moods. (See also PSYCHOSIS.)

afferent (af′er-ent) conducting toward a center or specific site of reference.

a. loop syndrome, chronic partial obstruction of the proximal loop (duodenum and jejunum) after gastrojejunostomy, resulting in duodenal distention, pain, and nausea following ingestion of food.

a. nerve, any nerve that transmits impulses from the periphery toward the central nervous system (see also NEURON).

affinity (ah-fin′ĭ-te) attraction; a tendency to seek out or unite with another object or substance.

chemical a., the force that unites atoms of different substances.

elective a., the force that causes union of a substance with one substance rather than another.

afibrinogenemia (a-fi″brin-o-jĕ-ne′me-ah) absence or deficiency of fibrinogen in the circulating blood. Congenital afibrinogenemia—complete absence of fibrinogen—is a rare anomaly that is inherited. Acquired afibrinogenemia is actually a deficiency of fibrinogen (*hypofibrinogenemia*) and often is a serious complication in obstetrics, the primary cause being excessive maternal use of fibrinogen during an abnormal pregnancy. The condition may be seen in association with malignancies of the bone and prostate and with leukemia. It also may follow transfusion of incompatible blood and sometimes may complicate thoracic and abdominal surgery.

SYMPTOMS. As would be expected in a deficiency

of fibrinogen, which plays an important role in the blood clotting mechanism, the chief symptom is generalized bleeding, external or internal. In obstetric or surgical patients suffering from this condition there is frequently sudden and uncontrollable hemorrhage.

TREATMENT. Fibrinogen is administered intravenously to supply the body with this essential substance; transfusions of whole blood may also be indicated. In patients with cancer of the prostate the fibrinogen level often returns to normal after administration of estrogens. In obstetric patients the fibrinogen level returns to normal after the uterus has been emptied.

African sleeping sickness African TRYPANOSOMIASIS.

afterbirth (af'ter-berth") the special tissues associated with the development of a fetus in the uterus that are expelled after the birth of a baby. These are the PLACENTA, or the structure attached to the wall of the uterus through which nourishment passes from the mother of the fetus, and the UMBILICAL CORD, which attaches the fetus to the placenta.

afterbrain (af'ter-brān) metencephalon.

afterhearing (af"ter-hēr'ing) hearing of sounds after the stimulus has ceased.

afterimage (af'ter-im"ij) a retinal impression remaining after cessation of the stimulus causing it.

afterpain (af'ter-pān") pain that follows expulsion of the placenta, due to contraction of the uterus.

afterperception (af"ter-per-sep'shun) perception of aftersensations.

aftersensation (af"ter-sen-sa'shun) sensation persisting after cessation of the stimulus that caused it.

aftersound (af'ter-sownd") sensation of a sound after cessation of the stimulus causing it.

aftertaste (af'ter-tāst") sensation of taste continuing after the stimulus has ceased.

A-G ratio the ratio of albumin to globulin in blood serum, plasma, or urine.

Ag chemical symbol, *silver* (L. argentum); antigen.

agalactia (ag"ah-lak'she-ah) absence or failure of secretion of milk.

agammaglobulinemia (a"gam-ah-glob"u-lin-e'me-ah) absence or severe deficiency of the plasma protein gamma globulin. There are three main types: transient, congenital, and acquired. The transient type occurs in early infancy, because gamma globulins are not produced in the fetus and the gamma globulins derived from the maternal blood are soon depleted. This temporary deficiency of gamma globulin lasts for the first 6 to 8 weeks, until the infant begins to synthesize the protein. Congenital agammaglobulinemia is a rare condition, occurring in males, and resulting in decreased production of antibodies. Acquired agammaglobulinemia is secondary to other disorders and is usually a hypogammaglobulinemia, that is, a deficiency rather than total absence of this plasma protein. It is often secondary to malignant diseases such as leukemia, myeloma, and lymphoma, and to diseases associated with hypoproteinemia such as nephrosis and liver disease. Some patients have a family history of rheumatoid arthritis or allergies. This seems to indicate the presence of genetic factors in the development of agammaglobulinemia.

SYMPTOMS. Because gamma globulin is so important in the production of antibodies and thus in the body's ability to defend itself against infection, it follows that a deficiency or absence of gamma globulin would result in severe and recurrent infections. The infections are usually bacterial rather than viral in origin and are extremely difficult to eliminate. The condition is often complicated by local damage to tissues because of scarring and repeated infection. Disorders of connective tissue such as scleroderma, arthritis, and lupus erythematosus are also frequent complications.

TREATMENT. Replacement therapy with human gamma globulin is effective in preventing severe infections. The aim is to maintain the gamma globulin level above 150 mg. per 100 ml. of blood. The patient is given an initial dose of 0.2 gm. per kilogram of body weight and a maintenance dose of 0.1 gm. per kilogram every 4 weeks. Antibiotics are also given and are continued until all signs of infection have disappeared.

aganglionic (a-gang"gle-on'ik) lacking ganglion cells.

aganglionosis (ah-gang"gle-on-o'sis) congenital absence of parasympathetic ganglion cells.

agar (ag'ar) a dried hydrophilic, colloidal substance extracted from various species of red algae. It is used in cultures for bacteria and other microorganisms, in making emulsions, and as a supporting medium for immunodiffusion and immunoelectrophoresis. Because of its bulk it is also used in medicines to promote peristalsis and relieve constipation.

agastric (ah-gas'trik) having no stomach.

age (āj) 1. the duration, or the measure of time of the existence of a person or object. 2. to undergo change as a result of passage of time.

achievement a., proficiency in study expressed in terms of the chronologic age of a normal child showing the same degree of attainment.

chronologic a., the actual measure of time elapsed since a person's birth.

mental a., the age level of mental ability of a person as gauged by standard intelligence tests.

aged (a'jed) persons of advanced age. It is convenient for statisticians to define everyone 65 or over as "aged"; however, there is no known definite age at which individuals become "old." Improvements in public health, nutrition, surgery, drugs, and medical care since 1900 have added years to life expectancy in the United States, resulting in an ever larger "aging" population. According to present figures, the average white, male American who has reached the age of 65 will live for another dozen years, and the average woman will live for another 14.

CAUSES OF THE AGING PROCESS. The reasons why we age are complex and only partially understood. It is evident that the aging process is a combination of many factors.

The body is contantly replacing its worn-out cells, literally by the millions, every day of our lives. As the years pass, this rate of replacement slows down very gradually, beginning at about the time the body has reached its full growth. This is such a gradual change, in fact, that in some of the body's functions there is remarkably little difference between people in their forties and those in their sixties. The part of the body that ages least, and maintains its vigor into the latest years, is the brain.

Hereditary factors play a part in determining how durable a person may be. It is known, for example, that people born to long-living parents and grandparents tend to be longer-lived themselves. It is also believed that the capacity to withstand or adjust to such stresses and strains of living as disease, infection, and worry comes in part from hereditary make-up.

The process of aging may also be hastened by environment, disease, emotional stress, and such lifetime habits as boredom, laziness, or faulty diet. The physical exhaustion and malnutrition of poverty are two prime causes of early aging.

EFFECTS OF AGING. Old age brings certain physical changes as a normal aspect of aging. They may be discomforting, even limiting, but they are not necessarily incapacitating. The body has less strength and less endurance as it ages, and needs more repair work. Its speed of reaction and its agility are slowed. The basal metabolism, or rate of energy production in the body cells, is gradually lowered, so that people tire more easily, and are more sensitive to weather changes. Sexual desire and ability decline although they need never entirely end for either sex. The capacity to bear children ends in women with MENOPAUSE, but many men apparently retain their reproductive function into the late years. Those who never used eyeglasses usually need them in later years, or their regular glasses will need changing to bifocals (see also PRESBYOPIA). Hearing changes also come with greater age. Older people hear low tones fairly well, but their ability to perceive the high tones declines. The capacity of tissue and bone to repair itself is slowed, as is cellular growth and division. Bones are more brittle. Skin becomes drier and loses some of its elasticity. Artificial teeth may become necessary. Few people reach the age of 65 with a full set of natural teeth.

Much of the disability and discomfort that used to be considered a part of normal aging can now be prevented with proper medical care and health habits.

DISEASES OF OLD AGE. No disease is caused by old age, but certain diseases are more likely to occur in old age. ARTHRITIS, CATARACT, CORONARY OCCLUSION (heart attack), CEREBRAL VASCULAR ACCIDENT (stroke), DIABETES MELLITUS, SENILITY, and others are diseases that tend to develop after decades of living. Worry, poor habits such as overeating, malnutrition, and lack of proper preventive attention to early signs very likely accelerate onset of these diseases of the aged.

In the majority of cases, the disease originates during the middle years. This is why the habit of periodic health examinations is so important and becomes increasingly important after middle age.

AGE AND MENTAL POWERS. In most people aging has little effect upon mental powers. It is one of the joys of old age that long after the body slows down and begins to limit physical activity, the mind can continue to seek and explore.

In older persons memory of recent events declines while important memories from long ago remain intact. This has been found to be largely a matter of interest and attention rather than an inability to remember. If the memory changes at all, it tends to become more accurate. Older people do not learn new things as quickly as younger people, but once something has been learned, they remember it better and more accurately. Older persons have the further benefit of long experience and seasoned judgment to apply to the solution of new problems.

SOME RULES OF HEALTH AND HYGIENE FOR THE AGED

Periodic Health Examinations. The diseases that make invalids of old people, such as diabetes mellitus and heart disease, begin unnoticed in middle age; with regular checkups they can be detected in their early stages when they are easier to treat. The physician can also give good advice on exercise, diet, and rest needs through the years.

Proper Nutrition. Poor eating habits may stem from childhood but they begin to have their effects as people grow older. Poor nutrition has been demonstrated to have a definite adverse effect upon mental and physical vigor. Proper food can prolong life as well as preserve the strength and ability to fight off disease. Good nutrition is a vital aspect of successful aging.

Many older people subsist on poor diets because they live alone and the preparation of proper meals requires too much effort. Some suffer from poor teeth or dentures that interfere with chewing. Others are victims of poor diet habits or lack of interest, or, in some cases, misinformation.

The aged need the same nutrients as those that must be supplied at any age. They must have all basic food elements every day, and this means not overloading the menu with any single type of food. The only kind of food that can be safely reduced in the diet is fat. Because of a gradual decrease in the amount of fat-digesting enzymes in the digestive tract of an older person, the aging body manages fat less well. In general, the older person's diet tends to include too little of the foods that supply vitamin C, iron, vitamin A, vitamin B (thiamine), and vitamin B_2 (riboflavin).

Some older people believe that acid-containing foods such as citrus fruits and tomatoes, which are prime sources of vitamin C, cause acidity in the body. Actually, these acid-containing fruits are excellent alkalizers and rich sources of necessary vitamins and minerals as well, and should be included in the diet. Another common mistake is the belief that milk is only for children. It is an excellent food for adults too. Milk (whole or skimmed) contains protein, calcium, and riboflavin, and is readily digested and tolerated by most people of all ages.

If an older person has difficulty chewing, some foods will have to be chopped, strained, or cooked soft for his special requirements, but foods with important nutrient values must not be eliminated from the diet. (See also NUTRITION.)

Exercise. Proper exercise promotes good circulation and appetite, and helps to maintain good mental and physical functioning. Older people should be as active as possible, although never to the point of strain or exhaustion.

Rest. Rest becomes increasingly important in the later years. It is of great value to rest for half an hour after meals, and at intervals during the day. Older people whose work does not permit them to lie down should take advantage of "breaks" or rest periods to relax as completely as possible, with their feet elevated, perhaps on a chair, if at all feasible.

Avoidance of Inactivity. Following an illness, when the physician says it is time to get out of bed, his instructions should be followed. A prolonged unnecessary stay in bed is harmful at all ages but especially in later years.

RETIREMENT PROBLEMS. Although many people look forward to retirement, it is not uncommon to hear of someone who, having worked hard all his life with that goal in mind, begins to fail mentally and physically the moment he actually reaches it. Successful retirement depends on far more than money in the bank. There must be a reserve of interests that make life worth living. Hobbies and recreational activities are important because they can be continued in later years. As Dr. George Lawton, an authority on gerontology, the scientific study of aging, puts it: "To grow old successfully, a man must learn to push around, not his body, but his mind. If his speed, strength, and endurance decline with the years, then he must train in advance skills which will hold up with age and even improve."

agenesis (a-jen'ĕ-sis) absence of an organ due to nonappearance of its primordium in the embryo.

agenitalism (a-jen'ĭ-tal-izm") a condition due to lack of secretion of the testes or ovaries.

agenosomia (ah-jen"o-so'me-ah) imperfect development of reproductive organs.

agent (a'jent) a person or substance by which something is accomplished.

alkylating a., a compound with two or more end (alkyl) groups that combine readily with other molecules.

chelating a., a compound that combines with metals to form weakly dissociated complexes in which the metal is part of a ring, and used to extract certain elements from a system.

chimpanzee coryza a., respiratory syncytial virus.

Eaton a., *Mycoplasma pneumoniae.*

surface-active a., a substance that exerts a change on the surface properties of a liquid, especially one, such as a detergent, that reduces its surface tension. Called also surfactant.

ageusia (ah-gu'ze-ah) absence or impairment of the sense of taste.

agger (aj'er), pl. *ag'geres* [L.] an elevation.

a. na'si, an elevation at the anterior free margin of the middle nasal concha.

agglutinable (ah-gloo'tĭ-nah- b'l) capable of agglutination.

agglutinant (ah-gloo'tĭ-nant) 1. acting like glue. 2. a substance that promotes union of parts.

agglutination (ah-gloo"tĭ-na'shun) aggregation of separate particles into clumps of masses; especially the clumping together of bacteria by the action of certain antibodies. adj., **agglutina'tive.**

group a., agglutination of an organism by an agglutinin specific for other, related organisms.

platelet a., clumping together of platelets due to the action of platelet agglutinins.

agglutinin (ah-gloo'tĭ-nin) a specific antibody formed in the blood in response to the presence of an invading agent and capable of causing a clumping together (agglutination) of cells. Agglutinins are proteins (GAMMA GLOBULINS) and function as part of the immune mechanism of the body. When the invading agents that bring about the production of agglutinins are bacteria, the agglutinins produced bring about agglutination of the bacterial cells.

Erythrocytes also may agglutinate when agglutinins are formed in response to the entrance of noncompatible blood cells into the bloodstream. A transfusion reaction is an example of the result of agglutination of blood cells brought about by agglutinins produced in the recipient's blood in response to incompatible or foreign cells (the donor's blood). Anti-Rh agglutinins are produced in cases of Rh incompatibility and can result in a condition known as ERYTHROBLASTOSIS FETALIS when the maternal blood is Rh negative and the fetal blood is Rh positive (see also RH FACTOR).

cold a., one that acts only at low temperature.

group a., one that has a specific action on certain organisms, but will agglutinate other species as well.

H a., one that is specific for flagellar antigens of the motile strain of an organism.

immune a., a specific agglutinin found in the blood after recovery from the disease or injection of the microorganism.

incomplete a., one that at appropriate concentrations fails to agglutinate the homologous antigen.

normal a., a specific agglutinin found in the blood of an animal or of man that has neither had the associated disease nor been injected with the causative organism.

O a., one specific for somatic antigens of a microorganism.

partial a., one present in agglutinative serum which acts on organisms closely related to the specific antigen, but in a lower dilution.

warm a., an incomplete antibody that sensitizes and reacts optimally with erythrocytes at 37° C.

agglutinogen (ag"loo-tin'o-jen) a substance (antigen) that stimulates the animal body to form agglutinin (antibody).

aggregation (ag"rĕ-ga'shun) 1. massing or clumping of materials together. 2. a clumped mass of material.

familial a., the occurrence of more cases of a given disorder in close relatives of a person with the disorder than in control families.

platelet a., platelet agglutination.

aglaucopsia (ah"glaw-kop'se-ah) inability to distinguish green tints.

aglossia (ah-glos'e-ah) congenital absence of the tongue.

aglossostomia (ah"glos-o-sto'me-ah) congenital absence of the tongue and the mouth opening.

aglucone (a-gloo'kōn) aglycone.

aglutition (ag"loo-tish'un) inability to swallow.

aglycemia (a"gli-se'me-ah) absence of sugar from the blood. (See also HYPOGLYCEMIA.)

aglycone (a-gli'kōn) the noncarbohydrate portion of a glycoside molecule.

aglycosuric (ah-gli"ko-su'rik) free from glycosuria.

agnathia (ag-na'the-ah) congenital absence of the lower jaw.

agnogenic (ag"no-jen'ik) of unknown origin.

agnosia (ag-no'ze-ah) inability to recognize the import of sensory impressions; the varieties correspond with several senses and are distinguished as auditory (acoustic), gustatory, olfactory, tactile, and visual.

finger a., loss of ability to indicate one's own or another's fingers.

time a., loss of comprehension of the succession and duration of events.

-agogue (ah-gog') word element [Gr.], *something that leads or induces.*

agonad (ah-go'nad) an individual having no sex glands (gonads).

agonadal (ah-gon'ah-dal) having no sex glands; due to absence of sex glands.

agonal (ag′ŏ-nal) pertaining to death or extreme suffering.

agonist (ag′o-nist) a muscle which in contracting to move a part is opposed by another muscle (the antagonist).

agony (ag′o-ne) 1. death struggle. 2. extreme suffering.

agoraphobia (ag″o-rah-fo′be-ah) fear of open or public spaces.

-agra (ag′rah) word element [Gr.], *attack; seizure.*

agranular reticulum smooth-surfaced endoplasmic reticulum.

agranulocyte (a-gran′u-lo-sīt″) a nongranular leukocyte.

agranulocytosis (a-gran″u-lo-si-to′sis) an acute disease in which there is a sudden drop in the production of leukocytes, leaving the body defenseless against bacterial invasion. A great majority of the cases of agranulocytosis are caused by sensitization to drugs or chemicals that affect the bone marrow and thereby depress the formation of granulocytes.

SYMPTOMS. The first manifestations of this disorder are usually produced by a severe infection and include high fever, chills, prostration, and ulcerations of mucous membrane such as in the mouth, rectum, or vagina. Laboratory tests reveal a profound leukopenia (low leukocyte count).

TREATMENT. Treatment is aimed at immediate withdrawal of the drug or chemical causing the disorder, and control of infection. In most cases control can be achieved by the administration of antibiotics, usually penicillin, streptomycin, or oxytetracycline. If the bone marrow is not irreparably damaged, the prognosis is good, with proper treatment, and the patient will recover as the production of granulocytes resumes. Rarely, the leukocyte-producing tissues are damaged beyond repair, and death ensues.

agranuloplastic (a-gran″u-lo-plas′tik) forming nongranular cells only.

agranulosis (a-gran″u-lo′sis) agranulocytosis.

agraphia (a-graf′e-ah) loss of ability to express thoughts in writing.

ague (a′gu) 1. malaria. 2. a chill.

agyria (ah-ji′re-ah) a malformation in which the gyri of the cerebral cortex are not normally developed; called also lissencephaly.

A.H.A. American Heart Association; American Hospital Association.

AHF antihemophilic factor (clotting factor VIII).

AHG antihemophilic globulin (clotting factor VIII).

ailurophobia (i-lu″ro-fo′be-ah) morbid fear of cats.

ainhum (ān′hum) a condition of unknown origin, occurring chiefly in dark-skinned races, leading to spontaneous amputation of the fourth of fifth toe.

air (ār) the gaseous mixture that makes up the atmosphere.

a. hunger, a distressing dyspnea occurring in paroxysms, characteristic of diabetic acidosis and coma; called also Kussmaul's respiration.

airway (ār′wa) 1. the passage by which air enters and leaves the lungs. 2. a mechanical device used for securing unobstructed respiration during general anesthesia or other occasions in which the patient is not ventilating or exchanging gases properly.

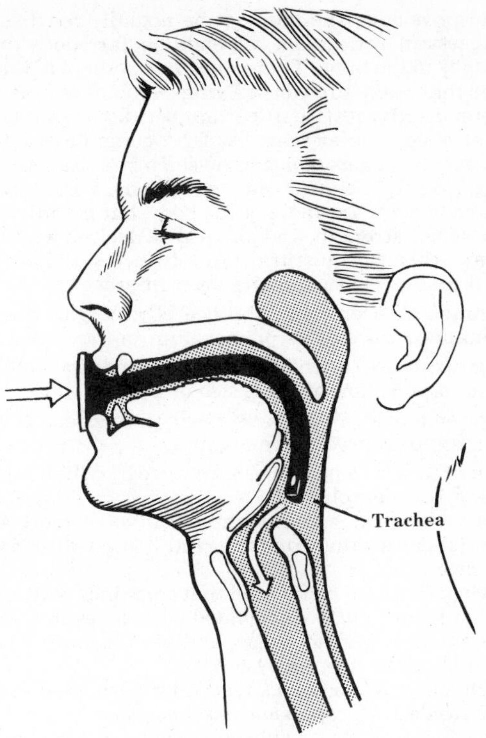

Oral airway.

In order to provide and maintain an open airway when there is cessation of breathing, the head should be tilted back as far as possible, hyperextending the neck. This is accomplished by placing one hand under the neck and lifting up, while the other hand is placed on the forehead, pressing back. This simple technique frequently is all that is needed to provide an open airway for spontaneous resumption of breathing.

OROPHARYNGEAL AIRWAY. This device is a hollow tube inserted into the mouth and back of the throat to prevent the tongue from slipping back into the throat and closing off the passage of air. It should not be used on alert or semiconscious patients as it invariably stimulates the gag reflex and causes vomiting unless the patient is deeply unconscious.

Selection of proper size is essential because an airway that is too short cannot lift the tongue away from the oropharynx. The airway should be gently inserted so as to avoid trauma to the mucous membranes. It must be inserted so that the tongue is not displaced back into the pharynx, where it will obstruct the air passage.

ENDOTRACHEAL TUBE. This inflatable tube is inserted into the mouth or nose and passed down into the trachea. It is used for the administration of anesthetics and may be left in place after the completion of surgery until the patient is no longer in danger of asphyxiation. The endotracheal tube can be connected to a mechanical ventilator when necessary.

S-TUBE AIRWAY. This tube may be used to maintain a patent airway and to keep the mouth open during emergency resuscitation efforts. It does not, however, provide an adequate seal around the mouth, and may induce vomiting if not used properly.

TRACHEOSTOMY. This involves a surgical incision

into the trachea to relieve obstruction of the respiratory tract above the level of the incision. A metal or plastic tracheostomy tube is inserted into the incision. (See also TRACHEOSTOMY.)

A.J.C.C.S. American Joint Committee on Cancer Staging and End Results Reporting.

akaryocyte (ah-kar′e-o-sīt″) a non-nucleated cell, e.g., an erythrocyte.

akaryote (ah-kar′e-ōt) 1. non-nucleated. 2. a non-nucleated cell.

akathisia (ak″ah-the′ze-ah) a condition marked by motor restlessness and anxiety.

akinesia (a″ki-ne′ze-ah) 1. abnormal absence or poverty of movements. 2. the temporary paralysis of a muscle by the injection of procaine.

a. al′gera, paralysis due to the intense pain of muscular movement.

akinesthesia (ah-kin″es-the′ze-ah) absence of movement sense.

akinetic (a″ki-net′ik) affected with akinesia.

Akineton (a″ki-ne′ton) trademark for preparations of biperiden, an anticholinergic used in the treatment of Parkinson's disease and certain forms of spasticity.

Al chemical symbol, *aluminum.*

ala (a′lah), pl. *a′lae* [L.] a winglike process. adj., **a′late.**

a. na′si, the cartilaginous flap on the outer side of either nostril.

alalia (ah-la′le-ah) impairment of the ability to speak.

alanine (al′ah-nēn, al′ah-nin) a naturally occurring, nonessential amino acid.

alar (a′lar) 1. pertaining to or like a wing. 2. pertaining to the axilla.

alarm reaction (ah-larm′) the response of the adrenal cortex in times of stress or emergency, resulting in the production of certain adrenocortical hormones (corticosteroids); called also stress response. The exact mechanism is not known; it is believed that the release of epinephrine from the adrenal medulla triggers the production of ACTH, which in turn stimulates the adrenal cortex to release its hormones. Another theory is that the cortiscosteroids are released independently of ACTH and are a direct response to impulses from the sympathetic nervous system. The corticosteroids provide the body with glucose and amino acids for energy and tissue repair, elevate the blood pressure, and help maintain a normal fluid and electrolyte balance.

alastrim (ah-las′trim) variola minor.

alba (al′bah) [L.] white.

Albamycin (al′bah-mi″sin) trademark for preparations of novobiocin, an antibiotic.

Albers-Schönberg disease (al′berz shān′berg) a rare hereditary, congenital condition in which there are bandlike areas of condensed bone at the epiphyseal lines of long bones and condensation of the edges of smaller bones. Fractures occur frequently and deformities of the head, chest, or spine develop. There is no treatment and the prognosis is unfavorable. Called also osteopetrosis and marble bones.

albicans (al′bĭ-kans) [L.] white.

albiduria (al″bĭ-du′re-ah) the discharge of white or pale urine.

Albini's nodules (al-be′nēz) gray nodules of the size of small grains, sometimes seen on the free

edges of the atrioventricular valves of infants; they are remains of fetal structures.

albinism (al′bĭ-nizm) congenital absence of normal pigmentation in the body (hair, skin, eyes).

albino (al-bi′no) a person affected with albinism.

albinuria (al″bĭ-nu′re-ah) albiduria.

Albl's ring a ring-shaped shadow in radiographs of the skull, caused by aneurysm of a cerebral artery.

Albright's syndrome (awl′brīts) a group of symptoms, including distortion of bone with fibrous changes in the bone marrow spaces, brownish pigmentation of the skin and precocious puberty in females, of unknown cause. Called also polyostotic fibrous dysplasia. The bone lesions may cause the bones to become bowed or shortened, resulting in difficulty in walking, and may make them more susceptible to fractures. Treatment is concerned with the complications of the disorder—fractures and deformities. Corrective orthopedic surgery is often indicated.

albuginea (al″bu-jin′e-ah) 1. a tough, whitish layer of fibrous tissue investing a part or organ. 2. the tunica albuginea.

albumin (al-bu′min) a simple protein found in most animal and vegetable tissues; it is soluble in water and coagulable by heat. Albumin is a plasma protein, formed principally in the liver and constituting about four-sevenths of the 6 to 8 per cent protein concentration in the plasma. Albumin is responsible for much of the osmotic force of the blood, and thus is a very important factor in regulating the exchange of water between the plasma and the intercellular compartment (space between the cells). Because of hydrostatic pressure, water is forced through the walls of the capillaries into the tissue spaces. This flow of water continues until the osmotic pull of protein (albumin) molecules causes it to stop. A drop in the amount of albumin in the plasma leads to an increase in the flow of water from the capillaries into the intercellular compartment. This results in an increase in tissue fluid which, if severe, becomes apparent as edema. Albumin serves also as a transport substance.

The presence of albumin in the urine (albuminuria) indicates malfunction of the kidney, and may accompany kidney disease or heart failure. A person with severe renal disease may lose as much as 20 to 30 gm. of plasma proteins in the urine in one day.

The normal amount of albumin in the blood is 4.5 to 5.5 gm. per milliliter of serum. A decrease in serum albumin may, as stated, occur with severe disease of the kidney. Other conditions such as liver disease, malnutrition, and extensive burns may result in serious decrease of plasma proteins.

a.-globulin ratio, the ratio of albumin to globulin in blood serum, plasma, or urine.

egg a., the white of eggs.

normal human serum a., a sterile solution of the serum albumin constituent from healthy donors.

radioiodinated serum a., normal human serum albumin treated with iodine-131, used for measuring blood volume and cardiac output.

serum a., albumin of the blood.

albuminate (al-bu′mĭ-nāt) a compound of albumin with a base.

albuminimeter (al-bu″mĭ-nim′ĕ-ter) an instrument for determining the proportion of albumin present.

albuminocholia (al-bu″mĭ-no-ko′le-ah) presence of protein in the bile.

albuminoid (al-bu′mĭnoid) 1. resembling albumin. 2. an albumin-like substance; the term is sometimes applied to scleroproteins.

albuminolysis (al-bu″mĭ-nol′ĭ-sis) the splitting up of albumins.

albuminoptysis (al-bu″mĭ-nop′tĭ-sis) albumin in the sputum.

albuminous (al-bu′mĭ-nus) charged with or resembling albumin.

albuminuria (al-bu″mĭ-nu′re-ah) the presence in the urine of serum albumin. adj. **albuminu′ric.**

Albumisol (al-bu′mĭ-sol) trademark for a preparation of normal human serum albumin.

Alcaligenes (al″kah-lij′ĕ-nēz) a genus of bacteria found in the intestines of vertebrates or in dairy products.

alcapton (al-kap′ton) alkapton.

alcaptonuria (al-kap″to-nu′re-ah) alkaptonuria.

Alcock's canal (al′koks) a tunnel formed by a splitting of the obturator fascia, which encloses the pudendal vessels and nerve.

alcohol (al′ko-hol) 1. a colorless, volatile liquid obtained by fermentation of carbohydrates by yeast. 2. a compound of hydrocarbon with hydroxyl (OH).

absolute a., alcohol free from water and impurities.

benzyl a., a colorless liquid used as a local anesthetic.

cetyl a., a solid alcohol used in making ointment bases.

denatured a., ethyl alcohol made unfit for consumption by the addition of substances known as denaturants. Although it should never be taken internally, denatured alcohol is widely used on the skin as a cooling agent and skin disinfectant.

ethyl a., the major ingredient of alcoholic beverages; called also ethanol and grain alcohol. It is sometimes used medically to stimulate the appetite of convalescent, weak, or elderly patients.

isopropyl a., a transparent, volatile colorless liquid used as a rubbing compound; called also isopropanol.

methyl a., a mobile, colorless liquid used as a solvent; called also wood alcohol or methanol. It is a useful fuel, but is poisonous if taken internally. Consumption may lead to blindness or death.

phenylethyl a., an alcohol used as an antibacterial and preservative.

primary a., an alcohol that on oxidation forms a corresponding aldehyde and acid having the same number of carbon atoms.

propyl a., a colorless fluid of alcoholic taste and fruity odor.

stearyl a., a mixture of solid alcohols, used as an ingredient of various pharmaceutic or cosmetic preparations.

wood a., methyl alcohol.

alcoholic (al″ko-hol′ik) 1. containing or pertaining to alcohol. 2. a person suffering from alcoholism.

alcoholism (al′ko-hol″izm) drunkenness (acute alcoholism); or long-continued, excessive consumption of alcohol (chronic alcoholism). Generally, the term refers to chronic alcoholism. The chronic alcoholic is a person who drinks compulsively and in such a way that his drinking is damaging to himself, to his way of life, and to those about him. It is the compulsive character of his drinking that sets the alcoholic apart from the heavy or occasionally excessive drinker. His craving for alcohol is deeply rooted, and he cannot govern that craving even if he is aware of its destructive consequences.

CAUSES. There is no accepted explanation to account for the fact that one person becomes an alcoholic while another does not. Generally speaking, a person is more likely to become an alcoholic if his environment emphasizes drinking, presenting it as a fashionable, or indeed indispensable, social pastime. Also, the heavy social drinker has a good chance of becoming an alcoholic. Psychologic factors play an important role in the development of alcoholism in an individual. Unresolved conflicts, loneliness, financial difficulties, or marital problems may contribute to alcoholism.

Once a person becomes an alcoholic, whatever the cause or causes, he has something in common with all other alcoholics: he cannot stop drinking by a simple act of will. It is the recognition of this fact that forms the basis of modern treatment for alcoholics. The alcoholic is regarded not as depraved or weak but as sick. He is unable to cure himself. His problem is not moral but medical.

COMPLICATIONS. Alcoholism is all the more a medical matter because it is often complicated by other diseases which afflict both body and mind. Nervous and mental disorders are common in the alcoholic. DELIRIUM TREMENS (DT's) is an acute condition that is particularly apt to occur if the alcoholic is suddenly deprived of drink. The body trembles and there are frightening hallucinations. In KORSAKOFF'S SYNDROME, the memory is impaired, sometimes permanently. Deterioration of the powers of reasoning is a real possibility in alcoholics. In alcoholic polyneuritis, there may be persistent nerve changes. Cirrhosis of the liver, in which the liver becomes swollen with fatty and fibrous tissue, is not limited to alcoholics but often does occur in those with alcoholism of several years' standing. Alcoholic amblyopia, or dimness of vision, is a result of alcohol's toxic effect on the optic nerve. The heart and kidneys may be impaired as an indirect result of alcoholism. Gastric disturbances, excessive bowel activity, and circulatory disorders may affect the alcoholic. The chronic alcoholic may suffer from severe malnutrition, including vitamin deficiencies. Habitual drinking usually lowers resistance to infectious diseases such as pneumonia.

TREATMENT. There is no simple remedy for alcoholism. To be helped, the alcoholic must drastically alter his approach to life and destroy a pattern of habits that has been firmly established, perhaps for years. He must stop drinking altogether, for there is little possibility that he will recover the ability to take a drink or two with restraint. Successful treatment is possible only if the alcoholic wants to stop drinking, and this happens only when he has been brought to recognize the seriousness of his condition and the prospect of help. Since he has probably created many difficulties and problems in his life, he will feel guilty and despondent, wishing more for oblivion than for rehabilitation. Condemnation, sermonizing, and the like will only reinforce his conviction that life is not worth the trouble.

The first step is to place the alcoholic under the care of a competent physician. He will recommend one or more of the following modes of treatment:

Vitamin and Other Nutritional Therapy. Some of the diseases that complicate alcoholism are due to nutritional deficiencies because the alcoholic often eats improperly or not at all.

Tranquilizers and Sedatives. These are used during withdrawal of alcohol to aid in relaxation and sleep.

Hospitalization. This is advised when withdrawal must be subject to controlled conditions, when the patient's health is bad, or when the patient is a criminal risk.

Disulfiram (Antabuse). This is a compound that renders the body so sensitive to alcohol that one drink produces breathlessness, flushing, rapid heartbeat, and later nausea, vomiting, and fall in blood pressure. Although far from a cure, it is useful in abolishing impulsive drinking. In some cases it is possible through long-continued use of disulfiram to create in the alcoholic, by means of reflex conditioning, a lasting aversion to alcohol. The preparation must be administered only under a doctor's supervision and with the full knowledge and consent of the patient.

Alcoholics Anonymous. A.A. is an organization of individuals who have conquered or are trying to conquer their own habitual drinking. From their own experiences, these people have learned how to encourage and stimulate others in their desire to stop drinking. Meetings and discussions provide the individual with an opportunity to air his own problems as well as to learn from the experiences of others. Hundreds of thousands of alcoholics have been helped by A.A. since the organization was founded in 1935, and membership today totals about 350,000. Help in locating a local group and information about A.A. and alcoholism can be obtained from Alcoholics Anonymous, P.O. Box 459, Grand Central Station, New York, N.Y. 10017.

Psychotherapy. This is advisable when a personality disorder is at the root of the problem.

PATIENT CARE. Education of the public as to the true nature of alcoholism as an illness is the responsibility of all members of the health team. Each person concerned with the care of an alcoholic should evaluate his/her own feelings toward alcoholism and avoid a self-righteous and disdainful attitude toward the alcoholic. Although alcoholics can be and often are difficult patients to care for, they are suffering from a serious and crippling illness that affects their physical well-being, family life, economic status, and social relationships.

Hospital treatment of alcoholism is often necessary and alcoholic patients are sometimes admitted to a medical unit if no other facilities are available. They are often boisterous and belligerent and may disrupt the routine of the unit, but their acute illness demands all the attention afforded any patient in this condition. During the acute state of alcoholism the patient requires serenity and physical rest. Attendants must be alert for early symptoms of withdrawal from alcohol as the patient is denied the drug. These symptoms include irritability, insomnia, or extreme restlessness. Convulsions and delirium tremens can usually be avoided if adequate sedation is given when the withdrawal symptoms first appear. If delirium tremens does occur, the patient becomes truly frightened and terrified by auditory or visual hallucinations. He must be reassured and offered emotional support and understanding during these trying times.

Adequate fluid intake and a high-protein, high-vitamin diet are necessary because most acute alcoholics are dehydrated and poorly nourished. An accurate record of intake and output of fluids should be kept during the acute phase of this illness.

Diversional activities, such as reading, watching television, and visiting with other patients, help relieve the boredom and restlessness felt by the alcoholic during his convalescence. The alcoholic is likely to feel shame and remorse during this time and often indicates a desire to talk with someone about his problems. The attending staff must do much more than merely tolerate his presence. They should be good listeners, allowing him to express his feelings and anxieties without fear of reprisal or reprimand. An attitude of understanding will do much toward helping the alcoholic seek help in coping with his problem.

alcoholometer (al″ko-hol-om′ĕ-ter) an instrument for determining the amount of alcohol present.

alcoholuria (al″ko-hol-u′re-ah) the presence of alcohol in the urine.

alcoholysis (al″ko-hol′ĭ-sis) a process analogous to hydrolysis, but in which alcohol takes the place of water.

Aldactazide (al-dak′tah-zīd) trademark for a preparation of spironolactone with hydrochlorothiazide.

Aldactone (al-dak′tōn) trademark for a preparation of spironolactone, an aldosterone antagonist used as a diuretic.

aldehyde (al′dĕ-hīd) any of a large class of chemical compounds derived from the primary alcohols by oxidation and containing the monovalent group —CHO.

aldopentose (al″do-pen′tōs) any one of a class of sugars that contain five carbon atoms and an aldehyde group (—CHO).

aldose (al′dōs) a sugar containing an aldehyde group (—CHO).

aldosterone (al-dos′ter-ōn) an electrolyte-regulating hormone of the adrenal cortex; the principal MINERALOCORTICOID.

aldosteronism (al-dos′ter-ōn-izm″) hyperaldosteronism.

Aldrich syndrome (awl′drich) Wiskott-Aldrich syndrome.

alecithal (ah-les′ĭ-thal) having no distinct yolk.

Aleppo boil (ah-lep′o) cutaneous leishmaniasis, a type of ulcer or sore caused by *Leishmania tropica,* which is usually transmitted by a bite from the sandfly. The lesion is characterized by cutaneous granulation which has a tendency to become chronic. It occurs principally in Asian and African countries and is known by various names, such as Delhi sore, Baghdad sore, oriental sore.

aleukemia (ah″lu-ke′me-ah) 1. absence or deficiency of leukocytes in the blood. 2. aleukemic leukemia.

aleukia (ah-lu′ke-ah) leukopenia; absence of leukocytes from the blood.

aleukocytosis (ah-lu″ko-si-to′sis) diminished proportion of leukocytes in the blood.

Alevaire (al′ĕ-vār) trademark for a mucolytic solution that is administered by nebulizer in respiratory disorders.

alexia (ah-lek′se-ah) visual aphasia.

alexic (ah-lek′sik) 1. pertaining to alexia. 2. having the properties of an alexin.

alexin (ah-lek′sin) a nonspecific thermolabile substance which in the presence of specific sensitizer exerts a lytic action on bacteria and other cells (see also COMPLEMENT).

aleydigism (ah-li′dig-izm) absence of secretion of the interstitial cells of the testis (Leydig cells).

Alflorone (al′flo-rōn) trademark for preparations of fludrocortisone, a synthetic corticoid.

ALG antilymphocyte globulin.

algae (al′je) a group of plants living in the water, including all seaweeds, and ranging in size from microscopic cells to fronds hundreds of feet long.

algefacient (al″jĕ-fa′shent) cooling or refrigerant.

algesia (al-je′ze-ah) sensitiveness to pain; hyperesthesia. adj., **alge′sic, alget′ic.**

algesimetry (al″jĕ-sim′ĕ-tre) measurement of sensitivity of pain.

algesthesis (al″jes-the′sis) a painful sensation.

-algia (al′je-ah) word element [Gr.], *pain.*

algicide (al′jĭ-sīd) 1. destructive to algae. 2. an agent that destroys algae.

algid (al′jid) chilly; cold.

alginate (al′jĭ-nāt) a salt of alginic acid, a colloidal substance from brown seaweed; used, in the form of calcium, sodium, or ammonium alginate, as foam, clot, or gauze for absorbable surgical dressings.

algo- (al′go) word element [Gr.], *pain; cold.*

algogenic (al″go-jen′ik) 1. causing pain. 2. lowering temperature.

algometer (al-gom′ĕ-ter) a device used in testing the sensitiveness of a part.

algometry (al-gom′ĕ-tre) estimation of the sensitivity to painful stimuli.

algophobia (al″go-fo′be-ah) morbid dread of pain.

algor (al′gor) chill or rigor; coldness.

a. mor′tis, the cooling of the body after death, which proceeds at a definite rate, influenced by the environmental temperature and protection of the body.

Alidase (al′ĭ-dās) trademark for a preparation of hyaluronidase for injection, used as a spreading agent to promote diffusion and hasten absorption.

alienia (ah″li-e′ne-ah) absence of the spleen.

aliform (al′ĭ-form) shaped like a wing.

aliment (al′ĭ-ment) food; nutritive material.

alimentary (al″ĭ-men′tar-e) pertaining to or caused by food, or nutritive material.

a. canal, all the organs making up the route taken by food as it passes through the body from mouth to anus; it comprises the esophagus, stomach, and small and large intestines. Called also digestive tract. (See also DIGESTIVE SYSTEM and Plate 9.)

a. tract, alimentary canal.

alimentation (al″ĭ-men-ta′shun) giving or receiving of nourishment.

alinasal (al″ĭ-na′zal) pertaining to either of the cartilaginous flaps of the nose.

aliphatic (al″ĭ-fat′ik) pertaining to or derived from fat; having an open-chain structure.

aliquot (al′ĭ-kwot) 1. a sample that is representative of the whole. 2. a number that will divide another without a remainder; e.g., 2 is an aliquot of 6.

alizarin (ah-liz′ah-rin) a red coloring principle obtained from coal tar or madder, the root of the herb *Rubia tinctoria.*

alkalemia (al″kah-le′me-ah) abnormal alkalinity, or increased pH, of the blood.

alkali (al′kah-li) any one of a class of compounds such as sodium hydroxide that form salts with acids and soaps with fats; a base, or substance capable of neutralizing acids. Other properties include a bitter taste and the ability to turn litmus paper from red to blue. Alkalis play a vital role in maintaining the normal functioning of the body chemistry. (See also ACID-BASE BALANCE and BASE.)

a. reserve, the ability of the combined buffer systems of the blood to neutralize acid. The pH of the blood normally is slightly on the alkaline side, between 7.35 and 7.45. Since the principal buffer in the blood is bicarbonate, the alkali reserve essentially is represented by the plasma bicarbonate concentration. However, hemoglobin, phosphates, and other bases also act as buffers against acids. A lowered alkali reserve means a state of acidosis; increased reserve indicates alkalosis. Measurement of the alkali reserve is done by means of the CARBON DIOXIDE COMBINING POWER, expressed as the number of milliliters of carbon dioxide that can be bound as bicarbonate by 100 ml. of blood plasma. Normal values range from 53 to 78 ml. of carbon dioxide, sometimes stated as 53 to 78 volumes per cent.

alkali-ash diet a therapeutic diet prescribed to dissolve uric acid and cystine urinary calculi. This type of diet changes the urinary pH so that certain salts are kept in solution and excreted in the urine. Emphasis is placed on fruits, vegetables, and milk. Meat, eggs, bread, and cereals are restricted.

alkalimetry (al″kah-lim′ĕ-tre) measurement of alkalinity of a compound or of the alkali in a mixture.

alkaline (al′kah-līn) having the reactions of an alkali.

a. phosphatase, a phosphatase that is active in an alkaline environment.

alkalinity (al″kah-lin′ĭ-te) 1. the quality of being alkaline. 2. the combining power of a base, expressed as the maximum number of equivalents of acid with which it reacts to form a salt.

alkalinuria (al″kah-lin-u′re-ah) an alkaline condition of the urine.

alkalization (al″kah-lĭ-za′shun) the act of making alkaline.

alkalizer (al″kah-līz′er) an agent that causes alkalization.

alkaloid (al′kah-loid) one of a large group of organic, basic substances found in plants. They are usually bitter in taste and are characterized by powerful physiologic activity. Examples are morphine, cocaine, atropine, quinine, nicotine, and caffeine. The term is also applied to synthetic substances that have structures similar to plant alkaloids, such as procaine.

alkalosis (al″kah-lo′sis) a pathologic condition resulting from accumulation of base, or from loss of acid without comparable loss of base in the body fluids, and characterized by decrease in hydrogen ion concentration (increase in pH). Alkalosis is the opposite of ACIDOSIS. (See also ACID-BASE BALANCE.)

compensated a., a condition in which compensatory mechanisms have returned the pH toward normal.

hypochloremic a., a metabolic acidosis in which gastric losses of chloride are disproportionately greater than sodium loss because of corresponding increase in potassium loss.

hypokalemic a., a metabolic alkalosis due to losses of potassium level.

metabolic a., a disturbance in which the acid-base status shifts toward the alkaline because of uncompensated loss of acids, ingestion or retention of excess base, or potassium depletion. The condition can occur in any patient who is vomiting frequently or has gastric suction, is taking a diuretic, or has hyperadrenocortical disease.

Metabolic alkalosis is characterized by a blood serum pH above 7.45, an increase of serum Co_2 above 32 mEq/L, and an unchanged Pco_2 when the lungs are compensating for the alkalosis. These values are determined by BLOOD GAS ANALYSIS. The symptoms may be mild at first, with muscle weakness, irritability, confusion, and muscle twitching. Respirations are shallow and slow as the lungs attempt to compensate by building up carbonic acid stores. If the condition progresses unchecked, the symptoms increase in severity and the patient lapses into coma. Convulsive seizures may occur. Respiratory paralysis can develop if potassium loss is great.

TREATMENT AND PATIENT CARE. The best control of metabolic alkalosis is careful monitoring of the patient because the condition is most often brought on by medication, especially diuretics, and by postoperative loss of acids through vomiting or gastric suctioning. One of the most frequent sources of increased alkali intake is the overzealous self-administration of antacids, particularly bicarbonate of soda, which is a systemic alkalizer. Education of the public in the hazards of such practices can do much to prevent metabolic alkalosis. Patients on diuretic therapy also must be taught to be alert for, and to report to their physician the signs of potassium depletion and alkalosis.

The primary aim in the treatment of metabolic alkalosis is to reestablish fluid and electrolyte balance. Administration of potassium chloride and normal saline usually will correct the problem.

Vital signs should be checked frequently; hypotension and tachycardia may indicate potassium deficit, a decreased respiratory rate suggests compensation by the lungs. A record of intake and output is helpful in planning fluid and electrolyte replacement. Signs of neural irritability, such as Trousseau's sign, are helpful in detecting early stages of tetany due to calcium deficiency. Muscle weakness and energy loss should be reported, as they may be symptomatic of hypokalemia. Precautions are taken to prevent injury should disorientation or CONVULSIONS develop.

respiratory a., an alkalotic state occurring as a result of excessive blowing off of carbon dioxide through HYPERVENTILATION. The condition can be brought on by anoxia, high environmental temperture, fever, drug poisoning, hysteria, and overzealous use of mechanical VENTILATORS.

The condition is characterized by deep, rapid breathing, tingling of the fingers, pallor around the mouth, dizziness, and carpopedal spasm. It is usually the least common and least serious type of alkalosis, but it can produce major difficulties if left unchecked.

TREATMENT AND PATIENT CARE. Treatment is primarily aimed at removal of the underlying cause, particularly in cases of hyperventilation due to hysteria. Rebreathing carbon dioxide in a paper sack is helpful, as is encouraging the patient to hold his breath. The patient who has anoxia caused by pulmonary infection or congestive heart failure should be given oxygen to reduce respiratory effort and the resultant blowing off of carbon dioxide. If there is CNS involvement, sedation which suppresses activity of the respiratory center may be indicated.

alkalotic (al″kah-lot′ik) pertaining to or characterized by alkalosis.

alkapton (al-kap′tōn) a class of substances with an affinity for alkali, found in the urine and causing the condition known as alkaptonuria. The compound commonly found, and most commonly referred to by the term, is homogentisic acid.

alkaptonuria (al-kap″to-nu′re-ah) excretion in the urine of homogentisic acid and its oxidation products as a result of a genetic disorder of phenylalanine-tyrosine metabolism.

alkavervir (al″kah-ver′vir) a mixture of alkaloids extracted from *Veratrum viride,* used to lower blood pressure.

alkyl (al′kil) the radical that results when an aliphatic hydrocarbon loses one hydrogen atom.

alkylate (al′kĭ-lāt) to treat with an alkylating agent.

alkylating agent (al′kĭ-lāt-ing) a synthetic compound containing two or more end (alkyl) groups that combine readily with other molecules. Their action seems to be chiefly on the deoxyribonucleic acid (DNA) in the nucleus of the cell. They are used in chemotherapy of cancer although they do not damage malignant cells selectively, but also have a toxic action on normal cells. Locally they cause blistering of the skin and damage to the eyes and respiratory tract. Systemic toxic effects are nausea and vomiting, reduction in both leukocytes and erythrocytes, and hemorrhagic tendencies. Among the agents of this group used in therapy are the NITROGEN MUSTARDS, including mechlorethamine hydrochloride, chlorambucil and triethylenemelamine, and busulfan and cyclophosphamide.

all(o)- (al′o) word element [Gr.], *other; deviating from normal.*

allachesthesia (al″ah-kes-the′ze-ah) allesthesia.

allantochorion (ah-lan″to-ko′re-on) the allantois and chorion as one structure.

allantoid (ah-lan′toid) 1. sausage-shaped. 2. pertaining to the allantois.

allantoin (ah-lan′to-in) a crystalline substance from allantoic fluid and fetal urine; used topically to promote wound healing.

allantoinuria (ah-lan″to-ĭ-nu′re-ah) allantoin in the urine.

allantois (ah-lan′to-is) a ventral outgrowth of the hindgut of the early embryo, which is a conspicuous component of the developing umbilical cord. adj., **allanto′ic.**

allele (ah-lēl′) one of two or more alternative forms of a gene at the same site in a chromosome, which determine alternative characters in inheritance. adj., **allel′ic.**

silent a., one that produces no detectable effect.

allelotaxis (ah-le″lo-tak′sis) development of an organ from several embryonic structures.

Allen's law (al'enz) the more carbohydrates a diabetic takes, the less he utilizes.

Allen-Doisey test one for detection of estrogenic activity.

allergen (al'er-jen) a substance capable of inducing hypersensitivity. adj., **allergen'ic.** Almost any substance in the environment can become an allergen. The list of known allergens—that is, substances to which individual patients have become sensitive—includes plant and tree pollens, spores of mold, animal hairs, dust, foods, feathers, dyes, soaps, detergents, cosmetics, plastics, some valuable medicines, including penicillin, and even sunlight. Allergens can enter the body by being inhaled, swallowed, touched, or injected. The allergen is not directly responsible for the allergic reaction, but sets off the chain of events that brings it about.

When a foreign substance enters the body, the system reacts by producing ANTIBODIES that attack the substance and render it harmless. When their work is done, the antibodies attach themselves to tissue surfaces, where they remain in reserve, ready to be called into action if the same substance should enter the body again. Should the substance do so, the antibodies again enter into the immune reaction which is part of the body's valuable natural defense against invading disease germs.

A variety of allergic reactions can take place almost anywhere in the body; the cells affected may be destroyed or injured, and they release chemicals such as heparin, leukotaxine, and especially histamine that cause systemic symptoms characteristic of an ALLERGY, which may range from sneezing and slight local edema to fatal ANAPHYLACTIC SHOCK.

allergid (al'ler-jid) a papular or nodular allergic skin reaction.

allergist (al'er-jist) a physician specializing in the diagnosis and treatment of allergic conditions.

allergization (al″er-jĭ-za'shun) active sensitization by introduction of allergens into the body.

allergy (al'er-je) an abnormal and individual hypersensitivity to substances that are ordinarily harmless. For example, the pollen of plants is not generally harmful, yet many people are acutely sensitive to its presence in the atmosphere. adj., **aller'gic.**

An allergy cannot occur on the first contact with a potential ALLERGEN because antibodies have not yet been produced by the body. It may occur on the second contact, when antibodies have been produced and are in reserve in the body tissues, but it does not necessarily do so. In some cases, it may not occur until late in life when, after repeated contact with the allergen, a person suddenly develops a sensitivity.

COMMON ALLERGIES. The most common allergies affect the respiratory passages and the skin, although other areas such as the digestive tract, nervous system, joints, kidneys, and blood vessels can be affected. HAY FEVER symptoms are stuffed-up and running nose, spasms of sneezing and itching, and watery eyes. ASTHMA is an allergy characterized by shortness of breath, coughing, and wheezing. The allergies of the skin include URTICARIA (hives), or itchy swellings, and ECZEMA, an itchy rash. CONTACT DERMATITIS, a rash similar to eczema, occurs as a result of direct contact of the skin with the allergen. Skin eruptions, resulting from INSECT BITES AND STINGS and from contact with poisonous plants, such as POISON IVY, OAK, AND SUMAC, also are true allergic reactions. Not everyone is sensitive to poison ivy, oak, or sumac, and some people are comparatively unaffected by mosquito and other insect bites. Usually the stings of bees and wasps will produce more severe reactions in the allergic than in the nonallergic person. Some people react so strongly that the whole system is affected, and there is a risk of their suffering ANAPHYLACTIC SHOCK.

Emotional factors also have a role in allergy. There is as yet no evidence that allergy can be caused by emotional upset, but it is known that anxiety, fear, anger, and strong excitement may set off an allérgic attack.

TREATMENT. In most cases allergy is dealt with by identifying the responsible allergen and then avoiding it. In some instances, the victim himself knows what is causing his suffering, but usually it is more difficult to track down. In order to identify the harmful substance, a series of tests conducted by a physician may be necessary. The tests are not foolproof, but they are usually successful. In some cases, they reveal not only the guilty substance but the degree of sensitivity to it.

A minute quantity of various suspected allergens is applied to the skin of the patient's forearm, either to the skin surface by means of a saturated adhesive patch (patch test) or under the skin by injection or by applying the substance to a small scratch (scratch test). (See also SKIN TEST.) When the substance so applied is the offending allergen, a mild allergic reaction takes place at the test site. As many as 30 tests may be necessary before the allergen or allergens are identified, so the test series may be an inconvenience to the patient, but it is certainly worthwhile if it means the end to allergic discomfort. The tests are not painful.

In some cases it is not an easy matter to avoid the offending substance. Hay fever and asthma sufferers sometimes have to move to a different locale at certain seasons to escape an airborne allergen. If an important food such as milk is the offender, the doctor may have to design a special diet. If the allergen

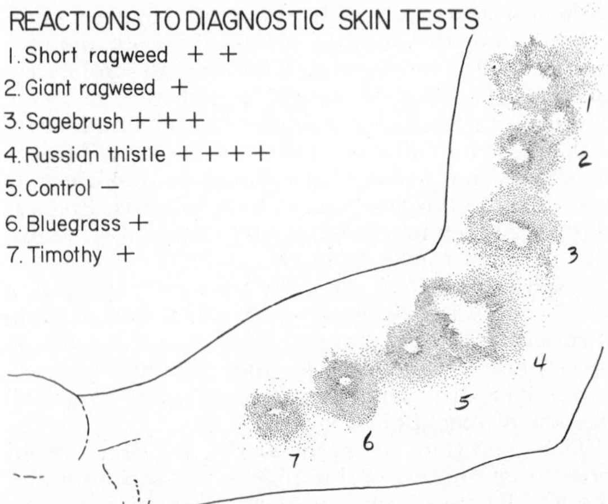

The results of a scratch test. In this case, the patient has reacted violently to Russian thistle and badly to sagebrush and short ragweed. The control and the other tests show no reaction. (Courtesy of Abbott Laboratories.)

is animal hair from a household pet, the pet may have to be given away.

An allergy that is resistant to cure may be controlled with medication. Some useful medications are ANTIHISTAMINES, EPINEPHRINE, ephedrine, aminophylline, and varieties of steroids of the cortisone and ACTH type. In many instances the patient can be cured of the allergy by a series of desensitization treatments, in which the patient is exposed to gradually increasing amounts of the allergen until his resistance is built up to immunity. The series is time consuming. A new "one-shot" treatment that may eliminate this inconvenience is being evaluated.

More information concerning allergy can be obtained by writing to the Allergy Foundation of America, 801 Second Avenue, New York, N.Y. 10017.

allesthesia (al″es-the′ze-ah) sensation of touch experienced at a point remote from the point touched.

allobarbital (al″o-bar′bĭ-tal) diallylbarbituric acid, an intermediate- to long-acting sedative and hypnotic.

allocheiria (al″o-ki′re-ah) allesthesia.

allochromasia (al″o-kro-ma′ze-ah) change in color of hair or skin.

allodiploidy (al″o-dip′loi-de) the state of having two sets of chromosomes derived from different ancestral species.

alloerotism (al″o-er′o-tizm) direction of libido toward another person.

allogeneic (al′o-jĕ-ne′ik) denoting individuals of the same species but of different genetic constitution (antigenically distinct).

allograft (al′o-graft) a graft between allogeneic individuals.

allolalia (al″o-la′le-ah) any defect of speech of central origin.

alloploidy (al″o-ploi′de) the state of having any number of chromosome sets derived from different ancestral species.

allopolyploidy (al″o-pol′e-ploi″de) the state of having more than two sets of chromosomes derived from different ancestral species.

allopsychic (al″o-si′kik) pertaining to the mind in its relation to the external world.

allopurinol (al″o-pūr′ĭ-nol) a drug that inhibits uric acid production and reduces serum and urinary uric acid levels; used in prevention of acute attacks of gout.

allorhythmia (al″o-rith′me-ah) irregularity of the pulse.

allosteric (al″o-ster′ik) denoting a macromolecule (an enzyme) whose reactivity with another molecule is altered by combination with a third molecule; also, denoting the enzyme inhibition exercised by such alteration.

a. site, that subunit of an enzyme molecule which binds with a nonsubstrate molecule, inducing a conformational change that results in inactivation of the enzyme for its substrate.

allotherm (al′o-therm) an organism whose body temperature changes with its environment.

allotriogeustia (ah-lot″re-o-gōōs′te-ah) perverted sense of taste.

allotropic (al″o-trop′ik) 1. exhibiting allotropism. 2. concerned with others: said of a type of personality that is more preoccupied with others than with self.

allotropism (ah-lot′ro-pizm) existence of an element in two or more distinct forms.

allotropy (ah-lot′ro-pe) 1. allotropism. 2. direction of one's interest more toward others than toward one's self.

alloxan (ah-lok′san) an oxidized product of uric acid which tends to destroy the islet cells of the pancreas, thus producing diabetes. It has been obtained from intestinal mucus in diarrhea and has been used in nutrition experiments and as an antineoplastic.

alloxuremia (ah-lok″su-re′me-ah) the presence of purine bases in the blood.

alloxuria (al″ok-su′re-ah) the presence of purine bases in the urine.

alloy (al′oi) a solid mixture of two or more metals or metalloids that are mutually soluble in the molten condition.

Almén tests tests for detection of albumin, blood, blood pigment, or dextrose in solutions, such as urine.

alogia (ah-lo′je-ah) inability to speak, due to a central lesion.

aloin (al′o-in) a mixture of active principles obtained from the plant aloe, used as a cathartic.

alopecia (al″o-pe′she-ah) loss of hair; baldness. The cause of simple baldness is not yet fully understood, although it is known that the tendency to become bald is limited almost entirely to males, runs in certain families and is more common in certain racial groups than in others. Baldness is often associated with aging. The maintenance of general good health may help postpone the onset of baldness; however, it is impossible to cure ordinary baldness once it has occurred.

a. area′ta, hair loss in sharply defined areas, usually the scalp or beard.

a. cap′itis tota′lis, loss of all the hair from the scalp.

cicatricial a., a. cicatrisa′ta, irreversible loss of hair associated with scarring, usually on the scalp.

a. congenita′lis, complete or partial absence of the hair at birth.

a. limina′ris, hair loss at the hairline along the front and back edges of the scalp.

male-pattern a., loss of scalp hair genetically determined and androgen-dependent, beginning with frontal recession and progressing symmetrically to leave ultimately only a sparse peripheral rim of hair.

a. medicamento′sa, hair loss due to ingestion of a drug.

symptomatic a., a. symptomat′ica, loss of hair due to systemic or psychogenic causes, such as general ill health, infections of the scalp or skin, nervousness, or a specific disease such as typhoid fever, or to stress. The hair may fall out in patches, or there may be diffuse loss of hair instead of complete baldness in one area.

a. tota′lis, loss of hair from the entire scalp.

a. universa′lis, loss of hair from the entire body.

aloxidone (ah-lok′sĭ-dōn) an anticonvulsive agent.

Alper's disease (al′perz) poliodystrophia cerebri.

alpha (al′fah) first letter of the Greek alphabet, α; used in names of chemical compounds to distinguish the first in a series of isomers, or to indicate position of substituting atoms or groups.

a. particles, a type of emission produced by the disintegration of a radioactive substance. The atoms of radioactive elements such as uranium and radium are very unstable; they are continuously breaking apart with explosive violence and emitting particulate and nonparticulate types of radiation. The alpha particles, consisting of two protons and two neutrons, have an electrical charge and form streams of tremendous energy when they are released from the disintegrating atoms. These streams of energy (alpha rays) are used to advantage in the treatment of various malignancies. (See also RADIATION and RADIOTHERAPY.)

Alphadrol (al′fah-drol) trademark for a preparation of fluprednisolone, a corticosteroid and anti-inflammatory agent.

alphaprodine (al″fah-pro′dēn) a compound used as an analgesic and narcotic.

Alport's syndrome (al′ports) a hereditary disorder marked by progressive nerve deafness, progressive pyelonephritis or glomerulonephritis, and occasionally ocular defects.

ALS antilymphocyte serum.

alseroxylon (al″ser-ok′sĭ-lon) a purified extract of *Rauwolfia serpentina,* used as a tranquilizer and sedative.

altitude sickness (al′tĭ-tūd) a syndrome caused by exposure to altitude high enough to cause significant hypoxia, or lack of oxygen. At high altitudes the atmospheric pressure is decreased and consequently arterial oxygen content is also lowered.

Acute altitude sickness may occur after a few hours' exposure to a high altitude. Mental functions may be affected, and there may be lightheadedness and breathlessness. Eventually headache and prostration may occur. Older persons and those with pulmonary or cardiovascular disease are most likely to be affected. After a few hours or days of acclimation the symptoms will subside.

Chronic altitude sickness (sometimes called Monge's disease or Andes disease) occurs in those living in the high Andes above 15,000 feet. It resembles POLYCYTHEMIA, but is completely relieved if the patient is moved to sea level.

alum (al′um) a substance used, in the form of colorless crystals or white powder, as a styptic or hemostatic because of its astringent action. It also may be given by mouth to induce vomiting. Large doses may cause gastrointestinal disturbances.

aluminum (ah-loo′mĭ-num) a chemical element, atomic number 13, atomic weight 26.982, symbol Al. (See table of ELEMENTS.)

a. acetate solution, a preparation of aluminum subacetate and glacial acetic acid, used for its antiseptic and astringent action on the skin; called also Burow's solution.

a. chloride, a deliquescent, crystalline powder used topically as an astringent solution and antiperspirant.

a. hydroxide gel, an aluminum preparation, available in suspension or in dried form, used as an antacid in the treatment of peptic ulcer and gastric hyperacidity.

a. phosphate gel, a water suspension of aluminum phosphate and some flavoring agents; used as a gastric antacid, astringent, and demulcent.

a. subacetate, a compound used as an astringent, diluted with water.

a. sulfate, a compound used as an astringent solution and antiperspirant.

Alurate (al′ūr-āt) trademark for a preparation of aprobarbital, an intermediate-acting sedative and hypnotic.

alveolectomy (al″ve-o-lek′to-me) surgical excision of part of the alveolar process.

alveolodental (al-ve″o-lo-den′tal) pertaining to teeth and the alveolar process.

alveolotomy (al″ve-o-lot′o-me) incision of the alveolar process.

alveolus (al-ve′o-lus), pl. *alve′oli* [L.] a little hollow, as the socket of a tooth, a follicle of an acinous gland, or one of the thin-walled chambers of the lungs (pulmonary alveoli), surrounded by networks of capillaries through whose walls exchange of carbon dioxide and oxygen takes place. adj., **alve′olar.**

dental alveoli, the cavities or sockets of either jaw, in which the roots of the teeth are embedded.

alverine (al′vĕ-rēn) an anticholinergic agent; alverine citrate is used as a smooth muscle relaxant and antispasmodic.

alveus (al′ve-us), pl. *al′vei* [L.] a canal or trough.

Alvodine (al′vo-dīn) trademark for preparations of piminodine ethanesulfonate, a narcotic analgesic.

alymphia (ah-lim′fe-ah) absence or lack of lymph.

alymphocytosis (a-lim″fo-si-to′sis) deficiency of lymphocytes in the blood.

alymphoplasia (a-lim″fo-pla′ze-ah) failure of development of lymphoid tissue.

thymic a., congenital agammaglobulinemia in which there is thymic hypoplasia, sparsity of lymphocytes in the thymus, spleen, lymph nodes, and intestines, absence of plasma cells, and absence of Hassall's corpuscles.

Alzheimer's disease (altz′hi-merz) a presenile dementia of unknown etiology beginning at middle age and affecting nerve cells of the frontal and temporal lobes of the cerebrum. Among its effects are speech defects and progressive loss of mental faculties. There is as yet no effective treatment.

Am chemical symbol, *americium.*

A.M.A. American Medical Association.

amacrine (am′ah-krīn) 1. without long processes. 2. a branched retinal structure, considered a modified nerve cell.

Amadil (am′ah-dil) trademark for a preparation of acetaminophen, an analgesic and antipyretic.

amalgam (ah-mal′gam) an alloy of mercury with another metal.

emotional a., an unconscious attempt to bind, neutralize, deny, or counteract anxiety.

amantadine (ah-man′tah-dēn) an antiviral compound; the hydrochloride salt used in the prophylaxis and treatment of influenza A.

amastia (ah-mas′te-ah) congenital absence of one or both mammary glands.

amaurosis (am″aw-ro′sis) loss of sight without apparent lesion of the eye, as from disease of the optic nerve, spine, or brain.

a. fu′gax, sudden temporary or fleeting blindness.

a. congen′ita of Leber, Leber's congenital a., hereditary blindness occurring at or shortly after birth, associated with an atypical form of diffuse pigmentation and commonly with optic atrophy and attenuation of the retinal vessels.

amaurotic (am″aw-rot′ik) pertaining to, or of the nature of, amaurosis.

a. familial idiocy, a group of hereditary disorders due to an inborn defect of lipid metabolism, in which sphingolipids accumulate in the brain. They are characterized by cerebromacular degeneration, blindness, progressive dementia, and progressive and unremitting paralysis, usually of the spastic type. There is no cure and the prognosis is extremely poor. The disorders in this group are classified according to age of onset: TAY-SACHS DISEASE is the infantile form; BIELSCHOWSKY'S DISEASE is the late infantile form; SPIELMEYER-VOGT DISEASE is the juvenile form; and KUFS' DISEASE is the late juvenile, or adult form.

ambenonium (am″be-no′ne-um) a cholinesterase inhibitor used to increase muscular strength in myasthenic patients.

ambidextrous (am″bĭ-deks′trus) able to use either hand with equal dexterity.

ambilateral (am″bĭ-lat′er-al) pertaining to or affecting both sides.

ambilevous (am″bĭ-le′vus) unable to use both hands with equal dexterity.

ambiopia (am″be-o′pe-ah) diplopia.

ambisexual (am″bĭ-seks′u-al) denoting sexual characteristics common to both sexes, e.g., pubic hair.

ambivalence (am-biv′ah-lens) simultaneous existence of conflicting emotional attitudes toward a goal, object, or person. adj., **ambiv′alent.**

amblyacousia (am″ble-ah-ku′se-ah) dullness of hearing.

amblyaphia (am″ble-a′fe-ah) bluntness of the sense of touch.

amblygeustia (am″ble-gōōs′te-ah) dullness of the sense of taste.

Amblyomma (am″ble-om′ah) a genus of ticks, comprising approximately 100 species, which are vectors of various disease-producing organisms.

A. america′num, a species of ticks widely distributed in the United States and Central and South America; a vector of Rocky Mountain spotted fever.

A. cajennen′se, a tick widely distributed in North, Central, and South America; a vector of São Paulo fever, a form of typhus.

A. macula′tum, a tick widely distributed in the United States and Central and South America.

amblyopia (am″ble-o′pe-ah) dimness of vision not due to organic defect or refractive errors, adj., **amblyop′ic.**

color a., dimness of color vision due to toxic or other influences.

amblyoscope (am′ble-o-skōp″) an instrument for training an amblyopic eye to take part in vision.

ambo (am′bo) ambon.

amboceptor (am′bo-sep″tor) hemolysin, particularly its double receptors, the one combining with the blood cell, the other with complement.

Ambodryl (am′bo-dril) trademark for preparations of bromodiphenhydramine, an antihistamine.

ambon (am′bon) the edge of the socket in which the head of a long bone is lodged.

ambulant, ambulatory (am′bu-lant), (am′bu-lah-tor″e) walking or able to walk; not confined to bed.

ameba (ah-me′bah), pl. *ame′bae, ame′bas* [L.] a minute, one-celled protozoan. The common laboratory example is *Amoeba proteus.* The usual cause of human amebic infection is *Entamoeba histolytica.*

amebiasis (am″e-bi′ah-sis) infection with amebas, especially with *Entamoeba histolytica* (see also AMEBIC DYSENTERY).

amebic (ah-me′bik) pertaining to, caused by, or of the nature of, an ameba.

a. abscess, an abscess cavity of the liver resulting from liquefaction necrosis due to entrance of *Entamoeba histolytica* into the portal circulation in amebiasis; amebic abscesses may affect the lung, brain, and spleen.

a. dysentery, a form of dysentery caused by *Entamoeba histolytica* and spread by contaminated food, water, and flies; called also amebiasis. Amebic dysentery was once thought to be a purely tropical disease, but it is now known that many cases occur throughout the United States. Symptoms are diarrhea, fatigue, and intestinal bleeding. Complications include involvement of the liver, liver abscess, and pulmonary abscess. For treatment several drugs are availale, for example, emetine hydrochloride and chloroquine, which may be used singly or in combination.

amebicide (ah-me′bĭ-sīd) destructive to amebas.

amebocyte (ah-me′bo-sīt) a cell showing ameboid movement.

ameboid (ah-me′boid) resembling an ameba.

ameboma (am″e-bo′mah) a tumor-like mass caused by granulomatous reaction in the intestines in amebiasis.

amelia (ah-me′le-ah) a developmental anomaly with absence of the limbs.

amelification (ah-mel″ĭ-fĭ-ka′shun) the development of ameloblasts into enamel.

ameloblast (ah-mel′o-blast) a cell that takes part in forming dental enamel.

ameloblastoma (ah-mel″o-blas-to′mah) a locally invasive, highly destructive tumor of the jaw. **pituitary a.**, craniopharyngioma.

amelodentinal (am″ĕ-lo-den′tĭ-nal) pertaining to dental enamel and dentin.

amelogenesis (ah-mel″o-jen′ĕ-sis) formation of dental enamel.

a. imperfec′ta, imperfect formation of enamel, resulting in brownish coloration and friability of the teeth.

amelogenic (am″ĕ-lo-jen′ik) forming enamel.

amelus (am′ĕ-lus) an individual exhibiting amelia.

amenorrhea (a-men″o-re′ah) absence of the menses. adj., **amenorrhe′al.** Primary amenorrhea refers to absence of the onset of menstruation at puberty. It may be caused by underdevelopment or malformation of the reproduction organs or by glandular disturbances. When menstruation has begun and then ceases, the term secondary amenorrhea is used. The most common cause is usually a disturbance of the endocrine glands concerned with the menstrual process. General ill health, a change in climate or living conditions, emotional shock or, frequently, either the hope or fear of becoming pregnant can sometimes stop the menstrual flow.

amensalism (a-men′sal-izm) interaction between coexisting populations of different species, one of which is adversely affected and the other unaffected.

amentia (a-men′she-ah) 1. congenital mental retardation of varying extent. 2. a mental disorder characterized by marked mental confusion.

nevoid a., Sturge-Weber syndrome.

American Nurses' Association A.N.A., the national organization and official spokesman for registered nurses. The A.N.A. was founded in 1896 and exists for the purposes of improving the standards of nursing and promoting the general welfare of professional nurses. The association is a federation of 54 local organizations in the 50 states, District of Columbia, Panama Canal Zone, Puerto Rico, and the Virgin Islands. The local organizations serve to implement the goals and carry out the functions of the national organization. The official publication of the A.N.A. is the *American Journal of Nursing.* Offices of the organization are located at 2420 Pershing Road, Kansas City, MO 64108.

americium (am″er-ish′e-um) a chemical element, atomic number 95, atomic weight 243, symbol Am. (See table of ELEMENTS.)

ametria (ah-me′tre-ah) congenital absence of the uterus.

ametropia (am″ĕ-tro′pe-ah) a condition of the eye in which parallel rays fail to come to a focus on the retina. adj., **ametrop′ic.**

amicrobic (ah″mi-kro′bik) not produced by microorganisms.

amicron (ah-mi′kron) a particle so small it is just visible with the ultramicroscope.

amidase (am′ĭ-dās) a deamidizing ferment.

amide (am′īd) any compound derived from ammonia by substitution of an acid radical for hydrogen, or from an acid by replacing the —OH group by $—NH_2$.

amido (am′ĭ-do) the monovalent radical NH_2 united with an acid radical.

amidopyrine (am″ĭ-do-pi′rēn) aminopyrine.

Amigen (am′ĭ-jen) trademark for protein hydrolysate preparation for intravenous injection.

amimia (a-mim′e-ah) loss of the power of expression by the use of signs or gestures.

aminacrine (am″in-ak′rin) an anti-infective agent used externally as the hydrochloride salt.

amine (am′in, ah′mēn) an organic compound containing nitrogen.

amino (am′ĭ-no, ah-me′no) the monovalent radical NH_2, when not united with an acid radical.

a. acid, any one of a class of organic compounds containing the amino (NH_2) and the carboxyl (COOH) group, occurring naturally in plant and animal tissues and forming the chief constituents of protein.

More than 20 different amino acids are commonly found in proteins. Some of them can be produced within the body, but there are eight that the human organism cannot manufacture; these essential amino acids must be provided by protein foods in the diet. The essential amino acids are isoleucine, leucine, lysine, methionine, phenylalanine, threonine, tryptophan, and valine. Histidine and arginine, which may be manufactured in the body under certain circumstances, are also sometimes considered essential.

Protein foods that provide large amounts of essential amino acids are known as complete proteins and include proteins from animal sources, such as meat, eggs, fish, and milk. Proteins that cannot supply the body with all the essential amino acids are known as incomplete proteins; these are the vegetable proteins most abundantly found in peas, beans, and certain forms of wheat.

aminoacetic acid (ah-me′no-ah-se′tik) glycine.

aminoacidemia (am″ĭ-no-as″ĭ-de′me-ah) an excess of amino acids in the blood.

aminoaciduria (am″ĭ-no-as″ĭ-du′re-ah) an excess in the urine of amino acids.

***p*-aminobenzoic acid** (par″ah-am″ĭ-no-ben-zo′ik) a member of the B group of vitamins, a growth factor for certain organisms, and used in the treatment of certain rickettsial infections, including scrub typhus; called also PABA. (See also para-AMINOBENZOIC ACID.)

ϵ-aminocaproic acid (ep′sĭ-lon am″ĭ-no-kah-pro′ik) an amino acid that is a potent inhibitor of plasminogen and plasmin and indirectly of fibrinolysis; used as a hemostatic.

aminoglutethimide (am″ĭ-no-gloo-teth′ĭ-mīd) an anticonvulsant used in the treatment of most forms of epilepsy.

aminohippuric acid (am″ĭ-no-hĭ-pu′rik) an acid used in renal function tests (see also PARA-AMINOHIPPURIC ACID).

aminolysis (am″ĭ-nol′ĭ-sis) the splitting up of amines.

aminometradine, aminometramide (am″ĭ-no-met′rah-dēn; am″ĭ-no-met′rah-mīd) a compound used to increase urine formation and in treatment of edema of heart failure.

aminopentamide (am″ĭ-no-pen′tah-mīd) a compound used as an anticholinergic and applied locally to the eye for dilatation of the pupil.

aminophylline (am″ĭ-no-fil′in) a mixture of theophylline and ethylenediamine; used as a respiratory stimulant, smooth muscle relaxant, myocardial stimulant, and diuretic. Administration of the drug may be by mouth, intramuscularly, intravenously, or rectally. If given too rapidly by vein it may produce circulatory collapse. Intramuscular administration should be performed with caution because aminophylline is very irritating to the tissues. It also may cause gastric or urinary irritation when taken by mouth. Dose depends on the route of administration and the effect desired.

aminopterin (am″in-op′ter-in) a folic acid antagonist used in the treatment of leukemia.

aminopyrine (am″ĭ-no-pi′rēn) white odorless crystals used as an analgesic and antipyretic, somewhat more potent than aspirin. This drug must be given with caution because it may cause a sudden serious and even fatal leukopenia and agranulocytosis. This reaction in hypersensitive persons can occur without warning and after they have taken the drug previously without incident. Aminopyrine was formerly used in many patent medicines dispensed as "headache preparations," but because of its toxicity, it is now dispensed only by prescription.

***p*-aminosalicylic acid** (par″ah-am″ĭ-no-sal″ĭ-sil′ik) an acid with antibacterial properties used in the treatment of tuberculosis (see also PARA-AMINOSALICYLIC ACID).

Aminosol (ah-me′no-sol) trademark for an amino acid preparation for intravenous injection.

aminuria (am″ĭ-nu′re-ah) an excess of amines in the urine.

amisometradine (am-i″so-met′rah-dēn) a compound used as diuretic.

amitosis (am″ĭ-to′sis) direct cell division; simple cleavage of the nucleus without the formation of a spireme spindle figure or chromosomes. adj., **amitot′ic.**

amitriptyline (am″ĭ-trip′tĭ-lēn) a compound used as an antidepressant.

ammeter (am′me-ter) an instrument for measuring in amperes the strength of a current flowing in a circuit.

ammoaciduria (am″o-as″ĭ-du′re-ah) an excess of ammonia and amino acids in the urine.

ammonia (ah-mo′ne-ah) a colorless alkaline gas, NH_3, with a pungent odor and acrid taste, and soluble in water.

ammoniate (ah-mo′ne-āt) to combine with ammonia.

ammoniated mercury (ah-mo′ne-āt″ed mer′ku-re) a compound used as an antiseptic skin and ophthalmic ointment. It should be applied with caution, as excessive use may irritate the skin and cause a dermatitis.

ammoniemia (ah-mo″ne-e′me-ah) the presence of ammonia or its compounds in the blood.

ammonium (ah-mo′ne-um) a hypothetical radical, NH_4, forming salts analogous to those of the alkaline metals.

a. acetate, a diaphoretic and diuretic.

a. bromide, a crystalline compound used as a central nervous system depressant.

a. carbonate, a mixture of ammonium compounds used as a liquefying expectorant in the treatment of chronic bronchitis and similar lung disorders. It is sometimes used as a reflex stimulant in "smelling salts" because of the strong ammonia odor it gives off.

a. chloride, colorless or white crystals, with a cool, salty taste, used as an expectorant because it liquefies bronchial secretions. In the body it is changed to urea and hydrochloric acid, and thus is useful in acidifying the urine and increasing the rate of urine flow. Excessive dosage may produce ACIDOSIS.

a. iodide, a resolvent and expectorant.

a. mandelate, a urinary antiseptic.

ammoniuria (ah-mo″ne-u′re-ah) excess of ammonia in the urine.

amnalgesia (am″nal-je′ze-ah) abolition of pain and memory of a painful procedure by the use of drugs or hypnosis.

amnesia (am-ne′ze-ah) pathologic impairment of memory. adj., **amnes′tic.** Amnesia is usually the result of physical damage to areas of the brain from injury, disease, or alcoholism. It may also be caused by a decreased supply of blood to the brain, a condition that may accompany senility. Another cause is psychologic. A shocking or unacceptable situation may be too painful to remember, and the situation is then retained only in the subconscious mind. The technical term for this is repression.

Rarely is the memory completely obliterated. When amnesia results from a single physical or psychologic incident, such as a concussion suffered in an accident or a severe emotional shock, the victim may forget only the incident itself; he may be unable to recall events occurring before or after the incident or the order of events is confused, with recent events imputed to the past and past events to recent times. In another form, only certain isolated events are lost to memory.

Amnesia victims usually have a good chance of recovery if there is no irreparable brain damage. The recovery is often gradual, the memory slowly reclaiming isolated events while others are still missing. Psychotherapy may be necessary when the amnesia is due to a psychologic reaction.

Amnesia takes different forms depending upon the area of the brain affected and how extensive the damage is. In auditory amnesia, or word deafness, the patient is unable to interpret spoken language. Words come to him as a jumble of sounds which he is unable to associate meaningfully with ideas. Similarly, in visual amnesia, or word blindness, the written language is forgotten. Tactile amnesia is the inability to recognize once familiar objects by the sense of touch.

anterograde a., amnesia for events subsequent to the episode precipitating the disorder.

retrograde a., amnesia for events prior to the episode precipitating the disorder.

amniocentesis (am″ne-o-sen-te′sis) transabdominal perforation of the amniotic sac for the purpose of obtaining a sample of amniotic fluid. This is a relatively new procedure and is safely done only by trained personnel and in well equipped medical centers.

The procedure is particularly valuable in the diagnosis of inherited disorders, for example, chromosomal defects such as DOWN'S SYNDROME, inborn errors of metabolism such as PKU, and hemoglobinopathies such as SICKLE CELL ANEMIA. It is currently possible to detect the presence of about 40 different types of inherited disorders in embryos and fetuses as young as 12 weeks.

A common indication for amniocentesis is the suspected occurrence of ERYTHROBLASTOSIS FETALIS, which results in incompatibility of the fetal and maternal blood. In order to forestall the effects of erythroblastosis the physician needs to know how much destruction of the fetal cells is taking place while the fetus is in utero. Samples of amniotic fluid obtained by amniocentesis are analyzed for concentrations of protein and bilirubin. The higher the concentration the stronger the evidence that erythrocytes are being destroyed.

Another use for amniocentesis is in determining the maturity of the lungs and the possibility that the infant will suffer from HYALINE MEMBRANE DISEASE after birth. A favorable ratio of lecithin to sphingomyelin indicates sufficient lung maturity.

The physician obtains the sample of amniotic fluid through a long pudendal needle that is introduced into the mother's abdomen and then guided through the uterine wall and into the amniotic cavity between the fetus and the placenta. Local anesthesia may be used and the patient must be cautioned not to move during the procedure lest the needle become displaced.

Following amniocentesis the patient is observed for changes in blood pressure. Hemorrhage from the placenta must be considered a possibility if the blood pressure begins to drop. Increased fetal activity or other signs of fetal distress such as changes in the fetal heart rate must be reported to the physician at once as they may warrant immediate measures such as delivery of the infant if it is considered to be viable.

amniochorial (am″ne-o-ko′re-al) pertaining to amnion and chorion.

amniogenesis (am″ne-o-jen′ĕ-sis) the development of the amnion.

amniography (am″ne-og′rah-fe) roentgenography of the gravid uterus.

amnion (am′ne-on) the innermost membrane enclosing the developing fetus and the fluid in which the fetus is bathed.

a. nodo′sum, a nodular condition of the fetal surface of the amnion, observed in oligohydramnios associated with absence of the kidneys in the fetus.

amnionitis (am″ne-o-ni′tis) inflammation of the amnion.

amniorrhea (am″ne-o-re′ah) escape of the amniotic fluid.

amniorrhexis (am″ne-o-rek′sis) rupture of the amnion.

amnioscope (am′ne-o-skōp″) an endoscope that, by passage through the abdominal wall into the amniotic cavity, permits direct visualization of the fetus and amniotic fluid.

amniote (am′ne-ōt) any animal with amnion.

amniotic (am″ne-ot′ik) pertaining to the amnion.

a. fluid, the albuminous fluid contained in the amniotic sac; called also liquor amnii and "waters." The fetus floats in the amniotic fluid, which serves as a cushion against injury from sudden blows or movements and helps maintain a constant body temperature for the fetus. Normally the amniotic fluid is clear and slightly alkaline. Discoloration or excessive cloudiness of the fluid may indicate fetal distress or disease, as in erythroblastosis fetalis in which the amniotic fluid is usually a greenish yellow color. The amount varies from 500 to 1500 ml.

An excessive amount of amniotic fluid is called polyhydramnios; the amount may be as much as several gallons. The cause of this condition is unknown but it frequently accompanies multiple pregnancy or some congenital defect of the fetus, especially hydrocephalus and meningocele.

An abnormally small amount of amniotic fluid is referred to as oligohydramnios. In this condition there may be less than 100 ml. of fluid present. The cause is unknown. The condition may produce pressure deformities of the fetus, such as clubfoot or torticollis (wryneck). Adhesions may result from direct contact of the fetus with the amnion.

The technique for removal of a sample of amniotic fluid from the pregnant uterus is called AMNIOCENTESIS.

a. sac, the amnion; the sac enclosing the fetus suspended in the amniotic fluid.

amniotome (am′ne-o-tōm) an instrument for cutting the fetal membranes.

amniotomy (am″ne-ot′o-me) surgical rupture of the fetal membranes.

amobarbital (am″o-bar′bĭ-tal) one of the barbiturates, used as a short-acting hypnotic and sedative. Effects develop rapidly and the drug is eliminated more quickly than other barbiturates. Regular use may lead to habituation, and overdosage can produce narcosis and death.

amodiaquine (am″o-di′ah-kwin) a drug used as the hydrochloride salt in treatment of malaria, especially falciparum malaria, and of amebic abscess.

Amoeba (ah-me′ba) a genus of amebae.

amolanone (ah-mo′lah-nōn) a chemical used for parasympathetic blockade, relaxation of spasm of the urinary tract, and as a topical anesthetic, particularly for urologic diagnostic procedures.

amorph (a′morf) an amorphous mutant gene.

amorphia, amorphism (a-mor′fe-ah; a-mor′fizm) state of being amorphous.

amorphous (ah-mor′fus) having no definite form; shapeless.

amotio (ah-mo′she-o) [L.] a removing.

a. ret′inae, detachment of the retina.

amoxicillin (ah-moks″ĭ-sil′in) a penicillin analogue similar in action to ampicillin but more efficiently absorbed from the gastrointestinal tract and therefore requiring less frequent dosage and not as likely to cause diarrhea.

AMP adenosine monophosphate.

amp. ampere, ampule.

ampere (am′pēr) a unit of electric current strength, the current yielded by one volt of electromotive force against one ohm of resistance.

Amphedroxyn (am″fe-drok′sin) trademark for a preparation of methamphetamine, an adrenergic, central nervous system stimulant.

amphetamine (am-fet′ah-mēn) a white crystalline powder used as a central nervous system stimulant. It is odorless and has a slightly bitter taste.

Amphetamine has the temporary effect of increasing energy and apparent mental alertness. It is used in some cases of mental depression and alcoholism, in the chronic rigidity following encephalitis, in attacks of narcolepsy, and to control the appetite in the overweight. It is also used to overcome the depressant effects of barbiturates.

Caution must be exercised in using amphetamine in persons hypersensitive to stimulants, those suffering from coronary or cardiovascular disease or hypertension, or women in the early stages of pregnancy. The drug should be used only with a doctor's prescription and never by normal persons as "pep pills" to increase their working capacity.

amphi- (am′fe) word element [Gr.], *both; on both sides.*

amphiarthrosis (am″fe-ar-thro′sis) a joint in which the surfaces are connected by disks of fibrocartilage, as between vertebrae.

amphiaster (am′fĭ-as″ter) the double star figure formed by achromatin fibers in karyokinesis; called also diaster.

Amphibia (am-fib′e-ah) a class of animals living both on land and in water.

amphibolic (am″fĭ-bol′ik) 1. uncertain. 2. having both an anabolic and catabolic function.

amphicelous (am″fĭ-se′lus) concave on either side or end.

amphicentric (am″fĭ-sen′trik) beginning and ending in the same vessel.

amphichroic, amphichromatic (am″fĭ-kro′ik; am″fĭ-kro-mat′ik) affecting both red and blue litmus.

amphidiarthrosis (am″fĭ-di″ar-thro′sis) a joint having the nature of both ginglymus and arthrodia, as that of the lower jaw.

amphitrichous (am-fit′rĭ-kus) having flagella at each end.

amphocyte (am′fo-sīt) a cell staining with either acid or basic dyes.

ampholyte (am′fo-līt) an organic or inorganic substance capable of acting as either an acid or a base.

amphophil (am′fo-fil) an amphophilic cell or element.

amphophilic (am″fo-fil′ik) staining with either acid or basic dyes.

amphoric (am-for′ik) pertaining to a bottle; resembling the sound made by blowing across the neck of a bottle.

amphoteric (am″fo-ter′ik) capable of acting as both an acid and a base; capable of neutralizing either bases or acids.

amphotericin B (am″fo-ter′ĭ-sin) an antifungal antibiotic used to treat deep-seated mycotic infections, especially histoplasmosis. It is of no benefit in the treatment of bacterial infections. It may be applied topically or administered intravenously. Toxic effects from the drug have not been clearly established but anorexia, chills, fever, and headache may occur. Renal damage with evidence of renal tubular acidosis occurs, but usually clears when the drug is discontinued.

amphotericity (am″fo-ter-is′ĭ-te) the power to unite with either positively or negatively charged ions, or with either basic or acid substances.

amphoterism (am-fo′ter-izm) the possession of both acid and basic properties.

amphotony (am-fot′o-ne) hypertonia of the entire autonomic nervous system.

ampicillin (am″pĭ-sil′in) a broad-spectrum penicillin of synthetic origin, used in treatment of a number of infections, and available in oral preparations as well as ampules for intramuscular injections. It is active against many of the gram-negative pathogens, in addition to the usual gram-positive ones that are affected by penicillin.

amplification (am″plĭ-fĭ-ka′shun) the process of making larger, as the increase of an auditory or visual stimulus, as a means of improving its perception.

amplitude (am′plĭ-tūd) largeness, fullness; wideness or breadth of range or extent.

a. of accommodation, the total amount of accommodative power of the eye.

amprotropine (am″pro-tro′pēn) an anticholinergic drug that acts like atropine in its depression of the parasympathetic impulses, but is much less potent. It is used in the treatment of peptic ulcer and cases of hypermotility of the intestinal tract, and is available in combination with a barbiturate.

ampule (am′pūl) a small, hermetically sealed glass flask, e.g., one containing medication for parenteral administration.

ampulla (am-pul′ah), pl. *ampul′lae* [L.] a flasklike dilatation of a tubular structure, especially of the expanded ends of the semicircular canals of the ear.

a. chy′li, receptaculum chyli.

a. duc′tus deferen′tis, the enlarged and tortuous distal end of the ductus deferens.

Henle's a., ampulla ductus deferentis.

hepatopancreatic a., ampulla of Vater; a flasklike cavity in the major duodenal papilla into which the common bile duct and pancreatic duct open.

Lieberkühn's a., the blind termination of the lacteals in the villi of the intestines.

ampul′lae membrana′ceae, the dilatations at one end of each of the three semicircular ducts.

ampul′lae os′seae, the dilatations at one of the ends of the semicircular canals.

phrenic a., the dilatation at the lower end of the esophagus.

a. of rectum, the dilated portion of the rectum just proximal to the anal canal.

a. of Thoma, one of the small terminal expansions of an interlobar artery in the pulp of the spleen.

a. of uterine tube, the longest and widest portion of the uterine tube, between the infundibulum and the isthmus of the tube.

a. of Vater, hepatopancreatic ampulla; the term "ampulla of Vater" is often mistakenly used instead of "papilla of Vater," or major duodenal papilla.

amputation (am″pu-ta′shun) the removal of a limb or other appendage or outgrowth of the body. The most common indication for amputation of an upper limb is severe trauma. Blood vessel disorders such as ARTERIOSCLEROSIS, often secondary to DIABETES MELLITUS, account for the greatest percentage of

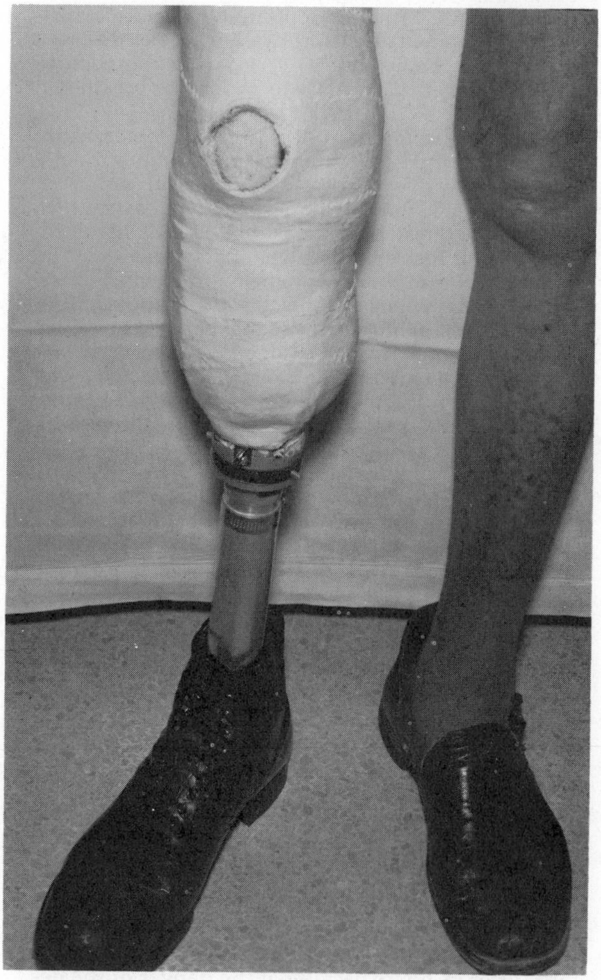

Immediate postsurgical prosthesis in place after below-knee amputation for occlusive arterial disease. Note rigid dressing, pylon, and foot-ankle assembly. (From Fairbairn, J. F., II, Juergens, J. L., and Spittell, J. A., Jr.: Peripheral Vascular Diseases, 4th ed. Philadelphia, W. B. Saunders Co., 1972.)

leg amputations. Other indications may include malignancy, infection, and gangrene.

There are two general types of surgical procedure for amputation: (1) the closed or "flap" amputation; and (2) the open or guillotine procedure, which is often required when infection is present and there is a need for free drainage from the operative site. A second surgical procedure involving stump revision or closure is needed after the guillotine procedure. This is done only after the infection has been eliminated.

PATIENT CARE. The goal of patient care for the amputee is total rehabilitation with attainment of full function and normal active life. Such total rehabilitation is not always possible because of physical and mental limitations of the patient. It requires that the patient be physically and psychologically able to accept and adapt to a PROSTHESIS and that each member of the health care team fulfill his responsibilities in preventing complications and in preparing the patient for optimum use of an artificial limb. Some patients, because of age or disease, do not have the necessary energy, muscular coordination, or mental capacity to undertake prosthetic training.

Preoperative Care. Unless time is a factor, as in emergency cases demanding immediate surgery, the preoperative care of the potential amputee should include emotional and vocational aspects as well as the physical. If the patient is fully involved in plans for his rehabilitation, understands what is expected of him, and knows the regimen of exercise and skills he will need to develop, his chances of full recovery and achievement of independence will be greatly enhanced. Much emotional support and encouragement can be offered by other amputees who are successfully mastering their prosthesis and making progress toward their goal of total rehabilitation.

In general, physical preparation of the patient undergoing surgical amputation includes measures to promote optimum health and well-being, to establish nutritional and fluid balances, and to increase muscular strength and endurance levels. A program of exercises may be started to help the patient develop skill in using crutches and a walker and transferring himself from wheelchair to bed.

Immediately prior to surgery the affected limb is shaved and thoroughly cleansed with an antiseptic. Special wrapping of the limb with sterile towels is sometimes requested by the surgeon.

Postoperative Care. Patient care during the immediate postoperative period is primarily centered on care of the stump and prevention of such complications as hemorrhage and edema at the operative site. There should be a large tourniquet at the bedside at all times in case excessive bleeding develops. The stump is elevated on a pillow for 24 to 48 hours to hasten venous return and control edema. Elevation of the stump of a lower extremity is discontinued after 48 hours because of the danger of the development of a hip contracture.

Fitting of a prosthesis may be *delayed* or *immediate* depending on the condition of the patient, the reason for the amputation, and the preference of the surgeon. In recent years there has been increased interest in immediate fitting of a prosthetic device in the operating room at the time of surgery. This technique has certain advantages and alters somewhat the kind of care needed by the patient during the postoperative period.

Immediate fitting of a prosthesis involves the application of a rigid plastic dressing which serves to protect the stump and prevent edema. The dressing is similar to a cast and the patient will require CAST care. The temporary prosthetic device is applied at the time of surgery and includes a pylon and foot-ankle assembly.

Early ambulation is a major advantage of immediate fitting of a prosthesis. Other benefits arise from the local compression exerted by the dressing. This serves to inhibit bleeding, to mold the stump and help shrink it, and to reduce phantom sensations, pain, and contractures. Unfortunately, not all amputees are candidates for immediate fitting. The technique is not advised for amputations above the knee or above the elbow, for weak and debilitated patients, or for those who are mentally or emotionally unable to cooperate with efforts at rehabilitation. The procedure also requires the services of prosthetic experts who may not be available in smaller medical facilities and rural areas.

The more conventional, and probably more frequently chosen, technique of delayed prosthetic fitting requires special care of the stump and a gradual preparation of the patient for weight-bearing and ambulation.

During the immediate postoperative period the stump dressings are changed or reinforced as ordered. The stump usually is wrapped with elastic bandages or covered with stump socks. The bandages are checked frequently for signs of bleeding and for slippage which may lead to a tourniquet effect and the occlusion of blood supply.

Exercises are started as soon as possible to strengthen the muscles and prevent contractures. Early ambulation is encouraged to promote wound healing and facilitate fitting of a prosthesis. If all goes well and no complications develop, the patient may be fitted for a temporary prosthesis during the second or third postoperative week. He is allowed to gradually increase weight-bearing on the stump until it can tolerate his full weight. By the tenth or twelfth week a permanent prosthesis can be fitted to the stump of the lower extremity. Crutch walking is begun as soon as the patient's condition allows.

The patient with amputation of an upper extremity also may receive immediate or delayed fitting of a prosthesis. When the surgeon has chosen the delayed fitting technique, the patient requires stump care similar to that of the lower extremity except that an upper extremity stump is bandaged more loosely, especially when trauma has necessitated removal of the limb. Exercises are begun the day after surgery and within ten to fourteen days the patient is fitted with a temporary prosthesis.

Chopart's a., amputation of the foot, with the calcaneus, talus, and other parts of the tarsus being retained.

closed a., flap amputation; one in which flaps are made from skin and subcutaneous tissue and sutured over the bone end of the stump.

congenital a., absence of a limb at birth, attributed to constriction of the part by an encircling band during intrauterine development.

a. in contiguity, amputation at a joint.

a. in continuity, amputation of a limb elsewhere than at a joint.

diaclastic a., amputation in which the bone is broken by osteoclast and the soft tissues divided by an écraseur.

Dupuytren's a., amputation of the arm at the shoulder joint.

flap a., closed amputation.

Gritti-Stokes a., amputation of the leg at the knee through condyles of the femur.

guillotine a., open amputation; one in which the entire cross-section is left open (flapless) for dressing.

Hey's a., amputation of the foot between the tarsus and metatarsus.

interpelviabdominal a., amputation of the thigh with excision of the lateral portion of the pelvic girdle.

interscapulothoracic a., amputation of the arm with excision of the lateral portion of the shoulder girdle.

Lisfranc's a., amputation of the foot between the metatarsus and tarsus.

open a., guillotine amputation.

racket a., one in which there is a single longitudinal incision continuous below with a spiral incision on either side of the limb.

spontaneous a., loss of a part without surgical intervention, as in leprosy, etc.

Syme's a., disarticulation of the foot with removal of both malleoli.

Trippier's a., amputation of the foot through the calcaneus.

Amsustain (am'sus-tān) trademark for a preparation of dextroamphetamine, an adrenergic, central nervous system stimulant.

amusia (a-mu'ze-ah) loss of ability to produce (motor amusia) or to recognize (sensory amusia) musical sounds.

A.M.W.A. American Medical Writers' Association.

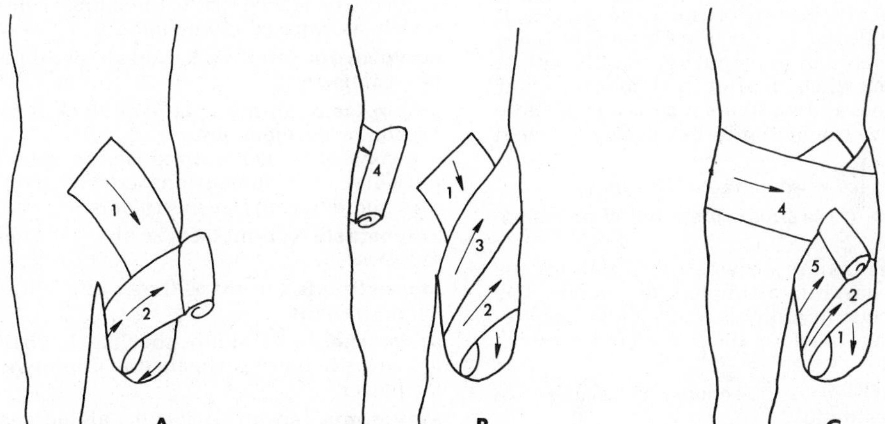

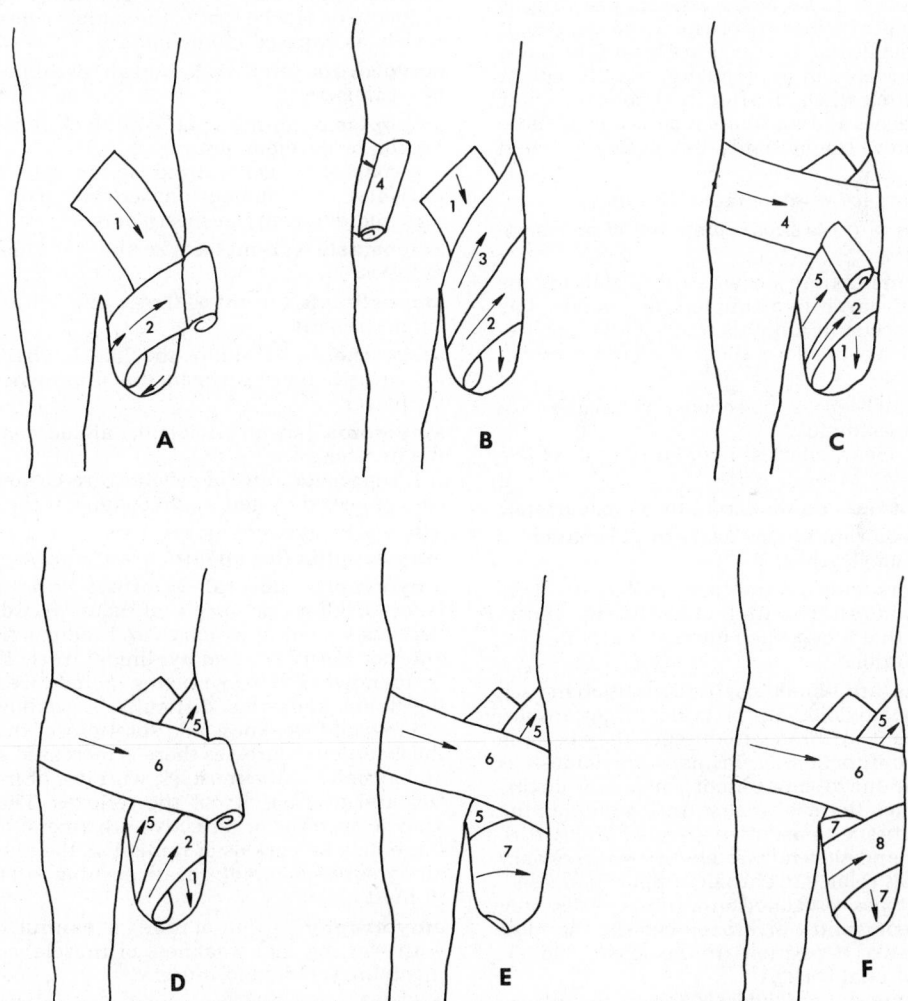

Bandaging an above-knee amputation stump. A, Use 6″ elastic bandage. Enclose medial, distal end of stump. Apply pressure via bandage to end of stump. Use diagonal, not circular, turns. B, Turn No. 3 must be high in groin and then turn made around waist to hold No. 3 in place. Do not pull hip into flexion. (A second 6″ roll may be needed.) C, Turn No. 5 must be high in groin and a loop made around waist again. D, See diagram. E, Enclose lateral, distal end of stump. (A 4″ roll may be needed.) Continue diagonal and figure-of-8 turns around stump. F, Continue turns to shape end of stump. (Courtesy of University of Washington Department of Prosthetics, from booklet *Prosthetics-Orthotics*.)

amyelia (a″mi-e′le-ah) congenital absence of the spinal cord.

amyelinic (ah-mi″ĕ-lin′ik) without myelin.

amyelonic (ah-mi″ĕ-lon′ik) 1. having no spinal cord. 2. having no marrow.

amyelus (ah-mi′ĕ-lus) a fetus with no spinal cord.

amygdala (ah-mig′dah-lah) 1. a tonsil. 2. a lobule of the cerebellum. 3. almond.

amygdalin (ah-mig′dah-lin) a glycoside from bitter almonds.

amygdaline (ah-mig′dah-līn) 1. like an almond. 2. pertaining to tonsils.

amygdalolith (ah-mig′dah-lo-lith″) a calculus in a tonsil.

amyl nitrite (am′il ni′trīt) a vasodilator often used in the treatment of ANGINA PECTORIS because of its quick relief of the pain. Presumably it relaxes the smooth muscles of the coronary arteries, bringing about dilation of these blood vessels. The drug is dispensed in pearls that are crushed and inhaled. It acts very quickly and its effects are brief. The blood pressure is lowered by amyl nitrite, and the patient should be sitting when inhaling its vapors. Irregular pulse, headache, and dizziness may occur. If these symptoms prove troublesome, the physician should be notified.

amyl(o)- (am′ĭ-lo) word element [Gr.], *starch.*

amylaceous (am″ĭ-la′shus) composed of or resembling starch.

amylase (am′ĭ-lās) an enzyme that catalyzes the hydrolysis of starch into simpler compounds. The α-amylases occur in animals and include pancreatic and salivary amylase; the β-amylases occur in higher plants.

amylene (am′ĭ-lēn) a poisonous hydrocarbon; a dangerous anesthetic.

a. hydrate, clear, colorless liquid used as a vehicle in pharmacy.

amylobarbitone (am″ĭ-lo-bar′bĭ-tōn) amobarbital.

amylogenesis (am″ĭ-lo-jen′ĕ-sis) the formation of starch. adj., **amylogen′ic.**

amyloid (am′ĭ-loid) 1. starchlike; amylaceous. 2. an optically homogeneous, waxy, translucent, abnormal protein that is deposited intercellularly in a variety of conditions.

amyloidosis (am″ĭ-loi-do′sis) the deposition in various tissues of amyloid. This protein is almost insoluble and once it infiltrates the tissues they become waxy and nonfunctioning. Primary amyloidosis is thought to be due to some obscure metabolic disturbance in which there is an abnormal protein in the plasma; the tissues most often affected are cardiac and smooth and skeletal muscle tissue. Secondary amyloidosis is related to chronic suppuration, especially those types associated with tuberculosis, lung abscess, osteomyelitis, or bronchiectasis; the most common sites of deposition are the spleen, kidney, liver, and adrenal cortex.

The symptoms of amyloidosis appear insidiously and progress slowly. They depend on the specific organ affected, and frequently in secondary amyloidosis they are overshadowed by symptoms of the disease causing the disorder. Primary systemic amyloidosis is treated symptomatically; there is no cure, and death usually occurs within 3 years of the onset. Heart failure is the most common cause of death. Secondary amyloidosis is best treated by eliminating the underlying cause. This includes control of suppuration by effective use of antibiotic drugs. There has been a reduction in incidence of secondary amyloidosis in recent years because of the development of drugs that are successful in controlling infection and suppuration.

amylolysis (am″ĭ-lol′ĭ-sis) digestive change of starch into sugar. adj., **amylolу′tic.**

amylopectin (am″ĭ-lo-pek′tin) the insoluble constituent of starch; the soluble constituent is amylose.

amylopectinosis (am″ĭ-lo-pek′tĭ-no′sis) glycogenosis (type IV) in which deficiency of the brancher enzyme amylo-1:4,1:6-transglucoside results in cirrhosis of the liver, hepatosplenomegaly, and progressive hepatic failure and death. Called also Andersen's disease.

amylopsin (am″ĭ-lop′sin) α-amylase; a pancreatic enzyme that converts starch to maltose.

amylorrhea (am″ĭ-lo-re′ah) the presence of an abnormal amount of starch in the stools.

amylose (am′ĭ-lōs) 1. any carbohydrate other than a glucose or saccharose. 2. the soluble constituent of starch, as opposed to amylopectin.

amyocardia (ah-mi″o-kar′de-ah) weakness of the heart muscle.

amyoplasia (ah-mi″o-pla′ze-ah) lack of muscle formation or development.

a. congen′ita, generalized lack in the newborn of muscular development and growth, with contracture and deformity at most joints.

amyostasia (ah-mi″o-sta′ze-ah) a tremor of the muscles.

amyosthenia (ah-mi″os-the′ne-ah) failure of muscular strength.

amyosthenic (ah-mĭ-os-then′ik) 1. characterized by amyosthenia. 2. an agent that diminishes muscular power.

amyotonia (ah-mi″o-to′ne-ah) atonic condition of the muscles.

a. congen′ita, any of several rare congenital diseases marked by general hypotonia of the muscles; called also Oppenheim's disease.

amyotrophia (ah-mi″o-tro′fe-ah) amyotrophy.

amyotrophic lateral sclerosis (ah-mi″o-trof′ik lat′er-al sklĕ-ro′sis) a type of motor disorder of the nervous system in which there is destruction of the anterior horn cells and pyramidal tract. The cause is unknown. Early symptoms include weakness of the hands and arms, difficulty in swallowing and talking, and weakness and spasticity of the legs. As the disorder progresses there is increased spasticity and atrophy of the muscles, with loss of motor control and overactivity of the reflexes. There is no known specific or effective treatment. Although there may be periods of remission, the disease usually progresses rapidly, death ensuing in 2 to 5 years in most cases.

amyotrophy (ah″mi-ot′ro-fe) a painful condition with wasting and weakness of muscle, commonly involving the deltoid muscle.

Amytal (am′ĭ-tal) trademark for amobarbital, a short-acting hypnotic and sedative.

amyxia (ah-mik′se-ah) absence of mucus.

amyxorrhea (ah-mik″so-re′ah) absence of mucous secretion.

An chemical symbol, *actinon.*

An. anisometropia; anode.

A.N.A. American Nurses' Association.

ana (an'ah) [Gr.] of each, used in prescription writing; abbreviated āā.

ana- (an'ah) word element [Gr.], *upward; again; backward; excessively.*

anabasis (ah-nab'ah-sis) the stage of increase in a disease.

anabiosis (an"ah-bi-o'sis) restoration of life processes after their apparent cessation.

anabolism (ah-nab'o-lizm) the constructive phase of metabolism, in which the body cells synthesize protoplasm for growth and repair. adj., **anabol'ic.** The manner in which this synthesis takes place is directed by the genetic code carried by the molecules of deoxyribonucleic acid (DNA). The "building blocks" for this synthesis of protoplasm are obtained from amino acids and other nutritive elements in the diet.

anachoresis (an"ah-ko-re'sis) preferential collection or deposit of particles at a site, as of bacteria or metals that have localized out of the bloodstream in areas of inflammation.

anacidity (an"ah-sid'ĭ-te) abnormal lack or deficiency of acid.

gastric a., achlorhydria.

anaclitic (an"ah-klit'ik) denoting the dependence of the infant on the mother or mother substitute for his sense of well being.

anacousia (an"ah-koo'ze-ah) anakusis.

anacrotism (ah-nak'rŏ-tizm) a pulse anomaly evidenced by the presence of a prominent notch on the ascending limb of the pulse tracing. adj., **anacrot'ic.**

anadipsia (an"ah-dip'se-ah) intense thirst.

anadrenalism (an"ah-dre'nal-izm) absence or failure of adrenal function.

Anadrol (an'ah-drol) trademark for a preparation of oxymetholone, an anabolic-androgenic steroid that promotes retention of nitrogen, phosphorus, and calcium.

anaerobe (an-a'er-ōb) an organism that lives and grows in the absence of molecular oxygen. adj., **anaero'bic.**

facultative a., a microorganism that can live and grow with or without molecular oxygen.

obligate a., an organism that can grow only in the complete absence of molecular oxygen.

anaerobiosis (an-a"er-o-bi-o'sis) life without free oxygen.

anaerogenic (an-a"er-o-jen'ik) suppressing the formation of gas by gas-producing bacteria.

anaerosis (an"a-er-o'sis) interruption of the respiratory function.

anakatadidymus (an"ah-kat"ah-did'ĭ-mus) a twin monster, separate above and below, but united in the trunk.

anakusis (an"ah-ku'sis) total deafness.

anal (a'nal) relating to the anus.

analbuminemia (an"al-bu"mĭ-ne'me-ah) absence or deficiency of serum albumins.

analeptic (an"ah-lep'tik) 1. a drug that acts as a stimulant to the central nervous system, such as caffeine and amphetamine. 2. a restorative medicine.

Analexin (an"ah-lek'sin) trademark for preparations of phenyramidol, an analgesic.

analgesia (an"al-je'ze-ah) absence of sensibility to pain, particularly the relief of pain without loss of consciousness.

continuous caudal a., continuous injection of an anesthetic solution into the sacral and lumbar plexuses within the epidural space to relieve the pain of childbirth; also used in general surgery to block the pain pathways below the navel (see also CAUDAL ANESTHESIA).

infiltration a., paralysis of the nerve endings at the site of operation by subcutaneous injection of an anesthetic.

surface a., local analgesia produced by an anesthetic applied to the surface of such mucous membranes as those of the eye, nose, throat, larynx, and urethra.

analgesic (an"al-je'sik) 1. relieving pain. 2. pertaining to analgesia. 3. a drug that relieves pain.

analgia (an-al'je-ah) painlessness. adj., **anal'gic.**

analogous (ah-nal'o-gus) resembling or similar in some respects, as in function or appearance, but not in origin or development.

analogue (an'ah-log) 1. a part or organ having the same function as another, but of different evolutionary origin. 2. a chemical compound having a structure similar to that of another but differing from it in respect to a certain component; it may have similar or opposite action metabolically.

analogy (ah-nal'o-je) the quality of being analogous; resemblance or similarity in function or appearance, but not in origin or development.

analysand (ah-nal'ĭ-sand) a person undergoing psychoanalysis.

analysis (ah-nal'ĭ-sis) 1. separation into component parts. 2. psychoanalysis. adj., **analyt'ic.**

qualitative a., determination of the nature of the constituents of a compound.

quantitative a., determination of the proportionate quantities of the constituents of a compound.

vector a., analysis of a moving force to determine both its magnitude and its direction, e.g., analysis of the scalar electrocardiogram to determine the magnitude and direction of the electromotive force for one complete cycle of the heart.

anamnesis (an"am-ne'sis) 1. the faculty of memory. 2. the past history of a patient and his family.

anamnestic (an"am-nes'tik) 1. pertaining to anamnesis. 2. aiding the memory.

anamniotic (an"am-ne-ot'ik) having no amnion.

ananabolic (an"an-ah-bol'ik) characterized by absence of anabolism.

anaphase (an'ah-fāz) the third stage of division of the nucleus of a cell in either meiosis or mitosis.

anaphia (an-a'fe-ah) lack or loss of the sense of touch.

anaphoresis (an"ah-fo-re'sis) diminished activity of the sweat glands.

anaphoria (an"ah-fo're-ah) the tendency to tilt the head downward, with visual axes deviating upward, on looking straight ahead.

anaphrodisia (an"af-ro-diz'e-ah) absence or loss of sexual desire.

anaphrodisiac (an"af-ro-diz'e-ak) 1. repressing sexual desire. 2. a drug that represses sexual desire.

anaphylactic shock (an"ah-fi-lak'tik) a serious and profound state of shock brought about by hypersensitivity (anaphylaxis) to an ALLERGEN, such as a drug, foreign protein, or toxin. Insect bites and stings in hypersensitive persons may produce anaphylactic shock. Early symptoms are typical of an allergic reaction, e.g., sneezing, edema, or itching at the site of injection or sting. The symptoms increase in severity very rapidly and progress to dyspnea, cyanosis, and shock. The blood pressure drops rapidly, the pulse becomes weak and thready, and convulsions and loss of consciousness may occur. Severe anaphylactic shock can be fatal if immediate emergency measures are not taken.

PREVENTION AND TREATMENT. Prevention of anaphylactic shock requires a thorough knowledge of the person's history and various allergies. If there is a history of allergy, a sensitivity test should be done before he receives injections of animal serum or other proteins or drugs. Any person who has been given an injection of animal serum or an antigen should be watched closely for 30 minutes after the injection. If early symptoms of a reaction occur, a physician should be notified immediately.

The drug most often used to counteract the effects of anaphylactic shock is epinephrine. Further treatment is aimed at combating shock and relieving dyspnea. In some cases tracheostomy may be necessary.

PATIENT CARE. Because of the serious nature of anaphylactic shock, alertness to this possibility is required in the administration of drugs and foreign proteins. Immunizing agents are particularly dangerous to hypersensitive persons. If a patient says he has a history of an allergy the medication should be withheld until the physician is notified.

Nursing measures that may be taken to combat shock once the reaction takes place include placing the patient in Trendelenburg position and maintaining body heat. An emergency tray containing needle, syringe, and epinephrine should be kept on hand, and a tracheostomy set should be readily available.

anaphylactogen (an″ah-fi-lak′to-jen) a substance that produces anaphylaxis.

anaphylactogenesis (an″ah-fi-lak″to-jen′ĕ-sis) the production of anaphylaxis. adj., **anaphylactogen′ic.**

anaphylatoxin (an″ah-fi″lah-tok′sin) a substance produced in blood serum during complement fixation which serves as a mediator of inflammation by inducing mast cell degranulation and histamine release; on injection into animals, it causes anaphylactic shock.

anaphylaxis (an″ah-fi-lak′sis) 1. an exaggerated reaction of an organism to foreign protein or other substances to which it has previously been sensitized. 2. anaphylactic shock. adj., **anaphylac′tic.**

acquired a., that in which sensitization is known to have been produced by administration of a foreign protein.

active a., that produced by injection of a foreign protein.

antiserum a., passive anaphylaxis.

heterologous a., passive anaphylaxis induced by transfer of serum from an animal of a different species.

homologous a., passive anaphylaxis induced by transfer of serum from an animal of the same species.

indirect a., that induced by an animal's own protein modified in some way.

passive a., that resulting in a normal person from injection of serum of a sensitized person.

passive cutaneous a. (PCA), localized anaphylaxis passively transferred by intradermal injection of an antibody and, after a latent period (about 24 to 72 hours), intravenous injection of the homologous antigen and Evans blue dye; blueing of the skin at the site of the intradermal injection is evidence of the permeability reaction. Used in studies of antibodies causing immediate hypersensitivity reactions.

reverse a., that following injection of antigen, succeeded by injection of antiserum.

anaplasia (an″ah-pla′ze-ah) loss of differentiation of cells, an irreversible alteration in adult cells toward more primitive (embryonic) cell types; a characteristic of tumor cells.

anaplastic (an″ah-plas′tik) 1. restoring a lost or absent part. 2. characterized by anaplasia.

anapophysis (an″ah-pof′ĭ-sis) an accessory vertebral process.

anaptic (an-ap′tik) pertaining to or characterized by loss of the sense of touch.

anarithmia (an″ah-rith′me-ah) inability to count, due to a lesion of the brain.

anarthria (an-ar′thre-ah) severe dysarthria resulting in speechlessness.

a. litera′lis, stuttering.

anasarca (an″ah-sar′kah) generalized massive edema.

anastalsis (an″ah-stal′sis) 1. an upward-moving wave of contraction without a preceding wave of inhibition, occurring in the alimentary canal in addition to the peristaltic wave. 2. styptic action.

anastaltic (an″ah-stal′tik) styptic; highly astringent.

anastole (ah-nas′to-le) retraction, as of the lips of a wound.

anastomosis (ah-nas″to-mo′sis) 1. communication between two tubular organs. 2. surgical, traumatic, or pathologic formation of a connection between two normally distinct structures. adj., **anastomot′ic.**

arteriovenous a., anastomosis between an artery and a vein.

crucial a., an arterial anastomosis in the upper part of the thigh.

heterocladic a., one between branches of different arteries.

intestinal a., establishment of a communication between two formerly distant portions of the intestine.

anat. anatomy.

anatomic, anatomical (an″ah-tom′ik), (an″ah-tom′ĭ-kal) pertaining to anatomy, or to the structure of the body.

anatomist (ah-nat′o-mist) one skilled in anatomy.

anatomy (ah-nat′o-me) the science dealing with the form and structure of living organisms.

comparative a., description and comparison of the form and structure of different animals.

developmental a., structural embryology.

gross a., macroscopic a., that dealing with structures visible with the unaided eye.

microscopic a., histology.

morbid a., pathologic a., anatomy of diseased tissues.

radiologic a., x-ray anatomy.

special a., anatomy devoted to study of particular organs or parts.

topographic a., that devoted to determination of relative positions of various body parts.

x-ray a., study of organs and tissues based on their visualization by x-rays in both living and dead bodies.

anatriptic (an″ah-trip′tik) a medicine applied by rubbing.

anatropia (an″ah-tro′pe-ah) upward deviation of the visual axis of one eye when the other eye is fixing. adj., **anatrop′ic.**

anchorage (ang′kŏ-rāj) fixation, e.g., surgical fixation of a displaced viscus or, in operative dentistry, fixation of fillings, or of artificial crowns or bridges. In orthodontics, the support used for a regulating apparatus.

anchylo- for words beginning thus, see those beginning *ankylo-*.

ancipital (an-sip′ĭ-tal) two-edged.

anconad (ang′ko-nad) toward the elbow or olecranon.

anconal, anconeal (ang′ko-nal; ang-ko′ne-al) pertaining to the elbow.

anconitis (an″ko-ni′tis) inflammation of the elbow joint.

ancylo- for words beginning thus, see also those beginning *ankylo-*.

Ancylostoma (an″sĭ-los′to-mah) a genus of nematode parasites (HOOKWORMS).

A. america′num, *Necator americanus.*

A. brazilien′se, a species parasitic in dogs and cats in tropical and subtropical regions; its larvae may cause creeping eruption in man.

A. cani′num, the common hookworm of dogs and cats.

a. duodena′le, a common hookworm, parasitic in the small intestine.

ancylostomiasis (an″sĭ-los″to-mi′ah-sis) infection by worms of the genus *Ancylostoma* or by other hookworms (*Necator americanus*). See HOOKWORM.

Ancylostomidae (an″sĭ-lo-sto′mĭ-de) a family of nematode parasites having two ventrolateral cutting plates at the entrance to a large buccal capsule, and small teeth at its base; the hookworms.

Andersen's disease (an′der-senz) glycogenosis (type IV); see also AMYLOPECTINOSIS.

andr(o)- word element [Gr.], *male; masculine.*

androblastoma (an″dro-blas-to′mah) 1. a rare benign tumor of the testis histologically resembling the fetal testis; there are three varieties: diffuse stromal, mixed (stromal and epithelial), and tubular (epithelial). The epithelial elements contain Sertoli cells, which may produce estrogen and thus cause feminization. 2. arrhenoblastoma.

androgen (an′dro-jen) any substance that stimulates male characteristics. The two main androgens are androsterone and testosterone. adj., **androgen′ic.**

The androgenic hormones are internal endocrine secretions circulating in the bloodstream and manufactured mainly by the testes under stimulation from the PITUITARY GLAND. To a lesser extent, androgens are produced by the adrenal glands in both sexes, as well as by the ovaries in women. Thus women normally have a small percentage of male hormones, in the same way that men's bodies contain some female sex hormones, the estrogens.

The androgens are responsible for the secondary sex characteristics, such as the beard and the deepening of the voice at puberty. They also stimulate the growth of muscle and bones throughout the body and thus account in part for the greater strength and size of men as compared to women.

android (an′droid) resembling a man.

androphobia (an″dro-fo′be-ah) morbid dread of the male sex.

androstane (an′dro-stān) the hydrocarbon nucleus, $C_{19}H_{32}$, from which androgens are derived.

androstanediol (an″dro-stān′de-ol) an androgen, $C_{19}H_{32}O_2$, prepared by reducing androsterone.

androstanedione (an″dro-stān′de-ōn) an androgen formed in the testes.

androstene (an′dro-stēn) an unsaturated cyclic hydrocarbon, $C_{19}H_{30}$, forming the nucleus of testosterone and certain other androgens.

androstenediol (an″dro-stēn′de-ol) a crystalline androgenic steroid, $C_{19}H_{30}O_2$.

androsterone (an-dros′tĕ-rōn) an androgenic hormone, $C_{19}H_{30}O_2$, occurring in urine or prepared synthetically.

anectasis (an-ek′tah-sis) congenital atelectasis due to developmental immaturity.

Anectine (an-ek′tin) trademark for preparations of succinylcholine, a skeletal muscle relaxant.

anemia (ah-ne′me-ah) reduction below normal of the number of erythrocytes (red blood cells), the quantity of hemoglobin, or the volume of packed red cells in the blood.

Anemia is not a disease; it is a symptom of a number of different diseases or disorders. It may be caused by poor diet, loss of blood, industrial poisons, diseases of the bone marrow, or any of several other conditions. Careful diagnosis is very important, since treatment varies according to the cause of the anemia.

SYMPTOMS. Mild degrees of anemia often cause only slight and vague symptoms, perhaps nothing more than a lack of energy. The anemic person may also become fatigued more often and more easily. In more severe cases of anemia, exertion causes shortness of breath. This may be accompanied by pounding of the heart and a rapid pulse and heart action. These symptoms are caused by the inability of anemic blood to supply the body tissues with enough oxygen.

Pallor, particularly in the palms of the hands, the fingernails, and the conjunctiva (the lining of the eyelids), may also indicate anemia. In very advanced cases, swelling of the ankles and other evidence of heart failure may appear.

DIAGNOSIS. Anemia is diagnosed by means of blood tests. A sample of the patient's blood is examined under a microscope, and the number, size, color, and shape of the erythrocytes are determined; the amount of hemoglobin in the sample is also measured. If these studies of the blood indicate signs of anemia, other tests, such as STERNAL PUNCTURE or other bone marrow examinations, may be necessary.

A thorough physical examination is also done to evaluate the person's state of general health and to rule out possible sources of blood loss.

COMMON CAUSES OF ANEMIA

Loss of Blood. If there is massive bleeding from a wound or other lesion, the body may lose enough blood to cause severe anemia. This acute anemia is often accompanied by shock. Immediate transfusions are generally required to replace the lost blood. Chronic blood loss, such as excessive menstrual flow or slow loss of blood from an ulcer or cancer of the stomach or intestines, may also lead to anemia.

These anemias disappear when the cause has been found and corrected. To help the blood rebuild itself, the physician may prescribe medicines containing iron, which is necessary to build hemoglobin, and foods with high iron content, such as kidney and navy beans, liver, spinach, and wholewheat bread.

Diet Deficiency. Anemia may develop if the diet does not provide enough iron, protein, vitamin B_{12}, and other vitamins and minerals needed in the production of hemoglobin and the formation of erythrocytes. The combination of poor diet and chronic loss of blood makes for particular susceptibility to severe anemia. For example, a child suffering from hookworm disease, living on an inadequate diet, is doubly likely to suffer from anemia.

A good basic diet is the best way to combat diet-deficiency anemia (see also NUTRITION). So-called "blood tonics" containing iron or other vitamins or minerals are not necessary unless the physician prescribes them.

PATIENT CARE. Rest is one of the first considerations in the care of the patient with anemia. Mild exercise is usually desirable but overexertion places an added and unnecessary strain on the heart and lungs.

Observation for signs of blood loss through the intestinal tract or urinary tract may assist the physician in his diagnosis of the cause of anemia. Tarry stools or hazy brown urine should be recognized as evidence of internal bleeding and should be reported.

Combating a lack of appetite and disinterest in food may be a problem in patients with anemia. Fatigue, weakness, or soreness of the mouth must be considered as contributing factors. The patient may need to overcome poor eating habits developed through ignorance or indifference to the nutritional values of food.

Special mouth care is required when mouth and gums are tender and bleed easily. Brushing of the teeth is usually too traumatic and frequent cleansing of the mouth with cotton-tipped applicators dipped in a mild mouthwash can be substituted. The lips are kept lubricated with mineral oil or some other emollient to prevent dryness and cracking.

Extra warmth in the form of blankets and warm clothing usually must be provided because many anemia patients suffer from poor circulation and are easily chilled. The poor circulation also brings about decreased sensitivity to heat and these patients may be burned if care is not taken with hot water bottles and heating pads.

achrestic a., megaloblastic anemia morphologically resembling pernicious anemia, but with multiple other causes.

aplastic a., anemia due to disease of the bone marrow—a tumor or cancer—or to destruction of bone marrow by certain agents, particularly chemical compounds of various sorts. Treatment consists of removal of the cause, if possible, regular transfusions and sometimes injections of cortisone. The prognosis is not good. (See also APLASTIC ANEMIA.)

Cooley's a., the homozygous form of β-THALASSEMIA.

erythroblastic a., the homozygous form of β-THALASSEMIA.

hemolytic a., that due to shortened survival of mature erythrocytes and inability of the bone marrow to compensate for their decreased life span; it may be hereditary or acquired, as that resulting from infection or chemotherapy or occurring as part of an autoimmune process (see also HEMOLYTIC ANEMIA).

hypochromic a., anemia in which the decrease in hemoglobin is proportionately much greater than the decrease in number of erythrocytes.

hypoplastic a., anemia due to incapacity of blood-forming organs.

hypoplastic a., congenital, 1. idiopathic progressive anemia occurring in the first year of life, without leukopenia and thrombocytopenia; it is unresponsive to hematinics and requires multiple blood transfusions to sustain life. Called also erythrogenesis imperfecta. 2. Fanconi's syndrome.

iron-deficiency a., a form characterized by low or absent iron stores, low serum iron concentration, low transferrin saturation, elevated transferrin, low hemoglobin concentration or hematocrit, and hypochromic, microcytic red blood corpuscles. (See also IRON.)

Lederer's a., an acute hemolytic anemia of short duration and unknown etiology.

macrocytic a., anemia in which the erythrocytes are much larger than normal.

Mediterranean a., the homozygous form of β-THALASSEMIA.

megaloblastic a., anemia characterized by the presence of megaloblasts in the bone marrow.

microcytic a., anemia characterized by decrease in size of the erythrocytes.

myelopathic a., myelophthisic a., anemia due to destruction or crowding out of hematopoietic tissues by space-occupying lesions.

normochromic a., that in which the hemoglobin content of the red cells as measured by the MCHC is in the normal range.

normocytic a., anemia characterized by proportionate decrease in hemoglobin, packed red cell volume, and number of erythrocytes per cubic millimeter of blood.

pernicious a., a serious anemia that results from lack of secretion by the gastric mucous membrane of a factor (intrinsic factor) essential to formation of erythrocytes and absorption of vitamin B_{12}. This deficiency may be secondary to an illness or idiopathic, that is, from unknown causes. Treatment consists of regular administration, usually by injection, of vitamin B_{12}, which must be continued for life. (See also PERNICIOUS ANEMIA.)

a. pseudoleuke'mica infan'tum, a syndrome caused by many factors, e.g., malnutrition, chronic infection, malabsorption, etc., with anisocytosis, poikilocytosis, peripheral red cell immaturity, leukocytosis, lymphadenopathy, and hepatosplenomegaly; once considered to be a specific entity in children under age 3. Called also von Jaksch's disease.

sickle cell a., a genetically determined defect of hemoglobin synthesis associated with poor physical development and skeletal anomalies, occurring usually in Negroes. (See also SICKLE CELL ANEMIA.)

anemic (ah-ne'mik) pertaining to anemia.

anencephaly (an"en-sef'ah-le) congenital absence of the cranial vault, with the cerebral hemispheres completely missing or reduced to small masses. adj., **anacephal'ic.**

anenzymia (an"en-zi'me-ah) absence of an enzyme normally present in the body.

a. catala'sea, acatalasia.

anergasia (an″er-ga′se-ah) psychosis due to organic lesions of the central nervous system.

anergy (an′er-je) diminished reactivity to specific antigen(s). adj., **aner′gic.**

anerythropsia (an″er-ĭ-throp′se-ah) inability to distinguish red colors.

anesthecinesia (an-es″the-sĭ-ne′ze-ah) combined sensory and motor paralysis.

anesthesia (an″es-the′ze-ah) loss of feeling or sensation. Artificial anesthesia may be produced by a number of agents capable of bringing about partial or complete loss of sensation (see also ANESTHETIC).

PATIENT CARE. The patient recovering from general anesthesia must be watched constantly until he has reacted. The vital signs and blood pressure are checked regularly; any sudden change is reported immediately. The patient must be observed to see that the airway is clear at all times. If vomiting occurs, the head is turned to the side to prevent aspiration of vomitus into the respiratory tract.

In addition to the physical effects of general anesthesia, the emotional and psychologic aspects must also be considered. Fear of being "put to sleep" or rendered unconscious is common among patients. During recovery from anesthesia noise should be kept at a minimum, as all sounds may be exaggerated to the patient. It is important to remember that conversations held within hearing of the patient may be misunderstood by him since he is not capable of interpreting words and phrases clearly as long as he is under the effects of the anesthetic. When the patient is awakening from general anesthesia he may be extremely restless, attempting to get out of bed or even striking out at those around him because he is afraid and disoriented.

Patients who have had local anesthesia of the throat for diagnostic procedures or minor surgery should not be given food or liquids until the effects of the anesthesia have worn off and the gag reflex has returned. Otherwise these substances may be aspirated into the respiratory tract.

Some local anesthetics produce violent allergic reactions or anaphylactic shock in certain hypersensitive persons; for this reason, skin tests are done before these drugs are administered. An emergency tray containing hypodermic needles, syringes, and ampules of a stimulant such as epinephrine should be on hand whenever a local anesthetic is to be used.

basal a., narcosis produced by preliminary medication so that the inhalation of anesthetic necessary to produce surgical anesthesia is greatly reduced.

block a., regional anesthesia. See also BLOCK.

caudal a., injection of an anesthetic into the sacral canal to relieve the pain of childbirth (see also CAUDAL ANESTHESIA).

central a., lack of sensation caused by disease of the nerve centers.

closed a., that produced by continuous rebreathing of a small amount of anesthetic gas in a closed system with an apparatus for removing carbon dioxide.

crossed a., loss of sensation on one side of the face and loss of pain and temperature sense on the opposite side of the body.

dissociated a., dissociation a., loss of perception of certain stimuli while that of others remains intact.

electric a., anesthesia induced by passage of an electric current.

endotracheal a., anesthesia produced by introduction of a gaseous mixture through a tube inserted into the trachea.

frost a., abolition of feeling or sensation as a result of topical refrigeration produced by a jet of a highly volatile liquid.

general a., a state of unconsciousness and insusceptibility to pain, produced by an anesthetic agent.

infiltration a., local anesthesia produced by injection of the anesthetic solution directly into the area of terminal nerve endings.

inhalation a., anesthesia produced by the respiration of a volatile liquid or gaseous anesthetic agent.

insufflation a., anesthesia produced by introduction of a gaseous mixture into the trachea through a slender tube.

local a., that confined to a limited area.

mixed a., that produced by use of more than one anesthetic agent.

open a., general inhalation anesthesia in which there is no rebreathing of the expired gases.

peripheral a., lack of sensation due to changes in the peripheral nerves.

rectal a., anesthesia produced by introduction of the anesthetic agent into the rectum.

refrigeration a., local anesthesia produced by chilling the part to near freezing temperature.

regional a., insensibility caused by interrupting the sensory nerve conductivity of any region of the body; it may be produced by (1) field block, encircling the operative field by means of injections of a local anesthetic; or (2) nerve block, making injections in close proximity to the nerves supplying the area.

segmental a., loss of sensation in a segment of the body due to a lesion of a nerve root.

spinal a., 1. anesthesia due to a spinal lesion. 2. anesthesia produced by injection of the agent beneath the membrane of the spinal cord.

splanchnic a., block anesthesia for visceral operation by injection of the anesthetic agent into the region of the celiac ganglia.

surgical a., that degree of anesthesia at which operation may safely be performed.

tactile a., loss of the sense of touch.

topical a., that produced by application of a local anesthetic directly to the area involved.

twilight a., twilight sleep.

anesthesimeter (an″es-thĕ-sim′ĕ-ter) 1. an instrument for testing the degree of anesthesia. 2. a device for regulating the amount of anesthetic given.

Anesthesin (ah-nes′the-sin) trademark for a preparation of benzocaine, a topical anesthetic.

anesthesiologist (an″es-the″ze-ol′o-jist) a physician who specializes in anesthesiology.

anesthesiology (an″es-the″ze-ol′o-je) that branch of medicine concerned with administration of anesthetics and the condition of the patient while under anesthesia.

anesthetic (an″es-thet′ik) 1. pertaining to, characterized by, or producing anesthesia. 2. an agent that produces anesthesia. There are two types of anesthetics: general anesthetics, which produce a sound sleep; and regional anesthetics, which render a specific area insensible to pain.

GENERAL ANESTHETICS. The inhalant types are the most widely used general anesthetics. Ether, one of the best known, is administered by means of a face mask in amounts controlled by the anesthesiologist or anesthetist.

Chloroform is now little used, principally because

it may damage the liver. Nitrous oxide, so-called laughing gas, is used for short surgical procedures, or, in the case of long operations, before the patient is given ether. Nitrous oxide is also used by dentists for extractions, especially when the patient is allergic to or has a distaste for a local anesthetic such as procaine.

Cyclopropane and halothane are more recently discovered inhalants, as is ethylene, a gas that produces a light sleep resembling that caused by nitrous oxide.

Intravenous anesthetics are also used for light general anesthesia or in advance of an inhalant anesthetic. The best known of these is a barbiturate, thiopental sodium (Pentothal sodium).

Some anesthetics are administered rectally, for example, paraldehyde, which is often prescribed for alcoholics, psychotics, and extremely apprehensive patients. Given in the form of a retention enema, the substance is absorbed into the system and takes effect rapidly.

REGIONAL ANESTHETICS. Regional anesthetics are administered by injection or by topical application to the skin or mucous membranes. Spinal anesthetics are injected into the subarachnoid space of the spinal canal. For short procedures, procaine is the anesthetic of choice; for longer ones, tetracaine or dibucaine is used. This type of regional anesthesia may be used for operations on the lower part of the body.

A variant of spinal anesthesia is caudal anesthesia, which is used in childbirth. The anesthetic, usually procaine, is dripped in through a needle inserted into the spinal canal at the sacrum. In continuous caudal anesthesia, the needle is left in place throughout the delivery while the anesthetic drips in gradually. (See also CAUDAL ANESTHESIA.)

Various local anesthetics are used for operations on the skin or the tissues immediately beneath, and in dentistry for many tooth fillings and most extractions. Cocaine was once popular for this type of minor surgery, but today it has been replaced by derivatives such as procaine. After injection, the sensory nerves in the area become insensitive and may remain so for several hours.

In some parts of the body where a main nerve is accessible, the anesthetic is injected directly into or adjacent to that nerve, in this way desensitizing all the adjacent tissue. This is called nerve block or block anesthesia, and is often used in dental surgery on the lower jaw.

Certain anesthetics have enough penetrating power to relieve pain when they are applied directly to a body surface, a technique known as topical (or surface) anesthesia. One such anesthetic, butacaine sulfate, is often applied to the surface of the eye before eye operations. Tetracaine is also used on the eye, as well as on membranes of the nose and throat. Some surface anesthetics, such as benzocaine, can be safely applied directly on wounds and ulcers for the relief of pain.

OTHER TECHNIQUES. The search continues for other anesthetics that will be safe, agreeable, quick, and effective. In some cases hypnosis has been used successfully without the necessity of any anesthetic substance whatsoever. There have also been experiments with electric anesthesia.

Another technique is cooling of the body, either wholly or in part. In hypothermia, the temperature of the entire body is lowered. The patient is first anesthetized by a general anesthetic and is then placed for about an hour in an ice blanket, through which cold alcohol circulates. At the resulting low temperature, the heart action and other body functions are slowed to a very low rate. Although this has an anesthetic effect, the real purpose is to permit heart and blood vessel operations with greater general safety, and particularly with less danger of hemorrhage.

Similar means are used to lower the temperature of specific parts of the body such as the foot in cases of amputation. A tourniquet is employed to reduce the circulation, and then cold is applied by ice packs or an electrical unit until the operative area is desensitized. This type of local anesthetic is called refrigeration anesthesia and although the idea is not entirely new, it is now being used in new ways.

Recently, interest has been shown in ACUPUNCTURE as a form of anesthesia.

anesthetist (ah-nes′thĕ-tist) a person trained in administering anesthetics.

anesthetization (ah-nes″thĕ-tĭ-za′shun) production of anesthesia.

anethole (an′ĕ-thōl) a colorless or faintly yellow liquid used as a flavoring agent for drugs.

anetoderma (ah-ne″to-der′mah) looseness and atrophy of the skin.

aneuploidy (an″u-ploi′de) the state of having chromosomes in a number that is not an exact multiple of the haploid number. adj., **an′euploid.**

aneurin (ah-nu′rin) thiamine (vitamin B_1).

aneurysm (an′u-rizm) a sac formed by localized dilatation of the walls of a blood vessel, usually an artery. adj., **aneurys′mal.** There are two types of aneurysms: true aneurysm, in which the wall of the sac consists of one or more of the layers that make up the wall of the blood vessel, and false aneurysm, in which all the layers of the vessel are ruptured and the blood is retained by surrounding tissues.

Aneurysms occur when the blood vessel wall becomes weakened, by a physical injury to the vessel, a congenital defect, or a disease. They may occur in any vein or artery, but they most commonly are located in the abdomen or chest. Certain infections may attack and weaken the tissues of the blood vessels; however, atherosclerosis is a common cause. A less common cause is syphilis. A person may have a small aneurysm for years without being aware of it; such aneurysms are often identified only accidentally, on x-ray examination for another purpose. An aneurysm may form a pulsating tumor which can be painful to the sufferer, especially if it is large enough to press against some other organ in the body.

Aneurysms tend to increase in size, and there is a risk of rupture. If rupture occurs in the heart or brain or any other vital organ of the body, the results can be very serious.

Great advances are being made in surgical methods of repairing aneurysms. If an aneurysm occurs in a small blood vessel, the vessel can be tied off and the flow of blood transferred to another vessel. There is also a more complex operation which involves removing the segment of widened blood vessel and replacing it with a plastic graft or an artery or vein from a vascular bank. This is a serious operation, but more physicians are recommending it when there is a danger that the aneurysm may rupture or may produce dangerous effects from blood clots.

arteriovenous a., an abnormal communication between an artery and a vein in which the blood flows directly into a neighboring vein or is carried into the vein by a connecting sac.

atherosclerotic a., one arising as a result of weakening of the tunica media in severe atherosclerosis.

berry a., a small outpouching of the inner lining of a blood vessel, usually at an angle of bifurcation of the cerebral arteries.

cirsoid a., dilatation and tortuous lengthening of part of an artery.

compound a., one in which some of the layers of the wall of the vessel are ruptured and some merely dilated.

dissecting a., one in which rupture of the inner coat has permitted blood to escape between layers of the vessel wall.

fusiform a., a spindle-shaped aneurysm.

mixed a., compound aneurysm.

racemose a., cirsoid aneurysm.

sacculated a., a saclike aneurysm.

varicose a., one formed by rupture of an aneurysm into a vein.

aneurysmectomy (an″u-riz-mek′to-me) excision of an aneurysm.

aneurysmoplasty (an″u-riz′mo-plas″te) plastic repair of an artery for aneurysm.

aneurysmorrhaphy (an″u-riz-mor′ah-fe) suture of an aneurysm.

anfractuous (an-frak′tu-us) convoluted; sinuous.

angi(o)- (an″je-o) word element [Gr.], *vessel* (*channel*).

angiectasis (an″je-ek′tah-sis) dilatation of a vessel. adj., **angiectat′ic.**

angiectomy (an″je-ek′to-me) excision of part of a blood or lymph vessel.

angiitis (an″je-i′tis) inflammation of the coats of a vessel, chiefly blood or lymph vessels.

angina (an′jĭ-nah, an-ji′nah) any disease marked by spasmodic suffocative attacks, especially angina pectoris. adj., **an′ginal.**

agranulocytic a., agranulocytosis.

a. cru′ris, intermittent lameness with cyanosis of the affected limb; due to arterial obstruction.

intestinal a., generalized cramping abdominal pain occurring shortly after a meal and persisting for one to three hours, due to ischemia of the smooth muscle of the bowel.

a. ludovi′ci, Ludwig's a., a. lud′wigi, purulent inflammation around the submaxillary gland (see also LUDWIG'S ANGINA).

a. parotid′ea, mumps.

a. pec′toris, acute pain in the chest resulting from decreased blood supply to the heart muscle. The attacks frequently occur during periods of physical activity or emotional stress which place an added burden on the heart and increase the need for additional blood supply to the myocardium. Some patients can predict the kinds of events which will precipitate an attack while others are unaware of any relationship between the onset of an attack and any particular situation in their lives.

Angina pectoris occurs more frequently in men than in women, and in older than in younger persons. It is not a disease entity but a symptom of an underlying disease of the arteries, especially ATHEROSCLEROSIS and ARTERIOSCLEROSIS.

SYMPTOMS. The chief symptom of angina pectoris is chest pain, usually of an unmistakable nature and readily distinguished by the patient as different from other types of pain which may be caused by indigestion. It is generally described as a feeling of tightness, strangling, heaviness, or suffocation. The pain is usually concentrated on the left side, beginning just under the sternum; it sometimes radiates to the neck, throat, and lower jaw and down the left arm, and, more rarely, to the stomach, back, or across to the right side of the chest.

The pain seldom lasts more than fifteen minutes and is usually relieved by rest and relaxation. If the pain is not relieved in 10 to 15 minutes, the physician should be notified and the patient taken to a hospital with cardiac monitoring equipment. The decreased blood supply to the heart makes it especially vulnerable to arrhythmias and MYOCARDIAL INFARCTION, which can be fatal. About one-half of all those who suffer from angina pectoris die suddenly, while about one-third succumb to a myocardial infarction.

TREATMENT AND PATIENT CARE. Relief from pain by rest and prevention of attacks by avoiding situations which precipitate them are the first steps in the treatment of the patient with angina. In most cases the patients are eager to learn about the disease process causing the pain and want to know how they can participate in control of their attacks.

Several medications bring immediate relief from the pain. Nitroglycerin may be given sublingually in doses of 0.3 to 0.6 mg. Amyl nitrite, which comes in ampules that are broken into a cloth and inhaled, acts more rapidly than nitroglycerin but is less commonly used. Drugs that produce prolonged dilation of the coronary arteries also may be prescribed. Another effective drug is the beta-adrenergic blocking agent propranolol (Inderal), which blocks reflex constriction of the coronary vessels.

Surgical procedures involving arterial transplants are becoming more common as a form of treatment of certain types of ischemic heart disease and resulting angina pectoris. These surgical procedures attempt to bypass the diseased portion of the coronary artery by suturing a vein graft from the aorta to one or more coronary arteries beyond the area of obstruction. In most instances the graft is obtained from the patient's saphenous vein.

An attitude of calmness and efficiency is most important when caring for a person suffering from an attack of angina pectoris. His pain produces emotional reactions and the strongest of these is fear. Most of these patients know that their pain is resulting from an insufficient supply of oxygen to the heart and they frequently have a feeling of impending death. Much anxiety and pain can be eliminated if the patient is assured that someone will stay with him and is reminded that the pain will eventually subside. It usually helps to raise the patient to a sitting position so that he may breathe without difficulty. The prompt administration of nitroglycerin or the specific drug ordered by the physician usually shortens the attack and relieves pain. Above all, the calm presence of someone who knows how to care for him can do much to reassure the patient and help him relax, thus lessening the severity of the attack.

Prinzmetal's a., a variant of angina pectoris in which the attacks occur during rest, exercise capacity is well preserved, and attacks are associated electrocardiographically with elevation of the ST-segment.

variant a., Prinzmetal's angina.

Vincent's a., gingivostomatitis caused by extension to the oral mucosa of necrotizing ulcerative gingivitis (TRENCH MOUTH) (see also VINCENT'S ANGINA).

anginoid (an'jĭ-noid) resembling angina.

anginophobia (an"jĭ-no-fo'be-ah) morbid dread of angina pectoris.

anginose (an'jĭ-nōs) characterized by angina.

angioblast (an'je-o-blast") 1. the earliest formative tissue from which blood cells and blood vessels arise. 2. an individual vessel-forming cell. adj., **angioblast'ic.**

angioblastoma (an"je-o-blas-to'mah) a term applied to certain blood-vessel tumors of the brain: those arising in the cerebellum (cerebellar angioblastoma) may be cystic and associated with von Hippel-Lindau disease; also, a blood-vessel tumor arising from the meninges of the brain or spinal cord (angioblastic meningioma).

angiocardiogram (an"je-o-kar'de-o-gram") the film produced by angiocardiography.

angiocardiography (an"je-o-kar"de-og'rah-fe) roentgenography of the heart and great vessels after introduction of an opaque contrast medium into a blood vessel or one of the cardiac chambers.

angiocardiokinetic (an"je-o-kar"de-o-ki-net'ik) pertaining to movements of the heart and blood vessels.

angiocardiopathy (an"je-o-kar"de-op'ah-the) disease of the heart and blood vessels.

angiocarditis (an"je-o-kar-di'tis) inflammation of the heart and blood vessels.

angioedema (an"je-o-ĕ-de'mah) angioneurotic edema.

angioendothelioma (an"je-o-en"do-the"le-o'mah) hemangioendothelioma.

angiofibroma (an"je-o-fi-bro'mah) angioma containing fibrous tissue.

nasopharyngeal a., a relatively benign tumor of the nasopharynx composed of fibrous connective tissue with abundant endothelium-lined vascular spaces, usually occurring during puberty, most commonly in boys. It is marked by nasal obstruction which may become total, adenoid speech, discomfort in swallowing, and auditory tube obstruction.

angiogenesis (an"je-o-jen'ĕ-sis) the development of blood vessels in the embryo.

angioglioma (an"je-o-gli-o'mah) a form of vascular glioma.

angiogram (an'je-o-gram") a roentgenogram of a blood vessel.

angiography (an"je-og'rah-fe) roentgenography of vessels of the body (arteriography, lymphangiography, or phlebography).

angiohemophilia (an"je-o-he"mo-fil'e-ah) a congenital hemorrhagic diathesis with bleeding from the skin and mucosal surfaces, due to abnormal blood vessels with or without platelet defects or deficiencies of clotting factor VIII or IX. Called also pseudohemophilia and von Willebrand's disease.

angiohyalinosis (an"je-o-hi"ah-lĭ-no'sis) hyaline degeneration of the muscular coat of blood vessels.

angioid (an'je-oid) resembling blood vessels.

angiokeratoma (an"je-o-ker"ah-to'mah) a dermatosis marked by telangiectasia with secondary epithelial changes, including acanthosis and hyperkeratosis.

a. corpo'ris diffu'sum, a hereditary disorder of phospholipid metabolism affecting many of the body systems, chiefly the blood vessels, marked by purpuric cutaneous lesions and associated with cardiovascular disease, renal abnormalities, and hypertension. Called also Fabry's disease or syndrome.

angiokinetic (an"je-o-ki-net'ik) vasomotor.

angiolipoma (an"je-o-lĭ-po'mah) angioma containing fatty tissue.

angiolith (an'je-o-lith") a calcareous deposit in the wall of a blood vessel. adj., **angiolith'ic.**

angiology (an"je-ol'o-je) scientific study or description of the blood and lymph vessels.

angiolupoid (an"je-o-lu'poid) a tuberculous skin lesion consisting of small, oval red plaques, chiefly on the side of the nose.

angiolysis (an"je-ol'ĭ-sis) retrogression or obliteration of blood vessels, as in embryologic development.

angioma (an"je-o'mah) a benign tumor made up of blood (hemangioma) or lymph vessels (lymphangioma). adj., **antiom'atous.**

a. caverno'sum, cavernous a., cavernous HEMANGIOMA.

a. serpigino'sum, a skin disease marked by minute vascular points arranged in rings on the skin.

telangiectatic a., an angioma made up of dilated blood vessels.

angiomatosis (an'je-o-mah-to'sis) the presence of multiple angiomas.

a. of retina, diseased retinal blood vessels with subretinal hemorrhages.

angiomegaly (an"je-o-meg'ah-le) enlargement of blood vessels, especially a condition of the eyelid marked by great increase in its volume.

angiomyolipoma (an"je-o-mi"o-lĭ-po'mah) a benign tumor containing vascular, adipose, and muscle elements, occurring most often in the kidney with smooth muscle elements.

angiomyoma (an"je-o-mi-o'mah) a hamartoma composed of blood vessels and smooth muscle.

angiomyoneuroma (an"je-o-mi"o-nu-ro'mah) glomangioma.

angiomyosarcoma (an"je-o-mi"o-sar-ko'mah) angioma blended with myoma and sarcoma.

angioneurectomy (an"je-o-nu-rek'to-me) excision of vessels and nerves.

angioneuroma (an"je-o-nu-ro'mah) glomangioma.

angioneuromyoma (an"je-o-nu"ro-mi-o'mah) glomangioma.

angioneurosis (an"je-o-nu-ro'sis) any neurosis affecting primarily the blood vessels; a disorder of the vasomotor system, as angioparalysis or angiospasm.

angioneurotic (an"je-o-nu-rot'ik) caused by or of the nature of an angioneurosis.

a. edema, a local condition characterized by the sudden and temporary appearance of large edematous areas (wheals) of the skin and mucous membranes accompanied by intense itching. Occasionally the viscera are involved. Called also angioedema, giant urticaria, and Quincke's disease. It may be an acute or chronic inflammatory reaction and is of allergic, neurotic, or unknown origin. Common causes are food, drugs, insect bites, parasitic infection, and emotional disturbances.

angioparalysis (an″je-o-pah-ral′ĭ-sis) vasomotor paralysis of blood vessels.

angiopathy (an″je-op′ah-the) any disease of the vessels.

angioplasty (an′je-o-plas″te) plastic repair of blood vessels or lymphatic channels.

angiopoiesis (an″je-o-poi-e′sis) the formation of blood vessels. adj., **angiopoiet′ic.**

angiorrhaphy (an″je-or′ah-fe) suture of a blood vessel.

angiosarcoma (an″je-o-sar-ko′mah) a malignant tumor of vascular tissue; called also hemangiosarcoma.

angiosclerosis (an″je-o-sklĕ-ro′sis) hardening of the walls of blood vessels.

angioscotoma (an″je-o-sko-to′mah) a defect in the visual field caused by the shadow of the retinal blood vessels.

angiospasm (an′je-o-spazm″) spasmodic contraction of the walls of a blood vessel. adj., **angiospas′tic.**

angiostrongyliasis (an″je-o-stron″jĭ-li′ah-sis) infection by nematodes of the genus *Angiostrongylus.*

Angiostrongylus (an″je-o-stron′jĭ-lus) a genus of nematode parasites.

A. cantonen′sis, a species reported in cases of human meningoencephalitis in Hawaii and in other areas in the Pacific and in Asia.

A. vaso′rum, a species of worms parastic in the pulmonary arteries of dogs.

angiotelectasis (an″je-o-tel-ek′tah-sis) dilation of blood vessels.

angiotensinase (an″je-o-ten′sĭ-nās) any of a group of peptidases in plasma and tissues that inactivate angiotensin.

angiotensin (an″je-o-ten′sin) a polypeptide formed by action of renin and angiotensinogen in blood plasma. The inactive form, angiotensin I, is in turn acted upon by a peptidase to form angiotensin II, a vasopressor and stimulator of aldosterone secretion by the adrenal cortex.

angiotensinogen (an″je-o-ten′sin-o-jen) a serum α_2-globulin secreted in the liver which, on hydrolysis by renin, gives rise to angiotensin.

angiotomy (an″je-ot′o-me) incision of a blood vessel or lymphatic channel.

angiotonic (an″je-o-ton′ik) increasing vascular tension.

angiotribe (an′je-o-trīb″) a strong forceps for crushing tissue containing an artery, for the purpose of checking hemorrhage.

angiotripsy (an′je-o-trip″se) hemostasis by means of an angiotribe.

angiotrophic (an″je-o-trof′ik) pertaining to the nutrition of vessels.

angle (ang′g'l) the space or figure formed by two diverging lines, measured as the number of degrees one would have to be moved to coincide with the other.

acromial a., that between the head of the humerus and the clavicle.

alpha a., that formed by intersection of the visual axis with the optic axis.

cardiodiaphragmatic a., that formed by the junction of the shadows of the heart and diaphragm in posteroanterior roentgenograms of the heart.

costovertebral a., the angle formed on either side of the vertebral column between the last rib and the lumbar vertebrae.

filtration a., a. of the iris, the angle between the iris and cornea at the periphery of the anterior chamber of the eye, through which the aqueous humor readily permeates.

a. of jaw, the junction of the lower edge with the posterior edge of the lower jaw.

meter a., the angle formed by intersection of the visual axis and the perpendicular bisector of the line joining the centers of rotation of the two eyes when viewing a point one meter distant (small meter angle) or the angle formed by intersection of the visual axes of the two eyes in the midline at a distance of one meter (large meter angle).

optic a., visual angle.

a. of pubis, that between the pubic bones at the symphysis.

sternoclavicular a., that between the sternum and the clavicle.

visual a., the angle between two lines passing from the extremities of an object seen, through the nodal point of the eye, to the corresponding extremities of the image of the object seen.

Angle's classification (ang′elz) a classification of dental MALOCLUSION based on mesiodistal (anteroposterior) position of the mandibular dental arch and teeth relative to the maxillary dental arch and teeth.

angstrom (ang′strom) the unit of wavelength, equivalent to 0.1 millimiçron (10^{-7} mm. or 10^{-10} meters); abbreviated A or Å.

angulation (ang″gu-la′shun) the formation of a sharp obstructive angle as in the intestine, the ureter, or similar tubes.

angulus (ang′gu-lus), pl. *an′guli* [L.] angle; used in names of anatomic structures or landmarks.

anhedonia (an″he-do′ne-ah) inability to experience pleasure.

anhidrosis (an″hĭ-dro′sis) absence of sweating.

anhidrotic (an″hĭ-drot′ik) 1. checking the flow of sweat. 2. an agent that suppresses perspiration.

anhydrase (an-hi′drās) an enzyme that catalyzes the removal of water from a compound.

carbonic a., an enzyme that catalyzes the decomposition of carbonic acid into carbon dioxide and water, facilitating transfer of carbon dioxide from tissues to blood and from blood to alveolar air.

anhydration (an″hi-dra′shun) the condition of not being hydrated.

anhydremia (an″hi-dre′me-ah) diminution of the fluid content of the blood.

anhydride (an-hi′drīd) a compound derived from an acid by removal of a molecule of water.

anhydrous (an-hi′drus) containing no water.

anideus (ah-nid′e-us) a parasitic fetus consisting of a shapeless mass of flesh.

anidrosis (an″ĭ-dro′sis) anhidrosis.

anileridine (an″ĭ-ler′ĭ-dēn) a compound used as a narcotic, analgesic, or sedative.

aniline (an′ĭ-lēn) an oily liquid from coal tar and indigo or prepared by reducing nitrobenzene; the parent substance of colors or dyes derived from coal tar. It is an important cause of serious industrial poisoning associated with bone marrow depression as well as methemoglobinemia.

anilism (an'ĭ-lizm) aniline poisoning.

anility (ah-nil'ĭ-te) the state of being like an old woman.

anima (an'ĭ-mah) 1. the soul. 2. Jung's term for the unconscious, or inner being, of the individual, as opposed to the personality he presents to the world (persona). In psychoanalysis, the more feminine soul or inner being of a man (see also ANIMUS.)

animal (an'ĭ-mal) 1. a living organism having sensation and the power of voluntary movement and requiring for its existence oxygen and organic food. 2. of or pertaining to such an organism.

a. bite, a wound caused by the bite of an animal (see also BITE).

control a., an untreated animal otherwise identical in all respects to one that is used for purposes of experiment; used for checking results of treatment.

animalcule (an"ĭ-mal'kūl) a minute animal organism.

animation (an"ĭ-ma'shun) the quality of being full of life.

suspended a., temporary suspension or cessation of the vital functions.

animus (an'ĭ-mus) in psychoanalysis, the more male soul or inner being of a woman (see also ANIMA).

anion (an'i-on) an ion carrying a negative charge; the element that in electrolysis passes to the positive pole.

anion-exchange resin ion-exchange resin.

aniridia (an"ĭ-rid'e-ah) congenital absence of the iris.

anis(o)- (an-i'so) word element [Gr.], *unequal.*

aniseikonia (an"ĭ-si-ko'ne-ah) inequality of the retinal images of the two eyes.

anisindione (an"is-in-de'ōn) an anticoagulant.

anisochromatic (an-i"so-kro-mat'ik) not of the same color throughout.

anisocoria (an-i"so-ko're-ah) inequality in size of the pupils of the eyes.

anisocytosis (an-i"so-si-to'sis) the presence in the blood of erythrocytes showing abnormal variations in size.

anisokaryosis (an-i"so-kar"e-o'sis) inequality in the size of the nuclei of cells.

anisomastia (an-i"so-mas'te-ah) inequality in size of the breasts.

anisometropia (an-i"so-mĕ-tro'pe-ah) inequality in the refractive power of the two eyes, of considerable degree. adj., **anisometrop'ic.**

anisopiesis (an-i"so-pi-e'sis) difference in blood pressure recorded in corresponding arteries on the right and left sides of the body.

anisosthenic (an-i"sos-then'ik) not having equal power; said of muscles.

anisotonic (an-i"so-ton'ik) 1. varying in tonicity or tension. 2. having different osmotic pressure; not isotonic.

anisotropic (an-i"so-trop'ik) 1. having unlike properties in different directions. 2. doubly refracting, or having a double polarizing power.

anisotropy (an"i-sot'ro-pe) the quality of being anisotropic.

anisuria (an"i-su're-ah) alternating oliguria and polyuria.

ankle (ang'k'l) the part of the leg just above the foot; the joint between the leg and the foot. The ankle joint is a hinge joint and is formed by the junction of the tibia and fibula with the talus, or ankle bone. The bones are cushioned by cartilage and connected by a number of ligaments, tendons, and muscles that strengthen the joint and enable it to be moved.

Because it is in almost constant use, the ankle is particularly susceptible to injuries, such as SPRAIN and FRACTURE. It is also often one of the first joints to be affected by ARTHRITIS or GOUT.

Edema or swelling of the tissues around the ankles is a fairly common occurrence in overweight people and pregnant women and is usually relieved by elevating the feet. It may, however, be a symptom of serious heart or renal disease.

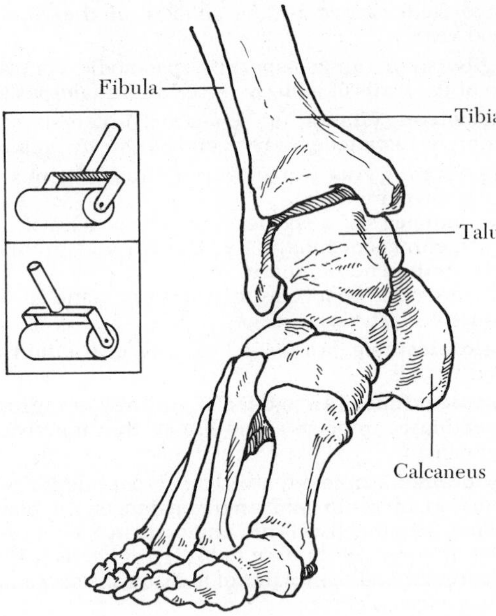

Ankle.

a. jerk, plantar extension of the foot elicited by a tap on the Achilles tendon, preferably while the patient kneels on a bed or chair, the feet hanging free over the edge; called also Achilles reflex and triceps surae reflex.

ankyl(o)- (ang'kĭ-lo) word element [Gr.], *bent; crooked; in the form of a loop; adhesion.*

ankyloblepharon (ang"kĭ-lo-blef'ah-ron) adhesion of the eyelids to each other.

ankylocheilia (ang"kĭ-lo-ki'le-ah) adhesion of the lips to each other.

ankyloglossia (ang"kĭ-lo-glos'e-ah) tongue-tie; abnormal shortness of the frenulum of the tongue, resulting in limitation of its motion.

a. superior, extensive adhesion of the tongue to the palate.

ankylopoietic (ang"kĭ-lo-poi-et'ik) producing ankylosis.

ankylosed (ang'kĭ-lōsd) affected with ankylosis.

ankylosis (ang"kĭ-lo'sis) abnormal immobility and consolidation of a joint. adj., **ankylot'ic.** Ankylosis may be caused by destruction of the membranes that line the joint or by faulty bone structure. It is most often a result of chronic rheumatoid arthritis, in which the affected joint tends to assume the least painful position and may become more or less permanently fixed in it.

Artificial ankylosis (arthrodesis), locking of a joint by surgical operation, is sometimes done in treatment of a severe joint condition.

bony a., union of the bones of a joint by proliferation of bone cells, resulting in complete immobility.

extracapsular a., that caused by rigidity of surrounding parts.

false a., fibrous a., reduced joint mobility due to proliferation of fibrous tissue.

intracapsular a., that caused by rigidity of structures within the joint.

spurious a., extracapsular ankylosis.

true a., bony ankylosis.

ankylotia (ang″kĭ-lo′she-ah) closure of the external meatus of the ear.

ankyroid (ang′kĭ-roid) hooklike.

anlage (ahn′lah-geh), pl. *anla′gen* [Ger.] primordium.

anneal (ah-nēl′) to soften a material, as a metal, by controlled heating and cooling, to make its manipulation easier.

annectent (ah-nek′tent) connecting; joining together.

Annelida (ah-nel′ĭ-dah) a phylum of metazoan invertebrates, the segmented worms, including leeches.

annular (an′u-lar) ring-shaped.

annulorrhaphy (an″u-lor′ah-fe) suture of a hernial ring or sac.

annulus (an′u-lus), pl. *an′nuli* [L.] a small ring or encircling structure; also spelled anulus.

anococcygeal (a″no-kok-sij′e-al) pertaining to the anus and coccyx.

anode (an′ōd) the positive electrode or pole to which negative ions are attracted. adj., **ano′dal.**

anodontia (an″o-don′she-ah) congenital absence of some or all of the teeth.

anodyne (an′o-dīn) 1. relieving pain. 2. a medicine that eases pain.

anodynia (an″o-din′e-ah) freedom from pain.

anoia (ah-noi′ah) idiocy.

anomalopia (ah-nom″ah-lo′pe-ah) a slight anomaly of color vision.

anomaloscope (ah-nom′ah-lo-skōp″) an apparatus used to detect anomalies of color vision.

anomaly (ah-nom′ah-le) marked deviation from normal. adj., **anom′alous.**

developmental a., absence, deformity, or excess of body parts as the result of faulty development of the embryo.

anomia (ah-no′me-ah) loss of power of naming objects or of recognizing names.

anonychia (an″o-nik′e-ah) absence of the nails.

Anopheles (ah-nof′ĕ-lēz) a widely distributed genus of mosquitoes, comprising over 300 species, many of which are important vectors of MALARIA.

anophthalmia, anophthalmos (an″of-thal′me-ah; an″of-thal′mos) a developmental anomaly marked by complete absence of one or both eyes or the presence of rudimentary eyes.

anoplasty (a′no-plas″te) plastic repair of the anus.

anopsia (an-op′se-ah) 1. nonuse or suppression of vision in one eye. 2. hypertropia.

anorchid (an-or′kid) a person with no testes or with cryptorchidism (undescended testes).

anorchidism, anorchism (an-or′kĭ-dizm; an-or′kizm) congenital absence of one or both testes.

anorectic (an″o-rek′tik) 1. pertaining to anorexia. 2. an agent that diminishes the appetite for food.

anorectum (a″no-rek′tum) the distal portion of the digestive tract, including the entire anal canal and the distal 2 cm. of the rectum. adj., **anorec′tal.**

anorexia (an″o-rek′se-ah) lack or loss of appetite for food. APPETITE is psychologic, dependent on memory and associations, as compared with hunger, which is physiologically aroused by the body's need for food. Anorexia can be brought about by unattractive food, surroundings, or company.

a. nervo′sa, loss of appetite due to emotional states, such as anxiety, irritation, anger, and fear. In true anorexia nervosa there is no real loss of appetite, but rather a refusal to eat or an aberration in eating patterns; hence, the term anorexia is probably a misnomer. The condition should be differentiated from restricted food intake such as that occurring in various psychiatric disorders.

The syndrome was first described more than 100 years ago and was once thought to be exceedingly rare. It is rapidly increasing throughout the world in developed countries as diverse as Russia, Japan, Australia, and the United States. The condition occurs mainly in girls around the age of puberty, and the prevalence may be as high as one in a hundred.

CAUSE. The cause of anorexia nervosa is unknown, but it is generally thought to be a disorder of psychologic origins. These patients have delusions of proportion in body image; that is, they tend to overestimate the width of their own bodies, seeing themselves as wider and fatter than they really are. Starvation is self-imposed to reduce body size, and although the patient is skeleton-like in appearance, she vigorously defends her condition as not too thin.

There is some evidence that anorexia nervosa is a hypothalamic disorder owing to the fact that during the course of the disease gonadotropins are not released from the anterior pituitary, there is a drop in the ovarian production of estrogens, and ovulation fails to occur. These conditions often persist long after the nutritional status has been improved. In some cases menstruation ceases *before* the weight loss occurs. These factors indicate that the endocrine disturbance is not simply a sequel to malnutrition. In males there is a corresponding endocrine disorder with a drop in the level of gonadotropins and testosterone in the blood.

SYMPTOMS. Manifestations of anorexia nervosa, other than those previously mentioned, include signs of psychological maladjustment. There may be a history of difficulty in making friends, fear of meeting strangers, and changes in temperament consisting of irritability and depression.

The refusal to eat leads to malnutrition that may last for months or years. The diet often is limited to small amounts of fruits and vegetables and on some days only black coffee is taken. On occasion the fasting period may be alternated with eating sprees, usually at night, after which the patient forces herself to vomit.

Most patients resist their parents' suggestions that they see a physician, insisting that they are not ill, in spite of progressive malnutrition and emaciation.

TREATMENT. The treatment of anorexia nervosa is difficult and lengthy. The primary goals are restitution of normal nutrition and resolution of the underlying psychological problems. Hospital admission may be necessary to avoid serious complications from malnutrition and electrolyte imbalance, but it should not be compulsory except as a last resort because, ultimately, success of treatment depends on the patient's cooperation.

Weight gain alone cannot be considered a sign of true progress. Relapses requiring readmission to the hospital occur in about half the cases. Psychotherapy utilizing techniques of behavior modification is employed to correct the emotional problems underlying the condition. Family counseling and therapy are sometimes helpful in resolving familial conflicts that may have contributed to the development of the disorder.

anorexic (an″o-rek′sik) anorectic.

anorexigenic (an″o-rek″sĭ-jen′ik) 1. producing anorexia. 2. an agent that diminishes or controls the appetite.

anorthography (an″or-thog′rah-fe) loss of the ability to write.

anorthopia (an″or-tho′pe-ah) asymmetrical or distorted vision.

anorthosis (an″or-tho′sis) absence of penile erectility.

anoscope (a′no-skōp) a speculum or endoscope used in direct visual examination of the anal canal.

anoscopy (a-nos′ko-pe) examination of the anal canal with an anoscope.

anosigmoidoscopy (a″no-sig-moi″dos′ko-pe) endoscopic examination of the anus and sigmoid.

anosmia (an-oz′me-ah) absence of the sense of smell. adj., **anosmat′ic, anos′mic.**

anosognosia (an″o-sog-no′ze-ah) failure to recognize one's own disease or defect.

anospinal (a″no-spi′nal) pertaining to the anus and spinal cord.

anostosis (an″os-to′sis) defective formation of bone.

anotia (an-o′she-ah) congenital absence of the external ears.

anovaginal (a″no-vaj′ĭ-nal) pertaining to or communicating with the anus and vagina.

anovarism (an-o′var-izm) absence of the ovaries.

anovesical (a″no-ves′ĭ-kal) pertaining to the anus and bladder.

anovular, anovulatory (an-ov′u-lar), (an-ov′u-lah-tor″e) not associated with ovulation.

anoxemia (an″ok-se′me-ah) lack of sufficient oxygen in the blood. adj., **anoxe′mic.**

anoxia (an-ok′se-ah) absence or deficiency of oxygen, as reduction of oxygen in body tissues below physiologic levels. The condition is accompanied by deep respirations, cyanosis, increased pulse rate, and impairment of coordination. adj., **anox′ic.**

anemic a., reduction of oxygen in body tissues because of diminished oxygen-carrying capacity of the blood.

anoxic a., reduction of oxygen in body tissues due to interference with the oxygen supply.

histotoxic a., condition resulting from diminished ability of cells to utilize available oxygen.

stagnant a., condition due to interference with the flow of blood and its transport of oxygen.

ansa (an′sah), pl. *an′sae* [L.] a looplike structure.

a. cervica′lis, a nerve loop in the neck attached in front and above to the hypoglossal nerve and behind to the upper cervical spinal nerves. Its hypoglossal attachment is misleading since this part of the loop ultimately rejoins the upper spinal nerves.

a. of Henle, Henle's loop.

a. hypoglos′si, ansa cervicalis.

a. lenticula′ris, a small nerve fiber tract arising in the globus pallidus and joining the anterior part of the ventral thalamic nucleus.

an′sae nervo′rum spina′lium, loops of spinal nerves joining the anterior spinal nerves.

a. peduncula′ris, a complex grouping of nerve fibers connecting the amygdaloid nucleus, piriform area, and anterior hypothalamus, and various thalamic nuclei.

Ansolysen (an″so-li′sen) trademark for preparation of pentolinium tartrate, used as an antihypertensive.

Anspor (an′spōr) trademark for preparations of cephradine, a cephalosporin antibiotic.

Antabuse (an′tah-būs) trademark for a preparation of disulfiram, used in the treatment of alcoholism.

antacid (ant-as′id) 1. counteracting acidity. 2. an agent that counteracts acidity. Substances that act as antacids include sodium bicarbonate, aluminum hydroxide gel, magnesium hydroxide, magnesium trisilicate, magnesium oxide, and calcium carbonate. They are often used in the treatment of peptic ULCER.

antagonist (an-tag′o-nist) 1. a muscle that counteracts the action of another muscle, its agonist. 2. a substance that tends to nullify the action of another, as of an enzyme, hormone, or drug. 3. a tooth in one jaw that articulates with one in the other jaw.

antarthritic (ant″ar-thrit′ik) 1. alleviating arthritis. 2. an agent that alleviates arthritis.

antazoline hydrochloride (ant-az′o-lēn) a drug that blocks the action of histamine, which is present in large amounts in individuals who are hypersensitive and suffering from various allergies. The drug relieves the symptoms of itching, nasal and conjunctival edema and inflammation, and urticaria of skin allergies. Another antazoline compound is antazoline phosphate, which is also an antihistamine.

Both drugs are likely to produce drowsiness, excessive dryness of the mouth and throat, lassitude, and other side effects of an antihistaminic drug. They are available in tablet form and in a 0.5 per cent solution to be used as eye drops or in a nebulizer.

ante (an′te) [L.] preposition, *before.*

ante- word element [L.], *before* (in time or space).

antebrachium (an″te-bra′ke-um) the forearm. adj., **antebra′chial.**

antecedent (an″te-se′dent) a precursor.

plasma thromboplastic a., PTA; clotting factor XI.

antecurvature (an″te-kur′vah-tūr) a slight anteflexion.

antefebrile (an″te-feb′ril) preceding fever.

anteflexion (an″te-flek′shun) the bending of an organ so that its top is thrust forward.

ante mortem (an′te mor′tem) [L.] before death.

antemortem (an″te-mor′tem) performed or occurring before death.

antenna (an-ten'ah) one of the appendages on the head of arthropods.

Antepar (an'te-par) trademark for preparations of piperazine citrate and piperazine phosphate, anthelmintics.

antepartal (an"te-par'tal) occurring before childbirth.

ante partum (an'te par'tum) [L.] before parturition.

antepartum (an"te-par'tum) performed or occurring before parturition.

antephase (an'te-fāz) the portion of interphase immediately preceding mitosis (or meiosis), when energy is being produced and stored for mitosis (or meiosis) and chromosome reproduction is taking place.

antepyretic (an"te-pi-ret'ik) occurring before the stage of fever.

anterior (an-tēr'e-or) situated at or directed toward the front; opposite of posterior.

a. chamber, the part of the aqueous humor–containing space of the eyeball between the cornea and the iris.

antero- (an'ter-o) word element [L.], *anterior; in front of.*

anterograde (an'ter-o-grād") extending or moving forward.

anteroinferior (an"ter-o-in-fēr'e-or) situated in front and below.

anterolateral (an"ter-o-lat'er-al) situated in front and to one side.

anteromedian (an"ter-o-me'de-an) situated in front and on the midline.

anteroposterior (an"ter-o-pos-tēr'e-or) directed from the front toward the back.

anterosuperior (an"ter-o-su-pēr'e-or) situated in front and above.

anteversion (an"te-ver'zhun) the tipping forward of an entire organ.

anteverted (an"te-vert'ed) tipped or bent forward.

anthelix (ant'he-liks) the semicircular ridge on the ear anterior and parallel to the helix.

anthelmintic (ant"hel-min'tik) 1. destructive to worms. 2. an agent destructive to worms. Examples of anthelmintic drugs include: piperazine and hexylresorcinol for the treatment of the roundworm *Ascaris lumbricoides;* quinacrine hydrochloride and aspidium oleoresin for the treatment of tapeworms; and oxytetracycline hydrochloride and emetine hydrochloride for protozoan infection such as amebic dysentery. The newer drug mebendazole is effective against a variety of intestinal worms.

Many anthelmintic drugs are toxic and should be given with care. The toxic effects of a specific drug should be known prior to administration and the patient observed carefully for these effects after the drug is given.

anthelone (ant-he'lon) see ENTEROGASTRONE (anthelone E) and UROGASTRONE (anthelone U).

anthocyanin (an"tho-si'ah-nin) any of a class of glycoside pigments of blue, red, and violet flowers.

anthracene (an'thrah-sēn) a crystalline hydrocarbon, $C_{14}H_{10}$, from coal tar.

anthracoid (an'thrah-koid) resembling anthrax.

anthracometer (an"thrah-kom'ĕ-ter) an instrument for measuring carbon dioxide in the air.

anthracosilicosis (an"thrah-ko-sil"ĭ-ko'sis) a lung disease due to inhalation of coal dust (anthracosis) and fine particles of silica (silicosis).

anthrocosis (an"thrah-ko'sis) a lung disease due to inhalation of coal dust not containing silica (see also PNEUMOCONIOSIS).

anthralin (an'thrah-lin) a yellowish brown cyrstalline powder used topically in eczema and psoriasis.

anthramycin (an"thrah-mi'sin) an antibiotic having antineoplastic activity, produced by *Streptomyces refuineus.*

anthraquinone (an"thrah-kwin'ōn) a yellow substance from anthracene, used in the manufacture of certain dyes.

anthrax (an'thraks) an infectious disease of cattle, horses, mules, sheep, and goats, due to ingestion of spores of *Bacillus anthracis;* sometimes acquired by man through contact with infected animals or their byproducts, such as carcasses or skins.

Anthrax in humans usually occurs as a malignant pustule or malignant edema of the skin. In rare instances it can affect the lungs if the spores of the bacillus are inhaled, or it can involve the intestinal tract when infected meat is eaten. The condition often is accompanied by hemorrhage, as the exotoxins from the bacillus attack the endothelium of small blood vessels. The condition is treated by the use of antibiotics such as penicillin, the tetracyclines, and chloramphenicol. The disorder is also known by a variety of names, including woolsorters' disease, ragpickers' disease, and charbon.

cutaneous a., anthrax due to lodgment of the causative organisms in wounds or abrasions of the skin, producing a black crusted pustule on a broad zone of edema.

pulmonary a., infection of the respiratory tract resulting from inhalation of dust or animal hair containing spores of *Bacillus anthracis;* an occupational disease usually affecting those who handle and sort wools and fleeces (woolsorters' disease).

anthropo- (an'thro-po) word element [Gr.], *man (human being).*

anthropocentric (an"thro-po-sen'trik) with a human bias; considering man the center of the universe.

anthropoid (an'thro-poid) resembling man; the anthropoid apes are tailless apes, including the chimpanzee, gibbon, gorilla, and orang-utan.

Anthropoidea (an"thro-poi'de-ah) a suborder of Primates, including monkeys, apes, and man, characterized by a larger and more complicated brain than the other suborders.

anthropology (an"thro-pol'o-je) the science that treats of man, his origins, historical and cultural development, and races.

criminal a., that branch of anthropology that treats of criminals and crimes.

cultural a., that branch of anthropology that treats of man in relation to his fellows and to his environment.

physical a., that branch of anthropology which treats of the physical characteristics of man.

anthropometer (an"thro-pom'e-ter) an instrument especially designed for measuring various dimensions of the body.

anthropometry (an"thro-pom'e-tre) the science that deals with the measurement of the size, weight, and proportions of the human body. adj., **anthropomet′ric.**

anthropomorphism (an″thro-po-mor′fizm) the attribution of human characteristics to nonhuman objects.

anthropophilic (an″thro-po-fil′ik) preferring human beings to animals; said of certain mosquitoes.

anthropophobia (an″thro-po″fo′be-ah) morbid dread of society.

anthropozoonosis (an″thro-po-zo″o-no′sis) a disease of either animals or man that may be transmitted from one species to the other.

anti- (an′ti, an′te) word element [Gr.], *counteracting; effective against.*

antiadrenergic (an″te-ah″dren-er″jik) 1. sympatholytic: opposing the effects of impulses conveyed by adrenergic postganglionic fibers of the sympathetic nervous system. 2. an antiadrenergic agent.

antiagglutinin (an″te-ah-gloo′tĭ-nin) a substance that opposes the action of an agglutinin.

antialexin (an″te-ah-lek′sin) a substance that opposes the action of alexin (complement).

antiamebic (an″te-ah-me′bik) 1. destroying or suppressing the growth of amebas. 2. an agent that destroys or suppresses the growth of amebas.

antianaphylaxis (an″te-an″ah-fi-lak′sis) a condition in which the anaphylaxis reaction does not occur because of free antigens in the blood; the state of desensitization to antigens.

antiandrogen (an″te-an′dro-jen) any substance capable of inhibiting the biological effects of androgenic hormones.

antianemic (an″te-ah-ne′mik) counteracting anemia.

antiantibody (an″te-an′tĭ-bod″e) a substance that counteracts the effect of an antibody.

antiarrhythmic (an″te-ah-rith′mik) 1. preventing or alleviating cardiac arrhythmias. 2. an agent that prevents or alleviates cardiac arrhythmias.

antiarthritic (an″te-ar-thrit′ik) 1. effective in treatment of arthritis. 2. an agent used in treatment of arthritis.

antibacterial (an″tĭ-bak-te′re-al) 1. destroying or suppressing the growth or reproduction of bacteria. 2. an agent having such properties.

antibechic (an″tĭ-bek′ik) 1. relieving cough. 2. an agent that relieves cough.

antibiosis (an″tĭ-bi-o′sis) an association between two populations of organisms that is detrimental to one of them.

antibiotic (an″tĭ-bi-ot′ik) a chemical compound produced by and obtained from certain living cells, especially bacteria, yeasts, and molds, or an equivalent synthetic compound, which is antagonistic to some other form of life, especially pathogenic or noxious organisms. Their action is biostatic or biocidal.

Penicillin, the first widely used antibiotic, was accidentally discovered in 1929 by Sir Alexander Fleming when bacteria in a laboratory dish were killed by mold spores floating in the air. In World War II it prevented many deaths from wound infection and disease. When penicillin was found to be ineffective against many types of disease, especially those caused by viruses, worldwide search in soil and other natural sources yielded new medicines such as chlortetracycline hydrochloride (Aureomycin), chloramphenicol and oxytetracycline (Terramycin), called the broad-spectrum antibiotics because they are effective against a wide range of bacterial infections, and also some viruses. Some antibiotics are now produced synthetically.

The antibiotics have now largely controlled pneumonia, mastoiditis, and peritonitis, have reduced the danger of many other diseases, and are frequently used to prevent infection in surgery and injury. They are powerful substances and should never be used except under a physician's care. Unless an antibiotic is properly prescribed, pathogenic organisms can develop resistance to the drug, and then the value of this weapon against disease is destroyed.

antibiotin (an″tĭ-bi′o-tin) avidin, a protein that renders biotin inactive.

antiblennorrhagic (an″tĭ-blen″o-raj′ik) 1. preventing or relieving gonorrhea. 2. an agent that prevents or relieves gonorrhea.

antibody (an′tĭ-bod″e) a modified soluble protein (an immunoglobulin molecule) having a specific amino acid sequence, which property gives each antibody the ability to adhere to and interact only with the ANTIGEN that induced its synthesis. This antigen-specific property of the antibody is the basis of the antigen-antibody reaction that is essential to an immune response. The antigen-antibody reaction begins as soon as substances interpreted as foreign invaders gain entrance into the body. (See also IMMUNITY.)

Antibodies, also called immune bodies, are synthesized by the plasma cells formed when antigen-specific groups (*clones*) of B-lymphocytes respond to the presence of antigen. The developmental process of antibody production begins when stem cells are transformed into B-lymphocytes, so called because they resemble the bursa-derived lymphocytes of birds. This transformation usually is completed a few months after birth, at which time the lymphocytes migrate to lymphoid tissue primarily located in the lymph nodes, but also found in the spleen, gastrointestinal tract, and bone marrow. Hence it is the lymphocyte that functions as the prime mover in antibody formation.

Antibody production, its interaction with a specific antigen, and the activation of complement (C), an interrelated group of eleven proteins, are the major components of the *humoral* system of IMMUNITY. Fortunately, the immune response of antibody and complement can be transferred passively from one individual to another, as, for example, the transfer of maternal antibody across the placental barrier to the fetus, who has not yet developed a mature immune system.

Antibodies are classified according to their mode of action as they react to and set about defending the body against foreign invaders. Some cause clumping together of bacterial cells (agglutination) and are called *agglutinins.* Agglutination also takes place when blood cells of one type are mixed with those of a different type. Those antibodies which cause bacterial cells to dissolve or liquefy are called *bacteriolysins.* This activity is assisted by COMPLEMENT, which interacts with the antigen-antibody complex in such a way that the cell ruptures and there is dissolution (*lysis*) of the cell body. *Opsonins* coat the outside of bacteria making them more attractive to phagocytes. Other types of antibodies include those which neutralize the toxins of antigens (*antitoxins*), and those which cause precipitation of antigens in a fluid medium (*precipitins*). (See also IMMUNOGLOBULIN.)

anaphylactic a., a substance formed as a result of the first injection of a foreign anaphylactogen and responsible for the anaphylactic symptoms following the second injection of the same anaphylactogen.

blocking a., an antibody which possesses the same specificity as one from another source and interferes with the reactivity of the other by combining with available epitopes of homologous specificity.

complete a., Wiener's term for the Rh antibody that is capable of directly agglutinating Rh-positive erythrocytes in physiologic saline, and implying that the antibody is multivalent, that is, possesses two or more reactive groups. The definition may be extended to include a number of other globulins with similar agglutinating, but not necessarily type-specific, features.

cross-reacting a., one that combines with an antigen other than the one that induced its production.

cytotropic a., any of a class of antibodies that attach to tissue cells (such as mast cells and basophils) through their Fc segments to induce the release of histamine and other vasoconstrictive amines important in immediate hypersensitivity reactions. In man, this antibody, also known as *reagin,* is of the immunoglobulin class known as IgE. Called also cytophilic antigen.

incomplete a., 1. an antibody which combines with antigen without producing an observable reaction (i.e., without precipitation); such antibodies are present in serum of patients with asthma, hay fever, eczema, and similar allergic diseases and are called *reagins* in these conditions. 2. a gamma globulin, described earlier as a univalent antibody combining specifically with Rh-positive erythrocytes without causing visible agglutination, but which, in the presence of antihuman globulin (Coombs) serum or high molecular weight media, e.g., albumin, will cause red cell clumping. Other red cell coating proteins, not group specific, may demonstrate similar properties.

natural a's, serum proteins present in low titer with the structural properties of immunoglobulins, which can react specifically with their antigens, even though the individuals in which they have formed have had no known previous exposure to those antigens. They may result from unknown exposure to naturally occurring antigens, e.g., food and bacterial flora.

neutralizing a., one that reduces or destroys infectivity of a homologous infectious agent by partial or complete destruction of the agent.

protective a., one responsible for immunity to an infectious agent, observed in passive immunity.

Rh a's, those directed against Rh antigen(s) of human erythrocytes. Not normally present, they may be produced when Rh-negative persons receive Rh-positive blood by transfusion or when an Rh-negative person is pregnant with an Rh-positive fetus.

antibrachium (an″tĭ-bra′ke-um) antebrachium, or forearm.

anticariogenic (an″tĭ-kār″e-o-jen′ik) effective in suppressing caries production.

anticholagogue (an″tĭ-ko′lah-gog) an agent that inhibits secretion of bile. adj., **anticholagog′ic.**

anticholinergic (an″tĭ-ko″lin-er′jik) blocking the

passage of impulses through the parasympathetic nerves; parasympatholytic.

anticholinesterase (an″tĭ-ko″lin-es′ter-ās) a substance that inhibits the action of cholinesterase.

anticoagulant (an″tĭ-ko-ag′u-lant) 1. serving to prevent the coagulation of blood. 2. any substance that, *in vivo* or *in vitro,* suppresses, delays, or nullifies coagulation of the blood.

Anticoagulant therapy often is employed in the treatment of patients in which thromboembolism exists or threatens, as in cases of acute thrombophlebitis, myocardial infarction, cardiac failure, cardiac surgery, and major fractures.

Anticoagulant agents include those drugs that interfere with the formation of clots (*antithrombotics*), for example, heparin and the coumarin compounds, and those that are capable of disintegrating thrombi that have already formed (*thrombolytics*), for example, streptokinase and urokinase. A third group of anticoagulant agents, the anti-platelet–aggregating agents, are currently under investigation in the hope that they will prove effective in preventing a primary step in the formation of thrombi, that is, the clumping together of platelets. These agents are classified as *antithrombocytics* and are not to be confused with or used as a substitute for other types of anticoagulants.

PATIENT CARE. The major difficulties that may arise during the course of anticoagulant therapy are hemorrhage and drug interaction. Obervation of the patient for early signs of internal as well as external spontaneous bleeding is of primary importance. Health care personnel responsible for the care of these patients must be knowledgeable about the various laboratory tests and interpretation of their results in the administration of anticoagulant drugs and assessment of the patient.

The effects of anticoagulants can be enhanced or inhibited by a variety of drugs and chemical compounds, especially the salicylates, barbiturates, and antibiotics. Ambulatory patients must be cautioned against taking any other drugs in combination with an anticoagulant agent without first consulting with the physician who prescribed the drug. This includes nonprescription or "over-the-counter" drugs as well as prescription drugs. Dietary restrictions such as fasting diets or those that limit the intake or utilization of the fat-soluble vitamin K can result in increased pharmacologic action of an anticoagulant.

The patient and his family should be given adequate instruction in the purposes of anticoagulant therapy, the effects and side effects of other drugs and dietary intake on anticoagulant agents, and the need for regular contact with members of the health care team so that adequate monitoring of the patient's status can be continued as long as he is receiving an anticoagulant.

anticoagulin (an″tĭ-ko-ag′u-lin) a substance that suppresses, delays, or nullifies coagulation of the blood.

anticodon (an″tĭ-ko′don) a triplet of nucleotides in transfer RNA that is complementary to the codon in messenger RNA which specifies the amino acid.

anticomplement (an″tĭ-kom′plĕ-ment) a substance that counteracts a complement.

anticonvulsant (an″tĭ-kon-vul′sant) 1. inhibiting convulsions. 2. an agent that suppresses convulsions. Drugs that act as anticonvulsants include diphenylhydantoin (Dilantin), mephenytoin (Mesantoin), and trimethadione (Tridione). They are used in the treatment of epilepsy and in psychomotor and myoclonic seizures.

anticus (an-ti′kus) anterior.

anticytolysin (an″tĭ-si-tol′ĭ-sin) a substance that counteracts cytolysin.

anticytotoxin (an″tĭ-si″to-tok′sin) a substance that counteracts cytotoxin.

antidepressant (an″tĭ-de-pres′ant) 1. effective against depressive illness. 2. an agent that is effective against depressive psychologic illness. The many antidepressant drugs used in the treatment of the various psychologic depressions include amitriptyline (Elavil), desipramine hydrochloride (Norpramin, Pertofrane), imipramine hydrochloride (Tofranil), isocarboxazid (Marplan), and nialamide (Niamid).

antidiarrheal (an″tĭ-di″ah-re′al) 1. counteracting diarrhea. 2. an agent that counteracts diarrhea.

antidinic (an″tĭ-din′ik) relieving giddiness or vertigo.

antidiuresis (an″tĭ-di″u-re′sis) the suppression of secretion of urine by the kidneys.

antidiuretic (an″tĭ-di″u-ret′ik) 1. pertaining to or causing suppression of urine. 2. an agent that causes suppression of urine.

a. hormone, vasopressin; a hormone that suppresses the excretion of urine; it has a specific effect on the epithelial cells of the renal tubules, stimulating the reabsorption of water independently of solids, and resulting in concentration of urine. Stored and released by the posterior lobe of the PITUITARY GLAND, it also has vasopressor activity. Abbreviated ADH.

antidote (an′tĭ-dōt) an agent that counteracts a poison. adj., **antido′tal.**

chemical a., one that neutralizes the poison by changing its chemical nature.

mechanical a., one that prevents absorption of the poison.

physiologic a., one that counteracts the effects of the poison by producing opposing effects.

universal a., a mixture formerly recommended as an antidote when the exact poison is not known. There is, in fact, no known universal antidote. Activated charcoal is now being used for many poisons.

antidromic (an″tĭ-drom′ik) conducting impulses in a direction opposite to the normal.

antidysenteric (an″tĭ-dis″en-ter′ik) counteracting dysentery.

antiemetic (an″te-e-met′ik) 1. useful in the treatment of vomiting. 2. an agent that relieves vomiting.

antienzyme (an″te-en′zīm) a substance that prevents or retards enzyme activity.

antiepileptic (an″te-ep″ĭ-lep′tik) 1. combating epilepsy. 2. a remedy for epilepsy.

entiepithelial (an″te-ep″ĭ-the′le-al) destructive to epithelial cells.

antiestrogen (an″te-es′tro-jen) any agent that inhibits the biological effects of estrogen.

antifebrile (an″tĭ-feb′ril) counteracting fever.

antifibrinolysin (an″tĭ-fi″brĭ-nol′ĭ-sin) antiplasmin.

antifibrinolytic (an″tĭ-fi″brĭ-no-lit′ik) inhibiting fibrinolysis.

antifungal (an″tĭ-fung′gal) 1. destructive to or checking the growth of fungi. 2. an agent that destroys or checks the growth of fungi.

antigalactic (an″tĭ-gah-lak′tik) 1. diminishing the secretion of milk. 2. an agent that so acts.

antigen (an′tĭ-jen) any substance which is capable, under appropriate conditions, of inducing the formation of ANTIBODY and of reacting specifically in some detectable manner with the antibody so induced. adj., **antigen′ic.** Antigens may be soluble substances, such as toxins and foreign proteins, or particulate, such as bacteria and tissue cells. Human cells that may function as antigens include those of another individual, as in blood transfusions of an incompatible blood type, organ transplants, and grafts. Or, they may be cells that arise within the host, such as malignant cells and cells that are not recognized as "self," as in AUTOIMMUNE DISEASE. (See also IMMUNITY.)

Au a., Australian a., an antigen found in the sera of patients with acute serum hepatitis and rarely in patients with infectious hepatitis; it is also found in the sera of large numbers of apparently normal people in the tropics and southeast Asia. So named because it was first detected in the serum of an Australian aborigine.

flagellar a., H antigen.

Forssman a., a heterogenetic antigen inducing the production of antisheep hemolysin, occurring in various unrelated species, mainly in the organs but not in the erythrocytes (guinea pig, horse), but sometimes only in the erythrocytes (sheep), and occasionally in both (chicken).

H a., (Ger. *Hauch,* film), the antigen that occurs in the flagella of motile bacteria.

heterogenetic a., heterophil a., one capable of stimulating the production of antibodies that react with tissues from other animals or even plants.

HL-A a's, histocompatibility antigens on the surface of nucleated cells determined by a single major chromosomal locus, the HL-A locus; they are important in cross-matching for transplantation procedures.

O a. (Ger. *ohne Hauch,* without film), the antigen that occurs in the bodies of bacteria.

partial a., an antigen that does not produce antibody formation, but gives specific precipitation when mixed with the antibacterial immune serum.

V a., Vi a., an antigen contained in the sheath of a bacterium, as *Salmonella typhosa* (the typhoid bacillus), and thought to contribute to its virulence.

antigenemia (an″tĭ-jĕ-ne′me-ah) the presence of antigens in the blood.

antigenicity (an″tĭ-jĕ-nis′ĭ-te) ability of a substance to stimulate antibody formation.

antihelix (an″tĭ-he′liks) anthelix.

antihelmintic (an″tĭ-hel-min′tik) anthelmintic.

antihemolysin (an″tĭ-he-mol′ĭ-sin) a substance that counteracts hemolysin.

antihemophilic (an″tĭ-he″mo-fil′ik) 1. effective against the bleeding tendency in hemophilia. 2. an agent that counteracts the bleeding tendency in hemophilia.

a. factor, AHF, one of the clotting factors, deficiency of which causes classic, sex-linked hemophilia; called also factor VIII and antihemophilic globulin. It is available in a preparation for preventive and therapeutic use.

antihemorrhagic (an″tĭ-hem″o-raj′ik) 1. exerting a hemostatic effect and counteracting hemorrhage. 2. an agent that prevents or checks hemorrhage.

antihistamine (an″tĭ-his′tah-min) a drug that counteracts the effects of histamine, a normal body chemical that is believed to cause the symptoms of persons who are hypersensitive to various allergens. Antihistamines are used to relieve the symptoms of allergic reactions, especially hay fever and other allergic disorders of the nasal passages. Some antihistamines have an antinauseant action that is useful in the relief of motion sickness. Others have a sedative and hypnotic action and may be used as tranquilizers.

Patients for whom an antihistamine has been prescribed should be warned of the side effects of these drugs, including drowsiness, dizziness, and muscular weakness. These side effects present a special hazard in driving an automobile or operating heavy machinery. Other side effects include dryness of the mouth and throat and insomnia.

antihistaminic (an″tĭ-his″tah-min′ik) 1. counteracting the pharmacologic effects of histamine. 2. an antihistamine.

antihormone (an″tĭ-hōr′mōn) a substance that counteracts a hormone.

antihypercholesterolemic (an″tĭ-hi″per-ko-les′-ter-ol-e″mik) 1. effective against hypercholesterolemia. 2. an agent that prevents or relieves hypercholesterolemia.

antihypertensive (an″tĭ-hi″per-ten′siv) 1. effective against hypertension. 2. an agent that reduces high blood pressure.

anti-immune (an″te-ĭ-mūn′) preventing immunity.

anti-infective (an″te-in-fek′tiv) 1. counteracting infection. 2. a substance that counteracts infection.

anti-inflammatory (an″te-in-flam′ah-to-re) 1. counteracting or suppressing inflammation. 2. an agent that so acts.

antiketogenesis (an″tĭ-ke″to-jen′ĕ-sis) inhibition of the formation of ketone bodies.

antiketogenic (an″tĭ-ke″to-jen′ik) preventing or suppressing the development of ketones (ketone bodies) and thus preventing development of ketosis.

antilewisite (an″tĭ-lu′ĭ-sīt) dimercaprol, a chelating agent used in poisoning with arsenic, gold, and mercury.

antilithic (an″tĭ-lith′ik) 1. preventing calculus formation. 2. an agent that prevents calculus formation.

antilysin (an″tĭ-li′sin) an antibody that inactivates a lysin.

antimalarial (an″tĭ-mah-la′re-al) 1. therapeutically effective against malaria. 2. an agent that is therapeutically effective against malaria.

antimere (an′tĭ-mēr) one of the segments of the body bounded by planes at right angles to the long axis of the body.

antimetabolite (an″tĭ-mĕ-tab′o-līt) a substance bearing a close structural resemblance to one required for normal physiological functioning, and exerting its effect by interfering with the utilization of the essential metabolite.

antimetropia (an″tĭ-mĕ-tro′pe-ah) hyperopia of one eye, with myopia in the other.

antimongoloid (an″tĭ-mon′go-loid) opposite to that characteristic of Down's syndrome (mongolism), e.g., antimongoloid slant of the palpebral fissures.

antimony (an′tĭ-mo″ne) a chemical element, atomic number 51, atomic weight 121.75, symbol Sb. (See table of ELEMENTS.) Antimony compounds are used in medicine as anti-infective agents in the treatment of tropical diseases, especially those of protozoan origin. All antimony compounds are potentially poisonous and must be used with caution. adj., **antimo′nial.**

a. potassium tartrate, a compound used in treatment of parasitic infections, e.g., schistosomiasis or leishmaniasis.

antimorphic (an″tĭ-mor′fik) in genetics, antagonizing or inhibiting normal activity (antimorphic mutant gene).

antimycotic (an″tĭ-mi-kot′ik) destructive to fungi.

antinarcotic (an″tĭ-nar-kot′ik) relieving narcotic depression.

antinauseant (an″tĭ-naw′se-ant) 1. counteracting nausea. 2. an agent that counteracts nausea.

antineoplastic (an″tĭ-ne″o-plas′ik) 1. inhibiting the maturation and proliferation of malignant cells. 2. an agent having such properties.

a. therapy, a regimen of treatment aimed at destruction of malignant cells and utilizing a variety of chemical agents that directly affect cellular growth and development. Antineoplastic therapy is but one of a variety of methods available in the treatment of CANCER. Chemotherapy is especially successful in curing choriocarcinoma, a highly malignant form of cancer that originates in the placenta, and Burkitt's lymphoma, a malignancy common among African children. Combinations of drugs have successfully controlled acute LEUKEMIA in children and in persons with advanced stages of Hodgkin's disease.

TYPES OF ANTINEOPLASTIC AGENTS. The chemicals and drugs used in the treatment of cancer may be divided into three groups. The first group, the *alkylating* agents are capable of damaging the DNA of cells, thereby interfering with the process of replication. Among these drugs are chlorambucil (Leukeran), cyclophosphamide (Cytoxan, Endotoxan), mechlorethamine nitrogen mustard (Mustargen, HN2), and triethylene thiophosphamide (thiotepa). The antibiotic actinomycin D is also included in this group.

The second type of drugs used in cancer chemotherapy is comprised of the *antimetabolites.* As the name suggests, these drugs interfere with the cancer cell's metabolism. Some replace essential metabolites without performing their function, while others compete with essential components by mimicking their functions and thereby inhibiting the manufacture of protein in the cell. Included in this group are cytosine arabinoside (Ara-C, Cytosar), flouridine (FUDR), fluorouracil (5-FU, and Efudex, which is for external use), mercaptopurine, methotrexate, and thioguanine.

The third group of chemicals employed in the treatment of cancer are "*natural products*" that directly affect the mechanism of cell division. The plant alkaloids, for example, vincristine and vinblastine, stop cell division at metaphase (a subphase in cell mitosis). The enzymes, for example, L-asparaginase, starve tumor cells by catabolizing substances (e.g., asparagine) which they need for survival. Hormones change cell metabolism by making the cellular environment unfavorable for growth of certain tumors.

Patient Care. The drugs used in antineoplastic therapy are highly toxic and likely to produce troublesome and sometimes extremely dangerous reactions. They may be given singly or in combination, depending on the type of malignancy and the stage of its development. The complexity of this type of therapy, particularly when used in conjunction with surgery or radiation therapy, demands a team of specialists, including radiotherapists, nurse clinicians, and clinical pharmacologists, working cooperatively to accomplish the goals of the prescribed regimen.

It is especially important that members of the team be aware of and capable of dealing with the toxicity inherent in antineoplastic therapy. The management of drug toxicities requires a delicate balance between effective dosage to destroy malignant cells and the individual patient's tolerance of drug and dosage. Anorexia, nausea, and vomiting are among the milder but more troublesome effects of antibiotics, alkylating agents, and antimetabolites. It is necessary to work with each patient and help him establish a routine that will incorporate administration of the drug, taking an antiemetic, and spacing meals so that adequate nutrition is provided and excessive weight loss is avoided. STOMATITIS and DIARRHEA are also likely to appear as early signs of toxicity from antimetabolic and antibiotic drug therapy.

Drugs that suppress bone marrow function produce leukopenia, which in turn increases susceptibility to infection. If the patient is also receiving an immunosuppressant such as prednisone, his resistance to infection is further compromised. He will need adequate rest, good nutrition, good habits of personal cleanliness, and avoidance of contact with persons who have infectious diseases. If an infection does develop, it should receive prompt attention to minimize its effects and inhibit its progress. It may be necessary to alter the dosage of the antineoplastic drug until the infection subsides.

Bone marrow-suppressing drugs can also affect the platelet count, reducing it to a level at which bleeding can readily occur. Normal clotting is impaired by some cancer therapeutic agents and there is therefore the danger of internal bleeding anywhere in the body. Should the situation become severe, the drug dosage may need to be reduced or stopped altogether and platelet transfusions may be given.

Hormonal therapy frequently is accompanied by fluid retention. Measurement of intake and output, daily weight measurement, and observation for signs of surface edema or congestive heart failure are essential parts of patient care. Care of the patient with EDEMA must include meticulous skin care. If DIURETICS are given, the patient must be watched for signs of potassium depletion. Another side-effect of hormonal therapy may be changes in secondary sexual characteristics. These can be particularly embarrassing and emotionally disturbing to the patient.

Neurologic disorders may result from treatment with the plant alkaloids. These conditions may manifest themselves as impaired sensation, loss of coordination, and severe constipation. Although these neurological effects usually are reversible, especially if caught in the early stages, it may take months for the nerve cells to recover and resume normal function.

As research in antineoplastic therapy continues it is expected that newer, less hazardous and more effective chemical agents will be developed. Many drugs now available are still in the investigational stage and must be approved by a human experimentation committee before they can be used in an accredited hospital. Drugs that are investigational are monitored by the Cooperative Clinical Cancer Research Program of the National Cancer Institute. Any person involved in the implementation of antineoplastic therapy should be aware of the status of the drugs being administered. It is also imperative that one read current literature and attend educational activities that are planned to keep practitioners abreast of the latest developments in this method of cancer therapy.

antinephritic (an″tĭ-nĕ-frit′ik) effective against nephritis.

antineuralgic (an″tĭ-nu-ral′jik) relieving neuralgia.

antineuritic (an″tĭ-nu-rit′ik) relieving neuritis.

antinion (an-tin′e-on) the frontal pole of the head.

antiovulatory (an″te-ov′u-lah-to″re) suppressing ovulation.

antioxidant (an″te-ok′sĭ-dant) a substance that in small amount will inhibit the oxidation of other compounds.

antioxidation (an″te-ok″sĭ-da′shun) prevention of oxidation.

antiparasitic (an″tĭ-par″ah-sit′ik) 1. destroying parasites. 2. an agent that destroys parasites.

antipediculotic (an″tĭ-pĕ-dik″u-lot′ik) 1. effective against lice and in treatment of pediculosis. 2. an agent that is effective against lice.

antipepsin (an″tĭ-pep′sin) an antienzyme that counteracts pepsin.

antiperistalsis (an″tĭ-per″ĭ-stal′sis) upward waves of contraction sometimes occurring normally in the lower ileum, competing with the normal downward peristalsis and retarding passage of intestinal contents into the cecum. adj., **antiperistal′tic.**

antiplasmin (an″tĭ-plaz′min) a principle in the blood that inhibits plasmin.

antiplastic (an″tĭ-plas′tik) unfavorable to healing.

antiprotease (an″tĭ-pro′te-ās) a substance that checks the proteolytic action of enzymes.

antiprothrombin (an″tĭ-pro-throm′bin) a substance that retards the conversion of prothrombin into thrombin.

antipruritic (an″tĭ-proo-rit′ik) 1. preventing or relieving itching. 2. an agent that counteracts itching.

antipyretic (an″tĭ-pi-ret′ik) 1. effective against fever. 2. an agent that relieves fever. Cold packs, aspirin, and quinine are all antipyretics. Antipyretic drugs dilate the blood vessels near the surface of the skin, thereby allowing more blood to flow through the skin, where it can be cooled by the air. Also, an antipyretic can increase perspiration, the evaporation of which cools the body.

antipyrine (an″tĭ-pi′rēn) a crystalline analgesic and antipyretic compound.

antipyrotic (an″tĭ-pi-rot′ik) 1. effective in the treatment of burns. 2. an agent used in the treatment of burns.

antirachitic (an″tĭ-rah-kit′ik) therapeutically effective against rickets.

antirheumatic (an″tĭ-roo-mat′ik) counteracting rheumatism.

antirickettsial (an″tĭ-rĭ-ket′se-al) 1. effective against rickettsiae. 2. an agent effective against rickettsiae.

antiscabietic (an″tĭ-ska″be-et′ik) 1. effective against scabies. 2. an agent effective against scabies.

antiscorbutic (an″tĭ-skor-bu′tik) 1. preventing or relieving scurvy. 2. an agent that prevents or cures scurvy.

antisepsis (an″tĭ-sep′sis) prevention of sepsis by destruction of microorganisms and infective matter.

antiseptic (an″tĭ-sep′tik) 1. preventing sepsis. 2. any substance that inhibits the growth of bacteria, in contrast to a germicide, which kills bacteria outright. Antiseptics are not considered to include antibiotics, which are usually taken internally. The term antiseptic includes disinfectants, although most disinfectants are too strong to be applied to body tissue and are generally used to clean inanimate objects such as floors and bathroom fixtures.

Antiseptics are divided into two types: physical and chemical. The most important physical antiseptic is heat, applied by boiling, autoclaving, flaming, or burning. These are among the oldest and most effective methods of disinfecting contaminated objects, water, and food.

Antiseptics have many applications. They are used in treating wounds and infections, in sterilizing, as before an operation, and in general hygiene. Antiseptics also have an application in the preservation of food and in the purification of sewage. The wide variety of antiseptics, their strength and the speed at which they work are all factors that influence the choice of which one to use for a specific job.

urinary a., a drug that is excreted mainly by way of the urine and performs its antiseptic action in the bladder. These drugs may be given before examination of or operation on the urinary tract, and they are sometimes used to treat urinary tract infections.

antiserum (an″tĭ-se′rum) a serum containing antibodies. It may be obtained from an animal that has been subjected to the action of antigen either by injection into the tissues or blood or by infection. (See also IMMUNITY and IMMUNIZATION.)

antisialagogue (an″tĭ-si-al′ah-gog) an agent that inhibits the flow of saliva.

antisialic (an″tĭ-si-al′ik) checking the flow of saliva.

antispasmodic (an″tĭ-spaz-mod′ik) 1. preventing or relieving spasms. 2. an agent that prevents or relieves spasms.

Antistine (an-tis′tin) trademark for preparations of antazoline, an antihistamine.

antistreptococcic (an″tĭ-strep″to-kok′sik) counteracting streptococcal infection.

antisudorific (an″tĭ-soo″dor-if′ik) 1. inhibiting perspiration. 2. an agent that inhibits perspiration.

antisyphilitic (an″tĭ-sif″ĭ-lit′ik) 1. counteracting syphilis. 2. a remedy for syphilis.

antithenar (an″tĭ-the′nar) placed opposite to the palm or sole.

antithrombin (an″tĭ-throm′bin) any naturally occurring or therapeutically administered substance that neutralizes the action of thrombin and thus limits or restricts blood coagulation.

antithrombocytic (an″tĭ-throm″bo-sit′ik) 1. preventing the aggregation of blood platelets (thrombocytes). 2. an antithrombocytic agent.

antithromboplastin (an″tĭ-throm″bo-plas′tin) any agent or substance that prevents or interferes with the interaction of blood clotting factors as they generate prothrombinase (thromboplastin).

antithrombotic (an″tĭ-throm-bot′ik) 1. preventing or interfering with the formation of thrombi. 2. an agent that interferes with thrombus formation.

antithyroid (an″tĭ-thi′roid) suppressing thyroid activity.

antitoxin (an″tĭ-tok′sin) a particular kind of ANTIBODY produced in the body in response to the presence of a toxin (see also IMMUNITY). adj., **antitox′ic.**

diphtheria a., preparation from the blood serum or plasma of healthy animals immunized against diphtheria toxin, used as a passive immunizing agent.

gas gangrene a., a sterile solution of antitoxic substances from blood of healthy animals immunized against gas-producing organisms of the genus *Clostridium.*

scarlet fever streptococcus a., sterile solution of antitoxic substances from blood serum of healthy animals immunized against toxin produced by the streptococcus causing scarlet fever.

tetanus a., preparation from the blood serum or plasma of healthy animals immunized against tetanus toxin, used as a passive immunizing agent.

antitragus (an″tĭ-tra′gus) a projection on the ear opposite the tragus.

antitrope (an′tĭ-trōp) one of two structures that are similar but oppositely oriented, like a right and a left glove.

antitrypsin (an″tĭ-trip′sin) an antienzyme counteracting the action of trypsin. adj., **antitryp′tic.**

antituberculotic (an″tĭ-tu-ber″ku-lot′ik) counteracting tuberculosis.

antitussive (an″tĭ-tus′iv) 1. effective against cough. 2. an agent that suppresses coughing.

antivenereal (an″tĭ-vĕ-ne′re-al) counteracting venereal disease.

antivenin (an″tĭ-ven′in) a material used to neutralize the venom of a poisonous animal.

black widow spider a., an antitoxin to the venom of a black widow spider (*Latrodectus mactans*).

a. (Crotalidae) polyvalent, a preparation containing globulins effective in neutralizing venoms of most pit vipers (rattlesnake, copperhead, water moccasin, fer-de-lance) throughout the world.

antiviral (an″tĭ-vi′ral) 1. effective against viruses. 2. an agent effective against viruses.

antivitamin (an″tĭ-vi′tah-min) a substance that inactivates a vitamin.

antixerotic (an″tĭ-ze-rot′ik) preventing dryness.

antr(o)- (an′tro) word element [L.], *chamber; cavity;* often used with specific reference to the maxillary antrum or sinus.

antrectomy (an-trek′to-me) excision of an antrum.

Antrenyl (an′trĕ-nil) trademark for a preparation of oxyphenonium, an anticholinergic.

antritis (an-tri′tis) inflammation of an antrum, especially of the antrum of Highmore (maxillary sinus).

antroatticotomy (an″tro-at″ĭ-kot′o-me) atticoantrotomy.

antrocele (an′tro-sēl) accumulation of fluid in the maxillary antrum (sinus).

antronasal (an″tro-na′zal) pertaining to the maxillary antrum (sinus) and nasal fossa.

antroscope (an′tro-skōp) an instrument for inspecting the maxillary antrum (sinus).

antrostomy (an-tros′to-me) incision of an antrum with drainage.

antrotomy (an-trot′o-me) incision of an antrum.

antrotympanic (an″tro-tim-pan′ik) pertaining to the tympanic (mastoid) antrum and tympanum.

antrum (an′trum) pl. *an′tra* [L.] a cavity or chamber. adj., **an′tral.**

a. of Highmore, maxillary sinus.

mastoid a., an air space in the mastoid portion of the temporal bone communicating with the middle ear and the mastoid cells.

a. maxilla′re, maxillary a., maxillary sinus.

pyloric a., a. pylor′icum, the proximal, expanded portion of the pyloric part of the stomach.

tympanic a., a. tympan′icum, mastoid antrum.

Anturane (an′tu-rān) trademark for a preparation of sulfinpyrazone, a uricosuric agent used in the management of gout.

anuclear (a-nu′kle-ar) having no nucleus.

anulus (an′u-lus) pl. *an′uli* [L.] alternate spelling of *annulus;* used in names of certain ringlike or encircling structures of the body.

anuresis (an″u-re′sis) 1. retention of urine in the bladder. 2. anuria. adj., **anuret′ic.**

anuria (ah-nu′re-ah) complete suppression of urine formation by the kidney. adj., **anu′ric.**

anus (a′nus) the opening of the rectum on the body surface.

imperforate a., congenital absence of the normal opening of the rectum.

anvil (an′vil) incus; the middle of the three bones of the ear.

anxiety (ang-zi′ĕ-te) a feeling of uneasiness, apprehension, or dread. This may be rational, such as the anxiety about making good in a new job, about one's own or someone else's illness, about passing an examination or about moving to a new community. People also feel realistic anxiety about world dangers, such as the possiblity of nuclear war, and about social and economic changes that may affect their livelihood or way of living. Modern mass communications tend to intensify normal anxieties about large issues by dramatizing minor incidents as though they were major crises.

A certain amount of unrealistic and irrational anxiety also is part of most people's experience. Some degree of generalized anxiety seems to be an unavoidable part of the human personality, since life is full of uncertainties and human beings have an awareness of past and future. Certain periods of life also generate increased anxiety; adolescence and middle age are especially anxious times for many. Persons who spend much of their time alone are likely to suffer more anxiety than those who live and work with others.

Most persons find healthy ways to deal with their normal quota of anxiety. They seek out friends and interesting activities; they take their minds off their own anxious feelings by listening to and doing things for other people. The enjoyment of art, music, and literature, especially when it is shared, is an antidote to anxiety. The physical activity of games and sports, preferably with companions and out of doors, is one of the best antidotes. A good walk often dissipates an anxious mood.

Overindulgence in alcohol does not alleviate anxiety but only makes it worse. When a cause of anxiety is real, then the healthy step is to take realistic measures against it; for example, a real anxiety about money should be dealt with by improving money management or income or both.

When anxiety is chronic and not traceable to any specific cause, or when it interferes with normal activity, then it is neurotic, and the sufferer is in need of some wholesome self-examination and possible expert help.

Anxiety that needs attention can often be readily recognized by family or friends or by the family physician. Parents should be alert to symptoms of anxiety in their children. For instance, a child may develop compulsive habits, like overeating, or he may lose his appetite for no apparent reason. He may seem to want to spend an abnormal amount of time on his own; he may have difficulty with his schoolwork, or he may develop frequent headaches or stomachaches as a result of anxiety about school or friends. In a younger child, excessive thumbsucking or an unusual attachment to a particular plaything can sometimes be a sign of the kind of anxiety that needs professional help. Any important change in a young child's life, such as moving to a new home or the illness or absence of a parent, can give rise to behavior problems stemming from anxiety. Similarly in adults, insomnia, recurrent headaches, or the development of compulsive habits may be signs of chronic anxiety.

Whether it is purely psychologic or arises from a real situation, severe anxiety can often be controlled by the proper use of medications, such as tranquilizers, under a physician's care. PSYCHOTHERAPY is frequently the most effective method to relieve cases of chronic anxiety.

a.-equivalent, translation of anxiety into a kind of emotional activity, e.g., the experiencing or expression of angry feelings.

free-floating a., fear in the absence of known cause for anxiety.

a. neurosis, a neurosis characterized by anxiety or extreme fear without apparent cause. Anxiety is regarded as pathologic when the individual cannot control his emotions and the anxiety interferes with effectiveness in living and the achievement of desired goals or satisfactions. The neurosis may be manifest as organic pain or physical illness.

separation a., apprehension due to removal of significant persons or familiar surroundings, common in infants 6 to 10 months old.

aorta (a-or′tah) pl. *aor′tae, aor′tas* [Gr.] the great artery arising from the left ventricle, being the main trunk from which the systemic arterial system proceeds. (See Table of ARTERIES for parts of aorta, and see also CIRCULATORY SYSTEM.)

overriding a., a congenital anomaly occurring in tetralogy of Fallot, in which the aorta is displaced to the right so that it appears to arise from both ventricles and straddles the ventricular septal defect.

aortalgia (a″or-tal′je-ah) pain in the region of the aorta.

aortic (a-or′tik) pertaining to the aorta.

a. arch syndrome, any of a group of disorders leading to occlusion of the arteries arising from the aortic arch; such occlusion may be caused by atherosclerosis, arterial embolism, etc. (See also PULSELESS DISEASE.)

a. bodies, small neurovascular structures on either side of the aorta in the region of the aortic arch, containing chemoreceptors that play a role in reflex regulation of respiration.

a. septal defect, a congenital anomaly in which there is abnormal communication between the ascending aorta and the pulmonary artery just above the semilunar valves.

a. valve, a semilunar valve that guards the orifice between the left ventricle and the aorta.

aortitis (a″or-ti′tis) inflammation of the aorta.

aortogram (a-or′to-gram) the film produced by aortography.

aortography (a″or-tog′rah-fe) roentgenography of the aorta after introduction into it of a contrast material.

aortopathy (a″or-top′ah-the) any disease of the aorta.

aortorrhaphy (a″or-tor′ah-fe) suture of the aorta.

aortosclerosis (a-or″to-sklĕ-ro′sis) sclerosis of the aorta.

aortostenosis (a-or″to-stĕ-no′sis) narrowing of the aorta.

aortotomy (a″or-tot′o-me) incision of the aorta.

Apamide (ap′ah-mīd) trademark for a preparation of acetaminophen, an analgesic and antipyretic.

apancreatic (ah-pan″kre-at′ik) due to absence of the pancreas.

aparalytic (ah″par-ah-lit′ik) characterized by absence of paralysis.

apathic (ah-path′ik) without sensation or feeling.

apathism (ap′ah-thizm) slowness of response to stimuli.

apathy (ah′pah-the) reactive absence of emotions. adj., **apathet′ic.**

APC abbreviation for acetylsalicylic acid, acetophenetidin, and caffeine, used as an analgesic or antipyretic.

APE anterior pituitary extract.

aperient (ah-pe′re-ent) 1. mildly cathartic. 2. a gentle purgative.

aperistalsis (ah″per-ĭ-stal′sis) absence of peristaltic action.

apertura (ap″er-tu′rah) pl. *apertu′rae* [L.] aperture.

aperture (ap′er-chūr) an opening.

numerical a., an expression of the measure of efficiency of a microscope objective.

apex (a′peks) pl. *a′pices* [L.] the pointed end of a cone-shaped part. adj., **ap′ical.**

root a., the terminal end of the root of the tooth.

Apgar Score (ap′gar) a method for determining an infant's condition at birth by scoring the heart rate, respiratory effort, muscle tone, reflex irritability, and color. The infant is rated from 0 to 2 on each of the five items, the highest possible score being 10. Each of the factors is rated 60 seconds after birth and again five minutes later. The Apgar Score is useful as a predictive measure of neonatal difficulties. It is estimated that of the infants with scores of 2 or less at birth, 78 per cent will not survive the neonatal period; of those with scores of 8 or greater, only about 1 per cent will die in the first 28 days of life.

A.P.H.A. American Public Health Association.

aphagia (ah-fa′je-ah) loss of the power of swallowing.

aphakia (ah-fa′ke-ah) absence of the lens of an eye, occurring congenitally or as a result of trauma or surgery. adj., **apha′kic.**

aphalangia (ah″fah-lan′je-ah) absence of fingers or toes.

aphasia (ah-fa′ze-ah) defect or loss of the power of expression by speech, writing, or signs, or of comprehension of spoken or written language, due to disease or injury of the brain centers. adj., **apha′sic.**

amnestic a., anomic aphasia.

anomic a., amnestic or nominal aphasia; inability to name objects, qualities, or conditions.

ataxic a., expressive aphasia.

auditory a., loss of ability to comprehend spoken language; word deafness.

Broca's a., expressive aphasia.

conduction a., aphasia due to a lesion of the pathway between the sensory and motor speech centers.

expressive a., that in which the patient understands written and spoken words and knows what he wants to say, but cannot utter the words. Called also ataxic, Broca's, or motor aphasia.

fluent a., that in which speech is well articulated and grammatically correct but is lacking in content.

global a., total aphasia involving all the functions that go to make up speech and communication.

jargon a., paraphasia; aphasia characterized by utterance of meaningless phrases.

mixed a., combined expressive and receptive aphasia.

motor a., expressive aphasia.

nominal a., anomic aphasia.

nonfluent a., that in which little speech is produced and is uttered slowly, with great effort and poor articulation; due to a lesion in Broca's area.

receptive a., inability to understand written, spoken, or tactile speech symbols.

sensory a., receptive aphasia.

visual a., loss of ability to comprehend written language.

aphasiologist (ah-fa″ze-ol′o-jist) a specialist in aphasiology.

aphasiology (ah-fa″ze-ol′o-je) scientific study of aphasia and specific neurologic lesions producing it.

aphemia (ah-fe′me-ah) loss of the power of speech due to a central lesion.

aphonia (a-fo′ne-ah) loss of the voice; inability to produce vocal sounds.

a. clerico′rum, loss of the voice from overuse, as by clergymen.

aphonic (a-fon′ik) 1. pertaining to aphonia. 2. without audible sound.

aphose (ah′fōz) any subjective visual sensation due to absence or interruption of light sensation.

aphrasia (ah-fra′ze-ah) inability to speak.

aphrenia (ah-fre′ne-ah) dementia.

aphrodisiac (af″ro-diz′e-ak) 1. arousing sexual desire. 2. a drug that arouses sexual desire.

aphtha (af′thah), pl. *aph′thae* [L.] (usually plural) small ulcers, especially the whitish or reddish spots in the mouth characteristic of aphthous stomatitis. adj., **aph′thous.**

aphthosis (af-tho'sis) a condition marked by presence of aphthae.

aphylaxis (ah"fi-lak'sis) absence of phylaxis or immunity. adj., **aphylac'tic.**

apical (ap'ĭ-kal) pertaining to an apex.

apicectomy (a"pĭ-sek'to-me) excision of the apex of the petrous portion of the temporal bone.

apicitis (a"pĭ-si'tis) inflammation of the apex of the lung or of the root of a tooth.

apicoectomy (a"pĭ-ko-ek'to-me) excision of the apical portion of the root of a tooth through an opening in overlying tissues of the jaw.

apicolysis (a"pĭ-kol'ĭ-sis) surgical collapse of the apex of the lung to obliterate the apical cavity.

A.P.L. trademark for a preparation of human chorionic gonadotropin.

aplacental (a"plah-sen'tal) having no placenta.

aplanatic (ap"lah-nat'ik) correcting or not affected by spherical aberration.

aplasia (ah-pla'ze-ah) defective development or complete absence of an organ due to failure of development of the embryonic primordium.

aplastic (a-plas'tik) pertaining to or characterized by aplasia; having no tendency to develop into new tissue.

a. anemia, the medical name given to anemia caused by disease of the bone marrow, which produces most of the blood cells. In addition to the usual symptoms of anemia, there is frequently bleeding from the nose and mouth and "black and blue" spots on the skin.

Aplastic anemia may be caused by a tumor or cancer of the bone marrow, or by destruction of the bone marrow by other agents, including excessive radiation, some antibiotics, sulfonamides, phenylbutazone, mephytoin, insecticides or weed killers, benzene, certain hair dyes, and medicines containing heavy metals such as gold, mercury, and bismuth. The physician will question the patient very closely about possible contact with such substances, since determining the cause of the disorder may be crucial in treating it.

Aplastic anemia is serious, and should be treated in a hospital. The most effective treatment is removal of the cause, if possible. Regular transfusions of blood are almost always necessary. In some cases, injections of cortisone have appeared to relieve the condition.

Individual cases of aplastic anemia vary a great deal, and may respond to treatment so successfully that transfusions can be stopped. Generally, however, the outlook for a patient with aplastic anemia is not good, although better than was thought in the past.

See ANEMIA for patient care.

apnea (ap'ne-ah) 1. temporary cessation of breathing. 2. asphyxia. adj., **apne'ic.**

apneumia (ap-nu'me-ah) congenital absence of the lungs.

apneusis (ap-nu'sis) sustained inspiratory effort, even to the point of asphyxia. adj., **apneu'stic.**

apo- word element [Gr.], *away from; separated.*

apochromatic (ap"o-kro-mat'ik) free from chromatic aberration.

apocrine (ap'o-krin) denoting that type of glandular secretion in which the secretory products become concentrated at the free end of the secreting cell and are thrown off, along with the portion of the cell where they have accumulated, as in the mammary gland; cf. holocrine and merocrine.

apodia (ah-po'de-ah) congenital absence of the feet.

apoenzyme (ap"o-en'zīm) the protein component of an enzyme that requires the presence of the prosthetic group (coenzyme) to form the functioning enzyme.

apoferritin (ap"o-fer'ĭ-tin) a colorless protein occurring in the mucosal cells of the small intestine, forming a compound with iron called ferritin.

apogee (ap'o-je) the state of greatest severity of a disease.

apolar (ah-po'lar) having neither poles nor processes; without polarity.

apomorphine (ap"o-mor'fēn) an alkaloid from morphine.

a. hydrochloride, a crystalline alkaloid that is a prompt and effective emetic; used to induce vomiting in certain kinds of poisoning.

aponeurectomy (ap"o-nu-rek'to-me) excision of an aponeurosis.

aponeurorrhaphy (ap"o-nu-ror'ah-fe) suture of an aponeurosis.

aponeurosis (ap"o-nu-ro'sis), pl. *aponeuro'ses* [Gr.] a sheetlike tendinous expansion, mainly serving to connect a muscle with the parts it moves. adj., **aponeurot'ic.**

aponeurositis (ap"o-nu-ro-si'tis) inflammation of an aponeurosis.

aponeurotomy (ap"o-nu-rot'o-me) incision of an aponeurosis.

apophyseal (ap"o-fiz'e-al) pertaining to an apophysis.

apophysis (ah-pof'ĭ-sis), pl. *apoph'yses* [Gr.] any outgrowth or swelling, especially a bony outgrowth that has never been entirely separated from the bone of which it forms a part, such as a process, tubercle, or tuberosity.

apophysitis (ah-pof"ĭ-si'tis) inflammation of an apophysis.

apoplectiform, apoplectoid (ap"o-plek'tĭ-form; ap"o-plek'toid) resembling apoplexy.

apoplexy (ap'o-plek"se) copious extravasation of blood into an organ; often used alone to designate such extravasations into the brain (cerebral apoplexy) after rupture of an intracranial blood vessel; stroke. The term is extended by some to include occlusive cerebrovascular lesions. (See also CEREBRAL VASCULAR ACCIDENT.) adj., **apoplec'tic.**

aporepressor (ap"o-re-pres'or) a repressor that is inactive until it combines with a corepressor.

apostasis (ah-pos'tah-sis) 1. an abscess. 2. the end or crisis of an attack or disease.

aposthia (ah-pos'the-ah) congenital absence of the prepuce.

apothecaries' weights and measures (ah-poth'ĕ-ka"rēz) a system used for measuring and weighing drugs and solutions. This system of measurement was brought to the United States from England during the colonial period; it is gradually being replaced by the metric system.

In the apothecaries' system fractions are used to designate portions of a unit of measure: e.g., one-fourth grain is written gr. 1/4. The fraction 1/2 is written ss.

There are two symbols in this system which are sometimes confused and always must be written clearly. These are the symbols for drams and ounces. Small Roman numerals are used after the symbols. For example, ʒiss reads drams one and one-half; ℥iii reads ounces three. (See also Table of Weights and Measures in the Appendix.)

apothecary (ah-poth′ĕ-ka″re) a pharmacist; a person who compounds and dispenses drugs.

apotripsis (ap″o-trip′sis) removal of a corneal opacity.

apparatus (ap″ah-ra′tus) an arrangement of a number of parts acting together to perform a special function.

Abbe-Zeiss a., a device for counting blood cells.

Golgi a., an irregular complex of parallel membranes and vesicles in a cell; it plays a role in the secretory activity of the cell.

Wangensteen's a., a nasal suction apparatus connected with a duodenal tube for aspirating gas and fluid from stomach and intestine.

appendage (ah-pen′dij) a less important portion of an organ, or an outgrowth, such as a tail. Also, a limb or limblike structure.

appendectomy (ap″en-dek′to-me) excision of the vermiform appendix.

appendicectomy (ah-pen″dĭ-sek′to-me) appendectomy.

appendicitis (ah-pen″dĭ-si′tis) inflammation of the vermiform appendix. Appendicitis is a serious disease, usually requiring surgery. When performed early by a competent surgeon, the operation is comparatively simple and safe. When the appendix becomes inflamed and infected, rupture may occur within a matter of hours. Rupture of the appendix leads to PERITONITIS, one of the most serious of all diseases, although its danger has been reduced by antibiotics.

CAUSE. If the tubelike appendix becomes plugged by a hard bit of fecal matter or by intestinal worms, or becomes inflamed from other causes, normal drainage cannot take place. The appendix then becomes susceptible to bacterial infection. Streptococci, *Escherichia coli* (colon bacilli), and other types of germs multiply and cause inflammation which will spread into the peritoneal cavity unless (1) the body's defenses overcome the infection or (2) a surgeon removes the infected appendix before it ruptures.

SYMPTOMS. There are usually three main symptoms: (1) nausea, (2) abdominal pain, which may localize in the lower right abdomen over the appendix area, and (3) mild fever in adults, sometimes high fever in young children. There may also be vomiting, constipation, or diarrhea.

The physician looks for positive evidence of an inflamed appendix. There may be tenderness over the appendix when pressure is exerted there. Sometimes pain is experienced in the region of the appendix during an examination through the rectum, or through the vagina in a female. A laboratory test, the leukocyte count, is also helpful in making the diagnosis. The physician always searches for other diseases that are sometimes mistaken for appendicitis, such as gallbladder attacks or kidney infection on the right side. The onset of pneumonia, rheumatic fever, or diabetic coma may imitate appendicitis. In women, there is the possibility of a ruptured ECTOPIC PREGNANCY, a twisted ovarian cyst, or a hemorrhaging ovarian follicle at the middle of the menstrual cycle.

PATIENT CARE. When appendicitis is suspected because of symptoms exhibited by the patient, a physician should be notified immediately. The patient should lie down and remain as quiet as possible. It is best to give him nothing by mouth, and because of the danger of aggravating the condition and possibly causing rupture of the apendix, cathartics and laxatives are contraindicated. Applications of heat are contraindicated for the same reasons. After the patient has been seen by the physician and

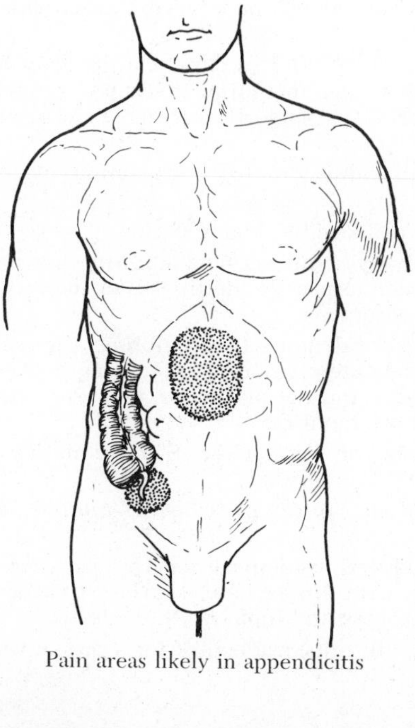
Pain areas likely in appendicitis

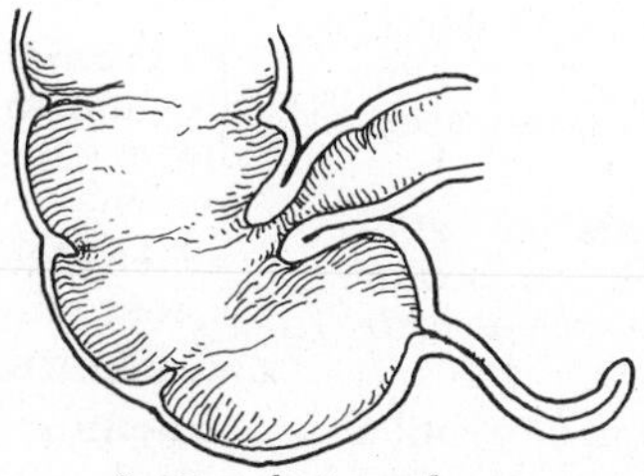
Sectional view of cecum and appendix

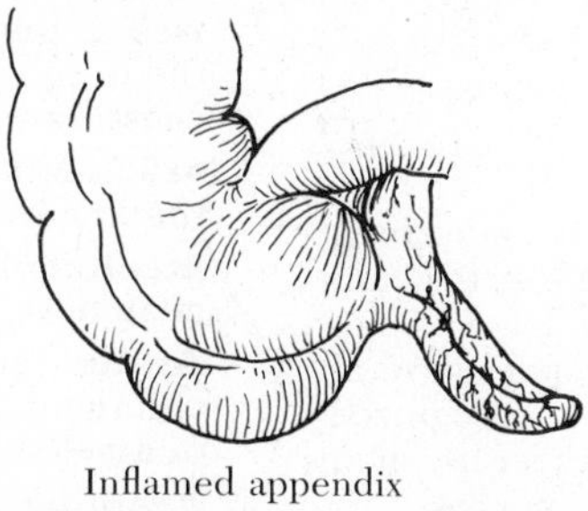
Inflamed appendix

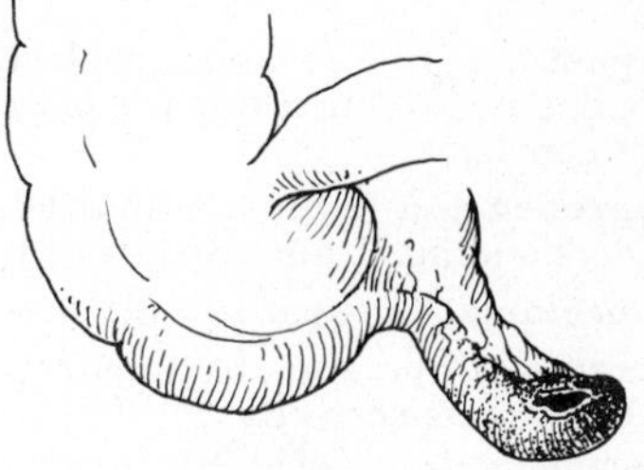
Ruptured appendix

a diagnosis of appendicitis has been established, surgical removal of the appendix (appendectomy) will probably be performed as soon as possible. Routine PREOPERATIVE CARE is then indicated.

appendicolithiasis (ah-pen″dĭ-ko-lĭ-thi′ah-sis) formation of calculi in the vermiform appendix.

appendicolysis (ah-pen″dĭ-kol′ĭ-sis) surgical separation of adhesions binding the appendix.

appendicostomy (ah-pen″dĭ-kos′to-me) surgical creation of an opening into the vermiform appendix.

appendicular (ap″en-dik′u-lar) 1. pertaining to an appendix or appendage. 2. pertaining to the limbs.

appendix (ah-pen′diks), pl. *appen′dices* [L.] 1. a slender outgrowth or appendage. 2. the vermiform appendix, a small appendage near the juncture of the small intestine and the large intestine (ileocecal valve). An apparently useless structure, it can be the source of a serious illness, APPENDICITIS. adj., **appendic′eal.**

apperception (ap″er-sep′shun) conscious perception of a sensory stimulus.

appestat (ap′pĕ-stat) a brain center (probably in the hypothalamus) concerned in controlling the appetite.

appetite (ap′ĕ-tīt) the desire for food. It is stimulated by the sight, smell, or thought of food and accompanied by the flow of saliva in the mouth and gastric juice in the stomach. The stomach wall also receives an extra blood supply in preparation for its digestive activity.

Appetite is psychologic, dependent on memory and associations, as compared with hunger, which is physiologically aroused by the body's need for food. Appetite can be discouraged by unattractive food, surroundings, or company, and by emotional states such as anxiety, irritation, anger, and fear.

Chronic loss of appetite is known as anorexia. It may be a symptom of physical disorders, or it may be related to emotional disturbances, in which case it is known as ANOREXIA NERVOSA. Excessive appetite may be an indication of metabolic disorders or may be caused by emotional disturbances. This latter condition is especially common among children, particularly girls, who may develop a habit of compulsive eating to compensate for a feeling of insecurity.

applanometer (ap″lah-nom′ĕ-ter) a mechanical or electronic instrument for determining intraocular pressure in the detection of glaucoma (see also TONOMETER).

apposition (ap″o-zish′un) the placement or position of adjacent structures or parts so that they can come into contact.

apprehension (ap″re-hen′shun) 1. perception and understanding. 2. anticipatory fear or anxiety.

approximal (ah-prok′sĭ-mal) close together.

apraxia (ah-prak′se-ah) impairment of the ability to use objects correctly.

amnestic a., loss of ability to carry out a movement on command due to inability to remember the command.

motor a., loss of ability to make proper use of an object, although its proper nature is recognized.

sensory a., loss of ability to make proper use of an object due to lack of perception of its purpose.

Apresoline (ah-pres′o-lēn) trademark for preparations of hydralazine hydrochloride, an antihypertensive drug.

aprobarbital (ap″ro-bar′bĭ-tal) a crystalline powder, an intermediate-acting sedative and hypnotic.

aproctia (ah-prok′she-ah) imperforate anus.

aprosopia (ap″ro-so′pe-ah) a developmental anomaly with partial or complete absence of the face.

aptyalism (ap-ti′ah-lizm) deficiency or absence of saliva.

apus (a′pus) an individual without feet.

apyogenous (ah″pi-oj′ĕ-nus) not caused by pus.

apyretic (ah″pi-ret′ik) without fever.

apyrexia (ah-pi-rek′se-ah) absence of fever.

apyrogenic (ah-pi″ro-jen′ik) not producing fever.

aq. [L.] *aq′ua* (water).

aq. dest., *aq′ua destilla′ta* (distilled water).

aqua (ak′wah) [L.] 1. water, H_2O. 2. a saturated solution of a volatile oil or other aromatic or volatile substance in purified water.

aquaphobia (ak″wah-fo′be-ah) morbid fear of water.

Aquatag (ak′wah-tag) trademark for a preparation of benzthiazide, an orally effective diuretic and antihypertensive.

aqueduct (ak′wĕ-dukt″) any canal or passage.

cerebral a., a narrow channel in the midbrain connecting the third and fourth ventricles and containing cerebrospinal fluid.

a. of cochlea, a foramen in the temporal bone for a vein from the cochlea.

a. of Fallopius, the canal for the facial nerve in pars petrosa of the temporal bone.

sylvian a., a. of Sylvius, ventricular a., cerebral aqueduct.

aqueous (a′kwe-us) watery; prepared with water.

a. humor, the fluid produced in the eye, occupying the anterior and posterior chambers, and diffusing out of the eye into the blood; regarded as lymph of the eye, its composition varies from that of lymph in the body generally.

Ar chemical symbol, *argon.*

arachnephobia (ah-rak″nĕ-fo′be-ah) arachnophobia.

Arachnida (ar-ak′nĭ-dah) a class of animals of the phylum Arthropoda, including 12 orders, comprising such forms as spiders, scorpions, ticks, and mites.

arachnidism (ah-rak′nĭ-dizm) poisoning from a spider bite.

arachnitis (ar″ak-ni′tis) arachnoiditis.

arachnodactyly (ah-rak″no-dak′tĭ-le) extreme length and slenderness of the fingers or toes, as in Marfan's syndrome.

arachnoid (ah-rak′noid) 1. resembling a spider's web. 2. the delicate membrane interposed between the dura mater and the pia mater, and with them constituting the meninges.

arachnoiditis (ah-rak″noid-i′tis) inflammation of the arachnoid membrane.

arachnophobia (ah-rak″no-fo′be-ah) morbid fear of spiders.

Aralen (ar′ah-len) trademark for a preparation of chloroquine, an antimalarial used also in treatment of amebic abscess and lupus erythematosus.

Aramine (ar′ah-min) trademark for a preparation

of metaraminol, a sympathomimetic and vasopressor.

Aran-Duchenne disease (ar-ahn' du-shen') spinal muscular atrophy.

araphia (ah-ra'fe-ah) failure of closure of the embryonic neural tube, the spinal cord developing as a flat plate. adj., **ara'phic.**

arbor (ar'bor), pl. *arbo'res* [L.] a tree.

a. vi'tae, 1. treelike outlines seen on median section of the cerebellum. 2. a series of ridges within cervix uteri.

arborescent (ar"bo-res'ent) branching like a tree.

arborization (ar"bor-ĭ-za'shun) a collection of branches, as the branching terminus of a nerve-cell process.

arbovirus (ar"bo-vi'rus) a group of viruses that are transmitted to man by mosquitoes and ticks. (See also VIRUS.)

A.R.C. American Red Cross.

arc (ark) a part of the circumference of a circle, or a regularly curved line.

binauricular a., the arc across the top of the head from one auricular point to the other.

reflex a., the circuit traveled by impulses producing a reflex action: receptor organ, afferent nerve, nerve center, efferent nerve, effector organ in a muscle. (See also REFLEX and Plate 12.)

arcate (ar'kāt) curved; bow-shaped.

arch (arch) a structure of bowlike or curved outline.

abdominothoracic a., the lower boundary of the front of the thorax.

a. of aorta, the curving portion between the ascending aorta and the descending aorta, giving rise to the brachiocephalic trunk, the left common carotid and the left subclavian artery.

aortic a's, paired vessels arching from the ventral to the dorsal aorta through the branchial clefts of fishes and amniote embryos. In mammalian development, arches 1 and 2 disappear; 3 joins the common to the internal carotid artery; 4 becomes the arch of the aorta and joins the aorta and subclavian artery; 5 disappears; 6 forms the pulmonary arteries and, until birth, the ductus arteriosus.

branchial a's, four pairs of mesenchymal and later cartilaginous arches of the embryo in the region of the neck.

dental a., the curving structure formed by the crowns of the teeth in their normal position, or by the residual ridge after loss of the teeth.

a's of foot, the longitudinal and transverse arches of the foot. The longitudinal arch comprises the pars medialis, formed by the calcaneus, talus, and the navicular, cuneiform, and the first three tarsal bones; and the pars lateralis formed by the calcaneus, the cuboid bone, and the lateral two metatarsal bones. The transverse arch comprises the navicular, cuneiform, cuboid, and five metatarsal bones.

lingual a., a wire appliance that conforms to the lingual aspect of the dental arch, used to secure movement of the teeth in orthodontic work.

mandibular a., the first branchial arch, being the rudiment of the maxillary and mandibular regions.

neural a., vertebral arch.

palatal a., the arch formed by the roof of the mouth from the teeth on one side to those on the other.

pubic a., the arch formed by the conjoined rami of the ischium and pubis of the two sides of the body.

pulmonary a's, the most caudal of the aortic arches, which become the pulmonary arteries.

tendinous a., a linear thickening of fascia over some part of a muscle.

vertebral a., the dorsal bony arch of a vertebra, composed of the laminae and pedicles of a vertebra.

zygomatic a., the arch formed by the processes of the zygomatic and temporal bones.

arch(i)- (ar'ke) word element [Gr.], *ancient; beginning; first; original.*

archencephalon (ark"en-sef'ah-lon) the primitive brain from which the midbrain and forebrain develop.

archenteron (ark-en'ter-on) the central cavity that is the provisional gut in the gastrula; the primitive digestive cavity of the embryo.

archeokinetic (ar"ke-o-ki-net'ik) relating to the primitive type of motor nerve mechanism as seen in the peripheral and ganglionic nervous systems.

archetype (ar'kĕ-tīp) in psychology, a type unconsciously considered to be the universal standard or ideal.

archinephron (ar"kĭ-nef'ron) the pronephros.

archipallium (ar"kĭ-pal'e-um) that portion of the pallium, or cerebral cortex, which phylogenetically is the first to show the characteristic layering of the cellular elements.

arciform (ar'sĭ-form) arcuate.

arctation (ark-ta'shun) narrowing of an opening or canal.

arcuate (ar'ku-āt) bent like a bow.

arcuation (ar"ku-a'shun) a bending or curvature.

arcus (ar'kus), pl. *ar'cus* [L.] arch; bow.

a. adipo'sus, arcus senilis.

a. juveni'lis, a condition identical to arcus senilis but occurring in young persons.

a. seni'lis, an opaque line partially surrounding the margin of the cornea, usually occurring bilaterally in persons of 50 years or older as a result of lipoid degeneration.

area (a're-ah), pl. *a'reae, areas* [L.] a limited space or plane surface.

association a's, areas of the cerebral cortex (excluding primary areas) connected with each other and with the neothalamus; they are responsible for higher mental and emotional processes, including memory, learning, etc.

Broca's motor speech a., an area comprising parts of the opercular and triangular portions of the inferior frontal gyrus; injury to this area may result in expressive APHASIA.

Broca's parolfactory a., see under B.

Brodmann's a's, specific occipital and preoccipital areas of the cerebral cortex, distinguished by differences in the arrangement of their six cellular layers, and identified by numbering each area. They are considered to be the seat of specific functions of the brain.

germinal a., a. germinati'va, embryonic disk.

Kiesselbach's a., an area on the anterior part of the nasal septum, richly supplied with capillaries, and a common site of epistaxis (nosebleed).

motor a., that area of the cerebral cortex which, on brief electrical stimulation, shows the lowest threshold and shortest latency for the production of muscle movement.

primary a., areas of the cerebral cortex comprising the motor and sensory regions.

psychomotor a., motor a.

silent a., an area of the brain in which pathologic conditions may occur without producing symptoms.

a. subcallo'sa, subcallosal a., Broca's parolfactory area.

vocal a., the part of the glottis between the vocal cords.

areflexia (ah″re-flek'se-ah) absence of the reflexes.

areola (ah-re'o-lah), pl. *are'olae* [L.] 1. a narrow zone surrounding a central area, e.g., the darkened area surrounding the NIPPLE of the mammary gland. 2. any minute space or interstice in a tissue.

Chaussier's a., the indurated area encircling a malignant pustule.

areolar (ah-re'o-lar) 1. containing minute spaces. 2. pertaining to an areola.

Arfonad (ar'fon-ad) trademark for a preparation of trimethaphan, a ganglion-blocking agent and antihypertensive.

Argas (ar'gas) a genus of ticks parasitic in poultry and other birds and sometimes man.

Argasidae (ar-gas'ĭ-de) a family of arthropods made up of the soft-bodied ticks.

argentaffin (ar-jen'tah-fin) staining readily with silver; see also under CELL.

argentaffinoma (ar″jen-taf″fĭ-no'mah) a tumor arising from argentaffin cells, most frequently in the terminal ileum or the appendix; called also carcinoid. Such tumors produce CARCINOID SYNDROME.

argentum (ar-jen'tum) [L.] silver (symbol Ag).

argillaceous (ar″jĭ-la'shus) composed of clay.

arginase (ar'jĭ-nās) an enzyme of the liver that splits arginine into urea and ornithine.

arginine (ar'jĭ-nin) a basic amino acid produced by the hydrolysis or digestion of proteins.

argininosuccinic acid (ar″-jĭ-ne'no-suk-sin″ik) a compound normally formed in urea formation in the liver, but not normally present in urine.

argininosuccinicaciduria (ar″jĭ-ne″no-suk-sin″ik-as″ĭ-du're-ah) excretion in the urine of argininosuccinic acid, a feature of an inborn error of metabolism marked also by mental retardation.

argon (ar'gon) a chemical element, atomic number 18, atomic weight 39.948, symbol Ar. (See table of ELEMENTS.)

Argyll Robertson pupil (ar-gīl' rob'ert-son) a pupil that is miotic and responds to accommodative effort, but not to light.

argyria (ar-ji're-ah) poisoning by silver or its salts; chronic argyria is marked by a permanent ashen-gray discoloration of the skin, conjunctiva, and internal organs.

argyric (ar-ji'rik) pertaining to silver.

argyrism (ar'jĭ-rizm) argyria.

Argyrol (ar'jĭ-rol) trademark for a preparation of mild silver protein that is used as an antiseptic on mucous membranes.

argyrophil (ar-ji'ro-fil) easily impregnated with silver.

argyrosis (ar″jĭ-ro'sis) argyria.

arhinia (ah-rin'e-ah) congenital absence of the nose.

Arias-Stella reaction nuclear and cellular hypertrophy of the endometrial epithelium, associated with ectopic pregnancy.

ariboflavinosis (a-ri″bo-fla″vĭ-no'sis) deficiency of RIBOFLAVIN (vitamin B_2) in the diet, a condition marked by lesions in the corners of the mouth, on the lips, and around the nose and eyes, malaise, weakness, weight loss and, in severe cases, corneal or other eye changes and seborrheic dermatitis.

Aristocort (ah-ris'to-cort) trademark for a preparation of triamcinolone, a prednisolone derivative used as an anti-inflammatory steroid.

Arlidin (ar'lĭ-din) trademark for a preparation of nylidrin, a peripheral vasodilator.

arm (arm) 1. the upper extremity, from shoulder to elbow; often used to denote the entire extremity, from shoulder to wrist. 2. an armlike part, e.g., the portion of the chromatid extending in either direction from the centromere of a mitotic chromosome.

brawny a., a hard, swollen condition of the arm following mastectomy.

armamentarium (ar″mah-men-ta're-um) the entire equipment of a practitioner, such as medicines, instruments, books.

arnica (ar'nĭ-kah) dried flowerheads of *Arnica montana*, used topically as a tincture for contusions, sprains, and superficial wounds.

Arnold's ganglion (ar'noldz) a parasympathetic ganglion immediately below the foramen ovale; its postganglionic fibers supply the parotid gland. Called also otic ganglion.

Arnold-Chiari malformation (deformity, syndrome) (ar'nold-ke-ar'e) a congenital anomaly in which the cerebellum and medulla oblongata protrude down into the cervical spinal canal through the foramen magnum; it is almost always associated with meningomyelocele and hydrocephalus.

aromatic (ar″o-mat'ik) 1. having a spicy fragrance. 2. a stimulant, spicy medicine. 3. denoting a compound characterized by the benzene ring.

arrector (ah-rek'tor), pl. *arrecto'res* [L.] raising, or that which raises; an erector muscle.

arrest (ah-rest') sudden cessation or stoppage.

cardiac a., sudden cessation of beating of the heart (see also CARDIAC ARREST).

epiphyseal a., premature arrest of the longitudinal growth of bone due to fusion of the epiphysis and diaphysis.

maturation a., interruption of the process of development, as of blood cells, before the final stage is reached.

arrheno- (ah-re'no) word element [Gr.], *male; masculine.*

arrhenoblastoma (ah-re″no-blas-to'mah) a rare ovarian tumor that sometimes causes virilization.

arrhinia (ah-rin'e-ah) arhinia.

arrhythmia (ah-rith'me-ah) variation from the normal rhythm, especially of the heartbeat. adj., **arrhyth'mic.**

sinus a., the physiologic cyclic variation in heart rate related to vagal impulses to the sinoatrial node; it occurs commonly in children and in the aged.

arseniasis (ar″sĭ-ni'ah-sis) arsenical poisoning.

arsenic (ar'sĕ-nik) a chemical element, atomic number 33, atomic weight 74.92, symbol As. (See table of ELEMENTS.) Arsenic compounds have been widely used in medicine; however, they have been replaced for the most part by antibiotics, which are less toxic and equally effective. Some of the arsenicals are used for infectious diseases, especially those caused by protozoa, and some skin disorders and blood dyscrasias also are treated with arsenic compounds. Since arsenic is highly toxic it must be administered with caution. The antidote for arsenic poisoning is DIMERCAPROL (BAL).

a. trioxide, white a., white, odorless powder used as an irritant and escharotic.

arsenical (ar-sen′ĭ-kal) 1. pertaining to arsenic. 2. a compound containing arsenic.

arsenoblast (ar-sen′o-blast) the male element of a zygote; a male pronucleus.

arsine (ar′sēn) a toxic gas, compounds of which have been used in warfare.

arsphenamine (ars-fen′ah-min) a light yellow powder containing 30 to 32 per cent of arsenic; formerly used intravenously in syphilis, yaws, and other protozoan infections.

arsthinol (ars′thĭ-nol) an arsenical preparation used for the treatment of intestinal amebiasis.

Artane (ar′tān) trademark for preparations of trihexyphenidyl hydrochloride, used as an anticholinergic in treatment of Parkinson's disease.

artefact (ar′tĕ-fakt) artifact.

arteria (ar-te′re-ah), pl. *arter′riae* [L.] artery.

a. luso′ria, an abnormally situated vessel in the region of the aortic arch.

arterial (ar-te′re-al) pertaining to an artery or to the arteries.

a. thrombosis, the presence of a thrombus in an artery. (See also arterial THROMBOSIS.)

arterialization (ar-te″re-al-ĭ-za′shun) the conversion of venous into arterial blood by the absorption of oxygen.

arteriectasis (ar-te″re-ek′tah-sis) dilatation of an artery.

arteriectomy (ar-te″re-ek′to-me) excision of an artery.

arterio- (ar-te′re-o) word element [L., Gr.], *artery.*

arteriogram (ar-te′re-o-gram″) a roentgenogram of an artery.

arteriography (ar-te″re-og′rah-fe) roentgenography of an artery or arterial system after injection of a contrast medium in the bloodstream.

catheter a., roentgenography of vessels after introduction of contrast material through a catheter inserted into an artery.

selective a., roentgenography of a specific vessel that is opacified by a medium introduced directly into it, usually via a catheter.

arteriol(o)- (ar-te″re-o′lo) word element [L.], *arteriole.*

arteriola (ar-te″re-o′lah), pl. *arterio′lae* [L.] arteriole.

arterio′lae rec′tae re′nis, branches of the arcuate arteries of the kidney that supply the renal pyramids.

arteriole (ar-te′re-ōl) a minute arterial branch. adj. **arterio′lar.**

arteriolith (ar-te′re-o-lith″) a chalky concretion in an artery.

arteriolitis (ar-te″re-o-li′tis) inflammation of arterioles.

arteriology (ar-te″re-ol′o-je) sum of knowledge regarding the arteries.

arteriolonecrosis (ar-te″re-o″lo-nĕ-kro′sis) necrosis or destruction of arterioles.

arteriolosclerosis (ar-te″re-o″lo-sklĕ-ro′sis) sclerosis and thickening of the walls of arterioles. The hyaline form may be associated with nephrosclerosis, the hyperplastic with malignant hypertension, nephrosclerosis, and scleroderma. adj., **arteriolosclerot′ic.**

arteriomotor (ar-te″re-o-mo′tor) involving or causing dilation or constriction of arteries.

arteriomyomatosis (ar-te″re-o-mi″o-mah-to′sis) growth of muscular fibers in the walls of an artery, causing thickening.

arterionecrosis (ar-te″re-o-nĕ-kro′sis) necrosis of arteries.

arteriopathy (ar-te″re-op′ah-the) any disease of an artery.

hypertensive a., widespread involvement of the smaller arteries and arterioles, associated with hypertension and characterized primarily by hypertrophy of the tunica media.

arterioplasty (ar-te′re-o-plas″te) plastic repair of an artery.

arteriopressor (ar-te″re-o-pres′or) increasing arterial blood pressure.

arteriorrhaphy (ar-te″re-or′ah-fe) suture of an artery.

arteriorrhexis (ar-te″re-o-rek′sis) rupture of an artery.

arteriosclerosis (ar-te″re-o-sklĕ-ro′sis) an arterial disease of three main types characterized by thickening and loss of elasticity of the arterial walls; popularly called "hardening of the arteries." adj. **arteriosclerot′ic.**

The three main forms of arteriosclerosis are: (1) ATHEROSCLEROSIS, in which plaques of fatty deposits form in the inner layer (intima) of the blood vessels; (2) Mönckeberg's arteriosclerosis, also called *medial arteriosclerosis* because of involvement of the middle layer (medial coat) of the arteries, in which there is destruction of the muscle and elastic fibers of the medial coat and calcium deposits; and (3) *arteriolar sclerosis* (arteriolosclerosis) which affects the small arteries (arterioles).

All three forms of arteriosclerosis may be present in the same patient, but in different blood vessels. Of the three types, atherosclerosis is the most common. When reference is made to hardening of the arteries, in most instances it is atherosclerosis that is meant. Frequently, the two terms are used interchangeably.

Arteriosclerosis is one of the major killers and disablers in the United States. The formation of fatty deposits (atheromas) in intimal arteriosclerosis can lead to scarring and calcification. These deposits encroach upon the lumen of the blood vessel and gradually obstruct the flow of blood. Calcification leads to loss of elasticity of the vessel walls, with increase in blood pressure. HYPERTENSION accelerates the process of arteriosclerosis.

CAUSES. The exact causes of arteriosclerosis are not yet known. However, several factors are thought to contribute to the disease. Heredity appears to play some part; men in certain families have been found to be more susceptible than the average. The fact that women are seldom affected by arteriosclerosis before menopause suggests that the sex hormones have a connection with the disease. Arteriosclerosis may also arise in connection with other diseases.

Persons suffering from DIABETES MELLITUS are especially susceptible and tend to develop the disease earlier in life than nondiabetics. Other conditions which may lead to arteriosclerosis include HYPERTENSION, hypothyroidism, and certain disorders of metabolism, such as gout.

One factor being investigated is the relationship of CHOLESTEROL, a fatty substance found in most tissues in the body, to atherosclerosis. There is evidence that a high cholesterol level in the blood often accompanies arteriosclerosis. Also, cholesterol levels appear to be higher when the fat in the diet contains an excess of saturated fatty acids, which are found in significant quantities in such foods as milk, dairy products, eggs, and meat fats. For this reason, the American Heart Association has recommended that people balance their intake of these foods with foods containing unsaturated and polyunsaturated FATS. Unsaturated fats are found abundantly in vegetable oils; fish and poultry are also good sources. In recent years some extravagant claims have been made for food products which contain unsaturated fats.

SYMPTOMS. The symptoms of arteriosclerosis depend on which arteries are most affected. Early symptoms may include coldness or numbness in the feet, dizziness, shortness of breath, headache, and a tendency to tire easily. If the arteries in the legs are affected, there may be cramps, aches, and sharp pains after even slight exercise. If the arteries that supply the brain are affected, mental symptoms, such as loss of memory, may develop. The symptoms of KIDNEY disease may follow hardening of the renal arteries and especially the arterioles.

ARTERIOSCLEROSIS AS A CAUSE OF OTHER DISEASES. As a major cause of HEART disease and other disorders, arteriosclerosis may manifest itself in various ways. If the coronary arteries, which supply blood to the heart muscle, are partly blocked, the result may be ANGINA PECTORIS, a pain or feeling of tightness in the chest. Sometimes the roughened lining of an affected artery can cause the blood to clot as it flows past. The blood flow may be obstructed, or the clot may break away from the artery wall and be carried through the bloodstream until it lodges and blocks the flow of blood elsewhere. More frequently an atheromatous plaque is the site of the formation of a blood clot. If this occurs in the coronary arteries, it can cause CORONARY OCCLUSION or CORONARY THROMBOSIS, often called a heart attack. If the arteries supplying the brain are blocked suddenly, a cerebral thrombosis, or CEREBRAL VASCULAR ACCIDENT (stroke), can result. If the clot has formed in an artery of the neck, it can sometimes be removed surgically. In the arteries of or leading to the legs, a blockage, or peripheral thrombosis, can cut off circulation to the affected limb.

TREATMENT AND PREVENTION. At present there is no treatment that can reverse the effects of advanced arteriosclerosis. Once they have become hardened, there is no way to make the walls of the arteries more elastic or to get rid of the minerals and fats that have accumulated inside them. Instead, treatment concentrates on preventing the condition from becoming worse, or on allowing other arteries to enlarge as they make up for some of the lost blood supply. Nitroglycerin and related medicines help relieve the pain of angina pectoris. Chronic reduction of circulation by narrowing or weakening of the abdominal aorta or distal arteries in the lower extremities often can be corrected by vascular surgery and replacement of the diseased arterial segment. In cases of thrombosis it is sometimes possible to remove the clot by surgery.

Because of the suspected relationship between blood cholesterol and the development of arteriosclerosis, the patient may be placed on a diet low in cholesterol and saturated fats.

Rest and relaxation are also important. Regular exercise will probably be prescribed by the physician and should be followed. Smoking should be stopped or greatly curtailed. If the legs are seriously involved, shoes and clothing must be properly fitted to avoid blocking circulation further, and the feet should be carefully protected from cold, dampness, and infection. Several drugs that may be helpful in treating arteriosclerosis are still in the experimental stage. Diseases such as diabetes mellitus, hypertension, and gout that predispose to arteriosclerosis should be treated and controlled to slow their effect on the arteries.

Since the causes of arteriosclerosis are not fully understood, it is not certain whether taking precautions can prevent the onset of the disease. In part, the disease may be a natural effect of aging. However, avoiding obesity is very important for good health in general, and seems to help retard arteriosclerosis as well. Men over 35 should take special care to control their weight and their intake of the saturated fats found in meat and dairy products. Several small meals a day are probably better than one or two large ones.

Mönckeberg's a., arteriosclerosis characterized by calcification of the middle coat (tunica media) of the artery.

a. oblit'erans, arteriosclerosis in which proliferation of the intima has caused complete obliteration of the lumen of the artery.

arteriospasm (ar-te're-o-spazm") spasm of an artery.

arteriostenosis (ar-te"re-o-stĕ-no'sis) constriction of an artery.

arteriosympathectomy (ar-te"re-o-sim"pah-thek'to-me) periarterial sympathectomy.

arteriotony (ar-te"re-ot'o-ne) blood pressure.

arteriovenous (ar-te"re-o-ve'nus) both arterial and venous; pertaining to both artery and vein.

arteritis (ar"ter-i'tis) inflammation of an artery.

giant cell a., temporal arteritis.

a. oblit'erans, endarteritis obliterans.

rheumatic a., generalized inflammation of arterioles and arterial capillaries occurring in rheumatic fever.

temporal a., a chronic disease of older persons, largely involving the carotid arterial system, marked by proliferative inflammation, often with giant cells and granulomas, and by headache, constitutional symptoms, and ocular involvement.

Takayasu's a., pulseless disease.

artery (ar'ter-e) a vessel through which the blood passes away from the heart to various parts of the body. The wall of an artery consists typically of an outer coat (tunica adventitia), a middle coat (tunica media), and an inner coat (tunica intima); see Plate 8. (For named arteries of the body, see table, p. 72.)

end a., one that undergoes progressive branching without development of channels connecting with other arteries.

arthr(o)- (ar′thro) word element [Gr.], *joint; articulation.*

arthragra (ar-thrag′rah) gouty pain in a joint.

arthralgia (ar-thral′je-ah) pain in a joint.

arthrectomy (ar-threk′to-me) excision of a joint.

arthritide (ar′thrĭ-tīd) a skin eruption of gouty origin.

arthritis (ar-thri′tis) inflammation of a joint. adj. **arthrit′ic.** The term is frequently used by the public to indicate any disease involving pain or stiffness of the musculoskeletal system and is considered by many to be synonymous with rheumatism. In medical terminology arthritis is restricted to those types of rheumatic disease in which there is an inflammatory condition involving the joints. The term rheumatic diseases is a broader term, referring to conditions in which there are changes in connective tissues, including muscle, tendons, bursae, joints, and fibrous tissue.

Arthritis and the rheumatic diseases in general constitute the major cause of chronic disability in the United States. It is estimated that 16 million persons in this country have a crippling disease which they call "arthritis" and which is severe enough to interfere with their daily activities of living.

The American Rheumatic Association and The Arthritis Foundation have grouped rheumatic diseases and arthritis into 13 different categories (see Table).

The two main types of arthritis are OSTEOARTHRITIS and rheumatoid arthritis. In general, the treatment and care of those suffering from rheumatic diseases is the same, regardless of the specific clinical diagnosis. These subjects are included here under rheumatoid arthritis (see below), the most common, the most virulent, and one of the most disabling of the rheumatic diseases.

acute a., arthritis marked by pain, heat, redness, and swelling.

acute rheumatic a., swelling, tenderness, and redness of many joints of the body, accompanying rheumatic fever.

hypertrophic a., rheumatoid arthritis marked by hypertrophy of the cartilage at the edge of the joints; OSTEOARTHRITIS.

juvenile rheumatoid a., rheumatoid arthritis of children, with swelling, tenderness, and pain involving one or more joints, leading to impaired growth and development, limitation of movement, and ankylosis and flexion contractures of the joints. It is frequently accompanied by systemic manifestations which may include spiking fever, transient rash on the trunk and extremities, hepatosplenomegaly, generalized lymphadenopathy, and anemia. Called also Still's disease. See also rheumatoid ARTHRITIS.

psoriatic a., that associated with severe psoriasis, classically affecting the terminal interphalangeal joints.

rheumatoid a., a chronic systemic disease with inflammatory changes occurring throughout the body's connective tissues. As such, it is classified as a COLLAGEN DISEASE.

This form of arthritis strikes during the most productive years of adulthood, with the majority of cases beginning between the ages of 20 and 40. No age is spared, however, and the disease may affect infants as well as the very old. For some reason the disease affects men and women about equally in number, but three times as many women as men develop symptoms severe enough to require medical attention.

ETIOLOGY. The cause of rheumatoid arthritis is unknown and it is doubtful that there is one specific cause. It is regarded by some researchers as an AUTOIMMUNE disease, in which the body produces abnormal antibodies against its own cells and tissues. Evidence to support this theory is found in the fact that there is an abnormally high level of certain types of IMMUNOGLOBULINS in the blood of patients suffering

(Text continued on page 87.)

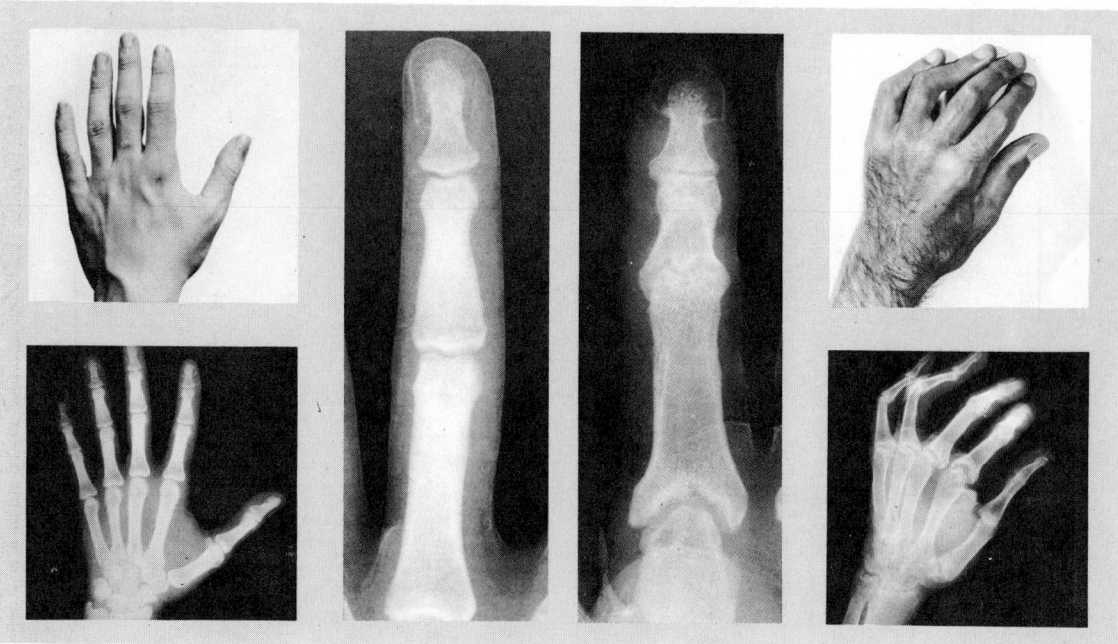

Arthritis of the fingers. Left, normal hand and finger. Right, arthritic hand and finger, with ankylosis, or "locking" of the joint by bone and scar tissue. (Courtesy of Bergman Associates.)

TABLE OF ARTERIES

COMMON NAME*	NA EQUIVALENT†	ORIGIN*	BRANCHES*	DISTRIBUTION
accompanying a. of sciatic nerve. *See* sciatic a.				
acromiothoracic a. *See* thoracoacromial a.				
alveolar a's, anterior superior	aa. alveolares superiores anteriores	infraorbital a.	dental branches	incisor and canine regions of upper jaw, maxillary sinus
alveolar a., inferior	a. alveolaris inferior	maxillary a.	dental, mylohyoid branches, mental a.	lower jaw, lower lip, chin
alveolar a., posterior superior	a. alveolaris superior posterior	maxillary a.	dental branches	molar and premolar regions of upper jaw, maxillary sinus, buccinator muscle
angular a.	a. angularis	facial a.		lacrimal sac, lower eyelid, nose
aorta	aorta	left ventricle		
abdominal aorta	aorta abdominalis	lower portion of descending aorta, from aortic hiatus of diaphragm to bifurcation into common iliac a's	inferior phrenic, lumbar, median sacral, superior and inferior mesenteric, middle suprarenal, renal, and testicular or ovarian a's, celiac trunk	
arch of aorta	arcus aortae	continuation of ascending aorta	brachiocephalic trunk, left common carotid and left subclavian a's; continues as descending (thoracic) aorta	
ascending aorta	aorta ascendens	proximal portion of aorta, arising from left ventricle	right and left coronary a's; continues as arch of aorta	
descending aorta. *See* thoracic aorta; abdominal aorta	aorta descendens	continuation of arch of aorta		
thoracic aorta	aorta thoracica	proximal portion of descending aorta, continuing from arch of aorta to aortic hiatus of diaphragm	bronchial, esophageal, pericardiac, and mediastinal branches, superior phrenic a's, posterior intercostal a's [III–XI], subcostal a's, continues as abdominal aorta	

*a. = artery; a's = (pl.) arteries.
†a. = [L.] arteria; aa. = [L. (pl.)] arteriae.

appendicular a.	a. appendicularis	ileocolic a.		vermiform appendix
arcuate a. of foot	a. arcuata pedis	dorsalis pedis a.	deep plantar branch, dorsal metatarsal a's	foot, toes
arcuate a's of kidney	aa. arcuatae renis	interlobar a.	interlobar a's, straight arterioles of kidney	parenchyma of kidney
auditory a., internal. *See* a. of labyrinth				
auricular a., deep	a. auricularis profunda	maxillary a.		skin of auditory canal, tympanic membrane, temporomandibular joint
auricular a., posterior	a. auricularis posterior	external carotid a.	auricular and occipital branches, stylomastoid a.	middle ear, mastoid cells, auricle, parotid gland, digastric and other muscles
axillary a.	a. axillaris	continuation of subclavian a.	subscapular branches, highest thoracic, thoracoacromial, lateral thoracic, subscapular, and anterior and posterior circumflex humeral a's	upper limb, axilla, chest, shoulder
basilar a.	a. basilaris	from junction of right and left vertebral a's	pontine branches, anterior inferior cerebellar, labyrinthine, superior cerebellar, posterior cerebral a's	brain stem, internal ear, cerebellum, posterior cerebrum
brachial a.	a. brachialis	continuation of axillary a.	superficial and deep brachial, nutrient of humerus, superior and inferior ulnar collateral, radial, ulnar a's	shoulder, arm, forearm, hand
brachial a., deep	a. profunda brachii	brachial a.	nutrient to humerus, deltoid branch, middle and radial collateral a's	humerus, muscles and skin of arm
brachial a., superficial	a. brachialis superficialis	variant brachial a., taking a more superficial course than usual	see *brachial a.*	see *brachial a.*
brachiocephalic trunk	truncus brachiocephalicus	arch of aorta	right common carotid, right subclavian a's	right side of head and neck, right arm
buccal a.	a. buccalis	maxillary a.		buccinator muscle, oral mucous membrane
a. of bulb of penis	a. bulbi penis	internal pudendal a.		bulbourethral gland, bulb of penis
a. of bulb of urethra. *See* a. of bulb of penis				
a. of bulb of vestibule of vagina	a. bulbi vestibuli vaginae	internal pudendal a.		bulb of vestibule of vagina, Bartholin glands
carotid a., common	a. carotis communis	brachiocephalic trunk (right), arch of aorta (left)	external and internal carotid a's	see *carotid a., external* and *carotid a., internal*

TABLE OF ARTERIES – *Continued*

COMMON NAME*	NA EQUIVALENT†	ORIGIN*	BRANCHES*	DISTRIBUTION
carotid a., external	a. carotis externa	common carotid a.	superior thyroid, ascending pharyngeal, lingual, facial, sternocleidomastoid, occipital, posterior auricular, superficial temporal, maxillary a's	neck, face, skull
carotid a., internal	a. carotis interna	common carotid a.	caroticotympanic branches, ophthalmic, posterior communicating, anterior choroid, anterior cerebral, middle cerebral a's	middle ear, brain, hypophysis, orbit, choroid plexus of lateral ventricle
caudal a. *See* sacral a., median				
celiac trunk	truncus celiacus	abdominal aorta	left gastric, common hepatic, splenic a's	esophagus, stomach, duodenum, spleen, pancreas. liver, gallbladder
central a. of retina	a. centralis retinae	ophthalmic a.		retina
cerebellar a., inferior, anterior	a. cerebelli inferior anterior	basilar a.	a. of labyrinth	lower anterior cerebellum, inner ear
cerebellar a., inferior, posterior	a. cerebelli inferior posterior	vertebral a.		lower part of cerebellum, medulla, choroid plexus of fourth ventricle
cerebellar a., superior	a. cerebelli superior	basilar a.		upper part of cerebellum, midbrain, pineal body, choroid plexus of third ventricle
cerebral a., anterior	a. cerebri anterior	internal carotid a.	cortical (orbital, frontal, parietal), anterior choroidal, and central branches (including medial striate a.), and anterior communicating a.	orbital, frontal, and parietal cortex, corpus callosum, diencephalon, corpus striatum, internal capsule, choroid plexus of lateral ventricle
cerebral a., middle	a. cerebri media	internal carotid a.	cortical (orbital, frontal, parietal, temporal) and central (striate) branches	orbital, frontal, parietal, and temporal cortex, corpus striatum, internal capsule
cerebral a., posterior	a. cerebri posterior	terminal bifurcation of basilar a.	cortical (temporal, occipital, parieto-occipital), central, and choroid branches	occipital and temporal lobes, basal ganglia, choroid plexus of lateral ventricle, thalamus, midbrain
cervical a., ascending	a. cervicalis ascendens	inferior thyroid a.	spinal branches	muscles of neck, vertebrae, vertebral canal
cervical a., deep	a. cervicalis profunda	costocervical trunk		deep neck muscles
cervical a., transverse	a. transversa colli	subclavian a.	deep and superficial branches	root of neck, muscles of scapula
choroid a., anterior	a. choroidea anterior	internal carotid or middle cerebral a.		choroid plexus of lateral ventricle and adjacent parts

ciliary a's, anterior	aa. ciliares anteriores	ophthalmic and lacrimal a's	episcleral and anterior conjunctival a's	iris, conjunctiva
ciliary a's, posterior, long	aa. ciliares posteriores longae	ophthalmic a.		iris, ciliary processes
ciliary a's, posterior, short	aa. ciliares posteriores breves	ophthalmic a.		choroid coat of eye
circumflex femoral a., lateral	a. circumflexa femoris lateralis	deep femoral a.	ascending, descending, and transverse branches	hip joint, thigh muscles
circumflex femoral a., medial	a. circumflexa femoris medialis	deep femoral a.	deep, ascending, transverse, and acetabular branches	hip joint, thigh muscles
circumflex humeral a., anterior	a. circumflexa humeri anterior	axillary a.		shoulder joint and head of humerus, long tendon of biceps, tendon of greater pectoral muscle
circumflex humeral a., posterior	a. circumflexa humeri posterior	axillary a.		deltoid, shoulder joint, teres minor and triceps muscles
circumflex iliac a., deep	a. circumflex ilium profunda	external iliac a.	ascending branches	iliac region, abdominal wall, groin
circumflex iliac a., superficial	a. circumflexa ilium superficialis	femoral a.		groin, abdominal wall
circumflex a. of scapula	a. circumflexa scapulae	subscapular a.		inferolateral muscles of scapula
coccygeal a. *See* sacral a., median				
colic a., left	a. colica sinistra	inferior mesenteric a.		descending colon
colic a., middle	a. colica media	superior mesenteric a.		transverse colon
colic a., right	a. colica dextra	superior mesenteric a.		ascending colon
colic a., right, inferior. *See* ileocolic a.				
colic a., superior accessory. *See* colic a., middle				
collateral a., middle	a. collateralis media	deep brachial a.		triceps muscle, elbow joint
collateral a., radial	a. collateralis radialis	deep brachial a.		brachioradial and brachial muscles
collateral a., inferior ulnar	a. collateralis ulnaris inferior	brachial a.		arm muscles at back of elbow
collateral a., superior ulnar	a. collateralis ulnaris superior	brachial a.		elbow joint, triceps muscle
communicating a., anterior	a. communicans anterior cerebri	interconnects anterior cerebral a's		
communicating a., posterior	a. communicans posterior cerebri	interconnects internal carotid and posterior cerebral a's		

TABLE OF ARTERIES – *Continued*

COMMON NAME*	NA EQUIVALENT†	ORIGIN*	BRANCHES*	DISTRIBUTION
conjunctival a's, anterior	aa. conjunctivales anteriores	anterior ciliary a's		conjunctiva
conjunctival a's, posterior	aa. conjunctivales posteriores	medial palpebral a.		lacrimal caruncle, conjunctiva
coronary a., left	a. coronaria sinistra	left aortic sinus	anterior interventricular and circumflex branches	left ventricle, left atrium
coronary a., right	a. coronaria dextra	right aortic sinus	posterior interventricular branch	right ventricle, right atrium
costocervical trunk	truncus costocervicalis	subclavian a.	deep cervical and highest intercostal a's	deep neck muscles, first two intercostal spaces, vertebral column, back muscles
cremasteric a.	a. cremasterica	inferior epigastric a.		cremaster muscle, coverings of spermatic cord
cystic a.	a. cystica	right branch of hepatic a., proper		gallbladder
deep brachial. *See* brachial a., deep				
deep a. of clitoris	a. profunda clitoridis	internal pudendal a.		clitoris
deep a. of penis	a. profunda penis	internal pudendal a.		corpus cavernosum penis
deep femoral a. *See* femoral a., deep				
deep lingual a. *See* profunda linguae a.				
deferential a. *See* a. of ductus deferens				
dental a's. *See* alveolar a's				
diaphragmatic a's. *See* phrenic a's				
digital a's, collateral. *See* digital a's, palmar, proper				
digital a's of foot, common. *See* metatarsal a's, plantar				
digital a's of foot, dorsal	aa. digitales dorsales pedis	dorsal metatarsal a's		dorsum of toes
digital a's of hand, dorsal	aa. digitales dorsales manus	dorsal metacarpal a's		dorsum of fingers
digital a's, palmar, common	aa. digitales palmares communes	superficial palmar arch	proper palmar digital a's	fingers
digital a's, palmar, proper	aa. digitales palmares propriae	common palmar digital a's		fingers

digital a's, plantar, common	aa. digitales plantares, communes	plantar metatarsal a's	proper plantar digital a's	toes
digital a's, plantar, proper	aa. digitales plantares propriae	common plantar digital a's		toes
dorsal a. of clitoris	a. dorsalis clitoridis	internal pudendal a.		clitoris
dorsal a. of foot. *See* dorsalis pedis a.				
dorsal a. of nose	a. dorsalis nasi	ophthalmic a.	lacrimal branch	dorsum of nose
dorsal a. of penis	a. dorsalis penis	internal pudendal a.		glans, corona, and prepuce of penis
dorsalis pedis a.	a. dorsalis pedis	continuation of anterior tibial a.	lateral and medial tarsal, and arcuate a's	foot, toes
a. of ductus deferens	a. ductus deferentis	umbilical a.	ureteral artery	ureter, ductus deferens, seminal vesicles, testes
duodenal a's. *See* pancreaticoduodenal a., inferior				
epigastric a., external. *See* circumflex iliac a., deep				
epigastric a., inferior	a. epigastrica inferior	external iliac a.	pubic branch, cremasteric a., a. of round ligament of uterus	abdominal wall
epigastric a., superficial	a. epigastrica superficialis	femoral a.		abdominal wall, groin
epigastric a., superior	a. epigastrica superior	internal thoracic a.		abdominal wall, diaphragm
episcleral a's	aa. episclerales	anterior ciliary a.		iris, ciliary processes
ethmoidal a., anterior	a. ethmoidalis anterior	ophthalmic a.	anterior meningeal a.	dura mater, nose, frontal sinus, anterior ethmoidal cells
ethmoidal a., posterior	a. ethmoidalis posterior	ophthalmic a.		posterior ethmoidal cells, dura mater, nose
facial a.	a. facialis	external carotid a.	ascending palatine, submental, inferior and superior labial and angular a's; tonsillar and glandular branches	face, tonsil, palate, submandibular gland
facial a., deep. *See* maxillary a.				
facial a., transverse	a. transversa faciei	superficial temporal a.		parotid region
fallopian a. *See* uterine a.				
femoral a.	a. femoralis	continuation of external iliac a.	superficial epigastric, superficial circumflex iliac, external pudendal, profunda femoris, and descending genicular a's	lower abdominal wall, external genitalia, lower limb
femoral a., deep	a. profunda femoris	femoral a.	medial and lateral circumflex femoral a's, perforating a's	thigh muscles, hip joint, gluteal muscles, femur

TABLE OF ARTERIES – *Continued*

COMMON NAME*	NA EQUIVALENT†	ORIGIN*	BRANCHES*	DISTRIBUTION
fibular a. *See* peroneal a.				
frontal a. *See* supratrochlear a.				
funicular a. *See* testicular a.				
gastric a., left	a. gastrica sinistra	celiac trunk	esophageal branches	esophagus, lesser curvature of stomach
gastric a., right	a. gastrica dextra	common hepatic a.		lesser curvature of stomach
gastric a's, short	aa. gastricae breves	splenic a.		upper part of stomach
gastroduodenal a.	a. gastroduodenalis	common hepatic a.	superior pancreaticoduodenal and right gastroepiploic a's	stomach, duodenum, pancreas, greater omentum
gastroepiploic a., left	a. gastroepiploica sinistra	splenic a.	epiploic branches	stomach, greater omentum
gastroepiploic a., right	a. gastroepiploica dextra	gastroduodenal a.	epiploic branches	stomach, greater omentum
genicular a., descending	a. genus descendens	femoral a.	saphenous and articular branches	knee joint, upper and medial part of leg
genicular a., inferior, lateral	a. genus inferior lateralis	popliteal a.		knee joint
genicular a., inferior, medial	a. genus inferior medialis	popliteal a.		knee joint
genicular a., middle	a. genus media	popliteal a.		knee joint, cruciate ligaments, patellar synovial and alar folds
genicular a., superior, lateral	a. genus superior lateralis	popliteal a.		knee joint, femur, patella, contiguous muscles
genicular a., superior medial	a. genus superior medialis	popliteal a.		knee joint, femur, patella, contiguous muscles
gluteal a., inferior	a. glutea inferior	internal iliac a.	sciatic a.	buttock, back of thigh
gluteal a., superior	a. glutea superior	internal iliac a.	superficial and deep branches	buttocks
helicine a's of penis	aa. helicinae penis	deep and dorsal a's of penis		erectile tissue of penis
hemorrhoidal a's. *See* rectal a's				
hepatic a., common	a. hepatica communis	celiac trunk	right gastric, gastroduodenal, proper hepatic a's	stomach, pancreas, duodenum, liver, gallbladder, greater omentum
hepatic a., proper	a. hepatica propria	common hepatic a.	right and left branches	liver, gallbladder
hyaloid a.	a. hyaloidea	fetal ophthalmic a.		fetal lens (usually not present after birth)

hypogastric a. *See* iliac a., internal				
ileal a's	aa. ilei	superior mesenteric a.		ileum
ileocolic a.	a. ileocolica	superior mesenteric a.	ascending, anterior, and posterior cecal branches, appendicular a.	ileum, cecum, vermiform appendix, ascending colon
iliac a., common	a. iliaca communis	abdominal aorta	internal and external iliac a's	pelvis, abdominal wall, lower limb
iliac a., external	a. iliaca externa	common iliac a.	inferior epigastric, deep circumflex iliac a's	abdominal wall, external genitalia, lower limb
iliac a., internal	a. iliaca interna	continuation of common iliac a.	iliolumbar, obturator, superior and inferior gluteal, umbilical, inferior vesical, uterine, middle rectal, and internal pudendal a's	wall and viscera of pelvis, buttock, reproductive organs, medial aspect of thigh
iliolumbar a.	a. iliolumbalis	internal iliac a.	iliac and lumbar branches, lateral sacral a's	pelvic muscles and bones, fifth lumbar vertebra, sacrum
infraorbital a.	a. infraorbitalis	maxillary a.	anterior superior alveolar a's	maxilla, maxillary sinus, upper teeth, lower eyelid, cheek, nose
innominate a. *See* brachiocephalic trunk				
intercostal a., highest	a. intercostalis suprema	costocervical trunk	posterior intercostal a's I and II	upper thoracic wall
intercostal a's, posterior, I and II	aa. intercostales posteriores I et II	highest intercostal a.	dorsal and spinal branches	upper thoracic wall
intercostal a's, posterior, III–XI	aa. intercostales posteriores III–XI	thoracic aorta	dorsal, lateral, and lateral cutaneous branches	thoracic wall
interlobar a's of kidney	aa. interlobares renis	renal a.	arcuate a's of kidney	lobes of kidney
interlobular a's of kidney	aa. interlobulares renis	arcuate a's of kidney		renal glomeruli
interlobular a's of liver	aa. interlobulares hepatis	right or left branch of proper hepatic a.		between lobules of liver
interosseous a., anterior	a. interossea anterior	posterior or common interosseous a.	median a.	deep parts of front of forearm
interosseous a., common	a. interossea communis	ulnar a.	anterior and posterior interosseous a's	antecubital fossa
interosseous a., posterior	a. interossea posterior	common interosseous a.	recurrent interosseous a.	deep parts of back of forearm
interosseous a., recurrent	a. interossea recurrens	posterior or common interosseous a.		back of elbow joint
intestinal a's		vessels arising from superior mesenteric a. and supplying intestines; they include pancreaticoduodenal, jejunal, ileal, ileocolic, and colic a's		
jejunal a's	aa. jejunales	superior mesenteric a.		jejunum
labial a., inferior	a. labialis inferior	facial a.		lower lip

TABLE OF ARTERIES—*Continued*

COMMON NAME*	NA EQUIVALENT†	ORIGIN*	BRANCHES*	DISTRIBUTION
labial a., superior	a. labialis superior	facial a.	septal and alar branches	upper lip and nose
a. of labyrinth	a. labyrinthi	basilar or anterior inferior cerebellar a.	vestibular and cochlear branches	internal ear
lacrimal a.	a. lacrimalis	ophthalmic a.	lateral palpebral a.	lacrimal gland, eyelids, conjunctiva
laryngeal a., inferior	a. laryngea inferior	inferior thyroid a.		larynx, trachea, esophagus
laryngeal a., superior	a. laryngea superior	superior thyroid a.		larynx
lingual a.	a. lingualis	external carotid a.	suprahyoid, sublingual, dorsal lingual, profunda linguae branches	tongue, sublingual gland, tonsil, epiglottis
lingual a., deep. *See* profunda linguae a.				
lumbar a's	aa. lumbales	abdominal aorta	dorsal and spinal branches	posterior abdominal wall, renal capsule
lumbar a., lowest	a. lumbalis ima	median sacral a.		sacrum, greatest gluteal muscle
malleolar a., anterior, lateral	a. malleolaris anterior lateralis	anterior tibial a.		ankle joint
malleolar a., anterior, medial	a. malleolaris anterior medialis	anterior tibial a.		ankle joint
mammary a., external. *See* thoracic a., lateral				
mammary a., internal. *See* thoracic a., internal				
mandibular a. *See* alveolar a., inferior				
masseteric a.	a. masseterica	maxillary a.		masseter muscle
maxillary a.	a. maxillaris	external carotid a.	pterygoid branches; deep auricular, anterior tympanic, inferior alveolar, middle meningeal, masseteric, deep temporal, buccal, posterior superior alveolar, infraorbital, descending palatine, and sphenopalatine a's, and a. of pterygoid canal	both jaws, teeth, muscles of mastication, ear, meninges, nose, paranasal sinuses, palate
maxillary a., external. *See* facial a.				
maxillary a., internal. *See* maxillary a.				
median a.	a. mediana	anterior interosseous a.		median nerve, muscles of front of forearm

meningeal a., anterior	a. meningea anterior	anterior ethmoidal a.		dura mater of anterior cranial fossa
meningeal a., middle	a. meningea media	maxillary a.	frontal, parietal, lacrimal, anastomotic, accessory meningeal, and petrous branches, and superior tympanic a.	cranial bones, dura mater
meningeal a., posterior	a. meningea posterior	ascending pharyngeal a.		bones and dura mater of posterior cranial fossa
mental a.	a. mentalis	inferior alveolar a.		chin
mesenteric a., inferior	a. mesenterica inferior	abdominal aorta	left colic, sigmoid, and superior rectal a's	descending colon, rectum
mesenteric a., superior	a. mesenterica superior	abdominal aorta	inferior pancreaticoduodenal, jejunal, ileal, ileocolic, right and middle colic a's	small intestine, proximal half of colon
metacarpal a's, dorsal	aa. metacarpeae dorsales	dorsal carpal rete and radial a.	dorsal digital a's	dorsum of fingers
metacarpal a's, palmar	aa. metacarpeae palmares	deep palmar arch		deep parts of metacarpus
metatarsal a's, dorsal	aa. metatarseae dorsales	arcuate a. of foot	dorsal digital a's	dorsum of foot, including toes
metatarsal a's, plantar	aa. metatarseae plantares	plantar arch	perforating branches, common and proper plantar digital a's	plantar surface of toes
musculophrenic a.	a. musculophrenica	internal thoracic a.		diaphragm, abdominal and thoracic walls
nasal a's, posterior, lateral and septal	aa. nasales posteriores laterales et septi	sphenopalatine a.		nasal cavity, nasal septum, adjacent sinuses
nutrient a's of humerus	aa. nutriciae humeri	brachial and deep brachial a's		humerus
obturator a.	a. obturatoria	internal iliac a.	pubic, acetabular, anterior and posterior branches	pelvic muscles, hip joint
obturator a., accessory	a. obturatoria accessoria	variant obturator a., arising from inferior epigastric instead of internal iliac a.		
occipital a.	a. occipitalis	external carotid a.	auricular, meningeal, mastoid, descending, occipital, and sternocleidomastoid branches	muscles of neck and scalp, meninges, mastoid cells
ophthalmic a.	a. ophthalmica	internal carotid a.	lacrimal and supraorbital a's, central a. of retina, ciliary, posterior and anterior ethmoidal, palpebral, supratrochlear, and dorsal nasal a's	eye, orbit, adjacent facial structures
ovarian a.	a. ovarica	abdominal aorta	ureteral branches	ureter, ovary, uterine tube
palatine a., ascending	a. palatina ascendens	facial a.		soft palate, wall of pharynx, tonsil, auditory tube
palatine a., descending	a. palatina descendens	maxillary a.	greater and lesser palatine a's	soft and hard palates, tonsil
palatine a., greater	a. palatina major	descending palatine a.		hard palate

TABLE OF ARTERIES—*Continued*

COMMON NAME*	NA EQUIVALENT†	ORIGIN*	BRANCHES*	DISTRIBUTION
palatine a's, lesser	aa. palatinae minores	descending palatine a.		soft palate, tonsil
palpebral a's, lateral	aa. palpebrales laterales	lacrimal a.		eyelids, conjunctiva
palpebral a's, medial	aa. palpebrales mediales	ophthalmic a.	posterior conjunctival a's	eyelids
pancreaticoduodenal a's, inferior	aa. pancreaticoduodenales inferiores	superior mesenteric a.		pancreas, duodenum
pancreaticoduodenal a., superior		gastroduodenal a.		pancreas, duodenum
perforating a's	aa. perforantes	deep femoral a.		adductor, hamstring, and gluteal muscles, femur
pericardiacophrenic a.	a. pericardiacophrenica	internal thoracic a.		pericardium, diaphragm, pleura
perineal a.	a. perinealis	internal pudendal a.		perineum, skin of external genitalia
peroneal a.	a. peronea	posterior tibial a.	perforating, communicating, calcaneal, and lateral and medial malleolar branches, calcaneal rete	lateral side and back of ankle, deep calf muscles
pharyngeal a., ascending	a. pharyngea ascendens	external carotid a.	posterior meningeal, pharyngeal, inferior tympanic branches	pharynx, soft palate, ear, meninges
phrenic a's, great. *See* phrenic a's, inferior				
phrenic a's, inferior	aa. phrenicae inferiores	abdominal aorta	superior suprarenal a's	diaphragm, suprarenal gland
phrenic a's, superior	aa. phrenicae superiores	thoracic aorta		upper surface of vertebral portion of diaphragm
plantar a., lateral	a. plantaris lateralis	posterior tibial a.	plantar arch, plantar metatarsal a's	sole of foot, toes
plantar a., medial	a. plantaris medialis	posterior tibial a.	deep and superficial branches	sole of foot, toes
popliteal a.	a. poplitea	continuation of femoral a.	lateral and medial superior genicular, middle genicular, sural, lateral and medial inferior genicular, anterior and posterior tibial a's; articular rete of knee, patellar rete	knee and calf
princeps pollicis a.	a. princeps pollicis	radial a.	radialis indicis a.	sides and palmar aspect of thumb
principal a. of thumb. *See* princeps pollicis a.				
profunda linguae a.	a. profunda linguae	lingual a.		tongue
a. of pterygoid canal	a. canalis pterygoidei	maxillary a.		roof of pharynx, auditory tube
pudendal a's, external	aa. pudendae externae	femoral a.	anterior scrotal or anterior labial branches, inguinal branches	external genitalia, upper medial thigh

pudendal a, internal	a. pudenda interna	internal iliac a.	posterior scrotal or posterior labial branches, inferior rectal, perineal, urethral a's, a. of bulb of penis or vestibule, deep a. and dorsal a. of penis or clitoris	external genitalia, anal canal, perineum
pulmonary trunk	truncus pulmonalis	right ventricle	right and left pulmonary a's	conveys unaerated blood toward lungs
pulmonary a., left	a. pulmonalis sinistra	pulmonary trunk	numerous branches named according to segments of lung to which they distribute unaerated blood	left lung
pulmonary a., right	a. pulmonalis dextra	pulmonary trunk	numerous branches named according to segments of lung to which they distribute unaerated blood	right lung
radial a.	a. radialis	brachial a.	palmar carpal, superficial palmar and dorsal carpal branches; recurrent radial a., princeps pollicis a., deep palmar arch	forearm, wrist, hand
radial a., collateral. *See* collateral a., radial				
radial a. of index finger. *See* radialis indicis a.				
radialis indicis a.	a. radialis indicis	princeps pollicis a.		index finger
radiate a's of kidney. *See* interlobular a's of kidney				
ranine a. *See* profunda linguae a.				
rectal a., inferior	a. rectalis inferior	internal pudendal a.		rectum, anal canal
rectal a., middle	a. rectalis media	internal iliac a.		rectum
rectal a., superior	a. rectalis superior	inferior mesenteric a.		rectum
recurrent a., radial	a. recurrens radialis	radial a.		brachioradial and brachial muscles, elbow region
recurrent a., tibial, anterior	a. recurrens tibialis anterior	anterior tibial a.		anterior tibial muscle and long extensor muscle of toes; knee joint, contiguous fascia and skin
recurrent a., tibial, posterior	a. recurrens tibialis posterior	anterior tibial a.		knee
recurrent a., ulnar	a. recurrens ulnaris	ulnar a.	anterior and posterior branches	elbow region
renal a.	a. renalis	abdominal aorta	ureteral branches, inferior suprarenal a.	kidney, suprarenal gland, ureter

TABLE OF ARTERIES – *Continued*

COMMON NAME*	NA EQUIVALENT†	ORIGIN*	BRANCHES*	DISTRIBUTION
renal a's. *See* arcuate, interlobar, and interlobular a's, and straight arterioles of kidney	aa. renis			
a. of round ligament of uterus	a. ligamenti teretis uteri	inferior epigastric a.		round ligament of uterus
sacral a's, lateral	aa. sacrales laterales	iliolumbar a.	spinal branches	structures about coccyx and sacrum
sacral a., median	a. sacralis mediana	central continuation of abdominal aorta, beyond origin of common iliac a's	lowest lumbar a.	sacrum, coccyx, rectum
scapular a., transverse. *See* suprascapular a.				
sciatic a.	a. comitans nervi ischiadici	inferior gluteal a.		accompanies sciatic nerve
sigmoid a's	aa. sigmoideae	inferior mesenteric a.		sigmoid colon
spermatic a., external. *See* cremasteric a.				
sphenopalatine a.	a. sphenopalatina	maxillary a.	lateral and septal posterior nasal a's	structures adjoining nasal cavity, nasopharynx
spinal a., anterior	a. spinalis anterior	vertebral a.		spinal cord
spinal a., posterior	a. spinalis posterior	vertebral a.		spinal cord
splenic a.	a. lienalis	celiac trunk	pancreatic and splenic branches, left gastroepiploic, short gastric a's	spleen, pancreas, stomach, greater omentum
straight arterioles of kidney	arteriolae rectae renis	arcuate a's of kidney		renal pyramids
stylomastoid a.	a. stylomastoidea	posterior auricular a.	mastoid and stapedial branches, posterior tympanic a.	middle ear walls, mastoid cells, stapedius
subclavian a.	a. subclavia	brachiocephalic trunk (right), arch of aorta (left)	vertebral, internal thoracic a's, thyrocervical and costocervical trunks	neck, thoracic wall, spinal cord, brain, meninges, upper limb
subcostal a.	a. subcostalis	thoracic aorta	dorsal and spinal branches	upper posterior abdominal wall
sublingual a.	a. sublingualis	lingual a.		sublingual gland
submental a.	a. submentalis	facial a.		tissues under chin
subscapular a.	a. subscapularis	axillary a.	thoracodorsal and circumflex scapular a's	scapular and shoulder region
supraorbital a.	a. supraorbitalis	ophthalmic a.		forehead, superior muscles of orbit, upper eyelid, frontal sinus

suprarenal a., inferior	a. suprarenalis inferior	renal a.		suprarenal gland
suprarenal a., middle	a. suprarenalis media	abdominal aorta		suprarenal gland
suprarenal a's, superior	aa. suprarenales superiores	inferior phrenic a.		suprarenal gland
suprascapular a.	a. suprascapularis	thyrocervical trunk	acromial branch	clavicular, deltoid, and scapular regions
supratrochlear a.	a. supratrochlearis	ophthalmic a.		anterior scalp
sural a's	aa. surales	popliteal a.		popliteal space, calf
sylvian a. *See* cerebral a., middle				
tarsal a., lateral	a. tarsea lateralis	dorsalis pedis a.		tarsus
tarsal a's, medial	aa. tarseae mediales	dorsalis pedis a.		side of foot
temporal a's, deep	aa. temporales profundae	maxillary a.		deep parts of temporal region
temporal a., middle	a. temporalis media	superficial temporal a.		temporal region
temporal a., superficial	a. temporalis superficialis	external carotid a.	parotid, anterior auricular, frontal and parietal branches; transverse facial, zygomaticoorbital, middle temporal a's	parotid and temporal regions
testicular a.	a. testicularis	abdominal aorta	ureteral branches	ureter, epididymis, testis
thoracic a., highest	a. thoracica suprema	axillary a.		axillary aspects of chest wall
thoracic a., internal	a. thoracica interna	subclavian a.	mediastinal, thymic, bronchial, sternal, perforating, lateral costal and anterior intercostal branches; pericardiacophrenic, musculophrenic, superior epigastric a's	anterior thoracic wall, mediastinal structures, diaphragm
thoracic a., lateral	a. thoracica lateralis	axillary a.	mammary branches	pectoral muscles, mammary gland
thoracoacromial a.	a. thoracoacromialis	axillary a.	clavicular, pectoral, deltoid, and acromial branches	deltoid, clavicular, thoracic regions
thoracodorsal a.	a. thoracodorsalis	subscapular a.		subscapular and teres major and minor muscles
thyrocervical trunk	truncus thyrocervicalis	subclavian a.	inferior thyroid, suprascapular and transverse cervical a's	deep neck, including thyroid gland, scapular region
thyroid a., inferior	a. thyroidea inferior	thyrocervical trunk	pharyngeal, esophageal, tracheal branches; inferior laryngeal, ascending cervical a's	thyroid gland and adjacent structures
thyroid a., lowest. *See* a. thyroidea ima				
thyroid a., superior	a. thyroidea superior	external carotid a.	hyoid, sternocleidomastoid, superior laryngeal, cricothyroid, muscular, and glandular branches	thyroid gland and adjacent structures
thyroidea ima a.	a. thyroidea ima	arch of aorta, brachiocephalic trunk or right common carotid a.		thyroid gland

Table of Arteries – *Concluded*

COMMON NAME*	NA EQUIVALENT†	ORIGIN*	BRANCHES*	DISTRIBUTION
tibial a., anterior	a. tibialis anterior	popliteal a.	posterior and anterior tibial recurrent a's, lateral and medial anterior malleolar a's, lateral and medial malleolar retes	leg, ankle, foot
tibial a., posterior	a. tibialis posterior	popliteal a.	fibular circumflex branch; peroneal, medial plantar, lateral plantar a's	leg, foot
transverse a. of face. *See* facial a., transverse				
transverse a. of neck. *See* cervical a., transverse				
transverse a. of scapula. *See* suprascapular a.				
tympanic a., anterior	a. tympanica anterior	maxillary a.		tympanic cavity
tympanic a., inferior	a. tympanica inferior	ascending pharyngeal a.		tympanic cavity
tympanic a., posterior	a. tympanica posterior	stylomastoid a.		tympanic cavity
tympanic a., superior	a. tympanica superior	middle meningeal a.		tympanic cavity
ulnar a.	a. ulnaris	brachial a.	palmar carpal, dorsal carpal, and deep palmar branches; ulnar recurrent and common interosseous a's; superficial palmar arch	forearm, wrist, hand
ulnar a., collateral. *See* collateral a., ulnar, inferior and collateral a., ulnar, superior				
umbilical a.	a. umbilicalis	internal iliac a.	a. of ductus deferens, superior vesical a's	ductus deferens, seminal vesicles, testes, urinary bladder, ureter
urethral a.	a. urethralis	internal pudendal a.		urethra
uterine a.	a. uterina	internal iliac a.	ovarian and tubal branches; vaginal a.	uterus, vagina, round ligament of uterus, uterine tube, ovary
vaginal a.	a. vaginalis	uterine a.		vagina, fundus of bladder
vertebral a.	a. vertebralis	subclavian a.	spinal and meningeal branches; posterior inferior cerebellar, basilar, anterior, and posterior spinal a's	muscles of neck, vertebrae, spinal cord, cerebellum, interior of cerebrum
vesical a., inferior	a. vesicalis inferior	internal iliac a.		bladder, prostate, seminal vesicles
vesical a's, superior	aa. vesicales superiores	umbilical a.		bladder, urachus, ureter
zygomaticoorbital a.	a. zygomaticoorbitalis	superficial temporal a.		lateral side of orbit

ARA Nomenclature and Classification of Arthritis and Rheumatism (Tentative)

I. Polyarthritis of unknown etiology
  A. Rheumatoid arthritis
  B. Juvenile rheumatoid arthritis (Still's disease)
  C. Ankylosing spondylitis
  D. Psoriatic arthritis
  E. Reiter's syndrome
  F. Others
II. "Connective tissue" disorders
  A. Systemic lupus erythematosus
  B. Polyarteritis nodosa
  C. Scleroderma (progressive systemic sclerosis)
  D. Polymyositis and dermatomyositis
  E. Others
III. Rheumatic fever
IV. Degenerative joint disease (osteoarthritis, osteoarthrosis)
  A. Primary
  B. Secondary
V. Nonarticular rheumatism
  A. Fibrositis
  B. Intervertebral disk and low back syndromes
  C. Myositis and myalgia
  D. Tendinitis and peritendinitis (bursitis)
  E. Tenosynovitis
  F. Fasciitis
  G. Carpal tunnel syndrome
  H. Others
  (See also shoulder-hand syndrome, VIII. E.)
VI. Diseases with which arthritis is frequently associated
  A. Sarcoidosis
  B. Relapsing polychondritis
  C. Henoch-Schönlein syndrome
  D. Ulcerative colitis
  E. Regional ileitis
  F. Whipple's disease
  G. Sjögren's syndrome
  H. Familial Mediterranean fever
  I. Others
  (See also psoriatic arthritis, I. D.)
VII. Associated with known infectious agents
  A. Bacterial
    1. Brucella
    2. Gonococcus
    3. Mycobacterium tuberculosis
    4. Pneumococcus
    5. Salmonella
    6. Staphylococcus
    7. Streptobacillus moniliformis (Haverhill fever)
    8. Treponema pallidum (syphilis)
    9. Treponema pertenue (yaws)
    10. Others
  B. Rickettsial
  C. Viral
  D. Fungal
  E. Parasitic
  (See also rheumatic fever, III.)
VIII. Traumatic and/or neurogenic disorders
  A. Traumatic arthritis (viz., the result of direct trauma)
  B. Lues (tertiary syphilis)
  C. Diabetes
  D. Syringomyelia
  E. Shoulder-hand syndrome
  F. Mechanical derangement of joints
  G. Others
  (See also degenerative joint disease, IV.; carpal tunnel syndrome, V. G.)
IX. Associated with known biochemical or endocrine abnormalities
  A. Gout
  B. Ochronosis
  C. Hemophilia
  D. Hemoglobinopathies (e.g., sickle cell disease)
  E. Agammaglobulinemia
  F. Gaucher's disease
  G. Hyperparathyroidism
  H. Acromegaly
  I. Hypothyroidism
  J. Scurvy (hypovitaminosis C)
  K. Xanthoma tuberosum
  L. Others
  (See also multiple myeloma, X. G.; Hurler's syndrome, XII. C.)
X. Tumor and tumor-like conditions
  A. Synovioma
  B. Pigmented villonodular synovitis
  C. Giant cell tumor of tendon sheath
  D. Primary juxta-articular bone tumors
  E. Metastatic
  F. Leukemia
  G. Multiple myeloma
  H. Benign tumors of articular tissue
  I. Others
  (See also hypertrophic osteoarthropathy, XIII. G.)
XI. Allergy and drug reactions
  A. Arthritis due to specific allergens (e.g., serum sickness)
  B. Arthritis due to drugs (e.g., hydralazine syndrome)
  C. Others
XII. Inherited and congenital disorders
  A. Marfan's syndrome
  B. Ehlers-Danlos syndrome
  C. Hurler's syndrome
  D. Congenital hip dysplasia
  E. Morquio's disease
  F. Others
XIII. Miscellaneous disorders
  A. Amyloidosis
  B. Aseptic necrosis of bone
  C. Behcet's syndrome
  D. Chondrocalcinosis (pseudogout)
  E. Erythema multiforme (Stevens-Johnson syndrome)
  F. Erythema nodosum
  G. Hypertrophic osteoarthropathy
  H. Juvenile osteochondritis
  I. Osteochondritis dissecans
  J. Reticulohistiocytosis of joints (lipoid dermato-arthritis)
  K. Tietze's disease
  L. Others

From the Committee of the American Rheumatism Association: Primer On Rheumatic Diseases. The Arthritis Foundation.

from rheumatoid arthritis. Other researchers contend that the disease may be due to infection, perhaps from an undefined virus or some other microorganism (e.g., *Mycoplasma*). There also is the possibility that rheumatoid arthritis is a genetic disorder in which one inherits a predisposition to the disease.

Physical and emotional STRESS also plays some part in the onset of acute attacks; however, psychological stress is implicated as a causative factor in the onset of many illnesses.

SYMPTOMS AND PATHOLOGY. In about 75 percent of patients the onset of rheumatoid arthritis is gradual with only mild symptoms at the beginning. Early symptoms include malaise, fever, weight loss, and morning stiffness of the joints. One or more joints may become swollen, painful, and inflamed. Some patients may experience only mild espisodes of acute symptoms with lengthy remissions. The more typical patient, however, experiences increasingly severe and frequent attacks with subsequent joint damage and deformity. The pattern of remissions and exacerbations continues throughout the course of the disease.

If untreated, and sometimes in spite of treatment, the joint pathology in rheumatoid arthritis goes through four stages: (1) proliferative inflammation of the synovium with increased exudate, which eventually leads to thickening of the synovium; (2) formation of a layer of granulation tissue (pannus) which erodes and destroys the cartilage and eventually spreads to contiguous areas, causing destruction of the bone capsule and parts of the muscles that control the joint; (3) fibrous ankylosis resulting from the invasion of the pannus by tough fibrous tissue; and (4) bony ankylosis as the fibrous tissue becomes calcified.

In addition to the joint changes there is atrophy of muscles, bones, and skin adjacent to the affected joint. The most characteristic lesions of rheumatoid arthritis are subcutaneous nodules, which may be present for weeks or months and are most commonly found over bony prominences, especially near the elbow.

Because rheumatoid arthritis is a systemic disease, there is involvement of connective tissues other than those in the musculoskeletal system. Degenerative lesions may be found in the collagen in the lungs, heart, blood vessels, and pleura.

Patients with rheumatoid arthritis appear undernourished and chronically ill. Most are anemic because of the effect of the disease on blood-forming organs. The erythrocyte sedimentation rate is elevated and the WBC may be slightly elevated.

TREATMENT AND PATIENT CARE. Management of rheumatoid arthritis is aimed at providing rest and freedom from pain, minimizing emotional stress, preventing or correcting deformities, and maintaining or restoring function so that the patient can enjoy as much independence and mobility as possible.

Rest and Exercise. It is recommended that the patient with rheumatoid arthritis allow himself from 10 to 12 hours sleep out of each 24. During the time the patient is lying in bed he should be careful to maintain good posture and avoid pillows or other devices that support the joints in a flexed position. A firm mattress is recommended, with only one pillow under the head. During periods of severe attacks, the patient may require continuous bed rest.

The purpose of rest is to allow the body's natural defenses against inflammation to work at optimal level. It is necessary, however, even in the acute phase to balance rest with prescribed exercises which take into account the severity of the case, the joints affected, and the patient's individual needs and tolerance.

Physical Therapy. The goals of physical therapy for the patient with rheumatoid arthritis are to prevent and correct deformities, control pain, strengthen weakened muscles, and improve function.

Therapeutic EXERCISE is of major importance in the physical therapy program established for the patient. It is necessary to enlist his cooperation, and this can be done most effectively by explaining the purposes of the exercises and teaching him ways to exercise which will not increase pain. In many instances proper exercise can actually diminish pain. The patient's tolerance for exercises must be carefully monitored. While it is expected that some discomfort may be present during exercise, there should not be persistent pain that continues for hours after the exercises have been done. If such pain and fatigue do occur, the exercise program should be reviewed and revised so that a good balance of rest and exercise is obtained. It should be remembered that overactivity can contribute to the inflammatory process.

Applications of HEAT or COLD may be used in the management of rheumatoid arthritis. Heat applications improve circulation, promote relaxation, and relieve pain. When used in conjunction with exercise, heat can allow more freedom of joint movement. Various forms of heat therapy may be used, including dry heat, moist heat, DIATHERMY, and ultrasound. For dry heat a therapeutic infrared heat lamp may be most convenient during home care. Hot water bottles or electric heating pads also may be used. For treatment of the hands, paraffin baths are effective. Wet heat can be applied by hot tub baths with the water temperature not exceeding 39° C. (102° F.) or by means of a towel dipped in hot water, wrung out, and applied to the joint. Whirlpool baths are effective, especially when prolonged treatment is indicated.

Relief from pain and stiffness can be provided for some patients by applications of cold packs to the affected joints. This can be done by placing ice packs directly over the joint.

When either heat or cold is used, care must be taken to protect the patient's skin. It should be remembered that rheumatoid arthritis affects the skin as well as other tissues.

Whenever it is necessary to handle the joints and limbs of a patient with rheumatoid arthritis, it is extremely important to move slowly and gently, avoiding sudden, jarring movements which stimulate muscle contraction and produce pain. The affected joints should be supported so that there is no excessive motion.

Medication. There is no drug that will cure arthritis. The physician does have a variety of medications that he may prescribe, depending on the individual patient, his needs and tolerance. It is important that the patient be advised of the expected results and possible undesirable side-effects that may accompany the ingestion of certain drugs. With this information at hand, he can work cooperatively with the physician in determining which drug or drugs can be most beneficial for treatment of his condition.

The least expensive, safest, and among the most useful medicines in the treatment of arthritis are the salts of salicylic acid. The most common of these are aspirin and sodium salicylate. There is some evidence that salicylates have beneficial effects as anti-inflammatory agents as well as providing relief from pain, and therefore should be taken on a regular basis as prescribed. For those who suffer stomach upset or other gastrointestinal side effects from aspirin, enteric-coated tablets or antacid mixtures of aspirin are available. The average dose of aspirin is 14 tablets (4.2 gm.) per day, taken in doses of three to four tablets with each of three meals per day and three tablets with an evening snack. Analgesics other than aspirin also may be prescribed to control pain.

Indomethacin (Indocin) is a relatively new analgesic anti-inflammatory drug that may be used in the treatment of rheumatoid arthritis. It is not considered to be more effective than aspirin and it produces numerous untoward effects related to the gastrointestinal and nervous systems. Other drugs which have similar effects are phenylbutazone (Butazolidin) and oxyphenbutazone (Tanderil). They are not used as major drugs in the treatment of rheumatoid arthritis because of their serious toxic effects.

Gold compounds may be prescribed for selected patients who cannot tolerate or are not responding well to more conservative methods of treatment.

The adrenocorticosteroids may be used in treating rheumatoid arthritis, but they are not a substitute for other forms of treatment. In some cases these drugs produce side effects that are more difficult to treat than arthritis. They also may worsen certain features of the disease rather than relieve them. Drugs included in this group are cortisone, hydrocortisone, prednisone, prednisolone, and dexamethasone.

Surgical Intervention and Orthopedic Devices. In the past, surgical intervention was reserved for patients who had already suffered severe joint deformity. There is presently a trend toward the use of surgery in the early stages of the disease so that deformities and serious mechanical abnormalities can be prevented or at least modified.

One surgical procedure employed is *synovectomy* (excision of the synovial membrane of a joint). The goal of this treatment is to interrupt the destructive inflammatory processes which eventually lead to ankylosis and invasion of surrounding cartilage and bone tissues.

Surgical repair of a hip joint (*arthroplasty*) may be performed when there is extensive damage and ambulation is not possible. The purpose of this procedure is to restore, improve, or maintain joint function. In cases in which it is not possible to restore the damaged hip joint there is a surgical procedure in which the diseased joint is completely replaced with a total hip prosthesis. The procedure is called a *total hip replacement.* A similar procedure involving total replacement of the knee can be done when there is extensive damage to the knee joint.

Braces, casts, or splints are sometimes used to immoblize the affected part so that it can rest during an active stage of the disease. Devices which immobilize the affected joint also may allow for motion of adjacent muscle, thereby improving muscle strength and permitting more independence on the part of the patient. Braces also may be used to prevent deformities by maintaining good position of the joints.

Patient Education. Unfortunately, arthritis is so widespread and such a crippling disease that its victims are easy prey for charlatans and promoters of miraculous "cures." The nature of the disease, with its unexplained remissions and relief of symptoms, makes it easy for unscrupulous individuals to convince the arthritic patient that some bizarre treatment they have used has indeed "cured" the arthritis. It is important that members of the health team recognize the need for patient education and work diligently with the patient and his family so that they can cooperatively participate in a program of care that is most effective for the individual patient.

Home care is an essential part of the management of arthritis. To help in the education of the public The Arthritis Foundation provides a number of pamphlets and other educational materials. The foundation also supports a broad program of research and education and helps finance improvement of local facilities for treatment of arthritis. The address of the foundation is The Arthritis Foundation, 1212 Avenue of the Americas, New York, New York 10036.

The Self-Help Device Office of the Institute of Physical Medicine and Rehabilitation, 400 East 34th Street, New York, New York 10016, can supply information on specifically designed self-help devices for arthritic patients. The office is maintained by a grant received from The Arthritis Foundation.

suppurative a., inflammation of a joint with a purulent effusion into the joint, due chiefly to bacterial infection.

arthrocele (ar′thro-sēl) a joint swelling.

arthrocentesis (ar″thro-sen-te′sis) surgical puncture of a joint cavity for aspiration of fluid.

arthrochondritis (ar″thro-kon-dri′tis) inflammation of the cartilage of a joint.

arthroclasia (ar″thro-kla′ze-ah) surgical breaking down of an ankylosis to permit a joint to move freely.

arthrodesis (ar″thro-de′sis) surgical fusion of a joint.

arthrodia (ar-thro′de-ah) a type of synovial joint

that allows only a gliding motion; called also gliding joint. adj., **arthro′dial.**

arthrodynia (ar″thro-din′e-ah) arthralgia.

arthrodysplasia (ar″thro-dis-pla′ze-ah) any abnormality of joint development.

arthroempyesis (ar″thro-em″pi-e′sis) suppuration within a joint.

arthroendoscopy (ar″thro-en-dos′ko-pe) inspection of the interior of a joint with an endoscope.

arthrography (ar-throg′rah-fe) roentgenography of a joint.

air a., pneumoarthrography.

arthrogryposis (ar″thro-grĭ-po′sis) 1. persistent flexion of a joint. 2. tetanoid spasm.

arthrolith (ar′thro-lith) a calculous deposit within a joint.

arthrology (ar-throl′o-je) scientific study or description of the joints.

arthrolysis (ar-throl′ĭ-sis) operative loosening of adhesions in an ankylosed joint.

arthrometer (ar-throm′ĕ-ter) an instrument for measuring the angles of movements of joints.

arthro-ophthalmopathy (ar″thro-of″thal-mop′ah-the) an association of degenerative joint disease and eye disease.

arthropathy (ar-throp′ah-the) any joint disease.

Charcot's a., neuropathic a., chronic progressive degeneration of the stress-bearing portion of a joint, with hypertrophic changes at the periphery; it is associated with neurologic disorders involving loss of sensation in the joint.

osteopulmonary a., clubbing of fingers and toes, and enlargement of ends of the long bones, in cardiac or pulmonary disease.

arthrophyma (ar″thro-fi′mah) a joint swelling.

arthrophyte (ar″thro-fīt) an abnormal growth in a joint cavity.

arthroplasty (ar′thro-plas″te) plastic repair of a joint.

arthropod (ar″thro-pod) an individual of the phylum Arthropoda.

Arthropoda (ar-throp′o-dah) a phylum of the animal kingdom including bilaterally symmetrical animals with hard, segmented bodies bearing jointed appendages; embracing the largest number of known animals, with at least 740,000 species, divided into 12 classes. It includes the arachnids, crustaceans, and insects.

arthrosclerosis (ar″thro-sklĕ-ro′sis) stiffening or hardening of the joints.

arthroscope (ar″thro-skōp) an endoscope for examining the interior of a joint.

arthroscopy (ar-thros′ko-pe) examination of the interior of a joint with an arthroscope.

arthrosis (ar-thro′sis) 1. a joint or articulation. 2. disease of a joint.

arthrostomy (ar-thros′to-me) surgical creation of an opening in a joint, as for drainage.

arthrosynovitis (ar″thro-sin″o-vi′tis) inflammation of the synovial membrane of a joint.

arthrotomy (ar-throt′o-me) incision of a joint.

arthroxesis (ar-throk′sĕ-sis) scraping of an articular surface.

articular (ar-tik′u-lar) pertaining to a joint.

articulare (ar-tik″u-la′re) the point of intersection of the dorsal contours of the articular process of the mandible and the temporal bone.

articulate (ar-tik′u-lāt) 1. to unite by joints; to join. 2. united by joints. 3. capable of expressing one's self orally.

articulatio (ar-tik″u-la′she-o), pl. *articulatio′nes* [L.] an articulation or joint.

articulation (ar-tik″u-la′shun) 1. a joint; the place of union or junction between two or more bones of the skeleton. 2. enunciation of words and sentences.

articulator (ar-tik′u-la″tor) a device for effecting a jointlike union.

dental a., a device that simulates movements of the temporomandibular joints or mandible, used in dentistry.

articulo mortis (ar-tik′u-lo mor′tis) at the point or moment of death.

artifact (ar′tĭ-fakt) a structure or appearance that is not natural, but is due to manipulation (man-made).

artificial (ar″tĭ-fish′al) made by art; not natural or pathologic.

a. eye, see under EYE.

a. limb, a replacement for a natural limb (see also PROSTHESIS).

a. organ, a mechanical device that can substitute temporarily or permanently for a body organ. The development of artificial organs represents one of the outstanding achievements of contemporary medicine. The field of organ substitution has progressed rapidly over a brief span of years. Most of the artificial organs in use today are hospital devices that are connected temporarily to patients in order to do the work of an organ that is either disabled or undergoing surgery. Recent advances in electronics (principally the development of the transistor and the low-drain battery), together with advances in surgical techniques, have made possible the development of miniature artificial organs that can be surgically implanted in a patient and function independently for long periods.

The development of artificial organs has paved the way for other medical advances in the field of organ TRANSPLANTATION, the replacement of a disabled organ with a healthy living organ from a "donor." The surgical techniques of artificial organ implantation and living organ transplantation have much in common. Also, it is often necessary to use an artificial organ to temporarily take over the functions of an organ undergoing transplantation surgery.

The HEART-LUNG MACHINE is a surgery aid that permits previously impossible operations on the heart, lungs, and great vessels, and also allows other kinds of surgery to be performed on seriously weakened patients without fear of heart failure.

Cardiac patients suffering from HEART BLOCK (a defect in the transmission of nerve impulses between the separate pumping chambers of the heart) are kept alive with an electronic heart stimulator called the artificial PACEMAKER. The device is also used in certain cardiac operations in which heart block is a possible complication. A compact version of the hospital pacemaker can be surgically implanted in the chest of a patient. Miniature pacemakers of this kind are keeping thousands of heart block victims alive today.

Researchers in cardiac disease are experimenting with several types of artificial hearts. It is hoped that a mechanical pump implanted permanently in a patient can match the output of a normal heart. Another experimental device along similar lines is called a "booster heart," designed to reduce the work load of the left ventricle.

Artificial heart valves are used to replace those damaged by disease. The mitral valve, which controls the passage of blood between the left atrium and left ventricle, is often impaired by rheumatic fever. Some cardiac disorders impair the aortic valve, which controls blood flow from the heart to the body. Artificial aortic and mitral valves have been successfully implanted in human hearts. Damaged blood vessels (which in the past could be replaced only by the difficult procedure of transplantation from donors who had died suddenly) are now replaced with tubes made of Teflon or Dacron.

Normal kidneys filter waste products from the blood, expelling these substances in the urine. When the kidneys fail, waste products can build up in the blood to poisonous levels, causing uremia. The only treatment available for this condition is the artificial kidney. A simple filtering device, the artificial kidney takes blood from the patient and circulates it through a coil of cellophane tubing which is immersed in a "rinsing" fluid. The process is complete only after all the patient's blood has been purified. (See also KIDNEY and PERITONEAL DIALYSIS.)

a. respiration, any method of forcing air into and out of the lungs to start breathing in a person whose breathing has stopped. Artificial respiration can be given with no equipment whatsoever, so that it is an ideal emergency first-aid procedure.

INDICATIONS. Artificial respiration can save a life whenever breathing has stopped but heartbeat has not, as in near-drowning, electric shock, choking, gas poisoning, drug poisoning, injury to the chest, or suffocation from other causes. Usually one can tell that breathing has stopped by noting the lack of up-and-down movement of the chest. Often the cause of the stoppage of breathing is obvious, as when a drowning person is pulled out of the water. But sometimes it is impossible to tell what stopped the breathing—accident or disease—and therefore whether artificial respiration would or would not be helpful. In such cases, the rule to follow is: when in doubt, give artificial respiration and continue until additional medical help is available.

WHAT TO DO. To be effective, artificial respiration must be begun immediately. A person dies in minutes after his beathing stops. A delay of seconds may be the difference between life and death. That is why it is so important to learn how to apply artificial respiration before an accident happens.

At the same time artificial respiration is begun someone should call a doctor or the local fire department, but if there is no one to send, artificial respiration should be given in preference to going for help.

Any obstruction in the victim's mouth that would interfere with the passage of air—mud, sand, chewing gum, or displaced false teeth, for example—is removed immediately. Clothing that is tight around the neck is loosened.

Once begun, artificial respiration should be continued until the victim begins to breathe regularly by himself, until a physician takes charge, or until it is obvious that the victim will not revive. Do not give up easily. Victims have recovered as long as 4

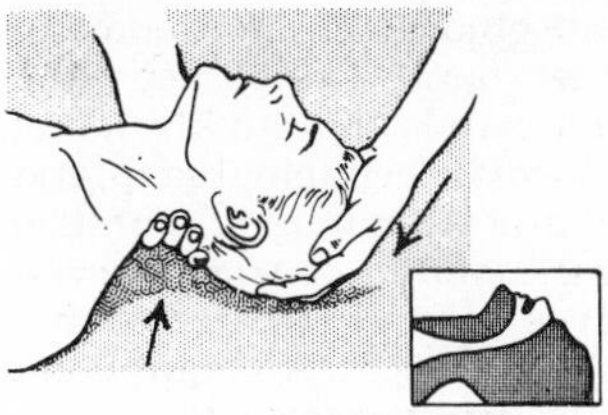

(1)

The operator takes his position at the patient's head.

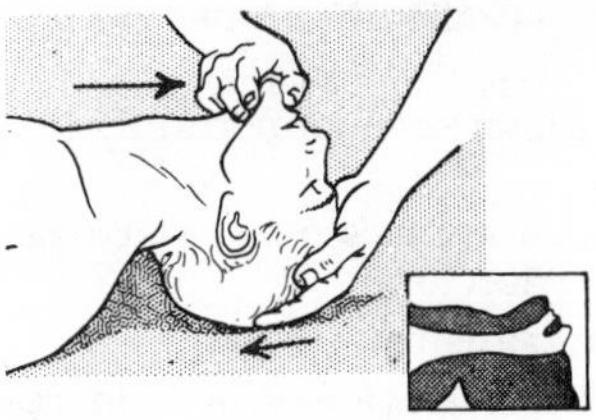

(2)

With the right thumb and index finger he displaces the mandible forward by pressing at its central portion, at the same time lifting the neck and tilting the head as far back as possible.

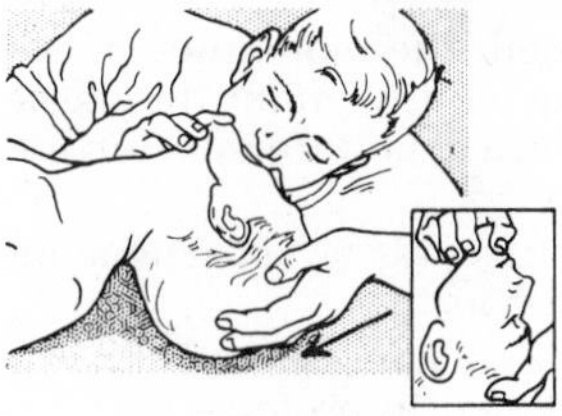

(3)

After taking a deep breath, the operator immediately seals his mouth around the mouth (or nose) of the victim and exhales until the chest of the victim rises.

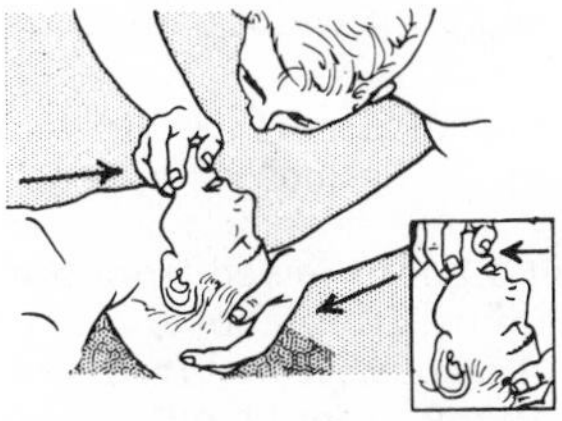

(4)

The victim's mouth is opened by downward and forward traction on the lower jaw or by pulling down the lower lip.

Technique of mouth-to-mouth resuscitation. (From Chatton, M. J., et al.: *Handbook of Medical Treatment.* 12th ed. Los Altos, Calif., Lange Medical Publishers, 1970.)

hours after artificial respiration was started. If cardiac arrest or weakness occurs, a second person who knows how should give CARDIAC MASSAGE. If only one person is present, he should provide both alternately. (See also CARDIOPULMONARY RESUSCITATION.)

When the victim has revived, he is kept quiet, covered to prevent chills, and given other first aid for SHOCK.

METHODS. There are three methods of artificial respiration: the mouth-to-mouth method, the chest pressure–arm lift (Silvester) method, and the back pressure–arm lift (Holger-Nielsen) method.

The mouth-to-mouth technique is recognized by authorities as the most effective method that can be given by an individual. Some persons feel squeamish at the thought of using it, but in an emergency such doubts usually vanish. Anyone who hesitates about putting his mouth on another person's, even in an emergency, can place a handkerchief over the victim's mouth. Air will pass readily through the cloth.

If the victim is a laryngectomee who has a stoma at the trachea, the lips of the rescuer are placed around the stoma so as to make a seal. The procedure is followed in the same manner as in mouth-to-mouth resuscitation.

The other two methods are recommended only (1) if a person cannot bring himself to use the mouth-to-mouth technique, (2) if circumstances (such as a severe mouth injury in the victim) prevent him from using it, or (3) if he feels more familiar with another method at the time of the emergency.

aryl- (ar′il) prefix, *a chemical radical belonging to the aromatic series.*

arytenoid (ar″ĭ-te′noid) shaped like a jug or pitcher, as the arytenoid cartilage or arytenoid muscle of the larynx.

arytenoidectomy (ar″ĭ-tĕ-noi-dek′to-me) excision of an arytenoid cartilage.

arytenoiditis (ar″ĭ-te-noi-di′tis) inflammation of the arytenoid muscle or cartilage.

arytenoidopexy (ar″ĭ-te-noi′do-pek″se) surgical fixation of arytenoid cartilage or muscle.

A.S. [L.] *au′ris sinis′tra (left ear).*

As chemical symbol, *arsenic.*

ASA acetylsalicylic acid (aspirin).

asbestiform (as-bes′tĭ-form) resembling asbestos.

asbestos (as-bes′tos) fibrous magnesium and calcium silicate, a nonburning compound used in roofing and insulating materials.

a. bodies, golden yellow bodies of various shapes in the sputum, lung secretions, and feces of patients with asbestosis, formed by deposition of calcium and iron salts and proteins on spicules of asbestos.

asbestosis (as″bes-to′sis) lung disease caused by inhalation of asbestos fibers (see also PNEUMOCONIOSIS).

ascariasis (as″kah-ri′ah-sis) infection with *Ascaris.*

ascaricide (as-kar′ĭ-sīd) an agent destructive to ascarids. adj., **ascarici′dal.**

ascarid (as′kah-rid) any of the phasmid nematodes of the Ascaridoidea, which includes the genera *Ascaridia, Ascaris, Toxocara,* and *Toxascaris.*

Ascaris (as′kah-ris) a genus of nematode parasites found in the intestines of man and other vertebrates.

A. lumbricoi′des, a species causing colicky pains and diarrhea, especially in children. (See also WORMS.)

A. su′is, a species morphologically similar to *A. lumbricoides,* but commonly found in pigs.

Aschheim-Zondek test (ash′hīm tson′dek) AZ test; a biologic test for pregnancy. Injection of urine from a pregnant woman into immature female mice produces marked changes in the appearance of their ovaries within 100 hours. The test is 95 to 99 per cent accurate. (See also PREGNANCY TESTS.)

Aschoff's bodies (nodules) (ash′ofs) submiliary collections of cells and leukocytes in the interstitial tissues of the heart in rheumatic myocarditis.

ascites (ah-si′tēz) abnormal accumulation of serous fluid in the peritoneal cavity, sometimes resulting in considerable and uncomfortable distention of the abdomen. adj., **ascit′ic.** Ascites can be caused by many conditions, including cirrhosis of the liver, heart and kidney disease, and inflammation and tumors within the abdominal cavity.

NURSING CARE. The position most comfortable for the patient is with the head of the bed elevated to facilitate breathing. When the patient is lying on his side a small pillow is used to support the rib cage. Skin care is given frequently to prevent the breakdown of edematous tissue associated with ascites.

Sodium restriction and diuretics are usually necessary as a part of the treatment of ascites. Potassium may be given to replace that lost through the kidneys. Intake and output must be measured and recorded accurately.

PARACENTESIS may be done to remove excess fluid from the abdominal cavity. The patient should void immediately before the procedure so as to eliminate the danger of injury to the urinary bladder. The amount and character of the fluid removed is observed and recorded on the patient's chart. The site of the puncture should be covered with a dry dressing after the procedure and observed periodically for drainage and signs of infection.

chylous a., the presence of milky fluid containing globules of fat in the peritoneal cavity owing to rupture of the thoracic duct or to extravasation through its wall.

Ascomycetes (as″ko-mi-se′tēz) a genus of fungi.

ascorbate (as-kor′bāt) a compound or derivative of ascorbic acid.

ascorbic acid (as-kor′bik) vitamin C, called also cevitamic acid; a substance found in many fruits and vegetables, especially citrus fruits, such as oranges and lemons, and tomatoes. Ascorbic acid is an essential element of the diet; lack of vitamin C can lead to SCURVY or to less severe conditions, such as delayed healing of wounds. Solutions of ascorbic acid deteriorate very rapidly and the vitamin is not stored in the body to any extent. Large doses of commercial preparations of ascorbic acid may cause gastrointestinal irritation. There is no general agreement as to the normal and therapeutic daily requirements of vitamin C. It is believed that ascorbic acid requirements in stress are abnormally high. Under moderate stress circumstances authorities recommend about 300 mg. daily.

ascospore (as′ko-spōr) a spore contained or produced in an ascus.

ascus (as′kus) the spore case of certain fungi.

-ase (ās) suffix used in forming the name of enzymes, affixed to a stem indicating the substrate (luciferase), the general nature of the substrate (proteinase), the type of reaction effected (hydrolase), or a combination of these (transaminase).

asemasia (as″e-ma′ze-ah) inability to make or comprehend signs or tokens of communication.

asepsis (a-sep′sis) absence of septic matter; freedom from infection or infectious material. adj., **asep′tic.**

MEDICAL ASEPSIS. Medical asepsis refers to destruction of organisms after they leave the body. This technique is used in the care of patients with infectious diseases to prevent reinfection of the patient and to avoid the spread of infection from one person to another. This is achieved by ISOLATION TECHNIQUE, in which the objects in the patient's environment are protected from contamination or disinfected as soon as possible after contamination.

SURGICAL ASEPSIS. Surgical asepsis refers to destruction of organisms before they enter the body. It is used in caring for open wounds and in surgical procedures. In surgical asepsis an object may be sterile (free from microorganisms) or unsterile. Measures that can be taken to provide surgical asepsis include absolute sterilization of all instruments, linens, or other inanimate objects that may come in contact with the surgical wound. The surgeon and his assistants wash their hands thoroughly for at least 5 minutes, using a special germicidal soap, and then don surgical gloves and other outer clothing to avoid contamination of the wound. In some operating rooms the air supply is specially treated so that organisms present can be destroyed. All equipment and other inanimate objects in the operating room must be kept clean and periodically treated with a disinfectant.

asexual (a-seks′u-al) without sex; not pertaining to or involving sex.

asexualization (a-seks″u-al-ĭ-za′shun) sterilization, as by castration or vasectomy.

asialia (ah″si-a′le-ah) aptyalism.

asiderosis (ah″sid-er-o′sis) deficiency of iron reserve of the body.

asparagine (ah-spar′ah-jēn) the monamide of aspartic acid, from asparagus and many kinds of seeds; used as a diuretic and as a culture medium for certain bacteria.

aspartate (ah-spahr′tāt) any salt of aspartic acid; aspartic acid in dissociated form.

aspartic acid (ah-spar′tik) a nonessential dibasic amino acid, widely distributed in proteins.

aspecific (ah″spĕ-sif′ik) not specific; not caused by a specific organism.

aspect (as′pekt) 1. that part of a surface viewed from a particular direction. 2. the look or appearance.

dorsal a., that surface of a body viewed from the back or, in veterinary anatomy, from above.

ventral a., that surface of a body viewed from the front or, in veterinary anatomy, from below.

aspergilloma (as″per-jil-o′mah) a tumor-like granulomatous mass formed by colonization of *Aspergillus* in a bronchus or pulmonary cavity; the organism may disseminate through the blood stream to the brain, heart, and kidneys.

aspergillosis (as″per-jil-o′sis) a disease caused by species of *Aspergillus,* marked by inflammatory granulomatous lesions in the skin, ear, orbit, nasal sinuses, lungs, and sometimes bones and meninges.

Aspergillus (as″per-jil′us) a genus of fungi (molds), several species of which are endoparasitic and opportunistic pathogens.

aspermia (ah-sper′me-ah) failure of formation or emission of semen.

asphyxia (as-fik′se-ah) a condition in which there is a deficiency of oxygen in the blood and an increase in carbon dioxide in the blood and tissues. adj., **ashyx′ial.** The symptoms include irregular and disturbed respirations, or a complete absence of breathing, and pallor or cyanosis. Asphyxia may occur whenever there is an interruption in the normal exchange of oxygen and carbon dioxide between the lungs and the outside air. Some common causes are drowning, electric shock, lodging of a foreign body in the air passages, inhalation of smoke and poisonous gases, and trauma to or disease of the lungs or air passages. Treatment includes immediate remedy of the situation by ARTIFICIAL RESPIRATION and removal of the underlying cause whenever possible.

asphyxiant (as-fik′se-ant) any substance capable of producing asphyxia.

asphyxiate (as-fik′se-āt) to suffocate; to deprive of oxygen for utilization by the tissues.

aspidium (as-pid′e-um) the dried products of a genus of plants known as male fern.

a. oleoresin, a dark green, thick liquid used as a vermifuge or anthelmintic in the treatment of tapeworm infection. It is toxic in large doses and may cause violent symptoms such as vomiting, weakness, convulsions, coma, permanent blindness, jaundice, and kidney damage. This drug is contraindicated in heart disease, liver and kidney disorders, and ulcerations of the gastrointestinal tract, and is seldom used today.

aspirate (as′pĭ-rāt) 1. to withdraw fluid by negative pressure, or suction. 2. the fluid obtained by aspiration.

aspiration (as″pĭ-ra′shun) 1. the act of inhaling. Pathologic aspiration of vomitus or mucus into the respiratory tract may occur when a person is unconscious or under the effects of a general anesthesia. This can be avoided by keeping the head turned to the side and removing foreign material such as vomitus, mucus, or blood from the air passages. 2. withdrawal of fluid by an aspirator. The method is widely used in hospitals, especially during surgery, to drain the area of the body being operated on and keep it clear of excess fluids. Sometimes after extensive surgery, suction drainage under the skin is used to speed the healing process.

aspirator (as″pĭ-ra′tor) an instrument for evacuating fluid by suction.

aspirin (as′pĭ-rin) acetylsalicylic acid, a common drug generally used to relieve pain and reduce fever, and specifically prescribed for rheumatic and arthritic disorders. Indiscriminate use of the drug may lead to toxic symptoms such as gastrointestinal disorders, ringing in the ears, headache, and, in severe toxicity, depression of the heart rate.

asplenia (ah-sple′ne-ah) absence of the spleen.

asporogenic (as″po-ro-jen′ik) not producing spores; not reproduced by spores.

asporous (ah-spo′rus) having no true spores.

assay (as′a) determination of the purity of a substance or the amount of any particular constituent of a mixture.

biological a., bioassay; determination of the potency of a drug or other substance by comparing the effects it has on animals with those of a reference standard.

immune a., immunoassay.

assimilation (ah-sim″ĭ-la′shun) 1. conversion of nutritive material into living tissue; anabolism. 2. psychologically, absorption of new experiences into the existing psychologic makeup.

association (ah-so″se-a′shun) close relation in time or space. In neurology, correlation involving a high degree of modifiability and also consciousness. In genetics, the occurrence together of two characteristics (e.g., blood group O and peptic ulcers) at a frequency greater than would be predicted on the basis of chance.

a. areas, areas of the cerebral cortex (excluding primary areas) connected with each other and with the neothalamus; they are responsible for higher mental and emotional processes, including memory, learning, etc.

free a., oral expression of one's ideas as they arrive spontaneously; a method used in psychoanalysis.

astasia (as-ta′ze-ah) motor incoordination with inability to stand. adj., **astat′ic.**

a.-aba′sia, inability or refusal to stand or walk although the legs are otherwise under control.

astatine (as′tah-tēn) a chemical element, atomic number 85, atomic weight 210, symbol At. (See table of ELEMENTS.)

asteatosis (as″te-ah-to′sis) any disease in which persistent dry scaling of the skin suggests scantiness or absence of sebum.

aster (as′ter) a cluster of raylike filaments extending from each daughter centriole at the beginning of division of the nucleus of a cell.

astereognosis (ah-ster″e-og-no′sis) inability to recognize familiar objects by feeling their shape.

asterixis (as″ter-ik′sis) a motor disturbance marked by intermittent lapses of an assumed posture as a result of intermittency of sustained contraction of groups of muscles; called liver flap because of its occurrence in coma associated with liver disease, but also observed in other conditions.

asternal (a-ster′nal) 1. not joined to the sternum. 2. pertaining to asternia.

asternia (ah-ster′ne-ah) congenital absence of the sternum.

asteroid (as′ter-oid) star-shaped.

Asterol (as′ter-ol) trademark for preparations of diamthazole, an antifungal.

asthen(o)- word element [Gr.], *weak; weakness.*

asthenia (as-the′ne-ah) debility; loss of strength and energy; weakness. adj., **asthen′ic.**

neurocirculatory a., a symptom complex characterized by breathlessness, giddiness, a sense of fatigue, pain in the region of the precordium, and palpitation. It occurs chiefly in soldiers in active war service, though it is also seen in civilians, and is a form of NEUROSIS.

tropical anhidrotic a., a condition due to generalized absence of sweating in conditions of high temperature, characterized by a tendency to overfatigability, irritability, anorexia, inability to concentrate, and drowsiness, with headache and vertigo.

asthenocoria (as″thĕ-no-ko′re-ah) sluggishness of the pupillary light reflex.

asthenometer (as″thĕ-nom′ĕ-ter) a device used in measuring the degree of muscular asthenia or of asthenopia.

asthenopia (as″thĕ-no′pe-ah) weakness or easy fatigue of the eye, with pain in the eyes, headache, dimness of vision, etc. adj., **asthenop′ic.**

accommodative a., asthenopia due to strain of the ciliary muscle.

muscular a., asthenopia due to weakness of the external ocular muscles.

asthenospermia (as″thĕ-no-sper′me-ah) reduced motility of spermatozoa in the semen.

asthma (az′mah) a condition marked by recurrent attacks of dyspnea, with wheezing due to spasmodic constriction of the bronchi. adj., **asthmat′ic.** It is also known as *bronchial asthma.* Attacks vary greatly from occasional periods of wheezing and slight dyspnea to severe attacks that almost cause suffocation. An acute attack that lasts for days or weeks is called *status asthmaticus.* This is a medical emergency that can be fatal.

CAUSES. Asthma can be classified into three types according to causative factors. *Extrinsic asthma* is due to an allergy to antigens; usually the offending allergens are suspended in the air in the form of pollen, dust, smoke and automobile exhaust, and animal dander. More than half of the cases of asthma in children and young adults is of this type.

Intrinsic asthma is usually secondary to chronic or recurrent infections of the bronchi, sinuses, or tonsils and adenoids. There is evidence that this type of asthma develops from a hypersensitivity to the bacteria causing the infection. The third type of asthma, *mixed,* is due to a combination of extrinsic and intrinsic factors.

There is an inherited tendency toward the development of asthma. It is related to a hypersensitivity reaction of the IMMUNE RESPONSE. The patient often gives a family medical history that includes allergies of one kind or another and a personal history of allergic disorders.

Secondary factors affecting the severity of an attack or triggering its onset include events that produce emotional stress, environmental changes in humidity and temperature, and exposure to noxious fumes or other airborne allergens.

SYMPTOMS. Typically, an attack of asthma is characterized by dyspnea and a wheezing type of respiration. The patient usually assumes a classical sitting position, leaning forward so as to use all the muscles of respiration. The skin is usually pale and moist with perspiration, but in a severe attack there may be cyanosis of the lips and nailbeds. In the early stages of the attack coughing may be dry; but as the attack progresses the cough becomes more productive of a thick, tenacious, mucoid sputum.

TREATMENT. The treatment of asthma begins with attempts to determine the allergens causing the attacks. The cooperation of the patient is needed to relate onset of attacks with specific environmental substances and emotional factors which trigger or intensify his symptoms.

Drugs given for the treatment of asthma are primarily used for the relief of symptoms. There is no cure for asthma but the disease can be controlled with an individualized regimen of rest, relaxation, and avoidance of causative factors. Bronchodilators such as epinephrine and aminophylline may be used to enlarge the bronchioles, thus relieving respiratory embarassment. Other drugs that thin the secretions and help in their ejection (expectorants) may also be prescribed.

The patient with status asthmaticus is very seriously ill and must receive special attention and medication to avoid excessive strain on the heart and severe respiratory difficulties that can be fatal.

PATIENT CARE. Because asthma is a chronic condition with an irregular pattern of remissions and exacerbations, education of the patient is essential to successful treatment. The care plan must be highly individualized to meet the needs of the patient and designed so that he can actively participate in his own care. He may need to adjust his life style so that he works and plays at a more leisurely pace and at the same time does not feel that he is an invalid who cannot lead a normal life. Most patients welcome the opportunity to learn more about their disorder and ways in which they can exert some control over the environmental and emotional events which are likely to precipitate an attack.

Exercises that improve posture are helpful in maintaining good air exchange. Special deep-breathing exercises can be taught to him so that he maintains elasticity and full expansion of lung and bronchial tissues. (See also LUNG and CHRONIC OBSTRUCTIVE PULMONARY DISEASE.) Some asthmatic patients have developed a protective breathing pattern that is shallow and ineffective because of a fear that deep breathing will bring on an attack of coughing and wheezing. They will need help in breaking this pattern and learning to breathe deeply and fully expand the bronchi and lungs.

The patient should be encouraged to drink large quantities of fluids unless otherwise contraindicated. The extra fluids are needed to replace those lost during respiratory distress and seizures of coughing. The increased intake of fluids also can help thin the bronchial secretions so that they are more easily removed by coughing and deep breathing.

The patient should be warned of the hazards of extremes in eating, exercise, and emotional events such as prolonged laughing or crying. The key words are modification and moderation to avoid overtaxing and overstimulating the body systems. Relaxation techniques can be very helpful, especially if the patient can find a method that works well for him in reducing tension.

Asthmatic patients fare better if they feel that they do have some control over their disease and are not necessarily helpless victims of a debilitating incurable illness. There is no cure for asthma but there are ways in which one can adjust to the illness and minimize its effects.

bronchial a., asthma.

cardiac a., a term applied to breathing difficulties due to pulmonary edema in heart disease.

astigmatism (ah-stig′mah-tizm) an error of refraction in which a ray of light is not sharply focused on the retina, but is spread over a more or less diffuse area; it is due to differences in curvature in various meridians of the refractive surfaces (cornea and lens) of the eye. adj., **astigmat′ic.** The exact cause of astigmatism is not known. Common types of astigmatism seem to run in families and are believed to be inherited. Probably everyone has some astigmatism, since it is rare to find perfectly shaped curves in the cornea and lens. The defect may not be serious enough to make treatment necessary; however, corrective lenses may be needed when the refractive error is troublesome.

compound a., that in which both principal meridians are hyperopic (compound hyperopic astigmatism) or myopic (compound myopic astigmatism).

corneal a., that due to the presence of abnormal curvatures on the anterior or posterior surface of the cornea.

hypermetropic a., hyperopic astigmatism.

hyperopic a., that in which the light rays are brought to a focus behind the retina.

irregular a., that in which the curvature varies in different parts of the same meridian or in which refraction in successive meridians differs irregularly.

lenticular a., astigmatism due to defect of the crystalline lens.

mixed a., that in which one principal meridian is hyperopic and the other myopic.

myopic a., that in which the light rays are brought to a focus in front of the retina.

regular a., that in which the refraction changes gradually in power from one principal meridian of the eye to the other, the two meridians always being at right angles; this condition is further classified as being *against the rule* when the meridian of greatest refractive power tends toward the horizontal, *with the rule* when it tends toward the vertical, and *oblique* when it lies 45 degrees from the horizontal and vertical.

astigmometer (as″tig-mom′ĕ-ter) an apparatus used in measuring astigmatism.

astomia (ah-sto′me-ah) congenital atresia of the mouth. adj., **asto′matous.**

astragalectomy (ah-strag″ah-lek′to-me) excision of the astragalus.

astragalus (ah-strag′ah-lus) talus. adj., **astrag′alar.**

astringent (ah-strin′jent) 1. causing contraction or arresting discharges. 2. an agent that causes contraction or arrests discharges. Astringents act as protein precipitants; they arrest discharge by causing shrinkage of tissue.

Some astringents, such as tannic acid, have been used in treating diarrhea; others, such as boric acid and sodium borate, help relieve the symptoms of inflammation of the mucous membranes of the throat or conjunctiva of the eye. Skin preparations such as shaving lotions often contain astringents such as aluminum acetate that help to reduce oiliness and excessive perspiration. Witch hazel is a common household astringent used to reduce swelling. Styptic pencils, used to stop bleeding from small cuts, contain astringents. Zinc oxide and calamine are astringents used in lotions, powders, and ointments to relieve itching and chafing in various forms of dermatitis. Astringents have some bacteriostatic properties, though they are not generally used as antiseptics.

astroblast (as′tro-blast) a cell that develops into an astrocyte.

astroblastoma (as″tro-blas-to′mah) an astrocytoma of Grade II, composed of cells with abundant cytoplasm and two or three nuclei.

astrocyte (as′tro-sīt) a neuroglial cell of ectodermal origin, characterized by fibrous or protoplasmic processes; collectively called astroglia, or macroglia.

astrocytoma (as″tro-si-to′mah) a tumor composed of astrocytes; classified in order of malignancy as: *Grade I,* consisting of fibrillary or protoplasmic astrocytes; *Grade II* (see ASTROBLASTOMA); *Grades III* and *IV* (see GLIOBLASTOMA MULTIFORME).

astroglia (ah-strog′le-ah) neuroglia tissue made up of astrocytes.

astrosphere (as′tro-sfēr) 1. the central mass of an aster, excluding the rays. 2. aster.

asymbolia (ah″sim-bo′le-ah) loss of ability to understand symbols, such as words, figures, gestures, signs.

asymmetry (a-sim′ĕ-tre) lack or absence of symmetry; dissimilarity in corresponding parts or organs on opposite sides of the body which are normally alike. In chemistry, lack of symmetry in the special arrangements of the atoms and radicals within the molecule or crystal. adj., **asymmet′rical.**

asymphytous (ah-sim′fĭ-tus) separate or distinct; not grown together.

asymptomatic (a″simp-to-mat′ik) showing no symptoms.

asynchronism (a-sin′kro-nizm) occurrence at different times; disturbance of coordination.

asynclitism (ah-sin′klĭ-tizm) 1. oblique presentation of the fetal head in labor, called anterior asynclitism when the anterior parietal bone is designated the point of presentation, and posterior asynclitism when the posterior parietal bone is so designated. 2. maturation at different times of the nucleus and of the cytoplasm of blood cells.

asyndesis (ah-sin′dĕ-sis) a language disorder in which related elements of a sentence cannot be welded together in a whole.

asynechia (ah″sĭ-nek′e-ah) absence of continuity of structure.

asynergia (a″sin-er′je-ah) lack of coordination among parts or organs normally acting in unison. adj., **asyner′gic.**

asynovia (ah″sĭ-no′ve-ah) absence or insufficiency of synovial secretion.

asyntaxia (a″sin-tak′se-ah) lack of proper and orderly embryonic development.

asystole (a-sis′to-le) cardiac standstill or arrest —absence of heartbeat. adj., **asystol′ic.**

At chemical symbol, *astatine.*

at. atomic.

Atabrine (at′ah-brin, at′ah-brēn) trademark for quinacrine, an antimalarial and anthelmintic preparation.

atactic (ah-tak′tik) pertaining to or characterized by ataxia; marked by incoordination or irregularity.

ataractic (at″ah-rak′tik) 1. pertaining to or characterized by ataraxia. 2. an agent that induces ataraxia; a tranquilizer.

ataralgesia (at″ar-al-je′ze-ah) combined sedation and analgesia intended to abolish mental distress and pain attendant on surgical procedures, with the patient remaining conscious and alert.

Atarax (at′ah-raks) trademark for preparations of hydroxyzine hydrochloride, a tranquilizer.

ataraxia (at″ah-rak′se-ah) a state of detached serenity with depression of mental faculties or impairment of consciousness.

atavism (at′ah-vizm) apparent inheritance of characters from remote ancestors. adj., **atavis′tic.**

ataxia (ah-tak′se-ah) failure of muscular coordination; irregularity of muscular action. adj., **atac′tic, atax′ic.**

cerebellar a., ataxia due to disease of the cerebellum.

Friedreich's a., the spinal form of hereditary sclerosis (see also FRIEDREICH'S ATAXIA).

frontal a., disturbance of equilibrium occurring in tumor of the frontal lobe.

hereditary a., Friedreich's ataxia.

locomotor a., tabes dorsalis.

sensory a., ataxia due to loss of proprioception (joint position sense), resulting in poorly judged movements and becoming aggravated when the eyes are closed.

a.-telangiectasia, hereditary progressive ataxia, associated with oculocutaneous telangiectasia, sinopulmonary disease with frequent respiratory infections, and abnormal eye movements. Called also Louis-Bar syndrome.

ataxiaphasia (ah-tak″se-ah-fa′ze-ah) inability to arrange words into sentences.

ataxophemia (ah-tak″so-fe′me-ah) lack of coordination of speech muscles.

atel(o)- word element [Gr.], *incomplete; imperfectly developed.*

atelectasis (at″ĕ-lak′tah-sis) a collapsed or airless state of the lung, which may be acute or chronic, and may involve all or part of the lung. adj., **atelectat′ic.** The primary cause of atelectasis is obstruction of the bronchus serving the affected area. In fetal atelectasis the lungs fail to expand normally at birth. This condition may be due to a variety of causes, including prematurity (and may accompany HYALINE MEMBRANE DISEASE), diminished nervous stimulus to breathing and crying, fetal hypoxia from any cause, including oversedation of the mother during labor and delivery and obstruction of the bronchus by a mucous plug.

SYMPTOMS. In acute atelectasis in which there is sudden obstruction of the bronchus, there may be pain in the affected side, dyspnea and cyanosis, elevation of temperature, a drop in blood pressure or shock. In the chronic form, the patient may experience no symptoms other than gradually developing dyspnea and weakness.

X-ray examination may show a shadow in the area of collapse. If an entire lobe is collapsed, the x-ray will show the trachea, heart, and mediastinum deviated toward the collapsed area, with the diaphragm elevated on that side.

TREATMENT. Atelectasis in the newborn is treated by suctioning the trachea to establish an open airway, positive-pressure breathing, and administration of oxygen (40 per cent concentration). High concentrations of oxygen given over a prolonged period tend to promote atelectasis and may lead to the development of retolental fibroplasia in premature infants.

Acute atelectasis is treated by removing the cause whenever possible. To accomplish this, coughing (sometimes using a cough-inducing machine), suctioning, and BRONCHOSCOPY may be employed. A detergent AEROSOL, used with a mist-producing apparatus, may be administered at regular intervals. Chronic atelectasis usually requires surgical removal of the affected segment or lobe of lung. Antibiotics are given to combat the infection that almost always accompanies secondary atelectasis.

congenital a., that present at (primary atelectasis) or immediately after birth (secondary atelectasis).

primary a., congenital atelectasis in which the alveoli have never been expanded with air.

secondary a., congenital atelectasis in which resorption of the contained air has led to collapse of the aveoli.

atelia (ah-te′le-ah) imperfect or incomplete development.

ateliosis (ah-te″le-o′sis) 1. a condition characterized by failure to develop completely. 2. hypophyseal infantalism.

atelocardia (at″ĕ-lo-kar′de-ah) imperfect development of the heart.

atelocephaly (at″ĕ-lo-sef′ah-le) imperfect development of the skull. adj., **atelocephal′ic, ateloceph′alous.**

atelomyelia (at″ĕ-lo-mi-e′le-ah) imperfect development of the spinal cord.

athelia (ah-the′le-ah) congenital absence of the nipples.

athermic (ah-ther′mik) without rise of temperature.

athermosystaltic (ah-ther″mo-sis-tal′tik) not contracting under the action of cold or heat.

atherogenesis (ath″er-o-jen′ĕ-sis) formation of atheromas in arterial walls. adj. **atherogen′ic.**

atheroma (ath″er-o′mah) an abnormal mass of fatty or lipid material with a fibrous covering, existing as a discrete, raised plaque within the intima of an artery. adj. **atherom′atous.**

atheromatosis (ath″er-o″mah-to′sis) the presence of multiple atheromas.

atherosclerosis (ath″er-o-sklĕ-ro′sis) a form of arteriosclerosis in which atheromas containing cholesterol, lipoid material, and lipophages are formed within the intima of large and medium-sized arteries. (See also ARTERIOSCLEROSIS.)

athetoid (ath′ĕ-toid) 1. resembling athetosis. 2. affected with athetosis.

athetosis (ath″ĕ-to′sis) repetitive involuntary, slow, sinuous, writhing movements.

athlete's foot (ath′lēts) a fungal infection of the skin of the foot; called also tinea pedis. Athlete's foot causes itching and often blisters and cracks, usually between the toes. Causative agents are *Candida albicans, Epidermophyton floccosum,* and species of *Trichophyton,* which thrive on warmth and dampness.

If not arrested, athlete's foot can cause a rash and itching in other parts of the body as well. It is likely to be recurrent, since the fungus survives under the toenails and reappears when conditions are favorable. Although athlete's foot is usually little more than an uncomfortable nuisance, its open sores provide excellent sites for more serious infections. Early treatment and medical advice insure correct diagnosis and prevention of complications. Specific diagnosis is made by microscopic examination or culture of skin scrapings for the fungus.

Prevention of athlete's foot includes keeping the feet dry and open to the air as much as possible, especially the areas between the toes. Small cotton pads may be used between the toes if this area is difficult to keep dry. A dusting powder may be used on the feet and sprinkled in the shoes to reduce the accumulation of moisture.

For treatment, there are a number of compounds that can be applied locally for both the acute and chronic stages. Resistant cases may need x-ray or grenz-ray therapy (by a specialist).

athrepsia (ah-threp′se-ah) marasmus. adj., **athrep′tic.**

athymia (ah-thi′me-ah) 1. dementia. 2. absence of functioning thymus tissue.

athymism (ah-thi′mizm) the condition induced by removal of the thymus.

athyreosis (ah-thi″re-o′sis) hypothyroidism. adj. **athyreot′ic.**

athyria (ah-thi′re-ah) 1. absence of functioning thyroid tissue. 2. hypothyroidism.

atlantal (at-lan′tal) pertaining to the atlas.

atlas (at′las) the first cervical vertebra, the uppermost segment of the backbone which supports the skull.

atloaxoid (at″lo-ak′soid) pertaining to the atlas and axis.

atmos (at′mos) atmosphere (2).

atmosphere (at′mos-fēr) 1. The entire gaseous envelope surrounding the earth, extending to an altitude of 10 miles. 2. a unit of pressure, equivalent to that on a surface at sea level, being about 14.7 lb. per square inch, or equivalent to that of a column of mercury 760 mm. high.

atmospheric (at″mos-fer′ik) of or pertaining to the atmosphere.

a. pressure, the pressure exerted by the atmosphere, about 14.7 lb. to the square inch at sea level.

at. no. atomic number.

atocia (ah-to′se-ah) sterility in the female.

atom (at′om) the smallest particle of an element that has all the properties of the element. adj., **atom′ic.** There are two main parts of an atom: the nucleus and the electron cloud. The nucleus is made up of protons, which carry a positive electrical charge, and (except in hydrogen) neutrons, which contain one proton and one electron and carry no electrical charge. The electron cloud is made up of particles called electrons, which carry a negative electrical charge and move in orbits or "shells" around the nucleus. Different atoms have different numbers of protons, neutrons, and electrons in their makeup.

In a chemical change, atoms do not break up but act as individual units. The chemical behavior of an atom is controlled by the number and spatial arrangement of electrons in orbit around the nucleus. The atoms of radioactive elements are very unstable and are capable of emitting nuclear particles in a stream or "ray." These are called radiations. (See also ELEMENT and RADIATION.)

The atomic number of an element is the number of free protons (those not in neutrons) in the nucleus; it is equal to the net positive charge of the nucleus.

The atomic weight is the weight of an atom of a substance as compared with the weight of an atom of carbon-12, which is taken as 12.

atomization (at″om-ĭ-za′shun) the act or process of breaking up a liquid into a fine spray.

atomizer (at′om-iz″er) an instrument for dispensing liquid in a fine spray.

atonia, atony (ah-to′ne-ah; at′o-ne) absence or lack of normal tone. adj., **aton′ic.**

atopen (at′o-pen) the antigen responsible for atopy.

atopic (ah-top′ik) 1. displaced; ectopic. 2. pertaining to atopy.

atopy (at′o-pe) a clinical hypersensitivity state or ALLERGY with a hereditary predisposition; i.e., the tendency to develop an allergy is inherited, but the specific clinical form (hay fever, asthma, etc.) is not. The antibody reagin is involved.

atoxic (ah-tok′sik) not poisonous; not due to a poison.

ATP adenosine triphosphate.

ATPase adenosine triphosphatase.

atraumatic (a″traw-mat′ik) not producing injury or damage.

atresia (ah-tre′ze-ah) congenital absence or closure of a normal body opening or tubular structure. adj., **atret′ic.**

a. a′ni, imperforate anus.

aortic a., absence of the opening from the left ventricle of the heart into the aorta.

biliary a., congenital obliteration or hypoplasia of one or more components of the bile ducts, resulting in persistent jaundice and liver damage.

esophageal a., congenital lack of continuity of the esophagus, commonly accompanied by tracheoesophageal fistula, and characterized by accumulations of mucus in the nasopharynx, gagging, vomiting when fed, cyanosis, and dyspnea. Treatment is by surgical repair by esophageal anastomosis and division of the fistula.

follicular a., a. follic′uli, degeneration and resorption of an ovarian follicle before it reaches maturity and ruptures.

tricuspid a., absence of the opening between the right atrium and right ventricle, circulation being made possible by an atrial septal defect.

atria (a′tre-ah) plural of *atrium.*

atrial (a′tre-al) pertaining to an atrium.

a. septal defect, a CONGENITAL HEART DEFECT in which there is persistent patency of the atrial septum, owing to failure of closure of the ostium primum or ostium secundum.

atrichia (ah-trik′e-ah) absence of hair or of flagella or cilia.

atrichous (ah-trik′us) 1. having no hair. 2. having no flagella.

atriomegaly (a″tre-o-meg′ah-le) abnormal enlargement of an atrium of the heart.

atrioseptopexy (a″tre-o-sep′to-pek″se) surgical correction of a defect in the interatrial septum.

atrioseptoplasty (a″tre-o-sep′to-plas″te) plastic repair of the interatrial septum.

atrioventricular (a″tre-o-ven-trik′u-lar) pertaining to an atrium and ventricle of the heart.

a. bundle, bundle of His.

a. canal, the common canal connecting the primitive atrium and ventricle; it sometimes persists as a congenital anomaly.

a. node, a mass of cardiac muscle fibers (Purkinje fibers) lying on the right lower part of the interatrial septum of the heart. Its function is the transmission of the cardiac impulse from the sinoatrial node to the muscular walls of the ventricles. The conductive system is organized so that transmission is slightly delayed at the atrioventricular node, thus allowing time for the atria to empty their contents into the ventricles before the ventricles begin to contract.

atrioventricularis communis (a″tre-o-ven-trik″u-la′ris kŏ-mu′nis) a congenital cardiac anomaly in which the endocardial cushions fail to fuse, the ostium primum persists, the atrioventricular canal is undivided, a single atrioventricular valve has anterior and posterior cusps, and there is a defect of the membranous interventricular septum.

atrium (a′tre-um), pl. *a′tria* [L.] a chamber affording entrance, especially the upper chamber (a′trium cor′dis) on either side of the heart, transmitting to the ventricle of the same side blood received (left atrium) from the pulmonary veins and (right atrium) from the venae cavae.

atrophia (ah-tro′fe-ah) [L.] atrophy.

atrophoderma (at″ro-fo-der′mah) atrophy of the skin.

atrophy (at′ro-fe) 1. decrease in size of a normally developed organ or tissue; wasting. 2. to undergo or cause atrophy. adj., **atroph′ic.**

acute yellow a., the shrunken, yellow liver which is a complication, usually fatal, of fulminant hepatitis with massive hepatic necrosis.

disuse a., atrophy of a tissue or organ as a result of inactivity or diminished function.

Leber's optic a., hereditary bilateral atrophy of the optic nerve affecting postpubertal males; there is rapid loss of vision resulting in permanent central scotoma.

myelopathic muscular a., muscular atrophy due to lesion of the spinal cord, as in spinal muscular atrophy.

progressive neuromuscular a., progressive neuropathic (peroneal) muscular a., hereditary muscular atrophy beginning in the muscles supplied by the peroneal nerves, progressing slowly to involve the muscles of the hands and arms. Called also Charcot-Marie-Tooth disease.

spinal muscular a., progressive degeneration of the motor cells of the spinal cord, beginning usually in the small muscles of the hands, but in some cases (scapulohumeral type) in the upper arm and shoulder muscles, and progressing slowly to the leg muscles. Called also Aran-Duchenne disease, Cruveilhier's disease, and Duchenne's disease.

atropine (at′ro-pēn) an anticholinergic alkaloid derived from belladonna, hyoscyamus, or stramonium, or produced synthetically, it is used in a variety of conditions. Actions include decrease of secretions, increased heart rate and rate of respirations, and relaxation of smooth muscle tissue. It may be used to dilate pupils, for general cerebral stimulation, for relief of gastrointestinal cramps and hypermotility, and locally to relieve pain. In various combinations with other drugs, atropine may be administered orally or intramuscularly, or applied topically. Atropine methylnitrate and atropine sulfate are soluble compounds of atropine, with similar uses.

a. poisoning, severe toxic reaction due to overdosage of atropine. Symptoms include dryness of mouth, thirst, difficulty in swallowing, dilated pupils, tachycardia, fever, delirium, stupor, and a rash on the face, neck, and upper trunk. Treatment consists of gastric suction or the inducement of vomiting to remove the poison from the stomach; the stomach is then washed with 2 to 4 liters of water containing activated charcoal. The lavage is followed with a solution of 30 gm. of sodium sulfate in 200 ml. of water, which is left in the stomach. Barbiturates may be used to control excitability. There may be a need for treatment of respiratory difficulty. Measures also are taken to reduce the high body temperature.

attenuation (ah-ten″u-a′shun) 1. the act of thinning or weakening. 2. the change in the virulence of a pathogenic microorganism induced by passage through another host species, decreasing its virulence for the native host and increasing it for the new host. This is the basis for the development of live vaccines. 3. the change in a beam of radiation as it passes through matter. The intensity of the electromagnetic radiation decreases as its depth of penetration increases. (See also ABSORPTION, RADIATION.)

attic (at′ik) a small upper space of the middle ear, containing the head of the malleus and the body of the incus.

atticoantrotomy (at″ĭ-ko-an-trot′o-me) surgical exposure of the attic and mastoid antrum.

atticotomy (at″ĭ-kot′o-me) incision into the attic.

attitude (at′ĭ-tūd) 1. a posture or position of the body; in obstetrics, the relation of the various parts of the fetal body to one another. 2. a pattern of mental views established by cumulative prior experience.

atto- a prefix signifying one quintillionth, or 10^{-18}; symbol a.

attraction (ah-trak′shun) the force or influence by which one object is drawn toward another.

capillary a., the force that causes a liquid to rise in a fine-caliber tube.

at. wt. atomic weight.

atypia (a-tip′e-ah) deviation from the normal or typical state.

atypical (a-tip′ĭ-kal) irregular; not conformable to the type.

A.U. 1. Angstrom unit. 2. both ears.

Au chemical symbol, *gold* (L. *aurum*).

audi(o)- word element [L.], *hearing.*

audioanalgesia (aw″de-o-an″al-je′ze-ah) reduction or abolition of pain by listening to recorded music to which has been added a background of so-called white sound.

audiogenic (aw″de-o-jen′ik) produced by sound.

audiogram (aw′de-o-gram″) a graphic record of the findings by audiometry.

audiologist (aw″de-ol′o-jist) an expert in audiology.

audiology (aw″de-ol′o-je) the science concerned with the sense of hearing, especially in the evaluation and measurement of impaired hearing and the rehabilatation of those with impaired hearing.

audiometer (aw″de-om′ĕ-ter) an apparatus used in audiometry.

audiometry (aw″de-om′ĕ-tre) measurement of the acuity of hearing for the various frequencies of sound waves.

audiosurgery (aw″de-o-ser′jer-e) surgery of the ear.

audition (aw-dish′un) perception of sound; hearing.

chromatic a., chromesthesia.

auditory (aw′dĭ-to″re) pertaining to the ear or the sense of hearing.

a. bulb, the membranous labyrinth and cochlea.

a. nerve, the eighth cranial nerve; called also VESTIBULOCOCHLEAR NERVE and acoustic nerve.

a. tube, the narrow channel connecting the middle ear and the nasopharynx (see also EUSTACHIAN TUBE).

augnathus (awg-nath′us) a fetus with a double lower jaw.

aura (aw′rah) a peculiar sensation preceding the appearance of more definite symptoms. An epileptic aura precedes the convulsive seizure and may involve visual disturbances, dizziness, numbness, or any of a number of sensations which the patient may find difficult to describe exactly. In epilepsy the aura serves a useful purpose in that it warns the patient of an impending attack and gives him time to seek privacy and a safe place to lie down before the seizure actually begins.

A migraine aura sometimes precedes migraine headache, warning the patient that an attack is imminent. When it occurs the patient should lie down in a quiet, darkened room. A warm bath before lying down sometimes increases relaxation and helps to prevent a severe attack.

aural (aw′ral) 1. pertaining to the ear. 2. pertaining to an aura.

aurantiasis (aw″ran-ti′ah-sis) yellowness of skin caused by intake of large amounts of food containing carotene.

Aureomycin (aw″re-o-mi′sin) trademark for chlortetracycline hydrochloride, a broad-spectrum antibiotic effective against many different types of microorganisms.

auriasis (aw-ri′ah-sis) chrysiasis.

auric (aw′rik) pertaining to gold.

auricle (aw′rĭ-k′l) 1. the flap of the ear. 2. the ear-shaped appendage of either atrium of the heart; formerly used to designate the entire atrium.

auricula (aw-rik′u-lah), pl. *auric′ulae* [L.] auricle.

auricular (aw-rik′u-lar) pertaining to an auricle or ear.

auricularis (aw-rik″u-la′ris) [L.] pertaining to the ear.

auriculotemporal (aw-rik″u-lo-tem′po-ral) pertaining to the ear and the temporal region.

auripuncture (aw′rĭ-pungk″tūr) myringotomy; surgical puncture of the tympanic membrane.

auris (aw′ris), pl. *au′res* [L.] ear.

auriscope (aw′rĭ-skōp) otoscope; an instrument for examining the ear.

aurotherapy (aw″ro-ther′ah-pe) use of gold salts in treatment of disease.

aurothioglucose (aw″ro-thi″o-gloo′kōs) a gold preparation used in treating rheumatoid arthritis.

aurothioglycanide (aw″ro-thi″o-gli′kah-nīd) a gold preparation used in treating rheumatoid arthritis.

aurum (aw′rum) [L.] gold (symbol Au).

auscultate (aw′skul-tāt) to examine by auscultation.

auscultation (aw″skul-ta′shun) listening for sounds produced within the body, chiefly to ascertain the condition of the thoracic or abdominal viscera and to detect pregnancy; it may be performed with the unaided ear (direct or immediate auscultation) or with a stethoscope (mediate auscultation).

auscultatory (aw-skul′tah-to″re) pertaining to auscultation.

aut(o)- (aw′to) word element [Gr.], *self.*

autacoid (aw′tah-koid) an organic substance produced in one organ and carried by the blood to other organs, on which the substance acts.

autism (aw′tizm) extreme self-absorption and egocentricity with failure to form interpersonal relationships.

akinetic c., coma vigil.

early infantile a., a syndrome beginning in infancy, marked by drastic inability to form interpersonal relationships and by severe obsessive-compulsive behavior; there are also peculiarities of thought and language.

infantile a., early infantile autism.

autistic (aw-tis′tik) pertaining to or exhibiting autism.

a. child, a child suffering from infantile autism.

autoagglutination (aw″to-ah-gloo″tĭ-na′shun) clumping together of an individual's cells due to a substance present in his own serum.

autoagglutinin (aw″to-ah-gloo′tĭ-nin) a factor in serum capable of causing clumping together of the subject's own cellular elements.

autoamputation (aw″to-am″pu-ta′shun) spontaneous detachment from the body and elimination of an appendage or an abnormal growth, such as a polyp.

AutoAnalyzer (aw″to-an′ah-līz″er) trademark for an instrument developed by the Technicon Instruments Corporation and used in the clinical laboratory to perform a sequence of operations for analysis of samples of serum. The procedures performed by automated analysis include measurement of the sample, separation of protein by dialysis, addition of reagents, heating and reaction timing, measurement of color, and calculation of results.

Using 2.5 ml. of blood in each sample, the instrument (also called the SMA—sequential multiple analyzer) evaluates and records on a printout sheet as many as 12 different readings on the chemicals in a sample of blood. The record is in the form of a graph. Shaded areas indicate normal ranges and a dark line shows the individual patient's reading. The chemicals tested by automated analysis can vary, but they usually include the electrolytes, albumin, blood urea nitrogen, bilirubin, glucose, and certain ezymes.

autoantibody (aw″to-an′tĭ-bod″e) an antibody formed in response to, and reacting against, an antigenic constituent of the individual's own tissues.

autoantigen (aw″to-an′tĭ-jen) a tissue constituent that stimulates production of autoantibodies in the organism in which it occurs.

autoantitoxin (aw″to-an″tĭ-tok′sin) antitoxin produced by tissues of the body to protect it from the homologous toxin.

autocatalysis (aw″to-kah-tal′ĭ-sis) catalysis in which a product of the reaction hastens or intensifies the catalysis.

autochthonous (aw-tok′tho-nus) 1. originating in the same area in which it is found. 2. denoting a tissue graft to a new site on the same individual.

autoclasis (aw-tok′lah-sis) destruction of a part by influences within itself.

autoclave (aw′to-klāv) a self-locking apparatus for the sterilization of materials by steam under pressure. The autoclave allows steam to flow around each article placed in the chamber. The vapor penetrates cloth or paper used to package the articles being sterilized. Autoclaving is one of the most effective methods for destruction of all types of microorganisms. The amount of time and degree of temperature necessary for sterilization depend on the articles to be sterilized and whether they are wrapped or left directly exposed to the steam.

Autoclip (aw′to-klip″) trademark for a stainless steel surgical clip inserted by means of a mechanical applier that automatically feeds a series of clips for wound closing.

autocytolysin (aw″to-si-tol′ĭ-sin) autolysin.

autocytolysis (aw″to-si-tol′ĭ-sis) autolysis.

autodigestion (aw″to-di-jes′chun) dissolution of tissue by its own secretions.

autodiploid (aw″to-dip′loid) 1. characterized by autodiploidy. 2. an autodiploid cell or individual.

autodiploidy (aw″to-dip′loi-de) the state of having two sets of chromosomes as the result of doubling of the haploid set.

autoecholalia (aw″to-ek″o-la′le-ah) repetition of one's own words.

autoeczematization (aw″to-ek-zem″ah-tĭ-za′shun) the spread, at first locally and later more generally, of lesions from an originally circumscribed focus of eczema.

autoeroticism, autoerotism (aw″to-ĕ-rot′ĭ-sizm)

(aw″to-er′o-tizm) erotic behavior directed toward one's self. adj., **autoerot′ic.**

autoerythrocyte sensitization syndrome (aw″-to-e-rith′ro-sīt) a purpuric reaction occurring chiefly in young women, in which spontaneous, painful, recurrent single or multiple ecchymoses occur on any part of the body without trauma or after insufficient trauma. Sensitivity to a component of the erythrocytes' structural framework is responsible in many cases, but in some cases the leukocytes seem to be responsible. Emotional upsets are believed to be a precipitating factor. Called also painful bruising syndrome.

autogeneic (aw″to-jĕ-ne′ik) arising from self; pertaining to an autograft.

autogenesis (aw″to-jen′ĕ-sis) self-generation; origination within the organism. adj., **autogenet′ic, autog′enous.**

autograft (aw′to-graft) a graft transferred from one part of the patient's body to another part.

autohemagglutination (aw″to-hem″ah-gloo″tĭ-na′-shun) agglutination of erythrocytes by a factor produced in the subject's own body.

autohemagglutinin (aw″to-hem″ah-gloo′tĭ-nin) a substance produced in a person's body that causes agglutination of his own erythrocytes.

autohemolysin (aw″to-he-mol′ĭ-sin) a hemolysin produced in the body of an animal which causes destruction of its own erythrocytes.

autohemolysis (aw″to-he-mol′ĭ-sis) hemolysis of the blood cells of an individual by his own serum. adj., **autohemolyt′ic.**

autohemotherapy (aw″to-he″mo-ther′ah-pe) treatment by reinjection of the patient's own blood.

autohypnosis (aw″to-hip-no′sis) self-induced hypnosis; the act or process of hypnotizing oneself.

autoimmune disease (aw″to-ĭ-mūn′) disease due to immunologic action of one's own cells or antibodies on components of the body.

The immunological mechanism of the body is dependent on two major factors: (1) the inactivation and rejection of foreign substances and (2) the ability to differentiate between the body's own material ("self") and that which is foreign ("nonself"). It is not yet known exactly what causes the body to fail to recognize proteins as its own and to react to them as if they were foreign. Several possibilities have been identified as pertinent to the development of autoimmunity.

1. There may be a leakage of normally *inaccessible* tissue antigen from its isolated location into an area where it comes into contact with the immunocompetent cells of the reticuloendothelial system (RES). These RES cells do not recognize the formerly inaccessible antigen as "self" and react accordingly.

2. The antigens that are normally accessible to the RES cells may suddenly stimulate the production of autoantibodies. It is thought that this occurs as a result of the emergence of "forbidden clones" (colonies) of cells. Normally these cells are inactivated as a result of adaptive changes that occur during fetal life. For reasons not yet fully explained, these "forbidden clones" survive and emerge to produce an autoimmune reaction. It is believed that they may be activated by injury, disease, or a metabolic change in the body, or there may be a mutation of the forbidden clone cells and immunologically competent cells.

3. Certain body proteins may be so altered by viral infection, by combination with a drug or chemical, or by extensive trauma (as in a severe burn and myocardial infarction) that they are not recognized by the body as "self" and are therefore rejected as foreign.

Diseases that may be classified as being autoimmune include *systemic lupus erythematosus, autoimmune hemolytic anemia, idiopathic thrombocytopenic purpura, rheumatoid arthritis,* and *postviral encephalomyelitis.* There is some controversy over this classification and in the classifying of scleroderma, glomerulonephritis, rheumatic fever, and multiple sclerosis as autoimmune diseases. Of these diseases, systemic lupus erythematosus, rheumatic fever, rheumatoid arthritis, and scleroderma also are called diffuse COLLAGEN DISEASES because they are characterized by changes in collagenous connective tissue throughout the body. In classifying these diseases as autoimmune, the reference is to the cause of the disease, whereas the classifying of them as collagen disease refers to the particular tissues involved in the disease process.

Treatment of autoimmune diseases varies with each specific disease, but in all cases the physician must strive to achieve a delicate balance between adequate suppression of the autoimmune reaction to avoid continued damage to the body tissues, and maintenance of sufficient functioning of the immune mechanism to protect the patient against foreign invaders.

In general, autoimmune diseases are treated by (1) the administration of corticosteroids to produce an anti-inflammatory effect, (2) the use of ionizing radiation to suppress the antigen-antibody reactions in the body, and (3) the administration of salicylates to provide symptomatic relief.

autoimmunity (aw″to-ĭ-mu′nĭ-te) a condition characterized by a specific humoral or cell-mediated immune response against the constituents of the body's own tissues (autoantigens); it may result in hypersensitivity reactions or, if severe, in AUTOIMMUNE DISEASE.

autoimmunization (aw″to-im″u-nĭ-za′shun) induction in an organism of an immense response to its own tissue constituents.

autoinoculation (aw″to-ĭ-nok″u-la′shun) inoculation with microorganisms from one's own body.

autointoxication (aw″to-in-tok″sĭ-ka′shun) poisoning by uneliminated material (toxins) formed within the body.

autoisolysin (aw″to-i-sol′ĭ-sin) a substance that lyses cells (e.g., blood cells) of the individual in which it is formed and also those of other individuals of the same species.

autokeratoplasty (aw″to-ker′ah-to-plas″te) grafting of corneal tissue from one eye to the other.

autokinesis (aw″to-ki-ne′sis) voluntary motion. adj., **autokinet′ic.**

autolesion (aw″to-le′zhun) a self-inflicted injury.

autologous (aw-tol′o-gus) related to self; belonging to the same organism.

autolysate (aw-tol′ĭ-sāt) a substance produced by autolysis.

autolysin (aw-tol′ĭ-sin) a lysin originating in an organism and capable of destroying its own cells and tissues.

autolysis (aw-tol′ĭ-sis) the disintegration of cells or tissues by endogenous enzymes. adj., **autolyt′ic.**

automatic (aw″to-mat′ik) spontaneous; done involuntarily; self-regulating.

automatism (aw-tom′ah-tizm) mechanical, often repetitive motor behavior performed without conscious control.

command a., uncritical response to commands, as in hypnosis and certain mental states.

autonomic (aw″to-nom′ik) not subject to voluntary control.

a. nervous system, the branch of the nervous system that works without conscious control. The voluntary nervous system governs the striated or skeletal muscles, whereas the autonomic nervous system governs the glands, the cardiac muscle, and the smooth muscles, such as those of the digestive system, the respiratory system, and the skin. The autonomic nervous system is divided into two subsidiary systems, the sympathetic system and the parasympathetic system. See Plate 14.

autonomotropic (aw″to-nom″o-trop′ik) having an affinity for the autonomic nervous system.

autopathy (aw-top′ah-the) idiopathic disease; one without apparent external causation.

autophagia (aw″to-fa′ge-ah) 1. eating or biting of one's own flesh. 2. nutrition of the body by consumption of its own tissues.

autophilia (aw″to-fil′e-ah) pathologic self-esteem; narcissism.

autoplasmotherapy (aw″to-plaz″mo-ther′ah-pe) therapeutic reinjection of one's own plasma.

autoplasty (aw′to-plas″te) 1. replacement or reconstruction of diseased or injured parts with tissues taken from another region of the patient's own body. 2. in psychoanalysis, instinctive modification within the psychic systems in adaptation to reality. adj., **autoplas′tic.**

autoploidy (aw″to-ploi′de) the state of having two or more chromosome sets as the result of doubling the haploid set. adj., **au′toploid.**

autopolymer resin (aw″to-pol′ĭ-mer) self-curing resin.

autopolyploidy (aw″to-pol″ĭ-ploi′de) the state of having more than two chromosome sets as a result of redoubling of the chromosomes of a haploid individual or cell. adj., **autopol′yploid.**

autoprecipitin (aw″to-pre-sip′ĭ-tin) an autoantibody with the characteristics of a precipitin.

autoprothrombin (aw″to-pro-throm′bin) an activation product of prothrombin.

autopsy (aw′top-se) examination of a body after death to determine the actual cause of death; called also postmortem examination and necropsy. An autopsy is ordered by a coroner or medical examiner whenever the cause of death is unknown or the death takes place under suspicious circumstances. Unless an autopsy is demanded by public authorities, it cannot be performed without the permission of the next of kin of the deceased. However, an autopsy examination is always undertaken in a dignified and respectful manner, and leading religious authorities are in favor of it when it is requested by the attending physician. Autopsies are also valuable sources of medical knowledge.

autopsychic (aw″to-si′kik) pertaining to one's ideas concerning his own personality.

autoradiograph (aw″to-ra′de-o-graf) the film produced by autoradiography.

autoradiography (aw″to-ra″de-og′rah-fe) the making of a radiograph of an object or tissue by recording on a photographic plate the radiation emitted by radioactive material within the object.

autoregulation (aw″to-reg″u-la′shun) control of certain phenomena by factors inherent in a situation; specifically, (1) maintenance by an organ or tissue of a constant blood flow despite changes in arterial pressure, and (2) adjustment of blood flow through an organ in accordance with its metabolic needs.

autosensitization (aw″to-sen″sĭ-tĭ-za′shun) development of sensitivity to one's own serum or tissues.

autosepticemia (aw″to-sep″tĭ-se′me-ah) septicemia from poisons developed within the body.

autoserodiagnosis (aw″to-se″ro-di″ag-no′sis) diagnostic use of autoserum.

autoserum (aw″to-se′rum) serum administered to the patient from whom it was derived.

autosite (aw′to-sīt) the larger, more normal member of asymmetrical conjoined twin fetuses, to which the other twin (the parasite) is attached.

autosome (aw′to-sōm) any of the 22 pairs of chromosomes in man not concerned with determination of sex.

autosplenectomy (aw″to-sple-nek′to-me) almost complete disappearance of the spleen due to progressive fibrosis and shrinkage.

autostimulation (aw″to-stim″u-la′shun) stimulation of an animal with antigenic material from its own tissues.

autosuggestion (aw″to-sug-jes′chun) suggestion arising in one's self.

autotomography (aw″to-to-mog′rah-fe) a method of body-section roentgenography involving movement of the patient instead of the x-ray tube.

autotopagnosia (aw″to-top-ag-no′se-ah) inability to orient correctly different parts of the body.

autotoxin (aw″to-tok′sin) a toxin developed within the body.

autotransfusion (aw″to-trans-fu′zhun) reinfusion of a patient's own blood.

autotransplantation (aw″to-trans″plan-ta′shun) transfer of tissue from one part of the body to another part.

autotroph (aw′to-trōf) an autotrophic organism.

autotrophic (aw″to-trof′ik) capable of synthesizing necessary nutrients if water, carbon dioxide, inorganic salts, and a source of energy are available.

autovaccination (aw″to-vak″sĭ-na′shun) treatment with autovaccine.

autovaccine (aw″to-vak′sēn) a vaccine prepared from cultures of organisms from the patient's own tissues or secretions.

autoxidation (aw″tok-sĭ-da′shun) the spontaneous reaction of a compound with molecular oxygen at room temperature.

auxesis (awk-se′sis) increase in size of an organism, especially that due to growth of its individual cells rather than increase in their number. adj. **auxet′ic.**

auxin (awk′sin) a growth-promoting plant hormone that acts by causing cell elongation rather than cell multiplication.

auxodrome (awk-so-drōm) the course of growth of a child as plotted on a specially devised graph (Wetzel grid).

auxotherapy (awk″so-ther′ah-pe) substitution therapy.

auxotroph (awk′so-trōf) an auxotrophic organism.

auxotrophic (awk″so-trof′ik) 1. requiring a growth factor not required by the parental or prototype strain; said of microbial mutants. 2. requiring specific organic growth factors in addition to the carbon source present in a minimal medium.

AV, A-V atrioventricular; arteriovenous.

av. avoirdupois.

avascular (a-vas′ku-lar) not vascular; bloodless.

avascularization (a-vas″ku-lar-ĭ-za′shun) diversion of blood from tissues, as by bandaging.

Avellis' syndrome (av-el′ēz) ipsilateral paralysis of the vocal cord and soft palate, loss of pain and temperature sensibility in the contralateral leg, trunk, arm, neck, and in the skin over the scalp.

aversive control (ah-ver′siv) in BEHAVIOR THERAPY, the use of unpleasant stimuli to change undesirable behavior.

Avertin (ah-ver′tin) trademark for tribromoethanol, used in the induction phase of anesthesia.

avidin (av′ĭ-din) a protein in egg white which combines with biotin to render the latter inactive.

avirulence (a-vir′u-lens) lack of virulence; lack of competence of an infectious agent to produce pathologic effects. adj., **avir′ulent.**

avitaminosis (a-vi″tah-mĭ-no′sis) disease due to deficiency of vitamins in the diet. adj., **avitaminot′ic.**

Avlosulfon (av″lo-sul′fon) trademark for a preparation of dapsone, used in the treatment of leprosy and dermatitis herpetiformis.

Avogadro's law (av″o-gad′rōz) equal volumes of perfect gases at the same temperature and pressure contain the same number of molecules.

Avogadro's number (av″o-gad′rōz) the number of particles of the type specified by the chemical formula of a certain substance in 1 gram-molecule of the substance. Called also Avogadro's constant.

avoidance (ah-void′ans) a conscious or unconscious defensive reaction intended to escape anxiety, conflict, danger, fear, or pain.

avoir. avoirdupois.

avoidupois (av′er-dŭ-poiz″) a system of weight used in English-speaking countries for all commodities except drugs, precious stones, and precious metals. (See also Table of Weights and Measures in the Appendix.)

avulsion (ah-vul′shun) the tearing away of a structure or part.

phrenic a., extraction of a portion of the phrenic nerve, producing one-sided paralysis of the diaphragm and partial collapse of the corresponding lung.

axenic (a-zen′ik) not contaminated by or associated with any foreign organisms; used in reference to pure cultures of microorganisms or to germ-free animals. (See also GNOTOBIOTIC.)

axilla (ak-sil′ah), pl. *axil′lae* [L.] the armpit.

axillary (ak′sĭ-ler″e) of or pertaining to the armpit.

axio- word element [L., Gr.] denoting relation to an axis; in dentistry, used in special reference to the long axis of a tooth.

axis (ak′sis), pl. *ax′es* [L., Gr.] 1. a line through a center of a body, or about which a structure revolves. 2. the second cervical vertebra. adj., **ax′ial.**

celiac a., celiac trunk.

a. cylinder, axon.

dorsoventral a., one passing from the back to the belly surface of the body.

electrical a. of heart, the resultant of the electromotive forces within the heart at any instant.

frontal a., an imaginary line running from right to left through the center of the eyeball.

a. of heart., a line passing through the center of the base of the heart and the apex.

optic a., 1. visual axis. 2. the hypothetical straight line passing through the centers of curvature of the front and back surfaces of a simple lens.

sagittal a., an imaginary line extending through the anterior and posterior poles of the eye.

visual a., an imaginary line passing from the midpoint of the visual field to the fovea centralis.

axolemma (ak″so-lem′ah) the surface membrane of an axon.

axolysis (ak-sol′ĭ-sis) degeneration of an axon.

axon (ak′son) the long outgrowth of the body of a nerve cell which conducts impulses away from the cell body; sometimes spelled axone. (See also NEURON and Plate 12.) adj., **ax′onal.**

axoneme (ak′so-nēm) a slender axial filament, such as the axial thread of a chromosome, or that forming the central core of a flagellum or cilium.

axonotmesis (ak″son-ot-me′sis) damage to nerve fibers causing complete peripheral degeneration, but not disturbing the epineurium and intimate supporting structures of the nerve, so that regeneration of fibers occurs, with spontaneous recovery.

axophage (ak′so-fāj) a glia cell occurring in excavations in the myelin in myelitis.

axoplasm (ak′so-plasm) the cytoplasm of an axon; called also hyaloplasm.

axopodium (ak″so-po′de-um) a more or less permanent type of pseudopodium, long and needlelike, characterized by an axial rod, composed of a bundle of fibrils inserted near the center of the body of the cell.

axospongium (ak″so-spun′je-um) the meshwork structure of the substance of an axon.

axostyle (ak′so-stīl) 1. the central supporting structure of an axopodium. 2. a supporting rod running through the body of a trichomonad and protruding posteriorly.

Ayerza's disease (ah-yer′thaz) a form of polycythemia vera marked by chronic cyanosis, chronic dyspnea, chronic bronchitis, bronchiectasis, hepatosplenomegaly, and hyperplasia of bone marrow, and associated with sclerosis of the pulmonary artery.

AZ test Aschheim-Zondek test (for pregnancy).

Az. azote (nitrogen).

azacyclonol (a″zah-si′klo-nol) an isomer of pipradol, used as a tranquilizer.

azapetine (a″zah-pet′ēn) an adrenergic-blocking agent used to dilate peripheral blood vessels.

azaribine (ah-zar′ĭ-bēn) an antimetabolite used in the treatment of psoriasis that does not respond to conventional therapy.

azaserine (a″zah-ser′ēn) an antibiotic used as an immunosuppressive agent in autoimmune disease.

azathioprine (a″zah-thi′o-prēn) a mercaptopurine derivative used as a cytotoxic and immunosuppressive agent in the treatment of leukemia and autoimmune diseases and in transplantation therapy.

azoospermia (a″zo-o-sper′me-ah) absence of spermatozoa in the semen.

azote (a″zōt) nitrogen.

azotemia (az″o-te′me-ah) the presence of nitrogen-containing compounds in the blood. adj., **azote′mic.**

azotenesis (az″o-tĕ-ne′sis) any disease due to excess nitrogen in system.

Azotobacter (ah-zo″to-bak′ter) a genus of nitrogen-fixing bacteria.

azotometer (az″o-tom′ĕ-ter) an instrument for measuring nitrogen content of compounds in solution.

azotorrhea (az″o-to-re′ah) discharge of excessive quantities of nitrogenous matter in the stools.

azoturia (az″o-tu′re-ah) excess of urea in the urine.

Azulfidine (ah-zul′fĭ-dēn) trademark for a preparation of salicylazosulfapyridine, used in the treatment of chronic ulcerative colitis.

azure (azh′ūr) any of the partially methylated homologues of the series of basic dyes extending from thionine to methylene blue, or to certain mixtures thereof; used in many staining procedures.

azuresin (azh″u-rez′in) a complex combination of azure A dye and carbacrylic cation–exchange resin used as a diagnostic aid in detection of gastric secretion.

azurophil (azh-u′ro-fil) an element or cell that stains easily with azure dye.

azurophilia (azh″u-ro-fil′e-ah) a condition in which the blood contains cells having azurophilic granules.

azurophilic (azh″u-ro-fil′ik) staining well with blue aniline dyes; pertaining to or characterized by azurophilia.

azygogram (az′ĭ-go-gram″) the film obtained by azygography.

azygography (az″ĭ-gog′rah-fe) roentgenography of the azygous venous system.

azygos (az′ĭ-gos) 1. any unpaired part, as the azygos vein. 2. unpaired.

a. vein, a vein beginning in the abdomen as a continuation of the ascending lumbar vein which is a tributary of the inferior vena cava. The azygos vein and its tributaries serve as vessels for the return of blood from the thorax to the superior vena cava. The azygos vein also serves as a connecting link, through the ascending lumbar vein, between the venae cavae returning blood from above and below the heart.

azygous (az′ĭ-gus) having no fellow; unpaired.

azymia (a-zim′e-ah) absence of enzyme.

azymic (ah-zim′ik) not giving rise to fermentation.

B

B chemical symbol, *boron.*

B. Baumé scale; boils at; buccal.

B.A. Bachelor of Arts.

Ba chemical symbol, *barium.*

Babcock's test one for determination of the fat content of milk.

Babès-Ernst granules (bah′bāz ernst) metachromatic granules, present in many bacterial cells.

Babinski reflex (bah-bin′ske) a reflex action of the toes, indicative of abnormalities in the motor control pathways leading from the cerebral cortex and widely used as a diagnostic aid in disorders of the central nervous system. It is elicited by a firm stimulus (usually scraping) on the sole of the foot, which results in dorsiflexion of the great toe and fanning of the smaller toes. Normally such a stimulus causes all the toes to bend downward. Called also Babinski's sign.

baby (ba′be) an infant; a child not yet able to walk.

blue b., an infant born with cyanosis due to a congenital heart lesion or to congenital atelectasis (see also BLUE BABY).

"cloud b.," an apparently well infant who, because of viruses and bacteria in the respiratory tract or elsewhere, is able to contaminate the surrounding atmosphere with clouds of bacteria, and thus may be responsible for nursery epidemics.

collodion b., an infant affected with LAMELLAR EXFOLIATION OF THE NEWBORN.

bacillary (bas′ĭ-ler″e) pertaining to bacilli or to rod-like structures.

bacillemia (bas″ĭ-le′me-ah) the presence of bacilli in the blood.

bacilli (bah-sil′i) plural of *bacillus.*

bacilliform (bah-sil′ĭ-form) having the appearance of a bacillus.

bacillin (bah-sil′in) an antibiotic substance isolated from strains of *Bacillus subtilis,* highly active on both gram-positive and gram-negative bacteria.

bacillosis (bas″ĭ-lo′sis) infection with bacilli.

bacillotherapy (bah-sil″o-ther′ah-pe) bacteriotherapy.

bacilluria (bas″ĭ-lu′re-ah) bacilli in the urine.

Bacillus (bah-sil′us) a genus of bacteria containing 33 species, two of which are pathogenic for humans.

B. an′thracis, the causative agent of anthrax.

B. co′li, *Escherichia coli.*

B. dysente′riae, *Shigella dysenteriae.*

B. enterit′idis, *Salmonella enteritidis.*

B. lep′rae, *Mycobacterium leprae.*

B. pneumo′niae, *Klebsiella pneumoniae.*

B. pyocya′neus, *Pseudomonas aeruginosa.*

B. sub′tilis, a common saprophytic soil and water form, often occurring as a laboratory contaminant, and rarely, in apparently causal relation to pathologic processes, such as conjunctivitis.

B. tet′ani, *Clostridium tetani.*

B. ty′phi, B. typho′sus, *Salmonella typhosa.*

B. welch′ii, *Clostridium perfringens.*

bacillus (bah-sil′us), pl. *bacilli* [L.] 1. an organism of the genus *Bacillus.* 2. a rod-shaped bacterium; any spore-forming, rod-shaped microorganism of the order Eubacteriales.

Bang's b., *Brucella abortus.*

Battey bacilli, unclassified mycobacteria that may produce tuberculosis-like disease in man.

Bordet-Gengou b., *Bordetella pertussis.*

Calmette Guérin b., *Mycobacterium bovis,* rendered completely avirulent by cultivation over a long period on bile-glycerol-potato medium (see BCG VACCINE).

colon b., *Escherichia coli.*

Friedländer's b., *Klebsiella pneumoniae.*

Gärtner's b., *Salmonella enteritidis.*

glanders b., *Pseudomonas mallei.*

Hansen's b., *Mycobacterium leprae.*

Klebs-Löffler b., *Corynebacterium diphtheriae.*

Koch-Weeks b., *Hemophilus aegyptius.*

Pfeiffer's b., *Hemophilus influenzae.*

tubercle b., *Mycobacterium tuberculosis.*

typhoid b., *Salmonella typhosa.*

bacitracin (bas″ĭ-tra′sin) an antibacterial substance elaborated by the licheniformis group of *Bacillus subtilis,* found in a contaminated wound, and named for the patient, Margaret Tracy; useful in a wide range of infections, applied topically or given intramuscularly.

zinc b., the zinc salt of bacitracin, used in an ointment as a topical antibacterial agent.

backache (bak′āk) any pain in the back, usually the lower part. The pain is often dull and continuous, but sometimes sharp and throbbing.

Backache, or lumbago, is one of the commonest ailments and can be caused by a wide variety of disorders, some serious and some not. Occasionally backache is a symptom of spinal arthritis, peptic ulcer, enlargement of the pancreas, SCIATICA, diseases of the kidney or other serious disorders, but usually backache is caused simply by strain of the back in such a way that the bones, ligaments, nerves or muscles of the spine are compressed or stretched. A sudden action, using muscles that are already fatigued or out of condition, is particularly likely to cause acute strain. In such cases, rest and time usually bring recovery, although a physician should always be consulted. A very sharp and persistent pain, following the use of unusual force against something—for example, when trying to open a jammed window—could indicate a slipped DISK or SACROILIAC strain.

TREATMENT. Aspirin and a heating pad or hot, wet towels may temporarily relieve backache, but persistent pain requires a thorough examination, perhaps including x-ray examination, for the disorders of the back are not only many in number, but often difficult to identify.

backbone (bak′bōn) the vertebral column.

back-cross (bak′cros) a mating between a heterozygote and a homozygote.

double b., the mating between a double heterozygote and a homozygote.

backflow (bak′flo) abnormal backward flow of fluids; regurgitation.

pyelovenous b., drainage from the renal pelvis into the venous system occurring under certain conditions of back pressure.

backscatter (bak′skat-er) in radiology, radiation deflected by scattering processes at angles greater than 90 degrees to the original direction of the beam of radiation.

bacter(io)- word element [Gr.], *bacteria.*

bacteremia (bak″ter-e′me-ah) the presence of bacteria in the blood.

bacteria (bak-te′re-ah) plural of *bacterium.* adj., **bacte′rial.**

bactericidal (bak-tēr″ĭ-si′dal) destructive to bacteria.

bactericide (bak-tēr′ĭ-sīd) an agent that destroys bacteria.

bacterid (bak′ter-id) a skin eruption due to bacterial infection elsewhere in the body.

bacteriemia (bak-tēr″e-e′me-ah) bacteremia.

bacteriocidin (bak-te″re-o-si′din) a bactericidal antibody.

bacterioclasis (bak-te″re-ok′lah-sis) bacteriolysis.

bacteriogenic (bak-te″re-o-jen′ik) 1. bacterial in origin. 2. producing bacteria.

bacteriologist (bak-te″re-ol′o-jist) an expert in the study of bacteria.

bacteriology (bak-te″re-ol′o-je) the scientific study of bacteria, adj., **bacteriolog′ic.**

bacteriolysin (bak-te″re-ol′ĭ-sin) an antibody that lyses bacterial cells.

bacteriolysis (bak-te″re-ol′ĭ-sis) destruction or dissolution of bacteria. adj., **bacteriolyt′ic.**

bacterio-opsonin (bak-te″re-o-op-so′nin) bacteriopsonin.

bacteriophage (bak-te′re-o-fāj″) a virus that destroys bacteria by lysis; several varieties exist, and usually each attacks only one kind of bacteria. Certain types of bacteriophages attach themselves to the cell membrane of the bacterium and instill a charge of DNA into the cytoplasm. DNA carries the genetic code of the virus, so that rapid multiplication of the virus can and does take place inside the bacterium. The growing viruses act as parasites, using the metabolism of the bacterial cell for growth and development. Eventually the bacterial cell bursts, releasing many more viruses capable of destroying similar bacteria. Called also bacterial virus. adj., **bacteriopha′gic.**

temperate b., one whose genetic material (PROPHAGE) becomes an intimate part of the bacterial GENOME, persisting and being reproduced through many cell division cycles; the affected bacterial cell is known as a LYSOGENIC BACTERIUM.

bacteriophagia (bak-te″re-o-fa′je-ah) destruction of bacteria by a lytic agent; bacteriolysis.

bacterioprecipitin (bak-te″re-o-pre-sip′ĭ-tin) any precipitin formed in the body in response to bacterial antigens.

bacterioprotein (bak-te″re-o-pro′te-in) a toxalbumin formed by bacteria.

bacteriopsonin (bak-te″re-op′so-nin) an opsonin that acts on bacteria.

bacteriosis (bak-te″re-o′sis) any bacterial disease.

bacteriostatic (bak-te″re-o-stat′ik) arresting the growth or multiplication of bacteria; also, an agent that so acts.

bacteriotherapy (bak-te″re-o-ther′ah-pe) treatment of disease by introducing bacteria into the system.

bacteriotoxin (bak-te″re-o-tok′sin) a toxin produced by or destructive to bacteria. adj., **bacteriotox′ic.**

Bacterium (bak-te′re-um) former name for a genus of schizomycetes the species of which are now assigned to other genera, e.g., *Aerobacter, Pseudomonas, Salmonella,* etc.

bacterium (bak-te′re-um), pl. *bacte′ria* [L., Gr.] in general, any schizomycete; formerly sometimes restricted to rod-shaped or to nonsporulating rod-shaped microorganisms. Popularly called germ. Bacteria are one-cell organisms visible only through a microscope. There are many varieties, only some of which cause disease; most are nonpathogenic, and many are useful.

Bacteria are forms of plant life, and are found almost everywhere. They reproduce about every 20 minutes, and would soon overrun the world if there were not other types of bacteria waiting to feed on them.

Bacteria are classified in three basic groups according to their shape. The rod-shaped bacteria are called bacilli, spiral-shaped bacteria spirilla, and dot-shaped bacteria cocci. The last-named may appear in pairs (diplococci), in chains like strings of beads (streptococci), or in clusters that resemble a bunch of grapes (staphylococci).

The great majority of bacteria coexist peacefully with mankind. Many are necessary to plant life. For example, certain bacteria in the soil convert dead matter such as leaves into humus, which is rich in the nitrates essential to plant growth. Other bacteria have the ability to take atmospheric nitrogen from the air and convert it to nutrients usable by plants.

Helpful bacteria existing in the human intestine feed on other microscopic organisms that might be harmful. They also produce some vitamins, including the vitamin B complex and vitamins C and K.

Most pathogenic bacteria that invade the body produce toxins. The body's defenses fight back against the invader by rushing leukocytes (white blood cells) and antitoxins to the area of infection; some of the leukocytes engulf the bacteria while the antitoxins neutralize the poisons. The extra blood supply contributes to the inflammatory process. The resulting fever and pain also help by enforcing rest and thus conserving the body's energies to fight off the invader.

DISEASES CAUSED BY BACTERIA. The different kinds of bacteria tend to affect different organs and systems of the body, producing infectious diseases, each with its own group of symptoms.

Staphylococci are generally found on the surface of the skin. When they invade the body tissue, for instance through a cut, they usually produce a local infection with inflammation and pus. Occasionally a strain of staphylococcus develops that can cause an infection affecting more than a local area of the body, but this is relatively rare.

The diseases produced by streptococci are often more serious. Streptococci tend to resist localization and may spread through the bloodstream. Among the diseases caused by streptococci are streptococcal sore throat (see also THROAT), RHEUMATIC FEVER, and SCARLET FEVER.

PNEUMONIA, MENINGITIS, and GONORRHEA are produced by different types of diplococci. The pneumococcus, which produces pneumonia, has its special effect on the lungs; the meningococcus has an affinity for the coverings, or meninges, of the brain and spinal cord. Both types of bacteria enter the body via the respiratory tract. The gonorrhea bacteria (gonococci) are usually spread by coitus.

CHOLERA, caused by a spirillum and spread by unsanitary water supplies, was formerly a dread epidemic disease. SYPHILIS, like gonorrhea, is spread most often by coitus. It also is caused by a spirillum.

Bacilli are responsible for many serious diseses, including PLAGUE, DIPHTHERIA, LEPROSY, TUBERCULOSIS, and TYPHOID FEVER. Prevention and control of the spread of many infectious diseases can be accomplished through IMMUNIZATION and proper sanitary conditions.

acid-fast b., one that is not readily decolorized by acids after staining, especially *Mycobacterium tuberculosis.*

coliform bacteria, see *Aerobacter, Escherichia,* and *Paracolobactrum.*

lactic acid bacteria, bacteria that, in suitable media, produce fermentation of carbohydrate materials to form lactic acid.

lysogenic b., any bacterial cell harboring in its GENOME the genetic material (PROPHAGE) of a TEMPERATE BACTERIOPHAGE and thus reproducing the bacteriophage in cell division; occasionally the prophage develops into the mature form, replicates, lyses the bacterial cell, and is free to infect other cells.

bacteriuria (bak-te″re-u′re-ah) bacteria in the urine.

bacteroid (bak′ter-oid) 1. resembling a bacterium. 2. a structurally modified bacterium.

Bacteroides (bak″tĕ-roi′dēz) a genus of bacteria occurring as normal flora in the mouth and large bowel, and often in necrotic tissue, probably as secondary invaders.

B. fundulifor′mis, a pathogen of animals, causing diphtheria with abscesses in cattle, gangrenous dermatitis in horses, necrotic lesions in hogs, cattle, and sheep, and abscesses and necrotic areas in rabbits; also found in chronic ulcer of the colon in man.

bacteroides (bak″tĕ-roi′dēz) 1. any highly pleomorphic rod-shaped bacteria. 2. an organism of the genus *Bacteroides.*

bacteruria (bak″ter-u′re-ah) bacteriuria.

bag (bag) a sac or pouch.

Barnes' b., a water-filled rubber bag for dilating the cervix uteri.

colostomy b., a receptable worn over the stoma by a COLOSTOMY patient, to receive the fecal discharge.

Douglas b., a receptacle for the collection of expired air, permitting measurement of respiratory gases.

ileostomy b., any of various plastic or latex pouches attached to the body for the collection of urine or fecal material following ileostomy or the establishment of an ileal bladder.

micturition b., a receptacle used for urine by ambulatory patients with urinary incontinence.

Politzer b., a soft bag of rubber for inflating the eustachian tube.

Voorhees' b., a rubber bag to be inflated with water to dilate the cervix uteri.

b. of waters, the membranes enclosing the AMNIOTIC FLUID and the developing fetus in utero.

bagassosis (bag″ah-so′sis) a lung disease due to inhalation of dust from the residue of cane after extraction of sugar (bagasse).

Baker's cyst (ba′kerz) a swelling about the knee, due to escape of synovial fluid that has become enclosed in a sac of membrane.

BAL dimercaprol (British antilewisite), a chelating agent used in poisoning with arsenic, gold, mercury, and certain other metals.

balance (bal′ans) 1. an instrument for weighing. 2. harmonious adjustment of different elements or parts; harmonious performance of functions.

acid-base b., the proportion of acid and base required to keep the blood and body fluids neutral (see also ACID-BASE BALANCE).

analytical b., a laboratory balance sensitive to variations of the order of 0.05 to 0.1 mg.

fluid b., the state of the body in relation to ingestion and excretion of water and electrolytes (see also FLUID BALANCE).

microchemical b., a laboratory balance sensitive to variations of the order of 0.001 mg.

nitrogen b., the state of the body in regard to ingestion and excretion of nitrogen. In negative nitrogen balance the amount of nitrogen excreted is greater than the quantity ingested. In positive nitrogen balance the amount excreted is smaller than the amount ingested.

semimicro b., a device for determining weight, sensitive to variations of 0.01 mg.

water b., fluid balance.

balanic (bah-lan′ik) pertaining to the glans penis or glans clitoridis.

balanitis (bal″ah-ni′tis) inflammation of the glans penis.

gangrenous b., erosion of the glans penis leading to rapid destruction, believed to be due to continually unhygienic conditions together with secondary spirochetal infection.

balanoposthitis (bal″ah-no-pos-thi′tis) inflammation of glans penis and prepuce.

balanopreputial (bal″ah-no-pre-pu′she-al) pertaining to the glans penis and prepuce.

balanorrhagia (bal″ah-no-ra′je-ah) balanitis with free discharge of pus.

balantidiasis (bal″an-tĭ-di′ah-sis) infection with organisms of the genus *Balantidium.*

Balantidium (bal″an-tid′e-um) a genus of ciliated protozoa, including many species found in the intestine in vertebrates and invertebrates.

B. co′li, a common parasite of swine, rarely in man, in whom it may cause dysentery.

Balarsen (bah-lar′sen) trademark for preparations of arsthinol, an arsenical used in the treatment of intestinal amebiasis.

baldness (bawld′nes) total or partial loss or absence of hair, especially absence of the hair from the scalp; called also ALOPECIA. Baldness is a common condition that occurs much more often in men than in women. Ordinary baldness is usually a permanent and incurable condition; symptomatic baldness occurs as a result of some other condition or disorder and usually is temporary.

Balkan frame (bawl′kan) an apparatus for continuous extension in treatment of fractures of the femur, consisting of an overhead bar, with pulleys attached, by which the leg is supported in a sling.

ball (bawl) a more or less spherical mass.
fungus b., aspergilloma.

ballismus (bah-liz′mus) violent flinging movements of the limbs, sometimes affecting only one side of the body (HEMIBALLISMUS).

ballistocardiogram (bah-lis″to-kar′de-o-gram″) the tracing made by ballistocardiography.

ballistocardiograph (bah-lis″to-kar′de-o-graf″) the apparatus used in ballistocardiography.

ballistocardiography (bah-lis″to-kar″de-og′rah-fe) graphic recording of forces imparted to the body by cardiac ejection of blood.

ballottement (bah-lot′maw) [Fr.] a palpatory maneuver to test for a floating object, especially a maneuver for detecting pregnancy by inserting two fingers into the vagina and pushing the fetal head or breech, causing the fetus to leave and quickly return to the fingers.

balm (bahm) 1. a balsam. 2. a soothing or healing medicine.

balneology (bal″ne-ol′o-je) the science dealing with baths and bathing.

balneotherapeutics (bal″ne-o-ther″ah-pu′tiks) scientific study of the use of baths in the treatment of disease.

balneotherapy (bal″ne-o-ther′ah-pe) use of baths in the treatment of disease.

balsam (bawl′sam) a semifluid, fragrant, resinous, vegetable juice. Balsams are resins combined with oils, used in various preparations to treat irritated or denuded areas of the skin and mucous membranes. Stains from these preparations are extremely difficult to remove. Friar's balsam, called also compound benzoin tincture, is used as a topical protectant. Balsam of Peru, or peruvian balsam, is used as a local protectant and rubefacient. Tolu balsam is used as an ingredient in compound benzoin and as an expectorant.

Balser's fatty necrosis (bahl′zerz) gangrenous pancreatitis with omental bursitis and disseminated patches of necrosis of fatty tissues.

Bamberger-Marie disease (bahm′ber-ger mah-re′) hypertrophic pulmonary osteoarthropathy.

bancroftosis (ban″krof-to′sis) infection with *Wuchereria bancrofti.*

band (band) a strip that constricts or binds a part. In dentistry, a thin strip of metal formed to encircle horizontally the crown of a natural tooth or its root.

bandage (ban′dij) 1. a strip or roll of gauze or other material for wrapping or binding any part of the body. 2. to cover by wrapping with such material. Bandages may be used to stop the flow of blood, to provide a safeguard against contamination, or to hold a medicated dressing in place. They may also be used to hold a splint in position or otherwise immobilize an injured part of the body to prevent further injury and to facilitate healing.

USE OF STERILE GAUZE SQUARE

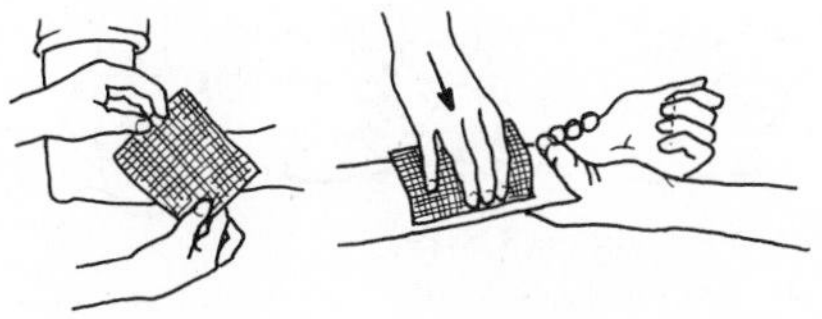

To cover wound
Fasten square over wound with tape or bandage.

To stop bleeding
Place square over wound and press down firmly.

USE OF ROLLER BANDAGE

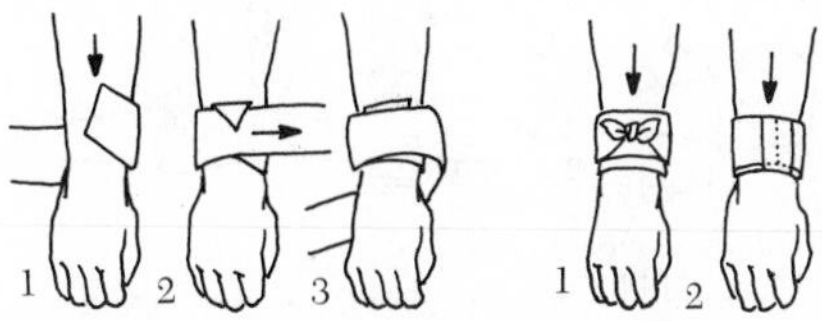

To anchor bandage
1. Place end on bias. 2. Fold down corner of end over first winding. 3. Cover corner with subsequent windings.

To fasten final end
1. Split into two ends and tie. 2. Or fasten with tape.

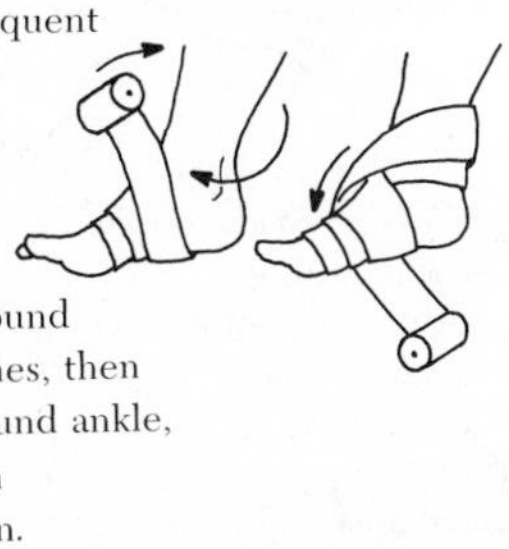

To bandage ankle
Wrap bandage around instep several times, then wind it twice around ankle, and bring it down under instep again.

USE OF ROLLER BANDAGE (CONTINUED)

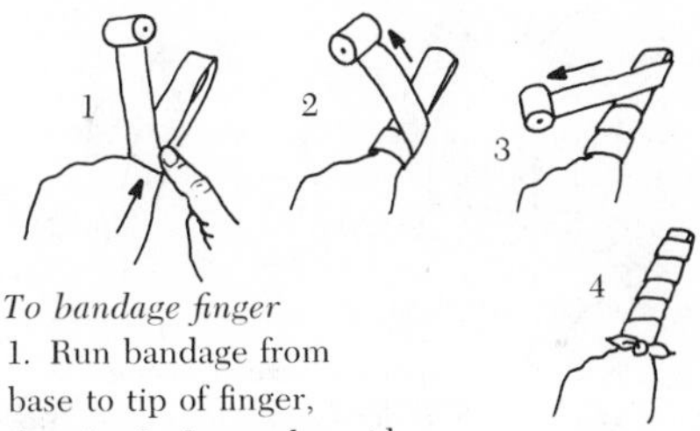

To bandage finger
1. Run bandage from base to tip of finger, then back along other side.
2. Wind around base several times.
3. Wind to tip of finger and back to base.
4. Split end and tie.

USE OF TRIANGULAR BANDAGE

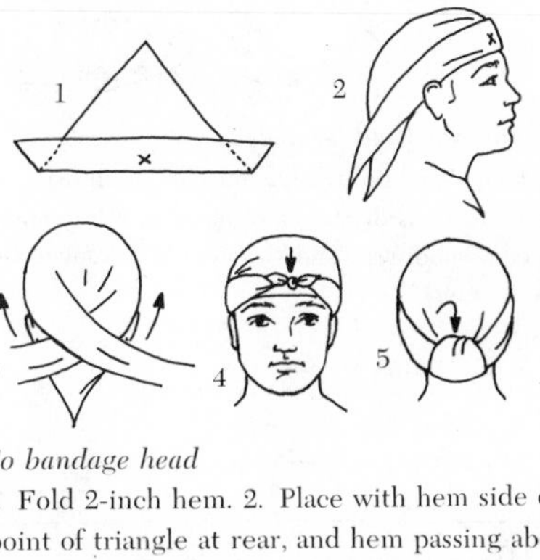

To bandage head
1. Fold 2-inch hem. 2. Place with hem side out, point of triangle at rear, and hem passing above ears. 3. Cross ends at back of head. 4. Bring to front and tie. 5. Tuck point of triangle under hem, or pin in place.

APPLICATION OF BANDAGES. In applying a bandage: (1) If the skin is broken a sterile pad or several thicknesses of gauze should be placed over the wound before tape or bandaging material is applied over the pad to hold it in place. Adhesive tape is never applied directly on a wound. (2) The bandage should not be made so tight that it interferes with circulation. A pressure bandage should be applied only for the purpose of arresting hemorrhage. (3) A bandage does not have to look good to be effective; in an emergency, that the bandage serves its purpose is more important than its appearance.

cravat b., one made by bringing the point of a triangular bandage to the middle of the base and then folding lengthwise to the desired width.

demigauntlet b., one that covers the hand, but leaves the fingers uncovered.

Esmarch's b. an India rubber bandage applied upward around (from the distal part to the proximal) a part in order to expel blood from it; the part is often elevated as the elastic pressure is applied.

figure-of-8 b., one in which the turns cross each other like the figure 8.

gauntlet b., one that covers the hands and fingers like a glove.

plaster b., a bandage stiffened with a paste of plaster of Paris.

pressure b., one for applying pressure, for the purpose of arresting hemorrhage; pressure is applied directly over the wound.

roller b., a tightly rolled, circular bandage of varying widths and materials, often prepared commercially. In an emergency, strips may be torn from a sheet or piece of yard goods and rolled. When more than a few inches of length is needed, rolling is essential for quick and clean bandaging.

sculteus b., sculteus binder.

tailed b., a square piece of cloth cut or torn into strips from the ends toward the center, with as large a center left as necessary. The bandage is centered over a compress on the wound and the ends are then tied separately. A four-tailed bandage is useful for wounds of the nose and chin.

triangular b., one made by folding or cutting a large square of cloth diagonally. It may form a sling for an injured arm, or can be folded several times into a cravat of any desired width.

Bandl's ring (ban'delz) a complication of prolonged labor marked by failure of relaxation of the circular fibers at the internal opening of the cervix, obstructing delivery of the infant; called also pathologic retraction ring.

bank (bank) a stored supply of human material or tissues for future use by other individuals, as BLOOD BANK, bone bank, skin bank, EYE BANK, etc.

Banthine (ban'thīn) trademark for preparations of methantheline bromide, an anticholinergic used to depress gastrointestinal activity.

USE OF TRIANGULAR BANDAGE (CONTINUED)

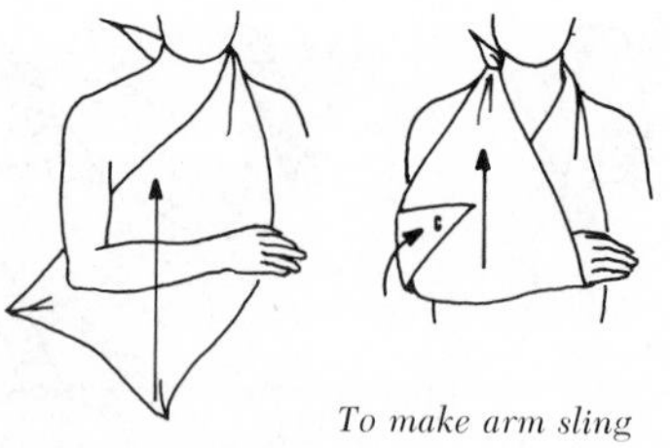

To make arm sling

Place triangle as shown so point extends a little beyond elbow. Bring lower end around arm and up. Tie ends behind neck. Pin point of triangle to front. Be sure fingers are visible and wrist is higher than elbow.

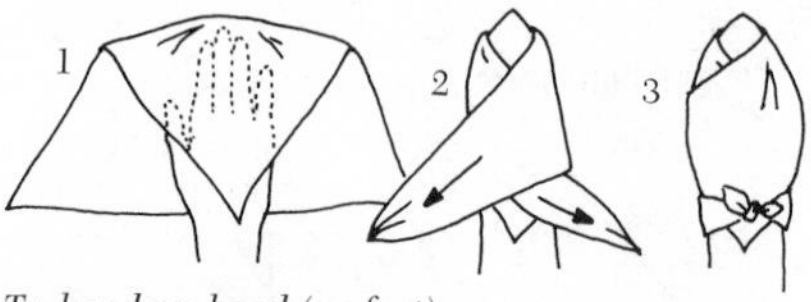

To bandage hand (or foot)

1. Place hand on triangle and fold as shown. 2. Cross ends over back of hand. 3. Wrap ends once around wrist and tie. Foot is bandaged in same way.

USE OF CRAVAT BANDAGE

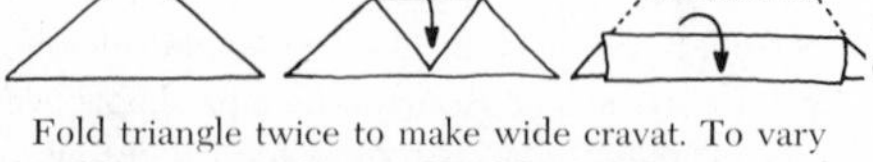

Fold triangle twice to make wide cravat. To vary width, vary number and width of folds.

USE OF CRAVAT BANDAGE (CONTINUED)

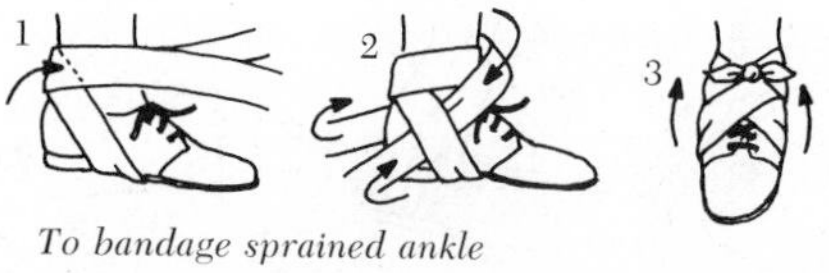

To bandage sprained ankle

1. Loosen shoelaces. With middle of cravat under shoe in front of heel, cross ends behind ankle and bring to front. 2. Cross ends and wrap them under and around diagonal parts of bandage. 3. Pull ends to front and tie.

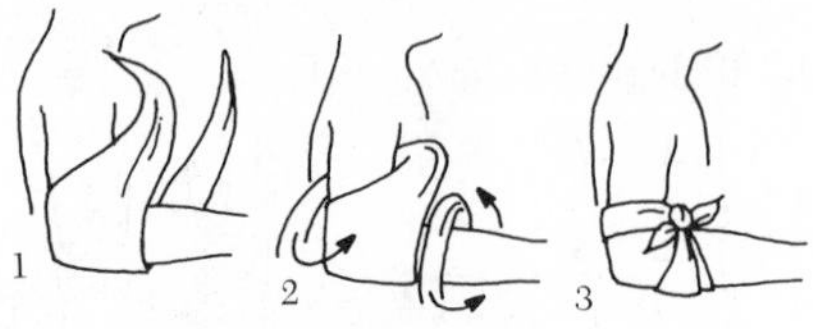

To bandage elbow (or knee)

1. Place middle of wide cravat under elbow of bent arm. 2. Cross ends and wind one around arm above elbow. 3. Tie.

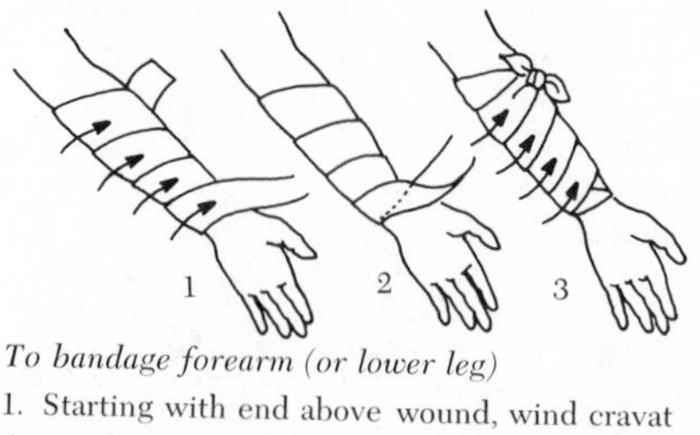

To bandage forearm (or lower leg)

1. Starting with end above wound, wind cravat diagonally over and past wound. 2. When wound is under middle of cravat, twist cravat and wind it back upward. 3. Tie ends above wound. Repeat, each time overlapping previous winding, until desired area is covered.

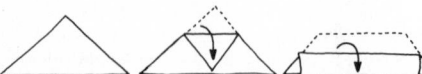

Banti's disease (ban'tēz) a disease originally described as a primary disease of the spleen with splenomegaly and pancytopenia, now considered secondary to portal hypertension.

Banting (ban'ting) Sir Frederick Grant (1891–1941). Canadian scientist. Born in Allison, Ontario, and educated at the University of Toronto, Banting undertook research on the internal secretion of the pancreas, and in 1921, with Charles Herbert Best, he discovered insulin. Banting and J. J. R. Macleod shared the Nobel prize for medicine in 1923. The Banting Research Foundation was established in 1924, and the Banting Institute was opened at Toronto in 1930. Banting was knighted in 1934.

Banting treatment (ban'ting) treatment of obesity by a low carbohydrate diet rich in nitrogenous matter.

bar (bahr) 1. a unit of pressure, being the pressure exerted by 1 megadyne per square cm. 2. a heavy wire or a wrought or cast metal segment, longer than its width, used to connect parts of a removable partial denture.

median b., a fibrotic formation across the neck of the prostate, producing obstruction of the urethra.

baragnosis (bar″ag-no'sis) impairment of the ability to perceive differences in weight or pressure.

barber's itch a contagious infection of the hair follicles on the face and neck, caused by staphylococci; called also SYCOSIS BARBAE.

barbital (bahr'bi-tahl) the first of the barbiturates, being a long-acting hypnotic and sedative.

barbiturate (bahr-bit'u-rāt) any of a group of organic compounds derived from barbituric acid, and commonly described as "sleeping pills." Available by prescription only, barbiturates may be used to induce sedation or sleep. The many types of barbiturates vary in their strength and in the rapidity and duration of their effect. In varying degrees, all serve to depress the central nervous system, depress respiration, affect the heart rate, and decrease blood pressure and temperature.

Barbiturates in the proper dosage may be helpful in several ways. As a sedative, a barbiturate such as phenobarbital, which is slowly absorbed by the system, may relieve tension, anxiety, and insomnia. Certain types of pruritus respond to the soothing effects of barbiturates. Dentists sometimes prescribe a mild dose to allay acute fear in an unusually apprehensive patient before dental work is begun. Barbiturates have proved effective in the controlling of epileptic convulsions.

Sometimes for brief operations a quick-acting barbiturate such as thiopental sodium (Pentothal sodium) may be used as an intravenous anesthetic. In essence, this has the effect of a powerful sleeping pill. The so-called "truth serum" is in reality a barbiturate adjusted to produce a state of semiconsciousness, much like a hypnotic trance.

Since barbiturates can become habit-forming, they should be used only by the person for whom they have been prescribed and only according to specific directions.

Barbiturate overdose can be fatal and should be treated with utmost promptness. It produces heavy, unnatural sleep, or a state resembling acute intoxication. A physician or the local emergency unit of the police or fire department should be called immediately. Until professional help arrives, the victim should be made to vomit by sticking a finger down his throat, but *only if he is awake;* he should be kept warm and his breathing should be facilitated by removing constricting clothing and proper positioning. (See also POISONING.)

barbituric acid (bahr″bi-tu'rik) a compound, $C_4H_4N_2O_3$, the parent substance of BARBITURATES.

barbotage (bahr″bo-tahzh') [Fr.] repeated alternate injection and withdrawal of fluid with a syringe, as in gastric lavage or administration of an anesthetic agent into the subarachnoid space by alternate injection of part of the anesthetic and withdrawal of cerebrospinal fluid into the syringe.

baresthesia (bar″es-the'ze-ah) sensibility for weight or pressure.

baresthesiometer (bar″es-the″ze-om'ĕ-ter) an instrument for estimating the acuteness of the sense of weight or pressure.

bariatrics (bar″e-at'riks) a field of medicine encompassing the study of overweight, its causes, prevention, and treatment.

barium (ba're-um) a chemical element, atomic number 56, atomic weight 137.34, symbol Ba. (See table of ELEMENTS.)

b. sulfate, a water-insoluble salt used as an opaque contrast medium for x-ray examination of the digestive tract.

b. test, x-ray examination using a barium mixture to help locate disorders in the esophagus, stomach, duodenum, and the small and large intestines. Such conditions as peptic ulcer, benign or malignant tumors, colitis, or enlargement of organs that might be causing pressure on the stomach may be readily identified with the use of barium tests.

Barium sulfate is a harmless chalky, water-insoluble compound that does not permit x-rays to pass through it. Taken before or during an examination, it causes the intestinal tract to stand out in silhouette when viewed through a fluoroscope or seen on an x-ray film.

Two main types of tests are conducted with the use of barium: the barium meal and the barium enema.

BARIUM MEAL. The patient, who has fasted since the previous evening, reports to the x-ray laboratory in the morning. He swallows a substance known as the "barium meal" (barium sulfate mixed with water and perhaps a flavoring). By fluoroscopy the radiologist watches the barium pass through the esophagus into the stomach, with the patient positioned so that the stomach and duodenum can be seen in various profiles. Then x-ray films are taken. If the small bowel is being studied it may be necessary to take additional x-rays during subsequent hours as the barium progresses through the digestive tract. The test is therefore often referred to as an "upper G.I. series" (gastrointestinal series). The patient is given no food until the series is completed.

The barium mixture may be constipating, and sometimes a laxative is given afterward. The patient is told to expect white barium in his stool during the following few days.

BARIUM ENEMA. The barium enema is valuable in examining the colon. The patient is given no food after a light evening meal. He may be given a cathartic to clear the colon of its contents, and an enema is usually given the morning of the test.

On the examination table, the patient is asked to relax on his side as the rectal tube is inserted. He is then helped to turn on his back. He is examined under the fluoroscope while the barium is being injected. For better views, the patient may be asked to turn from side to side. Usually enough of the barium mixture is administered to fill the entire colon. The films are taken, and the patient is allowed to evacuate in the bathroom. After another x-ray film is taken the test is finished.

barognosis (bar″og-no′sis) conscious perception of weight; the faculty by which weight is recognized.

baro-otitis (bar″o-o-ti′tis) barotitis.

barophilic (bar″o-fil′ik) growing best under high atmospheric pressure; said of bacteria.

baroreceptor (bar″o-re-sep′tor) a sensory nerve terminal that is stimulated by changes in pressure, as those in blood vessel walls.

barosinusitis (bar″o-si″nŭ-si′tis) a symptom complex due to differences in environmental atmospheric pressure and the air pressure in the paranasal sinuses.

barotaxis (bar″o-tak′sis) stimulation of living matter by change of atmospheric pressure.

barotitis (bar″o-ti′tis) a morbid condition of the ear due to exposure to differing atmospheric pressures.

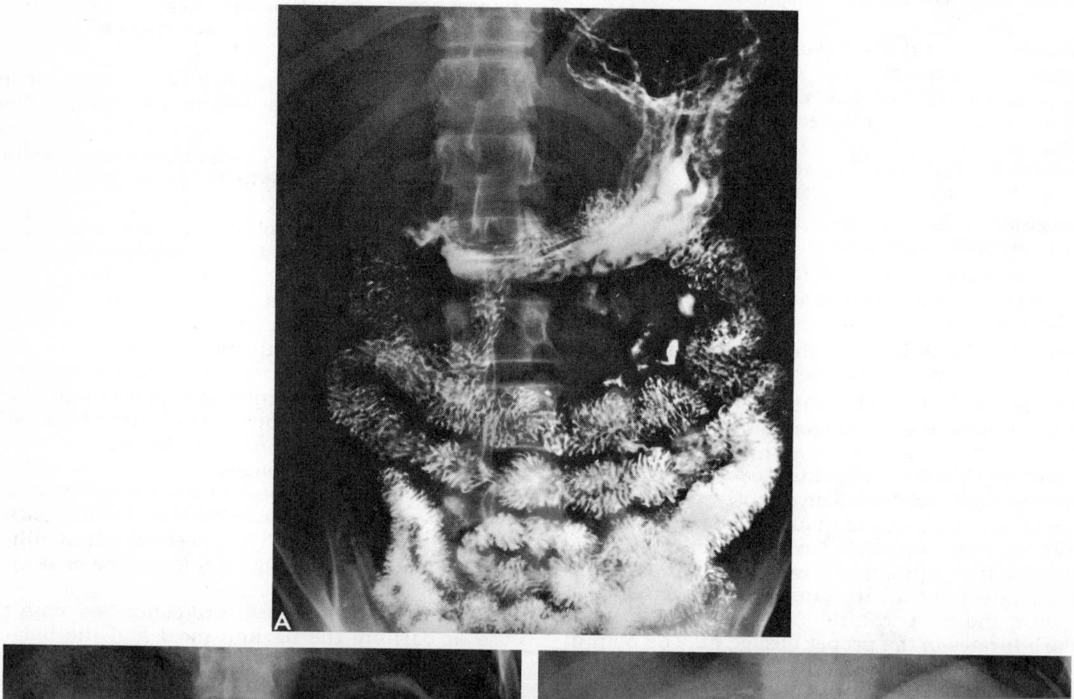

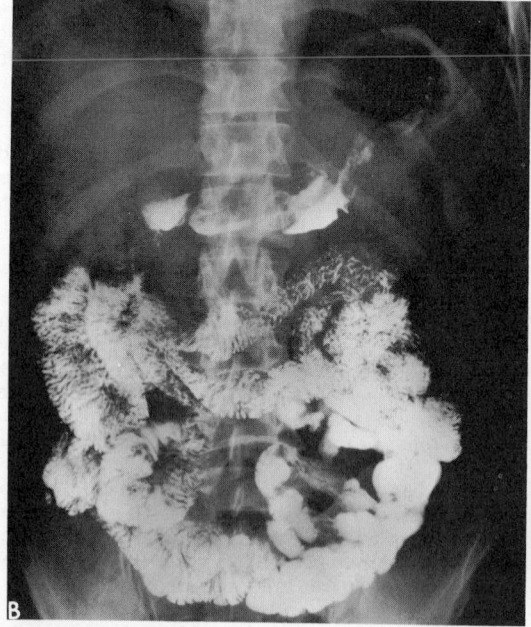

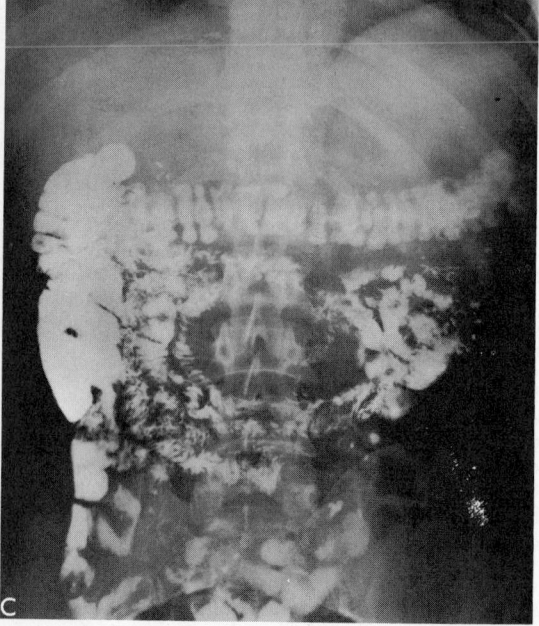

Frequent-interval film and fluoroscopy method for examination of the small intestine. *A*, At 1 hour after administration of the barium; *B*, at 2 hours; *C*, at 3 hours. (From Meschan, I.: Radiographic Positioning and Related Anatomy. Philadelphia, W. B. Saunders Co., 1968.)

b. me'dia, a symptom complex due to difference between the atmospheric pressure of the environment and air pressure in the middle ear.

barotrauma (bar"o-traw'mah) injury due to pressure, as to structures of the ear, in high-altitude flyers, owing to differences between atmospheric and intratympanic pressures. (See also BAROTITIS and BAROSINUSITIS.)

Barr body (bahr) sex chromatin; the persistent mass of the material of the inactivated X chromosome in cells of normal females.

Barron ligation (bar'on) surgical treatment of hemorrhoids by binding them with rubber ligatures so that the ligated portion sloughs away after several days.

Bartholin cyst (bar'to-lin) a retention cyst affecting a Bartholin gland, and usually developing as a consequence of an earlier infection of the gland.

Bartholin's duct (bar'to-linz) the larger of the sublingual glands, which opens into the submandibular duct.

Bartholin's glands (bar'to-linz) two small glands, one on each side of the vaginal orifice, that secrete mucus; their ducts open on the vulva. Called also the vulvovaginal glands. Their exact function is not clear but they are believed to secrete large amounts of mucus during sexual excitement, thereby providing lubrication for the vagina during coitus. The Bartholin glands are homologues of the bulbourethral glands in the male.

bartholinitis (bar"to-lin-i'tis) inflammation of the Bartholin glands.

Barton (bar"ton) Clara (1821–1912). Founder and first president of American National Red Cross. Born in North Oxford, Massachusetts, she distributed supplies for the relief of wounded soldiers during the Civil War, and at its close organized a bureau of records in Washington to aid in the search of missing men. She assisted in organizing military hospitals when the Franco-Prussian War started in 1870, and began at once to establish an American Red Cross Society upon her return to the United States in 1873.

Barton's fracture (bar'tunz) fracture of the distal end of the radius into the wrist joint.

Bartonella (bar"to-nel'lah) a genus of the family Bartonellaceae.

B. bacilliform'is, the etiologic agent of Carrión's disease.

Bartonellaceae (bar"to-nel-la'se-e) a family of the order Rickettsiales, occurring as pathogenic parasites in the erythrocytes of man and other animals.

bartonellemia (bar"to-nel-le'me-ah) the presence in the blood of organisms of the genus *Bartonella.*

bartonellosis (bar"to-nel-lo'sis) Carrión's disease.

Bartter's syndrome (bar'terz) a hereditary disorder marked by juxtaglomerular cell hyperplasia, hyperaldosteronism, hypokalemic alkalosis, increased concentrations of plasma renin in the absence of hypertension, and by mental retardation and short stature.

baryesthesia (bar"e-es-the'ze-ah) baresthesia.

barylalia (bar"e-la'le-ah) indistinct, thick speech, resulting from a lesion of the central nervous system.

baryphonia (bar"e-fo'ne-ah) deepness and hoarseness of the voice.

basal (ba'sal) pertaining to or situated near a base; in physiology, pertaining to the lowest possible level.

b. metabolism test, a method of measuring the body's expenditure of energy by recording its rate of oxygen intake and consumption. Once a major test of THYROID GLAND function, it is being replaced by diagnostic tests requiring less extensive preparation and capable of producing more accurate test results, e.g., the PROTEIN-BOUND IODINE test (PBI) and RADIOACTIVE IODINE UPTAKE test.

The basal metabolic rate (BMR) is calculated from the patient's rate of metabolism while he is at complete rest and in a fasting state. The BMR usually is expressed as a percentage that indicates how far it varies from the average. For example, a BMR of plus 15 would mean that the patient's basal metabolic rate was 15 percent higher than the average for someone of his age, sex, and size. A variation between plus 20 and minus 20 is considered within normal range. A reading above the normal range is interpreted as overactivity of the thyroid gland, or HYPERTHYROIDISM; one below normal usually indicates a thyroid deficiency, or HYPOTHYROIDISM.

The basal metabolic rate also can be determined by use of a metabolic scale designed to make highly accurate measurements of the patient's weight while he is lying in his hospital bed. The measurement is taken during a period of 30 to 60 minutes when no food or liquids are taken in and there is no output of urine or feces. Thus the very small amount of weight lost through the evaporation of water from the lungs and skin (insensible weight loss) can be measured. The amount of insensible weight loss is proportional to the metabolic rate. By measuring the weight lost in 1 hour, and multiplying this amount in grams by 54.4, the basal metabolic rate can be calculated.

base (bās) 1. the lowest part or foundation of anything (see also BASIS). 2. the main ingredient of a compound. 3. the nonacid part of a salt; a substance that combines with acids to form salts. In the chemical processes of the body, bases are essential to the maintenance of a normal ACID-BASE BALANCE. Excessive concentration of bases in the body fluids leads to ALKALOSIS.

nitrogenous b., an aromatic, nitrogen-containing molecule that serves as a proton acceptor, e.g., purine or pyrimidine.

purine b's, a group of compounds of which purine is the base, including uric acid, adenine, xanthine, and theobromine.

pyrimidine b's, a group of chemical compounds of which pyrimidine is the base, including uracil, thymine, and cytosine, which are common constituents of nucleic acids.

Basedow's disease (bas'ĕ-dōz) exophthalmic goiter.

Basedow's goiter (bas'ĕ-dōz) a colloid goiter which has become hyperfunctioning after administration of iodine.

baseline (bās'līn) a known value or quantity used to measure or assess an unknown, as a baseline urine sample.

basement membrane (bās'ment) the delicate layer of extracellular condensation of mucopolysaccharides and proteins underlying the epithelium of mucous membranes and secreting glands.

basic (ba'sik) 1. pertaining to or having properties of a base. 2. capable of neutralizing acids.

basicity (ba-sis'ĭ-te) 1. the quality of being a base, or basic. 2. the combining power of an acid.

Basidiobolus (bah-sid"e-ob'o-lus) a genus of fungi of the group Phycomycetes, including *B. hapto-spo'rus,* the cause of subcutaneous phycomycosis.

basidiospore (bah-sid'e-o-spōr") a spore of certain higher fungi formed on a basidium following karyogamy and meiosis.

basidium (bah-sid'e-um), pl. *basid'ia* [L.] the club-like organ bearing basidiospores.

basihyoid (ba"se-hi'oid) the body of the hyoid bone.

basilad (bas'ĭ-lad) toward the base.

basilar (bas'ĭ-lar) pertaining to a base or basal part.

basilateral (ba"sĭ-lat'er-al) both basilar and lateral.

basilemma (ba"sĭ-lem'ah) basement membrane.

basiloma (bas"ĭ-lo'mah) a basal cell carcinoma.

basion (ba'se-on) the midpoint of the anterior border of the foramen magnum.

basipetal (bah-sip'ĕ-tal) descending toward the base; developing in the direction of the base, as a spore.

basis (ba'sis) the lower, basic, or fundamental part of an object, organ, or substance. In anatomic nomenclature, used as a general term to designate the base of a structure or organ, or the part opposite to or distinguished from the apex.

basisphenoid (ba"sĭ-sfe'noid) an embryonic bone that becomes the back part of the body of the sphenoid.

basoerythrocyte (ba"so-ĕ-rith'ro-sīt) an erythrocyte containing basophil granules.

basophil (ba'so-fil) 1. any structure, cell, or histologic element staining readily with basic dyes. 2. a granular leukocyte with an irregularly shaped, relatively pale-staining nucleus that is partially constricted into two lobes, and with cytoplasm containing coarse bluish black granules of variable size.

basophile (ba'so-fīl) basophilic.

basophilia (ba"so-fil'e-ah) 1. the reaction of relatively immature erythrocytes to basic dyes whereby the stained cells appear blue, gray, or grayish-blue, or bluish granules appear. 2. abnormal increase of basophilic leukocytes in the blood. 3. basophilic leukocytosis.

basophilic (ba"so-fil'ik) staining readily with basic dyes.

basophilism (ba-sof'ĭ-lizm) abnormal increase of basophilic cells.

Cushing's b., pituitary b., Cushing's syndrome.

basoplasm (ba'so-plazm) cytoplasm that stains with basic dyes.

bath (bath) 1. a medium, e.g., water, vapor, sand, or mud, with which the body is washed or in which the body is wholly or partially immersed for therapeutic or cleansing purposes; application of such a medium to the body. 2. the equipment or apparatus in which a body or object may be immersed.

colloid b., a bath prepared by adding soothing agents, such as gelatin, starch, bran, or similar substances, to the bath water, for the purpose of relieving skin irritation and pruritus. The patient is dried by patting rather than rubbing the skin. Care must be taken to avoid chilling.

contrast b., alternate immersion of a part in hot water and cold water.

cool b., one in water from 60° to 75° F. (15° to 24° C.).

emollient b., a bath in a soothing and softening liquid, used in various skin disorders.

hot b., one in water from 98° to 112° F. (36° to 44° C.).

sitz b., immersion of only the hips and buttocks. Sitz baths are used to relieve pain and discomfort following rectal surgery, cystoscopy, or vaginal surgery; they also may be ordered for patients with cystitis or infections within the pelvic cavity. Temperature for a hot sitz bath is started at 95° F. (35° C.), and gradually increased to 105° to 110° F. (41° to 43° C.); the patient must be watched for fatigue and faintness, and an attendant must remain within calling distance. Cool compresses to the head or cool drinks during the bath promote comfort and relieve faintness.

sponge b., one in which the patient's body is not immersed but is wiped with a wet cloth or sponge. Sponge baths are most often employed for reduction of body temperature in the presence of a fever, in which case the water used is ice cold and may contain alcohol to increase evaporation of moisture from the skin.

tepid b., one in water 85° to 92° F. (30° to 33° C.).

MEDICATED BATHS

TYPE	PURPOSE	PREPARATION
Mustard	To stimulate peripheral circulation and promote muscle relaxation	Mustard is dissolved in tepid water and added to bath water. For adult use 1 tsp. dry mustard to 1 gal. water; for child use ½ tsp. dry mustard to 1 gal. water
Oatmeal	As soothing agent in skin disorders	3 cups oatmeal boiled in 2 qt. water. Add 1 cup sodium bicarbonate (baking soda) and pour in cheesecloth bag. Tie bag securely and put in bath water; use swirling action to mix thoroughly
Paraffin	To apply heat to inflamed joints; especially useful in the treatment of arthritis	Melt 3 to 4 lb. paraffin with 1 lb. petrolatum; take care to *keep away from open flame.* Cool mixture until a thin crust appears on the surface
Saline (salt)	As stimulant to skin, to lessen pain of sprains and contusions	Mix sodium chloride in sufficient water to make 2% solution (8 lb. table salt to 30 gal. water)
Sodium bicarbonate	To relieve pruritus in various skin disorders	Dissolve sodium bicarbonate (baking soda) in hot water and add to bath to make a 5% solution (20 lb. sodium bicarbonate to 30 gal. water)

warm b., one in water 90° to 104° F. (32° to 40° C.).

whirlpool b., one in which the water is kept in constant motion by mechanical means. It has a gentle massaging action that promotes relaxation.

bathrocephaly (bath″ro-sef′ah-le) a developmental anomaly marked by a steplike posterior projection of the skull, caused by excessive growth of the lambdoid suture.

bathy- word element [Gr.], *deep.*

bathyanesthesia (bath″e-an″es-the′ze-ah) loss of deep sensibility.

bathyesthesia (bath″e-es-the′ze-ah) deep sensibility.

bathyhyperesthesia (bath″ĭ-hi″per-es-the′ze-ah) abnormally increased sensitiveness of deep body structures.

bathyhypesthesia (bath″ĭ-hi″pes-the′ze-ah) abnormally diminished deep sensibility.

bathypnea (bath″ĭ-ne′ah) deep breathing.

Bayle's disease (bālz) progressive general paralysis of the insane.

Bazin's disease (bah-zaz′) erythema induratum; a chronic necrotizing vasculitis, usually occurring on the calves of young women; it was thought to be a form of tuberculosis of the skin complicated by vasculitis, but now the role of tuberculosis is in dispute.

BCG vaccine bacille Calmette Guérin vaccine, a tuberculosis vaccine, containing living, avirulent, bovine-strain tubercle bacilli (*Mycobacterium bovis*). The vaccine is administered by a special technique using a multiple-puncture disk. It cannot be given when the patient is reactive to tuberculin, when acute infectious disease is present, or when there is any skin disorder. It offers some protection against tuberculosis, but cannot be relied on for total control of the disease. In a high percentage of cases the vaccine causes local ulcers at the site of administration. Public health officials in this country recommend the use of BCG vaccine only for those persons living in communities having a high rate of tuberculosis cases. After vaccination with BCG, the patient will have a positive response to the tuberculin test.

Be chemical symbol, *beryllium.*

beaker (bēk′er) a round laboratory vessel of various materials, usually with parallel sides and often with a pouring spout.

beat (bēt) a throb or pulsation, as of the heart or of an artery.

apex b., the beat felt over the apex of the heart, normally in the fifth left intercostal space.

capture b's, occasional ventricular responses to a sinus impulse that reaches the atrioventricular node in a nonrefractory phase.

ectopic b., a heartbeat originating at some point other than the sinus node.

escaped b's, heart beats that follow an abnormally long pause.

forced b., an extrasystole produced by artificial stimulation of the heart.

premature b., an extrasystole.

Beau's lines (bōz) transverse furrows on the fingernails, usually a sign of a systemic disease but also due to other causes.

bechic (bek′ik) pertaining to cough.

Bechterew's disease (bek-ter′yefs) rheumatoid spondylitis.

Beck's triad (beks) rising venous pressure, falling arterial pressure, and small quiet heart; characteristic of cardiac compression.

bed (bed) 1. a supporting structure or tissue. 2. a couch or support for the body during sleep.

capillary b., the capillaries of a tissue, area, or organ considered collectively, and their volume capacity; see Plate 8.

b. cradle, a frame placed over the body of a bed patient for application of heat or cold or for protecting injured parts from coming into contact with the bed clothes. Cradles vary in size according to their intended purpose and can be used over the entire body or over one or more extremities.

fracture b., a bed for the use of patients with broken bones.

Gatch b., a bed fitted with jointed springs, which may be adjusted to various positions.

nail b., the area of modified epithelium beneath the nail.

bedbug (bed′bug) a bug of the genus *Cimex,* a flattened, oval, reddish insect that inhabits houses, furniture, and neglected beds and feeds on man, usually at night.

bedpan (bed′pan) a shallow vessel used for defecation or urination by patients confined to bed.

bedsore (bed′sōr) an ulcerlike sore caused by prolonged pressure of the patient's body against the bed (see also DECUBITUS ULCER).

bed-wetting (bed′wet-ing) enuresis. Most small children wet their beds occasionally; although it is a nuisance it is no cause for alarm. Only when a child persists in regularly wetting his bed after the age of 6, when he can reasonably be expected to have stopped, or when a child who has stopped bed-wetting reverts to it, should a physical or emotional disorder be sought.

bee sting injury caused by the venom of a bee. The pain from a bee sting can be relieved by sodium bicarbonate, a few drops of ammonia, or calamine lotion. A paste made from unseasoned meat tenderizer is effective in breaking down the protein of the venom from the bee sting and in diminishing its harmful effects. Cold compresses help prevent swelling. The skin should not be scratched as this may lead to infection. The insect's "stinger" should be scraped out with a fingernail or removed with tweezers held flat against the skin. If the pain or swelling persists, or if the sting is on the tongue or in the mouth, a physician should be consulted at once. Symptoms of a severe allergic reaction, such as collapse or swelling of the body, indicate ANAPHYLACTIC SHOCK and require that medical help be sought immediately.

behavior (be-hāv′yer) the manner in which an individual acts or performs. adj., **behav′ioral.**

automatic b., automatism.

invariable b., activity whose character is determined by innate structure, such as reflex action.

b. modification, an approach to correction of undesirable conduct that focuses on changing observable actions. Modification of the behavior is accomplished through systematic manipulation of the environmental and behavioral variables related to the specific behavior to be changed. The principles and techniques of behavior modification have been utilized in the treatment of both physical and mental disorders; for example, in control of alcoholism, smoking, obesity, and stress. (See also CONDITIONING.)

b. therapy, a therapeutic technique in which an attempt is made to change the patient's behavior directly, rather than correct the basic cause of the undesirable behavior. Examples of techniques that may be used in behavior therapy include token economy, shaping, aversive control, and instrumental CONDITIONING.

variable b., behavior that is modified by individual experience.

behaviorism (be-hāv'yer-izm) a theory of psychology based upon objectively observable, tangible, and measurable data, rather than subjective phenomena, such as ideas and emotions.

Behçet's syndrome (ba'sets) severe uveitis and retinal vasculitis, optic atrophy, and aphtha-like lesions of the mouth and genitalia, and often with other signs and symptoms suggestive of a diffuse vaculitis; it most often affects young males. Called also Behçet's disease.

Behring's law (ba'ringz) blood and serum of an immunized person, when transferred to another subject, will render the latter immune.

bejel (bej'el) NONVENEREAL SYPHILIS occurring in the Middle East.

bel (bel) a unit used to express the ratio of two powers, usually electric or acoustic powers; an increase of 1 bel in intensity approximately doubles loudness of most sounds (see also DECIBEL).

belching (belch'ing) eructation.

belemnoid (be-lem'noid) 1. dart-shaped. 2. the styloid process.

Bell's palsy (belz) neuropathy of the facial nerve, resulting in paralysis of the muscles of the face, usually on one side. The victim usually is unable to close his mouth, so that he drools and cannot whistle. If he is unable to close the eye on the affected side, it may become tearful and inflamed.

Bell's palsy is often no more than a temporary condition lasting a few days or weeks. Occasionally facial paralysis results from a tumor pressing on the nerve, or from physical trauma to the nerve. In this event, recovery will depend on the success in treating the tumor or injury. More often, however, the cause is unknown. In many cases the deformity can be reduced by plastic surgery.

belladonna (bel"ah-don'ah) 1. *Atropa belladonna* (deadly nightshade), a plant that is the source of various alkaloids, e.g., atropine, hyoscyamine, etc. 2. belladonna leaf; the dried leaves and fruiting tops of *Atropa belladonna,* used as an anticholinergic in the management of peptic ulcer and other gastrointestinal disorders.

b. poisoning, a severe toxic condition due to overdosage of belladonna or accidental ingestion of large amounts of the drug. Symptoms include dryness of the mouth, thirst, dilated pupils, flushed skin or rash on the face, neck, and upper trunk, tachycardia, fever, delirium, and stupor. Treatment consists of removal of the poison from the stomach by inducing vomiting or gastric suction. This is followed by gastric lavage with water containing activated charcoal and an instillation of a solution of 200 ml. of water and 30 gm. of sodium sulfate. Barbiturates such as Seconal are administered to reduce excitability. Respiratory difficulties may require administration of oxygen or in extreme cases tracheostomy. Measures are also taken to reduce high body temperature and maintain an adequate blood pressure.

belly (bel'e) 1. the abdomen. 2. the fleshy, contractile part of a muscle.

bemegride (bem'ĕ-grīd) an analeptic used especially in the treatment of barbiturate poisoning. The drug may cause muscle twitching and convulsions; if so, it is discontinued and thiopental is given as an antidote. Bemegride is administered intravenously.

benactyzine (ben-ak'tĭ-zēn) an ataractic, used as the hydrochloride salt. It is contraindicated in patients with severe psychosis.

Benadryl (ben'ah-dril) trademark for diphenhydramine, an antihistamine.

Bence Jones protein (bens jōnz) a low–molecular weight, heat-sensitive urinary protein found in patients with multiple myeloma, which coagulates on heating to 45°–55° C. and redissolves partially or wholly on boiling.

bendroflumethiazide (ben"dro-floo"mĕ-thi'ah-zīd) a diuretic and antihypertensive; it enhances the excretion of sodium and chloride.

bends (bendz) decompression sickness; a condition resulting from a too-rapid decrease in atmospheric pressure, as when a deep-sea diver is brought too hastily to the surface. The term bends is derived from the bodily contortions its victims undergo when atmospheric pressure is abruptly changed from a high pressure to a relatively lower one. Aqualung divers and underwater construction workers are particularly susceptible to this condition (see also CAISSON DISEASE). A form of altitude sickness suffered by aviators who ascend too rapidly to high altitudes is similar to bends. Bends may also be a complication in a type of oxygen therapy called HYPERBARIC OXYGENATION, in which the patient is placed in a high-pressure chamber to increase the oxygen content of his blood. Nursing personnel, physicians, and the patient within the chamber must be protected from bends when they emerge from the high-pressure chamber.

CAUSE. The phenomenon of bends is explained in terms of a law of physics: The greater the atmospheric pressure, the greater the amount of gas that can be dissolved in a liquid. The gas involved in bends is the air we breathe, composed chiefly of nitrogen and oxygen. Under normal atmospheric pressure (about 15 lb. per square inch), nitrogen is present in the blood in dissolved form. If the atmospheric pressure is substantially increased, a proportionately greater amount of nitrogen will be dissolved in the blood. The same is true of oxygen, and this is the basis for hyperbaric oxygenation in the treatment of oxygen deficiency.

The increase in pressure causes no ill effects. Nor will there be any ill effects if the pressure is gradually brought back to normal. When the decrease in pressure is slow, the nitrogen escapes safely from the blood as it passes through the lungs to be exhaled. If the pressure drops abruptly back to normal, the nitrogen is suddenly released from its state of solution in the blood and forms bubbles. Although the body is now under normal air pressure, expanding bubbles of nitrogen are present in the circulation and force their way into the capillaries, blocking the normal passage of the blood. This blockage (or embolism) starves cells dependent on a constant supply of oxygen and other blood nutrients. Some of these cells may be nerve cells located in the limbs or in the spinal cord. When they are deprived of blood, an attack of bends occurs.

The oxygen in the blood reacts similarly when abnormal pressure is abruptly relieved. But because oxygen is dissolved more easily than nitrogen, and because some of the oxygen combines chemically with hemoglobin, the oxygen released in decompression forms fewer bubbles, and is therefore less troublesome.

SYMPTOMS AND TREATMENT. The symptoms of bends include joint pain, dizziness, staggering, visual disturbances, dyspnea, and itching of the skin. Partial paralysis occurs in severe cases; collapse and insensibility are also possible. Only rarely is the condition itself fatal, although a diver while in this condition may suffer a fatal accident unless he is rescued.

Bends is treated by placing the victim in a decompression chamber where the air pressure is at the level to which he was originally exposed. If the victim is a diver, this is the pressure at the depth where he was working. Pressure in the chamber is then reduced to normal at a safe rate.

Benedict's solution (ben′ĕ-dikts) a chemical solution used to determine the presence of glucose in the urine; called also Benedict's reagent. It is prepared by dissolving 173 gm. of sodium citrate and 100 gm. of anhydrous sodium carbonate in 800 ml. of water; the solution in filtered and to the filtrate is added 17.3 gm. of copper sulfate in 100 ml. of water. Water is then added to make a total of 1 liter of prepared solution.

Benedict's test (ben′ĕ-dikts) a laboratory test for determining the presence of sugar in the urine. Eight drops of urine and 5 ml. of Benedict's solution are mixed in a test tube and then held over a flame and allowed to boil for 5 minutes. The color of the solution after boiling determines the amount of sugar present. Blue indicates no glucose; green a trace, or 1 plus; yellow, up to 0.5 per cent or 2 plus; orange, 0.5 to 1.5 per cent or 3 plus; red, 1.5 per cent and over or 4 plus.

Benedikt's syndrome (ben′ĕ-dikts) ipsilateral oculomotor paralysis, contralateral hyperkinesia, contralateral tremor and paralysis of the arm and leg, and ipsilateral ataxia; due to damage to the third cranial nerve with involvement of the nucleus ruber and corticospinal tract.

Benemid (ben′ĕ-mid) trademark for probenecid, a uricosuric agent used mainly in the treatment of chronic gout and also for some forms of arthritis.

benign (be-nīn) not malignant; not recurrent; favorable for recovery.

Bennett's fracture (ben′ets) fracture of the base of the first metacarpal bone running into the carpometacarpal joint, complicated by subluxation.

Benoquin (ben′o-kwin) trademark for a preparation of monobenzone, a depigmenting agent.

benoxinate (ben-ok′sĭ-nāt) a surface anesthetic for the eye.

Benson's disease (ben′sunz) a unilateral condition of unknown origin, sometimes occurring with age, characterized by spherical and stellate opacities in the vitreous body, which appear to sparkle when illuminated by an examining light. Called also asteroid hyalitis.

bentonite (ben′to-nīt) a native colloidal hydrated aluminum silicate that swells in water; used as a bulk laxative and in preparations for use on the skin.

benzaldehyde (ben-zal′dĕ-hīd) artificial essential oil of almond; used as a flavoring agent.

benzalkonium chloride (ben″zal-ko′ne-um) a mixture of alkylbenzyldimethylammonium chlorides; used as a topical antiseptic in 1:750 to 1:10,000 solution.

Benzedrex (ben′zĕ-dreks) trademark for a propylhexedrine inhaler, used as a vasoconstrictor to decongest the nasal mucosa.

Benzedrine (ben′zĕ-drēn) trademark for amphetamine, a central nervous system stimulant.

benzene (ben′zēn) a liquid hydrocarbon, C_6H_6, from coal tar; used as a solvent.

b. hexachloride, a substance occurring in 5 isomeric forms, the gamma isomer (GAMMA BENZENE HEXACHLORIDE) is a powerful insecticide.

b. ring, the closed hexagon of carbon atoms in benzene, from which the different benzene compounds are derived by replacement of the hydrogen atoms.

benzestrol (ben-zes′trol) a synthetic estrogenic compound administered orally in the treatment of menopausal symptoms, to depress lactation, to relieve the symptoms of prostatic cancer, and in the relief of certain forms of vaginitis.

benzethonium (ben″zĕ-tho′ne-um) an ammonium derivative, used as a local anti-infective in the form of the hydrochloride salt.

benzhexol (benz-hek′sol) trihexyphenidyl, an anticholinergic used in treatment of Parkinson's disease.

benzhydramine (benz-hi′drah-mēn) diphenhydramine, an antihistamine.

benzidine (ben′zĭ-dēn) a compound used as a test for traces of blood (benzidine test).

benzin, benzine (ben′zin; ben′zēn) petroleum benzene; a purified distillate from petroleum, a solvent for organic compounds.

benzoate (ben′zo-āt) a salt of benzoic acid.

benzoated (ben′zo-āt″ed) containing or combined with benzoic acid.

benzocaine (ben′zo-kān) a local anesthetic for topical use.

benzodiazepine (ben″zo-di-az′ĕ-pēn) any of a group of minor tranquilizers, e.g., chlordiazepoxide, diazepam, and oxazepam, having similar molecular structure.

benzoic acid (ben-zo′ik) an acid from benzoin and other resins and from coal tar, used as an antifungal agent in pharmaceutical preparations and as a germicide. The sodium salt of benzoic acid, sodium benzoate, is used as an antifungal agent in pharmaceutical preparations, and may be used as a test for liver function.

benzoin (ben′zo-in, ben-zo′in) a balsamic resin from *Styrax benzoin* and other *Styrax* species, used chiefly as a topical protectant and antiseptic. Benzoin acts as an expectorant and thus is sometimes used in steam inhalations in treating respiratory disorders.

benzol (ben′zol) benzene.

benzonatate (ben-zo′nah-tāt) an antitussive drug that depresses cough without affecting respiration. It is administered orally in capsule or tablet form, but should not be chewed or dissolved in the mouth because the local anesthetic action may cause numbness of the oral mucosa.

benzononatine (ben-zo″no-na′tin) benzonatate.

benzphetamine (benz-fet′ah-mēn) a sympathomimetic amine, used as an anorexiant in the form of the hydrochloride salt.

benzquinamide (benz-kwin′ah-mīd) an antiemetic, particularly beneficial in treating patients who cannot tolerate such other antiemetics as prochlorperazine.

benzthiazide (benz-thi′ah-zīd) an orally effective diuretic and antihypertensive.

benztropine (benz′tro-pēn) a parasympatholytic agent, used as the mesylate salt in Parkinson's disease.

benzyl (ben′zil) the hydrocarbon radical, C_7H_7.

b. alcohol, a colorless liquid used as a bacteriostatic in solutions for injection, and also topically as a local anesthetic.

b. benzoate, a clear, oily liquid used as a scabicide and with dimercaprol as an antidote in metal poisoning.

benzylpenicillin (ben′zil-pen-ĭ-sil′in) penicillin G.

Berger rhythm (ber′ger) alpha rhythm.

Bergeron's chorea (disease) (berzh′ronz) electric chorea of childhood, characterized by violent rhythmic spasms, but running a benign course.

beriberi (ber″e-ber′e) an endemic form of polyneuritis due to an unbalanced diet, chiefly a lack of vitamin B_1, or thiamine. The disease is more common in areas in which refined rice is the main staple in the diet; however, improved refining processes and dietary habits have decreased the incidence of this disease.

In the United States, mild forms of the disease sometimes occur in persons who are on extremely restricted diets. Alcoholics, who tend to decrease food intake drastically during periods of drinking, may show signs of beriberi. The disease also occurs in persons whose diet consists of highly refined and overcooked food.

Berkefeld's filter (ber′ke-feldz) a filter composed of diatomaceous earth, impermeable to ordinary bacteria.

berkelium (ber-ke′le-um) a chemical element, atomic number 97, atomic weight 247, symbol Bk. (See table of ELEMENTS.)

Berubigen (be-roo′bĭ-jen) trademark for preparations of vitamin B_{12} (cyanocobalamin).

berylliosis (bĕ-ril″e-o′sis) a morbid condition caused by exposure to fumes or finely divided dust of beryllium salts, marked by formation of granulomas, usually involving the lungs and, rarely, the skin, subcutaneous tissues, lymph nodes, liver, and other organs.

beryllium (bĕ-ril′e-um) a chemical element, atomic number 4, atomic weight 9.012, symbol Be. (See table of ELEMENTS.)

Besnier-Boeck disease (bez′ne-a bek) sarcoidosis.

Best's disease (bests) congenital macular degeneration.

bestiality (bes-te-al′ĭ-te) sexual connection with an animal.

beta (ba′tah) second letter of the Greek alphabet, β; used in names of chemical compounds to distinguish one of two or more isomers or to indicate position of substituting atoms or groups.

b. particles, negatively charged particles emitted by radioactive elements. These particles are the result of the disintegration of neutrons, their source being the unstable atoms of radioactive metals such as radium and uranium. There are three general types of emissions from radioactive substances: alpha and beta particles and gamma rays. Beta particles are less penetrating than gamma rays and may be used to treat certain conditions on or near the surface of the body. (See also RADIATION and RADIOTHERAPY.)

betacism (ba′tah-sizm) excessive use of the *b* sound in speaking.

Betadine (ba′tah-dēn) trademark for preparations of providone-iodine, which have a longer antiseptic action than most iodine solutions.

betahistine (ba″tah-his′tēn) a vasodilator that has histamine-like activity.

betaine (be′tah-in) an agent used in the form of the hydrochloride salt as a lipotropic agent and as a substitute for hydrochloric acid in achlorhydria.

beta-ketobutyric acid (ba″tah-ke″to-bu-tir′ik) acetoacetic acid.

Betalin (ba′tah-lin) trademark for preparations of the vitamin B complex.

betamethasone (ba″tah-meth′ah-sōn) a synthetic glucocorticoid, the most active of the anti-inflammatory steroids; available as a cream or tablet for topical or oral use.

betanaphthol (ba″tah-naf′thol) a form of naphthol used as a topical antiseptic.

beta-oxybutyric acid (ba″tah-ok″se-bu-tir′ik) one of the KETONE BODIES, occurring in abnormal amounts in diabetic ketoacidosis and in starvation due to fatty acid oxidation.

betatron (ba′tah-tron) an apparatus for accelerating electrons to millions of electron volts by magnetic induction.

Betaxin (be-tak′sin) trademark for preparations of thiamine hydrochloride, used as a vitamin supplement.

betazole (ba′tah-zōl) an analogue of histamine used in place of it in gastric function tests to stimulate gastric secretion. There is no accompanying fall in blood pressure with the administration of benzole as there is with histamine. Epinephrine should be on hand at the time betazole is given in the event an untoward reaction occurs. Called also gastramine.

bethanechol (bĕ-tha′nĕ-kol) a derivative of a choline-like substance, the chloride salt is used as a cholinergic in the treatment of abdominal distention and urinary retention. Hypotension and dyspnea may occur as side effects; if they do, the patient is placed in Fowler's position and atropine is usually administered.

bethanidine (bĕ-than′ĭ-dēn) an adrenergic blocking agent used in the treatment of essential hypertension, especially the malignant phase.

Betz cells (betz) large pyramidal cells forming a layer of the gray matter of the brain.

Bev billion electron volts (3.82×10^{-11} gram (small) calorie, or 1.6×10^{-3} erg).

Bevidox (bev′ĭ-doks) trademark for a solution of vitamin B_{12} (cyanocobalamin).

bezoar (be′zōr) a mass formed in the stomach by

compaction of repeatedly ingested material that does not pass into the intestine.

BFP biologic false-positive reaction; a positive finding in serologic tests for syphilis when syphilis does not exist.

Bi chemical symbol, *bismuth.*

bi- (bi) word element [L.], *two.*

biarticular (bi″ar-tik′u-lar) affecting two joints.

biarticulate (bi″ar-tik′u-lāt) having two joints.

bibasic (bi-ba′sik) having two hydrogen atoms that may react with bases.

bibliotherapy (bib″le-o-ther′ah-pe) use of books and the reading of them in treatment of nervous disorders.

bicameral (bi-kam′er-al) having two chambers or cavities.

bicapsular (bi-kap′su-lar) having two capsules.

bicarbonate (bi-kar′bon-āt) any salt containing the HCO_3^- anion.

blood b., plasma b., the bicarbonate of the blood plasma, an index of the ALKALI RESERVE.

b. of soda, sodium bicarbonate.

bicaudal, bicaudate (bi-kaw′dal; bi-kaw′dāt) having two tails.

bicellular (bi-sel′u-lar) made up of two cells.

bicephalus (bi-sef′ah-lus) a two-headed monster.

biceps (bi′seps) a muscle having two heads. The biceps muscle of the arm flexes and supinates the forearm; the biceps muscle of the thigh flexes and rotates the leg laterally and extends the thigh. (See table of MUSCLES.)

Bichat's fissure (be-shaz′) transverse fissure.

Bichat's tunic (be-shaz′) tunica intima.

bichloride (bi-klo′rīd) a chloride containing two equivalents of chlorine.

Bicillin (bi′sĭ-lin) trademark for a preparation of benzathine penicillin G.

bicipital (bi-sip′ĭ-tal) having two heads; pertaining to a biceps muscle.

biconcave (bi-kon′kāv) having two concave surfaces.

biconvex (bi-kon′veks) having two convex surfaces.

bicornate, bicornuate (bi-kor′nāt) (bi-kor′nu-āt) having two horns, or cornua.

bicorporate (bi-kor′po-rāt) having two bodies.

bicuspid (bi-kus′pid) 1. having two cusps. 2. bicuspid (mitral) valve. 3. a premolar tooth.

b.i.d. [L.] *bis in di′e* (twice a day).

biduous (bid′u-us) lasting two days.

Bielschowsky's disease (be″el-show′skēz) the late infantile form of AMAUROTIC FAMILIAL IDIOCY, differing from the infantile form (TAY-SACHS DISEASE) in that it occurs between 3 and 4 years of age, progresses more slowly, and the cherry-red retinal spot is frequently absent, but there are pigmentary changes of the retina.

Bielschowsky-Jansky disease (be″el-show′ske yan′ske) Bielschowsky's disease.

bifid (bi′fid) cleft into two parts or branches.

bifocal eyeglasses (bi-fo′kal) eyeglasses in which each lens is made up of two segments of different refractive powers, or strength. Generally, the upper part of the lens is used for ordinary or distant vision, and the smaller, lower section for near vision, for close work such as reading or sewing. Bifocal eyeglasses are often prescribed for PRESBYOPIA, which may occur as part of the aging processes. For advanced cases of presbyopia, and for special purposes such as watchmaking, trifocal glasses are available.

biforate (bi-fo′rāt) having two perforations or foramina.

bifurcate (bi-fur′kāt) divided into two branches.

bifurcation (bi-fur-ka′shun) 1. a division into two branches. 2. the point at which division into two branches occurs.

bilateral (bi-lat′er-al) having two sides; pertaining to both sides.

bile (bīl) a clear yellow or orange fluid produced by the liver. It is concentrated and stored in the gallbladder, and is poured into the small intestine via the bile ducts when needed for digestion. Bile helps in alkalinizing the intestinal contents and plays a roll in the emulsification, absorption, and digestion of fat; its chief constitutents are conjugated bile salts, cholesterol, phospholipid, bilirubin, and electrolytes. The bile salts emulsify fats by breaking up large fat globules into smaller ones so that they can be acted on by the fat-splitting enzymes of the intestine and pancreas. A healthy liver produces bile according to the body's needs and does not require stimulation by drugs. Infection or disease of the liver, inflammation of the gallbladder, or gallstones can interfere with the flow of bile.

b. acids, glycocholic acid and taurocholic acid, formed in the liver and secreted in the bile.

b. ducts, the canals or passageways that conduct bile. There are three bile ducts: the hepatic duct drains bile from the liver; the cystic duct is an extension of the gallbladder and conveys bile from the gallbladder. These two ducts may be thought of as branches which drain into the "trunk," or common bile duct. The common bile duct passes through the wall of the small intestine at the duodenum and joins with the pancreatic duct to form the hepatopancreatic ampulla, or ampulla of Vater. At the opening into the small intestine there is a sphincter that automatically controls the flow of bile into the intestine.

The bile ducts may become obstructed by GALLSTONES, benign or malignant tumors, or a severe local infection. Various disorders of the GALLBLADDER or bile ducts are often diagnosed by CHOLECYSTOGRAPHY and CHOLANGIOGRAPHY, i.e., x-ray examination of the gallbladder and bile ducts, using a special contrast medium so that these hollow structures can be clearly outlined on the x-ray film.

b. pigment, any one of the coloring matters of the bile; they are bilirubin, biliverdin, bilifuscin, biliprasin, choleprasin, bilihumin, and bilicyanin.

bilharziasis (bil″har-zi′ah-sis) schistosomiasis.

bili- (bil′ĭ) word element [L], *bile.*

biliary (bil′e-a″re) pertaining to the bile, to the bile ducts, or to the gallbladder.

b. tract, the organs, ducts, etc., participating in secretion (the liver), storage (the gallbladder), and delivery (hepatic and bile ducts) of bile into the duodenum.

bilicyanin (bil″ĭ-si′ah-nin) a blue pigment derived by oxidation from biliverdin.

bilifuscin (bil″ĭ-fus′in) one of a class of compounds related to the bile pigments (but produced in constructive metabolism in the body), found in human bile and gallstones; chiefly responsible for the color of the feces.

biligenesis (bil″ĭ-jen′ĕ-sis) production of bile.

biligenic (bil″ĭ-jen′ik) producing bile.

bilihumin (bil″ĭ-hu′min) an insoluble ingredient of gallstones.

bilin (bi′lin) any of a group of yellow bile pigments, including stercobilin and urobilin.

biliousness (bil′yus-nes) a symptom complex comprising nausea, abdominal discomfort, headache, and constipation, formerly attributed to excessive bile secretion.

biliprasin (bil″ĭ-pra′sin) a green pigment from bile.

bilirachia (bil″ĭ-ra′ke-ah) the presence of bile pigments in the spinal fluid.

bilirubin (bil″ĭ-roo′bin) an orange bile pigment produced by the breakdown of heme and reduction of biliverdin; it normally circulates in plasma and is taken up by liver cells and conjugated to form bilirubin diglucuronide, the water-soluble pigment excreted in the bile. Failure of the liver cells to excrete bile, or obstruction of the BILE DUCTS, can cause an increased amount of bilirubin in the body fluids and thus lead to OBSTRUCTIVE JAUNDICE.

Another type of jaundice results from excessive destruction of erythrocytes (HEMOLYTIC JAUNDICE). The more rapid the destruction of red blood cells and the degradation of hemoglobin, the greater the amount of bilirubin in the body fluids.

Laboratory tests for the determination of bilirubin content in the blood are of value in diagnosising liver dysfunction and in evaluating HEMOLYTIC ANEMIAS. Bilirubin may be classified as indirect ("free" or unconjugated) while en route to the liver from its site of formation by reticuloendothelial cells, and direct (bilirubin diglucuronide) after its conjugation in the liver.

Normally the body produces a total of about 260 mg. of bilirubin per day. Almost 99 per cent of this is excreted in the feces; the remaining 1 per cent is excreted in the urine as UROBILINOGEN. A test for bilirubin in the blood is called the VAN DEN BERGH TEST. Normal range for this test is 0.0 to 0.1 mg. per 100 ml. of serum for direct bilirubin, and 0.2 to 1.4 mg. per 100 ml. of serum for total bilirubin. The only preparation required for the van den Bergh test is that the patient be in a fasting state when the blood is drawn.

bilirubinemia (bil″ĭ-roo″bĭ-ne′me-ah) the presence of bilirubin in the blood.

bilirubinuria (bil″ĭ-roo″bĭ-nu′re-ah) the presence of bilirubin in the urine.

biliuria (bil″e-u′re-ah) the presence of bile acids in the urine.

biliverdin (bil″ĭ-ver′din) a green bile pigment formed by catabolism of hemoglobin and converted to bilirubin in the liver; it may also arise from oxidation of bilirubin.

Billroth's operation (bil′rōts) gastrectomy.

bilobate (bi-lo′bāt) having two lobes.

bilobular (bi-lob′u-lar) having two lobules.

bilocular (bi-lok′u-lar) having two compartments.

bimanual (bi-man′u-al) with both hands.

bimastoid (bi-mas′toid) pertaining to both mastoid processes.

binary (bi′nah-re) made up of two elements, or of two equal parts); denoting a number system with a base of two.

b. fission, the halving of the nucleus and then of the cytoplasm of the cell, as in protozoa.

binaural (bi-naw′ral, bin-aw′ral) pertaining to both ears.

binauricular (bin″aw-rik′u-lar) pertaining to both auricles of the ears.

binder (bīnd′er) a girdle or large bandage for support of the abdomen or breast.

abdominal b., one applied to the abdomen after childbirth to support relaxed abdominal walls.

breast b., one used to give support and hold the breasts firmly in proper position.

double T b., one used for male patients to hold perineal or rectal dressings in place.

obstetric b., an abdominal girdle or bandage chiefly for women in labor who have pendulous abdomen.

sculteus b., a many-tailed bandage applied with the tails overlapping each other and held in position by safety pins.

T b., one used to hold perineal or rectal dressings in place.

Binet's test, Binet-Simon test, a method of ascertaining a child's or youth's mental age by asking a series of questions adapted to, and standardized on, the capacity of normal children at various ages.

binocular (bin-ok′u-lar) 1. pertaining to both eyes. 2. having two eyepieces, as in a microscope.

binomial (bi-no′me-al) composed of two terms, e.g., names of organisms formed by combination of genus and species names.

binotic (bin-ot′ik) binaural.

binovular (bin-ov′u-lar) pertaining to or derived from two distinct ova.

Binswanger's dementia (bins′wang-erz) dementia due to demyelination of the subcortical white matter of the brain with sclerotic changes in the blood vessels supplying it.

binuclear (bi-nu′kle-ar) having two nuclei.

binucleation (bi″nu-kle-a′shun) formation of two nuclei within a cell through division of the nucleus without division of the cytoplasm.

binucleolate (bi-nu′kle-o-lāt) having two nucleoli.

bio- (bi′o) word element [Gr.], *life; living.*

bioassay (bi″o-as′a) determination of the active power of a drug sample by comparing its effects on a live animal or an isolated organ preparation with those of a reference standard.

bioastronautics (bi″o-as″tro-naw′tiks) scientific study of effects of space and interplanetary travel on biologic systems.

bioavailability (bi″o-ah-vāl″ah-bil′ĭ-te) the degree to which a drug or other substance becomes available to the target tissue after administration.

biochemistry (bi″o-kem′is-tre) the chemistry of living organisms and of vital processes.

biocidal (bi″o-si′dal) destructive to living organisms.

bioclimatologist (bi″o-kli″mah-tol′o-jist) one skilled in bioclimatology.

bioclimatology (bi″o-kli″mah-tol′o-je) scientific study of effects on living organisms of conditions of natural environment (rainfall, daylight, temperature, etc.) prevailing in specific regions of the earth.

biocolloid (bi″o-kol′oid) a colloid from animal, plant, or microbial tissue.

biodegradable (bi″o-de-grād′ah-b′l) susceptible of degradation by biological processes, as by bacterial or other enzymatic action.

biodegradation (bi″o-deg″rah-da′shun) the series of processes by which living systems render chemicals less noxious to the environment.

biodynamics (bi″o-di-nam′iks) scientific study of the nature and determinants of all organismic (including human) behavior.

bioelectricity (bi″o-e″lek-tris′ĭ-te) electrical phenomena apparent in living cells.

bioelectronics (bi″o-e″lek-tron′iks) the study of the role of intermolecular transfer of electrons in biological regulation and defense.

biofeedback (bi″o-fēd′bak) the provision of visual or auditory evidence to a person of the status of an autonomic body function as a method of teaching control of certain visceral responses previously thought to be exclusively dictated by the autonomic nervous system and therefore involuntary or unconscious.

Examples of the kinds of biological feedback that can be provided include information about changes in skin temperature, muscle tonicity, cardiovascular activities, blood pressure, and brain wave activities. With the aid of such sensitive electronic equipment as the electrocardiogram, electromyelogram, and electroencephalogram, it is possible for the person to become consciously aware of the response being measured and to learn to control it. The feedback may be presented in the form of musical tones, lights, or direct visualization of scales or meters which indicate variance in the response.

In clinical biofeedback, the patient must practice the particular desired response many times under the supervision of professional persons who are skilled in the techniques of psychophysiology and have a thorough understanding of sophisticated electronics. An example in which biofeedback may be used clinically is in the treatment of RAYNAUD'S DISEASE, in which the patient learns to consciously raise skin temperature in the extremities and thus reduce vasoconstriction.

While clinical biofeedback is still an emerging field, encouraging results have been reported in the treatment of a variety of diseases, particularly those considered to be PSYCHOSOMATIC. Examples would include modifying insomnia and phobias, the control of certain types of epileptic seizures, and cardiac arrhythmias. It has also been used in muscle retraining in cases of hemiplegia, paralysis, and spasticity.

bioflavonoid (bi″o-fla′vo-noid) a generic term for a group of compounds widely distributed in plants and concerned with maintenance of a normal state of the walls of small blood vessels.

biogenesis (bi″o-jen′ĕ-sis) 1. origin of life, or of living organisms. 2. the theory that living organisms originate only from other living organisms.

biogeography (bi″o-je-og′rah-fe) the scientific study of the geographic distribution of living organisms.

biokinetics (bi″o-ki-net′iks) the science of movements within developing organisms.

biologic (bi″o-loj′ik) pertaining to biology.

biological (bi″o-loj′ĭ-kal) 1. pertaining to biology. 2. a medicinal preparation made from living organisms and their products; these include serums, vaccines, etc.

b. clock, the physiologic mechanism that governs the rhythmic occurrence of certain biochemical, physiologic, and behavioral phenomena in living organisms. (See also biological RHYTHM.)

biologist (bi-ol′o-jist) a specialist in biology.

biology (bi-ol′o-je) scientific study of living organisms. adj., **biolog′ic, biolog′ical.**

molecular b., study of molecular structures and events underlying biological processes, including relation between genes and the functional characteristics they determine.

radiation b., scientific study of the effects of ionizing radiation on living organisms.

bioluminescence (bi″o-lu″mĭ-nes′ens) chemoluminescence occurring in living cells.

biolysis (bi-ol′ĭ-sis) decomposition of organic matter by living organisms.

biolytic (bi″o-lit′ik) 1. pertaining to or characterized by biolysis. 2. destructive to life.

biomass (bi′o-mas) the entire assemblage of living organisms of a particular region, considered collectively.

biomathematics (bi″o-math″ĕ-mat′iks) mathematics as applied to the phenomena of living things.

biome (bi′ōm) a large, distinct, easily differentiated community of organisms arising as a result of complex interactions of climatic factors, biota, and substrate; usually designated, according to kind of vegetation present, as tundra, coniferous or deciduous forest, grassland, etc.

biomechanics (bi″o-mĕ-kan′iks) the application of mechanical laws to living structures.

biomedicine (bi″o-med′ĭ-sin) clinical medicine based on the principles of the natural sciences (biology, biochemistry, etc.) adj., **biomed′ical.**

biometeorologist (bi″o-me″te-or-ol′o-jist) one skilled in biometeorology.

biometeorology (bi″o-me″te-or-ol′o-je) scientific study of effects on living organisms of the extraorganic aspects (temperature, humidity, barometric pressure, rate of air flow, and air ionization) of the physical environment, whether natural or artificially created, and also their effects in closed ecological systems, as in satellites or submarines.

biometer (bi-om′ĕ-ter) an instrument for measuring carbon dioxide given off by living tissue.

biometrics, biometry (bi″o-met′riks; bi-om′ĕ-tre) the application of statistical methods to biological facts.

biomicroscope (bi″o-mi′kro-skōp) a microscope for examining living tissue in the body.

biomicroscopy (bi″o-mi-kros′ko-pe) microscopic examination of living tissue in the body.

bion (bi′on) an individual living organism.

bionecrosis (bi″o-nĕ-kro′sis) necrobiosis.

bionergy (bi-on′er-je) the life force; the force exercised in the living organism.

bionics (bi-on′iks) scientific study of functions, characteristics, and phenomena observed in the living world, and application of knowledge gained therefrom to nonliving systems.

bionucleonics (bi″o-nu″kle-on′iks) scientific study of biological applications of radioactive and rare stable isotopes.

biophysics (bi″o-fiz′iks) the science dealing with

the application of physical methods and theories to biological problems.

biophysiology (bi″o-fiz″e-ol′o-je) that portion of biology including organogenesis, morphology, and physiology.

bioplasm (bi′o-plazm) 1. protoplasm. 2. the more vital or essential part of protoplasm. adj. **bioplas′mic.**

biopsy (bi′op-se) removal and examination, usually microscopic, of tissue from the living body. Biopsies are usually done to determine whether a tumor is malignant or benign; however, a biopsy may be a useful diagnostic aid in other disease processes such as infections.

aspiration b., biopsy in which tissue is obtained by application of suction through a needle attached to a syringe.

endoscopic b., removal of tissue by appropriate instruments through an endoscope.

excisional b., biopsy of tissue removed from the body by surgical cutting.

incisional b., biopsy of a selected portion of a lesion.

needle b., biopsy in which tissue is obtained by puncture of a tumor, the tissue within the lumen of the needle being detached by rotation, and the needle withdrawn.

punch b., biopsy in which tissue is obtained by a punch.

sternal b., biopsy of bone marrow of the sternum removed by puncture or trephining (see also STERNAL PUNCTURE).

biorhythm (bi′o-rith″m) biologic RHYTHM.

bios (bi′os) any of a group of growth factors for single-celled organisms such as yeast. Bios occurs in yeast, leaves of plants, bran, and the outer coating of seeds, and is probably a mixture of B vitamins and pantothenic acid.

b. I, inositol.

b. II, biotin.

bioscience (bi″o-si′ens) the study of biology wherein all the applicable sciences (physics, chemistry, etc.) are applied.

bioset (bi′o-set) a grouping of biological components.

biospectrometry (bi″o-spek-trom′ĕ-tre) the spectrometry of the quantity of a substance in living tissue.

biospectroscopy (bi″o-spek-tros′ko-pe) the spectroscopy of living tissue.

biosphere (bi′o-sfēr) 1. that part of the universe in which living organisms are known to exist, comprising the atmosphere, hydrosphere, and lithosphere. 2. the sphere of action between an organism and its environment.

biostatistics (bi″o-stah-tis′tiks) vital statistics.

biosynthesis (bi″o-sin′thĕ-sis) creation of a compound by physiologic processes in a living organism. adj., **biosynthet′ic.**

biota (bi-o′tah) all the living organisms of a particular area; the combined flora and fauna of a region.

biotaxis (bi″o-tak′sis) the selecting and arranging powers of living cells.

biotaxy (bi″o-tak′se) 1. biotaxis. 2. taxonomy.

biotelemetry (bi″o-tel-em′ĕ-tre) the recording and measuring of certain vital phenomena occurring in living organisms that are at a distance from the measuring device.

biotic (bi-ot′ik) pertaining to life or living organisms. 2. pertaining to the biota.

biotics (bi-ot′iks) the functions and qualities peculiar to living organisms, or the sum of knowledge regarding these qualities.

biotin (bi′o-tin) a member of the vitamin B complex, required by or occurring in all forms of life tested.

biotomy (bi-ot′o-me) 1. study of animal and plant life by dissection. 2. vivisection.

biotoxication (bi″o-tok″sĭ-ka′shun) intoxication due to a biotoxin.

biotoxicology (bi″o-tok″sĭ-kol′o-je) scientific study of poisons produced by living organisms, their cause, detection, and effects, and treatment of conditions produced by them.

biotoxin (bi″o-tok′sin) a poisonous substance produced by a living organism.

biotransformation (bi″o-trans″for-ma′shun) the series of chemical alterations of a compound (e.g., a drug) occurring within the body, as by enzymatic activity.

biotype (bi′o-tīp) 1. a group of individuals having the same genotype. 2. any of a number of strains of a species of microorganisms having differentiable physiologic characteristics.

biovular (bi-ov′u-lar) binovular.

biparental (bi″pah-ren′tal) derived from two parents, male and female.

biparous (bip′ah-rus) producing two ova or offspring at one time.

bipenniform (bi-pen′ĭ-form) doubly feather-shaped; said of muscles whose fibers are arranged on each side of a tendon like barbs on a feather shaft.

biperiden (bi-per′ĭ-den) a synthetic anticholinergic used to reduce the tremors of parkinsonism and certain other forms of spasticity. Side effects are minor and include dryness of the mouth, blurring of vision, drowsiness, and nausea. Biperiden is contraindicated in patients with epilepsy and should be given with great care to patients with glaucoma.

bipolar (bi-po′lar) 1. having two poles. 2. pertaining to both poles.

bipotentiality (bi″po-ten″she-al′ĭ-te) ability to develop or act in either of two different ways.

biramous (bi-ra′mus) having two branches.

birefractive (bi″re-frak′tiv) doubly refractive.

birefringence (bi″re-frin′jens) the quality of transmitting light unequally in different directions.

birth (berth) a coming into being; the act or process of being born.

b. canal, the canal through which the fetus passes in birth.

b. certificate, a written, authenticated record of the birth of a child, required by state laws throughout the United States. After a birth is registered, a birth certicate is issued which represents legal proof of parentage, age, and citizenship, and is of great personal and legal importance. A birth certificate is required for many legal and business or personal transactions. Whether the child is born at home or at the hospital, the physician, midwife, or other attendant must report the birth to the local or state registrar. The report becomes a permanent record, and a certificate is issued to the parents. If a child dies during birth, an immediate report and certification of the birth and death are required, containing a statement of the cause of death.

b. control, the concept of limiting the size of families by measures designed to prevent conception. The movement of that name began in modern times as a humanitarian reform to conserve the health of mothers and the welfare of children, especially among the poor. More recently it has been superseded by the term "planned parenthood," which means planning the arrival of children to correspond with the desire and resources of the married couple and to provide greater happiness for the children. (See also CONTRACEPTION.) Planned parenthood is concerned not only with controlling fertility but also with overcoming apparent sterility in those couples who want a child but have been unsuccessful in having one.

multiple b., the birth of two or more offspring produced in the same gestation period.

premature b., expulsion of the fetus from the uterus before termination of the normal gestation period, but after independent existence has become a possibility. (See also PREMATURE INFANT.)

b. rate, the number of births during one year for the total population (crude birth rate), for the female population (refined birth rate), or for the female population of childbearing age (true birth rate), that is, between the ages of 15 and 45.

birthmark (berth′mark) a congenital blemish or spot on the skin, usually visible at birth or shortly after. Those appearing later occur at the location of a skin defect present at birth. The cause is unknown. (See also NEVUS.)

physiologic b., one so common as to be considered normal; once applied to nevus flammeus in the suboccipital region.

vascular b., one caused by an unusual clustering of small blood vessels near the surface of the skin; called also HEMANGIOMA. These birthmarks include "strawberry" or "raspberry" marks, "port-wine stains," and an elevated type called cavernous hemangiomas.

bisacodyl (bis-ak′o-dil) a cathartic.

bisacromial (bis″ah-kro′me-al) pertaining to the two acromial processes.

bisalbuminemia (bis″al-bu″mĭ-ne′me-ah) a congenital abnormality marked by the presence of two distinct serum albumins that differ in mobility on electrophoresis.

bisection (bi-sek′shun) division into two parts by cutting.

bisexual (bi-seks′u-al) 1. having gonads of both sexes. 2. hermaphrodite. 3. both heterosexual and homosexual.

bisferious (bis-fe′re-us) dicrotic; having two beats.

bishydroxycoumarin (bis″hi-drok″se-koo′mahrin) a white crystalline powder used as an anticoagulant. It interferes with the production, in the liver, of prothrombin, so that the prothrombin content of the blood is decreased and the prothrombin time is lengthened. It prevents clotting within the blood vessels and reduces the formation of emboli and thrombi, and is used in the treatment of coronary thrombosis and thrombophlebitis and in the prevention of emboli. Average dose depends on the results of a daily prothrombin time test and varies greatly from one patient to another. In overdosage, which can be accompanied by severe hemorrhage, intravenous injections of vitamin K and transfusions of whole fresh blood may be necessary to restore the normal prothrombin content of the blood.

bisiliac (bis-il′e-ak) pertaining to the two iliac bones or to any two corresponding points on them.

bis in die (bis in de′a) [L.] twice a day; abbreviated b.i.d.

bismuth (biz′muth) a chemical element, atomic number 83, atomic weight 208.980, symbol Bi. (See table of ELEMENTS.) Its salts have been much used in inflammatory diseases of the stomach and intestines and in syphilis.

b. glycolylarsanilate, glycobiarsol, used in treatment of intestinal amebiases.

b. subcarbonate, a basic salt used as a topical protectant, intestinal astringent, and antacid.

b. subgallate, a bright yellow, amorphous powder, applied locally in skin diseases.

b. subnitrate, a basic salt, used as an antacid.

bismuthosis (biz″muth-o′sis) chronic bismuth poisoning, with anuria, stomatitis, dermatitis, and diarrhea.

bistoury (bis′too-re) a long, narrow, straight or curved surgical knife used in opening sinuses and fistulas, incisioning abscesses, etc.

bisulfate (bi-sul′fāt) an acid sulfate.

bite (bīt) 1. seizure with the teeth. 2. a wound or puncture made by a living organism. 3. an impression made by closure of the teeth upon some plastic material, e.g., wax. 4. occlusion (2).

ANIMAL BITE. Any animal bite that breaks the skin should be treated rapidly and with care. The wound should be washed at once with soap and water. A physician should be consulted so that necessary steps may be taken to prevent the development of RABIES.

Every effort should be made to catch an animal that has bitten someone, so that it may be confined and examined by the health department for signs of rabies. Whenever possible the animal should be caught alive because evidence of rabies disappears rapidly after death. If the animal is not caught, the bitten person is given antirabies treatment immediately.

HUMAN BITE. Any human bite that penetrates the skin should be considered dangerous. The wound should be washed immediately with soap and water and a physician should be consulted. Antibiotics may be needed as there is a serious danger of infection, a danger that is more serious with human bites than with animal bites since many of the organisms carried by animals do not affect humans.

over-b., overbite.

bitemporal (bi-tem′po-ral) pertaining to both temples or temporal bones.

biteplate (bīt′plāt) an appliance, usually plastic or wire, worn in the palate as a diagnostic or therapeutic adjunct in orthodontics or prosthodontics.

bite-wing (bīt′wing) a wing or fin attached along the center of the tooth side of a dental x-ray film and bitten on by the patient, permitting production of images of the corona of the teeth in both dental arches and their contiguous peridontal tissues.

Bitot's spot (be′tōz) foamy gray, triangular spots of keratinized epithelium on the conjunctiva, associated with vitamin A deficiency.

bitrochanteric (bi-tro″kan-ter′ik) pertaining to

both trochanters on one femur or to both greater trochanters.

bitumen (bĭ-too'men) any of various natural or artificial dry petroleum products.

bituminosis (bĭ-too"mi-no'sis) a form of PNEUMOCONIOSIS due to dust from soft coal.

biuret (bi'u-ret) a urea derivative; its presence is detected after addition of sodium hydroxide and copper sulfate solutions by a pinkish-violet color (protein test) or a pink and finally a bluish color (urea test).

bivalent (bi-va'lent, biv'ah-lent) 1. having a valence of two. 2. denoting homologous chromosomes associated in pairs during the first meiotic prophase.

biventral (bi-ven'tral) 1. having two bellies. 2. digastric muscle.

bizygomatic (bi-zi"go-mat'ik) pertaining to the two most prominent points of the two zygomatic arches.

Bk chemical symbol, *berkelium.*

black eye (blak i) a bruise of the tissue around the eye marked by discoloration, swelling, and pain. Cold compresses, if applied immediately, help to slow the bleeding under the skin and thus reduce swelling and discoloration. Later, warm wet towels should be applied in order to hasten the absorption of discoloring fluids. Any of the complications of a bruise, such as a clot, may develop, in which case medical attention will be necessary. A black eye resulting from an unusually violent blow may be accompanied by injury to the skull or damage to the eye itself.

blackhead (blak'hed) comedo; a plug of keratin and sebum within the dilated orifice of a hair follicle. The color of blackheads is caused not by dirt but by the discoloring effect of air on the sebum in the clogged pore. Infection may cause the comedo to develop into a pustule or boil. (See also ACNE VULGARIS.)

blackout temporary loss of vision and momentary unconsciousness due to diminished circulation to the brain and retina. Blackout refers specifically to a condition which sometimes occurs in aviators resulting from increased acceleration, which causes a decrease in blood supply to the brain cells. The term can also refer to other forms of temporary loss of consciousness and to FAINTING, as well as to temporary loss of memory and to certain forms of VERTIGO.

blackwater fever a dangerous and poorly understood complication of falciparum malaria, characterized by the passage of dark red to black urine, severe toxicity, and high mortality, especially for Europeans.

bladder (blad'er) a membranous sac, such as one serving as receptacle for a secretion, especially the urinary bladder. The urinary bladder is a hollow container with muscular walls in the anterior part of the pelvic cavity. It is joined to the kidneys by the ureters and to the exterior of the body by the urethra. Urine passes to the bladder from the kidneys every few seconds, and it remains there until it is voided. Voiding occurs when the sphincters (circular muscles) at the juncture of the bladder and urethra are relaxed and the muscular walls of the bladder contract, forcing the urine out. In the adult the sphincters can prevent urination even when the bladder is uncomfortably full, but in children full bladder control is slow to develop. BED-WETTING may normally continue to the age of 3 or 4 years.

DISORDERS OF THE BLADDER. Infections of the bladder are fairly common, especially in women and girls, since the female urethra is shorter than that of the male and permits easier entry of infectious agents. Most infections yield readily to treatment with antibiotics.

Inflammation of the bladder, or CYSTITIS, may be caused by many different agents, and can vary greatly in seriousness. Its most usual symptoms are a persistent desire to urinate, and a burning sensation at urination.

Various deformations of the bladder are found. The most common and least serious is the formation of an outpocketing or diverticulum. The pocket may be caused by pressure from inside the bladder, when for some reason the urine is obstructed, or it may have existed from birth.

An abnormal opening in the bladder causes a fistula, which conducts escaping urine to other parts of the body, or to the exterior through the skin. The most common varieties are those in which the fistulas lead into the intestine or directly into the vagina (vesicovaginal fistula). They occur sometimes after childbirth or after diverticulitis of the colon. The condition may be remedied by surgery.

Stones (calculi) may form in the bladder and often lead to painful and difficult urination. They are usually caused by obstructions in the mouth of the bladder, brought about, for example, by an enlarged prostate. If necessary, they can be removed by surgery.

Tumors may also form in the bladder, especially in later life. These may be benign or cancerous. The benign tumors do not spread, but may require removal to relieve other symptoms. The most common symptom of tumor of the bladder is the presence of blood in the urine unaccompanied by pain. In malignancy, surgery is likely to be necessary.

Atonic bladder is a condition marked by a dilated, poorly contracting urinary bladder without any evidence of a lesion of the central nervous system. Cord, or automatic, bladder refers to defective bladder function from a lesion in the sacral portion of the spinal cord that interrupts the reflex arc controlling the bladder. Neurogenic bladder refers to any disturbance of the bladder due to a lesion of the nervous system. A nonfunctioning neurogenic bladder can result from SPINA BIFIDA, MULTIPLE SCLEROSIS, PARAPLEGIA, or QUADRIPLEGIA. Urinary flow in these patients can sometimes be managed by insertion of an indwelling Foley catheter via the urethra to the bladder, or a suprapubic catheter inserted directly into the bladder. If chronic urinary infection persists, surgical intervention may be necessary to divert the urinary flow through a cutaneous URETEROSTOMY or a ureteroileostomy.

SURGERY OF THE BLADDER. The two most common types of major surgery of the bladder are cystotomy and cystectomy. Cystotomy is surgical incision into the bladder for removal of bladder stones or as a part of the surgical procedure known as suprapubic PROSTATECTOMY.

Tumors of the bladder are the most frequent indication for surgery of the bladder. Large tumors involving several layers of the bladder wall require partial or complete removal of the bladder. Cystectomy is done when widespread malignant disease or severe physical trauma has destroyed much of the bladder wall. Removal of the entire bladder requires diversion of the urinary flow by transplantation of the ureters to the surface of the abdomen (ureterostomy) or to the bowel (ureteroenterostomy).

Small, superficial tumors of the bladder may be treated by fulguration, with the use of a cystoscope and an electric cautery. Normally, after fulguration there is minimal bleeding and the patient is usually allowed to go home within a few days.

Cystostomy is an operation in which an opening is made through the abdominal wall for draining of the bladder.

Patient Care. In any type of surgery of the bladder or ureters it is extremely important that there be constant maintenance of the flow of urine. Urine is secreted by the kidneys continuously and normally dribbles in a constant stream down the ureters into the bladder. If for any reason the flow of urine from the ureters is obstructed, there is a damming up of urine in the kidney and hydronephrosis results. To be aware of this eventuality it is necessary to observe carefully and at frequent intervals any drainage from CATHETERS inserted before or after surgery. Should there be evidence of obstruction to the urine flow the surgeon should be notified at once.

The urine is also observed for signs of hemorrhage, presence of clots or bits of tissue, and unusual odor or concentration. These observations are important in the preoperative as well as the postoperative period. The amount of urinary output must be measured with extreme care and recorded accurately.

Infection is always a possibility after surgery of the urinary system. To guard against this complication care must be taken in the handling of catheters or other drainage tubes. If dressings are applied they should be changed frequently to reduce the hazard of infection and the unpleasant odor that usually is caused by the leakage of urine.

The intake of fluids is prescribed by the physician as part of the treatment and the fluids should be considered medication. Explaining to the patient and his family the need to restrict or force fluids usually insures their cooperation.

Providing for adequate collection and disposal of urine for patients with total cystectomy and cystostomy is accomplished by cutaneous URETEROSTOMY or ureteroileostomy. Care of the patient with a urinary STOMA requires special knowledge to meet the needs of each individual patient.

b. training, a program designed to assist the patient having difficulties controlling the flow of urine. The training program and techniques used will depend on the optimal neural and muscular control that can be realistically expected, as in PARAPLEGIA and HEMIPLEGIA, and on the mental and emotional status of the patient. The cause of urinary incontinence must be known and the specific symptoms manifested by the patient clearly defined. This would include information about difficulty in initiating voiding, degree of awareness of the need to void, ability to empty the bladder completely and amount of residual urine, signs of distention and dribbling of overflow, night incontinence, stress incontinence, and usual times for voiding.

Spinal cord injuries and lesions produce what is known as a cord bladder or neurogenic bladder. Patients with disorders of this type are not aware of the need to void and must be trained in techniques to initiate voiding and empty the bladder. If the lesion is above the 2nd, 3rd, and 4th sacral segment of the spinal cord, it is sometimes possible for the bladder to empty partially by reflex, and so training is centered on techniques to improve emptying of the bladder. This is done because pooling of residual urine in the bladder can lead to infection and the formation of bladder stones. If the lesion is located at the site of the 2nd, 3rd, and 4th sacral segment, the bladder is flaccid because of interference with the reflex arc. Bladder training in these cases is concerned with emptying the bladder to prevent distention and the dribbling of overflow.

Some urinary problems can be relieved by a simple scheduling of times to void, getting the patient up to the bathroom, or offering the bedpan at regular intervals. Many elderly patients wet the bed at night because they are not fully awake and are not aware of the need to void. Noting the time of bedwetting and offering the bedpan or urinal about 30 minutes before that time each night can avoid this type of night incontinence. This same technique can be used to control so-called "incontinence" during the day. It is especially important not to assume that an incontinent patient cannot be helped. With diligence and genuine interest, the problem often can be resolved.

Those patients with neural damage and paralysis require more intensive training for bladder control. An indwelling catheter is inserted at the onset of incontinence and some patients may never become catheter free. This does not mean, however, that every effort should not be made to teach urinary control so that whenever possible the patient can achieve some degree of independence and avoid the hazards that an indwelling catheter presents.

When bladder training is begun the catheter is removed and specific techniques planned for the individual patient are initiated. The usual procedure on the first day of the program is to force fluids at the rate of 200 ml. hourly so that after several hours the bladder contains about 300 ml. of urine. The catheter is then removed and the patient is encouraged to void using a toilet or portable commode whenever possible. Aids to stimulate voiding are used for those patients who have difficulty initiating voiding. These aids are chosen according to each patient's response and are highly individualistic. They usually are found by the trial and error method; one patient responding to simply concentrating on the act of voiding, another to the stimulus produced by stroking the inner aspect of the thigh, and so on. The CREDÉ TECHNIQUE for manual expression of urine often is successful in removing urine from a flaccid bladder.

If the patient is successful in voiding, the attempts to void are repeated throughout the day. The hourly intake of fluids is continued until about 8:00 P.M. and the time of successful urination is noted so that a pattern of voiding for the individual patient can be established. An unsuccessful attempt at voiding does not mean that bladder control cannot be achieved. The plan is revised, the catheter is reinserted and the residual urine measured. After a wait of several days the catheter is removed and the patient tries again. It is important that he not be allowed to become discouraged by failure at the first try.

Blakemore-Sengstaken tube (blāk′mōr-sengz′-ta-ken) Sengstaken-Blakemore tube.

Blalock-Taussig operation (bla′lok taw′sig) anastomosis of the subclavian artery to the pulmonary artery to shunt some of the systemic circulation into the pulmonary circulation; done in congenital pulmonary stenosis.

blanch (blanch) to become pale.

blast (blast) 1. an immature stage in cellular development before appearance of the definitive characteristics of the cell; used also as a word termination, as in ameloblast, etc. 2. the wave of air pressure produced by the detonation of high-explosive bombs or shells or by other explosions; it causes pulmonary damage and hemorrhage (lung blast, blast chest), laceration of other thoracic and abdominal viscera, ruptured eardrums, and effects in the central nervous system. 3. see BLASTO-.

blastema (blas-te′mah) 1. the primitive substance from which cells are formed. 2. a group of cells that will give rise to a new individual, in asexual reproduction, or to an organ or part, in either normal development or in regeneration.

blasto- word element [Gr.], *a bud; budding.*

blastocoele (blas′to-sēl) the fluid-filled central segmentation cavity of the mass of the blastula.

blastocyst (blas′to-sist) the mammalian conceptus in the post-morula stage, consisting of the trophoblast and an inner cell mass.

blastocyte (blas′to-sīt) an undifferentiated embryonic cell.

blastocytoma (blas″to-si-to′mah) blastoma.

blastoderm (blas′to-derm) the single layer of cells forming the wall of the blastula, or the cellular cap above the floor of segmented yolk in the discoblastula of telolecithal ova.

blastodisc (blas′to-disk) the convex structure formed by the blastomeres at the animal pole of an ovum undergoing incomplete cleavage.

blastogenesis (blas″to-jen′ĕ-sis) 1. development of an individual from a blastema, i.e., by asexual reproduction. 2. transmission of inherited characters by the germ plasm. 3. morphological transformation of small lymphocytes into larger cells resembling blast cells on exposure to phytohemagglutin, or to antigens to which the donor is immunized.

blastolysis (blas-tol′ĭ-sis) destruction, or splitting of the germ substance. adj., **blastolyt′ic**.

blastoma (blas-to′mah) a neoplasm composed of embryonic cells derived from the blastema of an organ or tissue. adj., **blasto′matous**.

blastomatosis (blas″to-mah-to′sis) the formation of blastomas; tumor formation.

blastomere (blas′to-mēr) one of the cells produced by cleavage of a fertilized ovum, forming the blastoderm.

Blastomyces (blas″to-mi′sēz) a genus of pathogenic fungi growing as mycelial forms at room temperature and as yeastlike forms at body temperature; applied to the yeasts pathogenic for man and animals.

B. brasilien′sis, *Paracoccidioides brasiliensis.*

B. dermatit′idis, the species causing North American blastomycosis.

blastomycete (blas″to-mi′sēt) any organism of the genus *Blastomyces*; also, any yeastlike organism.

blastomycosis (blas″to-mi-ko′sis) 1. infection with *Blastomyces.* 2. infection with any yeastlike organism.

North American b., a chronic infection caused by *Blastomyces dermatitidis,* marked by suppurating tumors in the skin (cutaneous blastomycosis) or by lesions in the lungs, bones, subcutaneous tissues, liver, spleen, and kidneys (systemic blastomycosis).

South American b., paracoccidioidomycosis.

blastopore (blas′to-pōr) the opening of the archenteron to the exterior of the embryo at the GASTRULA stage.

blastospore (blas′to-spōr) a spore formed by budding, as in yeast.

blastula (blas′tu-lah) the usually spherical body produced by cleavage of a fertilized ovum, consisting of a single layer of cells (blastoderm) surrounding a fluid-filled cavity (blastocoele); it follows the morula stage.

blastulation (blas″tu-la′shun) conversion of the morula to the blastula by development of a blastocoele.

bleb (bleb) a large flaccid vesicle, usually at least 1 cm. in diameter.

bleeder (blēd′er) 1. the popular term for a person who bleeds freely, especially one suffering from a condition in which the blood fails to clot properly; a hemophiliac (see also HEMOPHILIA). 2. any large blood vessel cut during surgery.

bleeding (blēd′ing) 1. the escape of blood, as from an injured vessel. (See also HEMORRHAGE.) 2. the purposeful withdrawal of blood from a vessel of the body; venesection; phlebotomy.

functional b., bleeding from the uterus when no organic lesions are present.

implantation b., that occurring at the time of implantation of the fertilized ovum in the decidua.

occult b., escape of blood in such small quantity that it can be detected only by chemical tests or by microscopic or spectroscopic examination.

placentation b., bleeding from the uterus during the early weeks of pregnancy, when the maternal blood vessels are being eroded.

b. time, the time required for a small pinpoint wound to cease bleeding. If done properly, the test can be helpful in determining the functional capacity of platelets and of vasoconstriction. The test for bleeding time involves making a small cut with a lancet into a fingertip, earlobe (Duke method), or forearm (Ivy method). The Ivy method is generally considered to be the most accurate: a blood pressure cuff is placed on the arm and a pressure of 40 mm. of mercury is maintained. A small puncture wound is made on the inner surface of the forearm. Normally, bleeding will cease in 3 to 6 minutes. A prolonged bleeding time is found in patients with vascular abnormalities, with deficiencies in the platelet count, and with conditions in which there is a deficiency of fibrinogen.

blenn(o)- word element [Gr.], *mucus.*

blennadenitis (blen″ad-ĕ-ni′tis) inflammation of mucous glands.

blennogenic (blen″o-jen′ik) producing mucus.

blennoid (blen′oid) resembling mucus.

blennorrhagia (blen″o-ra′je-ah) 1. any excessive discharge of mucus; blenorrhea. 2. gonorrhea.

blennorrhea (blen″o-re′ah) any free discharge of mucus, especially a gonorrheal discharge from the urethra or vagina; gonorrhea.

inclusion b., inclusion conjunctivitis.

blennostasis (blĕ-nos′tah-sis) suppression of an abnormal mucous discharge, or correction of an excessive one. adj., **blennostat′ic**.

blennothorax (blen″o-tho′raks) an accumulation of mucus in the chest.

blennuria (blen-u′re-ah) mucus in the urine.

bleomycin (ble″o-mi′sin) a polypeptide antibiotic mixture having antineoplastic properties, derived from *Streptomyces verticillus*, or the same substance produced by other means; it is active in the Hodgkin's disease, lymphomas, certain squamous cell carcinomas of the head and neck region, and testicular tumors.

blephar(o)- word element [Gr.], *eyelid; eyelash.*

blepharadenitis (blef″ar-ad″ĕ-ni′tis) inflammation of the meibomian glands.

blepharal (blef′ar-al) pertaining to the eyelids.

blepharectomy (blef″ar-ek′to-me) partial or complete excision of an eyelid.

blepharism (blef′ah-rizm) spasm of the eyelid; continuous blinking.

blepharitis (blef″ah-ri′tis) inflammation of the eyelids.

angular b., inflammation involving the outer angle of the eyelids.

squamous b., that in which the edge of the eyelid is covered with small white or gray scales.

ulcerative b., that marked by small ulcerated areas along the eyelid margin, multiple, suppurative lesions, and loss of lashes.

blepharoadenitis (blef″ah-ro-ad″ĕ-ni′tis) blepharadenitis.

blepharoatheroma (blef″ah-ro-ath″er-o′mah) an encysted tumor or sebaceous cyst of an eyelid.

blepharochalasis (blef″ah-ro-kal′ah-sis) hypertrophy and loss of elasticity of the skin of the upper eyelid.

blepharoconjunctivitis (blef″ah-ro-kon-junk″tĭ-vi′tis) inflammation of the eyelids and conjunctiva.

blepharoncus (blef″ar-ong′kus) a tumor on the eyelid.

blepharophimosis (blef″ah-ro-fi-mo′sis) abnormal narrowness of the palpebral fissures.

blepharoplasty (blef′ah-ro-plas″te) plastic surgery of an eyelid.

blepharoplegia (blef″ah-ro-ple′je-ah) paralysis of an eyelid.

blepharoptosis (blef″ar-op-to′sis) drooping of an upper eyelid; ptosis.

blepharorrhaphy (blef″ah-ror′ah-fe) 1. suture of an eyelid. 2. tarsorrhaphy.

blepharospasm (blef′ah-ro-spazm″) spasm of the orbicular muscle of the eyelid.

blepharostat (blef′ah-ro-stat″) an instrument for holding the eyelids apart.

blepharostenosis (blef″ah-ro-stĕ-no′sis) blepharophimosis.

blepharosynechia (blef″ah-ro-sĭ-nek′e-ah) growing together or adhesion of the eyelids.

blepharotomy (blef″ah-rot′o-me) surgical incision of an eyelid; tarsotomy.

blind (blīnd) not having the sense of sight.

b. spot, the area marking the site of entrance of the optic nerve on the retina; it is not sensitive to light.

blindness (blīnd′nes) lack or loss of ability to see; lack of perception of visual stimuli. Legally, less than 20/200 vision with eyeglasses (vision of 20/200 is the ability to see only at 20 feet what the normal eye can see at 200 feet). It is estimated that there are more than 350,000 legally blind persons in the United States. Of these, over half are 65 or older.

CAUSES. A major cause of blindness is CATARACT, clouding of the lens of the eye. Removal of the clouded lens from the eye restores sight to most cataract patients.

A second major cause is chronic GLAUCOMA, an increase in the fluid pressure inside the eyeball. This disease, which can usually be cured or controlled if discovered and treated early enough, often causes no pain and gives no warning. People over 35 are more susceptible to glaucoma than younger persons, and there is a familial tendency toward the disease.

DETACHMENT OF RETINA is a condition in which pieces of the retina become separated from the underlying tissues. It once led to incurable blindness, but now can often be repaired by a delicate surgical operation.

Scarring of the cornea may result from a local infection and can usually be checked by medical treatment. If it becomes so severe as to interfere seriously with vision, the condition may require a cornea transplant.

TRACHOMA, a viral infection of the conjunctiva, was once a major cause of blindness in the United States, and still is in many of the developing countries. Sulfonamide drugs and antibiotics can halt the disease.

In the last 30 years, two of the greatest causes of blindness in newborn children have been virtually eliminated. One, ophthalmia neonatorum, is caused by gonococci and is transmitted to the infant during passage through the birth canal. The practice of instilling silver nitrate or an antibiotic in the eyes of every child at the time of birth has greatly reduced its incidence. The second disease, RETROLENTAL FIBROPLASIA, was found to occur most often in premature infants. Investigation proved excessive administration of oxygen during the neonatal period to be the cause of this disorder. With revised procedures in the administration of oxygen to newborn infants the incidence of retrolental fibroplasia has decreased greatly.

Blindness may also come as an effect of various infectious diseases, including scarlet fever, smallpox, and syphilis. Modern techniques of IMMUNIZATION and the development of antibiotics have brought most of these diseases under control. There is still grave danger to the sight of the child whose mother contracts rubella (German measles) during the early months of pregnancy.

About 3 per cent of all cases of blindness in the United States are the result of accidental injury on the job.

Some cases of blindness are caused by hereditary factors. Little is known about this aspect of heredity, but an increasing amount of research is being done.

The National Society for the Prevention of Blindness estimates that more than half of all cases of blindness could be prevented or cured with our present knowledge. An eye examination every 2 years is recommended for early detection and prompt treatment.

EDUCATION AND TRAINING. Today a blind person is no longer thought of as helpless or dependent on others for everything. New methods of education and recreation have made it possible for more than half the blind children in school to attend schools with children having normal eyesight. Many colleges provide special funds to enable blind students to hire readers and tape recorders to help them in their studies.

The Library of Congress, in Washington, D.C., lends records and recording machines without charge to the blind, and maintains a wide selection of recordings. Tape-recorded textbooks and other educational material are available from a private organization, Recording for the Blind, 121 East 58th Street, New York, N.Y. 10022.

Those of working age who are legally blind are entitled to special counseling, vocational training, and placement through joint state and federal programs. Other programs provide work for blind people who are home-bound, visiting teachers for those who want to learn to read and write Braille, and recreation facilities, including swimming pools and bowling alleys.

The American Foundation for the Blind publishes many excellent pamphlets to help those who must deal with the special problems involved in blindness.

PATIENT CARE. The patient who is blind often presents a special challenge to those assigned to his care. They must strive to know the patient well and quickly learn his degree of dependence and his attitude toward his loss of vision. Their handling of the situation will depend on whether the patient has been deprived of his sight recently or has been blind for several years. If he is to adjust to a recent loss of vision, they must delicately balance sympathy with a sincere desire to help him adjust to a new life in which he must learn again the simple activities of daily living. A patient who has been blind for years and has adjusted to his handicap most often wishes to be treated as any other patient.

Feeding the Blind Patient. A blind person should be told what different types of food he has on his tray. Before he is given hot foods or iced liquids he should be warned that they are hot or cold. Liquids are usually easier for the blind patient to handle if they are served in a cup, without a straw. The cup is placed in his hand so that he can drink from it himself. Solid foods are given to the patient in the same manner in which one would eat them oneself, with variety and combining of foods that go well together. The patient should be allowed to feed himself "finger foods" and liquids.

The Ambulatory Patient. When walking with a blind patient it is best to hold his arm and walk at his side. Directions are given in advance so that he will know to turn to the left or right or go down steps, as well as how many steps. The prevention of accidents is an important part of the care of the blind patient who is up and about. Aside from the physical effects of bumping into objects or falling over them, the blind person also suffers from a loss of self-confidence and security if he cannot move about safely and independently. Doors should be kept closed or completely open. They must never be left ajar. If it is necessary to move a piece of furniture in the patient's room, he should be told of its new location.

Other rules that should be observed in caring for the blind include:

1. Remember that the person is blind, not deaf. There is no reason to shout at him or address him as if he were a child or mentally retarded. Speak normally and naturally.

2. Speak to the blind person as you enter his room and do not touch him until after you have spoken to him. Otherwise he may be startled or frightened if he has not heard you enter his room.

3. When you leave the room tell the patient you are going. He will not then resume the conversation later and find that he is talking to someone who is not there.

4. Pity is neither expected nor appreciated by the blind. They want to be treated as normal people, and would rather ask for help than have someone do everything for them. It is important to remember that there are no such things as "extra senses of blindness," which many people mistakenly believe blind people are given to compensate for their loss of sight. Whatever a blind person has learned about living with his blindness he has accomplished through hard work and determination.

blue b., tritanopia.

blue-yellow b., 1. tritanopia. 2. tetartanopia (2).

color b., popular term for any deviation from normal perception of color (see also COLOR BLINDNESS).

day b., defective vision in bright light.

green b., deuteranopia.

night b., failure or imperfection of vision in conditions of diminished illumination (see also NIGHT BLINDNESS).

red b., protanopia.

snow b., dimness of vision, usually temporary, due to the glare of the sun upon snow.

blister (blis'ter) a vesicle, especially a bulla.

blood b., a vesicle having bloody contents, as may be caused by a pinch or bruise.

fever b., a lesion on the skin or mucous membrane, due to infection with the virus of HERPES SIMPLEX, which often accompanies fever, and is most common about the lips or nose. Called also herpes fibrilis.

block (blok) 1. an obstruction or stoppage. 2. regional anesthesia.

bundle-branch b., a form of HEART BLOCK involving obstruction in one of the branches in the bundle of His.

epidural b., anesthesia produced by injection of the anesthetic between the vertebral spines and beneath the ligamentum flavum into the extradural space.

field b., regional anesthesia obtained by blocking conduction in nerves with chemical or physical agents.

heart b., impairment of conduction in heart excitation; often applied specifically to ATRIOVENTRICULAR HEART BLOCK (see also HEART BLOCK).

mental b., obstruction to thought or memory, particularly that produced by emotional factors.

nerve b., regional anesthesia secured by injection of an anesthetic in close proximity to the appropriate nerve.

paracervical b., anesthesia of the inferior hypogastric plexus and ganglia produced by injection of the local anesthetic into the lateral fornices of the vagina.

parasacral b., regional anesthesia produced by injection of a local anesthetic around the sacral nerves as they emerge from the sacral foramina.

paravertebral b., infiltration of the cervicothoracic ganglion with procaine hydrochloride.

perineural b., regional anesthesia produced by injection of the anesthetic agent close to the nerve.

presacral b., anesthesia produced by injection of the local anesthetic into the sacral nerves on the anterior aspect of the sacrum.

pudendal b., anesthesia produced by blocking the pudendal nerves, accomplished by injection of the local anesthetic into the tuberosity of the ischium.

sacral b., anesthesia produced by injection of the local anesthetic into the extradural space of the spinal canal.

saddle b., the production of anesthesia in a region corresponding roughly with the areas of the buttocks, perineum, and inner aspects of the thighs, by introducing the anesthetic agent low in the dural sac.

subarachnoid b., anesthesia produced by the injection of a local anesthetic into the subarachnoid space around the spinal cord.

vagal b., vagus nerve b., blocking of vagal impulses by injection of a solution of local anesthetic into the vagus nerve at its exit from the skull.

Blockain (blok'ān) trademark for preparations of propoxycaine, a local anesthetic.

blocking (blok'ing) 1. interruption of an afferent nerve pathway (see BLOCK). 2. inhibition of an intracellular biosynthetic process, as by injection of dactinomycin. 3. difficulty in recollection, or interruption of a train of thought or speech, due to emotional factors, usually unconscious.

blood (blud) the fluid that circulates through the heart, arteries, capillaries, and veins. Blood is the chief means of transport within the body. It transports oxygen from the lungs to the body tissues, and carbon dioxide from the tissues to the lungs. It carries foods from the digestive system to the tissues, removes waste products to the kidneys and carries fluid to and from the tissues, helping to maintain the fluid balance of the body.

In an emergency, blood cells and antibodies carried in the blood are brought to a point of infection, or blood-clotting substances are carried to a break in a blood vessel. The blood distributes hormones from the endocrine glands to the organs they influence. And it helps in the regulation of body temperature by carrying excess heat from the interior of the body to the surface layers of the skin, where the heat is dissipated to the surrounding air.

Blood varies in color from a bright red in the arteries to a duller red in the veins. The total quantity of blood within an individual depends upon his body weight. A person who weighs 150 lbs. has about 5 quarts of blood in his body.

Blood is composed to two main parts: (1) plasma, the fluid portion, consisting mainly of water in which are dissolved the substances carried by the blood to and from the tissues; and (2) solid particles, including blood cells and blood platelets, suspended in the fluid.

PLASMA. The plasma accounts for about 55 per cent of the total volume of the blood. It consists of about 92 per cent water, 7 per cent proteins, and less than 1 per cent inorganic salts, organic substances other than proteins, dissolved gases, hormones, antibodies, and enzymes. Plasma from which the fibrinogen has been removed is called serum.

Dissolved in the plasma are many important proteins such as serum albumin, gamma globulin, and fibrinogen. Serum albumin is important in the nutrition of the body. It probably originates in the liver, as does the fibrinogen. Fibrinogen is essential in the clotting process. Gamma globulin, which is formed in the lymphoid tissues and reticuloendothelial system, contains almost all of the antibodies important in establishing IMMUNITY.

Plasma volume is sometimes measured in order to calculate the total BLOOD VOLUME. The most common method for determining plasma volume is by injection of a dye (T-1824, called Evans blue) into the circulating blood and later calculating the total blood volume.

BLOOD CELLS AND PLATELETS. The suspended particles of the blood comprise the other 45 per cent of the total volume of blood. They include erythrocytes (red blood cells), leukocytes (white blood cells), and platelets (thrombocytes). The red and white blood cells are also known as corpuscles (Latin for "little bodies").

Erythrocytes (Red Blood Cells). The great majority of the cells in the blood are red blood cells. There are about 5 million red blood cells in a speck of blood the size of a pinhead, and about 35 trillion of them in the average adult. Although microscopic in size, these cells have a total surface area almost the size of a football gridiron. This vast surface area is important in the blood's task of carrying oxygen from the lungs to the tissues, because the exchange of oxygen in both places takes place across the cell surfaces and must be accomplished quickly as the blood flows by.

The erythrocytes owe their oxygen-carrying ability to the protein HEME, which contains iron and gives the blood its red color. Heme combines with another protein, GLOBIN, and forms HEMOGLOBIN, a major part of the red blood cell. Hemoglobin has the special ability of attracting and forming a loose connection with free oxygen, and its presence enables blood to absorb some 60 times the amount of oxygen that the plasma by itself absorbs.

Red blood cells are stored in the SPLEEN, which acts as a reservoir for the blood system and discharges the cells into the blood as required. The spleen also discharges extra red blood cells into the blood during emergencies such as hemorrhage or shock.

Red blood cells originate in the red bone marrow of the ribs, sternum, skull, pelvic bone, vertebrae, and the ends of the long bones of the limbs. The average red cell has a life of 110 to 120 days. It then disintegrates, and is removed in the spleen and the LIVER. About 180 million red blood cells are destroyed every minute. Since the number of cells in the blood remains more or less constant, this means that about 180 million red blood cells are manufactured every minute. The hemoglobin of destroyed cells is decomposed and carried to the liver. There the iron is stored and the rest of the chemicals are passed on to be excreted from the body in the bile, the feces, and the urine.

Determination of the red blood cell volume is usually done as a preliminary step in the determination of the total BLOOD VOLUME. A radioactive substance, usually chromium, is used to "tag" cells of a sample of blood drawn from the patient. The sample is then reintroduced into the circulating blood and subsequent samples are taken to be evaluated for degree of radioactivity. The degree of dilution is used to calculate total blood volume.

Leukocytes (White Blood Cells). The leukocytes are the body's primary defense against infections. They have no hemoglobin and thus are colorless and, unlike red blood cells, they can move about under their own power. White blood cells are larger than red blood cells and fewer in number. Normally the blood has about 8000 white blood cells per cubic millimeter.

Of the several types of leukocytes, the neutrophils are the most numerous, forming about 70 per cent of the total number; lymphocytes make up about 20 per cent of the total. The neutrophils, the lymphocytes, and most other white blood cells are phagocytic—that is, they have the ability to engulf and destroy bacteria. Leukocytes multiply rapidly when the body is invaded by bacteria. The cells migrate rapidly to the site of the infection, surround the bacteria and overwhelm them. Under a microscope, as many as 15 or 20 bacteria can be seen within a single white blood cell. Leukocytes originate in the red bone marrow, except for the lymphocytes, which are formed in lymphoid tissue.

Platelets. Platelets are small, clear, disk-shaped bodies about one-third the size of red blood cells or even smaller, which initiate blood clotting and are concerned in contraction of a clot. When they encounter a leak in a blood vessel, they disintegrate and adhere to the edges of the injured tissue. There are about 250,000 platelets per cubic millimeter of blood.

BIOCHEMICAL TESTS. Chemical analyses of various substances in the blood are invaluable aids in (1) the prevention of disease by alerting the patient and physician to potentially dangerous levels of blood constituents that could lead to more serious conditions, (2) diagnosis of pathologic conditions already present, (3) assessment of the patient's progress when a disturbance in blood chemistry exists, and (4) assessment of the patient's status by establishing a baseline or "normal" levels for each individual patient.

In recent years, with the increasing attention to preventive medicine and rapid progress in technology and automation, the use of a battery of screening tests performed by automated instruments has become quite common. These instruments are capable of performing simultaneously a variety of blood chemistry tests on as many as 60 patients. One such instrument, the AUTOANALYZER, is designed with a multi-channel system in which the blood sample is divided among flow patterns for a desired set of tests. Analyzing 2.5 ml. of blood in each sample, the instrument evaluates and records on a print-out sheet as many as 12 different readings on the sample.

Some of the more common screening tests performed on samples of blood include evaluation of ELECTROLYTES, ALBUMIN, and BILIRUBIN levels, blood urea notrigen (BUN), CHOLESTEROL, total protein, and such enzymes as lactic dehydrogenase (LDH) and serum glutamic oxaloacetic transaminase (SGOT).

Another relatively new method of analysis of blood components is that of ELECTROPHORESIS. The principle of electrophoresis is most widely applied to the separation of proteins. The procedure derives its name from the use of an electric field across which various protein particles or ions "migrate" in a characteristic way and at a characteristic speed. As the members of each group of proteins move in their own way across the electric field, the volume and activity of each protein can be distinguished from other proteins. Studies of this type are valuable in diagnosing and treating of many diseases in which the protein constituents of blood have been affected. The technique of electrophoresis also is used in separating and identifying types of human HEMOGLOBIN.

Blood urea nitrogen (BUN) tests measure the blood's content of urea, one of the nitrogenous waste products of protein metabolism (see also UREA NITROGEN). Measurement of nonprotein NITROGEN (NPN) also may be used as a test of kidney function, after severe injury or extended infection or when the body is overloaded with fluid; a high level of NPN may indicate poisoning, hormonal disorders, or shock.

Analysis of blood gases is quite useful in the care of patients having difficulty with oxygen and carbon dioxide transport and maintenance of a normal ACID-BASE BALANCE. BLOOD GAS ANALYSIS determines oxygen and carbon dioxide levels and their partial pressure in arterial and venous blood. The pH or hydrogen ion concentration as determined by blood gas analysis is extremely important in evaluating a patient's status in regard to states of ACIDOSIS and ALKALOSIS.

Determinations of glucose as in a GLUCOSE TOLERANCE TEST are helpful in identifying diseases of the liver and disorders of carbohydrate metabolism.

Iron determinations may be used to identify and differentiate certain anemias. In cases of iron deficiency, a test of the blood's iron-binding capacity can indicate the extent to which the patient will be helped by increasing his intake of iron, either by diet or by taking iron preparations.

central b., blood from the pulmonary venous system; sometimes applied to splanchnic blood, or blood obtained from chambers of the heart or from bone marrow.

citrated b., blood treated with sodium citrate to prevent its coagulation.

cord b., that contained in the umbilical vessels at the time of delivery of the infant.

defibrinated b., whole blood from which fibrin has been separated during the clotting process.

occult b., that present in such small amounts as to be detectable only by chemical tests or by spectroscopic or microscopic examination.

peripheral b., that obtained from acral areas, or from the circulation remote from the heart; the blood in the systemic circulation.

splanchnic b., that circulating in thoracic, abdominal, and pelvic viscera, further distinguished on the basis of specific organ, e.g., pulmonary, hepatic, splenic.

whole b., that from which none of the elements has been removed, especially that drawn from a selected donor under aseptic conditions, containing citrate ion or heparin.

blood bank 1. a place of storage for blood. 2. an organization that collects, processes, stores, and transfuses blood. In most health agencies the blood bank is located in the pathology laboratory. It is operated under the direction of a medical technologist.

blood-brain barrier the barrier that prevents or delays the entry into brain tissue of certain substances in the blood. Presumably it consists of the walls of the blood vessels of the central nervous system and the surrounding glial membranes.

blood clotting, coagulation see CLOTTING.

blood count the number of blood cells in a given sample of blood, usually expressed as the number of cells in a cubic millimeter of blood (as red blood cell, white blood cell, or platelet count). A differential white cell count determines the number of various types of leukocytes in a sampling of blood. The cell count is useful in the diagnosis of various blood dyscrasias, infections or other abnormal conditions of

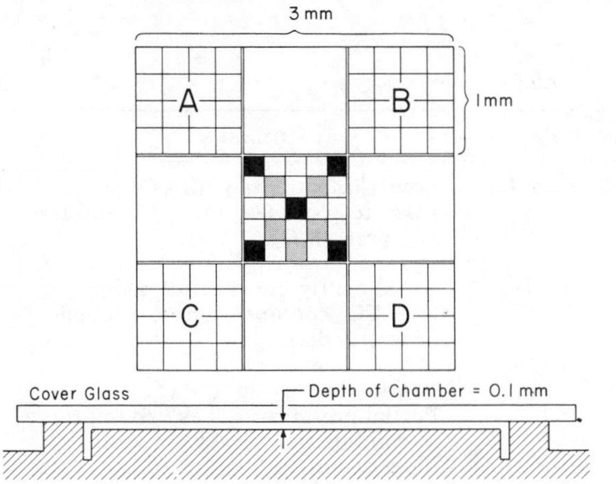

The upper figure is a diagram of the improved Neubauer ruling; this is etched on the surface of each side of the hemacytometer. The large corner squares, A, B, C, and D, are used for leukocyte counts. The five black squares in the center (colored only for purposes of illustration) are used for red cell counts or for platelet counts, and the 10 black plus checked squares for platelet counts. Actually, each of the 25 squares within the central sq. mm. has within it 16 smaller squares for convenience in counting.

The lower figure is a side view of the chamber with the cover glass in place. (From Davidsohn, I., and Henry, J. B.: Todd-Sanford Clinical Diagnosis by Laboratory Methods. 15th ed. Philadelphia, W. B. Saunders Co., 1974.)

the body and is one of the most common tests done on the blood. For normal ranges and significance of changes in the blood count see the table of normal values under BLOOD.

blood gas analysis laboratory studies of arterial and venous blood for the purpose of measuring oxygen and carbon dioxide levels and pressure or tension, and hydrogen ion concentration (pH). (See accompaning table.) Analyses of blood gases provide the following information:

Pa_{O_2}—partial pressure (P) of oxygen (O_2) in the arterial blood (a)

Sa_{O_2}—percentage of available hemoglobin that is saturated (Sa) with oxygen (O_2)

Pa_{CO_2}—partial pressure (P) of carbon dioxide (CO_2) in the arterial blood (a)

pH—an expression of the extent to which the blood is alkaline or acidic

The Pa_{CO_2} is related to the pH of arterial blood because of the chemical reaction of carbon dioxide and water which results in the formation of carbonic acid. The presence of an elevated Pa_{CO_2} results in an excess of hydrogen ions which indicates a lowered pH and ACIDOSIS. (See also pH.)

Analysis of blood gases and determination of pH levels are useful in assessing patient status in conditions affecting the transport of oxygen and hemoglobin, as in respiratory and circulatory disorders, and in those cases in which there is a disturbance in fluid and electrolyte imbalance and malfunction of the body's buffer systems. Because the lungs and kidneys act as regulators of the ACID-BASE BALANCE, care of a patient with any disorder seriously affecting the functions of either of these organs would include periodic blood gas analyses.

The manner in which specimens of blood for blood gas analysis are obtained is important to the accuracy of the test results. Arterial blood samples may be taken from an indwelling arterial catheter or by a femoral puncture performed by a physician. Because peripheral venous blood does not usually present a true pH, electrolyte, or gaseous picture, it is recommended that a sample of venous blood collected for analysis of these factors be drawn from a CENTRAL VENOUS CATHETER or from a catheter in the pulmonary artery.

During the process of drawing blood for gas analyses care is taken to avoid getting any air bubbles into the sample. The amount drawn may vary from 0.5 ml. to 2.5 ml., depending on the type of analyzer used in the laboratory. The sample usually is collected in a heparinized vacuum tube or plastic syringe. Heparin is used because unclotted blood is needed for the analyses; care is exercised in the strength and amount of heparin used because heparin in excessive amounts will cause falsely low blood pH values.

It is extremely important that the container for the blood sample be labeled correctly. Values and norms for venous and arterial blood differ. Therefore, the container should indicate the source of the blood sample and this information also should be written on the report of the results.

Measurements of the Pa_{O_2} and Sa_{O_2} are both concerned with oxygen transport in the blood. Pa_{O_2} represents the oxygen dissolved in the blood, which is a very small amount, and oxygen in combination with hemoglobin (oxyhemoglobin), the form in which most of the oxygen in the blood occurs. Adequate oxygen transport therefore depends on a normal amount of hemoglobin and normally *functioning* hemoglobin. Both Pa_{O_2} and Sa_{O_2} levels must be examined to determine adequacy of oxygenation.

It is important to remember that, although the normal Pa_{O_2} is 80 to 104 mm. Hg, some patients with CHRONIC OBSTRUCTIVE PULMONARY DISEASE can tolerate a Pa_{O_2} as low as 70 mm. Hg without appearing hypoxic. In caring for patients with this condition it is important to know that attempts to elevate the Pa_{CO_2} level to normal laboratory range can be dangerous and even fatal. It is best to establish a "normal" level for each individual patient before supplementary oxygen is administered, and then to assess his condition and the effectiveness of therapy according to that baseline.

Measures that will raise the Pa_{O_2} level include the administration of oxygen and changing body position so that there is improvement in pulmonary circulation with increased oxygenation of blood returning to the heart from the lungs.

The Pa_{CO_2} defines adequacy of ventilation. If carbon dioxide, which is the end product of all body metabolism, accumulates in the body because it is not "blown off" by the lungs, the patient will develop acidosis.

Pa_{O_2} and Pa_{CO_2} both refer to partial pressure or tension of oxygen and carbon dioxide, respectively. Determination of partial pressure allows for a comparison of the amount of gas available and is dependent upon the barometric pressure and the fraction of the specific gas present. The word "partial" is used because it refers only to the amount of

BLOOD GAS ANALYSIS

TERM	DEFINITION	NORMAL RANGE	REMARKS
Pa_{O_2}	Partial pressure of oxygen in arterial blood	80–100 mm. Hg	Lower in patients with COPD. Rises to about 600 mm. if breathing 100 percent O_2.
Pa_{CO_2}	Partial pressure of carbon dioxide in arterial blood	36–44 mm. Hg	Bears nearly linear relationship to total CO_2 content. Defines adequacy of ventilation.
Sa_{O_2}	Percent saturation of hemoglobin with oxygen in arterial blood	93–98%	Bears relationship to Pa_{O_2}. Partial pressure acts as driving force in combination of oxygen with hemoglobin.
Total CO_2 content of plasma (venous)	Carbon dioxide obtainable from bicarbonate, dissolved CO_2, carbamino compounds, and H_2CO_3 (carbonic acid)	26–30 mEq/L 58–67 vol. %	Reflects either metabolic or respiratory disturbances in acid-base balance.
pH (arterial)	Expression of hydrogen ion concentration. Negative logarithm (p) of hydrogen (H) ion	7.38–7.44	Determined by ratio of bicarbonate ion concentration to CO_2 concentration, low pH indicates acidity. Inversely, low hydrogen ion concentration, high pH indicates alkalinity.

pressure being exerted by a particular gas in a mixture of gases. Information about the partial pressure of oxygen and carbon dioxide is useful in determining the facility with which they can be transported across the tissues of the alveoli.

blood group the phenotype of erythrocytes defined by one or more cellular antigenic structural groupings under the control of allelic genes. In clinical practice there are four main blood types or groups: A, B, O, and AB. In addition to this major grouping there is an Rh-hR system that is important in the prevention of ERYTHROBLASTOSIS FETALIS resulting from incompatibility of blood groups in mother and fetus.

The ABO blood group system was first introduced in 1900 by Karl Landsteiner; in 1920 group AB was discovered by van Descatello and Sturli. Identification of these four major blood groups represented a major step toward resolving the problem of blood transfusion reactions resulting from donor-recipient incompatibility. In 1938 Landsteiner and Weiner discovered another blood factor related to maternal-fetal incompatibility. The factor was named Rh because the researchers were using rhesus monkeys in their studies. Further research has uncovered additional factors in the Rh group.

Although more than 90 factors have been identified, many of these are not highly antigenic and are not, therefore, a cause for concern in the typing of blood for clinical purposes.

The term *factor,* in reference to blood groups, is synonymous with antigen and the reaction occurring between incompatible blood types is an ANTIGEN-ANTIBODY reaction. In cases of incompatibility, the antigen, located on the red blood cells, is an agglutinogen and the specific antibody, located in the serum, is an agglutinin. These are so named because whenever red blood cells with a certain factor come in contact with the agglutinin specific for it, there is agglutination or clumping of the erythrocytes.

In determining blood group, a sample of blood is taken and mixed with specially prepared sera. One serum, anti-A agglutinin, causes blood of group A to agglutinate; another serum, anti-B agglutinin, causes blood of group B to agglutinate. Thus, if anti-A serum alone causes clumping, the blood is group A; if anti-B serum alone causes clumping, it is group B. If both cause clumping, the blood group is AB, and if it is not clumped by either, it is identified as group O.

blood plasma see BLOOD.

blood poisoning septicemia.

blood pressure the pressure of the blood against the walls of the blood vessels. The term usually refers to the pressure of the blood within the arteries, or arterial blood pressure. This pressure is determined by several factors, including the pumping action of the heart, the resistance to the flow of blood in the arterioles, the elasticity of the walls of the main arteries, the quantity of blood within the blood vessels, and the blood's viscosity, or thickness.

The pumping action of the heart refers to how hard the heart pumps the blood (force of heartbeat) and how much blood it pumps and how efficiently it does the job. Contraction of the heart, which forces blood through the arteries, is the phase known as systole. Relaxation of the heart between contractions is called diastole.

The main arteries leading from the heart have walls with strong elastic fibers capable of expanding and absorbing the pulsations generated by the heart. At each pulsation the arteries expand and absorb the momentary increase in blood pressure. As the heart relaxes in preparation for another beat, the aortic valves close to prevent blood from flowing back to the heart chambers, and the artery walls spring back, forcing the blood through the body between contractions. In this way the arteries act as dampers on the pulsations and thus provide a steady flow of blood through the blood vessels.

HUMAN BLOOD GROUP SYSTEMS AND ERYTHROCYTIC ANTIGENIC DETERMINANTS

Antigenic determinants are systematized according to observed and assumed independent assortment of their responsible genes. Within many systems, alleles are responsible for differing combinations of antigenic determinants.

BLOOD GROUP SYSTEM	ANTIGENIC DETERMINANTS*
ABO	A, A_1, B
H	H
I	I, i, I^T, I^D, I^F
MN	M, N, S, s, U, Cl^a, Far, He, Hill, Hu, M^A, M^C, M^e, M^g, M_1, Mi^a, Mt^a, Mur, M^v, Ny^a, Ri^a, S^B, Sj, St^a, Sul, Tm, U^B, Vr, Vw, N^A, Z
P	P1, P2 (Tj^a), P3 (P^K)
Rh	Rh1 (D, Rh_0), Rh2 (C, rh′), Rh3 (E, rh″), Rh4 (c, hr′), Rh5 (e, hr″), Rh6 (f, ce, hr), Rh7 (Ce, rh_i), Rh8 (C^w, rh^{w1}), Rh9 (C^x, rh^x), Rh10 (V, ce^s, hr^v), Rh11 (E^w, rh^{w2}), Rh12 (G, rh^G), Rh13 (Rh^A), Rh14 (Rh^B), Rh15 (Rh^C), Rh16 (Rh^D), Rh17 (Hr_0), Rh18 (Hr), Rh19 (hr^s), Rh20 (VS, e^s), Rh21 (C^G), Rh22 (CE), Rh23 (D^w), Rh24 (E^T), Rh26, Rh27 (cE), Rh28 (hr^H), Rh29 (RH), Rh30 (Go^a), Rh31 (hr^B), Rh32, Rh33
Lutheran	Lu^a (Lu1), Lu^b (Lu2), Lu^{ab} (Lu3), Lu4, Lu5, Lu6, Lu7, Lu8, Lu9, Lu10, Lu11, Lu12, Lu13, Lu14 (Sw^a)
Kell	K1 (K), K2 (k), K3 (Kp^a), K4 (Kp^b), K5 (Ku), K6 (Js^a), K7 (Js^b), K8 (kw), K9 (KL), K10 (Ul^a), K11, K12, K13, K14, K15, K16
Lewis	Le^a (Le1), Le^b (Le2), Le^x (Le^{ab}, Le3), Mag (Le4), Le^c (Le5), Le^d
Duffy	Fy^a (Fy1), Fy^b (Fy2), Fy^{ab} (Fy3), Fy4
Kidd	Jk^a (Jk1), Jk^b (Jk2), Jk^{ab} (Jk3)
Cartwright	Yt^a, Yt^b
Xg	Xg^a
Dombrock	Do^a, Do^b
Auberger	Au^a
Cost-Sterling	Cs^a, Yk^a
Wright	Wr^a, Wr^b
Diego	Di^a, Di^b
Vel	Vel 1, Vel 2
Sciana	Sm, Bu^a
Bg	Bg^a, Bg^b, Bg^c, Ho, Ho-like, Ot, Sto, DBG (similar to HL-A7 of lymphocytes)
Gerbich	Ge1, Ge2, Ge3 (anti-Gel = M.Y.; anti-Ge1,2 = Ge; anti-Ge1,2,3 = Yus)
Coltan	Co^a, Co^b
Stoltzfus	Sf^a

Low-incidence antigenic determinants not thus far associated with a blood group system:

Be^a, Bec, Bi, Big Charles, Bp^a, Bx^a, By, Cad, Chr^a, Coates, Craig, Dahl, Donaviesky, Driver, Duch, Evans, Evelyn, Fin, Fuerhart, Gf^a, Gilbraith, Good, Green, Hands, Heibel, Hil, Ht^a, Je^a, Jn^a, Job, Kam, Ken, Kosis, Lev, Lw^a, McCall, Man, Mar, Mo^a, Nij, Orr, Pt^a, Rd^a, Reid, Rm, Skjelbred, Th^a, To^a, Tr^a, Ven, Wb, Weeks, Wu, Yh^a, Za, 754

High-incidence antigenic determinants not thus far associated with a blood group system:

An^a, At^a, Bou, Bra, Car, Chido (Gursha), Cip, Dp, El, En^a, Fuj, Gn^a Go^b, Gy^a, Hen, Hy, Jo^a, Jr, Kelly, Knops, Lan, MZ443, Ola, Pea,Savior, Sch, Sd^a, Simon, Ters, Todd, Vennera, Wil, Winbourne

Antigenic determinants that depend on gene interactions:

ABO/I	IH, IA, IB, iH
P/I	IP1, IP2(IT_j^a), I^TP1, iP1
Lewis/I	ILe^{bh}
Lewis/ABO	A_1Le^b
P/ABO	Luke
Xor/Duffy	Fy5
Rh/LW	Rh25 (LW)

*Symbols within parentheses are those of alternative nomenclatures. (Compiled by Dr. Fred H. Allen, Jr.)

Because of this, there are actually two blood pressures within the blood vessels during one complete beat of the heart; a higher blood pressure during *systole* (contraction phase) and a lower blood pressure during *diastole* (relaxation phase). These two blood pressures are known as the systolic pressure and the diastolic pressure, respectively.

MEASUREMENT OF THE BLOOD PRESSURE. The blood pressure is usually measured in the artery of the upper arm, with a sphygmomanometer. This consists of a rubber cuff connected to a glass tube containing a column of mercury. Alongside the glass tube are numbers that indicate the height of the column of mercury in millimeters (25 mm. equals 1 inch). In some sphygmomanometers the mercury column is replaced by a gauge. The rubber cuff is wrapped about the patient's arm, and then air is pumped into the cuff by means of a rubber bulb. As the pressure inside the rubber cuff increases, the flow of blood through the artery is momentarily checked. The pressure within the cuff causes the mercury to rise or the gauge's needle to move.

A stethoscope is then placed over the artery at the elbow and the air pressure within the cuff is slowly released. The pressure begins to fall slowly. As soon as blood begins to flow through the artery again, tapping sounds can be heard through the stethoscope. This is the pulse. When the first tapping sound is heard, the systolic pressure is noted.

As the air pressure continues to escape from the

cuff, the tapping sounds grow louder. A point is reached at which the sounds change suddenly to very soft and then disappear entirely. The point on the mercury column at which the sound disappears entirely is the diastolic pressure.

The blood pressure is usually written and spoken of as one number over another—for example, 120/80, or "one-twenty over eighty." The first number represents the systolic pressure and the second is the diastólic pressure, both recorded in millimeters of mercury.

The blood pressure can vary considerably between the sexes, among different age groups, and even between two persons of the same age and sex. At birth, the systolic blood pressure is about 80 mm. of mercury. In young people it varies normally from 100 to 140 mm., and in people at 60 years of age from 140 to about 170 mm.

Blood pressure also varies according to the time of day and the kind of activity a person is engaged in. It is usually lowest just before awakening in the morning. Strenuous physical activity can increase the systolic blood pressure 60 to 80 mm. above normal. Excitement, nervous tension or fright raises the systolic blood pressure. Increased weight tends to lead to increased blood pressure. See also HYPERTENSION and HYPOTENSION.

Errors in blood pressure measurement can result from failure of the cuff to reach and compress the artery. The cuff diameter should be 20 percent greater than the diameter of the limb, the bladder of the cuff must be centered over the artery, and the cuff must be wrapped smoothly and snugly to assure proper inflation. When a mercury gauge is used the meniscus should be at eye level to avoid a false reading.

Critically ill patients who require continuous monitoring of the blood pressure may have a catheter inserted into an artery and attached to a catheter-monitor-transducer system. The blood pressure is displayed on an oscilloscope at the bedside so that the patient's pressure can be determined at a glance. This intra-arterial technique of blood pressure monitoring provides accurate, objective, and continuous data on the patient's status.

blood serum see BLOOD.

blood transfusion see TRANSFUSION.

blood type 1. blood group. 2. the phenotype of an individual with respect to a blood group system.

blood vessel any of the vessels conveying the blood; an artery, arteriole, vein, venule or capillary.

blood volume the total quantity of blood in the body. The regulation of blood volume in the circulatory system is affected by the intrinsic mechanism for fluid exchange at the capillary membranes and by hormonal influences and nervous reflexes that affect the excretion of fluids by the kidneys. A rapid decrease in the blood volume, as in hemorrhage, greatly reduces the cardiac output and creates a condition called SHOCK or circulatory shock. Conversely, an increase in blood volume, as when there is retention of water and salt in the body because of renal failure, results in an increase in cardiac output. The eventual outcome of this situation is increased arterial blood pressure.

The blood volume in the pulmonary circulation is approximately 12 percent of the total blood volume. Such conditions as left-sided heart failure and mitral stenosis can greatly increase the pulmonary blood volume while decreasing the systemic volume. As would be expected, right-sided heart failure has the opposite effect. The latter condition has less serious effects because the volume of the systemic circulation is about seven times that of the pulmonary circulation and it is therefore better able to accommodate a change in fluid volume.

Measurement of blood volume is accomplished by using substances that combine with red blood cells, for example, iron, chromium, and phosphate, or substances that combine with plasma proteins. In either case the measurement of the blood volume is based on the "dilution" principle. That is, the volume of any fluid compartment can be measured if a given amount of a substance is dispersed evenly in the fluid within the compartment, and then the extent of dilution of the substance is measured.

For example, a small amount of radioactive chromium (^{51}Cr), which is widely used to determine blood volume, is mixed with a sample of blood drawn from the patient. After about 30 minutes the ^{51}Cr will have entered the red blood cells. The sample with the tagged red blood cells is then returned by injection into the patient's blood stream. About 10 minutes later a sample is removed from the patient's circulating blood and the radioactivity level of this sample is measured. The total blood volume is calculated according to this formula:

$$\text{volume in ml.} = \frac{\text{quantity of test substance instilled}}{\text{concentration per ml. of dispersed fluid}}$$

When *plasma volume* is used to arrive at the total blood volume, a dye (usually T-1824, also known as Evans blue) is injected into the circulating blood. The dye immediately combines with the blood proteins and within 10 minutes is dispersed throughout the circulatory system. A sample of blood is then drawn and the exact quantity of dye is measured. Using the information about plasma volume obtained by applying the above formula, the total blood volume can be calculated, provided the hematocrit is also known. The formula for this calculation is:

$$\text{blood volume} = \text{plasma volume} \times \frac{100}{100 - 0.87 \text{ hematocrit}}$$

Blount's disease (bluntz) aseptic necrosis of the medial condyle of the tibia, sometimes causing lateral bowing of the legs.

blowpipe (blo′pīp) a tube through which a current of air is forced upon a flame to concentrate and intensify the heat.

blue baby an infant born with cyanosis, with a bluish color that is due to abnormally low concentration of oxygen in the circulating blood. The term is commonly used to designate an infant born with congenital atelectasis or with one or more defects of the heart and great vessels (see also CONGENITAL HEART DEFECT).

blue dome cyst a benign retention cyst of the breast that shows a brown to blue color (see also CYSTIC DISEASE OF BREAST). Called also Schimmelbusch's disease.

Blumberg's sign (blum′bergz) pain on abrupt release of steady pressure (rebound tenderness) over the site of a suspected abdominal lesion, indicative of peritonitis.

blush (blush) sudden, brief erythema of the face and neck, resulting from vascular dilatation due to emotion or heat.

B.M.A. British Medical Association.

BMR basal metabolic rate.

BNA Basle Nomina Anatomica, a system of anatomic nomenclature adopted at the annual meeting of the German Anatomic Society in 1895; superseded by NOMINA ANATOMICA.

body (bod'e) 1. the trunk, or animal frame, with its organs. 2. the largest and most important part of any organ. 3. any mass or collection of material.

acetone b's, ketone bodies.

alkapton b's, a class of substances with an affinity for alkali, found in the urine and causing the condition known as alkaptonuria. The compound commonly found, and most commonly referred to by the term, is homogentisic acid.

amygdaloid b., a small mass of subcortical gray matter within the tip of the temporal lobe, anterior to the inferior horn of the lateral ventricle of the brain.

aortic b's, small neurovascular structures on either side of the aorta in the region of the aortic arch, containing chemoreceptors that play a role in reflex regulation of respiration.

asbestos b's, golden yellow bodies of various shapes in sputum, lung secretions, and feces of patients with asbestosis (see also ABESTOS BODIES).

Aschoff's b's, submiliary collections of cells and leukocytes in the interstitial tissues of the heart in rheumatic myocarditis; called also Aschoff's nodules.

asteroid b., an irregularly star-shaped inclusion body found in the giant cells in sarcoidosis and other diseases.

Barr b., sex chromatin; the persistent mass of the material of the inactivated X-chromosome in cells of normal females.

carotid b's, a small neurovascular structure lying in the bifurcation of the right and left carotid arteries, containing chemoreceptors that monitor oxygen content in blood and help to regulate respiration.

ciliary b., the thickened part of the vascular tunic of the eye, connecting the choroid and iris (see also CILIARY BODY).

Donovan b's, *Donovania granulomatis.*

elementary b., 1. a blood platelet. 2. an inclusion body.

fimbriate b., corpus fimbriatum.

foreign b., a mass of material that is not normal to the place where it is found.

geniculate b's, lateral, two metathalamus eminences, one on each side just lateral to the medial geniculate bodies, marking the termination of the optic tract.

geniculate b's, medial, two metathalamus eminences, one on each side, just lateral to the superior colliculi, concerned with hearing.

Howell's b's, Howell-Jolly b's, smooth, round remnants of nuclear chromatin seen in erythrocytes when stains are added to fresh blood and found in various anemias and leukemias and after splenectomy.

inclusion b's, round, oval, or irregular-shaped bodies in the cytoplasm and nuclei of cells, as in disease caused by viral infection, such as rabies, smallpox, herpes, etc.

ketone b's, acetone, acetoacetic acid, and β-hydroxybutyric acid; except for acetone (which may arise spontaneously from acetoacetic acid), they are normal products of lipid metabolism within the liver, and are oxidized by muscles (see also KETONE BODIES).

Lafora's b's, intracytoplasmic inclusions consisting of a complex of glycoprotein and acid mucopolysaccharide; widespread deposits are found in myoclonus epilepsy.

Leishman-Donovan b's, round or oval bodies found in the reticuloendothelial cells, especially those of the spleen and liver, in kala-azar; they are nonflagellate intracellular forms of *Leishmania donovani.* Also used to designate similar forms of *L. tropica* found in macrophages in lesions of cutaneous leishmaniasis.

mamillary b., either of the pair of small spherical masses in the interpeduncular fossa of the midbrain, forming part of the hypothalamus.

Negri b's, oval or round bodies in the nerve cells of animals dead of rabies.

Nissl b's, large granular bodies that stain with basic dyes, forming the reticular substance of the cytoplasm of neurons. Ribonucleoprotein is one of the main constituents.

olivary b., a rounded elevation, lateral to the upper part of each pyramid of the medulla oblongata. Called also olive.

para-aortic b's, enclaves of chromaffin cells near the sympathetic ganglia along the abdominal aorta, which serve as chemoreceptors responsive to oxygen, carbon dioxide, and hydrogen in concentration and which help control respiration. Tumors of these structures produce symptoms similar to those of PHEOCHROMOCYTOMA. Called also organs of Zuckerkandl.

pineal b., a small, conical structure attached by a stalk to the posterior wall of the third ventricle of the cerebrum (see also PINEAL BODY).

pituitary b., pituitary gland.

psammoma b's, usually microscopic, laminated masses of calcareous material, occurring in both benign and malignant epithelial and connective-tissue tumors, and sometimes associated with chronic inflammation. (See also PSAMMOMA.)

quadrigeminal b's, corpora quadrigemina.

striate b., corpus striatum.

trachoma b's, inclusion bodies found in clusters in the cytoplasm of the epithelial cells of the conjunctiva in trachoma.

vitreous b., the transparent gel filling the inner portion of the eyeball between the lens and retina. Called also vitreous and vitreous humor.

wolffian b., mesonephros.

Boeck's sarcoid (beks) sarcoidosis.

Bohr effect (bor) displacement of the oxyhemoglobin dissociation curve by a change in carbon dioxide tension.

boil (boil) a painful nodule formed in the skin by circumscribed inflammation of the corium and subcutaneous tissue, enclosing a central slough or "core." Called also furuncle. Boils occur most frequently on the neck and buttocks, although they may develop wherever friction or irritation, or a scratch or break in the skin, allows the bacteria resident on the surface to penetrate the outer layer of the skin. A CARBUNCLE is a group of interconnected boils and is more serious than a simple boil.

CAUSE. When bacteria gain entrance into the skin, the infection settles in the hair follicles or the sebaceous glands. To combat the infection, large numbers of leukocytes travel to the site and attack the invading bacteria. Some bacteria and white cells are killed and they and their liquefied products form pus. The body's defenses may succeed in overcoming the invaders so that the boil subsides by itself, or the pus may build up pressure against the skin surface so that it ruptures, drains and heals.

Boils may afflict healthy persons but often their appearance is a sign that the resistance is low, usually as a result of poor nutrition or illness. Persons suffering from dermatitis or untreated DIABETES MELLITUS are particularly susceptible to boils.

TREATMENT. In most cases, a single boil is not serious and will respond to careful treatment, but there are some important exceptions. Medical attention is necessary if the patient is an infant, a young child, or an elderly person. A boil on or above the upper lip, on the nose or scalp or in the outer ear can be very serious because in these areas infection has easy access to the brain. Other danger zones are the armpit, the groin, and the breast of a woman who is nursing. If bacteria from a boil enter the bloodstream, septicemia may result.

bolometer (bo-lom′ĕ-ter) 1. an instrument for measuring the force of the heart beat. 2. an instrument for measuring minute degrees of radiant heat.

boloscope (bo′lo-skōp) an apparatus for locating metallic foreign bodies in the tissues.

bolus (bo′lus) 1. a rounded mass of food or pharmaceutical preparation ready to be swallowed, or such a mass passing through the gastrointestinal tract. 2. a concentrated mass of pharmaceutical preparation, e.g., an opaque contrast medium, given intravenously. 3. a mass of scattering material, such as wax or paraffin, placed between the radiation source and the skin to achieve a precalculated isodose pattern in the tissue irradiated.

alimentary b., the mass of food, made ready by mastication, that enters the esophagus at one swallow.

bond (bond) the linkage between atoms or radicals of a chemical compound, or the symbol representing this linkage and indicating the number and attachment of the valencies of an atom in constitutional formulas, represented by a pair of dots on a line between atoms, e.g., H—O—H, H—C≡C—H or H:O:H, H:C:::C:H.

covalent b., chemical bonds in which electrons can be shared, as the peptide bonds in proteins.

high-energy b., a chemical bond the hydrolysis of which yields high levels of free energy; such bonds involve phosphate (high-energy phosphate bond) or sulfur (high-energy sulfur bond) or other mixed anhydride types of chemical structure.

hydrogen b., a weak, primarily electrostatic, bond between a hydrogen atom bound to a highly electronegative element (such as oxygen or nitrogen) in a given molecule, or part of a molecule, and a second highly electronegative atom in another molecule or in a different part of the same molecule.

peptide b., a ·CO·NH· group produced in linking amino acids to form peptides.

bone (bōn) 1. the hard, rigid form of connective tissue constituting most of the skeleton of vertebrates, composed chiefly of calcium salts. 2. any distinct piece of the skeleton of the body. See table of BONES for regional listing and alphabetical listing of common names of bones of the body, and see Plates 1 and 2.

There are 206 separate bones in the human body. Collectively they form the SKELETAL SYSTEM, a structure bound together by ligaments at the joints and set in motion by the muscles, which are secured to the bones by means of tendons. Bones, ligaments, muscles, and tendons are the tissues of the body responsible for supporting and moving the body.

Some bones have chiefly a protective function. An example is the skull, which encloses the brain, the back of the eyeball, and the inner ear. Some, such as the pelvis, are mainly supporting structures. Other bones, such as the jaw and the bones of the fingers, are concerned chiefly with movement. The MARROW contained in bones manufactures the blood cells. The bones themselves act as a storehouse of calcium, which must be maintained at a certain level in the blood for the body's normal chemical functioning.

STRUCTURE AND COMPOSITION. Bone is not uniform in structure but is composed of several layers of different materials. The outermost layer, the periosteum, is a thin, tough membrane of fibrous tissue. It gives support to the tendons that secure the muscle to the bone and also serves as a protective sheath. This membrane encloses all bones completely except at the joints where there is a layer of cartilage. Beneath the periosteum lie the dense, hard layers of bone tissue called compact bone. Its composition is fibrous rather than solid and it gives bone its resiliency. Encased within these layers is the tissue that makes up most of the volume of bone, called cancellous or spongy bone because it contains little hollows like those of a sponge. The innermost portion of the bone is a hollow cavity containing marrow. Blood vessels course through every layer of bone, carrying nutritive elements, oxygen, and other products. Bone tissue also contains a large number of nerves. The basic chemical in bone, which gives bone its hardness and strength, is calcium phosphate.

DEVELOPMENT. Cartilage forms the major part of bone in the very young; this accounts for the great flexibility and resiliency of the infant skeleton. Gradually, calcium phosphate collects in the cartilage, and it becomes harder and more brittle. Some of the cartilage cells break loose, so that channels develop in the bone shaft. Blood vessels enter the channels, bearing with them small cells of connective tissue, some of which become osteoblasts, cells that form true bone. The osteoblasts enter the hardened cartilage, forming layers of hard, firm bone. Other cells, called osteoclasts, work to tear down old or excess bone structure, allowing the osteoblasts to rebuild with new bone. This renewal continues throughout life, although it slows down with age.

Cartilage formation and the subsequent replacement of cartilage by hard material is the mechanism by which bones grow in size. During the period of bone growth, cartilage grows over the hardened portion of bone. In time, this layer of cartilage hardens as calcium phosphate is added, and a fresh layer grows over it, and it too hardens. The process continues until the body reaches full growth. Long bones grow in length because of special cross-sectional layers of cartilage located near the flared ends of the bone. These harden and new cartilage is produced by the same process as previously described.

BONE DISORDERS. FRACTURE, a break in the bone, is the most common injury to the bone; it may be closed, with no break in the skin, or open, with penetration of the skin and exposure of portions of the broken bone.

OSTEOPOROSIS is excessive brittleness and porosity of bone in the aged. OSTEOMYELITIS is a bone infection similar to a boil on the skin, but much more serious because the infection can destroy the bone and invade other body tissues. OSTEOMALACIA is the term used for RICKETS when it occurs in adults. In these diseases there is softening of the bones, due to inadequate concentration of calcium or phosphorus in the body. The usual cause is deficiency of vitamin D, which is required for utilization of calcium and phosphorus by the body.

In OSTEITIS FIBROSA CYSTICA, bone is replaced by fibrous tissue because of abnormal calcium metabolism. The condition usually is due to overactivity of the parathyroid glands.

OSTEOMA refers to abnormal new growth, either benign or malignant, of the tissue of the bones. Although it is not common, it may occur in any of the bones of the body, and at any age.

ankle b., talus.

brittle b's, osteogenesis imperfecta.

cancellated b., cancellous b., bone composed of thin intersecting lamellae, usually found internal to compact bone.

cartilage b., bone developing within cartilage, ossification taking place within a cartilage model.

cheek b., zygomatic bone.

collar b., clavicle.

compact b., bone substance that is dense and hard.

cortical b., the compact bone of the shaft of a bone that surrounds the marrow cavity.

flat b., one whose thickness is slight, sometimes consisting of only a thin layer of compact bone, or of two layers with intervening cancellated bone and marrow; usually curved rather than flat.

heel b., calcaneus.

incisive b., the portion of the maxilla bearing the incisors; developmentally, it is the premaxilla, which in humans later fuses with the maxilla, but in most other vertebrates persists as a separate bone.

jaw b., the mandible or maxilla, especially the mandible.

jugal b., zygomatic bone.

lingual b., hyoid bone.

long b., one whose length far exceeds its breadth and thickness.

malar b., zygomatic bone.

marble b's, osteopetrosis.

mastoid b., the mastoid process.

membrane b., bone that develops within a connective tissue membrane.

pelvic b., hip bone.

petrous b., the petrous portion of the temporal bone; pars petrosa.

pneumatic b., bone that contains air-filled spaces.

premaxillary b., premaxilla.

pterygoid b., pterygoid process.

rider's b., localized ossification sometimes seen on the inner aspect of the lower end of the tendon of the adductor muscle of the thigh in horseback riders.

shin b., tibia.

short b., one of approximately equal length, width, and thickness.

solid b., compact bone.

spongy b., cancellous bone.

squamous b., the upper forepart of the temporal bone, forming an upright plate.

sutural b's, variable and irregularly shaped bones in the sutures between the bones of the skull.

thigh b., femur.

turbinated b., nasal conchae.

tympanic b., the part of the temporal bone surrounding the middle ear.

wormian b's, sutural bones.

bonelet (bōn′let) an ossicle, or small bone.

bone marrow (mar′o) the soft, organic, spongelike material in the cavities of bones, which has as its principal function the manufacture of erythrocytes, leukocytes, and platelets. (See also MARROW.)

Bonine (bo′nēn) trademark for preparations of meclizine, an antinauseant.

Bonner's position (bon′erz) flexion, abduction, and outward rotation of the thigh in coxitis.

Bonnevie-Ullrich syndrome pterygium colli, lymphangiectatic edema of the hands and feet, ocular hypertelorism, short stature, and other developmental anomalies.

Boophilus (bo-of′ĭ-lus) a genus of hard-bodied ticks primarily parasitic on cattle.

booster dose (bo͞ost′er dōs) see under DOSE.

boot (bo͞ot) an encasement for the foot; a protective casing or sheath.

Gibney b., an adhesive tape support used in treatment of sprains and other painful conditions of the ankle, the tape being applied in a basket-weave fashion with strips placed alternately under the sole of the foot and around the back of the leg.

Unna's paste b., a dressing for varicose ulcers, consisting of a paste made from gelatin, zinc oxide, and glycerin, and spiral bandages. The entire leg is covered with paste and bandage, applied in alternate layers until they make a rigid boot.

borate (bōr′āt) any salt of boric acid.

borax (bōr′aks) sodium borate.

borborygmus (bor″bor-ig′mus) a rumbling noise caused by propulsion of gas through the intestines.

border (bor′der) a bounding line, edge, or surface.

brush b., a specialization of the free surface of a cell, consisting of minute cylindrical processes (microvilli) that greatly increase the surface area.

vermilion b., the exposed red portion of the upper or lower lip.

Bordet-Gengou phenomenon (bor-da′-zhaw-goo′) complement fixation.

Bordetella (bor″dĕ-tel′ah) a genus of bacteria.

B. parapertussis, a species found occasionally in whooping cough (pertussis).

B. pertussis, the causative agent of whooping cough (pertussis).

boric acid (bōr′ik) a crystalline powder used as a buffer. It was formerly used as a household antiseptic for treating minor irritations of the skin and eyes. Because the powder is highly poisonous when taken internally, and since other antiseptics are more effective, boric acid is no longer recommended. Boric acid ointment (for external use only) is occasionally helpful in cases of mild skin irritations or in keeping a gauze dressing from sticking to a wound.

borism (bōr′izm) poisoning by a boron compound.

Bornholm disease (born′hōm) epidemic pleurodynia, an epidemic disease due to cocksackievirus

(Text continued on page 143.)

Table of Bones, Listed by Regions of the Body

REGION	NAME	TOTAL NUMBER
Axial skeleton		
	Skull	21
	(eight paired – 16)	
	inferior nasal concha	
	lacrimal	
	maxilla	
	nasal	
	palatine	
	parietal	
	temporal	
	zygomatic	
	(five unpaired – 5)	
	ethmoid	
	frontal	
	occipital	
	sphenoid	
	vomer	
	Ossicles of each ear	6
	incus	
	malleus	
	stapes	
	Lower jaw	
	mandible	1
	Neck	
	hyoid	1
	Vertebral column	26
	cervical vertebrae (7)	
	(atlas)	
	(axis)	
	thoracic vertebrae (12)	
	lumbar vertebrae (5)	
	sacrum (5 fused)	
	coccyx (4–5 fused)	
	Chest	
	sternum	1
	ribs (12 pairs)	24

REGION	NAME	TOTAL NUMBER
Upper limb (×2)		64
Shoulder	scapula	
	clavicle	
Upper arm	humerus	
Lower arm	radius	
	ulna	
Wrist	carpal (8)	
	(capitate)	
	(hamate)	
	(lunate)	
	(pisiform)	
	(scaphoid)	
	(trapezium)	
	(trapezoid)	
	(triquetral)	
Hand	metacarpal (5)	
Fingers	phalanges (14)	
Lower limb (×2)		62
Pelvis	hip bone (1)	
	(ilium)	
	(ischium)	
	(pubis)	
Thigh	femur	
Knee	patella	
Leg	tibia	
	fibula	
Ankle	tarsal (7)	
	(calcaneus)	
	(cuboid)	
	(cuneiform, medial)	
	(cuneiform, intermediate)	
	(cuneiform, lateral)	
	(navicular)	
	(talus)	
Foot	metatarsal (5)	
Toes	phalanges (14)	

TABLE OF BONES

COMMON NAME*	NA EQUIVALENT†	REGION	DESCRIPTION	ARTICULATIONS
astragalus. *See* talus				
atlas	atlas	neck	first cervical vertebra, ring of bone supporting the skull	with occipital b. and axis
axis	axis	neck	second cervical vertebra, with thick process (odontoid process) around which first cervical vertebra pivots	with atlas above and third cervical vertebra below
calcaneus	calcaneus	foot	the "heel bone," of irregularly cuboidal shape, largest of the tarsal bones	with talus and cuboid b.
capitate b.	o. capitatum	wrist	third from thumb side of 4 bones of distal row of carpal b's	with second, third, and fourth metacarpal b's, and hamate, lunate, trapezoid, and scaphoid b's
carpal b's	oss. carpi	wrist	see *capitate, hamate, lunate, pisiform b's, scaphoid, trapezium, trapezoid,* and *triquetral b's*	
clavicle	clavicula	shoulder	elongated, slender, curved bone (collar bone) lying horizontally at root of neck, in upper part of thorax	with sternum and ipsilateral scapula and cartilage of first rib
coccyx	o. coccygis	lower back	triangular bone formed usually by fusion of last 4 (sometimes 3 or 5) (coccygeal) vertebrae	with sacrum
concha, inferior nasal	concha nasalis inferior	skull	thin, rough plate of bone attached by one edge to side of each nasal cavity, the free edge curling downward	with ethmoid and ipsilateral lacrimal and palatine b's and maxilla
cuboid b.	o. cuboideum	foot	pyramidal bone, on lateral side of foot, in front of calcaneus	with calcaneus, lateral cuneiform b., fourth and fifth metatarsal b's, occasionally with navicular b.
cuneiform b., intermediate	o. cuneiforme intermedium	foot	smallest of 3 cuneiform b's, located between medial and lateral cuneiform b's	with navicular, medial and lateral cuneiform b's, and second metatarsal b.
cuneiform b., lateral	o. cuneiforme laterale	foot	wedge-shaped bone at lateral side of foot, intermediate in size between medial and intermediate cuneiform b's	with cuboid, navicular, intermediate cuneiform b's and second, third, and fourth metatarsal b's

*b. = bone; b's = (pl.) bones.
†o. = os; oss. = (L. pl.) ossa.

TABLE OF BONES – *Continued*

COMMON NAME*	NA EQUIVALENT†	REGION	DESCRIPTION	ARTICULATIONS
cuneiform b., medial	o. cuneiforme mediale	foot	largest of 3 cuneiform b's, at medial side of foot	with navicular, intermediate cuneiform, and first and second metatarsal b's
epistropheus. *See* axis				
ethmoid b.	o. ethmoidale	skull	unpaired bone in front of sphenoid b. and below frontal b., forming part of nasal septum and superior and medial conchae of nose	with sphenoid and frontal b's, vomer, and both lacrimal, nasal, and palatine b's, maxillae, and inferior nasal conchae
fabella		knee	sesamoid b. in lateral head of gastrocnemius muscle	with femur
femur	femur	thigh	longest, strongest, heaviest bone of the body (thigh b.)	proximally with hip b., distally with patella and tibia
fibula	fibula	leg	lateral and smaller of 2 bones of leg	proximally with tibia, distally with tibia and talus
frontal b.	o. frontale	skull	unpaired bone constituting anterior part of skull	with ethmoid and sphenoid b's, and both parietal, nasal, lacrimal, and zygomatic b's, and maxillae
hamate b.	o. hamatum	wrist	most medial of 4 bones of distal row of carpal b's	with fourth and fifth metacarpal b's and lunate, capitate, and triquetral b's
hip b.	o. coxae	pelvis and hip	broadest bone of skeleton, composed orginally of 3 bones which become fused together in acetabulum: *ilium,* broad, flaring, uppermost portion; *ischium,* thick, three-sided part behind and below acetabulum and behind obturator foramen; *pubis,* consisting of body (expanded anterior portion), inferior ramus (extending backward and fusing with ramus of ischium) and superior ramus (extending from body to acetabulum)	with femur, anteriorly with its fellow (at symphysis pubis), posteriorly with sacrum
humerus	humerus	arm	long bone of upper arm	proximally with scapula, distally with radius and ulna
hyoid b.	o. hyoideum	neck	U-shaped bone at root of tongue, between mandible and larynx	none; attached by ligaments and muscles to skull and larynx
ilium	o. ilium	pelvis	see *hip b.*	
incus	incus	ear	middle ossicle of chain in the middle ear, so named because of its resemblance to an anvil	with malleus and stapes
innominate b. *See* hip b.				

ischium	o. ischii	pelvis	see *hip b.*	
lacrimal b.	o. lacrimale	skull	thin, uneven scale of bone near rim of medial wall of each orbit	with ethmoid and frontal b's, and ipsilateral inferior nasal concha and maxilla
lunate b.	o. lunatum	wrist	second from thumb side of 4 bones of proximal row of carpus	with radius, and capitate, hamate, scaphoid, and triquetral b's
malleus	malleus	ear	most lateral ossicle of chain in middle ear, so named because of its resemblance to a hammer	with incus; fibrous attachment to tympanic membrane
mandible	mandibula	lower jaw	horseshoe-shaped bone carrying lower teeth	with temporal b's
maxilla	maxilla	skull (upper jaw)	paired bone, below orbit and at either side of nasal cavity, carrying upper teeth	with ethmoid and frontal b's, vomer, fellow maxilla, and ipsilateral inferior nasal concha and lacrimal, nasal, palatine, and zygomatic b's
maxilla, inferior. *See* mandible				
maxilla, superior, *See* maxilla				
metacarpal b's	oss. metacarpalia	hand	five miniature long bones of hand proper, slightly concave on palmar surface	first–trapezium and proximal phalanx of thumb; second–third metacarpal b., trapezium, trapezoid, capitate, and proximal phalanx of index finger (second digit); third–second and fourth metacarpal b's, capitate and proximal phalanx of middle finger (third digit); fourth–third and fifth metacarpal b's, capitate, hamate, and proximal phalanx of ring finger (fourth digit); fifth–fourth metacarpal b., hamate b. and proximal phalanx of little finger (fifth digit)
metatarsal b's	oss. metatarsalia	foot	five miniature long bones of foot, concave on plantar and slightly convex on dorsal surface	first–medial cuneiform b., proximal phalanx of great toe, and occasionally with second metatarsal b.; second–medial, intermediate, and lateral cuneiform b's, third and occasionally with first metatarsal b., and proximal phalanx of second toe; third–lateral cuneiform b., second and fourth metatarsal b's and proximal phalanx of third toe; fourth–lateral cuneiform b., cuboid b., third and fifth metatarsal b's, and proximal phalanx of fourth toe; fifth–cuboid b., fourth metatarsal b., and proximal phalanx of fifth toe

TABLE OF BONES—*Continued*

COMMON NAME*	NA EQUIVALENT†	REGION	DESCRIPTION	ARTICULATIONS
multangulum majus. *See* trapezium; trapezoid				
nasal b.	o. nasale	skull	paired bone, the two uniting in median plane to form bridge of nose	with frontal and ethmoid b's, fellow of opposite side, and ipsilateral maxilla
navicular b.	o. naviculare	foot	bone at medial side of tarsus, between talus and cuneiform b's	with talus and 3 cuneiform b's, occasionally with cuboid b.
occipital b.	o. occipitale	skull	unpaired bone constituting back and part of base of skull	with sphenoid b. and atlas and both parietal and temporal b's
os magnum. *See* capitate b.				
palatine b.	o. palatinum	skull	paired bone, the two forming posterior portion of bony palate	with ethmoid and sphenoid b's, vomer, fellow of opposite side, and ipsilateral inferior nasal concha and maxilla
parietal b.	o. parietale	skull	paired bone between frontal and occipital b's, forming superior and lateral parts of skull	with frontal, occipital, sphenoid, fellow parietal, and ipsilateral temporal b's
patella	patella	knee	small, irregularly rectangular compressed (sesamoid) bone over anterior aspect of knee (kneecap)	with femur
phalanges (proximal middle and distal phalanges)	oss. digitorum (phalanx proximalis, phalanx media, and phalanx distalis)	fingers and toes	miniature long bones, two only in thumb and great toe, three in each of other fingers and toes	proximal phalanx of each digit with corresponding metacarpal or metatarsal b., and phalanx distal to it; other phalanges with phalanges proximal and distal (if any) to them
pisiform b.	o. pisiforme	wrist	medial and palmar of 4 bones of proximal row of carpal b's	with triquetral b.
pubic b.	o. pubis	pelvis	see *hip b.*	
radius	radius	forearm	lateral and shorter of 2 bones of forearm	proximally with humerus and ulna; distally with ulna and lunate and scaphoid b's
ribs	costae	chest	12 pairs of thin, narrow, curved long bones, forming posterior and lateral walls of chest	all posteriorly with thoracic vertebrae; upper 7 pairs (true ribs) with sternum; lower 5 pairs (false ribs), by costal cartilages, with rib above or (lowest 2—floating ribs) unattached anteriorly.

sacrum	o. sacrum	lower back	wedge-shaped bone formed usually by fusion of 5 vertebrae below lumbar vertebrae, constituting posterior wall of pelvis	with fifth lumbar vertebra above, coccyx below, and with ilium at each side
scaphoid	o. scaphoideum	wrist	most lateral of 4 bones of proximal row of carpal b's	with radius, trapezium, and trapezoid, capitate and lunate b's
scapula	scapula	shoulder	wide, thin, triangular bone (shoulder blade) opposite second to seventh ribs in upper part of back	with ipsilateral clavicle and humerus
sesamoid b's	oss. sesamoidea	chiefly hands and feet	small, flat, round bones related to joints between phalanges or between digits and metacarpal or metatarsal b's; include also 2 at knee (fabella and patella)	
sphenoid b.	o. sphenoidale	base of skull	unpaired, irregularly shaped bone, constituting part of sides and base of skull and part of lateral wall of orbit	with frontal, occipital, and ethmoid b's, vomer and both parietal, temporal, palatine, and zygomatic b's
stapes	stapes	ear	most medial ossicle of chain in middle ear, so named because of its resemblance to a stirrup	with incus; ligamentous attachment to fenestra vestibuli
sternum	sternum	chest	elongated flat bone, forming anterior wall of chest, consisting of 3 segments: *manubrium* (topmost segment), *body* (in youth composed of 4 separate segments joined by cartilage), and *xiphoid process* (lowermost segment)	with both clavicles and upper 7 pairs of ribs
talus	talus	ankle	the "ankle bone," second largest of tarsal b's	with tibia, fibula, calcaneus, and navicular b.
tarsal b's	oss. tarsi	ankle and foot	see *calcaneus, cuboid, intermediate, lateral,* and *medial cuneiform b's, navicular b.,* and *talus*	
temporal b.	o. temporale	skull	irregularly shaped bone, one on either side, forming part of side and base of skull, and containing middle and inner ear	with occipital, sphenoid, mandible, and ipsilateral parietal and zygomatic b's
tibia	tibia	leg	medial and larger of 2 bones of lower leg (shin b.)	proximally with femur and fibula, distally with talus and fibula
trapezium	o. trapezium	wrist	most lateral of 4 bones of distal row of carpal b's	with first and second metacarpal b's and trapezoid and scaphoid b's
trapezoid b.	o. trapezoideum	wrist	second from thumb side of 4 bones of distal row of carpal b's	with second metacarpal b. and capitate, trapezium, and scaphoid b's
triquetral b.	o. triquetrum	wrist	third from thumb side of 4 bones of proximal row of carpal b's	with hamate, lunate, and pisiform b's and articular disk

TABLE OF BONES – *Concluded*

COMMON NAME*	NA EQUIVALENT†	REGION	DESCRIPTION	ARTICULATIONS
turbinate b., inferior. *See* concha, inferior nasal				
ulna	ulna	forearm	medial and longer of 2 bones of forearm	proximally with humerus and radius, distally with radius and articular disk
vertebrae (cervical, thoracic [dorsal], lumbar, sacral, and coccygeal)	vertebrae (vertebrae cervicales, vertebrae thoracicae, vertebrae lumbales, vertebrae sacrales, vertebrae coccygeae)	back	separate segments of vertebral column; about 33 in the child; uppermost 24 remain separate as true, movable vertebrae; the next 5 fuse to form the sacrum; the lowermost 3-5 fuse to form the coccyx	except first cervical (atlas) and fifth lumbar, each vertebra articulates with adjoining vertebrae above and below; the first cervical articulates with the occipital b. and second cervical vertebra (axis); the fifth lumbar with the fourth lumbar verbetra and sacrum; the thoracic vertebrae articulate also with the heads of the ribs
vomer	vomer	skull	thin bone forming posterior and posteroinferior part of nasal septum	with ethmoid and sphenoid b's and both maxillae and palatine b's
zygomatic b.	o. zygomaticum	skull	bone forming hard part of cheek and lower, lateral portion of rim of each orbit	with frontal and sphenoid b's and ipsilateral maxilla and temporal b.

B, and marked by a sudden attack of violent pain in the chest or epigastrium, fever of brief duration, and a tendency to recrudescence on the third day; called also devil's grip, epidemic myalgia, and epidemic myositis.

boron (bōr′on) a chemical element, atomic number 5, atomic weight 10.811, symbol B. (See table of ELEMENTS.)

Borrelia (bo-rel′e-ah) a genus of bacteria.

B. recurren′tis, a causative agent of relapsing fever, trasmitted by the human body louse.

B. vincen′tii, a species parasitic in the human mouth, occurring in large numbers with a fusiform bacillus in necrotizing ulcerative gingivitis (trench mouth) and in necrotizing ulcerative gingivostomatitis.

boss (bos) a rounded eminence.

bosselated (bos′ĕ-lāt″ed) marked or covered with bosses.

botryoid (bot′re-oid) shaped like a bunch of grapes.

botuliform (bot-u′lĭ-form) sausage-shaped.

botulin (bot′u-lin) a neurotoxin produced by *Clostridium botulinum* sometimes found in imperfectly preserved or canned foods.

botulism (bot′u-lizm) an extremely severe form of food poisoning due to a neurotoxin (botulin) produced by *Clostridium botulinum,* sometimes found in improperly canned or preserved foods.

The symptoms include vomiting, abdominal pain, headache, weakness, constipation, and nerve paralysis, which causes difficulty in seeing, breathing, and swallowing. Death is usually due to paralysis of the respiratory organs.

This is a highly dangerous form of food poisoning, and to prevent it home canning and preserving of all nonacid foods—that is, all foods other than fruits and tomatoes—must be done according to proper specific directions.

Treatment consists of removing unabsorbed toxin from the intestinal tract through gastric lavage and induced emesis, administration of antitoxin to neutralize the circulating toxin (care should be taken in considering the risk of ANAPHYLACTIC SHOCK), and providing required respiratory support.

Bouchard's nodes (boo-sharz′) cartilaginous and bony enlargements of the proximal interphalangeal joints of the fingers in degenerative joint disease.

bougie (boo′zhe) a slender, flexible, hollow or solid, cylindrical instrument for introduction into the urethra or other tubular organ, usually for calibrating or dilating constricted areas.

filiform b., a bougie of very slender caliber.

soluble b., a bougie composed of a substance that becomes fluid *in situ.*

bougienage (boo″zhĕ-nahzh′) passage of a bougie.

Bouillaud's syndrome (boo-e-yōz) the coincidence of pericarditis and endocarditis in acute articular rheumatism.

bouquet (boo-ka′) a structure resembling a cluster of flowers.

Bourneville's disease (boor′nĕ-vēz) tuberous sclerosis.

bouton (boo-taw′) [Fr.] button.

boutonneuse fever (boo-ton-ez′) a tickborne disease endemic in the Mediterranean area, Crimea, Africa, and India, due to infection with *Rickettsia conorii,* with chills, fever, primary skin lesion (tache noire), and rash appearing on the second to fourth day.

bovine (bo′vīn) pertaining to, characteristic of, or derived from the ox (cattle).

bowel (bow′el) the intestine.

b. training, a program designed to assist the patient having difficulty with the regulation and control of defecation. A program of this type may be indicated in a variety of cases ranging from chronic constipation to paralysis, as in PARAPLEGIA and HEMIPLEGIA. Patients who suffer from lesions or congenital anomalies of the intestinal tract also may benefit from a program of training.

Before planning a program of bowel control it is necessary to determine the cause of the difficulty, the patient's former bowel habits, and his specific symptoms. The plan devised will depend on the patient's needs and his physical, mental, and emotional capacities for cooperation in the planning and implementation of the program. It is necessary to know whether he can realistically be expected to achieve complete control, or if neural damage or anatomical and structural changes in the intestine prevent his reaching this goal. For example, a COLOSTOMY patient cannot achieve complete control over his bowel movements, but regulation of his diet and fluid intake can affect the number and consistency of the stools, giving him some sense of security. Diet also is important in all other types of bowel training in which the goal is regularity of defecation and stools of normal consistency.

It is important that the patient participate as much as possible in planning the program. He will need to give an accurate history of his bowel habits, his former use of laxatives and enemas, his usual time of day for bowel movements, and the frequency, and whether or not he is aware of the urge to defecate. As the program is carried out, revisions may be necessary as the patient learns which techniques are most helpful to him.

The major components of a bowel training program are choosing the location to ensure some degree of privacy, getting the patient into a sitting position, having him attempt defecation at a specific time that is most natural for him, regulating the food and fluid intake, and establishing some plan of regular exercise and physical activity.

In some cases of paralysis it may be necessary to stimulate bowel function through the use of suppositories and digital stimulation. Enemas, laxatives, and bulk-forming medications are used only if necessary, not on a regular basis if at all possible. These measures may be necessary, however, at the beginning of a bowel training program to remove constipated stool and FECAL IMPACTION.

Bowen's disease (bo′enz) intraepidermal squamous cell carcinoma, often occurring in multiple sites.

bowleg (bo′leg) an outward curvature of one or both legs near the knee; genu varum.

Bowman's capsule (bo′manz) malpighian capsule.

Bowman's disk (bo′manz) one of the flat, disklike plates making up a striated muscle fiber.

Bowman's glands (bo′manz) small mucous glands in olfactory mucosa; called also olfactory glands.

Boyle's law (boilz) at a constant temperature and mass the volume of a perfect gas varies inversely with pressure; that is, as increasing pressure is applied, the volume decreases. Conversely, as pressure is reduced, volume is increased.

Bozeman's position (böz′manz) the knee-elbow position with straps used for support.

B.P. 1. blood pressure. 2. boiling point. 3. British Pharmacopoeia, a publication of the General Medical Council, describing and establishing standards for medicines, preparations, materials, and articles used in the practice of medicine, surgery, or midwifery.

b.p. boiling point.

Br chemical symbol, *bromine.*

brace (brās) an orthopedic appliance or apparatus (ORTHOSIS), usually made of metal or leather, applied to the body, particularly the trunk and lower extremities, to support the weight of the body, to correct deformities, to prevent deformities, or to control involuntary movements, such as occur in spastic conditions. In some cases bracing is needed after remedial surgery. Back braces are used to treat certain kinds of backache.

Dental braces are used to support the teeth or to change their position in treatment of malocclusion.

brachi(o)- word element [L., Gr.], *arm.*

brachial (bra′ke-al) pertaining to the arm.

b. plexus, a nerve plexus originating from the ventral branches of the last four cervical and the first thoracic spinal nerves. It gives off many of the principal nerves of the shoulder, chest, and arms.

brachialgia (bra″ke-al′je-ah) pain in the arm.

brachiation (bra″ke-a′shun) locomotion in a position of suspension by means of the hands and arms, as by monkeys swinging from branch to branch.

brachiocephalic (bra″ke-o-sĕ-fal′ik) pertaining to the arm and head.

brachiocrural (bra′ke-o-kroo′ral) pertaining to the arm and leg.

brachiocubital (bra″ke-o-ku′bĭ-tal) pertaining to the arm and forearm.

brachiocyrtosis (bra″ke-o-ser-to′sis) crookedness of the arm.

brachium (bra′ke-um), pl. *bra′chia* [L.] 1. the arm; specifically the arm from shoulder to elbow. 2. any armlike process or structure.

b. conjuncti′vum cerebel′li, the superior cerebellar peduncle, a fibrous band extending from each hemisphere of the cerebellum upward over the pons, the two joining to form the sides and part of the roof of the fourth ventricle.

b. pon′tis, the brachium of the pons, the middle cerebellar peduncle.

brachy- word element [Gr.], *short.*

brachybasia (brak″e-ba′ze-ah) a slow, shuffling, short-stepped gait.

brachycardia (brak″e-kar′de-ah) bradycardia.

brachycephalic (brak″e-sĕ-fal′ik) having a short wide head, with a cephalic index of 81.0 to 85.4.

brachycephaly (brak″e-sef′ah-le) the state of being brachycephalic.

brachycheilia (brak″e-ki′le-ah) shortness of the lip.

brachydactyly (brak″e-dak′tĭ-le) abnormal shortness of the fingers and toes.

brachygnathia (brak″ig-na′the-ah) abnormal shortness of the mandible.

brachymetacarpia (brak″e-met″ah-kar′pe-ah) abnormal shortness of the metacarpal bones.

brachymetatarsia (brak″e-met″ah-tar′se-ah) abnormal shortness of the metatarsal bones.

brachymetropia (brak″e-mĕ-tro′pe-ah) myopia. adj., **brachymetrop′ic.**

brachyphalangia (brak″e-fah-lan′je-ah) abnormal shortness of one of the phalanges.

Bradford frame (brad′ford) a rectangular structure of gas pipe across which are stretched two strips of canvas, used as a bed frame for patients with fractures or disease of the hip or spine.

brady- word element [Gr.], *slow.*

bradyacusia (brad″e-ah-ku′ze-ah) dullness of hearing.

bradyarrhythmia (brad″e-ah-rith′me-ah) bradycardia.

bradycardia (brad″e-kar′de-ah) slowness of the heart beat, as evidenced by slowing of the pulse rate to less than 60 per minute. adj., **bradycar′diac.** The condition may occur following an infectious or febrile disease or it may be a symptom of a disorder of the conduction system of the heart. It sometimes occurs with increased intracranial pressure, obstructive jaundice, and myxedema.

A heart rate and pulse of less than 60 beats per minute can occur in normal persons, particularly during sleep. Trained athletes usually have a slow pulse and heart rate.

bradyesthesia (brad″e-es-the′ze-ah) slowness or dullness of perception.

bradyglossia (brad″e-glos′e-ah) abnormal slowness of utterance.

bradykinesia (brad″e-kin-ne′ze-ah) abnormal slowness of movement; sluggishness of physical and mental responses. adj., **bradykinet′ic.**

bradykinin (brad″e-ki′nin) a kinin composed of a chain of amino acids liberated by the action of trypsin or certain snake venoms on a globulin of blood plasma.

bradylalia (brad″e-la′le-ah) abnormally slow utterance due to a central nervous system lesion; bradyphasia.

bradylexia (brad″e-lek′se-ah) abnormal slowness in reading, due neither to defect in intelligence or of vision, nor to ignorance of the alphabet.

bradylogia (brad″e-lo′je-ah) abnormal slowness of speech, due to slowness of thinking, as in a mental disorder.

bradyphagia (brad″e-fa′je-ah) abnormal slowness of eating.

bradyphasia (brad″e-fa′ze-ah) slow utterance of speech.

bradyphemia (brad″e-fe′me-ah) slowness of speech.

bradyphrasia (brad″e-fra′ze-ah) slowness of speech due to mental disorder.

bradypnea (brad″e-ne′ah) abnormal slowness of breathing.

bradyspermatism (brad″e-sper′mah-tizm) abnormally slow ejaculation of semen.

bradysphygmia (brad″e-sfig′me-ah) abnormal slowness of the pulse.

bradystalsis (brad″e-stal′sis) abnormal slowness of peristalsis.

bradytachycardia (brad″e-tak″e-kar′de-ah) alternating attacks of bradycardia and tachycardia.

bradytocia (brad″e-to′she-ah) slow parturition.

bradyuria (brad″e-u′re-ah) slow discharge of urine.

brain (brān) encephalon; that part of the central nervous system contained within the cranium, comprising the forebrain, midbrain, and hindbrain, and developed from the embryonic neural tube. It is connected at its base with the spinal cord. The brain is a mass of soft, spongy, pinkish gray nerve tissue which, in the human, weighs about 3 lbs. (See also Plate 13.)

The brain is made up of billions of nerve cells, intricately connected with each other. It contains centers (groups of NEURONS and their connections) which control many involuntary functions, such as circulation, temperature regulation, and respiration, and interpret sensory impressions received from the eyes, ears, and other sense organs. Consciousness, emotion, thought, and reasoning are functions of the brain. It also contains centers or areas for associative memory which allow for recording, recalling, and making use of past experiences.

CEREBRUM. The largest and main portion of the brain, the cerebrum is made up of an outer coating, or cortex, of gray cells, several layers deep, which covers the CEREBRAL HEMISPHERES. The cortex is the thinking and reasoning brain, the intellect, as well as the part of the brain that receives information from the senses and directs the conscious movements of the body.

In appearance the cortex is rather like a relief map, with one very deep valley (longitudinal fissure) dividing it lengthwise into symmetrical halves, and each of the halves again divided by two major valleys and many shallower folds. The longitudinal fissure runs from the brow to the back of the head, and deep within it is a bed of matted white fibers, the corpus callosum, which connects the left and right halves of the brain hemispheres.

The major folds of the cortex divide each hemisphere of the cerebrum into four sections or lobes: the occipital lobe at the back of the skull, the parietal lobe at the side, the frontal lobe at the forehead, and the temporal lobe at the temple.

The Senses. The major senses of sight and hearing are well mapped in the cortex; the center for vision is at the back, in the occipital lobe, and the center for hearing is at the side, in the temporal lobe. Two other areas have been carefully explored; these are the sensory and motor areas for the body, which parallel each other along the fissure of Rolando.

In the sensory strip are located the brain cells that register all sensations. In the motor strip are the nerves that control the voluntary muscles. In both, the parts of the body are represented in an orderly way.

It is in the sensory areas of the brain that all perception takes place. Here sweet and sour, hot and cold, and the form of an object held in the hand are recognized. Here are sorted out the sizes, colors, depth, and space relationships of what the eye sees, and the timbre, pitch, intensity, and harmony of what the ear hears. The significance of these perceptions is interpreted in the cortex and other parts of the brain. A face is not merely seen; it is recognized as familiar or interesting or attractive. Remembering takes place at the same time as perception, so that other faces seen in the past, or experiences linked to that face are called up. Emotions may also be stirred. For this type of association the cortex draws on other parts of the brain by way of the communicating network of nerves.

A large part of the cortex that remains unmapped is thought to be involved in associative response. Factual knowledge and technical skills depend upon a background of experience and relationships between one kind of thing and another. Whether the mind is daydreaming, thinking rationally, or experiencing a surge of emotion, it draws upon an intensely personal and private background of association. The richer a person's life is in experiences that have made their imprint on thought and feeling, the richer will be the patterns upon which the conscious mind can draw.

Until recently, the frontal lobe, which particularly distinguishes man's brain from that of the lower orders, was thought to be an associative area. It was called a "silent" area because it seemed to have no specific function. This appears to be true for most of the frontal area, but it has been learned that in the frontal lobe, close to the small center for the sense of smell, is the center for speech.

Memory. In the temporal lobe, near the auditory area, is a recently discovered center for memory. This center appears to be a storehouse where memories are filed. When this area alone is stimulated, a particular event, a piece of music, or an experience long forgotten or deeply buried is brought to the individual's mind, complete in every detail. This is a very mechanical type of memory; when the stimulation is removed the memory ends. When it is applied again, the memory begins again, not where it left off, but from the beginning. (See also MEMORY.)

BRAIN STEM. This is the stemlike portion of the brain connecting the cerebral hemispheres with the spinal cord, and comprising midbrain, pons, and medulla oblongata. Some consider it to include the diencephalon.

Thalamus. Beneath the cortex, deep within the cerebral hemispheres, lies the THALAMUS. This organ is a relay station for body sensations; it also integrates these sensations on their way to the cortex. The thalamus is an organ of crude consciousness and of sensations of rough contact and extreme temperatures, either hot or cold. It is principally here that pain is felt. In the thalamus, responses are of the all-or-nothing sort; even mild stimuli would be felt as acutely painful if they were not graded and modified by the cortex.

Hypothalamus. Below the thalamus, at the base of the cerebrum, is the HYPOTHALAMUS. This organ, no larger than a lump of sugar, takes part in such vital activities as the ebb and flow of the body's fluids and the regulation of metabolism, blood sugar levels, and body temperature. It directs the body's many rhythms, including those of activity and rest, appetite and digestion, sexual desire, and menstrual and reproductive cycles. The hypothalamus is also the body's emotional brain. It is the integrating center of the autonomic NERVOUS SYSTEM, with its sympathetic and parasympathetic branches, and is situated close to the PITUITARY GLAND.

Midbrain. Just below the thalamus is the short narrow pillar of the MIDBRAIN. This contains a center for visual reflexes, such as moving the head and eyes, as well as a sound-activated center, obsolete in man, for pricking up the ears.

Medulla Oblongata. Below the midbrain is the medulla oblongata, the continuation upward of the spinal cord. In the medulla, the great trunk nerves, both motor and sensory, cross over, left to right and right to left, producing the puzzling phenomenon by which the left hemisphere of the cerebrum controls the right half of the body, while the right hemisphere controls the left half of the body. This portion of the brain also contains the centers that activate the heart, blood vessels, and respiratory system.

CEREBELLUM. The cerebellum, or "little brain," is attached to the back of the brain stem, under the curve of the cerebrum. It is connected, by way of the midbrain, with the motor area of the cortex and with the spinal cord, as well as with the SEMICIRCULAR CANALS, the organs of balance.

The function of the cerebellum appears to be to blend and coordinate motion of the various muscles involved in voluntary movements. It does not direct these movements; that is the function of the cortex. The cortex, however, operates in terms of movements, not of muscles. As a conscious function the cortex may, for example, direct the arm to pick up a glass of water; the cerebellum, which operates entirely below the level of consciousness, then translates this instruction into detailed actions by the 32 different muscles in the hand, plus several more in the arm and shoulder. When the cerebellum is injured, the patient's movements are jerky and uncoordinated.

CRANIAL NERVES. From the brain stem there emerge on their separate pathways the CRANIAL NERVES. They arise within the skull and, with one important exception, the VAGUS NERVE, serve the head and neck.

PROTECTION OF THE BRAIN. The brain is protected by the bony skull and by three layers of membranes, the meninges. Between the middle and inner layer is a space filled with CEREBROSPINAL FLUID, which serves as a shock absorber. The same system of membranes and fluid protects the spinal cord.

The brain is protected from harmful substances in the bloodstream by a barrier (the BLOOD-BRAIN BARRIER) that keeps some of the substances out of the brain entirely and delays the entry of others for hours or even days after they have penetrated the rest of the body.

DISORDERS OF THE BRAIN. In spite of protection of the brain by the skull and membranes and by the blood-brain barrier, a number of functional disorders and diseases may affect the brain.

Concussion or fracture of the skull may occur as a result of a severe shock or blow to the head (see also HEAD SURGERY). An interruption to the flow of blood to the brain may result from hemorrhage from one of the blood vessels serving the brain, or an obstruction caused by formation of a thrombus. Cerebral vascular accident (stroke) occurs when brain cells are deprived of their supply of blood.

Several diseases attack the brain specifically, including epilepsy, meningitis, and encephalitis.

Hydrocephalus, or "water on the brain," is caused by an abnormal accumulation of cerebrospinal fluid in the head.

Cerebral palsy is a name given to a motor disorder that results in inability to control muscle movement. It is usually the result of brain damage before, during, or immediately after birth.

Many diseases that originate in other parts of the body may affect the brain and nerves. Rabies and tetanus (lockjaw) are two examples of diseases that can cause brain damage. Others are syphilis, rheumatic fever, and alcoholism.

Brain Abscess. Brain abscess is a localized suppurative lesion within the intracranial cavity. The majority of cases are secondary to middle ear infections. Other causes include compound fracture of the skull with contamination of the brain tissue, sinusitis, and infections of the face, lung or heart. Symptoms include fever, malaise, irritability, severe headache, convulsions, vomiting, and other signs of intracranial hypertension. Treatment consists of surgical removal of the infected area and administration of antibiotic drugs.

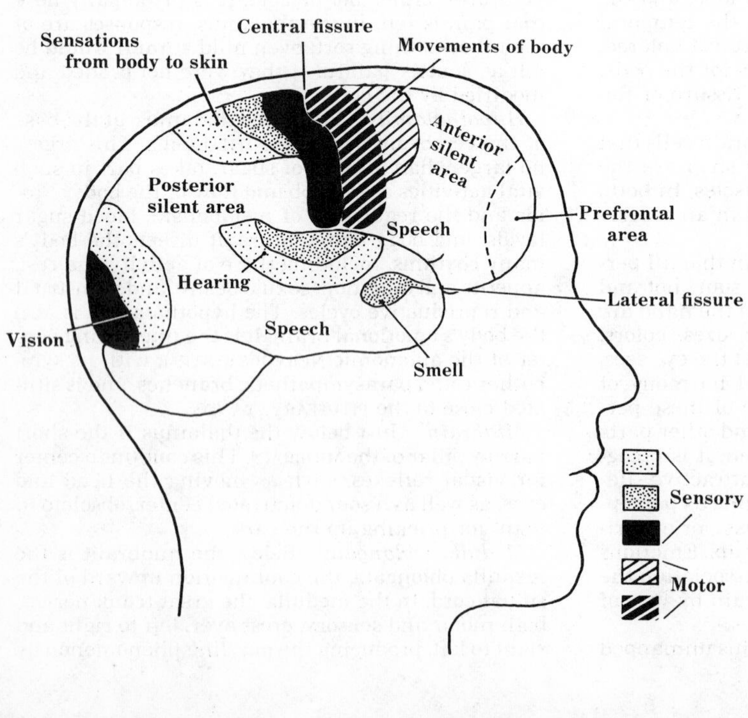

Projection areas of the brain.

Brain Tumor. Any abnormal growth within the skull creates a special problem because it is in a confined space and will press on normal brain tissue and interfere with the functions of the body controlled by the affected parts. This is true whether the tumor itself is benign or malignant. Fortunately, the functions of certain areas of the brain are well known, and a disturbance of some specific function guides physicians readily to the affected area. If diagnosed early, a benign tumor often can be removed surgically with a good chance of recovery. Malignant tumors are more difficult to remove.

The causes of brain tumor are not known. It is not a common disease, but it can occur at any age, and it can appear in any part of the brain. It may originate in the brain or may metastasize from a tumor in another part of the body.

The symptoms of brain tumor vary. Headache together with nausea is sometimes the first sign. The headache can be generalized or localized in one part of the head, and the pain is usually intense. Vomiting can be significant if it is sudden and without nausea. Disturbances of vision, loss of coordination in movement, weakness, and stiffness on one side of the body are also possible symptoms. Loss of sight, hearing, taste, or smell may result from brain tumor. A tumor can also cause a distortion of any of these senses, such as seeing flashes at the sides of the field of vision, or smelling odors or hearing sounds that do not exist. It can affect the ability to speak clearly or to understand the speech of others. Varying degrees of weakness or paralysis in the arms or legs may appear. A tumor may cause convulsions.

Changes in personality or mental ability are rare in cases of brain tumor. When such changes occur they may take the form of lapses of memory or absent-mindedness, mental sluggishness, or loss of initiative.

Brain tumor is treated surgically. As a result of recent progress in the methods of brain surgery, many cases of brain tumor can now be operated on successfully.

BRAIN SURGERY. There are two types of brain surgery—that which corrects damage to the brain itself, and that which seeks to remedy a condition in another part of the body. The first type includes operations to relieve tumors, brain injuries, abscesses, and infections, hydrocephalus, and PARKINSON'S DISEASE. The second includes surgery for severe neuralgia and MENIÈRE'S DISEASE.

Patient Care. Before surgery the patient's condition may be evaluated by such diagnostic tests as MYELOGRAPHY, PNEUMOENCEPHALOGRAPHY, BRAIN SCANNING, and other techniques used to determine the type and location of the lesion present. In addition to these tests it is important to establish baseline data on the patient's vital signs, personality, and speech characteristics, and to assess visual and other sensory responses and the patient's strength and coordination of motor activities. These data are then available as a basis for comparison in the detection of change postoperatively.

Physical preparation includes shaving the head, which may be done in the operating room after the patient has been anesthetized. If an enema is ordered preoperatively, the patient is cautioned not to strain, as this may cause increased intracranial pressure. The patient is instructed in the kinds of activity that will be allowed after surgery during the immediate postoperative period; for example, he may be required to lie with his head elevated and instructed not to cough or move vigorously. He and his family should be told the purpose of each procedure and kind of equipment expected to be used during the postoperative period. Knowledge of what to expect and how they may cooperate can do much to relieve apprehension and anxiety.

The patient's unit is prepared well in advance of his expected return from the recovery room. There should be assembled at the bedside a suction apparatus with catheters, a padded tongue depressor, equipment for measuring blood pressure and other vital signs, a lumbar puncture set, and a tray with syringes and needles and emergency drugs such as caffeine sodium benzoate and amobarbital. The bed is made so that the patient's head is at the foot of the bed to facilitate observation of the operative site and the changing of dressings. Side rails are applied to the bed.

Postoperatively, the patient will require constant attendance during the first 24 hours. Observations should include checking and recording the vital signs as ordered, usually every 15 minutes until they stabilize and then every 2 hours. The dressings are checked for drainage and if necessary reinforced with sterile dressings and towels. A clear, yellowish drainage may indicate leakage of cerebrospinal fluid and should be reported immediately. The pupils are observed for irregularity in size or fixation with failure to respond to light. The level of CONSCIOUSNESS is determined periodically as is the patient's reaction to stimuli.

As the patient progresses he is allowed a diet as tolerated and may be ambulatory if the surgeon deems this advisable.

brain death syndrome irreversible coma.

Brain's reflex (brānz) quadrupedal extensor reflex.

brain scanning a diagnostic technique for the detection of pathologic lesions in the intracranial cavity, based on the tendency of certain tumors and blood vessel lesions to accumulate radioactive substances more readily than does normal tissue. A radioisotope is given intravenously or injected into the subarachnoid space by lumbar or cisternal puncture. A scintillation detector (scanner) is passed over the head, and areas of isotopic concentration are recorded. Brain scanning is a valuable tool in the detection of tumors, cerebral vascular disorders, and obstruction to the flow of cerebrospinal fluid, as in hydrocephalus.

The patient and his family should be told that the procedure is simple and painless and there is no danger from the radioactive material used. A booklet available from the Mallinckrodt Chemical Works, St. Louis, Missouri, entitled "What You Can Expect from Your Brain Scan" can do much to alleviate fears and relieve anxiety in the patient and his family.

brain stem (brān′stem) the stemlike portion of the brain connecting the cerebral hemispheres with the spinal cord, and comprising the pons, medulla oblongata, and midbrain; considered by some to include the diencephalon.

brainwashing mental conditioning of a captive designed to secure attitudes conformable to the wishes of the captors.

branch (branch) ramus; a division or offshoot from a main stem, especially of blood vessels, nerves, or lymphatics.

bundle b., see BUNDLE BRANCH.

branchial (brang′ke-al) pertaining to, or resembling, gills of a fish or derivatives of homologous parts in higher forms.

b. arches, paired arched columns that bear the gills in lower aquatic vertebrates and which, in embryos of higher vertebrates, become modified into structures of the ear and neck.

b. clefts, the clefts between the branchial arches of the embryo, formed by rupture of the membrane separating corresponding entodermal pouch and ectodermal groove.

b. cyst, a cyst formed deep within the neck from an incompletely closed branchial cleft, usually located between the second and third branchial arches. The branchial arches develop during the first 2 months of embryonic life and are separated by four clefts, which correspond to the gills of a fish. As the fetus develops, these arches grow to form structures within the head and neck. Two of the arches grow together and enclose the cervical sinus, a cavity in the neck. A branchial cyst may develop within the cervical sinus. Called also branchiogenic or branchiogenous cyst.

b. groove, an external furrow lined with ectoderm, occurring in the embryo between two branchial arches.

branchiogenic (brang″ke-o-jen′ik) gill-forming; forming a branchial cleft.

Branham's sign (bran′hamz) bradycardia produced by digital closure of an artery proximal to an arteriovenous fistula.

brash (brash) a burning sensation in the stomach.

weaning b., diarrhea in infants occurring as a result of weaning.

Braxton Hicks contractions (braks′ton hiks) light, usually painless, irregular contractions of the uterus throughout pregnancy, gradually increasing in intensity and frequency and becoming more rhythmic during the third trimester; are often mistaken for true labor, and sometimes referred to as "false labor." They may be stimulated by the descent of the head of the fetus into the pelvic inlet. Braxton Hicks contractions are not as regular and rhythmic as are true LABOR contractions.

breast (brest) the front of the chest, especially the modified cutaneous, glandular structure it bears, the mamma. In women the breasts are secondary sex organs with the function of producing milk after childbirth. The term breast is less commonly used to refer to the breasts of the human male, which neither function nor develop.

At the tip of each breast is an area called the areola, usually reddish in color; at the center of this area is the NIPPLE. About 20 separate lactiferous ducts empty into a depression at the top of the nipple. Each duct leads from alveoli within the breast called lobules, where the milk is secreted. Along their length, the ducts have widened areas that form reservoirs in which milk can be stored. The ducts and lobules form the glandular tissue of which the breasts are chiefly composed. Connective tissue covers the glandular tissue and is itself sheathed in a layer of fatty tissue. The fatty tissue gives the breast its smooth outline and contributes to its size and firmness.

ABNORMALITIES AND DISORDERS OF THE BREAST. Amastia is the absence of one or both breasts at birth. Hypomastia is abnormal smallness of the

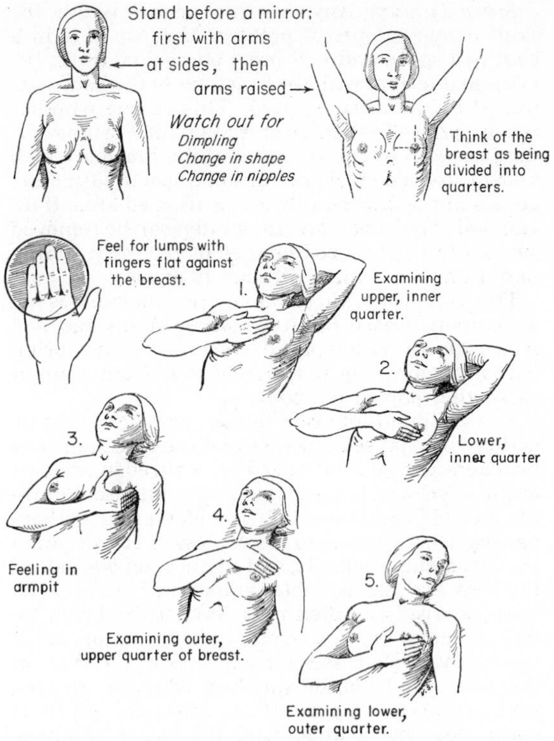

Self-examination of the breast. (From Dowling, H. F., and Jones, T.: That the Patient May Know. Philadelpha, W. B. Saunders Co., 1959.)

breasts. Hypertrophy of the breasts, abnormal enlargement of the breasts, is often a symptom of an endocrine disorder. Enlargement of the breasts in the male is called gynecomastia and is a not uncommon occurrence during adolescence. Polymastia is the presence of more than two breasts; it is more common in men than in women.

MASTITIS, inflammation of the breast, may occur in a variety of forms and in varying degrees of severity. Persistent cases may require mastectomy, but usually medical treatment suffices.

Breast Tumor. Benign tumors are growths of breast tissue that are usually encapsulated, do not metastasize, and usually can be removed by surgery without difficulty. Once removed, they do not recur. The most common of these is fibroadenoma, which is found most frequently in women between 21 and 25, although it can develop during and after menopause. This tumor grows rapidly during pregnancy, is seldom painful, and can be removed surgically. Another benign breast tumor is intraductal papilloma. It occurs most frequently in women between 35 and 55. Its symptons are discharge of blood or fluid containing blood from the nipples when the breast is compressed.

Breast cancer is one of the two most common types of cancer among women. Malignant tumors are rare among men, but can occur, usually in those between the ages of 50 and 60.

Breast cancer first appears as a small, painless lump, most frequently in the outer, upper portion of the breast. If the lump is near the surface, there is often a visible dimpling of the skin. If a malignant tumor is suspected, a biopsy is usually done to confirm the diagnosis. Surgery is usually indicated for malignant tumors, and is often followed by radiation therapy and sometimes by administration of hormones.

Recent improvements in x-ray techniques have made it possible to diagnose breast tumors in the beginning stages; however, the interpretation of the films must be done by an experienced radiologist. The term used for x-ray study of the breast is mammography. Another technique involves the use of infrared rays and is called thermography.

SELF-EXAMINATION OF THE BREAST. Women should train themselves to perform a simple self-examination of the breasts, described in the accompanying diagrams. The best time for this is just after menstruation when the breasts are normally soft. If any lump in the breast can be felt, a physican should be consulted immediately.

SURGERY OF THE BREAST. Surgical operations of the breast may be done for a variety of reasons. Mammoplasty refers to reconstructive surgery of the breast and is usually done for the purpose of reducing the size of large, pendulous breasts. Mastectomy is surgical removal of breast tissue and is most often done to treat cancer of the breast. Simple mastectomy is the surgical removal of breast tissue only; radical mastectomy involves removal of the entire breast and neighboring tissues such as the underlying pectoral muscles and axillary lymph nodes.

Patient Care. The psychologic aspects of surgery of the breast must always be considered. The breast is a symbol of femininity, motherhood, and sexual attractiveness; thus, a surgical procedure involving its partial or complete removal will always bring about some degree of emotional upheaval for the patient. Many women, out of fear of multilation or even death, resist surgical treatment of the breast even though the procedure may be necessary to save their lives. The patient should be reassured that modern prostheses and specially designed brassieres eliminate many of the outward signs of the loss of a breast.

Before the operation the surgeon usually explains the procedure to the patient and her family, stressing the need for surgery and the type of operation that will be performed. Diagnostic tests, such as x-ray examination and electrocardiography, are done to determine the extent of metastasis, if any, and to rule out heart disease. If there is doubt that the tumor is malignant, a biopsy is performed in the operating room so that, if cancer is present, mastectomy may be performed immediately. Since there is danger of spreading malignant cells once the tumor has been incised for biopsy, most surgeons prefer to perform the necessary surgery as soon as the sample tissue has been removed, examined and found to be malignant. For this reason, preoperative physical preparation of the skin should include complete cleansing and shaving of the entire breast and axilla.

After the operation dressings must be checked at frequent intervals for signs of excessive bleeding. The patient is placed on her back immediately after surgery; however, it is important to turn the patient gently, and to inspect the back on the operative side frequently to be sure blood is not seeping through. Although the dressings will be snug to reduce the loss of blood, they should not be so tight as to restrict circulation. Numbness and tingling or paralysis of the arm or hand should be reported at once.

Pulmonary complications are prevented by having the patient cough and breathe deeply at frequent intervals. This may produce discomfort in the operative site but is necessary. Pain may be quite severe the first few days after surgery, requiring frequent administration of analgesics as ordered by the physician.

Most surgeons wish to have the patient out of bed and walking the first day after mastectomy. Loss of balance is quite common immediately after this operation because of reduction in body weight on one side of the chest and restriction of arm movement on the affected side. The patient will need assistance and supervision while getting up and walking until she has adjusted to this change in her body structure.

Special exercises are essential to recovery from mastectomy. They are begun as soon as ordered by the surgeon and should be continued after the patient has returned home. Combing and brushing the hair, buttoning clothes at the back, "wall climbing" with the fingers, and arm-swinging exercises are all useful in preserving muscle tone and preventing contracture of the joints. The pamphlet "Help Yourself to Recovery," published by the American Cancer Society, is a useful guide for the patient during the convalescent period.

A program called "Reach to Recovery," sponsored by the American Cancer Society, is designed to help the patient adjust to the effects of mastectomy. The

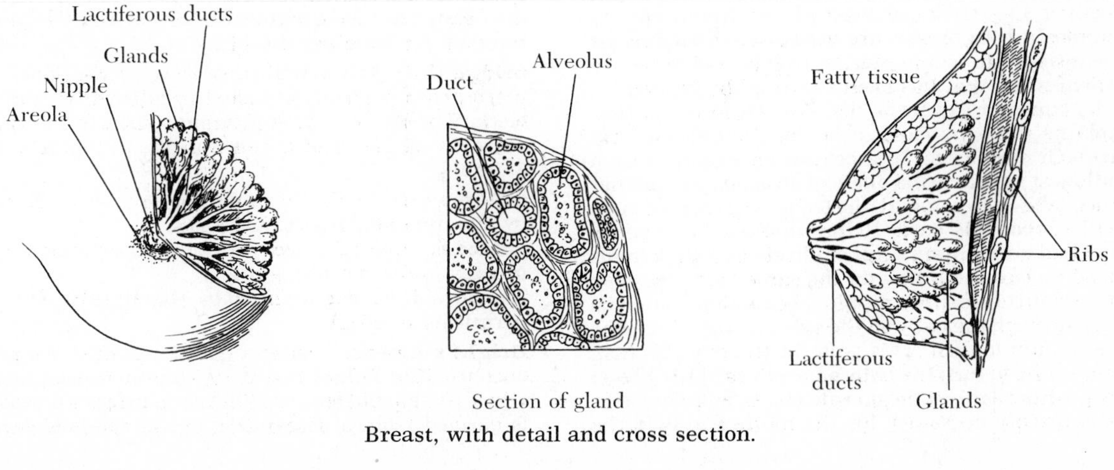

Breast, with detail and cross section.

attending physician's permission must be obtained before this rehabilitation program is begun. Volunteers, who usually have experienced a mastectomy themselves, visit the patient in the hospital and offer help in learning exercises, obtaining a breast prosthesis and brassiere, making suggestions for clothing, and offering more personal advice and counsel if requested by the patient.

chicken b., pectus carinatum.

breast feeding the method of feeding a baby with milk directly from the mother's breasts rather than from a bottle. Most physicians agree that breast feeding is usually better for baby and mother physically and emotionally, although there are conditions in which bottle feeding proves more satisfactory; sometimes a combination of both methods is the best solution.

ADVANTAGES. Breast milk is easily digested by the baby, for whom nature especially made it. It is safe and clean and contains practically everything the baby needs during the first months of his life. Babies who are breast fed are less susceptible to certain types of infections than bottle-fed babies. Also, the act of nursing helps to satisfy some of their emotional needs.

For the mother, nursing causes contraction of the muscles of the uterus, encouraging its rapid return to normal size. It makes her feel close to the baby, satisfying her emotional needs. It is less expensive and is not dependent on obtaining supplies. Nursing mothers need not gain any weight even though they eat well and drink a quart of milk a day (skimmed milk is suitable and is less fattening than whole milk). If the mother does not gain weight, and if she wears a good supporting brassiere, the appearance of her breasts is not appreciably altered. Nursing does not interfere with her health.

The LALECHE LEAGUE is a voluntary organization that encourages breast feeding and offers support and guidance to nursing mothers.

Women who feel a real revulsion toward the act of nursing a baby (and not just an objection on the grounds that it will be a nuisance) should not force themselves to do so. Nursing is a little better than bottle feeding, but there is not enough difference to matter significantly.

NURSING THE BABY. Breast feeding can be a very simple and satisfactory way to feed a baby. The mother should be relaxed about it, because tension or fatigue can inhibit the milk supply.

The breasts require little care. Just before each feeding, the hands are washed and the nipple (or nipples if both breasts are used at each feeding) is cleansed with some sterile cotton moistened in warm water that has been sterilized by boiling.

The mother can lie on one side while she nurses, holding the baby close to her in the curve of her arm. Or she can sit in a comfortable chair with a pillow at her back and one foot on a stool so that her knee will help support the baby; her curved arm will support his back. If the nipple or a finger is touched to the infant's lips or cheek, he will turn his head toward the breast on the same side and open his mouth to grasp the nipple. The mother should be sure to touch the baby on the side toward which she wants him to turn. This is an instinctive reaction, and trying to turn the baby's face toward the breast by pushing against the oposite cheek will not work. It is usually necessary for the mother to hold the breast back from the baby's nose with her free hand so that it will not interfere with his breathing.

As a rule, the baby nurses at one breast at a feeding, and the breasts are alternated with each feeding. In this way the breast is emptied completely; this prevents the milk from diminishing. Some babies nurse rapidly and some slowly. They usually get most of the milk during the first few minutes, but should be allowed to continue. The average nursing time is 15 to 20 minutes at first, but after 2 to 3 weeks, when the milk begins to flow more rapidly and the baby sucks more efficiently, the time may be reduced to as little as 10 minutes.

Menstruation usually does not interfere with nursing. Also, nursing is not, as some believe, an effective contraceptive measure.

breath (breth) the air taken in and expelled by the expansion and contraction of the thorax.

breathing (brēth'ing) the alternate inspiration and expiration of air into and out of the lungs (see also RESPIRATION).

frog b., glossopharyngeal b., respiration unaided by the primary or ordinary accessory muscles of respiration, the air being "swallowed" rapidly into the lungs by use of the tongue and the muscles of the pharynx; used by patients with chronic muscle paralysis to augment their vital capacity.

intermittent positive pressure b., IPPB, the active inflation of the lungs during inspiration under positive pressure from a cycling valve; a principle used in the operation of certain types of RESPIRATORS.

Breckinridge (brek'in-rij) Mary (1881-1965). American nurse, founder of the Frontier Nursing Service, a primarily midwifery service for women in remote areas of Kentucky. The Service, originally the Kentucky Committee for Mothers and Babies, was founded in 1925.

Breda's disease (bra'dahz) yaws.

breech (brēch) the buttocks.

b. presentation, presentation of the buttocks or feet of the fetus in labor (see also PRESENTATION).

bregma (breg'mah) the point on the surface of the skull at the junction of the coronal and sagittal sutures. adj. **bregmat'ic.**

brevicollis (brev'ĭ-kol'is) shortness of the neck.

Brevital (brev'ĭ-tal) trademark for a preparation of methohexital, an ultrashort-acting barbiturate.

Bricker procedure (brik'er) use of a segment of the ileum as a stoma for the diversion of urinary flow from the ureters (see also ILEAL CONDUIT).

Brickner's position (brik'nerz) the wrist is tied to the head of the bed to obtain abduction and external rotation, for shoulder disability.

bridge (brij) 1. a dental prosthesis bearing one or more artificial teeth attached to adjacent natural teeth. 2. pons. 3. a protoplasmic structure uniting adjacent elements of a cell, similar in plants and animals.

bridgework (brij'werk) a partial denture retained by attachments other than clasps.

fixed b., one retained with crowns or inlays cemented to the natural teeth.

removable b., one retained by attachments which permit its removal.

Bright's disease (brīts) a broad descriptive term once used for kidney disease with proteinuria, usually GLOMERULONEPHRITIS. The name Bright's disease is derived from a description of the diseases published in 1827 by Richard Bright, an English physician.

Brill's disease (brilz) recrudescent typhus.

Brill-Symmers disease (bril sim′erz) giant follicular lymphadenopathy.

Brill-Zinsser disease (bril zin′ser) recrudescent typhus.

brim (brim) the edge of the superior strait of the pelvis.

brisement (brēz-maw′) [Fr.] a crushing, especially the breaking up of an ANKYLOSIS.

British antilewisite BAL; dimercaprol, a chelating agent used against poisoning with arsenic, gold, mercury, and certain other metals.

British thermal unit B.T.U., a unit of heat being the amount necessary to raise the temperature of 1 pound of water from 39° to 40° F., generally considered the equivalent of 252 calories.

Broca's aphasia (bro′kahz) expressive aphasia.

Broca's center (bro′kahz) speech center.

Broca's gyrus (bro′kahz) the inferior frontal gyrus.

Broca's motor speech area (bro′kahz) an area comprising parts of the opercular and triangular portions of the inferior frontal gyrus; injury to this area may result in expressive APHASIA.

Broca's parolfactory area (bro′kahz) an area of the cortex on the medial surface of each cerebral hemisphere, immediately in front of the gyrus subcallosus. Called also area subcallosa.

Brock syndrome (brok) middle lobe syndrome.

Brodmann's areas (brod′manz) specific occipital and preoccipital areas of the cerebral cortex, distinguished by differences in the arrangement of their six cellular layers, and identified by number. They are considered to be the seat of specific functions of the brain.

bromatotherapy (bro″mah-to-ther′ah-pe) dietotherapy.

bromatoxism (bro″mah-tok′sizm) food poisoning.

bromelain (bro′mĕ-lān) any of a group of proteolytic and milk-clotting enzymes derived from the pineapple plant, *Ananas sativus.* In the plural, a concentrate of these enzymes, used as an anti-inflammatory agent. Also used in tenderizing meat, preparing protein hydrolysates, and chill-proofing beer.

bromhidrosis (bro″mĭ-dro′sis) the secretion of foul-smelling perspiration.

bromide (bro′mīd) a binary compound of bromine. Many of these compounds have a depressant effect on the nervous system and can be used as sedatives. Since bromides are slowly eliminated and may cumulate in the body to reach toxic amounts, their use is of questionable value and many hospital formularies have omitted them. Patent medicines and drugs sold over the counter frequently contain bromides, and bromide poisoning (BROMINISM) is relatively common.

bromidrosis (bro″mĭ-dro′sis) bromhidrosis.

bromine (bro′mēn) a chemical element, atomic number 35, atomic weight 79.909, symbol Br. (See table of ELEMENTS.)

brominism (bro′min-izm) poisoning by excessive use of bromine or its compounds. This condition occurs when the bromine concentration in the body fluids is high enough to have a toxic and depressant action on the central nervous system. The toxic level varies with each individual and is also somewhat dependent on chloride intake because the bromide ion and the chloride ion are equally absorbed and distributed throughout the same fluid compartments. This means that in a person with a limited salt intake bromine accumulates more quickly and severe poisoning can occur after ingestion of an amount of bromine that would be relatively harmless for a person with a normal or high salt intake.

Many cases of brominism result from indiscriminate use of patent medicines advertised as "nerve tonics" and "headache remedies" containing bromide. The early symptoms may be similar to the symptoms for which the patient is taking the patent medicine, and correct diagnosis and treatment of the condition may be delayed. The symptoms of bromine poisoning include acne, coldness of arms and legs, fetid breath, sleeplessness, impotence, headache, irritability, emotional instability, malaise, and mental aberrations such as hallucinations, amnesia, and disorientation.

Treatment consists of immediate curtailment of bromine ingestion and efforts to eliminate the substance from the body. Mercurial diuretics aid in bromine removal. Enteric-coated tablets of ammonium and sodium chloride are prescribed if they are not contraindicated by cardiac or renal disease. The removal of bromine from the system may take as long as several months. In severe, acute poisoning the bromine may be removed by DIALYSIS.

When an emotional disturbance or mental illness is the primary cause of brominism, psychotherapy is indicated.

bromisovalum (brōm″i-so-val′um) a mild, quick-acting sedative and hypnotic of moderately long action. It does not belong to the barbiturate group. Long-term use can lead to BROMINISM.

bromochlorotrifluoroethane (bro″mo-klo″ro-tri-flu″o-ro-eth′ān) halothane, a general anesthetic.

bromocriptine (bro″mo-krip′tēn) a dopamine agonist, a derivative of ergot alkaloids used to suppress prolactin secretion. It raises serum growth hormone levels in normal persons, but lowers them in persons with acromegaly.

bromoderma (bro″mo-der′mah) a skin eruption due to use of bromides.

bromodiphenhydramine (bro″mo-di″fen-hi′drah-mēn) a compound used as an antihistamine in the form of the hydrochloride salt.

bromomania (bro″mo-ma′ne-ah) a mental disorder induced by misuse of bromides.

bromomenorrhea (bro″mo-men″o-re′ah) menstruation characterized by an offensive odor.

5-bromouracil (bro″mo-u′rah-sil) a pyrimidine analogue with mutagenic properties.

brompheniramine (brōm″fen-ir′ah-mēn) a pyridine derivative used as an antihistamine in the form of the maleate salt.

Bromsulphalein (brōm-sul′fah-lin) trademark for sulfobromophthalein, a dye used in testing liver function; abbreviation BSP. In the laboratory test, the dye is introduced into the circulatory system and a blood sample is withdrawn 30 or 45 minutes later, depending on the dose injected. The parenchymal cells remove almost all of the dye within this time if they are functioning normally. The rate of removal is influenced by the blood flow through the portal circulation, the functioning capacity of the liver cells, and the patency of the biliary tract.

The patient must be in a fasting state for the test. A blood sample is taken, and then the Bromsulphalein is given by vein very slowly. The amount given is determined by body weight (2 or 5 mg. per kilogram of body weight). While the dye is being administered the patient should be watched closely for signs of an allergic reaction. Thirty minutes after the injection (or 45 minutes if 5 mg. per kilogram of body weight was given) a blood sample is taken from a vein in the opposite arm. Normally the liver cells remove about 95 per cent of the dye in that period of time, leaving about 5 per cent in the circulating blood.

Bromural (brōm-u'ral) trademark for preparations of bromisovalum, a sedative and hypnotic.

bronchadenitis (brongk"ad-ĕ-ni'tis) inflammation of the bronchial glands.

bronchi (brong'ki) plural of *bronchus.*

bronchial (brong'ke-al) pertaining to or affecting one or more bronchi.

b. asthma, asthma.

b. calculus, see LUNG CALCULUS.

b. spasm, bronchospasm.

b. tree, the bronchi and their branching structures.

bronchiarctia (brong"ke-ark'she-ah) bronchostenosis.

bronchiectasis (brong"ke-ek'tah-sis) chronic dilatation of the bronchi and bronchioles with secondary infection, usually involving the lower lobes of the lung. The condition may occur as a congenital malformation of the alveoli with resultant dilation of the terminal bronchi. Most often it is an acquired disease secondary to partial obstruction of the bronchi with necrotizing infection. Primary diseases leading to bronchiectasis include chronic sinusitis, allergy, whooping cough, pneumonia, influenza, tuberculosis, and lung tumor. The presence of a foreign body in the respiratory tract can produce bronchiectasis.

SYMPTOMS. The most immediate symptom of bronchiectasis is persistent coughing. The coughing may be mild, often occurring when the patient first gets up in the morning. In severe cases, the coughing becomes more violent as the walls of the bronchial tubes thicken and secrete quantities of mucus. The muscles may become so weak that even violent coughing fails to expel the mucus. Pus may also be secreted, and the cilia destroyed. In advanced cases the sputum and breath may become foul-smelling, and the patient may suffer loss of appetite, anemia, fever, intermittent attacks of pneumonia, and a general lowering of resistance to infection.

TREATMENT. To maintain the strength and general health of the patient, fresh air and sunshine, a good diet, and plenty of rest are essential. A move to a mild climate may be of great benefit. Cigarette smoking should be stopped. If the disease is fairly well localized, it may be relieved by surgery. Penicillin or other antibiotics are sometimes useful, particularly in controlling other infections, which may weaken the patient and further lower his resistance.

Long-term care is essentially the same as for any patient with CHRONIC OBSTRUCTIVE PULMONARY DISEASE.

bronchiloquy (brong-kil'o-kwe) high-pitched pectoriloquy due to lung consolidation.

bronchiocele (brong'ke-o-sēl") dilatation or swelling of a bronchiole.

bronchiogenic (brong"ke-o-jen'ik) bronchogenic.

bronchiole (brong'ke-ōl) one of the successively smaller channels into which the segmental bronchi divide within the bronchopulmonary segments. adj., **bronchi'olar.**

respiratory b., the final branch of a bronchiole, communicating directly with the alveolar ducts; a subdivision of a terminal bronchiole, it has alveolar outcroppings and itself divides into several alveolar ducts. (See Plate 6.)

bronchiolectasis (brong"ke-o-lek'tah-sis) dilatation of the bronchioles.

bronchiolitis (brong"ke-o-li'tis) inflammation of the bronchioles; bronchopneumonia.

acute obliterating b., cirrhosis of the lung due to hardening of the walls of the bronchioles.

b. exudati'va, exudative b., inflammation of the bronchioles with exudation of Curschmann's spirals (coiled mucinous fibrils) and gray, tenacious sputum; often associated with asthma.

b. fibro'sa oblit'erans, bronchiolitis marked by in-growth of connective tissue from the wall of the terminal bronchi, with occlusion of their lumina.

vesicular b., bronchopneumonia.

bronchiolus (brong-ki'o-lus), pl., *bronchi'oli* [L.] bronchiole.

bronchiospasm (brong'ke-o-spazm") bronchospasm.

bronchiostenosis (brong"ke-o-stĕ-no'sis) bronchostenosis.

bronchitis (brong-ki'tis) inflammation of one or more bronchi. adj., **bronchit'ic.** Bronchitis may be either an acute or chronic disorder and frequently involves the trachea as well as the bronchi (tracheobronchitis). The acute stage of the disease often is an extension of an upper respiratory infection which is usually viral in origin. Causes other than infectious agents are physical and chemical irritants that are inhaled in air polluted by dust, automobile exhaust, industrial fumes, and tobacco smoke.

ACUTE BRONCHITIS. Acute bronchitis is most often encountered in small children and in the elderly or the debilitated. It is particularly serious in infants and small children because their bronchi are smaller and more easily obstructed. The elderly and debilitated are prime targets for complications of bronchitis because they are more susceptible to secondary infections.

Symptoms of acute bronchitis include the early symptoms of an upper respiratory infection or common cold which progress to chest pain, fever, and a dry, irritating cough. Later the cough becomes more productive of mucopurulent to purulent sputum. There may be moderate fever with accompanying chills, muscle soreness, and headache.

The condition is treated conservatively, with antibiotics being administered only as indicated by a positive sputum culture. Symptoms may be relieved through the use of humidifying devices that produce either warm or cool moist air, cough mixtures and AEROSOLS to reduce coughing and soothe the irritated tracheal and bronchial mucosa, and bed rest to promote healing and minimize the effects of the inflammation. Fluids are forced and a well-balanced bland diet is recommended.

Acute bronchitis and tracheobronchitis require a period of convalescence to avoid development of a chronic condition. Although the disease in its acute form occurs most often in the winter months, repeated bouts indicate a chronic bronchitis.

CHRONIC BRONCHITIS. This condition is characterized by increased secretion from the bronchial mucosa and obstruction of the respiratory passages. It is a stubborn disease that interferes with the flow of air to and from the lungs, causes shortness of breath, induces persistent coughing and expectoration, breeds infection, and causes necrosis and fibrosis of the respiratory tract.

The symptoms and treatment of chronic bronchitis are the same as those of any CHRONIC OBSTRUCTIVE PULMONARY DISEASE. There is no cure for the disorder and its management requires long-range planning involving patient education and cooperation in carrying out the prescribed regimen.

bronchocandidiasis (brong″ko-kan″dĭ-di′ah-sis) candidiasis of the respiratory tree, occurring in a mild afebrile form manifested as chronic bronchitis, and in a usually fatal form resembling tuberculosis.

bronchocavernous (brong″ko-kav′er-nus) both bronchial and cavitary.

bronchocele (brong′ko-sēl) localized dilatation of a bronchus.

bronchoconstriction (brong″ko-kon-strik′shun) bronchostenosis.

bronchoconstrictor (brong″ko-kon-strik′tor) 1. narrowing the lumina of the air passages of the lungs. 2. an agent that causes such constriction.

bronchodilatation (brong″ko-dil″ah-ta′shun) a dilated state of a bronchus, or the site at which a bronchus is dilated.

bronchodilator (brong″ko-di-la′tor) 1. expanding the lumina of the air passages of the lungs. 2. an agent that causes dilation of the bronchi. Epinephrine is one of the most powerful bronchodilators and can be administered by INJECTION or by AEROSOL. Isoproterenol (Isuprel) affects the bronchi by relieving bronchospasm through its action on smooth muscle. It is one of the most widely used aerosol bronchodilators. Other drugs used to enlarge the lumen of the bronchi and thereby facilitate breathing and removal of secretions are isoetharine, atropine, and aminophylline.

bronchoesophageal (brong″ko-e-sof″ah-je′al) pertaining to or communicating with a bronchus and the esophagus.

bronchoesophagology (brong″ko-e-sof″ah-gol′o-je) the branch of medicine concerned with the air passages (bronchi) and esophagus.

bronchoesophagoscopy (brong″ko-e-sof″ah-gos′ko-pe) instrumental examination of the bronchi and esophagus.

bronchogenic (brong″ko-jen′ik) originating in the bronchi.

bronchogram (brong′ko-gram) the film obtained by bronchography.

bronchography (brong-kog′rah-fe) radiography of the lungs after instillation of an opaque medium in the bronchi.

broncholith (brong′ko-lith) a bronchial calculus.

broncholithiasis (brong″ko-lĭ-thi′ah-sis) a condition in which calculi are present within the lumen of the tracheobronchial tree.

bronchology (brong-kol′o-je) the study and treatment of diseases of the tracheobronchial tree. adj. **broncholog′ic.**

bronchomalacia (brong″ko-mah-la′she-ah) a deficiency in the cartilaginous wall of the trachea or a bronchus that may lead to atelectasis or obstructive emphysema.

bronchomoniliasis (brong″ko-mo″nĭ-li′ah-sis) bronchocandidiasis.

bronchomotor (brong″ko-mo′tor) affecting the caliber of the bronchi.

bronchopathy (brong-kop′ah-the) any disease of the bronchi.

bronchophony (brong-kof′o-ne) the sound of the voice as heard through the stethoscope applied over a healthy large bronchus.

bronchoplasty (brong′ko-plas″te) plastic surgery of a bronchus; surgical closure of a bronchial fistula.

bronchoplegia (brong″ko-ple′je-ah) paralysis of the muscles of the walls of the bronchial tubes.

bronchopleural (brong″ko-ploor′al) pertaining to a bronchus and the pleura, or communicating with a bronchus and the pleural cavity.

bronchopneumonia (brong″ko-nu-mo′ne-ah) inflammation of the bronchi and lungs, usually beginning in the terminal bronchioles. (see also PNEUMONIA).

bronchopneumopathy (brong″ko-nu-mop′ah-the) disease of the bronchi and lung tissue.

bronchopulmonary (brong″ko-pul′mo-ner″e) pertaining to the bronchi and lungs.

b. segment, one of the smaller divisions of the lobe of a lung, separated from others by a connective tissue septum and supplied by its own branch of the bronchus leading to the particular lobe.

bronchorrhagia (brong″ko-ra′je-ah) hemorrhage from the bronchi.

bronchorrhaphy (brong-kor′ah-fe) suture of a bronchus.

bronchorrhea (brong″ko-re′ah) excessive discharge of mucus from the bronchi.

bronchoscope (brong′ko-skōp) an endoscope especially designed for passage through the trachea to permit inspection of the interior of, or for removal of foreign bodies from, the tracheobronchial tree. adj., **bronchoscop′ic.**

bronchoscopy (brong-kos′ko-pe) inspection of the interior of the tracheobronchial tree through a bronchoscope. Bronchoscopy is used as a diagnostic aid and therapeutically.

As an aid to diagnosis the bronchoscope allows for visualization of the bronchial mucosa and removal of tissue for biopsy. Bronchial washings and collection of secretions are done at the time of bronchoscopy to obtain samples for culture and cytological examination. Therapeutically, the bronchoscope permits removal of foreign bodies that have been aspirated into the bronchial tree and also may be used to facilitate suctioning of the lower airway. The latter technique is done at the bedside and anesthesia is not considered necessary.

PATIENT CARE. If the fiberoptic bronchoscope is used at the bedside as an adjunct to bronchial hygiene and removal of secretions, it should be used only by health care personnel who have been trained in the technique. It has the advantage of allowing for more precise suctioning with less trauma to the respiratory tract, because it is possible to visualize the areas needing suctioning and to reach lower segments not accessible to the larger suction catheter.

Bronchoscopy as a surgical diagnostic procedure requires preparation and instruction of the patient in regard to the purpose of the procedure, what he can expect to be done, and how he may cooperate during the procedure. A topical anesthetic is used most often, but in some cases the patient may have general anesthesia.

Food and fluids are withheld for 8 hours before bronchoscopy is performed. The patient should brush his teeth and wash out his mouth carefully before the procedure to lessen the danger of introducing bacteria from the mouth into the bronchi. Dentures are removed and any loose teeth are brought to the attention of the physician. A mild sedative such as one of the barbiturates may be given prior to the bronchoscopy. This medication plus instructions to the patient and a full explanation of what is going to be done will help him relax and make the passing of the bronchoscope into the bronchi easier and less traumatic.

After bronchoscopy, fluids and food are withheld until the effects of the local anesthetic have worn off and the gag reflex has returned completely. The patient must be observed for signs of bleeding from the throat and respiratory embarrassment. Since swelling of the larynx may necessitate a TRACHEOSTOMY, the equipment should be readily at hand. The patient should be kept quiet and discouraged from talking or coughing.

bronchospasm (brong'ko-spazm) bronchial spasm; spasmodic contraction of the muscular coat of the smaller divisions of the bronchi, such as occurs in asthma.

bronchospirography (brong"ko-spi-rog'rah-fe) the recording of bronchospirometry results.

bronchospirometry (brong"ko-spi-rom'ĕ-tre) determination of vital capacity, oxygen intake, and carbon dioxide excretion of a single lung, or simultaneous measurements of the function of each lung separately.

differential b., measurement of the function of each lung separately.

bronchostaxis (brong"ko-stak'sis) bleeding from the bronchial wall.

bronchostenosis (brong"ko-stĕ-no'sis) stricture or cicatricial diminution of the caliber of a bronchial tube.

spasmodic b., a spasmodic contraction of the walls of the bronchi.

bronchostomy (brong-kos'to-me) surgical creation of an opening through the chest wall into the bronchus.

bronchotomy (brong-kot'o-me) incision of a bronchus.

bronchotracheal (brong"ko-tra'ke-al) pertaining to the bronchi and trachea.

bronchovesicular (brong"ko-vĕ-sik'u-ler) pertaining to the bronchi and alveoli.

bronchus (brong'kus), pl. *bron'chi* [L.] any of the larger passages conveying air to (right or left principal bronchus) and within the lungs (lobar and segmental bronchi). (See also RESPIRATION and plate 5.)

bronze diabetes (bronz di"ah-be'tēz) a disorder of iron metabolism, with deposits of iron-containing pigments in the body tissues, with bronze pigmentation of the skin, diabetes mellitus, and cirrhosis of the liver; called also hemochromatosis and iron storage disease.

brow (brow) the forehead, or either lateral half of it.

Brown-Séquard's syndrome (brown-sa-karz') paralysis and loss of descriminatory and joint sensation on one side of the body and of pain and temperature sensation on the other, due to a lesion involving one side of the spinal cord.

Brucella (broo-sel'ah) a genus of bacteria.

B. abor'tus, the causative agent of infectious abortion in cattle and the commonest cause of BRUCELLOSIS in man.

B. meliten'sis, the causative agent of BRUCELLOSIS, occurring primarily in goats as the reservoir of infection.

B. su'is, a species found in swine that is capable of producing severe disease in man.

brucella (broo-sel'ah), pl. *brucel'lae.* any member of the genus *Brucella.* adj. **brucel'lar.**

Brucellergen (broo-sel'er-jen) trademark for a solution of nucleoproteins derived from *Brucella*; used in a skin test for brucella infection.

brucellosis (broo"sel-o'sis) a generalized infection involving primarily the reticuloendothelial system, marked by remittent undulant fever, malaise, headache, and anemia. It is caused by various species of *Brucella* and is transmitted to man from domestic animals such as pigs, goats, and cattle, especially through infected milk or contact with the carcass of an infected animal.

The disease is also called undulant fever because one of the major symptoms in man is a fever that fluctuates widely at regular intervals. The symptoms in the beginning stages are difficult to notice and include loss of weight and increased irritability. As the illness advances, headaches, chills, diaphoresis, and muscle aches and pains appear. It is possible for these symptoms to persist for years, either intermittently or continuously, although most patients recover completely within 2 to 6 months. Diagnosis is confirmed by blood tests.

Treatment consists of bed rest, antibiotics, and a high intake of vitamins.

Prevention is best accomplished by the pasteurization of milk and a program of testing, vaccination, and elimination of infected animals.

Brudzinski's sign (brood-zin'skēz) 1. in meningitis, bending the patient's neck usually produces flexion of the knee and hip. 2. in meningitis, passive flexion of the lower limb on one side causes a similar movement in the opposite limb.

Brugia (broo'je-ah) a genus of filarial worms.

B. mala'yi, a species similar to, and often found in association with, *Wuchereria bancrofti,* which causes human filariasis and elephantiasis throughout Southeast Asia, the China Sea, and eastern India.

bruise (bro͞oz) superficial discoloration due to hemorrhage into the tissues from ruptured blood vessels beneath the skin surface, without the skin itself being broken; called also CONTUSION.

bruit (brwe, bro͞ot) [Fr.] a sound or murmur heard in auscultation, especially an abnormal one.

aneurysmal b., a blowing sound heard over an aneurysm.

placental b., a soft, blowing auscultatory sound

supposed to be produced by the blood current in the placenta. Called also placental souffle.

Brunner's glands (brun'erz) glands in the submucosa of the duodenum, opening into the glands of the small intestine; called also duodenal glands.

brush border (brush bor'der) a specialization of the free surface of a cell, consisting of minute cylindrical processes (microvilli) that greatly increase the surface area.

bruxism (bruk'sizm) grinding of the teeth, especially during sleep.

B.S. Bachelor of Surgery; Bachelor of Science; breath sounds; blood sugar.

BSA body surface area.

BSP Bromsulphalein, a dye used in the study of liver function.

B.T.U., B.Th.U. British thermal unit.

buba (boo'bah) 1. mucocutaneous leishmaniasis. 2. yaws.

bubo (bu'bo) an enlarged and inflamed lymph node, particularly in the axilla or groin, resulting from absorption of infective material and occurring in various diseases, e.g., lymphogranuloma venereum, plague, syphilis, gonorrhea, chancroid, and tuberculosis.

indolent b., a hard, nearly painless bubo that shows no tendency to break.

bubonalgia (bu″bo-nal'je-ah) pain in the groin.

bubonic (bu-bon'ik) characterized by or pertaining to buboes.

b. plague, a highly contagious and severe disease caused by the bacillus *Pasteurella pestis* carried in infected rats and transmitted to man by fleas (see also PLAGUE).

bubonocele (bu-bon'o-sēl) inguinal or femoral hernia forming a swelling in the groin.

bucardia (bu-kar'de-ah) extreme enlargement of the heart (see also COR BOVINUM).

bucca (buk'ah) [L.] the cheek.

buccal (buk'al) pertaining to or directed toward the cheek.

bucco- word element [L.], *cheek.*

Buck's extension (bukz) extension of fractured leg by weights, the foot of the bed being raised so that the body makes counterextension.

buclizine (bu'klĭ-zēn) a minor tranquilizer having antiemetic, antihistaminic, and anticholinergic activities; used as the dihydrochloride salt.

bucnemia (buk-ne'me-ah) diffuse, tense, inflammatory swelling of the leg.

bud (bud) a structure resembling the bud of a plant, especially a protuberance in the embryo from which an organ or part develops.

end b., the remnant of the embryonic primitive knot, from which arises the caudal part of the trunk.

limb b., one of the four lateral swellings appearing in vertebrate embryos, which develop into the two pairs of limbs.

tail b., 1. the primordium of the caudal appendage. 2. end bud.

taste b's, end organs of the gustatory nerve containing the receptor surfaces for the sense of TASTE.

ureteric b., an outgrowth of the mesonephric duct giving rise to all but the nephrons of the permanent kidney.

b. of urethra, bulb of urethra.

budding (bud'ing) gemmation; asexual reproduction in which a portion of the cell body is thrust out and then becomes separated, forming a new individual.

Buerger's disease (ber'gerz) a disease affecting the medium-sized blood vessels, particularly the arteries of the legs, which can cause severe pain and in serious cases lead to gangrene; called also thromboangiitis obliterans, a term that refers to the clotting, pain, and inflammation occurring in this disease and to the fact that it can obliterate, or destroy, blood vessels.

The cause of this violent reaction has been thought to be excessive use of tobacco over a long period of time. The number of cases has diminished strikingly in recent years.

The intense pain that is a symptom of the disease is caused by the formation of blood clots, or THROMBOSIS, in the lining of the arterial blood vessels.

When the clots grow larger, the blood flow slows and may stop entirely. Since every part of the body depends on the continuous flow of blood, affected areas such as fingers and toes, for example, soon begin to atrophy or develop ulcers. If the causes of the disease are not completely arrested, amputation may be necessary.

To treat the disease, the patient must stop smoking at once and entirely. This generally results in the partial healing of the affected membrane with a renewed flow of blood. However, more blood may have to be brought to damaged tissue by surgical methods of channeling detours or making canals in the clot itself.

Special exercises called BUERGER-ALLEN EXERCISES are sometimes used to empty the engorged blood vessels and stimulate collateral circulation. These exercises can be done at home by the patient and are usually prescribed to be done several times during the day. The patient is also instructed to avoid wearing any tight clothing, such as tight girdles, rolled garters, constricting belts, and other items that may impair circulation. He should also avoid sitting or standing in one position for long periods of time. Care should be used in the selection of shoes and stockings so that they fit properly and do not cause pressure against the blood vessels. The patient should be told to avoid walking barefoot or otherwise subjecting himself to the hazards of trauma to the feet and legs. Should such an accident occur, no matter how minor it may seem, he must notify the physician so that treatment may be begun and infection and ulceration can be prevented.

Buerger-Allen exercises (ber'ger al'en) specific exercises intended to improve circulation to the feet and legs. The lower extremities are elevated to a 45 to 90 degree angle and supported in this position until the skin blanches (appears dead white). The feet and legs are then lowered below the level of the rest of the body until redness appears (care should be taken that there is no pressure against the back of the knees); finally, the legs are placed flat on the bed for a few minutes. The length of time for each position varies with the patient's tolerance and the speed with which color change occurs. Usually the exercises are prescribed so that the legs are elevated for 2 to 3 minutes, down 5 to 10 minutes, and then flat on the bed for 10 minutes.

buffer (buf'er) a substance that, by its presence in solution, increases the amount of acid or alkali necessary to produce a unit change in pH.

buffy coat (buf'e) reddish gray layer observed above packed red cells in centrifuged blood.

bulb (bulb) a rounded mass or enlargement. adj., **bul'bar.**

b. of aorta, the enlargement of the aorta at its point of origin from the heart.

auditory b., the membranous labyrinth and cochlea.

b. of eye, the eyeball.

gustatory b's, taste buds.

hair b., the bulbous expansion at the proximal end of a hair, in which the hair shaft is generated.

Krause's b's, end-bulbs.

olfactory b., the bulblike expansion of the olfactory tract on the under surface of the frontal lobe of each cerebral hemisphere.

b. of penis, bulb of urethra.

taste b's, taste buds.

b. of urethra, the enlarged proximal part of the corpus spongiosum.

b. of vestibule, vestibulovaginal b., a body consisting of paired masses of erectile tissue, situated one on either side of the vaginal orifice.

bulbiform (bul'bĭ-form) bulb-shaped.

bulbitis (bul-bi'tis) inflammation of the bulb of the urethra.

bulbourethral (bul"bo-u-re'thral) pertaining to the bulb of the urethra.

b. glands, two glands embedded in the substance of the sphincter of the male urethra, just posterior to the membranous part of the urethra. Their secretion, which is slippery and viscous, lubricates the urethra. Called also bulbocavernous glands and Cowper's glands.

bulbous (bul'bus) having the form or nature of a bulb; bearing or arising from a bulb.

bulbus (bul'bus), pl., *bul'bi* [L.] bulb.

b. aor'tae bulb of the aorta.

b. carot'icus carotid sinus.

b. oc'uli, the bulb, or globe, of the eye.

b. olfacto'rius olfactory bulb.

b. ure'thrae bulb of the urethra.

b. vestib'uli vagin'nae, bulb of the vestibule.

bulimia (bu-lim'e-ah) abnormal increase in the sensation of hunger. adj., **bulim'ic.**

bulla (bul'ah), pl., *bul'lae* [L.] a blister; a circumscribed, fluid-containing, elevated lesion of the skin, usually more than 5 mm. in diameter. adj., **bul'late, bul'lous.**

bullosis (bul-lo'sis) the production of, or a condition characterized by, bullous lesions.

BUN blood urea nitrogen (see UREA NITROGEN).

bundle (bun'd'l) a collection of fibers or strands, as of muscle fibers, or a fasciculus or band of nerve fibers.

atrioventricular b., bundle of His.

fundamental b., ground b., that part of the white matter of the spinal cord bordering the gray matter and containing fibers that travel for a distance of only a few segments of the cord.

b. of His, a band of cardiac muscle connecting the atria with the ventricles of the heart; called also atrioventricular bundle.

Keith's b., sinoatrial b., a bundle of fibers in the wall of the atrium of the heart between the venae cavae.

Thorel's b., a bundle of muscle fibers in the human heart connecting the sinoatrial and atrioventricular nodes.

b. of Vicq d'Azyr, a band of fibers from the mamillary body to the anterior nucleus of the thalamus.

bundle branch (bun'd'l branch) a branch of the bundle of His.

bunion (bun'yun) an abnormal prominence on the inner aspect of the first metatarsal head, with bursal formation, and resulting in lateral or valgus displacement of the great toe. Bunions are almost always caused by wearing shoes that are too tight and that force the toes together. They are also often associated with flat or weak feet. In mild cases, the pain can be relieved by heat, and the condition will clear by itself after properly fitting shoes have been worn for some time. In more severe cases a physician should be consulted; he may recommend special corrective shoes or a simple surgical operation (bunionectomy) to correct the condition.

bunionectomy (bun"yun-ek'to-me) excision of a bunion.

bunionette (bun"yun-et') enlargement of the lateral aspect of the fifth metatarsal head.

buphthalmos (būf-thal'mos) abnormal enlargement of the eyes; see infantile GLAUCOMA.

bur, burr (bur) a form of drill used for creating openings in bone or similar hard material.

buret, burette (bu-ret') a glass tube with a capacity of the order of 25 to 100 ml. and graduation intervals of 0.05 to 0.1 ml., with stopcock attachment, used to deliver an accurately measured quantity of liquid.

burimamide (bu-rim'ah-mīd) an antagonist to histamine, competing for the histamine$_2$ receptor site on cells.

Burkitt's lymphoma (tumor) (berk'itz) a form of undifferentiated malignant lymphoma, usually found in central Africa, but also reported from other areas, and manifested most often as a large osteolytic lesion in the jaw or as an abdominal mass; called also *African lymphoma.*

The Epstein-Barr virus (EB virus), a herpesvirus, has been isolated from Burkitt's lymphoma cells in culture, and has been implicated as a causative agent.

burn (bern) injury to tissues caused by contact with dry heat (fire), moist heat (steam or liquid), chemicals, electricity, lightning, or radiation.

Burns have been classified traditionally according to degree. A first-degree burn involves a reddening of the skin area. In a second-degree burn the skin is blistered. A third-degree burn is the most serious type, involving damage to the deeper layers of the skin. In some cases the growth cells of the tissues in the burned area may be destroyed.

In recent literature burn wounds may be described as *partial-thickness wounds* in which the epithelializing elements remain intact, and *full-thickness wounds* in which all of the epithelializing elements and those lining the sweat glands, hair follicles, and sebaceous glands are destroyed. A *deep thermal* burn is a deep partial-thickness wound which often has the white, waxy appearance of a full-thickness burn.

It is difficult to determine the depth of a wound at first glance, but any burn involving more than 15 percent of the body surface is considered serious. Because surface area as well as depth is important in evaluating a burned patient's status, a method called the Rule of Nines has been developed to determine surface area involvement. The head and each arm are figured at 9 percent. The anterior and posterior trunk and each leg comprise 18 or (2×9) percent each, and the perineum is figured as 1 percent.

In a burn the *crust* is the dry, scablike covering that forms over a superficial burn. *Eschar* is a hard layer of tissue that results from full-thickness injury. The eschar is considered to be a protective covering over the wound, serving as a barrier to bacterial invasion. Recent research indicates that the eschar may be a viable tissue that can contribute to healing and the prevention of scarring.

IMMEDIATE TREATMENT. The following steps should be taken for prompt and effective treatment of the various types of burns.

Major Burns. The victim of a serious burn should lie down to lessen shock, and a physician or emergency unit should be called. The head and chest should be kept lower than the rest of the body, and the legs should be elevated, if possible. In shock, the liquid part of the blood rushes to the burned area, and there may not be enough left to maintain normal function of the heart, brain, and other vital organs. Therefore these organs should be lowered so that gravity will help send them a supply of blood.

With attention to cleanliness to prevent contamination, dry dressings of sterile gauze are applied over the burned areas. If sterile dressings are not available, at least four layers of clean cotton cloth should be used. To protect the burn from air, the dressings are covered with a layer of tightly woven cloth; protecting a burn from air helps to relieve pain, and the application of a sterile dressing reduces the danger of infection. In case of an extensive burn, the victim should be wrapped in a clean sheet and transported to a hospital.

Attempts should *not* be made to remove clothing from a burned area; the clothing should be cut around the area. Absorbent cotton, oily substances, and antiseptics are *not* used on a burn. Blisters are *not* opened or disturbed in any way.

If the victim is conscious and can swallow, he is given fluids to quench his thirst. If medical aid is not available quickly, he should be given, at 15 minute intervals, a solution of ½ teaspoonful of salt and ½ teaspoonful of sodium bicarbonate (baking soda) dissolved in a quart of water. This is discontinued if it causes nausea.

Minor Burns. For a small first-degree burn, the reddened area is immersed in clean cold water or ice cubes are applied. This relieves the pain. Or a sterile gauze pad or clean cloth soaked in a solution of 2 tablespoonfuls of sodium bicarbonate (baking soda) dissolved in a quart of lukewarm water is applied and bandaged loosely. Or a paste of baking soda and water, or petroleum jelly, may be applied and covered with sterile gauze.

Even first-degree burns are extremely serious if they involve a large area. They should receive prompt medical attention. Death may result if a first-degree burn covers as much as two-thirds of the body area. On a child such burns are dangerous on a smaller area of the skin.

Chemical and Other Burns. For chemical burns, such as those caused by acids, the affected area should be bathed immediately with water, using plenty of water and continuing bathing the area until all of the chemical has been washed away. A physician should be called and first-aid treatment should be given as for any similar heat burn. If the burned area is extensive, the victim should lie down and be treated for shock.

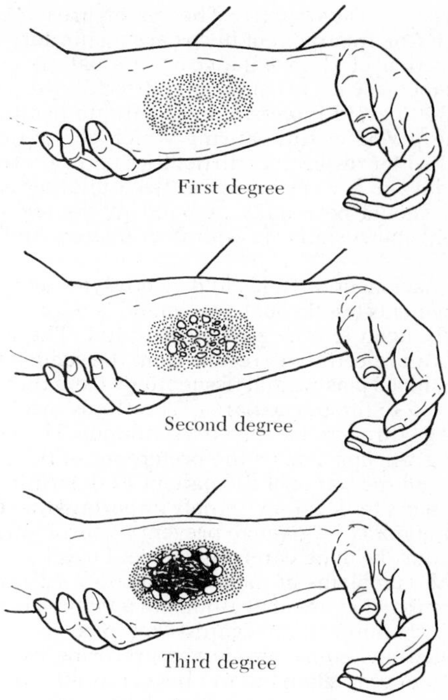

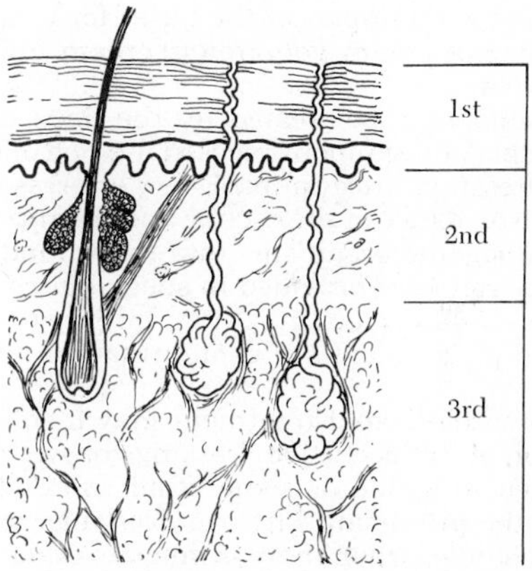

First-degree burns damage the epidermis; second-degree burns damage both epidermis and dermis; third-degree burns damage the epidermis, dermis, and subcutaneous tissue.

If the area affected is the eye, it is held open and flushed gently but thoroughly with water. Then it is covered with a sterile dressing and medical aid is sought immediately.

In electrical burns, shock is the main danger. It may be necessary to use ARTIFICIAL RESPIRATION. This should be begun as soon as contact with the current has been broken. A person struck by lightning also requires artificial respiration if the shock has been severe enough to interfere with normal breathing.

Safety measures in the home and on the job are extremely important in the prevention of burns.

HOSPITAL TREATMENT. The major areas of concern in the treatment of burns are respiratory care, restoration of fluid balance to combat SHOCK, replacement of ELECTROLYTES, and local care of the wound to avoid infection and facilitate healing.

The period of time during which the patient is watched for respiratory difficulties can vary from a few days to a week or more. Resuscitation equipment should be readily at hand in the event the patient shows signs of respiratory distress and hypoxia.

Replacement of fluids and electrolytes and blood components lost through the wound is begun immediately upon entrance to the hospital. The loss of fluids and electrolytes results from the sudden shifting of blood plasma and tissue fluids from their normal site to the burned area. The fluids are lost by seepage through the open burn wounds. The type of fluid given depends on the preference of the physician and the status of the patient as determined by laboratory tests. It is extremely important that sufficient quantity be given to prevent hypovolemia, but this must be done carefully to avoid overhydration and the problems of increased BLOOD VOLUME.

The major cause of death in burn victims is infection. Immunization against tetanus is recommended and some physicians prescribe hyperimmune gamma globulin and hyperimmune plasma. A vaccine against pseudomonal infection, a common complication of burn wounds, is under development.

Antibiotics may be given systemically and applied topically. Examples of the latter form are silver sulfadiazine cream, gentamicin cream, and Sulfamylon cream.

The wound may be treated by the open or the closed method. In the open, exposed method of treatment no dressings are applied. Every effort is made to avoid disturbance of the eschar and the introduction of pathogenic organisms into the wound. The type of environment provided in special burn units of large medical centers may vary, but the overriding concern is avoiding contamination of the wound.

The closed method of treatment may involve the application of dry occlusive dressings or wet dressings soaked in saline or some other solution preferred by the physician. The wet dressings require frequent changes when there is much exudate from the wound.

Tubbing is especially helpful in cleansing the wound, removing debris and caked creams, and facilitating EXERCISES which are essential to avoid orthopedic deformities. (See also HYDROTHERAPY.)

Patient Care. The primary concerns in patient care are prevention of infection, avoidance of a fluid and electrolyte imbalance, and prevention of such orthopedic deformities as contractures and ankylosis. If the patient is confined to a bed or frame, all the hazards of immobility must be guarded against. In addition to these measures it is especially important that good sanitation practices and sterile technique be carried out faithfully. Handwashing is of vital importance.

The patient must be protected from extremes of heat and cold as when dry or wet dressings are used. Dry dressngs which do not allow for circulation of air can cause a build-up of body heat, especially in a febrile patient. The patient receiving wet dressings must be protected from drafts and other conditions that could produce chilling.

GRAFTING of skin is done very soon after the initial injury to the skin and underlying tissues. The donor skin is best taken from the patient, but when this is not possible, the skin of another person can be used. In recent years porcine skin has been used for skin grafts but its use has not yet been universally accepted.

Careful and accurate taking and recording of vital signs is done periodically and any significant change reported immediately. An accurate record of intake and output is of primary importance. Because large amounts of body fluids and many essential minerals and salts can escape through burn wounds, it is imperative that a record be kept of fluids excreted through the kidneys or intestinal tract or by emesis. Observations should include not only the amount but also the color, concentration, unusual odor, or any other characteristic of the urine, emesis, or liquid stool.

A high-protein diet with supplemental vitamins and minerals is prescribed to aid in the repair of damaged tissue. Ingenuity and imagination may be needed to convince the patient that he must eat all of his meals as well as the between-meal feedings prescribed for him.

The patient who has suffered some disfigurement from burns will have additional emotional problems as he adjusts to a new body image. Burn therapy can be long and tedious for the patient and his family. They will need emotional and psychological support and attention to their spiritual needs as they work their way through the many problems created by the physical and emotional trauma of a major burn.

Burow's solution (bo͞or′ovz) a preparation of aluminum subacetate, glacial acetic acid, and water; used topically on the skin as an astringent, and as a topical antiseptic and antipruritic in various skin disorders. Called also aluminum acetate solution.

bursa (ber′sah), pl. *bur′sae, bursas* [L.] a small fluid-filled sac or saclike cavity situated in places in tissues where friction would otherwise occur. adj., **bur′sal**. Bursae function to facilitate the gliding of muscles or tendons over bony or ligamentous surfaces. They are numerous and are found throughout the body; the most important are located at the shoulder, elbow, knee, and hip. Inflammation of a bursa is known as BURSITIS.

b.-dependent, requiring interaction with the bursa of Fabricius in birds (see also B-lymphocyte [under LYMPHOCYTE]).

b.-equivalent, requiring interaction with human tissue analogous to the bursa of Fabricius in birds (see also B-lymphocyte [under LYMPHOCYTE]).

b. of Fabricius, an epithelial outgrowth of the cloaca in chick embryos, with develops in a manner similar to that of the thymus in mammals, atrophying after 5 or 6 months and persisting as a fibrous remnant in sexually mature birds. It contains lymphoid follicles, and before involution is a site of formation of lymphocytes associated with humoral IMMUNITY.

b. mucosa, synovial b., a closed synovial sac interposed between surfaces that glide upon each other; it may be subcutaneous, submuscular, subfascial, or subtendinous in location.

bursectomy (ber-sek′to-me) excision of a bursa.

bursitis (ber-si′tis) inflammation of a bursa. The bursa of the shoulder is most commonly affected, but inflammation may develop in almost any bursa in the body. Excessive use of the joint or chilling or a draft on the joint may be the cause.

Acute bursitis comes on suddenly; severe pain and limitation of motion of the affected joint are the principal symptoms. Resting the joint in a sling and applications of moist heat frequently are sufficient treatment. In some cases it may be necessary to aspirate fluid and calcium salts from the inflamed area. Steroids, such as cortisone, hydrocortisone, and ACTH, injected into the joint, may be effective in relieving acute attacks. X-ray therapy is also frequently effective.

Chronic bursitis may follow the acute attacks. There is continued pain and limitation of motion around the joint. X-ray examination will usually reveal the deposit of calcium salts. If rest, heat, and medications do not relieve the condition, x-ray therapy or surgery may be required to remove the calcium deposits or free the area of chronic inflammation.

bursolith (ber'so-lith) a calculus in a bursa.

bursopathy (ber-sop'ah-the) any disease of a bursa.

bursotomy (ber-sot'o-me) incision of a bursa.

Busse-Buschke disease (bo͞os'ĕ bo͞osh'ke) cryptococcosis.

busulfan (bu-sul'fan) an alkylating agent that acts selectively on the bone marrow, depressing granulocyte formation, and therefore used in the treatment of myelocytic (granulocytic) leukemias. Side effects include nausea and vomiting, and heavy doses may lead to excessive bone marrow depression. Complete blood counts (including platelet counts) must be done frequently while the drug is being administered and are used as a guide to dosage and effects on bone marrow production.

butabarbital (bu″tah-bar'bĭ-tal) a short- to intermediate-acting barbiturate; the sodium salt is used as a sedative and hypnotic.

butacaine (bu'tah-kān) a local anesthetic; the sulfate salt is used as a topical anesthetic in the eye and on mucous membranes, in solution or ointment.

butalbital (bu-tal'bĭ-tal) an intermediate-acting barbiturate used as a sedative and hypnotic.

butallylonal (bu″tah-lil'o-nal) an intermediate-acting barbiturate used as a central nervous system depressant.

butamben (bu-tam'ben) butyl aminobenzoate, a topical anesthetic.

butane (bu'tān) an aliphatic hydrocarbon, C_4H_{10}, from petroleum.

Butazolidin (bu″tah-zol'ĭ-din) trademark for a preparation of phenylbutazone, an analgesic, anti-inflammatory, and antipyretic.

Butesin (bu-te'sin) trademark for a preparation of butyl aminobenzoate, a topical anesthetic.

butethamine (bu-teth'ah-mēn) a local anesthetic; used in dentistry in the form of the hydrochloride salt.

Butisol (bu'tĭ-sol) trademark for preparations of butabarbital, a short- to intermediate-acting barbiturate.

buttock (but'ok) either of the two fleshy prominences formed by the gluteal muscles on the lower part of the back.

butyl (bu'til) a hydrocarbon radical, C_4H_9.

b. aminobenzoate, a white crystalline powder used as a local anesthetic. Excessive amounts may be absorbed if applied to broken skin and can produce systemic toxic effects. The drug is available in powder, ointment, suppository, or lozenge forms.

butylene (bu'tĭ-lēn) a gaseous hydrocarbon, C_4H_8.

butyraceous (bu″tĭ-ra'shus) of a buttery consistency.

butyrate (bu'tĭ-rāt) a salt of butyric acid.

butyric acid (bu-tir'ik) a saturated fatty acid found in butter.

butyrin (bu'tĭ-rin) a triglyceride of butyric acid.

butyroid (bu'tĭ-roid) resembling butter.

butyrophenone (bu″tĭ-ro-fe'nōn) a chemical class of major tranquilizers especially useful in the treatment of manic and moderate to severe agitated states and in the control of the vocal utterances and tics of Gilles de la Tourette's syndrome.

butyrous (bu'tĭ-rus) resembling butter.

bypass (bi'pas) an auxiliary flow; a shunt; a surgically created pathway circumventing the normal anatomical pathway, as an aortoiliac or an intestinal bypass.

aortocoronary b., a section of saphenous vein or suitable substitute grafted between the aorta and a coronary artery distal to an obstructive lesion in the latter.

aortoiliac b., insertion of a vascular prosthesis from the abdominal aorta to the femoral artery to bypass intervening atherosclerotic segments.

cardiopulmonary b., diversion of the flow of blood from the entrance to the right atrium directly to the aorta, usually via a pump oxygenator, avoiding both the heart and the lungs; a form of extracorporeal circulation used in HEART surgery.

femoropopliteal b., insertion of a vascular prosthesis from the femoral to the popliteal artery to bypass occluded segments.

intestinal b., jejunoileal b., a surgical procedure in which all but a few inches of the proximal jejunum and terminal ileum are bypassed; done to bring about malabsorption of digested food for the purpose of correcting obesity (see also INTESTINAL BYPASS).

left heart b., diversion of the flow of blood from the pulmonary veins directly to the aorta, avoiding the left atrium and the left ventricle.

partial b., the deviation of only a portion of the blood flowing through an artery.

right heart b., diversion of the flow of blood from the entrance of the right atrium directly to the pulmonary arteries, avoiding the right atrium and right ventricles.

byssinosis (bis″ĭ-no'sis) pneumoconiosis due to inhalation of cotton dust.

C

C 1. chemical symbol, *carbon.* 2. in the electrocardiogram, C stands for chest (precordial) lead; see PRECORDIAL LEAD. 3. symbol for *complement.*

C. cathode (cathodal); Celsius or centigrade (scale); cervical; clearance; clonus; closure; contraction; cylinder.

c. contact; curie.

CA chronologic age.

Ca chemical symbol, *calcium;* cathode (cathodal); cancer.

cac(o)- word element [Gr.], *bad; ill.*

cacanthrax (kak-an′thraks) anthrax.

cacao (kah-ka′o) 1. cocoa. 2. the seeds of the tropical tree *Theobroma cacao.*

cacesthesia (kak″es-the′ze-ah) disordered sensibility.

cachet (kah-sha′) [Fr.] a dish-shaped wafer or capsule enclosing a dose of medicines.

cachexia (kah-kek′se-ah) a profound and marked state of constitutional disorder; general ill health and malnutrition. adj. **cachec′tic.**

c. hypophysiopri′va, the train of syptoms resulting from total deprivation of pituitary function, including loss of sexual function, bradycardia, hypothermia, apathy, and coma.

malarial c., the physical signs resulting from antecedent attacks of severe malaria, including anemia, sallow skin, yellow sclera, splenomegaly, hepatomegaly, and, in children, retardation of growth and puberty.

pituitary c., that due to diminution or absence of pituitary function (see also PANHYPOPITUITARISM and SIMMONDS′ DISEASE).

cachinnation (kak″ĭ-na′shun) excessive, hysterical laughter.

cacodyl (kak′o-dil) a poisonous arsenical compound, which is flammable when exposed to air.

cacodylate (kak′o-dil″āt) any salt of cacodylic acid.

cacodylic acid (kak″o-dil′ik) a crystalline deliquescent solid used as an herbicide.

cacogenics (kak″o-jen′iks) racial deterioration resulting from the mating and propagation of inferior individuals. adj., **cacogen′ic.**

cacogeusia (kak″o-gu′se-ah) a bad taste.

cacomelia (kak″o-me′le-ah) congenital deformity of a limb.

cacosmia (kak-oz′me-ah) 1. foul odor; stench. 2. a hallucination of unpleasant odor.

cactinomycin (kak″tĭ-no-mi′sin) actinomycin C, an antibiotic from *Streptomyces chrysomallus,* composed of a mixture of actinomycins; used as an antineoplastic.

cacumen (kah-ku′men), pl. *cacu′mina* [L.] 1. the top or apex of an organ. 2. the top of a plant. 3. the anterior and upper part of the monticulus cerebelli; called also culmen.

cadaver (kah-dav′er) a dead body; generally applied to a human body preserved for anatomical study. adj., **cadav′eric, cadav′erous.**

cadaverine (kah-dav′er-in) a relatively nontoxic ptomaine, $C_5H_{14}N_2$, formed by decarboxylation of lysine; it is sometimes one of the products of *Vibrio proteus* and of *V. cholerae,* and occasionally found in the urine in cystinuria.

cadmiosis (kad″me-o′sis) pneumoconiosis due to inhalation of and tissue reaction to CADMIUM dust.

cadmium (kad′me-um) chemical element, atomic number 48, symbol Cd; its salts are poisonous. (See table of ELEMENTS.) Inhalation of cadmium fumes causes pulmonary edema, followed by proliferative interstitial pneumonia, and is associated with various degrees of lung damage; poisoning may also be due to ingestion of foods contaminated by cadmium-plated containers, causing violent gastrointestinal symptoms.

c. sulfide, a salt used, in a 1 per cent suspension, in treatment of seborrheic dermatitis of the scalp (dandruff).

caduceus (kah-du′se-us) the wand of Hermes or Mercury; used as a symbol of the medical profession and as the emblem of the Medical Corps of the U.S. Army. Another symbol of medicine is the staff of Æsculapius, which is the official insignia of the American Medical Association.

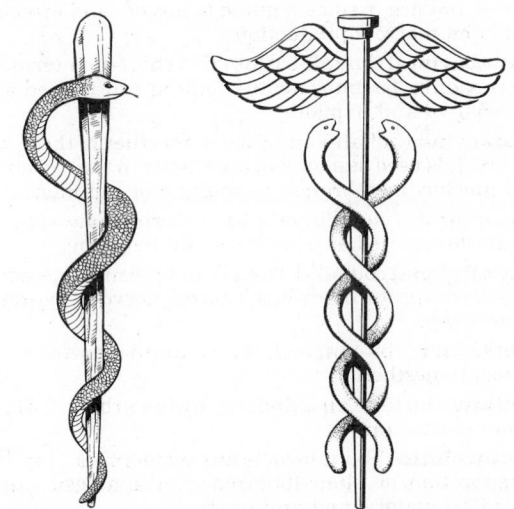

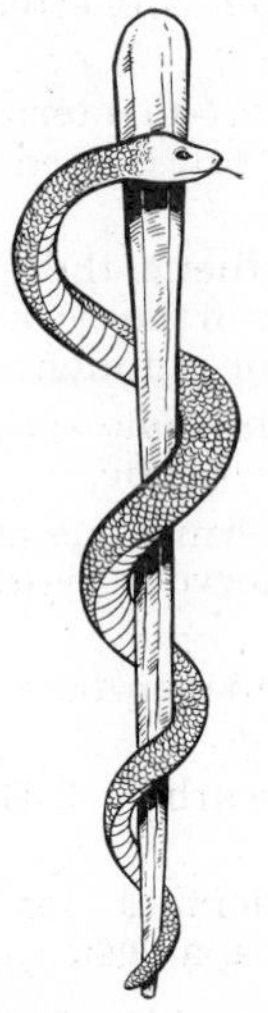

Staff of Æsculapius.

Caduceus.

cae- for words beginning thus, see also those beginning *ce-.*

caelotherapy (se″lo-ther′ah-pe) the therapeutic use of religion and religious symbols.

café au lait spot (kah-fa′o-la′) pigmented macules of a distinctive light brown color, like coffee with milk, as in neurofibromatosis and Albright′s syndrome.

caffeine (kaf′ēn, kaf′fe-in) a central nervous system stimulant from coffee, tea, guarana, and maté; it also acts as a mild diuretic.

citrate c., citrated c., a mixture of caffeine and

citric acid, used as a central nervous system stimulant.

c. sodium benzoate, a mixture of equal parts of anhydrous caffeine and sodium benzoate, used as a central nervous system stimulant; overdosage may produce nervousness and wakefulness.

caffeinism (kaf'ēn-izm) an agitated state induced by excessive ingestion of caffeine.

Caffey's disease (kaf'fēz) infantile cortical hyperostosis.

caisson disease (ka'son) decompression sickness, a condition occurring in underwater workers, and caused by too-rapid decrease in atmospheric pressure. The condition is named after the pressurized, watertight compartments (caissons) in which underwater construction men work. The main symptoms are dizziness, staggering, muscle spasms, difficulty in breathing, abdominal pain, and partial paralysis. Caisson disease is a form of BENDS.

Cal. large calorie (kilogram calorie).

cal. small calorie (gram calorie).

calamine (kal'ah-mīn) a preparation of zinc and ferric oxides, used topically as a protectant and astringent.

calcaneoapophysitis (kal-ka"ne-o-ah-pof"ĭ-si'tis) inflammation of the posterior part of the calcaneus, marked by pain and swelling.

calcaneoastragaloid (kal-ka"ne-o-ah-strag'ah-loid) pertaining to the calcaneus and astragalus.

calcaneodynia (kal-ka"ne-o-din'e-ah) pain in the heel.

calcaneum, calcaneus (kal-ka'ne-um; kal-ka'ne-us) the irregular quadrangular bone at the back of the tarsus; called also heel bone and os calcis. (See also table of BONES.)

calcar (kal'kar) a spur or spur-shaped structure.

c. a'vis, the lower of two medial elevations in the lateral cerebral ventricle, produced by the lateral extension of the calcarine sulcus; called also hippocampus minor.

calcareous (kal-kăr'e-us) pertaining to or containing lime; chalky.

calcarine (kal'kar-in) 1. spur-shaped. 2. pertaining to the calcar avis.

c. sulcus, a sulcus of the medial surface of the occipital lobe, separating the cuneus from the lingual gyrus.

calcariuria (kal-kăr"e-u're-ah) the presence of lime (calcium) salts in the urine.

calcemia (kal-se'me-ah) excessive calcium in the blood; hypercalcemia.

calcibilia (kal"sĭ-bil'e-ah) the presence of calcium in the bile.

calcic (kal'sik) of or pertaining to lime or calcium.

calcicosis (kal"sĭ-ko'sis) a lung disease due to inhalation of marble dust.

calciferol (kal-sif'er-ol) 1. see VITAMIN D. 2. ergocalciferol.

calcific (kal-sif'ik) forming lime.

calcification (kal"sĭ-fĭ-ka'shun) the deposit of calcium salts in a tissue. The normal absorption of calcium is facilitated by parathyroid hormone and by vitamin D. When there are increased amounts of parathyroid hormone in the blood (as in HYPERPARATHYROIDISM), there is deposition of calcium in the alveoli of the lungs, the renal tubules, the thyroid gland, the gastric mucosa, and the arterial walls. Normally calcium is deposited in the bone matrix to insure stability and strength of the bone. In OSTEOMALACIA there is decalcification of bone because of a failure of calcium and phosphorus to be deposited in the bone matrix.

dystrophic c., the deposition of calcium in abnormal tissue, such as scar tissue or atherosclerotic plaques, without abnormalities of blood calcium.

calcine (kal'sīn) to reduce to a dry powder by heat.

calcinosis (kal"sĭ-no'sis) a condition characterized by abnormal deposition of calcium salts in the tissues.

c. circumscrip'ta, localized deposition of calcium in small nodules in subcutaneous tissues or muscle.

c. universa'lis, widespread deposition of calcium in nodules or plaques in the dermis, panniculus, and muscles.

calcipenia (kal"sĭ-pe'ne-ah) deficiency of calcium in the system.

calcipexis, calcipexy (kal"sĭ-pek'sis; kal'sĭ-pek"se) fixation of calcium in the tissues. adj., **calcipec'tic, calcipex'ic.**

calciphilia (kal"sĭ-fil'e-ah) a tendency to calcification.

calciphylaxis (kal"sĭ-fi-lak'sis) the formation of calcified tissue in response to administration of a challenging agent after induction of a hypersensitive state. adj., **calciphylac'tic.**

calciprivia (kal"sĭ-priv'e-ah) deprivation or loss of calcium. adj., **calcipriv'ic.**

calcitonin (kal"sĭ-to'nin) a polypeptide hormone elaborated by the parafollicular cells of the thyroid gland in response to hypercalcemia; it lowers plasma calcium and phosphate levels, inhibits bone resorption, and serves as an antagonist to parathyroid hormone. Called also thyrocalcitonin.

calcium (kal'se-um) a chemical element, atomic number 20, atomic weight 40.08, symbol Ca. (See table of ELEMENTS.) Calcium is the most abundant mineral in the body. In combination with phosphorus it forms calcium phosphate, the dense, hard material of the bones and teeth.

A constant level of a small amount of calcium in the blood is required for certain important body functions, including maintenance of the heartbeat, clotting of blood (in which it is considered CLOTTING factor IV), and normal functioning of muscles and nerves.

The body obtains calcium from food sources. Milk and cheese are the readiest sources, and other dairy products are rich in calcium. Molasses, turnip greens, and dandelion greens also provide calcium. In addition, vitamin D is necessary to put the calcium to use.

Calcium deficiency diseases may be due to an insufficient amount of calcium food sources in the diet, to a lack of vitamin D, or occasionally to a disorder of the parathyroid glands.

The most familiar calcium deficiency disease is RICKETS, in which the bones and teeth soften. Calcium deficiency may also impair blood clotting, and cause nervous and muscular disturbances. Tetany, a disorder characterized by convulsive muscle cramps, is due to underactivity of the parathyroid glands, which causes the level of blood calcium to fall.

c. benzoylpas, a tuberculostatic drug.

c. carbonate, a compound occurring naturally in

bone, shells, etc., and prepared artificially (precipitated) as a source of calcium. Precipitated calcium carbonate may be prepared by reaction of a soluble calcium salt with a soluble carbonate; used as an antacid.

c. chloride, a salt used in solution to restore electrolyte balance.

c. cyclamate, a noncaloric sweetener.

c. disodium edetate, edetate c. disodium, see EDETATE CALCIUM DISODIUM.

c. gluconate, a calcium replenisher.

c. glycerophosphate, a calcium and phosphorus dietary supplement.

c. hydroxide, an astringent compound used topically in solution or lotions.

c. ipodate, a diagnostic radiopaque medium used in cholangiography and cholecystography.

c. lactate, a calcium supplement.

c. levulinate, a calcium supplement.

c. mandelate, a white, odorless powder used as a urinary antiseptic.

c. oxalate, a compound occurring in the urine in crystals and in certain calculi.

c. oxide, lime (1).

c. oxytetracycline, an antibacterial.

c. pantothenate, a calcium salt of the dextrorotatory isomer of pantothenic acid; used as a growth-promoting vitamin.

c. phosphate, one of three salts containing calcium and the phosphate radical: dibasic and tribasic calcium phosphate are used as sources of calcium; monobasic calcium phosphate is used in fertilizer and as a calcium and phosphorus supplement.

c. saccharin, a non-nutritive sweetener.

c. sulfate, a compound of calcium and sulfate, occurring as GYPSUM or as PLASTER OF PARIS.

calciuria (kal″se-u′re-ah) calcium in the urine.

calcospherite (kal″ko-sfēr′it) one of the minute globular bodies formed during calcification by chemical union of calcium particles and albuminous matter of cells.

calculifragous (kal″ku-lif′rah-gus) breaking up calculi.

calculogenesis (kal″ku-lo-jen′ĕ-sis) the formation of calculi.

calculosis (kal″ku-lo′sis) a condition characterized by the presence of calculi; lithiasis.

calculus (kal′ku-lus), pl. *cal′culi* [L.] an abnormal concretion, usually composed of mineral salts, occurring within the animal body, chiefly in the hollow organs or their passages. Called also stones, as in kidney stones (see also KIDNEY) and GALLSTONES. adj., **cal′culous.**

biliary c., a gallstone.

bronchial c., lung calculus.

dental c., calcium phosphate and carbonate, with organic matter, deposited on tooth surfaces.

lung c., a concretion formed in the bronchi (see also LUNG CALCULUS).

renal c., a calculus occurring in the kidney.

urinary c., a calculus in any part of the urinary tract.

vesical c., one in the urinary bladder.

Caldwell-Moloy classification (kald′wel-mŏ-loi′) the classification of female pelves as gynecoid, android, anthropoid, and platypelloid (see also PELVIS and accompanying illustration).

calefacient (kal″ĕ-fa′shent) causing a sensation of warmth; an agent that so acts.

calf (kaf) sura; the fleshy back part of the leg below the knee.

caliber (kal′ĭ-ber) the diameter of the lumen of a canal or tube.

calibration (kal″ĭ-bra′shun) determination of the accuracy of an instrument, usually by measurement of its variation from a standard, to ascertain necessary correction factors.

calibrator (kal″ĭ-bra′ter) an instrument for dilating a tubular structure or for determining the caliber of such a structure.

calicectasis (kal″ĭ-sek′tah-sis) dilatation of a calix of the kidney.

calicectomy (kal″ĭ-sek′to-me) excision of a calix of the kidney.

calices (kal′ĭ-sēs) plural of *calix.*

caliculus (kah-lik′u-lus) a small cup or cup-shaped structure.

California disease coccidioidomycosis.

californium (kal″ĭ-fōr′ne-um) a chemical element, atomic number 98, atomic weight 249, symbol Cf. (See table of ELEMENTS.)

calipers (kal′ĭ-perz) an instrument with two bent or curved legs used for measuring thickness or diameter of a solid.

calisthenics (kal″is-then′iks) systematic exercise for attaining strength and gracefulness.

calix (ka′liks), pl. *cal′ices* [L.] a cuplike organ or cavity, e.g., one of the recesses of the kidney pelvis which enclose the pyramids. adj., **calice′al.**

Calliphora (kal-lif′o-rah) a genus of flies, the blowflies or bluebottle flies, which deposit their eggs in decaying matter, on wounds, or in body openings; the maggots are a cause of myiasis.

callosity (kah-los′ĭ-te) a callus (1).

callosum (kah-lo′sum) corpus callosum.

callous (kal′us) of the nature of a callus; hard.

callus (kal′us) 1. localized hyperplasia of the horny layer of the epidermis due to pressure or friction. 2. an unorganized network of woven bone formed about the ends of a broken bone; it is absorbed as repair is completed (provisional callus), and ultimately replaced by true bone (definitive callus).

calmative (kal′mah-tiv, kah′mah-tiv) 1. sedative; allaying excitement. 2. an agent having such effects.

calomel (kal′o-mel) a heavy white powder, mercurous chloride; used rarely as a cathartic. It increases peristalsis and glandular secretions, especially of bile. It is also used rarely as an intestinal antiseptic and to reduce edema, or in an ointment as a local antibacterial agent.

calor (kal′er) [L.] heat; one of the cardinal signs of inflammation.

caloric (kah-lor′ik) pertaining to heat or to calories.

calorie (kal′o-re) a unit of heat; commonly used alone to designate small CALORIE. One calorie is the amount of heat required to raise the temperature of 1 kilogram of water by 1 degree Celsius (C.). (This is about the same as the amount of heat required to raise the temperature of 1 lb. of water by 4 degrees Fahrenheit.) It is possible to calculate the amount of energy contained in a particular food by measuring the amount of heat units, or calories, in that food. Every bodily process—the building up of cells, motion of the muscles, the maintenance of body tem-

CALORIE CHART

FOOD AND MEASURES*	APPROXIMATE CALORIES
Apple, baked, 1 large and 2 tbs. sugar	200
fresh, 1 large	100
Asparagus, fresh or canned, 5 stalks, 5 in. long	15
Avocado, 1/2 4-in. pear	265
Bacon, 2-3 long slices, cooked	100
Banana, 1 medium, 6 in. long	90
Beans, lima, fresh or canned, 1/2 cup	100
green or yellow, fresh or canned, 1/2 cup	25
canned with pork, 1/2 cup	175
Beef (cooked), corned, 1 slice 4 by 1 1/2 in. by 1 in.	100
hamburger, 3 oz.	300
round, lean, 1 medium slice (2 oz.)	125
sirloin lean, 1 average slice (3 oz.)	250
tongue, 2 oz.	125
Beets, fresh or canned, 2, 2-in. in diam.	50
Bread, corn (1 egg), 1, 2-in. square	120
rye, 1 slice, 1/2 in. thick	70–75
white, enriched, 1 slice, average	75
whole wheat, 100%, 1 slice average	75
Broccoli, 3 stalks, 5 1/2 in. long	100
Brussels sprouts, 6 sprouts, 1 1/2 in. diam.	50
Butter, 1 tbs.	95
Cabbage, cooked, 1/2 cup	40
raw, 1 cup	25
Cake, angel, 1/10 large cake	
choc, or vanilla, with icing	155
2 by 1 1/2 by 2 in.	200
cupcake (med.), choc. icing	250
Cantaloupe, 1/2 5 1/2-in. melon	50
Carrot, 4 in. long	25
Cauliflower, 1/4 of head, 4 1/2 in. in diam.	25
Celery, 2 stalks	15
Cheese, American cheddar, 1 cube 1 1/8 in. square	110
cottage, 5 tbs.	100
cream, 2 tbs.	100
Chicken, 1/2 med. broiler	270
Chocolate, milk, sweetened 1 oz.	140
malted milk, fountain size	460
syrup, 1/4 cup	200
Cocoa, half milk, half water, 1 cup	150
Cod steak, 1 piece, 3 1/2 by 2 by 1 in.	100
Cola soft drinks, 6-oz. bottle	75
Collards, 1/2 cup, cooked	50
Corn, 1/2 cup	70
Corn flakes, 1 cup	80
Cracker, graham, 1 square	35
saltine, 2-in. square	15
Cream, light, 2 tbs.	65
heavy, 2 tbs.	120
whipped, 3 tbs.	100
Custard, 1/2 cup	130
Eggs, medium	75
Eggplant, 3 slices, 4 in. diam., 1/2 in. thick, raw	50
Flour, 1 tbs., unsifted	35
Frankfurter	125
Gelatin, fruit flavored, ready to serve, 1/2 cup	85
Grapefruit juice, unsweetened, 1 cup	100
Grape juice, 1/2 cup	80
Griddle cake, 4 in. diam.	75
Halibut, 1 piece, 3 by 1 3/8 by 1 in.	100
Ham, lean, 1 slice, 4 1/4 by 4 by 1/2 in.	265
Hominy grits, cooked, 3/4 cup	100
Ice cream, 1/2 cup	200
Ice cream soda, fountain size	325
Jellies and jams, 1 rounded tbs.	100
Lamb, roast, 1 slice, 3 1/2 by 4 1/2 by 1/8 in.	100
Lettuce, 2 large leaves	5
Liver, 1 slice, 3 by 3 by 1/2 in.	100
Liverwurst, 2 oz.	130
Macaroni, cooked, 3/4 cup	100
Maple syrup, 1 tbs.	70
Margarine, 1 tbs.	100
Milk, buttermilk, 1 cup	85
condensed, 1 1/2 tbs.	100
evaporated, 1/2 cup	160
skim, 1 cup	85
whole, 1 cup	170
yogurt, plain, 1 cup	120–160
Mushrooms, 10 large	10
Noodles, cooked, 3/4 cup	75
Oatmeal, cooked, 3/4 cup	110
Oil, corn, cottonseed, olive, peanut, 1 tbs.	100
Olives, green, 6 medium	50
ripe, 4-5 medium	50
Onions, 3-4 medium	100
Orange, 1 medium	80
juice, 1 cup	125
Parsnip, 7 in. long	100
Peach, fresh, 1 medium	50
canned in syrup, 2 lg. halves, 3 tbs. juice	100
Peanut butter, 1 tbs.	100
Peanuts, shelled, 10	50
Pear, fresh, 1 medium	50
canned in syrup, 3 halves, 3 tbs. juice	100
Peas, canned, 1/2 cup	65
fresh, shelled, 3/4 cup	100
Pepper, green, 1 medium	20
Pie, apple, 3-in. sector	200
mincemeat, 3-in. sector	300
Pineapple, fresh, 1 slice, 3/4 in. thick	50
canned, unsweetened, 1 slice, 1/2 in. thick, 1 tbs. juice	50
juice, unsweetened, 1 cup	135
Pork chop, lean, 1 medium	200
Potato chips, 8-10 large	100
Potato salad with mayonnaise, 1/2 cup	200
Potatoes, mashed, 1/2 cup	100
sweet, 1/2 medium	100
white, 1 medium	100
Prunes, dried, 4 medium	100
Pumpkin, 1/2 cup	50
Raisins, 1/4 cup	90
Rice, cooked, 3/4 cup	100
Rutabagas, 1/2 cup	30
Salad dressing, French, 1 tbs.	90
mayonnaise, 1 tbs.	100
Salmon, canned, 1/2 cup	100
Sauerkraut, 1/2 cup	15
Soup, condensed, 11-oz. can,	
mushroom	360
tomato	230
vegetable	200
Spaghetti, cooked, 3/4 cup	100
Spinach, cooked, 1/2 cup	20
Squash, summer, cooked, 1/2 cup	20
winter, cooked, 1/2 cup	50
Sugar, brown, 1 tbs.	50
granulated, 1 tbs.	50
Tapioca, uncooked, 1 tbs.	50
Tomato juice, 1 cup	60
Tomatoes, canned, 1/2 cup	25
fresh, 1 medium	30
Tuna fish, canned, 1/4 cup, drained	100
Turnip, 1, 1 3/4 in. diam.	25
Veal, roast, 1 slice, 3 by 3 3/4 by 1/2 in.	120
Waffle, 6 in. in diam.	250
Wheat flakes, 3/4 cup	100
Alcoholic Beverages	
Beer, 8 oz.	120
Gin, 1 1/2 oz.	120
Rum, 1 1/2 oz.	150
Whisky, 1 1/2 oz.	150
Wines	
champagne, 4 oz.	120
port, 1 oz.	50
sherry, 1 oz.	40
table, red or white, 4 oz.	95

*1 cup equals 8 ounces (oz.); 3 teaspoons (tsp.) equal 1 tablespoon (tbs.); 4 tablespoons (tbs.) equal 1/4 cup.
Courtesy of the Metropolitan Life Insurance Company.

perature—requires energy, and the body derives this energy from the food it consumes. Digestive processes reduce food to usable "fuel," which the body "burns" in the complex chemical reactions that sustain life.

The amount of energy required for these chemical processes varies. Factors such as weight, age, activity, and metabolic rate determine a person's daily calorie requirement. Nutrition experts have computed daily calorie requirements in terms of age and other factors. These tabulations serve only as guides; they cannot, of course, embrace all individual variations.

Average Calorie Requirements

Adult male	2900 calories
Adult female	2000 calories
Adolescent male	3400 calories
Adolescent female	2400 calories
Retired male	2200 calories
Retired female	1600 calories

From its daily intake of energy foods, the body uses only the amount it needs for energy purposes. The remainder is stored as fat; hence the utility of calorie counting in weight control. If the average adult male consumes more than his 2900-calorie daily requirement, he will gain weight. However, if he consumes less than 2900 calories, the body will supplement its energy sources by drawing upon fat which the body has stored away, and he will lose weight.

A person can usually gain or lose weight as he wishes by keeping to a daily diet with a calorie count above or below his daily requirement.

gram c., small calorie.

kilogram c., large calorie.

large c., the calorie used in metabolic studies, being the amount of heat required to raise the temperature of 1 kg. of water 1 degree Celsius (C.). Abbreviated Cal.

small c., the amount of heat required to raise the temperature of 1 gm. of water 1 degree Celsius (C.). Abbreviated cal.

standard c., small calorie.

calorifacient (kah-lor″ĭ-fa′shent) producing heat.

calorific (kal″o-rif′ik) producing heat.

calorigenic (kah-lor″ĭ-jen′ik) producing or increasing production of heat or energy; increasing oxygen consumption.

calorimeter (kal″o-rim′ĕ-ter) an instrument for measuring the amount of heat produced in any system or organism.

calorimetry (kal″o-rim′ĕ-tre) measurement of the heat eliminated or stored in any system.

calusterone (kal-us′ter-on) an antineoplastic androgenic steroid used in relief of symptoms of advanced inoperable breast cancer and associated metastases.

calvacin (kal′vah-sin) an antineoplastic substance derived from the fungus *Calvatia gigantea.*

calvaria, calvarium (kal-va′re-ah; kal-va′re-um) the domelike superior portion of the cranium, comprising the superior portions of the frontal, parietal, and occipital bones.

Calvé-Perthes disease (kal-va′ per′tēz) osteochondrosis of the epiphysis at the head of the femur.

calx (kalks) 1. lime or chalk. 2. the hindmost part of the foot; the heel.

calyculus (kah-lik′u-lus) caliculus.

Calymmatobacterium (kah-lim″mah-to-bak-te′re-um) a genus of bacteria made up of gram-negative rods.

calyx (ka′liks) calix.

camera (kam′er-ah), pl. *cam′erae* [L.] a cavity or chamber.

Camoquin (kam′o-kwin) trademark for a preparation of amodiaquine, used as an antimalarial and to treat amebic abscess of the liver.

camphor (kam′fer) a ketone derived from a cinnamon tree, *Cinnamomum camphora,* or produced synthetically; used topically as an antipruritic agent.

camphorated (kam′fer-āt″ed) containing or tinctured with camphor.

camptocormia (kamp″to-kor′me-ah) a static deformity consisting of forward flexion of the trunk.

camptodactyly (kamp″to-dak-tĭ-le) permanent flexion of one or more fingers.

camptospasm (kamp′to-spazm) camptocormia.

Canada-Cronkhite syndrome (kan′ah-dah krong′kīt) familial polyposis of the gastrointestinal tract associated with alopecia, nail dystrophy, and hyperpigmentation of the skin.

canal (kah-nal′) a relatively narrow tubular passage or channel.

adductor c., Hunter's canal.

Alcocks' c., a tunnel formed by a splitting of the obturator fascia, which encloses the pudendal vessels and nerve.

alimentary c., the digestive tube from mouth to anus (see also ALIMENTARY CANAL).

anal c., the terminal portion of the alimentary canal, from the rectum to the anus.

atrioventricular c., the common canal connecting the primitive atrium and ventricle; it sometimes persists as a congenital anomaly.

birth c., the canal through which the fetus passes in birth.

carotid c., one in the pars petrosa of the temporal bone, transmitting the internal carotid artery to the cranial cavity.

cervical c., the part of the uterine cavity lying within the cervix.

condylar c., an occasional opening in the condylar fossa for transmission of the transverse sinus; called also posterior condyloid foramen.

c. of Corti, a space between the outer and inner rods of Corti.

femoral c., the cone-shaped medial part of the femoral sheath lateral to the base of Gimbernat's ligament.

haversian c., any of the anastomosing channels of the haversian system in compact bone, containing blood and lymph vessels, and nerves.

Hunter's c., a fascial tunnel in the middle third of the medial part of the thigh, containing the femoral vessels and saphenous nerve. Called also adductor canal.

hypoglossal c., an opening in the occipital bone, transmitting the hypoglossal nerve and a branch of the posterior meningeal artery; called also anterior condyloid foramen.

infraorbital c., a small canal running obliquely through the floor of the orbit, transmitting the infraorbital vessels and nerve.

inguinal c., the oblique passage in the lower anterior abdominal wall on either side, through which passes the round ligament of the uterus in the female, and the spermatic cord in the male.

medullary c., 1. spinal canal. 2. the cavity, containing marrow, in the diaphysis of a long bone; called also marrow or medullary cavity.

optic c., a passage for the optic nerve and ophthalmic artery at the apex of the orbit; called also optic foramen.

pulp c., root canal.

root c., that part of the pulp cavity extending from the pulp chamber to the apical foramen. Called also pulp canal.

sacral c., the continuation of the spinal canal through the sacrum.

Schlemm's c., the venous sinus of the sclera, a circular canal at the junction of the sclera and cornea (see also venous SINUS of sclera).

semicircular c's, the long canals (anterior, lateral, and posterior) of the bony labyrinth of the ear (see also SEMICIRCULAR CANALS).

spinal c., vertebral c., the canal formed by the series of vertebral foramina together, enclosing the spinal cord and meninges.

Volkmann's c's, canals communicating with the haversian canals, for passage of blood vessels through bone.

canaliculus (kan″ah-lik′u-lus), pl. *canalic′uli* [L.] an extremely narrow tubular passage or channel. adj., **canalic′ular.**

bile canaliculi, fine tubular channels forming a three-dimensional network within the parenchyma of the liver.

lacrimal c., the short passage in an eyelid, beginning at the lacrimal point and draining tears from the lacrimal lake to the lacrimal sac; called also lacrimal duct. (See also LACRIMAL APPARATUS.)

mastoid c., a small channel in the temporal bone transmitting the tympanic branch of the vagus nerve.

canalis (kah-na′lis), pl. *cana′les* [L.] a canal or channel.

canalization (kan″al-ĭ-za′shun) 1. the formation of canals, natural or morbid. 2. the surgical establishment of canals for drainage.

canaloplasty (kah-nal′o-plas″te) plastic reconstruction of a passage, as of the external acoustic meatus.

Canavan's disease (kan′ah-vanz) see spongy DEGENERATION of central nervous system.

canavanine (kah-nav′ah-nin) a naturally occurring amino acid, isolated from soybean meal.

cancellated (kan′sel-āt″ed) having a lattice-like structure.

cancellous (kan′sĕ-lus) of a reticular, spongy, or lattice-like structure; said mainly of bone tissue.

cancellus (kan-sel′us), pl. *cancel′li* [L.] the lattice-like structure in bone; any structure arranged like a lattice.

cancer (kan′ser) any malignant, cellular tumor. adj., **can′cerous.** Cancer is a group of neoplastic diseases, in which there is new growth of abnormal cells. Normally the cells that compose body tissues grow in response to a normal stimulus. Worn-out body cells are regularly replaced by new cell growth which stops when the cells are replaced; new cells form to repair tissue damage and stop forming when healing is complete. Why they stop forming is unknown, but clearly the body in its normal processes regulates cell growth. In cancer, cell growth is unregulated. The cells continue to reproduce until they form a mass of tissue known as a tumor. Not all tumors are malignant; those which are noncancerous are referred to as benign tumors. Benign tumors vary in size, and may grow so large that they obstruct organs or cause ulceration and bleeding. They are encapsulated, do not metastasize, and usually can be removed by surgery without difficulty.

Malignant tumors grow in a disorganized fashion, interrupting body functions and robbing normal cells of their food and blood supply. The malignant cells may spread to other parts of the body by (1) direct extension into adjacent tissue, (2) permeation along lymphatic vessels, (3) traveling in the lymph stream to the lymph nodes, (4) entering the blood circulation, and (5) invasion of a body cavity by diffusion.

CAUSES. Cancer is many different diseases and no one factor can be pinpointed as the cause of the various types of malignant growths. Environmental, hereditary, and biological factors are all known to play a role in the development of cancer.

Environmental causes are believed to account for at least 50 per cent and perhaps, in some types, as much as 80 per cent of all cancers. For example, cigarette smoking is directly related to approximately 90 per cent of all cancers of the lung. Other environmental carcinogens include industrial pollutants and radiation. Among the chemical carcinogens are arsenic from mining and smelting industries; asbestos from insulation, at construction sites and power plants; benzene from oil refineries, solvents, and insecticides; and products from coal combustion in steel and petrochemical industries. Each year new products that in all probability are carcinogenic are being produced by industrial operations. A major concern is the occupational and environmental hazards these chemicals present to those who work in or live near these plants.

Radiation from prolonged exposure to the ultraviolet rays from the sun and from injudicious use of diagnostic and therapeutic procedures involving x-rays and radioactive substances is also a significant factor in the incidence of cancer, particularly in the development of cancer of the skin, bone marrow, and thyroid.

Hormones, especially the synthetic estrogens given to forestall the effects of menopause and to prevent spontaneous abortion, are directly related to some cancers of the female reproductive organs.

Viruses as causal agents in the development of cancers have been subjected to intensive research efforts in recent years, and, while a number of cancers can be produced in experimental laboratory animals, there is still no irrefutable evidence that cancers in humans are caused by viruses. An exception may be the Epstein-Barr virus, which may have a causal association with Burkitt's lymphoma and certain cases of nasopharyngeal cancer. There remains, however, the intriguing fact that viruses are capable of introducing new genetic material into a normal cell and transforming it into a malignant one, and that cell reproduction may be altered when viruses interact with such carcinogens as chemicals and radiation. It is not known exactly how these properties enhance the ability of malignant cells to thrive under adverse conditions and to metastasize to other parts of the body and produce another cancerous tumor. Recent studies have shown that an extracellular enzyme plays an important role in the transmission of genetic information to the cell and thereby facilitates the reproduction of cancer cells. The enzyme is called reverse transcriptase because it reverses the usual mechanism for replication of genetic information; that is, whereas in normal cellular replication the DNA is the template for RNA copies, in the presence of the enzyme, RNA serves as the template for DNA copies.

The incidence of cancer in certain populations suggests that other factors are important in its development. It is known, for example, that some families show a high incidence of malignancy among its members, but there is no definite hereditary pattern. There also is a high incidence of cancer in persons receiving drugs for immunosuppression, yet cancer itself is immunosuppressive. It is suggested that prolonged suppression of the body's immune response may eventually impair its ability to distinguigh between self and nonself and thus render it unable to destroy malignant cells. When cancer itself acts to suppress the immune response, it may be the result of an overwhelming demand on the body to destroy more foreign cells than it is prepared to cope with at any given time.

CLASSIFICATION. Cancers are classified on the basis of two factors: the type of tissue and the type of cell in which they arise. Using this classification system, it is possible to identify over 150 types of cancer in humans. In the classification of cancers according to the type of tissue from which they evolve, there are two main groups: SARCOMAS and CARCINOMAS. Sarcomas are of mesenchymal origin and affect such tissues as the bones and muscles. They tend to grow rapidly and to be very destructive. The carcinomas are of epithelial origin and make up the great majority of the glandular cancers and cancers of the breast, stomach, uterus, skin, and tongue.

Cell type affects the appearance, rate of growth, and degree of malignancy. Thus, classification of tumors according to the type of cell from which they are derived is important in deciding the course of treatment for a specific malignancy.

Staging. A new approach to describing and categorizing malignant tumors is evolving from the work of the International Union Against Cancer (U.I.C.C.) and the American Joint Committee on Cancer Staging and End Results Reporting (A.J.C.C.S.). It is hoped that by standardizing the classification and staging of tumors, treatment protocols can be established and end-results reporting can be utilized to determine the effectiveness of the suggested treatment.

Whereas classification of tumors refers to the anatomical and histological descriptions of the tumor (see above), staging refers to the extent of the tumor. The three basic components of the staging system are the primary tumor (T), regional nodes (N), and metastasis (M). Subscripts may be used to describe the extent to which the malignancy has increased in size, its involvement of regional nodes, and its metastatic development (see Table). For example, a tumor may be described $T_1N_2M_0$.

At the present time, the U.I.C.C. system differs slightly from that of the A.J.C.C.S. in describing the staging of certain tumors. For this reason, it is important that one is very clear about which system is used to describe the malignancy of a specific patient.

Precancers. Some potentially dangerous cancers appear first in the form of harmless changes in the body's tissues. Their danger lies in the fact that they have a tendency to become malignant. Hence they are known as precancers. Among these are sores that appear as thickened white patches (leukoplakia) in the mouth and on the vulva, some moles, and any chronically irritated area on the skin or the mucous membranes of the mouth and tongue. Polyps also are possible precancers, as are some forms of lymphomas.

Hodgkin's Disease. This disease is generally considered a form of cancer. It usually afflicts young people, causing a progressive enlargement of the lymph nodes, in most cases starting in the neck, groin, or armpit. Treatment may be by surgery, radiotherapy, use of certain chemicals, or a combination of these (see HODGKIN'S DISEASE).

Leukemias. In these diseases, abnormal leukocytes are produced in enormous quantities. The leukemias respond to much the same treatment as cancer and are commonly considered cancers (see LEUKEMIA).

TNM STAGING SYSTEM

TUMOR	
T_0	No evidence of primary tumor
TIS	Carcinoma in situ
T_1 T_2 T_3 T_4	Progressive increase in tumor size and involvement
T_X	Tumor cannot be assessed
NODES	
N_0	Regional lymph nodes not demonstrably abnormal
N_1 N_2 N_3	Increasing degrees of demonstrable abnormality of regional lymph nodes. (For many primary sites, the subscript "a," e.g., $N1_a$, may be used to indicate that metastasis to the node is not suspected; and the subscript "b," e.g., $N1_b$, may be used to indicate that metastasis to the node is suspected or proved.)
N_X	Regional lymph nodes cannot be assessed clinically
METASTASIS	
M_0	No evidence of distant metastasis
M_1 M_2 M_3	Ascending degrees of distant metastasis, including metastasis to distant lymph nodes

American Joint Committee for Cancer Staging and End Results Reporting, and adapted from Clinical Staging System for Carcinoma of the Esophagus, CA: A Cancer Journal for Clinicians. Vol. 25, No. 2, March-April, 1975.

PREVENTION. Until specific causal agents can be identified for the various forms of malignancy, there can be no preventive measures guaranteed to eliminate cancer from the list of ailments that plague mankind. Efforts at reduction of the incidence of cancer must be aimed primarily at those individuals known to be at greater risk for developing cancer, monitoring them frequently for early signs of malignancy and reducing whenever possible their exposure to substances believed to contribute to the development of the disease.

Early detection of cancer before symptoms become severe can be a major deterrent to its crippling and all too often fatal effects. Of all persons found to have a malignant tumor, about 66 percent already have had some metastasis from the original site at the time of diagnosis. If the primary tumor is detected before the symptoms develop (they usually develop after metastasis), the chances for cure are excellent. The availability of more sophisticated technology in diagnosis of cancer is expected to improve the cure rate for cancer because of earlier detection and prompt treatment.

SYMPTOMS OF CANCER. There are seven early warning signs of cancer. *These signs do not necessarily signify cancer, but should they occur, a physician should be consulted and an examination is advisable.* Other symptoms depend on location and type of malignancy present.

EARLY DANGER SIGNS OF CANCER

1. Any lump or thickening, especially in the breast, lip, or tongue.
2. Any irregular or unexplained bleeding. Blood in the urine or bowel movements. Blood or bloody discharge from the nipple or any body opening. Unexplained vaginal bleeding or discharge, or any bleeding after the menopause.
3. A sore that does not heal, particularly around the mouth, tongue, or lips, or anywhere on the skin.
4. Noticeable changes in the color or size of a wart, mole, or birthmark.
5. Loss of appetite or continual indigestion.
6. Persistent hoarseness, cough, or difficulty in swallowing.
7. Persistent change in normal elimination (bowel habits).

Special Note: Pain is not usually an early warning sign of cancer.

Stomach cancer: continued lack of appetite; persistent indigestion; pain after eating; loss of weight; vomiting; anemia.

Cancer of the rectum: changes in bowel habits, such as periods of constipation followed by episodes of diarrhea; abdominal cramps and a sensation of incomplete elimination or a feeling that there is a mass in the rectum; rectal pain and bleeding.

Cancer of the uterus: increased or irregular vaginal discharges; return of vaginal bleeding after the menopause; bleeding between menstrual periods or after coitus.

Cancer of the breast: painless lumps in the breast; bleeding or discharging from the nipple. Many kinds of lumps in the breast are innocent, but since this form of cancer is now the leading cause of death from cancer among women, any breast nodule or tumor should be examined by a physician.

Skin cancer: sores and ulcers that do not heal; sudden changes in color, size, and texture in moles, warts, scars, and birthmarks.

Lung cancer: a persistent cough that lasts beyond 2 weeks; wheezing or other noises in the chest; coughing up of blood or bloody sputum; shortness of breath not caused by obvious exertion, such as climbing stairs or running; chest ache or pain.

Cancer of the mouth, tongue, and lips: any sore that does not heal in 2 weeks; any white patch taking the place of the normal pink color of the tongue or inside of the mouth; hoarseness lasting more than 2 weeks.

Cancer of the larynx: persistent hoarseness.

Kidney, bladder, and prostate cancers: bloody urine or reddish or pink urine; difficulty in starting urination; increasing frequency of urination during the night.

Brain tumors and cancers: headaches; changes in vision; dizziness; nausea and vomiting; paralysis.

DIAGNOSIS. The detection of cancer can be accomplished by a number of tests and examinations. By palpation, a tumor can be felt as a lump or nodule below the surface of the skin or mucous membrane. By visualization of the hollow organs with instruments such as the cystoscope, proctoscope, or bronchoscope, abnormal growths of cells can be seen. Laboratory examination of the cells removed by BIOPSY can determine whether a tumor is malignant or benign. This test is considered the most accurate and dependable aid to diagnosis of cancer.

The PAPANICOLAOU SMEAR TEST is used for diagnosing early cancers of the uterine cervix, mouth, bronchi, stomach, and other organs lined with mucous membrane. In this technique washings or scrapings from the mucous membrane are removed by the physician, placed on a glass slide and sent to a laboratory for cytologic examination. Radiologic studies, using x-ray films and fluoroscopy, can reveal tumors which may not be detected by other means. In addition to gastrointestinal studies, chest x-rays and pyelography, radiologic studies for cancer include angiography and mammography. Radioisotopes and photoscanners may be used to locate tumors of the brain, pancreas, thyroid, liver, and kidney. In this method the radioactive compound is introduced into the body orally or by injection. The compound travels through the body and localizes in a specific organ. Special instruments are used to trace and "photograph" the abnormal collection of radioisotopes, thereby pinpointing the location of the tumor. Other diagnostic techniques include ultrasonography, xerography, and thermography.

There is at present no general chemical test of the blood by which malignant growths can be distinguished from benign. The blood can be tested chemically for cancer of the prostate and for a rare malignancy of the bone marrow called MULTIPLE MYELOMA. A blood count can also help in the diagnosis of leukemias.

TREATMENT AND PATIENT CARE. The current methods of treating cancer are surgery, RADIOTHERAPY, and chemotherapy or ANTINEOPLASTIC THERAPY. These forms of treatment may be used singly or in combination depending on the type of cancer present and the condition of the individual patient.

Surgical removal of the tumor and the areas to which it has metastasized is aimed at removal of all cancerous and potentially cancerous tissue. This method of treatment is most successful when the growth is small and localized and is situated in areas where adjacent tissues, particularly lymphatic tissues, also can be excised.

Patient care is concerned with physical and psychological preparation of the patient. At this time, he is told the purpose and expected outcome of the surgical procedure and he is given an explanation of his role and what is expected of him. If the surgical procedure involves mastectomy, (see surgery of the BREAST), COLOSTOMY, AMPUTATION, or some other alteration in body image or adjustment of life style, plans for rehabilitation should be started before surgery is done. Before and after surgery, the patient and his family should be involved in a cooperative effort with all members of the health care team to achieve maximum rehabilitation. There is still some controversy as to whether a patient should be told that he has a malignancy, but the consensus is that the patient has a right to know and should be encouraged to participate in planning and carrying out the prescribed regimen.

Therapeutic radiation utilizes ionizing radiations to destroy cells by inhibiting their ability to multiply. Radiation damages tissue, particularly tissue that is growing rapidly, and because malignant tissue does grow more rapidly than normal tissue, it is more readily affected by radiation. Cells vary in their susceptibility to radiation and not all malignancies respond to this form of treatment.

Radiation therapy techniques vary in respect to the source of radiation and method of delivery. X-ray therapy utilizes high voltage x-ray machines. In TELETHERAPY the source of radiation is a radioactive element that is housed in a shielded unit located some distance from the patient. Interstitial therapy requires placement or implantation of a radioactive substance directly into the tissues of the malignant growth.

Although normal tissue can be damaged by x-ray radiation, instruments that deliver high voltage x-rays and techniques that pinpoint the beams of energy keep that damage to a minimum.

Whenever any type of radiation is used it is necessary to explain to the patient where the radiation comes from and how he and others are protected from excessive radiation exposure. Most lay persons are familiar with some of the hazards of radiation but do not understand how it can be used in a beneficial way. Many are apprehensive about receiving radiotherapy because they believe that once treated, they are sources of radiation themselves. In cases of x-ray therapy and teletherapy there is no danger that the patient will become a source of radiation or hazardous to those with whom he comes in contact. However, when radioactive materials are implanted in the body tissues, those materials do emit radiations that could be harmful to others. (See also RADIATION.)

In caring for a patient receiving x-ray therapy, meticulous skin care is essential. Before each treatment the skin is washed and all powders and ointments, particularly those with a metallic base, for example zinc oxide, are removed to avoid burning the skin. After a series of treatments has begun the skin is likely to become progressively drier and more irritated and more susceptible to trauma and breakdown. The "ports" of entry for the x-rays are marked on the skin by the radiologist and are not removed until the series of treatment is completed.

Of the chemicals and drugs used in treating cancer there are two general classes: (1) cytotoxic drugs that kill or injure malignant cells in dosages sufficient to affect these cells and at the same time not destroy large numbers of normal cells, and (2) drugs that alter the environment of cancer cells so that growth is retarded or stopped altogether. Most ANTINEOPLASTIC drugs are limited in their usefulness and therefore are given in combinations that act on cells in different ways. Various drugs may be prescribed simultaneously or in sequence so that malignant cells are destroyed at different stages of development, normal cell damage is kept at a minimum, and resistance to a single drug is not likely to develop.

All chemical agents presently used for treatment of cancer have serious toxic effects. They demand careful monitoring of patient status by laboratory testing throughout the course of therapy, and they should be administered only by physicians and other medical care personnel trained in the techniques of administration and familiar with the hazards of this mode of therapy. The drugs may be given systemically by the oral route or by intravenous or intramuscular injection, regionally as by arterial infusion, or locally by instillation into a body cavity. Specially designed infusion pumps and infusion controllers aid in administering proper dosage and rate of flow of chemotherapeutic agents.

When drug therapy is continued on an out-patient basis, the patient and his family are to be advised about the reportable toxic reactions of the drugs, expected side effects, and the importance of returning to a clinical laboratory for blood studies and other tests that assess progress of the disease and effects of the drugs.

Adjuncts to chemotherapy with toxic agents must include other drugs and techniques to improve the patient's well-being by restoring normal tissue function, replacing blood elements, encouraging reossification of bone lesions, and removing pressure and obstruction of blood vessels, lymphatic vessels, and neural pathways.

canceremia (kan″ser-e′me-ah) the presence of cancer cells in the blood.

cancericidal (kan″ser-ĭ-si′dal) destructive to cancer cells.

cancerigenic (kan″ser-ĭ-jen′ik) giving rise to a malignant tumor.

cancerophobia, cancerphobia (kan″ser-o-fo′be-ah; kan″ser-fo′be-ah) carcinophobia; morbid dread of cancer.

cancriform (kang′frĭ-form) resembling cancer.

cancroid (kang′kroid) 1. cancer-like. 2. a skin cancer of a low grade of malignancy.

cancrum (kang′krum) [L.] canker.

c. o′ris, see NOMA.

c. puden′di, see NOMA.

Candeptin (kan-dep′tin) trademark for a preparation of candicidin, an antifungal agent.

candicidin (kan″di-si′din) an antifungal agent derived from *Streptomyces griseus,* used principally to treat candidal vaginitis.

Candida (kan′dĭ-dah) a genus of yeastlike fungi that are commonly part of the normal flora of the mouth, skin, intestinal tract, and vagina, but can cause a variety of infections (see also CANDIDIASIS).

C. al'bicans, the usual pathogen in human infection.

candidemia (kan"dĭ-de'me-ah) the presence in the blood of fungi of the genus *Candida.*

candidiasis (kan"dĭ-di'ah-sis) infection by fungi of the genus *Candida,* generally *C. albicans,* most commonly involving the skin, oral mucosa (thrush), respiratory tract, and vagina; rarely there is a systemic infection or endocarditis.

candidid (kan'dĭ-did) a secondary skin eruption that is an expression of hypersensitivity to infection with *Candida* elsewhere on the body.

candidin (kan'dĭ-din) a skin test antigen derived from *Candida albicans,* used in testing for the development of delayed-type hypersensitivity to the microorganism.

candidosis (kan"dĭ-do'sis) candidiasis.

canine (ka'nīn) 1. pertaining to or characteristic of dogs. 2. pertaining to a canine tooth (cuspid).

canker (kang'ker) an ulceration, especially of the lip or oral mucosa.

cannabinoid (kah-nab'ĭ-noid) any of the active principles of *Cannabis,* the two most active being the tetrahydrocannabinols.

cannabinol (kah-nab'ĭ-nol) a physiologically inactive principle from *Cannabis;* its tetrahydro derivatives are active.

Cannabis (kan'ah-bis) a genus of plants, hemp.

C. in'dica, an Asiatic variety of common hemp; preferred for medicinal use.

C. sati'va, the common hemp (see CANNABIS).

cannabis (kan'ah-bis) the dried flowering tops of hemp plants (*Cannabis sativa*), which have euphoric principles (tetrahydrocannabinols); classified as a hallucinogen and prepared as bhang, ganja, hashish, and marihuana.

cannabism (kan'ah-bizm) a morbid state produced by misuse of cannabis.

Cannon's ring (kan'unz) a focal contraction seen radiographically at the mid-third of the transverse colon, marking an area of overlap between the superior and inferior nerve plexuses.

cannula (kan'u-lah) a tube for insertion into a duct or cavity; during insertion its lumen is usually occupied by a trocar.

cannulate (kan'u-lat) to introduce a cannula, which may be left in place.

cannulation (kan"u-la'shun) introduction of a cannula into a tubelike organ or body cavity.

canthectomy (kan-thek'to-me) excision of a canthus.

canthitis (kan-thi'tis) inflammation of a canthus.

cantholysis (kan-thol'ĭ-sis) surgical section of a canthus or a canthal ligament.

canthoplasty (kan'tho-plas"te) plastic surgery of a canthus.

canthorrhaphy (kan-thor'ah-fe) the suturing of the palpebral fissure at either canthus.

canthotomy (kan-thot'o-me) incision of a canthus.

canthus (kan'thus), pl. *can'thi* [L.] the angular junction of the eyelids at either corner of the eyes. adj., **can'thal**.

Cantil (kan'til) trademark for a preparation of mepenzolate, an anticholinergic used to relieve abdominal pain, gaseous distention, and diarrhea associated with colonic disease.

capacitance (kah-pas"ĭ-tans) 1. the property of being able to store an electric charge. 2. the ratio of charge to potential in a conductor.

capacitation (kah-pas"ĭ-ta'shun) the process by which spermatozoa become capable of fertilizing an ovum after it reaches the ampullar portion of the uterine tube.

capacitor (kah-pas'ĭ-tor) a device for holding and storing charges of electricity.

capacity (kah-pas'ĭ-te) the power to hold, retain, or contain, or the ability to absorb; usually expressed numerically as the measure of such ability.

functional residual c., the amount of gas remaining at the end of normal quiet respiration.

heat c., thermal capacity.

inspiratory c., the volume of gas that can be taken into the lungs in a full inspiration, starting from the resting inspiratory position; equal to the tidal volume plus the inspiratory reserve volume.

maximal breathing c., the greatest volume of gas that can be breathed per minute by voluntary effort.

thermal c., the amount of heat absorbed by a body in being raised 1° C.

total lung c., the amount of gas contained in the lung at the end of a maximal inspiration.

vital c., the volume of gas that can be expelled from the lungs from a position of full inspiration, with no limit to duration of exspiration; equal to inspiratory capacity plus expiratory reserve volume.

capillarectasia (kap"ĭ-lār"ek-ta'ze-ah) dilatation of capillaries.

Capillaria (kap"ĭ-la're-ah) a genus of parasitic nematodes.

C. hepat'ica, a species parasitic in the liver of rats and other mammals, including man.

C. philippinen'sis, a species found in the human intestine in Luzon, causing severe diarrhea, malabsorption, and high mortality.

capillariasis (kap"ĭ-lah-ri'ah-sis) infection with nematodes of the genus *Capillaria,* especially *C. philippinensis.*

capillariomotor (kap"ĭ-lār"e-o-mo'tor) pertaining to the functional activity of the capillaries.

capillaritis (kap"ĭ-lār-i'tis) inflammation of the capillaries.

capillarity (kap"ĭ-lār'ĭ-te) the action by which the surface of a liquid where it is in contact with a solid, as in a capillary tube, is elevated or depressed.

capillary (kap'ĭ-ler"e) 1. pertaining to or resembling a hair. 2. one of the minute vessels connecting arterioles and venules, the walls of which act as a semipermeable membrane for interchange of various substances beetween the blood and tissue fluid. (See Plate 8 and see CIRCULATORY SYSTEM.) The walls consist of thin endothelial cells through which dissolved substances and the body fluids can pass. At the arterial end, the blood pressure within the capillary is higher than the pressure in the surrounding tissues, and the blood fluid and some dissolved solid substances pass outward through the capillary wall. At the venous end of the capillary, the pressure within the tissues is higher and waste material and fluids from the tissues pass into the capillary, to be carried away for disposal.

capillus (kah-pil'us), pl. *capil'li* [L.] a hair; used in the plural to designate the aggregate of hair on the scalp.

capitation (kap″ĭ-ta′shun) the annual fee paid to a physician or group of physicians by each participant in a health plan.

capitular (kah-pit′u-lar) pertaining to a capitulum or the head of a bone.

capitulum (kah-pit′u-lum), pl. *capit′ula* [L.] a small eminence on a bone, as on the distal end of the humerus, by which it articulates with another bone.

Capla (kap′lah) trademark for a preparation of mebutamate, an antihypertensive agent.

capnohepatography (kap″no-hep″ah-tog′rah-fe) radiography of the liver after intravenous injection of carbon dioxide gas.

capotement (kah-pōt-maw′) [Fr.] a splashing sound heard in dilatation of the stomach.

capping (kap′ing) the provision of a protective or obstructive covering.

pulp c., the covering of an exposed dental pulp with some material to provide protection against external influences and to encourage healing.

Capsebon (kap′se-bon) trademark for a suspension of cadmium sulfide, used in treatment of dandruff.

capsicum (kap′sĭ-kum) dried ripe fruit of various species of *Capsicum* (pepper plants), used as an irritant and carminative.

capsid (kap′sid) the shell of protein that protects the nucleic acid of a virus; it is composed of structural units, or capsomers. According to the number of subunits possessed by capsomers, they are called dimers (2), trimers (3), pentamers (5), or hexamers (6).

capsitis (kap-si′tis) inflammation of the capsule of the crystalline lens.

capsomer, capsomere (kap′so-mer; kap′so-mēr) a morphological unit of the capsid of a virus.

capsula (kap′su-lah), pl. *cap′sulae* [L.] capsule.

capsulation (kap″su-la′shun) enclosure in a capsule.

capsule (kap′sūl) 1. an enclosing structure, as a soluble container enclosing a dose of medicine. 2. a cartilaginous, fatty, fibrous, or membranous structure enveloping another structure, organ, or part. adj., **cap′sular**.

articular c., the saclike envelope that encloses the cavity of a synovial joint by attaching to the circumference of the articular end of each involved bone.

bacterial c., a gelantinous envelope surrounding a bacterial cell, usually polysaccharide but sometimes polypeptide in nature; it is associated with the virulence of pathogenic bacteria.

Bowman's c., malpighian capsule.

c's of the brain, two layers of white matter in the substance of the brain; external capsule and internal capsule.

external c., the layer of white fibers between the putamen and claustrum.

Glisson's c., a sheath of connective tissue accompanying the hepatic ducts and vessels through the hepatic portal.

glomerular c., malpighian capsule.

c. of heart, pericardium.

internal c., the fanlike mass of white fibers separating the lentiform nucleus laterally from the head of the caudate nucleus, the dorsal thalamus, and the tail of the caudate nucleus medially.

joint c., articular capsule.

c. of lens, the elastic sac enclosing the lens of the eye.

malpighian c., the globular dilatation forming the beginning of a uriniferous tubule within the kidney, and surrounding the glomerulus. Called also Bowman's capsule and glomerular capsule.

renal c., adipose, the investment of fat surrounding the fibrous capsule of the kidney, continuous at the hilus with the fat in the renal sinus.

renal c., fibrous, the connective tissue investment of the kidney, which continues through the hilus to line the renal sinus.

Tenon's c., the connective tissue enveloping the posterior eyeball.

capsulectomy (kap″su-lek′to-me) excision of a capsule, especially a joint capsule or lens capsule.

capsulitis (kap″su-li′tis) inflammation of a capsule, as that of the lens.

adhesive c., adhesive inflammation between the joint capsule and the peripheral articular cartilage of the shoulder, with obliteration of the subdeltoid bursa; it is characterized by increasing pain, stiffness, and limitation of motion.

capsulolenticular (kap″su-lo-len-tik′u-lar) pertaining to the lens of the eye and its capsule.

capsuloma (kap″su-lo′mah) a capsular or subcapsular tumor of the kidney.

capsuloplasty (kap′su-lo-plas″te) plastic repair of a joint capsule.

capsulorrhaphy (kap″su-lor′ah-fe) suture of a joint capsule.

capsulotomy (kap″su-lot′o-me) incision of a capsule, as that of the lens or of a joint.

captodiamine (kap″to-di′ah-mēn) an antihistaminic, sedative, and tranquilizer.

captodramin (kap″to-dram′in) captodiamine.

caput (kap′ut), pl. *cap′ita* [L.] the head; a general term applied to the expanded or chief extremity of an organ or part.

c. medu′sae, the dilated cutaneous veins around the umbilicus, seen mainly in the newborn and in patients suffering from cirrhosis of the liver.

c. succeda′neum, edema occurring in and under the fetal scalp during labor.

caramel (kar′ah-mel) a concentrated solution obtained by heating sugar or glucose until it is a uniform dark brown mass; used as a coloring agent for pharmaceuticals.

caramiphen (kah-ram′ĭ-fen) an anticholinergic, used as an antispasmodic and in treatment of parkinsonism.

caraway (kar′ah-wa) dried ripe fruit of *Carum carvi;* used as a flavoring agent.

carbachol (kar′bah-kol) white or yellowish crystals, a parasympathomimetic (cholinergic) agent used topically to relieve intraocular pressure in GLAUCOMA.

carbamate (kar′bah-māt) any ester of carbamic acid.

ethyl c., urethan.

carbamazepine (kar″bam-az′ĕ-pin) a drug used in the U.S. as an analgesic in the management of trigeminal neuralgia, and in other countries as an anticonvulsant.

carbamic acid (kar-bam′ik) the parent acid of urethan.

carbamide (kar-bam′īd) urea in anhydrous, lyophilized, sterile powder form; injected intravenously in dextrose or invert sugar solution to induce diuresis.

carbaminohemoglobin (kar-bam″ĭ-no-he″mo-glo′bin) a combination of carbon dioxide and hemoglobin, CO_2HHb, being one of the forms in which carbon dioxide exists in the blood.

carbamoyl (kar′bah-moil) the radical NH_2—CO—; see CARBAMOYLTRANSFERASE.

carbamylcholine (kar″bah-mil-ko′lēn) carbachol.

carbamoyltransferase (kar″bah-moil-trans′fer-ās) an enzyme that catalyzes the transfer of carbamoyl, as from carbamoylphosphate to L-ornithine to form orthophosphate and citrulline in the synthesis of urea.

carbarsone (kar′bar-sōn) an arsenical compound used as an antiamebic agent.

carbenicillin (kar″ben-ĭ-sil′in) a semisynthetic antibiotic of the penicillin group, prepared as both the disodium and the potassium salt and used in urinary tract infections.

carbetapentane (kar-ba″tah-pen′tān) an antitussive agent; used as the hydrochloride salt.

carbidopa (kar-bĭ-do′pah) a decarboxylase inhibitor used in combination with levodopa to control the symptoms of PARKINSON'S DISEASE. In the presence of carbidopa, levodopa enters the brain in larger quantities, thus avoiding the need for excessively high doses of it.

carbinoxamine (kar″bin-ok′sah-mēn) a pyridine derivative used as an antihistamine in the form of the hydrochloride salt.

Carbocaine (kar′bo-kān) trademark for a preparation of mepivacaine, a local anesthetic.

carbocholine (kar″bo-ko′lēn) carbachol.

carbocyclic (kar″bo-si′klik) having, or pertaining to, a closed chain or ring formation which includes only carbon atoms; said of chemical compounds.

carbohemia (kar″bo-he′me-ah) the presence of carbon monoxide in the blood.

carbohemoglobin (kar″bo-he″mo-glo′bin) carbaminohemoglobin.

carbohydrase (kar″bo-hi′drās) any of a group of enzymes that catalyze the hydrolysis of higher carbohydrates to lower forms.

carbohydrate (kar″bo-hi′drāt) a compound of carbon, hydrogen, and oxygen, the latter two usually in the proportions of water $(CH_2O)_n$. They are classified into mono-, di-, tri-, poly-, and heterosaccharides. Carbohydrates in food are an important and immediate source of energy for the body; 1 gm. of carbohydrate yields 4 calories. They are present, at least in small quantities, in most foods, but the chief sources are the sugars and starches. The sugars include granulated sugar, maple sugar, honey, and molasses. The simple sugars (MONOSACCHARIDES) include glucose, called also dextrose or grape sugar, and fructose, called also levulose or fruit sugar. Galactose is a simple sugar produced by the digestion or hydrolysis of lactose (milk sugar). The double sugars (DISACCHARIDES) include sucrose, which is found in sugar cane or sugar beet, maltose or malt sugar, and lactose or milk sugar. All ripe fruits and many vegetables contain some natural sugars. The starches are present in such foods as rice, wheat, and potatoes.

Carbohydrates may be stored in the body as glycogen for future use. If they are eaten in excessive amounts, however, the body changes them into fats and stores them in that form.

carbohydraturia (kar″bo-hi″drah-tu′re-ah) excess of carbohydrates in the urine.

carbolic acid (kar-bol′ik) a caustic poison obtained by distillation of coal tar or produced synthetically; used as an antiseptic and disinfectant (see also PHENOL [1]).

carbolism (kar′bo-lizm) phenol (carbolic acid) poisoning (see PHENOL [1]).

carbolize (kar′bo-līz) to treat with phenol (carbolic acid).

carboluria (kar″bo-lu′re-ah) phenol (carbolic acid) in the urine.

carbomer (kar′bo-mer) a polymer of acrylic acid, cross-linked with a polyfunctional agent; a suspending agent.

carbomycin (kar″bo-mi′sin) a crystalline monobasic antibiotic isolated from the elaborated products of *Streptomyces halstedii* or produced by other means; it is bacteriostatic for gram-positive organisms.

carbon (kar′bon) a chemical element, atomic number 6, atomic weight 12.011, symbol C. (See table of ELEMENTS.)

^{13}C, a natural isotope of carbon, atomic mass 13, used as a tracer in chemical reactions in living tissue.

^{14}C, a radioactive isotope of carbon, atomic mass 14, used in cancer and metabolic research.

c. cycle, the steps by which carbon (in the form of CARBON DIOXIDE) is extracted from the atmosphere by living organisms and ultimately returned to the atmosphere (see also carbon CYCLE).

carbon dioxide an odorless, colorless gas, CO_2, resulting from oxidation of carbons, formed in the tissues and eliminated by the lungs; used with oxygen to stimulate respiration and in solid form (CARBON DIOXIDE SNOW) as an escharotic.

c. d. combining power, the ability of blood plasma to combine with carbon dioxide; indicative of the ALKALI RESERVE and a measure of the acid-base balance of the blood. In determination of the carbon dioxide combining power, actually the plasma bicarbonate is measured, since it is virtually impossible to determine the plasma carbon dioxide concentration in a clinical laboratory.

c. d. content, the amount of carbonic acid and bicarbonate in the blood; reported in millimoles per liter. Normal range is 24–30 mM/l.

c. d. narcosis, respiratory acidosis.

c. d. snow, solid carbon dioxide, formed by rapid evaporation of liquid carbon dioxide; it gives a temperature of about −110° F. (−79° C.), and is used as an escharotic in various skin diseases. Called also dry ice.

c. d. tension, the partial pressure of carbon dioxide in the blood; noted as pCO_2 in BLOOD GAS ANALYSIS. (See also RESPIRATION.)

carbon monoxide a colorless, odorless, tasteless gas, CO, formed by burning carbon or organic fuels with a scanty supply of oxygen; inhalation causes central nervous system damage and asphyxiation. Carbon monoxide is present in the exhaust of gasoline engines, in the smoke of wood and coal fires, in manufactured gas such as that used in the household, and wherever carbon burns without a sufficient supply of oxygen.

c. m. poisoning, poisoning by carbon monoxide;

one of the most common types of gas poisoning. When carbon monoxide is inhaled, it comes in contact with the blood and combines with hemoglobin. Since carbon monoxide combines more readily with hemoglobin than does oxygen, it takes the place of oxygen in the erythrocytes, and the tissues are thus deprived of their normal oxygen supply. Death from asphyxia results if a large enough quantity of carbon monoxide is inhaled.

SYMPTOMS AND TREATMENT. The symptoms of carbon monoxide poisoning are dizziness, headache, weakness, shortness of breath, possibly nausea, and then unconsciousness. The skin and mucous membranes become cherry red in color.

Emergency treatment consists of opening doors and windows, and turning off the source of the gas, if possible. The victim should be dragged or carried out into the air. If breathing has stopped or is irregular, ARTIFICIAL RESPIRATION should be undertaken immediately. The police or fire department or the hospital should be called and the nature of the accident described so that emergency equipment to administer oxygen may be rushed to the scene. The victim is kept lying down.

PREVENTION. Cases of carbon monoxide poisoning are usually accidental. It should be remembered that carbon monoxide has no odor and its presence may not be detected unless other gases, such as exhaust fumes from an automobile motor, are also escaping. Care should be taken to ensure proper ventilation of working and sleeping areas. It is extremely dangerous to leave an automobile motor running in a closed garage. Stoves and furnaces should be kept in good repair. Burners using gas, especially in a bedroom, should have a ventilator pipe to carry the exhaust to the outside.

carbon tetrachloride a clear, colorless, mobile liquid; the inhalation of its vapors can depress central nervous system activity and cause degeneration of the liver and kidneys.

carbonate (kar′bon-āt) a salt of carbonic acid.
ferrous c., a hematinic useful in the treatment of iron deficiency anemia but extremely irritating to the gastric mucosa.

carbonemia (kar″bo-ne′me-ah) carbohemia.

carbonic acid (kar-bon′ik) aqueous solution of carbon dioxide, H_2CO_3.
c. a. anhydrase, an enzyme that catalyzes the decomposition of carbonic acid into carbon dioxide and water, facilitating transfer to carbon dioxide from tissues to blood and from blood to alveolar air.

carbonize (kar′bo-nīz) to char or to convert into charcoal.

carbonuria (kar″bo-nu′re-ah) the presence in the urine of carbon dioxide or other carbon compounds.

carbonyl (kar′bo-nil) the bivalent organic radical, C:O, characteristic of aldehydes, ketones, carboxylic acid, and esters.
c. chloride, phosgene, a poisonous gas developed for war use.

carboxyhemoglobin (kar-bok″se-he″mo-glo′bin) a compound formed from hemoglobin on exposure to carbon monoxide.

carboxyl (kar-bok′sil) the monovalent radical, —COOH, found in those organic acids termed carboxylic acids.

carboxylase (kar-bok′sĭ-lās) an enzyme that catalyzes the removal of carbon dioxide from the carboxyl group of alpha amino keto acids.

carboxylation (kar-bok″sil-a′shun) the addition of a carboxyl group, as to pyruvate to form oxaloacetate.

carboxylesterase (kar-bok″sil-es′ter-ās) an enzyme that catalyzes the hydrolysis of the esters of carboxylic acids.

carboxylic acid (kar-bok-sil′ik) a compound of carboxyl with another radical, a hydrocarbon.

carboxyltransferase (kar-bok″sil-trans′fer-ās) an enzyme that catalyzes carboxylation.

carboxy-lyase (kar-bok′se-li′ās) any of a group of lyases that catalyze the removal of a carboxyl group; it includes the carboxylases and decarboxylases.

carboxymyoglobin (kar-bok″se-mi″o-glo′bin) a compound formed from myoglobin on exposure to carbon monoxide.

carboxypeptidase (kar-bok″se-pep′tĭ-dās) an exopeptidase that acts only on the peptide linkage of a terminal amino acid containing a free carboxyl group.

carboxypolypeptidase (kar-bok″se-pol″e-pep′tĭ-dās) an exopeptidase that attacks the peptide linkage of a terminal amino acid possessing a free carboxyl group, releasing a free amino acid from a polypeptide.

carbromal (kar-bro′mal) a sedative and hypnotic.

carbuncle (kar′bung-k′l) a necrotizing infection of skin and subcutaneous tissue composed of a cluster of BOILS (furuncles), usually due to *Staphylococcus aureus,* with multiple formed or incipient drainage sinuses. They are often a symptom of poor health. adj., **carbunc′ular.**

Like boils, carbuncles are caused by pus-forming bacteria. These organisms are often present on the skin but are unable to do any damage unless resistance is lowered by such conditions as irritating friction, cuts, poor health, nutritional deficiency, or diabetes mellitus.

Treatment includes administration of antibiotics and incision and drainage when necessary to remove exudate. Efforts are made to determine the cause of the carbuncles so that it can be eliminated.
malignant c., anthrax.

carbunculoid (kar-bung′ku-loid) resembling a carbuncle.

carbunculosis (kar-bung″ku-lo′sis) a condition marked by the formation of numerous carbuncles.

carbutamide (kar-bu′tah-mīd) a hypoglycemic agent.

carcass (kar′kas) a dead body; generally applied to other than a human body.

Carcholin (kar′ko-lin) trademark for a preparation of carbachol, applied topically to the conjunctiva to constrict the pupil.

carcinogen (kar-sin′o-jen) a substance that causes cancer. adj., **carcinogen′ic.**

carcinogenesis (kar″sĭ-no-jen′ĕ-sis) production of cancer.

carcinogenicity (kar″sĭ-no-jĕ-nis′ĭ-te) the ability or tendency to produce cancer.

carcinoid (kar′sĭ-noid) a tumor of the gastrointestinal tract formed from the argentaffin cells of the enteric canal and producing CARCINOID SYNDROME. Called also argentaffinoma.
c. syndrome, a symptom complex associated with carcinoid tumors (argentaffinomas), marked by at-

tacks of severe cyanotic flushing of the skin lasting from minutes to days and by diarrheal watery stools, bronchoconstrictive attacks, sudden drops in blood pressure, edema, and ascites; it is caused by a variety of catecholamines secreted by the agentaffinoma cells.

carcinolysis (kar″sĭ-nol-ĭ-sis) destruction of cancer cells. adj., **carcinolyt′ic.**

carcinoma (kar″sĭ-no′mah) a malignant new growth made up of epithelial cells tending to infiltrate surrounding tissues and to give rise to metastases. A form of CANCER, carcinoma makes up the majority of the cases of malignancy of the breast, uterus, intestinal tract, skin, and tongue.

adenocystic c., adenoid cystic c., carcinoma marked by cylinders or bands of hyaline or mucinous stroma separated or surrounded by nests or cords of small epithelial cells, occurring in the mammary and salivary glands, and mucous glands of the respiratory tract. Called also cylindroma.

alveolar c., alveolar adenocarcinoma.

basal cell c., an epithelial tumor of the skin that seldom metastasizes but has potentialities for local invasion and destruction.

basosquamous c., carcinoma that histologically exhibits both basal and squamous elements.

bronchogenic c., carcinoma of the lung, so called because it arises from the epithelium of the bronchial tree.

chorionic c., choriocarcinoma.

colloid c., mucinous carcinoma.

cylindrical cell c., carcinoma in which the cells are cylindrical or nearly so.

embryonal c., a highly malignant primitive form of carcinoma, probably of germinal cell or teratomatous derivation, usually arising in a gonad.

epidermoid c., that in which the cells tend to differentiate in the same way as those of the epidermis; i.e., they tend to form prickle cells and undergo cornification.

giant cell c., carcinoma containing many giant cells.

Hürthle cell c., Hürthle cell tumor.

c. in si′tu, a neoplastic entity wherein the tumor cells have not invaded the basement membrane but are still confined to the epithelium of origin; popularly applied to such cells in the uterine cervix.

medullary c., that composed mainly of epithelial elements with little or no stroma.

mucinous c., adenocarcinoma producing significant amounts of mucin.

oat cell c., a radiosensitive tumor composed of small, oval, undifferentiated cells that are intensely hematoxyphilic and typically bronchogenic.

papillary c., carcinoma in which there are papillary excrescences; called also papillocarcinoma.

scirrhous c., carcinoma with a hard structure owing to the formation of dense connective tissue in the stroma.

renal cell c., carcinoma of the renal parenchyma, composed of tubular cells in varying arrangements.

c. sim′plex, an undifferentiated carcinoma.

spindle cell c., squamous cell carcinoma marked by fusiform development or rapidly proliferating cells.

squamous cell c., that arising from squamous epithelium and having cuboid cells.

carcinomatosis (kar″sĭ-no″mah-to′sis) the condition of widespread dissemination of cancer throughout the body.

carcinomatous (kar″sĭ-no′mah-tus) pertaining to or of the nature of cancer; malignant.

carcinophilia (kar″sĭ-no-fil′e-ah) special affinity for cancerous tissue. adj., **carcinophil′ic.**

carcinophobia (kar″sĭ-no-fo′be-ah) morbid dread of cancer.

carcinosarcoma (kar″sĭ-no-sar-ko′mah) a malignant tumor composed of carcinomatous and sarcomatous tissues.

embryonal c., a rapidly developing, malignant mixed tumor of the kidneys, made up of embryonal elements, and occuring chiefly in children before the fifth year; called also Wilms' tumor.

carcinosis (kar″sĭ-no′sis) carcinomatosis.

miliary c., that marked by development of numerous nodules resembling miliary tuberculosis.

cardamom (kar′dah-mom) the fruit of *Elettaria cardamomum*, a plant of tropical Asia, the source of a seed and oil used as flavoring agents.

Cardarelli's sign (kar-dar-el′ēz) transverse pulsation of the laryngotracheal tube in aneurysms and in dilatation of the arch of the aorta.

cardi(o)- word element [Gr.], *heart.*

cardia (kar′de-ah) 1. the cardiac opening. 2. the cardiac part of the stomach; that part of the stomach surrounding the esophagogastric junction, distinguished by the presence of cardiac glands.

cardiac (kar′de-ak) 1. pertaining to the heart. 2. pertaining to the cardia.

c. arrest, sudden and often unexpected stoppage of effective heart action. Either the periodic impulses which trigger the coordinated heart muscle contractions cease or ventricular fibrillation or flutter occurs in which the individual muscle fibers have a rapid irregular twitching. If resuscitation is not undertaken within minutes of the occurrence of cardiac arrest, permanent damage to other organs will result from insufficient blood supply, and the death of the individual is probable. Resuscitation involves not only use of CARDIAC MASSAGE (external or internal), but also ARTIFICIAL RESPIRATION by the mouth-to-mouth method or by mechanical respirator (see also CARDIOPULMONARY RESUSCITATION). The use of a defibrillator or artificial pacemaker will depend on the cause of the arrest, usually determined by electrocardiography.

c. catheterization, passage of a long, fine catheter through a vein in an arm or leg or the neck and into the chambers of the heart, permitting the securing of blood samples, determination of intracardiac pressure, and detection of cardiac anomalies. This procedure is carried out under direct visualization with a FLUOROSCOPE. Samples of blood are taken from the right and left chambers of the heart and from the pulmonary artery, and later tested for measurement of the hematocrit and oxygen saturation. Pressures within the heart chambers are also measured and recorded. The findings obtained from these tests help determine valvular insufficiencies and stenosis, deformities of the heart chambers and pulmonary artery, and other disorders and malfunctions of the heart.

c. massage, an emergency measure to empty the ventricles of the heart in an effort to circulate the blood, and also to stimulate the heart so that it will resume its pumping action. In both external and internal cardiac massage, mouth-to-mouth resuscitation must be carried out at the same time the heart is being massaged. If available, an automatic resuscitator with mask and rebreathing bag can be used. (See also CARDIOPULMONARY RESUSCITATION.)

CLOSED OR EXTERNAL CARDIAC MASSAGE. This closed-chest method of cardiopulmonary resuscitation is a rhythmic massage of the heart between the lower sternum in the front and the vertebral column in the back. It is a drastic measure that should be undertaken only by trained personnel because of the risk of causing injuries such as rib fractures, damage to the heart and liver, and puncture of the lungs or blood vessels that can lead to internal bleeding, fat emboli, and other serious complications.

OPEN OR INTERNAL CARDIAC MASSAGE. This involves a surgical incision directly over the heart and manual massage of the heart or stimulation with an electric current.

cardialgia (kar″de-al′je-ah) cardiodynia.

cardioaccelerator (kar″de-o-ak-sel′er-a″tor) quickening the heart action; an agent that so acts.

cardioactive (kar″de-o-ak′tiv) having an effect on the heart.

cardioangiology (kar″de-o-an″je-ol′o-je) the medical specialty dealing with the heart and blood vessels.

cardiocele (kar′de-o-sēl″) hernial protrusion of the heart through a fissure of the diaphragm or through a wound.

cardiocentesis (kar″de-o-sen-te′sis) surgical puncture of the heart.

cardiochalasia (kar″de-o-kah-la′ze-ah) relaxation or incompetence of the sphincter action of the cardiac opening of the stomach.

cardiocirrhosis (kar″de-o-sĭ-ro′sis) cirrhosis of the liver complicating heart disease, with recurrent intractable congestive heart failure.

cardiodiaphragmatic (kar″de-o-di″ah-frag-mat′ik) pertaining to the heart and the diaphragm.

cardiodilator (kar″de-o-di′la-tor) an instrument for dilating the cardia.

cardiodiosis (kar″de-o-di-o′sis) dilatation of the cardiac opening of the stomach.

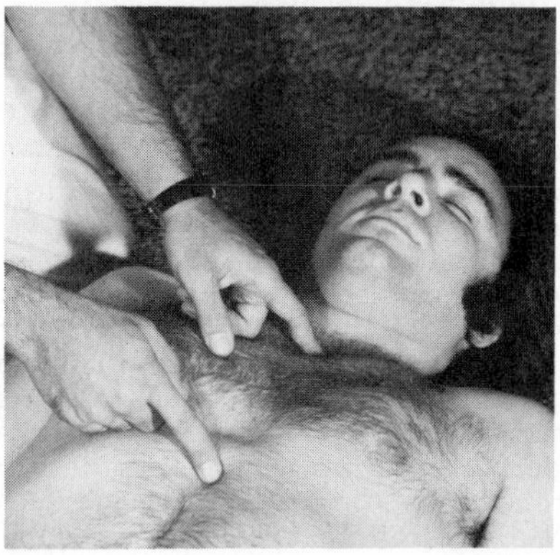

(1)

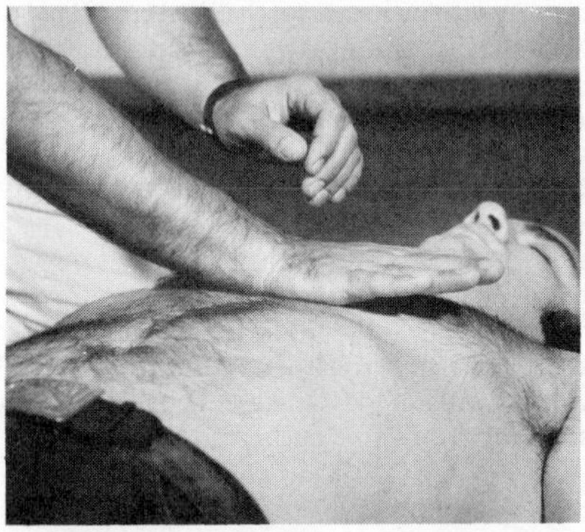

(2)

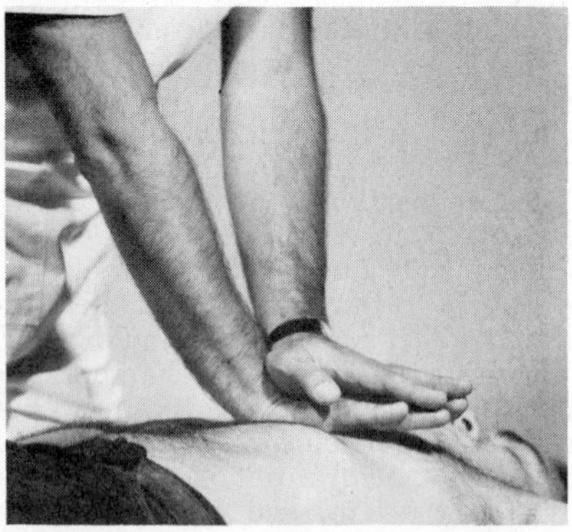

(3)

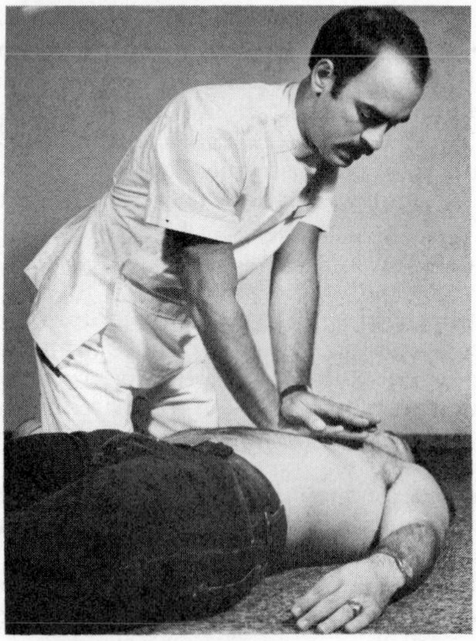

(4)

Closed cardiac massage. (1) Locate lower half of sternum. (2) Apply heel of one hand over lower half of sternum 1–1½ inches above the tip of the sternum. (3) Place second hand over first, bringing shoulders directly over victim's sternum. (4) Apply pressure so that sternum is depressed 1½–2 inches. (From American Journal of Nursing. Feb., 1975.)

cardiodynamics (kar″de-o-di-nam′iks) study of the forces involved in the heart's action.

cardiodynia (kar″de-o-din′e-ah) pain in the heart.

cardiogenesis (kar″de-o-jen′ĕ-sis) development of the heart in the embryo.

cardiogenic (kar″de-o-jen′ik) originating in the heart.

cardiogram (kar′de-o-gram″) a tracing of a cardiac event produced by cardiography (see also ELECTROCARDIOGRAM).

cardiograph (kar′de-o-graf″) an instrument for recording some element of the heart beat.

cardiography (kar″de-og′rah-fe) the graphic recording of a physical or functional aspect of the heart, e.g., electrocardiography, kinetocardiography, phonocardiography, vibrocardiography.

apex c., graphic recording of low-frequency pulsations at the anterior chest wall over the apex of the heart.

ultrasonic c., echocardiography.

vector c., vectorcardiography.

Cardio-Green (kar′de-o-grēn″) trademark for a preparation of indocyanine green, a dye used intravenously as a diagnostic aid in the determination of blood volume, cardiac output, and hepatic function.

cardiohepatic (kar″de-o-hĕ-pat′ik) pertaining to the heart and liver.

cardioinhibitor (kar″de-o-in-hib′ĭ-tor) an agent that restrains the heart's action.

cardioinhibitory (kar″de-o-in-hib′ĭ-to-re) restraining or inhibiting the heart movements.

cardiokinetic (kar″de-o-ki-net′ik) 1. exciting or stimulating the heart. 2. an agent that excites or stimulates the heart.

cardiolipin (kar″de-o-lip′in) a substance extracted from fresh beef hearts which, when combined with lecithin and cholesterol, forms an antigen for use in flocculation and precipitation tests for syphilis.

cardiologist (kar″de-ol′o-jist) a physician skilled in the diagnosis and treatment of heart disease.

cardiology (kar″de-ol′o-je) study of the heart and its functions.

cardiolysin (kar″de-ol′ĭ-sin) a lysin that acts on the heart muscle.

cardiolysis (kar″de-ol′ĭ-sis) the operation of freeing the heart from its adhesions to the sternal periosteum in adhesive mediastinopericarditis.

cardiomalacia (kar″de-o-mah-la′she-ah) morbid softening of the muscular substance of the heart.

cardiomegaly (kar″de-o-meg′ah-le) hypertrophy of the heart.

cardiomelanosis (kar″de-o-mel″ah-no′sis) melanosis of the heart.

cardiometer (kar″de-om′ĕ-ter) an instrument for estimating the power of the heart's action.

cardiomotility (kar″de-o-mo-til′ĭ-te) the movement of the heart; motility of the heart.

cardiomyoliposis (kar″de-o-mi″o-lĭ-po′sis) fatty degeneration of the heart muscle.

cardiomyopathy (kar″de-o-mi-op′ah-the) a general diagnostic term designating primary myocardial disease.

cardiomyopexy (kar″de-o-mi′o-pek″se) surgical removal of the epicardium and application of a pedicled flap of adjacent muscle to the denuded myocardium and pericardium, as a means of supplying collateral circulation to the heart.

cardionector (kar″de-o-nek′tor) the structures that regulate the heart beat, comprising the sinoatrial node, bundle of His, and atrioventricular node.

cardionephric (kar″de-o-nef′rik) pertaining to the heart and kidney.

cardioneural (kar″de-o-nu′ral) pertaining to the heart and nervous system.

cardioneurosis (kar″de-o-nu-ro′sis) neurocirculatory asthenia.

cardio-omentopexy (kar″de-o-o-men′to-pek″se) suture of a portion of the omentum to the heart.

cardiopaludism (kar″de-o-pal′u-dizm) heart disease due to malaria.

cardiopathy (kar″de-op′ah-the) any disorder or disease of the heart.

cardiopericardiopexy (kar″de-o-per″ĭ-kar′de-o-pek″se) surgical establishment of adhesive pericarditis, for relief of coronary disease.

cardiopericarditis (kar″de-o-per″ĭ-kar-di′tis) inflammation of the heart and pericardium.

cardiophobia (kar″de-o-fo′be-ah) morbid dread of heart disease.

cardioplasty (kar′de-o-plas″te) esophagogastroplasty.

cardioplegia (kar″de-o-ple′je-ah) interruption of myocardial contraction, as by use of chemical compounds or cold in cardiac surgery.

cardiopneumatic (kar″de-o-nu-mat′ik) pertaining to the heart and respiration.

cardiopneumograph (kar″de-o-nu′mo-graf) an apparatus for registering cardiopneumatic movements.

cardioptosis (kar″de-o-to′sis) downward displacement of the heart.

cardiopulmonary (kar″de-o-pul′mo-ner″e) pertaining to the heart and lungs.

c. resuscitation, the reestablishing of heart and lung action as indicated for cardiac arrest or "sudden death" resulting from cardiovascular collapse, electric shock, drowning, respiratory arrest, and other causes. The technique is used as an emergency first aid procedure to provide basic life support until more advanced life support is available.

Since the late 1960's cardiopulmonary resuscitation has become an integral part of the broader field of emergency care. In 1973 a National Conference on Standards for Cardiopulmonary Resuscitation (CPR) and Emergency Cardiac Care (ECC) was sponsored by the American Heart Association and the National Academy of Sciences. At this conference standards for CPR and ECC were developed and recommended. The standards relate to principles and techniques for basic and advanced life support, CPR training and certification, training of medical and allied health personnel, the role of the American National Red Cross and other agencies in training the lay public, and medicolegal aspects of CPR and ECC.

It is recognized that the standards developed by this conference group for the training and performance of CPR may be subject to change as research in this area continues. These standards were intended as a guide for the proper training and performance of CPR. The procedure is not without its hazards and can be completely ineffective if not performed by trained and knowledgeable persons.

For this reason it is strongly recommended that those interested in mastering the technique enroll in an approved course of instruction that is conducted according to standards set by the American Heart Association.

INDICATIONS FOR CPR. Prompt action is essential to the successful outcome of the procedure. At the moment breathing and heart action stop, "clinical death" occurs. Within four to six minutes the cells of the brain, which are most sensitive to lack of oxygen, begin to deteriorate. If breathing and circulation are not restored in this period of time, irreversible damage to the brain cells occurs and "biological death" takes place.

Although CPR is strongly recommended as a life-saving measure, it is not without danger; specifically, there is risk of rib fracture, damage to the heart and liver, and puncture of the lungs and blood vessels. Since these dangers are present whenever vigorous cardiac massage is carried out, CPR is begun only when three signs are present: (1) absence of pulse, (2) absence of breathing, and (3) dilated pupils that do not react to light. Failure of the pupils to constrict in the presence of light indicates lack of oxygen supply to the brain cells.

CPR TECHNIQUE. The victim is positioned on his back on the ground or floor. If he is lying on a soft surface, a board is placed under his back. The two major components of cardiopulmonary resuscitation are ARTIFICIAL RESPIRATION and external CARDIAC MASSAGE. The recommended type of artificial respiration is mouth-to-mouth resuscitation at the rate of once every five seconds or about 12 times a minute.

The first step is providing an open airway so that nothing obstructs the passage of air to and from the lungs. The head is tilted back, hyperextending the neck so that the chin is pointed upward and the air passages straightened. This may be the only maneuver necessary for breathing to resume spontaneously. If foreign material is obstructing the airway, it must be removed.

After blowing into the victim's lungs the rescuer turns his head to take another deep breath and to look at the victim's chest to see that it is falling into a relaxed position and air is being exhaled. If there is no evidence of air exchange, the mouth and throat are checked for obstruction. The cycle of blowing into and allowing for exchange of air from the lungs is repeated regularly once every five seconds until the victim breathes on his own or a mechanical respirator is available. The head is maintained in position throughout the procedure. Variations of the ventilation technique are necessary for infants and small children, for accident victims, and for laryngectomees and others with tracheostomy tubes or stomas.

Cardiac compression is instituted immediately after the first three to five breaths are blown into the lungs. The first step in cardiac compression is to locate the lower half of the sternum. The area can be located by pressing on the upper abdomen. The point at which the softer abdominal wall and the harder tip of the sternum come together is identified. The heel of one hand is then placed directly over the lower half of the sternum (NOT on the xiphoid process), and the heel of the other hand is placed over the first. The fingers of both hands are held as high as possible to avoid contact with the ribs.

The rescuer giving external massage should position himself directly over the victim so that pressure can be applied downward vertically, thus using the weight of the upper part of his body to compress the heart. The arms are kept straight and firm heavy pressure is applied. The amount of pressure varies with the anatomy of the victim; the goal is to push the sternum down $1\frac{1}{2}$ to 2 inches in order to squeeze the heart against the spinal column. The sternum is pressed down and held about one-half second and then quickly released. The heel of the hand is not removed from the sternum and the rhythm is not interrupted. If interruption is necessary, as in transporting the victim, interruption should never exceed 15 seconds.

Compression is applied once every second or 60 to 80 times a minute for adults. Children and infants require a faster rate of 100 to 120 times per minute. External cardiac compression is always accompanied by artificial ventilation.

It is possible for one person to administer CPR without assistance. The first step is to blow into the victim's mouth three times. The rescuer then quickly shifts position and applies cardiac compression fifteen times. He then starts a cycle of 2 breaths to 15 compressions.

When two persons are available, the first rescuer immediately clears the airway and blows into the lungs three times. The second person then begins cardiac compression. The two rescuers work together in a rhythmic cycle of one blow into the lungs *between* every fifth and sixth compression (5:1 ratio). The compression of the heart is NOT stopped to allow ventilation. The person giving the massage counts while the one ventilating the victim periodically feels for the carotid pulse to assure that blood is being circulated by the compression. When resuscitation efforts are prolonged, the two rescuers can switch positions so that neither becomes unduly fatigued.

THE PRECORDIAL THUMP. Delivering a sharp blow to the sternum to revive heart action is useful in specific types of cardiac arrest cases. The precordial thump is recommended in cases of witnessed cardiac arrest, with patients who are being monitored during advanced life support, and those with known atrioventricular block. In delivering the precordial thump one should strike a single, sharp and quick blow over the midportion of the sternum. The blow is delivered with the bottom, fleshy portion of the fist, striking from 8 to 12 inches over the chest. If there is no immediate response from the heart, CPR is begun at once.

cardiopuncture (kar″de-o-pungk′tūr) cardiocentesis.

cardiopyloric (kar″de-o-pi-lor′ik) pertaining to the cardiac opening of the stomach and the pylorus.

cardiorenal (kar″de-o-re′nal) pertaining to the heart and kidneys.

cardiorrhaphy (kar″de-or′ah-fe) suture of the heart muscle.

cardiorrhexis (kar″de-o-rek′sis) rupture of the heart.

cardiosclerosis (kar″de-o-skle-ro′sis) fibrous induration of the heart.

cardiospasm (kar′de-o-spazm″) achalasia of the esophagus.

cardiosphygmograph (kar″de-o-sfig′mo-graf) a combination of the cardiograph and sphygmograph for recording the movements of the heart and an arterial pulse.

cardiosplenopexy (kar″de-o-splen′o-pek″se) suture of the parenchyma of the spleen to the denuded surface of the heart for revascularization of the myocardium.

cardiotachometer (kar″de-o-tah-kom′ĕ-ter) an instrument for continuously portraying or recording the heart rate.

cardiotachometry (kar″de-o-tah-kom′ĕ-tre) continuous recording of the heart rate for long periods.

cardiotherapy (kar″de-o-ther′ah-pe) the treatment of diseases of the heart.

cardiotomy (kar″de-ot′o-me) 1. surgical incision of the heart. 2. surgical incision into the cardia.

cardiotonic (kar″de-o-ton′ik) having a tonic effect on the heart; an agent that so acts.

cardiotoxic (kar″de-o-tok′sik) having a poisonous or deleterious effect upon the heart.

cardiovalvular (kar″de-o-val′vu-lar) pertaining to the valves of the heart.

cardiovalvulotome (kar″de-o-val′vu-lo-tōm″) an instrument for incising a heart valve.

cardiovascular (kar″de-o-vas′ku-lar) pertaining to the heart and blood vessels.

cardioversion (kar′de-o-ver″zhun) the restoration of sinus rhythm by electrical shock.

cardioverter (kar′de-o-ver″ter) an energy-storage capacitor-discharge type of condenser that is discharged with an inductance; it delivers a direct-current shock which restores sinus rhythm in atrial fibrillation.

carditis (kar-di′tis) inflammation of the heart; MYOCARDITIS.

cardivalvulitis (kar″dĭ-val″vu-li′tis) inflammation of the heart valves.

Cardrase (kar′drās) trademark for a preparation of ethoxzolamide, a diuretic used mainly in edema, glaucoma, and epilepsy.

Carey-Coombs murmur (kār′e-ko͞omz) a rumbling mid-diastolic murmur occurring in the early stages of rheumatic fever.

caries (ka′re-ēz, kār′ēz) decay, as of bone or teeth. adj., **ca′rious.**

dental c., a destructive process causing decalcification of the tooth enamel and leading to continued destruction of enamel and dentin, and cavitation of the tooth.

Decayed and infected teeth can be the source of other infections throughout the body, and decayed or missing teeth can interfere with the proper chewing of food, leading to nutrition deficiencies or to disorders of digestion.

CAUSES. The causes of tooth decay are not completely understood, but certain facts are known. Tooth decay seems to be a disease of civilization, possibly associated with refined foods. A lack of dental cleanliness is also closely associated with tooth decay.

Decay occurs where bacteria and food adhere to the surface of the teeth, especially in pits or crevices, and form plaques. It is believed that the action of the bacteria on sugars and starches creates lactic acid, which can quickly and permanently dissolve the enamel that covers the teeth. The acid produced in just half an hour when sugar comes into contact with the plaque is enough to begin the process of dissolving tooth enamel. In most people this process and its resulting decay occur whenever sweet foods are eaten. It is for this reason that sweet or starchy foods between meals and at bedtime can be so harmful to the teeth unless the teeth are thoroughly brushed and rinsed immediately afterward.

Decay that is not treated will progress through the tooth enamel and the dentin just below it into the pulp of the tooth, which contains the nerves. When it reaches the pulp, it can cause intense pain. There is no relief until the pulp dies or is removed, or the tooth is extracted.

TREATMENT. The only treatment for tooth decay is regular dental care. Enamel that has been destroyed does not grow back. The decay must be removed, and the cavity filled. The fillings, or restorations, may be of gold foil, baked porcelain, synthetic cements, silver amalgam, or cast gold inlays.

When decay has reached the pulp of a tooth, it may be necessary to extract the tooth. Whenever possible, however, the exposed pulp is re-covered, or capped, and the tooth is then filled. New techniques of root canal therapy are saving many teeth that would formerly have been lost.

PREVENTION. There is no cure for tooth decay. Prevention is the only real answer to the problem. This means scrupulous cleanliness and removal of plaques. The teeth should be thoroughly brushed at least once a day, and preferably after every meal. Dental floss or tape should be used to remove any particles of food from between the teeth. If teeth cannot be brushed after every meal, the mouth should be thoroughly rinsed with water.

Diet, too, plays a most important part in the prevention of tooth decay. Sugars and starches (the carbohydrates) should be limited, especially between meals. This applies particularly to those which are sticky and tend to cling to the teeth.

FLUORIDATION of drinking water is also proving effective in combating tooth decay. In communities where fluoride is not added to the water supply, a dentist may apply a fluoride solution directly to a child's teeth. Fluoride drops or tablets may also be prescribed in small amounts, to be mixed with milk or other fluids, but this treatment must always be carefully supervised by a doctor or dentist.

dry c., c. sic′ca, a form of tuberculous caries of the joints and ends of bones.

carina (kah-ri′nah), pl. *cari′nae* [L.] a ridgelike structure.

c. tra′cheae, a downward and backward projection of the lowest tracheal cartilage, forming a ridge between the openings of the right and left principal bronchi.

c. urethra′lis vagi′nae, the column of rugae in the lower anterior wall of the vagina, immediately below the urethra.

cariogenesis (kār″e-o-jen′ĕ-sis) the development of caries.

cariogenic (kār″e-o-jen′ik) conducive to caries.

carisoprodol (kar″i-so′pro-dol) an analgesic and skeletal muscle relaxant.

carminative (kar-min′ah-tiv) 1. relieving flatulence. 2. an agent that relieves flatulence.

carnitine (kar′nĭ-tēn) a vitamin of the B complex present in meat extracts.

carnivore (kar′nĭ-vōr) any animal that eats primarily flesh, particularly mammals of the order Carnivora, which includes cats, dogs, bears, etc. adj., **carniv'orus.**

carnosinase (kar'no-sĭ-nās) an enzyme that hydrolyzes carnosine (amino-acyl-L-histidine) and other dipeptides containing L-histidine into their constituent amino acids.

carnosine (kar'no-sin) a dipeptide composed of beta-alanine and histidine, found in skeletal muscle of vertebrates.

carnosinemia (kar"no-sĭ-ne'me-ah) excessive amounts of carnosine in the blood; it has been associated with a progressive neurologic disease characterized by severe mental defect and myoclonic seizures, and is probably due to a genetic deficiency of carnosinase in the serum.

carnosinuria (kar"no-sĭ-nu're-ah) an aminoaciduria characterized by excess of carnosine in the urine; it occurs in carnosinemia or may be dietary in origin, especially in young children.

carotenase (kar-ot'ĕ-nās) an enzyme that converts carotene into vitamin A.

carotene (kar'o-tēn) a yellow or red pigment from carrots, sweet potatoes, milk and body fat, egg yolk, etc.; it is a chromolipoid hydrocarbon existing in several forms (α-, β-, and γ-carotene), which can be converted into vitamin A in the body.

carotenemia (kar"o-tĕ-ne'me-ah) the presence of carotene in the blood; sometimes occurring in sufficient amounts to cause yellowing of the skin.

carotenodermia (kah-rot"ĕ-no-der'me-ah) yellowness of the skin due to carotenemia.

carotenoid (kah-rot'ĕ-noid) 1. any member of a group of red, orange, or yellow pigmented polyisoprenoid lipids found in carrots, sweet potatoes, green leaves, and some animal tissues; examples are the carotenes, lycopene, and xanthophyll. 2. marked by yellow color. 3. lipochrome.

carotenosis (kar"o-tĕ-no'sis) deposition of carotene in tissues, especially the skin.

caroticotympanic (kah-rot"ĭ-ko-tim-pan'ik) pertaining to the carotid canal and tympanum.

carotid (kah-rot'id) relating to the carotid artery, the principal artery of the neck (see table of ARTERIES).

c. body, a small neurovascular structure lying in the bifurcation of the right and left carotid arteries, containing chemoreceptors that monitor oxygen content in blood and help to regulate respiration.

c. canal, a canal in the pars petrosa of the temporal bone, transmitting the internal carotid artery to the cranial cavity.

c. sinus, a dilatation of the proximal portion of the internal carotid or distal portion of the common carotid artery, containing in its wall pressoreceptors which are stimulated by changes in blood pressure.

c. sinus reflex, slowing of the heart beat when pressure is exerted on the carotid artery at the level of the cricoid cartilage.

c. sinus syndrome, syncope sometimes associated with convulsive seizures due to overactivity of the carotid sinus reflex. In certain susceptible persons the carotid sinus is too easily stimulated and symptoms are produced by sudden turning of the head or the wearing of a tight collar. Transient attacks of numbness or weakness of the face, arm, or leg, headache, and in some cases aphasia may also occur. Diagnosis can be confirmed by a gentle massage of the carotid sinus area, which will cause an attack. Drugs used to terminate attacks or to prevent their occurrence include atropine sulfate, ephedrine sulfate with phenobarbital, and amphetamine sulfate.

carotidynia (kah-rot"ĭ-din'e-ah) tenderness along the course of the carotid artery.

carotin (kar'o-tin) carotene.

carpal (kar'pal) pertaining to the carpus, or wrist.

c. tunnel, the osseofibrous passage for the median nerve and the flexor tendons, formed by the flexor retinaculum and the carpal bones.

c. tunnel syndrome, a symptom complex resulting from compression of the median nerve in the carpal tunnel, with pain and burning or tingling paresthesias in the fingers and hand, sometimes extending to the elbow. The disorder is found most often in middle-aged women. Excessive wrist movements, arthritis, hypertrophy of the bone and connective tissue in ACROMEGALY, and swelling of the wrist can produce the carpal tunnel syndrome. Treatment is usually conservative and consists of splinting the wrist to immobilize it for several weeks until the irritation of the median nerve has healed. In severe cases surgical resection of the carpal ligament is helpful.

carpectomy (kar-pek'to-me) excision of a carpal bone.

carphenazine (kar-fen'ah-zēn) a major tranquilizer; used as the maleate salt.

carphology (kar-fol'o-je) involuntary picking at the bedclothes, seen in states of great exhaustion and grave fevers.

carpometacarpal (kar"po-met"ah-kar'pal) pertaining to the carpus and metacarpus.

carpopedal (kar"po-pe'dal) affecting the wrist and foot.

carpophalangeal (kar"po-fah-lan'je-al) pertaining to the carpus and phalanges.

carpoptosis (kar"po-to'sis) wristdrop.

carpus (kar'pus) the joint between the arm and hand, made up of eight bones; the WRIST. (See also table of BONES.)

carrageen, carragheen (kar'ah-gēn) the dried and bleached plant of the seaweed *Chondrus crispus* or *Gigartina mammillosa*, containing a valuable polysaccharide widely used as a gel, thickening agent, and emulsifier; it also has demulcent properties.

carrier (kăr'e-er) 1. one who harbors disease organisms in his body without manifest symptoms, thus acting as a carrier or distributor of infection. 2. a heterozygote, i.e., one who carries a recessive gene, autosomal or sex-linked, together with its normal allele.

carrier-free (kar'e-er-fre") a term denoting a radioisotope of an element in pure form, i.e., essentially undiluted with a stable isotope carrier.

Carrión's disease (kar-e-ōnz') an infectious disease of South America due to *Bartonella bacilliformis*, and transmitted by the sandfly *Phlebotomus verrucarum*; an acute febrile anemic stage (Oroya fever) is followed by the appearance of a nodular cutaneous eruption (verruga peruana). Called also bartonellosis.

cartilage (kar'tĭ-lij) a specialized, fibrous connective tissue present in adults, and forming most of the temporary skeleton in the embryo, providing a model in which most of the bones develop, and constituting an important part of the organism's growth mechanism; the three most important types are hyaline cartilage, elastic cartilage, and fibrocartilage. Also, a general term for a mass of such tissue in a particular site in the body.

alar c's, the cartilages of the wings of the nose.

aortic c., the second costal cartilage on the right side.

arthrodial c., articular c., that lining the articular surfaces of synovial joints.

arytenoid c's, two pyramid-shaped cartilages of the larynx.

connecting c., that connecting the surfaces of an immovable joint.

costal c., a bar of hyaline cartilage that attaches a rib to the sternum in the case of true ribs, or to the immediately above rib in the case of the upper false ribs.

cricoid c., a ringlike cartilage forming the lower and back part of the larynx.

diarthrodial c., articular cartilage.

elastic c., cartilage that is more opaque, flexible, and elastic than hyaline cartilage, and is further distinguished by its yellow color. The ground substance is penetrated in all directions by frequently branching fibers that give all of the reactions for elastin.

ensiform c., xiphoid process.

fibrous c., fibrocartilage.

floating c., a detached portion of semilunar cartilage in the knee joint.

hyaline c., flexible, somewhat elastic, semitransparent cartilage with an opalescent bluish tint, composed of a basophilic fibril-containing substance with cavities in which the chondrocytes occur.

permanent c., cartilage that does not normally become ossified.

reticular c., elastic cartilage.

semilunar c., one of the two interarticular cartilages of the knee joint.

temporary c., cartilage that is normally destined to be replaced by bone.

thyroid c., the shield-shaped cartilage of the larynx.

vomeronasal c., either of the two narrow strips of cartilage, one on each side, of the nasal septum supporting the vomeronasal organ.

yellow c., elastic cartilage.

cartilaginiform (kar″tĭ-lah-jin′ĭ-form) resembling cartilage.

cartilaginous (kar″tĭ-laj′ĭ-nus) consisting of or of the nature of cartilage.

cartilago (kar″tĭ-lah′go), pl. *cartilag′ines* [L.] cartilage.

caruncle (kar′ung-k'l) a small fleshy eminence, often abnormal.

hymenal c's, small elevations of mucous membrane around the vaginal opening, being relics of the ruptured hymen.

lacrimal c., the red eminence at the medial angle of the eye.

sublingual c., an eminence on either side of the frenulum of the tongue (frenulum linguae), on which the major duct of the sublingual gland and the duct of the submandibular gland open.

urethral c., a small red eminence in the mucous membrane of the female urinary meatus, sometimes causing difficulty in voiding.

caruncula (kah-rung′ku-lah), pl. *carun′culae* [L.] caruncle.

caryo- for words beginning thus, see those beginning *karyo-*.

casanthranol (kah-san′thrah-nōl) a purified mixture of the anthranol glycosides derived from cascara sagrada; a cathartic.

cascade (kas-kād′) a series of steps or stages (as of a physiological process) which, once initiated continues to the final step by virtue of each step being triggered by the preceding one, sometimes with cumulative effect.

cascara (kas-kār′ah) bark.

c. sagra′da, dried bark of *Rhamnus purshiana*, used as a cathartic.

case (kās) a particular instance of disease; as a case of leukemia; sometimes used incorrectly to designate the patient with the disease.

casease (ka′se-ās) a protease from bacterial cultures, capable of dissolving albumin and the casein of milk and cheese.

caseation (ka″se-a′shun) 1. the precipitation of casein. 2. a form of necrosis in which tissue is changed into a dry, amorphous mass resembling cheese.

casein (ka′se-in) a phosphoprotein, the principal protein of milk, the basis of curd and of cheese. NOTE: In British nomenclature casein is called caseinogen, and paracasein is called casein.

caseinogen (ka″se-in′o-jen) the British term for casein.

caseous (ka′se-us) resembling cheese or curd; cheesy.

Casoni's test (kah-so′nēz) intradermal injection of hydatid fluid followed by production of wheal-flare reaction denotes hydatid infection.

cassette (kah-set′) [Fr.] a light-proof housing for x-ray film, containing front and back intensifying screens, between which the film is placed; a magazine for film or magnetic tape.

cast (kast) 1. a positive copy of an object, e.g., a mold of a hollow organ (a renal tubule, bronchiole, etc.), formed of effused plastic matter and extruded from the body, as a urinary cast; named according to constituents, as epithelial, fatty, waxy, etc. 2. a positive copy of the tissues of the jaws, made in an impression, and over which denture bases or other restorations may be fabricated. 3. to form an object in a mold. 4. a stiff dressing or casing, usually made of plaster of Paris, used to immobilize body parts. 5. strabismus.

PATIENT CARE. If the patient is confined to bed after a plaster of Paris cast is applied, it is necessary to provide a firm mattress protected by a waterproof material. Several small pillows should be available for placing under the curves of the cast to prevent remolding or cracking of the plaster and to provide adequate support of the patient. When handling a wet cast only the palm or flat of the hand is used so that the fingertips will not make indentations that might produce pressure against the patient's skin.

While the cast is drying it is left uncovered to allow sufficient circulation of air around it. The parts of the body not included in the cast are covered with a sheet or light blanket to avoid chilling. Extreme heat should not be used to hasten drying as this may produce burns under the cast. The patient is turned frequently to insure proper drying and to avoid prolonged pressure on any one area.

Parts of the cast that may become soiled by urine or feces can be covered with a plastic material which can be changed as necessary. To minimize crumbling of the edges and irritation of the skin around and under the cast, a strip of stockinette or adhesive tape is applied so that the rim of the cast is thoroughly covered. Observation of the patient for signs of impaired circulation or pressure against a nerve is extremely important. Any numbness, recurrent pain, or tingling should be reported at once. If an extremity is enclosed in a cast it should be elevated to reduce swelling. Cyanosis or blanching of the fingers or toes extending from a cast usually indicates impaired blood flow which may lead to serious complications if not corrected immediately.

castor oil (kas′tor) a fixed oil obtained from the seed of the castor bean plant (*Ricinus communis*); it has an irritant effect on the intestines and acts as a powerful purgative. Castor oil is a powerful CATHARTIC, and should not be used as a treatment for constipation or any digestive disorder. It is used primarily in the preparation of the bowel for diagnostic tests and surgery. Its unpleasant taste and texture can be disguised if it is given in iced orange juice. Castor oil is also used externally as an emollient in seborrheic dermatitis and other skin diseases.

castrate (kas′trāt) 1. to deprive of the gonads, rendering the individual incapable of reproduction. 2. a castrated individual.

castration (kas-tra′shun) excision of the gonads, or their destruction, as by radiation or parasites.

female c., removal of the ovaries, or bilateral OOPHORECTOMY; spaying.

male c., removal of the testes, or bilateral ORCHIECTOMY. It may be employed in therapy of metastatic cancer of the prostate.

casualty (kaz′u-al-te) 1. an accident; an accidental wound; death or disablement from an accident; also the person so injured. 2. in the armed forces, one missing from his unit as a result of death, injury, illness, capture, because his whereabouts are unknown, or other reasons.

casuistics (kaz″u-is′tiks) the recording and study of cases of disease.

CAT computerized axial tomography (see computerized transverse axial TOMOGRAPHY).

cat(a)- word element [Gr.], *down; lower; under; against; along with; very.*

catabasis (kah-tab′ah-sis) the stage of decline of a disease. adj., **catabat′ic.**

catabiosis (kat″ah-bi-o′sis) the natural senescence of cells. adj., **catabiot′ic.**

catabolin (kah-tab′o-lin) a product of destructive metabolism; a catabolite.

catabolism (kah-tab′o-lizm) any destructive process by which complex substances are converted by living cells into simpler compounds, with release of energy (see also METABOLISM). adj., **catabol′ic.**

catabolite (kah-tab′o-lit) a compound produced in catabolism.

catacrotism (kah-tak′rŏ-tizm) a pulse anomaly in which a small additional wave or notch appears in the descending limb of the pulse tracing. adj., **catacrot′ic.**

catadicrotism (kat″ah-di′krŏ-tizm) a pulse anomaly in which two small additional waves or notches appear in the descending limb of the pulse tracing. adj., **catadicrot′ic.**

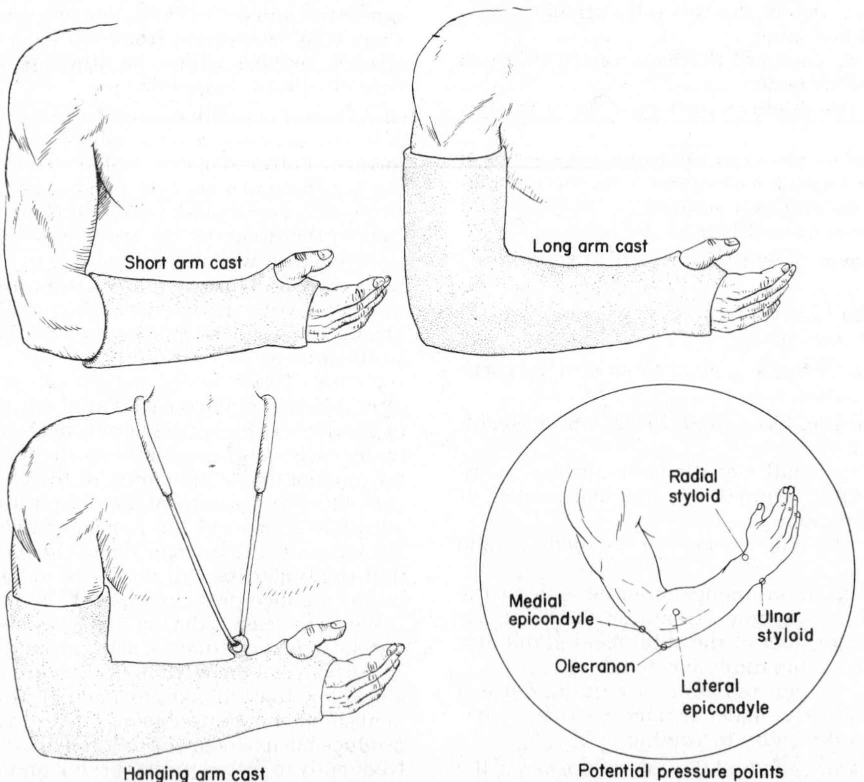

Some types of arm casts and potential pressure points in a casted arm. (From Luckmann, J., and Sorensen, K. C.: Medical-Surgical Nursing. Philadelphia, W. B. Saunders Co., 1974.)

catadioptric (kat″ah-di-op′trik) deflecting and reflecting light at the same time.

catagenesis (kat″ah-jen′ĕ-sis) involution or retrogression.

catalase (kat′ah-lās) a crystalline enzyme that specifically catalyzes the decomposition of hydrogen peroxide and is found in almost all cells except certain anaerobic bacteria. adj., **catalat′ic.**

catalepsy (kat′ah-lep″se) a condition of diminished responsiveness usually characterized by a trance-like state and constantly maintained immobility, often with flexibilitas cerea. The patient with catalepsy may remain in one position for minutes, days, or even longer. adj., **catalep′tic.**

Catalepsy may occur in several mental illnesses. It is most common and indeed considered typical in cases of catatonic SCHIZOPHRENIA. The patient may sit with his hands flat on his knees and his head bowed, or may remain in an awkward and uncomfortable position. He is not necessarily unaware of what is going on, but he does not respond. This apathetic condition may end as suddenly as it begins.

Treatment depends on the underlying disturbance and requires psychiatric examination. It may consist of PSYCHOTHERAPY, medications, SHOCK THERAPY, or a combination of methods.

PATIENT CARE. Regular skin care and exercise of the muscles and joints are necessary to prevent circulatory complications in the patient with catalepsy. Attention must also be given to his nutritional status and an adequate diet provided. Even though the patient may not be able to respond to spoken directions or conversation and is physically unable to move, he cannot be left in one position for long periods of time any more than can the patient who is physically paralyzed. The patient's mental state is such that he cannot recognize numbness or pain, nor can he communicate his need for attention.

Care must be used in conversations held within

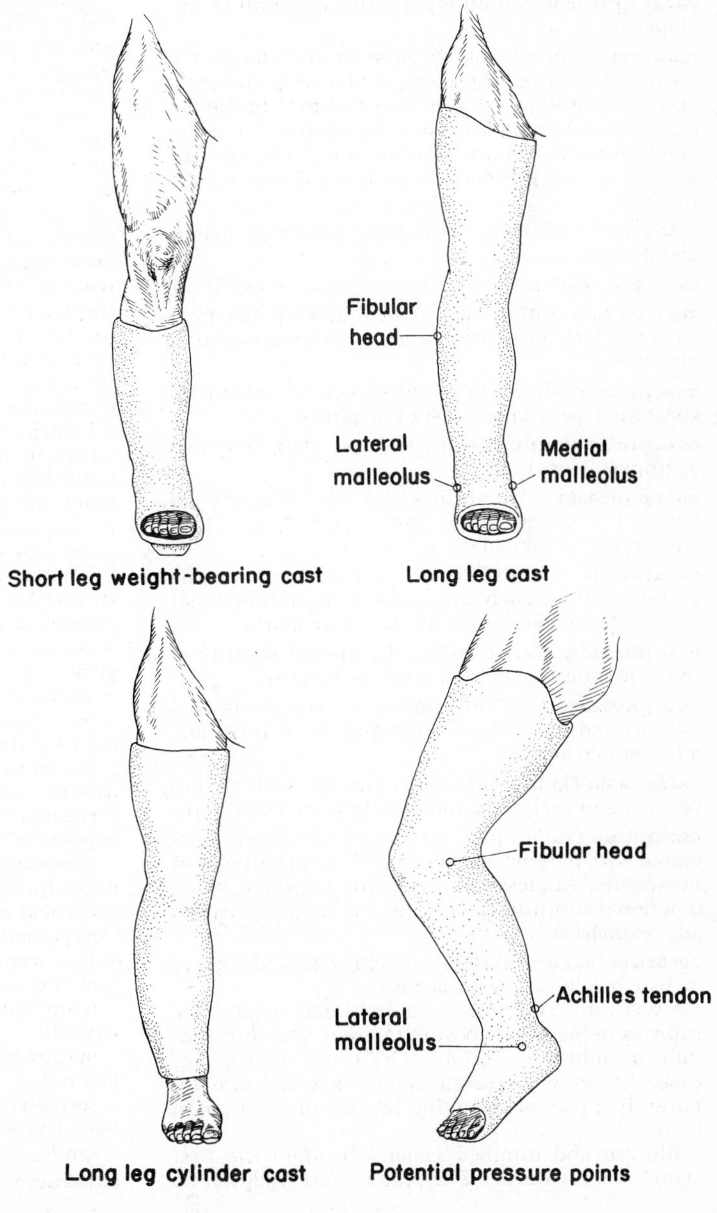

Some types of leg casts and potential pressure points in a casted leg. (From Luckmann, J., and Sorensen, K. C.: Medical-Surgical Nursing. Philadelphia, W. B. Saunders Co., 1974.)

the patient's hearing. His total apathy does not mean that he cannot hear or see what is going on around him. Sometimes it is of great help to this type of patient to have someone sit quietly beside him so that he is aware that someone cares and is genuinely interested in his welfare. Above all, he should not be ignored simply because he is quiet and undemanding of the staff's time and attention.

A sudden change in the patient's condition, with increased activity, may indicate his progression from one state of extreme emotion to another. Restlessness or talkativeness usually do not indicate that his mental condition has dramatically improved. When the patient becomes more active the staff should be alert to the possibility of SUICIDE and attempts at self-mutilation. A person who has exhibited symptoms as severe as catalepsy is very ill and will need continued and long-term care to help him overcome his serious emotional problems.

cataleptiform (kat″ah-lep′tĭ-form) resembling catalepsy.

catalysis (kah-tal′ĭ-sis) increase in the velocity of a chemical reaction or process produced by the presence of a substance that is not consumed in the net chemical reaction or process; negative catalysis denotes the slowing down or inhibition of a reaction or process by the presence of such a substance. adj., **cataly′tic.**

catalyst (kat′ah-list) any substance that brings about catalysis.

catalyze (kat′ah-līz) to cause or produce catalysis.

catamnesis (kat″am-ne′sis) the follow-up history of a patient after he is discharged from treatment or a hospital.

cataphasia (kat″ah-fa′ze-ah) speech disorder with constant repetition of a word or phrase.

cataphora (kah-taf′ŏ-rah) lethargy with intervals of imperfect waking.

cataphoresis (kat″ah-fo-re′sis) the passage of charged particles toward the negative pole (cathode) in ELECTROPHORESIS.

cataphoria (kat″ah-fo′re-ah) a downward turning of the visual axes of both eyes after visual functional stimuli have been removed. adj., **cataphor′ic.**

cataphrenia (kat″ah-fre′ne-ah) mental debility of the dementia type which tends to recovery.

cataphylaxis (kat″ah-fi-lak′sis) movement of leukocytes and antibodies to the site of an infection. adj., **cataphylac′tic.**

cataplasia (kat″ah-pla′ze-ah) atrophy with tissues reverting to earlier, or more embryonic conditions.

cataplexy (kat′ah-plek″se) a condition, often associated with narcolepsy; marked by abrupt attacks of muscular weakness and hypotonia triggered by an emotional stimulus, such as mirth, anger, fear, etc. adj., **cataplec′tic.**

cataract (kat′ah-rakt) opacity of the lens of the eye or its capsule. adj., **catarac′tous.**

CAUSES AND SYMPTOMS. Cataract may result from injuries to the eye, exposure to great heat or radiation, or inherited factors. The great majority of cases, however, are senile cataracts, which are apparently a part of the aging process of the human body.

Blurred and dimmed vision are often the first symptoms of cataract. The patient may find that he needs a brighter reading light, or must hold objects closer to his eyes. The continued clouding of the lens may cause double vision. Finally a need for frequent changes of eyeglasses may be caused by the presence of cataract. These symptoms do not necessarily indicate cataract, but if any of them are present, an ophthalmologist should be consulted immediately.

TREATMENT. The only known effective treatment for cataract is surgical removal of the lens (lens extraction or cataract extraction). In most cases, the procedure of choice is intracapsular extraction, which involves total removal of the lens within its capsule. At one time it was believed that senile cataracts could be removed only after they had become "ripe," that is, after they had reached the mature stage when the lens could be easily separated from the capsule. With the technique of intracapsular extraction it is no longer necessary to wait for maturity of the cataract.

Cryoextraction is a relatively new procedure in which a supercooled metal probe is used to form a bond with the lens capsule; then the lens and its capsule are gently removed. This surgical technique is less traumatic than removal with forceps and has the advantage of allowing removal of immature cataracts. Another surgical technique for cataract extraction is PHACOEMULSIFICATION.

The lens of the eye serves only to focus light rays upon the retina. After cataract extraction the loss of the natural lens is conpensated for by either special eyeglasses or contact lenses.

PATIENT CARE. There is no special care required preoperatively other than administration of eye drops to produce mydriasis and vasoconstriction. Because the patient may have extremely poor eyesight, care should be taken that he does not injure himself in the unfamiliar hospital environment. Local anesthesia is usually preferred for the surgical procedure and preoperative medications are given to produce drowsiness.

Restrictions on movement after surgery are less stringent than they once were. The surgeon may order bed rest for the first 24–48 hours, or he may allow the patient to be ambulatory with care. The patient should be instructed to avoid sudden movements, sneezing or coughing, or squeezing the eyelids together, as these motions place stress on the suture line. Before discharge from the hospital, the patient is instructed to move with caution and to avoid strenuous activity for several weeks after surgery.

after-c., 1. any membrane of the pupillary area after extraction or absorption of the lens. 2. secondary cataract (1).

brown c., brunescent c., senile cataract appearing as a brown opacity.

capsular c., one consisting of an opacity of the capsule of the lens.

complicated c., a cataract occurring secondarily to other intraocular disease.

cortical c., an opacity in the cortex of the lens.

hypermature c., one in which the entire lens capsule is wrinkled and the contents have become solid and shrunken, or soft and liquid.

lenticular c., opacity of the lens not affecting the capsule.

mature c., one in which the lens is completely opaque.

secondary c., 1. one that forms after most of the lens has been removed. 2. complicated cataract.

senile c., the cataract of old persons.

cataracta (kat″ah-rak′tah) [L.] cataract.

cataractogenic (kat″ah-rak″to-jen′ik) tending to induce the formation of cataracts.

catarrh (kah-tahr′) inflammation of a mucous membrane (particularly of the head and throat), with free discharge, adj., **catar′rhal.**

catathymic (kat″ah-thi′mik) pertaining to psychic disorders marked by perseveration.

catatonia (kat″ah-to′ne-ah) SCHIZOPHRENIA marked by excessive and sometimes violent motor activity and excitement, or by generalized inhibition. Called also catatonic schizophrenia. adj., **cataton′ic.**

catatricrotism (kat″ah-tri′kro-tizm) a pulse anomaly in which three small additional waves or notches appear in the descending limb of the pulse tracing. adj., **catatricrot′ic.**

catatropia (kat″ah-tro′pe-ah) a downward turning of the visual axes of both eyes in the presence of visual fusional stimuli.

cat-bite fever an infectious disease of man transmitted by the bite of a cat, caused by *Pasteurella multocida* and marked by the formation of an abscess at the site of inoculation. NOTE: Not to be confused with CAT-SCRATCH DISEASE.

catechol (kat′ĕ-kol) a compound, *o*-dehydroxybenzene, used as a reagent and comprising the aromatic portion in the synthesis of catecholamines.

catecholamine (kat″ĕ-kol-ah-mēn″) any of a group of sympathomimetic amines (including dopamine, epinephrine, and norepinephrine), the aromatic portion of whose molecule is catechol.

catechu (kat′ĕ-ku) a powerful astringent extracted from the leaves and twigs of *Ourouparia gambir.*

black c., an astringent from the heartwood of *Acacia catechu.*

Catenabacterium (kah-te″nah-bak-te′re-um) a genus of anaerobic, gram-positive bacteria (tribe Lactobacilleae) found in the intestinal tract and occasionally associated with purulent infections.

catgut (kat′gut) an absorbable sterile strand obtained from collagen derived from healthy mammals, used as a surgical ligature.

catharsis (kar-thar′sis) 1. a cleansing or purgation. 2. the bringing into consciousness and the emotional reliving of a forgotten (repressed) painful experience as a means of releasing anxiety and tension. (See also ABREACTION.)

cathartic (kah-thar′tik) 1. causing bowel evacuation; an agent that so acts. 2. producing catharsis.

bulk c., one stimulating bowel evacuation by increasing fecal volume.

lubricant c., one that acts by softening the feces and reducing friction between them and the intestinal wall.

saline c., one that increases fluidity of intestinal contents by retention of water by osmotic forces, and indirectly increases motor activity.

stimulant c., one that directly increases motor activity of the intestinal tract.

cathectic (kah-thek′tik) pertaining to cathexis.

cathepsin (kah-thep′sin) a proteinase found in most cells, which takes part in cell autolysis and self-digestion of tissues.

catheter (kath′ĕ-ter) a tubular, flexible instrument, passed through body channels for withdrawal of fluids from (or introduction of fluids into) a body cavity.

arterial c., one inserted into an artery and utilized as part of a catheter-transducer-monitor system to continuously observe the BLOOD PRESSURE of critically ill patients. An arterial catheter also may be inserted for x-ray studies of the arterial system and for delivery of chemotherapeutic agents directly into the arterial supply of malignant tumors.

cardiac c., a long, fine catheter especially designed for passage, usually through a peripheral blood vessel, into the chambers of the heart under fluoroscopy. (See also CARDIAC CATHETERIZATION and ANGIOCARDIOGRAPHY.)

central venous c., a long, fine catheter inserted into a vein for the purpose of administering through a large blood vessel parenteral fluids (as in HYPERALIMENTATION), antibiotics, and other therapeutic agents. This type of catheter is also used in the measurement of CENTRAL VENOUS PRESSURE. (See also CENTRAL VENOUS CATHETERIZATION.)

de Pezzer's c., Pezzer's catheter.

double-current c., one having two channels; one

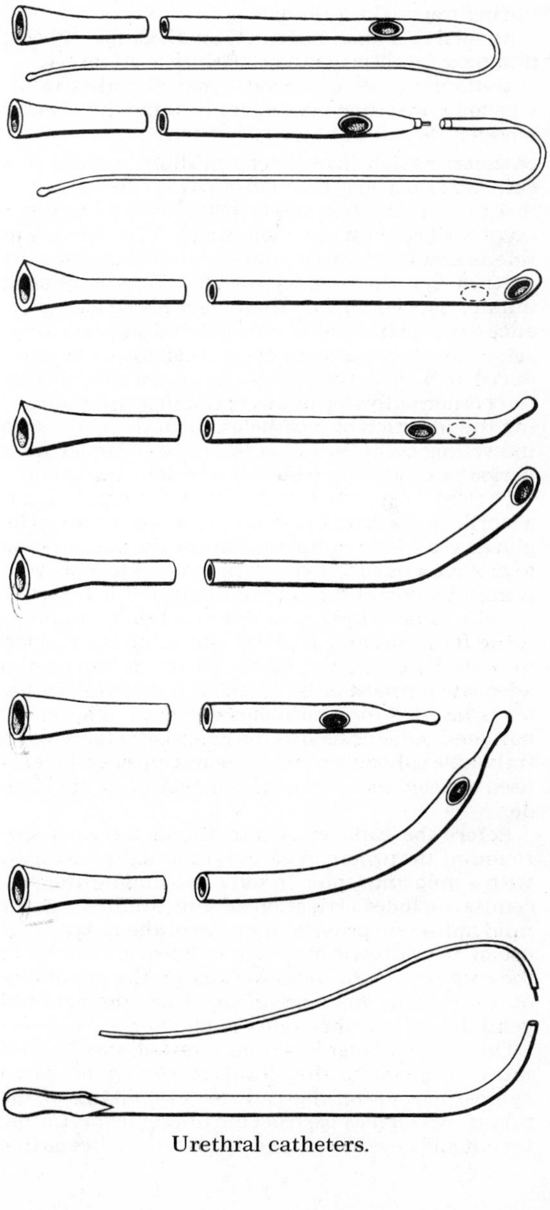

Urethral catheters.

for injection and one for removal of fluid.

elbowed c., a catheter bent at an angle near the beak; used principally in cases of enlarged prostate.

eustachian c., one for inflating the eustachian tube.

faucial c., a eustachian catheter for passage through the fauces.

indwelling c., one especially designed so that it is held in place in the urethra for the purpose of draining urine from the bladder.

nasal c., oropharyngeal c., one made of soft flexible rubber or plastic with several holes in the terminal 1 inch; used for the administration of oxygen.

Pezzer's c., a self-retaining catheter with a bulbous extremity.

prostatic c., one with a short, angular tip.

self-retaining c., one so constructed as to be retained at will in the bladder, effecting constant drainage.

tracheal c., one with small holes at the terminal 1 inch, especially designed for removal of secretions during tracheal SUCTIONING.

ureteral c., a long, extremely small gauge catheter designed for insertion directly into a ureter.

urethral c., any of various types of catheters designed for insertion via the urethra into the urinary bladder. (See also CATHETERIZATION.)

catheterization (kath″ĕ-ter-ĭ-za′shun) passage of a catheter into a body channel or cavity. (See also CARDIAC CATHETERIZATION and CENTRAL VENOUS CATHETERIZATION.) The most common usage of the term is in reference to the introduction of a catheter via the urethra into the urinary bladder. This is often a nursing procedure, one that demands strict adherence to the principles of medical and surgical asepsis so that pathogenic microorganisms are not introduced into the urinary system. Since the urinary tract is normally sterile, any break in technique during the insertion of a catheter, or in the care of an indwelling catheter that is left in the bladder for a period of time, may result in a serious infection.

PATIENT CARE. As stated above, catheterization is a sterile procedure. The therapist must wear sterile gloves, use sterile equipment, drape the patient so as to provide a sterile field on which to work, and avoid contamination of the catheter before it is inserted.

If the catheterization is done to obtain a sample of urine for laboratory analysis, the urine is collected in a sterile container; 60 to 100 ml. is considered adequate for most tests. When an indwelling catheter is inserted for continuous drainage, a specially designed catheter such as the Foley catheter with an inflatable balloon, or a mushroom-tipped catheter is used to avoid its accidental removal from the bladder.

Before the catheter is introduced, the area surrounding the urinary meatus is thoroughly cleansed with a mild antiseptic. In some institutions the procedure includes irrigation of the urethra with a mild antiseptic prior to insertion of the catheter, or use of an antibiotic ointment to lubricate the tip of the catheter. These measures reduce the possibility of transferring microorganisms from the external genitalia and urethra into the bladder.

Once the catheter has been inserted, special care must be given to the drainage tubing to guard against tension on the catheter or kinking of the tubing, which may obstruct the flow of urine. Catheters should never be pinned to the bed clothes as this may result in accidental removal or unnecessary pulling when the patient moves about in bed. The tubing leading from the catheter to the collecting bottle must *always* be kept below the level of the bladder to avoid backflow or urine and introduction of bacteria into the urinary tract. When changing the tubing, or disconnecting it for irrigations or to empty the drainage bottle, the nurse must be careful to avoid contamination of the catheter and inside of the tubing. Cleansing the open end of the catheter and the end of the connecting tubing with 70 per cent alcohol is recommended as a means of reducing the possibility of contamination. The urine may be collected by way of an open drainage system (in which there is more danger of infection) or a closed drainage system. The type of system used will depend on hospital policy and the instructions from the attending physician.

Patient care must also include attention to the area surrounding the urinary meatus. At least twice daily, or more often if necessary, the genital area should be washed gently with soap and water and dried thoroughly. Crusts and secretions around the catheter may be removed by gentle wiping with a gauze or cotton square saturated with a mild antiseptic. These measures will reduce the possibility of infection and insure the comfort of the patient by eliminating unpleasant odors and irritation.

catheterize (kath′ĕ-ter-iz″) to introduce a catheter into a body cavity, usually into the urinary bladder for the withdrawal of urine.

cathexis (kah-thek′sis) the charge or attachment of mental or emotional energy upon an object or idea. adj., **cathec′tic.**

cathode (kath′ōd) 1. the negative electrode, from which electrons are emitted and to which positive ions are attracted. 2. the electrode through which current leaves a nerve or other substance.

cathodic (kah-thod′ik) pertaining to or emanating from a cathode.

Cathomycin (kath′o-mi″sin) trademark for preparations of novobiocin, an antibiotic.

cation (kat′i-on) a positively charged ion.

cation-exchange resin ion-exchange resin.

cat-scratch disease (fever) a benign, subacute, regional lymphadenitis resulting from a scratch or bite of a cat or a scratch from a surface contaminated by a cat.

No specific causative agent has been isolated, but a viral etiology is suspected. Cats thought to be associated with human infection show no signs of illness, and probably act only as vectors of the disease, conveying the causative agent on claws or teeth.

In half the cases, after several days there is a persistent sore at the site of the scratch, and fever and other symptoms of infection may develop. There is also swelling of the lymph nodes draining the infected part.

In milder cases, the symptoms soon disappear, with no aftereffects. Sometimes the attack is more serious and the glands may require surgical incision and drainage. Occasionally meningoencephalitis is a serious complication. The disease is generally mild and lasts for about 2 weeks. In rare cases, it may persist for a period of up to 2 years.

No specific remedy exists for cat-scratch disease, although certain antibiotics appear to shorten its course. The main treatment consists simply of keeping the patient as comfortable as possible. The disease can, however, usually be prevented by avoiding cat scratches or bites or by thoroughly washing and disinfecting any wound that does occur. NOTE: Not to be confused with CAT-BITE FEVER.

cauda (kaw′da), pl. *cau′dae* [L.] a tail or tail-like appendage.

c. equi′na, the collection of spinal roots descending from the lower spinal cord and occupying the vertebral canal below the cord.

caudad (kaw′dad) directed toward the tail or distal end; opposite of cephalad.

caudal (kaw′dal) 1. pertaining to a cauda. 2. situated more toward the cauda, or tail, than some specified reference point; toward the inferior (in humans) or posterior (in animals) end of the body.

c. anesthesia, a type of regional anesthesia used in childbirth in which the anesthetizing solution, usually procaine, is injected into the caudal area of the spinal canal through the lower end of the sacrum. It affects the caudal nerve roots, and renders the cervix, vagina, and perineum insensitive to pain. In continuous caudal anesthesia, the needle is left in place throughout the delivery and the anesthetic is allowed to drip in gradually. Care must be taken to ensure that the solution does not enter higher in the spinal canal, and use of the procedure requires constant attendance by an obstetrician, anesthesiologist, or trained anesthetist. It is used in only a small percentage of patients.

caudate (kaw′dat) having a tail.

caudatum (kaw-da′tum) the caudate nucleus.

caul (kawl) a part of the amnion that sometimes envelops the head of the fetus at birth.

cauliflower ear (kaw′lĭ-flow″er) a thickened and deformed ear caused by the accumulation of fluid and blood clots in the tissue following repeated injury. It is most commonly seen in boxers, for whom it is almost an occupational hazard. A cauliflower ear will not recover its normal shape but it can be restored to normal by means of plastic surgery.

caumesthesia (kaw″mes-the′ze-ah) a sensation of burning heat even though the body temperature is not elevated.

causalgia (kaw-zal′je-ah) a burning pain often associated with trophic skin changes in the hand or foot, caused by peripheral nerve injury. The syndrome may be aggravated by the slightest stimuli or it may be intensified by the emotions. Causalgia usually begins several weeks after the initial injury and the pain is described as intense, with the patient sometimes taking elaborate precautions to avoid any stimulus he knows to be capable of causing a flare-up of symptoms. He often will go to great extremes to protect the affected limb and becomes preoccupied with such protection.

Any one of a variety of injuries to the hand, foot, arm, or leg can lead to causalgia, but in most cases there has been some injury to the median or the sciatic nerve. Sympathectomy may be necessary to eliminate the severe pain, and in the majority of cases it is quite successful. Psychotherapy may be necessary when emotional instability is suspected. Emotional problems may have been present before the initial injury, or they may result from the intense suffering characteristic of severe causalgia.

caustic (kaws′tik) 1. burning or corrosive; destructive to tissue. 2. having a burning taste. 3. a corrosive or escharotic agent.

cauterant (kaw′ter-ant) 1. any caustic material or application. 2. caustic.

cauterization (kaw″ter-ĭ-za′shun) destruction of tissue with a cautery.

cautery (kaw′ter-e) 1. the application of a caustic agent, a hot iron, an electric current, or other agent to destroy tissue. 2. an agent used for such purpose.

cold c., cauterization by carbon dioxide, called also cryocautery.

cava (ka′vah) [L.] 1. plural of *cavum.* 2. a vena cava.

caverna (ka-ver′nah), pl. *caver′nae* [L.] a cavity.

cavernitis (kav″er-ni′tis) inflammation of the corpora cavernosa or corpus spongiosum of the penis.

cavernoma (kav″er-no′mah) cavernous hemangioma (see also HEMANGIOMA).

cavernositis (kav″er-no-si′tis) cavernitis.

cavernostomy (kav″er-nos′to-me) operative drainage of a pulmonary abscess of the lung.

cavernous (kav′er-nus) pertaining to a hollow, or containing hollow spaces.

cavitary (kav′ĭ-ta″re) characterized by the presence of a cavity or cavities.

cavitas (kav′ĭ-tas), pl. *cavita′tes* [L.] cavity.

cavitation (kav″ĭ-ta′shun) the formation of cavities; also, a cavity.

cavitis (ka-vi′tis) inflammation of a vena cava.

cavity (kav′ĭ-te) a hollow or space, or a potentional space, within the body or one of its organs. In dentistry, the lesion produced by CARIES.

abdominal c., the cavity of the body between the diaphragm above and the pelvis below, containing the abdominal organs.

amniotic c., the closed sac betwen the embryo and the amnion, containing the amniotic fluid.

cranial c., the space enclosed by the bones of the cranium.

glenoid c., a depression in the lateral angle of the scapula for articulation with the humerus.

medullary (marrow) c., the cavity, containing marrow, in the diaphysis of a long bone; called also medullary canal.

nasal c., the proximal part of the respiratory tract, within the nose, separated by the nasal septum and extending from the nares to the pharynx.

oral c., the cavity of the mouth, bounded by the jaw bones and associated structures (muscles and mucosa).

pelvic c., the space within the walls of the pelvis.

pericardial c., the potential space between the epicardium and the parietal layer of the serous pericardium.

peritoneal c., the potential space between the parietal and the visceral peritoneum.

pleural c., the potential space between the parietal and the visceral pulmonary pleura.

pulp c., the pulp-filled central chamber in the crown of a tooth.

serous c., a celomic cavity, like that enclosed by the pericardium, peritoneum, or pleura, not communicating with the outside of the body, the lining membrane of which secretes a serous fluid.

tension c., cavities of the lung in which the air pressure is greater than that of the atmosphere.

thoracic c., the portion of the ventral body cavity situated between the neck and the diaphragm.

tympanic c., the middle ear.

uterine c., the flattened space within the uterus

communicating proximally on either side with the uterine tubes and below with the vagina.

cavum (ca′vum), pl. *ca′va* [L.] cavity.

cavus (ka′vus) [L.] hollow.

CBC complete blood (cell) count (see also BLOOD COUNT).

cc. cubic centimeter.

c.cm. cubic centimeter.

C.D. curative dose; that which is sufficient to restore normal health.

C.D.$_{50}$ median curative dose.

Cd 1. chemical symbol, *cadmium*. 2. caudal or coccygeal.

Ce chemical symbol, *cerium*.

cebocephalus (se″bo-sef′ah-lus) a fetus exhibiting cebocephaly.

cebocephaly (se″bo-sef′ah-le) a monkey-like deformity of the head, with the eyes close together and the nose defective.

cecal (se′kal) pertaining to the cecum.

cecectomy (se-sek′to-me) excision of the cecum.

cecitis (se-si′tis) inflammation of the cecum.

ceco- word element [L.], *cecum*.

cecocele (se′ko-sēl) a hernia containing part of the cecum.

cecocolopexy (se″ko-ko′lo-pek″se) an operation for fixation or suspension of the cecum and ascending colon.

cecocolostomy (se″ko-ko-los′to-me) surgical anastomosis of the cecum and the colon.

cecoileostomy (se″ko-il″e-os′to-me) ileocecostomy; surgical anastomosis of the ileum to the cecum.

Cecon (se′kon) trademark for preparations of ascorbic acid (vitamin C).

cecopexy (se′ko-pek″se) fixation or suspension of the cecum to correct excessive mobility.

cecoplication (se″ko-pli-ka′shun) plication of the cecal wall to correct ptosis or dilatation.

cecorrhaphy (se-kor′ah-fe) suture or repair of the cecum.

cecosigmoidostomy (se″ko-sig″moi-dos′to-me) formation, usually by surgery, of an opening between the cecum and sigmoid.

cecostomy (se-kos′to-me) surgical creation of an artificial opening or fistula into the cecum.

cecotomy (se-kot′o-me) incision of the cecum.

cecum (se′kum) 1. the first or proximal part of the large intestine, forming a dilated pouch distal to the ileum and proximal to the colon, and giving off the vermiform appendix. 2. any blind pouch.

Cedilanid (se″dĭ-lan′id) trademark for a preparation of lanatoside C; used as a cardiotonic where digitalis is recommended.

Cefadyl (sef′ah-dil) trademark for a preparation of cephapirin, an analogue of cephalosporin.

Celbenin (sel′bĕ-nin) trademark for a preparation of methicillin, a semisynthetic penicillin.

-cele word element [Gr.], *tumor; hernia; cavity*.

celi(o)- word element [Gr.], *abdomen; through the abdominal wall*.

celiac (se′le-ak) pertaining to the abdomen.

c. disease, a comparatively uncommon malabsorption syndrome affecting both children and adults, in which there is an inability to digest and utilize fats, starches, and sugars. Called also nontropical sprue and gluten enteropathy.

CAUSE. Celiac disease is precipitated by ingestion of gluten-containing foods; its etiology is unknown but a hereditary factor has been implicated. Pathologically, the proximal intestinal mucosa loses its structure, surface epithelial cells exhibit degenerative changes, and the absorptive function of these cells is severely impaired.

SYMPTOMS. The disease is characterized by flatulence and by large, very foul-smelling, bulky, frothy, and pale-colored stools containing much fat. There are recurrent attacks of diarrhea, with possible accompanying stomach cramps, alternating with constipation. There is abdominal distention as in severe malnutrition, and weight loss, asthenia, deficiency of vitamins B, D, and K, and electrolyte depletion.

In the infantile form the onset is insidious, and is marked by irritability, loss of appetite, weakness, extreme wasting, growth retardation, and CELIAC CRISIS. The adult form is marked by extreme lassitude, fatigue, difficulty in breathing, clubbing of the fingers, bone pain, muscle cramping, tetany, abdominal distention during the day, megacolon, tympanitis, and skin pigmentation. Until recently it was thought that the infantile form and the adult form were different entities, but it is now believed that they are the same.

TREATMENT. Treatment usually depends on a diet high in protein and free from gluten and fat. Fruit sugars are used to replace the milk sugars and other sugars, and the main content of the diet is made up of milk protein or skimmed milk, the white of eggs, lean meat, fish, liver, and protein-rich vegetables such as peas and beans. After the patient has done well on this for 6 months, a full diet is gradually achieved by adding one food at a time. The last foods to be added are starchy foods. While on the diet the patient is given vitamin supplements, especially vitamin B complex, to combat the anemia and nutritional deficiencies.

Full recovery from this disease may take 1 to 2 years, and relapses may occur if the diet is disregarded. During severe relapses, intravenous feeding may be necessary to combat acidosis, dehydration, and symptoms of starvation.

Death from uncomplicated celiac disease is rare, and the symptoms usually disappear in later childhood and adolescence, although in a few cases the condition may be permanent, or the symptoms may reappear in the third to sixth decade of life, with the onset of adult celiac disease.

c. crisis, an attack of severe watery diarrhea and vomiting producing dehydration and acidosis, which sometimes occurs in the infantile form of CELIAC DISEASE.

celiectomy (se″le-ek′to-me) 1. excision of the celiac branches of the vagus nerve. 2. excision of an abdominal organ.

celiocentesis (se″le-o-sen-te′sis) puncture into the abdominal cavity.

celiocolpotomy (se″le-o-kol-pot′o-me) incision into the abdomen through the vagina.

celioenterotomy (se″le-o-en″ter-ot′o-me) incision through the abdominal wall into the intestine.

celiogastrotomy (se″le-o-gas-trot′o-me) incision through the abdominal wall into the stomach.

celioma (se″le-o′mah) a tumor of the abdomen.

celiomyomectomy (se″le-o-mi″o-mek′to-me) myomectomy by abdominal incision.

celiomyositis (se″le-o-mi″o-si′tis) inflammation of the abdominal muscles.

celioparacentesis (se″le-o-par″ah-sen-te′sis) paracentesis of the abdominal cavity.

celiopathy (se″le-op′ah-the) any abdominal disease.

celiorrhaphy (se″le-or′ah-fe) suture of the abdominal wall.

celioscope (se′le-o-skōp″) an endoscope for use in celioscopy.

celioscopy (se″le-os′ko-pe) examination of a body cavity, especially the abdominal cavity, through a celioscope.

celiotomy (se″le-ot′o-me) incision into the abdominal cavity.

vaginal c., incision into the abdominal cavity through the vagina.

cell (sel) 1. any of the minute protoplasmic masses making up organized tissue. Although cells may be widely differentiated and highly specialized in their function, they all have the same basic structure; that is, they have an outer covering called the membrane, a main substance called the cytoplasm, and a control center called the nucleus. The cytoplasm and the substance of the nucleus (nucleoplasm or karyoplasm) are collectively referred to as protoplasm. In some low forms of life, e.g., bacteria, a morphological nucleus is absent, although nucleoproteins (and genes) are present. 2. a small, more or less closed space.

Cell membranes are capable of selection in the passage of substances into and out of the cell. These substances can pass through a cell membrane by DIFFUSION, by active transport, and by pinocytosis, a mechanism by which the membrane engulfs some of the extracellular fluid and its contents. Another method of ingestion by the cell is phagocytosis, whereby the cell ingests large particles such as a bacterium or a particle of degenerating tissue. Gases such as oxygen and carbon dioxide readily pass through the cell membrane. Because of this semipermeability of the cell membrane it is possible for cells to receive nutrition and dispose of waste products.

Metabolism of the cell, which includes all the physical and chemical reactions within the cell, takes place in the protoplasm. These reactions are essential to the life of the cell and the normal functioning of the body. They include the synthesis of protein, lipid secretion, oxidation with release of energy, and the release of glucose from glycogen stores of the cells.

The control center of the cell is the nucleus. The chemical reactions of cellular metabolism are controlled in the nucleus, and it is this part of the cell that contains DEOXYRIBONUCLEIC ACID (DNA), which effects reproduction of the cell. The nucleus, then, influences growth, repair, and reproduction of the cell.

Cells of the body are organized into tissues and tissues into organs. The fluid within the cell (60 to 90 per cent of the protoplasm is water) is called intracellular fluid. The fluid surrounding the cell and within the tissues is called interstitial fluid or tissue fluid. The molecules and ions in these fluids are essential to the life of the cell. (See also FLUIDS and ELECTROLYTES.)

alpha c's, 1. cells in the islands of Langerhans that secrete glucagon and contain large granules that are insoluble in alcohol. 2. acidophilic cells of the anterior pituitary.

argentaffin c's, cells containing cytoplasmic granules capable of reducing silver compounds, located throughout the gastrointestinal tract, chiefly in the basilar portions of the gastric glands and the crypts of Lieberkühn.

band c., a neutrophil in which the nucleus is not lobulated but in the form of a continuous band, horseshoe shaped, twisted, or coiled. Called also band-form granulocyte.

basal c., an early keratinocyte, present in the basal layer of the epidermis.

beta c's, 1. basophilic cells in the pancreas that secrete insulin and make up most of the bulk of the islands of Langerhans; they contain granules that are soluble in alcohol. 2. basophilic cells of the anterior pituitary.

Betz c's, large pyramidal ganglion cells forming a layer of the gray matter of the brain.

blast c., the least differentiated blood cell type.

blood c., one of the formed elements of the blood (see also BLOOD).

bone c., a nucleated cell in the lacunae of bone.

chromaffin c's, cells whose cytoplasm shows fine brown granules when stained with potassium bichromate, occurring in the adrenal medulla and in scattered groups in various organs and throughout the body.

cleavage c., any of the cells derived from the fertilized ovum by mitosis; a blastomere.

daughter c., a cell formed by division of a mother cell.

foam c., a cell with a vacuolated appearance due to the presence of complex lipoids; seen in xanthoma.

ganglion c., a large nerve cell, especially one of those of the spinal ganglia.

Gaucher's c., a large cell characteristic of Gaucher's disease (see also GAUCHER'S CELLS).

germ c., an ovum or spermatozoon.

giant c., a very large, multinucleate cell; applied to megakaryocytes of bone marrow and to giant cells occurring in the lesions of tuberculosis and other infectious granulomas and about foreign bodies.

glia c's, neuroglia cells.

Golgi's c's, Golgi neurons.

granular c., one containing granules, such as a keratinocyte in the stratum granulosum of the epidermis, when it contains a dense collection of darkly staining granules.

heart failure c's, heart-lesion c's, iron-containing, rust-colored macrophages found in the pulmonary alveoli and sputum in congestive heart failure.

HeLa c's, cells of the first continuously cultured carcinoma strain, descended from a human cervical carcinoma.

Hürthle c's, large eosinophilic cells sometimes found in the thyriod gland. (See also HÜRTHLE CELL TUMOR.)

interstitial c's, the cells of the connective tissue of the ovary or of the testis (Leydig's cells) which furnish the internal secretion of those structures.

islet c's, cells composing the islands of Langerhans.

juxtaglomerular c's, specialized cells, containing secretory granules, located in the tunica media of the afferent glomerular arterioles, thought to stimulate aldosterone secretion and to play a role in renal autoregulation.

Kupffer's c's, large, stellate or pyramidal, intensely phagocytic cells lining the walls of the hepatic sinusoids and forming part of the reticuloendothelial system.

L.E. c., a mature neutrophilic polymorphonuclear leukocyte characteristic of lupus erythematosus (see also L.E. CELL).

Leydig's c's, interstitial cells of the testis, which secrete testosterone.

lutein c's, the plump, pale-staining, polyhedral cells of the corpus luteum.

lymph c., lymphocyte.

lymphoid c's, lymphocytes and plasma cells.

mast c., a connective tissue cell capable of elaborating basophilic, metachromatic cytoplasmic granules that contain histamine, heparin, and, in some species, serotonin.

mastoid c's, air spaces of various size and shape in the mastoid process of the temporal bone.

mother c., a cell that divides to form new, or daughter, cells.

myeloma c., a cell found in bone marrow and sometimes in peripheral blood in multiple myeloma.

nerve c., any cell of the nervous system; a NEURON.

neuroglia c's, neuroglial c's, the branching non-neural cells of the supporting tissue (the neuroglia) of the central nervous system; they are of three types: astroglia (macroglia), oligodendroglia, and microglia.

olfactory c's, a set of specialized cells of the mucous membrane of the nose; the receptors for smell.

parafollicular c's, cells found in the follicular epithelium and interfollicular spaces of the thyroid gland, which elaborate calcitonin (thyrocalcitonin).

Pick's c's, round, oval, or polyhedral cells with foamy, lipid-containing cytoplasm found in the bone marrow and spleen in Niemann-Pick disease.

pigment c's, cells containing granules of pigment.

plasma c., a spherical or ellipsoidal cell with a single nucleus containing chromatin, an area of perinuclear clearing, and generally abundant, sometimes vacuolated cytoplasm. Plasma cells are involved in the synthesis, storage, and release of antibody. Called also plasmacyte and plasmocyte.

prickle c., a dividing keratinocyte of the prickle-cell layer of the epidermis, with delicate radiating process connecting with other similar cells.

primordial germ c's, the earliest germ cells, at first located outside the gonad but migrating to the gonad in early embryonic development.

Purkinje's c's, large branching cells of the middle layer of the cerebellar cortex.

red c., red blood c., erythrocyte.

reticular c's, the cells forming the reticular fibers of connective tissue; those forming the framework of lymph nodes, bone marrow, and spleen form part of the reticuloendothelial system and may differentiate into macrophages.

reticuloendothelial c., a cell of the RETICULOENDOTHELIAL SYSTEM.

Sertoli c's, elongated cells in the tubules of the testes to which the spermatids become attached; they provide support, protection, and, apparently, nutrition until the spermatids are transformed into mature spermatozoa.

sickle c., a crescentic or sickle-shaped erythrocyte, the abnormal shape caused by the presence of varying proportions of hemoglobin S (see also SICKLE CELL ANEMIA).

signet-ring c., a cell in which the nucleus has been pressed to one side by an accumulation of intracytoplasmic mucin (see also KRUKENBERG'S TUMOR).

somatic c's, the cells of the somatoplasm; undifferentiated body cells.

squamous c's, flat, scalelike epithelial cells.

stellate c., any star-shaped cell, as a Kupffer cell or astrocyte, having many filaments extending in all directions.

Sternberg's giant c's, Sternberg-Reed c's, enlarged, atypical histiocytes with multiple or hyperlobulated nucleoli; a characteristic feature of Hodgkin's disease.

stipple c., an erythrocyte containing granules that take a basic or bluish stain with Wright's stain.

target c., an abnormally thin erythrocyte showing, when stained, a dark center and a peripheral ring of hemoglobin, separated by a pale, unstained zone containing less hemoglobin; seen in various anemias and other disorders.

tart c., a macrophage or monocytoid reticuloendothelial cell containing a phagocytized nucleus with well preserved nuclear structure.

taste c's, cells in the taste buds associated with the nerves of taste.

totipotential c., an embryonic cell that is capable of developing into any variety of body cell.

visual c's, the neuroepithelial elements of the retina.

wandering c's, cells capable of ameboid movement, e.g., macrophages, lymphocytes, etc.

white c., white blood c., leukocyte.

cell division the process by which cells reproduce; fission of a cell.

direct c.d., see AMITOSIS.

indirect c. d., see MEIOSIS and MITOSIS.

cellobiase (sel″lo-bi′ās) β-glucosidase (see GLUCOSIDASE).

cellular (sel′u-lar) pertaining to, or made up of, cells.

cellularity (sel″u-lar′ĭ-te) the state of a tissue or other mass as regards the number of its constituent cells.

cellulicidal (sel″u-lĭ-si′dal) destroying cells.

cellulitis (sel″u-li′tis) a diffuse inflammatory process within solid tissues, characterized by edema, redness, pain, and interference with function. It may be caused by infection with streptococci, staphylococci, or other organisms.

Cellulitis usually occurs in the loose tissues beneath the skin, but may also occur in tissues beneath mucous membranes or around muscle bundles or surrounding organs.

ERYSIPELAS, a surface cellulitis of the skin, is characterized by patches of skin that are red with sharply defined borders and that feel hot to the touch. Other types of skin cellulitis are also characterized by hot red patches, but the borders are less clearly defined. Red streaks extending from the patch indicate that the lymph vessels have been infected. Ludwig's angina is a cellulitis of the tissues of the floor of the mouth and neck, in the area around the submaxillary gland. Orbital cellulitis is an acute inflammation of the eye socket. Pelvic cellulitis involves the tissues surrounding the uterus and is called parametritis.

Cellulitis is potentially dangerous but usually can be treated successfully with antibiotics or sulfonamides. Any cellulitis on the face must be given special attention because the infection may extend directly to the cavernous sinuses of the brain.

cellulofibrous (sel″u-lo-fi′brus) partly cellular and partly fibrous.

celluloid (sel′u-loid) a plastic compound of pyroxylin and camphor.

celluloneuritis (sel″u-lo-nu-ri′tis) inflammation of neurons.

cellulose (sel′u-lōs) a carbohydrate forming the skeleton of most plant structures and plant cells.
absorbable c., oxidized c., an absorbable oxidation product of cellulose, applied locally to stop bleeding.

Celontin (se-lon′tin) trademark for a preparation of methsuximide, an anticonvulsant.

celoschisis (se-los′kĭ-sis) congenital fissure of the abdominal wall.

celoscope (se′lo-skōp) celioscope.

celosomia (se″lo-so′me-ah) congenital fissure or absence of the sternum, with hernial protrusion of the viscera.

celothelioma (se″lo-the″le-o′mah) mesothelioma.

celozoic (se″lo-zo′ik) inhabiting the intestinal canal of the body; said of parasites.

Celsius scale (sel′se-us) a temperature scale with the ice point at 0 and the normal boiling point of water at 100 degrees (100° C.). (For equivalents of Celsius and Fahrenheit temperatures, see Appendix.)

Celsius thermometer (sel′se-us) a centigrade thermometer employing the Celsius scale. The abbreviation 100° C. should be read "one hundred degrees Celsius."

cement (se-ment′) 1. a substance that produces a solid union between two surfaces. 2. in dentistry, a filling material used to aid the retention of gold castings and to insulate the tooth pulp. 3. cementum.
dental c., cementum.
intercellular c., a mucilaginous substance that holds cells, especially epithelial cells, together.
muscle c., the myoglia.
nerve c., the neuroglia.

cementicle (se-men′tĭ-k′l) a small, discrete globular mass of cementum in the region of a tooth root.

cementoblast (se-men′to-blast) a large cuboidal cell, found between fibers on the surface of cementum, which is active in the formation of cementum.

cementoblastoma (se-men″to-blas-to′mah) an odontogenic fibroma whose cells are developing into cementoblasts and in which there is only a small proportion of calcified tissue.

cementoclasia (se-men″to-kla′ze-ah) disintegration of the cementum of a tooth.

cementocyte (se-men′to-sīt) a cell found in lacunae of cellular cementum, frequently having long processes radiating from the cell body toward the periodontal surface of the cementum.

cementogenesis (se-men″to-jen′ĕ-sis) development of cementum on the root dentin of a tooth.

cementoma (se″men-to′mah) a mass of cementum lying free at the apex of a tooth, probably a reaction to injury.

cementosis (se″men-to′sis) proliferation of cementum.

cementum (se-men′tum) the bonelike connective tissue covering the root of a tooth and assisting in tooth support.

cenesthesia (sen″es-the′ze-ah) the general feeling or sense of conscious existence; the sense of normal functioning of body organs. adj., **cenesthe′sic, cenesthet′ic.**

ceno- word element [Gr.], *new; empty;* or denoting relationship to a common feature.

cenosis (se-no′sis) a morbid discharge. adj., **cenot′ic.**

cenosite (se′no-sīt) coinsite.

cenotype (sen′o-tīp) the original from which other types have arisen.

censor (sen′sor) 1. a member of a committee on ethics or for critical examination of a medical or other society. 2. the psychic influence which prevents unconscious thoughts and wishes coming into consciousness.

center (sen′ter) a point from which a process starts, especially a plexus or ganglion giving off nerves that control a function.
accelerating c., one in the brain stem involved in acceleration of heart action.
apneustic c., a nerve center in the brain stem controlling normal respiration.
auditory c., the center for hearing, in the more anterior of the transverse temporal gyri.
Broca's c., speech center.
cardioinhibitory c., one in the medulla oblongata that exerts an inhibitory influence on the heart.
deglutition c., swallowing center.
germinal c., the area in lymphoid tissue where mitotic figures are observed, differentiation and formation of lymphocytes occur, and elements related to antibody synthesis are found.
gustatory c., the cerebral center supposed to control taste.
health c., 1. a community health organization for providing ambulatory health care and coordinating the efforts of all health agencies. 2. an educational complex consisting of a medical school and various allied health professional schools.
medullary respiratory c., one in the medulla oblongata that coordinates respiratory movements.
motor c., any center that originates, controls, inhibits, or maintains motor impulses.
nerve c., a collection of nerve cells in the central nervous system that are associated together in the performance of some particular function.
c. of ossification, any point in bones at which ossification begins.
pneumotaxic c., one in the upper pons that rhythmically inhibits inspiration.
reflex c., any nerve center at which afferent sensory impressions are converted into efferent motor impulses.
respiratory c's, a series of the centers (the apneustic, pneumotaxic, and medullary respiratory centers) in the medulla and pons that coordinate respiratory movements.
speech c., one in the left (or right) inferior frontal gyrus concerned with the motor aspects of speech.
swallowing c., one in the floor of the fourth ventricle of the brain concerned in deglutition.
thermoregulatory c's, hypothalamic centers regulating the conservation and dissipation of heat.
Wernicke's c., the speech center in the cortex of the left temporo-occipital convolution.
word c., one concerned with the recognition of words, different areas being involved for recognition of written and of spoken words.

-centesis word element [Gr.], *puncture and aspiration of.*

centi- word element [L.], *hundred;* usually used in naming units of measurement to indicate one-hundredth (10^{-2}) of the unit designated by the root with which it is combined, e.g., centigram. Symbol c.

centigrade (sen'tĭ-grād) having 100 gradations (steps or degrees), as the Celsius scale; abbreviated C. (For equivalents of Celsius and Fahrenheit temperatures, see Appendix.)

centigram (sen'tĭ-gram) one-hundredth of a gram; abbreviated cg.

centiliter (sen"tĭ-le"ter) one-hundredth of a liter; abbreviated cl.

centimeter (sen'tĭ-me"ter) one-hundredth of a meter, or approximately 0.3937 inch; abbreviated cm.

cubic c., a unit of capacity, being that of a cube each side of which measures 1 cm.; abbreviated $cm.^3$, cu. cm. or cc.

centinormal (sen"tĭ-nor'mal) one-hundredth of normal strength.

centrad (sen'trad) toward a center.

central (sen'tral) pertaining to a center; located at the midpoint.

c. fissure, c. sulcus, fissure of Rolando.

c. nervous system, the portion of the NERVOUS SYSTEM consisting of the brain and spinal cord.

c. sulcus, fissure of Rolando.

c. venous catheterization, insertion of an indwelling catheter into a central vein for the purpose of administering fluid and medications and for the measurement of CENTRAL VENOUS PRESSURE. The most common sites of insertion are the jugular and subclavian veins; however, such large peripheral veins as the saphenous and femoral veins can be used in an emergency even though they offer some disadvantages. The procedure is performed under sterile conditions and placement of the catheter is verified by x-rays before fluids are administered or central venous pressure measurements are made.

Selection of a large central vein in preference to a smaller peripheral vein for the administration of therapeutic agents is based on the nature and amount of fluid to be injected. Central veins are able to accommodate large amounts of fluid when shock or hemorrhage demand rapid replacement. The larger veins are less susceptible to irritation from caustic drugs and from hypertonic nutrient solutions administered during HYPERALIMENTATION.

Long-term use of an indwelling venous catheter demands strict attention to technique to avoid contamination when fluids and medications are added. The site of insertion must be kept free from contamination; dressings must be sterile and be changed every two to three days. At this time the wound is cleaned with an antiseptic solution and an antimicrobial ointment is applied to the puncture site.

c. venous pressure, CVP; the pressure of blood in the right atrium. Measurement of central venous pressure is made possible by the insertion of a catheter through the median cubital vein to the superior vena cava. The distal end of the catheter is attached to a manometer on which can be read the amount of pressure being exerted by the blood inside the right atrium. The manometer is positioned at the bedside so that the zero point is at the level of the right atrium. Each time the patient's position is changed the zero point on the manometer must be reset.

The normal range for CVP is 0 to 5 mm. of water. A CVP of 15 to 20 mm. usually indicates inability of the right atrium to accommodate the current BLOOD VOLUME. However, the trend of response to rapid administration of fluid is more significant than the specific level of pressure. Normally the right heart can circulate additional fluids without an increase in CVP. If the CVP is elevated in response to the rapid administration of a small amount of fluid, there is indication that the patient is hypervolemic in relation to the pumping action of the right heart. Thus, the CVP is used as a guide to the safe administration of replacement fluids intravenously, particularly in patients who are subject to pulmonary EDEMA.

A high venous pressure may indicate congestive HEART FAILURE, hypervolemia (increased blood volume), cardiac tamponade in which the heart is unable to fill, or vasoconstriction, which affects the heart's ability to empty its chambers. Conversely, a low venous pressure indicates hypovolemia (low blood volume) and possibly a need to increase fluid intake.

centrencephalic (sen"tren-sĕ-fal'ik) pertaining to the center of the encephalon.

centric (sen'trik) pertaining to a center.

centriciput (sen-tris'ĭ-put) the central part of the upper surface of the head, located between the occiput and sinciput.

centrifugal (sen-trif'u-gal) moving away from a center.

centrifugate (sen-trif'u-gāt) material subjected to centrifugation.

centrifugation (sen-trif"u-ga'shun) the process of separating lighter portions of a solution, mixture, or suspension from the heavier portions by centrifugal force.

centrifuge (cen'trĭ-fūj) 1. to rotate, in a suitable container, at extremely high speed, to cause the deposition of solids in solution. 2. a laboratory device for subjecting substances in solution to relative centrifugal force up to 25,000 times gravity.

centrilobular (sen"trĭ-lob'u-lar) pertaining to the central portion of a lobule.

centriole (sen'tre-ōl) either of the two minute organelles that migrate to opposite poles of a cell during cell division and serve to organize the alignment of the spindles.

centripetal (sen-trip'ĕ-tal) moving toward a center.

centro- word element [L., Gr.], *center; central location.*

centrokinesia (sen"tro-ki-ne'se-ah) movement originating from central stimulation. adj., **centrokinet'ic.**

centrolecithal (sen"tro-les'ĭ-thal) having the yolk in the center.

centromere (sen'tro-mēr) the clear constricted portion of the chromosome at which the chromatids are joined and by which the chromosome is attached to the spindle during cell division. adj., **centromer'ic.**

centrosclerosis (sen"tro-sklĕ-ro'sis) osteosclerosis of the marrow cavity of a bone.

centrosome (sen'tro-sōm) a specialized area of condensed cytoplasm containing the centrioles and playing an important part in mitosis.

centrosphere (sen'tro-sfēr) centrosome.

centrostaltic (sen″tro-stal′tik) pertaining to a center of motion.

centrum (sen′trum), pl. *cen′tra* [L.] 1. a center. 2. the body of a vertebra.

c. commu′ne, the solar plexus.

cephal(o)- word element [Gr.], *head.*

cephalad (sef′ah-lad) toward the head.

cephalalgia (sef″al-al′je-ah) pain in the head; headache.

cephaledema (sef″al-ĕ-de′mah) edema of the head.

cephalexin (sef″ah-lek′sin) an oral cephalosporin used in the treatment of pneumococcal and Group-A streptococcal respiratory infections and infections of the urinary tract, skin, and soft tissue.

cephalhematocele (sef″al-he-mat′o-sēl) a hematocele under the pericranium, communicating with the sinuses of the dura mater.

cephalhematoma (sef″al-he″mah-to′mah) a localized effusion of blood beneath the periosteum of the skull of a newborn infant, due to disruption of the vessels during birth.

cephalic (sĕ-fal′ik) pertaining to the head, or to the head end of the body.

c. index, 100 times the maximal breadth of the skull divided by its maximal length.

cephalin (sef′ah-lin) 1. a monaminomonophosphatide in brain tissue, nerve tissue, and yolk of egg. 2. a crude phospholipid usually extracted from brain tissue, used as a clotting agent in blood coagulation work.

c.-cholesterol flocculation test, a liver function test based upon alterations in serum proteins; called also Hanger's test. The purpose of the test is to distinguish between jaundice due to liver disease and obstructive jaundice. When the liver cells are damaged they are unable to make certain changes in the serum proteins. Serum from the blood of a patient with liver damage shows distinct flocculation (collects in small lumps) when combined with a reagent. The reagent in this test is an emulsion of cholesterol, cephalin, and water. The emulsion is mixed with dilute serum and then checked at 24 and 48 hours for signs of flocculation. Normally flocculation will be negative; normal range for the test is negative to 2 plus.

Preparation of the patient requires fasting from midnight the evening before the test. Venous blood is used for the test.

cephalitis (sef″ah-li′tis) encephalitis.

cephalocele (sĕ-fal′o-sēl) protrusion of a part of the cranial contents.

cephalocentesis (sef″ah-lo-sen-te′sis) surgical puncture of the head.

cephalodynia (sef″ah-lo-din′e-ah) pain in the head; headache.

cephalogaster (sef″ah-lo-gas′ter) the anterior portion of the enteric canal of the embryo.

cephaloglycin (sef″ah-lo-gli′sin) an analogue of cephalosporin C used in urinary tract infections.

cephalogram (sef″ah-lo-gram) an x-ray image of the structures of the head; cephalometric radiograph.

cephalogyric (sef″ah-lo-ji′rik) pertaining to turning motions of the head.

cephalohematoma (sef″ah-lo-he″mah-to′mah) cephalhematoma.

cephalomelus (sef″ah-lom′ĕ-lus) a monster with an accessory limb growing from the head.

cephalometer (sef″ah-lom′ĕ-ter) an instrument for measuring the head; an orienting device for positioning the head for radiographic examination and measurement.

cephalometry (sef″ah-lom′ĕ-tre) scientific measurement of the dimensions of the head and face.

cephalomotor (sef″ah-lo-mo′tor) moving the head; pertaining to motions of the head.

cephalonia (sef″ah-lo′ne-ah) a condition in which the head is abnormally enlarged, with sclerotic hyperplasia of the brain.

cephalopathy (sef″ah-lop′ah-the) any disease of the head.

cephalopelvic (sef″ah-lo-pel′vik) pertaining to the relationship of the fetal head to the maternal pelvis.

cephaloridine (sef″ah-lor′ĭ-dēn) a broad-spectrum antibiotic of the cephalosporin group.

cephalosporin (sef″ah-lo-spōr′in) any of a group of broad-spectrum, penicillinase-resistant antibiotics from *Cephalosporium,* including cephalexin, cephaloridine, cephaloglycin, cephalothin, cephapirin, and cephradine, which share the nucleus 7-aminocephalosporanic acid.

c. C, a component of cephalosporin used as an antimicrobial.

c. P, an antibacterial steroid, the crude form of which contains at least five components (P_1, P_2, P_3, P_4, P_5,), P_1 being the major active substance.

Cephalosporium (sef″ah-lo-spo′re-um) a genus of soil-inhabiting fungi, some species of which are the source of a group of broad-spectrum antibiotics, the cephalosporins.

cephalostat (sef′ah-lo-stat″) a head-positioning device which assures reproducibility of the relations between an x-ray beam, a patient's head, and an x-ray film.

cephalothin (sef′ah-lo-thin) a semisynthetic analogue of the natural antibiotic cephalosporin C; used as the sodium salt against various bacteria, including many penicillin-resistant staphylococci.

cephalothoracic (sef″ah-lo-tho-ras′ik) pertaining to the head and thorax.

cephalothoracopagus (sef″ah-lo-tho″rah-kop′ah-gus) a double monster joined in the frontal plane, the fusion extending from the crown of the head to the middle abdominal region.

cephalotomy (sef″ah-lot′o-me) 1. the cutting up of the fetal head to facilitate delivery. 2. dissection of the fetal head.

cephalotropic (sef″ah-lo-trop′ik) having an affinity for brain tissue.

cephalotrypesis (sef″ah-lo-tri-pe′sis) trephination of the skull.

cephapirin (sef″ah-pi′rin) a cephalosporin antibiotic used parenterally in the form of the sodium salt.

cephradine (sef′rah-dēn) a cephalosporin antibiotic for oral administration.

ceptor (sep′tor) 1. in Ehrlich's side-chain theory, receptors that have been thrown off into the blood stream. 2. any nervous apparatus that receives external stimuli or impressions and transfers them to nerve centers.

cera (se′rah) [L.] wax.

ceramidase (ser-am′ĭ-dās) an enzyme occurring in

most mammalian tissue that catalyzes the reversible acylation-deacylation of ceramides.

ceramide (ser′ah-mīd) any of a group of naturally occurring sphingolipids in which the NH_2 group of sphingosine is acylated with a fatty acyl CoA derivative to form N-acylsphingosine.

c. glucoside, the major sphingolipid accumulated in Gaucher's disease.

c. trihexoside, the major sphingolipid accumulated in Fabry's disease.

cerasine (ser′ah-sīn) a red azo dye, used as a cytoplasmic stain.

cerate (sēr′āt) a medicinal preparation for external use, compounded of fat or wax, or both, intermediate in consistency between an ointment and a plaster.

ceratin (ser′ah-tin) keratin.

ceratitis (ser″ah-ti′tis) keratitis.

cerato- for words beginning thus, see also those beginning *kerato-*.

Ceratophyllus (ser-ah-tof′ĭ-lus) a genus of fleas.

cercaria (ser-ka′re-ah), pl. *cerca′riae* [Gr.] the final, free-swimming larval stage of a trematode parasite.

cerclage (ser-klahzh′) [Fr.] encircling of a part with a ring or loop, as for correction of an incompetent cervix uteri or fixation of the adjacent ends of a fractured bone.

cercus (ser′kus) a bristle-like structure.

cerebellar (ser″ĕ-bel′ar) pertaining to the cerebellum.

c. cortex, the superficial gray matter of the cerebellum.

cerebellitis (ser″ĕ-bel-i′tis) inflammation of the cerebellum.

cerebellum (ser″ĕ-bel′um) the part of the metencephalon situated on the back of the brain stem, to which it is attached by three cerebellar peduncles on each side; it consists of a median lobe (vermis) and two lateral lobes (the hemispheres). (See also BRAIN.)

cerebral (ser′ĕ-bral, sĕ-re′bral) pertaining to the cerebrum.

s. contusion, contusion of the brain following a HEAD INJURY (see also cerebral CONTUSION).

c. cortex, the convoluted layer of gray matter covering the cerebral hemispheres, which governs thought, reasoning, memory, sensation, and voluntary movement. (See also BRAIN.)

c. gigantism, gigantism in the absence of increased levels of growth hormone, attributed to a cerebral defect (see also cerebral GIGANTISM).

c. palsy, partial paralysis and lack of muscle coordination resulting from a defect, injury, or disease of the nerve tissue contained within the skull. The defects are generally thought to be caused at or near the time of birth and may be due to a lack of oxygen, premature delivery, blood type incompatibility, head injury, or infections of the brain or the meninges.

SYMPTOMS. The defect may affect one or more areas of the brain and produce a variety of muscular disorders. The largest majority of cerebral palsy cases are of three forms: (1) spastic type, in which there are exaggerated stretch reflexes, muscle spasm, and increased deep tendon reflexes; (2) athetoid, with purposeless, uncontrollable movements and muscle tension; and (3) atactic, in which the child has poor balance, poor coordination, and a staggering gait. Visual, hearing, and speech defects may be present. Mental retardation may or may not be a manifestation of the brain damage.

Often the parents or pediatrician can observe indications of cerebral palsy when an infant is only a few months old, but in mild cases the diagnosis may not be made until age 2 or 3.

TREATMENT. Treatment varies according to the nature and extent of brain damage. Muscle relaxants may help reduce spasms. Anticonvulsant drugs are necessary when seizures are among the symptoms of the disorder. Orthopedic surgery, casts, braces, and traction can be used to correct some types of disability associated with cerebral palsy. Early muscle training and special exercises often help the child lead a useful, productive life. If muscle training is not begun early, extensive rehabilitation may be necessary to correct faulty habits and poor muscle patterns established by the child. However, it is never too late for a complete evaluation of the condition of a patient with cerebral palsy. A rehabilitation program can produce good results later in life as well as in childhood.

c. vascular accident (CVA), a disorder of the blood vessels serving the cerebrum, resulting from an impaired blood supply to parts of the brain. Called also stroke; the resultant symptom complex of neurological damage is called stroke syndrome.

Cerebral vascular accidents are more common than is generally realized. It is estimated that by the age of 30, one out of four persons has sufficient change in the cerebral arteries to provide a setting for a stroke at any time. Autopsy studies show that nearly half of those who die from other causes have had minor strokes without ever having been aware of them.

Attacks that are sometimes called "little strokes" may last from a few minutes to almost 24 hours. These attacks have been termed transient cerebral ischemic attacks (TIA). The term arises from the nature of the attack, which is only temporary and leaves no noticeable residual effects, and from the ischemia or deficiency of blood supply to the cerebral tissues. These attacks are considered as warnings that a more severe attack will probably occur unless steps are taken to improve blood flow through the arteries. Those vessels most commonly affected are the extracranial arteries, particularly the carotid and vertebral arteries in the neck.

A second type of attack lasts for several days and then subsides with some minor residual effects. This type is termed TIA-IR (incomplete recovery). An attack of cerebral ischemia that presents the more severe symptoms usually associated with stroke is diagnosed as (CS) completed stroke.

CAUSES. There are three main causes of cerebral vascular accident, all of which are related to a pathological condition of the arteries and associated with cerebral infarction, i.e., a necrotic area in the brain tissue. They are cerebral embolism, cerebral thrombosis, and cerebral hemorrhage. Other causes include compression of cerebral vessels, as from tumor or edema, and arterial spasm.

Cerebral Embolism. An embolus is a small mass of material circulating in the blood vessels. It can consist of air, fat, or other material introduced into the circulatory system; or, as is most often the case, it is a detached portion of a thrombus that settles in a cerebral vessel. Damage from cerebral embolism is often less extensive and recovery more rapid than in strokes from thrombosis and cerebral hemorrhage.

Cerebral Thrombosis. A thrombus, or clot, in a blood vessel of the brain is by far the most common cause of stroke. Most often the thrombosis occurs where there is narrowing of the lumen of a vessel, usually caused by ATHEROSCLEROSIS. The thrombosis produces ischemia, edema, and congestion of the brain tissues surrounding the area. Symptoms appear more gradually in this type of stroke.

Cerebral Hemorrhage. A rupturing of a blood vessel, usually an artery, within the brain. The hemorrhage is frequently associated with preexisting HYPERTENSION. There often is weakening of the vessel wall as well. Healthy arteries can withstand considerable pressure because of their elasticity, but in persons with ARTERIOSCLEROSIS this elasticity is lost and the blood vessel may rupture from the increased pressure within it. In other situations the cerebral vessel wall may be weakened by an ANEURYSM, and thus is susceptible to rupture and hemorrhage into the brain tissues.

Stroke from cerebral hemorrhage is most common after the age of 50 and usually produces more extensive neurologic defects with slower recovery than does stroke from other causes.

SYMPTOMS. The symptoms of cerebral vascular accident vary widely, depending on its cause, location of ischemia, and extent of damage to brain cells. The onset is sudden in cerebral hemorrhage and cerebral embolism because the interruption of blood flow happens quickly. Its effects are noticed almost immediately. Strokes from cerebral hemorrhage occur most often in the daytime while the person is active. In cerebral thrombosis the clot gradually occludes the blood vessels, therefore the onset is gradual. A stroke caused by thrombosis tends to occur while the patient is sleeping or within an hour after arising.

There may be preliminary symptoms, particularly with thrombosis. The patient may experience dizziness, headache, mental confusion, and poor coordination. More often there is a sudden and dramatic onset with loss of consciousness; convulsions may occur. The unconsciousness may last for a few minutes or continue for weeks; it can terminate in a slow recovery or death. Sudden death rarely occurs as a result of stroke.

There usually are neurologic symptoms related to the site of ischemia; for example, hemiplegia, loss of sensation, and reflex changes. The area of paralysis is directly related to the area of cerebral ischemia. If the left side of the brain is affected, the paralysis of the face, arm, and leg will be present on the opposite or right side. Speech disturbances also are related to the area of brain cell damage; if the left side of the brain, which is the location of the speech center in right-handed persons, is affected, then aphasia as well as hemiplegia will be present.

Involvement of the region of the thalamus produces a sensation of pain in the hemiplegic area, especially the hand. The discomfort begins several weeks after the stroke.

Emotional disturbances also accompany thalamic involvement. The patient has difficulty controlling his emotions; he may laugh or cry with little or no provocation.

The symptoms of stroke are almost unlimited in type, severity, and permanency. Some may eventually subside, while others are never completely eliminated. Anyone concerned with the care of the stroke victim should be alert to all signs and symptoms that occur. These observations can be extremely helpful in establishing a definite diagnosis and planning a regimen of patient care.

PREVENTION AND TREATMENT. The overall goal in the prevention of stroke of any type is prevention or removal of the established primary cause; i.e., atherosclerosis, arteriosclerosis, aneurysm, and hypertension. Specific techniques in the prevention of stroke are related to the improvement of blood supply to the brain tissue within the limitations imposed by the particular pathologic condition producing either impaired blood flow or intracranial bleeding, the surgical techniques and medical care available, and the general condition of the patient and his potential for survival.

Surgical procedures employed to prevent stroke or lessen the severity of its effects once it has occurred include (1) endarectomy to remove thickened areas from the inner lining of the carotid or vertebral arteries in the neck, (2) patching with a graft a section of artery in which there is an aneurysm, or removal of a section of artery so affected, and (3) removal of a blood clot within the artery.

The choice of medical prevention and treatment is governed by the conditions which predispose the patient to cerebral vascular accident, and, in the event a stroke has already occurred, the potential of the individual patient to benefit from the treatment. ANTICOAGULANT drugs are employed only when hemorrhage has been ruled out as a possibility and clot formation has been found to be either the potential or actual cause of decreased blood flow. Antihypertensive drugs are used to reduce pressure within the blood vessel and thereby avoid rupture.

EMERGENCY AND ACUTE CARE. Emergency care consists of loosening all constricting clothing, especially around the neck, to improve respiration and circulation to the head. The patient's head should be turned to the affected side to prevent aspiration of saliva and mucus. He is kept calm and quiet and reassured that he is being cared for. If he is conscious he may sit up or his head may be elevated to lessen blood pressure within the head.

After admission and during the acute stage of cerebral vascular accident, it is extremely important to assess the patient's condition frequently to determine the neurologic effects of the stroke and to ascertain whether there is evidence of recurrent strokes. Observations of the patient are valuable in determining the cause of the stroke and the choice of treatment.

Maintenance of a patent AIRWAY and adequate oxygenation are critical. SUCTIONING may be necessary if paralysis prevents normal swallowing of saliva. An artificial airway is inserted if the patient cannot maintain an adequate airway on his own. In severe cases a TRACHEOSTOMY may be required.

The vital signs are taken and recorded at frequent intervals during the 24 hours of the day. An elevated temperature, with decrease in the pulse and respiratory rates, indicates a poor prognosis.

GENERAL CARE. In order to avoid complications that can develop very quickly in a stroke victim, it is necessary to attend to proper positioning, good body alignment, and frequent turning. The patient is turned at least every two to three hours. Because of poor circulation to the affected area, he should not be left to lie on his affected side for more than 20 minutes four times a day.

The amount of activity allowed the patient will depend on the cause of the stroke and the stage of illness. Those who have increased intracranial pressure from hemorrhage and edema will be placed on complete bed rest. Others who are comatose will require continuous care to avoid complications arising from inactivity (see also COMA).

Complications to be avoided in the patient who has suffered a stroke include DECUBITUS ULCERS, hypostatic PNEUMONIA, THROMBOSIS and other conditions resulting from circulatory stasis, kidney stones and urinary infections, and such orthopedic deformities as foot and wrist drop and CONTRACTURES. Unless contraindicated, the joints are put through their full range of motion at least once a day (see also EXERCISE). A program of PHYSICAL THERAPY is planned and started as soon as possible to assure maximum rehabilitation.

Nutrition is maintained by whatever means necessary, depending on the patient's ability to chew, handle food in his mouth, and swallow. In some cases TUBE FEEDING may be the only method by which food is administered. If the patient is able to swallow, but has difficulty moving the food about in his mouth, he should be turned to the affected side while he is being fed. Rinsing the mouth after meals and frequent mouth care help eliminate accumulation of food in the mouth and halitosis. The lips should be kept lubricated with cold cream or mineral oil to keep them from drying and cracking.

INCONTINENCE of urine and feces sometimes accompanies a cerebral vascular accident. A regular schedule of offering the bedpan, especially after each meal, may help establish a routine of elimination. It is also helpful to get the patient up to the bathroom or to a bedside commode whenever this is possible. In any event the patient must be kept clean and dry and skin care must be given frequently to avoid pressure areas and decubitus ulcers. Fecal impaction and urinary retention may occur and can be avoided by intelligent observation and recording of bowel movements and urinary output. The physician may order an enema to be given periodically if constipation becomes a problem. (See also BLADDER TRAINING and BOWEL TRAINING.)

Rehabilitation of the patient begins the moment he enters the hospital. This means that all measures taken to maintain bodily functions and to avoid complications are aimed at the ultimate goal of getting the patient back to a state as near normal as possible. His reaction to his illness, his family's attitude, the quality of care he receives, and the attitude of those caring for him will greatly affect the eventual outcome of his illness. There may be a tendency on the part of the hospital staff and the patient's family to do everything for the patient when he seems so helpless and handicapped. Certainly he should be helped with the things he cannot do for himself, but total dependence on others can become very demoralizing and for the patient's sake he must be encouraged to help himself. This may be a slow and demanding process, requiring much patience and optimism. One can begin by providing the means by which the patient can gradually begin to bathe, feed, and dress himself.

Special equipment, such as an overbed table made of cardboard or plywood, can be used so that the patient can reach the bath water, toilet articles, and other things he needs. His food should be prepared and arranged on his tray so that he can handle it without great difficulty. If his first movements are awkward and messy, no mention should be made of this and he must never be made to feel that he has caused an inconvenience to anyone through his efforts to help himself.

There has been much interest in the rehabilitation of cerebral vascular accident patients in recent years and there is a wealth of information and help available for the stroke victim and his family. Pamphlets dealing with the special problems of this illness are readily available from the American Heart Association and the American Red Cross.

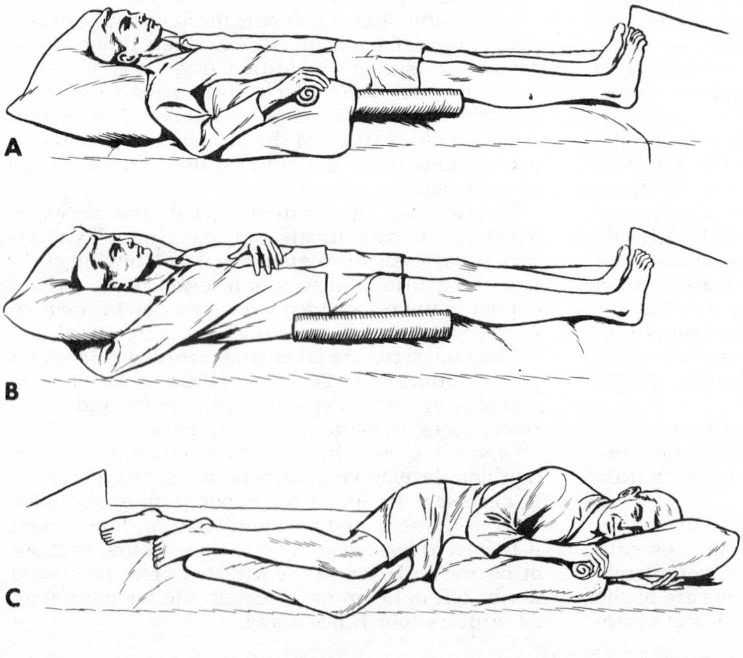

Positioning in cerebral vascular accident. *A*, A pillow is placed next to the body on the weak side. The weak arm is placed on the pillow. Make sure that the elbow points away from the body and that the lower arm and hand are placed alongside the body and about 12 inches away from it. A rolled napkin or small towel is placed under the weak hand to keep the fingers open. Note trochanter roll along affected side to keep hip from rotating. *B*, The affected arm is tucked under the pillow with hand flattened to prevent curling of the fingers. C. in this side-lying position, a pillow is used to support the weak arm. Another pillow is used to support the weak leg. (From Strike Back at Stroke. Washington, D.C., U.S. Government Printing Office.)

Centers for speech therapy, vocational rehabilitation, and homemaker services are located in many communities. The local health department can provide information as to the location of these centers and services they provide.

cerebration (ser″ĕ-bra′shun) functional activity of the brain.

cerebritis (ser″ĕ-bri′tis) inflammation of the cerebrum.

cerebrocuprein (ser″ĕ-bro-ku′pre-in) a copper protein isolated from the human and bovine brain.

cerebroid (ser′ĕ-broid) resembling brain substance.

cerebroma (ser″ĕ-bro′mah) any abnormal mass of brain substance.

cerebromalacia (ser″ĕ-bro-mah-la′she-ah) abnormal softening of the substance of the cerebrum.

cerebromeningitis (ser″ĕ-bro-men″in-ji′tis) meningoencephalitis.

cerebronic acid (ser″ĕ-bron′ik) a fatty acid derived from sphingomyelin, which is the principal hydroxy saturated acid from the brain.

cerebropathy (ser″ĕ-brop′ah-the) any brain disorder.

cerebrophysiology (ser″ĕ-bro-fiz″e-ol′o-je) the physiology of the brain.

cerebropontile (ser″ĕ-bro-pon′tīl) pertaining to the cerebrum and pons.

cerebrosclerosis (ser″ĕ-bro-sklĕ-ro′sis) morbid hardening of the substance of the cerebrum.

cerebrose (ser′ĕ-brōs) galactose (of cerebrosides).

cerebroside (sĕ-re′bro-sīd) a general designation for sphingolipids in which sphingosine is combined with galactose or glucose; found chiefly in nervous tissue.

cerebrosis (ser″ĕ-bro′sis) any disease of the cerebrum.

cerebrospinal (ser″ĕ-bro-spi′nal) pertaining to the brain and spinal cord.

c. fluid, the fluid within the subarachnoid space, the central canal of the spinal cord, and the four ventricles of the brain. The fluid is formed continuously by the choroid plexus in the ventricles, and, so that there will not be an abnormal increase in amount and pressure, it is reabsorbed into the blood by the arachnoid villi at approximately the same rate at which it is produced.

The cerebrospinal fluid aids in the protection of the brain, spinal cord, and meninges by acting as a watery cushion surrounding them to absorb the shocks to which they are exposed. There is a blood-cerebrospinal fluid barrier that prevents harmful substances, such as metal poisons, some pathogenic organisms, and certain drugs from passing from the capillaries into the cerebrospinal fluid.

The normal cerebrospinal fluid pressure is 5 mm. of mercury (100 mm. of water) when the individual is lying in a horizontal position on his side. Fluid pressure may be increased by a brain tumor or by hemorrhage or infection in the cranium. HYDROCEPHALUS, or excess fluid in the cranial cavity, can result from either excessive formation or poor absorption of cerebrospinal fluid. Blockage of the flow of fluid in the spinal canal may result from a tumor, blood clot, or severance of the spinal cord. The pressure remains normal or decreases below the point of obstruction but increases above that point.

Cell counts, bacterial smears, and cultures of samples of cerebrospinal fluid are done when an inflammatory process or infection of the meninges is suspected. Since the cerebrospinal fluid contains nutrient substances such as glucose, proteins, and sodium chloride, and also some waste products such as urea, it is believed to play a role in metabolism. The major constituents of cerebrospinal fluid are water, glucose, sodium chloride, and protein, and changes in their concentrations are helpful in diagnosis of brain diseases.

Samples of cerebrospinal fluid may be obtained by SPINAL PUNCTURE, in which a hollow needle is inserted between two lumbar vertebrae (below the lower end of the spinal cord), or into the cisterna cerebellomedullaris just below the occipital bone of the skull (cisternal puncture). Pressure of the cerebrospinal fluid is measured by a manometer attached to the end of the needle after it has been inserted.

cerebrotomy (ser″ĕ-brot′o-me) anatomy or dissection of the brain.

cerebrovascular (ser″ĕ-bro-vas′ku-lar) pertaining to the blood vessels of the cerebrum, or brain.

c. accident, cerebral vascular accident.

cerebrum (ser′ĕ-brum) the main portion of the brain, occupying the upper part of the cranial cavity; its two cerebral hemispheres, united by the corpus callosum, form the largest part of the central nervous system in man. The term is sometimes applied to the postembryonic forebrain and midbrain together or to the entire brain. (See also BRAIN.)

cerium (se′re-um) a chemical element, atomic number 58, atomic weight 140.12, symbol Ce. (See also table of ELEMENTS.)

ceroma (se-ro′mah) a tumor that has undergone amyloid (waxy) degeneration.

ceruloplasmin (sĕ-roo″lo-plaz′min) an alpha$_2$-globulin of the plasma, being the form in which most of the plasma copper is transported.

cerumen (sĕ-roo′men) a waxy secretion of the glands of the external acoustic meatus; ear wax. adj., **ceru′minal, ceru′minous.**

ceruminolysis (sĕ-roo″mĭ-nol′ĭ-sis) dissolution or disintegration of cerumen in the external acoustic meatus. adj., **ceruminolyt′ic.**

ceruminosis (sĕ-roo′mĭ-no′sis) excessive or disordered secretion of cerumen.

cervic(o)- word element [L.], *neck; cervix.*

cervical (ser′vĭ-kal) pertaining to the neck or to the cervix.

c. canal, the part of the uterine cavity lying within the cervix.

c. plexus, a network of nerve fibers formed by the first four cervical nerves and supplying the structures in the region of the neck. One important branch is the phrenic nerve, which supplies the diaphragm.

c. rib, a supernumerary rib arising from a cervical vertebra.

c. rib syndrome, pain over the shoulder, often extending down the arm or radiating up the back of the neck, due to compression of the nerves and vessels between a cervical rib and the anterior scalene muscle.

c. vertebrae, the upper seven vertebrae, constituting the skeleton of the neck.

cervicectomy (ser′vĭ-sek′to-me) excision of the cervix uteri.

cervicitis (ser″vĭ-si′tis) inflammation of the cervix uteri.

cervicobrachialgia (ser″vĭ-ko-brak″e-al′je-ah) pain in the neck radiating to the arm, due to compression of nerve roots of the cervical spinal cord.

cervicocolpitis (ser″vĭ-ko-kol-pi′tis) inflammation of the cervix uteri and vagina.

cervicofacial (ser″vĭ-ko-fa′shal) pertaining to the neck and face.

cervicoplasty (ser′vĭ-ko-plas″te) plastic surgery on the neck.

cervicovesical (ser″vĭ-ko-ves′ĭ-kal) relating to the cervix uteri and urinary bladder.

Cervilaxin (ser″vĭ-lak′sin) trademark for a preparation of relaxin.

cervix (ser′viks), pl. *cer′vices* [L.] neck; the front portion of the neck (collum), or a constricted part of an organ (e.g., CERVIX UTERI).

incompetent c., a cervix uteri that is abnormally prone to dilate before termination of the normal period of gestation, resulting in premature expulsion of the fetus.

c. u′teri, the narrow lower end of the uterus between the isthmus and the opening of the uterus into the vagina.

Cervical cancer is surpassed only by breast cancer as a cause of female cancer deaths in the United States. Its victims are usually women over 40. One of the first warning signs of cervical cancer is vaginal bleeding between menstrual periods, after coitus, or after menopause is established. There may also be increased vaginal discharge. The PAPANICOLAOU SMEAR TEST should be done routinely every year in women over 30 to rule out the possibility of cervical malignancy. This test identifies cancer in its earliest stages while the malignancy is still capable of relatively easy eradication. Treatment may include surgery or radiotherapy or both.

Cervical erosion refers to ulceration of the surface epithelium of the cervix resulting from trauma (as in childbirth) or infection. The condition is treated by cauterization and douches. Although the condition is not serious, it should be treated promptly to avoid possible development of malignancy in later years. Cervical lacerations are likely to occur during childbirth. Most small lacerations heal by themselves; more extensive tears in the cervix may require surgical repair. Cervical polyps are fleshy growths that may form on the cervix, causing bleeding. They are removed surgically.

c. ves′icae, the lower, constricted part of the urinary bladder, proximal to the opening of the urethra.

cesarean section (sĕ-sa′re-an) delivery of a fetus by incision through the abdominal wall and uterus. The procedure takes its name from the Latin word *caedere,* to cut, and has no relation to the birth of Caesar as is sometimes believed. Indications for cesarean section include dystocia, toxemia, hemorrhage from abruptio placentae or placenta praevia, fetal distress, and breech presentation.

cesium (se′ze-um) a chemical element, atomic number 55, atomic weight 132.905, symbol Cs. (See table of ELEMENTS.)

Cestan-Chenais syndrome (ses-tan′ shen-āz′) an association of contralateral hemiplegia, contralateral hemianesthesia, ipsilateral lateropulsion and hemiasynergia, Horner's syndrome, and ipsilateral laryngoplegia, due to scattered lesions of the pyramid, sensory tract, inferior cerebellar peduncle, nucleus ambiguus, and oculopupillary center.

cesticidal (ses″tĭ-si′dal) destructive to cestodes.

Cestoda (ses-to′dah) a subclass of Cestoidea comprising the true tapeworms, which had a head (scolex) and segments (proglottides). The adults are endoparasitic in the alimentary tract and associated ducts of various vertebrate hosts; their larvae may be found in various organs and tissues.

Cestodaria (ses″to-da′re-ah) a subclass of tapeworms, the unsegmented tapeworms of the class Cestoidea, which are endoparasitic in the intestines and coelom of various primitive fishes and rarely in reptiles.

cestode (ses′tōd) 1. any individual of the class Cestoidea, especially any member of the subclass Cestoda. 2. cestoid.

cestodology (ses″to-dol′o-je) the scientific study of cestodes.

cestoid (ses′toid) resembling a tapeworm.

Cestoidea (ses-toi′de-ah) a class of tapeworms (phylum Platyhelminthes), characterized by a noncellular cuticular layer covering their bodies and by the absence of a mouth and digestive tract. The true tapeworms are included in the subclass Cestoda.

cetylpyridinium (se″til-pi″rĭ-din′e-um) a pyridine derivative used as a local anti-infective in the form of the chloride salt.

Cevalin (se′vah-lin) trademark for preparations of ascorbic acid (vitamin C).

Cevex (se′veks) trademark for a liquid preparation of ascorbic acid (vitamin C).

Ce-Vi-Sol (se′vi-sol) trademark for a preparation of ascorbic acid (vitamin C).

cevitamic acid (se″vi-tam′ik) ascorbic acid.

Cf chemical symbol, *californium.*

cg. centigram.

C.G.S., c.g.s. centimeter-gram-second (system), a system of measurements based on the centimeter as the unit of length, the gram as the unit of mass, and the second as the unit of time.

Chaddock's sign (reflex) (chad′oks) dorsiflexion of the big toe when the foot is stroked around the lateral malleolus and along the dorsum laterally. It occurs in lesions of the pyramidal tract.

chafe (chāf) to irritate the skin by friction, usually from clothing, or the rubbing together of body surfaces, such as the thighs, when they are damp with perspiration, or the rubbing together of opposing skin folds. The skin folds of the obese are particularly subject to chafing. Tight shoes, badly fitting brassieres, and other clothing that binds, all cause chafing. Babies are particularly susceptible.

The irritation can usually be cleared up by keeping the parts dry, using a plain talcum powder, and, if necessary, substituting clothing that does not bind or rub. In some cases, a sterile dressing may be necessary to help relieve the rubbing. The best prevention is to keep the skin clean and dry and to wear clothing that fits properly.

Chagas' disease, Chagas-Cruz disease (chag′as, chag′as kruz) trypanosomiasis due to *Trypanosoma cruzi* (see also South American TRYPANOSOMIASIS).

chain (chān) a collection of objects linked together

in linear fashion, or end to end, as the assemblage of atoms or radicals in a chemical compound, or an assemblage of individual bacterial cells.

branched c., an open chain of atoms, usually carbon, with one or more side chains attached to it.

closed c., see closed-chain COMPOUND.

heavy c., any of the large polypeptide chains of five classes that, paired with the light chains, make up the antibody molecule. Heavy chains bear the antigenic determinants that differentiate the immunoglobulin classes. See also HEAVY-CHAIN DISEASE.

light c., either of the two small polypeptide chains (molecular weight 22,000) that, when linked to heavy chains by disulfide bonds, make up the antibody molecule; they are of two types, kappa and lambda, which are unrelated to immunoglobulin class differences.

open c., see open-chain COMPOUND.

side c., a chain of atoms attached to a larger chain or to a ring.

chalasia (kah-la′ze-ah) relaxation of a bodily opening, such as the cardiac sphincter (a cause of vomiting in infants).

chalazion (kah-la′ze-on) a small eyelid mass resulting from chronic inflammation of a meibomian gland. A chalazion can sometimes be treated at home with the application of hot compresses, but while this method is usually successful with a STY, a similar infection that has not yet formed a cyst, chalazion often requires incision and drainage, performed by a physician. Called also meibomian cyst.

chalcosis (kal-ko′sis) copper deposits in tissue.

chalicosis (kal″ĭ-ko′sis) pneumoconiosis due to inhalation of particles of stone.

chalybeate (kah-lib′e-āt) containing or charged with iron.

chamaecephaly (kam″ĕ-sef′ah-le) the condition of having a low, flat head, i.e., a cephalic index of 70 or less. adj., **chamaecephal′ic.**

chamber (chām′ber) an enclosed space.

anterior c., the part of the aqueous humor-containing space of the eyeball between the cornea and iris.

hyperbaric c., an enclosed space in which gas (oxygen) can be raised to greater than atmospheric pressure (see also HYPERBARIC OXYGENATION).

ionization c., an enclosure containing two or more electrodes between which an electric current may be passed when the enclosed gas is ionized by radiation; used for determining the intensity of x-rays and other rays.

posterior c., that part of the aqueous humor-containing space of the eyeball between the iris and the lens.

vitreous c., the vitreous humor-containing space in the eyeball, bounded anteriorly by the lens and ciliary body and posteriorly by the posterior wall of the eyeball.

Chamberlen forceps (chām′ber-len) the original form of obstetric forceps.

chancre (shang′ker) 1. the primary lesion of SYPHILIS, occurring at the site of entry of the infection. Called also hard, hunterian, or true chancre. 2. a papular lesion occurring at the site of entry of infection in tuberculosis of the skin or in sporotrichosis.

A true chancre begins as a papule which breaks down into a reddish ulcer. It is generally firm and accompanied by little or no pain. Although most frequently located on the external genitalia, it may be on the lips or fingers. In women, a chancre is sometimes concealed in the internal genitalia where it may not be seen or felt. Two or three may develop simultaneously. A chancre heals of its own accord without treatment, thus leading many persons infected with syphilis to believe they are cured. They are not, and if adequate medical treatment is not begun at this early and curable stage of syphilis, the disease will progress, doing irreparable damage.

chancroid (shang′kroid) a soft nonsyphilitic veneral sore caused by *Haemophilus ducreyi.* As in syphilis, the first symptom of the disease may be the appearance of a sore, but the sore is soft, as distinguished from the hard chancre of syphilis.

Chancroid is almost always spread by sexual contact, but in rare instances it may be transmitted indirectly from soiled dressings or towels. Three to five days after exposure one or more small soft sores appear on or near the external genitalia. These sores soon develop into ulcers with irregular edges and surrounding areas which become red and swollen. In many cases, the infection spreads to the lymph nodes of the groin, causing swelling and tenderness.

Chancroid is successfully treated with sulfonamides or the antibiotics tetracyclıne and streptomycin.

chancrous (shang′krus) of the nature of chancre.

Chaoul tube (showl) a tube used in x-ray therapy.

character (kar′ak-ter) a quality or attribute indicative of the nature of an object or an organism; in genetics, the expression of a gene or group of genes as seen in a phenotype.

acquired c., a noninheritable modification produced in an animal as a result of its own activities or of environmental influences.

dominant c., a mendelian character that is expressed when it is transmitted by a single gene.

mendelian c's, in genetics, the separate and distinct traits exhibited by an animal or plant and dependent on the genetic constitution of the organism.

primary sex c., those characters of the male and female directly concerned in reproduction.

recessive c., a mendelian character that is expressed only when transmitted by both genes (one from each parent) determining the trait.

secondary sex c., those characters specific to the male and female but not directly concerned in the reproduction.

sex-conditioned c., sex-influenced c., an autosomal trait whose full expression is conditioned by the sex of the individual, e.g., human baldness.

sex-linked c., one transmitted consistently to individuals of one sex only, being carried in the sex chromosome.

charcoal (char′kōl) carbon prepared by charring wood or other organic material.

activated c., the residue of destructive distillation of various organic materials, treated to increase its adsorptive power; used as a general purpose antidote.

animal c., charcoal prepared from bone, which is purified (purified animal charcoal) by removal of materials dissolved by hot hydrochloric acid and water; adsorbent and decolorizer.

Charcot's arthropathy (disease) (shar-kōz′) chronic progressive degeneration of the stress-bearing portion of a joint, with hypertrophic changes at the periphery; it is associated with neurologic disorders involving loss of sensation in the joint. Called also neuropathic arthropathy.

Charcot-Marie-Tooth disease (shar-ko′ mah-re′ tōōth) progressive neuropathic (peroneal) muscular atrophy.

charlatan (shar′lah-tan) a pretender to knowledge or skills not possessed; in medicine, a quack.

Charles' law (sharlz) at a constant pressure the volume of a given mass of perfect gas varies directly with the absolute temperature.

charleyhorse (char′le-hors) soreness and stiffness in a muscle, especially the quadriceps, due to overstrain or contusion. It usually occurs when muscles that have not been conditioned for hard use are put under a strain, with the result that some of the muscle fibers are strained or may actually tear. It is characterized by soreness, stiffness, and pain which often comes on very suddenly. Heat, particularly from warm baths, helps the condition, and aspirin is useful in relieving the pain. If the pain persists for several days, there may be some other muscle injury and a physician should be consulted.

chart (chart) a record of data in graphic or tabular form.

genealogical c., a graph showing various descendants of a common ancestor, used to indicate those affected by genetically determined disease.

reading c., a chart with material printed in gradually increasing type sizes, used in testing acuity of near vision.

Reuss' c's, charts with colored letters printed on colored backgrounds, used in testing color vision.

Snellen's c., a chart printed with block letters in gradually decreasing sizes, used in testing visual acuity.

charting (chart′ing) the keeping of a clinical record of the important facts about a patient and the progress of his illness. The patient's chart most often contains a medical history, results of a physical examination, laboratory reports, results of special diagnostic tests, and the observations of the nursing staff and the particular treatments and medications administered to the patient. (See also PROBLEM-ORIENTED RECORD.)

chauffage (sho-fahzh′) [Fr.] treatment with a low-heated cautery that is passed to and fro close to the tissue.

chaulmoogra oil (chawl-moo′grah) a fixed oil expressed from the ripe seeds of *Taraktogenos kurzii* and species of *Hydnocarpus,* which has been used in the treatment of leprosy. Because of its toxicity and tendency to cause local skin and mucous membrane irritation, it has been replaced by antibiotics and modern chemotherapeutic agents, especially the sulfones, and is virtually in disuse in most areas of the world. (See also ETHYL CHAULMOOGRATE.)

chaulmoogric acid (chawl-moo′grik) a cyclic fatty acid, from chaulmoogra oil.

Ch.B. [L.] *Chirur′giae Baccalau′reus* (Bachelor of Surgery).

Chédiak-Higashi syndrome a hereditary disorder marked by massive leukocytic inclusions, decreased pigmentation of the skin, hair, and eyes, photophobia, nystagmus, susceptibility to infections, and early death; it may be associated with a predisposition to leukemia and malignant lymphoma.

cheek (chēk) a fleshy, rounded protuberance, especially the fleshy portion of either side of the face. Called also bucca.

cleft c., congenital fissure of the cheek.

cheil(o)- word element [Gr.], *lip.*

cheilectropion (ki″lek-tro′pe-on) eversion of the lip.

cheilitis (ki-li′tis) inflammation of the lips.

actinic c., c. actin′ica, involvement of the lips after exposure to actinic rays, with pain and swelling, and development of a scaly crust on the vermilion border. (See also solar CHEILITIS.)

solar c., involvement of the lips after exposure to solar radiation; it may be acute (actinic cheilitis), or chronic, with alteration of the epithelium and sometimes fissuring or ulceration.

cheilognathopalatoschisis (ki″lo-na″tho-pal″ah-tos′kĭ-sis) cleft of the lip, upper jaw, and hard and soft palates.

cheiloplasty (ki′lo-plas″te) surgical repair of a lip defect.

cheilorrhaphy (ki-lor′ah-fe) suture of the lip; surgical repair of a harelip.

cheilosis (ki-lo′sis) fissuring and dry scaling of the vermilion surface of the lips and angles of the mouth, a characteristic of riboflavin deficiency.

cheilotomy (ki-lot′o-me) incision of the lip.

cheir(o)- word element [Gr.], *hand.* See also words beginning *chir(o)-*.

cheiralgia (ki-ral′je-ah) pain in the hand.

cheirarthritis (ki″rar-thri′tis) inflammation of the joints of the hand and fingers.

cheirognostic (ki″rog-nos′tik) pertaining to or characterized by the ability to distinguish stimuli as originating on the right or left side of the body.

cheirokinesthesia (ki″ro-kin″es-the′ze-ah) subjective perception of movements of the hand, especially in writing.

cheiroplasty (ki′ro-plas″te) plastic surgery on the hand.

cheiropodalgia (ki″ro-po-dal′je-ah) pain in the hands and feet.

cheiropompholyx (ki″ro-pom′fo-liks) pompholyx.

cheirospasm (ki′ro-spazm) spasm of the muscles of the hand.

chelate (ke′lāt) to combine with a metal in complexes in which the metal is part of a ring; by extension, a chemical compound in which a metallic ion is sequestered and firmly bound into a ring within the chelating molecule. Chelates are used in chemotherapy of metal poisoning.

Chel-Iron (kēl′i-ern) trademark for preparations of ferrocholinate, an iron preparation used as a hematinic.

cheloid (ke′loid) keloid.

chem(o)- word element [Gr.], *chemical; chemistry.*

chemabrasion (kēm″ah-bra′shun) superficial destruction of the epidermis and the upper layer of the dermis by application of a cauterant to the skin; done to remove scars, tattoos, etc. (See also PLANING.)

chemexfoliation (kēm″eks-fo″le-a′shun) chemabrasion.

chemical (kem′ĭ-kal) 1. pertaining to chemistry. 2. a substance composed of chemical elements, or obtained by chemical processes.

cheminosis (kem″ĭ-no′sis) any disease due to chemical agents.

chemist (kem′ist) 1. an expert in chemistry. 2. (British) pharmacist.

chemistry (kem′is-tre) the science that treats of the elements and atomic relations of matter, and of the various compounds of the elements.

colloid c., chemistry dealing with the nature and composition of colloids.

inorganic c., the scientific study of compounds not containing carbon.

organic c., the scientific study of carbon-containing compounds.

chemoautotroph (ke″mo-aw′to-trōf) a chemoautotrophic organism.

chemoautotrophic (ke″mo-au″to-trof′ik) capable of synthesizing cell constituents from carbon dioxide by means of energy derived from inorganic reactions.

chemobiotic (ke″mo-bi-ot′ik) a compound of a chemotherapeutic agent and an antibiotic.

chemocautery (ke″mo-kaw′ter-e) cauterization by application of a caustic substance.

chemodectoma (ke″mo-dek-to′mah) any tumor of the chemoreceptor system, e.g., a carotid body tumor.

chemokinesis (ke″mo-ki-ne′sis) increased activity of an organism caused by a chemical substance.

chemoluminescence (ke″mo-loo″mĭ-nes′ens) luminescence produced by the direct transformation of chemical energy into light energy.

chemolysis (ke-mol′ĭ-sis) chemical decomposition. adj., **chemolyt′ic.**

chemomorphosis (ke″mo-mor-fo′sis) change of form due to chemical action.

chemonucleolysis (ke″mo-nu″kle-ol′ĭ-sis) dissolution of a portion of the nucleus pulposus by injection of a chemolytic agent for treatment of a herniated intervertebral disk.

chemopallidectomy (ke″mo-pal″ĭ-dek′to-me) destruction of tissue of the globus pallidus by a chemical agent.

chemoprophylaxis (ke″mo-pro″fĭ-lak′sis) prevention of disease by chemical means.

chemopsychiatry (ke″mo-si-ki′ah-tre) the treatment of mental and emotional disorders by the use of drugs.

chemoreceptor (ke″mo-re-sep′tor) any of the special cells or organs adapted for excitation by chemical substances and located outside the central nervous system. There are chemoreceptors in the large arteries of the thorax and the neck; these are called carotid and aortic bodies. These receptors are responsive to changes in the oxygen, carbon dioxide, and hydrogen ion concentration in the blood. When oxygen concentration falls below normal in the arterial blood, the chemoreceptors send impulses to stimulate the respiratory center so that there will be an increase in alveolar ventilation, and consequently, an increase in the intake of oxygen by the lungs.

Other chemoreceptors are the taste buds, which are sensitive to chemicals in the mouth, and the olfactory cells of the nose, which detect certain chemicals in the air.

chemosensitive (ke″mo-sen′sĭ-tiv) sensitive to changes in chemical composition.

chemosensory (ke″mo-sen′so-re) relating to the perception of chemical substances, as in odor detection.

chemoserotherapy (ke″mo-se″ro-ther′ah-pe) treatment of infection by means of drugs and serum.

chemosis (ke-mo′sis) edema of the conjunctiva of the eye.

chemosterilant (ke″mo-ster′ĭ-lant) a chemical compound that upon ingestion causes sterility of an organism.

chemosurgery (ke″mo-ser′jer-e) the destruction of tissue by chemical agents for therapeutic purposes; originally applied to chemical fixation of malignant, gangrenous, or infected tissue, with use of frozen sections to facilitate systematic microscopic control of its excision.

chemosynthesis (ke″mo-sin′thĕ-sis) the building up of chemical compounds under the influence of chemical stimulation, specifically the formation of carbohydrates from carbon dioxide and water as a result of energy derived from chemical reactions. adj., **chemosynthet′ic.**

chemotaxis (ke″mo-tak′sis) taxis in response to the influence of chemical stimulation. adj., **chemotac′tic.**

leukocyte c., the response of leukocytes to products formed in immunologic reactions, wherein leukocytes are attracted to and accumulate at the site of the reaction; a part of the inflammatory response. (See also INFLAMMATION.)

chemotherapy (ke″mo-ther′ah-pe) the treatment of illness by chemical means; that is, by medication. adj., **chemotherapeu′tic.** The term was first applied to the treatment of infectious diseases, but it now is used to include treatment of mental illness and cancer with drugs.

chemotic (ke-mot′ik) 1. pertaining to or affected with chemosis. 2. an agent tha increases lymph production in the ocular conjunctiva.

chemotropism (ke-mot′ro-pizm) tropism in response to the influence of chemical stimulation.

cherry-red spot the choroid appearing as a red circular area surrounded by gray-white retina, as viewed through the fovea centralis in Tay-Sachs disease. Called also Tay's spot.

cherubism (cher′oo-bizm) hereditary and progressive bilateral swelling at the angle of the mandible, sometimes involving the entire jaw, imparting a cherubic look to the face, in some cases enhanced by upturning of the eyes.

chest (chest) the thorax; the part of the body enclosed by the ribs and sternum, especially its anterior aspect.

flail c., one whose wall moves paradoxically with respiration, owing to multiple fractures of the ribs (see also FLAIL CHEST).

funnel c., depression of the sternum and rib cartilage; PECTUS EXCAVATUM.

pigeon c., prominence of the sternum and rib cartilage; PECTUS CARINATUM.

c. tube, a tube inserted into the thoracic cavity for the purpose of removing air or fluid, or both. In some cases more than one tube is inserted so that both fluid and air can be removed. Chest tubes are attached to a closed drainage system so that normal pressures within the alveoli and the pleural cavity can be restored. These pressures are essential to adequate expansion and deflation of the lung.

Chest tubes are indicated when the normally airtight pleural space has been penetrated through surgery or trauma, when a defect in the alveoli allows air to enter the intrapleural space, and when there is an accumulation of fluid, as from PLEURAL EFFUSION.

The effect of excessive amounts of air and fluid within the pleural space is collapse of the lung and the danger of MEDIASTINAL SHIFT.

PATIENT CARE. It is important that those responsible for the personal care of a patient who has chest tubes inserted understand the basic mechanics of lung inflation and deflation (see MECHANICS OF INFLATION and DEFLATION, under LUNG), and the purpose of the tubes and their location in each patient. In some cases one tube is inserted higher in the thorax (usually in the 2nd intercostal space) to remove air, and a second tube is placed lower (in the 8th or 9th intercostal space) to drain off fluids.

Chest tubes may be connected to a variety of closed drainage systems: a water-seal drainage system with one, two, or three bottles; and a Pleur-evac, a self-contained system. Whatever the type, the purpose of the system is to allow for drainage from the pleural cavity to the outside and at the same time prevent the entry of atmospheric air into the pleural cavity.

Precautions that must be taken in the maintenance of the drainage system are:

1. The bottles and collection apparatus of the system must be kept below the level of the chest to prevent backflow.

2. The lumens of the tubes must be kept open to allow for drainage. If they are obstructed there will be no fluctuation of the fluid level in the glass tube that is connected to the chest tube at one end and kept under water in the bottle at the other end. In the Pleur-evac, the liquid in the chamber should rise on the right side and fall on the left side. If there is evidence that the system is not working properly, this must be attended to immediately. Occlusion of the tubes can lead to a buildup of air and fluids in the pleural cavity and creation of a tension PNEUMOTHORAX.

3. The system must be a *closed* system. There can be no leaks around connections, and the lower end of the glass tube must remain under water in the bottle.

The amount, color, and consistency of the fluid drainage should be checked at least once each hour for the first 24 hours after surgery. The chest tubes should be milked and stripped every one to two hours to assure patency and adequate drainage. The amount of air being removed is indicated by occasional bubbling in the water-seal chamber. Excessive bubbling may indicate air leaks in the tubing.

An important aspect of patient care is proper positioning to maintain adequate drainage. The positions allowed and the amount of mobility permitted will depend on the patient's surgical diagnosis, the placement of the tube(s), and preference of the attending physician. Frequent turning, coughing, and deep breathing are instituted on a regular basis to avoid serious pulmonary complications. An exception to the rule of turning is the pneumonectomy patient, who is placed in high Fowler's position and not turned for at least 24 hours after surgery. Chest physical therapy and intermittent positive pressure breathing (IPPB) treatments usually are ordered for all patients with chest tubes. Some patients may require a VENTILATOR during the immediate postoperative period.

The patient is observed for signs of respiratory distress and a buildup of air and fluid within the pleural cavity. Early correction of this condition can prevent mediastinal shift.

Removal of chest tubes is done by the physician. The wound is promptly sealed with a sterile petroleum jelly dressing to occlude the opening and prevent entry of air into the pleural space.

Cheyne-Stokes respiration (chān′ stōks) breathing characterized by rhythmic waxing and waning of the depth of respiration; the patient breathes deeply for a short time and then breathes very slightly or stops breathing altogether. The pattern occurs over and over again every 45 seconds to 3 minutes. Periodic breathing of this type is caused by disease affecting the respiratory centers, usually heart failure or brain damage.

chiasm (ki′azm) a decussation or X-shaped crossing.

optic c., a structure in the forebrain formed by the decussation of fibers of the optic nerve from each half of each retina.

chiasma (ki-az′mah) chiasm; in genetics, the points at which members of a chromosome pair are in contact during the prophase of meiosis and because of which recombination, or crossing over, occurs on separation.

c. formation, the process by which a chiasma is formed; it is the cytologic basis of genetic recombination, or crossing over.

chickenpox (chik′en-poks) an acute, highly contagious, viral disease, with mild constitutional symptoms and a maculopapular vesicular skin eruption; called also varicella. It is a common childhood disease, and is rarely severe, but in infants and adults it may be accompanied by severe symptoms. Although there is no preventive inoculation for chickenpox, one attack usually gives immunity.

The varicella virus is usually spread either by contact with blisters, or by droplet infection. The incubation period is 2 to 3 weeks. The period of contagion lasts about 2 weeks, beginning 2 days before the rash appears. The same virus that causes chickenpox also causes HERPES ZOSTER (shingles); the differences in the two diseases probably reflect differences in the response to the virus.

SYMPTOMS. Chickenpox may begin with a slight fever, headache, backache, and loss of appetite. At the same time, or a day or two later, small red spots appear, usually on the back and chest first. Within a few hours the spots enlarge and a vesicle filled with a clear fluid appears in the center of each spot, surrounded by an area of reddened skin. After a day or two, the fluid turns yellow and a crust or scab forms. This crust peels off in from 5 to 20 days. During this period the patient experiences severe itching.

The vesicles do not appear all at once, but in crops, the number of crops depending on the severity of the case. Usually the eruptions are concentrated on the back and chest, with only a few appearing on the arms, legs, and face, but in severe cases they may cover almost all of the body.

TREATMENT. Most cases of chickenpox are mild and require no special treatment except rest in bed and forcing fluids during the fever stage. For severe itching, emollient baths, calamine lotion, or other applications offer some relief. Since scratching the scabs may result in permanent scars and opens the way for other infections, the child's fingernails should be cut short and his hands washed often. Petrolatum applied to the sores reduces itching, keeps the scabs soft, and reduces the possibility of scarring. The clothes and bedding should be kept fresh and clean.

The child should be kept in bed during the period of acute illness and isolated during the period of communicability, or until about 12 days after the first appearance of the blisters. Isolation should continue until the last vesicle has dried, which may be as long as 20 days after the rash first appears.

chigger (chig′er) the six-legged red larva of mites of the family Trombiculidae (e.g., *Eutrombicula alfreddugèsi, E. splendens, Trombicula autumnalis*), which attach to their host's skin, and whose bite produces a wheal, usually with intense itching and severe dermatitis. Some species are vectors of the rickettsiae of scrub typhus. Called also harvest mite and red bug.

chigoe (chig′o) the sand flea, *Tunga penetrans,* of tropical and subtropical America and Africa. The pregnant female flea burrows into the skin of the feet, legs, or other part of the body, causing intense irritation and resulting in ulceration, sometimes leading to spontaneous amputation of a digit, if untreated.

chilblain (chil′blān) one of the mildest forms of cold injury, characterized by recurrent localized itching, swelling, painful erythema, and sometimes blistering and ulceration, caused by exposure to cold and dampness. It occurs chiefly on the fingers, toes, ears, and face, but may involve other areas of the body. Called also pernio. The basic cause of chilblain is sensitivity to cold, sometimes resulting from circulatory disturbances, which may be corrected in part by exercise and proper diet; severe cases require medical attention. Extreme heat or cold applications should not be applied directly to chilblains. This condition should not be confused with FROSTBITE, another type of skin damage caused by exposure to cold.

child (chīld) the human young, from infancy to puberty.

c. abuse, the nonaccidental use of physical force or the nonaccidental act of omission by a parent or other custodian responsible for the care of a child. Cases of child abuse account for at least 750 deaths annually in the United States. Many thousand more children are traumatized physically or psychologically by their parents or guardians. Examples of physical battering range from burns or exposure to extreme cold to beating, poisoning, strangulation, and withholding food and water. Psychological abuse is limited only by the imagination of the abuser.

Battering parents come from all socioeconomic groups and are usually found to have been battered children themselves. They typically engage in role reversal with their children and look to the child for protection and loving response while at the same time denying the child satisfaction of his own needs.

In recent years there has been formed a self-help group of former abusers similar to Alcoholics Anonymous. The organization is called Parents Anonymous and its purpose is to provide individual and group therapy, homemaker services, and a telephone crisis line that parents can use when they feel the need for help. The National Parent Chapter is located in Redondo Beach, California.

Members of the health care team should be alert for signs of child abuse and aware of the proper procedure for reporting suspected cases to local authorities.

childbed (chīld-bed) the puerperal state or period.

c. fever, puerperal fever.

childbirth (chīld′berth) the act or process of giving birth to a child (see also LABOR).

natural c., a term used to describe an approach to labor and delivery in which the parents are prepared for the event so that the mother is awake and cooperative and the father is able to assume an active and supportive role during the birth of their child (see also NATURAL CHILDBIRTH).

chill (chil) a sensation of cold, with convulsive shaking of the body. A true chill, or rigor, results from an increase in chemical activity within the body and usually ushers in a considerable rise in body temperature. The pallor and coldness of a chill, and the goose flesh that often accompanies it, are caused by constriction of the peripheral blood vessels. Chills are symptomatic of a wide variety of diseases. They usually do not accompany well localized infections.

PATIENT CARE. During a chill sufficient heat should be applied to maintain normal body temperature. Since the patient will most likely begin to have a sharp rise in body temperature immediately after or during the chill, it is best to use only a light blanket and several hot water bottles of moderate temperature to alleviate the sensation of cold. In addition to this the patient's temperature should be taken every 30 minutes until it is stabilized or further orders are obtained from the physician.

Chilomastix (ki″lo-mas′tiks) a genus of parasitic protozoa found in the intestines of vertebrates.

C. mesnil′i, a very common, widely distributed species found as a commensal in the human cecum and colon.

Chilopoda (ki-lop′o-dah) a class of the phylum Arthropoda embracing the centipedes.

chimera (ki-me′rah) an organism whose body contains different cell populations derived from different zygotes of the same or different species, occurring spontaneously or produced artificially.

heterologous c., one in which the foreign cells are derived from an organism of a different species.

homologous c., one in which the foreign cells are derived from an organism of the same species, but of a different genotype.

isologous c., one in which the foreign cells are derived from a different organism having the identical genotype, as from an identical twin.

radiation c., an organism with immunologic characteristics of host and donor after a bone marrow graft from an antigenically different donor, the host having first been subjected to irradiation to inhibit his immune response.

chimerism (ki′mer-izm) the state of being a chimera; the presence in an individual of cells of different origin.

chin (chin) the anterior prominence of the lower jaw; the mentum.

Chinese restaurant syndrome transient arterial dilatation due to ingestion of monosodium glutamate, which is used liberally in seasoning Chinese food, marked by throbbing head, light-headedness, tightness of the jaw, neck, and shoulders, and backache.

chionablepsia (ki″o-nah-blep′se-ah) snow blindness.

chir(o)- word element [Gr.], *hand.* See also words beginning *cheir(o)-.*

chiropodist (ki-rop′ŏ-dist) former name for podiatrist.

chiropractic (ki″ro-prak′tik) a system of treating disease by manipulation of the vertebral column. Chiropractic is based on the theory that most diseases are caused by pressure on the nerves because of faulty alignment of the bones, especially the vertebrae, and that the nerves are thus prevented from transmitting to various organs of the body the neural impulses for proper functioning. Medical science has never found a scientific basis for this theory.

Acting on this theory, the chiropractor manipulates various parts of the spine in treating the complaint. If the patient is suffering from a displaced vertebra, the manipulation may bring relief. If he has some other disorder or disease, however, manipulation will have little if any effect.

Chiropractors are licensed to practice in 44 states and the District of Columbia. They are not physicians and hence are forbidden by law to dispense prescription medicines.

chiropractor (ki″ro-prak′tor) a practitioner in chiropractic.

chirurgery (ki-rer′jer-e) surgery.

chitin (ki′tin) a horny polysaccharide, the principal constituent of shells of arthropods and shards of beetles, and found in certain fungi.

chlamydemia (klah-mĭ-de′me-ah) the presence of chlamydiae in the blood.

Chlamydia (klah-mid′e-ah) a genus of the family Chlamydiaceae, occurring as two species, both pathogenic for man.

C. psitta′ci, a species, strains of which cause psittacosis, ornithosis, and a variety of diseases in animals.

C. tracho′matis, a species, various strains of which cause trachoma, inclusion conjunctivitis, urethritis, bronchopneumonia of laboratory mice, proctitis, and lymphogranuloma venereum.

chlamydia (klah-mid′e-ah), pl. *chlamyd′iae.* any member of the genus *Chlamydia.*

Chlamydiaceae (klah-mid″e-a′se-e) a family of bacteria of the order Chlamydiales, containing a single genus, *Chlamydia.*

Chlamydiales (klah-mid′e-al-ēz) an order of coccoid, gram-negative, parasitic microorganisms that multiply only within the cytoplasm of vertebrate host cells by a unique development cycle.

chlamydiosis (klah-mid″e-o′sis) any infection or disease caused by *Chlamydia.*

chlamydospore (klam′ĭ-do-spōr″) a thick-walled intercalary or terminal asexual spore formed by the rounding-up of a cell; it is not shed.

chloasma (klo-az′mah) hyperpigmentation in circumscribed areas of the skin; called also melasma.

c. gravida′rum, melasma gravidarum.

c. hepat′icum, discoloration of the skin allegedly due to disorder of the liver.

c. uteri′num, melasma gravidarum.

chlophedianol (klo″fĕ-di′ah-nol) an antitussive agent, used as the hydrochloride salt.

chloracne (klōr-ak′ne) an acneiform eruption, caused by exposure to chlorine compounds.

chloral (klor′al) 1. an oily liquid with a pungent, irritating odor, prepared by the mutual action of alcohol and chlorine; used in the manufacture of chloral hydrate and DDT. 2. chloral hydrate.

c. betaine, an adduct formed by the reaction of chloral hydrate with betaine; used as a sedative.

c. hydrate, a hypnotic and sedative with mild action as a pain reliever but used most commonly to induce sleep. It is given when barbiturates are not desirable, as in patients who have poor kidney function and who might have difficulty excreting barbiturates, or in the elderly, who react poorly to barbiturates. It is also used for patients undergoing withdrawal from alcohol, morphine, or barbiturates, and in cases of delirium tremens. Overdoses can be extremely poisonous.

Chloral hydrate is available in liquid and in capsule form. It may be habit forming. It should not be given with alcohol.

chloralism (klor′al-izm) a morbid condition due to excessive use of chloral.

chlorambucil (klor-am′bu-sil) a nitrogen mustard derivative used as an antineoplastic agent.

chloramphenicol (klor″am-fen′ĭ-kol) a broad-spectrum antibiotic with specific therapeutic activity against rickettsiae and many different bacteria. Side effects include serious, even fatal, blood dyscrasias in certain patients. Frequent blood tests are recommended during therapy.

chlorate (klor′āt) a salt of chloric acid.

chlorbutol (klor′bu-tol) chlorobutanol.

chlorcyclizine (klor-si′klĭ-zēn) an antihistamine, used as the hydrochloride salt.

chlordane (klor′dān) a poisonous substance of the chlorinated hydrocarbon group, used as an insecticide.

chlordantoin (klor-dan′to-in) a topical antifungal agent.

chlordiazepoxide (klor″di-a″ze-pok′sīd) a minor tranquilizer.

chlorellin (klŏ-rel′in) a bacteriostatic substance derived from the fresh-water algae *Chlorella.*

chloremia (klo-re′me-ah) hyperchloremia.

Chloretone (klor′ĕ-tōn) trademark for a preparation of chlorobutanol, an antibacterial preservative for solutions and dental analgesic.

chlorhexidene (klor-heks′ĭ-dēn) an anti-infective, used as the hydrochloride salt.

chlorhydria (klor-hi′dre-ah) an excess of hydrochloric acid in the stomach.

chloride (klor′īd) a salt of hydrochloric acid; any binary compound of chlorine in which the latter carries a negative charge of electricity.

ferric c., $FeCl_3$, used as a reagent and topically as an astringent and antiseptic.

chloridimetry (klor″ĭ-dim′ĕ-tre) measurement of the chloride content of a fluid.

chloriduria (klor″ĭ-du′re-ah) an excess of chlorides in the urine.

chlorinated (klor′ĭ-nāt″ed) charged with chlorine.

chlorination (klor″ĭ-na′shun) the addition of chlorine to water or sewage to kill germs. Liquid chlorine has been found to be the most effective water disinfectant, and is almost invariably used in the United States for the purification of both public water supplies and swimming pools. This addition of chlorine is harmless, since enough chlorine to affect the health of those using the chlorinated water would also make the water too unpalatable to drink.

chlorine (klor'ēn) a gaseous chemical element, atomic number 17, atomic weight 35.453, symbol Cl. (See table of ELEMENTS.) It is a disinfectant, decolorizer, and irritant poison. It is used for disinfecting, fumigating, and bleaching, either in an aqueous solution or in the form of chlorinated lime.

chlorisondamine (klor″i-son'dah-mēn) a ganglionic blocking agent used as an antihypertensive agent.

chlorite (klor'īt) a salt of chlorous acid; disinfectant and bleaching agent.

chlormadinone (klor-mah'dĭ-nōn) a progestin, used in combination with an estrogen as a contraceptive.

chlormerodrin (klor-mer'o-drin) a mercurial diuretic.

chlormezanone (klor-mez'ah-nōn) a muscle relaxant and tranquilizer.

chlorobutanol (klor″o-bu'tah-nol) an antibacterial preservative for solutions and dental analgesic.

chloroform (klor″o-form) a colorless, mobile liquid with an ethereal odor and sweet taste, used as a solvent; once used widely as an inhalation anesthetic and analgesic, and as an antitussive, carminative, and counterirritant.

chlorolabe (klor'o-lāb) the pigment in retinal cones that is more sensitive to the green portion of the spectrum than are the other pigments (cyanolabe and erythrolabe).

chloroleukemia (klor″o-lu-ke'me-ah) myelogenous leukemia in which no specific tumor masses are observed at autopsy, but the body organs and fluids show a definite green color.

chlorolymphosarcoma, chloroma (klor″o-lim″fo-sar-ko'mah; klŏ-ro'mah) a malignant, green-colored tumor arising from myeloid tissue, associated with myelogenous leukemia, and occurring anywhere in the body.

Chloromycetin (klor″o-mi-se'tin) trademark for preparations of chloramphenicol, a broad-spectrum antibiotic.

chloromyeloma (klor″o-mi″ĕ-lo'mah) chloroma with multiple growths in bone marrow.

chloropexia (klor″o-pek″se-ah) the fixation of chlorine in body tissues.

chlorophane (klor'o-fān) a green-yellow pigment from the retina.

chlorophenol (klor″o-fe'nol) a topical antiseptic prepared by the action of chlorine on phenol.

chlorophenothane (klor″o-fe'no-thān) DDT; a once widely used insecticide, now used chiefly as a pediculicide.

chlorophyll (klor'o-fil) the green coloring matter of plants by which photosynthesis is accomplished.

chlorophyllin (klor'o-fil″in) any of the water-soluble salts obtained by alkaline hydrolysis of chlorophyll with replacement of the methyl and phytyl ester groups by sodium or potassium.

chloroplast (klor'o-plast) the photosynthetic unit of a plant cell, containing all the chlorophyll.

chloroprivic (klor″o-pri'vik) deprived of chlorides; due to loss of chlorides.

chloroprocaine (klor″o-pro'kān) a local anesthetic, used as the hydrochloride salt.

chloropsia (klŏ-rop'se-ah) a defect of vision in which objects appear to have a greenish tinge.

chloroquine (klor'o-kwin) an antimalarial and lupus erythematosus suppressant.

chlorosis (klŏ-ro'sis) a disorder, generally of pubescent females, characterized by greenish yellow discoloration of the skin and hypochromic erythrocytes; believed to be related to iron deficiency. adj., **chlorot'ic.**

chlorothen (klor'o-then) a pyridine derivative used as an antihistamine in the form of the chloride salt.

chlorothiazide (klor″o-thi'ah-zīd) a diuretic drug that also has an antihypertensive effect. It is used in treatment of the edema of congestive heart failure, liver disease, etc., and of hypertension. Possible side effects include potassium depletion and other electrolyte imbalances; bone marrow depression with a lowering of the platelet and leukocyte counts, agranulocytosis, and aplastic anemia are rare side reactions.

chlorothymol (klor″o-thi'mol) a topical antibacterial.

chlorotrianisene (klor″o-tri-an'ĭ-sēn) a synthetic estrogenic compound used especially in relieving menopausal symptoms.

chlorpheniramine (klor″fen-ir'ah-mēn) a pyridine derivative used as an antihistamine in the form of the maleate salt.

chlorphenoxamine (klor″fen-ok'sah-mēn) an agent used to reduce muscular rigidity in parkinsonism.

chlorpromazine (klor-pro'mah-zēn) a phenothiazine used as a major tranquilizer in rectal suppositories; the hydrochloride salt is used orally, intramuscularly, and intravenously. Side effects include drowsiness and slight hypotension. In prolonged therapy the patient should be observed for jaundice.

chlorpropamide (klor-pro'pah-mīd) an oral hypoglycemic drug useful in the treatment of diabetes mellitus in the adult whose condition is stabilized. The drug is contraindicated in patients with impairment of renal, thyroid, or hepatic function. Dosage is individually adjusted.

chlorprophenpyridamine (klor″pro-fen-pi-rid'-ah-mēn) chlorpheniramine.

chlorprothixene (klor″pro-thiks'ēn) a major tranquilizer.

chlorquinaldol (klor-kwin'al-dol) a keratoplastic, bactericidal, and fungicidal agent used topically in dermatoses.

chlortetracycline (klor″tet-rah-si'klēn) a broad-spectrum antibiotic obtained from *Streptomyces aureofaciens,* used in the form of the hydrochloride salt as an antibacterial (effective against both gram-positive and gram-negative bacteria) and as an antiprotozoal. It is available in capsules, in ampules for intravenous injection, and in ointment for topical use. Side effects include gastrointestinal disturbances, especially diarrhea.

chlorthalidone (klor″thal'ĭ-dōn) a diuretic and antihypertensive.

Chlor-Trimeton (klor-tri'mĕ-ton) trademark for preparations of chlorpheniramine, an antihistamine.

chloruresis (klor″u-re′sis) excretion of chlorides in the urine. adj., **chloruret′ic.**

chloruria (klor-u′re-ah) an excess of chlorides in the urine.

chlorzoxazone (klor-zok′sah-zōn) a skeletal muscle relaxant.

Ch.M. [L.] *Chirur′giae Ma′gister* (Master of Surgery).

choana (ko-a′nah), pl. *choa′nae* [L.] 1. any funnel-shaped cavity or infundibulum. 2. [pl.] the paired openings between the nasal cavity and the nasopharynx.

Choanotaenia (ko-a″no-te′ne-ah) a genus of tapeworms.

choke (chōk) 1. to interrupt respiration by obstruction or compression, or the condition resulting from such interruption. 2. [pl.] a burning sensation in the substernal region, with uncontrollable coughing, occurring during decompression.

chol(o)- word element [Gr.], *bile.*

cholagogue (ko′lah-gog) an agent that stimulates gallbladder contraction to promote bile flow. adj., **cholagog′ic.**

cholalic acid (ko-lal′ik) an acid formed in the liver from cholesterol that plays, with other bile acids, an important role in digestion; called also cholic acid.

Cholan-DH (ko′lan) trademark for preparations of dehydrocholic acid.

cholangiectasis (ko-lan″je-ek′tah-sis) dilatation of a bile duct.

cholangiocarcinoma (ko-lan″je-o-kar″sĭ-no-mah) adenocarcinoma of the bile ducts.

cholangioenterostomy (ko-lan″je-o-en″ter-os′to-me) surgical anastomosis of a bile duct to the intestine.

cholangiogastrostomy (ko-lan″je-o-gas-tros′to-me) surgical anastomosis of a bile duct to the stomach.

cholangiogram (ko-lan′je-o-gram″) the film obtained by cholangiography.

cholangiography (ko-lan″je-og′rah-fe) x-ray examination of the bile ducts, using a radiopaque dye as a contrast medium. In the intravenous method, the dye is administered intravenously and is excreted by the liver into the bile ducts. X-ray films are taken at 10-minute intervals as the dye is excreted via the cystic, hepatic, and common bile ducts into the intestinal tract. The excretion is usually completed within 4 hours. Preparation of the patient for the intravenous method requires restriction of fluids to concentrate the dye and also cleansing of the intestinal tract with castor oil and enemas so that fecal material and gas will not obscure the biliary tract.

Sometimes cholangiography is done after surgery of the gallbladder and biliary tract. In this method the radiopaque dye is injected directly into a tube that has been left in the biliay tract since the time of surgery. Films are taken immediately after the dye is injected. If no obstruction is present, the biliary structures fill readily and rapidly empty into the intestinal tract.

When it is necessary for the surgeon to locate gallstones or other obstructive conditions at the time that surgery is being performed, the dye may be injected directly into the bile ducts. Films are taken in the operating room, and obstructions not otherwise discernible can be located and corrected while the patient is still anesthetized. This procedure may also be performed in the x-ray department prior to the contemplated surgery to evaluate the cause of jaundice.

cholangiole (ko-lan′je-ōl) one of the fine terminal elements of the bile duct system. adj., **cholangi′olar.**

cholangiolitis (ko-lan″je-o-li′tis) inflammation of the cholangioles. adj., **cholangiolit′ic.**

cholangioma (ko-lan″je-o′mah) a tumor of the bile ducts.

cholangiostomy (ko″lan-je-os′to-me) fistulization of a bile duct.

cholangiotomy (ko″lan-je-ot′o-me) incision into a bile duct.

cholangitis (ko″lan-ji′tis) inflammation of a bile duct. adj., **cholangit′ic.**

cholanopoiesis (ko″lah-no-poi-e′sis) the synthesis of bile acids or of their conjugates and salts by the liver.

cholanopoietic (ko″lah-no-poi-et′ik) 1. promoting cholanopoiesis. 2. an agent that promotes cholanopoiesis.

cholate (ko′lāt) a salt or ester of cholic acid.

chole- word element [Gr.], *bile.*

cholebilirubin (ko″le-bil″ĭ-ru′bin) a pigment, differing from bilirubin, occurring in gallbladder bile; it gives a direct reaction to the VAN DEN BERGH TEST.

cholecalciferol (ko″le-kal-sif′er-ol) vitamin D_3, an oil-soluble antirachitic vitamin (see also VITAMIN D and table of the principal VITAMINS).

cholecystagogue (ko″le-sis′tah-gog) an agent that promotes evacuation of the gallbladder.

cholecystalgia (ko″le-sis-tal′je-ah) biliary colic.

cholecystectasia (ko″le-sis″tek-ta′ze-ah) distention of the gallbladder.

cholecystectomy (ko″le-sis-tek′to-me) excision of the gallbladder (see also surgery of the GALLBLADDER).

cholecystenterostomy (ko″le-sis″ten-ter-os′to-me) formation of a new communication between the gallbladder and the intestine.

cholecystic (ko″le-sis′tik) pertaining to the gallbladder.

cholecystitis (ko″le-sis-ti′tis) inflammation of the GALLBLADDER, acute or chronic.

ACUTE CHOLECYSTITIS. The most frequent cause of acute cholecystitis is GALLSTONES. Other causes include typhoid fever and a malignant tumor obstructing the biliary tract. The inflammation may be secondary to a systemic staphylococcal or streptococcal infection.

The symptoms of a mild inflammation may be very slight and include indigestion, moderate pain and tenderness in the upper right quadrant of the abdomen that is usually aggravated by deep breathing, malaise, and a low-grade fever. When gallstones or other disorders cause complete obstruction of the bile ducts, the symptoms are much more extreme. The pain becomes unbearable, the temperature may rise to 104° F. (40° C.), and there is nausea and vomiting.

Treatment of acute cholecystitis may entail either cholecystectomy or cholecystostomy. In some cases the surgery may be postponed until the attack subsides, the initial treatment consisting of administration of antibiotics and parenteral fluids and, after a period of no oral intake, administration of a special gallbladder diet.

CHRONIC CHOLECYSTITIS. Chronic cholecystitis progresses more slowly than acute cholecystitis, but it also is usually the result of gallstones or other conditions that lead to obstruction of the bile ducts and impaired gallbladder function. It is the most common disorder of the gallbladder.

The characteristic symptom of chronic cholecystitis is indigestion manifested by discomfort after eating, with flatulence and nausea. If the meal has been larger than usual, or high in fat content, the symptoms are more pronounced and there is eructation (belching) and regurgitation. There may also be vomiting and some pain in the upper right quadrant of the abdomen. It is not unusual for patients to suffer repeated episodes before seeking medical attention. Neglect of the situation may lead to permanent damage to the gallbladder and liver.

Diagnosis of cholecystitis is aided by the use of CHOLECYSTOGRAPHY, x-ray examination after administration of a radiopaque dye that is concentrated by the gallbladder.

The preferred treatment of chronic cholecystitis with gallstones is cholecystectomy. If surgery is contraindicated for some reason, then the symptoms may be controlled to some extent by low-fat diet, restriction of alcohol intake and spacing of meals so that large amounts of food are avoided and there is not a long interval between meals.

emphysematous c., that due to gas-producing organisms, marked by gas in the gallbladder lumen, often infiltrating into the gallbladder wall and surrounding tissues.

cholecystocolostomy (ko″le-sis″to-ko-los′to-me) surgical anastomosis of the gallbladder and the colon.

cholecystoduodenostomy (ko″le-sis″to-du″o-dĕ-nos′to-me) surgical anastomosis of the gallbladder and the duodenum.

cholecystogastrostomy (ko″le-sis″to-gas-tros′to-me) surgical anastomosis between the gallbladder and stomach.

cholecystogram (ko″le-sis′to-gram) a roentgenogram of the gallbladder.

cholecystography (ko″le-sis-tog′rah-fe) roentgenography of the gallbladder, using a radiopaque dye as contrast medium. adj., **cholecystograph′ic.** The purpose of the examination is to determine the ability of the gallbladder to fill, concentrate bile, and empty. The dye is administered in tablets the evening before the x-ray films are made.

Preparation of the patient requires enemas and a mild cathartic to cleanse the intestinal tract of fecal material and gas which can prevent adequate visualization of the gallbladder. The evening before the test the patient is given a fat-free meal. The tablets are administered after the meal, usually at 5-minute intervals until six tablets have been taken. The patient is then given nothing by mouth until the x-ray filming is completed.

In the morning films are made of the gallbladder, which should be filled with the dye. The patient is then given a fatty meal to stimulate emptying of the gallbladder and further x-ray films are made to evaluate the functioning of the gallbladder.

cholecystojejunostomy (ko″le-sis″to-je-ju-nos′to-me) surgical anastomosis of the gallbladder and jejunum.

cholecystokinin (ko″le-sis″to-ki′nin) a hormone secreted in the small intestine, which stimulates gallbladder contraction and secretion of pancreatic enzymes.

cholecystolithiasis (ko″le-sis″to-lĭ-thi′ah-sis) cholelithiasis.

cholecystopexy (ko″le-sis′to-pek″se) surgical suspension or fixation of the gallbladder.

cholecystorrhaphy (ko″le-sis-tor′ah-fe) suture or repair of the gallbladder.

cholecystostomy (ko″le-sis-tos′to-me) the creation of an opening into the gallbladder for drainage.

cholecystotomy (ko″le-sis-tot′o-me) incision of the gallbladder.

choledochal (kol′ĕ-dok″al) pertaining to the common bile duct.

choledochectomy (kol″ĕ-do-kek′to-me) excision of part of the common bile duct.

choledochitis (kol″ĕ-do-ki′tis) inflammation of the common bile duct.

choledocho- word element [Gr.], *common bile duct.*

choledochoduodenostomy (ko-led″ŏ-ko-du″o-dĕ-nos′to-me) surgical anastomosis of the common bile duct to the duodenum.

choledochoenterostomy (ko-led″ŏ-ko-en″ter-os′to-me) surgical anastomosis of the common bile duct to the intestine.

choledochogastrostomy (ko-led″ŏ-ko-gas-tros′to-me) surgical anastomosis of the common bile duct to the stomach.

choledochojejunostomy (ko-led″ŏ-ko-je-ju-nos′to-me) surgical anastomosis of the common bile duct to the jejunum.

choledocholithiasis (ko-led″ŏ-ko-lĭ-thi′ah-sis) calculi in the common bile duct.

choledocholithotomy (ko-led″ŏ-ko-lĭ-thot′o-me) incision into the common bile duct for removal of stone.

choledochoplasty (ko-led′ŏ-ko-plas″te) plastic repair of the common bile duct.

choledochorrhaphy (ko-led″o-kor′ah-fe) suture or repair of the common bile duct.

choledochostomy (ko″led-o-kos′to-me) creation of an opening into the common bile duct for drainage.

choledochotomy (ko″led-o-kot′o-me) incision into the common bile duct.

choledochus (ko-led′o-kus) the common bile duct.

Choledyl (kōl′ĕ-dil) trademark for a preparation of oxtriphylline, a bronchodilator.

choleic (ko-le′ik) pertaining to the bile.

cholelith (ko′lĕ-lith) gallstone.

cholelithiasis (ko″le-lĭ-thi′ah-sis) the presence or formation of GALLSTONES. adj., **cholelith′ic.**

cholelithotomy (ko″le-lĭ-thot′o-me) incision of the biliary tract for removal of gallstones.

cholelithotripsy, cholelithotrity (ko″le-lith′o-trip″se; ko″le-lĭ-thot′rĭ-te) crushing of a gallstone.

cholemesis (ko-lem′ĕ-sis) vomiting of bile.

cholemia (ko-le′me-ah) bile or bile pigment in the blood. adj., **chole′mic.**

choleperitoneum (ko″le-per″ĭ-to-ne′um) the presence of bile in the peritoneum.

cholepoiesis (ko″le-poi-e′sis) the formation of bile in the liver. adj., **cholepoiet′ic.**

choleprasin (ko″le-pra′sin) one of the bile pigments isolated from gallstones.

cholera (kol′er-ah) Asiatic cholera; an acute infectious enteritis endemic and epidemic in Asia, caused by *Vibrio cholerae,* marked by severe diarrhea and vomiting, with extreme fluid and electrolyte depletion, and by muscle cramps and prostration.

INCIDENCE. Immunization and modern methods of sanitation have all but eliminated cholera epidemics in the United States and Europe, but they are still a danger in many other parts of the world, e.g., in the tropics, and particularly in India. Travelers to cholera-ridden areas should protect themselves by vaccination, but this does not provide complete immunity. The local drinking water should be boiled and uncooked foods avoided. Food should be protected from flies, and fruits and vegetables peeled and the rinds discarded.

TRANSMISSION. *Vibrio cholerae,* a spiral microorganism, is carried in the cholera victim's feces, urine, and vomitus, and transmitted to others in contaminated water or food. Once it has reached the intestines, the intestinal lining becomes inflamed and the passages distended with a thin, watery fluid.

SYMPTOMS. Symptoms begin to appear at any time from a few hours to 5 days after contact; the usual incubation period is 3 days. When the disease is at its peak, diarrhea and vomiting occur with such frequency and abundance that dehydration results very rapidly. The skin is cyanotic and shriveled, the eyes are sunken and the voice is feeble. There may be painful muscular cramps throughout the body.

TREATMENT. Because alkaline substances are lost in the vomitus and feces, ACIDOSIS as well as dehydration must be combated. The fluids and electrolytes are replaced by intravenous infusions. Acid intoxication may require intravenous administration of sodium bicarbonate.

PATIENT CARE. Measures must be taken to maintain normal body temperature because of the loss of body heat, which often causes the body temperature to drop dangerously low. Warmth by blankets, hot-water bottles, and electric pads may be necessary. Antiemetic drugs are given to reduce vomiting.

Victims of cholera (and proved carriers of the disease) should be isolated. The vomitus, urine, and feces of the patient must be promptly and thoroughly disinfected. Eating utensils, dishes, and all other contaminated articles must be disinfected or burned. (See also COMMUNICABLE DISEASE and ISOLATION TECHNIQUE.)

Asiatic c., see CHOLERA.

c. infan′tum, a noncontagious diarrhea occurring in infants; formerly common in the summer months.

choleragen (kol′er-ah-jen) the exotoxin produced by the cholera vibrio, which is thought to stimulate electrolyte and water secretion into the small intestine and to block the absorption of sodium.

choleraic (kol″ĕ-ra′ik) of or pertaining to cholera, or of the nature of cholera.

choleresis (ko-ler′ĕ-sis) the secretion of bile by the liver.

choleretic (ko″ler-et′ik) 1. stimulating bile production by the liver. 2. an agent that stimulates bile production by the liver.

choleriform (ko-ler′ĭ-form) resembling cholera.

cholerine (kol′er-ēn) 1. the earliest stage of cholera. 2. a relatively mild form of cholera.

choleroid (kol′er-oid) resembling cholera.

cholestasis (ko″le-sta′sis) stoppage or suppression of bile flow, due to factors within (intrahepatic cholestasis) or outside the liver (extrahepatic cholestasis). adj., **cholestat′ic.**

cholesteatoma (ko″lĕ-ste″ah-to′mah) a cystlike mass with a lining of stratified squamous epithelium, filled with desquamating debris frequently including cholesterol, which occurs in the meninges, central nervous system, and bones of the skull, but most commonly in the middle ear and mastoid region.

cholesteatosis (ko″lĕ-ste″ah-to′sis) fatty degeneration due to cholesterol esters.

cholesteremia (ko-les″ter-e′me-ah) hypercholesterolemia.

cholesterin (ko-les′ter-in) cholesterol.

cholesterinemia (ko-les″ter-in-e′me-ah) hypercholesterolemia.

cholesterinuria (ko-les″ter-in-u′re-ah) cholesteroluria.

cholesterol (ko-les′ter-ol) 1. a monatomic alcohol, found in animal fats and oils, bile, blood, brain tissue, milk, egg yolk, myelin sheaths of nerve fibers, liver, kidneys, and adrenal glands. It is a precursor of all the steroid hormones. 2. a preparation of cholesterol used as a pharmaceutic aid.

Research has suggested the possibility that eating foods high in cholesterol may be a contributing factor in heart and circulatory disease, particularly in the formation of fatty deposits in the arteries (atherosclerosis). However, the reason why such deposits form is still unknown. Some investigators believe that the fatty deposits accumulate from an excess of fatty particles in the blood brought about by eating foods rich in cholesterol. Others reject this theory and claim that no relationship exists between the amount of cholesterol eaten and the amount of cholesterol found in the blood.

It is also thought that the saturated fats found in animal fat, which are low in linoleic acid, may contribute to the formation of cholesterol in the body. Experiments have indicated that unsaturated fats (called also polyunsaturates), which are high in linoleic acid, help to reduce the amount of cholesterol in the blood. These unsaturated fats are found in large quantities in vegetable oils such as corn oil.

The body's own normal production of cholesterol is essential to the functioning of certain systems, for example, the nervous system. The medical approach in controlling tendencies to atherosclerosis and high blood pressure is to keep cholesterol formation in the body at its lowest normal levels.

It seems likely that a relationship exists between tension and the cholesterol level of the blood. When a person is under stress, his cholesterol level tends to rise. It is also known that the obese usually have higher than normal levels of cholesterol in their blood, and that they are more subject to coronary occlusion ("heart attack") than are lean people. As a result, the American Heart Association has suggested that reducing the amount of food containing large amounts of cholesterol, and maintaining the weight within reasonable limits, are possible ways of preventing atherosclerosis and decreasing the risk of coronary occlusion.

Blood Cholesterol. A laboratory test for determination of the blood cholesterol level is often included in liver function studies because the liver plays an important role in the metabolism of cholesterol and an unusually high blood cholesterol may indicate liver disease. It also may be indicative of the metabolic rate since the cholesterol level tends to be low in hyperthyroidism and high in hypothyroidism. The normal ranges for blood cholesterol tests are: Cholesterol esters, from 95 to 200 mg. per 100 ml. of serum; total cholesterol, from 135 to 260 mg. per 100 ml. of serum. The patient must be in a fasting state for this test.

cholesterolemia (ko-les″ter-ol-e′me-ah) hypercholesterolemia.

cholesteroluria (ko-les″ter-ol-u′re-ah) the presence of cholesterol in the urine.

cholesterosis (ko-les″ter-o′sis) a condition in which cholesterol is deposited in tissues in abnormal amounts.

cholestyramine resin (ko″les-ti′rah-mēn) a synthetic, strongly basic anion-exchange resin in the chloride form which chelates bile salts in the intestine, thus preventing their reabsorption; used in the symptomatic relief of pruritus associated with bile stasis.

choletherapy (ko″le-ther′ah-pe) treatment by administration of bile salts.

choleuria (ko″le-u′re-ah) choluria.

cholic acid (ko′lik, kol′ik) an acid formed in the liver from cholesterol that plays, with other bile acids, an important role in digestion; called also cholalic acid.

choline (ko′lēn) a quaternary ammonium compound that is an essential component of the diet of mammals and is therefore sometimes included among the vitamins. It is derivable from many animal and some vegetable tissues. It prevents the deposition of fat in the liver and is required for the synthesis of acetylcholine, a compound concerned with the transmission of nerve impulses at the myoneural junction.

Synthetic preparations of choline derivatives are used as parasympathetic stimulants and act to increase the heart rate, contract smooth muscle tissue, contract the pupil of the eye, and increase secretions of most of the glands.

c. acetylase, c. acetyltransferase, an enzyme that brings about the synthesis of acetylcholine.

cholinergic (ko″lin-er′jik) 1. parasympathomimetic; activated or transmitted by acetylcholine; said of nerve fibers that liberate acetylcholine at a synapse when a nerve impulse passes, i.e., the parasympathetic fibers. 2. an agent that resembles acetylcholine or simulates its action.

c. receptors, receptor sites on effector organs which are innervated by cholinergic nerve fibers and which respond to the acetylcholine secreted by these fibers.

cholinesterase (ko″lin-es′ter-ās) an enzyme that splits acetylcholine into acetic acid and choline. Called also acetylcholinesterase. This enzyme is present throughout the body, but is particularly important at the myoneural junction, where the nerve fibers terminate and become embedded in muscle fibers. Acetylcholine, which is formed when a nerve impulse reaches a myoneural junction, acts as a stimulant to the muscle fibers, causing them to contract. Immediately after acetylcholine has sparked a contraction it must be removed so that the muscle fiber will repolarize, or recharge itself; otherwise, it would not be ready to contract the next time it is stimulated. Cholinesterase performs this service by splitting acetylcholine into its components, thus rendering it ineffective. The end products of the metabolism of acetylcholine are eventually resynthesized into acetylcholine, which can once again act as a stimulant.

The drugs neostigmine, physostigmine, and pyridostigmine combine chemically with cholinesterase to deactivate it. Some authorities believe that the muscular weakness of MYASTHENIA GRAVIS is due to excessive amounts of cholinesterase at the myoneural junction. They base this theory on the fact that the symptoms of this disorder respond to the administration of these drugs. The relief is only temporary and lasts no more than several hours in most cases.

cholinolytic (ko″lin-o-lit′ik) 1. blocking the action of acetylcholine, or of cholinergic agents. 2. an agent that blocks the action of acetylcholine in cholinergic areas, i.e., areas supplied by parasympathetic nerves, and voluntary muscles.

cholinomimetic (ko″lin-o-mi-met′ik) having an action similar to that of choline.

cholochrome (ko′lo-krōm) a bile pigment.

Cholografin (ko″lo-gra′fin) trademark for preparations of iodipamide, used in cholecystography.

cholohemothorax (ko″lo-he″mo-tho′raks) the presence of bile and blood in the thorax.

chololithiasis (ko″lo-lĭ-thi′ah-sis) cholelithiasis.

cholothorax (ko″lo-tho′raks) cholohemothorax.

choluria (ko-lu′re-ah) the presence of bile in the urine; discoloration of the urine with bile pigments. adj., **cholu′ric.**

chondodendron tomentosum extract (kon″do-den′dron to″men-to′sum) a curare derivative used as a strong skeletal muscle relaxant.

chondr(o)- word element [Gr.], *cartilage.*

chondral (kon′dral) pertaining to cartilage.

chondralgia (kon-dral′je-ah) pain in a cartilage.

chondrectomy (kon-drek′to-me) excision of a cartilage.

chondrification (kon″drĭ-fĭ-ka′shun) conversion into cartilage.

chondrin (kon′drin) a protein, resembling gelatin, from cartilage; considered to be a mixture of gelatin and mucin.

chondrio- word element [Gr.], *cartilage; granule.*

chondriome (kon′dre-ōm) the total mitochondrial content of a cell.

chondriosome (kon′dre-o-sōm″) mitochondrion.

chondritis (kon-dri′tis) inflammation of a cartilage.

chondroadenoma (kon″dro-ad″ĕ-no′mah) adenochondroma.

chondroangioma (kon″dro-an″je-o′mah) a benign mesenchymoma containing chondromatous and angiomatous elements.

chondroblast (kon′dro-blast) an immature cartilage-producing cell.

chondroblastoma (kon″dro-blas-to′mah) a benign

tumor arising from young chondroblasts in the epiphysis of a bone.

chondrocalcinosis (kon″dro-kal″sĭ-no′sis) 1. deposition of calcium in cartilage. 2. pseudogout.

chondroclast (kon′dro-klast) a giant cell believed to be concerned in absorption of cartilage.

chondrocostal (kon″dro-kos′tal) pertaining to the ribs and costal cartilages.

chondrocranium (kon″dro-kra′ne-um) the cartilaginous cranial structure of the embryo from the seventh week to the middle of the third month, when it is a unified cartilaginous mass without clear boundaries indicating the limits of future bones.

chondrocyte (kon′dro-sīt) a mature cartilage cell. adj., **chondrocyt′ic.**

chondrodermatitis (kon″dro-der″mah-ti′tis) an inflammatory process involving cartilage and skin; used almost exclusively to mean chondrodermatitis nodularis chronica helicis, a condition marked by a painful nodule on the helix of the ear.

chondrodynia (kon″dro-din′e-ah) pain in a cartilage.

chondrodysplasia (kon″dro-dis-pla′ze-ah) enchondromatosis.

chondrodystrophia, chondrodystrophy (kon″dro-dis-tro′fe-ah; kon″dro-dis′tro-fe) a disorder of cartilage formation.

chondroendothelioma (kon″dro-en″do-the″le-o′mah) an endothelioma containing cartilage tissue.

chondroepiphysitis (kon″dro-ep″ĭ-fiz-i′tis) inflammation of the epiphyseal cartilages.

chondrofibroma (kon″dro-fi-bro′mah) a fibroma with cartilaginous elements.

chondrogen (kon′dro-jen) a substance regarded as the basis of cartilage and of corneal tissue.

chondrogenesis (kon″dro-jen′ĕ-sis) formation of cartilage.

chondrogenic (kon″dro-jen′ik) giving rise to or forming cartilage.

chondroid (kon′droid) resembling cartilage.

chondroitic acid (kon″dro-it′ik) chondroitin-sulfuric acid.

chondroitin (kon-dro′ĭ-tin) a mucopolysaccharide, the sulfate ester of which is widespread in connective tissue, particularly cartilage, and in the cornea.

c.-sulfuric acid a compound of high molecular weight in skin and connective tissue and, combined with collagen, constituting 20 to 40 per cent of cartilage.

chondroitinuria (kon″dro-ĭ-tin-u′re-ah) the presence of chondroitin-sulfuric acid in the urine.

chondrolipoma (kon″dro-lĭ-po′mah) a tumor containing cartilaginous and fatty tissue.

chondroma (kon-dro′mah) a tumor or tumor-like growth of cartilage cells. It may remain in the interior or substance of a cartilage or bone (true chondroma, or enchondroma), or may develop on the surface of a cartilage and project under the periosteum of a bone (ecchondroma, or ecchondrosis).

chondromalacia (kon″dro-mah-la′she-ah) abnormal softening of cartilage.

chondromatosis (kon″dro-mah-to′sis) formation of multiple chondromas.

synovial c., a rare condition in which cartilage is formed in the synovial membrane of joints, tendon sheaths, or bursae, sometimes becoming detached and producing a number of loose bodies.

chondromere (kon′dro-mēr) a cartilaginous vertebra of the fetal vertebral column.

chondrometaplasia (kon″dro-met″ah-pla′ze-ah) a condition characterized by metaplastic activity of the chondroblasts.

chondromucin, chondromucoid (kon″dro-mu′sin; kon″dro-mu′koid) a compound of chondroitin-sulfuric acid and mucin forming the intercellular substance of cartilage.

chondromucoprotein (kon′dro-mu″ko-pro′te-in) the principal constituent of the ground substance of cartilage, a copolymer of a mucoprotein, chondroitin-4-sulfate (chondroitin sulfate A), and chondroitin-6-sulfate (chondroitin sulfate C).

chondromyoma (kon″dro-mi-o′mah) a benign tumor with myomatous and cartilaginous elements.

chondromyxoma (kon″dro-mik-so′mah) myxoma with cartilaginous elements.

chondromyxosarcoma (kon″dro-mik″so-sar-ko′mah) a sarcoma containing cartilaginous and mucous tissue.

chondro-osseous (kon″dro-os′e-us) composed of cartilage and bone.

chondro-osteodystrophy (kon″dro-os″te-o-dis′tro-fe) Morquio's disease.

chondropathy (kon-drop′ah-the) any disease of cartilage.

chondroplasia (kon″dro-pla′ze-ah) the formation of cartilage by specialized cells (chondrocytes).

chondroplast (kon′dro-plast) chondroblast.

chondroplasty (kon′dro-plas″te) plastic repair of cartilage.

chondroporosis (kon″dro-po-ro′sis) the formation of sinuses or spaces in cartilage.

chondroprotein (kon″dro-pro′te-in) any of a series of glycoproteins occurring in cartilage.

chondrosamine (kon-dro′sam-in) a galactosamine which results from hydrolysis of chondrosin.

chondrosarcoma (kon″dro-sar-ko′ma) a malignant tumor derived from cartilage cells or their precursors.

central c., one in the interior of a bone.

chondrosin (kon′dro-sin) a disaccharide, the most common aldohexuronic acid in nature occurring as a structural unit; obtained by hydrolysis of chondroitins and chondroitin sulfates.

chondrosis (kon-dro′sis) the formation of cartilage.

chondrosteoma (kon″dros-te-o′mah) osteochondroma.

chondrosternal (kon″dro-ster′nal) pertaining to the costal cartilages and sternum.

chondrosternoplasty (kon″dro-ster′no-plas″te) surgical correction of pectus excavatum (funnel chest).

chondrotomy (kon-drot′o-me) the dissection or the surgical divison of cartilage.

chondroxiphoid (kon″dro-zif′oid) pertaining to the xiphoid process.

chondrus (kon′drus) the dried, sun-bleached plant of the seaweed *Chondrus crispus;* used as a protective agent for the skin.

chord (kord) cord.

chorda (kor′dah), pl. *chor′dae* [L.] a cord or sinew. adj., **chor′dal.**

c. mag'na, Achilles tendon.

chor'dae tendin'eae, tendinous cords connecting the two atrioventricular valves to the appropriate papillary muscles in the heart ventricles.

c. tym'pani, a nerve originating from the facial nerve, distributed to the submandibular, sublingual, and lingual glands and the anterior two-thirds of the tongue; it is a parasympathetic and special senory nerve.

c. umbilica'lis, umbilical cord.

c. voca'lis, vocal cord.

Chordata (kor-da'tah) a phylum of the animal kingdom comprising all animals having a notochord during some developmental stage.

chordate (kor'dāt) 1. an animal of the Chordata. 2. having a notochord.

chordee (kor'de) downward deflection of the penis, due to a congenital anomaly (hypospadias) or to urethral infection.

chorditis (kor-di'tis) inflammation of vocal or spermatic cords.

chordoma (kor-do'mah) a malignant tumor arising from embryonic remains of the notochord.

chordotomy (kor-dot'o-me) surgical division of the anterolateral tracts of the spinal cord.

chorea (ko-re'ah) the ceaseless occurrence of rapid, jerky involuntary movements. adj., **chore'ic.**

acute c., Sydenham's chorea.

Bergeron's c., electric chorea of childhood (see also BERGERON'S CHOREA).

chronic c., Huntington's chorea.

Dubini's c., an acute fatal form of electric chorea (see also DUBINI'S CHOREA).

electric c., a variety with violent and sudden movements.

c. gravida'rum, Sydenham's chorea occurring in early pregnancy, with or without a previous history of rheumatic fever.

Henoch's c., chronic progressive electric chorea.

hereditary c., Huntington's c., a hereditary disease marked by chronic progressive chorea and mental deterioration (see also HUNTINGTON'S CHOREA).

Sydenham's c., an acute, usually self-limited disorder, chiefly occurring between the ages of 5 and 15, or during pregnancy, closely linked with rheumatic fever, and marked by involuntary movements that gradually become severe, affecting all motor activities (see also SYDENHAM'S CHOREA).

choreiform (ko-re'ĭ-form) resembling chorea.

choreoathetosis (ko″re-o-ath″ĕ-to'sis) a condition characterized by choreic and athetoid movements. adj., **choreoath'etoid.**

chorioadenoma (ko″re-o-ad″ĕ-no'mah) adenoma of the chorion.

c. destru'ens, a form of hydatidiform mole in which molar chorionic villi penetrate into the myometrium and/or parametrium or are transported to distant sites, most often the lungs.

chorioallantois (ko″re-o-ah-lan'to-is) an extraembryonic structure formed by union of the chorion and allantois, which by means of vessels in the associated mesoderm serves in gas exchange; in many mammals, it forms the placenta. adj., **chorioallanto'ic.**

chorioamnionitis (ko″re-o-am″ne-o-ni'tis) bacterial infection of the fetal membranes.

chorioangioma (ko″re-o-an″je-o'mah) an angioma of the chorion.

choriocapillaris (ko″re-o-kap″ĭ-la'ris) the capillary layer of the choroid.

choriocarcinoma (ko″re-o-kar″sĭ-no'mah) a malignant neoplasm of trophoblastic cells formed by abnormal proliferation of the placental epithelium, without production of chorionic villi.

choriocele (ko're-o-sēl″) protrusion of the chorion through an aperture.

chorioepithelioma (ko″re-o-ep″ĭ-the″le-o'mah) choriocarcinoma.

choriogenesis (ko″re-o-jen'ĕ-sis) the development of the chorion.

chorioid (ko're-oid) choroid.

chorioma (ko″re-o'mah) any trophoblastic proliferation, benign or malignant.

choriomeningitis (ko″re-o-men″in-ji'tis) cerebral meningitis with lymphocytic infiltration of the choroid plexus.

lymphocytic c., a form of viral meningitis, usually occurring in adults between the ages of 20 and 40, during the fall and winter months.

chorion (ko're-on) the outermost of the fetal membranes, composed of trophoblast lined with mesoderm; it develops villi, becomes vascularized by allantoic vessels, and forms the fetal part of the placenta.

c. frondo'sum, the part of the chorion covered by villi.

c. lae've, the smooth, membranous part of the chorion.

chorionic (ko″re-on'ik) pertaining to the chorion.

c. gonadotropin, a hormone with properties similar to those of luteinizing hormone; it is secreted in large amounts by the placenta during gestation. It stimulates the formation of interstitial cells in the testes of the fetus and causes the secretion of testosterone. It is found in substantial amounts in human pregnancy urine (see PREGNANCY TESTS). It is used in treatment of underdevelopment of the gonads.

chorioretinal (ko″re-o-ret'ĭ-nal) pertaining to the choroid and retina.

chorioretinitis (ko″re-o-ret″ĭ-ni'tis) inflammation of the choroid and retina.

chorioretinopathy (ko″re-o-ret″ĭ-nop'ah-the) a noninflammatory process involving both the choroid and retina.

chorista (ko-ris'tah) defective development due to, or marked by, displacement of the primordium.

choristoma (ko″ris-to'mah) a mass of histologically normal tissue in an abnormal location.

choroid (ko'roid) the middle, vascular coat of the eye, between the sclera and the retina. adj., **choroid'al.** It contains an abundant supply of blood vessels and a large amount of brown pigment which serves to reduce reflection or diffusion of light when it falls on the retina. Adequate nutrition of the eye is dependent upon blood vessels in the choroid.

c. plexus, vascular fringelike folds in the pia mater in the third, fourth, and lateral ventricles of the brain; concerned with formation of cerebrospinal fluid.

choroidea (ko-roi'de-ah) choroid.

choroideremia (ko-roi″der-e'me-ah) hereditary (X-linked) primary choroidal degeneration which, in males, eventually leads to blindness as degeneration of the retinal pigment epithelium progresses to complete atrophy; in females, it is nonprogressive and vision is usually normal.

choroiditis (ko″roi-di′tis) inflammation of the choroid.

choroidocyclitis (ko-roi″do-si-kli′tis) inflammation of the choroid and ciliary processes.

choroidoiritis (ko-roi″do-i-ri′tis) inflammation of the choroid and iris.

choroidoretinitis (ko-roi″do-ret″ĭ-ni′tis) inflammation of the choroid and retina.

Christian-Weber disease (kris′chan web′er) nodular nonsuppurative panniculitis.

Christmas disease (kris′mas) a hereditary hemorrhagic diathesis clinically similar to hemophilia A (classic hemophilia) but due to deficiency of clotting factor IX; called also hemophilia B.

chrom(o)- word element [Gr.], *color.*

chromaffin (kro-maf′in) taking up and staining strongly with chromium salts; said of certain cells occurring in the adrenal and coccygeal glands and the carotid bodies, along with the sympathetic nerves, and in various organs.

chromaffinoma (kro-maf″ĭ-no′mah) 1. any tumor containing chromaffin cells. 2. pheochromocytoma.

chromaffinopathy (kro-maf″ĭ-nop′ah-the) disease of the chromaffin system.

chromaphil (kro′mah-fil) chromaffin.

chromat(o)- word element [Gr.], *color; chromatin.*

chromate (kro′māt) any salt of chromic acid.

chromatelopsia (kro″mat-el-op′se-ah) imperfect perception of colors.

chromatic (kro-mat′ik) 1. pertaining to color; stainable with dyes. 2. pertaining to chromatin.

chromatid (kro′mah-tid) either of two parallel filaments joined at the centromere which make up a chromosome, and which divide in cell division, each going to a different pole of the dividing cell and each becoming a chromosome of one of the two daughter cells.

chromatin (kro′mah-tin) the more readily stainable portion of the cell nucleus, composed of DNA attached to a protein base; it is the carrier of the genes.

sex c., Barr body; the persistent mass of the material of the inactivated X chromosome in cells of normal females.

chromatin-negative (kro′mah-tin-neg′ah-tiv) lacking sex chromatin; characteristic of the nuclei of cells in a normal male.

chromatin-positive (kro′mah-tin-poz′ĭ-tiv) containing sex chromatin; characteristic of the nuclei of cells in a normal female.

chromatism (kro′mah-tizm) 1. hallucinatory perception of color. 2. abnormal pigmentation.

chromatogenous (kro″mah-toj′ĕ-nus) producing color or coloring matter.

chromatogram (kro-mat′o-gram) the record produced by chromatography.

chromatograph (krom-mat′o-graf) 1. to analyze by chromatography. 2. the apparatus used in chromatography.

chromatography (kro″mah-tog′rah-fe) a technique for analysis of chemical substances. The term *chromatography* literally means color writing, and denotes a method by which the substance to be analyzed is poured into a vertical glass tube containing an adsorbent, the various components of the substance moving through the adsorbent at different rates of speed, according to their degree of attraction to it, and producing bands of color at different levels of the adsorption column. The term has been extended to include other methods utilizing the same principle, although no colors are produced in the column.

The mobile phase of chromatography refers to the passage of the substances through the adsorptive material. The stationary phase (or adsorbent) refers to the solid material that takes up the particles of the substance passing through it. Kaolin, alumina, silica, and activated charcoal have been used as adsorbing substances or stationary phases.

Classification of chromatographic techniques tends to be confusing because it may be based on the type of stationary phase, the nature of the adsorptive force, the nature of the mobile phase, or the method by which the mobile phase is introduced.

The technique is a valuable tool for the research biochemist and is readily adaptable to investigations conducted in the clinical laboratory. For example, chromatography is used to detect and identify in body fluids certain sugars and amino acids associated with inborn errors of metabolism.

adsorption c., the technique in which the adsorptive force is provided by molecules adhering to the surface of a solid that is packed in a column, spread as a thin film on a glass or plastic sheet, or as a coating inside a tube.

column c., the technique in which the various solutes of a solution are allowed to travel down a column, the individual components being adsorbed by the stationary phase. The most strongly adsorbed component will remain near the top of the column; the other components will pass to position farther and farther down the column according to their affinity for the adsorbent. If the individual components are naturally colored, they will form a series of colored bands or zones.

Column chromatography has been employed to separate vitamins, steroids, hormones, and alkaloids. Clinically, it is particularly useful in determining the amount of these substances in samples of body fluids.

filter paper c., paper chromatography.

gas c., that in which an inert gas is used to move the vapors of the material to be separated. The method has been applied in the clinical laboratory to separate and quantify steroids, barbiturates, and lipids.

gas-liquid c., that in which the substances to be separated are moved by an inert gas along a tube filled with a finely divided inert solid coated with a nonvolatile oil; each component migrates at a rate determined by its solubility in oil and its vapor pressure.

paper c., a form of chromatography in which a sheet of blotting paper, usually filter paper, is substituted for the adsorption column. After separation of the components as a consequence of their differential migratory velocities, they are stained to make the chromatogram visible. In the clinical laboratory paper chromatography is employed to detect and identify sugars and amino acids. Called also filter paper chromatography.

partition c., a form of separation of solutes utilizing the partition of the solutes between two liquid phases, namely the original solvent and the film of solvent on the adsorption column.

thin-layer c., chromatography through a thin layer of inert material, such as cellulose.

chromatokinesis (kro″mah-to-ki-ne′sis) movement of chromatin during the life and division of a cell.

chromatolysis (kro″mah-tol′ĭ-sis) 1. the solution and disintegration of the chromatin of cell nuclei. 2. disintegration of the Nissl bodies of a neuron as a result of injury, fatigue, or exhaustion.

chromatometer (kro″mah-tom′ĕ-ter) an instrument for measuring color or color perception.

chromatophil (kro-mat′o-fil) a cell or structure that stains easily. adj., **chromatophil′ic.**

chromatophore (kro-mat′o-fōr) any pigmentary cell or color-producing plastid.

chromatopsia (kro″mah-top′se-ah) perversion of color vision, in which objects are seen as abnormally colored.

chromatoptometer (kro″mah-top-tom′ĕ-ter) a device for measuring color perception.

chromatoptometry (kro″mah-top-tom′ĕ-tre) measurement of color perception.

chromaturia (kro″mah-tu′re-ah) abnormal coloration of the urine.

chromesthesia (kro″mes-the′ze-ah) association of imaginary color sensations with actual sensations of taste, hearing, or smell.

chromhidrosis (krōm″hĭ-dro′sis) secretion of colored sweat.

chromic acid (kro′mik) 1. a dibasic acid, H_2CrO_4; its salts are called chromates. 2. chromium trioxide.

chromicize (kro′mĭ-sīz) to treat with chromium.

chromidiosis (kro-mid″e-o′sis) outflow of chromatin and nuclear substance from the nucleus to the cytoplasm of a cell.

chromidium (kro-mid′e-um), pl. *chromid′ia.* a granule of extranuclear chromatin in the cytoplasm of a cell.

chromidrosis (kro″mĭ-dro′sis) chromhidrosis.

chromium (kro′me-um) a chemical element, atomic number 24, atomic weight 51.996, symbol Cr. (See table of ELEMENTS.)

c. trioxide, chromic acid, a powerful oxidizing agent and caustic; formerly used in solutions as an astringent, topical antiseptic, and corrosive.

chromoblast (kro′mo-blast) an embryonic cell that develops into a pigment cell.

chromoblastomycosis (kro″mo-blas″to-mi-ko′sis) chromomycosis.

chromocyte (kro′mo-sīt) any colored cell or pigmented corpuscle.

chromocystoscopy (kro″mo-sis-tos′ko-pe) cystoscopy of the ureteral orifices after oral administration of a dye which is excreted in the urine.

chromodacryorrhea (kro″mo-dak″re-o-re′ah) the shedding of bloody tears.

chromogen (kro′mo-jen) any substance giving origin to a coloring matter.

chromogenesis (kro″mo-jen′ĕ-sis) the formation of color or pigment.

chromogenic (kro″mo-jen′ik) producing color or pigment.

chromolipoid (kro″mo-lip′oid) lipochrome.

chromolysis (kro-mol′ĭ-sis) chromatolysis.

chromomycosis (kro″mo-mi-ko′sis) a chronic fungal infection of the skin, producing wartlike nodules or papillomas that may ulcerate. Called also chromoblastomycosis.

chromomere (kro′mo-mēr) 1. any of the beadlike granules occurring in series along a chromonema. 2. granulomere.

chromonema (kro″mo-ne′mah), pl. *chromone′mata* [Gr.] any of the coiled threads in anaphase and telophase chromosomes, later giving rise to the spireme. adj., **chromone′mal.**

chromopectic (kro″mo-pek′tik) pertaining to, characterized by, or promoting chromopexy.

chromopexy (kro′mo-pek″se) the fixation of pigment, especially by the liver in the formation of bilirubin.

chromophane (kro′mo-fān) a retinal pigment.

chromophil (kro′mo-fil) any easily stainable structure. adj., **chromophil′ic.**

chromophobe (kro′mo-fōb) any cell, structure, or tissue that does not stain readily; applied especially to the chromophobe cells of the anterior lobe of the pituitary gland.

chromophobia (kro″mo-fo′be-ah) the quality of staining poorly with dyes. adj., **chromopho′bic.**

chromophore (kro′mo-fōr) any chemical group whose presence gives a decided color to a compound and which unites with certain other groups (auxochromes) to form dyes; called also color radical.

chromophoric (kro″mo-fōr′ik) 1. bearing color. 2. pertaining to a chromophore.

chromophose (kro′mo-fōz) a subjective sensation of color.

chromoplasm (kro′mo-plazm) chromatin.

chromoplastid (kro″mo-plas′tid) any pigment-producing cell other than a chloroplast.

chromoprotein (kro″mo-pro′te-in) a colored conjugated protein, for example, the red hemoglobin of higher animals, which has a respiratory function and is closely related to the chlorophyll of higher plants.

chromopsia (kro-mop′se-ah) chromatopsia.

chromoscopy (kro-mos′ko-pe) the diagnosis of renal function by the color of urine following the administration of dyes.

gastric c., diagnosis of gastric function by the color of the gastric contents: a test for achylia gastrica.

chromosome (kro′mo-sōm) in animal cells, a structure in the nucleus, containing a linear thread of DEOXYRIBONUCLEIC ACID (DNA), which transmits genetic information and is associated with RIBONUCLEIC ACID and histones. adj., **chromoso′mal.** During cell division the material composing the chromosome is compactly coiled, making it visible with appropriate staining and permitting its movement in the cell with minimal entanglement. Each organism of a species is normally characterized by the same number of chromosomes in its somatic cells, 46 being the number normally present in man, including 22 pairs of autosomes and the two sex chromosomes (XX or XY), which determine the sex of the organism. (See also HEREDITY.) In bacterial genetics, a closed circle of double-stranded DNA which contains the genetic material of the cell and is attached to the cell membrane; the bulk of this material forms a compact bacterial nucleus.

CLASSIFICATION. Human chromosomes are difficult to classify into exactly 23 pairs; for practical purposes however, the so-called Denver Classification is frequently used. The chromosomes are classified on the basis of size and centromere position. Ideally, the 23 pairs of chromosomes are classified individually, but usually the best that can be done is to arrange them into seven groups, labeled A to G, in the order of decreasing length. The word karyotype is used to identify this classification (see illustration). The karyotyping of chromosomes is useful in determining whether or not they are normal in number and structure.

CHROMOSOMAL ERRORS. Abnormalities in the number and structure of chromosomes in the human cell recently have become the subject of much research and widespread interest. In 1959 it was shown that children with DOWN'S SYNDROME have an extra chromosome per cell. Since that time chromosomal aberrations in number or structure have been shown to be a significant cause of mental and physical defects.

Trisomy is the term used to describe the state of having an extra chromosome. If a chromosome is missing, the individual is said to be monosomic for that particular chromosome.

The causes of chromosomal errors are not completely understood. In some conditions such as Down's syndrome, late maternal age seems to be a factor. Other factors may include the predisposition of chromosomes to nondisjunction (failure to separate during meiosis), exposure to radiation, and viruses.

homologous c's, the chromosomes of a matching pair in the diploid complement that contain alleles of specific genes.

Ph^2 c., Philadelphia c., an abnormality of chromosome 21, characterized by shortening of its long arms, seen in the leukocytes of most patients with chronic leukemia.

ring c., a chromosome in which both ends have been lost (deletion) and the two broken ends have reunited to form a ring-shaped figure.

sex c's, the chromosomes responsible for determination of the sex of the individual that develops from a zygote, in mammals constituting an unequal pair, the X and the Y chromosome.

somatic c., autosome.

X c., the female sex chromosome, being carried by half the male gametes and all female gametes; female diploid cells have two X chromosomes.

Y c., the male sex chromosome, being carried by half the male gametes and none of the female gametes; male diploid cells have an X and a Y chromosome.

chromotoxic (kro″mo-tok′sik) destructive to hemoglobin, or due to destruction of hemoglobin.

chromotropic (kro″mo-trop′ik) turning to or attracting color or pigment.

chron(o)- word element [Gr.], *time.*

chronaxie, chronaxy (kro′nak-se) the minimum time at which an electric current must flow at a voltage twice the rheobase to cause a muscle to contract.

chronic (kron′ik) persisting for a long time; applied to a morbid state, designating one showing little change or extremely slow progression over a long period.

c. obstructive pulmonary disease (COPD), a functional category designating a chronic condition of persistent obstruction of bronchial air flow. Called also chronic obstructive lung disease (COLD) and diffuse obstructive lung disease (DOLD). ASTHMA, CHRONIC BRONCHITIS, and PULMONARY EMPHYSEMA are the diseases mainly associated with this condition; others are BRONCHIECTASIS, pulmonary TUBERCULOSIS, and SILICOSIS.

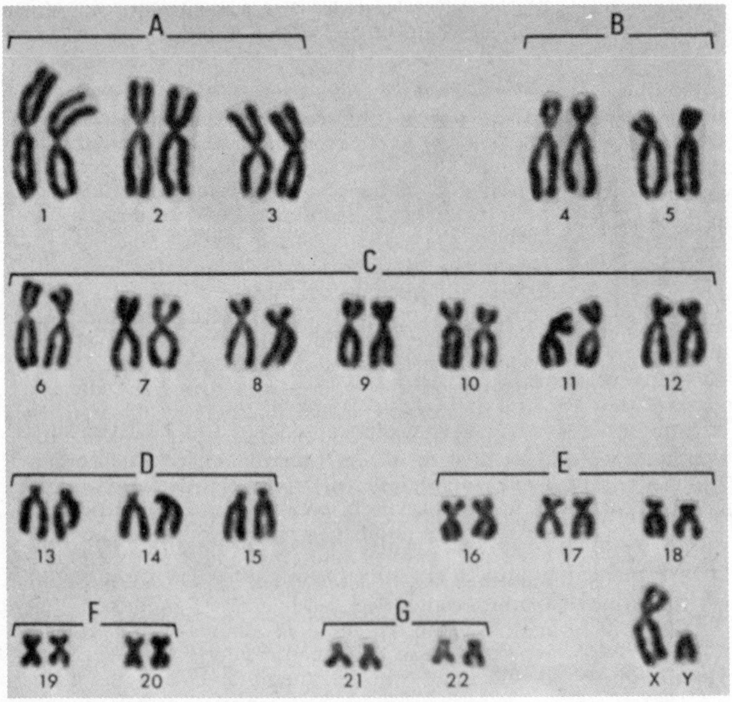

Human metaphase chromosomes from a leukocyte culture, arranged in a standard classification known as a karyotype. (Courtesy of D. H. Carr; from Thompson, J. S., and Thompson, M. W.: Genetics in Medicine. Philadelphia, W. B. Saunders Co., 1973.)

COPD is the most significant chronic pulmonary disorder in the United States in regard to morbidity rate, and is the second most common cause of hospital admissions in this country. It is difficult to estimate the exact incidence of COPD because most diseases of the respiratory tract are not reportable and there is some confusion in definition of terms related to diseases of this type. However, the Social Security Administration reports that COPD ranked only second to heart disease as the cause of disability in men over the age of 40.

The incidence of COPD is increasing and, although the specific cause is not known, factors contributing to its development and affecting its degree of severity have been identified. Of these known factors heavy cigarette smoking appears to be most important; other factors are related to industrial pollution and occupational exposure to irritating inhalants, allergy, autoimmunity, genetic predisposition, and chronic infections.

Prevention of COPD is best accomplished through education of the public about the hazards of cigarette smoking and air pollution and the need for early detection and prompt treatment of respiratory disorders that could become chronic in nature. The American Lung Association is particularly interested in education of lay persons in these matters and in the prevention of all types of respiratory disorders. This agency, which has local offices distributed throughout the country, is an excellent source of information about prevention and the latest developments in the treatment of respiratory diseases.

SYMPTOMS. COPD is an insidious disease that can develop into advanced lung damage almost before its victim is aware that his condition is serious. The early symptoms are shortness of breath upon exertion, a mild cough, sometimes called "smoker's cough," which occurs most often in the morning, and easy fatigability that follows even minimal physical effort. Prompt treatment of these symptoms can forestall the more serious effects of extensive lung damage; however, the destruction of lung tissue and bronchial mucosa damage that has already occurred by the time these symptoms appear is irreversible.

As COPD progresses, the symptoms of dyspnea, weakness, and cough become more severe. The patient has difficulty expelling air from his lungs and his cough becomes more productive of thick, tenacious sputum. He looks anxious and drawn and may speak in short, hesitant sentences. Symptoms related to disturbances of the respiratory and circulatory systems and ACID-BASE BALANCE may appear as these complications develop.

COMPLICATIONS. Destructive involvement of respiratory structures and the resultant impairment of circulatory function can produce serious life-threatening complications in patients with COPD. Among these are acute respiratory failure, disturbance in the acid-base balance (which can occur either as uncompensated respiratory ACIDOSIS or metabolic ALKALOSIS), bronchopulmonary infections, COR PULMONALE (occurring as a result of increased resistance in the pulmonary circulation), PULMONARY EMBOLISM (especially if polycythemia is severe), and peptic ULCER.

PATHOLOGY. In COPD there is an irreversible change in the structure and function of the bronchi and bronchioles, and in the lungs and the blood vessels that serve them. The bronchial mucosa becomes swollen, cilia are destroyed, and the mucus-producing glands hypertrophy. These changes bring about difficulty in removal of mucus and increased obstruction of the air passages.

The walls of the alveoli break down, resulting in large, nonfunctioning air spaces and enlargement of the surviving alveoli. The destruction of alveoli is accompanied by a loss of the capillaries serving them, thus diminishing the diffusion of gases and exchange of carbon dioxide and oxygen. Loss of the capillary bed also interferes with pulmonary circulation, which in turn increases the work load of the right side of the heart. The normal elasticity of the lungs, which allows for their expansion during inspiration and return to normal volume during expiration, is severely impaired.

DIAGNOSIS. A history of heavy cigarette smoking over a period of years or long-term exposure to air pollutants is almost invariably found in patients with COPD. In addition the patient may have suffered from a chronic allergy manifested by respiratory symptoms, a chronic respiratory infection, or a congenital lung defect.

The triad of dyspnea, cough, and easy fatigability is strongly indicative of COPD. A more definitive diagnosis is made through laboratory studies and pulmonary function tests.

Physical examination using palpation, percussion, and auscultation usually reveals symptoms of pathologic changes that are confirmed by x-ray films and FLUOROSCOPY. PULMONARY FUNCTION TESTS include total lung capacity (total amount of air in the lung at peak inspiration), maximum breathing capacity (greatest amount of air moved in and out of the lungs with maximal effort), and vital capacity (maximum amount of air expelled following maximal inspiration).

In COPD the maximum breathing capacity is reduced below normal levels in proportion to the degree of obstructive change in the airways. The vital capacity may be normal or decreased, depending on the extent of obstruction. The volume of air remaining in the lungs at the end of maximal expiration (residual volume) is reduced. Other more sophisticated measurements utilizing complex machinery may be done in large medical centers where the facilities and personnel are readily available. (See also SPIROMETRY.)

BLOOD GAS ANALYSIS is helpful in evaluating effectiveness of blood gas exchange across alveolar walls. In severe COPD, the Pa_{CO_2} level is high while the Pa_{O_2} and the Sa_{O_2} is low.

TREATMENT AND PATIENT CARE. In general, the treatment of COPD is concerned with restoring and maintaining existing lung function, relieving symptoms, and planning a program of rehabilitation tailored to accommodate the individual patient's physiologic needs, physical stamina, vocational needs, life style, and personality.

Specific measures of patient care are concerned with (1) initial and periodic evaluation of patient status, (2) maintenance of general health insofar as possible, (3) prevention and control of infection, (4) improvement of ventilation, and (5) patient education.

COPD is a chronic disease for which there is no cure. The nature of the disease demands an on-going program of assessment and long-term care that is planned and revised as the patient's needs dictate. Whatever the patient care setting—acute care facility, out-patient clinic, convalescent center, or home—the elements of care presented below are essential to the effective management of COPD.

Evaluation. Patient assessment begins with the taking of the patient's history and performing physical examination and lung function tests at the time the diagnosis is established. These measures, along with blood gas analysis at rest and after exercise, provide a baseline for periodic evaluation of the patient's status to determine the progress of the disease and the effectiveness of treatment.

When patients are informed about the purpose of the tests they are more likely to participate in the planned regimen of care and to become motivated to continue carrying out their responsibilities in the management of their illness. Those who work with the patient should clarify for him the goals to be achieved and offer encouragement when he makes progress toward those goals, no matter how slight the improvement might be. This implies, of course, that all members of the health care team have an understanding of the disease, the meaning of various test values, and the purpose of each aspect of care.

Maintenance of Health Status. It is important to communicate to the patient the concept of health status, particularly in regard to his position on the health-illness continuum. He cannot be completely healthy again or restored to his former state of health, before the development of COPD. He can, however, hold his own against the ravages of the disease for periods of time and even make progress toward a better state of health.

Adequate nutrition can be assured by careful planning of well-balanced meals, spacing them so that the stomach is not overloaded at any one time, perhaps as five small meals a day. If POSTURAL DRAINAGE or deep breathing exercises are a part of his daily routine, they should be scheduled for a time when the stomach is not full. Each time these procedures are done they should be followed by good oral hygiene measures to remove the unpleasant taste of sputum and thereby reduce anorexia and nausea.

Physical activity may be severely limited by COPD because of inadequate ventilation and decreased circulation. As with all other aspects of patient care, plans to increase exercise tolerance and promote physical activity should be designed according to the patient's cardiopulmonary status. Techniques that promote muscular relaxation and breathing control are the first step, followed by gradual increase in activity as the patient's progress and general physical condition permit.

Adequate rest is essential, but the well-known hazards of immobility must be avoided, especially in patients who are fearful that any physical activity may precipitate an exhausting episode of coughing and dyspnea. The goal is to provide sufficient rest so that the body's natural restorative processes can work, but to avoid long periods of sleeping and lying in bed during the day.

When the patient's cardiopulmonary condition is such that bed rest is prescribed, care is taken to avoid complete physical inactivity, which will only serve to increase problems of inadequate ventilation and muscle weakness. Proper positioning is essential and should be such that the neck is extended, with the chin well off of the chest. Support under the thighs, while the patient is supine, will release tension on the abdominal muscles, thereby facilitating movement of the diaphragm for deep breathing and effective coughing. The arms and hands should also be supported on pillows and positioned away from the sides to allow for maximum lung expansion without elevation of the upper chest. A foot board is placed so as to maintain good posture, promote comfort, and ensure good muscle tone in the legs and feet.

Prevention and Control of Infection. Acute respiratory infection can be fatal in patients with COPD. Chronic infections inflict further damage to the respiratory structures, lead to increased debilitation, and increase the likelihood of severe complications. Both acute and chronic infections produce increased secretions in the air passages, which further restrict the flow of air.

Contact with others who have an upper respiratory infection should be avoided, as should being in large crowds during the season when such infections are common. A high level of resistance should be maintained through good personal hygiene and adequate nutrition. Vaccines to guard against influenza are recommended.

Because the lungs of the patient with COPD are never entirely free of bacteria, he is a prime candidate for severe bacterial infections. He should be taught to watch for changes in color and amount of sputum. If a change in sputum or any other symptoms of infection appear, he should report to his physician for medication and reassessment of his condition. A small maintenance dose of antibiotics may be prescribed during the winter season as a prophylactic measure. Should an infection develop, the physician may increase the dosage or switch to another drug to avoid the development of drug-resistant organisms.

Improvement of Ventilation. It is obvious that measures to improve ventilation in the patient with COPD are of primary importance, and perhaps that is why so many ways have been devised to facilitate the flow of air to and from the lungs. One should bear in mind that the patient has most of his difficulty during the expiratory phase, he is likely to have air trapped in his lungs, and he most certainly must contend with copious bronchial secretions. In addition, the bronchial walls are weakened in patients with emphysema and are subject to collapse. All of these factors contribute to anxiety and apprehension, which further compound the dyspnea and fatigabiity.

Before employing any of the techniques described below, the therapist must take into account the patient's ability to cooperate and follow instructions. His physical condition at the time the technique is used will affect the choice of method and its effectiveness.

Hydration is considered especially valuable in improvement of ventilation. Inhaled air should be moist so as to thin the secretions for removal and soothe the irritated mucous membranes. This can be accomplished through the use of vaporizers and humidifiers, either for environmental humidification in his room or in conjunction with oxygen therapy and the administration of AEROSOLS. Although many other agents can be used for humidification, water remains the most effective. The patient is encouraged to maintain a daily intake of fluids equal to 10–12 glasses daily.

BRONCHODILATORS in the form of aerosols, oral medications, injections, or rectal suppositories are usually prescribed. The method of aerosol delivery depends on the ability of the patient to breathe deeply so that the medication reaches the lower segments of the respiratory tract. Research studies show that intermittent positive pressure breathing machines (VENTILATORS) are not superior to other devices for the delivery of bronchodilating drugs, as long as the patient can breathe deeply.

Controlled deep breathing patterns are especially helpful in emptying the lungs and providing adequate ventilation. The patient with COPD is taught to expand his lower chest and to use his abdominal muscles and diaphragm to improve his breathing pattern. He must be trained in the performance of these breathing patterns because he probably is not in the habit of breathing in the most effective manner, making optimum use of his remaining pulmonary function.

He is taught slow, controlled, and steady breathing, using his abdominal muscles during expiration and relaxing them during inspiration. His efforts should be concentrated on slow expiratory flow, through parted or pursed lips. During the instruction he is watched for signs of exhaustion and warned against overdoing the deep breathing until he has adjusted to it.

A correct breathing pattern should be coordinated with all of the patient's daily activities so that it becomes habitual and he does it without too much thought. Exercises that strengthen the abdominal muscles are valuable in developing a correct deep breathing pattern.

Effective coughing does not come easily to the patient with COPD. He may have experienced too many episodes in which a dry hacking cough exhausted him; he then became more dyspneic and the tenacious sputum remained in his air passages. As a consequence, over a period of time he may have developed defenses against coughing. He must be convinced that, when done correctly, coughing can remove mucus plugs and relieve rather than produce dyspnea.

The patient is instructed to assume a position that will lead to effective coughing: sitting upright with his feet on the floor or on a footstool, his head flexed, and shoulder rolled forward slightly. He should then drop his head and bend forward slowly and, while doing so, exhale slowly through pursed lips. This maneuver may be sufficient to move secretions upward along the airway and produce a natural cough reflex. If it does not lead to a cough, the patient is told to exhale as fully as possible and at the end of expiration to give a small cough. He is warned not to produce a very large explosive cough, as this will not be as effective and can lead to exhaustion. Instead he is told that the objective is to gradually move secretions upward and to cough them out a little at a time.

When the patient is physically unable to undertake deep breathing and coughing maneuvers, it is necessary to use a mechanical ventilator. Extremely weak patients may require SUCTIONING. This procedure is particularly effective when done correctly, but should be undertaken only by persons thoroughly trained in the technique and fully aware of its inherent dangers.

POSTURAL DRAINAGE is also valuable in facilitating the removal of mucus from the air passages. The various maneuvers involved in this procedure are designed to take advantage of gravity flow as a means of clearing specified segments of the air passages when normal air flow is not sufficient to move secretions or stimulate the cough reflex. Chest percussion and vibration may be employed during postural drainage to loosen secretions.

OXYGEN THERAPY is used as a supportive measure when there is decreased oxygenation of arterial blood. Blood gas analysis is an excellent guide in determining the need for initiating oxygen therapy and for monitoring dosage.

Patient Education. As with all chronic diseases that require long-term planning and management, patient education is of primary importance in successful execution of the plan. Each of the measures previously described involve instruction of the patient and his family, particularly when care is carried out on an out-patient basis. The patient should be told *why* it is necessary for him to stop smoking, avoid other irritating inhalants, carry out good heath practices, take his medication only as prescribed, and faithfully perform techniques to improve ventilation.

It is especially important that the patient be made to feel that he is a worthwhile person, that he is a partner in his care, that he is considered capable of understanding what is being taught to him, and that his opinions and evaluations of his progress and the effectiveness of therapy are valuable contributions to the successful management of his illness. We all need to feel that we have some control over our lives and what is happening to us. The patient, too, has this need and it cannot be met unless he is given instructions and attention to his needs as he perceives them.

chronobiology (kron″o-bi-ol′o-je) the scientific study of the effect of time on living systems.

chronognosis (kron″og-no′sis) perception of the lapse of time.

chronograph (kron′o-graf) an instrument for recording small intervals of time.

chronoscope (kron′o-skōp) an instrument for measuring small intervals of time.

chronotropic (kron″o-trop′ik) affecting the time or rate.

chronotropism (kro-not′ro-pizm) interference with regularity of a periodical movement, such as the heart's action.

chrys(o)- word element [Gr.], *gold.*

chrysarobin (kris″ah-ro′bin) a mixture of neutral principles derived from Goa powder; used in treatment of psoriasis and other chronic skin diseases.

chrysiasis (krĭ-si′ah-sis) deposition of gold in living tissue.

chrysoderma (kris″o-der′mah) permanent pigmentation of the skin due to gold deposit.

Chrysops (kris′ops) a genus of bloodsucking tropical flies, the grove flies, including *C. disca′lis* (deer fly), a vector of tularemia in the western U.S., and *C. sila′cea,* an intermediate host of *Loa loa.*

chrysotherapy (kris″o-ther′ah-pe) treatment with gold salts.

chthonophagia (thon″o-fa′je-ah) the habit of eating clay or earth; geophagia.

Chvostek's sign, Chvostek-Weiss sign (vos′teks; vos′tek vīs) a spasm of the facial muscles resulting from tapping the muscles or the branches of the facial nerve; seen in tetany.

chylangioma (ki-lan″je-o′mah) a tumor of intestinal lymph vessels filled with chyle.

chyle (kīl) the milky fluid taken up by the lacteals from the intestine during digestion, consisting of lymph and triglyceride fat (chylomicrons) in a stable emulsion, and conveyed by the thoracic duct to empty into the venous system.

chylemia (ki-le'me-ah) the presence of chyle in the blood.

chylifaction, chylification (ki"lĭ-fak'shun; ki"lĭ-fĭ-ka'shun) the formation of chyle.

chyliform (ki'lĭ-form) resembling chyle.

chylocele (ki'lo-sēl) distention of the tunica vaginalis testis with effused chyle.

chyloderma (ki"lo-der'mah) elephantiasis filariensis.

chylology (ki-lol'o-je) the study of chyle.

chylomediastinum (ki"lo-me"de-ah-sti'num) the presence of effused chyle in the mediastinum.

chylomicron (ki"lo-mi'kron) a stable droplet containing principally triglyceride fat, but also cholesterol, phospholipids, and protein; found in intestinal lymphatics (lacteals) and blood during and after meals.

chylomicronemia (ki"lo-mi"kro-ne'me-ah) an excess of chylomicrons in the blood.

chylopericardium (ki"lo-per"ĭ-kar'de-um) the presence of effused chyle in the pericardium.

chyloperitoneum (ki"lo-per"ĭ-to-ne'um) the presence of effused chyle in the peritoneal cavity.

chylopneumothorax (ki"lo-nu"mo-tho'raks) the presence of effused chyle and air in the pleural cavity.

chylopoiesis (ki"lo-poi-e'sis) chylification. adj., **chylopoiet'ic.**

chylothorax (ki"lo-tho'raks) the presence of effused chyle in the pleural cavity.

chylous (ki'lus) pertaining, mingled with, or of the nature of chyle.

chyluria (ki-lu're-ah) the presence of chyle in the urine, giving it a milky appearance.

Chymar (ki'mar) trademark for preparations of chymotrypsin, used as an anti-inflammatory agent.

chymase (ki'mās) an enzyme of the gastric juice that hastens the action of the pancreatic juice.

chyme (kīm) the semifluid, homogeneous, creamy or gruel-like material produced by action of the gastric juice on ingested food and discharged through the pylorus into the duodenum.

chymification (ki"mĭ-fĭ-ka'shun) conversion of food into chyme; gastric digestion.

chymosin (ki-mo'sin) rennin.

chymotrypsin (ki"mo-trip'sin) an endopeptidase with action similar to that of trypsin, produced in the intestine by activation of chymotrypsinogen; a product crystallized from an extract of the pancreas of the ox has been used clinically as an anti-inflammatory agent and for other purposes.

chymotrypsinogen (ki"mo-trip-sin'o-jen) the inactive precursor of chymotrypsin, the form in which it is secreted by the pancreas.

Ci abbreviation for *curie* recommended by the International Commission on Radiological Units and Measurements.

cib. [L.] *ci'bus* (food).

cicatrectomy (sik"ah-trek'to-me) excision of a cicatrix.

cicatricial (sik"ah-trish'al) pertaining to a cicatrix.

cicatrix (sik'ah-triks, sĭ-ka'triks), pl. *cica'trices* [L.] the fibrous tissue left after the healing of a wound; a scar.

cicatrization (sik"ah-trĭ-za'shun) the formation of a cicatrix or scar; scarring.

cicutoxin (sik"u-toks'in) a very poisonous principle from plants of the genus *Cicuta,* including the water hemlocks *C. maculata* and *C. virosa.*

-cide word element [L.], *destruction or killing* (homicide); *an agent that kills or destroys* (germicide). adj., **-ci'dal.**

cili(o)- word element [L.], *cilia; ciliary (body).*

cilia (sil'e-ah), sing. *cil'ium* [L.] 1. the eyelashes. 2. minute, motile, hairlike processes attached to the free surface of a cell.

ciliariscope (sil"e-ar'ĭ-skōp) an instrument for examining the ciliary region of the eye.

ciliarotomy (sil"e-ar-ot'o-me) surgical division of the ciliary zone.

ciliary (sil'e-er"e) pertaining to or resembling cilia; used particularly in reference to certain eye structures, as the ciliary body or muscle.

c. body, the thickened part of the vascular tunic of the eye, connecting choroid and iris, make up of the ciliary muscle and the ciliary processes. These processes radiate from the ciliary muscle and give attachment to ligaments supporting the lens of the eye.

c. glands, sweat glands that have become arrested in their development, situated at the edges of the eyelids.

c. muscle, the muscle that forms the main part of the ciliary body and functions in accommodation of the eye (see also table of MUSCLES).

c. reflex, the movement of the pupil in accommodation.

Ciliata (sil"e-a'tah) a class of protozoa (subphylum Ciliophora) whose members possess cilia throughout the life cycle; a few species are parasitic.

ciliate (sil'e-āt) 1. having cilia. 2. any individual of the Ciliata.

ciliated (sil'e-āt"ed) provided with cilia.

ciliectomy (sil"e-ek'to-me) 1. excision of a portion of the ciliary body. 2. excision of the portion of the eyelid containing the roots of the eyelashes.

Ciliophora (sil"e-of'o-rah) a subphylum of Protozoa, including two major groups, the ciliates and suctorians, and distinguished from the other subphyla by the presence of cilia at some stage in the existence of the member organisms.

cilium (sil'e-um) [L.] singular of cilia.

Cillobacterium (sil"o-bak-te're-um) a genus of bacteria found in the intestinal tract and occasionally associated with purulent infections.

cillosis (sil-o'sis) spasmodic quivering of the eyelid.

cimbia (sim'be-ah) a white band running across the ventral surface of the crus cerebri.

cimetidine (si-met'ĭ-dēn) an antagonist to histamine H_2 receptors; it inhibits gastric acid secretion and is effective especially in the treatment of peptic ulcer.

Cimex (si'meks) a genus of blood-sucking insects (order Hemiptera), the bedbugs.

C. lectula'rius, the common bedbug of temperate regions; other species are limited to tropical and subtropical areas and feed on other animals as well as man.

cinchona (sin-ko′nah) the dried bark of the stem or root of various South American trees of the genus *Cinchona;* it is the source of quinine, cinchonine, and other alkaloids.

cinchonine (sin′ko-nēn) an alkaloid obtained from cinchona, used like quinine as an antimalarial agent.

cinchonism (sin′ko-nizm) the morbid or injurious effects of the injudicious use of cinchona bark or its alkaloids.

cine- word element [Gr.], *movement;* see also words beginning *kine-*.

cineangiocardiography (sin″e-an″je-o-kar″de-og′rah-fe) the photographic recording of fluoroscopic images of the heart and great vessels by motion picture techniques.

cineangiography (sin″e-an″je-og′rah-fe) the photographic recording of fluoroscopic images of the blood vessels by motion picture techniques.

cinefluorography (sin″ĕ-floo′or-og′rah-fe) cineradiography.

cinematics (sin″ĕ-mat′iks) kinematics.

cinematography (sin″ĕ-mah-tog″rah-fe) the taking of motion pictures.

cinematoradiography (sin″ĕ-mah-to-ra″de-og′rah-fe) cineradiography.

cinemicrography (sin″ĕ-mi-krog′rah-fe) the making of motion pictures of a small object through the lens system of a microscope.

cinephlebography (sin″ĕ-flĕ-bog′rah-fe) cineradiography of the veins after administration of a contrast medium. In ascending functional cinephlebography, the contrast medium is introduced into a vein in a foot and its progress is observed as it courses through the tibial, popliteal, and iliac veins.

cineplasty (sin′e-plas″te) kineplasty.

cineradiography (sin″ĕ-ra″de-og′rah-fe) the making of a motion picture record of successive images appearing on a fluoroscopic screen.

cinerea (sĭ-ne′re-ah) the gray matter of the nervous system. adj., **cine′real.**

cineroentgenofluorography (sin″ĕ-rent″gen-o-floo″or-og′rah-fe) cineradiography.

cinesi- for words beginning thus, see those beginning *kinesi-*.

cineto- for words beginning thus, see those beginning *kineto-*.

cingulectomy (sing″gu-lek′to-me) bilateral extirpation of the anterior half of the gyrus cinguli.

cingulotomy (sing″gu-lot′o-me) the creation of lesions in the cingulum of the frontal lobe for relief of intractable pain.

cingulum (sing′gu-lum), pl. *cingula* [L.] 1. an encircling part or structure; a girdle. 2. a bundle of association fibers partly encircling the corpus callosum not far from the median plane, interrelating the cingulate and hippocampal gyri. 3. the lingual lobe of an anterior tooth. adj., **cing′ulate.**

circadian (ser″kah-de′an, ser-ka′de-an) denoting a period of about 24 hours.

c. rhythm, the regular recurrence of certain phenomena in cycles of approximately 24 hours, e.g., biologic activities that occur at about the same time each day (or night) regardless of constant darkness or other conditions of illumination.

circinate (ser′sĭ-nāt) resembling a ring, or circle.

circle (ser′k'l) a round figure, structure, or part.

Berry's c's, charts with circles on them for testing stereoscopic vision.

Minsky's c., a device for the graphic recording of eye lesions.

sensory c., a body area within which it is impossible to distinguish separately the impressions arising from two sites of stimulation.

c. of Willis, the anastomatic loop of vessels near the base of the brain.

CircOlectric bed (ser″ko-lek′trik) an electrically operated frame similar in principle to the STRYKER FRAME. The bed can be rotated so that the patient may be placed in a prone, supine, or sitting position, or an erect position. It may be utilized to facilitate turning of a patient with severe burns, a patient in traction, or a patient with various types of spinal injuries.

circulation (ser-ku-la′shun) movement in a regular or circuitous course, returning to the point of origin, as the circulation of the blood through the heart and blood vessels (see also CIRCULATORY SYSTEM).

collateral c., that carried on through secondary channels after obstruction of the principal channel supplying the part.

coronary c., that within the coronary vessels; which supply the muscle of the heart.

extracorporeal c., circulation of blood outside the body, as through an ARTIFICIAL KIDNEY or a HEART-LUNG MACHINE.

fetal c., circulation of blood through the body of the fetus and to and from the placenta through the umbilical cord (see also FETAL CIRCULATION).

portal c., a general term denoting the circulation of blood through larger vessels from the capillaries of one organ to those of another; applied especially to the passage of blood from the gastrointestinal tract and spleen through the portal vein to the liver.

pulmonary c., the flow of blood from the right ventricle through the pulmonary artery to the lungs, where carbon dioxide is exchanged for oxygen, and back through the pulmonary vein to the left artrium (see also PULMONARY CIRCULATION).

systemic c., the flow of blood from the left ventricle through the aorta, carrying oxygen and nutrient material to all the tissues of the body, and returning through the superior and inferior venae cavae to the right atrium.

c. time, the time required for blood to flow between two given points. It is determined by injecting a substance into a vein and then measuring the time required for it to reach a specific site, for example, arm-to-tongue time.

circulatory (ser′ku-lah-tor″e) pertaining to circulation.

c. collapse, SHOCK; circulatory insufficiency without congestive heart failure.

c. system, the major system concerned with the movement of blood and lymph; it consists of the heart, blood vessels, and lymph vessels. (See also Plates 7 and 8.) The circulatory system transports to the tissues and organs of the body the oxygen, nutritive substances, immune substances, hormones, and chemicals necessary for normal function and activities of the organs; it also carries away waste products and carbon dioxide. It equalizes body temperature and helps maintain normal water and electrolyte balance.

An adult has an average of 5 quarts of blood in his body; the circulatory system carries this entire quantity on one complete circuit through the body every minute. In the course of 24 hours, 7200 quarts of blood passes through the heart.

The rate of blood flow through the vessels depends upon several factors: force of the heartbeat, rate of the heartbeat, venous return, and control of the arterioles and capillaries by chemical, neural, and thermal stimuli.

PULMONARY AND SYSTEMIC CIRCULATION. There are in reality two independent circulatory systems within the body, each with its own pump inside the sheathing of the heart. In one of these systems, called the pulmonary circulation, the right side of the heart pumps blood through the lungs. In the lungs, the blood gives up its carbon dioxide and absorbs a fresh supply of oxygen. The reoxygenated blood than flows to the left side of the heart, and is pumped out again to all the systems and organs of the body. This major circulatory system is called the systemic circulation.

The circulation of blood through the fetus bypasses the pulmonary circuit (see also FETAL CIRCULATION).

ARTERIAL SYSTEM. Blood pumped from the left side of the heart enters the aorta, the main arterial trunk of the systemic circulation. The aorta, which is about 1 inch in diameter, arches upward and toward the left side of the body. Just above the heart two coronary arteries branch off from the aorta. These arteries supply the muscles of the heart with blood.

Branching from the top of the aortic arch are three large arteries which supply the upper part of the body, the brachiocephalic trunk (which divides into the right carotid and right subclavian arteries) and the left carotid and left subclavian arteries. The carotid arteries supply the head and neck; the subclavian arteries supply the arms. The aorta then turns downward and passes through the trunk of the body, close to the vertebral column. Smaller arteries branch off from the aorta to supply the lungs, stomach, spleen, pancreas, kidneys, intestines, and other organs of the body. At about the level of the umbilicus, the aorta divides into two branches, the two iliac arteries, which supply the vessels of the pelvic organs and the legs.

The arteries so far named are the main conducting arteries. They consist of a smooth inner lining covered largely by elastic fibers that absorb the pulsations of the heart. As the heart beats the elastic arterial walls damp the strong pulsations into a more nearly constant blood pressure.

Distributing arteries branch out from the conducting arteries. These arteries are composed largely of muscle fibers that encircle the smooth inner lining of the blood vessels and have the ability to contract and relax. The distributing arteries in turn branch out into arterioles, or little arteries, which are barely visible to the eye. The elastic walls of the arterioles and distributing arteries are under the control of the AUTONOMIC NERVOUS SYSTEM. The arterioles lead directly to the capillaries.

Blood passes through the aorta at the speed of

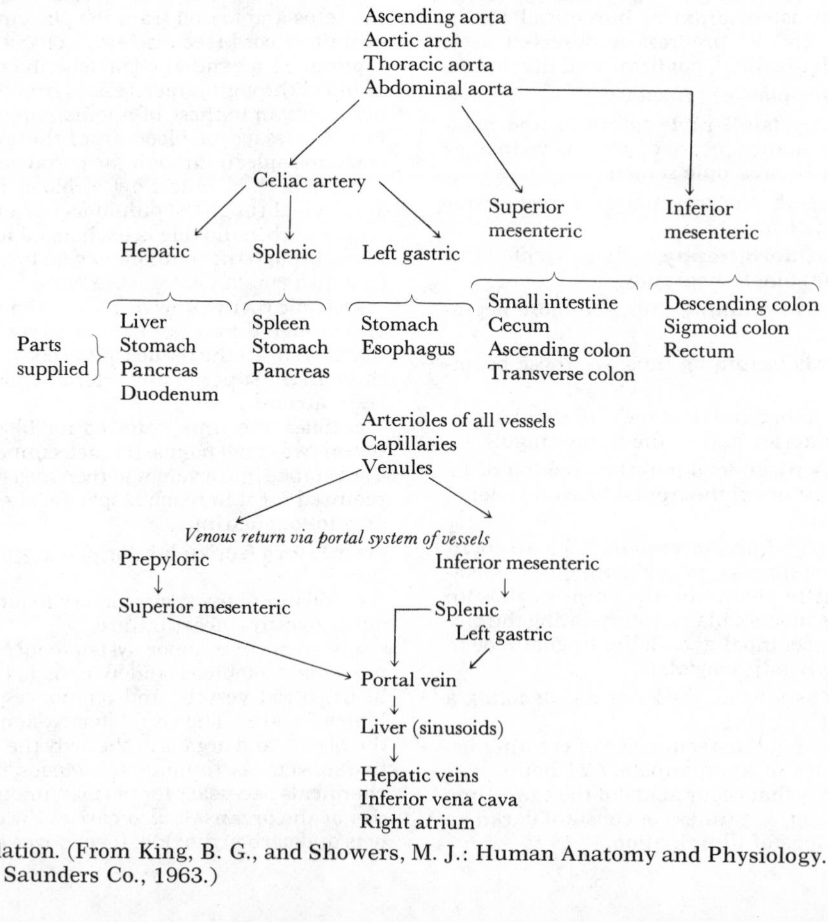

Portal circulation. (From King, B. G., and Showers, M. J.: Human Anatomy and Physiology. 5th ed. Philadelphia, W. B. Saunders Co., 1963.)

about 15.6 inches per second when the body is at rest, and at a faster rate when it is active. As the blood spreads through the distributing arteries and arterioles, its speed gradually diminishes. By the time the blood has reached the capillaries, it has slowed to a speed about one-eightieth of that in the arteries.

CAPILLARIES. The complex network of innumerable and microscopically small capillaries distributed throughout the tissues supplies blood to all cells in the body. Each capillary is about 10 microns in diameter, about the size of a single blood cell, and the blood cells must make their way through the capillaries in single file.

Despite their minute size, the capillaries have a vast total area. The capillary "lake" can be called the climax of the circulatory system, for it is here that the vital work of the circulatory system is carried out. Nutrients leaving the blood capillaries enter the capillary lake, a collection of tissue fluid which bathes each cell. From there the nutrients permeate the walls of the cells. Waste products of cell metabolism enter the capillary lake and eventually pass through the capillary wall and into the blood circulation. The capillary walls are selective; i.e., they permit the exchange of special nutrients and chemicals and bar the passage of unwanted substances. For example, the cells making up the walls of the capillaries in the brain bar the passage of many substances that might injure the brain cells, and the capillaries in the placenta also act as a barrier against substances that might be harmful to the developing fetus.

VENOUS SYSTEM. From the capillaries the blood returns to the heart via the veins, which together make up the venous system. The blood flows from the capillaries to minute venules, and then to the veins, in a network of blood vessels of ever increasing size that parallels in reverse the branching of the arterial system. The walls of the veins, however, are thinner, less elastic and less muscular than those of the arteries. And whereas the arteries are for the most part buried deep within the body for protection, the venous system has many superficial veins that run close to the surface of the skin. If an arterial blood vessel is cut, the blood flows from the cut in spurts, whereas blood from a cut vein flows steadily.

The blood returning to the heart collects into two main veins. Blood returning from the arms, head and upper chest flows into the superior vena cava; blood returning from the rest of the body flows into the inferior vena cava. Both these veins return the blood to the right side of the heart.

The blood from the lower part of the body must return to the heart against the force of gravity, since all the pressure built up by the heart has been dissipated in the capillaries. This is accomplished in several ways. The veins themselves contain one-way venous valves which work in pairs. When the blood is flowing in the correct direction, the venous valves are pressed against the walls of the veins, permitting unobstructed flow. If the blood should tend to flow backward, however, the venous valves fall inward and press against each other, effectively stopping the backward flow of blood. The blood is "milked" upward toward the heart principally by the massaging action of the abdominal and leg muscles as they press against the veins. Inspirations of air also force the blood through the venous system, as do the movements of the intestines. If the leg muscles do not move for long periods of time, the blood collects in the lower part of the body and the amount available for the brain is decreased.

SYSTEMIC CIRCUITS. The circulatory system has been discussed so far as if the blood flowed through the body in a simple circular path. In fact, the blood can take one of several circuits through the body. Among these circuits are the coronary circuit through the arteries and veins of the heart; a circuit through the neck, head, and brain; a circuit through the digestive organs; and the renal circuit through the kidneys. The importance of the renal circulation lies in the fact that the kidneys act as the cleansing filter of the circulatory system, removing a variety of products that have been cast off from the cells and body tissues. At any given time, about one-quarter of all the blood pumped through the body is passing through the renal circuit.

The most complex circuit (portal circulation) is that which flows through the digestive system, picking up proteins, carbohydrates, fats, and chemicals from the intestines and delivering them to the tissues. Separate distributing arteries conduct the blood to the lower intestine, upper intestine, stomach, spleen, and pancreas. The veins leading from these organs combine to form the portal vein, which leads to the liver. Within the liver, the artery leading to the liver (the hepatic artery) and the portal vein subdivide themselves into a complex network of capillary-like vessels called sinusoids which bring the blood into closer contact with the cells of the liver. The liver cells withdraw glucose from the blood for storage as glycogen or release it as needed, and remove from the blood many harmful substances that might be toxic to body tissues. The blood leaving the liver flows to the inferior vena cava.

LYMHATIC SYSTEM. The cells, chemicals, and other components of the blood are suspended within the blood vessels in plasma. Similar fluid also fills the spaces between the tissue cells. Nutrients reaching the cells are carried there by this tissue fluid, and it also carries waste products from the cells to the capillaries. One function of the lymphatic system is to collect and return this fluid via the lymphatic vessels to the circulatory system. When this tissue fluid is within the lymphatic system, it is called lymph. In addition to draining off excess tissue fluid, the lymphatic capillaries also transport some waste products as well as dead blood cells, pathogenic organisms in case of infection, and malignant cells from cancerous growths. From the lymphatic capillaries the lymph is carried into larger lymphatic vessels which contain one-way valves similar to those in the veins. Lymph nodes are interspersed among the lymph vessels and filter their fluids. Eventually large lymph ducts (the thoracic duct and right lymphatic duct) empty into the right and left subclavian veins. The lymph is propelled by the same massaging action that causes the blood to circulate through the venous system. There are larger masses of lymphatic tissue called lymphatic organs, and among them are the SPLEEN, TONSILS, and THYMUS. These organs produce specialized leukocytes (lymphocytes) that help protect the body against infections (see also IMMUNITY).

CONTROL OF CIRCULATION. The organs and systems of the body vary greatly in the quantity of blood they require at different times. The needs of the brain are constant; the demands of the muscles are more varied. Heavy physical exertion may increase the rate of blood flow to the muscles eight times above the normal resting rate. In hot weather, a larger percentage of blood flows through the skin to cool the body. After every meal an extra supply of blood is required by the stomach to help digest and absorb the meal.

These changes in blood supply are accomplished automatically by the autonomic nervous system, which acts through the muscle fibers that surround the distributing arteries and arterioles. These muscle fibers either contract or relax according to the specific nerve signal transmitted to them by the medulla oblongata in the deepest part of the brain. As these muscle fibers contract or relax, they alter the diameter of the blood vessels and, therefore, the rate of blood flow. Certain chemicals, such as epinephrine, ephedrine, histamine, and alcohol, as well as tobacco, can also affect the size of the blood vessels. These changes in the size of the blood vessels are entirely reflexive and the individual has no conscious control over them at all. Ordinarily, the autonomic nervous system maintains the muscles surrounding the arteries in a state of mild tension, which keeps the blood pressure at its normal level.

The brain requires a constant, unvarying supply of blood. Except for the presence of a special control system, this would be impossible to maintain, since every time a person moved or shifted position the quantity of blood flowing to the brain would change. The control system consists of the action of two nerves, one located in the aorta and the other in the carotid artery in the neck, which, acting together, register any changes in the blood pressure and cause the autonomic nervous system to change the rate of heartbeat and the size of the blood vessels to maintain the correct blood pressure.

circum- word element [L.], *around.*

circumcision (ser″kum-sizh′un) surgical removal of all or part of the foreskin, or prepuce, of the penis. The operation is done for hygienic and medical reasons and also is the oldest known religious rite. In the Jewish faith circumcision is a ritual that is performed by a *mohel* (ordained circumciser) on the eighth day after birth whenever possible. The circumcision is followed by a religious ceremony during which the baby also receives his name.

Circumcision is most often performed in infancy, usually before the baby leaves the delivery room, provided the infant is full-term, in good health, and not jaundiced. Most physicians advocate the practice of circumcision, though there are some who do not consider it a necessary procedure unless phimosis, infection, or other difficulties develop.

The incidence of cancer of the penis is much higher in uncircumcised males, and cancer of the prostate less common in circumcised males. The wives of uncircumcised males have a higher incidence of cancer of the cervix than do wives of circumcised men.

Patient Care. Preoperative care for the older child or adult undergoing circumcision includes laboratory tests to determine coagulation or clotting time and a general checkup to assure that the patient is in good health. A mild sedative may be given, though newborn infants usually do not receive any special preoperative care or sedation.

The patient is watched closely after the operation for signs of bleeding; however, excessive bleeding is extremely rare. Other observations include watching for signs of infection, difficulty in urination, and jaundice.

A sterile gauze dressing with ointment is usually placed over the penis when surgery is completed. The dressing is changed each time the diaper is changed, or, in young children and adults, after each urination. When the Plastibell method of circumcision is used, the penis and attached ring is cleansed with sterile water each time the diaper is changed. Healing usually takes place in five to seven days.

circumclusion (ser″kum-kloo′zhun) compression of an artery by a wire and pin.

circumduction (ser″kum-duk′shun) circular movement of a limb or of the eye.

circumflex (ser′kum-fleks) curved like a bow.

circumscribed (ser′kum-skrībd) bounded or limited; confined to a limited space.

circumstantiality (ser″kum-stan″she-al′ĭ-te) think-

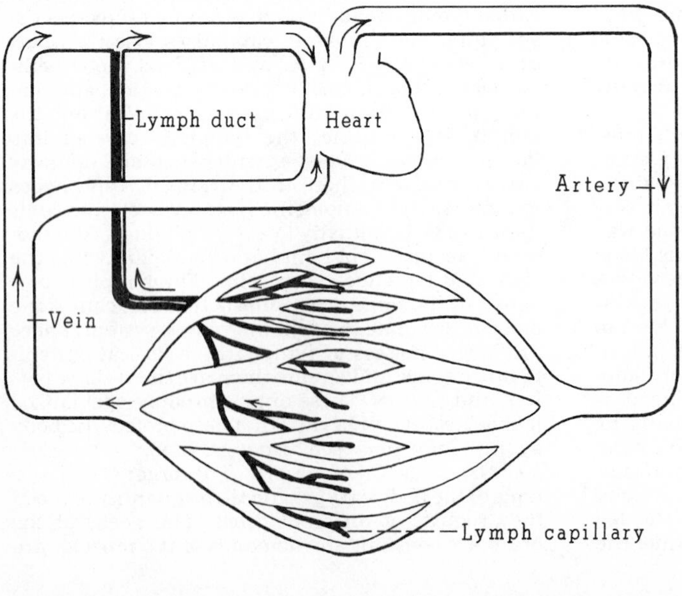

Diagram of lymphatic system, showing its relationship to the circulatory system. (From Jacob, S. W., and Francone, C. A.: Structure and Function in Man. 3rd ed. Philadelphia, W. B. Saunders Co., 1974.)

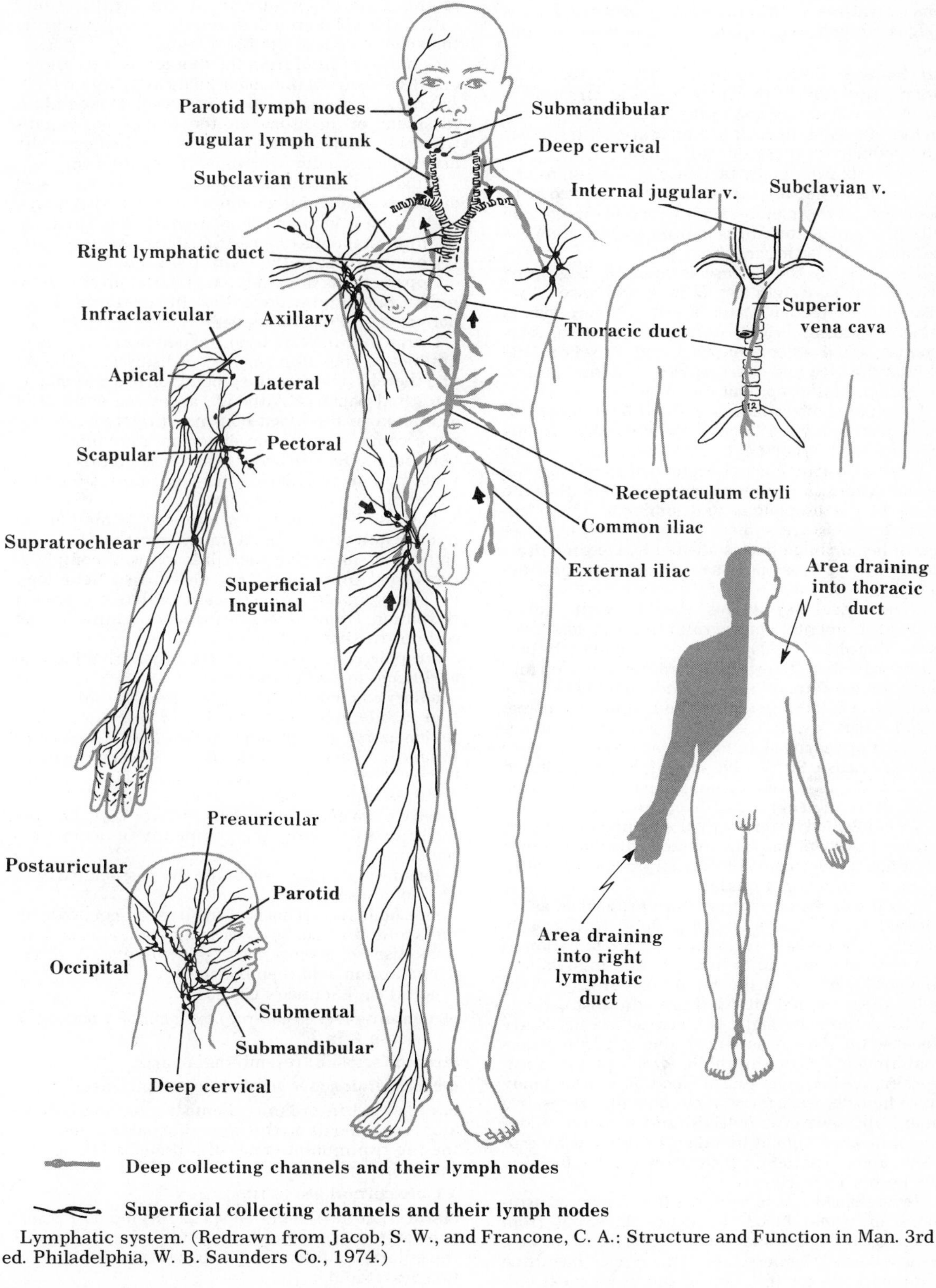

Lymphatic system. (Redrawn from Jacob, S. W., and Francone, C. A.: Structure and Function in Man. 3rd ed. Philadelphia, W. B. Saunders Co., 1974.)

ing or conversation characterized by unnecessary elaboration of trivial details.

circumvallate (ser″kum-val′āt) surrounded by a ridge or trench, as the vallate (circumvallate) papillae.

cirrhosis (si-ro′sis) interstitial inflammation of an organ, particularly the liver. Hepatic cirrhosis is marked by degeneration of the liver cells resulting in loss of normal hepatic architecture, with fibrosis and nodular regeneration. adj., **cirrhot′ic.**

SYMPTOMS AND COURSE OF DISEASE. The signs and symptoms of hepatic cirrhosis are associated with disorders in the metabolism of food elements and vitamins and disturbances in fluid and ELECTROLYTE balance and clotting mechanisms.

The onset of the disease is gradual, beginning with anorexia, weight loss, fatigue, and lowered resistance to infection. Later, there are more visible signs including bright red palms (palmar erythema), small spider-shaped blood vessels in the skin of the face and chest (spider angioma), loss of body hair, and atrophy of the testicles.

Eventually, disturbances in the fluid and electrolyte balance and inefficient metabolism of nutrients produce ASCITES, EDEMA, HYPOGLYCEMIA, and HYPOPROTEINEMIA. Obstruction to the return of blood from the portal system causes increased pressure within the veins of the esophagus and stomach. These engorged vessels are subject to rupture with subsequent hemorrhage that is abetted by clotting disorders. JAUNDICE develops as a result of biliary obstruction.

Neurological symptoms begin with subtle changes in mental acuity, mild memory loss, poor reasoning ability, and irritability. Tremor of the outstretched hands (asterixis) is common. These symptoms become more severe and may eventually progress to delirium, suicidal tendencies, and coma.

TREATMENT AND PATIENT CARE. Treatment of cirrhosis is primarily symptomatic as there is no cure for the disease. Supportive measures are instituted to help the liver rebuild and repair its damaged cells. Prevention of further deterioration of the cells is accomplished by removing the primary cause; for example, restriction of the intake of alcohol or other toxic agent, treatment of infection, and providing an adequate nutritional intake.

Specific forms of treatment are prescribed as indicated by the status of the patient. In the early stages of the disease, rest and adequate nutrition in the form of a normal to high-protein, high-caloric diet are essential to the repair of damaged liver cells; supplemental vitamins are administered.

Observations for signs of bleeding are necessary because the liver is no longer able to produce normal amounts of prothrombin, which plays an important role in the clotting of blood. The patient may have hematemesis, tarry stools, bleeding gums, frequent and severe nosebleeds, and bleeding under the skin. Care should be taken in the brushing of teeth, and the patient is instructed to avoid blowing his nose with force.

Severe blood loss is compensated for by transfusions of whole blood. Excessive bleeding from esophageal varices may necessitate insertion of a Sengstaken-Blakemore tube. This device has three channels: one for inflation of the esophageal balloon, one for inflation of the gastric balloon, and a third for aspiration of stomach contents.

Relief of portal hypertension sometimes is accomplished by a surgical procedure called a portacaval shunt. The portal vein is surgically connected to the inferior vena cava, thus allowing for drainage of excessive amounts of blood from the portal system to the general circulation. A similar procedure called the splenorenal shunt involves connecting the splenic vein to the renal vein.

Removal of fluid from the thoracic cavity (THORACENTESIS) or from the abdominal cavity (PARACENTESIS) may be necessary to relieve respiratory embarrassment or pressure on the abdominal organs caused by ascites. The patient is watched carefully after this procedure for signs of hepatic coma.

Fluid and electrolyte in patients with advanced cirrhosis are carefully monitored. A record of intake and output is kept and the patient is weighed daily. Sodium intake may be restricted and DIURETICS prescribed to assist in the control of edema.

Hepatic coma demands total restriction of protein intake, but a high-caloric diet utilizing fats and carbohydrates is recommended.

Drugs that may be used include broad-spectrum antibiotics, such as neomycin, to disinfect the bowel and thereby decrease the production of ammonia by intestinal bacteria. Although an increased level of ammonia in the blood does not directly cause hepatic coma, a reduction of serum ammonia has a beneficial effect. In order to accomplish this L-arginine monohydrochloride may be administered intravenously.

The semi-comatose or completely comatose patient requires continued monitoring of the vital signs and supportive measures to avoid complications from immobility. (See also COMA.) Neurological symptoms demand constant vigilance to protect the patient from injury due to mental confusion and self-destructive tendencies.

atrophic c., cirrhosis marked by shriveling and shrinkage in size of the liver.

biliary c., cirrhosis of the liver from chronic retention of bile, due to obstruction or infection of the major extra- or intrahepatic bile ducts (secondary biliary cirrhosis), or of unknown etiology (primary biliary cirrhosis), and sometimes occurring after administration of certain drugs.

fatty c., a form in which the liver cells become infiltrated with fat; seen commonly in acute alcoholism.

Laënnec's c., cirrhosis of the liver associated with alcohol abuse.

metabolic c., cirrhosis of the liver associated with metabolic disease, such as hemochromatosis, Wilson's disease, glycogenosis, galactosemia, or disorder of amino acid metabolism.

portal c., Laennec's cirrhosis.

cirsectomy (ser-sek′to-me) excision of a portion of a varicose vein.

cirsoid (ser′soid) resembling a varix.

cirsomphalos (ser-som′fah-los) caput medusae.

cis (cis) [L.] in organic chemistry, having certain atoms or radicals on the same side; in genetics, having the two mutant genes of a pseudoallele on the same chromosome.

11-*cis* retinal see RETINAL (2).

cistern (sis′tern) a closed space serving as a reservoir for lymph or other body fluids, especially one of the enlarged subarachnoid spaces containing cerebrospinal fluid.

cisterna (sis-ter′nah), pl. *cister′nae* [L.] cistern.

c. cerebellomedulla′ris, the enlarged subarachnoid

space between the undersurface of the cerebellum and the posterior surface of the medulla oblongata; called also cisterna magna.

c. chy'li, the dilated portion of the thoracic duct at its origin in the lumbar region; called also receptaculum chyli.

cisternal (sis-ter'nal) pertaining to a cistern, especially the cisterna cerebellomedullaris.

c. puncture, puncture of the cisterna cerebellomedullaris with a hollow needle inserted just between the occipital bone, to obtain a specimen of CEREBROSPINAL FLUID (see also SPINAL PUNCTURE).

Preparation of the patient for this procedure should include a detailed explanation, because insertion of a needle so close to the brain may cause apprehension. The physician may request that the back of the neck be shaved. The patient is positioned on his side with his head bent forward and held firmly by an attendant. Complications seldom occur, but the patient should be observed for signs of dyspnea or cyanosis during and immediately after the procedure. A cisternal puncture is often done in the out-patient clinic, and the patient is allowed to go home soon after it is completed.

cistron (sis'tron) the smallest unit of genetic material that must be intact to function as a transmitter of genetic information; as traditionally construed, approximately synonymous with gene.

citrate (sit'rāt, si'trāt) any salt of citric acid.

citrated (sit'rāt-ed) treated with or containing a citrate, especially potassium citrate.

citreoviridin (sĭ"tre-o-vir'ĭ-din) a toxic principle from the fungus *Penicillium citreoviride.*

citric acid (sit'rik) a crystalline acid from citrus fruits and other plant and animal sources or produced by fermentation of sugars; it is antiscorbutic, refrigerant, and diuretic. Citric acid is used as a flavoring agent. Its sodium salt (sodium citrate) is used chiefly as an anticoagulant for blood that is to be fractionated or stored; its potassium salt (potassium citrate) is used in potassium deficiencies and as a systemic alkalizer, sudorific, diuretic, and expectorant.

c. a. cycle, tricarboxylic acid cycle.

citrinin (sit'rĭ-nin) a toxic antibiotic produced by the fungus *Penicillium citrinum* and some species of *Aspergillus;* active against gram-positive bacteria.

citronella (sit"ron-el'ah) a fragrant grass, the source of a volatile oil (citronella oil) used in perfumes and insect repellents.

citrovorum factor (sit-rov'or-um) folinic acid, a factor necessary for the growth of *Leuconostoc citrovorum.*

citrulline (sit-rul'ēn) an alpha amino acid involved in urea production.

citrullinuria (sit-rul"ĭ-nu're-ah) the presence in the urine of large amounts of citrulline, with increased levels also in both plasma and cerebrospinal fluid.

cittosis (sĭ-to'sis) pica.

Cl chemical symbol, *chlorine.*

cladosporiosis (klad"o-spo"re-o'sis) any infection with *Cladosporium.*

Cladosporium (klad"o-spo're-um) a genus of fungi, including *C. herbarum,* which produces "black spot" on meat in cold storage, growing at a temperature of 18° F. (–8° C.); and *C. carrioni* an agent of chromomycosis.

clairvoyance (klār-voi'ans) [Fr.] a form of extrasensory perception in which knowledge of objective events is acquired without the use of the senses.

clamp (klamp) a surgical device for compressing a part or structure.

clap (klap) gonorrhea.

clapotement (klah-pōt-maw') [Fr.] a splashing sound, as in succussion.

clarificant (klah-rif'ĭ-kant) a substance that clears a liquid of turbidity.

Clark's rule (klarks) the dose of a drug for a child is obtained by multiplying the adult dose by the child's weight in pounds and dividing the result by 150.

Clarke-Hadfield syndrome (klark had'fēld) congenital pancreatic infantilism, with hepatomegaly, bulky stools, and extensive atrophy of the pancreas in an undersized and underweight child.

clasmatocyte (klaz-mat'o-sīt) a macrophage.

class (klas) 1. a taxonomic category subordinate to a phylum and superior to an order. 2. a group of variables all of which show a value falling between certain limits.

clastic (klas'tik) 1. undergoing or causing division. 2. separable into parts.

clastothrix (klas'to-thriks) trichorrhexis nodosa.

clathrate (klath'rāt) 1. having the shape or appearance of a lattice; pertaining to clathrate compounds. 2. [pl.] clathrate compounds: inclusion complexes in which molecules of one type are trapped within cavities of the crystalline lattice of another substance.

Claude's syndrome (klawdz) paralysis of the third (oculomotor) nerve on one side and asynergia on the other side, together with dysarthria.

claudication (klaw"dĭ-ka'shun) limping or lameness.

intermittent c., a complex of symptoms characterized by absence of pain or discomfort in a limb when at rest, the commencement of pain, tension, and weakness after walking is begun, intensification of the condition until walking is impossible, and the disappearance of symptoms after the limb has been at rest. It is seen in occlusive arterial disease of the limbs.

venous c., intermittent claudication caused by venous stasis.

claustrophilia (klaws"tro-fil'e-ah) an abnormal desire to be in a closed room or space.

claustrophobia (klaws"tro-fo'be-ah) morbid fear of closed places.

claustrum (klaws'trum), pl. *claus'tra* [L.] the thin layer of gray matter lateral to the external capsule of the brain, separating it from the white matter of the insula.

clavacin (klav'ah-sin) patulin.

Claviceps (klav'ĭ-seps) a genus of parasitic fungi that infest various seed plants.

C. purpu'rea, the source of ergot.

clavicle (klav'ĭ-k'l) an elongated, slender, curved bone lying horizontally at the root of the neck, in the upper part of the thorax; called also collar bone. adj., **clavic'ular.** (See also table of BONES.)

clavicotomy (klav"ĭ-kot'o-me) surgical division of the clavicle.

clavicula (klah-vik′u-lah), pl. *clavic′ulae* [L.] the clavicle.

claviformin (klav′ĭ-for′min) patulin.

clavus (kla′vus) a corn.

c. hyster′icus, a sensation as if a nail were being driven into the head.

clawfoot (klaw′foot) a high-arched foot with the toes hyperextended at the metatarsophalangeal joint and flexed at the distal joints.

clawhand (klaw′hand) flexion and atrophy of the hand and fingers.

clearance (klēr′ans) the act of clearing; specifically, complete removal by the kidneys of a solute or substance from a specific volume of blood per unit of time.

blood-urea c., the volume of the blood cleared of urea per minute by renal elimination.

creatinine c., the volume of plasma cleared of creatinine in a unit of time by the kidney system. (See also CREATININE.)

inulin c., an expression of the renal efficiency in eliminating inulin from the blood, a measure of glomerular function.

urea c., blood-urea clearance.

cleavage (klēv′ij) 1. division into distinct parts. 2. the early successive splitting of a fertilized ovum into smaller cells (blastomers) by mitosis.

cleft (kleft) a fissure or longitudinal opening, especially one occurring during embryonic development.

branchial c's, the clefts between the branchial arches of the embryo, formed by rupture of the membrane separating corresponding entodermal pouch and ectodermal groove.

c. lip, c. palate, congenital fissure, or split, of the lip (cleft lip) or of the roof of the mouth (cleft palate).

Cleft palate and cleft lip occur in about one birth per thousand and are sometimes associated with clubfoot (talipes) or other anatomic defects. They have no connection with mental retardation. Although poor health of the mother during pregnancy may have some effect on the development of her child, the old superstition that psychologic experiences of the pregnant mother can cause cleft palate and cleft lip has no scientific basis. However, it is true that parents who were born with cleft palate or cleft lip are somewhat more likely than other parents to have children with these defects.

Cleft palate and cleft lip result from failure of the two sides of the face to unite properly at an early stage of prenatal development. The defect may be limited to the outer flesh of the upper lip (the term harelip, suggesting the lip of a rabbit, is both inaccurate and unkind), or it may extend back through the midline of the upper jaw through the roof of the palate. Sometimes only the soft palate, located at the rear of the mouth, is involved.

The infant with a cleft palate is unable to suckle properly, because the opening between mouth and nose through the palate prevents suction. Feeding must be done by other means, with a dropper, a cup, a spoon, or an obturator, a device inserted in the mouth to close the cleft while the baby is sucking. Cleft palate allows food to get into the nose, and it causes difficulty in chewing and swallowing. Later it will hinder speech, because consonants such as *g, b, d,* and *f,* which are normally formed by pressure against the roof of the mouth, are distorted by resonance in the nasal cavity. The cleft may also prevent movements of the soft palate essential in clear speech.

TREATMENT. Treatment of cleft palate and cleft lip is by surgery, followed by measures to improve speech. A cleft palate should be reconstructed by plastic surgery when the child is about 18 months old, before he learns to talk. The corrective work usually requires only one operation. After surgery, the child often needs special training in speech to prevent his being handicapped and developing inferiority feelings.

Cleft lip usually can be corrected by surgery when the child reaches a weight of 12 to 15 lb., generally at the age of 2 to 3 months. Successful surgery often leaves only a thin scar and a greatly improved ability to form the *p, b,* and *m* sounds.

A child born with a moderate degree of cleft palate or cleft lip can look forward to a normal life—in appearance, speech, and manner—if proper action is taken early. This means consulting and carefully following the advice of competent specialists in medicine, surgery, dentistry, and speech.

The child should be patiently encouraged to overcome his handicap. He must not be pushed so hard as to become resentful or discouraged, nor should he be allowed to become too self-conscious or dependent. He needs opportunities to play normally with other children and to talk freely with adults. As he makes progress at a reasonable rate, his confidence will increase.

PATIENT CARE. The main concerns during the preoperative period are maintenance of adequate nutrition, prevention of respiratory infections, and speech therapy to prevent development of bad habits of speech.

Postoperative care must be aimed at prevention of trauma to or infection of the operative site. The child is not allowed to lie on his stomach until the incision is completely healed. Elbow restraints are used to keep the fingers and hands away from the mouth. The patient is usually fed with a special syringe with a rubber tip as long as he is on a liquid diet (about 7 to 10 days postoperatively). When he is given a soft diet care must be taken that the spoon or other eating utensils do not damage the suture line.

Mouth care is given frequently to keep the mouth clean and reduce the danger of infection. Dental caries often occurs in cleft palate and regular visits to the dentist are needed.

Tender loving care, always a part of pediatric care, is even more necessary when caring for these children. They must be reassured and kept quiet so that crying and restlessness do not undo the work done by the surgeon.

c. tongue, a tongue whose anterior portion is divided by a longitudinal fissure.

cleid(o)- word element [Gr.], *clavicle.*

cleidocranial (kli″do-kra′ne-al) pertaining to the clavicles and head.

c. dysostosis, a rare hereditary condition in which there is defective ossification of the cranial bones; complete or partial absence of the clavicles, so that the shoulders may be brought together in front; and dental and vertebral anomalies.

cleidotomy (kli-dot′o-me) surgical division of the clavicle of the fetus in difficult labor to facilitate delivery.

clemizole (klem′ĭ-zōl) an antihistaminic.

click (klik) a brief, sharp sound, especially any of the short, dry clicking heart sounds during systole, indicative of various heart conditions.

clidinium bromide (klĭ-din′e-um) an anticholinergic.

climacteric (kli-mak′ter-ik, kli″mak-ter′ik) the complex of endocrine, somatic, and psychic changes occurring at the end of the female reproductive period (menopause); it may also accompany normal diminution of sexual activity in the male.

climatotherapy (kli″mah-to-ther′ah-pe) treatment of disease by means of a favorable climate.

climax (kli′maks) the period of greatest intensity, as in the course of a disease.

clindamycin (klin″dah-mi′sin) a semisynthetic antibiotic derivative of lincomycin; used as an antibacterial and antiparasitic agent.

clinic (klin′ik) 1. a clinical lecture; examination of patients before a class of students; instruction at the bedside. 2. an establishment where patients are admitted for special study and treatment by a group of physicians practicing medicine together.

clinical (klin′ĭ-k′l) pertaining to a clinic or to the bedside; pertaining to or founded on actual observation and treatment of patients, as distinguished from theoretical or experimental.

clinician (klĭ-nish′an) an expert clinical physician and teacher.

clinicopathologic (klin″ĭ-ko-path″o-loj′ik) pertaining to both symptoms of disease and to its pathology.

clinidine (klin′ĭ-dēn) a moderate antihypertensive which, when combined with a diuretic, can be used to control severe hypertension.

Clinistix (klin′ĭ-stiks) trademark for an enzyme-impregnated strip of plastic used to test for sugar in the urine. The strip is dipped into the urine and results of positive or negative are indicated by the color of the strip. This test is not as accurate as the Clinitest or Benedict's test.

Clinitest (klin′ĭ-test) trademark for reagent tablets containing copper sulfate, used to test for the presence of sugar in the urine. Ten drops of water and 5 of urine are placed in a test tube. The tablet, which generates heat, is added and the solution is allowed to boil. Within a few moments the color of the solution is compared to a color chart similar to the one used for Benedict's test.

clinocephaly (kli″no-sef′ah-le) congenital flatness or concavity of the vertex of the head.

clinodactyly (kli″no-dak′til-e) permanent deviation or deflection of one or more fingers.

clinoscope (kli′no-skōp) an instrument for measuring the paralysis of the ocular muscles as shown by torsion of the eyeballs.

clip (klip) a metallic device for approximating the edges of a wound or for the prevention of bleeding from small individual blood vessels.

Clistin (klis′tin) trademark for preparations of carbinoxamine, an antihistamine.

clition (klit′e-on) the midpoint of the anterior border of the clivus.

clitoridectomy (klit″o-rĭ-dek′to-me) excision of the clitoris.

clitoriditis (klit″o-rĭ-di′tis) clitoritis.

clitoridotomy (klit″o-rĭ-dot′o-me) incision of the clitoris.

clitoris (klit′o-ris) the small, elongated, erectile body in the female, situated at the anterior angle of the rima pudendi, and homologous with the penis in the male.

clitorism (klit′o-rizm) 1. hypertrophy of the clitoris. 2. persistent erection of the clitoris.

clitoritis (klit″o-ri′tis) inflammation of the clitoris.

clivus (kli′vus), pl. *cli′vi* [L.] a bony surface in the surface of the posterior cranial fossa sloping upward from the foramen magnum to the dorsum sellae.

cloaca (klo-a′kah), pl. *cloa′cae* [L.] 1. a common passage for fecal, urinary, and reproductive discharge in most lower vertebrates. 2. the terminal end of the hindgut before division into rectum, bladder, and genital primordia in mammalian embryos. 3. an opening in the involucrum of a necrosed bone. adj., **cloa′cal.**

cloacogenic (klo″ah-ko-jen′ik) originating from the cloaca or from persisting cloacal remnants; said of a group of rare transitional-cell nonkeratinizing epidermoid anal cancers.

clofazimine (klo-faz′ĭ-mēn) an antibacterial used as a tuberculostatic and leprostatic; investigational in the United States.

clofibrate (klo-fi′brāt) an anticholesterolemic.

clomiphene (klo′mĭ-fēn) a nonsteroid estrogen analogue used as the citrate salt to stimulate ovulation.

clonazepam (klo-naz′ĕ-pam) a benzodiazepine derivative used as an oral anticonvulsant.

clone (klōn) 1. the asexual progeny of a single cell. 2. a strain of cells descended in culture from a single cell; the establishment or initiation of such a strain. 3. to establish or initiate such a strain. adj., **clo′nal.**

clonic (klon′ik) pertaining to or characterized by clonus.

clonicity (klo-nis′ĭ-te) the condition of being clonic.

clonicotonic (klon″ĭ-ko-ton′ik) both clonic and tonic.

clonidine (klo′nĭ-dēn) a centrally acting antihypertensive agent.

clonism (klon′izm) a succession of clonic spasms.

clonograph (klon′o-graf) an instrument for recording spasmodic movements of parts and tendon reflexes.

Clonorchis (klo-nor′kis) a genus of Asiatic liver flukes.

clonospasm (klon′o-spazm) clonic spasm.

clonus (klo′nus) alternate involuntary muscular contraction and relaxation in rapid succession.

ankle c., foot c., a series of abnormal reflex movements of the foot, induced by sudden dorsiflexion, causing alternate contraction and relaxation of the triceps surae muscle.

toe c., abnormal rhythmic contraction of the great toe, induced by sudden passive extension of its first phalanx.

wrist c., spasmodic contraction of the hand muscles, induced by forcibly extending the hand at the wrist.

Clopane (klo′pān) trademark for preparations of cyclopentamine, a sympathomimetic amine used as a nasal decongestant in the form of the hydrochloride salt.

Clostridium (klo-strid′e-um) a genus of anaerobic

spore-forming bacteria (family Bacillaceae).

C. bifermen'tans, a species common in feces, sewage, and soil, and associated with gas gangrene.

C. botuli'num, the agent causing botulism in man.

C. histolyt'icum, a species found in feces and soil.

C. no'vyi, a species that is an important cause of gas gangrene.

C. perfrin'gens, the most common causative agent of gas gangrene.

C. sep'ticum, a species commonly occurring in animal intestines and soil, strikingly pathogenic for various animals and sometimes associated with gaseous infections in man. Called also vibrion septique.

C. tet'ani, a common inhabitant of soil and human and horse intestines, and the cause of TETANUS in man and domestic animals.

C. welch'ii, British name for *C. perfringens.*

clostridium (klo-strid'e-um), pl. *clostrid'ia* [Gr.] any individual of the genus *Clostridium.*

clot (klot) 1. a semisolidified mass, as of blood or lymph. 2. to form such a mass.

c. retraction, the drawing away of a blood clot from a vessel wall, a function of blood platelets.

clotrimazole (klo-trim'ah-zōl) a synthetic broad-spectrum antifungal agent applied topically in the treatment of diseases caused by dermatophytes and yeasts.

clotting (klot'ing) the formation of a jellylike substance over the ends or within the walls of a blood vessel, with resultant stoppage of the blood flow. Clotting is one of the natural defense mechanisms of the body when injury occurs. A clot will usually form within 5 minutes after a blood vessel wall has been damaged. The exact process of clotting is not known; however, it is believed that the mechanism is triggered by the platelets, which disintegrate as they pass over rough places in the injured surface. As they disintegrate they release serotonin and thromboplastin. Serotonin causes constriction of the blood vessels and reduction of local blood pressure. Thromboplastin unites with calcium ions and other substances which promote the formation of fibrin. When examined under a microscope, a clot consists of a mesh of fine threads of fibrin in which are embedded erythrocytes and leukocytes and small amounts of fluid (serum).

Twelve factors essential to normal blood clotting, whose absence, diminution, or excess may lead to abnormality of the clotting mechanism, have been described; they are designated by Roman numerals (I to V and VII to XIII; VI is no longer considered to have a clotting function): *factor I,* a high-molecular-weight plasma protein that is converted to fibrin through the action of thrombin and that participates in stages 3 and 4 of blood clotting. Deficiency results in afibrogenemia or hypofibrinogenemia. Called also fibrinogen. *factor II,* a glycoprotein present in the plasma that is converted into thrombin by extrinsic thromboplastin during the second stage of blood clotting. Deficiency leads to hypoprothrombinemia. Called also prothrombin. *factor III,* a material that has a number of sources in the body and is important in the formation of extrinsic thromboplastin; called also tissue thromboplastin. *factor IV,* an appellation that is, in the scheme of hemostasis, assigned to calcium, because of its requirement in the first, second, and probably the third stages of blood clotting. *factor V,* a heat- and storage-labile material, present in plasma and not in serum, and functioning in the formation of intrinsic and extrinsic thromboplastins. Deficiency leads to parahemophilia. Called also accelerator globulin and proaccelerin. *factor VI,* a factor previously called accelerin and thought to be an intermediate product of prothrombin conversion; it no longer is considered in the scheme of hemostasis, and hence it is assigned neither a name or a function. *factor VII,* a heat- and storage-stable material, present in serum but not in plasma and participating only in the formation of extrinsic thromboplastin. Deficiency, either hereditary or acquired (VITAMIN K deficiency), leads to hemorrhagic tendency. Called also prothrombinogen and serum prothrombin conversion accelerator, SPCA. *factor VIII,* a relatively storage-labile material present in plasma and not in serum, and participating only in the formation of extrinsic thromboplastin. Deficiency, a sex-linked recessive trait, results in classical hemophilia. Called also antihemophilic factor (AHF) and antihemophilic globulin (AHG). *factor IX,* a relatively storage-stable substance, present in normal serum but not in plasma, that is involved in the generation of intrinsic thromboplastin; a deficiency of this factor results in a hemorrhagic syndrome called hemophilia B or Christmas disease, which is similar to classical hemophilia A; called also plasma thromboplastin component, PTC. *factor X,* a heat-labile material with limited storage stability at room temperature, present in serum but not in plasma, that functions in the formation of both intrinsic and extrinsic thromboplastin. Deficiency may result in a systemic coagulation disorder. Called also Stuart factor. *factor XI,* a stable factor, present in both serum and plasma, that together with factor XII forms a complex that activates factor IX in the formation of intrinsic thromboplastin. Deficiency results in hemophilia C. Called also plasma thromboplastin antecedent, PTA. *factor XII,* a stable factor, present in plasma and serum, that is activated by contact with glass or other foreign substances and initiates the process of blood coagulation *in vitro;* its precise role during *in vivo* hemostasis remains unclear; called also Hageman factor. *factor XIII,* a factor that polymerizes fibrin monomers. Deficiency causes a clinical hemorrhagic diathesis. At least four platelet factors also exist that have a part in clotting.

It is possible for a clot to form within a blood vessel if the inner wall of the vessel has been roughened by injury or disease. Clots may form in conditions such as arteriosclerosis, varicose veins, and thrombophlebitis. An internal clot that remains at the place where it forms is called a thrombus; the general condition is called THROMBOSIS. If the clot (or pieces of it) breaks loose and flows through the blood vessels, it is called an embolus, and the condition is called EMBOLISM.

Clotting of the blood can be hastened by contact with injured tissue, by warming, by adding such coagulants as calcium, or by combination with thromboplastin and thrombin. The process can be retarded by cooling, by dilution, by adding oxalates and citrates, or by administration of substances such as HEPARIN and dicumarol, called ANTICOAGULANTS.

c. time, the time required for blood to clot in a glass tube. Called also coagulation time.

cloxacillin (kloks″ah-sil'in) a semisynthetic penicillin; its sodium salt is used in treating staphylococcal infections due to penicillinase-positive organisms.

clubbing (klub′ing) proliferation of soft tissue about the terminal phalanges of fingers or toes, without osseous change.

clubfoot (klub′foot) a deformity in which the foot is twisted out of normal position. The medical term for this condition is talipes. The deformity is usually congenital but a few cases of clubfoot in older children may have been caused by injury or poliomyelitis. There are several types of clubfoot; the foot may be turned inward, outward, upward, or downward. Sometimes a combination of these defects may be present. (See also illustration accompanying TALIPES.)

There are several theories as to the cause of clubfoot. A familial tendency or arrested growth during fetal life may contribute to its development, or it may be caused by a defect in the ovum. It sometimes accompanies meningomyelocele as a result of paralysis. In mild clubfoot there are slight changes in the structure of the foot; more severe cases involve orthopedic deformities of both the foot and leg.

Treatment varies according to the severity of the deformity. Milder cases may be corrected with casts that are changed periodically, the foot being manipulated into position each time the cast is changed so that it gradually assumes normal position. A specially designed splint also may be used. It is made of two plates attached to shoes with a crossbar between the plates and special, set screws so that the angulation of the foot can be changed as necessary. More severe deformities require surgery of the tendons and bones, followed by the application of a cast to maintain proper position of the joint.

clubhand (klub′hand) deformity of the hand, resembling that of the foot in clubfoot; talipomanus.

clumping (klump′ing) the aggregation of particles, such as bacteria or other cells, into irregular masses.

cluneal (kloo′ne-al) pertaining to the buttocks.

clunis (kloo′nis), pl. *clu′nes* [L.] buttock.

clysis (kli′sis) the administration other than orally of any of several solutions to replace lost body fluid, supply nutriment, or raise blood pressure; also, the solution so administered.

clyster (klis′ter) an enema.

C.M. [L.] *Chirur′giae Ma′gister* (Master in Surgery).

Cm chemical symbol, *curium.*

cm. centimeter.

cm.^{2} square centimeter.

cm.^{3} cubic centimeter.

C.M.A. Canadian Medical Association.

c./min. cycles per minute.

c.mm. cubic millimeter.

C.N.A. Canadian Nurses' Association.

cnemial (ne′me-al) pertaining to the shin.

C.N.M. Certified Nurse-Midwife.

C.N.S. central nervous system.

Co chemical symbol, *cobalt.*

CoA coenzyme A.

coacervate (ko-as′er-vāt) a collection of less fully hydrated particles of a colloid system, with less solvent bound to them than they had before.

coacervation (ko-as″er-va′shun) the formation of coacervates in a colloid system.

coadaptation (ko″ad-ap-ta′shun) the mutual, correlated, adaptive changes in two interdependent organs.

coagglutination (ko″ah-gloo″tĭ-na′shun) the aggregation of particulate antigens combined with agglutinins of more than one specificity.

coagglutinin (ko″ah-gloo′tĭ-nin) partial agglutinin.

coagulability (ko-ag″u-lah-bil′ĭ-te) the state of being capable of forming or of being formed into clots.

coagulant (ko-ag′u-lant) promoting, accelerating, or making possible coagulation of blood; also, an agent that so acts.

coagulase (ko-ag′u-lās) an antigenic substance of bacterial origin, produced chiefly by staphylococci, which may be causally related to thrombus formation.

coagulate (ko-ag′ū-lāt) 1. to cause to clot. 2. to become clotted.

coagulation (ko-ag″u-la′shun) 1. formation of a clot. 2. in surgery, the disruption of tissue by physical means to form an amorphous residuum, as in electrocoagulation and photocoagulation.

c. factors, factors essential to normal blood clotting, whose absence, diminution, or excess may lead to abnormality of the clotting; 12 factors, commonly designated by Roman numerals, have been described. (See also CLOTTING.)

c. time, clotting time.

coagulopathy (ko-ag″u-lop′ah-the) any disorder of blood coagulation.

consumption c., a disorder characterized by reduction in elements involved in blood coagulation due to their utilization in excessive blood clotting, usually in disseminated intravascular coagulation.

coagulum (ko-ag′u-lum), pl. *coag′ula* [L.] a clot.

coalescence (ko″ah-les′ens) a fusion or blending of parts.

coal tar (kōl tar) a by-product obtained in destructive distillation of bituminous coal; used in ointment or solution in treatment of eczema.

coapt (ko′apt) to approximate, as the edges of a wound.

coarctate (ko-ark′tāt) 1. to press close together; contract. 2. pressed close together; restrained.

coarctation (ko″ark-ta′shun) stricture or narrowing.

c. of aorta, a localized malformation characterized by deformity of the tunica media of the aorta, causing narrowing, usually severe, of the lumen of the vessel.

reversed c., pulseless disease.

coat (kōt) a membrane or other tissue covering or lining an organ; in anatomic nomenclature called also tunica.

buffy c., the thin yellowish layer of leukocytes overlying the packed erythrocytes in centrifuged blood.

Coats' disease (kōts) chronic progressive retinopathy usually affecting male children, in which the fundus reveals an exudative retinal detachment associated with telangiectatic blood vessels and multiple hemorrhages; it may lead to total retinal detachment, iritis, glaucoma, and cataract.

cobalamin (ko-bal′ah-min) a cobalt-containing complex common to all members of the vitamin B_{12} group.

cobalt (ko′bawlt) a chemical element, atomic number 27, atomic weight 58.933, symbol Co. (See table of ELEMENTS.) RADIOISOTOPES of cobalt, such as cobalt 60 (^{60}Co), are used for implantation in the treatment of various forms of malignancy and also serve as the radioactive source in teletherapy machines.

Cobelli's glands (ko-bel′lēz) mucous glands in the esophageal mucosa just above the cardia.

cocaine (ko-kān′, ko′kān) an alkaloid obtained from the leaves of various species of *Erythroxylon* (coca plants) or produced synthetically; used as an anesthetic, applied topically or administered as a local or spinal anesthetic. Cocaine has limited use in its pure form but its derivatives are widely used. The drug must be administered with caution because of frequent idiosyncrasy even in small doses. Toxic effects include excitement, dizziness, headache, convulsions, and hypotension. Barbiturates are sometimes given prior to the administration of cocaine to allay the side effects. If a reaction to cocaine does occur during its administration the drug is stopped immediately and barbiturates are given.

cocainism (ko′kān-izm) the morbid condition produced by misuse of cocaine.

cocainize (ko-kān′īz) to put under the influence of cocaine.

cocarboxylase (ko″kar-bok′sĭ-lās) phosphorylated thiamine.

cocarcinogen (ko″kar-sin′o-jen) an agent that increases the effect of a carcinogen by direct concurrent local effect on the tissue.

cocarcinogenesis (ko-kar″sĭ-no-jen′ĕ-sis) the development, according to one theory, of cancer only in preconditioned cells as a result of conditions favorable to its growth.

cocci (kok′si) plural of *coccus*.

Coccidia (kok-sid′e-ah) an order of sporozoa commonly parasitic in epithelial cells of the intestinal tract, but also found in the liver and other organs; it includes two genera, *Eimeria* and *Isospora*.

coccidia (kok-sid′e-ah) plural of *coccidium*.

coccidial (kok-sid′e-al) of, pertaining to, or caused by Coccidia.

coccidian (kok-sid′e-an) 1. pertaining to Coccidia. 2. any member of the Coccidia; coccidium.

Coccidioides (kok-sid″ĕ-oi′dēz) a genus of pathogenic fungi.

C. immit′is, the etiologic agent of coccidioidomycosis.

coccidioidin (kok-sid″e-oi′din) a sterile preparation containing by-products of growth products of *Coccidioides immitis*, injected intracutaneously as a test for coccidioidomycosis.

coccidioidoma (kok-sid″e-oi-do′mah) residual pulmonary granulomatous nodules seen roentgenographically as solid round foci in coccidioidomycosis.

coccidioidomycosis (kok-sid″e-oi″do-mi-ko′sis) a fungal disease caused by infection with *Coccidioides immitis*. This fungus grows in hot, dry areas, especially in the southwestern United States, Mexico, and parts of Central and South America. The disease occurs in a primary and in a secondary form. The primary form, due to inhalation of windborne spores, varies in severity from that of the common cold to symptoms resembling those of influenza; called also desert fever, desert rheumatism, and San Joaquin Valley fever. The secondary form is a virulent and severe, chronic, progressive, granulomatous disease resulting in involvement of cutaneous and subcutaneous tissues, viscera, central nervous system, and lungs.

Treatment consists primarily of rest. Antibiotics may be given to prevent secondary bacterial infection. Amphotericin B has been used parenterally in treating the disease.

coccidioidosis (kok-sid″e-oi-do′sis) coccidioidomycosis.

coccidiosis (kok-sid″e-o′sis) infection by coccidia. In man, applied to the presence of *Isospora belli* in stools; such infection is often asymptomatic, rarely causing a severe watery mucous diarrhea.

coccidium (kok-sid′e-um), pl. *coccid′ia* [L.] any member of the Coccidia; coccidian.

coccobacillus (kok″o-bah-sil′us) an oval bacterial cell intermediate between the coccus and bacillus forms. adj., **coccobac′illary.**

coccobacteria (kok″o-bak-te′re-ah) a common name for spheroid bacteria, or for various bacterial cocci.

coccoid (kok′oid) resembling a coccus.

cocculin (kok′u-lin) picrotoxiin.

coccus (kok′us), pl. *coc′ci* [L.] a spherical bacterium, usually slightly less than 1μ in diameter, belonging to the Micrococcaceae family. It is one of the three basic forms of bacteria, the other two being bacillus (rod-shaped) and spirillum (spiral-shaped). Almost all of the pathogenic cocci are either staphylococci, which occur in clusters, or streptococci, which occur in short or long chains. Both staphylococci and streptococci are gram-positive and do not form spores.

The staphylococci are responsible for many serious infections, especially *Staphylococcus aureus*, which is the causative agent in boils, abscesses, osteomyelitis, and a large variety of other infections. The staphylococcus has received much attention in recent years because of the ability of most strains to develop a resistance to antibiotics.

The most dangerous streptococci are those of the beta-hemolytic type. Various species of streptococci cause sore throat, scarlet fever, mastoiditis, and septicemia.

coccyalgia, coccydynia (kok″se-al′je-ah; kok″sĭ-din′e-ah) coccygodynia.

coccygeal (kok-sij′e-al) pertaining to or located in the region of the coccyx.

coccygectomy (kok″sĭ-jek′to-me) excision of the coccyx.

coccygeus (kok-sij′e-us) pertaining to the coccyx.

coccygodynia (kok″sĭ-go-din′e-ah) pain in the coccyx and neighboring region.

coccygotomy (kok″sĭ-got′o-me) incision of the coccyx.

coccyx (kok′siks) the small bone caudad to the sacrum in man, formed by the union of four (sometimes five or three) rudimentary vertebrae, and forming the caudal extremity of the vertebral column; called also os coccygis.

cochineal (koch′ĭ-nēl) dried female insects of *Coccus cacti*, enclosing young larvae; used as a coloring agent for pharmaceuticals and as a biological stain.

cochlea (kok′le-ah) a spiral tube forming part of the inner ear, shaped like a snail shell, which is the essential organ of hearing. (See also Plate 15.) adj., **coch'lear.** The cochlea is filled with fluid and is connected with the middle ear by two membrane-covered openings, the oval window (fenestra vestibuli) and the round window (fenestra cochleae). Inside the cochlea is the organ of Corti, a structure of highly specialized cells that translate sound vibrations into nerve impulses. The cells of this organ have tiny hairlike strands (cilia) that protrude into the fluid of the cochlea.

Sound vibrations are relayed from the tympanic membrane (eardrum) by the bones of hearing in the middle ear of the oval window of the cochlea, where they set up corresponding vibrations in the fluid of the cochlea. These vibrations move the cilia of the organ of Corti, which then sends nerve impulses to the brain. (See also HEARING.)

cochleariform (kok″le-ar′ĭ-form) spoon-shaped.

cochleitis (kok″le-i′tis) inflammation of the cochlea.

cochleovestibular (kok″le-o-ves-tib′u-lar) pertaining to the cochlea and vestibule of the ear.

coconsciousness (ko-kon′shus-nes) consciousness secondary to the main stream of consciousness.

cocontraction (ko″kon-trak′shun) coordination of antagonistic muscles.

coctolabile (kok″to-la′bil) capable of being destroyed or altered by heating to the boiling point of water.

coctoprecipitin (kok″to-pre-sip′ĭ-tin) a precipitin produced by injecting a heated serum or other antigen.

coctostabile (kok″to-sta′bil) incapable of being altered by heating to the boiling point of water.

cod liver oil an oil pressed from the fresh liver of the cod and purified. It is one of the best-known natural sources of vitamin D, and a rich source of vitamin A. Because cod liver oil is more easily absorbed than other oils, it was formerly widely used as a nutrient and tonic, but it is rarely used today since more efficient sources are available. (See also VITAMIN.)

code (kōd) 1. a set of rules governing one's conduct. 2. a system by which information can be communicated.

genetic c., the arrangement of nucleotides in the polynucleotide chain of a chromosome that governs the transmission of genetic information to proteins, i.e., determines the sequence of amino acids in the polypeptide chain making up each protein synthesized by the cell (see also GENETIC CODE).

triplet c., the three-base sequence (nucleotide) in the DNA molecule which codes for an amino acid.

codeine (ko′dēn) an alkaloid obtained from opium or prepared from morphine by methylation; used as a narcotic analgesic and antitussive.

c. phosphate, c. sulfate, water-soluble preparations administered orally or parenterally for relief of pain.

Codivilla's extension (ko″di-vil′ahz) extension for fractures made by a weight pulling on calipers or a nail passed through the lower end of the bone.

codon (ko′don) a series of three adjacent bases in one polynucleotide chain of a DNA or RNA molecule, which codes for a specific amino acid.

coe- for words beginning thus, see also those beginning *ce-*.

coefficient (ko″ĕ-fish′ent) 1. an expression of the change or effect produced by the variation in certain factors, or of the ratio between two different quantities. 2. in chemistry, a number or figure put before a chemical formula to indicate how many times the formula is to be multiplied.

absorption c., 1. the ratio of the linear rate of change of roentgen rays in a homogenous material to the intensity at a given point (A.M.A.). 2. a number indicating the volume of a gas absorbed by a unit volume of a liquid at 0° C. and at a pressure of 760 mm. Hg.

Bunsen c., absorption coefficient (2).

phenol c., a measure of the bactericidal activity of a compound in relation to phenol (see also PHENOL COEFFICIENT).

-coele word element [Gr.], *cavity; space.*

Coelenterata (se-len″ter-a′tah) a phylum of invertebrates including the hydras, jellyfish, sea anemones, and corals.

coelenterate (se-len′ter-āt) 1. pertaining or belonging to Coelenterata. 2. an individual member of the phylum Coelenterata.

coeloblastula (se″lo-blas′tu-lah) the common type of blastula, consisting of a hollow sphere composed of blastomeres.

coelom (se′lom) body cavity, especially the cavity in the mammalian embryo between the somatopleure and splanchnopleure, which is both intra- and extraembryonic; the principal cavities of the trunk arise from the intraembryonic portion. adj., **coelom′ic.**

coelosomy (se″lo-so′me) a developmental anomaly characterized by protrusion of the viscera from and their presence outside the body cavity.

coenzyme (ko-en′zīm) an organic molecule, usually containing phosphorus and some vitamins, sometimes separable from the enzyme protein; a coenzyme and an apoenzyme must unite in order to function (as a holoenzyme).

c. A, a coenzyme essential for carbohydrate and fat metabolism; among its constitutents are PANTOTHENIC ACID and a terminal SH group, which forms thioester linkages with various acids, e.g., acetic acid (acetyl CoA).

c. Q, any of a group of related quinones with isoprenoid units in the side chains (the ubiquinones), occurring in the lipid fraction of mitochondria and serving, along with the cytochromes, as an intermediate in electron transport; they are similar in structure and function to vitamin K_1.

c. I, nicotinamide-adenine dinucleotide.

c. II, nicotinamide-adenine dinucleotide phosphate.

coeur (ker) [Fr.] heart.

c. en sabot (on să-bo′), a heart whose shape on a radiograph vaguely resembles that of a wooden shoe; noted in tetralogy of Fallot.

cofactor (ko′fak-tor) an element or principle, e.g., a coenzyme, with which another must unite in order to function.

Cogentin (ko-jen′tin) trademark for preparations of benztropine.

cognition (kog-nish′un) that operation of the mind process by which we become aware of objects of thought and perception, including all aspects of perceiving, thinking, and remembering. adj., **cog′nitive.**

cohesion (ko-he′zhun) the force causing various particles to unite. adj., **cohe′sive.**

Cohnheim's theory (kōn′hīmz) 1. the emigration of leukocytes is the essential feature of inflammation. 2. tumors develop from embryonic rests which do not participate in the formation of normal surrounding tissue.

coil (koil) a winding structure or spiral; called also helix.

coinosite (koi′no-sīt) a free commensal organism.

coition (ko-ish′un) coitus.

coitophobia (ko″ĭ-to-fo′be-ah) morbid fear of coitus.

coitus (ko′ĭ-tus) sexual union by vagina between male and female; usually applied to the mating process in human beings.

c. incomple′tus, c. interrup′tus, coitus in which the penis is withdrawn from the vagina before ejaculation.

c. reserva′tus, coitus in which ejaculation of semen is intentionally suppressed.

colation (ko-la′shun) the process of straining or filtration, or the product of such a process.

colchicine (kol′chĭ-sēn) a poisonous alkaloid from *Colchicum autumnale* (meadow saffron), used in treatment of gout and usually effective in terminating an attack of acute gout. Side effects include gastrointestinal symptoms and hypotension.

cold (kold) 1. an acute and highly contagious virus infection of the upper respiratory tract (see also COMMON COLD). 2. a relatively low temperature; the lack of heat. A total absence of heat is absolute zero, at which all molecular motion ceases.

A body temperature below 94° F. (34.5° C.) results in impairment of the heat-regulating center in the hypothalamus. As the temperature drops, sleepiness and coma develop, and as a result the central nervous system heat-control mechanism is depressed and shivering (a means of heat production) is prevented. FROSTBITE is a local freezing of a surface area of the body and results from exposure to extremely low temperatures. Circulatory disturbances and gangrene can result from frostbite.

Induced HYPOTHERMIA, in which the body temperature is deliberately lowered and maintained below 90° F. (32° C.), is sometimes used during heart and other types of surgery when it is necessary to stop the heart action for several minutes. This type of prolonged cooling does not have any seriously harmful effects on the body.

USE OF COLD APPLICATIONS

Effects. The primary effect of cold on the surface of the body is constriction of the blood vessels. Cold also causes contraction of the involuntary muscles of the skin. These actions result in a reduced blood supply to the skin and produce a marked pallor. If cold is prolonged there may be damage to the tissues because of the decreased blood supply.

Cold acts as a depressant to the activity of the cells and slows the heart action and pulse rate. By causing constriction of the blood vessels it may elevate the blood pressure. Intense cold numbs the sensory nerve endings so that impulses are not transmitted and sensations such as pain and taste are lost.

The secondary effects of cold are the opposite of its primary action. There is increased cell activity, dilatation of the blood vessels, and increased sensitivity of the nerve endings. The outward appearance of the skin is a characteristic mottled blue or purple color, and there is stiffness and numbness of the affected part.

Purposes. Cold applications may be used to control bleeding or to check an inflammatory process. Application of cold may inhibit the swelling and relieve pain and loss of motion in an inflamed area; however, it will not reduce edema that is already present in the tissues. Because cold slows down activity of all living cells it may be used to check the growth of bacteria in a local infection.

Cold applications are used in the emergency treatment of burns because the cold reduces the loss of fluids from the blood vessels into the tissue spaces and thus controls edema.

Cool sponge baths, using cool water or alcohol, are often used to lower the body temperaure when FEVER is present.

Methods. Cold is applied locally by the use of ice caps, ice collars, and cold wet compresses. Ice caps are applied to the head for the relief of headache and treatment of fever, delirium, and some types of head injury. An ice cap may also be used to check an inflammatory process within the pelvic or abdominal cavity, or to treat certain cardiac conditions. An ice cap usually is not left on for more than 1 hour and is used for less than an hour if the patient complains of cold or numbness or the area appears mottled. Unless otherwise ordered by the physician, ice caps and ice collars are always covered with a cotton cloth or towel before they are applied.

Ice collars are used to control bleeding and reduce swelling after tonsillectomy or other surgical conditions of the throat. They also may be applied to relieve nausea or to reduce discomfort from the passage of a nasogastric tube.

Cold compresses are most often applied to the eyes for relief of swelling and inflammation. They also may be used to relieve the symptoms of hemorrhoids.

cold sore (kold′sōr) a lesion caused by the virus of HERPES SIMPLEX, usually on the border of the lips or nares.

colectomy (ko-lek′to-me) excision of the colon or of a portion of it.

colibacillemia (ko″lĭ-bas″ĭ-le′me-ah) the presence of *Escherichia coli* in the blood.

colibacillosis (ko″lĭ-bas″ĭ-lo′sis) infection with *Escherichia coli.*

colibacilluria (ko″lĭ-bas″ĭ-lu′re-ah) the presence of *Escherichia coli* in the urine.

colibacillus (ko″le-bah-sil′us) *Escherichia coli.*

colic (kol′ik) 1. pertaining to the colon. 2. acute paroxysmal abdominal pain.

Colic usually refers to an attack of abdominal pain caused by spasmodic contractions of the intestine, most common during the first 3 months of life. The infant may pull up his arms and legs, cry loudly, turn red-faced, and expel gas from the anus or belch it up from the stomach.

The exact cause of infant colic is not known but several factors may contribute to its occurrence. These include excessive swallowing of air, too rapid feeding or overfeeding, overexcitement, and an anxious or easily disturbed mother. The infant can usually be relieved by being picked up, "bubbled" gently, and given some warm water to drink. To relieve his tenseness he should be held and soothed with tender loving care. His condition is not serious and most infants gain weight and are healthy in spite of the colic.

biliary c., colic due to passage of gallstones along the bile duct.

lead c., colic due to lead poisoning.

menstrual c., dysmenorrhea.

renal c., intermittent and acute pain usually resulting from the presence of one or more calculi in the kidney or ureter. The pain begins in the kidney region and radiates forward and downward to envelop the abdomen, genitalia, and legs. Other symptoms include nausea, vomiting, diaphoresis, and a desire to urinate frequently.

colicky (kol′ik-e) pertaining to or affected by colic.

colicoplegia (kol″ĭ-ko-ple′je-ah) combined colic and paralysis produced by lead poisoning.

coliform (kol′ĭ-form) resembling or being *Escherichia coli.*

coliplication (ko″lĭ-pli-ka′shun) coloplication.

colipuncture (ko″lĭ-pungk′tūr) colocentesis.

colisepsis (ko″lĭ-sep′sis) infection with *Escherichia coli.*

colistimethate (ko-lis″tĭ-meth′āt) a colistin derivative; the sodium salt is used in the treatment of infections, particularly those of the urinary tract.

colistin (ko-lis′tin) an antibiotic produced by *Bacillus polymyxa* var. *colistinus,* or the same substance produced by other means; it is related chemically to polymyxin, and used in the treatment of urinary tract infections.

c. sulfate, a water-soluble salt of colistin, effective against several gram-negative bacilli, but not against *Proteus;* used as an intestinal antibacterial.

colitides (ko-lit′ĭ-dēz) plural of *colitis;* inflammatory disorders of the colon considered collectively.

colitis (ko-li′tis) inflammation of the colon. The most common form of colitis is mucous colitis, called also spastic colitis, irritable colon, or functional bowel distress.

SYMPTOMS. In the early phase of mucous colitis, spasms occur in the lower portion of the bowel. They may be accompanied by cramplike pain in the upper stomach. Frequently there is constipation, sometimes alternating with diarrhea. As the disturbance progresses, mucus is secreted more readily, and diarrhea becomes more likely.

CAUSES. The most common cause of mucous colitis is emotional stress or anxiety. This indicates that at least part of the treatment should be psychologic. The patient must learn to control his tension and anxiety so that they will not affect his physical well-being. Unwise eating habits, including too much roughage in the diet, and overdosing with laxatives can also cause some forms of colitis.

TREATMENT. Changes in diet and eating habits are recommended for the treatment of mucous colitis. The diet change depends on the symptoms. In most cases a bland diet with a minimum of roughage is advised. Food to which a patient has previously shown an intolerance should be totally excluded. Laxatives also should be excluded. Irritant substances such as strong seasonings, alcohol, coffee, tea, and tobacco should be avoided. Meals should be serene, leisurely, and as pleasant and attractive as possible. Proper exercise, a regular routine of daily living, and the avoidance of emotional conflicts are all important. Mild sedatives and antispasmodic drugs may also be prescribed.

ulcerative c., a chronic ulceration in the colon producing diarrhea, loss of weight, and sometimes anemia; it is less common and more serious than mucous colitis (see also ULCERATIVE COLITIS).

colitoxicosis (ko″lĭ-tok″sĭ-ko′sis) toxemia caused by *Escherichia coli.*

colitoxin (ko″lĭ-tok′sin) a toxin from *Escherichia coli.*

coliuria (ko″le-u′re-ah) the presence of *Escherichia coli* in the urine.

collagen (kol′ah-jen) an albuminoid, a main supportive protein of skin, tendon, bone, cartilage, and connective tissue. adj., **collag′enous.**

c. diseases, a group of diseases having in common certain clinical and histological features that are manifestations of involvement of CONNECTIVE TISSUE, i.e., those tissues that provide the supportive framework (musculoskeletal structures) and protective covering (skin and mucous membranes and vessel linings) for the body.

The basic components of connective tissue are cells and extracellular protein fibers embedded in a matrix or ground substance of large carbohydrate molecules and carbohydrate-protein complexes called mucopolysaccharides.

For the sake of clarity and organization, collagen diseases may be divided into two major groups: (1) those that are genetically determined and are a result of structural and biochemical defects, and (2) those that are acquired and in which immmunological and inflammatory reactions are taking place within the tissues. Among the first group are those diseases caused by a lack of a specific enzyme necessary for proper storage and excretion of one or more mucopolysaccharides. Also included in this group are osteogenesis imperfecta, Ehlers-Danlos syndrome, and Marfan's syndrome. These disorders are distinguished by structural defects affecting the formation of the extracellular fibers called collagen.

Acquired connective tissue diseases are believed to develop as a result of at least two causative factors: a genetic factor and an abnormal immunological response. The exact role of these factors in the development of connective tissue diseases has not been firmly established, but there is strong evidence that immunological mechanisms are involved. Examples of collagen diseases that are most probably the result of an aberration of the immunological reactions that mitigate injury and inflammation of connective tissues are systemic lupus erythematosus, scleroderma, rheumatoid arthritis, rheumatic fever, polymyositis, and dermatomyositis.

collagenase (kol-laj′ĕ-nās) an enzyme that hydrolyzes peptides containing proline, including collagen and gelatin.

collagenation (kol-laj″ĕ-na′shun) the appearance of collagen in developing cartilage.

collagenic (kol″ah-jen′ik) 1. producing collagen. 2. pertaining to collagen.

collagenoblast (kol-laj′ĕ-no-blast″) a cell arising from a fibroblast and which, as it matures, is associated with collagen production; it may also form cartilage and bone by metaplasia.

collagenocyte (kol-laj′ĕ-no-sīt″) a mature collagen-producing cell.

collagenogenic (kol-laj″ĕ-no-jen′ik) pertaining to or characterized by collagen production; forming collagen or collagen fibers.

collagenolysis (kol″ah-jĕ-nol′ĭ-sis) dissolution or digestion of collagen. adj., **collagenolyt′ic.**

collagenosis (kol″ah-jĕ-no′sis) collagen disease.

collapse (kŏ-laps′) 1. a state of extreme prostration and depression, with failure of circulation. 2. abnormal falling in of the walls of a part or organ.

circulatory c., shock; circulatory insufficiency without congestive heart failure.

c. therapy, operative collapse and immobilization of the lung in treatment of pulmonary disease; artificial pneumothorax (see also surgery of the LUNG).

collateral (kŏ-lat′er-al) 1. secondary or accessory; not direct or immediate. 2. a small side branch, as of a blood vessel or nerve.

c. fissure, c. sulcus, a longitudinal fissure on the inferior surface of the cerebral hemisphere between the fusiform and parahippocampal gyri.

Colles' fracture (kol′ēz) a break in the lower end of the radius, the distal fragment being displaced backward (see illustration accompanying FRACTURE). If the lower fragment is displaced forward, it is a reversed Colles' fracture.

Colles' law (kol′ēz) a child affected with congenital syphilis, the mother showing no signs of the disease, will not infect the mother.

colliculectomy (kŏ-lik″u-lek′to-me) excision of the seminal colliculus.

colliculitis (kŏ-lik″u-li′tis) inflammation about the seminal colliculus.

colliculus (kŏ-lik′u-lus), pl. *collic′uli* [L.] a small elevation.

seminal c., a prominent portion of the male urethral crest, on which are the opening of the prostatic utricle and, on either side of it, the orifices of the ejaculatory ducts; called also verumontanum.

collimation (kol″ĭ-ma′shun) in microscopy, the process of making light rays parallel; the adjustment of two or more optical axes with respect to each other. In radiology, the elimination of the more divergent portion of an x-ray beam.

colliquation (kol″ĭ-kwa′shun) liquefactive degeneration of tissue.

colliquative (kŏ-lik′wah-tiv) characterized by excessive liquid discharge, or by liquefaction of tissue.

collodiaphyseal (kol″o-di″ah-fiz′e-al) pertaining to the neck and shaft of a long bone, especially the femur.

collodion (kŏ-lo′de-on) a syrupy liquid compounded of pyroxylin dissolved in ether and alcohol, which dries to a clear tenacious film; used as a topical protectant.

flexible c., a mixture of collodion, camphor, and castor oil; used topically as a protectant.

salicylic acid c., flexible collodion containing salicylic acid, used topically as a keratolytic.

colloid (kol′oid) 1. gluelike. 2. the translucent, yellowish, gelatinous substance resulting from colloid degeneration. 3. a state of matter composed of single large molecules or groups of smaller molecules in a solid, liquid, or gaseous state, dispersed (subdivided) in a continuous medium (disperse medium) which may also be solid, liquid, or gas. Different types of colloids (colloid systems) are designated by their dispersed and dispersing phases. For example, if the dispersed phase is a solid and the dispersing phase a liquid, the system is called a sol, such as glue. Milk is an example of an emulsion, in which both phases are liquid, one an oil and one water. Colloids do not dissolve into true solutions and are not capable of passing through a semipermeable membrane, as in DIALYSIS. The physical opposite of a colloid is a crystalloid.

c. bath, a bath containing gelatin, bran, starch or similar substances, to relieve skin irritation and pruritus.

c. degeneration, the assumption by the tissues of a gumlike or gelatinous character.

colloidal (kŏ-loi′dal) of the nature of a colloid.

c. gold test, a test of cerebrospinal fluid based on alterations in the albumin-globulin ratios that occur in certain disorders of the central nervous system. Normal spinal fluid, when diluted and added to a colloidal gold suspension, will not precipitate the colloidal gold. The extent of precipitation is indicative of various diseases such as multiple sclerosis, poliomyelitis, and encephalitis. A positive reaction also occurs in the presence of neurosyphilis. The sample of spinal fluid must not contain blood because this will cause a false-positive reaction.

colloidin (kŏ-loi′din) a jelly-like principle produced in colloid degeneration.

colloidoclasia (kŏ-loi″do-kla′ze-ah) breaking up of the physical equilibrium of the colloid of the body, producing ANAPHYLACTIC SHOCK; called also colloidoclastic shock.

collum (kol′um), pl. *col′la* [L.] the neck, or a necklike part.

c. distor′tum, torticollis.

c. val′gum, coxa valga.

collutory (kol′u-to″re) mouthwash or gargle.

collyrium (kŏ-lir′e-um), pl. *collyr′ia* [L.] a lotion for the eyes; an eye wash.

colo- word element [Gr.], *colon.*

coloboma (kol″o-bo′mah) an apparent absence or defect of some ocular tissue, usually due to failure of a part of the fetal fissure to close; it may affect the choroid, ciliary body, eyelid (palpebral coloboma, colobo′ma palpebra′le), iris (colobo′ma i′ridis), lens (colobo′ma len′tis), optic nerve, or retina (colobo′ma ret′inae).

colocecostomy (ko″lo-se-kos′to-me) cecocolostomy.

colocentesis (ko″lo-sen-te′sis) surgical puncture of the colon.

coloclysis (ko-lok′lĭ-sis) irrigation of the colon.

coloclyster (ko″lo-klis′ter) an enema introduced into the colon through the rectum.

colocolostomy (ko″lo-ko-los′to-me) surgical formation of an anastomosis between two portions of the colon.

colocutaneous (ko″lo-ku-ta′ne-us) pertaining to the colon and skin, or communicating with the colon and the cutaneous surface of the body.

colocynth (kol′o-sinth) the dried pulp of the unripe but full-grown fruit of *Citrullus colocynthis;* used as a drastic cathartic.

coloenteritis (ko″lo-en″ter-i′tis) enterocolitis.

colofixation (ko″lo-fik-sa′shun) the fixation of the colon in cases of ptosis.

Cologel (kol′o-jel) trademark for a preparation of methylcellulose, which acts as a mild laxative by increasing intestinal bulk.

coloileal (ko″lo-il′e-al) ileocolic.

colon (ko′lon) the part of the large intestine extending from the cecum to the rectum. adj., **colon′ic.** The colon is divided as follows: the ascending colon, which passes upward from the cecum to the lower edge of the liver, where it bends and becomes the transverse colon. This section lies across the abdominal cavity from right to left, below the stomach, and then bends downward to become the descending colon. The descending colon extends downward along the left side of the abdomen. At the brim of the pelvis the colon extends in an S-shaped curve down to the sacrum where it becomes the rectum. The curved portion of the colon is called the sigmoid colon. (See also DIGESTIVE SYSTEM and Plates 9 and 10.)

irritable c., spastic c., see COLITIS.

colonitis (ko″lon-i′tis) inflammation of the colon; colitis.

colonopathy (ko″lon-op′ah-the) any disese or disorder of the colon.

colonorrhagia (ko″lon-o-ra′je-ah) hemorrhage from the colon.

colonorrhea (ko″lon-o-re′ah) mucous colitis.

colonoscope (ko-lon′o-skōp) an elongated flexible fiberoptic endoscope which permits visual examination of the entire colon.

colonoscopy (ko″lon-os′ko-pe) endoscopic examination of the colon, either transabdominally during laparotomy, or transanally by means of a colonoscope.

colony (kol′o-ne) a discrete group of organisms, as a collection of bacteria in a culture.

colopexy (kol′o-pek″se) surgical fixation or suspension of the colon.

coloplication (ko″lo-pli-ka′shun) the operation of taking a reef in the colon.

coloproctectomy (ko″lo-prok-tek′to-me) surgical removal of the colon and rectum.

coloproctitis (ko″lo-prok-ti′tis) inflammation of the colon and rectum; colorectitis.

coloproctostomy (ko″lo-prok-tos′to-me) anastomosis of the colon to the rectum.

coloptosis (ko″lop-to′sis) downward displacement of the colon.

colopuncture (ko′lo-pungk″tūr) colocentesis.

color (kul′er) 1. a property of a surface or substance due to absorption of certain light rays and reflection of others within the range of wavelengths (roughly 370 to 760 mμ) adequate to excite the retinal receptors. 2. radiant energy within the range of adequate chromatic stimuli of the retina, i.e., between the infrared and ultraviolet. 3. a sensory impression of one of the rainbow hues.

c. blindness, inability to distinguish between certain colors. Genuine color blindness, a complete inability to see colors, is quite rare, affecting only one person in 300,000. Generally the term describes some form of deficiency of color vision. The most common form is red-green confusion, which affects approximately 8 million people in the United States. There is no known cure for color deficiency.

Color vision is a function of the cones in the retina of the eye, which are stimulated by light and transmit impulses to the brain. It is now thought that there are three types of cones, each type stimulated by one of the primary colors in light (red, green, and violet). Most cases of color deficiency affect either the red or green receptors, so that the two colors do not appear distinct from each other.

Color vision is usually tested with cards called pseudoisochromatic color plates. These have a letter, number, or symbol printed in dots of one color in the midst of dots of gray or other colors. The normal person can see the symbol with no difficulty, but the person with color deficiency cannot distinguish it from the background.

Although color deficiency may occasionally result from injuries, diseases, or certain drugs, most cases are hereditary. The deficiency is most often inherited by males through the mother, who carries the trait from her father although she is not color-deficient herself. In some cases, if the grandfather is color-dificient and the mother carries the trait, a daughter may inherit the disability. The ratio of men to women affected with inherited color deficiency is about 20 to 1.

c. index, an expression of the relative amount of hemoglobin contained in an erythrocyte compared with that of a normal individual of the patient's age and sex. The percentage of hemoglobin is divided by the percentage of erythrocytes.

c. radical, chromophore.

Colorado tick fever a nonexanthematous febrile disease occurring in the Rocky Mountain regions of the United States where the tick vector (*Dermacentor andersoni*) of the causative virus is prevalent.

colorectitis (ko″lo-rek-ti′tis) inflammation of the colon and rectum; coloproctitis.

colorectostomy (ko″lo-rek-tos′to-me) coloproctostomy.

colorectum (ko″lo-rek′tum) the distal 10 inches (25 cm.) of the bowel, including the distal portion of the colon and the rectum, regarded as a unit. adj., **colorec′tal.**

colorimeter (kul″er-im′ĕ-ter) an instrument for measuring color differences; especially one for measuring the color of the blood in order to determine the proportion of hemoglobin.

colorrhaphy (ko-lor′ah-fe) suture of the colon.

colosigmoidostomy (ko″lo-sig″moi-dos′to-me) the surgical anastomosis of a formerly remote portion of the colon to the sigmoid.

colostomy (ko-los′to-me) an artificial opening (stoma) created in the large intestine and brought to the surface of the abdomen for the purpose of evacuating the bowels; also the opening (STOMA) so created. Conditions necessitating colostomy include INTESTINAL OBSTRUCTION, perforation of the bowel, CANCER, and birth defects. The operation may be required in occasional cases of ulcerative colitis.

The artificial anus created by colostomy may be permanent or temporary, depending on the primary condition being treated. The most common types of colostomy are transverse, descending, and sigmoid, the name being derived from the site of the disorder and the location of the stoma.

A transverse colostomy may be located on the right, left, or midline of the abdomen. This type of colostomy usually is done as a temporary measure, allowing for discharge of feces while the diseased portion of the intestine returns to normal. Later, the two ends are anastomosed to restore continuity of the bowel. In most transverse colostomies a loop of the colon is brought out through an abdominal incision and an opening made through the intestine. Observation of the stoma as it functions can determine which side of the colostomy leads from the functioning colon and which side leads to the lower, nonfunctioning segment.

A double-barrelled colostomy is one in which

there are two separate stomas. The proximal or tight-sided stoma provides an opening for the active segment of the colon; the distal or left-sided stoma opens into the inactive segment. The double-barrelled colostomy may later be joined by anastomosis and returned to the abdominal cavity.

Descending and sigmoid colostomies usually are permanent. The colostomy is formed and the diseased portion of the colon and anus are removed (abdominoperineal resection) in a single operation. The stoma created in the descending colon and in the sigmoid colon is usually located on the left side of the abdomen.

PATIENT CARE. Unless otherwise prohibited by physical weakness or mental incompetence, colostomy care is directed toward helping the patient become totally self-sufficient in the care of his colostomy. He is taught to care for the physical aspects of his colostomy and is assisted in adjusting psychologically to a new method of handling solid body waste. This is accomplished in stages, doing for the patient those things he cannot do, showing him the way they can be done, and encouraging him to accept responsibility for his own care. Once having overcome initial shock and revulsion at the prospect of colostomy care, most patients welcome the opportunity to care for themselves in privacy.

Prior to surgery the operative procedure is explained to the patient and he is encouraged at this time to ask questions that are of concern to him. The idea of an artificial anus in the abdominal wall may well be overwhelming to someone who has never heard of the operation. It is best to be open and matter-of-fact in discussing this with the patient, remembering that he cannot be expected to absorb too much information at one time. He should be assured that his questions will be answered as they occur to him, that there will be someone to listen to him when he wants to talk, and that there are many sources of information available to help him through his adjustment.

When the patient is ready to learn about caring for his own colostomy, printed information and teaching aids can be obtained through local offices of national health agencies. For example, the Rehabilitation Program of the American Cancer Society publishes a pamphlet entitled *Colostomies: A Guide,* and the United Ostomy Association provides pamphlets, audiovisual material, a quarterly bulletin, and a monthly newsletter. Many times it is helpful to have the patient talk with someone who has a colostomy and is living a normal active life. A new member of the health team, the certified Enterostomal Therapist, is specially trained to work with colostomy patients and others who have permanent stomas.

Devices for collection of waste passing through the stoma vary in design according to the patient's progress. An open-ended bag is needed until bowel control is developed and then a closed pouch is used. Eventually the patient may need nothing more than a simple dressing over the stoma. Selection of a drainage pouch should be based on the size of the stoma. As the stoma shrinks following surgery, the pouch size is changed so that it fits correctly, not so small as to constrict the stoma, and not so large as to permit leakage around the stoma.

Skin care around the stoma is planned so the area is kept clean and protected from the enzymes and acid in the digestive fluid. The area is washed with soap and water, dried thoroughly, and then a medicated skin barrier such as karaya gum is applied.

Irrigation of a colostomy is prescribed on an individual basis. Not all patients require irrigation to regulate fecal discharge. When irrigation is needed, the newer cone-shaped device is less hazardous and easier for most patients to use. Catheters sometimes cause difficulties in that the patients do not know how far to insert them, they may perforate the intestine, and there often is leakage of the irrigating fluid around the catheter during irrigation. As soon as possible the patient is taught to irrigate his colostomy on a regular schedule based on his previous bowel habits and the availability of time and facilities to perform the procedure in privacy after discharge from the hospital.

The diet of a patient with a colostomy need not be severely restricted. He will need to notice which foods produce gas, diarrhea, and constipation and then adjust his diet to reduce difficulties arising from his own individual problems with certain foods.

Odors may be a source of worry for the patient until he learns to control them with cleanliness, avoidance of gas-producing foods, and the use of deodorants within the pouch. Commercially produced deodorants are available, but if these cannot be found it is possible to eliminate much of the odor by placing four aspirin tablets in the pouch.

colostrum (ko-los′trum) the thin, yellow, milky fluid secreted by the mammary gland a few days before or after parturition.

colotomy (kŏ-lot′o-me) incision of the colon.

colotyphoid (ko″lo-ti′foid) typhoid fever with follicular ulceration of the colon, with extensive lesions in the small intestine.

colovaginal (ko″lo-vaj′ĭ-nal) pertaining to or communicating with the colon and vagina.

colovesical (ko″lo-ves′ĭ-kal) pertaining to or communicating with the colon and urinary bladder.

colp(o)- word element [Gr.], *vagina.*

colpalgia (kol-pal′je-ah) pain in the vagina.

colpatresia (kol″pah-tre′ze-ah) atresia, or occlusion of the vagina.

colpectasia (kol″pek-ta′ze-ah) distention or dilation of the vagina.

colpectomy (kol-pek′to-me) excision of the vagina.

colpeurysis (kol-pu′rĭ-sis) operative dilatation of the vagina.

colpitis (kol-pi′tis) inflammation of the vaginal mucosa; vaginitis.

colpocele (kol′po-sēl) vaginal hernia.

colpocleisis (kol″po-kli′sis) surgical closure of the vaginal canal.

colpocystitis (kol″po-sis-ti′tis) inflammation of the vagina and bladder.

colpocystocele (kol″po-sis′to-sēl) hernia of the bladder into the vagina.

colpocytogram (kol″po-si′to-gram) a differential listing of the cells observed in smears from the vaginal mucosa.

colpocytology (kol″po-si-tol′o-je) the quantitative and differential study of cells exfoliated from the epithelium of the vagina.

colpomicroscope (kol″po-mi′kro-skōp) an instrument for examining stained tissues of the cervix *in situ.*

colpomicroscopy (kol″po-mi-kros′ko-pe) examination by means of a colpomicroscope.

colpoperineoplasty (kol″po-per″ĭ-ne′o-plas″te) plastic repair of the vagina and perineum.

colpoperineorrhaphy (kol″po-per″ĭ-ne-or′ah-fe) suture of the ruptured vagina and perineum.

colpopexy (kol′po-pek″se) suture of a relaxed vagina to the abdominal wall.

colpoplasty (kol′po-plas″te) plastic surgery involving the vagina.

colpoptosis (kol″pop-to′sis) prolapse of the vagina.

colporrhaphy (kol-por′ah-fe) 1. suture of the vagina. 2. the operation of denuding and suturing the vaginal wall to narrow the vagina.

colporrhexis (kol″po-rek′sis) laceration of the vagina.

colposcope (kol′po-skōp) a speculum for examining the vagina and cervix by means of a magnifying lens.

colpospasm (kol′po-spazm) vaginal spasm.

colpostenosis (kol″po-stĕ-no′sis) contraction or narrowing of the vagina.

colpostenotomy (kol″po-stĕ-not′o-me) a cutting operation for stricture of the vagina.

colpotomy (kol-pot′o-me) incision of the vagina with entry into the cul-de-sac.

colpoxerosis (kol″po-ze-ro′sis) abnormal dryness of the vulva and vagina.

columella (kol″u-mel′ah), pl. *columel′lae* [L.] a little column.

c. na′si, the fleshy external termination of the septum of the nose.

column (kol′um) an anatomical part in the form of a pillar-like structure; anything resembling a pillar.

anal c's, vertical folds of mucous membrane at the upper half of the anal canal; called also rectal columns.

anterior c., the anterior portion of the gray substance of the spinal cord, in transverse section seen as a horn.

gray c., the longitudinally oriented parts of the spinal cord in which the nerve cell bodies are found, comprising the gray matter of the spinal cord.

lateral c., the lateral portion of the gray substance of the spinal cord, in transverse section seen as a horn; present only in the thoracic and upper lumbar regions.

posterior c., the posterior portion of the gray substance of the spinal cord, in transverse section seen as a horn.

rectal c's, anal columns.

spinal c., vertebral c., the rigid structure in the midline of the back, composed of the vertebrae. (See also SPINE.)

columna (ko-lum′nah), pl. *colum′nae* [L.] column.

Coly-Mycin (kol′e-mi″sin) trademark for preparations of colistimethate, an antibiotic.

coma (ko′mah) a state of unconsciousness from which the patient cannot be aroused, even by powerful stimuli. In the 1960's, the Harvard Medical School Ad Hoc Committee to Examine the Definition of Brain Death established criteria for determining irreversible coma or brain death. These criteria are often used to complement the traditional criteria for determining DEATH.

PATIENT CARE. The patient in coma requires meticulous care and almost constant surveillance to maintain the integrity and function of all body organs. In the absence of gagging and swallowing reflexes, he must be fed intravenously or by TUBE FEEDING; SUCTIONING is necessary to remove secretions from the mouth and throat and maintain an open AIRWAY. In some cases TRACHEOSTOMY may be performed and a mechanical VENTILATOR used to maintain adequate respiration.

The comatose patient should be turned at least every two hours to relieve pressure on the skin and prevent decubitus ulcers, to aerate the lungs and avoid hypostatic pneumonia, and to maintain good circulation in an effort to prevent formation of blood clots within the blood vessels. In order to minimize the danger of orthopedic deformities he must be positioned so that the body is in good alignment, and his joints are kept functional by range of motion EXERCISES at least once daily.

Incontinence of urine usually is handled by an indwelling catheter and drainage apparatus. Loss of bowel control requires initiating a basic bowel program to prevent fecal impaction. This involves regular digital removal of stool from the rectum or the insertion of a rectal suppository at the same time each day.

The vital signs are taken and recorded at regular intervals throughout the day and night. If the patient is in an intensive care unit, electronic monitoring equipment may be used. A very important part of assessment of the status of the comatose patient is determination of the level of CONSCIOUSNESS. This is done periodically by noting his response to various kinds of stimuli.

In carrying out the many details of the physical care and assessment of the comatose patient, health care personnel must not lose sight of the fact that the patient is a fellow human being and a member of a family. One cannot always be sure exactly how much the patient is aware of the quality of care he is receiving, the gentleness with which he is handled, or the courtesy and respect with which he is treated. Whether he is aware of or totally oblivious to what is being done to and for him, he deserves the same respect afforded an alert and aware patient. Members of his family can be greatly reassured and supported in their ordeal by the knowledge that he is receiving the best of care. With the life support devices now available it is possible for persons in deep coma to live for months and even years.

alcoholic c., stupor accompanying severe alcoholic intoxication.

diabetic c., the coma of severe diabetic ACIDOSIS (see also DIABETES MELLITUS).

hepatic c., coma accompanying cerebral damage resulting from degeneration of liver cells, especially that associated with CIRRHOSIS of the liver.

hyperglycemic hyperosmolar nonketotic c., see under HYPERGLYCEMIC.

irreversible c., coma in which for a period of 24 hours there is complete unreceptivity and unresponsivity even to the most intensely painful stimuli, no spontaneous movement or breathing, absence of elicitable reflexes, and a flat electroencephalogram. Called also brain death syndrome.

Kussmaul's c., the coma and air hunger of diabetic ACIDOSIS (see also DIABETES MELLITUS).

c. vigil, apparent wakefulness with absent or grossly diminished response to outside stimuli; called also akinetic autism.

comatose (ko′mah-tōs) pertaining to or affected with coma.

combustion (kom-bus′chun) rapid oxidation with emission of heat.

comedo (kom′ĕ-do), pl. *comedo′nes.* a blackhead; a plug of keratin and sebum within the dilated orifice of a hair follicle (see also ACNE VULGARIS).

comedomastitis (kom″ĕ-do-mas-ti′tis) a condition characterized chiefly by dilation of the collecting ducts of the mammary gland, inspissation of breast secretion, and inflammation within and around the ducts; called also mammary duct ectasia.

comes (ko′mēz), pl. *com′ites* [L.] an artery or vein accompanying a nerve trunk.

commensal (kŏ-men′sal) 1. living on or within another organism, and deriving benefit without harming or benefiting the host individual. 2. a parasitic organism that causes no harm to the host.

commensalism (kŏ-men′sal-izm) symbiosis in which one population (or individual) is benefited and the other is neither benefited nor harmed.

comminuted (kom′ĭ-nūt″ed) broken or crushed into small pieces, as a comminuted fracture.

comminution (kom″ĭ-nu′shun) the act of breaking, or condition of being broken, into small fragments.

commissura (kom″ĭ-su′rah), pl. *commissu′rae* [L.] commissure.

commissure (kom′ĭ-shūr) a site of union of corresponding parts, as the angle of the lips or eyelids; used also with specific reference to the sites of junction between adjacent cusps of the heart valves.

anterior c., the band of fibers connecting the parts of the two cerebral hemispheres.

middle c., a band of gray matter joining the optic thalami; it develops as a secondary adhesion and may be absent.

posterior c., a large fiber bundle crossing from one side of the cerebrum to the other dorsal to where the aqueduct opens into the third ventricle.

commissurorrhaphy (kom″ĭ-shūr-or′ah-fe) suture of the components of a commissure, to lessen the size of the orifice.

commissurotomy (kom″ĭ-shūr-ot′o-me) surgical incision or digital disruption of the components of a commissure to increase the size of the orifice.

mitral c., the breaking apart of the adherent leaves (commissure) of the mitral valve. This surgical procedure is indicated when the leaflets of the mitral valve have become scarred as a result of inflammation, usually as a complication of rheumatic fever. Normally, these leaflets of the valve open with each pulsation of the heart and allow blood to flow from the left atrium into the left ventricle. They then close as the ventricle fills again, and thus prevent a backward flow of blood. Inflammation and scarring of these leaflets prevents their opening and closing as they should (mitral stenosis) and there is a resultant increase of pressure with the pulmonary artery and hypertrophy of the left ventricle.

Commissurotomy may or may not involve open heart surgery. In one surgical procedure the surgeon feels rather than sees the diseased valve, and breaks apart the adhering leaflets with a finger or dilator. This closed cardiac surgery does not involve the use of the heart-lung machine because the heart is not emptied of blood and the heartbeat is not stopped.

In an open-heart surgical procedure the surgeon can see the diseased valve and he can release the stenosed valve leaflets with his finger or with an instrument called a valvulotome. In this procedure the heart is emptied of blood and circulation of the patient's blood is maintained by a HEART-LUNG MACHINE.

There usually is a dramatic relief of symptoms following mitral commissurotomy. In some cases, however, the valve is badly scarred or there are large deposits of calcium which prevent proper function of the valve and only partial relief can be obtained by surgery. Reoperation may be necessary in some cases when stenosis of the valve recurs.

commmon cold an acute and highly contagious virus infection of the upper respiratory tract; called also acute rhinitis. At least 20 identifiable viruses have been found to cause colds, and they may attack anyone with lowered resistance. Cold viruses are resistant to present antibiotics. Nor is there a really effective preventive vaccine as yet that will work against them in all situations for all people. Having a cold confers only a brief immunity.

SYMPTOMS. All colds are not identical, because of different causative agents and individual reactions. Usually the common cold starts with a runny nose, sneezing, a stuffy feeling in the head, slight headache, watering of the eyes, general aching and listlessness, inability to concentrate, and perhaps a slight fever. The affected membranes swell until the nasal passages are blocked. Often the inflammation spreads to the throat, causing sore throat and cough. The senses of smell and taste are blunted so that the patient hardly knows or cares what he is eating. He has no energy or ambition and just wants to lie down, as in fact he should.

A cold usually begins to subside after several days. The nasal discharge lessens, the membranous swelling decreases and the patient is able to breathe through his nose again. The average cold lasts from 7 to 14 days.

If at any stage the cold shows signs of getting worse—for example, if there are prolonged chills, noticeable fever (above 103° F.), aches in the chest, ears, or face, shortness of breath, coughing up of blood-streaked or rust-colored mucus, or persistent hoarseness—then a physician should be consulted.

TREATMENT. To help avoid complications of all kinds, it is best to take a cold seriously from the beginning. Going to bed at the first signs will accomplish the dual purpose of speeding recovery and preventing the passing on of the cold to others. If it is not possible to stay in bed, extra hours of rest or sleep at night are important. During the "runny" stage, the patient should keep warm and avoid changing temperatures as much as possible. He should drink plenty of liquids and eat moderately of anything that appeals to him. The nose should be blown gently, to avoid forcing the infection into the sinuses and ears.

Aspirin brings the quickest and safest relief. Antibiotics are *not* helpful for colds. They may be prescribed if complications occur. Among the complications that may accompany a cold is SINUSITIS, which occurs when the infection spreads and causes inflammation of the membranes of the paranasal sinuses. The infection may also affect the membranes of the middle ear.

Other complications may occur if the infection

enters the lower respiratory system, including laryngitis, bronchitis, and pneumonia.

communicable disease (kŏ-mu′nĭ-kah-b′l) a disease the causative agents of which may pass or be carried from one person to another directly or indirectly. Modes of transmission include (1) direct contact with body excreta or discharges from an ulcer, open sore, etc.; (2) indirect contact with inanimate objects such as drinking glasses, toys, bedclothing, etc.; (3) vectors—flies, mosquitoes, or other insects capable of spreading the disease.

PATIENT CARE. The goals of patient care include identification of the causative organism, control of the spread of the disease, protection of others from contamination, and specific measures to combat the disease and provide symptomatic relief. Specific techniques of disinfection of contaminated objects and isolation of the patient vary according to the type of causative organism and mode of transmission. (See also ISOLATION TECHNIQUE.)

compaction (kom-pak′shun) a complication of labor in twin births in which there is simultaneous full engagement of the leading fetal poles of both twins, so that the true pelvic cavity is filled and further descent is prevented.

Compazine (kom′pah-zēn) trademark for preparations of prochlorperazine, a major tranquilizer and antiemetic.

compensation (kom″pen-sa′shun) the counterbalancing of any defect of structure or function. In psychoanalysis, the mechanism by which an approved character trait is put forward to hide from the ego the existence of an opposite trait. In cardiology, the maintenance of an adequate blood flow without distressing symptoms. adj., **compen′satory.**

complement (kom′plĕ-ment) a complex series of enzymatic proteins occurring in normal serum that interact to combine with the antigen-antibody complex, producing lysis when the antigen is an intact cell. Complement comprises eleven discrete proteins, or nine functioning components symbolized as C1 through C9, with C1 being divided into subcomponents C1q, C1r, and C1s. Components C3 and C5 are involved in the generation of anaphylatoxin and in the promotion of leukocyte chemotaxis, the result of these two activities being the inflammatory response. C1 and C4 are involved in the neutralization of viruses. The components also combine in various sequences to participate in other biological activities, including antibody-mediated immune lysis, phagocytosis, opsonization, and anaphylaxis. The complement system is known to be activated by the IMMUNOGLOBULINS IgM and IgG. Called also alexin.

c. fixation, when antigen unites with its specific ANTIBODY, complement, if present, is taken into the combine and becomes inactive or fixed. Its presence or absence as free, active complement can be shown by adding sensitized blood cells to the mixture. If free complement is present, hemolysis occurs; if not, no hemolysis is observed. This reaction is the basis of many serologic tests for infection, including the Wassermann test for syphilis, and reactions for gonococcus infection, glanders, typhoid fever, tuberculosis, and amebiasis. Called also Bordet-Gengou phenomenon. (See also IMMUNITY and FIXATION.)

complex (kom′pleks) 1. the sum or combination of various things, like or unlike, as a complex of symptoms. 2. a group of associated, partially or wholly repressed ideas, usually outside of awareness, which can evoke emotional forces that influence an individual's behavior. 3. that portion of an electrocardiographic tracing that represents the systole of an atrium or ventricle.

Electra c., libidinous fixation of a daughter toward her father. (See also OEDIPUS COMPLEX.)

Golgi c., a complex of membranes and vesicles in the cytoplasm; it plays a role in the cell's secretory activities.

inferiority c., unconcious feelings of inferiority, producing timidity or, as a compensation, exaggerated agressiveness and expression of superiority (superiority complex).

Oedipus c., libidinous fixation of a son toward his mother (see also OEDIPUS COMPLEX.)

superiority c., see INFERIORITY COMPLEX.

complexion (kom-plek′shun) the color and appearance of the skin of the face.

compliance (kom-pli′ans) the quality of yielding to pressure or force without disruption, or an expression of the measure of ability to do so, as an expression of the distensibility of an air- or fluid-filled organ, e.g., the lung or urinary bladder, in terms of unit of volume per unit of pressure.

complication (kom″plĭ-ka′shun) 1. a disease(s) concurrent with another disease. 2. the occurrence of two or more disease in the same patient.

compos mentis (kom′pos men′tis) [L.] sound of mind; sane.

compound (kom′pownd) 1. made up of diverse elements or ingredients. 2. a substance made up of two or more materials. 3. in chemistry, a substance made up of two or more elements in union. The elements are united chemically, which means that each of the original elements loses its individual characteristics once it has combined with the other element(s). When elements combine they do so in definite proportions by weight; this is why the union of hydrogen and oxygen always produces water. Sugar, salt, and vinegar are examples of compounds.

Organic compounds are those containing carbon atoms; inorganic compounds are those that do not contain carbon atoms.

acyclic c., aliphatic c., open-chain compound.

closed-chain c., an organic compound in which the carbon atoms are linked together to form a ring.

cyclic c., closed-chain compound.

heterocyclic c., a closed-chain compound in which the ring is made up of dissimilar atoms.

open-chain c., an organic compound in which the carbon atoms are united to form a straight chain; i.e., they do not form a ring.

compress (kom′pres) a square of gauze or similar dressing, for application of pressure or medication to a restricted area, or for local applications of heat or cold.

compression (kom-presh′un) 1. the act of pressing upon or together; the state of being pressed together. 2. in embryology, the shortening or omission of certain developmental stages.

compulsion (kum-pul′shun) an overwhelming urge to perform an irrational act or ritual. adj., **compul′sive.**

computerized axial tomography (CAT) a noninvasive radiologic technique utilizing an x-ray source, an x-ray detector, and a computer to obtain a cross-sectional view of the body (see also computerized transverse axial TOMOGRAPHY).

conarium (ko-na're-um) the pineal body.

conation (ko-na'shun) in psychology, the power that impels effort of any kind; the conscious tendency to act.

conative (kon'ah-tiv) pertaining to the basic strivings of a person, as expressed in his behavior and actions.

concanavalin (kon"kah-nav'ah-lin) either of two phytohemagglutinins isolated along with canavalin from the meal of the Jack bean (*Canavalia ensiformis* and other species of *Canavalia*), which agglutinate the blood of mammals as a result of reaction with polyglucosans. Concanavalin A has been shown to inhibit the growth of ascites tumors.

Concato's disease (kon-ka'tōs) progressive malignant polyserositis with large effusions into the pericardium, pleura, and peritoneum.

concave (kon'kāv) rounded and somewhat depressed or hollowed out.

concavity (kon-kav'ĭ-te) a depression or hollowed surface.

concentrate (kon'sen-trāt) 1. to bring to a common center; to gather at one point. 2. to increase the strength by diminishing the bulk of, as of a liquid; to condense. 3. a drug or other preparation that has been strengthened by evaporation of its nonactive parts.

concentration (kon"sen-tra'shun) 1. increase in strength by evaporation. 2. the ratio of the mass or volume of a solute to the mass or volume of the solution or solvent.

hydrogen ion c., an expression of the degree of acidity or alkalinity (pH) of a solution. (See also ACID-BASE BALANCE.)

c. test, a test of renal function based on the patient's ability to concentrate urine.

concept (kon'sept) the image of a thing held in the mind.

conception (kon-sep'shun) 1. fertilization of the ovum by the spermatozoon. Also, the implantation of the blastocyst in the endometrium. 2. concept.

conceptus (kon-sep'tus) the whole product of conception at any stage of development, from fertilization of the ovum to birth, including extraembryonic membranes as well as the embryo or fetus.

concha (kong'kah), pl. *con'chae* [L.] a shell-shaped structure.

c. of auricle, the hollow of the auricle of the external ear, bounded anteriorly by the tragus and posteriorly by the antihelix.

nasal c., inferior, a bone forming the lower part of the lateral wall of the nasal cavity.

nasal c., middle, the lower of two bony plates projecting from the inner wall of the ethmoidal labyrinth and separating the superior from the middle meatus of the nose.

nasal c., superior, the upper of two bony plates projecting from the inner wall of the ethmoidal labyrinth and forming the upper boundary of the superior meatus of the nose.

nasal c., supreme, a third thin bony plate occasionally found projecting from the inner wall of the ethmoidal labyrinth, above the two usually found.

sphenoidal c., a thin curved plate of bone at the anterior and lower part of the body of the sphenoid bone, on either side, forming part of the roof of the nasal cavity.

conchitis (kong-ki'tis) inflammation of a concha.

conchotomy (kong-kot'o-me) incision of a nasal concha.

conclination (kon"klĭ-na'shun) inward rotation of the upper pole of the vertical meridian of each eye.

concordance (kon-kor'dans) in genetics, the occurrence of a given trait in both members of a twin pair. adj., **concor'dant.**

concrescence (kon-kres'ens) a growing together of parts originally separate.

concretio (kon-kre'she-o) [L.] concretion.

c. cor'dis, adhesive pericarditis in which the pericardial cavity is obliterated.

concretion (kon-kre'shun) 1. a calculus or inorganic mass in a natural cavity or in tissue. 2. abnormal union of adjacent parts. 3. a process of becoming harder or more solid.

concussion (kon-kush'un) a violent jar or shock, or the condition that results from such an injury.

c. of the brain, loss of consciousness, transient or prolonged, due to a blow to the head; there may be transient amnesia, vertigo, nausea, and weak pulse. Breathing often is unusually rapid or slow. Outward evidence of the injury may include bleeding and contusions (bruises). When he regains consciousness, the victim is likely to have severe headache, and he may have blurred vision. If severely injured, he may lapse into a coma.

FIRST AID. The patient is kept lying down and quiet. He should be covered with a blanket or coat, and medical assistance should be obtained. Artificial respiration is given if breathing stops. Stimulants or drugs that may be depressants, e.g., pain relievers, should not be given; these drugs may mask the symptoms and make an accurate diagnosis difficult. (See also HEAD INJURY.)

condensation (kon"den-sa'shun) 1. the act of rendering, or the process of becoming, more compact. 2. the fusion of events, thoughts, or concepts to produce a new and simpler concept. 3. the process of passing from a gaseous to a liquid or solid phase.

condenser (kon-den'ser) 1. a vessel or apparatus for condensing gases or vapors. 2. a device for illuminating microscopic objects. 3. an apparatus for concentrating energy or matter.

condition (kon-dish'un) to train; to subject to conditioning.

conditioned response (kon-dish'und) a response that does not occur naturally in the animal but that may be developed by regular association of some physiologic function with an unrelated outside event, such as ringing of a bell or flashing of a light. Soon the physiological function starts whenever the outside event occurs. Called also conditioned reflex. (See also CONDITIONING.)

conditioning (kon-dish'un-ing) a form of learning in which a response is elicited by a neutral stimulus which previously had been repeatedly presented in conjunction with the stimulus that originally elicited the response. Called also classical and respondent conditioning.

The concept had its beginnings in experimental techniques for the study of reflexes. The traditional procedure is based on the work of Ivan P. Pavlov, a Russian physiologist. In this technique the experimental subject is a dog that is harnessed in a sound-shielded room. The neutral stimulus is the sound of a metronome or bell which occurs each time the dog is presented with food, and the response is the production of saliva by the dog. Eventually the sound of the bell or metronome produces salivation, even though the stimulus that originally elicited the response (the food) is no longer presented.

In the technique just described, the conditioned stimulus is the sound of the bell or metronome, and the conditioned response is the salivation that occurs when the sound is heard. The food, which was the original stimulus to salivation, is the unconditioned stimulus and the salivation that occurred when food was presented is the unconditioned response.

Reinforcement is said to take place when the conditioned stimulus is appropriately followed by the unconditioned stimulus. If the unconditioned stimulus is withheld during a series of trials, the procedure is called extinction because the frequency of the conditioned response will gradually decrease when the stimulus producing the response is no longer present. The process of extinction eventually results in a return of the preconditioning level of behavior.

classical c., see CONDITIONING.

instrumental c., operant c., learning in which a particular response is elicited by a stimulus because that response produces desirable consequences (reward).

Instrumental conditioning differs from classical conditioning in that the reinforcement takes place only after the subject performs a specific act that has been previously designated. If no unconditioned stimulus is used to bring about this act, the desired behavior is known as an operant. Once the behavior occurs with regularity the behavior may be called a conditioned response. The classic example of instrumental or operant conditioning involves the use of the Skinner box, named after B. F. Skinner, an American behavioral psychologist. In this example the subject, a rat, is kept in the box and becomes conditioned to press a bar by being rewarded with food pellets each time its early random movements caused it to press against the bar.

The principles and techniques related to instrumental conditioning are used clinically in BEHAVIOR THERAPY to help patients eliminate undesirable behavior and substitute for it newly learned behavior that is more appropriate and acceptable.

respondent c., see CONDITIONING.

condom (kon′dum) a sheath or cover worn over the penis in coitus, to prevent impregnation or infection.

conductance (kon-duk′tans) ability to conduct or transmit, as electricity or other energy or material; in studies of respiration, an expression of the amount of air reaching the avleoli per unit of time per unit of pressure, the reciprocal of resistance.

conduction (kon-duk′shun) conveyance of energy, as of heat, sound, or electricity.

aerial c., air c., conduction of sound waves to the organ of hearing through the air.

bone c., conduction of sound waves to the inner ear through the bones of the skull.

conductivity (kon″duk-tiv′ĭ-te) capacity for conduction.

condylarthrosis (kon″dil-ar-thro′sis) a modification of the spheroidal form of synovial joint, in which the articular surfaces are ellipsoidal rather than spheroid.

condyle (kon′dīl) a rounded projection on a bone, usually for articulation with another bone.

condylectomy (kon″dil-ek′to-me) excision of a condyle.

condylion (kon-dil′e-on) the most lateral point on the surface of the head of the mandible.

condyloid (kon′dĭ-loid) resembling a condyle.

condyloma (kon″dĭ-lo′mah) an elevated wartlike lesion of the skin. adj., **condylo′matous.**

c. acumina′tum, a small, pointed papilloma of viral origin, usually occurring on the skin or mucous surfaces of the external genitalia or perianal region.

flat c., c. la′tum, a wide, flat, syphilitic condyloma occurring on moist skin, especially about the genitals and anus.

condylotomy (kon″dĭ-lot′o-me) transection of a condyle.

condylus (kon′dĭ-lus), pl. *con′dyli* [L.] condyle.

cone (kōn) 1. a solid figure or body having a circular base and tapering to a point, especially one of the conelike structures of the retina, which, with the retinal rods, form the light-sensitive elements of the retina. The cones make possible the perception of color. 2. in radiology, a conical or open-ended cylindrical structure used as an aid in centering the radiation beam and as a guide to source-to-film distance.

ether c., a cone-shaped device used over the face in administration of ether for anesthesia.

c. of light, the triangular reflection of light seen on the tympanic membrane.

pressure c., the area of compression exerted by a mass in the brain, as in transtentorial herniation.

retinal c′s, see CONE (1).

conexus (kŏ-nek′sus) a connecting structure.

confabulation (kon-fab″u-la′shun) the recitation of imaginary experiences to fill gaps in memory.

configuration (kon-fig″u-ra′shun) 1. the general form of a body. In chemistry, the arrangement in space of the atoms of a molecule. 2. see GESTALT and GESTALTISM.

confinement (kon-fīn′ment) restraint within a specific area; used especially to designate the termination of pregnancy with delivery of an infant.

conflict (kon′flikt) a painful state of consciousness caused by presence of opposing emotional forces or desires and failure to resolve them, found to a certain extent in all persons.

confluence (kon′floo-ens) a running together; a meeting of streams.

c. of sinuses, the dilated point of confluence of the superior sagittal, straight, occipital, and two transverse sinuses of the dura mater.

confusion (kon-fu′zhun) disturbed orientation in regard to time, place, or person, sometimes accompanied by disordered consciousness.

congener (kon′jĕ-ner) something closely related to another thing, as a chemical compound closely related to another in composition and exerting similar or antagonistic effects. adj., **congen′erous.**

congenital (kon-jen′ĭ-tal) present at and existing from the time of birth.

c. heart defect, a structural defect of the heart or

great vessels or both, present at birth. Any number of defects may occur, singly or in combination. They result from improper development of the heart and blood vessels during the prenatal period. Between 30,000 and 40,000 children with one or more heart defects are born annually in the United States.

A fairly common defect is TETRALOGY OF FALLOT, so-called because it involves four major defects and was first described by Fallot. It can, in some instances, be corrected by surgery. Another defect, PATENT DUCTUS ARTERIOSUS, involves the persistent presence of a passage, the ductus arteriosus, between the aorta and pulmonary artery. Normally this passage closes at birth.

VENTRICULAR SEPTAL DEFECT is an opening between the ventricles, often described by laymen as a "hole in the heart." This defect results in a flow of blood directly from one ventricle to the other, resulting in a bypassing of the pulmonary circulation and producing varying degrees of cyanosis because of oxygen deficiency. Defective valves affecting the flow of blood to and from the heart may be associated.

A rarer congenital condition is transposition of the great vessels. In this defect the position of the chief blood vessels of the heart is reversed. The aorta rises from the right ventricle instead of the left, and the pulmonary artery emerges from the left ventricle rather than from the right. The result of this circulatory confusion is that oxygen-poor blood returning from the systemic circulation to the right side of the heart is pumped back into the general circulation instead of being transported to the lungs. Meanwhile, oxygen-rich blood flows aimlessly to and from the lungs. Transposition of the great vessels can sometimes be corrected by surgery.

Another congenital defect results when the ostium primum or ostium secundum, openings in the septum primum of the embryonic heart, fails to close completely after birth. This condition is called atrial septal defect. When an opening remains between the atria, some of the oxygen-rich blood from the left atrium passes into the right atrium and travels back to the lungs without being first transported through the body. Coarctation of the aorta is a narrowing of a portion of the aorta.

In many cases—depending on the severity of the defect and the physical condition of the patient—these congenital conditions can be treated by surgery. Some congenital defects are so minor that they do not significantly affect the action of the heart; these kinds of defects do not require surgery.

The cause of most congenital abnormalities is unknown. In a small number of cases, rubella (German measles) when contracted by the mother during the first 2 or 3 months of pregnancy can cause congenital defects in the baby.

congestion (kon-jes′chun) abnormal accumulation of blood in a part.

congestive (kon-jes′tiv) pertaining to or associated with congestion.

conglobation (kon″glo-ba′shun) the act of forming, or the state of being formed, into a rounded mass.

conglutinant (kon-gloo′tĭ-nant) promoting union, as of the lips of a wound.

conglutination (kon-gloo″tĭ-na′shun) 1. the adherence of tissues to each other. 2. agglutination of erythrocytes that is dependent upon both complement and antibodies.

Congo red (kong′go) a synthetic dye, a derivative of benzidine and naphthionic acid. It is used for differential staining of elastic fibers for microscopic examination. Congo red undergoes a change in hue with acidity and thus can be used as an indicator of pH, turning red in the presence of alkalies (bases) and blue when exposed to acids.

C. r. test, a laboratory test used in the diagnosis of AMYLOIDOSIS. A measured amount of the dye is injected intravenously in one arm and, after a four-minute interval, a blood sample is withdrawn from the opposite arm. Because of the dye's affinity for amyloid, it is removed from the blood stream and deposited in the body tissues of the patient with amyloidosis in greater quantities in a given period of time than in normal persons.

coniofibrosis (ko″ne-o-fi-bro′sis) pneumoconiosis with exuberant growth of connective tissue in the lungs.

coniosis (ko″ne-o′sis) a diseased state due to inhalation of dust.

coniosporosis (ko″ne-o-spo-ro′sis) a condition characterized by asthmatic symptoms and acute pneumonitis, caused by inhalation of spores of *Coniosporium corticale,* a fungus growing under the bark of certain trees; observed in workers engaged in peeling logs.

coniotoxicosis (ko″ne-o-tok″sĭ-ko′sis) pneumoconiosis in which the irritant affects the tissues directly.

conization (ko″nĭ-za′shun) the removal of a cone of tissue, as in partial excision of the cervix uteri.

conjugata (kon″ju-ga′tah) the conjugate diameter of the pelvis (see also PELVIC DIAMETERS).

conjugate (kon′ju-gāt) 1. paired, or equally coupled; working in union. 2. a conjugate diameter of the pelvic inlet; used alone usually to denote the true conjugate diameter (see also PELVIC DIAMETERS).

conjugation (kon″ju-ga′shun) a joining. In unicellular organisms, a form of sexual reproduction in which two individuals join in temporary union to transfer genetic material. In biochemistry, the joining of a toxic substance with some natural substance of the body to form a detoxified product for elimination from the body.

conjunctiva (kon″junk-ti′vah), pl. *conjuncti′vae* [L.] the delicate membrane lining the eyelids and covering the eyeball. adj., **conjuncti′val.**

conjunctivitis (kon-junk″tĭ-vi′tis) inflammation of the conjunctiva. The disorder may be caused by bacteria or a virus, or by allergic, chemical, or physical factors. Its infectious form (of bacterial or viral origin) is highly contagious. The type known as pinkeye, or acute contagious conjunctivitis, is an example of a highly contagious conjunctivitis and must be handled with extreme care to prevent its spread. It is caused by *Hemophilus aegypticus.*

gonorrheal c., a severe form due to infection with gonococci.

inclusion c., conjunctivitis primarily affecting newborn infants, caused by a strain of *Chlamydia trachomatis,* beginning as acute purulent conjunctivitis and leading to papillary hypertrophy of the palpebral conjunctiva.

conjunctivoma (kon-junk″tĭ-vo′mah) a tumor of the eyelid composed of conjunctival tissue.

conjunctivoplasty (kon″junk-ti′vo-plas″te) plastic repair of the conjunctiva.

Conn's syndrome (konz) primary hyperaldosteronism.

connective tissue (kō-nek′tiv) a fibrous type of body tissue with varied functions. The connective tissue system supports and connects internal organs, forms bones and the walls of blood vessels, attaches muscles to bones, and replaces tissues of other types following injury.

Connective tissue consists mainly of long fibers embedded in noncellular matter, the ground substance. The density of these fibers and the presence or absence of certain chemicals make some connective tissues soft and rubbery and others hard and rigid. Compared with most other kinds of tissue, connective tissue has few cells. The fibers contain a protein called collagen.

Connective tissue can develop in any part of the body, and the body uses this ability to help repair or replace damaged areas. Scar tissue is the most common form of this substitute. (See also COLLAGEN DISEASES.)

consanguinity (kon″sang-gwin′ĭ-te) blood relationship; kinship.

conscious (kon′shus) capable of responding to sensory stimuli and having subjective experiences; awake; aware.

consciousness (kon′shus-nes) the state of being conscious; responsiveness of the mind to impressions made by the senses.

levels of c., the somewhat loosely defined states of awareness of and response to stimuli, generally considered an integral component of the assessment of an individual's neurologic status. Levels of consciousness range from behavioral wakefulness and a capacity to respond appropriately to stimuli (fully conscious), to COMA which is complete unconsciousness.

Consciousness depends upon close interaction between the intact cerebral hemispheres and the central gray matter of the upper brain stem. Although the hemispheres contribute most of the specific components of consciousness (memory, intellect, and learned responses to stimuli), there must be arousal or activation of the cerebral cells before they can function. For this reason, it is suggested that a detailed description of the patient's response to specific auditory, visual, and tactile stimuli will be more meaningful to those concerned with neurologic assessment than would the use of such terms as "stuperous," "semiconscious," or other equally subjective terms.

Examples of the kinds of stimuli that may be used to determine a patient's responsiveness as a measure of consciousness include calling him by name, producing a sharp noise, giving simple commands, gentle shaking, pinching the biceps, and application of a blood pressure cuff. Responses to stimuli should be reported in specific terms relative to how the patient responded, whether the response was appropriate, and what occurred immediately after the response.

consolidation (kon-sol″ĭ-da′shun) solidification; the process of becoming solidified or the condition of being solid; said especially of the lung as it fills with exudate in pneumonia.

constipation (kon″stĭ-pa′shun) ordinarily a condition in which the waste matter in the bowels is too hard to pass easily, or in which bowel movements are so infrequent that discomfort or uncomfortable symptoms result. Many people also use the term when referring to a sense of incomplete evacuation or when they feel they should have more frequent bowel movements. The frequency of bowel movements varies according to individual body make-up, type of intestine, eating habits, physical activity, and custom.

CAUSES. An organic cause of constipation may be a disease such as hypothyroidism. Or there may be a structure or obstruction that prevents wastes from being passed through the intestines, as in the case of hernia, tumor, or cancerous growth. Often constipation from such obstructions comes on suddenly.

SYMPTOMS. Prolonged constipation, called obstipation, can cause such uncomfortable symptoms as nausea, heartburn, headache, or distress in the rectum or intestines, which may last until the stool is passed. These symptoms are not due to the absorption of poisons from the waste material, as some people believe. Rather they are a reaction of the nerves when the rectum is distended by the matter it contains. This condition is uncomfortable rather than harmful.

PREVENTION AND TREATMENT. Elimination is largely a matter of habit. Therefore it is desirable to establish a regular routine for it. Sensible living can also help to prevent or combat constipation. Emotional tension and strain can cause constipation. Therefore, it is important to avoid unnecessary tensions and worry, including concern over constipation itself.

When constipation does not respond to roughage added to the diet and an effort to improve bowel habits, an enema may be advisable, or a mild laxative such as petroleum and agar, aromatic cascara sagrada, or milk of magnesia may be taken. Laxatives should be resorted to only after the bowels have been given a chance to function by themselves. The frequent and often unnecessary use of laxatives can be the cause of constipation, rather than its cure. Cathartics, such as castor oil, which are more powerful in their purgative action than laxatives, should never be used unless prescribed by a physician. (See also BOWEL TRAINING.)

constitution (kon″stĭ-tu′shun) 1. the make-up or functional habit of the body. 2. the order in which the atoms of a molecule are joined together.

constitutional (kon″stĭ-tu′shun-al) 1. affecting the whole constitution of the body; not local. 2. pertaining to the constitution.

constriction (kon-strik′shun) 1. a narrowing or compression of a part; a stricture. 2. a diminution in range of thinking or feeling, associated with diminished spontaneity.

constrictor (kon-strik′tor) that which causes constriction.

consultant (kon-sul′tant) a physician or surgeon whose opinion on diagnosis or treatment is sought by the physician originally attending a patient.

consultation (kon″sul-ta′shun) a deliberation of two or more physicians about diagnosis or treatment in a particular case.

consumption (kon-sump′shun) 1. the act of consuming, or the process of being consumed. 2. a wasting away of the body; once applied especially to pulmonary tuberculosis.

contact (kon′takt) 1. a mutual touching of two bodies or persons. 2. an individual known to have been sufficiently near an infected person to have been exposed to the transfer of infectious material.

c. dermatitis, a skin rash marked by itching, swelling, blistering, oozing, and scaling. It is caused by direct contact between the skin and a substance to which the person is allergic or sensitive. The rash usually occurs only on that area of the body that has come into contact with the irritating substance. The most common form of contact dermatitis is that caused by POISON IVY, OAK, or SUMAC. Other plants, too, sometimes cause an allergic reaction. Contact dermatitis may also be caused by industrial oils, medicines, cosmetics, perfumes, mouthwashes, deodorants, rubber, plastics, metals, and clothing made of various materials and treated with certain preservatives and dyes. A nonallergic form, primary-irritant dermatitis, may be induced by a substance acting as an irritant rather than as a sensitizer or allergen. Some soaps, detergents, and other cleansing products can cause a condition of the hands often referred to as "housewives' dermatitis" (or "dishpan hands"). (See also DERMATITIS.)

direct c., immediate c., the contact of a healthy person with a person having a communicable disease, the disease being transmitted as a result.

indirect c., that achieved through some intervening medium, as propagation of a communicable disease through the air or by means of fomites.

c. lenses, corrective lenses that fit directly over the cornea of the eye, for correction of refractive errors. They do not actually touch the surface of the eye, but float on a thin layer of the fluid that naturally moistens the eyeball. Contact lenses are made of glass or plastic, and are invisible when in place. Their invisibility is one of their chief advantages. There are certain disadvantages to contact lenses. It takes time to become accustomed to wearing them, and even with practice most people cannot wear them for more than 6 or 8 hours at a time without irritation to the eyes. Since they must be molded to the exact shape of the patient's corneas, they are quite expensive. A soft, hydrophilic contact lens is also available.

mediate c., indirect contact.

contactant (kon-tak′tant) an allergen capable of inducing delayed contact-type hypersensitivity of the epidermis after one or more episodes of contact.

contagion (kon-ta′jun) 1. the spread of disease from one person to another. 2. a contagious disease.

contagiosity (kon-ta″je-os′ĭ-te) the quality of being contagious.

contagious (kon-ta′jus) capable of being transmitted from person-to-person.

contaminant (kon-tam′ĭ-nant) something that causes contamination.

contamination (kon-tam″ĭ-na′shun) 1. the soiling or making inferior by contact or mixture, as by introduction of organisms into a wound. 2. the deposition of radioactive material in any place where it is not desired.

content (kon′tent) that which is contained within a thing.

latent c., the part of a dream that is hidden in the unconsciousness.

manifest c., the part of a dream that is remembered after awakening.

continence (kon′tĭ-nens) the ability to exercise voluntary control over natural impulses, such as the urge to defecate or urinate. adj., **con′tinent.**

contra- word element [L.], *against; opposed.*

contra-aperture (kon″trah-ap′er-tūr) a second opening made in an abscess to facilitate the discharge of its contents.

contraception (kon″trah-sep′shun) prevention of conception or impregnation. Contraception may be achieved by several methods. (See also BIRTH CONTROL.)

RHYTHM METHOD. This is called the natural method since it uses no artificial means and is based on the natural cycle of ovulation in the female. The period of possible conception usually lasts from 2 days before ovulation through 1 day after it, or 3 days in all; during these days if conception is to be prevented the woman must abstain from coitus. The other days of the cycle constitute the so-called "safe period." In practice, however, the safe period is considered to be shorter, since ovulation generally occurs between the twelfth and sixteenth days of the cycle, so that any of these days must be counted as days of possible conception. (The first day of the cycle in the first day of menstruation.)

To calculate the fertile period, it is necessary to keep an accurate record of menstrual cycles for 8 to 12 months. The length of the longest and shortest cycles must be carefully noted over this time.

It is also possible to determine when ovulation takes place by daily readings of body temperature since the temperature is elevated after ovulation takes place.

OVULATION METHOD. Recent research into "rhythm failures" has led to the development of a more reliable technique of natural contraception, the ovulation method. It is based on an awareness of days of "dryness" and days of "wetness" during the menstrual cycle, and recognition of the significance of a unique "fertile mucus" which appears in the vaginal area at the time of ovulation. According to proponents of this method, appearance of the mucus signals the onset of the period during which impregnation can occur.

Success of the ovulation method depends on the female's ability to observe and recognize the characteristics of a vaginal discharge which gives warning of the period of ovulation. The cycle begins with the onset of menstruation. Following menses there are "early dry days" during which no mucus is seen or felt in the vaginal area. With the ripening of the ovum just prior to ovulation, there is production of some opaque and sticky mucus which is generally yellow or white. As the menstrual cycle proceeds and hormonal changes take place, the blood estrogen level reaches a critical stage, at which point the cervical glands begin to produce the fertile mucus. This mucus usually appears three days prior to ovulation, though the time may vary with individuals. It is cloudy at first and then becomes clear, similar in appearance and consistency to the white of an uncooked egg. The vaginal area has a sensation of wetness or lubrication. The egg is released from the follicle within 24–48 hours of the peak of wetness.

It is recommended that those persons using the ovulation method of contraception refrain from sexual intercourse from the first appearance of the fertile mucus through the height of the sensation of wetness and then for an additional 72 hours. The reason for this precaution is that the fertile mucus produced by the glands at the time of ovulation helps keep the sperm alive and active and facilitates penetration of the ovum. Should there be sperm present before ovulation occurs, the mucus can help maintain their potency until the egg is released from the follicle and is available for impregnation.

The life span of the sperm is in part determined by the presence of the fertile mucus, therefore an additional 72 hours after the period of wetness assures that the ovum has been released and expelled through the vaginal tract without becoming impregnated.

One of the major advantages of this method over the rhythm method is that it can be used by women with irregular menstrual cycles and does not rely on extensive keeping of accurate records of menstrual cycles.

ORAL CONTRACEPTIVES. Considered to be the most reliable of all nonsurgical methods of contraception, and popularly referred to as "the pill," this method involves taking, for a set number of days each month, an oral form of hormone or hormone-like products that duplicate the action of estrogen and progesterone in women. Oral contraceptives can be obtained by prescription only, as they may produce serious side effects in women with such disorders as cardiovascular and renal disease, diabetes, epilepsy, migraine headaches, and others, including mental depression. The average woman in good health may experience some minor side effects including nausea, a feeling of fullness, or weight gain.

Other hormonal contraceptives are currently being tested. These include the once-a-month pill, the morning-after pill, and the every-three-month injection. Research on hormonal contraceptives for the male is currently being conducted.

PERMANENT STERILIZATION. Irreversible contraceptive techniques involving surgical procedures include salpingectomy, tubal ligation, and vasectomy. Newer techniques utilizing endoscopy include hysteroscopic, culdoscopic, and laparoscopic STERILIZATION.

MECHANICAL AND CHEMICAL MEANS

Condom and Cervical Diaphragm. The condom is a thin flexible sheath worn over the penis to prevent entry of spermatozoa into the vagina during coitus. The diaphragm is a cup-shaped device of molded rubber or other soft plastic material, with a flexible spring forming the circular outer edge. It is inserted in the vagina in such a position that it covers the cervix uteri and prevents entry of spermatozoa. The diaphragm is used in conjunction with a spermicidal cream or jelly.

Jellies, Creams, and Foams. A number of contraceptive jellies, or gels, creams, and aerosol foams are made to be used without any mechanical device. These are more powerful in their spermicidal effects than the creams and jellies to be used with diaphragms. Doubt has been cast on their reliability and there have also been objections to them on esthetic grounds.

INTRAUTERINE DEVICES. These consist of a ring, spiral, coil, loop, T, or other shape that is permanently placed inside the uterine cavity. Although the mechanism is not completely understood, it is believed that these devices do not interfere with fertilization but rather in some way render implantation of the fertilized ovum impossible. The advantage of the intrauterine device is that once it has been inserted by the physician it can be left in place for as long as a year, after which it can be removed for a short pĕriod and then reinserted. (See also INTRAUTERINE CONTRACEPTIVE DEVICES.)

ANTIZYGOTIC AGENTS. Experimental work is being carried on with agents that will inhibit the development of the ovum; to date the experiments have been confined to laboratory animals. Antispermatogenic agents, which would inhibit the development of sperm, are also being studied.

contraceptive (kon″trah-sep′tiv) 1. diminishing the likelihood of or preventing conception. 2. an agent that diminishes the likelihood of or prevents conception. (See also CONTRACEPTION.)

contractile (kon-trak′til) having the power or tendency to contract in response to a suitable stimulus.

contractility (kon″trak-til′ĭ-te) a capacity for becoming short in response to suitable stimulus.

contraction (kon-trak′shun) a drawing together; a shortening or shrinkage.

Braxton Hicks c's, light, usually painless, irregular uterine contractions during pregnancy, gradually increasing in intensity and frequency and becoming more rhythmic during the third trimester (see also BRAXTON HICKS CONTRACTIONS.)

carpopedal c., the condition resulting from chronic shortening of the muscles of the fingers, toes, arms, and legs in tetany.

Dupuytren's c., Dupuytren's contracture.

Hicks c's, Braxton Hicks contractions.

isometric c., see ISOMETRIC CONTRACTION.

isotonic c., see ISOTONIC CONTRACTION.

postural c., the state of muscular tension and contraction that just suffices to maintain the posture of the body.

tetanic c., tonic c., sustained muscular contraction with alternating relaxation.

Volkmann's c., Volkmann's contracture.

contracture (kon-trak′tūr) abnormal shortening of muscle tissue, rendering the muscle highly resistant to stretching. A contracture can lead to permanent disability. It can be caused by fibrosis of the tissues supporting the muscle or the joint, or by disorders of the muscle fibers themselves.

Improper support and positioning of joints affected by arthritis or injury, and inadequate exercising of joints in patients with paralysis can result in contractures. For example, a patient with arthritis or severe burns may assume a position most comfortable for him and will resist changing position because motion is painful. If the joints are allowed to remain in this position, the muscle fibers that normally provide motion will stretch or shorten to accommodate the position and eventually they will lose their ability to contract and relax.

In many cases contractures can be prevented by proper exercise (active or passive), and by adequate support of the joints to eliminate constant shortening or stretching of the muscles and surrounding tissues.

Dupuytren's c., a flexion deformity of the fingers or toes, due to shortening, thickening, and fibrosis of the palmar or plantar fascia.

ischemic c., muscular contracture and degeneration due to interference with the circulation due to pressure or to injury or cold.

Volkmann's c., contraction of the fingers and sometimes of the wrist, or of analogous parts of the foot, with loss of power, after severe injury or improper use of a tourniquet or cast in the region of the elbow.

contrafissure (kon″trah-fish′er) a fracture in a part opposite the site of the blow.

contraindication (kon″trah-in″dĭ-ka′shun) any condition that renders a particular line of treatment improper or undesirable.

contralateral (kon″trah-lat′er-al) pertaining to, situated on, or affecting the opposite side.

contrast medium (kon′trast) a radiopaque substance used in roentgenography to permit visualization of internal body structures.

contrecoup (kon″truh-koo′) [Fr.] denoting an injury, as to the brain, occurring at a site opposite to the point of impact.

control (kon-trōl′) 1. the governing or limitation of certain objects or events. 2. a standard against which experimental observations may be evaluated, as a procedure identical to the experimental procedure except for the absence of the one factor being studied. Also, any individual of the group exhibiting the standard characteristics.

birth c., regulation of childbearing by measures designed to prevent conception (see also BIRTH CONTROL and CONTRACEPTION).

contuse (kon-tūz′) to bruise; to injure without breaking the skin.

contusion (kon-too′zhun) injury to tissues without breakage of skin; a bruise. In a contusion, blood from the broken vessels accumulates in surrounding tissues, producing pain, swelling, and tenderness. A discoloration appears as a result of blood seepage under the surface of the skin.

Most contusions heal without special treatment, but cold compresses may reduce bleeding, and thus reduce swelling and discoloration, and relieve pain. If a contusion is unusually severe, the injured part should be rested and slightly elevated. Later the application of heat may hasten the absorption of blood.

Serious complications may develop in some cases of contusion. Normally blood is drawn off from the bruised area in a few days, but there is a possibility that blood clotted in the area will form a cyst or calcify and require surgical treatment. The contusion may also be complicated by infection.

cerebral c., contusion of the brain following a HEAD INJURY. It may occur with extradural or subdural collections of blood, in which case the patient may be left with neurologic defects or EPILEPSY. (See also cranial HEMATOMA.)

conus (ko′nus), pl. *co′ni* [L.] 1. a cone or cone-shaped structure. 2. posterior staphyloma of the myopic eye.

c. arterio′sus, the anterosuperior portion of the right ventricle of the heart, at the entrance to the pulmonary trunk.

c. medulla′ris, the cone-shaped lower end of the spinal cord, at the level of the upper lumbar vertebrae.

convalescence (kon″vah-les′ens) the stage of recovery from an illness, operation, or injury.

convalescent (kon″vah-les′ent) 1. pertaining to or characterized by convalescence. 2. a patient who is recovering from a disease, operation, or injury.

convection (kon-vek′shun) the act of conveying or transmission; specifically, transmission of heat in a liquid or gas by circulation of heated particles.

convergence (kon-ver′jens) 1. a moving together, or inclination toward a common point; the coordinated movement of the two eyes toward fixation of the same near point. 2. the point of meeting of convergent lines. adj., **conver′gent.**

conversion (kon-ver′zhun) 1. the act of changing into something of different form or properties. 2. the transformation of emotions into physical manifestations. 3. manipulative correction of malposition of a fetal part during labor.

c. reaction, a mental mechanism that is unconsciously employed by an individual to solve a strong emotional conflict. In conversion reaction the patient "converts" his emotional distress into any of a wide variety of physical symptoms, none of which have any organic basis. Among the symptoms which may develop are deafness, blindness, and paralysis of a limb. The symptom chosen by the patient can be related to his particular emotional conflict, and his reaction to the symptom appears to be one of indifference. This is not surprising when one realizes that the patient is using the symptom to obtain relief from a distressing conflict in his mind, and that such a symptom often provokes sympathy and a solicitous attitude from the person or persons involved in the conflict. Treatment of conversion reaction is aimed at helping the patient find more realistic ways of solving his emotional conflict.

convex (kon′veks) having a rounded, somewhat elevated surface.

convolution (kon″vo-lu′shun) a tortuous irregularity or elevation caused by the infolding of a structure upon itself.

convulsion (kun-vul′shun) an involuntary contraction or series of contractions of voluntary muscles. In general there are three types of convulsions: clonic, in which opposing muscles contract and relax alternately, producing rhythmic movements; tonic, in which all the muscles tighten until the victim becomes rigid; and those that occur in jacksonian epilepsy, in which the muscular twitching begins in one area and spreads to another.

CAUSES. Convulsions may arise from any of a number of changes in the chemical balance of the body. Insufficient amounts of sugar, calcium, or various hormones in the blood may bring on seizures. Accumulation of waste products in the blood, such as occurs in uremia, or toxic conditions such as toxemia of pregnancy can produce convulsions. Disease or injury to the brain or central nervous system may also be severe enough to set off convulsions. Drug poisoning frequently produces convulsions. The seizures associated with EPILEPSY are a form or convulsion.

PATIENT CARE. Prevention of injury to the patient is the first concern. If convulsions are likely, side rails should be applied to the bed and then padded with cotton blankets. The head of the bed should be covered with a folded blanket or pillow to avoid trauma to the head during the seizure. A padded tongue depressor is kept at the bedside at all times. This is used to place between the patient's teeth so that he will not bite his tongue or the inside of his mouth during the convulsion. No restraint should be used.

Observations before and during the convulsion should include: The time the convulsion began; whether the patient had any warning or specific symptoms (AURA) just before the convulsion occurred, and the length of time it lasted; the type of convulsion and the area in which it began, and whether it was restricted to one part of the body or was generalized; whether the patient lost consciousness or was incontinent of urine or feces; the effects of the convulsion on the patient's pulse and respiration, and any other objective symptoms such as change in color or profuse perspiration.

convulsive (kon-vul′siv) pertaining to, characterized by, or of the nature of a convulsion.

Cooley's anemia (koo'lēz) the hemozygous form of β-THALASSEMIA.

Coolidge tube (koo'lij) a vacuum tube for the generation of roentgen rays in which the cathode consists of a spiral filament of incandescent tungsten, and the anode (the target) of massive tungsten.

Coombs tests (koomz) laboratory tests that reveal certain antigen-antibody reactions; used in differentiating between various types of hemolytic anemias, for determining minor blood types, including the RH FACTOR, and for testing for anticipated ERYTHROBLASTOSIS FETALIS.

direct C. t., the test used to detect the presence of antibodies that may damage erythrocytes but will not cause visible agglutination. Clinically its most important use is in early diagnosis of erythroblastosis fetalis and autoimmune HEMOLYTIC ANEMIAS. It is used also in crossmatching blood for transfusions. Venous blood or blood from the umbilical cord may be used.

indirect C. t., a test for detecting incompatibility in transfusions when the recipient has a greater than normal risk of TRANSFUSION REACTION. The test also can reveal the presence of anti-Rh antibodies in maternal blood during pregnancy. Either clotted blood or blood with an anticoagulant may be used.

coordination (ko-or"dĭ-na'shun) the harmonious functioning of interrelated organs and parts. Applied especially to the process of the motor apparatus of the brain which provides for the coworking of particular groups of muscles for the performance of definite adaptive useful responses.

COPD chronic obstructive pulmonary disease.

copiopia (ko"pe-o'pe-ah) eyestrain.

copolymer (ko-pol'ĭ-mer) a polymer containing monomers of more than one kind.

copper (kop'er) a chemical element, atomic number 29, atomic weight 63.54, symbol Cu. (See table of ELEMENTS.) It is necessary for bone formation and for the formation of blood because it acts as a catalyst in the transformation of inorganic iron into hemoglobin. There is little danger of deficiency in ordinary diets because of relatively abundant supply and minute daily requirements.

c. sulfate, cupric sulfate.

coprecipitin (ko"pre-sip'ĭ-tin) any of two or more precipitins in the same serum.

copremesis (kop-rem'ĕ-sis) the vomiting of fecal matter.

coproantibody (kop"ro-an'tĭ-bod-e) an antibody (chiefly IgA) present in the intestinal tract, associated with immunity to enteric infection.

coprolalia (kop"ro-la'le-ah) the utterance of obscene words, especially words relating to feces.

coprolith (kop'ro-lith) a hard fecal concretion in the intestine.

coprology (kop-rol'o-je) the study of the feces.

coprophagia (kop"ro-fa'je-ah) the ingestion of dung, or feces.

coprophilia (kop"ro-fil'e-ah) a psychopathologic interest in filth, especially in feces and defecation.

coprophilic (kop"ro-fil'ik) 1. pertaining to or characterized by coprophilia. 2. inhabiting dung or feces; said of bacteria.

coprophobia (kop"ro-fo'be-ah) abnormal repugnance to defecation and to feces.

coproporphyria (kop"ro'por-fir'e-ah) hereditary PORPHYRIA marked by excessive excretion of coproporphyrin, chiefly in the feces.

coproporphyrin (kop"ro'por'fĭ-rin) a porphyrin formed in the blood-forming organs and intestine and found in the urine and feces in coproporphyrinuria.

coproporphyrinogen (kop"ro-por"fĭ-rin'o-jen) the fully reduced, colorless compound giving rise to coproporphyrin by oxidation.

coproporphyrinuria (kop"ro-por"fĭ-rĭ-nu're-ah) the presence of coproporphyrin in the urine.

coprostasis (kop-ros'tah-sis) fecal impaction.

coprozoic (kop"ro-zo'ik) living in fecal matter.

copula (kop'u-lah) any connecting part or structure.

copulation (kop"u-la'shun) sexual union or coitus; usually applied to the mating process in animals lower than man.

cor (kor) [L.] heart.

c. bovi'num, a greatly enlarged heart due to a hypertropied left ventricle.

c. pulmona'le, a serious cardiac condition in which there is right ventricular heart failure due to pulmonary hypertension secondary to disease of the blood vessels of the lungs. Acute cor pulmonale is an emergency situation arising from a sudden dilatation of the right ventricle as a result of pulmonary embolism. Chronic cor pulmonale develops gradually and is associated with such CHRONIC OBSTRUCTIVE PULMONARY DISEASES as EMPHYSEMA, SILICOSIS, and fibrosis of the lung following an infection. These conditions impair pulmonary circulation and thus create a "damming" effect on the blood flowing through the pulmonary artery. This in turn slows down the flow of blood from the right ventricle, and the ventricle becomes hypertrophied and dilated.

SIGNS AND SYMPTOMS. Symptoms are similar to those of congestive heart failure from other causes: dyspnea, edema of the lower extremities, enlargement of the liver, and distention of the veins in the neck. The hematocrit is increased as the body attempts to compensate for impaired circulation by producing more erythrocytes.

TREATMENT. Treatment is ultimately aimed at relief of the lung disorder causing the condition and relieving the pulmonary insufficiency. This includes the administration of bronchodilators and the use of a mechanical VENTILATOR to reduce hypoxia and dyspnea. Severe polycythemia and hypervolemia may require phlebotomy to lower the blood volume and red cell count. The heart failure is treated with digitalis, diuretics, adequate rest, and dietary measures. (See also HEART FAILURE.)

coracoid (kor'ah-koid) 1. like a crow's beak. 2. the coracoid process, a projection from the upper part of the neck of the scapula, overhanging the shoulder joint.

Coramine (ko'rah-min) trademark for preparations of nikethamide, a central nervous system and respiratory stimulant.

cord (kord) any long, cylindrical, flexible structure.

spermatic c., the strucutre extending from the abdominal inguinal ring to the testis, comprising the pampiniform plexus, nerves, ductus deferens, testicular artery, and other vessels.

spinal c., that part of the central nervous system lodged in the spinal canal, extending from the foramen magnum to upper part of the lumbar region. (See Plates 12, 13, and 14.)

umbilical c., the structure connecting the fetus and placenta, and containing the channels through which fetal blood passes to and from the placenta (see also UMBILICAL CORD).

vocal c's, folds of mucous membrane in the larynx, the superior pair being called the false, and the inferior pair the true, vocal cords (see also VOCAL CORDS).

cordal (kor'dal) pertaining to a cord; used specifically in referring to the vocal cords.

cordate (kor'dāt) heart-shaped.

cordectomy (kor-dek'to-me) excision of a cord, as of a vocal cord.

corditis (kor-di'tis) inflammation of the spermatic cord.

cordopexy (kor'do-pek"se) surgical fixation of a vocal cord.

cordotomy (kor-dot'o-me) 1. section of a vocal cord. 2. chordotomy.

Cordran (kor'dran) trademark for preparations of flurandrenolide, a topical glucocorticoid.

core(o)- word element [Gr.], *pupil of the eye.*

corectasis (kor-ek'tah-sis) morbid dilatation of the pupil of the eye.

corectome (ko-rek'tōm) a cutting instrument for iridectomy.

corectomy (ko-rek'to-me) iridectomy.

corectopia (kōr"ek-to'pe-ah) abnormal location of the pupil of the eye.

coredialysis (ko"re-di-al'ĭ-sis) surgical separation of the external margin of the iris from the ciliary body.

corediastasis (ko"re-di-as'tah-sis) dilatation of the pupil.

corelysis (ko-rel'ĭ-sis) operative destruction of the pupil; especially detachment of adhesions of the pupillary margin of the iris from the lens.

coremorphosis (ko"re-mor-fo'sis) surgical formation of an artificial pupil.

corenclisis (ko"ren-kli'sis) iridencleisis.

coreometer (ko"re-om'ĕ-ter) pupillometer.

coreoplasty (kor're-o-plas"te) any plastic operation on the pupil.

corepressor (ko"re-pres'or) a substance (e.g., the product of a metabolic pathway) that activates a repressor by combining with it.

coretomy (ko-ret'o-me) iridotomy.

Cori's disease (ko'rēz) Forbes' disease.

corium (ko're-um) the dermis; true skin; the fibrous inner layer of the skin just beneath the epidermis, derived from the embryonic mesoderm, varying from 1/50 to 1/8 inch in thickness, well supplied with nerves and blood vessels and containing hair roots and sebaceous and sweat glands; on the palms and soles it bears ridges whose arrangement in whorls and loops is peculiar to the individual.

corn (korn) a circumscribed, conical, horny induration and thickening of the stratum corneum that causes severe pain by pressure on nerve endings in the corium. Corns are always caused by friction or pressure from poorly fitting shoes or hose. There are two kinds: the hard corn, usually located on the outside of the little toe or on the upper surfaces of the other toes; and the soft corn, found between the toes, usually the fourth and fifth toes, kept softened by moisture.

cornea (kor'ne-ah) the clear, transparent anterior covering of the EYE (see also Plate 15). The cornea is subject to injury by foreign bodies in the eye, bacterial infection, and viral infection, especially by the herpesvirus that causes HERPES SIMPLEX. The herpesvirus that causes HERPES ZOSTER (shingles), can also infect the cornea. Prompt treatment of any corneal injury or infection is essential to avoid ulceration and loss of vision.

corneal (kor'ne-al) pertaining to the cornea.

c. reflex, a reflex action of the eye resulting in automatic closing of the eyelid when the cornea is stimulated. The corneal reflex can be elicited in a normal person by gently touching the cornea with a wisp of cotton. Absence of the corneal reflex indicates deep coma or injury of one of the nerves carrying the reflex arc.

corneitis (kor"ne-i'tis) keratitis.

corneoiritis (kor"ne-o-i-ri'tis) inflammation of the cornea and iris, keratoiritis.

corneosclera (kor"ne-o-skle'rah) the cornea and sclera regarded as one organ.

corneous (kor'ne-us) hornlike or horny; consisting of keratin.

cornification (kor"nĭ-fĭ-ka'shun) 1. conversion into keratin, or horn. 2. conversion of epithelium to the stratified squamous type.

cornified (kor'nĭ-fīd) converted into horny tissue (keratin); keratinized.

cornu (kor'nu), pl. *cor'nua* [L.] horn; a hornlike excrescence or projection; an anatomic structure that appears horn-shaped, especially in section.

c. ammo'nis, hippocampus.

c. sacra'le, either of two hook-shaped processes extending downward from the arch of the last sacral vertebra.

cornual, cornuate (kor'nu-al; kor'nu-āt) pertaining to a horn, especially to the horns of the spinal cord.

corona (kŏ-ro'nah), pl. *coro'nae* [L.] a crown; in anatomic nomenclature, a crownlike eminence or encircling structure. adj., **coro'nal.**

c. radia'ta, 1. the radiating crown of projection fibers passing from the internal capsule to every part of the cerebral cortex. 2. an investing layer of radially elongated follicle cells surrounding the zona pellucida of the ovum.

coronary (kor'ŏ-nar-e) encircling in the manner of a crown; a term applied to vessels, ligaments, nerves, etc.

c. arteries, two large arteries that branch from the ascending aorta and supply all of the heart muscle with blood (see also table of ARTERIES).

c. insufficiency, decreased supply of blood to the myocardium resulting from constriction or obstruction of the coronary arteries, but not accompanied by necrosis of the myocardial cells. Called also myocardial ischemia.

c. occlusion, the occlusion, or closing off, of a coronary artery. The occlusion may result from formation of a clot (thrombosis), but it is most often caused by a narrowing of the lumen of the blood vessels by the plaques of ATHEROSCLEROSIS. If there is adequate collateral circulation to the heart muscle at the time of the occlusion, there may be little or no damage to the myocardial cells. When occlusion is complete, however, with no blood being supplied to an area of the myocardium, MYOCARDIAL INFARCTION results.

c. sinus, the terminal portion of the great cardiac vein, which lies in the cardiac sulcus between the left atrium and ventricle, and empties into the right atrium.

c. thrombosis, formation of a clot in a coronary artery. (See also MYOCARDIAL INFARCTION.)

coronavirus (kor″o-nah-vi′rus) any of a group of morphologically similar, ether-sensitive viruses, probably RNA, causing infectious bronchitis of birds, hepatitis in mice, gastroenteritis in swine, and respiratory infections in humans.

coroner (kor′o-ner) an official of a local community who holds inquests concerning sudden, violent, or unexplained deaths.

coronoidectomy (kor″o-noi-dek′to-me) surgical removal of the coronoid process of the mandible.

coroscopy (ko-ros′ko-pe) retinoscopy, or skiametry.

corotomy (ko-rot′o-me) iridotomy.

corpulency (kor′pu-len″se) undue fatness; OBESITY.

corpus (kor′pus), pl. *cor′pora* [L.] body.

c. albi′cans, white fibrous tissue that replaces the regressing corpus luteum in the human ovary in the latter half of pregnancy, or soon after ovulation when pregnancy does not supervene.

cor′pora amyla′cea, small hyaline masses of degenerate cells found in the prostate, neuroglia, etc.

c. amygdaloi′deum, a small mass of subcortical gray matter within the tip of the temporal lobe, anterior to the inferior horn of the lateral ventricle of the brain.

c. callo′sum, an arched mass of white matter in the depths of the longitudinal fissure, and made up of transverse fibers connecting the cerebral hemispheres.

c. caverno′sum, either of the two columns of erectile tissue forming the body of the penis or clitoris.

c. fimbria′tum, a band of white matter bordering the lateral edge of the lower cornu of the lateral ventricle of the brain.

c. genicula′tum, see GENICULATE BODIES, LATERAL, and GENICULATE BODIES, MEDIAL.

c. hemorrhag′icum, 1. an ovarian follicle containing blood. 2. a corpus luteum containing a blood clot.

c. lu′teum, a yellow glandular mass in the ovary formed by an ovarian follicle that has matured and discharged its ovum (see also OVULATION).

cor′pora quadrigem′ina, four rounded eminences on the posterior surface of the mesencephalon.

c. spongio′sum pe′nis, a column of erectile tissue forming the urethral surface of the penis, in which the urethra is found.

c. stria′tum, a subcortical mass of gray and white substance in front of and lateral to the thalmus in each cerebral hemisphere.

corpuscle (kor′pus′l) any small mass or body. adj., **corpus′cular.**

blood c's, formed elements in the BLOOD, i.e., erythrocytes and leukocytes.

colostrum c's, large rounded bodies in colostrum, containing droplets of fat and sometimes a nucleus.

Krause's c's, small, encapsulated nerve endings of sensory nerve fibers in skin, mucous membranes, muscles, and other areas. Called also end-buds and Krause's bulbs.

malpighian c., the funnel-like structure constituting the beginning of the structural unit of the kidney (nephron) and comprising the malpighian capsule and its partially enclosed glomerulus. Called also renal corpuscle.

Purkinje's c's, large, branched nerve cells composing the middle layer of the cortex of the cerebellum.

red blood c., erythrocyte.

renal c., malpighian corpuscle.

tactile c's, medium-sized nerve endings in the skin, chiefly in the palms and soles; called also tactile papillae.

white blood c., leukocyte.

correlation (kor″ĕ-la′shun) in neurology, the union of afferent impulses within a nerve center to bring about an appropriate response. In statistics, the degree of association of variable phenomena, as intelligence and birth order.

correspondence (kor″ĕ-spon′dens) the condition of being in agreement or conformity.

retinal c., the state concerned with the impingement of image-producing stimuli on the retinas of the two eyes.

Corrigan's pulse (kor′ĕ-ganz) a jerky pulse with full expansion and sudden collapse.

corrosive (kŏ-ro′siv) having a caustic and locally destructive effect; an agent having such effects.

Cortate (kor′tāt) trademark for preparations of desoxycorticosterone, a steroid.

Cort-Dome (kort′dōm) trademark for preparations of hydrocortisone, an adrenocortical steroid.

Cortef (kor′tef) trademark for preparations of hydrocortisone, an adrenocortical steroid.

cortex (kor′teks), pl. *cor′tices* [L.] an outer layer, as the bark of the trunk or root of a tree, or the outer layer of an organ or other structure, as distinguished from its inner substance. adj., **cor′tical.**

adrenal c., the outer, firm layer comprising the larger part of the ADRENAL GLAND; it secretes various hormones.

cerebellar c., the superficial gray matter of the cerebellum.

cerebral c., c. cer′ebri, the convoluted layer of gray matter covering each cerebral hemisphere (see also cerebral cortex of BRAIN).

renal c., the smooth-textured outer layer of the kidney, composed mainly of glomeruli and convoluted tubules, extending in columns between the pyramids constituting the renal medulla.

Corti's canal (kor′tēz) a space between the outer and inner rods of Corti.

Corti's ganglion (kor′tēz) the ganglion of the cochlear nerve, located within the modiolus, sending fibers peripherally to the organ of Corti and centrally to the cochlear nuclei of the brain stem. Called also spiral ganglion.

Corti's organ (cor′tēz) the terminal acoustic apparatus within the scala media of the inner ear, including the rods of Corti and the auditory cells, with their supporting elements. (See also Plate 15.)

Corti's rods (fibers) (kor′tēz) rodlike bodies in the inner ear, having their heads joined and their bases on the basilar membrane widely separated so as to form a spiral tunnel.

corticate (kor′tĭ-kāt) having a cortex or bark.

corticectomy (kor″tĭ-sek′to-me) excision of an area of cerebral cortex, as of a scar or microgyrus in the treatment of focal epilepsy.

corticifugal (kor″tĭ-sif′u-gal) proceeding, conducting, or moving away from the cortex.

corticipetal (kor″tĭ-sip′ĕ-tal) proceeding, conducting, or moving toward the cortex.

corticoadrenal (kor″tĭ-ko-ad-re′nal) pertaining to the adrenal cortex; adrenocortical.

corticobulbar (kor″tĭ-ko-bul′bar) pertaining to or connecting the cerebral cortex and the medulla oblongata.

corticoid (kor′tĭ-koid) a hormone of the adrenal cortex, or other natural or synthetic compound with similar activity.

corticopontine (kor″tĭ-ko-pon′tīn) pertaining to or connecting the cerebral cortex and the pons.

corticospinal (kor″tĭ-ko-spi′nal) pertaining to or connecting the cerebral cortex and spinal cord.

corticosteroid (kor″tĭ-ko-ste′roid) any of the hormones produced by the adrenal cortex; also, their synthetic equivalents. Called also adrenocortical hormone and adrenocorticosteroid. All the hormones are steroids having similar chemical structures, but quite different physiologic effects. Generally they are divided into GLUCOCORTICOIDS (cortisol, or hydrocortisone, and cortisone and corticosterone), MINERALOCORTICOIDS (aldosterone and desoxycorticosterone, and also corticosterone) and androgens.

At times of stress or emergency the adrenal cortex responds to a special alarm system which results in increased production of its hormones ALARM REACTION. The corticosteroids help supply the body with emergency materials such as amino acids, fatty acids, glucose, sodium, and water. These materials are used to provide energy, to increase resistance and aid in tissue repair and to maintain a normal fluid and electrolyte balance.

corticosterone (kor″tĭ-ko-stēr′ōn) a steroid hormone of the adrenal cortex; it is usually classified as a GLUCOCORTICOID, but it also has slight MINERALOCORTICOID activity.

corticotrophic (kor″tĭ-ko-trof′ik) corticotropic.

corticotrophin (kor″tĭ-ko-tro′fin) corticotropin.

corticotropic (kor″tĭ-ko-trop′ik) having a stimulating effect on the adrenal cortex; pertaining to corticotropin; adrenocorticotropic.

corticotropin (kor″tĭ-ko-tro′pin) 1. adrenocorticotropic hormone (see also ACTH). 2. a pharmaceutical preparation derived from the anterior pituitary of mammals is used to stimulate adrenal cortical activity in various conditions, such as allergy, hypersensitivity, and rheumatoid arthritis. It has also been used experimentally in a large number of disorders.

Cortifoam (kor′tĭ-fōm) trademark for an aerosol foam containing 10 per cent hydrocortisone acetate; used as an intrarectal anti-inflammatory.

cortisol (kor′tĭ-sol) a hormone from the adrenal cortex; the principal GLUCOCORTICOID. Called also 17-hydroxycorticosterone and, pharmaceutically, hydrocortisone. A synthetic preparation is used for its anti-inflammatory actions.

cortisone (kor′tĭ-sōn) a GLUCORTICOID with significant MINERALOCORTICOID activity, isolated from the adrenal cortex, largely inactive in man until it is converted to hydrocortisone (cortisol). Cortisone can be extracted from animals and prepared synthetically from plants; the acetate is used for its anti-inflammatory properties in various conditions.

Cortogen (kor′to-jen) trademark for preparations of cortisone.

Cortone (kor′tōn) trademark for preparations of cortisone.

Cortrophin (kor-tro′fin) trademark for preparations of corticotropin.

coruscation (kor″us-ka′shun) the sensation as of a flash of light before the eyes.

corybantism (kor″e-ban′tism) wild, frenzied, and sleepless delirium.

corymbiform (ko-rim′bi-form) clustered; said of lesions grouped around a single, usually larger, lesion.

Corynebacterium (ko-ri″ne-bak-te′re-um) a genus of bacteria.

C. **diphthe′riae**, the causative agent of diphtheria.

C. **minutis′simum**, the causative agent of erythrasma.

C. **pseudodiphtherit′icum**, a nonpathogenic microorganism present in the upper respiratory tract.

coryza (ko-ri′zah) profuse discharge from the mucous membrane of the nose.

coryzavirus (ko-ri″zah-vi′rus) rhinovirus.

cosmetic (koz-met′ik) 1. beautifying; tending to preserve, restore, or confer comeliness. 2. a beautifying substance or preparation.

cost(o)- word element [L.], *rib.*

costa (kos′tah), pl. *cos′tae* [L.] a rib. adj., **cos′tal.**

costalgia (kos-tal′je-ah) pain in the ribs.

costectomy (kos-tek′to-me) excision of a rib.

costive (kos′tiv) 1. pertaining to, characterized by, or producing constipation. 2. an agent that depresses intestinal motility.

costiveness (kos′tiv-nes) constipation.

costocervical (kos″to-ser′vĭ-kal) pertaining to the ribs and neck.

costochondral (kos″to-kon′dral) pertaining to a rib and its cartilage.

costoclavicular (kos″to-klah-vik′u-lar) pertaining to the ribs and clavicle.

costocoracoid (kos″to-kor′ah-koid) pertaining to the ribs and coracoid process.

costosternal (kos″to-ster′nal) pertaining to the ribs and sternum.

costosternoplasty (kos″to-ster′no-plas″te) surgical repair of funnel chest, a segment of rib being used to support the sternum.

costotomy (kos-tot′o-me) incision or division of a rib or costal cartilage.

costotransverse (kos″to-trans-vers′) lying between the ribs and the transverse processes of the vertebrae.

costovertebral (kos″to-ver′tĕ-bral) pertaining to a rib and a vertebra.

costoxiphoid (kos″to-zi′foid) connecting the ribs and xiphoid cartilage.

cosyntropin (ko″sin-tro′pin) a synthetic corticotropin used in the screening of adrenal insufficiency on the basis of plasma cortisol response after intramuscular or intravenous injection.

cot death sudden infant death syndrome.

Cothera (ko-ther′ah) trademark for preparations of dimethoxanate, an antitussive.

co-twin (ko′twin) one of a pair of twins.

cotton-wool spot white or gray soft-edged opacities in the retina composed of cytoid bodies; seen in hypertensive retinopathy, lupus erythematosus, and numerous other conditions.

cotyledon (kot″ĭ-le′don) any subdivision of the uterine surface of the placenta.

couching (kowch′ing) surgical displacement of the lens of the eye in cataract.

cough (kof) 1. a sudden noisy expulsion of air from the lungs. 2. to produce such an expulsion of air.

dry c., cough without expectoration.

productive c., cough attended with expectoration of material from the bronchi.

c. reflex, the sequence of events initiated by the sensitivity of the lining of the passageways of the lung and mediated by the medulla as a consequence of impulses transmitted by the vagus nerve, resulting in coughing, i.e., the clearing of the passageways of foreign matter.

whooping c., pertussis, an infectious disease caused by *Bordetella pertussis*, characterized by coryza, bronchitis, and a typical cough (see also WHOOPING COUGH).

coulomb (koo′lom) the unit of electrical charge, defined as the quantity of electrical charge transferred by 1 ampere in 1 second.

Coumadin (koo′mah-din) trademark for preparations of warfarin, an anticoagulant.

count (kownt) a numerical computation or indication.

Addis c., the determination of the number of erythrocytes, leukocytes, epithelial cells, casts, and the protein content in an aliquot of a 12-hour urine specimen.

blood c., determination of the number of formed elements in a measured volume of blood, usually a cubic millimeter (as of red blood cells, white blood cells, or platelet count).

differential c., a count on a stained blood smear, of the proportion of different types of leukocytes (or other cells), expressed in percentages.

direct platelet c., estimation of the number of platelets per cubic millimeter of blood.

filament-nonfilament c., determination of the number of juvenile and mature leukocytes, as in the differential blood count.

indirect platelet c., calculation of the total number of platelets per cubic millimeter of blood by determining the ratio of platelets to erythrocytes.

platelet c., the count of the total number of platelets per cubic millimeter of blood by counting the platelets on a stained blood film.

Schilling's c., a differential blood cell count in which the leukocytes are divided into four groups.

counter (kown′ter) an instrument or apparatus by which numerical value is computed; in radiology, a device for enumerating ionizing events.

Geiger c., Geiger-Müller c., an amplifying device that indicates the presence of ionizing particles.

scintillation c., a device for indicating the emission of ionizing particles, permitting determination of the concentration of radioisotopes in the body or other substance.

counterextension (kown″ter-eks-ten′shun) traction in a proximal direction coincident with traction in opposition to it.

counterimmunoelectrophoresis (kown″ter-im″u-no-e-lek″tro-fo-re′sis) abbreviated CIE; a laboratory technique in which an electric current is used to accelerate the migration of antibody and antigen through a buffered diffusion medium. Antigens in a gel medium in which the pH is controlled are strongly negatively charged and will migrate rapidly across the electric field toward the anode. The antibody in such a medium is less negatively charged and will migrate in an opposite or "counter" direction toward the cathode. If the antigen and antibody are specific for each other, they combine and form a distinct precipitin line.

The technique of CIE was first applied clinically in 1970 to detect hepatitis B antigen. With modification and refinement it is becoming increasingly more useful as a means of detecting antigens or antibodies specific for a variety of infectious diseases. It can be especially valuable as an aid to accurate diagnosis of clinical bacterial infections and the selection of specific therapeutic agents for control of infections once the causative organisms are identified.

counterincision (kown″ter-in-sizh′un) a second incision made to promote drainage or to relieve tension on the edges of a wound.

counterirritant (kown″ter-ir′ĭ-tant) producing counterirritation. 2. an agent that produces counterirritation.

counterirritation (kown″ter-ir″ĭ-ta′shun) superficial irritation intended to relieve some other irritation.

counteropening (kown″ter-o′pen-ing) a second incision made across an earlier one to promote drainage.

counterpulsation (kown″ter-pul-sa′shun) a technique for assisting the circulation and decreasing the work of the heart, by synchronizing the force of an external pumping device with cardiac systole and diastole.

counterpuncture (kown′ter-punk″chur) a second opening made opposite another.

counterstain (kown′ter-stān) a stain applied to render the effects of another stain more discernible.

countertraction (kown′ter-trak″shun) traction opposed to another traction; used in reduction of fractures.

countertransference (kown″ter-trans-fer′ens) in psychoanalysis, the emotional reaction aroused in the physician by the patient.

coup (koo) [Fr.] stroke.

c. de sabre (koo-duh-sahb′), a linear, circumscribed lesion of scleroderma on the forehead or scalp, so called because of its resemblance to the scar of a saber wound.

covalence (ko-va′lens) a chemical bond between two atoms in which electrons are shared between the two nuclei. adj., **cova′lent.**

covariance (ko-va′re-ans) the expected value of the product of the deviations of corresponding values of two random variables from their respective means.

coverglass (kuv′er-glas) a thin glass that covers a mounted microscopical object or a culture. Called also coverslip.

coverslip (kuv′er-slip) coverglass.

cowage (kow′aj) a perennial herb, *Mucuna pruriens*, of the East Indies. 2. the hairs of the cowage pods, which cause severe itching, are used medicinally as a vermifuge, anthelmintic, and counterirritant in admixture with such vehicles as honey. Also used as "itching powders" of joke-shop fame.

Cowper's glands (kow′pers) bulbourethral glands.

cowperitis (kow″per-i′tis) inflammation of the bulbourethral (Cowper's) glands, located in the urethral sphincter.

cowpox (kow′poks) a mild pustular eruption affecting milk cows, usually confined to the udder and teats, caused by the VACCINIA virus, and transmissible to man. Edward Jenner, in the 18th century, discovered that cowpox could be transmitted to humans who milked or tended cattle, and also noted that persons who contracted it in this way seldom contracted smallpox. This discovery led to VACCINATION against SMALLPOX.

coxa (kok′sah), pl. *cox′ae* [L.] the hip, loosely, the hip joint.

c. pla′na, flattening of the head of the femur resulting from osteochondrosis of its epiphysis.

c. val′ga, deformity of the hip joint with increase in the angle of inclination between the neck and shaft of the femur.

c. va′ra, deformity of the hip joint with decrease in the angle of inclination between the neck and shaft of the femur.

coxalgia (kok-sal′je-ah) 1. hip-joint disease. 2. pain in the hip.

Coxiella (kok″se-el′ah) a genus of microorganisms of the order Rickettsiales.

C. burnet′ii, the causative agent of Q fever.

coxitis (kok-si′tis) inflammation of the hip joint.

coxodynia (kok″so-din′e-ah) pain in the hip.

coxofemoral (kok″so-fem′o-ral) pertaining to the hip and thigh.

coxotuberculosis (kok″so-tu-ber″ku-lo′sis) tuberculosis of the hip joint; hip-joint disease.

coxsackievirus (kok-sak′e-vi″rus) one of a heterogeneous group of enteroviruses producing, in man, a disease resembling poliomyelitis, but without paralysis. Called also Coxsackie virus.

c. A disease, herpangina.

cozymase (ko-zi′mās) nicotinamide-adenine dinucleotide.

c.p.m. counts per minute, an expression of the particles emitted after administration of a radioactive material such as the isotope iodine-131 (^{131}I).

CPR cardiopulmonary resuscitation.

c.p.s. cycles per second.

CR conditioned reflex (response).

Cr chemical symbol, *chromium.*

Crabtree effect (krab′tre) the inhibition of oxygen consumption on the addition of glucose to tissues or microorganisms having a high rate of aerobic glycolysis; the converse of the Pasteur effect.

cradle (kra′d′l) a frame placed over the body of a bed patient for application of heat or cold or for protecting injured parts from coming in contact with the bed clothes. Cradles vary in size according to their intended purpose and can be used over the entire body or over one or more extremities.

c. cap, an oily yellowish crust that sometimes appears on the scalp of nursing infants; also called milk crust (crusta lactea). The crust is caused by excessive secretion of the sebaceous glands in the scalp. Treatment consists of applications of oil or a bland ointment and frequent scalp shampoos until the crust is removed.

electric c., heat c., a tunnel- or hood-shaped cradle

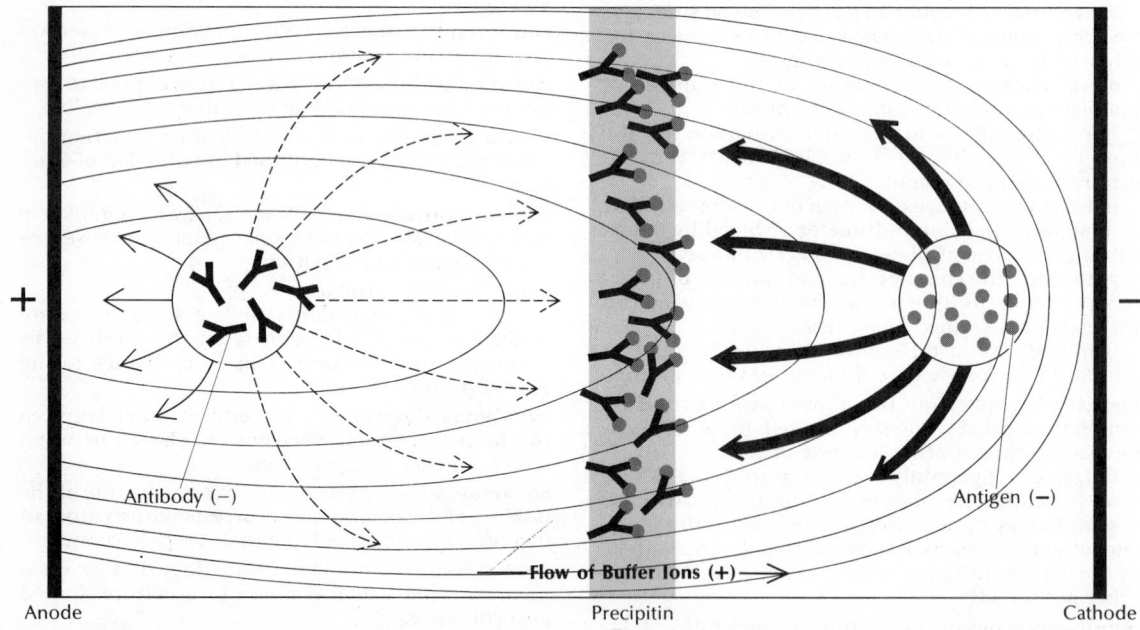

Counterimmunoelectrophoresis (CIE) test depends upon reactions to electric current of antibody and antigen molecules and buffer. At the pH used, antigen is strongly negative and migrates rapidly toward the anode. Although weakly negative antibody tends to migrate slowly toward the anode, it becomes swept along (dashed arrows) toward the cathode with positive buffer ions of the agar, in the "counter" motion of CIE. Antibody and antigen meet between wells (space here is exaggerated), combine, and precipitate if they are specific for each other, forming precipitin line characteristic of the test. (Drawing by A. Iselin, from Rytel, M. W.: Counterimmunoelectrophoresis in Diagnosis of Infectious Disease. *Hospital Practice,* Vol. 10, No. 10. Reprinted by permission.)

equipped with light bulbs, for applications of heat to the patient's body.

Craigia (kra′ge-ah) a genus of flagellate protozoa; its flagellate stages are thought by some to be *Chilomastix mesnili,* and its ameboid stages to be *Entamoeba coli.*

cramp (kramp) a painful spasmodic muscular contraction.

heat c., spasm accompanied by pain, weak pulse, and dilated pupils; seen in workers in intense heat.

recumbency c's, cramping in the muscles of the legs and feet occurring while resting or during light sleep.

writers' c., an occupational neurosis marked by spasmodic contraction of the muscles of the fingers, hand, and forearm, with neuralgic pain.

crani(o)- word element [L.], *skull.*

craniad (kra′ne-ad) in a cranial direction; toward the anterior (in animals) or superior (in humans) end of the body.

cranial (kra′ne-al) pertaining to the cranium or to the anterior (in animals) or superior (in humans) end of the body.

c. nerves, nerves that are attached to the brain and pass through the openings of the skull. There are 12 pairs of cranial nerves, symmetrically arranged so that they are distributed mainly to the structures of the head and neck. The one exception, the vagus nerve, extends beyond the head and carries among its fibers the motor fibers that go to the bronchi, stomach, gallbladder, small intestine, and part of the large intestine. It also carries the fibers that control the release of secretions of the gastric glands and the pancreas, and inhibitory fibers to the heart.

Some of the cranial nerves are both sensory and motor; i.e., they control motion as well as conduct sensory impulses. Others are sensory or motor only.

CRANIAL NERVES
(See also table of NERVES)

I	Olfactory	Sensory
II	Optic	Sensory
III	Oculomotor	Mixed
IV	Trochlear	Mixed
V	Trigeminal	
	Ophthalmic	Sensory
	Maxillary	Sensory
	Mandibular	Mixed
VI	Abducens	Motor
VII	Facial	Mixed
VIII	Vestibulocochlear	
	Cochlear	Sensory
	Vestibular	Sensory
IX	Glossopharyngeal	Mixed
X	Vagus	Mixed
XI	Accessory	Motor
XII	Hypoglossal	Motor

craniectomy (kra″ne-ek′to-me) excision of a segment of the skull.

craniocele (kra′ne-o-sēl″) protrusion of part of the brain through the skull.

craniocerebral (kra″ne-o-ser′ĕ-bral) pertaining to the skull and cerebrum.

cranioclasis (kra″ne-ok′lah-sis) craniotomy (2).

cranioclast (kra′ne-o-klast″) an instrument for performing craniotomy (2).

craniocleidodysostosis (kra″ne-o-kli″do-dis″os-to′sis) cleidocranial dysostosis.

craniodidymus (kra″ne-o-did′ĭ-mus) a monster with two heads.

craniofacial (kra″ne-o-fa′shal) of or pertaining to the cranium and face.

craniograph (kra′ne-o-graf″) an instrument for outlining the skull.

craniomalacia (kra″ne-o-mah-la′she-ah) abnormal softness of the bones of the skull.

craniometer (kra″ne-om′ĕ-ter) an instrument for use in craniometry.

craniometry (kra″ne-om′ĕ-tre) measurement of the skull and facial bones.

craniopagus (kra″ne-op′ah-gus) a double monster joined at the head.

craniopharyngeal (kra″ne-o-fah-rin′je-al) pertaining to the cranium and pharynx.

craniopharyngioma (kra″ne-o-fah-rin″je-o′mah) a tumor arising from the cell rests derived from the infundibulum of the hypophysis or Rathke's pouch.

cranioplasty (kra′ne-o-plas″te) any plastic operation on the skull.

craniopuncture (kra′ne-o-pungk″tūr) exploratory puncture of the brain.

craniorachischisis (kra″ne-o-rah-kis′kĭ-sis) congenital fissure of the skull and vertebral column.

craniosacral (kra″ne-o-sa′kral) pertaining to the skull and sacrum.

cranioschisis (kra″ne-os′kĭ-sis) congenital fissure of the skull.

craniosclerosis (kra″ne-o-sklĕ-ro′sis) abnormal calcification and thickening of the cranial bones.

cranioscopy (kra″ne-os′ko-pe) diagnostic examination of the head.

craniospinal (kra″ne-o-spi′nal) pertaining to the skull and spine.

craniostenosis (kra″ne-o-stĕ-no′sis) deformity of the skull due to premature closure of the cranial sutures.

craniostosis (kra″ne-os-to′sis) congenital ossification of the cranial sutures.

craniosynostosis (kra″ne-o-sin″os-to′sis) premature closure of the cranial sutures.

craniotabes (kra″ne-o-ta′bēz) reduction in mineralization of the skull, with abnormal softness of the bone, usually affecting the occipital and parietal bones along the lambdoidal sutures.

craniotome (kra′ne-o-tōm″) a cutting instrument used in craniotomy.

craniotomy (kra″ne-ot′o-me) 1. any operation on the cranium. 2. puncture of the skull and removal of its contents to decrease the size of the head of a dead fetus and facilitate delivery.

craniotympanic (kra″ne-o-tim-pan′ik) pertaining to the skull and tympanum.

cranium (kra′ne-um), pl. *cra′nia* [L.] the skeleton of the head, variously construed as including all of the bones of the head, all except the mandible, or the eight bones forming the vault lodging the brain.

crater (kra′ter) an excavated area surrounded by an elevated margin, such as is caused by ulceration.

craterization (kra″ter-ĭ-za′shun) excision of bone tissue to create a crater-like depression.

C-reactive protein (CRP) a globulin that forms a precipitate with the C-polysaccharide of the pneumococcus. For reasons not clearly understood, inflammation and tissue breakdown give rise to the C-reactive protein. Blood from patients with inflammatory conditions or disorders accompanied by necrosis gives a positive result with the test, and it is therefore of some use in diagnosing or determining the progress of such disorders as rheumatoid arthritis, acute rheumatic fever, widespread malignancy, and bacterial infections.

Creamalin (krēm′ah-lin) trademark for preparations of aluminum hydroxide gel, used as an antacid.

creatinase (kre-at′ĭ-nās) an enzyme that catalyzes the decomposition of creatine into urea and ammonia.

creatine (kre′ah-tin) a nonprotein substance synthesized in the body from three amino acids: arginine, glycine (aminoacetic acid), and methionine. Creatine readily combines with phosphate to form phosphocreatine, or creatine phosphate, which is present in muscle, where it serves as the storage form of high-energy phosphate necessary for muscle contraction.

phosphate c., phosphocreatine.

creatinemia (kre″ah-tĭ-ne′me-ah) excessive creatine in the blood.

creatinine (kre-at′ĭ-nin) a nitrogenous compound formed as a metabolic end product of creatine. It is formed in the muscle in relatively small amounts, passes into the blood and is excreted in the urine.

A laboratory test for the creatinine level in the blood may be used as a measurement of kidney function. Since creatinine is normally produced in fairly constant amounts as a result of the breakdown of phosphocreatine and is excreted in the urine; an elevation in the creatinine level in the blood indicates a disturbance in kidney function. Normal range for the creatinine level is 0.6 to 1.3 mg. per 100 ml. of serum. The patient must be in a state of rest for the test, but fasting is not necessary. If the dyes Bromsulphalein and phenolsulfonphthalein have been given to the patient within the previous 24 hours, the creatinine level may be elevated.

creatinuria (kre-at″ĭ-nu′re-ah) increased concentration of creatine in the urine.

Credé's technique (maneuver, method) (kra′dāz) a technique for manual expression of urine from the bladder used in BLADDER TRAINING for paralyzed patients: the hands are held flat against the abdomen, just below the umbilicus. A firm downward stroke toward the bladder is repeated six or seven times, followed by pressure from both hands placed directly over the bladder to manually remove all urine.

cremaster muscle (kre-mas′ter) the muscle that elevates the testis (see table of MUSCLES).

cremasteric (kre″mas-ter′ik) pertaining to the cremaster muscle.

crenate, crenated (kre′nāt; kre′nāt-ed) scalloped or notched.

crenation (kre-na′shun) the formation of abnormal notching around the edge of an erythrocyte; the notched appearance of an erythrocyte due to its shrinkage after suspension in a hypertonic solution.

crenocyte (kre′no-sīt) a crenated erythrocyte.

creosol (kre′o-sol) one of the active constituents of creosote.

creosote (kre′o-sōt) a mixture of phenols from wood tar; used externally as an antiseptic and internally in chronic bronchitis as an expectorant. A mixture of the carbonates of various constituents of creosote (creosote carbonate) is used the same as the base.

crepitant (krep′ĭ-tant) having a dry, crackling sound.

crepitation (krep″ĭ-ta′shun) a dry, crackling sound or sensation, such as that produced by the grating of the ends of a fractured bone.

crepitus (kre′ĭ-tus) 1. the discharge of flatus from the bowels. 2. crepitation. 3. a crepitant rale.

crescent (kres′ent) 1. shaped like a new moon. 2. a crescent-shaped structure. adj., **crescen′tic.**

Giannuzzi's c's, crescent-shaped patches of serous cells surrounding the mucous tubercles in mixed glands.

sublingual c., the crescent-shaped area on the floor of the mouth, bounded by the lingual wall of the mandible and the base of the tongue.

cresol (kre′sol) a phenol from coal or wood tar; a preparation consisting of a mixture of isomeric cresol from coal tar or petroleum is used as a disinfectant.

crest (krest) a projection, or projecting structure or ridge, especially one surmounting a bone or its border.

dental c., the maxillary ridge passing along the alveolar processes of the fetal maxillary bones.

iliac c., the thickened, expanded upper border of the ilium.

cresylic acid (krĕ-sil′ik) cresol.

cretin (kre′tin) a patient exhibiting cretinism.

cretinism (kre′tĭ-nizm) arrested physical and mental development with dystrophy of bones and soft tissues, due to congenital lack of thyroid gland secretion from hypofunctioning or absence of the gland. The child has a large head, short limbs, puffy eyes, a thick and protruding tongue, excessively dry skin, lack of coordination, and mental retardation. The acquired or adult form of thyroid deficiency is MYXEDEMA.

Administration of thyroid extract, which must be continued for life, can result in normal growth and mental developmment. If untreated, the child will become permanently dwarfed, probably mentally retarded, and sterile.

cretinoid (kre′tĭ-noid) resembling a cretin, or suggestive of cretinism.

cretinous (kre′tĭ-nus) affected with cretinism.

crevice (krev′is) a fissure.

gingival c., the space between the cervical enamel of a tooth and the overlying unattached gingiva.

crib death sudden infant death syndrome.

cribriform (krib′rĭ-form) perforated like a sieve.

cricoarytenoid (kri″ko-ar″ĭ-te′noid) pertaining to the cricoid and arytenoid cartilages.

cricoid (kri′koid) 1. ring-shaped. 2. the cricoid cartilage.

c. cartilage, a ringlike cartilage forming the lower and back part of the larynx.

cricoidectomy (kri″koi-dek′to-me) excision of the cricoid cartilage.

cricopharyngeal (kri″ko-fah-rin′je-al) pertaining to the cricoid cartilage and pharynx.

cricothyreotomy (kri″ko-thi″re-ot′o-me) incision through the cricoid and thyroid cartilages.

cricothyroid (kri″ko-thi′roid) pertaining to the cricoid and thyroid cartilages.

cricotomy (kri-kot′o-me) incision of the cricoid cartilage.

cricotracheotomy (kri″ko-tra″ke-ot′o-me) incision of the trachea through the cricoid cartilage.

cri du chat syndrome (kre-du-shah) [Fr.] a hereditary congenital syndrome characterized by hypertelorism, microcephaly, severe mental deficiency, and a plaintive catlike cry, due to deletion of the short arm of the chromosome of the B group.

Crigler-Najjar disease (syndrome) (krig′ler naj′er) a congenital hereditary non-hemolytic jaundice due to absence of the hepatic enzyme glucuronide transferase, marked by excessive amounts of unconjugated bilirubin in the blood, kernicterus, and severe central nervous system disorders.

crinogenic (kri″no-jen′ik, krin″o-jin′ik) causing secretion in a gland.

crisis (kri′sis), pl. *cri′ses* [L.] 1. the turning point of a disease for better or worse; especially a sudden change, usually for the better, in the course of an acute disease. 2. a sudden paroxysmal intensification of symptoms in the course of a disease.

addisonian c., symptoms of fatigue, nausea and vomiting, and weight loss accompanying an acute attack of Addison's disease.

celiac c., an attack of severe watery diarrhea and vomiting producing dehydration and acidosis, sometimes occurring in the infantile form of CELIAC DISEASE.

salt-losing c., see SALT-LOSING CRISIS.

tabetic c., a painful paroxysm occurring in tabes dorsalis.

thyroid c., thyrotoxic c., a sudden and dangerous increase of the symptoms of thyrotoxicosis.

crista (kris′tah), pl. *cris′tae* [L.] crest.

cris′tae cu′tis, ridges of the skin produced by the projecting papillae of the corium on the palm of the hand and sole of the foot, producing a fingerprint and footprint characteristic of the individual; called also dermal ridges.

c. gal′li, a thick, triangular process projecting upward from the cribriform plate of the ethmoid bone.

C.R.N.A. Certified Registered Nurse Anesthetist.

Crohn's disease (krōnz) inflammation of the terminal portion of the ileum; called also regional enteritis and regional ileitis. (See also ILEITIS.)

cromolyn (kro′mŏ-lin) a prophylactic antiasthmatic that has the advantage of reducing or eliminating the need for steroids and sympathomimetics. It is used in the form of the sodium salt, and is available as a dry powder aersol.

Crookes' tube (kruks) an early form of vacuum tube by use of which the roentgen rays were discovered.

cross (kros) 1. a cross-shaped figure or structure. 2. any organism produced by crossbreeding; a method of crossbreeding.

crossbite (kros′bīt) malocclusion in which the mandibular teeth are in buccal version (or completely lingual version in posterior segments) to the maxillary teeth.

crossbreeding (kros′brēd-ing) hybridization; the mating of organisms of different strains or species.

cross-eye STRABISMUS in which there is manifest deviation of the visual axis of one eye toward that of the other eye, resulting in diplopia. Called also esotropia and convergent strabismus.

crossing over (kros′ing o′ver) the exchanging of material between homologous chromosomes, during the first meiotic division, resulting in new combinations of genes.

cross matching (kros-mach′ing) a procedure vital in blood transfusions, testing for agglutination of donor erythrocytes by recipient's serum, and of recipient's red cells by donor serum (see also cross MATCHING).

crotamiton (kro″tah-mi′ton) an acaricide used in the treatment of scabies and as an antipruritic.

croton oil (kro′ton) the fixed oil of the seeds of the Asiatic plant *Croton tiglium*, which is a drastic purgative and counterirritant. Because of its high toxicity and extreme irritant effect on the intestinal membranes (see also CROTONISM), it has been deleted from the U.S.P. and replaced by equally effective but less dangerous drugs. It is used as a standard irritant in pharmacological research.

crotonism (kro′ton-izm) poisoning by croton oil, with burning of the mouth and sometimes emesis, followed by severe watery diarrhea and colic; sometimes accompanied by headache, somnolence, vertigo, prostration, and collapse. Death from circulatory or respiratory failure may occur.

croup (kro͞op) a condition resulting from acute obstruction of the larynx caused by allergy, foreign body, infection, or new growth, occurring chiefly in infants and children, adj., **croup′ous.**

CHARACTERISTICS. Croup in itself is not a disease but a group of symptoms of varied origin with the following general characteristics: (1) obstruction of the upper respiratory tract, usually at the level of the larynx or just below it in the trachea; (2) hoarseness; (3) a resonant cough, usually described as "barking"; and (4) a croaking sound, called stridor, during inspiration.

A typical attack of croup usually begins at night, and is often precipitated by exposure to cold air. The onset is sudden, with hoarse, "croupy" voice or cough, and what seems like difficult breathing. Spasms of choking that seem close to strangulation follow.

PATIENT CARE. An atmosphere of high humidity is provided to liquefy the secretions and reduce the spasm of the laryngeal muscles. Warm, moist air may be provided by a vaporizer and croup tent. Cool, moist air is provided by special equipment such as a Croupette which cools the air and converts it into a fine mist. Cool air is preferred if the patient has a fever because the warm, moist air tends to elevate the body temperature. While providing an atmosphere of high humidity, it is important to keep the patient dry and comfortable and prevent chilling.

An emetic, such as syrup of ipecac, may be ordered to induce vomiting and thereby reduce laryngeal spasms. The child must have someone in attendance until the vomiting has stopped and there is no further danger of aspiration of the vomitus.

An attitude of calm does much to help the patient relax and also reassures the parents of the child. Although croup is very frightening, with a sudden onset and dramatic symptoms of asphyxia, it is rarely fatal and the prognosis is very good.

Observations include rate and character of respirations, color of the skin, degree of restlessness and anxiety, and degree of prostration.

Crouzon's disease (kroo-zonz') craniofacial dysostosis.

crown (krown) 1. the topmost part of an organ or structure, e.g., the top of the head. 2. artificial crown.

anatomical c., the upper, enamel-covered part of a tooth.

artificial c., a metal, porcelain, or plastic reproduction of a crown affixed to the remaining natural structure of a tooth.

crowning (krown'ing) the appearance of the fetal scalp at the vaginal orifice in childbirth.

CRP C-reactive protein.

CRTT Certified Respiratory Therapy Technician.

crucial (kroo'shal) severe and decisive.

cruciate (kroo'she-āt) shaped like a cross.

crucible (kroo'sĭ-b'l) a vessel for melting refractory substances.

cruciform (kroo'sĭ-form) cross-shaped.

cruor (kroo'or) a blood clot.

crus (krus), pl. *cru'ra* [L.] 1. the leg, from knee to foot. 2. a leglike part.

c. cer'ebri, a structure comprising fiber tracts descending from the cerebral cortex to form the longitudinal fascicles of the pons.

c. of clitoris, the continuation of the corpus cavernosum of the clitoris, diverging posteriorly to be attached to the pubic arch.

crura of diaphragm, two fibroelastic bands that arise from the lumbar vertebrae and insert into the central tendon of the diaphragm.

crura of fornix, two flattened bands of white matter that unite to form the body of the fornix of the cerebrum.

c. of penis, the continuation of each corpus cavernosum of the penis, diverging posteriorly to be attached to the pubic arch.

crush syndrome (krush) the edema, oliguria, and other symptoms of renal failure that follow crushing of a part, especially a large muscle mass (see also lower nephron NEPHROSIS).

crust (krust) a formed outer layer, especially an outer layer of solid matter formed by drying of a bodily exudate or secretion.

crusta (krus'tah), pl. *crus'tae* [L.] 1. a crust. 2. crus cerebri.

Crustacea (krus-ta'she-ah) a class of arthropods including the lobsters, crabs, shrimps, wood lice, water fleas, and barnacles.

crutches (kruch'ez) artificial supports, made of wood or metal, used by those who need aid in walking because of injury, disease, or a birth defect.

TYPES. Crutches are made in different sizes suitable for persons of various heights. For the most part they are made of wood or tubular aluminum. The standard type is the tall crutch that fits under the armpits with double uprights and a small horizontal hand bar stretched between the uprights. The lower part is sometimes adjustable to allow for extensions. There always should be a rubber tip at the base, preferably a suction tip, to prevent slipping.

Gaining in popularity is the Lofstrand crutch, which consists of a single tube of aluminum surmounted by a metal cuff that fits around the forearm. The user supports his weight on a hand bar. He can release his hold on the handbar, as in grasping a handrail to climb stairs, without dropping the crutch. A variation of the Lofstrand crutch is the Canadian elbow extensor crutch, which goes farther up the arm.

In walking with crutches, the means of locomotion is transferred from the legs to the arms. The muscles of the arms, shoulders, back, and chest work together to manipulate the crutches. The kind of crutches used depends largely on the nature of the disability. In some cases, the legs may be partially able to function and bear some of the body's

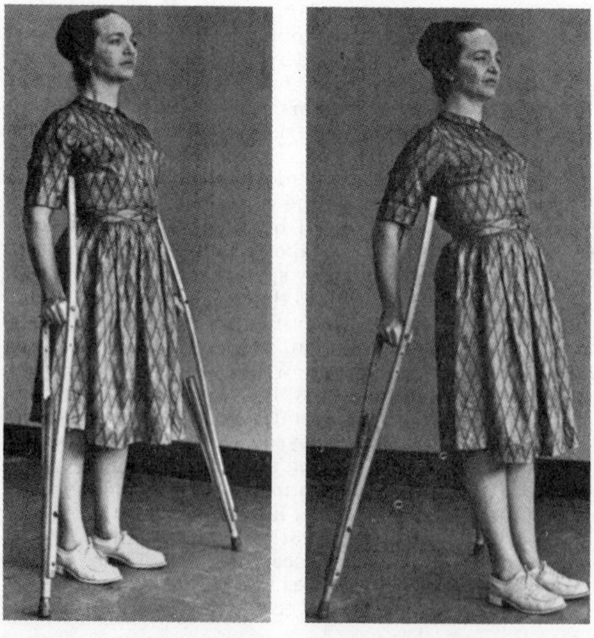

The swing-through gait is used mainly by paraplegics and severe arthritics who have good balance and muscle power in the arms and hands. From the tripod position, both crutches are brought forward, the patient bears down on the handpieces, lifts the body and swings it through the crutches into a reversed tripod position. To maintain balance in this gait, the pelvis moves first, then the shoulders and head.

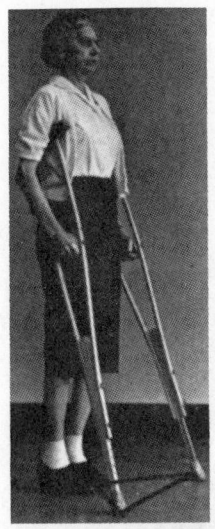

The four-point alternate gait is the slowest and safest crutch gait. It offers maximum balance and support because there are always three points of contact with the ground. From the left, it begins from the tripod position in which all gaits begin. The right crutch is brought forward, and then the left foot. The left crutch comes forward and then the right foot.

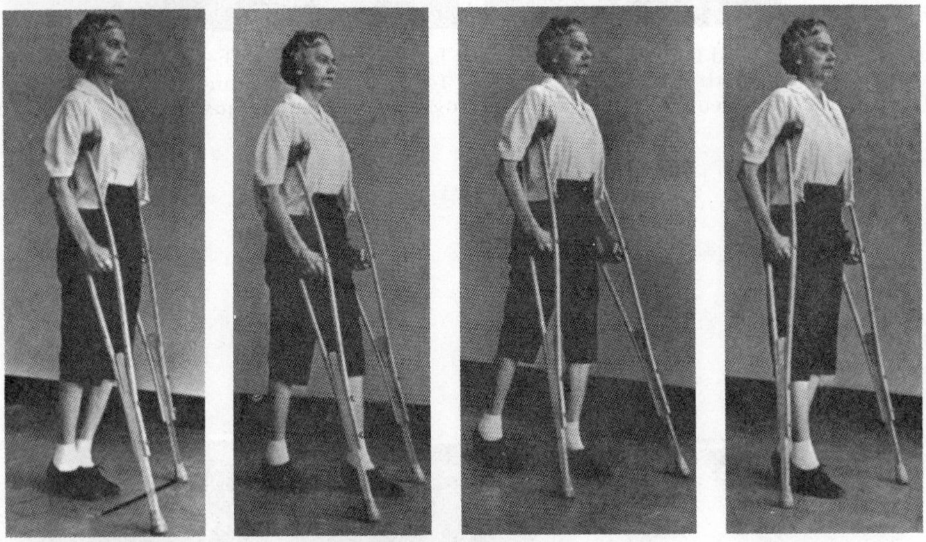

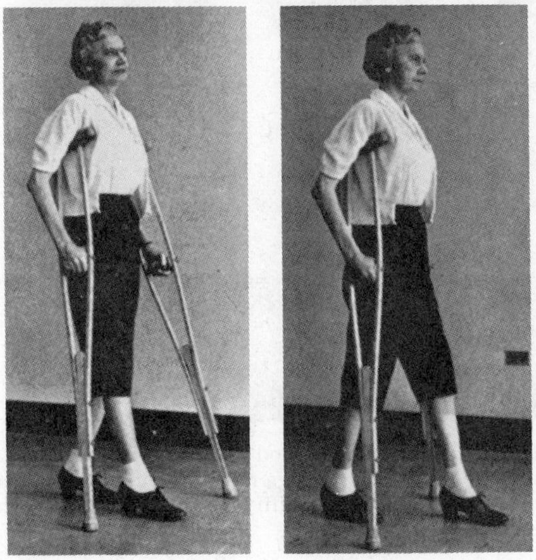

This three-point gait is used by patients who can bear some weight on the injured leg or foot. It begins from the tripod position. Then both crutches and the affected leg are brought forward at the same time. The patient must then rest lightly on the crutches while she moves the unaffected limb forward.

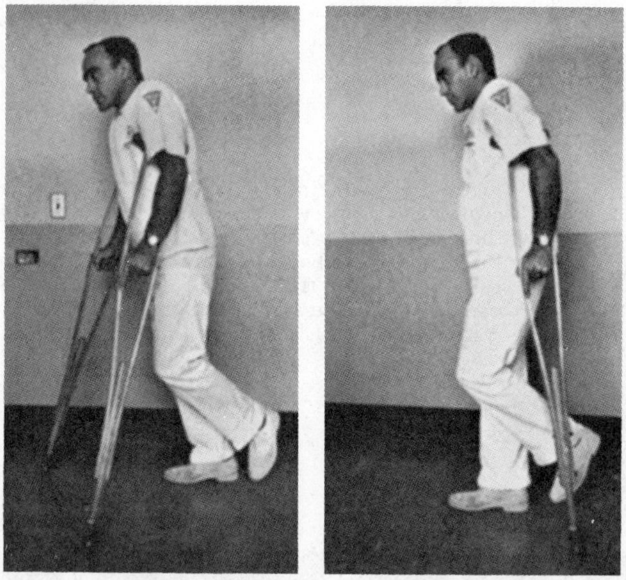

This three-point gait is used by patients who cannot bear any weight on the affected leg or foot. It begins from the tripod position. Both crutches are brought forward and the uninjured leg is brought forward through the crutches. The affected leg follows in a swinging movement because it is raised from the ground.

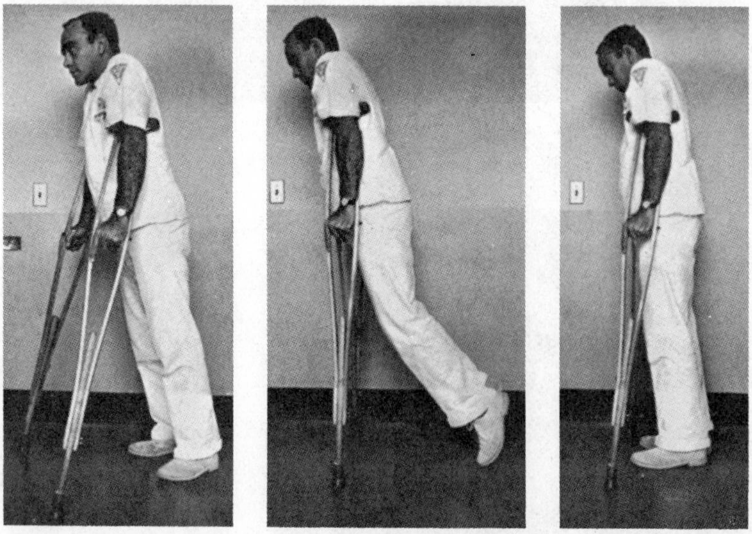

The swing-to gait is slower than the swing-through gait. From the tripod position, the patient places both crutches forward, either alternately or at the same time, and then swings his body ahead into a tripod position. The crutches and feet must never be even or the patient loses stability. In the drag-to gait, the patient slides his feet along the ground and does not raise them.

weight, so that there is less dependence on the crutches. In other cases, leg BRACES may be needed to supplement the crutches.

GAITS. The user is taught one of several standard methods or gaits, according to his condition. Eventually he should be able to master at least two gaits: a fast one for making speed in the open, and a slow one for crowded places, where the chief need is to maintain balance. A variety of gaits also helps to relieve fatigue because one set of muscles can rest while another works.

In describing a gait each foot and crutch is called a point, so that a two-point gait, for example, means that two points of the total of four are in contact with the ground during the performance of one step. A three-point gait may be used when one leg is stronger than the other, meaning that two crutches and the weaker leg hit the ground simultaneously while the next step is made by the stronger leg alone. There is also the so-called tripod gait, swinging gait, and variations of them. (See also GAIT ANALYSIS.)

Cruveilhier's disease (kroo-vāl-yāz′) 1. simple ulcer of the stomach. 2. spinal muscular atrophy.

Cruveilhier-Baumgarten murmur (kroo-vāl-ya′-bawm′gar-ten) a murmur heard at the abdominal wall over veins connecting the portal and caval systems.

Cruveilhier-Baumgarten syndrome (kroo-vāl-ya′bawm′gar-ten) cirrhosis of the liver with portal hypertension associated with congenital patency of the umbilical and paraumbilical veins.

cry(o)- word element [Gr.], *cold.*

cryalgesia (kri″al-je′ze-ah) pain on application of cold.

cryanesthesia (kri″an-es-the′ze-ah) loss of power of perceiving cold.

cryesthesia (kri″es-the′ze-ah) abnormal sensitiveness to cold.

cryobank (kri′o-bank″) a facility for freezing and preserving semen at low temperatures (usually –196.5° C.) for future use.

cryobiology (kri″o-bi-ol′o-je) the science dealing with the effect of low temperatures on biological systems.

cryocautery (kri″o-kaw′ter-e) cold cautery.

cryocrit (kri′o-krit) the percentage of the total volume of blood serum or plasma occupied by cryoprecipitates after centrifugation.

cryoextraction (kri″o-eks-trak′shun) application of extremely low temperature for the removal of a cataractous lens. (See also CATARACT.)

cryofibrinogen (kri″o-fi-brin′o-jen) an abnormal fibrinogen that precipitates at low temperatures and redissolves at 37° C.

cryofibrinogenemia (kri″o-fi-brin″o-jĕ-ne′me-ah) the presence of cryofibrinogen in the blood.

cryogenic (kri″o-jen′ik) producing low temperatures.

cryoglobulin (kri″o-glob′u-lin) an abnormal globulin that precipitates at low temperatures and redissolves at 37° C.

cryoglobulinemia (kri″o-glob″u-lin-e′me-ah) the presence of cryoglobulin in the blood.

cryohypophysectomy (kri-o-hi″po-fiz-ek′to-me) destruction of the pituitary gland by the application of cold.

cryometer (kri-om′ĕ-ter) a thermometer for measuring very low temperature.

cryophilic (kri″o-fil′ik) preferring or growing best at low temperatures; psychrophilic.

cryophylactic (kri″o-fi-lak′tik) resistant to very low temperatures; said of bacteria.

cryoprecipitate (kri″o-pre-sip′ĭ-tāt) any precipitate that results from cooling.

cryoprobe (kri′o-prōb) an instrument for applying extreme cold to tissue.

cryoprotein (kri″o-pro′te-in) a blood protein that precipitates on cooling.

cryoscopy (kri-os′ko-pe) examination of fluids based on the principle that the freezing point of a solution varies according to the amount and nature of the solute. adj., **cryoscop′ic**.

cryostat (kri′o-stat) 1. a device by which temperature can be maintained at a very low level. 2. in pathology and histology, a chamber containing a microtome for sectioning frozen tissue.

cryosurgery (kri″o-ser′jer-e) the destruction of tissue by application of extreme cold, as in the destruction of lesions in the thalamus for the treatment of Parkinson's disease and the treatment of certain malignant lesions of the skin and mucous membranes. The method has also been used successfully in some types of surgery of the eye, for example, in the removal of cataracts and the repair of retinal detachment.

cryothalamectomy (kri″o-thal″ah-mek′to-me) destruction of a portion of the thalamus by application of extreme cold.

cryotherapy (kri″o-ther′ah-pe) the therapeutic use of cold (see also HYPOTHERMIA).

cryotolerant (kri″o-tol′er-ant) able to withstand very low temperatures.

crypt (kript) a blind pit or tube on a free surface.

anal c's, furrows, with pouchlike recesses at the lower end, separating the rectal columns; call also anal sinuses.

c's of Lieberkühn, intestinal glands on the surface of the intestinal mucous membrane.

c's of tongue, deep, irregular invaginations from the surface of the lingual tonsil.

tonsillar c's, epithelium-lined clefts in the palatine tonsils.

crypt(o)- word element [Gr.], *concealed; pertaining to a crypt.*

cryptectomy (krip-tek′to-me) excision or obliteration of a crypt.

cryptenamine (krip-ten′ah-mīn) a mixture of alkaloids from an extract of *Veratrum viride,* used to lower blood pressure.

cryptesthesia (krip″tes-the′ze-ah) subconscious perception of occurrences not ordinarily perceptible to the senses.

cryptitis (krip-ti′tis) inflammation of the mucous membrane of the anal crypts.

cryptocephalus (krip″to-sef′ah-lus) a monster with an inconspicuous head.

cryptococcosis (krip″to-kok-o′sis) infection by *Cryptococcus neoformans,* having a predilection for the brain and meninges but also invading the skin, lungs, and other parts.

Cryptococcus (krip″to-kok′us) a genus of yeastlike fungi.

C. neofor'mans, a species of worldwide distribution, causing cryptococcosis in man.

cryptodidymus (krip"to-did'ĭ-mus) a twin monster, one fetus being enclosed within the body of the other.

cryptogenic (krip"to-jen'ik) of obscure or doubtful origin.

cryptoglioma (krip"to-gli-o'mah) a stage of retinal glioma in which the eyeball shrinks, masking the presence of the growth.

cryptolith (krip'to-lith) a concretion in a crypt.

cryptomenorrhea (krip"to-men"o-re'ah) the occurrence of menstrual symptoms without external bleeding, as in imperforate hymen.

cryptomerorachischisis (krip"to-me"ro-rah-kis'-kĭ-sis) spina bifida occulta.

cryptomnesia (krip"tom-ne'ze-ah) subconscious memory. adj., **cryptomne'sic.**

cryptophthalmia, cryptophthalmos, cryptophthalmus (krip"tof-thal'me-ah; krip"tof-thal'mos; krip"tof-thal'mus) congenital absence of the palpebral fissure, the skin extending from the forehead to the cheek, and the eye malformed or rudimentary.

cryptopodia (krip"to-po'de-ah) swelling of the lower leg and foot, covering all but the sole of the foot.

cryptorchid (krip-tor'kid) a person with undescended testes.

cryptorchidectomy (krip"tor-kĭ-dek'to-me) excision of an undescended testis.

cryptorchidism, cryptorchism (krip-tor'kĭ-dizm; krip-tor'kizm) failure of one or both of the testes to descend into the scrotum. As the unborn male child develops, the testes first appear in the abdomen at about the level of the kidneys. They develop at this site, and in approximately the seventh month of fetal life start to descend to the upper part of the groin. From there they move into the inguinal canal and then, normally, into the scrotum. In its descent, a testis may sometimes be halted in the abdomen or within the canal, becoming an undescended testis.

An improperly developed testis may never leave the abdomen, and it may not produce the hormones that induce secondary sex characters. A testis lodged in the canal may well produce these secondary sex characters, but cannot produce spermatozoa.

Cases in which both testes fail to descend are most uncommon. Usually only one testis is involved and the other produces sufficient numbers of spermatozoa.

TREATMENT. Often the undescended testis can be brought down into the scrotum by medical treatment with the gonadotropic hormone, and for physical and psychologic reasons this method is preferred.

Frequently, however, surgery is required. The operation is not particularly serious and is usually successful. It is best performed when the patient is 5 to 7 years old, since operating at a later age may involve more risk to the cells that produce spermatozoa. The procedure is called an ORCHIOPEXY.

cryptoxanthin (krip"to-zan'thin) a yellow carotenoid widely distributed in nature (egg yolk, green grass, yellow corn, etc.), which can be converted in the body into vitamin A.

cryptozygous (krip"to-zi'gus) having the calvaria wider than the face, so that the zygomatic arches are concealed when the head is viewed from above.

crystal (kris'tal) a naturally produced angular solid of definite form.

crystallin (kris'tah-lin) a globulin in the crystalline lens of the eye.

crystalline (kris'tah-lin) 1. resembling a crystal in nature or clearness. 2. pertaining to crystals.

c. lens, the transparent organ behind the pupil of the eye (see also LENS [2]).

crystallography (kris"tah-log'rah-fe) the science dealing with the study of crystals.

x-ray c., the determination of the three-dimensional structure of molecules by means of diffraction patterns produced by x-rays.

crystalloid (kris'tah-loid) 1. resembling a crystal. 2. a noncolloid substance. Crystalloids form true solutions and therefore are capable of passing through a semipermeable membrane, as in DIALYSIS. The physical opposite of a crystalloid is a COLLOID, which does not dissolve and does not form true solutions.

crystalluria (kris"tah-lu're-ah) the excretion of crystals in the urine, causing irritation of the kidney.

Crysticillin (kris"tĭ-sil'in) trademark for aqueous preparations of procaine penicillin G.

Crystodigin (kris"to-dij'in) trademark for preparations of crystalline digitoxin.

Crystoids (kris'toidz) trademark for hexylresorcinol, an anthelmintic.

CS completed stroke (see CEREBROVASCULAR ACCIDENT).

Cs chemical symbol, *cesium.*

C.S.F. cerebrospinal fluid.

C.S.M. cerebrospinal meningitis.

C-terminal (ter'min-al) the end of the peptide chain carrying the free alpha carboxyl group of the last amino acid, conventionally written to the right.

Cu chemical symbol, *copper* (L. *cuprum*).

cu. cubic.

cubitus (ku'bĭ-tus) 1. the elbow. 2. the upper limb distal to the humerus: the elbow, forearm, and hand. 3. ulna. adj., **cu'bital.**

c. val'gus, deformity of the elbow in which it deviates away from the midline of the body when extended.

c. va'rus, deformity of the elbow in which it deviates toward the midline of the body when extended.

cuboid (ku'boid) resembling a cube; applied particularly to a bone of the foot.

cu. cm. cubic centimeter.

cuffing (kuf'ing) formation of a cufflike surrounding border, as of leukocytes about a blood vessel observed in certain infections.

cuirass (kwe-ras') a covering for the chest.

cul-de-sac (kul-dĕ-sak') [Fr.] a blind pouch.

Douglas' c., a sac or recess formed by a fold of the peritoneum dipping down between the rectum and the uterus. Called also rectouterine excavation or pouch.

culdocentesis (kul"do-sen-te'sis) transvaginal puncture of Douglas' cul-de-sac for aspiration of fluid.

culdoscope (kul'do-skōp) an endoscope used in culdoscopy.

culdoscopy (kul-dos'ko-pe) direct visual examination of the female viscera through an endoscope introduced into the pelvic cavity through the posterior vaginal fornix.

Culex (ku′leks) a genus of mosquitoes found throughout the world; many species transmit various disease-producing agents, e.g., microfilariae, sporozoa, and viruses.

culicide (ku′lĭ-sīd) an agent that destroys mosquitoes.

culicifuge (ku-lis′ĭ-fūj) an agent that repels mosquitoes.

culicine (ku′lĭ-sin, ku′lĭ-sīn) 1. any member of the genus *Culex* or related genera. 2. pertaining to, involving, or affecting mosquitoes of the genus *Culex* or related species.

Cullen's sign (kul′enz) bluish discoloration around the umbilicus sometimes occurring in intraperitoneal hemorrhage, especially following rupture of the uterine tube in ectopic pregnancy. A similar discoloration is seen in acute hemorrhagic pancreatitis.

culmen (kul′men), pl. *cul′mina* [L.] the anterior and upper part of the monticulus cerebelli; called also cacumen.

cultivation (kul″tĭ-va′shun) the propagation of living organisms, applied especially to the growth of microorganisms or other cells in artificial media.

culture (kul′tūr) 1. the propagation of microorganisms or of living tissue cells in special media conducive to their growth. 2. to induce such propagation. 3. the product of such propagation. adj., **cul′tural.**

cell c., a growth of tissue cells *in vitro;* although the cells proliferate they do not organize into tissue.

continuous flow c., the cultivation of bacteria in a continuous flow of fresh medium to maintain bacterial growth in logarithmic phase.

hanging-drop c., a culture in which the material to be cultivated is inoculated into a drop of fluid attached to a coverglass inverted over a hollow slide.

c. medium, any substance or preparation used for the cultivation of living cells.

slant c., one made on the surface of solidified medium in a tube which has been tilted to provide a greater surface area for growth.

stab c., a culture into which the organisms are introduced by thrusting a needle deep into the medium.

streak c., one in which the medium is inoculated by drawing an infected wire across it.

tissue c., the cultivation of tissue cells *in vitro.*

type c., a culture of a species of microorganism usually maintained in a central collection of type or standard culture.

cu. mm. cubic millimeter.

cumulus (ku′mu-lus), pl. *cu′muli* [L.] a small elevation.

c. ooph′orus, a mass of follicular cells surrounding the ovum in the vesicular ovarian follicle.

cuneate (ku′ne-āt) wedge-shaped.

cuneiform (ku-ne′ĭ-form) wedge-shaped; applied particularly to three bones of the foot.

cuneus (ku′ne-us), pl. *cu′nei* [L.] a wedge-shaped lobule on the medial aspect of the occipital lobe of the cerebrum.

cuniculus (ku-nik′u-lus), pl. *cunic′uli* [L.] a burrow in the skin made by the itch mite, *Sarcoptes scabiei.*

cunnilingus (kun″ĭ-lin′gus) [L.] oral stimulation of the female genitals.

cup (kup) a depression or hollow.

eye c., eyecup.

glaucomatous c., a depression of the optic disk due to persistently increased intraocular pressure, broader and deeper than a physiologic cup, and occurring first at the temporal side of the disk.

physiologic c., a slight depression sometimes observed in the optic disk.

cupola (ku′pŏ-lah) cupula.

cupping (kup′ing) the formation of a cup-shaped depression.

cupric (ku′prik) pertaining to or containing divalent copper.

c. sulfate, a crystalline salt of copper used as an emetic, astringent, and fungicide.

cuprous (ku′prus) pertaining to or containing monovalent copper.

cupruresis (ku″proo-re′sis) the urinary excretion of copper.

cupula (ku′pu-lah), pl. *cu′pulae* [L.] a small, inverted cup or dome-shaped cap over a structure.

curare (koo-rah′re) any of a wide variety of highly toxic extracts from various botanical sources, including various species of *Strychnos,* a genus of tropical trees; used originally as arrow poisons in South America. A form extracted from the shrub, *Chondodendron tomentosum,* has been used as skeletal muscle relaxant.

curarization (koo″rar-i-za′shun) administration of curare (usually tubocurarine) to induce muscle relaxation by its blocking activity at the myoneural junction.

cure (kūr) 1. the course of treatment of any disease, or of a special case. 2. the successful treatment of a disease or wound. 3. a system of treating diseases. 4. a medicine effective in treating a disease.

curet (ku-ret′) 1. a spoon-shaped instrument for cleansing a diseased surface. 2. to use a curet.

curettage (ku″rĕ-tahzh′) [Fr.] the cleansing of a diseased surface, as with a curet.

curette (ku-ret′) curet.

curettement (ku-ret′ment) curettage.

curie (ku′re) a unit of radioactivity, defined as the quantity of any radioactive nuclide in which the number of disintegrations per second is 3.700×10^{10}; abbreviated Ci.

curiegram (ku′rĭ-gram) a photographic print made by radium emanation.

curie-hour (ku′re-our″) a unit of dose equivalent to that obtained by exposure for one hour to radioactive material disintegrating at the rate of 3.7×10^{10} atoms per second.

curietherapy (ku″re-ther′ah-pe) originally, radium or radon therapy; now applied to therapy given by emanations from any radioactive source.

curium (ku′re-um) a chemical element, atomic number 96, atomic weight 247, symbol Cm. (See table of ELEMENTS.)

Curling's ulcer (kur′lingz) an ulcer of the duodenum seen after severe burns of the body.

current (kur′ent) that which flows; electric transmission in a circuit.

alternating c., a current that periodically flows in opposite directions.

direct c., a current whose direction is always the same.

curvature (ker′vah-tūr) a nonangular deviation from a normally straight course.

greater c. of stomach, the left or lateral and inferior border of the stomach, marking the inferior junction of the anterior and posterior surfaces.

lesser c. of stomach, the right or medial border of the stomach, marking the superior junction of the anterior and posterior surfaces.

Pott's c., abnormal posterior curvature of the spine occurring as a result of Pott's disease.

spinal c., abnormal deviation of the vertebral column, as in KYPHOSIS, lordosis, and SCOLIOSIS.

curve (kerv) a line that is not straight, or that describes part of a circle, especially a line representing varying values in a graph.

frequency c., a curve representing graphically the probabilities of different numbers of recurrences of an event.

growth c., the curve obtained by plotting increase in size or numbers against the elapsed time.

Cushing's disease (koosh′ingz) Cushing's syndrome in which the hyperadrenocorticism is secondary to excessive pituitary excretion of adrenocorticotropic hormone.

Cushing's syndrome (koosh′ingz) a group of serious symptoms caused by overactivity of the cortices of the adrenal glands. This overactivity is commonly the result of an abnormal growth of the adrenal cortices, or it may be caused by a benign or malignant tumor of one of the adrenal glands. Very rarely the overactivity may be stimulated by a tumor of the pituitary gland or of an ovary.

Symptoms of Cushing's syndrome include painful, fatty swellings on the body (the buffalo hump), moonlike fullness of the face, distention of the abdomen, impotence (in males), amenorrhea, high blood presssure, and general weakness. There may also be an unusual growth of body hair (hirsutism) in females, and streaked purple markings on the body.

Treatment for the disorder is surgical removal of part of the adrenal glands, if their abnormal growth is the cause, or removal of the tumor if that is the source of the condition. The syndrome is named for Dr. Harvey Cushing, the celebrated American brain surgeon and endocrinologist, who in 1932 was the first to describe it.

cushingoid (koosh′ing-goid) resembling Cushing's syndrome, said of signs and symptoms.

cusp (kusp) a pointed or rounded projection, such as on the crown of a tooth, or a segment of a cardiac valve.

semilunar c., any of the semilunar segments of the aortic valve (having posterior, right, and left cusps) or the pulmonary valve (having anterior, right, and left cusps).

cuspid (kus′pid) 1. the third tooth on either side from the midline in each jaw; called also canine tooth. 2. having one cusp.

cuspis (kus′pis), pl. *cus′pides* [L.] a cusp.

cutaneous (ku-ta′ne-us) pertaining to the skin.

cutdown (kut′down) creation of a small incised opening, especially in a vein (venous cutdown), to facilitate venipuncture and permit the passage of a needle or cannula for withdrawal of blood or administration of fluids.

cuticle (ku′tĭ-k'l) 1. a layer of more or less solid substance covering the free surface of an epithelial cell. 2. the narrow band of epidermis extending from the nail wall onto the nail surface; called also eponychium.

cutin (ku′tin) 1. a waxy constituent of the cuticle of plants. 2. a preparation of ox gut used as suture material and as a wound dressing.

cutireaction (ku″tĭ-re-ak′shun) an inflammatory or irritative reaction of the skin, occurring in certain infectious diseases, or on application or injection of a preparation of the organism causing the disease.

cutis (ku′tis) the outer protective covering of the body; the skin.

c. anseri′na, transitory erection of the hair follicles due to contraction of the arrectores muscles, a reflection of sympathetic nerve discharge; goose flesh.

c. hyperelas′tica, Ehlers-Danlos syndrome.

c. lax′a, a hereditary disorder in which the skin and subcutaneous tissues hypertrophy, so that the skin hangs in folds.

cuvette (ku-vet′) [Fr.] a glass container generally having well defined characteristics (dimensions, optical properties), to contain solutions or suspensions for study.

CVA cerebral vascular accident.

CVP central venous pressure.

cwt. hundredweight.

cyan(o)- word element [Gr.], *blue.*

cyanhemoglobin (si″an-he″mo-glo′bin) a compound formed by the action of hydrocyanic acid on hemoglobin, which gives the bright red color to blood.

cyanide (si′ah-nīd) a binary compound of cyanogen. Some inorganic compounds, such as cyanide salts, potassium cyanide, and sodium cyanide, are important in industry for extracting gold and silver from their ores and in electroplating. Other cyanide compounds are used in the manufacture of synthetic rubber and textiles. Cyanides are also used in pesticides.

Most cyanide compounds are deadly poisons. Treatment for cyanide poisoning varies according to the nature of the poison. In the case of swallowed poison like hydrocyanic acid, the poison itself will cause vomiting. If the victim is able to swallow, milk or water may be given. A large dose of hydrocyanic acid will cause almost instant death.

If a gas such as hydrogen cyanide has been inhaled, the victim should be taken into open air and given artificial respiration.

cyanmethemoglobin (si″an-met″he-mo-glo′bin) a crystalline substance formed by the action of hydrocyanic acid on methemoglobin in the cold, or on oxyhemoglobin at body temperature; used in measuring hemoglobin in the blood.

cyanmetmyoglobin (si″an-met-mi″o-glo′bin) a compound formed from metmyoglobin by addition of the cyanide ion to yield reduction to the ferrous state.

cyanocobalamin (si″ah-no-ko-bal′ah-min) a substance having hematopoietic activity found in the liver, fish meal, eggs, and other natural sources, or produced from cultures of *Streptomyces griseus;* it combines with intrinsic factor for absorption and is needed for erythrocyte maturation. Absence of intrinsic factor leads to malabsorption of cyanocobalamin and results in pernicious anemia. Called also antianemia factor, extrinsic factor, and VITAMIN B_{12}.

radioactive c., cyanocobalamin containing radioactive cobalt of mass number 57 or 60, used in diagnosis of pernicious anemia.

cyanogen (si-an′o-jen) the radical CN—; also NCCN, the latter a very poisonous gas.

cyanolabe (si′ah-no-lāb″) the pigment in retinal cones that is more sensitive to the blue range of the spectrum than are chlorolabe and erythrolabe.

cyanopia, cyanopsia (si″ah-no′pe-ah; si-ah-nop′se-ah) a defect of vision in which objects appear tinged with blue.

cyanosed (si′ah-nōsd) cyanotic.

cyanosis (si″ah-no′sis) a bluish discoloration of the skin and mucous membranes due to excessive concentration of reduced hemoglobin in the blood. adj., **cyanot′ic.**

central c., that due to arterial unsaturation, the aortic blood carrying reduced hemoglobin.

enterogenous c., a syndrome due to absorption of nitrites and sulfides from the intestine, principally marked by methemoglobinemia and/or sulfhemoglobinemia associated with cyanosis, and accompanied by severe enteritis, abdominal pain, constipation or diarrhea, headache, dyspnea, dizziness, syncope, anemia, and, occasionally, digital clubbing and indicanuria.

peripheral c., that due to an excessive amount of reduced hemoglobin in the venous blood as a result of extensive oxygen extraction at the capillary level.

cybernetics (si″ber-net′iks) the science of communication and control in the animal and in the machine.

cycl(o)- word element [Gr.], *round; recurring; ciliary body of the eye.*

Cyclaine (si′klān) trademark for preparations of hexylcaine, a local anesthetic.

cyclamate (si′klah-māt) any salt of cyclamic acid.

cyclamic acid (si-klam′ik) an acid, the calcium and sodium salts of which have been used widely as non-nutritive sugar substitutes.

Cyclamycin (si′klah-mi″sin) trademark for preparations of troleandomycin, an antibiotic.

cyclandelate (si-klan′dĕ-lāt) a vasodilator for peripheral vascular disease.

cyclarthrosis (si″klar-thro′sis) a pivot joint.

cyclase (si′klās) an enzyme that catalyzes the formation of a cyclic phosphodiester.

adenyl c., adenylate c., an enzyme that catalyzes the conversion of adenosine triphosphate (ATP) to cyclic adenosine monophosphate (cyclic AMP) plus pyrophosphate, and is activated by many hormones.

cycle (si′k′l) a succession or recurring series of events.

carbon c., the steps by which carbon (in the form of CARBON DIOXIDE) is extracted from the atmosphere by living organisms and ultimately returned to the atmosphere. It comprises a series of interconversions of carbon compounds beginning with the production of carbohydrates by plants during photosynthesis, proceeding through animal consumption, and ending and beginning again in the decomposition of the animal or plant or in the exhalation of carbon dioxide by animals.

cardiac c., a complete cardiac movement, or heart beat, including systole, diastole, and the intervening pause.

citric acid c., tricarboxylic acid cycle.

estrous c., the recurring periods of heat (estrus) in adult females of most mammals and the correlated

changes in the reproductive tract from one period to another.

Krebs c., tricarboxylic acid cycle.

menstrual c., the period of the regularly recurring physiologic changes in the endometrium which culminate in its shedding (MENSTRUATION) (see also MENSTRUAL CYCLE).

nitrogen c., the steps by which nitrogen is extracted from the nitrates of soil and water, incorporated as amino acids and proteins in living organisms, and ultimately reconverted to nitrates: (1) conversion of nitrogen to nitrates by bacteria; (2) the extraction of the nitrates by plants and the building of amino acids and proteins by adding an amino group to the carbon compounds produced in photosynthesis; (3) the ingestion of plants by animals; and (4) the return of nitrogen to the soil in animal excretions or on the death and decomposition of plants and animals.

ovarian c., the sequence of physiologic changes in the ovary involved in ovulation (see also OVULATION and REPRODUCTION).

reproductive c., the cycle of physiologic changes in the reproductive organs, from the time of fertilization of the ovum through gestation and parturition (see also REPRODUCTION).

sex c., sexual c., 1. the physiologic changes recurring regularly in the reproductive organs of female mammals when pregnancy does not supervene. 2. the period of sexual reproduction in an organism that also reproduces asexually.

tricarboxylic acid c., the cyclic metabolic mechanism by which the complete oxidation of the acetyl moiety of acetyl-coenzyme A is effected; the process is the chief source of mammalian energy, during which carbon chains of sugars, fatty acids, and amino acid are metabolized to yield carbon dioxide, water, and high-energy phosphate bonds. Called also citric acid cycle and Krebs cycle.

urea c., a cyclic series of reactions that produce urea, a major route for removal of the ammonia produced in the metabolism of amino acids in the liver and kidney (see also UREA).

cyclectomy (si-klek′to-me) 1. excision of a piece of the ciliary body. 2. excision of a portion of the ciliary border of the eyelid.

cyclic (sik′lik) pertaining to or occurring in a cycle or cycles. The term is applied to chemical compounds that contain a ring of atoms in the nucleus.

cyclic AMP adenosine 3′:5′-cyclic phosphate.

cyclicotomy (si″klĭ-kot′o-me) cyclotomy.

cyclitis (si-kli′tis) inflammation of the ciliary body.

cyclizine (si′klĭ-zēn) an antihistamine used in the form of the hydrochloride salt as an antinauseant to prevent motion sickness.

cyclobarbital (si″klo-bar′bĭ-tal) a short- to intermediate-acting barbiturate used intravenously as an anesthetic and hypnotic.

cyclochoroiditis (si″klo-ko″roi-di′tis) inflammation of the ciliary body and choroid.

cyclocryotherapy (si″klo-kri″o-ther′ah-pe) freezing of the ciliary body; done in the treatment of glaucoma.

cyclocumarol (si″klo-koo′mah-rōl) a synthetic anticoagulant.

cyclodialysis (si″klo-di-al′ĭ-sis) creation of a communication between the anterior chamber of the eye and the suprachoroidal space, in glaucoma.

cyclodiathermy (si″klo-di″ah-ther′me) destruction of a portion of the ciliary body by diathermy.

cyclogram (si′klo-gram) a tracing of the visual field made with a cycloscope.

cycloguanil (si″klo-gwan′il) an antimalarial used as the pamoate salt.

Cyclogyl (si′klo-jil) trademark for a preparation of cyclopentolate, an anticholinergic, cycloplegic-mydriatic drug.

cycloid (si′kloid) 1. containing a ring of atoms; said of organic chemical compounds. 2. cyclothymic (2).

cycloisomerase (si″klo-i-som′er-ās) an enzyme that catalyzes intramolecular lyase reactions.

cyclokeratitis (si″klo-ker″ah-ti′tis) inflammation of the cornea and ciliary body.

cyclo-ligase (si″klo-li′gas) an enzyme that catalyzes the formation of carbon-nitrogen, C—N bonds, and the breakdown of a pyrophosphate bond, as of ATP.

cyclomethycaine (si″klo-meth′ĭ-kān) a local anesthetic.

cyclopentamine (si″klo-pen′tah-mēn) a sympathomimetic used as a nasal decongestant in the form of the hydrochloride salt.

cyclopentolate (si″klo-pen′to-lāt) an anticholinergic drug used as a topical cycloplegic and mydriatic in the form of the hydrochloride salt.

cyclophoria (si″klo-fo′re-ah) HETEROPHORIA in which there is deviation of the visual axis of one eye from the anteroposterior axis in the absence of visual fusional stimuli.

cyclophosphamide (si″klo-fos′fah-mīd) a neoplastic suppressant used in the treatment of lymphomas and leukemias.

cyclopia (si-klo′pe-ah) a developmental anomaly characterized by a single orbital fossa, with the globe absent or rudimentary, apparently normal, or duplicated, or the nose absent or present as a tubular appendix located above the orbit.

cycloplegia (si″klo-ple′je-ah) paralysis of the ciliary muscle; paralysis of accommodation.

cycloplegic (si″klo-ple′jik) 1. pertaining to, characterized by, or causing cycloplegia. 2. an agent that produces cycloplegia.

cyclopropane (si″klo-pro′pān) a powerful central nervous system depressent used as an inhalation ANESTHETIC. The drug can be given in small doses and is particularly useful in anesthetizing elderly or poor-risk patients. This gas is highly explosive and requires special handling and precautions against sparks or flames, which would result in an explosion.

Cyclops (si′klops) a genus of minute crustaceans, species of which act as hosts of *Diphyllobothrium* and *Dracunculus.*

cyclops (si′klops) a monster exhibiting cyclopia.

cycloscope (si′klo-skōp) a form of perimeter for mapping the visual fields.

cycloserine (si″klo-ser′ēn) a antibiotic substance elaborated by *Streptomyces orchidaceus* or produced synthetically, used as a tuberculostatic and in the treatment of urinary tract infections.

cyclosis (si-klo′sis) movement of the cytoplasm within a cell, without external deformation of the cell wall.

Cyclospasmol (si″klo-spaz′mol) trademark for preparations of cyclandelate, a peripheral vasodilator.

cyclothiazide (si″klo-thi′ah-zīd) a diuretic and antihypertensive agent.

cyclothymia (si″klo-thi′me-ah) a condition characterized by alternating moods of elation and dejection.

cyclothymic (si″ko-thi′mik) 1. pertaining to or characterized by cyclothymia. 2. a cyclothymic personality.

c. personality, a personality marked by alternate moods of elation and dejection.

cyclotomy (si-klot′o-me) incision of the ciliary muscle; cyclicotomy.

cyclotron (si′klo-tron) an apparatus for accelerating protons or deuterons to high energies by means of a constant magnet and an oscillating electric field.

cyclotropia (si″klo-tro′pe-ah) STRABISMUS in which there is permanent deviation of the eye around the anteroposterior axis in the presence of visual fusional stimuli, resulting in diplopia.

cycrimine (si′krĭ-mēn) an anticholinergic used as the hydrochloride salt in the treatment of parkinsonism.

cyesis (si-e′sis) pregnancy. adj., **cyet′ic.**

cylindroid (sil′in-droid) 1. shaped like a cylinder. 2. a urinary cast of various origins, which tapers to a slender tail that is often twisted or curled upon itself.

cylindroma (sil″in-dro′mah) 1. adenocystic carcinoma. 2. a benign skin tumor, usually on the face and scalp, in which the stroma has the form of elongated, twisted cords of hyaline material. adj., **cylindrom′atous.**

cylindruria (sil″in-droo′re-ah) the presence of cylindroids in the urine.

cymbocephaly (sim″bo-sef′ah-le) scaphocephaly.

cynanthropy (sin-an′thro-pe) a delusion in which the patient believes himself a dog.

cynophobia (sin″o-fo′be-ah) morbid fear of dogs.

cyotrophy (si-ot′ro-fe) nutrition of the fetus.

cyproheptadine (si″pro-hep′tah-dēn) a histamine and serotonin antagonist used as an antipruritic in the form of the hydrochloride salt.

cyrtometer (sir-tom′ĕ-ter) a device for measuring the curved surfaces of the body.

cyst (sist) 1. a closed epithelium-lined sac or capsule containing a liquid or semisolid substance. Most cysts are harmless. Nevertheless they should be removed when possible because they occasionally may change into malignant growths, become infected, or obstruct a gland. There are four main types of cysts: retention cysts, exudation cysts, embryonic cysts, and parasitic cysts. 2. a stage in the life cycle of certain parasites, during which they are enveloped in a protective wall.

alveolar c′s, dilatations of pulmonary alveoli, which may fuse by breakdown of their septa to form large air cysts (pneumatoceles).

blue dome c., a benign retention cyst of the breast that shows a blue color (see also CYSTIC DISEASE OF BREAST).

branchial c., branchiogenic c., branchiogenous c., one formed from an incompletely closed branchial cleft (see also BRANCHIAL CYST).

chocolate c., one filled with hemosiderin following local hemorrhage, such as may occur in the ovary in ovarian endometriosis.

daughter c., a small parasitic cyst developed from the walls of a larger cyst.

dermoid c., a tumor containing bone, hair, teeth, etc. (see also DERMOID CYST).

echinococcus c., hydatid cyst.

embryonic c., one developing from bits of embryonic tissue that have been overgrown by other tissues, or from developing organs that normally disappear before birth. An example is a BRANCHIAL CYST.

epidermal c., epidermal inclusion c., epidermoid c., one containing keratinized material and lined by keratinizing squamous epithelium, usually found in the skin.

exudation c., a cyst formed by the slow seepage of an exudate into a closed cavity.

follicular c., one due to occlusion of the duct of a follicle or small gland, especially one formed by enlargement of a graafian follicle as a result of accumulated transudate.

hydatid c., the larval stage of the tapeworms *Echinococcus granulosis* and *E. multilocularis* (see also HYDATID DISEASE).

keratin c., one arising in the pilosebaceous apparatus, lined by stratified squamous epithelium and containing largely macerated keratin and often sufficient sebum to render the contents greasy and often rancid.

meibomian c., chalazion.

myxoid c., a nodular lesion usually overlying a distal interphalangeal finger joint in the dorsolateral or dorsomesial position, consisting of focal mucinous degeneration of the collagen of the dermis; not a true cyst, lacking an epithelial wall, it does not communicate with the underlying synovial space.

Naboth's c's, nabothian c's, cystlike formations caused by occlusion of the lumina of glands in the mucosa of the uterine cervix, causing them to be distended with retained secretion. Called also Naboth's, or nabothian, follicles.

parasitic c., one forming around larval parasites (tapeworms, amebas, trichinae) that enter the body.

pilonidal c., a hair-containing sacrococcygeal dermoid cyst or sinus, often opening at a postanal dimple (see also PILONIDAL CYST).

retention c., a tumor-like accumulation of a secretion formed when the outlet of a secreting gland is obstructed. These cysts may develop in any of the secretory glands—the breast, pancreas, kidney, salivary or sebaceous glands, and mucous membranes.

sarcosporidian c's, cylindrical cysts containing parasitic spores, found in the muscles of those infected with *Sarcocystis.*

sebaceous c., a retention cyst of a sebaceous gland (see also SEBACEOUS CYST).

vitelline c., a congenital cyst lined with ciliated epithelium occurring along the gastrointestinal canal; the remains of the omphalomesenteric duct.

cyst(o)- word element [Gr.], *cyst; bladder.*

cystadenocarcinoma (sis-tad″ĕ-no-kar″sĭ-no′mah) adenocarcinoma with extensive cyst formation.

cystadenoma (sis-tad″ĕ-no′mah) cystoma blended with adenoma.

mucinous c., a multilocular tumor produced by ovarian epithelial cells and having mucin-filled cavities.

papillary c., any tumor producing patterns that are both papillary and cystic; called also papilloadenocystoma.

serous c., a cystic tumor of the ovary containing thin, clear yellow serum and some solid tissue.

cystalgia (sis-tal′je-ah) pain in the bladder.

cystectasia (sis″tek-ta′ze-ah) dilatation of the bladder.

cystectomy (sis-tek′to-me) 1. excision of a cyst. 2. excision or resection of the urinary bladder.

cysteic acid (sis-te′ik) an intermediate product in the oxidation of cysteine to taurine.

cysteine (sis′te-in) a sulfur-containing amino acid produced by enzymatic or acid hydrolysis of proteins, readily oxidized to cystine; sometimes found in urine.

cystencephalus (sis″ten-sef′ah-lus) a monster with a membranous sac in place of a brain.

cystic (sis′tik) 1. pertaining to or containing cysts. 2. pertaining to the urinary bladder or to the gallbladder.

c. disease of breast, a form of mammary dysplasia with formation of cysts containing a semitransparent, turbid fluid that imparts a brown to blue color to the unopened cysts (blue dome cysts). The condition is due to abnormal hyperplasia of the ductal epithelium and dilatation of the ducts of the mammary gland. Called also Schimmelbusch's disease.

c. duct, the excretory duct of the gallbladder (see also BILE DUCTS).

c. fibrosis, a generalized hereditary disorder associated with widespread dysfunction of the exocrine glands, with accumulation of excessively thick and tenacious mucus and abnormal secretion of sweat and saliva; called also cystic fibrosis of the pancreas, and mucoviscidosis. The disease is inherited as a recessive trait; both parents must be carriers. The cause of the disease is presumably the absence, insufficiency, or abnormality of some essential hormone or enzyme.

EFFECTS. Symptoms and severity of cystic fibrosis vary widely. Although it is congenital, it may not manifest itself to any appreciable degree during the early weeks or months of life, or it may cause intestinal obstruction and perforation in the newborn. The chief cause of complications in cystic fibrosis is the extremely thick mucus produced. Normal mucus bathes and protects internal surfaces and transports chemicals produced in one organ through intricate small ducts for use in another organ. Normal mucus flows easily, carrying with it bacteria, dirt, and wastes that will be eliminated from the body. The mucus of cystic fibrosis, in contrast, is highly adhesive. Bacteria and other matter stick to it, and it in turn clogs the lungs and usually interferes with the flow of digestive enzymes from the pancreas to the small intestine.

In the lungs, the mucus blocks the bronchioles, creating breathing difficulties. Infection develops, thereby increasing obstruction of the air passages. Air becomes trapped in the lungs (emphysema), and scattered small areas eventually collapse (patchy atelectasis). Repeated infections follow, inflaming and damaging lung tissue and leading to chronic lung disease. The organism that produces infection in cystic fibrosis is almost always a stahylococcus, but other organisms may be present in more severe cases.

When mucus prevents the pancreatic enzymes from reaching the duodenum (which occurs in approximately 80 per cent of cystic fibrosis patients), digestion is hindered. Fats especially are poorly digested and absorbed. The child may have a voracious appetite, yet fail to grow normally or gain weight. There may be marked signs of malnutrition. The outstanding symptom associated with pancreatic enzyme deficiency is frequent bulky, fatty, and foul-smelling feces.

Between 5 and 10 per cent of cystic fibrosis babies are born with intestines obstructed by putty-like intestinal secretions (meconium ileus) and die unless the condition is diagnosed promptly and relieved by surgery within the first few days of life. Such relief does not protect the child against the other manifestations of cystic fibrosis, although these may not appear until later.

Because cysts and scar tissue on the pancreas were observed during autopsy when the disease was first being differentiated from other conditions, it was given the name cystic fibrosis of the pancreas. Although this term describes a secondary rather than primary characteristic, it has been retained.

DIAGNOSIS. Sweat in cystic fibrosis is excessively salty. Collapse of cystic fibrosis patients from salt loss during a heat wave led, in 1953, to recognition of the sweat abnormality. A sweat test, introduced the next year, remains the cornerstone of diagnosis of cystic fibrosis. If either the chloride or sodium content of the sweat is from three to five times higher than in normal children, there is a strong basis for suspecting cystic fibrosis. Supporting evidence can confirm the sweat test finding.

TREATMENT. Under careful supervision by a physician or physical therapist, parents are taught the principles of home treatment of cystic fibrosis. The child may be required to sleep regularly in a plastic mist tent, into which a dense fog is pumped to help liquefy mucus and check infection. Aerosol therapy is generally prescribed. Extracts of animal pancreas taken with meals, which should be high in protein and low in fat, compensate for pancreatic deficiency. Physical therapy involving POSTURAL DRAINAGE together with "clapping" and "vibrating" by the physical therapist or parent aids in loosening the mucus so that it can be coughed up and expectorated.

It is estimated that in the United States cystic fibrosis occurs once in every few thousand births. Caucasians appear more subject to it than Negroes, and among Orientals it seems to be rare.

PATIENT CARE. Maintenance of the child's nutritional status may be difficult because of his tendency to cough and vomit frequently during feedings, and also because of difficulty in breathing. Small amounts of food, given slowly and at frequent intervals, are best for infants as well as for small children with cystic fibrosis.

Skin care is important, especially for infants and toddlers who are not yet toilet trained. The stools are likely to be copious and extremely irritating to the skin.

Frequent turning of the infant or bedridden child helps to prevent decubitus ulcers and lessens the danger of pneumonia, a constant threat to these children.

Prevention of infection is a most important aspect of the care of these children because of their extreme vulnerability to disorders of the respiratory tract.

Education of the parents must include the dietary regimen, use of the Croupette or AEROSOL therapy machine in the home, hygienic measures to prevent infections, and the need for continuous medical follow-up and administration of medications prescribed for the child by the physician.

cysticercosis (sis″tĭ-ser-ko′sis) infection with cysticerci.

cysticercus (sis″tĭ-ser′kus), pl. *cysticer′ci* [Gr.] a larval form of tapeworm.

cystiform (sis′tĭ-form) resembling a cyst.

cystigerous (sis-tij′er-us) containing cysts.

cystine (sis′tēn, sis′tin) a naturally occurring amino acid, the chief sulfur-containing component of the protein molecule. It is sometimes found in the urine and in the kidneys in the form of minute hexagonal crystals, frequently forming cystine calculus in the bladder.

c. storage d., Fanconi's syndrome (2).

cystinemia (sis″tĭ-ne′me-ah) the presence of cystine in the blood.

cystinosis (sis″tĭ-no′sis) Fanconi's syndrome (2).

cystinuria (sis″tĭ-nu′re-ah) the occurrence of cystine in the urine.

cystistaxis (sis″tĭ-stak′sis) oozing of blood from the mucous membrane into the bladder.

cystitis (sis-ti′tis) inflammation of the urinary bladder. The condition may result from an ascending infection coming from the exterior of the body by way of the urethra, or it may be caused by an infection descending from the kidney. A simple cystitis that does not involve the rest of the urinary tract is not as serious as the descending type in which the kidneys and ureters as well as the bladder are involved.

Often cystitis is not an isolated infection but is rather a result of some other physical condition. For example, urinary retention, calculi in the bladder, tumors, or neurologic diseases impairing the normal function of the bladder may lead to cystitis.

SYMPTOMS AND TREATMENT. The most common symptoms of cystitis are dysuria, frequency and urgency of urination, and in some cases hematuria. Chills and fever indicate involvement of the entire urinary tract and are not symptomatic of uncomplicated cystitis.

Treatment of acute cystitis consists of antibiotics, forcing of fluids, and bed rest. Hot sitz baths give some relief of the discomfort, and spasms of the bladder wall may respond to an antispasmodic drug such as hyoscyamine. Chronic cystitis is more difficult to cure and may require surgical dilatation of the urethra and antiseptic bladder instillations. In many cases removal of the underlying cause, such as chronic vaginal infection, relieves the cystitis.

cystitomy (sis-tit′o-me) surgical division of the capsule of the crystalline lens.

cystocarcinoma (sis″to-kar″sĭ-no′mah) carcinoma associated with cysts.

cystocele (sis′to-sēl) herniation of the urinary bladder into the vagina.

cystodynia (sis″to-din′e-ah) pain in the bladder; cystalgia.

cystoelytroplasty (sis″to-el′ĭ-tro-plas″te) surgical repair of a vesicovaginal fistula.

cystoepithelioma (sis″to-ep″ĭ-the″le-o′mah) a tumor with cystic and epitheliomatous elements.

cystofibroma (sis″to-fi-bro′mah) a fibroma containing cysts.

cystogastrostomy (sis″to-gas-tros′to-me) surgical anastomosis of a pancreatic cyst to the stomach for drainage.

cystogram (sis′to-gram) the film obtained by cystography.

voiding c., a radiogram of the urinary tract made while the patient is urinating.

cystography (sis-tog′rah-fe) roentgenography of the urinary bladder using a contrast medium, so that the outline of the organ can be seen clearly. This type of examination frequently is part of a complete x-ray study of the kidneys and ureters as well as the bladder. (See also PYELOGRAPHY.) It is useful in diagnosing tumors or other defects in the bladder wall, or calculi or other pathologic conditions of the bladder, especially when cystoscopy is impossible.

cystoid (sis′toid) 1. resembling a cyst. 2. a cystlike, circumscribed collection of softened material, having no enclosing capsule.

cystojejunostomy (sis″to-je-joo-nos′to-me) surgical anastomosis of a pancreatic cyst to the jejunum.

cystolith (sis′to-lith) a vesical calculus.

cystolithectomy (sis″to-lĭ-thek′to-me) surgical removal of a vesical calculus.

cystolithiasis (sis″to-lĭ-thi′ah-sis) formation of vesical calculi.

cystolithic (sis″to-lith′ik) pertaining to a vesical calculus.

cystolithotomy (sis″to-lĭ-thot′o-me) cystolithectomy.

cystoma (sis-to′mah) a tumor containing cysts of neoplastic origin; a cystic tumor.

cystometer (sis-tom′ĕ-ter) an instrument for studying the neuromuscular mechanism of the bladder by means of measurements of pressure and capacity.

cystometrogram (sis″to-met′ro-gram) the record obtained by cystometrography.

cystometrography (sis″to-mĕ-trog′rah-fe) the graphic recording of intravesical volumes and pressures.

cystomorphous (sis″to-mor′fus) resembling a cyst or bladder.

cystopexy (sis′to-pek″se) fixation of the bladder to the abdominal wall.

cystoplasty (sis′to-plas″te) plastic repair of the bladder.

cystoplegia (sis″to-ple′je-ah) paralysis of the bladder.

cystoproctostomy (sis″to-prok-tos′to-me) surgical creation of a communication between the urinary bladder and the rectum.

cystoptosis (sis″top-to′sis) prolapse of part of the inner coat of the bladder into the urethra.

cystopyelitis (sis″to-pi″ĕ-li′tis) inflammation of the bladder and renal pelvis.

cystopyelonephritis (sis″to-pi″ĕ-lo-nĕ-fri′tis) combined cystitis and pyelonephritis.

cystorrhaphy (sis-tor′ah-fe) suture of the bladder.

cystorrhea (sis″to-re′ah) mucous discharge from the bladder.

cystosarcoma (sis″to-sar-ko′mah) an unusually large fibroadenoma of the mammary gland, with a cellular, sarcoma-like stoma; it is locally aggressive and sometimes metastasizes.

cystoscope (sis′to-skōp) an endoscope especially designed for passing through the urethra into the bladder to permit visual inspection of the interior of that organ.

cystoscopy (sis-tos′ko-pe) examination of the bladder by means of a cystoscope, a hollow metal tube that is introduced into the urinary meatus and passed through the urethra and into the bladder. At the end of the cystoscope is an electric bulb that illuminates the bladder interior. By means of special lenses and mirrors the bladder mucosa is examined for inflammation, calculi, or tumors.

A catheter can be passed through the cystoscope into the bladder or, if necessary, beyond, into the ureters and kidneys. In this way samples of urine can be obtained for diagnostic purposes. Also, radiopaque fluids can be injected into the bladder or ure-

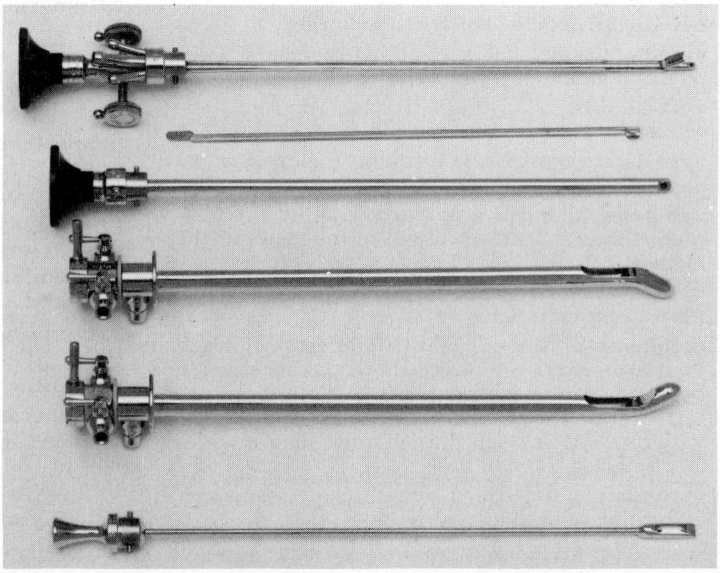

Cystoscope with lighting system. (Courtesy of American Cystoscope Makers, Inc.)

ters for x-rays of the urinary tract (see also PYELOGRAPHY).

cystostomy (sis-tos′to-me) surgical formation of an opening into the bladder.

cystotomy (sis-tot′o-me) incision of the bladder (see also VESICOTOMY).

cystoureteritis (sis″to-u-re″ter-i′tis) inflammation involving the urinary bladder and ureters.

cystoureterogram (sis″to-u-re′ter-o-gram″) a roentgenogram of the bladder and ureter.

cystourethroscope (sis″to-u-re′thro-skōp″) an instrument for examining the posterior urethra and bladder.

cyt(o)- word element [Gr.], *a cell.*

cytarabine (si-tār′ah-bēn) an antimetabolite that inhibits DNA synthesis, and hence has antineoplastic and antiviral properties.

-cyte (sīt) word element [Gr.], *a cell.*

cytoanalyzer (si″to-an″ah-li′zer) an electronic optical apparatus for the detection of malignant cells in smears.

cytoarchitectonic (si″to-ar″kĭ-tek-ton′ik) pertaining to the cellular structure or the arrangement of cells in tissue.

cytobiology (si″to-bi-ol′o-je) the biology of cells.

cytocentrum (si″to-sen′trum) centrosome.

cytochalasin (si′to-kal′ah-sin) any of a group of fungal metabolites that affect the motility of polymorphonuclear leukocytes.

cytochemistry (si″to-kem′is-tre) the identification and localization of the different chemical compounds and their activities within the cell.

cytochrome (si′to-krōm) any of a class of hemoproteins, widely distributed in animal and plant tissue, whose main function is electron transport; distinguished according to their prosthetic group as *a, b, c,* and *d.*

cytochylema (si″to-ki-le′mah) hyaloplasm (1).

cytocide (si′to-sīd) an agent that destroys cells. adj., **cytoci′dal.**

cytocinesia (si″to-si-ne′ze-ah) cytokinesis.

cytoclasis (si-tok′lah-sis) the destruction of cells. adj., **cytoclas′tic.**

cytodendrite (si″to-den′drīt) a dendrite.

cytodiagnosis (si″to-di″ag-no′sis) diagnosis based on examination of cells.

cytodieresis (si″to-di-er′ĕ-sis) cell division, i.e., meiosis or mitosis.

cytodistal (si″to-dis′tal) denoting that part of an axon remote from the cell body.

cytogene (si′to-jēn) a self-perpetuating cytoplasmic particle that traces origin to the genes of the nucleus.

cytogenesis (si″to-jen′ĕ-sis) the origin and development of the cell.

cytogenetics (si″to-jĕ-net′iks) that branch of genetics devoted to the cellular constituents concerned in heredity, i.e., the chromosomes.

clinical c., the branch of cytogenetics concerned with relations between chromosomal abnormalities and pathologic conditions.

cytogenic (si″to-jen′ik) 1. pertaining to cytogenesis. 2. forming or producing cells.

cytoglycopenia (si″to-gli″ko-pe′ne-ah) deficient glucose content of the body or blood cells.

cytohistogenesis (si″to-his″to-jen′ĕ-sis) development of the structure of cells.

cytokinesis (si″to-ki-ne′sis) the changes that occur in the cytoplasm during meiosis, mitosis, and fertilization.

cytokinin (si″to-ki′nin) any of a class of phytohormones (N^6-substituted adenines) whose principal functions are the induction of cell division (cytokinesis) and the regulation of differentiation of tissue (organogenesis).

cytologist (si-tol′o-jist) a specialist in cytology.

cytology (si-tol′o-je) the study of cells, their origin, structure, function, and pathology. adj., **cytolog′ic.**

exfoliative c., microscopic examination of cells desquamated from a body surface as a means of detecting malignant change.

cytolysin (si-tol′ĭ-sin) a substance or antibody that produces cytolysis.

cytolysis (si-tol′ĭ-sis) the dissolution of cells.

cytolysosome (si″to-li′so-sōm) a lysosome fused with mitochondria and other cell organelles and associated with cell autolysis.

cytomegalic inclusion disease (si″to-meg′ah-lik in-kloo′zhun) a disease, especially of newborns, due to infection with a cytomegalovirus, and characterized by hepatosplenomegaly and often by microcephaly and mental or motor retardation.

cytomegalovirus (si″to-meg″ah-lo-vi′rus) any of a group of highly host-specific herpesviruses infecting man, monkeys, or rodents, producing unique large cells with inclusion bodies; the virus specific for man causes cytomegalic inclusion disease.

Cytomel (si′to-mel) trademark for a preparation of sodium liothyronine, a thyroid hormone preparation.

cytometaplasia (si″to-met″ah-pla′ze-ah) change in function or form of cells.

cytometer (si-tom′ĕ-ter) a device for counting cells.

cytometry (si-tom′ĕ-tre) the counting of blood cells.

cytomitome (si″to-mi′tōm) a fibril or fibrillary structure in the cytoplasm.

cytomorphology (si″to-mor-fol′o-je) the morphology of body cells.

cytomorphosis (si″to-mor-fo′sis) the changes through which cells pass in development.

cyton (si′ton) the cell body of a neuron.

cytopathic (si″to-path′ik) pertaining to or characterized by pathologic changes in cells.

cytopathogenesis (si″to-path″o-jen′ĕ-sis) production of pathologic changes in cells. adj., **cytopathogenet′ic.**

cytopathology (si″to-pah-thol′o-je) the study of cells in disease; cellular pathology.

cytopenia (si″to-pe′ne-ah) deficiency in the cells of the blood.

cytophagy (si-tof′ah-je) the ingestion of cells by phagocytes.

cytophilic (si″to-fil′ik) having an affinity for cells.

cytophotometer (si″to-fo-tom′ĕ-ter) a photometer for measuring localization of organic compounds within cells by measuring the light intensity through selected stained areas of cytoplasm.

cytophylaxis (si″to-fi-lak′sis) 1. the protection of

cells against cytolysis. 2. increase in cellular activity.

cytophysics (si″to-fiz′iks) the physics of cell activity.

cytophysiology (si″to-fiz″e-ol′o-je) the physiology of cells.

cytopipette (si″to-pi-pet′) a pipette for taking cytological smears.

cytoplasm (si′to-plazm) the protoplasm of a cell surrounding the nucleus (nucleoplasm). adj., **cytoplas′mic.**

cytoscopy (si-tos′ko-pe) examination of cells.

cytosine (si′to-sēn) a pyrimidine base, one of the disintegration products of nucleic acid.

cytoskeleton (si″to-skel′ĕ-ton) a conspicuous internal reinforcement in the cytoplasm of a cell, containing minute filaments aggregated in bundles.

cytosol (si′to-sol) the liquid medium of the cytoplasm, e.g., cytoplasm minus organelles and nonmembranous insoluble components.

cytosome (si′to-sōm) the body of a cell apart from its nucleus.

cytospongium (si″to-spun′je-um) spongioplasm.

cytostatic (si″to-stat′ik) 1. suppressing the growth and multiplication of cells. 2. an agent that so acts.

cytotaxis (si″to-tak′sis) the movement and arrangement of cells with respect to a specific source of stimulation. adj., **cytotac′tic.**

cytothesis (si-toth′ĕ-sis) restitution of cells to their normal condition.

cytotoxic (si″to-tok′sik) having a deleterious effect upon cells.

cytotoxin (si″to-tok′sin) a toxin having a specific toxic action on cells of special organs.

cytotrophoblast (si″to-trof′o-blast) the cellular (inner) layer of the trophoblast.

cytotropism (si-tot′ro-pizm) 1. cell movement in response to external stimulation. 2. the tendency of viruses, bacteria, drugs, etc., to exert their effect upon certain cells of the body.

Cytoxan (si-tok′san) trademark for preparations of cyclophosphamide, an antineoplastic agent.

cytula (sit′u-lah) the impregnated ovum.

cyturia (sĭ-tu′re-ah) the presence of cells of any sort in the urine.

D

D chemical symbol, *deuterium*.

D- chemical prefix (small capital) specifying that the substance corresponds in chemical configuration to the standard substance D-glyceraldehyde. Opposed to L-. For carbohydrates, the configuration of the highest numbered asymmetric carbon atoms determines whether the substance is D- or L-; for amino acids, the lowest numbered asymmetric carbon atom is the key.

d- prefix, *dextro-*.

dacarbazine (dah-kar′bah-zēn) an antineoplastic used in the treatment of metastatic malignant melanoma.

dacry(o)- word element [Gr.], *tears* or *the lacrimal apparatus of the eye.*

dacryagogic (dak″re-ah-goj′ik) 1. inducing a flow of tears. 2. serving as a channel for discharge of secretion of the lacrimal glands.

dacryagogue (dak′re-ah-gog″) 1. an agent that induces a flow of tears. 2. a lacrimal duct.

dacryoadenalgia (dak″re-o-ad″ĕ-nal′je-ah) pain in a lacrimal gland.

dacryoadenectomy (dak″re-o-ad″ĕ-nek′to-me) excision of a lacrimal gland.

dacryoadenitis (dak″re-o-ad″ĕ-ni′tis) inflammation of a lacrimal gland.

dacryoblennorrhea (dak″re-o-blen″o-re′ah) mucous flow from the lacrimal apparatus.

dacryocele (dak′re-o-sēl″) dacryocystocele.

dacryocyst (dak′re-o-sist″) the lacrimal sac.

dacryocystalgia (dak″re-o-sis-tal′je-ah) pain in the lacrimal sac.

dacryocystectomy (dak″re-o-sis-tek′to-me) excision of the wall of the lacrimal sac.

dacryocystitis (dak″re-o-sis-ti′tis) inflammation of the lacrimal sac.

dacryocystoblennorrhea (dak″re-o-sis″to-blen″o-re′ah) chronic catarrhal inflammation of the lacrimal sac, with constriction of the lacrimal gland.

dacryocystocele (dak″re-o-sis′to-sēl) hernial protrusion of the lacrimal sac; dacryocele.

dacryocystoptosis (dak″re-o-sis″top-to′sis) prolapse of the lacrimal sac.

dacryocystorhinostenosis (dak″re-o-sis″to-ri″no-stĕ-no′sis) narrowing of the duct leading from the lacrimal sac to the nasal cavity.

dacryocystorhinostomy (dak″re-o-sis″to-ri-nos′to-me) surgical creation of an opening between the lacrimal sac and nasal cavity.

dacryocystorhinotomy (dak″re-o-sis″to-ri-not′o-me) passage of a probe through the lacrimal sac into the nasal cavity.

dacryocystostenosis (dak″re-o-sis″to-stĕ-no′sis) narrowing of the lacrimal sac.

dacryocystostomy (dak″re-o-sis-tos′to-me) surgical creation of a new opening into the lacrimal sac with drainage.

dacryocystotomy (dak″re-o-sis-tot′o-me) incision of the lacrimal sac and duct.

dacryohemorrhea (dak″re-o-he″mo-re′ah) the discharge of tears mixed with blood.

dacryolith (dak′re-o-lith″) a lacrimal calculus.

dacryolithiasis (dak″re-o-lĭ-thi′ah-sis) the presence of dacryoliths.

dacryoma (dak″re-o′mah) a tumor-like swelling due to obstruction of the lacrimal duct.

dacryon (dak′re-on) the point where the lacrimal, frontal, and upper maxillary bones meet.

dacryopyorrhea (dak″re-o-pi″o-re′ah) the discharge of tears mixed with pus.

dacryorrhea (dak″re-o-re′ah) excessive flow of tears.

dacryosolenitis (dak″re-o-so″lĕ-ni′tis) inflammation of a lacrimal duct.

dacryostenosis (dak″re-o-stĕ-no′sis) stricture or narrowing of a lacrimal duct.

dacryosyrinx (dak″re-o-sir′inks) 1. lacrimal duct. 2. a lacrimal fistula. 3. a syringe for irrigating the lacrimal ducts.

Dactil (dak′til) trademark for preparations of piperidolate, an anticholinergic.

dactinomycin (dak″tĭ-no-mi′sin) an antibiotic of the actinomycin complex (actinomycin D), produced by several species of *Streptomyces;* used as an antineoplastic agent.

dactyl (dak′til) a digit.

dactyl(o)- word element [Gr.], *a digit; a finger or toe.*

dactylitis (dak″tĭ-li′tis) inflammation of a finger or toe.

dactylography (dak″tĭ-log′rah-fe) the study of fingerprints.

dactylogryposis (dak″ti-lo-grĭ-po′sis) permanent flexion of the fingers.

dactylology (dak″tĭ-lol′o-je) communication between individuals by signs made with the hands and fingers.

dactylolysis (dak″tĭ-lol′ĭ-sis) 1. surgical correction of syndactyly. 2. loss or amputation of a digit.

dactylomegaly (dak″tĭ-lo-meg′ah-le) abnormally large fingers or toes.

dactyloscopy (dak″tĭ-los′ko-pe) examination of fingerprints for identification.

dactylus (dak′tĭ-lus), pl. *dac′tyli* [L.] a digit.

Dakin's solution (da′kinz) an aqueous solution containing sodium hypochlorite and sodium bicarbonate; used as a local antibacterial and to irrigate wounds.

Dalton's law (dawl′tonz) the pressure exerted by a mixture of nonreacting gases is equal to the sum of the partial pressures of the separate components.

daltonism (dawl′ton-izm) red-green color blindness.

dam (dam) a sheet of latex rubber used to isolate teeth from the fluids of the mouth during dental treatments; also used occasionally in surgical procedures to isolate certain tissues or structures. Called also rubber-dam.

damp (damp) foul air or noxious gas(es) in a mine. **black d., choke d.,** a gaseous mixture formed in a mine by the gradual absorption of the oxygen and the giving off of the carbon dioxide by the coal.

damping (damp′ing) steady diminution of the amplitude of successive vibrations of a specific form of energy, as of electricity.

danazol (dan′ah-zōl) a synthetic androgen that induces atrophy of the endometrium and amenorrhea; used in treatment of endometriosis.

D. and C. dilation (of cervix) and curettage (of uterus).

dander (dan′der) small scales from the hair or feathers of animals, which may be a cause of allergy in sensitive persons.

dandruff (dan′druf) 1. a scaly material shed from the scalp; applied to that normally shed from the scalp epidermis as well as to the excessive scaly material asssociated with disease. The condition may spread unless checked and in rare cases may extend to the eyebrows, ears, nose, and neck, causing a reddening of the skin in those areas. 2. SEBORRHEIC DERMATITIS of the scalp.

Dandy-Walker syndrome (dan′de-wok′er) congenital hydrocephalus due to obstruction of the foramina of Magendie and Luschka.

Dane particle (dān) a particle 42 nm. in diameter, containing hepatitis B (HB) antigen on its surface (HB_s) and in its core (HB_c).

Danilone (dan′ĭ-lōn) trademark for a preparation of phenindione, an anticoagulant.

danthron (dan′thron) a cathartic.

dantrolene (dan′tro-lēn) skeletal muscle relaxant producing its effect primarily on the myoneural junction and the muscle tissue, and only secondarily on the central nervous system.

dapsone (dap′sōn) an antibacterial used as a leprostatic and a dermatitis herpetiformis suppressant.

Daranide (dar′ah-nīd) trademark for a preparation of dichlorphenamide, a carbonic anhydrase inhibitor.

Daraprim (dar′ah-prim) trademark for a preparation of pyrimethamine, an antimalarial drug.

Darbid (dar′bid) trademark for a preparation of isopropamide, an anticholinergic.

Daricon (dar′ĭ-kon) trademark for a preparation of oxyphencyclimine, an anticholinergic.

Darier's disease (dar′e-āz) keratosis follicularis.

Darling's disease (dar′lingz) histoplasmosis.

darnel (dar′nel) a rye grass, *Lolium temulentum*, the seeds of which contain a narcotic poison; ingestion of contaminated flour may produce vertigo, staggering, vomiting, visual disturbances, burning pain in the mouth, and prostration.

Dartal (dar′tal) trademark for a preparation of thiopropazate, a major tranquilizer.

dartoid (dar′toid) resembling the dartos.

dartos (dar′tos) the contractile tissue under the skin of the scrotum; called also tunica dartos.

Darvon (dar′von) trademark for a preparation of propoxyphene, an analgesic.

darwinism (dar′wĭ-nizm) the theory of evolution according to which higher organisms have been developed from lower ones through the influence of natural selection.

daughter (daw′ter) 1. decay product. 2. arising from cell division, as a daughter cell.

db decibel.

DBI trademark for preparations of phenformin, a hypoglycemic drug.

D & C dilation (of cervix) and curettage (of uterus).

D.D.S. Doctor of Dental Surgery.

DDT dichloro-diphenyl-trichloroethane, a powerful insect poison; used in dilution as a powder or in an oily solution as a spray.

de- word element [L.] *down; from;* sometimes negative or privative, and often intensive.

deacidification (de″ah-sid″ĭ-fĭ-ka′shun) neutralization of acidity.

deactivation (de-ak″tĭ-va′shun) the process of making or becoming inactive.

deaf (def) lacking the sense of hearing or not having the full power of hearing; exhibiting DEAFNESS.

deafferentation (de-af″er-en-ta′shun) the elimination or interruption of afferent (sensory) nerve fibers.

deaf-mute (def′mūt) a person unable to hear or speak.

deafness (def′nes) lack or loss, complete or partial, of the sense of HEARING. Total deafness is quite rare, but partial deafness is common; an estimated 15 million Americans suffer from some degree of deafness, and of these, perhaps 2.5 million are children whose defective hearing is either congenital (from birth) or developed before the age of 5.

CAUSES. The two major types of deafness are conductive deafness and sensorineural (nerve) deafness. In some cases both types may be present; this is called mixed deafness.

In conductive deafness sound vibrations are interrupted in the outer or middle ear before they reach the nerve endings of the inner ear. In the outer ear, a foreign body or an accumulation of cerumen (earwax) may block the external acoustic meatus. These cases generally can be cured by removal of the obstruction. In the middle ear, infections, often entering through a perforated tympanic membrane (eardrum) or the eustachian tube, may fill the chamber with fluid, hampering the passage of vibrations. The small bones of the middle ear (ossicles) may be damaged by injury or fixed in place by otosclerosis.

In sensorineural deafness, the outer and middle ear function normally, but damage to the nerve endings of the inner ear, the cochlear portion of the vestibulocochlear (eighth cranial) nerve, or the hearing center in the brain causes either interruption or confusion of the sound messages. This damage may be caused by disease, head injury, tumor, excessively loud and sudden noise, or continuous loud noise.

A great many cases of congenital deafness are caused by infectious diseases, especially viral infections, contracted by the mother during pregnancy. Of these, rubella (German measles) is the most common.

Impaired hearing or a predisposition to ear diseases may be inherited. The laws of heredity with respect to deafness, though not yet fully understood, are the subject of continuing research.

Two of the greatest contributing factors to deafness are pride and neglect. Many ear diseases that can be cured if treated early are allowed to lead to deafness because of these two factors. Symptoms such as ringing in the ears, a feeling of pressure in the ear, or increasing hearing difficulty call for prompt medical consultation, if necessary with an ear specialist, or otologist.

Detection of Hearing Loss. In the infant and very young child hearing loss is evidenced by a lack of response to the sounds of his environment. As the infant matures and begins to talk there is a noticeable defect in his speech development and he may rely more on gestures than on words to communicate with others.

Emotional and behavioral disorders frequently are signs of hearing loss in children and in adults. The frustration they feel in trying to cope with their disability may be manifested by irritability, hyperactivity, hostility, and withdrawal from contact with others.

Special tests to determine hearing loss include the use of the tuning fork and the audiometer. The vibrating tuning fork produces sound waves that can be heard in both ears by a person with normal hearing when the stem of the fork is placed on the top of the head. The sound is heard louder in the affected ear in conductive hearing loss and softer in the affected ear in sensorineural loss. The audiometer produces sounds at varying levels of intensity and frequency. It is useful in determining the degree and type of hearing ability.

Treatment. Medical science has made great progress in the treatment of conditions that are capable of causing deafness. Middle ear infections now yield to the antibiotics and sulfonamide drugs. The greatest progress, however, has been in the field of microsurgery. Special binocular microscopes and miniature surgical instruments have enabled the surgeon to operate freely in the small crowded chambers of the ear. Two examples of this type of microsurgery are TYMPANOPLASTY and STAPEDECTOMY. In a stapedectomy the stapes, or stirrup, is removed and replaced by a piece of stainless steel wire or plastic, which allows the chain of transmission of sound vibrations to function again. Tympanoplasty in useful in correcting other types of conductive deafness as well. If chronic ear infection or injury has destroyed one or more of the ossicles, they can be rebuilt or replaced. Through plastic surgery and grafting techniques, the skilled surgeon can rebuild the entire middle ear.

Rehabilitation. There still remain many cases of deafness that cannot be improved by drugs or surgery. In particular, sensorineural deafness is not accessible to surgery because it involves parts deep in the inner ear or the brain itself.

For these patients, rehabilitation is required, with the aim of making the best use of what hearing remains. With proper training and the use of a suitable hearing aid where necessary, the deaf person can continue to lead a normal, useful life.

An important tool in rehabilitation is training in lip-reading. The patient is taught to use visual clues, such as the movements of the lips and tongue of the speaker, to supplement his hearing.

Another important tool is a correct HEARING AID. This should be selected with the help of an otologist, as different types of deafness require different instruments. Careful training in the use of the hearing aid also is necessary. After the silence of deafness, the patient may find it impossible at first to disregard the background noises that the instrument picks up. Also, some types of nerve deafness "scramble" sounds; training in the use of the hearing aid may enable the patient to distinguish among these sounds.

A third important component of rehabilitation is speech therapy. Since the deaf person is no longer able to hear his own voice, his speech often deteriorates. Proper training can help the patient prevent this deterioration, as well as correcting any speech defect that may already have developed.

Deafness in Children. The problems of a child who is deaf from birth or shortly afterward are somewhat different from those of a person who loses his hearing during adult life. Children learn to speak by imitating the sounds they hear; a child who cannot hear will be mute unless he is taught speech. This calls for special methods of teaching.

There are more than 350 schools and classes in the United States that specialize in teaching the partially and totally deaf child. These are located throughout the country, and many are publicly supported by taxes. There are also a number of summer camps that make it possible for the deaf child to continue his training throughout the year. Gallaudet College, in Washington, D.C., is the only college in the world devoted exclusively to educating the deaf. It is supported by the United States Government.

Agencies for the Deaf. The American Hearing Society is the best known of the organizations concerned with problems of the deaf. Located at 919 18th Street N.W., Washington, D.C. 20006, the society has affiliated agencies throughout the United States. The services offered by these branches include lip-reading classes, rehabilitation, and hearing aid clinics. The American Speech and Hearing Association, 1001 Connecticut Avenue N.W., Washington, D.C. 20006, is a professional association of specialists in speech and hearing therapy. The Alexander Graham Bell Association for the Deaf, 1537 35th Street N.W., Washington, D.C. 20007, has one of the world's finest libraries on deafness, and functions as an information center on the subject. The Deafness Research Foundation, 366 Madison Avenue, New York, N.Y. 10017, was founded several years ago to encourage medical research into the causes of deafness. The National Association of Hearing and Speech Agencies, 919 18th Street, N.W., Washington, D.C. 20006, has affiliates throughout the United States that offer many services to those with hearing difficulties. Among the federal agencies concerned with questions of the deaf are the Children's Bureau of the Department of Health, Education and Welfare and the Office of Vocational Rehabilitation. The Veterans Administration offers assistance and rehabilitation to those whose hearing was injured during military service. Many states have agencies that deal with problems of the handicapped, including the deaf. Interpreters for deaf patients often can be located by contacting the Registry of Interpreters for the Deaf, P.O. Box 1339, Washington, D.C. 20013.

cortical d., that due to disease of the cortical centers of the cerebrum.

hysterical d., that which may appear or disappear in a hysterical patient without an organic cause being present.

word d., auditory aphasia; receptive aphasia in which sounds are heard but convey no meaning to the mind.

deamidase (de-am'ĭ-dās) an enzyme that splits amides to form carboxylic acid and ammonia.

deamidization (de-am″ĭ-dĭ-za′shun) liberation of the ammonia from an amide.

deaminase (de-am′ĭ-nās) an enzyme causing deamination, or removal of an amino group from organic compounds, named according to its substrate as adenosine deaminase, cytidine deaminase, guanine deaminase, etc.

deamination (de-am″ĭ-na′shun) removal of the amino group, —NH_2, from a compound.

Deaner (de′ner) trademark for a preparation of deanol acetamidobenzoate.

deanol acetaminobenzoate (de′ah-nol as″et-am″ĭ-no-ben′zo-āt) a central stimulant with parasympathomimetic activity.

death (deth) the cessation of all physical and chemical processes that invariably occurs in all living organisms. There is at present no standardized diagnosis of clinical death, no precise definition of human death. The most widely known and commonly accepted means of determining death evolved from several medical conferences held in the late 1960's for the purpose of defining irreversible coma or nonfunctioning brain as a new criterion for death. The indications of deep irreversible COMA are: (1) unresponsivity to externally applied stimuli; (2) cessation of movement and breathing, including no spontaneous breathing for three minutes after an artificial respirator has been turned off; and (3) complete absence of cephalic reflexes. The pupils of the eyes must be dilated and unresponsive to direct light.

Use of the electroencephalogram is also recommended as being of value in confirmation of irreversible coma or death. If there is a flat electroencephalographic reading at the time of apparent death and a second flat reading 24 hours later, then the patient may be declared dead.

There are two exceptions to the above criteria. These are in regard to patients exhibiting marked hypothermia (body temperature below 32.2° C.), and those suffering from severe central nervous system depression as a result of drug overdose.

It is recognized that the above criteria are limited in that the notion of irreversibility is not readily agreed upon and may take on new meaning as medical technology advances. The criteria are especially helpful as complements to the traditional criteria of absence of heart beat and lack of spontaneous respiration as indications of death.

black d., bubonic plague.

clinical d., the absence of heart beat (no pulse can be felt) and cessation of breathing.

cot d., crib d., sudden infant death syndrome (SIDS).

d. rate, the number of deaths per stated number of person (100 or 10,000 or 100,000) in a certain region in a certain time period.

debility (de-bil′ĭ-te) lack or loss of strength; weakness.

débride (da-brēd′) [Fr.] to remove by débridement.

débridement (da-brēd-maw′) [Fr.] the removal of all foreign material and all contaminated and devitalized tissues from or adjacent to a traumatic or infected lesion until surrounding healthy tissue is exposed.

debris (dĕ-bre′) devitalized tissue or foreign matter. In dentistry, soft foreign matter loosely attached to the surface of a tooth.

debrisoquin (deb-ris′o-kwin) an antihypertensive agent, used as the sulfate salt.

deca- 1. word element [Gr.], *ten;* also spelled *deka-*. 2. used in naming units of measurement to indicate a quantity 10 times the unit designated by the root with which it is combined, e.g., decagram.

Decadron (dek′ah-dron) trademark for preparations of dexamethasone, an anti-inflammatory adrenocortical steroid.

Deca-Durabolin (de″ka-dur-ab′o-lin) trademark for a preparation of nandrolone, an androgenic, anabolic steroid.

decagram (dek′ah-gram) ten grams; 154.32 grains.

decalcification (de-kal″sĭ-fĭ-ka′shun) 1. the process of removing calcareous matter. 2. the loss of calcium salts from bone or teeth.

decalcify (de-kal′sĭ-fi) to deprive of calcium or its salts.

decaliter (dek′ah-le″ter) ten liters; 2.64 gallons.

decameter (dek′ah-me″ter) ten meters; 32.8 feet.

decamethonium (dek″ah-mĕ-tho′ne-um) a muscle relaxant used in surgical anesthesia and in electroshock treatment, in the form of its bromide or iodide salt.

decannulation (de-kan″nu-la′shun) the removal of a cannula.

decanormal (dek″ah-nor′mal) having ten times the strength of normal.

decantation (de″kan-ta′shun) the pouring of a clear supernatant liquid from a sediment.

decapitation (de-kap″ĭ-ta′shun) removal of the head, as of an animal, fetus, or bone.

decapsulation (de-kap″su-la′shun) removal of a capsule, especially the renal capsule.

decarboxylase (de″kar-bok′sĭ-lās) any of the lyase class of enzymes that catalyze the removal of a carbon dioxide molecule from a compound.

decarboxylation (de″kar-bok″sĭ-la′shun) removal of the carboxyl group from a compound.

decavitamin (dek″ah-vi′tah-min) a combination of vitamins in capsular or tablet form, each of which contains vitamins A and D, ascorbic acid, calcium pantothenate, cyanocobalamin, folic acid, niacinamide, pyridoxine hydrochloride, riboflavin, thiamine hydrochloride, and a suitable form of alpha tocopherol.

decay (de-ka′) 1. the gradual decomposition of dead organic matter. 2. the process or stage of decline, as in old age.

decerebrate (de-ser′ĕ-brāt) to eliminate cerebral function by transecting the brain stem or by ligating the common carotid arteries and basilar artery at the center of the pons; an animal so prepared, or a brain-damaged person with similar neurologic signs.

d. rigidity, see RIDIGITY.

decerebration (de-ser″ĕ-bra′shun) the act of decerebrating.

dechloridation (de-klo″rĭ-da′shun) the removal of chloride, or salt.

decholesterolization (de-ko-les″ter-ol-ĭ-za′shun) reduction of cholesterol levels in the blood.

Decholin (de′ko-lin) trademark for preparations of dehydrocholic acid.

deci- word element [L.], *one-tenth;* used to indicate

one-tenth (10^{-1}) of the unit designated by the root with which it is combined, e.g., decigram.

decibel (des′ĭ-bel) a unit used to express the ratio of two powers, usually electric or acoustic powers, equal to one-tenth of a bel; one decibel equals approximately the smallest difference in acoustic power the human ear can detect. Abbreviated db.

decidua (de-sid′u-ah) a name applied to the endometrium during pregnancy, which is shed after childbirth; called also the decidual, or deciduous, membrane. adj., **decid′ual.**

basal d., d. basa′lis, that portion on which the implanted ovum rests.

capsular d., d. capsula′ris, that portion directly overlying the implanted ovum and facing the uterine cavity.

menstrual d., d. menstrua′lis, the hyperemic uterine mucosa shed during menstruation.

parietal d., d. parieta′lis, true d., d. ver′ra, the decidua exclusive of the area occupied by the implanted ovum.

deciduate (de-sid′u-āt) characterized by shedding.

deciduation (de-sid″u-a′shun) the shedding of the decidua.

deciduitis (de-sid″u-i′tis) a bacterial disease leading to changes in the decidua.

deciduoma (de-sid″-u-o′mah) an intrauterine mass containing decidual cells.

deciduosis (de-sid″u-o′sis) the presence of decidual tissue or of tissue resembling the endometrium of pregnancy in an ectopic site.

deciduous (de-sid′u-us) falling off; subject to being shed, as deciduous teeth.

decigram (des′ĭ-gram) one-tenth of a gram; 1.54 grains.

deciliter (des′ĭ-le″ter) one-tenth of a liter; 3.38 fluidounces.

decimeter (des′ĭ-me″ter) one-tenth of a meter; 3.9 inches.

decinormal (des″ĭ-nor′mal) of one-tenth normal strength.

decipara (des″ĭ-pah′rah) a woman who has had ten pregnancies that resulted in viable offspring; para X.

declination (dek″lĭ-na′shun) cyclophoria.

declive (de-klīv′) a slope or a slanting surface. In anatomy, the part of the vermis of the cerebellum just caudal to the primary fissure.

declivis (de-kli′vis) [L.] declive.

Declomycin (dek′lo-mi″sin) trademark for preparations of demeclocycline, an antibiotic.

decoloration (de-kul″er-a′shun) 1. removal of color; bleaching. 2. lack or loss of color.

decolorizer (de-kul′or-iz″er) an agent that removes color, bleaches.

decompensation (de″kom-pen-sa′shun) inability of the heart to maintain adequate circulation; it is marked by dyspnea, venous engorgement, cyanosis, and edema.

decomposition (de-kom″po-zish′un) the separation of compound bodies into their constituent principles.

decompression (de″kom-presh′un) return to normal environmental pressure after exposure to greatly increased pressure.

cerebral d., removal of a flap of the skull and incision of the dura mater for the purpose of relieving intracranial pressure.

d. sickness, a disorder characterized by joint pains, respiratory manifestations, skin lesions, and neurologic signs, occurring as a result of rapid reduction in air pressure. Aviators flying at high altitudes and persons breathing compressed air in caissons and diving apparatus are particularly susceptible to this disorder (see also BENDS and CAISSON DISEASE).

decongestant (de″kon-jes′tant) 1. tending to reduce congestion or swelling. 2. an agent that reduces congestion or swelling, usually of the nasal membranes. Decongestants may be inhaled, taken as spray or nose drops, or used orally in liquid or tablet form. The medication acts by reducing swelling of the nasal membranes and thus opening up the nasal passages. Among the leading medications used as decongestants are epinephrine, ephedrine, and phenylephrine. Antihistamines, alone or in combination with decongestants, may also be effective.

A decongestant must be used several times a day to be helpful; but excessive use may cause headaches, dizziness, or other disorders and sometimes the medicine itself may cause reactive nasal swelling.

decongestive (de″kon-jes′tiv) reducing congestion.

decontamination (de″kon-tam-ĭ-na′shun) the freeing of a person or an object of some contaminating substance such as war gas, radioactive material, etc.

decortication (de-kor″tĭ-ka′shun) 1. removal of the outer covering from a plant, seed, or root. 2. removal of portions of the cortical substance of a structure or organ.

decrepitation (de-krep″ĭ-ta′shun) the explosion or crackling of certain substances (salt, crystals, etc.) upon heating.

decrudescence (de″kroo-des′ens) diminution or abatement of the intensity of symptoms.

decubitus (de-ku′bĭ-tus) 1. the act of lying down; the position assumed in lying down. 2. a decubitus ulcer. adj., **decu′bital.**

Andral's d., lying on the unaffected side in the early stages of pleurisy.

dorsal d., lying on the back.

lateral d., lying on one side, designated right lateral decubitus when the subject lies on the right side and left lateral decubitus when he lies on the left side.

d. ulcer, an ulcer due to local interference with the circulation; called also bedsore and pressure sore. The ulcer usually occurs over a bony prominence such as that of the sacrum, hip, heel, shoulder, or elbow. Excessive or prolonged pressure produced by the weight of the body or limb is the primary cause. Factors that may contribute to the development of an ulcer include wrinkling or unevenness of the bedclothes, accumulation of perspiration, and incontinence of urine or feces. The patients most likely to develop a decubitus ulcer are emaciated or diabetic patients, those confined to bed in traction or wearing a cast, and those with generalized edema. Although the term decubitus ulcer is derived from the Latin word meaning "lying down," these ulcerations can develop in patients who sit for long periods of time or are immobilized and unable to change positions on their own.

The prevention of a decubitus ulcer is far simpler and less costly than treatment and cure. It is estimated that each pressure sore adds $5,000.00 to the cost of medical care. Frequent changing of position of the patient who cannot move about in bed, thorough cleansing of the skin and gentle massage of the bony prominences to stimulate circulation are all important in avoiding pressure areas and ulcers. The use of sheepskin under the patient has been fairly successful in preventing pressure sores in patients confined to bed. Flotation pads and other support devices distribute pressure on the capillaries and thereby avoid restriction of circulation to any one area of the body. When a commercial flotation system is not available, an ordinary camper's air mattress partially filled with water is an effective alternative. Polyether urethan foam, a substance similar to foam rubber, can be used in large blocks as mattresses or in small squares with cut-out areas over the ulcer. These measures help relieve pressure and provide for increased circulation of blood to the affected area; they do not, however, replace such basic care as frequent turning, cleanliness, and massage of areas likely to develop decubitus ulcers.

Treatment of a decubitus ulcer is aimed at restoring circulation to the area as quickly and efficiently as possible, controlling secondary bacterial infection, and initiating measures to promote healing. The patient should be positioned so that the ulcer and surrounding area are completely relieved of pressure. Exposure to sunlight, ultraviolet rays, or heat lamp will aid in keeping the area dry and help promote healing.

Topical applications vary widely, depending on the preference of the physician. The diligence with which the prescribed regimen is carried out greatly affects its effectiveness. Remedies, both old and new, include granulated sugar, streptomycin-egg white mixtures, gold leaf, absorbable gelatin sponges (Gelfoam), and administration of oxygen under pressure. There remains much research to be done to find a universally successful cure for pressure sores. One of the most vital factors in the success of any form of treatment for these ulcers is a firm conviction on the part of the entire health care team that a specific prescribed treatment will work, and a concerted effort and dedication to assure that it does.

ventral d., lying on the stomach.

decussate (de-kus′āt) 1. to cross in the form of an X. 2. crossed like the letter X.

decussation (de″kus-sa′shun) a crossing over; the intercrossing of fellow parts or structures in the form of an X.

d. of pyramids, the anterior part of the lower medulla oblongata in which most of the fibers of each pyramid intersect as they cross the midline and descend as the lateral corticospinal tracts.

dedifferentiation (de-dif″er-en″she-a′shun) regression from a more specialized or complex form to a simpler state.

de-epicardialization (de″ep-ĭ-kar″dĭ-al-i-za′shun) a surgical procedure for the relief of intractable angina pectoris, in which epicardial tissue is destroyed by application of a caustic agent to promote development of collateral circulation.

deerfly fever (dēr′fli) tularemia.

def (de′e-ef) an expression of dental caries experience in deciduous teeth, *d* representing the number of teeth indicated for filling; *e* the number indicated for extraction; *f* the number of filled teeth.

defatted (de-fat′ed) deprived of fat.

defecation (def″ĕ-ka′shun) elimination of wastes and undigested food, as feces, from the rectum.

defect (de′fekt) an imperfection, failure, or absence.

filling d., an interruption in the contour of the inner surface of stomach or intestine revealed by roentgenography, indicating excess tissue or substance on or in the wall of the organ.

septal d., a defect in the cardiac septum resulting in an abnormal communication between opposite chambers of the heart. (See also AORTIC SEPTAL DEFECT, ATRIAL SEPTAL DEFECT, and VENTRICULAR SEPTAL DEFECT.)

defective (de-fek′tiv) 1. imperfect. 2. a person lacking in some physical, mental, or moral quality.

defeminization (de-fem″ĭ-nĭ-za′shun) loss of female sexual characteristics.

defense (de-fens′) behavior directed to protection of the individual from injury.

d. mechanism a mental mechanism by which psychic tension is diminished, e.g., repression, denial, overcompensation, rationalization, etc. Called also escape mechanism.

deferens (def′er-ens) [L.] deferent.

deferent (def′er-ent) conducting or progressing away, as from a center or specific site of reference.

deferentectomy (def″er-en-tek′to-me) excision of a ductus deferens.

deferential (def″er-en′shal) pertaining to the ductus deferens.

deferentitis (def″er-en-ti′tis) inflammation of the ductus deferens.

deferoxamine (de″fer-oks′ah-mēn) an iron-chelating agent isolated from *Streptomyces pilosus.*

defervescence (def″er-ves′ens) the period of abatement of fever.

defibrillation (de-fib″rĭ-la′shun) 1. termination of atrial or ventricular fibrillation, usually by electroshock. 2. separation of tissue fibers by blunt dissection.

defibrillator (de-fib′rĭ-la″tor) an apparatus used to produce defibrillation by application of brief electroshock to the heart, directly or through electrodes placed on the chest wall.

defibrination (de-fi″brĭ-na′shun) the destruction or removal of fibrin, as from the blood.

deficiency (de-fish′en-se) a lack or shortage; a condition characterized by the presence of less than the normal or necessary supply or competence.

d. disease, a condition caused by dietary or metabolic deficiency, including all diseases due to an insufficient supply of essential nutrients.

deficit (def′ĭ-sit) a lack or deficiency.

oxygen d., see ANOXEMIA, ANOXIA, HYPOXIA, and OXYGEN.

deflection (de-flek′shun) a turning aside. In psychoanalysis, an unconscious diversion of ideas from conscious attention. In the electrocardiogram, a deviation of the curve from the isoelectric baseline, that is, any wave or complex.

defluvium (de-floo′ve-um) [L.] a falling out, as of the hair.

defluxion (de-fluk′shun) 1. a sudden disappearance. 2. a copious discharge, as of catarrh. 3. a falling out, as of hair.

deformability (de-form″ah-bil′ĭ-te) the ability of cells, such as erythrocytes, to change shape as they pass through narrow spaces, such as the microvasculature.

deformation (de″for-ma′shun) 1. deformity. 2. the process of adapting in shape or form.

deformity (de-for′mĭ-te) distortion of any part or general disfigurement of the body; malformation.

defundation (de″fun-da′shun) excision of the fundus of the uterus.

degenerate 1. (de-jen′er-āt) to change from a higher to a lower form. 2. (de-jen′er-it) characterized by degeneration. 3. a person whose moral or physical state is below the normal.

degeneration (de-gen″ĕ-ra′shun) deterioration; change from a higher to a lower form, especially change of tissue to a lower or less functionally active form. When there is chemical change of the tissue itself it is true degeneration; when the change consists in the deposit of abnormal matter in the tissues, it is infiltration. adj., **degen′erative.**

albuminoid d., albuminous d., cloudy swelling, an early stage of degenerative change characterized by swollen, parboiled-appearing tissues which revert to normal when the cause is removed.

amyloid d., degeneration with deposit of lardacein in the tissues; indicative of impaired nutritive function, and seen in wasting diseases.

caseous d., caseation (2).

colloid d., degeneration with conversion of the tissues into a gelatinous or gumlike material.

congenital macular d., a congenital, hereditary form of macular degeneration, marked by the presence of a cystlike lesion that in the early stages resembles egg yolk.

cystic d., degeneration with formation of cysts.

fatty d., deposit of fat globules in a tissue.

fibroid d., degeneration into fibrous tissue.

hepatolenticular d., a hereditary disorder of copper metabolism, marked by a pigmented ring at the outer margin of the cornea, degenerative changes in the brain, cirrhosis of the liver, splenomegaly, tremor, rigidity, contractures, psychic disturbances, dysphagia, and increasing weakness and emaciation. Called also Wilson's disease.

hyaline d., a regressive change in cells in which the cytoplasm takes on a homogeneous, glassy appearance; also used loosely to describe the histologic appearance of tissues.

hydropic d., a form in which the epithelial cells absorb much water.

lattice d. of retina, a frequently bilateral, usually benign asymptomatic condition, characterized by patches of fine gray or white lines that intersect at irregular intervals in the peripheral retina, usually associated with numerous, round, punched-out areas of retinal thinning or retinal holes.

lipoid d., lipoidal d., a condition somewhat resembling fatty degeneration but in which the extraneous material is lipoid.

macular d., degenerative changes in the macula retinae.

mucoid d., degeneration with deposit of myelin and lecithin in the cells.

mucous d., degeneration with accumulation of mucus in epithelial tissues.

myxomatous d., degeneration with accumulation of mucus in connective tissues.

spongy d. of central nervous system, spongy d. of white matter, a rare hereditary form of leukodystrophy marked by early onset, widespread demyelination and vacuolation of the cerebral white matter giving rise to a spongy appearance, and by severe mental retardation, megalocephaly, atony of the neck muscles, spasticity of the arms and legs, and blindness; death usually occurs at about 18 months of age. Called also Canavan's disease.

subacute combined d. of spinal cord, degeneration of both the posterior and lateral columns of the spinal cord, producing various motor and sensory disturbances; it is due to vitamin B_{12} deficiency and usually associated with pernicious anemia. Called also Lichtheim's syndrome and Putnam-Dana syndrome.

wallerian d., fatty degeneration of a nerve fiber that has been severed from its nutritive source.

Zenker's d., Zenker's necrosis.

degloving (de-gluv′ing) intra-oral surgical exposure of the bony mandibular chin; it can be performed in the posterior region if necessary.

deglutition (deg″loo-tish′un) the act of swallowing.

degradation (deg″rah-da′shun) conversion of a chemical compound to one less complex, as by splitting off one or more groups of atoms.

degree (de-gre′) 1. a grade or rank awarded scholars by a college or university. 2. a unit of measure of temperature. 3. a unit of measure of arcs and angles, one degree being 1/360 of a circle.

degustation (de″gus-ta′shun) the act or function of tasting.

dehiscence (de-his′ens) a splitting open.

wound d. separation of all the layers of a surgical wound.

dehumidifier (de″hu-mid′ĭ-fi″er) an apparatus for reducing the content of moisture in the atmosphere.

dehydrase (de-hi′drās) a term once applied to both the dehydrogenases and the dehydratases.

dehydratase (de-hi′drah-tās) any enzyme of the lyase class that catalyzes the removal of H_2O, leaving double bonds (or adding groups to double bonds).

dehydration (de″hi-dra′shun) removal of water from the body or a tissue; or the condition that results from undue loss of water. Severe dehydration is a serious condition that may lead to fatal SHOCK, ACIDOSIS, and the accumulation of waste products in the body, as in UREMIA.

Water accounts for more than half the body weight. Under normal conditions, a certain amount of fluid is lost daily. About 1.5 liters is removed by urination, and another 90 ml. is lost from the digestive tract in the feces. Through vaporization another liter is given off through the skin and lungs. To make up for these losses, about 2.5 liters of fluid must be taken into the body in food and fluids, and the cells contribute another 250 ml. through chemical activities.

When the fluid intake is insufficient or the output is excessive, dehydration occurs.

CAUSES. Abnormal dehydration may occur as a result of prolonged fever, diarrhea, acidosis, and vomiting, and in severe injuries or surgical procedures in which there is loss of blood or body fluids. Dehydration is usually accompanied by a depletion of essential elecrolytes dissolved in the body fluids. Without a normal supply of these fluids and electrolytes the body processes are impaired and eventual shock and death can occur. (See also HYPERGLYCEMIC HYPEROSMOLAR NONKETONIC COMA.)

SYMPTOMS AND TREATMENT. The patient appears flushed and has dry skin and mucous membranes, cracked lips, loss of skin turgor, and oliguria. Mental confusion and hypotension indicate a very severe dehydration.

Treatment is aimed at replacement of fluids and specific electrolytes, and removal of the primary cause of dehydration.

PATIENT CARE. Accurate recording of fluid intake and fluid loss is essential. Special observations of profuse sweating, drainage from wounds, or any other visible loss of fluids are noted on the patient's chart. Daily weighing may be ordered to determine fluid loss or gain.

Intravenous administration of fluids must be done at the exact rate and in the amounts ordered. Rapid infusion of fluids to a dehydrated patient does not allow for proper diffusion into the tissues; thus, the vascular system is overloaded and added strain is placed on the heart. (See also FLUID BALANCE.)

dehydrocholesterol (de-hi″dro-ko-les′ter-ol) a sterol found in the skin which, when properly irradiated by ultraviolet rays, forms vitamin D.

activated 7-d., cholecalciferol.

11-dehydrocorticosterone (de-hi″dro-kor″tĭ-ko-stēr′ōn) a steroid from the adrenal cortex and produced synthetically, which has a slight effect on protein and carbohydrate metabolism; used like cortisone.

dehydrocholic acid (de-hi″dro-ko′lik) a white, fluffy, bitter, odorless powder used to increase output of bile by the liver and the filling of the gallbladder. Preparations of this acid are used to aid the digestion of fats and increase absorption of fat-soluble vitamins. Drugs containing dehydrocholic acid are contraindicated in cases of biliary obstruction. Because of its bitter taste on the tongue when injected into a vein, it is used to provide an end point for the measurement of arm-tongue circulation time.

dehydroepiandrosterone (de-hi″dro-ep″ĭ-an-dros′-ter-ōn) an androgen occurring in normal human urine and synthesized from cholesterol.

dehydrogenase (de-hi′dro-jen-ās″) an enzyme that mobilizes the hydrogen of a substrate so that it can pass to a hydrogen acceptor.

glucoce-6-phosphate d., an enzyme necessary for the oxidation of glucose-6-phosphate, an intermediate in carbohydrate metabolism. Hereditary deficiency of this enzyme in the erythrocytes is associated with a tendency toward hemolysis with certain antimalarial and sulfonamide drugs and fava beans (favism).

lactate d. (LDH), an enzyme that catalyzes the interconversion of lactate and pyruvate. It is widespread in tissues and is particularly abundant in kidney, skeletal muscle, liver, and myocardium. It appears in elevated concentrations when these tissues are injured.

dehydrogenate (de-hi′dro-jen-āt″) to remove hydrogen from.

dehydroretinal (de-hi″dro-ret′ĭ-nal) the aldehyde of dehydroretinol, derived from the visual pigment porphyropsin, found in fresh-water fishes and certain vertebrates and amphibians; its metabolic role is analogous to that of rhodopsin in other animals.

dehydroretinol (de-hi″dro-ret′ĭ-nol) vitamin A_2, the form, $C_{20}H_{28}O$, of vitamin A found in the retina and liver of fresh-water fishes and certain invertebrates and amphibians; it differs from retinol (vitamin A_1) in having one more conjugated double bond and has approximately one-third the biological activity of retinol. Called also retinol$_2$.

deionization (de-i″on-ĭ-za′shun) the production of a mineral-free state by the removal of ions.

déjà vu (da′zhah voo′) [Fr.] an illusion that a new situation is a repetition of a previous experience.

dejecta (de-jek′tah) excrement.

dejection (de-jek′shun) 1. a mental state marked by depression and melancholy. 2. discharge of feces; defecation. 3. excrement; feces.

Dejerine's disease (deh″zher-ēnz′) progressive hypertrophic interstitial neuropathy.

Dejerine-Sottas disease (deh″zher-ēn′ sot′tahz) progressive hypertrophic interstitial neuropathy.

delacrimation (de-lak″rĭ-ma′shun) excessive flow of tears.

delactation (de″lak-ta′shun) 1. weaning. 2. cessation of lactation.

Delalutin (del″ah-lu′tin) trademark for a preparation of hydroxyprogesterone, a long-acting progestational steroid.

Delatestryl (del″ah-tes′tril) trademark for a preparation of testosterone, a male sex hormone.

de-lead (de-led′) to induce the removal of lead from tissues and its excretion in the urine by the administration of chelating agents.

deleterious (del″ĕ-te′re-us) injurious; harmful.

deletion (de-le′shun) in genetics, loss from a chromosome of genetic material.

delinquent (de-ling′kwent) 1. lacking in some respect; characterized by antisocial, illegal, or criminal behavior. 2. a person exhibiting such behavior, especially a minor (juvenile delinquent).

deliquescence (del″ĭ-kwes′ens) the condition of becoming moist or liquified as a result of absorption of water from the air.

delirium (dĕ-lēr′e-um) a mental disturbance of relatively short duration usually reflecting a toxic state, marked by illusions, hallucinations, delusions, excitement, restlessness, and incoherence. Almost any acute illness accompanied by very high fever can bring on delirium. Other causes are physical and mental shock, exhaustion, fear and anxiety, alcoholism, drug overdose and insulin shock.

PATIENT CARE. The delirious patient must be protected from self-injury and carefully supervised so that accidental injury does not occur. The environment should be nonstimulating; the patient kept in a quiet secluded area free from noise, bright lights, and other stimuli. When the delirium is prolonged, measures must be taken to ensure adequate fluid intake to combat dehydration, and proper attention must be given to elimination from the bladder and bowels. Medications such as sedatives or tranquilizing drugs may be ordered to relieve the symptoms.

d. tre′mens, DT's, an acute mental disturbance marked by delirium with illusions and vivid hallucinations, extreme restlessness, agitation, uncontrollable shaking, sweating, gastrointestinal symptoms, precordial pain, and in general an increased body metabolism. The victim is extremely fearful and apprehensive because his illusions and hallucinations are very real to him. Delirium tremens is a form of alcoholic psychosis ordinarily seen after withdrawal from heavy alcohol intake. (See also AL-

COHOLISM and WITHDRAWAL.) It may also occur in narcotics addiction.

TREATMENT AND PATIENT CARE. The patient should be kept in a quiet, nonstimulating environment and approached in a calm, reassuring manner. He must be watched closely and protected from self-injury during the period of delirium and also when he is convalescing from his illness and is likely to feel great remorse and depression. He should be observed for signs of extreme fatigue, pneumonia, or heart failure. Respiratory infections are quite common in these patients because of their weakened condition and inattention to personal hygiene.

The diet should be of high fluid intake and high in protein and carbohydrate content and low in fats. Dietary supplements usually include vitamin preparations, especially the B complex vitamins. If the patient is unable to cooperate by taking fluids and food by mouth, tube feeding and intravenous fluids may be necessary. Tranquilizing agents and sedatives are useful for therapy.

deliver (de-liv′er) 1. to aid in childbirth. 2. to remove, as a fetus, placenta, or lens of the eye.

delivery (de-liv′er-e) expulsion or extraction of the child and fetal membranes at birth (see also LABOR).

abdominal d., delivery of an infant through an incision made into the uterus through the abdominal wall (cesarean section).

dellen (del′en) saucer-shaped excavations at the periphery of the cornea, usually on the temporal side.

delomorphous (del″o-mor′fus) having definitely formed and well-defined limits, as a cell or tissue.

Delphian node (del′fe-an) a lymph node encased in the fascia in the midline just anterior to the thyroid isthmus, so called because it is exposed first at operation and, if diseased, is indicative of disease of the thyroid gland.

delta (del′tah) 1. the fourth letter of the Greek alphabet, Δ or δ; used in chemical names to denote the fourth of a series of isomeric compounds or the carbon atom fourth from the carboxyl group, or to denote the fourth of any series. 2. a triangular area.

Delta-Cortef (del′tah-kor″tef) trademark for a preparation of prednisolone, a glucocorticoid.

deltacortisone (del″tah-kor′tĭ-sōn) prednisone, a glucocorticoid.

Deltalin (del′tah-lin) trademark for a preparation of synthetic vitamin D_2.

deltasone (del′tah-sōn) trademark for a preparation of prednisone, a glucocorticoid.

deltoid (del′toid) 1. triangular. 2. the deltoid muscle.

d. muscle, the muscular cap of the shoulder, an inverted triangle that abducts the arm. It is often used as a site for intramuscular injections. (See also table of MUSCLES).

Deltra (del′trah) trademark for a tablet containing prednisone, a glucocorticoid.

delusion (de-lu′zhun) a false belief inconsistent with an individual's own knowledge and experience. adj., **delu′sional.**

Delvinal (del′vĭ-nal) trademark for preparations of vinbarbital, an intermediate-acting barbiturate.

demecarium (dem″ĕ-ka′re-um) a cholinesterase inhibitor used as the bromide salt in the treatment of glaucoma and esotropia.

demeclocycline (dem″ĕ-klo-si′klēn) a broad-spectrum antibiotic produced by a mutant strain of *Streptomyces aureofaciens,* closely related to the other tetracyclines; the base and the hydrochloride salt are used as antibacterials. Called also demethylchlortetracycline.

demecycline (dem″ĕ-si′klēn) an antibacterial.

dementia (de-men′she-ah) organic loss of intellectual function.

Binswanger's d., dementia due to demyelination of the subcortical white matter of the brain, with sclerotic changes in the blood vessels supplying it.

paralytic d., d. paralyt′ica, a chronic meningoencephalitis characterized by degeneration of the cortical neurons, progressive dementia, and generalized paralysis, which, if untreated, is ultimately fatal; it results from antecedent syphilitic infection; called also general paresis.

d. prae′cox, in the U.S., a former name for schizophrenia; commonly used in Europe to denote process schizophrenia.

senile d., mental deterioration in old age (see also senile PSYCHOSIS).

Demerol (dem′er-ol) trademark for preparations of meperidine, a synthetic narcotic analgesic.

demethylchlortetracycline (de-meth″il-klor″tetrah-si′klēn) demeclocycline.

demilune (dem′ĭ-lūn) a crescent-shaped structure or cell.

demineralization (de-min″er-al-ī-za′shun) excessive elimination of mineral or organic salts from the tissues of the body.

demodectic (dem″o-dek′tik) pertaining to or caused by *Demodex.*

Demodex (dem′o-deks) a genus of mites parasitic within the hair follicles of the host, including the species *D. folliculo′rum* in man, and several other species in domestic and other animals.

demogram (de′mo-gram) a graphic representation of the population of a given area according to the time period and the age and sex of the individuals composing it.

demography (de-mog′rah-fe) the statistical science dealing with populations, including matters of health, disease, births, and mortality.

demorphinization (de-mor″fĭ-nĭ-za′shun) gradual withdrawal of morphine from one addicted to its use.

demucosation (de″mu-ko-za′shun) removal of the mucous membrane from a part.

demulcent (de-mul′sent) 1. soothing; bland. 2. a soothing mucilaginous or oily medicine or application.

de Musset's sign (dĕ-mu-sāz′) rhythmic jerky movements of the head; seen in cases of aortic aneurysm and aortic insufficiency. Called also Musset's sign.

demyelinate (de-mi′ĕ-lin-āt″) to destroy or remove the myelin sheath of a nerve or nerves.

demyelination (de-mi′ĕ-lin-a′shun) destruction or loss of the myelin sheath of a nerve or nerves.

denarcotize (de-nar′ko-tīz) to deprive of narcotics or of narcotic properties.

denaturant (de-na′chur-ant) a denaturing agent.

denaturation (de-na″chur-a′shun) a change in the usual nature of a substance, as by the addition of methanol or acetone to alcohol to render it unfit for drinking, or the change in molecular structure of proteins due to splitting of hydrogen bonds caused by heat or certain chemicals.

protein d., any nonproteolytic change in the chemistry, composition, or structure of a native protein which causes it to lose some or all of its unique or specific characteristics.

dendraxon (den-drak′son) a nerve cell whose axon splits up into terminal filaments immediately after leaving the cell.

dendric (den′drik) pertaining to a dendrite.

dendriform (den′drĭ-form) tree-shaped.

dendrite (den′drīt) any of the threadlike extensions of the cytoplasm of a neuron; dendrites, which typically branch into treelike processes, compose most of the receptive surface of a neuron.

dendritic (den-drit′ik) 1. branched like a tree. 2. pertaining to or possessing dendrites.

dendroid (den′droid) branched like a tree.

dendron (den′dron) dendrite.

dendrophagocytosis (den″dro-fag″o-si-to′sis) the absorption by microglia cells of broken portions of astrocytes.

denervation (de″ner-va′shun) interruption of the nerve connection to an organ or part.

dengue (deng′e; Spanish, dan′ga) a painful viral disease that flourishes in tropical climates throughout the world. The virus that causes the disease is carried by *Aedes* mosquitoes. Because of the intense pain in the bones, dengue is known also as "breakbone fever" and by other names based on the necessity of keeping the neck rigid, such as "dandy" and "giraffe." People who have had dengue are generally immunized against the disease for 5 years, and epidemics tend to recur at 5-year intervals. Occasional epidemics occur in the Gulf states of the United States.

SYMPTOMS. The symptoms of dengue begin within a week after the bite of the infected mosquito. The onset is marked by a severe headache and pain behind the eyes. Within hours the characteristic pain in the back and joints begins. Movement is difficult, and the temperature may rise as high as 106° F. (41° C.). A pink rash, congested eyeballs, and a flushed face are outward symptoms. The disease usually has two stages of about 3 days and 2 days separated by a period of 24 hours in which the symptoms disappear, raising hopes of the end of the attack. The second stage is marked by the earlier symptoms and in addition a red rash appears on the elbows, knees, and ankles, leading often to peeling skin. The total course of the disease is rarely more than 6 or 7 days. Although the sufferer is exhausted and less resistant to other diseases, dengue by itself is rarely fatal. Convalescence is slow.

TREATMENT AND PREVENTION. As there is no known remedy for dengue, the treatment is mainly palliative. An icecap to reduce the headache, analgesics to relieve the pain, and a large intake of liquid are the basic essentials.

The best method of preventing dengue is by controlling the mosquito, and in some areas this has been successful. In areas lacking mosquito control, protective clothing should be worn outside and mosquito netting used indoors to reduce the risk of infection.

denial (dĕ-ni′al) a defense mechanism in which the existence of intolerable actions, ideas, etc., are unconsciously denied.

denidation (de″ni-da′shun) the degeneration and expulsion, during menstruation, of certain epthelial elements, potentially the nidus of an embryo.

Denis Browne splint (den′is brown) a splint for the correction of clubfoot, consisting of two metal footplates connected by a crossbar.

dens (dens), pl. *den′tes* [L.] a tooth or toothlike structure.

densimeter, densitometer (den-sim′ĕ-ter; den″-sĭ-tom′ĕ-ter) an instrument for determining density or specific gravity of a liquid.

densitometry (den″sĭ-tom′ĕ-tre) determination of variations in density by comparison with that of another material or with a certain standard.

density (den′sĭ-te) 1. the ratio of the mass of a substance to its volume. 2. the quality of being compact. 3. the quantity of matter in a given space. 4. the quantity of electricity in a given area, volume, or time.

densography (den-sog′rah-fe) the exact determination of the contrast densities in a roentgenogram by a photoelectric cell.

dent(o)- word element [L.], *tooth; toothlike.*

dental (den′tal) pertaining to the teeth.

d. caries, tooth decay (see also CARIES).

d. hygienist, a dental health specialist whose primary concern is maintenance of dental health and the prevention of oral disease. Patient education in the area of proper brushing and flossing also is a major responsibility for the dental hygienist.

The registered dental hygienist (R.D.H.) must have completed an approved course of study in a four year college program offering a B.S. degree, and must successfully complete the written and practical examination required by the state in which the candidate wishes to practice. A two-year associate degree program prepares the student for dental hygiene certification.

The address of the American Dental Hygienists Association is 211 East Chicago Ave., Chicago, IL 60611.

dentalgia (den-tal′je-ah) toothache.

dentate (den′tāt) notched; tooth-shaped.

dentia (den′she-ah) a condition relating to development or eruption of the teeth.

d. prae′cox, premature eruption of the teeth; presence of teeth in the mouth at birth.

d. tar′da, delayed eruption of the teeth, beyond the usual time for their appearance.

dentibuccal (den″tĭ-buk′al) pertaining to the cheek and teeth.

denticle (den′tĭ-k′l) 1. a small toothlike process. 2. a distinct calcified mass within the pulp chamber or in the dentin of a tooth.

dentification (den″tĭ-fĭ-ka′shun) formation of tooth substance.

dentifrice (den″tĭ-fris) a preparation for cleansing and polishing the teeth.

dentigerous (den-tij′er-us) bearing teeth.

dentilabial (den″tĭ-la′be-al) pertaining to the teeth and lips.

dentilingual (den″tĭ-ling′gwal) pertaining to the teeth and tongue.

dentin (den′tin) the chief substance of the teeth, surrounding the tooth pulp and covered by the enamel on the crown and by cementum on the roots. adj., **den′tinal.**

dentinoblastoma (den″tĭ-no-blas-to′mah) dentinoma.

dentinogenesis (den″tĭ-no-jen′ĕ-sis) the formation of dentin.

d. imperfec′ta, a hereditary condition marked by imperfect formation and calcification of dentin, giving the teeth a brown or blue opalescent appearance.

dentinoma (den″tĭ-no′mah) tumor of odontogenic origin, consisting mainly of dentin; called also dentinoblastoma.

dentinosteoid (den″tin-os′te-oid) a tumor composed of or containing dentin and bone.

dentinum (den-ti′num) dentin.

dentist (den′tist) a person who has received a degree in dentistry and who is authorized to practice dentistry.

dentistry (den′tis-tre) 1. that branch of the healing arts concerned with the teeth and associated structures of the oral cavity, including prevention, diagnosis, and treatment of disease and restoration of defective or missing teeth. 2. the work done by dentists, e.g., the creation of restoration, crowns, and bridges, and surgical procedures performed in and about the oral cavity. 3. the practice of the dental profession collectively.

operative d., dentistry concerned with restoration of parts of the teeth that are defective as a result of disease, trauma, or abnormal development to a state of normal function, health, and esthetics.

preventive d., dentistry concerned with maintenance of a normal masticating mechanism by fortifying the structures of the oral cavity against damage and disease.

prosthetic d., prosthodontics.

dentition (den-tish′un) the teeth in the dental arch; ordinarily used to designate the natural teeth in position in the alveoli.

deciduous d., the complement of teeth that erupt first and are later succeeded by the permanent teeth.

mixed d., the complement of teeth in the jaws after eruption of some of the permanent teeth, but before all the deciduous teeth are shed.

permanent d., the complement of teeth that erupt and take their places after the deciduous teeth have been shed.

dentoalveolar (den″to-al-ve′o-lar) pertaining to a tooth and its alveolus.

dentoalveolitis (den″to-al″ve-o-li′tis) periodontitis.

dentofacial (den″to-fa′shal) of or pertaining to the teeth and alveolar process and the face.

dentulous (den′tu-lus) having natural teeth.

denture (den′tūr) a complement of teeth, either natural or artificial; ordinarily used to designate an artificial replacement for the natural teeth and adjacent tissues.

complete d., an appliance replacing all the teeth of one jaw, as well as associated structures of the jaw.

partial d., a removable (removable partial denture) or permanently attached (fixed partial denture) appliance replacing one or more missing teeth in one jaw and receiving support and retention from underlying tissues and some or all of the remaining teeth.

denucleated (de-nu′kle-āt″ed) deprived of the nucleus.

denudation (de″nu-da′shun) the stripping or laying bare of any part.

Denver classification (den′ver) the classification of human chromosomes on the basis of size and centromere position; the 23 pairs of chromosomes are arranged individually and numbered, or in seven groups (A to G), in order of decreasing length (see also CHROMOSOME and accompanying illustration).

deodorant (de-o′dor-ant) 1. destroying or masking odors. 2. an agent that masks offensive odors.

deodorize (de-o′dor-īz) to neutralize or absorb odor.

deodorizer (de-o′dor-īz″er) a deodorizing agent.

deorsumversion (de-or″sum-ver′zhun) the turning downward of a part, especially of the eyes.

deossification (de-os″ĭ-fĭ-ka′shun) loss or removal of the mineral elements of bone.

deoxidation (de-ok″sĭ-da′shun) the removal of oxygen from a chemical compound.

deoxy- a chemical prefix designating a compound containing one less atom of oxygen than the reference substance. For words beinning thus, see also those beginning *desoxy-*.

deoxycholic acid (de-ok″sĭ-ko′lik) one of the bile acids, capable of forming soluble, diffusible complexes with fatty acids, and thereby allowing for their absorption in the small intestine.

deoxycorticosterone (de-ok″sĭ-kor′tĭ-ko-stēr′ōn) desoxycorticosterone.

deoxygenation (de-ok″sĭ-jĕ-na′shun) the act of depriving of oxygen.

deoxypentosenucleic acid (de-ok″sĭ-pen″tōs-nu-kle′ik) deoxyribonucleic acid.

deoxyribonuclease (de-ok″sĭ-ri″bo-nu′kle-ās) an enzyme that catalyzes the hydrolysis (depolymerization) of deoxyribonucleic acid (DNA). Abbreviated DNase.

deoxyribonucleic acid (de-ok″sĭ-ri″bo-nu-kle′ik) DNA, a NUCLEIC ACID of complex molecular structure occurring in cell nuclei as the basic structure of the GENES. DNA is present in all body cells of every species, including unicellular organisms and DNA viruses. The structure of DNA was first described in 1953 by J. D. Watson and F. H. C. Crick.

The giant DNA molecules are composed of four basic nucleotides which have adenine, guanine, cytosine, and thymine as the nitrogen-containing bases, and deoxyribose as the sugar. In the DNA molecule there are two chains or strands of polynucleotides coiled around each other to form a double helix, with the bases of one strand being paired with complementary bases of the other strand. The paired bases are joined by hydrogen bonds, adenine being paired with thymine and guanine with cytosine. Each helix has a "backbone" consisting of a sequence of alternating molecules of sugar and phosphate.

The two strands of DNA are bound by loose and reversible bonds. This allows for the splitting apart of the two strands, an event that occurs many times during the course of their activities within the cell. One strand of the molecule is responsible for replication of the molecule, the other strand acts as a template (pattern) for the synthesis of several types of RIBONUCLEIC ACID (RNA). Thus DNA is directly responsible for replication of the cell and indirectly

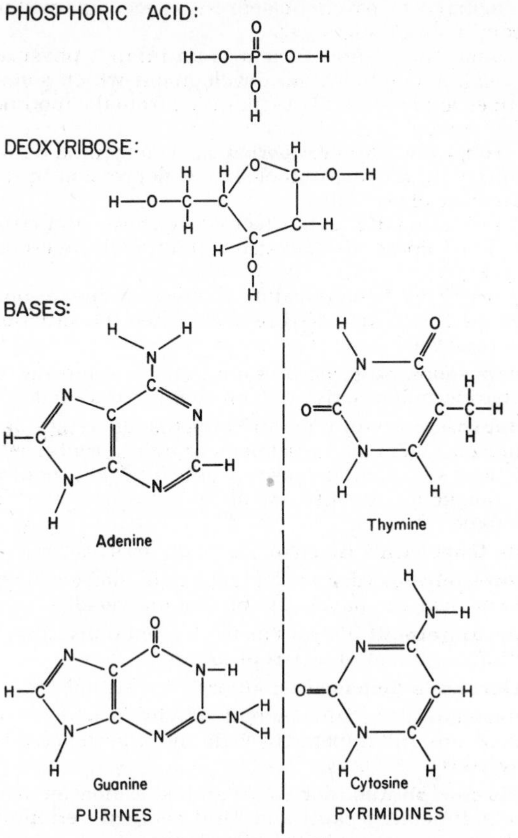

The basic building blocks of DNA. (From Guyton, Arthur C.: Textbook of Medical Physiology, 5th ed. Philadelphia, W. B. Saunders Co., 1976.)

responsible (through RNA) for the formation of structural proteins and the enzymes that promote all the chemical reactions which supply energy to the cell. (See also HEREDITY.)

deoxyribonucleoprotein (de-ok″sĭ-ri″bo-nu′kle-o-pro″te-in) a nucleoprotein in which the sugar is D-2-deoxyribose.

deoxyribonucleoside (de-ok″sĭ-ri″bo-nu′kle-o-sīd) a nucleoside having a purine or pyrimidine base bonded to deoxyribose.

deoxyribonucleotide (de-ok″sĭ-ri″bo-nu′kle-o-tīd) a nucleotide having a purine or pyrimidine base bonded to deoxyribose, which in turn is bonded to a phosphate group.

deoxyribose (de-ok″sĭ-ri′bōs) an aldopentose found in deoxyribonucleic acid, deoxyribonucleotides, and deoxyribonucleosides.

dependence (de-pen′dens) the total psychophysical state of a drug user, in which the usual or increasing doses of the drug are required to prevent the onset of WITHDRAWAL symptoms.

depersonalization (de-per″sun-al-ĭ-za′shun) feelings of unreality or strangeness concerning either the environment or the self or both.

de Pezzer's catheter Pezzer's catheter.

dephosphorylation (de-fos″for-ĭ-la′shun) removal of the phosphoryl, the trivalent PO group, from organic molecules.

depilate (dep′ĭ-lāt) to remove hair.

depilatory (de-pil′ah-tor″e) 1. having the power to remove hair. 2. an agent that removes or destroys the hair.

depolarization (de-po″lar-ĭ-za′shun) the process or act of neutralizing polarity.

depolymerization (de-pol″ĭ-mer-ĭ-za′shun) the conversion of a compound into one of smaller molecular weight and different physical properties without changing the percentage relations of the elements composing it.

deposit (de-poz′it) 1. sediment or dregs. 2. extraneous inorganic matter collected in the tissues or in an organ of the body.

depot (de′po, dep′o) a body area in which a substance, e.g., a drug, can be accumulated, deposited, or stored and from which it can be distributed.

fat d., a site in the body in which large quantities of fat are stored, as in adipose tissue.

Depo-Testosterone (de″po-tes-tos′ter-ōn) trademark for a sustained-action preparation of testosterone.

depressant (de-pres′ant) 1. diminishing any function or activity. 2. an agent that retards any function, especially a drug that slows a function of the body or calms and quiets nervous excitement; a sedative. Among the best-known depressants are barbiturates. Alcohol is also a depressant, although its first effect is sometimes stimulating. (See also TRANQUILIZER.)

depressed (de-prest′) carried below the normal level; associated with depression.

depression (de-presh′un) 1. a hollow or depressed area. 2. a lowering or decrease of functional activity. 3. in psychiatry, a morbid sadness, dejection, or melancholy, distinguished from grief, which is realistic

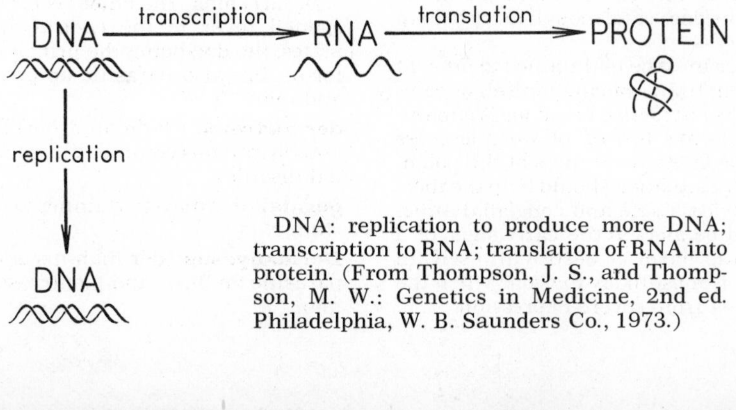

DNA: replication to produce more DNA; transcription to RNA; translation of RNA into protein. (From Thompson, J. S., and Thompson, M. W.: Genetics in Medicine, 2nd ed. Philadelphia, W. B. Saunders Co., 1973.)

and proportionate to a personal loss. Depression may be symptomatic of a psychiatric disorder or it may constitute the principal manifestation of a neurosis or psychosis. adj., **depres′sive.**

Treatment of depression is often very difficult, requiring in most cases intensive psychotherapy to help the patient understand the underlying cause of his depression. Antidepressant drugs such as imipramine hydrochloride (Tofranil) and amitriptyline (Elavil) are often used in the treatment of depression. They are not true stimulants of the central nervous system, but they do alter the function of the reticular system in the midbrain and of the nuclei of the thalamus. Monoamine oxidase (MAO) inhibitors are also used. When antidepressants fail, some form of shock therapy such as electric shock or insulin shock treatments is usually used in conjunction with the psychotherapy.

PATIENT CARE. The severely depressed patient usually expresses three basic feelings associated with his mental state. These are physical inactivity and a lack of desire to socialize, feelings of worthlessness, and loss of self-esteem and thoughts of self-injury or destruction. In planning the care of the depressed patient, one must always consider these attitudes and strive for some understanding as to why the patient behaves as he does. Although an optimistic approach should be used when helping the patient overcome his depression, one must guard against excessive cheerfulness and attempts to "jolly" the patient into a better mood. Only by gradually gaining his attention and pointing out to him encouraging signs of his progress can he be helped in his early attempts to return to reality and socialize with others. As he progresses out of his depression the patient may become overdependent on the therapist and then later show signs of hostility toward her. She must, however, remain consistent in her relationship with him, demonstrating warmth and a sincere interest in him no matter what type of behavior he may exhibit.

The patient's physical inactivity will require attention to adequate nutrition, a normal balance of fluid intake and output, proper elimination, and good skin care. He will need help in maintaining a pleasing personal appearance and good personal hygiene. At first it may be necessary for the hospital staff to initiate all such activities as bathing, dressing, and even eating and drinking. As his condition improves the patient should take over responsibility for his personal care and grooming. If he is severely depressed he may be totally out of touch with reality and completely unresponsive to anyone else's presence. In such instances the therapist may be able to do little more than sit with the patient, letting him know by her presence that she is interested in his problem and that she does care enough to try to help him.

Constant vigilance must be maintained to prevent the depressed patient from injuring himself or committing SUICIDE. Self-destructive behavior is a manifestation of the patient's feeling of worthlessness and loss of self-esteem. An awareness of the potential dangers in such a situation should help the therapist plan and provide a safe and congenial atmosphere. She should be alert to the early signs of a patient's intention to harm or destroy himself. In most cases suicide is most likely to occur when the patient is recovering from severe depression.

agitated d., psychotic depression accompanied by continuous restlessness.

anaclitic d., impairment of an infant's physical, social, and intellectual development which sometimes follows a sudden separation from the mothering person.

congenital chrondrosternal d., a congenital deformity with a deep, funnel-shaped depression in the anterior chest wall.

involutional d., an affective psychosis occurring in late middle life (see also involutional MELANCHOLIA).

reactive d., situational d., depression due to some external situation, and relieved when the situation is removed.

depressomotor (de-pres″o-mo′tor) 1. retarding or abating motor activity. 2. an agent that so acts.

depressor (de-pres′or) anything that depresses, as a muscle, agent, or instrument, or an afferent nerve, whose stimulation causes a fall in blood pressure.

tongue d., an instrument for pressing down the tongue.

de Quervain's disease see QUERVAIN'S DISEASE.

deradelphus (der″ah-del′fus) a twin monster fused at or near the navel, and having one head.

derangement (de-rānj′ment) 1. mental disorder. 2. disarrangment of a part or organ.

Dercum's disease (der′kumz) adiposis dolorosa.

dereism (de′re-izm) mental activity in which fantasy runs unhampered by logic and experience. adj., **dereis′tic.**

derencephalus (der″en-sef′ah-lus) a monster with a rudimentary skull and bifid cervical vertebrae, the brain resting in the bifurcation.

derepression (de″re-presh′un) 1. elevation of the level of an enzyme above the normal, either by lowering the corepressor concentration or by a mutation that decreases the formation of aporepressor or the response to the complete repressor. 2. the inhibition of the repressor substance produced by the regulator genes with the result that the operator gene is free to initiate the process of polypeptide formation.

derma (der′mah) the corium, or true skin.

dermabrasion (derm″ah-bra′shun) PLANING of the skin done by mechanical means, e.g., sandpaper, wire brushes, etc.

Dermacentor (der″mah-sen′tor) a genus of ticks parasitic on various animals, and vectors of disease-producing microorganisms.

D. anderso′ni, a species of tick common in the western United States, parasitic on numerous wild mammals, most domestic animals, and man. It is a vector of Rocky Mountain spotted fever, tularemia, Colorado tick fever, and Q fever in the United States, and is the cause of tick paralysis.

D. varia′bilis, the chief vector of Rocky Mountain spotted fever in the central and eastern United States, the dog being the principal host of the adult forms, but also parasitic on cattle, horses, rabbits, and man.

dermadrome (der′mah-drōm) a complex of cutaneous symptoms commonly associated with an internal disorder.

dermal (der′mal) pertaining to the true skin, or corium.

Dermanyssus (der″mah-nis′us) a genus of mites parasitic on birds and poultry, sometimes infesting man.

dermat(o)- word element [Gr.], *skin.*

dermatic (der-mat′ik) dermal.

dermatitides (der″mah-tit′ĭ-dēz) plural of *dermatitis;* inflammatory conditions of the skin considered collectively.

dermatitis (der″mah-ti′tis) inflammation of the skin. Dermatitis can result from various animal, vegetable, and chemical substances, from heat or cold, from mechanical irritation, from certain forms of malnutrition, or from infectious disease. In some cases, dermatitis may have a psychologic rather than a physical cause. The symptoms may include itching, redness, crustiness, blisters, watery discharges, fissures, or other changes in the normal condition of the skin. The treatment of dermatitis varies greatly and is determined by the cause.

TYPES OF DERMATITIS. One of the most common forms of the disorder, CONTACT DERMATITIS, results from contact of the skin with various substances. There are two types: allergic contact dermatitis and primary-irritant dermatitis. Familiar examples of the allergic type are POISON IVY, OAK, AND SUMAC, but many other substances may be the cause of an allergic reaction. These include rubber and plastics, industrial chemicals, cosmetics, clothing dyes, costume jewelry, some animals and plants, detergents, insecticides, and paints.

The second type of contact dermatitis is due to a direct irritating effect on the skin of certain chemical, physical, or mechanical agents. In contrast to the allergic type, which affects only people who have a specific sensitivity, these agents cause dermatitis in everyone upon sufficient exposure. Acids, alkalis, petroleum products, and mineral dusts are some of the chemical causes. A mild form is the familiar "dishpan hands," resulting from contact with strong soaps and detergents.

Such physical agents as excessive cold or heat may also cause inflammation of the skin. Prolonged exposure to extreme cold may result in CHILBLAINS or in FROSTBITE, and exposure to a hot sun may cause sunburn. When heat causes unusual sweating, miliaria (commonly called prickly heat) may result. All these familiar complaints are forms of dermatitis. Overexposure to x-rays is another factor which may cause skin inflammation. Mechanical agents, such as chafing, pressure, or scratching, are other common causes of dermatitis. Pressure and friction resulting from ill fitting shoes cause corns and calluses, and pressure on bony parts of the body incurred in extended bed rest may cause DECUBITUS ULCERS.

PATIENT CARE. The patient with dermatitis frequently is uncomfortable, irritable, and emotionally upset because of itching and the unsightly appearance produced by his condition. Efforts should be made to provide a quiet atmosphere that is conducive to rest, and to give the patient individual attention to help him feel acceptable to others.

If large areas of the skin are involved there will be increased sensitivity to cold, making the patient more susceptible to chilling. Care must be used to protect the patient and the bed linen from dampness when wet compresses are prescribed.

Bathing with ordinary soap and water is usually contraindicated and special colloid or medicated baths may be ordered to cleanse and soothe irritated or pruritic skin. After the bath the skin is dried by patting with a soft towel, *never* by rubbing. Scales, crusts, and other exudates are *not* removed without specific orders from the physician. The skin should be handled gently, and great care used in changing the bedclothes or the patient's clothing. Lotions and alcohol routinely used in the hospital for back rubs or as skin fresheners must not be applied to the skin of these patients without written directions from the physician because they may aggravate the skin disorder.

actinic d., d. actin′ica, that produced by exposure to actinic radiation, such as that from the sun, ultraviolet waves, or x- or gamma radiation.

atopic d., a chronic pruritic eruption of unknown etiology, although allergic, hereditary, and psychogenic factors appear to be involved.

contact d., acute dermatitis due to direct contact of the skin with various substances (see also CONTACT DERMATITIS and types of DERMATITIS, above).

d. exfoliati′va neonato′rum exfoliative dermatitis supervening in bullous impetigo of the newborn; called also Ritter's disease.

exfoliative d. virtually universal erythema, desquamation, scaling, and itching of the skin and loss of hair; it may result from internal medication with such drugs as penicillin, quinine, sulfonamides, gold salts, and iodides.

d. medicamento′sa, an eruption or solitary skin lesion caused by a drug taken internally.

photocontact d., allergic contact dermatitis caused by the action of sunlight on skin sensitized by contact with a substance capable of causing this reaction, such as a halogenated salicylanilide, sandalwood oil, or hexachlorophene.

primary-irritant d., dermatitis induced by a substance acting as an irritant rather than as a sensitizer or allergen (see also types of DERMATITIS above).

seborrheic d., d., seborrhe′ica, a chronic, usually pruritic, dermatitis with erythema, dry, moist, or greasy scaling, and yellow crusted patches on various areas, especially the scalp, with exfoliation of an excessive amount of dry scales (dandruff) (see also SEBORRHEIC DERMATITIS).

stasis d., an eczematous eruption of the lower legs, usually due to impeded circulation, with edema, pigmentation, and often chronic ulceration.

d. venena′ta, severe allergic contact dermatitis.

x-ray d., radiodermatitis.

Dermatobia (der″mah-to′be-ah) a genus of botflies, including *D. hominis,* whose larvae are parasitic in the skin of man, mammals, and birds.

dermatocele (der′mah-to-sĕl″) cutis laxa.

dermatofibroma (der″mah-to-fi-bro′mah) a fibrous tumor-like nodule of the skin.

dermatofibrosarcoma (der″mah-to-fi″bro-sar-ko′mah) a fibrosarcoma of the skin.

dermatogen (der-mat′o-jen) a skin antigen that may be associated with any skin disorder.

dermatoglyphics (der″mah-to-glif′iks) the study of the patterns of ridges of the skin of the fingers, palms, toes, and soles; of interest in anthropology and law enforcement as a means of establishing identity and in medicine, both clinically and as a genetic indicator, particularly of chromosomal abnormalities.

dermatographia (der″mah-to-graf′e-ah) urticaria due to physical allergy in which a pale, raised welt or wheal with a red flare on each side is elicited by stroking or scratching the skin with a dull instrument.

dermatoheteroplasty (der″mah-to-het′er-o-plas″-

te) the grafting of skin derived from an individual of another species.

dermatologic, dermatological (der″mah-to-loj′ik; der″mah-to-loj′ĭ-kal) pertaining to dermatology; of or affecting the skin.

dermatologist (der″mah-tol′o-jist) a physician who specializes in dermatology.

dermatology (der″mah-tol′o-je) the medical speciality concerned with the diagnosis and treatment of skin diseases.

dermatome (der′mah-tōm) 1. an instrument for cutting thin skin slices for grafting. 2. the area of skin supplied with afferent nerve fibers by a single posterior spinal root. 3. the lateral part of an embryonic somite.

dermatomegaly (der″mah-to-meg′ah-le) cutis laxa.

dermatomere (der′mah-to-mēr″) any segment of the embryonic integument.

dermatomycosis (der″mah-to-mi-ko′sis) a superficial fungal infection of the skin or its appendages.

dermatomyoma (der″mah-to-mi-o′mah) a dermal leiomyoma.

dermatomyositis (der″mah-to-mi″o-si′tis) an acute, subacute, or chronic disease marked by nonsuppurative inflammation of the skin, subcutaneous tissue, and muscles, with necrosis of muscle fibers. It is included among the group of illnesses known as COLLAGEN DISEASES.

Among a variety of symptoms that point to the onset of the disease are fever, loss of weight, skin lesions, and aching muscles. As the disease progresses there may be loss of the use of the arms and legs. Complications such as hardening may occur, similar to the changes seen in scleroderma. Occasionally steroids prove helpful in relieving symptoms, but the most beneficial treatment is physical therapy to maintain maximal use of the muscles.

dermatopathic (der″mah-to-path′ik) pertaining to or attributable to disease of the skin.

dermatopathology (der″mah-to-pah-thol′o-je) pathology that is especially concerned with lesions of the skin.

dermatopathy (der″mah-top′ah-the) any disease of the skin; dermopathy.

dermatophilosis (der″mah-to-fi-lo′sis) an actinomycotic disease caused by *Dermatophilus congolensis,* affecting cattle, sheep, horses, goats, deer, and sometimes man. In man, it is marked by nonpainful pustules on the hands and arms; the lesions break down and form shallow red ulcers which regress spontaneously, leaving some scarring.

Dermatophilus (der″mah-tof′ĭ-lus) 1. *Tunga.* 2. a genus of pathogenic actinomycetes.

D. congolen′sis, the etiologic agent of dermatophilosis.

dermatophyte (der′mah-to-fīt″) a fungus parasitic upon the skin, including *Microsporum, Epidermophyton,* and *Trichophyton.*

dermatophytid (der″mah-tof′ĭ-tid) a secondary skin eruption which is an expression of hypersensitivity to a dermatophyte, especially *Epidermophyton,* infection, occurring on an area remote from the site of infection.

dermatophytosis (der″mah-to-fi-to′sis) a fungal infection of the skin; often used to refer to ATHLETE'S FOOT (tinea pedis).

dermatoplasty (der′mah-to-plas″te) a plastic operation on the skin; operative replacement of lost skin. adj., **dermatoplas′tic.**

dermatosclerosis (der″mah-to-sklĕ-ro′sis) scleroderma.

dermatosis (der″mah-to′sis) any skin disorder, especially one not characterized by inflammation.

precancerous d., any skin condition in which the lesions—warts, nevi, or other excrescences—are likely to undergo malignant degeneration.

stasis d., a chronic, usually eczematous dermatitis almost always of the anteromesial aspect of the lower leg, and often complicated by ulceration; probably due to deficient venous return.

dermatotherapy (der″mah-to-ther′ah-pe) treatment of skin diseases.

dermatotropic (der″mah-to-trop′ik) having a specific affinity for the skin.

dermatozoon (der″mah-to-zo′on) any animal parasite on the skin; an ectoparasite.

dermis (der′mis) the true skin, or corium. adj., **der′mal, der′mic.**

dermoblast (der′mo-blast) the part of the mesoderm that develops into the true skin.

dermographia (der″mo-graf′e-ah) dermatographia.

dermoid (der′moid) 1. skinlike. 2. a dermoid cyst.

d. cyst, a tumor of developmental origin consisting of a fibrous wall lined with stratified epithelium and containing hair follicles, sweat glands, sebaceous glands, nerve elements, and teeth; a teratoma. When these cysts occur in the ovary they may present no symptoms, but their long pedicles may cause twisting, resulting in acute abdominal pain. Treatment is surgical removal.

dermoidectomy (der″moi-dek′to-me) excision of a dermoid cyst.

dermomycosis (der″mo-mi-ko′sis) dermatomycosis.

dermopathy (der-mop′ah-the) any skin disease; dermatopathy.

diabetic d., any of several cutaneous manifestations of diabetes.

dermophyte (der′mo-fīt) dermatophyte.

dermoskeleton (der″mo-skel′ĕ-ton) exoskeleton.

dermosynovitis (der″mo-sin″o-vi′tis) inflammation of the skin overlying an inflamed bursa or tendon sheath.

dermotropic (der″mo-trop′ik) dermatotropic.

dermovascular (der″mo-vas′ku-lar) pertaining to the skin and blood vessels of the skin.

derodidymus (der″o-did′ĭ-mus) a monster with two heads; dicephalus.

Deronil (der′o-nil) trademark for a preparation of dexamethasone, an anti-inflammatory adrenocortical steroid.

Descemet's membrane (des-ĕ-māz′) the posterior lining membrane of the cornea, a thin hyaline membrane between the substantia propria and the endothelial layer.

descensus (de-sen′sus), pl. *descen′sus* [L.] downward displacement or prolapse.

d. tes′tis, normal migration of the testis from its fetal position in the abdominal cavity to its location within the scrotum, usually during the last 3 months of gestation.

d. u'teri, prolapse of the uterus.

desensitization (de-sen″sĭ-tĭ-za′shun) 1. the reduction or abolition of sensitivity to a particular antigen; also, the condition of having undergone desensitization. 2. in psychiatry, the removal of a mental complex.

desensitize (de-sen′sĭ-tīz) 1. to deprive of sensation. 2. to subject to desensitization.

deserpidine (de-ser′pĭ-dēn) an antihypertensive and tranquilizer isolated from *Rauwolfia.*

desert fever, desert rheumatism the primary form of COCCIDIOIDOMYCOSIS.

desiccant (des′ĭ-kant) 1. promoting dryness. 2. an agent that promotes dryness.

desiccate (des′ĭ-kāt) to render thoroughly dry.

desiccation (des″ĭ-ka′shun) the act of drying.

desipramine (des-ip′rah-mēn) an antidepressant, used as the hydrochloride salt.

deslanoside (des-lan′o-sīd) a cardiotonic glycoside obtained from lanatoside C; used where digitalis is recommended.

desm(o)- word element [Gr.], *ligament.*

desmitis (des-mi′tis) inflammation of a ligament.

desmocranium (des″mo-kra′ne-um) the mass of mesoderm at the cranial end of the notochord in the early embryo, forming the earliest stage of the skull.

desmocyte (des′mo-sīt) fibroblast.

desmography (des-mog′rah-fe) a description of ligaments.

desmoid (des′moid) 1. fibrous or fibroid. 2. a lesion produced by progressive fibroblastic proliferation in striated muscle and sometimes in periosteum.

desmology (des-mol′o-je) the science of ligaments.

desmoma (des-mo′mah) desmoid tumor.

desmopathy (des-mop′ah-the) any disease of the ligaments.

desmoplasia (des″mo-pla′ze-ah) the formation and development of fibrous tissue. adj., **desmoplas′tic.**

desoxy- for words beginning thus, see also those beginning *deoxy-.*

desoxycorticosterone (des-ok″sĭ-kor″tĭ-ko-stēr′ōn) a MINERALCORTICOID precursor of corticosterone concerned in water and electrolyte metabolism; used in the form of the acetate and pivalate esters in adrenal insufficiency.

Desoxyn (des-ok′sin) trademark for preparations of methamphetamine, a central nervous system stimulant and pressor drug.

desquamation (des″kwah-ma′shun) the shedding of epithelial elements, chiefly of the skin, in scales or sheets. adj., **desquam′ative.**

desulfhydrase (de″sulf-hi′drās) an enzyme that splits cysteine into hydrogen sulfide, ammonia, and pyruvic acid.

desulfurase (de-sul′fu-rās) desulfhydrase.

DET diethyltryptamine.

detachment (de-tach′ment) the condition of being separated or disconnected.

d. of retina, retinal d., separation of the inner layers of the retina from the pigment epithelium, which remains attached to the choroid. The onset of symptoms may be gradual or sudden, depending on the cause, size, and location of the area involved. The patient may see flashes of light and then days or weeks later notice cloudy vision or loss of central vision. Another common symptom is the sensation of spots or moving particles in the field of vision. In severe retinal detachment there may be complete loss of vision.

The condition is treated surgically. Newer surgical procedures include the use of diathermy to seal the retinal break so that vitreous humor cannot leak between the retina and choroid. In some cases the vitreous is drained from the area in which it has accumulated so that the retina can be returned to its normal position. When sutures are used to hold the retina in place, the patient is confined to bed for 2 weeks postoperatively to avoid strain on the suture line. If one of the newer surgical techniques is used, the patient may be allowed out of bed the day after surgery but he must be warned to avoid vigorous movement of the head.

detergent (de-ter′jent) 1. purifying, cleansing. 2. an agent that purifies or cleanses.

determinant (de-ter′mĭ-nant) a factor that establishes the nature of an entity or event.

antigenic d., the structural component of an antigen molecule responsible for its specific interaction with antibody molecules elicited by the same or related antigen.

determination (de-ter″mĭ-na′shun) the establishment of the exact nature of an entity or event.

embryonic d., the loss of pluripotentiality in any embryonic part and its start on the way to an unalterable fate.

sex d., the process by which the sex of an organism is fixed, associated, in man, with the presence or absence of the Y chromosome.

determinism (de-ter′mĭ-nizm) the theory that all phenomena are the result of antecedent conditions and that nothing occurs by chance.

detoxicate (de-tok′sĭ-kāt) detoxify.

detoxication (de-tok″sĭ-ka′shun) detoxification.

detoxification (de-tok″sĭ-fĭ-ka′shun) 1. reduction of the toxic properties of a substance. 2. treatment designed to assist in recovery from the toxic effects of a drug.

metabolic d., reduction of the toxic properties of a substance by chemical changes induced in the body, producing a compound which is less poisonous or more readily eliminated.

detoxify (de-tok′sĭ-fi) to subject to detoxification.

detrition (de-trish′un) the wearing away, as of teeth, by friction.

detritus (de-tri′tus) particulate matter produced by or remaining after the wearing away or disintegration of a substance or tissue.

detruncation (de″trung-ka′shun) decapitation, especially of the fetus.

detrusor (de-tru′sor) a general term for a body part, e.g., a muscle, that pushes down.

detumescence (de″tu-mes′ens) the subsidence of congestion and swelling.

deutan (doo′tan) a person exhibiting deuteranomalopia or deuteranopia.

deuteranomalopia (doo″ter-ah-nom″ah-lo′pe-ah) a variant of normal color vision with imperfect perception of the green hues.

deuteranope (doo′ter-ah-nōp″) a person exhibiting deuteranopia.

deuteranopia, deuteranopsia (doo″ter-ah-no′pe-ah; doo″ter-ah-nop′se-ah) defective color vision, with confusion of greens and reds, and retention of the sensory mechanism for two hues only—blue and yellow. adj., **deuteranop′ic.**

deuterate (doo′ter-āt) to treat (combine) with deuterium (^2H).

deuterium (doo-te′re-um) the mass 2 isotope of hydrogen, symbol ^2H or D; it is available as a gas or HEAVY WATER (deuterium oxide) and is used as a tracer or indicator in studying fat and amino acid metabolism.

deuterohemophilia (doo″ter-o-he″mo-fil′e-ah) a group of hemorrhagic disorders resembling classical hemophilia, due to coagulation factor deficiencies or to the action of certain anticoagulants.

deuteron (doo″ter-on) the nucleus of deuterium atoms; deuterons are used as bombarding particles for nuclear disintegration.

deuteropathy (doo″ter-op′ah-the) a disease that is secondary to another disease.

deutoplasm (doo′to-plazm) the inactive materials in protoplasm, especially reserve foodstuffs, such as yolk.

devascularization (de-vas″ku-lar-ĭ-za′shun) interruption of circulation of blood to a part due to obstruction or destruction of blood vessels supplying it.

Devegan (dev′ĕ-gan) trademark for a preparation of acetarsone, an arsenical used in the treatment of amebic dysentery and trichomonas vaginalis.

development (de-vel′up-ment) the process of growth and differentiation.

psychosexual d., development of the psychological aspects of sexuality from birth to maturity.

developmental (de-vel″up-men′tal) pertaining to development.

d. anomaly, absence, deformity, or excess of body parts as the result of faulty development of the embryo.

deviant (de′ve-ant) 1. varying from a determinable standard. 2. a person with characteristics varying from what is considered standard or normal.

color d., a person whose color perception varies from the norm.

sexual d., a person exhibiting SEXUAL DEVIATION.

deviation (de″ve-a′shun) variation from the regular standard or course. In ophthalmology, a tendency for the visual axes of the eye to fall out of alignment owing to muscular imbalance.

sexual d., sexual behavior that varies from that normally considered biologically or socially acceptable.

standard d., the measure of variabilty of any frequency curve.

devil's grip epidemic pleurodynia.

devitalization (de-vi″tal-ĭ-za′shun) deprivation of vitality or life, as of tissue.

devitalize (de-vi′tal-īz) to deprive of life or vitality.

devitalized (de-vi′tal-īzed) devoid of vitality or life.

devolution (dev″o-lu′shun) the reverse of evolution; catabolic change.

dexamethasone (dek″sah-meth′ah-sōn) a glucocorticoid, used as an anti-inflammatory steroid with little salt-retaining action.

dexbrompheniramine (deks″brōm-fen-ir′ah-mēn) the dextrorotatory isomer of brompheniramine, used as an antihistaminic in the form of the maleate salt.

dexchlorpheniramine (deks″klōr-fen-i′rah-mēn) the dextrorotatory form of chlorpheniramine used as an antihistaminic in the form of the maleate salt.

Dexedrine (dek′sĕ-drēn) trademark for preparations of dextroamphetamine, a central nervous system stimulant.

Dexon (dek′son) trademark for a synthetic suture material, polyglycolic acid, a polymer that is completely absorbable and nonirritating.

Dexoval (dek′so-val) trademark for a preparation of methamphetamine, a central nervous system stimulant and pressor drug.

dexter (dek′ster) [L.] right; on the right side.

dextr(o)- word element [L.], *right.*

dextrality (dek-stral′ĭ-te) the preferential use, in voluntary motor acts, of the right member of the major paired organs of the body, as the right eye, hand, or foot.

dextran (dek′stran) a water-soluble polysaccharide of glucose (dextrose) produced by the action of *Leuconostoc mesenteroides* on sucrose; used as a plasma volume extender.

dextraural (dek-straw′ral) hearing better with the right ear.

dextriferron (deks″trĭ-fer′on) a complex of ferric hydroxide and partially hydrolyzed dextrin used in the treatment of iron-deficiency anemia.

dextrin (dek′strin) a carbohydrate formed during the hydrolysis of starch to sugar.

dextrin-1,6-glucosidase (deks″trin-glu-ko′sĭ-dās) dextrin 6-glucanohydrolase: an enzyme that catalyzes the hydrolysis of α-1-6-glucan links in dextrins containing short 1,6-linked side chains.

dextrinosis (dek″strĭ-no′sis) a condition characterized by accumulation in the tissues of an abnormal polysaccharide.

limit d., glycogenosis, type III (see also FORBES' DISEASE).

dextrinuria (dek″strin-u′re-ah) presence of dextrin in the urine.

dextroamphetamine (dek″stro-am-fet′ah-mēn) the dextrorotatory isomer of amphetamine, havng a more conspicuous stimulant effect on the central nervous system than the levorotatory (levamphetamine) racemic forms of amphetamine in the same dosage. Abuse of this drug may lead to dependence. (See also AMPHETAMINE.)

dextrocardia (dek″stro-kar′de-ah) location of the heart in the right side of the thorax, the apex pointing to the right.

mirror-image d., location of the heart in the right side of the chest, the atria being transposed and the right ventricle lying anteriorly and to the left of the left ventricle.

dextrocularity (dek″strok-u-lar′ĭ-te) having greater visual power in the right eye, therefore using it more than the left.

dextromanual (dek″stro-man′u-al) right-handed.

dextromethorphan (dek″stro-meth′or-fan) a synthetic morphine derivative used as an antitussive in the form of the hydrobromide salt.

dextropedal (dek-strop′ĕ-dal) right-footed.

dextroposition (dek″stro-po-zish′un) displacement to the right.

dextropropoxyphene (dek″stro-pro-pok′sĭ-fēn) propoxyphene, an analgesic.

dextrorotatory (dek″stro-ro′tah-tor″e) turning the plane of polarization, or rays of light, to the right.

dextrose (dek′strōs) a monosaccharide usually obtained by hydrolysis of starch. In biochemistry and physiology, dextrose is known as GLUCOSE. Dextrose is considered one of the most important carbohydrates because it makes up 80 per cent of all simple sugar absorbed into the blood. It is present in certain foodstuffs, especially sweet fruits, and in the blood of all animals. Through the process of metabolism, dextrose is used by the body to provide energy, or, in excess, it is converted into fat. The liver cells convert glucose into glycogen, so that it can be stored until needed. When the blood sugar drops below normal, there is increased production of epinephrine, which causes glycogen to be changed back into glucose and used for producing energy.

dextrosinistral (dek″stro-sin′is-tral) extending from right to left; also applied to a left-handed person trained to use the right hand in certain performances.

dextrosuria (dek″stro-su′re-ah) the presence of dextrose in the urine; called also glucosuria.

dextroversion (dek″stro-ver′zhun) 1. version to the right, especially movement of the eyes to the right. 2. location of the heart in the right chest, the left ventricle remaining in the normal position on the left, but lying anterior to the right ventricle.

DFP diisopropyl fluorophosphate (see ISOFLUROPHATE).

dg. decigram.

di- word element [Gr., L.], *two.*

dia- word element [Gr.], *through; between; apart; across; completely.*

diabetes (di″ah-be′tēz) any disorder characterized by excessive urine excretion, especially diabetes mellitus.

brittle d., diabetes that is difficult to control, characterized by unexplained oscillation between hypoglycemia and acidosis.

bronze d., a primary disorder of iron metabolism, with deposits of iron-containing pigments in the body tissues, and often with bronze pigmentation of the skin, diabetes mellitus, and cirrhosis of the liver; called also hemochromatosis and iron storage disease.

d. insip′idus, a metabolic disorder resulting from decreased activity of the posterior lobe of the pituitary gland. Normally, reabsorption of water from the renal tubules is promoted by vasopressin, or antidiuretic hormone, a hormone from the posterior pituitary lobe. A deficiency of this hormone leads to the symptoms of diabetes insipidus, which include excessive thirst and the passage of large amounts of urine with no excess of sugar. Treatment consists of administration of extracts of the posterior lobe of the pituitary gland or pure vasopressin.

d. melli′tus, a disorder of carbohydrate metabolism in which the ability to oxidize and utilize carbohydrates is lost as a result of disturbances in the normal insulin mechanism. A serious disruption of carbohydrate metabolism leads to abnormalities of protein and fat metabolism. The oxidation of fat is accelerated in diabetes, and thus there is an accumulation of the end products of fat metabolism in the blood and the development of the symptoms of ketosis, acidosis, and coma.

Factors leading to disturbances in the normal insulin mechanism and the onset of diabetes mellitus include insufficient production of insulin from the beta cells of the islands of Langerhans in the pancreas, an increase in the insulin requirement by the tissue cells, or a decrease in the effectiveness of insulin due to one or more insulin antagonists which can deactivate insulin. Any of these factors may produce the symptoms of diabetes mellitus.

Because the diabetic is unable to utilize the carbohydrates in his blood he is improperly nourished, no matter how much food he consumes. The accumulation of unused glucose leads to weakness, fatigue, and a spilling over of sugar into the urine. The high level of sugar in the blood makes the untreated diabetic particularly susceptible to infection. In a prolonged severe diabetic condition, the raised fat and glucose level of the blood may cause damage to blood vessels and to tissues and organs containing

FOOD EXCHANGE LISTS

List 1. Milk Exchanges

Carbohydrate – 12 gm., Protein 8 gm., Fat – 10 gm., Calories – 170

*Milk, whole – plain or homogenized	1 cup
Milk, evaporated	½ cup
*Milk, powdered	¼ cup
*Buttermilk	1 cup
*Milk, skim	1 cup

*Add 2 fat exchanges if fat free

List 2. Vegetable Exchanges

A. These vegetables may be used as desired in ordinary amounts. Carbohydrate, protein, and fat negligible. Servings: raw unlimited; cooked ½–1 cup.

Asparagus	*Greens	Mushrooms
*Broccoli	Beets	Okra
*Brussels Sprouts	Chard	*Pepper
	Collard	Radishes
Cabbage	Dandelion	Rhubarb
Cauliflower	Kale	Sauerkraut
Celery	Mustard	String Beans, young
*Chicory	Spinach	
Cucumbers	Turnip	Summer Squash
*Escarole		
Eggplant		*Tomatoes
Lettuce		*Watercress

B. Restricted vegetables: 1 Serving = ½ cup = 100 grams. Carbohydrate – 7 gm., Protein – 2 gm., Calories – 35

Beets	Peas, green	*Squash, winter
*Carrots	*Pumpkin	Turnip
Onions	Rutabaga	

*High vitamin A value. Use one daily.

List 3. Fruit Exchanges

Carbohydrate – 10 gm., Calories – 40

Fresh, dried, cooked, canned, frozen without sugar

Apple	1 sm. 2″ diam.
Applesauce	½ cup
Apricots, fresh	2 medium
Apricots, dried	4 halves
Banana	½ small
Berries; Strawberries, Raspberries, Blackberries	1 cup
Blueberries	⅔ cup
Canteloupe	¼ (6″ diam.)
Cherries	10 large
Dates	2
Figs, fresh	2 large

FOOD EXCHANGE LISTS *(Continued)*

Figs, dried	1 small
Grapefruit	1/2 small
Grapefruit Juice	1/2 cup
Grapes	12
Grape Juice	1/4 cup
Honeydew Melon	1/8 (7″ diam.)
Mango	1/2 small
Orange	1 small
Orange Juice	1/2 cup
Papaya	1/3 medium
Peach	1 medium
Pear	1 small
Pineapple	1/2 cup
Pineapple Juice	1/3 cup
Plums	2 medium
Prunes, dried	2 medium
Raisins	2 Tbsp.
Tangerine	1 large
Watermelon	1 cup

List 4. Bread Exchanges

Carbohydrate – 15 gm., Protein – 2 gm., Calories – 70

	Meas.
Bread	1 slice
Biscuit, Roll (2″ diam.)	1
Muffin (2″ diam.)	1
Cornbread (1½″ cube)	1
Flour	2½ Tbsp.
Cereal, cooked	1/2 cup
Cereal, dry (flake, puffed)	3/4 cup
Rice, Grits, cooked	1/2 cup
Spaghetti, Noodles, etc. cooked	1/2 cup
Crackers,	
Graham (2½″ sq.)	2
Oyster	20 (1/2 cup)
Saltines (2″ sq.)	5
Soda (2½″ sq.)	3
Round, thin (1½″ diam.)	6 to 8
Vegetables	
Beans and Peas, dried, cooked (lima, navy, split pea, cowpeas, etc.)	1/2 cup
Baked Beans, no pork	1/4 cup
Corn	1/3 cup
Parsnips	2/3 cup
Potatoes, white, baked, boiled	1 (2″ diam.)
Potatoes, white, mashed	1/2 cup
Potatoes, sweet, or Yams	1/4 cup
Sponge Cake, plain (1½″ cube)	1
Ice Cream (Omit 2 fat exchanges)	1/2 cup

List 5. Meat Exchanges

Protein – 7 gm., Fat – 5 gm., Calories – 75

Meat and Poultry (med. fat) (beef, lamb, pork, liver, chicken, etc.)	1 oz.
Cold Cuts (4½″ sq., 1/8″ thick)	1 slice
Frankfurter (8 to 9/lb.)	1
Fish: Cod, Mackerel, etc.	1 oz.
Salmon, Tuna, Crab	1/4 cup
Oysters, Shrimp, Clams	5 small
Sardines	3 med.
Cheese, cheddar, American	1 oz.
Cottage	1/4 cup
Egg	1
Peanut Butter*	2 Tbsp.

*Limit use or adjust carbohydrate.

List 6. Fat Exchanges

Fat – 5 gm., Calories – 45

Butter or Margarine	1 tsp.
Bacon, crisp	1 slice
Cream, light, 20%	2 Tbsp.
Cream, heavy, 40%	1 Tbsp.
Cream Cheese	1 Tbsp.
French Dressing	1 Tbsp.
Mayonnaise	1 tsp.
Oil or Cooking Fat	1 tsp.
Nuts	6 small
Olives	5 small
Avocado	1/8 (4″ diam.)

Foods Allowed as Desired

Negligible Carbohydrate, Protein and Fat

Vegetables, List 2A

Coffee	Rhubarb
Tea	Mustard
Clear Broth	Pickle, sour
Bouillon	Pickle, dill – unsweetened
Gelatin, unsweetened	Saccharine
Rennet Tablets	Pepper
Cranberries	Spices
Lemon	Vinegar

Composition of Food Exchanges

LIST	FOOD	MEAS.	GM.	C	P	F	CAL.
1	Milk Exchanges	1/2 pint	240	12	8	10	170
2b	Vegetable Exch.	1/2 cup	100	7	2	–	35
3	Fruit Exch.	varies	–	10	–	–	40
4	Bread Exch.	varies	–	15	2	–	70
5	Meat Exchanges	1 oz.	30	–	7	5	75
6	Fat Exchanges	1 tsp.	5	–	–	5	45

From Meal Planning with Exchange Lists, prepared by Committees of the American Diabetes Association, Inc., and The American Dietetic Association in cooperation with the Chronic Disease Program, Public Health Service, Department of Health, Education and Welfare.

Composition of Food Exchanges

Diet Prescription

Carbohydrate	180 grams
Protein	80 grams
Fat	80 grams
Calories	1800

Foods for the Day

1 pint	Milk	List 1
any amount	Vegetable Exchanges	List 2A
1	Vegetable Exchange	List 2B
3	Fruit Exchanges	List 3
8	Bread Exchanges	List 4
7	Meat Exchanges	List 5
5	Fat Exchanges	List 6

blood vessels. The resulting poor circulation may be a factor leading to other complications such as gangrene of the hands or feet. The heart or kidneys may suffer damage, difficulty with vision may develop, or the nervous system may be affected.

SYMPTOMS. Diabetes mellitus is characterized by elevated blood sugar (hyperglycemia), sugar in the urine (glycosuria), excessive urination (polyuria), increased thirst (polydipsia), increased appetite (polyphagia), and general weakness.

Although diabetes may develop in anyone, there

are four groups of people who are most susceptible to the disorder: those who are obese (about 80 per cent of diabetics have a history of obesity), those who are over 40 years of age, women, and those who have a history of diabetes in their families.

Diagnostic tests for diabetes mellitus include a urinalysis for sugar in the urine, and blood tests such as fasting blood sugar or the GLUCOSE TOLERANCE TEST, which indicates the ability of the body to utilize carbohydrates.

An insulin immunoassay, which involves tagging blood samples with radioactive iodine, is an effective means of detecting abnormalities in insulin secretion and utilization in the early stages of diabetes mellitus, before there is a significant rise in the blood sugar level.

TREATMENT. Treatment of diabetes depends on the severity of the disease, the age of the patient and the symptoms exhibited. Primarily the disease is controlled by diet, exercise, and the administration of INSULIN. Therapy is directed toward returning the carbohydrate metabolism as nearly as possible to normal. There is no cure for diabetes mellitus.

When diabetes develops in middle age or later, the disease can be controlled by diet alone in about 90 per cent of the cases. Early detection of the disease with a reduction in carbohydrate consumption can forestall many of the problems associated with diabetes. Oral hypoglycemic agents, used to treat diabetics with mild cases of maturity-onset diabetes, are now being questioned because of their toxicity, which can lead to heart disease, and their doubtful effectiveness.

Diet. The diabetic diet usually consists basically of foods high in nutritive value and low in concentrated sweets. The exact type of diet is prescribed by the physician and must be followed precisely by the diabetic. This does not imply severe restriction of the diabetic's meals, because most physicians prefer to give the patient an "exchange list" of foods which can be included, thereby providing a great variety for planning meals. The food-exchange lists prepared jointly by the American Diabetes Association, The American Dietetic Association and the Public Health Service are most often used. These lists are simple and easy to follow and can be obtained from The American Dietetic Association, 620 North Michigan Avenue, Chicago, Ill., 60611. The diet is explained to the patient by the physician, and detailed by the dietitian and nursing personnel. It should be stressed that all of the food must be eaten at the prescribed time, especially when insulin injections are given as part of the treatment.

EDUCATION OF THE PATIENT. The diabetic should be instructed in the nature of his disorder, the complications to be avoided, and the role he must play in the control of his disease. If insulin injections are part of the treatment, instructions must include self-administration of insulin. When a diabetic cannot or will not give himself the injections, a member of the family is usually taught the procedure. The patient should also know how to test his urine for sugar and acetone. Recent developments have made the testing of urine a relatively simple procedure for the diabetic (see CLINITEST, CLINISTIX, ACETEST).

The patient is also given directions for the regulation of his diet, and is taught the effects of exercise on carbohydrate and fat metabolism and insulin supply, and the early warning signs of diabetic acidosis and INSULIN SHOCK. When signs of impending diabetic coma first appear the diabetic is told to administer insulin to himself. When insulin shock occurs, the patient is taught to consume some form of simple sugar such as sweetened orange juice, lumps of sugar, or some candy. In both types of reaction the patient must call his physician immediately or go to a nearby hospital for emergency treatment. Special booklets written for the diabetic and useful in instruction of the patient and his family can be obtained from the American Diabetes Association or Eli Lilly & Co.

COMPLICATIONS. In general the complications of diabetes mellitus can be divided into emergency conditions and long-term disorders. The patient with severe diabetes who is taking insulin is particularly susceptible to the serious emergency situations of diabetic coma and insulin shock already mentioned. These disturbances in the normal glucose-insulin ratio in the blood can be brought about by dietary indiscretion, carelessness in the administration of insulin, infections, and emotional or physical shocks.

Other complications developing over a period of time are believed to be caused by poor fat metabolism which results in atherosclerosis. The coronary arteries may be damaged, thereby producing heart disease, or atherosclerosis of peripheral arteries may cause poor circulation in the lower extremities. Retinal changes, sclerosis of the renal capillaries, and nerve damage may also occur.

Because of poor circulation, a relatively high blood sugar level and decreased ability to repair damaged tissue, the diabetic may suffer serious complications from seemingly minor infections. Ulceration and gangrene, particularly of the lower extremities, are among these complications.

PATIENT CARE. The care of the diabetic patient will depend to some degree on the severity of his disease, his age, his general physical condition, and

SYMPTOMS OF DIABETIC COMA AND INSULIN REACTION

DIABETIC COMA	INSULIN REACTION
Gradual onset, may be more rapid in active children	Sudden onset, begins abruptly
Skin hot and dry, face may be flushed	Perspiration, skin pale, cold, and clammy
Deep, labored breathing	Shallow breathing
Nausea	Hunger
Drowsiness and lethargy	Mental confusion, strange behavior, nervousness
Fruity odor to breath	Double vision
Loss of consciousness	Loss of consciousness, convulsions (rarely)
Urine contains much sugar	There may be sugar in the urine, depending on the type of insulin and when it was taken
Blood sugar high	Blood sugar low

From Keane, C. B.: Essentials of Nursing. 2nd ed. Philadelphia, W. B. Saunders Co., 1969.

his ability to comprehend instructions and care for himself.

When the patient first learns he has diabetes he will need encouragement, moral support, and specific instructions about his disease. The basic principles of good personal hygiene, cleanliness, and prompt treatment of minor injuries or irritations of the skin must be stressed as important in the prevention of complications. Gangrene and possible loss of a lower limb can often be avoided by scrupulous foot care, including properly fitting shoes and stockings, correct trimming of the toenails, and avoidance of injury to the feet and legs.

The hospitalized diabetic often requires frequent injections of insulin, and urinalyses for sugar and acetone. These procedures must be done accurately and at the specific times ordered by the physician so that a normal blood sugar can be maintained. The patient is observed carefully for signs of impending diabetic coma or insulin shock, and prompt action must be taken should either condition occur. (See also HYPERGLYCEMIC HYPEROSMOLAR NONKETOTIC COMA.)

The meals of the diabetic are served at the exact times ordered and a record is kept of the amount and kinds of food and liquid accepted or refused by the patient.

diabetic (di″ah-bet′ik) 1. pertaining to or characterized by diabetes. 2. a person affected with diabetes.

diabetogenic (di″ah-bet″o-jen′ik) producing diabetes.

diabetogenous (di″ah-be-toj′ĕ-nus) caused by diabetes.

diabetometer (di″ah-be-tom′ĕ-ter) a polariscope for use in estimating the percentage of sugar in urine.

Diabinese (di-ab′ĭ-nēs) trademark for chlorpropamide, an oral hypoglycemic drug.

diabrotic (di″ah-brot′ik) 1. ulcerative; caustic. 2. a corrosive or escharotic substance.

diacetate (di-as′ĕ-tāt) any salt of diacetic acid (acetoacetic acid).

diacetic acid (di″ah-se′ik) acetoacetic acid.

diacetylmorphine (di″ah-se″til-mor′fēn) heroin; a highly addictive narcotic derived from opium.

diacrisis (di-ak′rĭ-sis) 1. diagnosis. 2. a disease characterized by a morbid state of the secretions. 3. a critical discharge or excretion.

diacritic (di″ah-krit′-ik) diagnostic; distinguishing.

diaderm (di′ah-derm) the blastoderm during the stage in which it consists of an ectoderm and an entoderm.

diadochokinesia (di″ah-do″ko-ki-ne′ze-ah) the function of arresting one motor impulse and substituting one that is diametrically opposite.

Diadol (di′ah-dol) trademark for a preparation of diallylbarbituric acid, an intermediate- to long-acting sedative and hypnotic.

Diafen (di′ah-fen) trademark for a preparation of diphenylpyraline, an antihistaminic.

Diagnex blue (di′ag-neks) trademark for a diagnostic agent for achlorhydria; it is a means of GASTRIC ANALYSIS based on the fact that free hydrochloric acid releases a dye (Azure A) from a resin base. Once the dye is released it is absorbed from the intestinal tract and excreted in the urine. If no hydrochloric acid is present in the stomach the dye will not appear in the urine.

The test is valuable as a screening device to rule out achlorhydria, and is much less disturbing than other methods of gastric analysis, which require the passage of a stomach tube. It does not, however, give conclusive evidence sufficient for diagnosis of cases in which there is no secretion of hydrochloric acid.

diagnose (di′ag-nōs) to identify or recognize a disease.

diagnosis (di″ag-no′sis) 1. determination of the nature of a case of a disease. 2. a concise technical description of the cause, nature, or manifestations of a condition, situation, or problem. adj., **diagnos′tic.**

clinical d., diagnosis based on signs, symptoms, and laboratory findings during life.

differential d., the determination of which one of several diseases may be producing the symptoms.

medical d., diagnosis performed by a physician and based on information gleaned from a variety of sources, including (1) findings from a physical examination, (2) interview with the patient or his family or both, (3) a medical history of the patient and his family, and (4) clinical findings as reported by pertinent laboratory tests and radiologic studies.

nursing d., a term that is relatively new to the health care field and at the present time remains somewhat controversial. It is generally understood to be a concise description of a health problem that can be treated by a professional nurse. The goal of a nursing diagnosis is management of the nursing care problem that has been identified and therefore excludes problems that are treated by surgery, prescription drugs, or other modes of treatment that are the reponsibility of the physician and are legally defined as medical practice. A nursing diagnosis is the outcome of patient assessment, a major component of the NURSING PROCESS.

physical d., diagnosis based on information obtained by inspection, palpation, percussion, and auscultation.

diagnostician (di″ag-nos-tish′an) an expert in diagnosis.

diagnostics (di″ag-nos′tiks) the science and practice of diagnosis of disease.

diagraph (di′ah-graf) an instrument for recording outlines, as in craniometry.

diakinesis (di″ah-ki-ne′sis) the stage of first meiotic prophase, in which the nucleolus and nuclear envelope disappear and the spindle fibers form.

diallylbarbituric acid (di-al″il-bar″bĭ-tūr′ik) allobarbital, a hypnotic and sedative of intermediate to long duration of action.

dialysance (di″ah-li′sans) the minute rate of net exchange of solute molecules passing through a membrane in dialysis.

dialysate (di-al′ĭ-sāt) the material passing through the membrane in dialysis.

dialysis (di-al′ĭ-sis) the diffusion of solute molecules through a semipermeable membrane, passing from the side of higher concentration to that of the lower; a method sometimes used in cases of defective renal function to remove from the blood elements that are normally excreted in the urine (hemodialysis). Most membranes of the body's cells are semipermeable; that is, they allow the passage of certain smaller molecules of such crystalloids as glucose and urea, but prevent the passage of larger molecules of such colloids as plasma proteins and protoplasm.

Many body processes, such as digestion, urine formation, respiration, and distribution of nutrients and waste by the blood, depend in part on dialysis. The principles of dialysis are utilized in the artificial KIDNEY (hemodialyzer) and in PERITONEAL DIALYSIS.

extracorporeal d., dialysis by artificial KIDNEY.

peritoneal d., dialysis through the peritoneum, the dialyzing solution being introduced into and removed from the peritoneal cavity, as either a continuous or an intermittent procedure (see also PERITONEAL DIALYSIS).

dialyzer (di′ah-līz″er) an apparatus for performing dialysis; a hemodialyzer.

diameter (di-am′ĕ-ter) the length of a straight line passing through the center of a circle and connecting opposite points on its circumference; hence the distance between the two specified opposite points on the periphery of a structure such as the cranium or pelvis.

cranial d's, craniometric d's, imaginary lines connecting points on opposite surfaces of the cranium; the most important are: biparietal, that joining the parietal eminences; bitemporal, that joining the extremities of the coronal suture; cervicobregmatic, that joining the center of the anterior fontanel and the junction of the neck with the floor of the mouth; frontomental, that joining the forehead and chin; occipitofrontal, that joining the external occipital protuberance and the most prominent midpoint of the frontal bone; occipitomental, that joining the external occipital protuberance and most prominent midpoint of the chin; suboccipitobregmatic, that joining the lowest posterior point of the occiput and the center of the anterior fontanel.

pelvic d., any of the diameters of the pelvis (see also PELVIC DIAMETER).

diamide (di-am′id) a double amide.

diamidine (di-am′ĭ-dēn) a compound that contains two amidine groups.

diamine (di-am′in, di′ah-min) a double amine.

diaminodiphenylsulfone (di-am″ĭ-no-di-fen″il-sul′fōn) dapsone, an antibacterial.

diaminuria (di-am″ĭ-nu′re-ah) diamines in the urine.

Diamox (di′ah-moks) trademark for preparations of acetazolamide, a diuretic.

diamthazole (di-am′thah-zōl) an antifungal agent, used as the dihydrochloride salt.

Dianabol (di-an′ah-bol) trademark for methandrostenolone, an anabolic hormone.

Diaparene (di-ap′ah-rēn) trademark for preparations of methylbenzethonium, a local anti-infective.

diapedesis (di″ah-pĕ-de′sis) the outward passage of blood cells through intact vessel walls.

diaphanometry (di″ah-fah-nom′ĕ-tre) measurement of the transparency of a liquid.

diaphanoscope (di″ah-fan′o-skōp) an instrument for transilluminating a body cavity.

diaphemetric (di″ah-fĕ-met′rik) pertaining to measurement of tactile sensibility.

diaphorase (di-af′o-rās) a flavoprotein that catalyzes the oxidation of nicotinamide-adenine dinucleotide (NAD) or nicotinaminide-adenine dinucleotide phosphate (NADP).

diaphoresis (di″ah-fo-re′sis) perspiration, especially profuse perspiration.

diaphoretic (di″ah-fo-ret′ik) 1. pertaining to, characterized by, or promoting diaphoresis. 2. an agent that promotes diaphoresis.

diaphragm (di′ah-fram) 1. the musculomembranous partition separating the thoracic and abdominal cavities. On its sides, it is attached to the six lower ribs; at the front, to the sternum; at the back, to the spine. The esophagus, the aorta and vena cava, and nerves pass through the diaphragm. When relaxed, the diaphragm is convex but it flattens as it contracts during inhalation, thereby enlarging the chest cavity and allowing for expansion of the lungs. (See also RESPIRATION.) 2. any separating membrane or structure. 3. a disk with one or more openings or with an adjustable opening, mounted in relation to a lens or source of radiation, by which part of the light or radiation may be excluded from the area. 4. contraceptive diaphragm. adj., **diaphragmat′ic.**

Bucky d., Bucky-Potter d., a device used in radiography to prevent scattered radiation from reaching the film, thereby securing better contrast and definition.

contraceptive d., a device of molded rubber or other soft plastic material, fitted over the cervix uteri to prevent entrance of spermatozoa. (See also CONTRACEPTION.)

pelvic d., the portion of the floor of the pelvis formed by the coccygeus muscles and the levator ani muscles, and their fascia.

urogenital d., the musculomembranous layer superficial to the pelvic diaphragm, extending between the ischiopubic rami and surrounding the urogenital ducts.

diaphragmatocele (di″ah-frag-mat′o-sēl) diaphragmatic hernia.

diaphragmitis (di″ah-frag-mi′tis) inflammation of the diaphragm.

diaphyseal (di″ah-fiz′e-al) pertaining to or affecting the shaft of a long bone (diaphysis).

diaphysectomy (di″ah-fĭ-zek′to-me) excision of part of a diaphysis.

diaphysial (di″ah-fiz′e-al) diaphyseal.

diaphysis (di-af′ĭ-sis), pl. *diaph′yses.* 1. the portion of a long bone between the ends or extremities, which are usually articular, and wider than the shaft; it consists of a tube of compact bone, enclosing the medullary cavity. Called also shaft. 2. the portion of a bone formed from a primary center of ossification.

diaplasis (di-ap′lah-sis) the setting of a fracture or reduction of a dislocation.

diapophysis (di″ah-pof′ĭ-sis) an upper transverse process of a vertebra.

diapyesis (di″ah-pi-e′sis) suppuration. adj., **diapyet′ic.**

diarrhea (di″ah-re′ah) rapid movement of fecal matter through the intestine resulting in poor absorption of water, nutritive elements, and electrolytes and producing abnormally frequent evacuation of watery stools. adj., **diarrhe′ic, diarrhe′al.** The major causes are local irritation of the intestinal mucosa by infectious or chemical agents (gastroenteritis), and emotional disorders which bring about increased peristalsis and increased secretion of mucus in the colon (psychogenic diarrhea or irritable colon) (see also COLITIS).

In all types of diarrhea there is rapid evacuation

of water and electrolytes resulting in a loss of these essential substances. Potassium supply especially is depleted by diarrhea, thus producing ACIDOSIS as well as DEHYDRATION.

SYMPTOMS. Diarrhea is accompanied by frequent and liquid bowel movements, abdominal cramps, and general weakness. The stools often contain mucus and may be blood streaked. In chronic diarrhea the patient is likely to be anemic and suffering from malnutrition.

TREATMENT. Mild cases of diarrhea of short duration can be treated conservatively with a bland diet, increased intake of liquids, and the administration of kaolin-pectin compounds to relieve the symptoms. Paregoric (camphorated tincture of opium) and other medicines are sometimes used to decrease peristalsis and relieve cramps.

More severe and chronic cases of diarrhea may be symptomatic of a wide variety of disorders including glandular disturbances, deficiency diseases, allergies, and tumors of the intestinal tract. Since diarrhea is a symptom rather than a disease, extensive diagnostic procedures and laboratory tests may be necessary to determine the underlying cause. In the meantime symptomatic treatment must be instigated to relieve the dehydration, nutritional deficiencies, and disturbances of acid-base balance produced by the loss of water, food elements, and electrolytes in the stools. Liquids and semisolids may be given orally at frequent intervals if they can be tolerated by the patient. In cases in which vomiting accompanies the diarrhea or the stools occur with serious frequency, the fluids may be given intravenously. Antidiarrheal drugs such as paregoric are usually ordered in small doses to be given after each stool.

When diarrhea is psychogenic, psychotherapy may be used in conjunction with other methods of management.

PATIENT CARE. The patient should be provided with an atmosphere conducive to rest and relaxation. Emotional factors must always be considered in cases of diarrhea, even though nervous tension may not always be the major cause of the disorder. The patient is likely to be embarrassed and inconvenienced by frequent trips to the bathroom or requests for the bedpan. The use of soap and warm water to cleanse the anal region after each bowel movement will help reduce local irritation and discomfort.

The number and character of each stool should be carefully noted and recorded on the patient's chart. Other observations include signs of DEHYDRATION and ACIDOSIS.

diarthric (di-ar′thrik) pertaining to or affecting two different joints; biarticular; diarticular.

diarthrodial (di″ar-thro′dĭ-al) of the nature of a diarthrosis.

diarthrosis (di″ar-thro′sis), pl. *diarthro′ses* [Gr.] a specialized form of articulation in which there is more or less free movement, the union of the bony elements being surrounded by an articular capsule enclosing a cavity lined by synovial membrane; called also synovial joint.

d. rotato′ria, a joint characterized by mobility in a rotary direction.

diarticular (di″ar-tik′u-lar) pertaining to two joints; diarthric.

diaschisis (di-as′kĭ-sis) loss of functional connection between various centers of neuron tracts forming one of the cerebral mechanisms.

diascope (di′ah-skōp) a glass plate pressed against the skin to permit observation of changes produced in the underlying areas after the blood vessels are emptied and the skin is blanched.

diascopy (di-as′ko-pe) 1. examination by means of a diascope. 2. transillumination.

Diasone (di′ah-sōn) trademark for a preparation of sodium sulfoxone, used as a leprostatic and dermatitis herpetiformis suppressant.

diastase (di′ah-stās) a combination of enzymes produced during germination of seeds, and contained in malt; it converts starch into maltose and then into dextrose.

diastasis (di-as′tah-sis) 1. dislocation or separation of two normally attached bones between which there is no true joint. 2. diastasis cordis, the rest period of the cardiac cycle, occurring just before systole.

diastema (di″ah-ste′mah) a space or cleft.

diastematocrania (di″ah-stem″ah-to-kra′ne-ah) congenital longitudinal fissure of the cranium.

diastematomyelia (di″ah-stem″ah-to-mi-e′le-ah) abnormal congenital division of the spinal cord by a bony spicule or fibrous band protruding from a vertebra or two, each of the halves being surrounded by a dural sac.

diastematopyelia (di″ah-stem″ah-to-pi-e′le-ah) congenital median fissure of the pelvis.

diaster (di-as′ter) the figure of chromatin fibers formed in karyokinesis, consisting of two asters joined by a spindle; called also amphiaster.

diastole (di-as′to-le) the phase of the cardiac cycle in which the heart relaxes between contractions; specifically, the period when the two ventricles are dilated by the blood flowing into them (see also BLOOD PRESSURE and HEART). adj., **diastol′ic.**

diataxia (di″ah-tak′se-ah) ataxia affecting both sides of the body.

diathermal, diathermic (di″ah-ther′mal; di″ah-ther′mik) pertaining to diathermy; permeable by heat waves.

diathermy (di′ah ther″me) the use of high-frequency electrical currents as a form of physical therapy and in surgical procedures. The term diathermy is derived from the Greek words *dia* and *therma,* and literally means "heating through."

Diathermy is used in physical therapy to deliver moderate heat directly to pathologic lesions in the deeper tissues of the body. Surgically, the extreme heat that can be produced by diathermy may be used to destroy neoplasms, warts, and infected tissues, and to cauterize blood vessels to prevent excessive bleeding. The technique is particularly valuable in neurosurgery and surgery of the eye.

The three forms of diathermy employed by physical therapists are shortwave, ultrasound, and microwave. The application of moderate heat by diathermy increases blood flow and speeds up metabolism and the rate of ion diffusion across cellular membranes. The fibrous tissues in tendons, joint capsules, and scars are more easily stretched when subjected to heat, thus facilitating the relief of stiffness of joints and promoting relaxation of the muscles and decrease of muscle spasms.

Short wave diathermy machines utilize two condenser plates that are placed on either side of the body part to be treated. Another mode of application is by induction coils that are pliable and can be molded to fit the part of the body under treatment. As the high-frequency waves travel through the body tissues between the condensers or the coils, they are converted into heat. The degree of heat and depth of penetration depend in part on the absorptive and resistance properties of the tissues that the waves encounter.

The frequency allowed for short wave diathermy operations is under the control of the Federal Communications Commission. The frequencies assigned for short wave diathermy operations are 13.66, 27.33, and 40.98 megacycles. Most commercial machines operate at a frequency of 27.33 megacycles and a wavelength of 11 meters.

Short wave diathermy usually is prescribed for treatment of deep muscles and joints that are covered with a heavy soft-tissue mass, for example, the hip. In some instances short wave diathermy may be applied to localize deep inflammatory processes, as in pelvic inflammatory disease.

Ultrasound diathermy employs high-frequency acoustic vibrations which, when propelled through the tissues, are converted into heat. This type of diathermy is especially useful in the delivery of heat to selected musculatures and structures because there is a difference in the sensitivity of various fibers to the acoustic vibrations; some are more absorptive and some are more reflective. For example, in subcutaneous fat, relatively little energy is converted into heat, but in muscle tissues there is a much higher rate of conversion to heat.

The therapeutic ultrasound apparatus generates a high-frequency alternating current, which is then converted into acoustic vibrations. The apparatus is moved slowly across the surface of the part being treated. Ultrasound is a very effective agent for the application of heat, but it should be used only by a therapist who is fully aware of its potential hazards and the contraindications for its use.

Microwave diathermy uses radar waves, which are of higher frequency and shorter wavelength than radio waves. Most, if not all, of the therapeutic effects of microwave therapy are related to the conversion of energy into heat and its distribution throughout the body tissues. This mode of diathermy is considered to be the easiest to use, but the microwaves have a relatively poor depth of penetration.

Microwaves cannot be used in high dosage on edematous tissue, over wet dressings, or near metallic implants in the body because of the danger of local burns. Microwaves and short waves cannot be used on or near persons with implanted electronic cardiac pacemakers.

As with all forms of heat applications, care must be taken to avoid burns during diathermy treatments, especially to patients with decreased sensitivity to heat and cold.

diathesis (di-ath′ĕ-sis) an unusual constitutional susceptibility or predisposition to a particular disease. adj., **diathet′ic.**

diatomic (di″ah-tom′ik) 1. containing two atoms. 2. dibasic.

diatrizoate (di″ah-tri-zo′āt) any salt of diatrizoic acid.

diatrizoic acid (di″ah-tri-zo′ik) a radiopaque medium, used as the sodium and meglumine salts.

diaxon (di-ak′son) a nerve cell with two axons.

diazepam (di-az′ĕ-pam) a minor tranquilizer and skeletal muscle relaxant.

diazo- (di-az′o) the group $—N_2—$.

diazotize (di-az′o-tīz) to introduce the diazo group into a compound.

diazoxide (di″az-ok′sīd) a rapid-acting antihypertensive having no diuretic activity. Diazoxide has a longer duration of action than other rapid-acting antihypertensives, and is used intravenously in the treatment of malignant hypertension.

dibasic (di-ba′sik) containing two replaceable hydrogen atoms, or furnishing two hydrogen ions.

dibenzylchlorethamine (di″ben-zil-klōr-eth′ah-mēn) an alpha-adrenergic blocking agent, used in the diagnosis of pheochromocytoma.

Dibenzyline (di-ben′zĭ-lēn) trademark for a preparation of phenoxybenzamine, an adrenergic-blocking agent.

Dibothriocephalus (di-both″re-o-sef′ah-lus) *Diphyllobothrium.*

dibucaine (di′bu-kān) a local anesthetic, used topically and intraspinally in the form of the base and as the hydrochloride salt; the latter is also used intramuscularly for infiltration anesthesia.

Dibuline (di′bu-lēn) trademark for a preparation of dibutoline.

dibutoline (di-bu′to-lēn) an anticholinergic; the sulfate salt is used as a mydriatic, cycloplegic, and gastrointestinal antispasmodic.

dicephalous (di-sef′ah-lus) having two heads.

dicephalus (di-sef′ah-lus) a monster with two heads.

dichlorisone (di-klōr′ĭ-sōn) a steroid used for topical antipruritic action.

dichloroisoproterenol (di-klo″ro-i″so-pro-ter′ĕ-nol) a beta-adrenergic blocking agent, used in the treatment of various cardiac disorders.

dichlorphenamide (di″klōr-fen′ah-mīd) a carbonic anhydrase inhibitor used to reduce intraocular pressure in glaucoma.

dichorial, dichorionic (di-ko′re-al; di-ko″re-on′ik) having two distinct chorions.

dichroic (di-kro′ik) characterized by dichroism.

dichroism (di′kro-izm) the quality or condition of showing one color in reflected and another in transmitted light.

dichromate (di-kro′māt) a salt containing the bivalent Cr_2O_7 radical.

dichromatic (di″kro-mat′ik) pertaining to or characterized by dichromatism.

dichromatism (di-kro′mah-tizm) 1. the quality of existing in or exhibiting two different colors. 2. dichromatopsia.

dichromatopsia (di″kro-mah-top′se-ah) a condition characterized by ability to perceive only two of the 160 colors discriminated by the normal eye.

dichromic (di-kro′mik) 1. showing only two colors. 2. containing two atoms of chromium.

dichromophilism (di″kro-mof′ĭ-lizm) capacity for double staining, i.e., with both acid and basic dyes.

Dick test (dik) an intracutaneous test for determination of susceptibility to scarlet fever.

dicloxacillin (di-kloks″ah-sil′in) a semisynthetic

penicillin used in infections with penicillin-resistant gram-positive organisms.

Dicodid (di-ko′did) trademark for preparations of hydrocodone, a synthetic analgesic.

dicoelous (di-se′lus) 1. hollowed on each of two sides. 2. having two cavities.

dicophane (di′ko-fān) chlorophenothane, or DDT, an insecticide.

dicoria (di-ko′re-ah) double pupil.

dicoumarin (di-koo′mah-rin) BISHYDROXYCOUMARIN, an anticoagulant.

Dicrocoelium (dik″ro-se′le-um) a genus of flukes.

D. dentrit′icum, a species of liver flukes that infest domestic animals and have been reported in man.

dicrotism (di′krŏ-tizm) the occurrence of two sphygmographic waves or elevations to one beat of the pulse. adj., **dicrot′ic.**

dictyoma (dik″te-o′mah) diktyoma.

Dicumarol (di-koo′mah-rol) trademark for a preparation of BISHYDROXYCOUMARIN, used as an anticoagulant.

Dicurin (di-kur′in) trademark for a preparation of merethoxylline, a mercurial diuretic.

dicylcic (di-si′klik) pertaining to or having two cycles; in chemistry, having two rings in the molecular structure.

dicyclomine (di-si′klo-mēn) an anticholinergic used as a gastrointestinal antispasmodic.

didactylism (di-dak′til-izm) the presence of only two digits on a hand or foot.

didelphia (di-del′fe-ah) the condition of having a double uterus.

didymalgia (did″ĭ-mal′je-ah) pain in a testis.

didymitis (did″ĭ-mi′tis) inflammation of a testis.

didymous (did′ĭ-mus) occurring in pairs.

didymus (did′ĭ-mus) a testis; also used as a word termination designating a fetus with duplication of parts or one consisting of conjoined symmetrical twins.

diecious (di-e′shus) sexually distinct; denoting species in which male and female genitals do not occur in the same individual. In botany, having staminate and pistillate flowers on separate plants.

dieldrin (di-el′drin) an insecticide.

diembryony (di-em′bre-on″e) the production of two embryos from a single egg.

diencephalon (di″en-sef′ah-lon) 1. the posterior part of the forebrain, consisting of the hypothalamus, thalamus, metathalamus, and epithalamus. 2. the posterior of the two brain vesicles formed by specialization of the prosencephalon in the developing embryo. (See also BRAIN stem.)

dienestrol (di″en-es′trol) an estrogen used in the treatment of menopausal symptoms and atrophic vaginitis and to suppress lactation.

Dientamoeba (di-en″tah-me′bah) a genus of amebas commonly found in the colon and appendix of man.

D. frag′ilis, a species that has been associated with diarrhea.

dieresis (di-er′ĕ-sis) 1. the division or separation of parts normally united. 2. the surgical separation of parts.

diet (di′et) the customary amount and kind of food and drink taken by a person from day to day; more narrowly, a diet planned to meet specific requirements of the individual, including or excluding certain foods.

acid-ash d., one of meat, fish, eggs, and cereals with little fruit or vegetables and no cheese or milk. (See also ACID-ASH DIET.)

alkali-ash d., one of fruit, vegetables, and milk with as little as possible of meat, fish, eggs, and cereals.

bland d., one that is free from any irritating or stimulating foods.

elimination d., one for diagnosis of food allergy, based on omission of foods that might cause symptoms in the patient.

Feingold d., a special diet used in the control of HYPERACTIVITY in children (see also FEINGOLD DIET).

high-calorie d., one that furnishes more calories than needed to maintain weight, often more than 3500–4000 calories per day.

high-fat d., ketogenic diet.

high-protein d., one containing large amounts of protein, consisting largely of meats, fish, milk, legumes, and nuts.

hospital d., a routine diet plan provided in a hospital that includes general, soft, and liquid diets and modifications of them to suit the needs of specific patients.

Karell d., a milk diet for nephritis and heart disease. (See also KARRELL TREATMENT.)

ketogenic d., one containing large amounts of fat (see also KETOGENIC DIET).

liquid d., a diet limited to liquids or to foods that can be changed to a liquid state (see also LIQUID DIET).

low-calorie d., one containing fewer calories than needed to maintain weight, e.g., less than 1200 calories per day for an adult.

low-fat d., one containing limited amounts of fat.

low-fiber d., low-residue d.

low-purine d., one for mitigation of gout, omitting meat, fowl, and fish and substituting milk, eggs, cheese, and vegetable protein.

low-residue d., one with a minimum of cellulose and fiber and restriction of connective tissue found in certain cuts of meat. It is prescribed for irritations of the intestinal tract, after surgery of the large intestine, in partial intestinal obstruction, or when limited bowel movements are desirable, as in colostomy patients. Called also low-fiber diet.

protein-sparing d., one consisting only of liquid protein or liquid mixtures of proteins, vitamins, and minerals, and containing no more than 600 calories; it is designed to maintain a favorable nitrogen balance.

purine-free d., low-purine diet.

Sippy d., a graduated diet for peptic ulcer and other conditions requiring a smooth diet (see also SIPPY DIET).

dietary (di′ĕ-ter″e) 1. pertaining to diet. 2. a course or system of diet.

dietetic (di″ĕ-tet′ik) pertaining to diet or proper food.

dietetics (di″ĕ-tet′iks) the science of diet and nutrition.

diethazine (di-eth′ah-zēn) an anticholinergic; the hydrochloride salt is used in the treatment of Parkinson's disease.

diethylcarbamazine (di-eth″il-kar-bam′ah-zēn) an antifilarial agent used as the citrate salt.

Types of Hospital Diets

	Clear Liquid Diet	Full Liquid Diet	Soft Diet	Regular–House General–Full
Characteristics	Temporary diet of clear liquids without residue; nonstimulating, nongas-forming, nonirritating	Foods liquid at room temperature or liquefying at body temperature	Normal diet modified in consistency to have no roughage Liquids and semisolid food; easily digested	Practically all foods; simple, easy-to-digest foods, simply prepared, palatably seasoned
Adequacy	Inadequate: deficient in protein, minerals, vitamins, calories	Can be adequate with careful planning: adequacy depends on liquids used	Entirely adequate liberal diet	Adequate and well balanced
Use	Acute illness and infections Postoperatively Temporary food intolerance To relieve thirst Reduce colonic fecal matter 1 to 2 hour feeding intervals	Transition between clear liquid and soft diets Postoperatively Acute gastritis and infections Febrile conditions Intolerance for solid food 2 to 4 hour feeding intervals	Between full liquid and light or regular diet Between acute illness and convalescence Acute infections Chewing difficulties Gastrointestinal disorders 3 meals with or without between-meal feedings	For uniformity and convenience in serving hospital patients Ambulatory patients Bed patients not requiring therapeutic diets
Foods	Water, tea, coffee, coffee substitutes Fat-free broth Carbonated beverages Synthetic fruit juices Ginger ale Plain gelatin Sugar	All liquids on clear liquid diet plus: All forms milk Soups, strained Fruit and vegetable juices Eggnogs Plain ice cream and sherbets Junket and plain gelatin dishes Soft custard Cereal gruels	All liquids Fine and strained cereals Cooked tender or pureed vegetables Cooked fruits without skins and seeds Ripe bananas Ground or minced meat, fish, poultry Eggs and mild cheeses Plain cake and puddings Moderately seasoned foods	All basic foods
Modification	Liberal clear liquid diet includes: fruit juices, egg white, whole egg, thin gruels	Consistency for tube feedings: foods that will pass through tube easily	Low residue–no fiber Bland–no chemical, thermal, physical stimulants Cold soft–tonsillectomy Mechanical soft–requiring no mastication	For a light or convalescent diet, fried foods, rich pastries, fat-rich foods, coarse vegetables, raw fruits may be omitted
			Light diet–intermediate between soft and regular Note: Because of trend toward more liberal interpretation of diets and foods, soft diet may be combined with light diet in some hospitals	

From Keane, C. B.: Saunders Review for Practical Nurses. Philadelphia, W. B. Saunders Co., 1966.

diethylpropion (di-eth″il-pro′pe-on) an appetite suppressant, used as the hydrochloride salt.

diethylstilbestrol (di-eth″il-stil-bes′trol) a synthetic estrogenic compound used in treating menopausal symptoms, vaginitis, and suppressed lactation.

diethyltoluamide (di-eth″il-tol-u′ah-mīd) an arthropod repellent.

diethyltryptamine (di-eth″il-trip′tah-mēn) a synthetic hallucinogenic substance closely related to dimethyltryptamine; abbreviated DET.

dietitian (di″ĕ-tish′an) one who is concerned with the promotion of good health through proper diet and with the therapeutic use of diet in the treatment of disease. The dietitian may work in a variety of settings, including hospitals and other health care agencies, schools, hotels, and other commercial institutions where her duties are primarily administrative, or she may choose to enter the fields of education and research. Some dietitians practice independently either as a consultant or private practitioner in the area of therapeutic dietetics.

A bachelor's degree with a major in foods and nutrition or institutional management is the minimal educational requirement for a dietitian. Membership in the American Dietetic Association (A.D.A.) requires satisfactory completion of either a one-year dietetic internship in a program approved by the Association, or three years' experience, two of which must have been served under the supervision of a member of the A.D.A. Additional education on the graduate level is necessary to qualify for positions in teaching, public health nutrition, and other specialty areas. The address of the American Dietetic Association is 620 No. Michigan Ave., Chicago, IL 60611.

dietotherapy (di″ĕ-to-ther′ah-pe) the scientific regulation of diet in treating disease, especially important in patients with inborn errors of metabolism and various other metabolic diseases.

differentiation (dif″er-en″she-a′shun) 1. the distinguishing of one thing from another. 2. the act or process of acquiring completely individual characteristics, such as occurs in the progressive diversification of cells and tissues in the embryo. 3. increase in morphological or chemical heterogeneity.

diffraction (dĭ-frakt′shun) the bending or breaking up of a ray of light into its component parts.

diffusate (dĭ-fu′zāt) material that has diffused through a membrane.

diffuse 1. (dĭ-fūs′) not definitely limited or localized. 2. (dĭ-fūz′) to pass through or to spread widely through a tissue or substance.

diffusion (dĭ-fu′zhun) 1. the state or process of being widely spread. 2. the spontaneous mixing of the molecules or ions of two or more substances resulting from random thermal motion; its rate is proportional to the concentrations of the substances and it increases with the temperature.

In the body fluids the molecules of water, gases, and the ions of substances in solution are in constant motion. As each molecule moves about, it bounces off other molecules and loses some of its energy to each molecule it hits, but at the same time it gains energy from the molecules that collide with it.

The rate of diffusion is influenced by the size of the molecules; larger molecules move less rapidly, because they require more energy to move about. Molecules of a solution of higher concentration move more rapidly toward those of a solution of lesser concentration; in other words, *the rate of movement from higher to lower concentration is greater than the movement in the opposite direction.*

Other factors influencing the rate of diffusion from one substance to another are the size of the chamber in which the diffusion is taking place and the temperature within the chamber. *The rate of diffusion increases as the size of the chamber increases.* Molecular motion never ceases except at absolute zero; as the temperature increases so does the rate of motion of molecules. Thus, *the higher the temperature, the greater the molecular activity and, consequently, the greater the rate of diffusion.*

Many of the substances passing through the cell membrane are transported actively or passively by the process of diffusion. Without this constant motion of molecules there would be no exchange of nutrients and end products of cellular metabolism between the intracellular and extracellular fluid and the cell could not survive. The diffusion of water across cell membranes is called OSMOSIS.

The diffusion of gases through the respiratory membrane is essential to normal respiration. The rapidity and ease with which oxygen and carbon dioxide are diffused through the membrane are affected by the thickness of the membrane and its surface area, the diffusion coefficient of the gas in the water within the membrane, and the difference between the partial pressures of the gases in the alveoli and the blood.

The respiratory membrane is at most only 1 micron in thickness, yet it is composed of three layers within the alveolus (surfactant and fluid layers and alveolar epithelium), an interstitial space between the alveolar epithelium and capillary membrane, and two layers in the capillary membrane. The thickness of the respiratory membrane can be affected by the presence of edematous fluid and by fibrotic changes in the membrane resulting from certain pulmonary diseases. An increase of fluid within the respiratory membrane and alveoli reduces the rate of diffusion because the gases must pass through the additional fluid as well as the other layers of the membrane. Thickening of the epithelial layers of the membrane, as in fibrosis, imposes additional restriction on the passage of gases.

The difference in the partial pressure of a gas in the alveoli and that same gas in the blood is a measure of the net tendency of that gas to pass through the respiratory membrane. The term partial pressure refers to the amount of pressure being exerted by a particular gas in a mixture of gases, the word *partial* referring to the part that is a particular gas in relation to the whole mixture. The partial pressure of oxygen, for example, reflects the number of oxygen molecules striking the surface of the membrane at any given point. The difference in the partial pressure refers to the difference in the amount of pressure being exerted by the oxygen molecules on the alveolar side of the membrane and the amount of pressure being exerted by the oxygen striking the same point from the opposite side. When the partial pressure of oxygen in the alveoli is greater than that of the oxygen in the blood, the oxygen molecules move across the membrane in the direction of the blood. The same is true in regard to carbon dioxide, which moves in the opposite direction when its partial pressure in the blood is greater than that in the alveoli. Partial pressures of oxygen and carbon dioxide are discussed in more detail under BLOOD GAS ANALYSIS.

d. capacity, the volume of gas that passes through a membrane each minute for a pressure difference of 1 mm. Hg. Average normal value for the diffusion capacity of oxygen is 20 ml./min./mm. Hg. If, during quiet breathing, the pressure difference of oxygen averages 11 mm. Hg, a total of approximately 220 ml. of oxygen diffuses through the respiratory membrane each minute. During strenous exercise or other conditions that increase pulmonary activity, the diffusion capacity may increase to three times as much as that during rest. Pulmonary diseases that damage the respiratory membrane greatly interfere with the capacity of the oxygen to pass through the membrane and oxygenate the blood.

d. coefficient, the number of milliliters of a gas that will diffuse at a distance of 0.001 mm. over a square centimeter surface per minute, at 1 atm. of pressure. The diffusion coefficient for any given gas is proportional to the solubility and molecular weight of the gas. The diffusion coefficient for oxygen is 1.0, for carbon dioxide it is 20.3, and for nitrogen it is 0.53. The diffusion capacity of a gas varies directly with the diffusion coefficient.

digastric (di-gas′trik) 1. having two bellies. 2. digastric muscle (see table of MUSCLES).

digenetic (di-jĕ-net′ik) having two stages of multiplication, one sexual in the mature forms, the other asexual in the larval stages.

digestant (di-jes′tant) 1. assisting or stimulating digestion. 2. an agent capable of aiding digestion.

digestion (di-jes′chun) 1. the act or process of converting food into chemical substances that can be absorbed into the blood and utilized by the body tissues. 2. the subjection of a substance to prolonged heat and moisture, so as to disintegrate and soften it.

Digestion is accomplished by physically breaking down, churning, diluting, and dissolving the food substances, and also by splitting them chemically into simpler compounds. Carbohydrates are eventually broken down to monosaccharides (simple sugars); proteins are broken down into amino acids; and fats are absorbed as fatty acids and glycerol (glycerin).

The digestive process takes place in the alimentary canal or DIGESTIVE SYSTEM. The salivary glands, liver, gallbladder, and pancreas are located outside the alimentary canal, but they are considered accessory organs of digestion because their secretions provide essential enzymes.

gastric d., digestion by the action of gastric juice.

intestinal d., digestion by the action of intestinal juices.

pancreatic d., digestion by the action of pancreatic juice.

peptic d., gastric digestion.

primary d., digestion occurring in the gastrointestinal tract.

salivary d., the change of starch into maltose by the saliva.

digestive (di-jes′tiv) pertaining to digestion.

d. system, the organs that have as their particular function the ingestion, digestion, and absorption of food or nutritive elements. They include the mouth, teeth, tongue, pharynx, esophagus, stomach, and intestines. The accessory organs of digestion, which contribute secretions important to digestion include the salivary glands, pancreas, liver, and gallbladder. (See also Plates 9 and 10.)

MOUTH. The entrance to the alimentary canal is the MOUTH, where the teeth, tongue, and jaws begin the process of digestion by mastication. Saliva is secreted into the mouth by three separate pairs of salivary glands located under the tongue, inside the lower jaw, and in the cheek. Saliva softens and lubricates the food, dissolves some of it, and begins the conversion of the starches into sugar by the action of ptyalin, the enzyme of the saliva. The saliva moistens the inside of the mouth, the tongue, and the teeth, and rinses them after the food has departed on the next stage of its journey.

Four passageways meet at the back of the throat: the oral and nasal passages, the larynx, and the esophagus. In the act of swallowing, the entrances to the nasal passages and the larynx are each sealed off momentarily by the soft palate and the epiglottis, so that the food can pass into the esophagus without straying into the respiratory tract.

STOMACH. Propelled by rhythmic muscular contractions called peristalsis, the food moves rapidly through the esophagus, past the cardiac sphincter—a circular muscle at the base of the esophagus—and into the STOMACH. Here the peristaltic motions are stronger and more frequent, occurring at the rate of three per minute, churning, liquefying, and mixing the foods with the gastric juice. In the juice are the enzymes pepsin and lipase and, in infants, rennin; a secretion called mucin, which coats and protects the stomach lining; and hydrochloric acid. Together the pepsin and hydrochloric acid begin the splitting of the proteins in the food. The lipase in the stomach is a rather weak fat-splitting enzyme, able to act only on fats that are already emulsified, such as those in cream and the yoke of egg; more powerful lipase is available in the intestine, where most fats are digested.

The average adult stomach holds $1\frac{1}{2}$ quarts. The stomach reaches its peak of digestive activity nearly 2 hours after a meal and may empty in 3 to $4\frac{1}{2}$ hours; a heavy meal may take as long as 6 hours to pass into the small intestine.

SMALL INTESTINE. The food leaves the stomach in the form of *chyme,* a thick, liquid mixture. It passes through the pylorus, a sphincter muscle opening from the lower part of the stomach into the duodenum. This sphincter is closed most of the time, opening each time a peristaltic wave passes over it. The stomach is much wider than the rest of the canal and also has a J-shaped curve at its bottom, so that the passage of food through the pylorus is automatically slowed until the food is of the right consistency to flow through the narrow opening into the intestine.

The small intestine is about 20 feet long. The lining of the small intestine has deep folds and finger-like projections called villi that give it a surface of about 100 square feet through which the absorption of food can take place.

The duodenum, a C-shaped curve with a length of about 10 inches, is the first and widest part of the small intestine. Into it flows the pancreatic juice, with enzymes that break down starch, protein, and fats. The common bile duct also empties into the duodenum. The bile emulsifies fats for the action of the fat-splitting enzymes.

Just below the duodenum is the jejunum, the lon-

1 Carbohydrates
Starch
Sugar

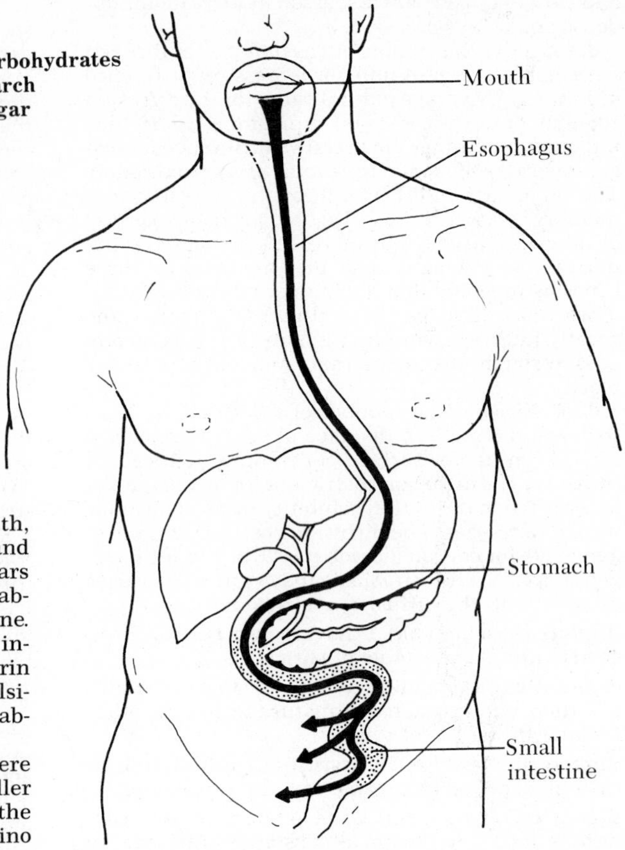

Digestion.

1. *Carbohydrates* are digested in the mouth, where saliva converts some starch into sugar, and in the small intestine, where all starches and sugars are converted into monosaccharides, which are absorbed into the bloodstream from the small intestine.

2. *Fats* are digested principally in the small intestine. Broken down into fatty acids and glycerin by the intestinal and pancreatic juices, and emulsified by bile from the gallbladder, they are then absorbed through the intestinal walls.

3. *Protein* digestion begins in the stomach, where the gastric juice breaks proteins down into smaller molecules. Pancreatic and intestinal juices in the small intestine convert the proteins into amino acids, which are then absorbed from the intestine.

2 Fats

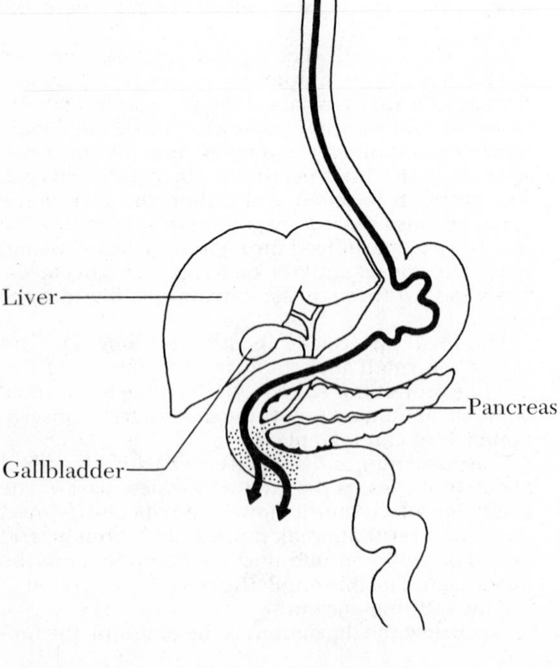

3 Proteins

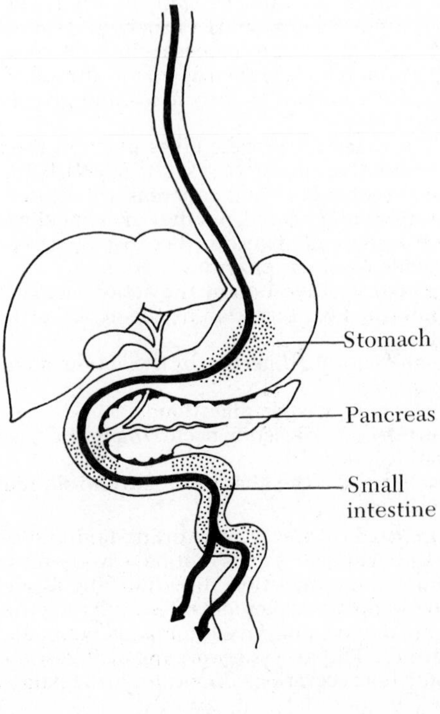

gest portion of the small intestine, and beyond that is the ileum, the last and narrowest section of the small intestine. Along this whole length, carbohydrates, proteins, and fats are broken down into sugars, amino acids, fatty acids, and glycerin. The lining of the small intestine absorbs these nutrient compounds as rapidly as they are produced. The bulky and unusable parts of the diet pass into the large intestine.

LARGE INTESTINE. At the junction of the small and large intestines is the ileocecal valve, so called because it is at the end of the ileum and the beginning of the cecum. A small blind tube called the vermiform appendix is attached to the cecum. The longer part of the large intestine is called the colon and is divided into the ascending, transverse, and descending colon, and the sigmoid flexure, an S-shaped bend at the distal end of the colon. The sigmoid colon empties into the rectum.

Along the $5\frac{1}{2}$ feet or so of the large intestine, the liquid in the waste is gradually reabsorbed through the intestinal walls. Thus the waste is formed into fairly solid feces and pushed down into the rectum for eventual evacuation. This takes from 10 to 20 hours. The evacuation consists of bacteria, cells cast off from the intestines, some mucus, and such indigestible substances as cellulose. The normal dark brown color of the stool is caused by bile pigments (see also FECES).

d. tract, alimentary canal.

digit (dij′it) a finger or toe. adj., **dig′ital.**

Digitaline nativelle (dij″ĭ-tal′ēn na″tĭ-vel′) trademark for preparations of digitoxin.

Digitalis (dij″i-tal′is) a genus of herbs.

D. lana′ta, a Balkan species that yields digoxin and lanatoside.

D. purpu′rea, the purple foxglove, whose leaves furnish digitalis.

digitalis (dij″ĭ-tal′is) dried leaf of *Digitalis purpurea;* used as a cardiotonic agent. All drugs prepared from this digitalis leaf are members of the same group and principles of administration are the same. The drugs vary according to speed of action and potency. They may cause intoxication, symptoms of which include nausea, vomiting, visual disturbances, and cardiac irregularity.

digitalization (dij″ĭ-tal-ĭ-za′shun) the administration of digitalis in a dosage schedule designed to produce and then maintain optimal therapeutic concentrations of its cardiotonic glycosides.

digitation (dij″ĭ-ta′shun) 1. a finger-like process. 2. surgical creation of a functioning digit by making a cleft between two adjacent metacarpal bones, after amputation of some or all of the fingers.

digitiform (dij′ĭ-tĭ-form″) finger-like.

digitonin (dij″ĭ-to′nin) a saponin from *Digitalis purpurea,* used as a reagent to precipitate cholesterol.

digitoxin (dij″ĭ-tok′sin) a cardiotonic glycoside obtained from *Digitalis purpurea* and other species of the same genus; used in the treatment of congestive heart failure. It has a slowly developing action and slow elimination. Parenteral solutions should be diluted when given by vein.

diglossia (di-glos′e-ah) bifid tongue.

diglyceride (di-glis′er-īd) a glyceride containing two fatty acid molecules in ester linkage.

dignathus (dig-na′thus) a fetus with two lower jaws.

digoxin (dĭ-jok′sin) a cardiotonic glycoside obtained from the leaves of *Digitalis lanata;* used in the treatment of congestive heart failure. It has a relatively rapid action and rapid elimination.

dihydric (di-hi′drik) having two hydrogen atoms in each molecule.

dihydrocodeinone (di-hi″dro-ko′de-ĭ-nōn) hydrocodone, a synthetic analgesic.

dihydroergotamine (di-hi″dro-er-got′ah-mēn) a product of the catalytic hydrogenation of ergotamine; used in the treatment of migraine.

dihydromorphinone (di-hi″dro-mor′fĭ-nōn) hydromorphone, a narcotic analgesic.

dihydrotachysterol (di-hi″dro-tah-kis′ter-ol) a synthetic steroid derived from ergosterol by irradiation; used as a blood-calcium regulator.

dihydroxyaluminum (di″hi-drok″se-ah-lu′mĭ-num) an aluminum compound having two hydroxyl groups in a molecule; available as dihydroxyaluminum aminoacetate and dihydroxyaluminum sodium carbonate, which are used as antacids.

dihydroxycholecalciferol (di″hi-drok″se-ko″le-kal-sif′er-ol) a group of active metabolites of cholecalciferol (vitamin D_3) numbered according to the carbon atom(s) on which a hydroxyl group is substituted; 1,25-dihydroxycholecalciferol is the most active form known.

3,4-dihydroxyphenylalanine (di″hi-drok″se-fen″-il-al′ah-nēn) dopa, an amino acid produced by oxidation of tyrosine by tyrosinase; it is the precursor of dopamine and an intermediate product in the biosynthesis of norepinephrine, epinephrine, and melanin. L-dopa, the naturally occurring form, and levodopa, the synthetic form, are used in parkinsonism and manganese poisoning.

diiodohydroxyquin (di″i-o″do-hi-drok′se-kwin) an antiamebic.

diiodotyrosine (di″i-o″do-ti′ro-sēn) an organic iodine-containing precursor of thyroxine, liberated from thyroglobulin by hydrolysis.

diisopropyl fluorophosphate (di-i″so-pro′pil floo″or-o-fos′fāt) isofluophate.

diktyoma (dik″te-o′mah) a tumor of the ciliary epithelium resembling embryonic retinal tissue in structure.

dilaceration (di-las″er-a′shun) a tearing apart, as of a cataract. In dentistry, an abnormal angulation or curve in the root or crown of a formed tooth.

Dilantin (di-lan′tin) trademark for phenytoin, an anticonvulsant used in the treatment of all forms of epilepsy except petit mal.

dilatation (dil″ah-ta′shun) 1. the condition, as of an orifice or tubular structure, of being dilated or stretched beyond normal dimensions. 2. the act of dilating or stretching.

d. of the heart, compensatory enlargement of the cavities of the heart, with thinning of the walls.

dilation (di-la′shun) 1. the act of dilating or stretching. 2. dilatation.

d. and curettage, expanding of the ostium uteri to permit scraping of the walls of the uterus; called also D and C.

dilator (di-la′tor) a structure (muscle) that dilates, or an instrument used to dilate.

Dilaudid (di-law′did) trademark for preparations of hydromorphone, a narcotic analgesic.

Diloderm (di′lo-derm) trademark for preparations of dichlorisone, an antipruritic.

diluent (dil′u-ent) 1. diluting. 2. an agent that dilutes or renders less potent or irritant.

dilution (di-lu′shun) 1. reduction of concentration of an active substance by admixture of a neutral agent. 2. a substance that has undergone dilution.

serial d., 1. the progressive dilution of a substance in a series of tubes in predetermined ratios. 2. a method of obtaining a pure bacterial culture by rapid transfer of an exceedingly small amount of material from one nutrient medium to a succeeding one of the same volume.

dimenhydrinate (di″men-hi′drĭ-nāt) an antihistaminic used as an antinauseant.

dimercaprol (di″mer-kap′rol) a colorless, liquid chelating agent used in the treatment of heavy metal poisoning; called also British antilewisite (BAL). The drug forms a relatively stable compound with arsenic,, mercury, gold, and certain other metals, thus protecting the vital enzyme systems of the cells against the effects of the metals. It is sometimes diluted with water and used to wash the stomach, some of the solution being permitted to remain in the stomach.

Side effects include tachycardia, hypertension, nausea and vomiting, severe headaches, and a sense of constriction of the chest. Barbiturates are usually ordered to relieve the symptoms, which should subside within an hour. The drug has a very disagreeable skunklike odor and should be handled carefully to avoid spilling.

Dimetane (di′mĕ-tān) trademark for preparations of brompheniramine, an antihistaminic.

dimethicone (di-meth′ĭ-kōn) a silicone oil used as a skin protective; available as an ointment, spray, and cream.

dimethindene (di″meth-in′dēn) an antihistaminic, used as the maleate salt.

dimethisoquin (di″mĕ-thi′so-kwin) a local anesthetic; used as the hydrochloride salt.

dimethisterone (di″mĕ-this′ter-ōn) a synthetic progestin, used as an oral contraceptive, either alone or in combination with ethinyl estradiol.

dimethoxanate (di-mĕ-thok′sĭ-nāt) a non-narcotic antitussive; used as the hydrochloride salt.

dimethyl- having two methyl groups in the molecule.

dimethylamine (di-meth″il-am′in) a ptomaine, from decaying gelatin, decomposing yeast, rotten fish, etc.

***p*-dimethylaminoazobenzene** (di-meth″il-am″ĭ-no-az″o-ben′zēn) a carcinogenic dye, used as a pH indicator.

Dimethylane (di-meth′ĭ-lan) trademark for preparations of promoxolane, a skeletal muscle relaxant and tranquilizer.

dimethyl phthalate (di-meth′il thal′āt) an insect repellent.

dimethyl sulfoxide (di-meth′il sul-fok′sid) DMSO, a powerful solvent which has the ability to penetrate animal and plant tissues and to preserve living cells during freezing; it has been proposed as a topical analgesic and anti-inflammatory agent and to increase penetrability of other substances.

dimethyltryptamine (di-meth″il-trip′tah-mēn) a hallucinogenic substance derived from the plant *Prestonia amazonica;* abbreviated DMT.

dimetria (di-me′tre-ah) a condition characterized by a double uterus.

Dimocillin (di″mo-sil′in) trademark for preparations of sodium methicillin.

dimorphism (di-mor′fizm) the quality of existing in two distinct forms. adj., **dimor′phous.**

sexual d., 1. physical or behavioral differences associated with sex. 2. having some properties of both sexes, as in the early embryo and in some hermaphrodites.

dineuric (di-nu′rik) having two neurons or axons.

Dinoflagellata (di″no-flaj″ĕ-la′tah) an order of minute, chiefly marine, plantlike protozoa; certain members sometimes flourish in numbers so vast as to cover and discolor the seawater (red tide), causing the death of many fish and invertebrates. Included are the genera *Gonyaulax* and *Gymnodinium.*

dinoflagellate (di″no-flaj′ĕ-lāt) 1. of or pertaining to the order Dinoflagellata. 2. any individual of the order Dinoflagellata.

dinoprost tromethamine (di′no-prost) a PROSTAGLANDIN administered intra-amniotically to induce abortion.

dinucleotide (di-nu′kle-o-tīd″) one of the cleavage products into which a polynucleotide may be split, itself composed of two mononucleotides, as flavin-adenine dinucleotide and nicotinamide-adenine dinucleotide.

Dioctophyma (di-ok″to-fi′mah) a genus of nematode parasites.

D. rena′le, the kidney worm, a species found in the kidney in various carnivorous animals, and sometimes in man; it is highly destructive to kidney tissue.

dioctyl calcium sulfosuccinate (di-ok′til kal′se-um sul″fo-suk′sĭ-nāt) a wetting agent and nonlaxative fecal softener.

dioctyl sodium sulfosuccinate (di-ok′til so′de-um sul″fo-suk′sĭ-nāt) a fecal softener, wetting agent, and cathartic.

Diodoquin (di″o-do′kwin) trademark for a preparation of diiodohydroxyquin, an antiamebic.

Diodrast (di′o-drast) trademark for a preparation of iodopyracet for injection, used for x-ray examination of the kidneys and urinary tract.

dioecious (di-e′shus) diecious.

diopter (di-op′ter) a unit adopted for calibration of lenses, being the reciprocal of the focal length when expressed in meters; symbol D.

dioptometry (di″op-tom′ĕ-tre) the measurement of ocular accommodation and refraction.

dioptric (di-op′trik) pertaining to refraction or to transmitted and refracted light; refracting.

dioptrics (di-op′triks) the science of refracted light.

diosgenin (di-os′jen-in) an aglycone of the saponin dioscin, obtained from yams of the genus *Dioscorea;* it is used as a precursor in the preparation of pregnenolone, progesterone,, and other steroids.

diovulatory (di-ov′u-lah-to″re) ordinarily discharging two ova in one ovarian cycle.

dioxide (di-ok′sīd) an oxide with two oxygen atoms.

dioxyline (di-ok′sĭ-lēn) a coronary and peripheral vasodilator; used as the phosphate salt.

Dipaxin (di-pak′sin) trademark for a preparation of diphenadione, an anticoagulant.

dipeptidase (di-pep′tĭ-dās) an enzyme that catalyzes the hydrolysis of the peptide linkage in a dipeptide.

dipeptide (di-pep′tīd) a peptide which, on hydrolysis, yields two amino acids.

diperodon (di-per′o-don) a surface anesthetic and analgesic; used as the hydrochloride salt.

Dipetalonema (di-pet″ah-lo-ne′mah) a genus of nematode parasites of the superfamily Filarioidea, including *D. per′stans* and *D. streptocer′ca,* species primarily parasitic in man, other primates serving as reservoir hosts.

diphallus (di-fal′us) a developmental anomaly characterized by duplication of the penis.

diphemanil (di-fe′mah-nil) an anticholinergic drug used to inhibit gastric mobility and secretion, relieve pylorospasm, control sweating, and relieve pruritus. Toxic symptoms are rare and include dry mouth, mydriasis, and fever. The drug is contraindicated in patients with glaucoma.

diphenadione (di-fen″ah-di′ōn) a yellow crystalline compound used as an anticoagulant; it is one of the most potent and long acting of these drugs, and is effective in relatively small doses.

diphenhydramine (di″fen-hi′drah-min) an antihistaminic used in treatment of allergic disorders in the form of the hydrochloride salt.

diphenicillin (di″fen-ĭ-sil′in) an acid- and penicillinase-resistant semisynthetic penicillin available as the sodium salt for oral and intramuscular use.

diphenoxylate (di″fen-ok′sĭ-lāt) an antidiarrheal, used as the hydrochloride salt.

diphenylhydantoin (di-fen″il-hi-dan′to-in) phenytoin, an anticonvulsant.

diphenylpyraline (di-fen″il-pi′rah-lēn) an antihistaminic, used as the hydrochloride salt.

diphonia (di-fo′ne-ah) the production of two different voice tones in speaking.

diphosphothiamin (di-fos″fo-thi′ah-min) the coenzyme that is involved in the decarboxylation of α-keto acids.

diphtheria (dif-the′re-ah) an acute, highly contagious childhood disease that generally affects the membranes of the throat and, less frequently, the nose; in rare instances it can affect other parts of the body, notably the skin, following an open wound. Caused by the bacillus *Corynebacterium diphtheriae,* it can be fatal if not treated promptly. adj., **diphthe′rial, diphther′ic, diphtherit′ic.**

Diphtheria spreads in droplets of moisture from the mouth, nose, or throat of an infected person. It may also be spread by handkerchiefs, towels, eating utensils, or any other object used by an infected person or sprayed by his coughing or sneezing. It may also be transmitted by a healthy person who is nevertheless a carrier of the disease or by someone who is convalescing from diphtheria. The incubation period of the disease is generally between 2 and 5 days, sometimes longer. An infected person may continue to have the bacilli in his throat from 2 to 4 weeks after he has recovered from its effects.

SYMPTOMS. The first symptoms of diphtheria usually include sore throat, fever, headache, and nausea. Patches of grayish or dirty-yellowish membrane form in the throat, and gradually grow into one membrane. This membrane, combined with swelling of the throat, may interfere with swallowing or breathing. In severe cases, when other measures fail, a tracheostomy may be necessary to restore breathing.

The diphtheria bacillus also produces a toxin that spreads throughout the body and may damage the heart and nerves permanently. Diagnosis of the disease can be verified by identifying the causative organisms from throat cultures. Susceptibilty to diphtheria is determined by the SCHICK TEST, which indicates the presence or absence of circulating antibodies to the diphtheria toxin.

TREATMENT. Diphtheria antitoxin is administered to counteract the toxic reaction from the bacillus. Prognosis depends on the severity of the infection and especially on how soon the antitoxin is given. Bed rest, antibiotics, and general hygienic measures are used to combat the infection. Oxygen is administered as necessary to relieve dyspnea and cyanosis. Heart complications are usually more severe in adults; thus the convalescent period is extended for these patients. ISOLATION TECHNIQUE must be employed during the entire period that the patient is considered capable of spreading infection.

PREVENTION. Repeated exposure to the causative organisms may provide a natural immunity. Immunization, artificially induced through the administration of weakened toxins, should be begun between the sixth and eighth week of life. These injections usually are given in combination with pertussis (whooping cough) and tetanus immunizing agents (DPT injections), and are given 1 month apart in three separate injections. Booster doses of diphtheria toxoid are given at the age of one and again before the child enters school. (See also table under IMMUNIZATION.)

Once one of the most fatal diseases of childhood, cases of diphtheria and death from the disease have become almost nonexistent in countries where mass immunization has been practiced.

diphtheroid (dif′thĕ-roid) 1. resembling diphtheria or the diphtheria bacillus. 2. pseudodiphtheria.

diphthongia (dif-thon′je-ah) the production of double vocal sounds.

diphyllobothriasis (di-fil″o-both-ri′ah-sis) infection with *Diphyllobothrium.*

Diphyllobothrium (di-fil″o-both′re-um) a genus of large TAPEWORMS.

D. la′tum, the broad or fish tapeworm, a species found in the intestines of man, dogs, cats, and other fish-eating mammals.

diphyodont (dif′e-o-dont″) having two dentitions, a deciduous and a permanent.

diplacusis (dip″lah-koo′sis) the perception of a single auditory stimulus as two separate sounds.

diplegia (di-ple′je-ah) paralysis of like parts on either side of the body. adj., **diple′gic.**

diplobacillus (dip″lo-bah-sil′us) a short, rod-shaped organism occurring in pairs; diplobacterium.

diplobacterium (dip″lo-bak-te′re-um) diplobacillus.

diploblastic (dip″lo-blas′tik) having two germ layers.

diplocardia (dip″lo-kar′de-ah) separation of the two halves of the heart.

Diplococcus (dip″lo-kok′us) a genus of bacteria (tribe Streptococceae).

D. pneumo′niae, pneumococcus, the commonest cause of lobar pneumonia, including some 80 serotypes distinguishable by the polysaccharide hapten of the capsular substance. Called also *Streptococcus pneumoniae.*

diplococcus (dip″lo-kok′us), pl. *diplococ′ci.* 1. any of the spherical, lanceolate, or coffee-bean-shaped bacteria occurring usually in pairs as a result of incomplete separation after cell division in a single plane. 2. any organism of the genus *Diplococcus.*

diplocoria (dip″lo-ko′re-ah) double pupil.

diploë (dip′lo-e) the spongy layer between the inner and outer compact layers of the flat bones of the skull. adj., **diploet′ic, diplo′ic.**

diplogenesis (dip″lo-jen′ĕ-sis) the production of a double monster.

diploid (dip′loid) 1. having a pair of each chromosome characteristic of a species (2n or, in man, 46). 2. a diploid individual or cell.

diploidy (dip′loi-de) the state of being diploid.

diplomyelia (dip″lo-mi-e′le-ah) lengthwise fissure and seeming doubleness of the spinal cord.

diplonema (dip″lo-ne′mah) the double chromosomes in the diplotene stage.

diploneural (dip″lo-nu′ral) having a double nerve supply.

diplopia (dĭ-plo′pe-ah) the perception of two images of a single object (double vision).

binocular d., perception of a separate image of a single object by each of the two eyes.

crossed d., horizontal diplopia in which the image belonging to the right eye is displaced to the left of the image belonging to the left eye (divergent strabismus).

direct d., horizontal diplopia in which the image belonging to the right eye appears to the right of the image belonging to the left eye (convergent strabismus).

horizontal d., diplopia in which the two images lie in the same horizontal plane, being either direct or crossed.

vertical d., diplopia in which one image appears above the other in the same vertical plane.

diplosomia (dip″lo-so′me-ah) a condition in which complete twins are joined at some part of their bodies.

diplotene (dip′lo-tēn) that stage of the first prophase of meiosis during which the paired bivalent chromosomes begin to repel one another.

dipole (di′pōl) 1. a molecule having charges of equal and opposite sign. 2. a pair of electric charges or magnetic poles separated by a short distance.

diprosopus (di-pros′o-pus) a monster with varying degrees of duplication of the face.

diprotrizoate (di″pro-tri′zo-āt) a compound used as a contrast medium in roentgenography of the urinary tract.

dipsomania (dip″so-ma′ne-ah) alcoholism.

dipsotherapy (dip″so-ther′ah-pe) the therapeutic limitation of the amounts of fluids ingested.

Diptera (dip′ter-ah) an order of insects, including flies, gnats, and mosquitoes.

dipterous (dip′ter-us) 1. having two wings. 2. pertaining to insects of the order Diptera.

dipygus (di-pi′gus) a fetus with a double pelvis.

dipylidiasis (dip″ĭ-lĭ-di′ah-sis) infection with *Dipylidium caninum.*

Dipylidium (dip″ĭ-lid′e-um) a genus of TAPEWORMS.

D. cani′num the dog tapeworm, parasitic in dogs and cats and occasionally found in man.

dipyridamole (di″pi-rid′ah-mol) a coronary vasodilator.

dipyrone (di′pi-rōn) an analgesic and antipyretic.

director (di-rek′tor) a grooved instrument for guiding a knife or other surgical instrument.

Dirofilaria (di″ro-fĭ-la′re-ah) a genus of nematode parasites of the superfamily Filarioidea.

dirofilariasis (di″ro-fil″ah-ri′ah-sis) infection with organisms of the genus *Dirofilaria.*

dis- word element [L.], *reversal* or *separation;* [Gr.], *duplication.*

disaccharidase (di-sak′ah-rĭ-dās″) an enzyme that catalyzes the hydrolysis of disaccharides.

disaccharide (di-sak′ah-rid, di-sak′ah-rīd) any of a class of sugars each molecule of which yields two molecules of monosaccharide on hydrolysis.

disarticulation (dis″ar-tik″u-la′shun) amputation or separation at a joint.

disassimilation (dis″ah-sim″ĭ-la′shun) catabolism.

disc (disk) disk.

discharge (dis-charj′) 1. a setting free, or liberation. 2. material or force set free. 3. an excretion or substance evacuated.

discission (dĭ-sizh″un) incision, or cutting into, as of a soft cataract.

discitis (dis-ki′tis) diskitis.

discogenic (dis″ko-jen′ik) caused by derangement of an intervertebral disk.

discography (dis-kog′rah-fe) diskography.

discoid (dis′koid) 1. disk-shaped. 2. a disklike medicated tablet.

discoplacenta (dis″ko-plah-sen′tah) a disk-shaped placenta.

discordance (dis-kor′dans) the occurrence of a given trait in only one member of a twin pair. adj., **discor′dant.**

discrete (dis-krēt′) made up of separated parts; characterized by lesions that do not become blended.

discus (dis′kus), pl. *dis′ci* [L.] disk.

d. ooph′orus, d. ovig′erus, d. prolig′erus, cumulus oophorus.

disdiaclast (dis-di′ah-klast) any of the doubly refracting elements of the contractile substance of muscle.

disease (dĭ-zēz′) a definite morbid process having a characteristic train of symptoms. It may affect the whole body or any of its parts, and its etiology, pathology, and prognosis may be known or unknown. For specific diseases, see under the specific name, as ADDISON'S DISEASE.

autoimmune d., any of a group of disorders in which tissue injury is associated with humoral or cell-mediated immune responses to body constituents; they may be systemic or organ-specific (see also AUTOIMMUNE DISEASE).

chronic granulomatous d., chronic suppurative lymphadenitis, eczematoid dermatitis, hepatosplenomegaly, and chronic pulmonary disease associated with a genetically determined defect in the intracellular bactericidal function of leukocytes.

collagen d's, a group of poorly understood diseases that have in common widespread pathologic changes in the connective tissues, including systemic lupus erythematosus, periarteritis nodosa, scleroderma, dermatomyositis, and perhaps rheumatoid arthritis and rheumatic fever (see also COLLAGEN DISEASES).

communicable d., a disease the causative agents of which may pass or be carried from one person to another directly or indirectly (see also COMMUNICABLE DISEASE).

complicating d., one that occurs in the course of some other disease as a complication.

constitutional d., one involving a system of organs or one with widespread symptoms.

contagious d., communicable disease.

cystine storage d., Fanconi's syndrome (2).

deficiency d., a condition due to dietary or metabolic deficiency, including all diseases caused by an insufficient supply of essential nutrients.

degenerative joint d., osteoarthritis.

demyelinating d., any condition characterized by destruction of myelin.

epizootic d., a disease that affects a large number of animals in some particular region within a short period of time.

extrapyramidal d., any of a group of clinical disorders marked by abnormal involuntary movements, alterations in muscle tone, and postural disturbances; it includes parkinsonism, chorea, athetosis, etc.

fifth venereal d., lymphogranuloma venereum.

focal d., a localized disease.

fourth d., Duke's disease.

fourth venereal d., gangrenous balanitis.

functional d., any disease involving body functions but not associated with detectable organic lesion or change.

glycogen d., glycogen storage d., glycogenosis.

heavy chain d., a monoclonal gammopathy in which there is elaboration of immunoglobulin IgG that lacks certain antigenic determinants. The resultant globulin fragment (molecular weight, 53,000), resembling the Fc fragment, is found in both serum and urine. Symptoms include recurring bacterial infections, anemia, enlargement of lymphoid organs, and edema of the palate. Histologically there is lymphoma, ranging from Hodgkin's disease to reticulum cell sarcoma. Heavy-chain disease involving the IgA and IgM systems has also been reported.

hemolytic d. of newborn, erythroblastosis fetalis.

hemorrhagic d. of newborn, see HEMORRHAGIC DISEASE OF NEWBORN.

hip-joint d., tuberculosis of the hip joint.

hookworm d., see HOOKWORM.

idiopathic d., one that exists without any connection with any known cause.

immune-complex d., a state in which circulating antigen-antibody complexes, formed by coexisting immune reactions, induce vascular injury.

infectious d., one due to organisms ranging in size from viruses to parasitic worms; it may be contagious in origin, result from nosocomial organisms, or be due to endogenous microflora from the nose and throat, skin, or bowel (see also COMMUNICABLE DISEASE).

intercurrent d., a disease occurring during the course of another disease with which it has no connection.

iron storage d., hemochromatosis.

Mediterranean d., the homozygous form of β-THALASSEMIA.

metabolic d., one caused by some defect in the chemical reactions of the cells of the body.

motor neuron d., any disease of the motor neurons, including spinal muscular atrophy, progressive bulbar paralysis, amyotrophic lateral sclerosis, and lateral sclerosis.

occupational d., a disease arising from various factors involved with the patient's occupation (see also OCCUPATIONAL DISEASES).

organic d., one due to or accompanied by structural changes.

periodontal d., any disease or disorder of the periodontium (see also PERIODONTITIS and PERIODONTOSIS).

secondary d., 1. a morbid condition subsequent to or a consequence of another disease. 2. a condition due to introduction of incompatible, immunologically competent cells into a host rendered incapable of accepting them by heavy exposure to ionizing radiation.

self-limited d., one that by its very nature runs a limited and definite course.

sixth venereal d., lymphogranuloma venereum.

storage d., a metabolic disorder in which a specific substance (a lipid, a protein, etc.) accumulates in certain cells in unusually large amounts.

systemic d., one affecting a number of tissues that perform a common function.

thyrocardiac d., thyrotoxic heart d., see THYROTOXIC HEART DISEASE.

venereal d., a contagious disease usually acquired in sexual intercourse or other genital contact, including SYPHILIS, GONORRHEA, CHANCROID, LYMPHOGRANULOMA VENEREUM, and GRANULOMA INGUINALE.

disengagement (dis″en-gāj′ment) emergence of the fetus, or part thereof, from the vaginal canal.

disequilibrium (dis″e-kwĭ-lib′re-um) unstable equilibrium.

disinfect (dis″in-fekt′) to free from pathogenic organisms, or to render them inert.

disinfectant (dis″in-fek′tant) 1. freeing from infection. 2. an agent that destroys infection-producing organisms. Heat and certain other physical agents such as live steam can be disinfectants, but in common usage the term is reserved for chemical substances such as mercury bichloride or phenol. Disinfectants are usually applied to inanimate objects since they are too strong to be used on living tissues. Chemical disinfectants are not always effective against spore-forming bacteria.

disinfection (dis″in-fek′shun) the act of disinfecting.

concomitant d., concurrent d., immediate disinfection and disposal of discharges and infective matter all through the course of a disease.

terminal d., disinfection of a sick room and its contents at the termination of a disease.

disinfestation (dis″in-fes-ta′shun) destruction of insects, rodents, or other animal forms present on the person or his clothes or in his surroundings, and which may transmit disease.

disinsectization (dis″in-sek″tĭ-za′shun) removal of insects; extermination of insects.

disintegrant (dis-in′tĕ-grant) an agent used in pharmaceutical preparation of tablets, which causes them to disintegrate and release their medicinal substances on contact with moisture.

disintegration (dis-in″tĕ-gra′shun) the process of breaking up or decomposing.

Disipal (dis′ĭ-pal) trademark for a preparation of orphenadrine, a skeletal muscle relaxant.

disjunction (dis-junk′shun) the act or state of being disjoined. In genetics, the moving apart of bivalent chromosomes at the first anaphase of meiosis.

disk (disk) a circular or rounded flat plate; often spelled disc in names of anatomic structures.

articular d., a pad of fibrocartilage or dense fibrous tissue present in some synovial joints.

Bowman's d., one of the flat, disklike plates making up a striated muscle fiber.

choked d., papilledema.

embryonic d., a flattish area in a cleaved ovum in which the first traces of the embryo are seen.

intervertebral d., the layer of fibrocartilage between the bodies of adjoining vertebrae (see also slipped DISK).

intra-articular d., articular disk.

optic d., the intraocular part of the optic nerve formed by fibers converging from the retina and appearing as a pink to white disk in the retina.

slipped d., the popular name for rupture of an intervertebral disk. The condition occurs most commonly in the lower back, occasionally in the neck, and rarely in the upper portion of the spine.

Pads of cartilage and fiber enclosing a rubbery tissue known as the nucleus pulposus lie between the vertebrae. They act as cushions between the vertebrae, absorbing ordinary shocks and strains and shifting position to accommodate the various movements of the spine. Excessive strain may weaken the cartilage to the extent that the nucleus pulposus protrudes through it and forms a bulge. This bulge may push against the nerve roots in the spinal canal, causing pain.

CAUSES AND SYMPTOMS. Rupture, or herniation, of the disks may be caused by injury or by sudden straining with the spine in an unnatural position. The condition may come on gradually as a result of a progressive deterioration of the disks.

EVALUATION OF LIQUID GERMICIDES (BACTERIA ONLY)

Compound	General Usefulness As		Effectiveness Against		Other Properties
	Disinfectants	*Antiseptics*	*TBC*[1]	*Spores*	
Mercurial compounds	None	Poor	None	None	Inact. by org. matter; bland
Phenolic compounds	Good	Poor	Good	Poor	Bad odor; irritating; not inact. by org. matter or soap; stable
Quaternary ammonium compounds ("Quats")	Good	Good	None	None	Neutr. by soap; rel. nontoxic; odorless; absorbed by gauze and fabrics
Chlorine compounds	Good[2]	Fair	Fair[2]	Fair[2]	Inact. by org. matter; corrosive
Iodine and iodophors	Good	Good	Good	Poor	Staining temporary; rel. nontoxic; corrosive
Alcohols	Good[3]	Very good[3]	Very good[3]	None	Volatile; strong conc. required; rapidly cidal; inact. by org. matter
Formaldehyde	Fair	None	Good[4]	Fair[4]	Toxic; irritating fumes
Glutaraldehyde	Good	None	Good	Good	Low protein coagulability; aqueous sol. useful for lens instruments and rubber articles; limited stability; corrodes carbon steel objects after 24 hours exposure
Combinations					
Iodine-alcohol	Fair	Very good	Very good	None	Stains fabrics
Formaldehyde-alcohol	Good[4]	None	Very good[4]	Good[4]	Toxic; irritating fumes; volatile

1. Tubercle bacillus
2. 4 to 5% conc.
3. 70 to 90% conc.
4. 5 to 8% formaldehyde (12 to 20% formalin)

From Evans, M. J.: Some contributions to prevention of infections. Nursing Clin. N. Amer., 3:641, 1968; modified from Spaulding, E. H.: J. Hosp. Res., 3:15, 1965.

Symptoms depend upon the location and the extent to which the disk material has been pushed out. Most cases involve the disks between the fourth and fifth lumbar vertebrae or between the fifth lumbar vertebra and the sacrum. There is severe pain in the lower back and difficulty in walking. The sciatic nerve, which originates in the lower part of the spinal cord, is affected, with resulting pain at the back of the thigh and lower leg. A cough, sneeze, or strain will send the pain along the course of the sciatic nerve to the calf or ankle.

When the disks of the cervical vertebrae are affected, severe pain in the back of the neck radiates down the arms to the fingers. Neck movements are restricted. Any neck motion, coughing, sneezing, or straining will accentuate the pain.

Diagnosis and Treatment. Careful examination, including laboratory tests and x-ray examination (myelography), is necessary to distinguish the condition from other disturbances of the spine. The x-rays may reveal pathologic changes in the spine and narrowing of the space between the vertebrae.

Treatment for slipped disk varies according to the seriousness of the condition. Conservative treatment for a ruptured disk of the lower back consists of bed rest on a firm mattress over a bed board and local application of heat, which should not be prolonged because it may aggravate the congestion, and muscle relaxants and analgesics to relieve pain. Traction may be applied to the legs or pelvis. In chronic cases the wearing of a surgical support may be helpful. Care must be taken to avoid aggravating the condition by excessive physical effort.

Cases of ruptured disk of the neck are treated in a similar manner with bed rest, heat, analgesics, and traction. A collar may be worn to immobilize the neck when the patient is out of bed.

If the response to these measures is poor or if the condition becomes disabling, surgery may be necessary to relieve the pressure on the injured disk (see LAMINECTOMY).

Patient Care. The patient receiving conservative treatment for a slipped disk must always have his spine in good alignment so as to avoid pressure on the adjacent nerves. In addition to the firm mattress and bed boards, he should be instructed in the proper method of turning himself by "log-rolling." To accomplish this the patient crosses his arms over his chest, flexes the knee opposite the side onto which he is to turn, and then rolls over in "one piece," being sure that his spine is not bent forward or twisted.

A footboard should be used to eliminate the weight of the bed clothes and also to prevent footdrop. A small bedpan is recommended for the patient's use so that he can roll onto it without discomfort. A folded towel or small pillow is placed under his lower back for support of the lumbar region. Measures must be taken to avoid constipation which is quite common and likely to cause increased pain as the patient strains to defecate. A nonconstipating diet may be sufficient; however, a mild laxative, such as one of the bulk laxatives, may also be necessary.

HEAT, in the form of a heating pad or infrared lamp, often relieves the pain caused by muscle spasms. Care should be taken in the application of heat because of the danger of burning the patient who has a loss of sensory perception because of nerve damage caused by the slipped disk.

Most physicians prescribe a special corset to be worn by the patient whenever he is out of bed. The corset is designed to give proper support to the vertebral column and to relieve tension on the back muscles. Support devices of this kind usually are discontinued after symptoms are relieved, because they weaken the musculature of the back. Training in good posture and body mechanics, especially during lifting or stooping, are important in preventing recurrence of acute episodes. Special exercises may be prescribed to strengthen the back muscles.

diskectomy (dis-kek′to-me) excision of an intervertebral disk.

diskiform (dis′kĭ-form) in the shape of a disk.

diskitis (dis-ki′tis) inflammation of a disk, especially of an intervertebral disk.

diskography (dis-kog′rah-fe) roentgenography of the vertebral column after injection of radiopaque material into an intervertebral disk.

dislocation (dis″lo-ka′shun) displacement of a bone from a joint. The most common dislocations are those involving a finger, thumb, or shoulder. Less common are those of the mandible, elbow, knee, or hip. Symptoms include loss of motion, temporary paralysis of the involved joint, pain and swelling, and sometimes shock.

A dislocation is usually caused by a blow or fall, although unusual physical effort may lead to this condition. Some dislocations, especially of the hip, are congenital, usually resulting from a faulty construction of the joint. Such a condition is best treated in infancy, with a cast and possibly surgery to correct the dislocation.

A dislocation should be treated as a fracture when

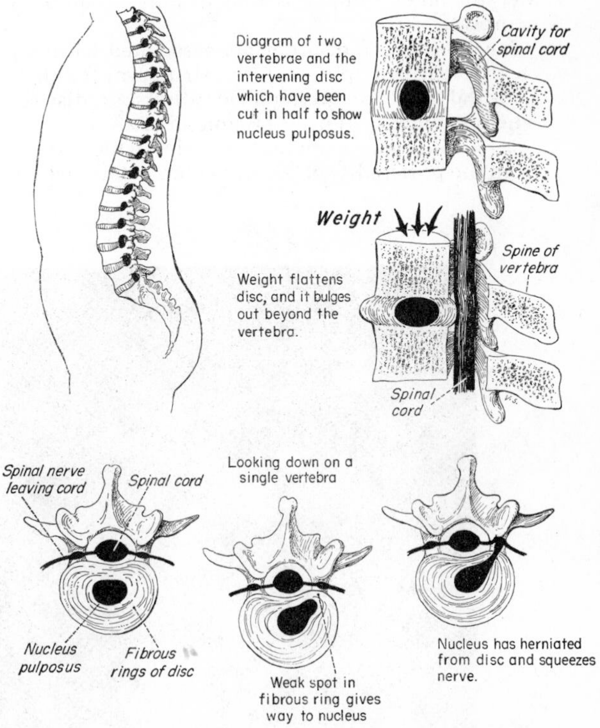

Slipped disk. (From Dowling, H. F., and Jones, T.: That the Patient May Know. Philadelphia, W. B. Saunders Co., 1959.)

first aid is administered. As soon as possible the dislocation is reduced by a surgeon. Traction, slight flexion, abduction, and rotation will often reduce a dislocation. The affected joint is then immobilized to allow for healing of the torn ligaments, tendons, and capsules. In some cases surgery may be necessary to stabilize the joint.

complete d., one in which the surfaces are entirely separated.

compound d., one in which the joint communicates with the outside air through a wound.

pathologic d., one due to disease of the joint or to paralysis of the muscles.

simple d., one in which there is no communication with the air through a wound.

dismemberment (dis-mem′ber-ment) amputation of a limb or a portion of it.

disodium edetate (di-so′de-um ed′ĕ-tāt) edetate disodium.

Disomer (di′so-mer) trademark for a preparation of dexbrompheniramine, an antihistaminic.

disomus (di-so′mus) a double-bodied monster.

disorder (dis-or′der) a derangement or abnormality of function; a morbid physical or mental state.

affective d's, the group of psychoses characterized chiefly by a predominant mood (extreme depression or elation) or by alternations between such moods, including involutional melancholia and manic-depressive psychosis.

character d., a mental disorder characterized by maladaptive behavior, emotional responses that are socially unacceptable, and minimal feelings of anxiety or other symptoms that usually accompany neuroses.

functional d., a disorder not associated with any clearly defined physical or structural change.

mental d., any psychiatric illness or disease, whether functional or of organic origin.

personality d., a mental disorder which stems from the personality of the individual and in which there is minimal feeling of subjective anxiety and little or no feeling of distress.

psychophysiologic d., psychosomatic d., a mental disorder in which physical symptoms are presumed to be of psychogenic origin.

disorganization (dis-or″gan-i-za′shun) the process of destruction of any organic tissue; any profound change in the tissues of an organ or structure which causes the loss of most or all of its proper characters.

disorientation (dis-o″re-en-ta′shun) the loss of proper bearings, or a state of mental confusion as to time, place, or identity.

dispensary (dis-pen′ser-e) 1. a place for dispensation of free or low-cost medical treatment. 2. any place where drugs or medicines are actually dispensed.

dispensatory (dis-pen′sah-tor″e) a book that describes medicines and their preparation and uses.

D. of the United States of America, a collection of monographs on unofficial drugs and drugs recognized by the Pharmacopeia of the United States, the Pharmacopoeia of Great Britain, and the National Formulary, also on general tests, processes, reagents, and solutions of the U.S.P. and N.F., as well as drugs used in veterinary medicine.

dispersate (dis′per-sāt) a suspension of finely divided particles of a substance.

disperse (dis-pers′) to scatter the component parts, as of a tumor or the fine particles in a colloid system; also, the particles so dispersed.

dispersion (dis-per′zhun) 1. the act of scattering or separating; the condition of being scattered. 2. the incorporation of one substance into another. 3. a colloid solution.

displacement (dis-plās′ment) removal to an abnormal location or position; in psychology, unconscious transference of an emotion from its original object onto a more acceptable substitute.

disproportion (dis″pro-por′-shun) a lack of the proper relationship between two elements or factors.

cephalopelvic d., abnormally large size of the fetal skull in relation to the maternal pelvis, leading to difficulties in delivery.

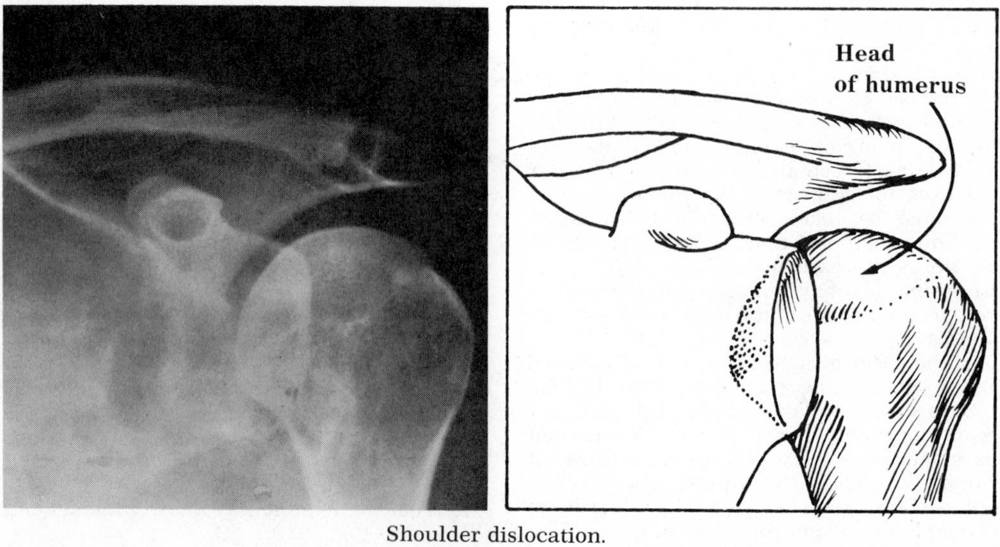

Shoulder dislocation.

dissect (dĭ-sekt′, di-sekt′) to cut apart, or separate; especially, the exposure of structures of a cadaver for anatomical study.

dissection (dĭ-sek′shun) 1. the act of dissecting. 2. a part or whole of an organism prepared by dissecting.

blunt d., separation of tissues along natural lines of cleavage, by means of a blunt instrument or finger.

sharp d., separation of tissues by means of the sharp edge of a knife or scalpel, or with scissors.

dissector (dĭ-sek′tor) 1. one who dissects. 2. a handbook used as a guide for dissecting.

disseminated (dĭ-sem′ĭ-nāt″ed) scattered; distributed over a considerable area.

dissimilation (dĭ-sim″ĭ-la′shun) catabolism.

dissociation (dĭ-so″se-a′shun) 1. the act of separating or the state of being separated. 2. an intrapsychic defense process in which one or more groups of mental processes become separated off from normal consciousness and then function as a unitary whole.

atrial d., independent beating of the left and right atria, each with normal rhythm or with various combinations of normal rhythm, atrial flutter, or atrial fibrillation.

atrioventricular d., control of the atria by one pacemaker and of the ventricles by another, independent pacemaker.

dissolution (dis″o-lu′shun) 1. the process in which one substance is dissolved in another. 2. separation of a compound into its components by chemical action. 3. liquefaction. 4. death.

dissolve (dĭ-zolv′) 1. to cause a substance to pass into solution. 2. to pass into solution.

distad (dis′tad) in a distal direction.

distal (dis′tal) remote; farther from any point of reference.

distance (dis′tans) the measure of space intervening between two objects or two points of reference.

focal d., focal length.

interocclusal d., the distance between the occluding surfaces of the maxillary and mandibular teeth with the mandible in physiologic rest position.

interocular d., the distance between the eyes, usually used in reference to the interpupillary distance (the distance between the two pupils when the visual axes are parallel).

target-skin d., the distance between the anode from which roentgen rays are reflected and the skin of the body surface interposed in their path.

distemper (dis-tem′per) a name for several infectious diseases of animals, especially canine distemper, a highly fatal viral disease of dogs, marked by fever, loss of appetite, and a discharge from the nose and eyes.

distention (dis-ten′shun) the state of being distended, or stretched out or enlarged; the act of distending.

distichia, distichiasis (dis-tik′e-ah; dis″tĭ-ki′ah-sis) the presence of a double row of eyelashes, one or both of which are turned against the eyeball.

distillate (dis′tĭ-lāt) a product of distillation.

distillation (dis″tĭ-la′shun) conversion of a liquid into vapors that then are reconverted to liquid form, as a means of eliminating contaminants from the original solution.

destructive d., decomposition of a solid at a high temperature in the absence of air so that combustion is prevented, as in the preparation of coal tar from coal.

fractional d., separation of volatilizable substances into a number of fractions, based on their different boiling points.

distobuccal (dis″to-buk′al) pertaining to or formed by the distal and buccal surfaces of a tooth, or by the distal and buccal walls of a tooth cavity.

distoclusion (dis″to-kloo′zhun) malrelation of the dental arches, with the lower jaw in a distal or posterior position in relation to the upper.

distomia (di-sto′me-ah) the presence of two mouths.

distomiasis (dis″to-mi′ah-sis) infection due to trematodes or flukes.

distortion (dĭ-stor′shun) the state of being twisted out of normal shape or position; in psychiatry, the conversion of material offensive to the superego into acceptable form.

distraction (dĭ-strak′shun) 1. diversion of attention. 2. separation of joint surfaces without rupture of their binding ligaments and without displacement.

distress (dĭ-stres′) physical or mental anguish or suffering.

disulfiram (di-sul′fĭ-ram) Antabuse; a compound that, when used in the presence of alcohol, produces distressing symptoms such a severe nausea and vomiting. It is a dangerous drug, should always be given under the supervision of a physician and is never given to a patient in a state of intoxication or without his full knowledge. Disulfiram acts as a blocking agent in the oxidation of alcohol, and stops the oxidation at the acetaldehyde stage, so that acetaldehyde accumulates in the body and produces nausea, vomiting, palpitation, dyspnea, lowered blood pressure, and occasionally profound collapse.

dithiazanine iodide (di″thi-az′ah-nēn) an anthelmintic used against strongylids and whipworms.

diurese (di″u-rēs) the act of effecting diuresis.

diuresis (di″u-re′sis) increased excretion of the urine.

diuretic (di″u-ret′ik) 1. increasing urine excretion or the amount of urine. 2. an agent that promotes urine secretion. Certain common substances such as tea, coffee, and water act as diuretics. The diuretic drugs are prescribed chiefly to rid the body of excess fluid when it accumulates in tissues and causes swelling, a condition known as EDEMA. The mercurial diuretics reduce the reabsorption of water via the renal tubules and increase the amount of sodium excreted. They are given by injection only and are considered highly effective but have been supplanted by the newer oral compounds. Orally active diuretics such as the thiazides, ethacrynic acid, and furosemide inhibit sodium and potassium reabsorption by the renal tubules, thereby increasing loss of fluid from the tissue. Acetazolamine (Diamox) is a diuretic that inhibits the reabsorption of sodium and bicarbonate. By increasing the loss of these salts from the body the diuretics cause an increase of excretion of body fluids as urine.

Diuretic drugs are used chiefly in the treatment of edema resulting from conditions other than kidney disease since the abnormal kidney rarely responds to them. They are most useful in relieving edema accompanying congestive heart failure or diminished plasma proteins.

Many diuretics, especially the thiazides, are used in the management of hypertension, particularly when used in conjunction with other kinds of antihypertensive agents.

PATIENT CARE. For all patients receiving diuretic drugs, fluid intake and output should be totaled and recorded at least every 24 hours. Daily weights are also recorded. Symptoms of DEHYDRATION and overhydration should be reported immediately. Because of the danger of potassium depletion and sodium loss resulting from the action of some diuretic drugs, the patient may suffer from an ACID-BASE IMBALANCE. To avoid this, extra potassium is usually given with the thiazides, and frequent laboratory determinations of serum potassium, sodium, chloride, and bicarbonate may be necessary.

Diuril (di'u-ril) trademark for preparations of chlorothiazide, a diuretic.

diurnal (di-er'nal) pertaining to or occurring during the daytime, or period of light.

divagation (di"vah-ga'shun) incoherent or wandering speech.

divalent (di-va'lent) 1. bivalent. 2. carrying an electronic charge of two units.

divergence (di-ver'jens) a moving apart, or inclination away from a common point. adj., **diver'gent.**

diverticular (di"ver-tik'u-lar) pertaining to or resembling a diverticulum.

diverticulectomy (di"ver-tik"u-lek'to-me) excision of a diverticulum.

diverticulitis (di"ver-tik"u-li'tis) inflammation of a diverticulum, especially inflammation involving diverticula of the colon. Weakness of the muscles of the colon, sometimes produced by chronic constipation, leads to the formation of diverticula, small blind pouches that form in the lining and wall of the colon. Inflammation may occur as a result of collections of bacteria or other irritating agents trapped in the pouches.

Symptoms of diverticulitis include muscle spasms and cramplike pains in the abdomen, especially in the lower left quadrant. Diagnosis is confirmed by barium enema (see BARIUM TEST), in which the diverticula are clearly shown.

Treatment consists of bed rest, cleansing enemas, a bland or low-residue diet, and drugs to reduce infection. In severe cases portions of the affected bowel may require surgical removal and a temporary *colostomy*.

diverticulogram (di"ver-tik'u-lo-gram") a roentgenogram of a diverticulum.

diverticulosis (di"ver-tik"u-lo'sis) the presence of diverticula.

diverticulum (di"ver-tik'u-lum), pl. *divertic'ula* [L.] a circumscribed pouch or sac occurring normally or created by herniation of the lining mucous membrane through a defect in the muscular coat of a tubular organ.

intestinal d., a pouch or sac formed by hernial protrusion of the mucous membrane through a defect in the muscular coat of the intestine.

Meckel's d., an occasional sacculation or appendage of the ileum, derived from an unobliterated yolk stalk.

pressure d., pulsion d., a sac or pouch formed by hernial protrusion of the mucous membrane through the muscular coat of the esophagus as a result of pressure from within.

traction d., a localized distortion, angulation, or funnel-shaped bulging of the esophageal wall, due to adhesions resulting from external lesion.

division (dĭ-vizh'un) the act of separating into parts.

cell d., fission of a cell, the process by which cells reproduce.

direct cell d., amitosis.

indirect cell d., meiosis or mitosis.

divulsion (dĭ-vul'shun) the act of separating or pulling apart.

divulsor (dĭ-vul'ser) an instrument for dilating the urethra.

Dix (diks) Dorothea Lynde (1802–1887). American humanitarian. Born in Hampden, Maine, Miss Dix contributed to the establishment and improvement of many insane asylums and prisons in the United States, Europe, and Japan, beginning with the establishment of the Boston Lunatic Asylum in 1839. During the Civil War she was appointed Superintendent of Female Nurses and organized the first nurse corps of the United States Army.

dizygotic (di"zi-got'ik) pertaining to or derived from two separate zygotes (fertilized ova); said of twins.

dizziness (diz'ĭ-nes) a disturbed sense of relationship to space; a sensation of unsteadiness and a feeling of movement within the head; vertigo is sometimes used erroneously as a synonym.

DL chemical prefix (small capitals) denoting that the substance is an equimolecular mixture of two enantiomorphs, one of which corresponds in configuration to D-glyceraldehyde, the other to L-glyceraldehyde.

D.M.D. Doctor of Dental Medicine.

D.M.F. *d*ecayed, *m*issing, *f*illed (teeth): an index used in dental surveys.

DMSO DIMETHYL SULFOXIDE, a powerful solvent.

DMT dimethyltryptamine.

DNA deoxyribonucleic acid.

DNase deoxyribonuclease.

D.O. Doctor of Osteopathy.

D.O.A. dead on admission (arrival).

Doca (do'kah) trademark for desoxycorticosterone, a mineralocorticoid.

Docibin (do'si-bin) trademark for a crystalline preparation of vitamin B_{12}.

doctor (dok'tor) a practitioner of the healing arts, as one graduated from a college of medicine, osteopathy, dentistry, or veterinary medicine, and licensed to practice.

dol (dōl) a unit of pain intensity.

DOLD diffuse obstructive lung disease (see CHRONIC OBSTRUCTIVE PULMONARY DISEASE).

dolich(o)- word element [Gr.], *long.*

dolichocephalic (dol"ĭ-ko-sĕ-fal'ik) long-headed; having a cephalic index below 75.

dolichofacial (dol"ĭ-ko-fa'shal) having a long face.

dolicomorphic (dol"ĭ-ko-mor'fik) having a long, thin, asthenic body type.

dolichopellic (dol"ĭ-ko-pel'ik) having a long pelvis from front to back, with a pelvic index of 95 or above.

Dolophine (do′lo-fēn) trademark for preparations of methadone, a narcotic analgesic.

dolor (do′lor) [L.] pain; one of the cardinal signs of inflammation.

d. cap′itis, headache.

dolorific (do″lor-if′ik) producing pain.

dolorimeter (do″lor-im′ĕ-ter) an instrument for measuring pain in dols.

dominance (dom′ĭ-nans) 1. the supremacy, or superior manifestation, in a specific situation of one of two or more competitive or mutually antagonistic factors. 2. the appearance, in the phenotype of a heterozygote, of one of two mutually antagonistic parental characters.

dominant (dom′ĭ-nant) 1. exerting a ruling or controlling influence; in genetics, capable of expression when carried by only one of a pair of homologous chromosomes. 2. a dominant allele or trait.

d. gene, one that produces an effect (the phenotype) in the organism regardless of the state of the corresponding allele. An example of a trait determined by a dominant gene is brown eye color (see also HEREDITY).

Donath-Landsteiner test (do′nath land′sti-ner) a test for paroxysmal cold hemoglobinuria based on the fact that the blood of patients with this disease contains isohemolysin and autohemolysin that unites with erythrocytes only at low temperatures (2° to 10° C.), hemolysis occurring only after warming with the complement to 37° C.

donor (do′ner) 1. an organism that supplies living tissue to be used in another body, as a person who furnishes blood for transfusion, or an organ for transplantation. 2. a substance or compound that contributes part of itself to another substance (acceptor).

universal d., a person with group O blood; such blood is sometimes used in emergency transfusion.

Donovan bodies (don′o-van) *Donovania granulomatis.*

Donovania granulomatis (don-o-va′ne-ah gran-u-lo′mah-tis) a gram-negative, pleomorphic, rod-shaped microorganism that cannot be cultured on nonviable mediums, but grows in the yolk, yolk sac, and amniotic fluid of the chick embryo. It is the causative organism of granuloma inguinale in man.

dopa (do′pah) 3,4-dihydroxyphenylalanine, produced by oxidation of tyrosine by tyrosinase; it is the precursor of dopamine and an intermediate product in the biosynthesis of norepinephrine, ephinephrine, and melanin. L-dopa, the naturally occurring form, and levodopa, the synthetic form, are used in PARKINSON'S DISEASE and manganese poisoning.

dopamine (do′pah-mēn) a compound, hydroxytyramine, produced by the decarboxylation of dopa; an intermediate product in the synthesis of norepinephrine.

dopaminergic (do′pah-mēn-er′jik) activated or transmitted by dopamine; pertaining to tissues or organs affected by dopamine.

dopa-oxidase (do′pah-ok′sĭ-dās) an enxyme that oxidizes dopa to melanin in the skin, producing pigmentation.

Doppler effect (dop′ler) the relationship of the apparent frequency of waves, as of sound, light, and radio waves, to the relative motion of the source of the waves and the observer, the frequency increasing as the two approach each other and decreasing as they move apart.

Dorbane (dor′bān) trademark for a preparation of danthron, a cathartic.

Doriden (dor′ĭ-den) trademark for preparations of glutethimide, a hypnotic and sedative.

dornase (dor′nās) a shortened term for *deoxyribonuclease;* also a word termination, as in strepto*dornase.*

pancreatic d., a stabilized preparation of deoxyribonuclease, prepared from beef pancreas; used as an aerosol to reduce tenacity of pulmonary secretions.

Dornavac (dor′nah-vak) trademark for a preparation of pancreatic dornase.

dors(o)- word element [L.], *the back; the dorsal aspect.*

Dorsacaine (dor′sah-kān) trademark for a preparation of benoxinate, a surface anesthetic for the eye.

dorsad (dor′sad) toward the back.

dorsal (dor′sal) directed toward or situated on the back surface; opposite the ventral.

dorsalgia (dor-sal′je-ah) pain in the back.

dorsalis (dor-sa′lis) [L.] dorsal.

dorsiflexion (dor″sĭ-flek′shun) backward flexion or bending, as of the hand or foot.

dorsocephalad (dor″so-sef′ah-lad) toward the back of the head.

dorsolateral (dor″so-lat′er-al) pertaining to the back and side.

dorsoventral (dor″so-ven′tral) 1. pertaining to the back and belly surfaces of a body. 2. passing from the back to the belly surface.

dorsum (dor′sum), pl. *dor′sa* [L.] 1. the back; the posterior or superior surface of a body or body part, as of the foot or hand. 2. the aspect of an anatomical structure or part corresponding in position to the back; posterior in the human.

dosage (do′sij) the determination and regulation of the size, frequency, and number of doses.

dose (dōs) the quantity to be administered at one time, as a specified amount of medication or a given quantity of radiation.

absorbed d., that amount of energy from ionizing radiations absorbed per unit mass of matter, expressed in rads.

air d., the intensity of a roentgen-ray or gamma-ray beam in air, expressed in roentgens.

booster d., an amount of immunogen (vaccine, toxoid, or other antigen preparation), usually smaller than the original amount, injected at an appropriate interval after primary immunization to sustain the immune response to that immunogen.

curative d., C.D., a dose that is sufficient to restore normal health.

curative d., median, $C.D._{50}$, a dose that abolishes symptoms in 50 per cent of test subjects.

divided d., a fraction of the total quantity of a drug prescribed to be given at intervals, usually during a 24-hour period.

erythema d., that amount of x-radiation which, when applied to the skin, causes temporary reddening.

fatal d., lethal dose.

infective d., I.D., that amount of pathogenic microorganisms that will cause infection in susceptible subjects.

infective d., median, I.D.$_{50}$, that amount of pathogenic microorganisms that will produce infection in 50 per cent of the test subjects.

lethal d., L.D., that quantity of an agent that will or may be sufficient to cause death.

lethal d., median, L.D.$_{50}$, the quantity of an agent that will kill 50 percent of the test subjects; in radiology, the amount of radiation that will kill, within a specified period, 50 per cent of individuals in a large group or population.

lethal d., minimum, 1. the amount of toxin that will just kill an experimental animal. 2. the smallest quantity of diphtheria toxin that will kill a guinea pig of 250-gm. weight in 4 to 5 days when injected subcutaneously.

maximum permissible d., the largest amount of ionizing radiation that one may safely receive according to recommended limits in radiation protection guides.

skin d., 1. the air dose of radiation at the skin surface, comprising the primary radiation plus backscatter. 2. the absorbed dose in the skin.

threshold erythema d., T.E.D., the single skin dose that will produce in 80 per cent of those tested, a faint but definite erythema within 30 days, and in the other 20 per cent, no visible reaction.

tolerance d., the largest quantity of an agent that may be administered without harm.

dosimeter (do-sim′ĕ-ter) an instrument used to detect and measure exposure to radiation.

dosimetry (do-sim′ĕ-tre) scientific determination of amount, rate, and distribution of radiation emitted from a source of ionizing radiation.

double-blind (dub′ul-blīnd′) denoting a study of the effects of a specific agent in which neither the administrator nor the recipient, at the time of administration, knows whether the active or an inert substance is given.

douche (dōōsh) [Fr.] a stream of water or air directed against a part of the body or into a cavity.

air d., a current of air blown into a cavity, particularly into the tympanum to open the eustachian tube.

vaginal d., irrigation of the vagina to cleanse the area, to apply medicated solutions to the vaginal mucosa and the cervix, or to apply heat in order to relieve pain, inflammation, and congestion. For the treatment to be effective the patient must be in the dorsal recumbent position with the hips level with the chest. Excessive pressure in administering the solution should be avoided so that the solution is not forced beyond the ostium uteri.

Douglas' cul-de-sac (pouch) (dug′las) a sac or recess formed by a fold of the peritoneum dipping down between the rectum and the uterus. Called also rectouterine excavation or pouch.

Douglas' fold (dug′las) a crescentic line marking the termination of the posterior layer of the sheath of the rectus abdominis muscle, just below the level of the iliac crest.

Down's syndrome (downz) a congenital condition characterized by physical malformations and some degree of mental retardation. The disorder was formerly known as mongolism because the patient's facial characteristics resemble those of persons of the Mongolian race. It is also called trisomy 21 syndrome because the disorder is concerned with a defect in the twenty-first chromosome.

The causes of Down's syndrome are not known. There is, however, a relatively high incidence of monogolism in children of mothers who are in the older childbearing age. A particular type of Down's syndrome that occurs in children of younger mothers seems to have a tendency to occur in certain families.

The term trisomy refers to the presence of three representative chromosomes in a cell instead of the usual pair. In Down's syndrome the twenty-first chromosome pair fails to separate when the germ cell (usually the ovum) is being formed. Thus the ovum contains 24 chromosomes, and when it is fertilized by a normal sperm carrying 23 chromosomes, the child is born with an extra chromosome (or total of 47) per cell.

Although all of the physical characteristics of Down's syndrome are not found in a child suffering from this disorder, there usually is a combination of several of them so that diagnosis can be made without difficulty at birth. These characteristics include a small, flattened skull, a short, flat-bridged nose, wide-set eyes, epicanthus, a protruding tongue that is furrowed and lacks a central fissure, short, broad hands and feet with a wide gap between the first and second toes, and a little finger that curves inward. The muscles are hypotonic and there is excessive mobility of the joints. The genitalia are often underdeveloped and congenital heart defects are not uncommon.

As the child grows older he remains below average in height and evidences some degree of mental retardation.

There is no cure for Down's syndrome. Depending on the level of intelligence, the child often can be helped to live productively. (See also MENTAL RETARDATION.)

doxapram (dok′sah-pram) a respiratory stimulant, used as the hydrochloride salt.

doxorubicin (dok″so-roo′bi-sin) an antineoplastic antibiotic; the hydrochloride salt is used intravenously to produce regression in various neoplastic conditions. The side effects include bone marrow depression, alopecia, and cardiac toxicity. Electroencephalogram monitoring is required during administration of the drug.

doxycycline (dok″sĕ-si′klēn) a broad-spectrum antibiotic, synthetically derived from oxytetracycline, active against a wide range of gram-positive and gram-negative organisms.

doxylamine (dok″sil-am′ēn) an antihistaminic, used as the bisuccinate salt.

D.P. Doctor of Pharmacy; Doctor of Podiatry.

D.P.H. Department of Public Health; Diplomate in Public Health; Doctor of Public Health.

DPT diphtheria, pertussis, and tetanus; used in reference to triple-antigen IMMUNIZATION against these diseases.

Dr. Doctor.

dr. dram.

drachm (dram) dram.

dracunculiasis, dracunculosis (drah-kung″ku-li′ah-sis; drah-kung″ku-lo′sis) infection by nematodes of the genus *Dracunculus.*

Dracunculus (drah-kung′ku-lus) a genus of nematode parasites.

D. medinen′sis, a threadlike worm widely distributed in North America, Africa, the Near East, East Indies, and India; frequently found in the subcutaneous and intermuscular tissues of man and certain other animals.

draft (draft) a potion or dose.

drain (drān) 1. to withdraw liquid gradually. 2. any device by which a channel or open area may be established for exit of fluids or purulent material from a cavity wound, or infected area.

cigarette d., Penrose d., a drain made by drawing a small strip of gauze or surgical sponge into a tube of gutta-percha.

drainage (drān'ij) systematic withdrawal of fluids and discharges from a wound, sore, or cavity.

capillary d., that effected by strands of hair, catgut, spun glass, or other material of small caliber which acts by capillary attraction.

closed d., drainage of an empyema cavity carried out with protection against the entrance of outside air into the pleural cavity.

open d., drainage of an empyema cavity through an opening in the chest wall into which one or more rubber drainage tubes are inserted, the opening not being sealed against the entrance of outside air.

postural d., therapeutic drainage in bronchiectasis, chronic bronchitis, and lung abscess by placing the patient head downward so that the trachea will be inclined downward and below the affected area (see also POSTURAL DRAINAGE).

tidal d., drainage of the urinary bladder by an apparatus that alternately fills the bladder to a predetermined pressure and empties it by a combination of siphonage and gravity flow.

dram (dram) a unit of weight in the avoirdupois (27.344 grains, $\frac{1}{16}$ ounce) or apothecaries' (60 grains, $\frac{1}{8}$ ounce) system; symbol ʒ.

fluid d., a unit of liquid measure of the apothecaries' system, containing 60 minims, and equivalent to 3.697 ml. (See also Table of Weights and Measures in the Appendix.) Abbreviated fl. dr.

Dramamine (dram'ah-mēn) trademark for preparation of dimenhydrinate, an antihistamine effective against nausea and vomiting, especially in motion sickness.

dream (drēm) a series of images, emotions, or thoughts occurring during SLEEP.

drepanocyte (drep'ah-no-sīt″) a sickle cell. adj., **drepanocyt'ic.**

drepanocytosis (drep″ah-no-si-to'sis) occurrence of drepanocytes (sickle cells) in the blood.

dressing (dres'ing) any of various materials used for covering and protecting a wound. A pressure dressing is used for maintaining constant pressure, as in the control of bleeding. A protective dressing is applied to shield a part from injury or from septic infection.

APPLICATION AND REMOVAL. All dressings applied should be sterile and must be handled with care to avoid contamination of the wound. Before applying or changing a dressing, assemble all equipment, ointments, salves, or other medications to be used. The wound is cleansed with a mild antiseptic each time a dressing is changed, unless otherwise directed by the physician. The hands are always washed with soap and running water immediately before changing dressings, even if sterile gloves are to be used.

A soiled dressing is removed by starting at the outer edges and releasing tape or other adhesive bandages, pulling *toward* the wound so as to avoid strain or damage to the healing tissues. This is done gently and slowly, and if there is dried exudate holding the dressing to the wound, sterile saline solution is applied until it loosens. All soiled dressings are placed in a paper bag, or wrapped in several thicknesses of newspaper. They are never left in the patient's room. They should be discarded in an incinerator or in a container provided for this purpose in the workroom.

If sterile technique is required for the changing of a dressing, sterile gloves are worn during the procedure. The first step is to open a sterile towel or wrapper and establish a sterile field from which to work. All principles of sterile technique must be observed when handling equipment. Containers of drugs to be applied are opened and the wrappings from dressings to be used are removed. After the equipment is ready and the soiled dressings are removed, the gloves are donned and the clean dressings applied.

Dressings may be held in place by a variety of tapes, bandages, or binders. The type chosen will depend on the location of the wound and the tolerance of the patient's skin to different adhesives. Special straps called Montgomery straps or tapes are best when dressings must be changed frequently. If there is profuse drainage from the wound, absorbent pads may be applied and then covered with a moisture-proof dressing. After the procedure is completed all equipment is removed and the patient's unit is left in order. The hands should be washed immediately after leaving the patient's room or unit.

drift (drift) a chance variation, as in gene frequency from one generation to another; the smaller the population, the greater are the random variations.

Drinalfa (drin-al'fah) trademark for preparations of methamphetamine, a central nervous system stimulant.

Drinker respirator (drink'er) a type of VENTILATOR that provides controlled, automatic breathing for a patient whose respiratory muscles are paralyzed (see also IRON LUNG).

drip (drip) the slow, drop-by-drop infusion of a liquid.

Murphy d., the continuous drop-by-drop administration per rectum of a saline solution.

postnasal d., drainage of excessive mucous or mucopurulent discharge from the postnasal region into the pharynx.

Drisdol (driz'dol) trademark for preparations of crystalline vitamin D (ergocalciferol).

drive (drīv) the force that activates human impulses.

Drolban (drol'ban) trademark for a preparation of dromostanolone.

dromostanolone (dro″mo-stan'o-lōn) an androgenic, anabolic steroid compound; used in the form of the propionate ester as an antineoplastic in the treatment of carcinoma of the breast.

dromotropic (dro″mo-trop'ik) affecting conductivity of a nerve fiber.

drop (drop) 1. a minute sphere of liquid as it hangs or falls. 2. a descent or falling below the usual position.

d. foot, a condition in which the foot hangs in a plantar-flexed position, due to lesion of the peroneal nerve.

droperidol (dro-per'ĭ-dol) a tranquilizer of the butyrophenone series, used as a narcoleptic preanesthetic and, in combination with fentanyl citrate, as a neuroleptanalgesic.

droplet infection (drop'let) infection due to inhalation of respiratory pathogens suspended on liquid particles exhaled from someone already infected.

dropper (drop'er) a pipet or tube for dispensing liquids in drops.

dropsical (drop'sĭ-kal) affected with or pertaining to dropsy.

dropsy (drop'se) an abnormal accumulation of serous fluid in a body cavity or in the cellular tissues; called also hydrops.

drowning (drown'ing) death from suffocation resulting from aspiration of water or other substance or fluid. Drowning occurs because the liquid prevents breathing. The lungs of a drowned person contain very little water or other liquid.

First-aid measures are begun as soon as the individual is rescued from the water. He should not be allowed to walk or remain standing if he has undergone a prolonged struggle to stay afloat because of the strain on his heart. Shock should be prevented by keeping the victim in a prone position with the head lower than the rest of the body. Blankets and other coverings are used only to prevent loss of body heat; the victim should not be kept overwarm. *No time should be lost in administering* ARTIFICIAL RESPIRATION *to anyone who has stopped breathing.* If the victim is unconscious but still breathing, he should be placed in a reclining position, preferably on his side. If the victim is not breathing and there is no evidence of a heart beat, CARDIOPULMONARY RESUSCITATION is begun immediately.

Dr.P.H. Doctor of Public Health.

drug (drug) 1. any medicinal substance. 2. a narcotic. 3. to administer a drug.

d. abuse, the use of one or more drugs for purposes other than those for which they are prescribed or recommended. The major groups of drugs and medicines generally considered to be most commonly misused in the United States are stimulants ("uppers"), depressants ("downers"), psychedelics, and narcotics.

The stimulants affect the central nervous system, producing increased physical and mental activity, excitability, and prevention of sleep. Among the more popular stimulants are the amphetamines, for example methamphetamine, or "speed." Prolonged use of these drugs can lead to acute toxic psychosis accompanied by hallucinations and delusions.

The depressant drugs favored by drug abusers are the babiturates, tranquilizers, and alcohol. Their effect is opposite to that of stimulants and they often are taken as a means of "coming down" from a "high" produced by a stimulant. Sudden withdrawal from depressants can cause convulsions and even death. Combinations of barbiturates and alcohol, which compound the effect of each other, frequently lead to death.

Probably the best known of the psychedelic drugs is LSD (lysergic acid diethylamide). Its use has declined in recent years because of public awareness of its long-term, if not permanent effects, on the psyche, producing "flashbacks" of an acute psychotic state, and its implication in chromosomal damage. Another popular psychedelic drug is mescaline, which is derived from the peyote cactus.

The narcotic drugs of choice for the addict or drug abuser are heroin and cocaine. Both of these drugs are extremely potent, highly addictive, and frequently present the complication of overdose.

MARIJUANA is a controversial drug that is thought by many authorities to be the least dangerous of all drugs commonly used by drug abusers. Extensive research has not as yet led to valid conclusions about the physical or mental health hazards presented by marijuana.

There is little evidence to substantiate the frequently heard claim that experimentation with "soft" drugs, such as marijuana, will lead to stronger drugs and narcotic addiction. There is no denying that many narcotic addicts do begin by abuse of milder drugs and experimentation with their effects on them. However, many factors enter into drug addiction, including individual personality, life style, social environment, and physical status. (See also HABITUATION.)

d. addiction, a state of periodic or chronic intoxication produced by the repeated consumption of a drug, characterized by (1) an overwhelming desire or need (compulsion) to continue use of the drug and to obtain it by any means, (2) a tendency to increase the dosage, (3) a psychological and usually a physical dependence on its effects, and (4) a detrimental effect on the individual and on society.

REASONS FOR ADDICTION. Addiction can result from extensive exposure to drugs for the relief of pain, although this is not common. The majority of persons who become addicted do so because of psychologic or emotional needs to avoid facing deep personal problems. The use of drugs can create a false sense of well-being that temporarily, if inadequately, helps the user to escape from his problems. The use of drugs for this purpose only adds to a person's difficulties, because he is faced with additional problems of obtaining a supply of drugs through illegal sources. The main purpose in an addict's life frequently centers on how to obtain the money necessary to purchase more drugs for his addiction. Because of this, many addicts resort to criminal acts in their effort to maintain their addiction.

WITHDRAWAL AND TREATMENT. There are differences of opinion on the treatment methods of withdrawal from narcotic addiction. The most extreme method, often known as "cold turkey," is abrupt and uncomfortable. It is the natural process that occurs when no more drugs are taken. This method often occurs in jail when the addict is arrested for possessing drugs. In such instances, facilities are usually not available for gradual withdrawal and the addict goes through abrupt withdrawal on his own.

If the narcotic addict's dosage has been mild, his withdrawal is equally mild and may include yawning, sneezing, watering eyes, perspiring, and running nose. In the case of the heavy user, the symptoms become increasingly severe. These include severe cramps, vomiting, diarrhea, and muscle spasms. Withdrawal in this manner lasts approximately 2 to 4 days. Since he cannot eat, an addict may lose 5 to 10 lb. during this period.

In the controlled withdrawal method, under the supervision of a physician, a synthetic drug, such as methadone, is substituted for the narcotic, and the dosage is gradually decreased over a period of about 10 days.

HELP FOR THE ADDICT. Help available to the addict who wants to be cured of his addiction varies throughout the United States. The federal government maintains two Public Health Service hospitals, at Fort Worth, Tex., and Lexington, Ky., where treatment for addiction to opiates or habituation to marijuana or cocaine is given to volunteer applicants. These institutions are augmented by community and private facilities. The majority of addicts are found in metropolitan areas where drugs are more likely to be available and the addict is less noticeable.

In most of the major cities treatment is available in the larger hospitals, in many of which beds are available for controlled withdrawal. The amount of help or treatment available varies greatly. Some hospitals maintain a staff of psychiatrists, psychologists, and social workers who offer the addict treatment for his psychologic addiction and help him to look realistically at some of the problems that drove him to drugs. Many of these treatment programs are known as "aftercare" because the addict returns regularly for additional care following his release from the hospital. For those addicts who are sent to prison, similar programs of individual and group treatment are offered to help him prepare for his return to the community.

The crucial period in the addict's adjustment following withdrawal is his attempt to find a place in community life. Job-hunting is difficult because he is often unable to explain his periods of unemployment and hospitalization. Many social service agencies offer treatment and support to these individuals during this period. It is often the difficulty in readjusting to community life that leads the addict to return to his previous habit of drug-taking.

d. eruption, dermatitis medicamentosa.

d. interaction, modification of the potency of one drug by another (or others) taken concurrently or sequentially. Some drug interactions are harmful and some may have therapeutic benefits. Present knowledge of drug interactions is limited and no single chart of drug interactions can be completely accurate in predicting the effects of a drug combination on an individual patient. For this reason any person responsible for administration of medications must be ever alert to the possibility of dangerous drug interaction any time drugs are given in combination. It is recommended that a clinical pharmacologist be consulted whenever the possibility of incompatibility is suspected in a multiple-drug regimen.

Additives, for example, in an intravenous infusion may produce an adverse chemical interaction. Factors influencing these interactions include pH and chemical composition, especially the various buffering, stabilizing, and preserving chemicals present in commercially prepared intravenous solutions. Due to the variety and volume of drugs and chemicals available and the high potential of incompatibility, it is recommended that admixtures be restricted to a single additive in each intravenous solution administered.

Drugs may also interact with various foods. In general, these interactions fall into three categories: (1) food malabsorption; (2) nutritional status; and (3) alteration of drug response by nutrients. In teaching patients self-care in the taking of prescribed medications, one should explain the need for meticulously following directions related to the intake of food and drink while the medication regimen is being followed.

d. rash, dermatitis medicamentosa.

druggist (drug'ist) pharmacist.

drum (drum) the cavity of the middle ear, closed by the TYMPANIC MEMBRANE, to which the term eardrum is commonly applied.

drusen (droo'sen) 1. hyaline excrescences in Bruch's membrane, the inner layer of the choroid of the eye, usually due to aging. 2. rosettes of granules occurring in the lesions of actinomycosis.

dry ice (dri īs) carbon dioxide snow.

duazomycin (du-az″o-mi'sin) an antibiotic substance with antineoplastic properties, produced by *Streptomyces ambofaciens.*

Dubin-Johnson syndrome (doo'bin jon'son) hereditary chronic nonhemolytic jaundice thought to be due to defective excretion of conjugated bilirubin and certain other organic anions by the liver; a brown coarsely granular pigment in hepatic cells is pathognomonic.

Dubini's chorea (disease) (du-be'nēz) an acute, fatal form of electric chorea caused by acute infection of the central nervous system.

Duchenne's disease (du-shenz') 1. spinal muscular atrophy. 2. bulbar paralysis. 3. tabes dorsalis.

Duchenne's muscular dystrophy (du-shenz') the childhood type of MUSCULAR DYSTROPHY.

Duchenne's paralysis (du-shenz') 1. Erb-Duchenne paralysis. 2. progressive bulbar paralysis.

Duchenne-Aran disease (du-shen' ar-ahn') spinal muscular atrophy.

Ducubee (doo'ko-be) trademark for preparations of vitamin B_{12}.

duct (dukt) a passage with well-defined walls, especially a tubular structure for the passage of excretions or secretions. adj., **duc'tal.**

alveolar d's, small passages connecting the respiratory bronchioles and the alveolar sacs.

d. of Bartholin, the larger and longer of the sublingual ducts.

bile d's, biliary d's, the passages for the conveyance of bile in and from the liver (see also BILE DUCTS).

cochlear d., a spiral membranous tube in the bony canal of the cochlea divided into the scala tympani, scala vestibuli, and spiral lamina.

common bile d., a duct formed by the union of the cystic and hepatic ducts (see also BILE DUCTS).

cystic d., the passage connecting the gallbladder neck and the common bile duct.

efferent d., any duct that gives outlet to a glandular secretion.

ejaculatory d., the duct formed by union of the ductus deferens and the duct of the seminal vesicles, opening into the prostatic urethra on the colliculus seminalis.

endolymphatic d., a canal connecting the membranous labyrinth of the ear with the endolymphatic sac.

excretory d., one through which the secretion is conveyed from a gland.

hepatic d., the excretory duct of the liver, or one of its branches in the lobes of the liver (see also BILE DUCTS).

lacrimal d., the excretory duct of the lacrimal gland (see also LACRIMAL CANALICULUS and LACRIMAL APPARATUS).

lacrimonasal d., nasal duct.

lactiferous d's, ducts conveying the milk secreted by the lobes of the breast to and through the nipples.

lymphatic d., left, thoracic duct.

lymphatic d., right, a vessel draining lymph from the upper right side of the body, receiving lymph from the right subclavian, jugular, and mediastinal trunks when those vessels do not open independently into the right brachiocephalic vein.

mammary d., lactiferous ducts.

mesonephric d., an embryonic duct of the mesonephros, which in the male becomes the ductus deferens and in the female is largely obliterated.

müllerian d., either of the two paired embryonic ducts developing into the vagina, uterus, and uterine tubes, and becoming largely obliterated in the male.

nasal d., nasolacrimal d., the downward continuation of the lacrimal sac, opening on the lateral wall of the inferior meatus of the nose (see also LACRIMAL APPARATUS).

pancreatic d., the main excretory duct of the pancreas, which usually unites with the common bile duct before entering the duodenum at the major duodenal papilla (see also BILE DUCTS).

papillary d's, the straight excretory or collecting portions of the renal tubules, which descend through the renal medulla to a renal papilla.

paramesonephric d., müllerian duct.

paraurethral d's, Skene's glands.

parotid d., the duct by which the parotid glands empty into the mouth (see also PAROTID DUCT).

prostatic d's, minute ducts from the prostate, opening into or near the prostatic sinuses on the posterior wall of the urethra.

salivary d's, the ducts of the salivary glands.

semicircular d's, the long ducts of the membranous labyrinth of the ear.

seminal d's, the passages for conveyance of spermatozoa and semen.

sublingual d's, the excretory ducts of the sublingual salivary glands.

submandibular d., submaxillary d., the duct that drains the submandibular gland and opens at the sublingual caruncle.

tear d., lacrimal duct.

thoracic d., a duct beginning in the cisterna chyli and emptying into the venous system at the junction of the left subclavian and left internal jugular veins. It acts as a channel for the collection of lymph from the portions of the body below the diaphragm and from the left side of the body above the diaphragm.

ductile (duk′til) susceptible of being drawn out without breaking.

ductless (dukt′les) having no excretory duct.

ductule (duk′tūl) a minute duct.

ductulus (duk′tu-lus), pl. *duc′tuli* [L.] ductule.

ductus (duk′tus), pl. *duc′tus* [L.] duct.

d. arterio′sus, a fetal blood vessel that joins the aorta and pulmonary artery.

d. arterio′sus, patent, abnormal persistence of an open lumen in the ductus arteriosus after birth (see also PATENT DUCTUS ARTERIOSUS).

d. def′erens, the excretory duct of the testis, which joins the excretory duct of the seminal vesicle to form the ejaculatory duct; called also vas deferens.

d. veno′sus, a major blood channel that develops through the embryonic liver from the left umbilical vein to the inferior vena cava.

Duke's disease (dūks) a febrile disease of childhood marked by an exanthematous eruption, probably a mild form of scarlet fever.

Dulcolax (dul′ko-laks) trademark for preparations of bisacodyl, a laxative.

dullness (dul′nes) a quality of sound elicited by percussion, being short and high-pitched with little resonance.

dumb (dum) unable to speak; mute.

dumping syndrome (dum′ping) nausea, weakness, sweating, palpitation, syncope, often a sensation of warmth, and sometimes diarrhea, occurring after ingestion of food in patients who have had partial gastrectomy (see also surgery of the STOMACH).

duodenal (du″o-de′nal) of or pertaining to the duodenum.

d. ulcer, peptic ulcer of the duodenum (see also ULCER).

duodenectomy (du″o-dĕ-nek′to-me) excision of the duodenum, total or partial.

duodenitis (du″o-dĕ-ni′tis) inflammation of the duodenum.

duodenocholedochotomy (du″o-de″no-ko-led″o-kot′o-me) incision of the duodenum and common bile duct.

duodenoenterostomy (du″o-de″no-en″ter-os′to-me) anastomosis of the duodenum to some other part of the small intestine.

duodenography (du″o-dĕ-nog′rah-fe) radiography of the duodenum.

duodenohepatic (du″o-de″no-hĕ-pat′ik) pertaining to the duodenum and liver.

duodenoileostomy (du″o-de″no-il″e-os′to-me) anastomosis of the duodenum to the ileum.

duodenojejunostomy (du″o-de″no-je″joo-nos′to-me) anastomosis of the duodenum to the jejunum.

duodenorrhaphy (du″o-dĕ-nor′ah-fe) suture of the duodenum.

duodenoscopy (du″o-dĕ-nos′ko-pe) examination of the duodenum by an endoscope.

duodenostomy (du″o-dĕ-nos′to-me) surgical formation of a permanent opening into the duodenum.

duodenotomy (du″o-dĕ-not′o-me) incision of the duodenum.

duodenum (du″o-de′num) the first or proximal portion of the small intestine, extending from the pylorus to the jejunum. It is about 10 inches long. It plays an important role in digestion of food because both the common bile duct and the pancreatic duct empty into it. (See also DIGESTIVE SYSTEM.) It is subject to various disorders, the most common of which are peptic ULCER and obstruction due to dilatation of the intestine and stasis of the duodenal contents. The duodenum also may be the site of diverticula, fistulas and, rarely, tumors.

Duphaston (du-fas′ton) trademark for a preparation of dydrogesterone, a progestin.

duplication (du-plĭ-ka′shun) a doubling; in genetics, the presence of an extra segment of chromosome.

dupp (dup) a syllable used to represent, or mimic the second sound heard at the apex of the heart in auscultation (see also LUBB-DUPP).

Dupuytren's contracture (du-pwe-trahnz′) a flexion deformity of the fingers or toes, due to shortening, thickening, and fibrosis of the palmar or plantar fascia.

Dupuytren's fracture (du-pwe-trahnz′) Pott's fracture.

Durabolin (du-rab′o-lin) trademark for a preparation of nandrolone, an androgenic, anabolic steroid.

Duracillin (du″rah-sil′in) trademark for preparations of crystalline procaine penicillin G.

dural (du′ral) pertaining to the dura mater.

dura mater (du′rah ma′ter) [L.] the outermost, toughest and most fibrous of the three membranes (meninges) covering the brain and spinal cord.

Durand-Nicolas-Favre disease (du-ran′ ne-ko-lah fav′r) lymphogranuloma venereum.

Durham's tube (dur′hamz) a jointed tracheotomy tube.

duroarachnitis (du″ro-ar″ak-ni′tis) inflammation of the dura mater and arachnoid.

Duroziez's disease (du-ro″ze-āz′) congenital mitral stenosis.

Duroziez's murmur (sign) (du-ro″ze-āz) in aortic insufficiency, a double murmur over the femoral artery or other large peripheral artery.

Duverney's fracture (du-ver-nāz′) fracture of the ilium just below the anterior inferior spine.

D.V.M. Doctor of Veterinary Medicine.

dwarf (dwarf) an abnormally undersized person.

dwarfism (dwar′fizm) the state of being a dwarf; underdevelopment of the body. Dwarfism may be the result of a developmental anomaly, of nutritional or hormone deficiencies, or of other diseases. The size of pygmies found in some parts of the world, such as the Philippines and equatorial Africa, is not the result of dwarfism; their small stature is a hereditary trait.

A dwarf in adulthood may be as small as 2½ feet tall. The proportions of body to head and limbs may be normal or abnormal. The dwarf may also be deformed, and may suffer from mental retardation, depending on the cause of his condition.

Achondroplasia is a developmental anomaly that affects the growth of the bones. The patient's trunk is usually normal, but his head is unusually large and his arms and legs unusually small. Most fetuses with achondroplasia are stillborn. Those who reach adulthood do not suffer any lessening of their mental or sexual abilities, and may have unusual muscular strength. Achondroplasia does not significantly shorten the patient's life span.

An infant who suffers from an insufficiency of thyroxine, a hormone secreted by the thyroid gland, may develop the symptoms of CRETINISM. These include an enlarged head, short limbs, puffy eyes, a thick and protruding tongue, very dry skin, and lack of coordination. Cretinism can be treated by giving the patient an extract of thyroxine; early treatment can result in normal growth and development. If the condition is not treated, however, the child will grow up dwarfed, mentally retarded, and sexually sterile.

Growth hormone, a hormone that plays a major role in the process of growth is produced in the pituitary gland. If this hormone is not produced in sufficient quantity, the patient's growth will be abnormally slight, although his head and limbs will be in normal proportion to his small torso. Administration of purified human growth hormone has been shown to induce skeletal growth in patients with pituitary dwarfism.

Dy chemical symbol, *dysprosium.*

Dyclone (di′klōn) trademark for preparations of dyclonine.

dyclonine (di′klo-nēn) a topical anesthetic, used as the hydrochloride salt.

dydrogesterone (di″dro-jes′ter-ōn) a synthetic progestin, used orally in treatment of amenorrhea and of abnormal uterine bleeding due to hormonal imbalance.

dye (di) any of various colored substances containing auxochromes and thus capable of coloring substances to which they are applied; used for staining and coloring, as test reagents, and as therapeutic agents.

Dymelor (di′mĕ-lor) trademark for acetohexamide, an oral hypoglycemic agent.

dynamic (di-nam′ik) pertaining to or manifesting force.

dynamics (di-nam′iks) 1. the scientific study of forces in action; a phase of mechanics. 2. the motivating or driving forces, physical or moral, in any field.

dynamograph (di-nam′o-graf) a self-registering dynamometer.

dynamometer (di″nah-mom′ĕ-ter) an instrument for measuring the force of muscular contraction.

dynamoneure (di-nam′o-nūr) a spinal neuron connected with the muscles.

dyne (dīn) the metric unit of force, being that amount which would, during each second, produce an acceleration of 1 cm. per second in a particle of 1 gram mass.

dyphilline (di-fil′lin) a theophylline compound used as a diuretic and as a bronchodilator and peripheral vasodilator.

dys- prefix [Gr.], *bad; difficult; disordered.*

dysacousia, dysacousis (dis″ah-koo′se-ah; dis″-ah-koo′sis) dysacusis.

dysacusis (dis″ah-koo′sis) 1. a hearing impairment in which the loss is not measurable in decibels, as in disturbances in discrimination of speech or tone quality, pitch, loudness, etc. 2. a condition in which certain sounds produce discomfort.

dysadrenalism, dysadrenia (dis″ad-re′nal-izm; dis″ah-dre′ne-ah) any disorder of adrenal function, whether of decreased or heightened function.

dysaphia (dis-a′fe-ah) impairment of the sense of touch.

dysarthria (dis-ar′thre-ah) imperfect articulation of speech due to disturbances of muscular control resulting from central or peripheral nervous system damage.

dysarthrosis (dis″ar-thro′sis) 1. deformity or malformation of a joint. 2. dysarthria.

dysaudia (dis-aw′de-ah) impaired hearing.

dysautonomia (dis″aw-to-no′me-ah) a hereditary condition marked by defective lacrimation, skin blotching, emotional instability, motor incoordination, and hyporeflexia.

dysbarism (dis′bar-izm) any clinical syndrome

caused by difference between the surrounding atmospheric pressure and the total gas pressure in the various tissues, fluids, and cavities of the body, including such conditions as barosinusitis, barotitis media, or expansion of gases in the hollow viscera.

dysbasia (dis-ba′ze-ah) difficulty in walking, especially that due to a nervous lesion.

dysbulia (dis-bu′le-ah) weakness or perversion of the will. adj., **dysbu′lic.**

dyscephaly (dis-sef′ah-le) malformation of the cranium and bones of the face. adj., **dyscephal′ic.**

dyschiria (dis-ki′re-ah) loss of power to tell which side of the body has been touched.

dyscholia (dis-ko′le-ah) a disordered condition of the bile.

dyschondroplasia (dis″kon-dro-pla′ze-ah) enchondromatosis.

dyschromatopsia (dis″kro-mah-top′se-ah) disorder of color vision.

dyschromia (dis-kro′me-ah) any disorder of pigmentation of the skin or hair.

dyschronism (dis-kro′nizm) separate in time; disturbance of any time relation.

dyscoria (dis-ko′re-ah) abnormality in shape or form of the pupil or in the reaction of the two pupils.

dyscorticism (dis-kor′tĭ-sizm) disordered functioning of the adrenal cortex.

dyscrasia (dis-kra′ze-ah) a morbid condition, usually referring to an imbalance of component elements. adj., **dyscrat′ic.**

blood d., any abnormal or pathologic condition of the blood.

dysdiadochokinesia (dis″di-ah-do″ko-ki-ne′ze-ah) derangement of the function of diadochokinesia. adj., **dysdiadochokinet′ic.**

dysembryoma (dis″em-bre-o′mah) teratoma.

dysentery (dis′en-ter″e) any of a number of disorders marked by inflammation of the intestine, especially of the colon, with abdominal pain, tenesmus, and frequent stools often containing blood and mucus. The causative agent may be chemical irritants, bacteria, protozoa, viruses, or parasitic worms. adj., **dysenter′ic.** Dysentery is less prevalent today than in years past because of improved sanitary facilities throughout the world; it was formerly a common occurrence in crowded parts of the world and it particularly plagued army camps. It can be dangerous to infants, children, the elderly, and others who are in a weakened condition.

In dysentery, there is an unusually fluid discharge of stool from the bowels, as well as fever, stomach cramps, and spasms of involuntary straining to evacuate, with the passage of little feces. The stool is often mixed with pus and mucus and may be streaked with blood.

amebic d., a form common in tropical countries but also found in temperate areas, including the United States; caused by the protozoon *Entamoeba hystolytica.* It is usually less acute and violent than bacillary dysentery, but it frequently becomes chronic and causes unexplained attacks of diarrhea over a long period of time. It rarely causes death, but complications may result, including involvement of the liver, liver abscess, and pulmonary abscess. Drugs used in treatment include emetine hydrochloride and chloroquine, among others.

bacillary d., the most common and violent form of the disease, caused by bacteria of the genus *Shigella.*

Bacillary dysentery is most common in the tropics, the subtropics, and the Orient. It can be fatal, especially among children. It can erupt anyplace where sanitation is poor and large groups of people, including carriers of the disease, are crowded together.

The disease is spread through the feces of carriers who have the bacteria in their intestines. These carriers may be suffering from diarrhea or dysentery, or they may seem perfectly well and still carry the disease. It is transmitted by eating or drinking from anything contaminated with the bacteria from the feces of these carriers. Even touching something contaminated and then touching the mouth can cause infection. Flies also spread the disease.

Attacks of bacillary dysentery are always acute after the incubation period of a few days. Temperature may rise as high as 104° F. (40° C.), sometimes with symptoms of dehydration, shock, and delirium. Bowel movements may be as many as 30 to 40 a day. Running its normal course, without special medicines, it is usually over within a few weeks from its outset, although an attack in a child may be more serious and last longer.

Antibiotics such as chlortetracycline (Aureomycin) and chloramphenicol are usually effective in relieving the symptoms and controlling bacillary dysentery in a day or two. They often completely cure it in that time. Sulfonamides, such as sulfadiazine, are less effective because of the emergence of resistant strains of bacteria. With proper care, a violent attack may be over in a few days.

The greatest threat of dysentery is from DEHYDRATION. This condition is combated with intravenous administration of fluids and electrolytes lost in the watery stools.

Although the usual dysenteric illness may last a few weeks if not treated with special medicines, symptoms of intestinal ulceration, diarrhea, and painful spasms in evacuating may in a few cases continue for a longer time.

viral d., a form caused by a virus, occurring in epidemics and marked by acute watery diarrhea. It is common in travelers who have eaten raw salads or fruit, or used contaminated tableware. With proper care, it should subside in 12 to 72 hours.

dyserethesia (dis″er-ĕ-the′ze-ah) impairment of sensibility.

dysergasia (dis″er-ga′ze-ah) a behavior disorder due to organic changes in the nervous system, with disorientation, hallucination, and delirious reactions.

dysergia (dis-er′je-ah) motor incoordination due to defect of efferent nerve impulse.

dysesthesia (dis″es-the′ze-ah) 1. impairment of any sense, especially of the sense of touch. 2. a painful, persistent sensation induced by a gentle touch of the skin.

dysfunction (dis-fungk′shun) disturbance, impairment, or abnormality of functioning of an organ.

dysgalactia (dis″gah-lak′she-ah) disordered milk secretion.

dysgammaglobulinemia (dis-gam″mah-glob″u-lin-e′me-ah) an immunological deficiency state marked by selective deficiencies of one or more, but not all, classes of immunoglobulins, resulting in heightened susceptibility to those infectious diseases vulnerable to immunoglobulin-associated defense mechanisms. adj., **dysgammaglobuline′mic.**

dysgenesis (dis-jen′ĕ-sis) defective development; malformation.

gonadal d., any of a variety of gonadal developmental anomalies, including gonadal dysplasia, Turner's syndrome, etc.

dysgenics (dis-jen′iks) the study of racial deterioration.

dysgerminoma (dis-jer″mĭ-no′mah) a solid, often radiosensitive, malignant ovarian neoplasm derived from undifferentiated germinal cells; the counterpart of seminoma of the testis.

dysgeusia (dis-gu′ze-ah) impairment of the sense of taste.

dysglobulinemia (dis-glob″u-lin-e′me-ah) any disorder of the serum globulins.

dysglycemia (dis″gli-se′me-ah) any disorder of blood sugar metabolism.

dysgnathia (dis-na′the-ah) any oral abnormality extending beyond the teeth to involve the maxilla or mandible, or both. adj., **dysgnath′ic.**

dysgnosia (dis-no′ze-ah) any abnormality of the intellect.

dysgonic (dis-gon′ik) seeding badly; said of bacterial cultures that grow poorly.

dysgraphia (dis-gra′fe-ah) inability to write properly; it may be part of a language disorder due to disturbance of the parietal lobe or of the motor system.

dyshematopoiesis (dis-hem″ah-to-poi-e′sis) defective blood formation. adj., **dyshematopoiet′ic.**

dyshidrosis (dis″hĭ-dro′sis) 1. a skin eruption on the sides of the digits or on the palms and soles (see also POMPHOLYX). 2. any disorder of the eccrine sweat glands.

dysjunction (dis-junk′shun) see DISJUNCTION.

dyskaryosis (dis″kar-e-o′sis) abnormality of the nucleus of a cell. adj., **dyskaryot′ic.**

dyskeratoma (dis″ker-ah-to′mah) a dyskeratotic tumor.

warty d., a solitary brownish red nodule with a soft, yellowish, central keratotic plug, most commonly occurring on the face, neck, scalp, or axilla, or in the mouth; histologically it resembles an individual lesion of keratosis follicularis.

dyskeratosis (dis″ker-ah-to′sis) abnormal, premature, or imperfect keratinization of the keratinocytes. adj., **dyskeratot′ic.**

dyskinesia (dis-ki-ne′ze-ah) impairment of the power of voluntary movement.

dyslalia (dis-la′le-ah) impairment of ability to speak associated with abnormality of external speech organs.

dyslexia (dis-lek′se-ah) impairment of ability to comprehend written language, due to a central lesion. adj., **dyslex′ic.**

dyslochia (dis-lo′ke-ah) disordered lochial discharge.

dyslogia (dis-lo′je-ah) impairment of the power of reasoning; also, impairment of speech, due to mental disorders.

dysmaturity (dis″mah-tūr′ĭ-te) the condition of being small or immature for gestational age; said of fetuses that are the product of a pregnancy involving placental dysfunction.

pulmonary d., Wilson-Mikity syndrome.

dysmelia (dis-me′le-ah) malformation of a limb or limbs due to disturbance in embryonic development.

dysmenorrhea (dis″men-ŏ-re′ah) painful menstruation. adj., **dysmenorrhe′al.** Dysmenorrhea is characterized by cramplike pains in the lower abdomen, and sometimes accompanied by headache, irritability, mental depression, malaise, and fatigue. There are a variety of causes, but in many cases the factors involved may be extremely elusive. Relief can often be obtained by simple hygienic measures such as adequate rest, avoidance of constipation, moderate exercise, applications of moderate heat to the abdomen, and removal of restricting clothing. Analgesics may be helpful. Hormone therapy may be required. Surgical procedures are rarely indicated unless a tumor or other demonstrable cause can be found.

congestive d., that accompanied by great congestion of the uterus.

essential d., painful menstruation for which there is no demonstrable cause.

inflammatory d., that due to inflammation.

membranous d., that marked by membranous exfoliation derived from the uterus.

obstructive d., that due to mechanical obstruction to the discharge of menstrual fluid.

dysmetria (dis-me′tre-ah) inability to properly direct or limit motions.

dysmimia (dis-mim′e-ah) impairment of the power to express thoughts by gestures.

dysmnesia (dis-ne′ze-ah) disordered memory.

dysmyotonia (dis″mi-o-to′ne-ah) muscular dystonia; abnormal tonicity.

dysodontiasis (dis″o-don-ti′ah-sis) defective, delayed, or difficult eruption of the teeth.

dysontogenesis (dis″on-to-jen′ĕ-sis) defective embryonic development. adj., **dysontogenet′ic.**

dysopia (dis-o′pe-ah) defective vision.

dysorexia (dis″o-rek′se-ah) impaired or deranged appetite.

dysosmia (dis-oz′me-ah) impairment of the sense of smell.

dysostosis (dis″os-to′sis) defective ossification; a defect in the normal ossification of fetal cartilages.

cleidocranial d., a hereditary condition in which there is defective ossification of the cranial bones, complete or partial absence of the clavicles, so that the shoulders may be brought together, or nearly together, in front, and dental and vertebral anomalies.

craniofacial d., a hereditary condition marked by acrocephaly, exophthalmos, hypertelorism, strabismus, parrot-beaked nose, and hypoplastic maxilla with relative mandibular prognathism. Called also Crouzon's disease.

mandibulofacial d., a hereditary disorder occurring in a complete form (Franceschetti's syndrome) with antimongoloid slant of the palpebral fissures, coloboma of the lower lid, micrognathia and hypoplasia of the zygomatic arches, and microtia, and in an incomplete form (Treacher Collins syndrome) with the same anomalies in lesser degree.

metaphyseal d., a skeletal abnormality in which the epiphyses are normal or nearly so, and the metaphyseal tissues are replaced by masses of cartilage, producing interference with endochondral bone formation and expansion and thinning of the metaphyseal cortices.

orodigitofacial d., orofaciodigital syndrome.

dyspancreatism (dis-pan′kre-ah-tizm″) disorder of function of the pancreas.

dyspareunia (dis″pah-ru′ne-ah) difficult or painful coitus in women.

dyspepsia (dis-pep′se-ah) impairment of the power or function of digestion; usually applied to epigastric discomfort after meals. adj., **dyspep′tic.**

acid d., dyspepsia associated with excessive acidity of the stomach.

dysphagia (dis-fa′je-ah) difficulty in swallowing.

dysphasia (dis-fa′ze-ah) impairment of speech consisting in lack of coordination and failure to arrange words in their proper order; due to a central lesion.

dysphemia (dis-fe′me-ah) stuttering or other speech disorder due to psychoneurosis.

dysphonia (dis-fo′ne-ah) any voice impairment; difficulty in speaking. adj., **dysphon′ic.**

d. clerico′rum loss of the voice from overuse, as by clergymen.

dysphoria (dis-fo′re-ah) disquiet; restlessness; malaise.

dysphrasia (dis-fra′ze-ah) imperfection of speech due to a central or cerebral defect.

dyspigmentation (dis″pig-men-ta′shun) any abnormality of pigmentation of the skin or hair.

dysplasia (dis-pla′ze-ah) an abnormality of development; in pathology, alteration in size, shape, and organization of adult cells. adj., **dysplas′tic.**

congenital alveolar d., respiratory distress of the newborn.

cretinoid d., a developmental abnormality characteristic of cretinism, consisting of retarded ossification and smallness of the internal and reproductive organs.

fibrous d. (of bone), thinning of the cortex of bone and replacement of bone marrow by gritty fibrous tissue containing bony spicules, causing pain, disability, and gradually increasing deformity; it may affect a single bone (monostotic fibrous dysplasia) or several or many bones (polyostotic fibrous dysplasia).

dyspnea (disp-ne′ah) labored or difficult breathing. adj., **dyspne′ic.** Dyspnea is a symptom of a variety of disorders and is primarily an indication of inadequate ventilation, or of insufficient amounts of oxygen in the circulating blood.

Physical exertion can produce dyspnea, as can hypoxia such as that experienced at high altitudes. Pathologic conditions that lead to dyspnea include: acute respiratory diseases and CHRONIC OBSTRUCTIVE PULMONARY DISEASE, such as asthma and bronchitis; defects in the lungs or chest wall which restrict lung expansion; and heart diseases, such as CONGESTIVE HEART FAILURE, which decrease the cardiac output.

There are certain respiratory neuroses that are accompanied by dyspnea. The most common of these is HYPERVENTILATION, which can lead to respiratory ALKALOSIS because of a "blowing off" of carbon dioxide.

functional d., respiratory distress not caused by organic disease and unrelated to exertion but associated with anxiety states.

paroxysmal nocturnal d., respiratory distress related to posture (especially reclining at night), usually attributed to congestive heart failure with pulmonary edema.

dyspragia (dis-pra′je-ah) painful performance of any function.

dyspraxia (dis-prak′se-ah) partial loss of ability to perform coordinated movements.

dysprosium (dis-pro′ze-um) a chemical element, atomic number 66, atomic weight 162.50, symbol Dy. (See table of ELEMENTS.)

dysproteinemia (dis-pro″te-in-e′me-ah) disorder of the protein content of the blood.

dysrhythmia (dis-rith′me-ah) disturbance of rhythm.

cerebral d., electroencephalographic d., disturbance or irregularity in the rhythm of the brain waves as recorded by electroencephalography.

dyssebacea (dis″sĕ-ba′she-ah) disorder of sebaceous follicles; specifically, a condition seen (but not exclusively) in riboflavin deficiency, marked by greasy, branny seborrhea on the midface, with erythema in the nasal folds, canthi, or other skin folds.

dysspermia (dis-sper′me-ah) impairment of the spermatozoa, or of the semen.

dysstasia (dis-sta′ze-ah) difficulty in standing. adj., **dysstat′ic.**

dyssynergia (dis″sin-er′je-ah) muscular incoordination.

d. cerebella′ris myoclon′ica, a condition characterized by cerebellar dyssynergia, myoclonus, and epilepsy.

d. cerebella′ris progressi′va, a condition marked by generalized tremors associated with disturbance of muscle tone and of muscular coordination; due to disorder of cerebellar function.

dystectia (dis-tek′she-ah) defective closure of the neural tube.

dysthymia (dis-thi′me-ah) mental depression; also, any intellectual abnormality.

dystocia (dis-to′se-ah) abnormal labor or childbirth.

fetal d., that due to shape, size, or position of the fetus.

maternal d., that due to some condition inherent in the mother.

placental d., difficult delivery of the placenta.

dystonia (dis-to′ne-ah) impairment of muscular tonus. adj., **dyston′ic.**

dystopia (dis-to′pe-ah) malposition; displacement. adj., **dystop′ic.**

dystrophia (dis-tro′fe-ah) [Gr.] dystrophy.

d. adiposogenita′lis, adiposogenital dystrophy.

d. epithelia′lis cor′neae, dystrophy of the corneal epithelium, with erosions.

d. myoton′ica, a rare, slowly pregressive, hereditary disease, marked by myotonia followed by muscular atrophy (especially of the face and neck), cataracts, hypogonadism, frontal balding, and cardiac disorders. Called also myotonia dystrophia.

d. un′guium, changes in the texture, structure, and/or color of the nails due to no demonstrable cause, but presumed by some to be attributable to some disturbance of nutrition.

dystrophoneurosis (dis-trof″o-nu-ro′sis) 1. any nervous disorder due to poor nutrition. 2. impairment of nutrition due to a nervous disorder.

dystrophy (dis'tro-fe) any disorder due to defective or faulty nutrition. adj., **dystroph'ic.**

adiposogenital d., a condition marked by adiposity of the feminine type, genital hypoplasia, changes in secondary sex characters, and metabolic disturbances; seen with lesions of the hypothalamus.

muscular d., progressive muscular d., a group of genetically determined, painless, degenerative myopathies marked by muscular weakness and atrophy without nervous system involvement (see also MUSCULAR DYSTROPHY).

pseudohypertrophic muscular d., muscular dystrophy affecting the shoulder and pelvic girdles, beginning in childhood and marked by increasing weakness, pseudohypertrophy of the muscles, followed by atrophy, and a peculiar swaying gait with the legs kept wide apart. Called also pseudohypertrophic paralysis.

myotonic d., dystrophia myotonica.

dysuria (dis-u're-ah) painful or difficult urination. adj., **dysu'ric.**

E

E. electromotive force, emmetropia, eye.

ear (ēr) the organ of hearing and of equilibrium. (See Plate 15.) The ear is made up of the outer (external) ear, the middle ear, and the inner (internal) ear.

The outer ear consists of the auricle, or pinna, and the external acoustic meatus. The auricle collects sound waves and directs them to the external acoustic meatus which conducts them to the tympanum (the cavity of the middle ear).

The tympanic membrane (eardrum) separates the outer ear from the middle ear. In the middle ear are the three ossicles, the malleus (hammer), incus (anvil), and stapes (stirrup), so called because of their resemblance to these objects. These three small bones form a chain across the middle ear from the tympanum to the oval window in the membrane separating the middle ear from the inner ear. The middle ear is connected to the nasopharynx by the eustachian tube, through which the air pressure on the inner side of the eardrum is equalized with the air pressure on its outside surface. The middle ear is also connected with the cells in the mastoid bone just behind the outer ear. Two muscles attached to the ossicles contract when loud noises strike the tympanic membrane, limiting its vibration and thus protecting it and the inner ear from damage.

In the inner ear (or labyrinth) is the cochlea, containing the nerves that transmit sound to the brain. The inner ear also contains the SEMICIRCULAR CANALS, which are essential to the sense of balance.

When a sound strikes the ear it causes the tympanic membrane to vibrate. The ossicles function as levers, amplifying the motion of the tympanic membrane, and passing the vibrations on to the cochlea. From there the vestibulocochlear (eighth cranial) nerve transmits the vibrations, translated into nerve impulses, to the auditory center in the brain. (See also HEARING.)

DISEASES OF THE EAR. Infections and inflammations of the ear include OTOMYCOSIS, a fungal infection of the outer ear; OTITIS MEDIA, an infection of the middle ear; and MASTOIDITIS, an infection of the mastoid cells. DEAFNESS may result from infection or from other causes such as old age, injury to the ear, or hereditary factors. Another cause of deafness is OTOSCLEROSIS. Disorders of equilibrium may be caused by imperfect functioning of the semicircular canals of the inner ear or from labyrinthitis, an inflammation of the inner ear. MENIÈRE'S DISEASE, believed to result from dilatation of the lymphatic channels in the cochlea, may also cause disturbances in balance.

SURGERY OF THE EAR. Surgical procedures on the ear usually are indicated when chronic infection has resulted in some destruction of the bones of the middle ear or mastoid. An exception is myringotomy, incision of the tympanic membrane, which is sometimes necessary to relieve pressure behind the eardrum and allow for drainage from an inflammatory process in the middle ear. Surgical procedures involving plastic reconstruction of the small bones of the middle ear are extremely delicate and have been made possible by the development of special instruments and technical equipment. STAPEDECTOMY and TYMPANOPLASTY are examples of this type of surgery, which has done much to preserve hearing that would otherwise be lost as a result of infectious destruction or sclerosis of these bones.

Within the past decade techniques have been developed for treatment of sensorineural hearing loss. Although these procedures are still in the experimental stage, it is hoped that such techniques as implantation of elelctronic receivers will offer relief to patients who have profound sensory deafness but some remaining functional nerve cells.

PATIENT CARE. Care following surgery of the ear is aimed at prevention of infection and promoting the comfort of the patient. Since the ear is so close to the brain, it is extremely important to avoid introducing pathogenic organisms into the operative site. The external ear and surrounding skin must be kept scrupulously clean. If the patient's hair is long it should be braided or arranged so that it does not come in contact with the patient's ear and side of the face. Aseptic technique must be used in all procedures carried out immediately before and after surgery.

The patient should be instructed to avoid nose blowing, especially after surgery, when there is a possibility that such an action can alter pressure within the ear. Observation of the patient after surgery of the ear includes watching for signs of injury to the facial nerve. The patient will not be able to wrinkle his forehead, close his eye, pucker his lips, or bare his teeth if the facial nerve has been damaged. This is often a temporary situation resulting from edema, and will subside as the edema is reduced. Some permanent damage may result, however, and signs of facial nerve damage should be reported to the surgeon. Vertigo is another common occurrence after surgery of the ear. It too is usually only temporary and will subside as the operative site heals. The situation does require special protective measures such as side rails, and support of the patient while he is up out of bed, so as to avoid falling and accidental injury.

Most surgeons prefer that the dressings around the ear not be changed during the immediate postoperative period. Should excessive drainage require more dressings, these can be applied over the basic dressing. Any drainage should be noted and recorded and excessive drainage reported immediately to the surgeon.

cauliflower e., a partially deformed auricle due to injury and subsequent perichondritis (see also CAULIFLOWER EAR).

earache (ēr'āk) pain in the ear; otalgia.

eardrum (ēr'drum) tympanic membrane.

earwax (ēr'waks) cerumen.

Eaton agent (e'ton) *Mycoplasma pneumoniae.*

E.B.A.A. Eye Bank Association of America (see EYE BANK.)

Ebner's glands (eb'nerz) serous glands at the back of the tongue near the taste buds.

Ebstein's anomaly (eb'stīnz) a malformation of

the tricuspid valve, usually associated with an atrial septal defect.

eburnation (e″ber-na′shun) conversion of bone into a hard, ivory-like mass.

EBV Epstein-Barr virus.

ecaudate (e-kaw′dāt) tail-less.

ecbolic (ek-bol′ik) oxytocic.

eccentro-osteochondrodysplasia (ek-sen″tro-os″-te-o-kon″dro-dis-pla′ze-ah) a condition in which ossification occurs from several centers instead of a single center, marked by dwarfing and bodily deformities.

ecchondroma, ecchondrosis (ek″kon-dro′mah; ek″-kon-dro′sis) a hyperplastic growth of cartilaginous tissue on the surface of a cartilage or projecting under the periosteum of a bone.

ecchymoma (ek″ĭ-mo′mah) swelling due to blood extravasation.

ecchymosis (ek″ĭ-mo′sis), pl. *ecchymo′ses* [Gr.] a hemorrhagic spot, larger than a petechia, in the skin or mucous membrane, forming a nonelevated, rounded or irregular, blue or purplish patch. adj., **ecchymot′ic.**

eccrine (ek′rin) exocrine, with special reference to ordinary sweat glands.

eccritic (ek-krit′ik) 1. promoting excretion. 2. an agent that promotes excretion.

eccyesis (ek″si-e′sis) ectopic pregnancy.

ECG electrocardiogram.

ecgonine (ek′go-nin) the final basic product obtained by hydrolysis of cocaine and several related alkaloids.

echinococcosis (e-ki″no-kok-o′sis) an infection, usually of the liver, caused by larval forms (hydatid cysts) of TAPEWORMS of the genus *Echinococcus,* marked by the development of expanding cysts (see also HYDATID DISEASE).

Echinococcus (e-ki″no-kok′us) a genus of small TAPEWORMS.

E. granulo′sis, a species parasitic in dogs and wolves and occasionally in cats; its larvae may develop in nearly all mammals, forming hydatid cysts in the liver, lungs, kidneys, and other organs.

E. multilocula′ris, a species whose adult forms usually parasitize the fox and wild rodents, although man is sporadically infected. It resembles *E. granulosis,* but the larvae form alveolar or multilocular rather than unilocular cysts.

echoacousia (ek″o-ah-koo′ze-ah) the subjective experience of hearing echoes after normally heard sounds.

echocardiogram (ek″o-kar′de-o-gram″) the record produced by echocardiography.

echocardiography (ek″o-kar″de-og′rah-fe) recording of the position and motion of the heart walls or internal structures of the heart and neighboring tissue by the echo obtained from beams of ultrasonic waves directed through the chest wall.

Echocardiography is based on the same principle as the oceanographic technique of depth-sounding; that is, it utilizes ultrasound to delineate anatomical structures by recording on a graph the echoes from the heart structures. It is particularly useful in demonstrating, without danger to the patient, valvular and other structural deformities of the heart which formerly required CARDIAC CATHETERIZATION or some other elaborate procedure for accurate diagnosis. (See also ULTRASONOGRAPHY.)

echoencephalogram (ek″o-en-sef′ah-lo-gram″) the record produced by echoencephalography.

echoencephalography (ek″o-en-sef′ah-log′rah-fe) a diagnostic technique in which pulses of ultrasonic waves are beamed through the head from both sides, and echoes from the midline structures of the brain are recorded graphically; shifts from any midline may indicate a centrally placed mass.

echogram (ek′o-gram) the record made by echography.

echography (ĕ-kog′rah-fe) the use of ultrasound as a diagnostic aid. Ultrasound waves are directed at the tissues, and a record is made, as on an oscilloscope, of the waves reflected back through the tissues, which indicate interfaces of different acoustic densities and thus differentiate between solid and cystic structures.

echolalia (ek″o-la′le-ah) automatic repetition by a patient of what is said to him.

echomimia (ek″o-mim′e-ah) echopraxia.

echomotism (ek″o-mo′tizm) echopraxia.

echopraxia (ek″o-prak′se-ah) the spasmodic and involuntary imitation of the movements of others.

echothiophate iodide (ek″o-thi′o-fāt) a cholinesterase inhibitor used to reduce intraocular pressure in glaucoma.

echovirus (ek′o-vi″rus) a group of viruses (enteroviruses) isolated from man, the name of which was derived from the first letters of the description "enteric cytopathogenic human orphan." At the time of the isolation of the viruses the diseases they caused were not known, hence the term "orphan," but it is now known that these viruses produce many different types of human disease, especially aseptic meningitis, and diarrhea and various respiratory diseases.

Eck's fistula (eks) an artificial communication made between the portal vein and the vena cava.

eclabium (ek-la′be-um) eversion of a lip.

eclampsia (e-klamp′se-ah) convulsions and coma, rarely coma alone, occuring in pregnant or puerperal women, associated with hypertension, edema, and/or proteiniuria. adj., **eclamp′tic.** Early prenatal care, including frequent blood pressure measurement and urinalysis, provides early detection of preeclampsia and adequate treatment to forestall the development of eclampsia.

TREATMENT. Recently there has been considerable controversy over the wisdom of treating preeclampsia with dietary restrictions, limited salt intake, and diuretics because of their effect on the developing fetus. Certainly efforts must be made to keep weight gain at a minimum utilizing a nutritious diet and to institute other measures to avoid extreme hypertension and edema. The hazards of "starvation" diets and the administration of medications during pregnancy are best avoided if the obese woman loses weight and is in optimal health *before* pregnancy. When these conditions are not met, the obstetrician is faced with the dilemma of choosing between treatment of the mother at the risk of damaging the fetus and inadequately controlling preeclampsia at the risk of endangering the life of both mother and child.

Hospitalization becomes necessary if the blood pressure continues to rise and cerebral, visual, and gastrointestinal symptoms develop. The patient is placed on bed rest, her calorie and sodium intake is monitored and diuretics may be administered. Medications that may be prescribed to control convulsive seizures include amobarbital (Amytal), chloral hydrate, paraldehyde, and morphine sulfate. The patient who develops HEART FAILURE or pulmonary EDEMA requires special medications and treatments to control these complications. If the eclampsia remains severe and progressive in spite of attempts to control it, and normal delivery of the infant is not expected within a reasonable period of time, the physician may decide to terminate the pregnancy.

PATIENT CARE. It is essential that the patient with preeclampsia be informed of the details of her care and that she is encouraged to cooperate in carrying out the regimen designed for the benefit of herself and her unborn baby. She should be made aware of the potential dangers of her condition, but not unduly frightened or threatened by it. Should all efforts fail to relieve the preeclamptic condition and symptoms become progressively worse, a state of full-blown eclampsia is almost inevitable.

The patient with eclampsia is critically ill; the maternal and infant mortality rate are extremely high. She is kept under constant surveillance and the vital signs are recorded at least every hour. Intake and output are carefully measured. Because these patients are extremely restless and often confused, padded side rails must be kept in place and the head board padded with a pillow or folded blanket. To avoid precipitation of a convulsion or aggravation of the patient's restlessness, a quiet and nonstimulating environment is provided (see CONVULSION). A precipitate delivery may occur during a convulsion. Recovery from eclampsia usually is rapid and complete once delivery of the infant has taken place.

puerperal e., that occurring after or during childbirth.

uremic e., eclampsia due to uremia.

eclampsism (e-klamp′sizm) preeclampsia.

eclamptogenic (e-klamp″to-jen′ik) causing eclampsia.

ecmnesia (ek-ne′ze-ah) forgetfulness of recent events with remembrance of more remote ones.

Ecolid (e′ko-lid) trademark for a preparation of chlorisondamine, an antihypertensive and ganglion-blocking agent.

ecologist (e-kol′o-jist) a person skilled in ecology.

ecology (e-kol′o-je) the science of organisms as affected by environmental factors; the study of the environment and the life history of organisms. adj., **ecolog′ic, ecolog′ical.**

ecomania (e″ko-ma′ne-ah) an attitude of mind that is dominating toward members of the family but humble toward those in authority.

Economo's encephalitis (a-kon′o-mōz) a form of epidemic encephalitis, the original type described by von Economo, marked by increasing languor, apathy, and drowsiness, passing into lethargy; observed in various parts of the world between 1915 and 1926. Called also lethargic encephalitis.

ecosystem (e″ko-sis′tem) the fundamental unit in ecology, comprising the living organisms and the nonliving elements interacting in a certain defined area.

ecphylaxis (ek″fi-lak′sis) a condition of impotency of the antibodies in the blood. adj., **ecphylac′tic.**

écraseur (a″krah-zer′) [Fr.] an instrument with a loop of chain or wire for removing a part by enclosing and dividing it.

E.C.T. electroconvulsive therapy.

ect(o)- word element [Gr.], *external; outside.*

ectasia (ek-ta′ze-ah) expansion, dilatation, or distention. adj., **ectat′ic.**

mammary duct e., comedomastitis.

ectental (ek-ten′tal) pertaining to the ectoderm and entoderm, and to their line of junction.

ecthyma (ek-thi′mah) a shallowly eruptive form of impetigo, chiefly on the shins and forearms.

ectoantigen (ek″to-an′tĭ-jen) 1. an antigen that seems to be loosely attached to the outside of bacteria. 2. an antigen formed in the ectoplasm (cell membrane) of a bacterium.

ectoblast (ek′to-blast) the ectoderm.

ectocardia (ek″to-kar′de-ah) congenital displacement of the heart; exocardia.

ectocervix (ek″to-ser′viks) portio vaginalis. adj., **ectocer′vical.**

ectocinerea (ek″to-sĭ-ne′re-ah) the cortical gray matter of the brain.

ectoderm (ek′to-derm) the outermost of the three primitive germ layers of the embryo; from it are derived the epidermis and epidermic tissues, such as the nails, hair, and glands of the skin, the nervous system, external sense organs (eye, ear, etc.) and mucous membrane of the mouth and anus. adj., **ectoder′mal, ectoder′mic.**

ectodermosis (ek″to-der-mo′sis) a disorder based on congenital maldevelopment of organs derived from the ectoderm.

ectoentad (ek″to-en′tad) from without inward.

ectoenzyme (ek″to-en′zīm) an extracellular enzyme.

ectogenous (ek-toj′ĕ-nus) originating outside the organism.

ectoglobular (ek″to-glob′u-lar) formed outside the blood cells.

ectogony (ek-tog′o-ne) the influence exerted on the mother by the developing embryo.

ectohormone (ek″to-hor′mon) a hormone secreted to the outside of the body, as a pheromone.

ectomere (ek′to-mēr) one of the blastomeres taking part in formation of the ectoderm.

ectomorph (ek′to-morf) an individual exhibiting ectomorphy.

ectomorphy (ek′to-mor″fe) a type of body build in which tissues derived from the ectoderm predominate; a somatotype in which both visceral and body structures are relatively slightly developed, the body being linear and delicate. adj. **ectomor′phic.**

-ectomy word element [Gr.], *excision; surgical removal.*

ectoparasite (ek″to-par′ah-sīt) a parasite living on the surface of the host's body. adj., **ectoparasit′ic.**

ectophyte (ek′to-fīt) a vegetable parasite living on the surface of the host's body.

ectopia (ek-to′pe-ah) [L.] ectopy.

e. cor′dis, congenital displacement of the heart outside the thoracic cavity.

ectopic (ek-top′ik) 1. pertaining to or characterized by ectopy. 2. located away from normal position.

e. pregnancy, pregnancy in which the fertilized ovum becomes implanted outside the uterus instead of in the wall of the uterus. Called also extrauterine pregnancy. The ovum may rarely develop in the abdominal cavity, ovary, or cervix uteri, but ectopic pregnancy is almost always found in one of the uterine (fallopian) tubes (see PREGNANCY). A spontaneous abortion may then occur, but more often the fetus will grow to a size large enough to burst the tube. This is an emergency situation requiring immediate treatment. The symptoms of a uterine tube ruptured by ectopic pregnancy are vaginal bleeding and severe pain in one side of the abdomen. Prompt surgery is necessary to remove the damaged tube and the fetus, and to stop the bleeding. Fortunately, the removal of one tube usually leaves the other one intact, so that future pregnancy is possible.

ectoplasm (ek′to-plazm) cell membrane.

ectoplastic (ek′to-plas″tik) having formative power on the surface, as ectoplastic cells.

ectopy (ek′to-pe) displacement or malposition, especially if congenital.

ectosteal (ek-tos′te-al) pertaining to or situated outside a bone.

ectostosis (ek″to-sto′sis) ossification beneath the perichondrium of a cartilage or the periosteum of a bone.

ectothrix (ek′to-thriks) a fungus that grows inside the shaft of a hair, but produces a conspicuous external sheath of spores.

extozoon (ek″to-zo′on) ectoparasite.

ectro- word element [Gr.], *miscarriage; congenital absence.*

ectrodactyly (ek″tro-dak′tĭ-le) congenital absence of all or part of a digit.

ectrogeny (ek-troj′ĕ-ne) congenital absence or defect of a part. adj. **ectrojen′ic.**

ectromelia (ek″tro-me′le-ah) gross hypoplasia or aplasia of one or more long bones of one or more limbs. adj., **ectromel′ic.**

ectromelus (ek-trom′ĕ-lus) an individual with rudimentary arms and legs.

ectropion (ek-tro′pe-on) eversion or turning outward, as of the margin of an eyelid.

ectrosyndactyly (ek″tro-sin-dak′tĭ-le) a condition in which some digits are absent and those that remain are webbed.

ectylurea (ek″til-u-re′ah) a urea compound used as a sedative.

eczema (ek′zĕ-mah) 1. a general term for any superificial inflammatory process involving primarily the epidermis, marked early by redness, itching, minute papules and vesicles, weeping, oozing, and crusting, and later by scaling, lichenification, and often pigmentation. 2. atopic dermatitis.

Eczema is a common allergic reaction in children but it also occurs in adults, usually in a more severe form. Childhood eczema often begins in infancy, the rash appearing on the face, neck, and folds of elbows and knees. It may disappear by itself when the offending food is removed from the diet, or it may become more extensive and in some instances cover the entire surface of the body. Severe eczema can be complicated by skin infections.

Childhood eczema may persist for several years or return after the child is older. A person who suffers eczema in childhood may develop some other allergic condition later, most commonly hay fever or asthma.

CAUSE AND TREATMENT. Eczema is frequently caused by an allergic sensitivity to foods such as milk, fish or eggs, or to dusts, pollens, or similar substances that are inhaled. Allergic eczema is cured or controlled by some of the methods used for other allergic disorders (see ALLERGY).

e. herpet′icum, disseminated herpes simplex (see KAPOSI'S VARICELLIFORM ERUPTION).

stasis e., stasis dermatitis.

e. vaccina′tum, disseminated vaccinia (see KAPOSI'S VARICELLIFORM ERUPTION).

eczematoid (ek-zem′ah-toid) resembling eczema.

eczematous (ek-zem′ah-tus) characterized by or of the nature of eczema.

edema (ĕ-de′mah) an abnormal accumulation of fluid in the intercellular spaces of the body. adj., **edem′atous.** Edema can be caused by a variety of factors, including hypoproteinemia, in which a lowered concentration of plasma proteins decreases the osmotic pressure, thereby permitting passage of abnormal amounts of fluid out of the blood vessels and into the tissue spaces. Some other causes are poor lymphatic drainage, increased capillary permeability (as in inflammation), and congestive HEART FAILURE.

Local edema due to inflammation or poor drainage through the lymph vessels may be relieved by elevation of the part and application of cold to the area. Generalized edema is treated by the administration of DIURETICS, which increase the loss of certain salts and thereby increase removal of tissue fluids, which are eliminated as urine. Sodium, which enhances retention of fluid in the tissues, is restricted in the diet of patients with edema.

PATIENT CARE. Edematous tissue breaks down quite readily because there is an interference with the normal exchange of nutrients and waste products within the tissue cells. Extreme care should be taken in handling edematous parts of the body, every effort should be made to keep the skin intact, and it is necessary to change the patient's position frequently to avoid the development of DECUBITUS ULCERS.

In dependent edema it is helpful to elevate the lower extremities periodically and promote drainage of fluid via the lymph and blood vessels.

Severe edema accompanying an allergic reaction may prove fatal if the respiratory passages become occluded. An emergency tracheostomy set and equipment for the administration of epinephrine should be kept at the patient's bedside in the event acute respiratory embarrassment develops.

In all types of generalized edema the patient's intake and output are recorded at least every 24 hours. The physician may also request daily weighing of the patient so that fluid gain or loss can be determined. The patient should be weighed at the same time each day, preferably before breakfast, and using the same scales.

angioneurotic e., temporary edema suddenly appearing in areas of skin or mucous membrane and occasionally in the viscera, of allergic, neurotic, or unknown origin (see also ANGIONEUROTIC EDEMA).

brain e., an excessive accumulation of fluid in the brain substance (wet brain).

cardiac e., a manifestation of congestive heart failure, due to increased venous and capillary pressures and often associated with renal sodium retention.

dependent e., edema affecting most severely the lowermost parts of the body.

e. neonato'rum, a disease of premature and feeble infants resembling sclerema, marked by spreading edema with cold, livid skin.

pitting e., edema in which pressure leaves a persistent depression in the tissues.

pulmonary e., diffuse extravascular accumulation of fluid in the tissues and air spaces of the LUNG due to changes in hydrostatic forces in the capillaries or to increased capillary permeability. Frequently a complication of congestive heart failure, the condition is a possibility in any patient with limited cardiac reserve, impaired kidney function, or an infection of the lung in which the pulmonary capillaries are affected. The risk of pulmonary edema is high in patients receiving intravenous therapy, and therefore must be considered in determining the rate of flow.

Early symptoms include moist rales and dyspnea. In severe cases the alveoli fill with fluid and signs of acute respiratory distress are evident.

edematogenic (ĕ-dem″ah-to-jen′ik) producing or causing edema.

edentia (e-den′she-ah) absence of the teeth.

edentulous (e-den′tu-lus) without teeth.

edetate (ed′ĕtāt) ethylenediaminotetraacetate (EDTA); any salt of edetic acid.

e. calcium disodium, calcium disodium e., a metal complexing agent used in the diagnosis and treatment of lead poisoning, and usually administered intravenously in saline or dextrose solution.

e. disodium or disodium e., a chelating agent used in poisoning with lead and other heavy metals and, because of its affinity for calcium, in the treatment of hypercalcemia and pathologic calcification. It is administered intravenously in saline or dextrose solution. Overuse may produce hypocalcemic tetany, convulsions, and respiratory and cardiovascular collapse.

edetic acid (e-det′ik) an acid whose salts are strong chelating agents (see also EDETATE).

edrophonium (ed″ro-fo′ne-um) a cholinergic used in the form of the chloride salt as a curare antagonist and diagnostic agent in myasthenia gravis.

EDTA see EDETATE.

EEG electroencephalogram.

E.E.N.T. eye-ear-nose-throat.

effacement (ĕ-fās′ment) the obliteration of form or features; applied to the cervix uteri during labor when it is so changed that only the ostium uteri remains.

effect (ĕ-fekt′) a result produced by an action.

additive e., the combined effect produced by the action of two or more agents, being equal to the sum of their separate effects.

Bohr e., displacement of the oxyhemoglobin dissociation curve by a change in carbon dioxide tension.

Crabtree e., the inhibition of oxygen consumption on the addition of glucose to tissues or microorganisms having a high rate of aerobic glycolysis; the converse of the Pasteur effect.

cumulative e., cumulation action.

Doppler e., the relationship of the apparent frequency of waves, as of sound, light, and radio waves, to the relative motion of the source of the waves and the observer, the frequency increasing as the two approach each other and decreasing as they move apart.

Pasteur e., the decrease in the rate of glycolysis and the suppression of lactate accumulation by tissues or microorganisms in the presence of oxygen.

position e., in genetics, the changed effect produced by alteration of the relative positions of various genes on the chromosomes.

pressure e., the sum of the changes that are due to obstruction of tissue drainage by pressure.

side e., a consequence other than that for which an agent is used, especially an adverse effect on another organ system.

effectiveness (ĕ-fek′tive-nes) the ability to produce a specific result or to exert a specific measurable influence.

relative biologic e., an expression of the effectiveness of other types of radiation in comparison with that of gamma or roentgen rays.

effector (ĕ-fek′tor) a muscle or gland that contracts or secretes, respectively, in direct response to nerve impulses.

effemination (ĕ-fem″ĭ-na′shun) feminization.

efferent (ef′er-ent) conducting or progressing away from a center or specific site of reference, as an efferent nerve.

e. nerve, any nerve that carries impulses from the central nervous system toward the periphery, as a motor nerve (see also NEURON).

effleurage (ef″lu-rahzh′) [Fr.] stroking movement in massage. In NATURAL CHILDBIRTH, a light circular stroke of the lower abdomen, done in rhythm to control breathing, to aid in relaxation of the abdominal muscles, and to increase concentration during a uterine contraction. The stroking is accomplished by moving the wrist only. Concentrating on the coordination of stroking and breathing is believed to block out some of the sensations created by the contracting uterus.

efflorescence (ef″lo-res′ens) 1. the quality of being efflorescent. 2. a rash or eruption.

efflorescent (ef″lo-res′ent) becoming powdery by losing the water of crystallization.

effluvium (ĕ-floo′ve-um), pl. *efflu′via* [L.] 1. an outflowing or shedding, as of the hair. 2. an exhalation or emanation, especially one of noxious nature.

effusion (ĕ-fu′zhun) 1. escape of a fluid into a part. 2. effused material.

pleural e., accumulation of fluid in the space between the membrane encasing the lung and that lining the thoracic cavity. The normal pleural space contains only a small amount of fluid to prevent friction as the lung expands and deflates. If, however, there is a disturbance in either the production of this fluid or its removal, the fluid accumulates and threatens collapse of the lung. In extreme cases there is total collapse of the lung and MEDIASTINAL SHIFT.

Excess fluid in the pleural space may be removed by THORACENTESIS or by insertion of CHEST TUBES to allow for drainage of the fluid and, through a closed-drainage system, gradual reexpansion of the lung.

Conditions that may lead to pleural effusion include infections, inflammatory processes, and malignancies affecting the pulmonary structures, and renal and cardiac disease. (See also PLEURISY.)

egesta (e-jes′tah) undigested material discharged from the body.

egestion (e-jes′chun) the casting out of undigested material.

egg (eg) an animal ovum or female reproduction cell, especially one that is normally extruded from the maternal body before development of the embryo, either before or after fertilization.

ego (e′go) in psychoanalytic theory, one of the three major parts of the personality, the others being the ID and the SUPEREGO. The word ego is Latin for "I," that is, self or individual as distinguished from other persons. The ego is represented by certain mental mechanisms, such as perception and memory, and specific defense mechanisms that are used to adjust to the demands of primitive instinctual drives (the id) and the demands of the external world (superego). The ego may be considered the psychologic aspect of one's personality, the id comprising the physiologic aspects and the superego the social aspects. The ego controls and directs an individual's actions and seeks compromises between the id impulses, social and parental prohibitions and the pressures of reality.

The word ego also is commonly used to express conceit or self-centeredness. This should not be confused with the psychiatric meaning described above.

e. ideal, the standard of perfection unconsciously created by a person for himself.

egocentric (e″go-sen′trik) having all one's ideas centered on one's self.

ego-dystonic (e″go-dis-ton′ik) denoting any impulse, idea, or the like, that is repugnant to and inconsistent with an individual's conception of himself.

egoism (e′go-izm) a self-seeking for advantage at the expense of others; overevaluation of the self.

egomania (e″go-ma′ne-ah) morbid self-esteem.

ego-syntonic (e″go-sin-ton′ik) denoting any impulse, idea, or the like, that is in harmony with an individual's conception of himself.

egotism (e′go-tizm) overevaluation of one's self.

egotropic (e″go-trop′ik) egocentric.

Ehlers-Danlos syndrome (a′lerz-dan′los) a congenital hereditary syndrome of joint hyperextensibility, hyperelasticity and fragility of the skin, poor wound healing leaving parchment-like scars, capillary fragility, and subcutaneous nodules after trauma. Called also cutis hyperelastica.

Ehrlich (ār′lik) Paul (1854–1915). German bacteriologist. Born in Silesia of Jewish parents, he studied medicine and was early drawn to research on aniline dyes. Ehrlich did vast work on the problems of serology and immunity, and is known preeminently for his discovery of salvarsan or "606," an arsenical compound now called arsphenamine, which is a cure for syphilis. He differentiated the leukemias, classified the leukocytes, described polychromatophilia, and is generally regarded the founder of hematology. In 1908 Ehrlich shared with Metchnikoff the Nobel prize for his work in immunology.

eidetic (i-det′ik) denoting exact visualization of events or objects previously seen; a person having such an ability.

eidogen (i′do-jen) in embryology, a substance elaborated by a second-grade inductor, which is capable of modifying the form of an embryonic organ already in the process of formation.

eidoptometry (i″dop-tom′ĕ-tre) measurement of the acuteness of visual perception.

einsteinium (īn-sti′ne-um) a chemical element, atomic number 99, atomic weight 254, symbol Es. (See table of ELEMENTS.)

Eisenmenger's syndrome (i′sen-meng″erz) ventricular septal defect with pulmonary hypertension and cyanosis due to right-to-left (reversed) shunt of blood. Sometimes defined as pulmonary hypertension (pulmonary vascular disease) and cyanosis with the shunt being at the atrial, ventricular, or great vessel area.

ejaculatio (e-jak″u-la′she-o) [L.] ejaculation.

e. prae′cox, premature ejaculation in coitus.

ejaculation (e-jak″u-la′shun) forcible, sudden expulsion; especially expulsion of semen from the male urethra, a reflex action that occurs as a result of sexual stimulation. adj., **ejac′ulatory.** The three components of semen are expelled in quick succession. First to emerge is a lubricating fluid produced by the bulbourethral glands in the penis. Next comes a fluid released into the urethral channel by the prostate; this fluid provides a neutral medium within which the sperm cells can swim. Lastly, the spermatic fluid, which has been stored in the seminal vesicles, is likewise injected into the urethral channel and ejaculated. (See also REPRODUCTION.)

ejecta (e-jek′tah) refuse cast off from the body.

EKG electrocardiogram.

EKY electrokymogram.

elaborate (e-lab′o-rāt) to produce complex substances out of simpler materials.

elastance (e-las′tans) the quality of recoiling on removal of pressure without disruption, or an expression of the measure of the ability to do so in terms of unit of volume change per unit of pressure change; it is the reciprocal of compliance.

elastase (e-las′tās) an enzyme capable of catalyzing the digestion of elastic tissue.

elastic (e-las′tik) capable of resuming normal shape after distortion.

e. cartilage, a substance that is more opaque, flexible, and elastic than hyaline cartilage, and is further distinguished by its yellow color. The ground substance is penetrated in all directions by frequently branching fibers that give all of the reactions for elastin.

e. tissue, connective tissue made up of yellow elastic fibers, frequently massed into sheets.

elasticity (e″las-tis′ĭ-te) the quality of being elastic.

elastin (e-las′tin) a yellow scleroprotein, the essential constituent of elastic connective tissue; it is brittle when dry, but flexible and elastic when moist.

elastofibroma (e-las″to-fi-bro′mah) a tumor consisting of both elastin and fibrous elements.

elastoidosis, nodular (e-las″toi-do′sis) a condition characterized by comedones and yellowish, circumscribed, thickened plaques around the orbits or the nose, or the nape.

elastoma (e″las-to′mah) a tumor or focal excess of elastic tissue fibers or abnormal collagen fibers of the skin.

elastometer (e″las-tom′ĕ-ter) an instrument for measuring the elasticity of tissues.

elastomucin (e-las″to-mu′sin) a polysaccharide component of elastic tissue.

elastorrhexis (e-las″to-rek′sis) a rupture of fibers composing elastic tissue.

elastosis (e″las-to′sis) degeneration of elastic tissue. adj., **elastot′ic.**

e. perfo′rans serpigino′sa, perforating e., an elastic tissue defect, occurring alone or in association with other disorders, including Down's syndrome and Ehlers-Danlos syndrome, in which elastomas are extruded through small keratotic papules in the epidermis; the lesions are usually arranged in arcuate serpiginous clusters on the sides of the nape, face, or arms.

elation (e-la′shun) emotional excitement marked by acceleration of mental and bodily activity.

Elavil (el′ah-vil) trademark for preparations of amitriptyline, an antidepressant.

elbow (el′bo) 1. the bend of the arm; the joint connecting the arm and forearm. 2. any angular bend.

The elbow joint connects the large bone of the upper arm, or humerus, with the two smaller bones of the lower arm, the radius and ulna. It is one of the body's more versatile joints, with a combined hinge and rotating action allowing the arm to bend and the hand to make a half turn. The flexibility of the elbow and shoulder joints together permits a nearly infinite variety of hand movements.

The action of the elbow is controlled primarily by the biceps and the triceps muscles. When the biceps contracts, the arm bends at the elbow. When the triceps contracts the arm straightens. In each action, the opposite muscle exerts a degree of opposing tension, moderating the movement so that it is smooth and even instead of sudden and jerky.

As in other joints, the ends of the bones meeting at the elbow have a smooth covering of cartilage, a tough rubbery substance that minimizes friction when the joint is moved. The elbow joint is lubricated with synovia. The bursa, a small sac of connective tissue, eases its movement. The bones forming the joint are held together by tough, fibrous ligaments.

The "funny bone" is not a bone but the ulnar

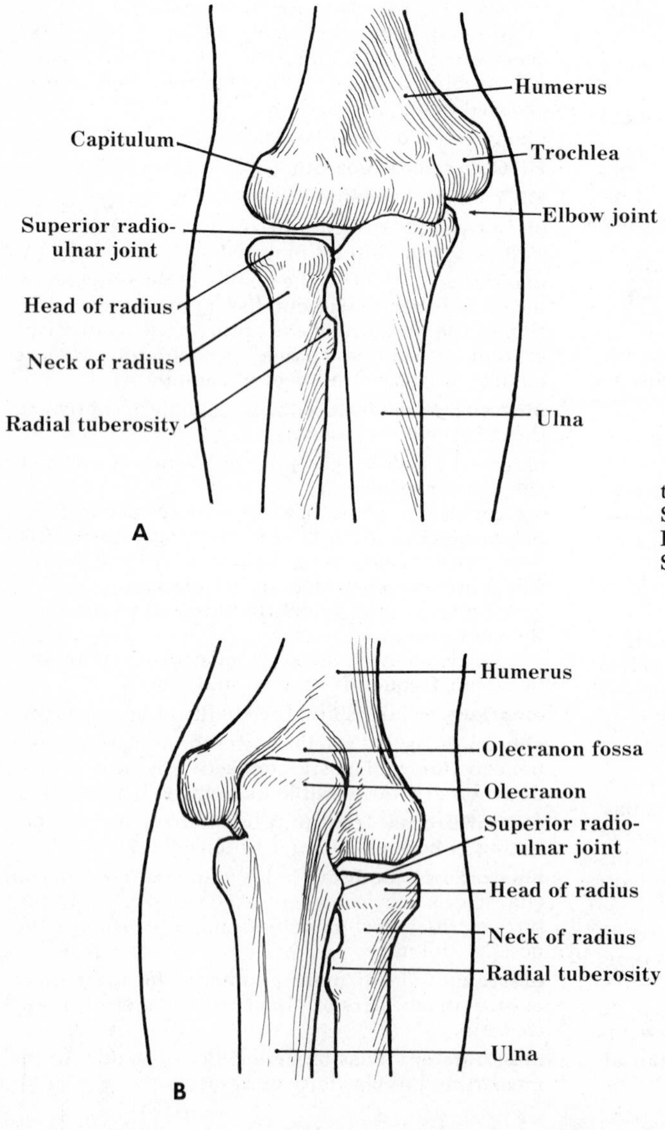

Elbow. *A*, Anterior view, right arm. *B*, Posterior view, right arm. (Redrawn from Jacob, S. W., and Francone, C. A.: Structure and Function in Man. 2nd ed. Philadelphia, W. B. Saunders Co., 1970.)

nerve, a vulnerable and sensitive nerve that lies close to the surface near the point of the elbow. Hitting it causes a tingling pain or sensation that may be felt all the way to the fingers.

DISORDERS OF THE ELBOW. The elbows, like the knees, are continually exposed to bumps, twists, and wrenches. A common injury of the elbow is a fracture of a bone near the joint. Another injury of the elbow is dislocation, in which the hinge joint is pulled apart by a violent twist or yank. Tendons and ligaments may be torn. In some cases, dislocation and fracture may occur together.

ARTHRITIS may affect the elbow and make it stiff or impossible to move. Special exercises, manipulation and heat therapy may be prescribed to help restore flexibility. BURSITIS can also cause pain in the elbow. It often results from excessive use of the joint. "Tennis elbow," which may affect people who never held a tennis racket, is a term often used for bursitis of the elbow but is more accurately a tendinitis, or inflammation of the tendons. Rest and heat therapy are usually effective in relieving the condition.

Electra complex (e-lek′trah) libidinous fixation of a daughter toward her father. (See also OEDIPUS COMPLEX.)

electric shock (e-lek′trik) shock caused by electric current passing through the body. The longer the contact with electricity, the smaller the chance of survival. The victim's breathing may stop, and his body may appear stiff.

In giving first aid for electric shock, first the electric contact is broken as quickly as possible; this must be done with care to avoid exposure to the current. The rescuer, keeping in mind that water and metals are conductors of electricity, stands on a *dry* surface and does not touch the victim or electric wire with his bare hands.

The victim may have stopped breathing and have no pulse. In this case CARDIOPULMONARY RESUSCITATION is begun immediately.

Electroshock, or electroconvulsive, therapy is sometimes used therapeutically for mental illness, especially depression, although recent development of new medications has displaced its use in some cases (see also SHOCK THERAPY).

electro- word element [Gr.], *electricity.*

electroaffinity (e-lek″tro-ah-fin′ĭ-te) the degree of tenacity with which a substance attracts electrons. Called also electronegativity.

electrobiology (e-lek″tro-bi-ol′o-je) the study of electric phenomena in living tissue.

electrobioscopy (e-lek″tro-bi-os′ko-pe) the determination of the presence or absence of life by means of an electric current.

electrocardiogram (e-lek″tro-kar′de-o-gram″) the record produced by ELECTROCARDIOGRAPHY; a tracing representing the heart's electrical action derived by amplification of the minutely small electrical impulses normally generated by the heart. Called also ECG and EKG.

electrocardiograph (e-lek″tro-kar′de-o-graf″) the apparatus used in electrocardiography.

electrocardiography (e-lek″tro-kar″de-og′rah-fe) the graphic recording from the body surface of the potential of electric currents generated by the heart, as a means of studying the action of the heart muscle. adj., **electrocardiograph′ic.** With the modern electrocardiograph, the current that accompanies the action of the heart is amplified 3000 times or

more, and it moves a small, sensitively balanced lever in contact with moving paper. The pattern of heart waves that is traced on the paper indicates the heart's rhythm and other actions.

The normal electrocardiogram is composed of a P wave, Q, R, and S waves known as the QRS COMPLEX, or QRS wave, and a T wave. The P wave occurs at the beginning of each contraction of the atria. The QRS wave occurs at the beginning of each contraction of the ventricles. The T wave seen in a normal electrocardiogram occurs as the ventricles recover electrically and prepare for the next contraction. There is a refractory period between these waves during which the muscle is inexcitable; this period is usually about 0.30 second.

The electric impulses in the heart muscle are picked up and conducted to the electrocardiograph by electrodes or leads connected to the body by small metal plates or other methods. The metal plates are moistened with a conductive paste and attached to the arms, legs, and chest (cardiac area) of the patient.

Electrocardiography is a valuable diagnostic tool, used in some routine physical examinations and when a heart disorder occurs or is suspected. It helps diagnose the damage that may have been inflicted on the heart muscle by a coronary occlusion, the progress of rheumatic fever, the presence of abnormal rhythms, or the effect of digitalis or other drugs. An electrocardiogram cannot always detect impending heart disease or all cardiovascular disorders. The readings are interpreted together with the results of other diagnostic tests.

electrocatalysis (e-lek″tro-kah-tal′ĭ-sis) catalysis produced by electricity.

electrocautery (e-lek″tro-kaw′ter-e) an apparatus for cauterizing tissue by means of a platinum wire heated by electric current.

electrochemistry (e-lek″tro-kem′is-tre) the study of chemical changes produced by electric action.

electrochromatography (e-lek″tro-kro″mah-tog′rah-fe) electrophoresis.

electrocoagulation (e-lek″tro-ko-ag″u-la′shun) coagulation of tissue by means of an electric current.

electrocontractility (e-lek″tro-kon″trak-til′ĭ-te) contractility in response to electric stimulation.

electroconvulsive therapy (e-lek″tro-kon-vul′siv) electroshock therapy; the induction of convulsions by the passage of an electric current through the brain, as in the treatment of affective disorders (see also SHOCK THERAPY).

electrocorticography (e-lek″tro-kor″tĭ-kog′rah-fe) electroencephalography with the electrodes applied directly to the cerebral cortex.

electrode (e-lek′trōd) either of two terminals of an electrically conducting system or cell.

active e., therapeutic electrode.

calomel e., one capable of both collecting and giving up chloride ions in neutral or acidic aqueous media, consisting of mercury in contact with mercurous chloride; used as a reference electrode in pH measurements.

depolarizing e., an electrode that has a resistance greater than that of the portion of the body enclosed in the circuit.

hydrogen e., an electrode made by depositing platinum black on platinum and then allowing it to absorb hydrogen gas to saturation; used in determination of hydrogen ion concentration.

indifferent e., one larger than a therapeutic electrode, dispersing electrical stimulation over a larger area.

point e., an electrode having on one end a metallic point; used in applying current.

therapeutic e., one smaller than an indifferent electrode, producing electrical stimulation in a concentrated area; called also active electrode.

electrodermal (e-lek″tro-der′mal) pertaining to the electrical properties of the skin, especially to changes in its resistance.

electrodessication (e-lek″tro-des″ĭ-ka′shun) destruction of tissue by dehydration, done by means of a high-frequency electric current.

electrodiagnosis (e-lek″tro-di″ag-no′sis) diagnosis by means of electric devices.

electrodialyzer (e-lek″tro-di″ah-li′zer) a blood dialyzer utilizing an applied electric field and semipermeable membranes for separating the colloids from the solution.

electroencephalogram (e-lek″tro-en-sef′ah-lo-gram″) the record produced by ELECTROENCEPHALOGRAPHY; a tracing of the electric impulses of the brain. Called also EEG.

electroencephalograph (e-lek″tro-en-sef′ah-lo-graf) the instrument used in electroencephalography.

electroencephalography (e-lek″tro-en-sef″ah-log′-rah-fe) the recording of changes in electric potentials in various areas of the brain by means of electrodes placed on the scalp or on or in the brain itself, and connected to a vacuum tube radio amplifier, which amplifies the impulses more than a million times. The impulses are of sufficient magnitude to move an electromagnetic pen that records the brain waves. adj., **electroencephalograph′ic.**

The rate, height, and length of the waves vary in different parts of the brain, and each individual has a unique and characteristic EEG pattern. Age and degree of consciousness also cause the wave patterns to differ. Most of the recorded waves in a normal adult's EEG are the occipital alpha waves, which are best obtained from the back of the head (occipital region) when the subject is resting quietly, but not asleep, with his eyes closed. These waves are blocked by excitement or by opening the eyes.

The beta waves, obtained from the central and front parts of the head are more closely related to the sensory-motor parts of the brain. These waves are blocked in the same way as are alpha waves, by opening the eyes. In a normal EEG the frequencies are predominately within the range of alpha and beta rhythms at the rate of 8 to 30 hertz (cycles per second). During sleep the brain cells generate higher voltage electrical waves, but the rhythm is slowed down to 2 or 3 hertz, sometimes with short "sleep" spindles of about 15 hertz. One should use the word "normal" with caution when speaking of EEG readings. Some persons with mild deviations from normal may have no evidence of cerebral dis-

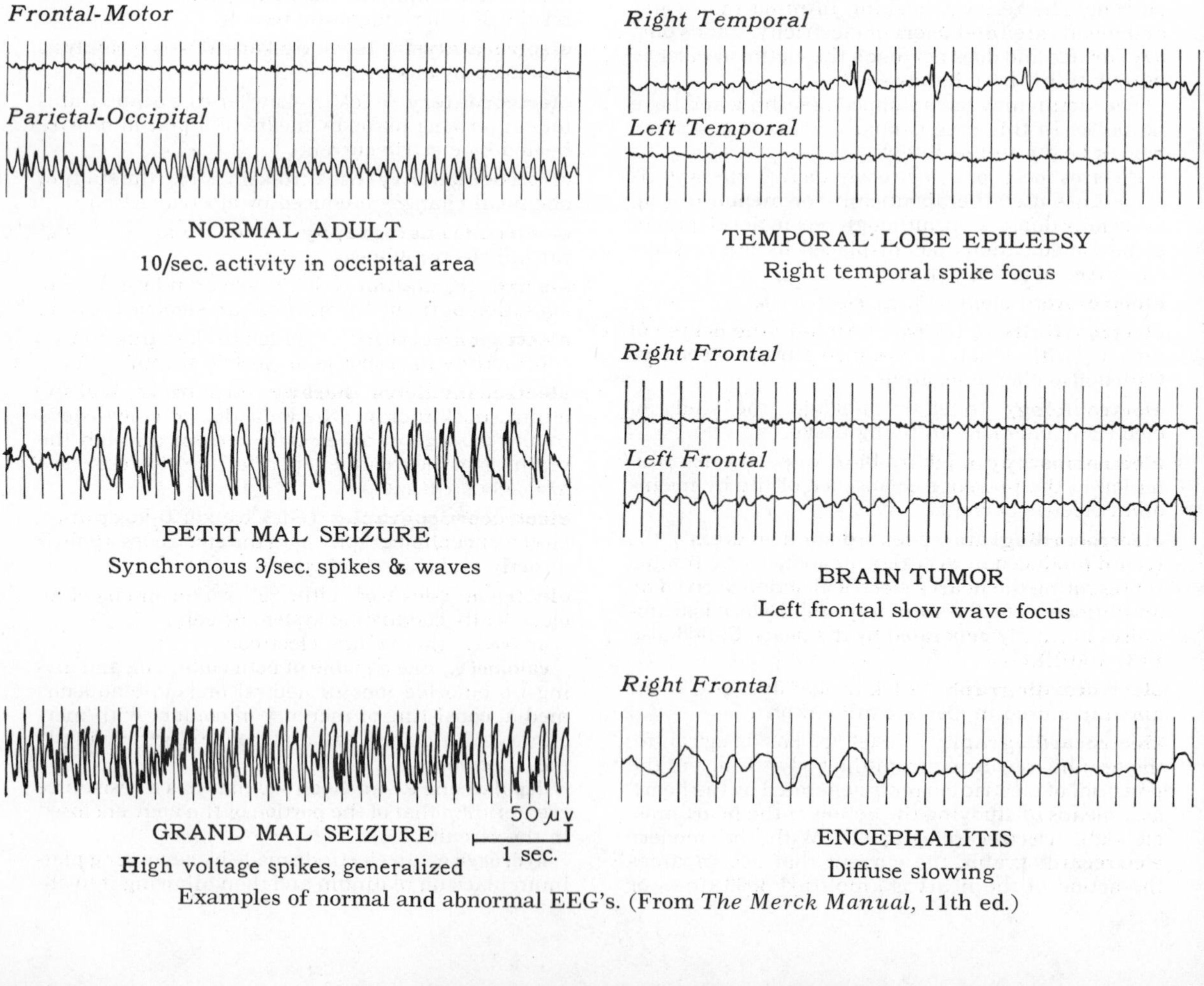

Examples of normal and abnormal EEG's. (From *The Merck Manual,* 11th ed.)

ease, while others with readings within normal ranges may be suffering from a serious disorder.

Irregular slow waves of 2 to 3 hertz, called delta waves or the delta pattern, are normally found in deep sleep and in infants and young children, but indicate an abnormality in the awake adult. Rhythmic slow waves of 4 to 7 hertz are called theta waves. "Electrical silence," or no evidence of brain activity, when demonstrated once and then again in 24 hours, has been taken as one of the criteria of DEATH.

Electroencephalography is widely used in studying brain function and in tracing the connections between the parts of the central nervous system. It is particularly valuable in diagnosing EPILEPSY, brain tumor, and other diseases of and injury to the brain.

An electroencephalogram is of little use in the study of those mental disorders and diseases that do not cause gross brain damage.

PATIENT CARE. The electroencephalograph is an extremely sensitive instrument and readings can be greatly influenced by the actions of the subject and his physiologic status. It is apparent, then, that the cooperation of the patient is needed, and that he is properly prepared physically and psychologically in order to obtain an accurate and useful record of brain activity. The patient is more likely to be cooperative if he has had adequate preparation in the purpose of the test, how the procedure will be carried out, and what will be expected of him during the testing. His fears about electricity and how it will be used must by allayed. He should know that the electrodes lead minute amounts of electrical charge *from* his body and that there is no danger of electric shock and no relationship of this procedure to electroshock therapy. In most instances the test is painless because the electrodes are attached to the scalp with collodion. If needle electrodes are to be used, however, he should be told there will be mild discomfort because the needles are extremely small.

A sleep recording usually is taken when a seizure disorder is suspected. The patient will be expected to go to sleep during the test. Some EEG technicians encourage the patient to stay up later than usual the evening before the test and to awaken early so he will be more likely to fall asleep during testing. Medications to produce sleep are given only as a last resort because these drugs alter brain wave patterns. Infants and small children are not allowed to nap before the test.

Other aspects of physical preparation include withholding all anticonvulsants, tranquilizers, and stimulants for at least 24 to 48 hours prior to testing. This includes coffee, tea, cola drinks, and alcohol. Hypoglycemia affects the brain wave patterns and so the patient is told not to skip any meals.

At the beginning of the test a baseline EEG reading is obtained by having the patient lie quietly in a dimly lit room with his eyes closed. He is cautioned to avoid movement of the eyelids, mouth, or tongue because these activities can be particularly disruptive. Provocative or "stressing" techniques are sometimes used during the EEG testing. These are particularly useful in the diagnosis of epilepsy because they can evoke seizure potentials on the EEG. The two techniques most often used are HYPERVENTILATION and "photic" stimulation which employs flickering lights to stimulate the brain. When these or any other techniques are anticipated, the patient should be informed so he can avoid becoming unduly apprehensive before and during the testing.

electrogastrograph (e-lek″tro-gas′tro-graf) an instrument for recording the electrical activity of the stomach by means of swallowed gastric electrodes.

electrogastrography (e-lek″tro-gas-trog′rah-fe) the recording of the electrical activity of the stomach as measured between its lumen and the body surface. adj., **electrogastrograph′ic.**

electrogram (e-lek′tro-gram) any record produced by changes in electric potential.

His bundle e., an intracardiac electrocardiogram of potentials in the bundle of His, done through a cardiac catheter.

electrohemostasis (e-lek″tro-he″mo-sta′sis) arrest of hemorrhage by electrocautery.

electrohysterography (e-lek″tro-his″ter-og′rah-fe) the recording of changes in electric potential associated with contractions of the uterine muscle.

electrokymogram (e-lek″tro-ki′mo-gram) the record produced by electrokymography.

electrokymograph (e-lek″tro-ki′mo-graf) the instrument used in electrokymography.

electrokymography (e-lek″tro-ki-mog′rah-fe) the photography on x-ray film of the motion of the heart or of other moving structures which can be visualized radiographically.

electrolysis (e″lek-trol′ĭ-sis) destruction by passage of a galvanic current, as in disintegration of a chemical compound in solution or removal of excessive hair from the body.

electrolyte (e-lek′tro-līt) a substance that dissociates into ions when fused or in solution, thus becoming capable of conducting electricity. Within the body, the electrolytes play an essential role in the workings of the cell, and in maintaining fluid balance and a normal ACID-BASE BALANCE.

The chief electrolyte ions are: sodium, a key regulator in water balance and also necessary to normal function of muscles and nerves; potassium, which is associated with acid-base balance and is one of the main constituents of cell protoplasm; and calcium, which plays an integral part in the clotting mechanism and is essential to normal muscle physiology. Magnesium and chloride also are considered to be vital electrolytes since they are essential to chemical changes necessary for normal body function.

Sodium and chloride are found in large amounts in the fluid outside the cell (extracellular fluid). Potassium, magnesium, and phosphate are found in large amounts in the fluid inside the cell (intracellular fluid). The difference in electrolyte composition of these fluids causes an electric charge to develop across the cell membrane. This electric charge allows for many electrochemical reactions necessary for regulation of the functions of the cells, for example, transmission of nerve impulses, contraction of muscle tissue, and secretion of glandular cells. Average electrolyte concentrations within each of the three major compartments of body fluids are given in the table.

electrolytic (e-lek″tro-lit′ik) pertaining to electrolysis or to an electrolyte.

electromagnet (e-lek″tro-mag′net) a piece of metal rendered temporarily magnetic by passage of electricity through a coil surrounding it.

electromagnetism (e-lek″tro-mag′nĕ-tizm) magnetism developed by an electric current.

electromotive force (e-lek″tro-mo′tiv) the force that, by reason of differences in potential, causes a

AVERAGE ELECTROLYTE CONCENTRATIONS OF THE BODY FLUIDS (mEq./L.)

	PLASMA	INTERSTITIAL FLUID	INTRA-CELLULAR FLUID
Cations			
Na^+ (Sodium)	142	147	15
K^+ (Potassium)	5	4	150
Ca^{++} (Calcium)	5	2.5	2
Mg^{++} (Magnesium)	2	1	27
	154	154.5	194
Anions			
Cl^- (Chloride)	103	114	1
HCO_3^- (Bicarbonate)	27	30	10
PO_4^{--} (Phosphate)	2	2	100
SO_4^{--} (Sulfate)	1	1	20
Organic acids	5	7.5	–
Proteinate	16	0	63
	154	154.5	194

From De Veber, G. A.: Fluid and electrolyte problems in the postoperative period. Nursing Clin. N. Amer., *1*:275, 1966; modified from Weisberg, H. F.: Water, Electrolyte, and Acid-Base Balance. 2nd ed. Baltimore, Md. 20202 U.S.A., The Williams & Wilkins Co., 1962.

flow of electricity from one place to another, giving rise to an electric current.

electromyogram (e-lek″tro-mi′o-gram) the record obtained by electromyography.

electromyograph (e-lek″tro-mi′o-graf) the instrument used in electromyography.

electromyography (e-lek″tro-mi-og′rah-fe) the recording and study of the intrinsic electrical properties of skeletal muscle. adj., **electromyograph′ic.** When it is at rest, normal muscle is electrically silent, but when the muscle is active, an electrical current is generated. In electromyography the electrical impulses are picked up by electrodes and amplified on an oscilloscope screen in the form of wavelike tracings. The visual recording may be accompanied by auditory monitoring in which the sounds are amplified.

Electromyography is useful in diagnosing disorders of the nerves supplying the muscle (as in amyotrophic lateral SCLEROSIS and POLIOMYELITIS) and in disorders affecting the muscle tissues. Recordings usually are obtained while the muscle is relaxed, during voluntary contraction, and during muscle activity that is produced by nerve stimulation. In this way it is possible to determine the presence of a disorder, localize the site, and identify the specific disease producing muscle weakness.

electron (e-lek′tron) any of the negatively charged particles arranged in orbits around the nucleus of an atom and determining all of the atom's physical and chemical properties except mass and radioactivity. Electrons flowing in a conductor constitute an electric current; when ejected from a radioactive substance, the beta particles.

The number of electrons revolving around the nucleus of an atom is equal to its atomic number. An atom of oxygen, for instance, which has an atomic number of 8, has eight electrons in orbit around the nucleus in a manner similar to the planets revolving around the sun in our solar system.

Electrons greatly influence the behavior of an atom toward other atoms. The combination of various ELEMENTS to form compounds is brought about by the losing or gaining of electrons; the process is sometimes called "sharing" of electrons. For example, the combination of the elements sodium and chlorine produce the compound sodium chloride (table salt). This is accomplished by the transfer of one electron from the outer orbit of the sodium atom to the outer orbit of the chlorine atom. This combining of elements by the loss or gain of electrons is called electrovalence. After the electron exchange, the atoms become charged particles called ions.

electronarcosis (e-lek″tro-nar-ko′sis) anesthesia produced by passage of an electric current through electrodes placed on the temples.

electron-dense (e-lek′tron-dens″) in electron microscopy, having a density that prevents electrons from penetrating.

electronegative (e-lek″tro-neg′ah-tiv) bearing a negative electric charge or an excess of electrons.

electronegativity (e-lek″tro-neg″ah-tiv′ĭ-te) electroaffinity.

electroneuromyography (e-lek″tro-nu″ro-mi-og′rah-fe) electromyography in which the nerve of the muscle under study is stimulated by application of an electric current.

electronic (e″lek-tron′ik) pertaining to or carrying electrons.

electronystagmograph (e-lek″tro-nis-tag′mo-graf) the instrument used in electronystagmography; abbreviated ENG.

electronystagmography (e-lek″tro-nis″tag-mog′rah-fe) electroencephalographic recordings of eye movements that provide objective documentation of induced and spontaneous nystagmus.

electro-oculogram (e″lek″tro-ok′u-lo-gram″) the electroencephalographic tracings made while moving the eyes a constant distance between two fixation points, inducing a deflection of fairly constant amplitude; abbreviated EOG.

electropherogram (e-lek″tro-fer′o-gram) electrophoretogram.

electrophoresis (e-lek″tro-fo-re′sis) the movement of charged particles suspended in a liquid on various media (e.g., paper, gel, liquid) under the influence of an applied electric field. adj., **electrophoret′ic.** The various charged particles of a particular substance migrate in a definite and characteristic direction—toward either the anode or the cathode—and at a characteristic speed. This principle has been widely used in the separation of proteins and is therefore valuable in the study of diseases in which the serum and plasma proteins are altered. The principle also has been applied in the separation and identification of various types of human hemoglobin.

electrophoretogram (e-lek″tro-fo-ret′o-gram) the record produced on or in a supporting medium by bands of material which have been separated by the process of electrophoresis.

electrophysiology (e-lek″tro-fiz″e-ol′o-je) the study of the effects of electric reactions of the body in health.

electropositive (e-lek″tro-poz′ĭ-tiv) bearing a positive electric charge.

electroresection (e-lek″tro-re-sek′shun) resection by electrosurgical means.

electroretinograph (e-lek″tro-ret′in-o-graf) an instrument for measuring the electrical response of the retina to light stimulation; abbreviated ERG.

electroscission (e-lek″tro-sish′un) cutting of tissue by means of the electric cautery.

electroscope (e-lek′tro-skōp) an instrument for measuring radiation intensity.

electroshock therapy (e-lek′tro-shok) electroconvulsive therapy; the induction of convulsions by the passage of an electric current through the brain, as in the treatment of affective disorders (see also SHOCK THERAPY).

electrostimulation (e-lek″tro-stim″u-la′shun) electric stimulation of tissues.

electrostriatogram (e-lek″tro-stri-a′to-gram) an electroencephalogram showing differences in electric potential recorded at various levels of the corpus striatum.

electrosurgery (e-lek″tro-ser′jer-e) surgery performed by electrical methods; the active electrode may be a needle, bulb, or disk. adj., **electrosur′gical.**

electrosynthesis (e-lek″tro-sin′thĕ-sis) the formation of a compound under the influence of electricity.

electrotaxis (e-lek″tro-tak′sis) taxis in response to electric stimuli.

electrotherapeutics, electrotherapy (e-lek″tro-ther-ah-pu′tiks; e-lek″tro-ther′ah-pe) treatment of disease by means of electricity. (See also DIATHERMY.)

electrotropism (e″lek-trot′ro-pizm) tropism in response to electric stimuli.

electrovalence (e-lek″tro-va′lens) the number of charges an atom acquires in a chemical reaction by gain or loss of electrons.

electroversion (e-lek″tro-ver′zhun) the act of electrically terminating a cardiac dysrhythmia.

electrovert (e-lek′tro-vert) to apply electricity to the heart or precordium to depolarize the heart and terminate a cardiac dysrhythmia.

electuary (e-lek′tu-a″re) a medicinal preparation consisting of a powdered drug made into a paste with honey or syrup.

eledoisin (el″ĕ-doi′sin) a decapeptide from the posterior salivary gland of a species of snail (*Eledone*), which is a precursor of a large group of biologically active peptides; it has vasodilator, hypotensive, and extravascular smooth muscle stimulant properties.

eleidin (el-e′ĭ-din) a substance, allied to keratin, found in the cells of the stratum lucidum of the skin.

element (el′ĕ-ment) 1. any of the primary parts or constituents of a thing. 2. in chemistry, a simple substance that cannot be decomposed by ordinary chemical means; the basic "stuff" of which all matter is composed.

Chemical elements are made up of atoms. Each atom consists of a nucleus with a cloud of negatively charged particles (ELECTRONS) revolving around it. The two major components of the nucleus are protons and neutrons. The number of protons in the atoms of a particular element is always the same, and therefore the physical and chemical properties of the element are always the same. It is possible, however, for a chemical element to exist in several different forms, the difference depending on the number of neutrons in the nucleus of its atoms. Different forms of the same element are called isotopes.

There are at least 105 different chemical elements known. The table lists the elements, and the symbol, atomic weight and atomic number of each. The atomic number of an element is determined by the number of protons in the nucleus of an atom of the element. The mass number of an isotope is determined by the total number of neutrons and protons in the nucleus.

STABLE CHEMICAL ELEMENTS. A stable chemical element is one that contains an optimal ratio or range of ratios between the number of protons and neutrons in the nucleus. A stable element does not spontaneously transmute into another element and therefore does not give off radiations. The stable elements are those that have an atomic number below 84, except for a few, such as potassium and rubidium, which are weakly radioactive.

RADIOACTIVE CHEMICAL ELEMENTS. A radioactive chemical element does not contain an optimal proton-to-neutron ratio in its atomic nuclei and therefore readily gives off nuclear particles until all nuclei have attained the optimal combination of protons and neutrons. The spontaneous releasing of its nuclear particles changes the radioactive atom into a new atom (transmutation).

As radioactive elements disintegrate and form new chemical elements, a tremendous amount of energy is released. This emission of energy and nuclear particles is called RADIATION. The radiations may be electrically charged particles having size and mass, such as ALPHA PARTICLES and BETA PARTICLES, or they may be nonparticulate and contain no electrical charges, such as GAMMA RAYS. Most radioactive elements give off either alpha or beta particles and at the same time emit gamma radiation.

formed e's (of the blood), erythrocytes, leukocytes, and platelets.

trace e., a chemical element present or needed in extremely small amount by plants and animals, such as manganese, copper, cobalt, zinc, iron.

ele(o)- word element [Gr.], *oil.*

eleoma (el″e-o′mah) a tumor or swelling caused by injection of oil into the tissues.

eleometer (el″e-om′ĕ-ter) an instrument for determining the percentage of oil in a mixture or the specific gravity of oils.

eleopten (el″e-op′ten) the more volatile constituent of a volatile oil.

eleotherapy (el″e-o-ther′ah-pe) oleotherapy.

elephantiasis (el″ĕ-fan-ti′ah-sis) a chronic filarial disease marked by inflammation and obstruction of the lymphatics and hypertrophy of the skin and subcutaneous tissues, chiefly affecting the legs and external genitals. The disease derives its name from

(*Text continued on page 334.*)

Table of Chemical Elements

Element (Date of Discovery)	Symbol	Atomic Number	Atomic Weight*	Valence	Sp. Gr. or Density (Grams/Liter)	Descriptive Comment
Actinium (1899)	Ac	89	[227]	....	10.07	radioactive element associated with uranium
Aluminum (1827)	Al	13	26.9815	3	2.6989	silvery-white metal, abundant in earth's crust, but not in free form
Americium (1944)	Am	95	[243]	3, 4, 5, 6	11.7	fourth transuranium element discovered
Antimony (prehistoric)	Sb	51	121.75	3, 5	6.691	exists in 4 allotropic forms
Argon (1894)	Ar	18	39.948	0?	1.7837 g./l.	colorless, odorless gas
Arsenic (1250)	As	33	74.9216	3, 5	5.73	(gray) semimetallic solid
					4.73	(black)
					1.97	(yellow)
Astatine (1940)	At	85	[210]	1, 3, 5, 7		radioactive halogen
Barium (1808)	Ba	56	137.34	2	3.5	silvery-white, alkaline earth metal
Berkelium (1949)	Bk	97	[247]	3, 4		fifth transuranium element discovered
Beryllium (1798)	Be	4	9.0122	2	1.848	light, steel-gray metal
Bismuth (1753)	Bi	83	208.980	3, 5	9.747	pinkish-white, crystalline, brittle metal
Boron (1808)	B	5	10.811	3	2.34, 2.37	crystalline or amorphous element, not occurring free in nature
Bromine (1826)	Br	35	79.909	1, 3, 5, 7	3.12	mobile, reddish-brown liquid, volatilizing readily
					7.59 g./l.	red vapor with disagreeable odor
Cadmium (1817)	Cd	48	112.40	2	8.65	soft, bluish-white metal
Calcium (1808)	Ca	20	40.08	2	1.55	metallic element, forming more than 3 per cent of earth's crust
Californium (1950)	Cf	98	[249]	....		sixth transuranium element discovered
Carbon (prehistoric)	C	6	12.01115	2, 3, 4	1.8–2.1	(amorphous) element widely distributed in nature
					1.9–2.3	(graphite)
					3.15–3.53	(diamond)
Cerium (1803)	Ce	58	140.12	3, 4	6.67–8.23	most abundant rare earth metal
Cesium (1860)	Cs	55	132.905	1	1.873	silvery-white, soft, alkaline metal
Chlorine (1774)	Cl	17	35.453	1, 3, 5, 7	3.214 g./l.	greenish-yellow gas of the halogen group
Chromium (1797)	Cr	24	51.996	2, 3, 6	7.18–7.20	steel-gray, lustrous, hard metal
Cobalt (1735)	Co	27	58.9332	2, 3	8.9	brittle, hard metal
Copper (prehistoric)	Cu	29	63.54	1, 2	8.96	reddish, lustrous, malleable metal
Curium (1944)	Cm	96	[247]	3	7	third transuranium element discovered
Dysprosium (1886)	Dy	66	162.50	3	8.536	rare earth metal with metallic bright silver luster

Einsteinium (1952)	Es	99	[254]	....		seventh transuranium element discovered
Erbium (1843)	Er	68	167.26	3	9.051	soft, malleable rare earth metal
Europium (1896)	Eu	63	151.96	2, 3	5.259	lustrous, silvery-white rare earth metal
Fermium (1953)	Fm	100	[253]	....		eighth transuranium element discovered
Fluorine (1771)	F	9	18.9984	1	1.696 g./l.	pale yellow, corrosive gas of the halogen group
Francium (1939)	Fr	87	[223]	1		product of alpha disintegration of actinium
Gadolinium (1880)	Gd	64	157.25	3	7.8, 7.895	lustrous, silvery-white rare earth metal
Gallium (1875)	Ga	31	69.72	2, 3	5.907	beautiful, silvery-appearing metal
Germanium (1886)	Ge	32	72.59	2, 4	5.323	grayish-white, brittle metal
Gold (prehistoric)	Au	79	196.967	1, 3	19.32	malleable yellow metal
Hafnium (1923)	Hf	72	178.49	4	13.29	gray metal associated with zirconium
Hahnium (1970)	Ha	105	[260]			twelfth transuranium element discovered
Helium (1895)	He	2	4.0026	0	0.177 g./l.	inert gas
Holmium (1879)	Ho	67	164.930	3	8.803	relatively soft and malleable rare earth metal
Hydrogen (1766)	H	1	1.00797	1	0.08988 g./l.	(gas) most abundant element in the universe
					0.070	(liquid)
Indium (1863)	In	49	114.82	1, 2?, 3	7.31	soft, silvery-white metal
Iodine (1811)	I	53	126.9044	1, 3, 5, 7	4.93, 11.27 g./l.	grayish-black, lustrous solid or violet-blue gas
Iridium (1803)	Ir	77	192.2	3, 4	22.42	white, brittle metal of platinum family
Iron (prehistoric)	Fe	26	55.847	2, 3, 4, 6	7.874	fourth most abundant element in earth's crust
Krypton (1898)	Kr	36	83.80	0	3.733 g./l.	inert gas
Lanthanum (1839)	La	57	138.91	3	5.98–6.186	silvery-white, ductile, rare earth metal
Lawrencium (1961)	Lw	103	[257]	....		tenth transuranium element discovered
Lead (prehistoric)	Pb	82	207.19	2, 4	11.35	bluish-white, lustrous, malleable metal
Lithium (1817)	Li	3	6.939	1	0.534	lightest of all metals
Lutetium (1907)	Lu	71	174.97	3	9.872	rare earth metal
Magnesium (1808)	Mg	12	24.312	2	1.738	silvery-white metallic element, eighth in abundance in earth's crust
Manganese (1774)	Mn	25	54.9380	1, 2, 3, 4, 6, 7	7.21–7.44	exists in 4 allotropic forms
Mendelevium (1955)	Md	101	[256]	....		ninth transuranium element discovered
Mercury (prehistoric)	Hg	80	200.59	1, 2	13.546	heavy, silvery-white metal, liquid at ordinary temperatures
Molybdenum (1782)	Mo	42	95.94	2, 3, 4?, 5?, 6	10.22	silvery-white, very hard metal
Neodymium (1885)	Nd	60	144.24	3	6.80, 7.004	exists in 2 allotropic forms
Neon (1898)	Ne	10	20.183	0?	0.89990 g./l.	inert gas
Neptunium (1940)	Np	93	[237]	3, 4, 5, 6	18.0–20.45	first transuranium element discovered
Nickel (1751)	Ni	28	58.71	0, 1, 2, 3	8.902	silvery-white, malleable metal
Niobium (1801)	Nb	41	92.906	2, 3, 4?, 5	8.57	shiny white, soft, ductile metal
Nitrogen (1772)	N	7	14.0067	3, 5	1.2506 g./l.	colorless, odorless, inert element, making up 78 per cent of the air
Nobelium (?) (1958)	No	102	[253]	....		acceptance of this element considered premature
Osmium (1803)	Os	76	190.2	2, 3, 4, 8	22.57	bluish-white, hard metal of platinum family
Oxygen (1774)	O	8	15.9994	2	1.429 g./l.	colorless, odorless gas, third most abundant element in the universe

TABLE OF CHEMICAL ELEMENTS (*Concluded*)

ELEMENT (DATE OF DISCOVERY)	SYMBOL	ATOMIC NUMBER	ATOMIC WEIGHT*	VALENCE	SP. GR. OR DENSITY (GRAMS/LITER)	DESCRIPTIVE COMMENT
Palladium (1803)	Pd	46	106.4	2, 3, 4	12.02	steel-white metal of the platinum family
Phosphorus (1669)	P	15	30.9738	3, 5	1.82	(white) waxy solid, transparent when pure
					2.20	(red)
					2.25–2.69	(black)
Platinum (1735)	Pt	78	195.09	1?, 2, 3, 4	21.45	silvery-white, malleable metal
Plutonium (1940)	Pu	94	[242]	3, 4, 5, 6	19.84	second transuranium element discovered
Polonium (1898)	Po	84	[210]	2, 4, 6	9.32	very rare natural element
Potassium (1807)	K	19	39.102	1	0.862	soft, silvery, alkali metal, seventh in abundance in earth's crust
Praseodymium (1885)	Pr	59	140.907	3, 4	6.782, 6.64	soft, silvery rare earth metal
Promethium (1941)	Pm	61	[147]	3		produced by irradiation of neodymium and praseodymium; identity established in 1945
Protactinium (1917)	Pa	91	[231]	4 or 5	15.37	bright lustrous metal
Radium (1898)	Ra	88	[226]	2	5(?)	brilliant white, radioactive metal
Radon (1900)	Rn	86	[222]	0	9.73 g./l.	heaviest known gas
Rhenium (1925)	Re	75	186.2	−1, 2, 3, 4, 5, 6, 7	21.02	silvery-white lustrous metal
Rhodium (1803)	Rh	45	102.905	−2, 3, 4, 5,	12.41	silvery-white metal of platinum family
Rubidium (1861)	Rb	37	85.47	1, 2, 3, 4	1.532	soft, silvery-white, alkali metal
Ruthenium (1844)	Ru	44	101.07	0, 1, 2, 3, 4, 5, 6, 7, 8	12.41	hard white metal of platinum family
Rutherfordium (1969)	Rf	104	[261]			eleventh transuranium element discovered
Samarium (1879)	Sm	62	150.35	2, 3	7.536–7.40	bright silver lustrous metal
Scandium (1879)	Sc	21	44.956	3	2.992	soft, silvery-white metal
Selenium (1817)	Se	34	78.96	2, 4, 6	4.79, 4.28	exists in several allotropic forms
Silicon (1823)	Si	14	28.086	4	2.33	a relatively inert element, second in abundance in earth's crust
Silver (prehistoric)	Ag	47	107.870	1, 2	10.50	malleable, ductile metal with brilliant white luster
Sodium (1807)	Na	11	22.9898	1	0.971	most abundant of alkali metals, sixth in abundance in earth's crust
Strontium (1808)	Sr	38	87.62	2	2.54	exists in 3 allotropic forms
Sulfur (prehistoric)	S	16	32.064	2, 4, 6	1.957, 2.07	exists in several isotopic and many allotropic forms
Tantalum (1802)	Ta	73	180.948	2?, 3, 4?, 5	16.6	gray, heavy, very hard metal
Technetium (1937)	Tc	43	[99]	3?, 4, 6, 7	11.50	first element produced artificially
Tellurium (1782)	Te	52	127.60	2, 4, 6	6.24	silvery-white, lustrous element

Terbium (1843)	Tb	65	158.924	3, 4	8.272	silvery-gray, malleable, ductile rare earth metal
Thallium (1861)	Tl	81	204.37	1, 3	11.85	very soft, malleable metal
Thorium (1828)	Th	90	232.038	4	11.66	silvery-white, lustrous metal
Thulium (1879)	Tm	69	168.934	2, 3		least abundant rare earth metal
Tin (prehistoric)	Sn	50	118.69	2, 4	5.75	(gray) malleable metal existing in 2 or 3 allotropic forms, changing from white to gray on cooling and back to white on warming
					7.31	(white)
Titanium (1791)	Ti	22	47.90	2, 3, 4	4.54	lustrous white metal
Tungsten (1783)	W	74	183.85	2, 3, 4, 5, 6	19.3	steel-gray to tin-white metal
Uranium (1789)	U	92	238.03	3, 4, 5, 6	18.95	heavy, silvery-white metal
Vanadium (1801)	V	23	50.942	2, 3, 4, 5	6.11	bright, white metal
Xenon (1898)	Xe	54	131.30	0?	5.887 g./l.	one of the so-called rare or inert gases
Ytterbium (1878)	Yb	70	173.04	2, 3	6.977, 6.54	exists in 2 allotropic forms
Yttrium (1794)	Y	39	88.905	3	4.45	rare earth metal with silvery metallic luster
Zinc (1746)	Zn	30	65.37	2	7.133	bluish-white, lustrous metal, malleable at 100–150° C.
Zirconium (1789)	Zr	40	91.22	4	6.4	grayish-white, lustrous metal

*Figures in brackets represent mass number of most stable isotope.

Table of Elements by Atomic Numbers

1 hydrogen	16 sulfur	31 gallium	46 palladium	61 promethium	76 osmium	91 protactinium
2 helium	17 chlorine	32 germanium	47 silver	62 samarium	77 iridium	92 uranium
3 lithium	18 argon	33 arsenic	48 cadmium	63 europium	78 platinum	93 neptunium
4 beryllium	19 potassium	34 selenium	49 indium	64 gadolinium	79 gold	94 plutonium
5 boron	20 calcium	35 bromine	50 tin	65 terbium	80 mercury	95 americium
6 carbon	21 scandium	36 krypton	51 antimony	66 dysprosium	81 thallium	96 curium
7 nitrogen	22 titanium	37 rubidium	52 tellurium	67 holmium	82 lead	97 berkelium
8 oxygen	23 vanadium	38 strontium	53 iodine	68 erbium	83 bismuth	98 californium
9 fluorine	24 chromium	39 yttrium	54 xenon	69 thulium	84 polonium	99 einsteinium
10 neon	25 manganese	40 zirconium	55 cesium	70 ytterbium	85 astatine	100 fermium
11 sodium	26 iron	41 niobium	56 barium	71 lutetium	86 radon	101 mendelevium
12 magnesium	27 cobalt	42 molybdenum	57 lanthanum	72 hafnium	87 francium	102 [*see* nobelium]
13 aluminum	28 nickel	43 technetium	58 cerium	73 tantalum	88 radium	103 lawrencium
14 silicon	29 copper	44 ruthenium	59 praseodymium	74 tungsten	89 actinium	104 rutherfordium
15 phosphorus	30 zinc	45 rhodium	60 neodymium	75 rhenium	90 thorium	105 hahnium

the symptoms, particularly swelling of the legs, which makes them look like those of an elephant. The term is often applied to hypertrophy and thickening of the tissues from any cause.

True elephantiasis, or elephantiasis filariensis, is most often caused by a slender, threadlike parasite, the filarial worm, *Wuchereria bancrofti,* which enters the lymphatic system, causing an obstruction to drainage. The disease, sometimes called FILARIASIS, is transmitted by mosquitoes or flies which carry blood infected with filaria larvae. Elephantiasis is most often encountered in Central Africa, in some Pacific Islands, and in other tropical and subtropical areas. It is rare or nonexistent in the temperate zone.

The first visible signs are inflamation of the lymph nodes, with temporary swelling in the affected area, red streaks along the leg or arm, pain, and tenderness. Specific drugs are administered for destruction of the parasites; bandages and elevation of the affected area help relieve the swelling. Sanitary control to eliminate the carrier insects is the most effective approach to elimination of this disease.

e. scro′ti, that in which the scrotum is the main seat of the disease.

elephantoid fever (el″ĕ-fan′toid) a recurrent acute febrile condition occurring with filariasis; it may be associated with elephantiasis or lymphangitis.

elimination (e-lim″ĭ-na′shun) discharge from the body of indigestible materials and of waste products of body metabolism.

e. diet, one for diagnosing food allergy, based on the sequential omission of foods that might cause the symptoms in the patient.

Elipten (e-lip′ten) trademark for a preparation of aminoglutethimide, an anticonvulsant.

elixir (e-lik′ser) a clear, sweetened, usually hydroalcoholic liquid containing flavoring substances and sometimes active medicinal ingredients, for oral use.

Elkosin (el′ko-sin) trademark for preparations of sulfisomidine, a sulfonamide.

elliptocyte (e-lip′to-sīt) an elliptical erythrocyte.

elliptocytosis (e-lip″to-si-to′sis) a hereditary disorder in which the erythrocytes are largely elliptical and which is characterized by increased red cell destruction and anemia.

Elorine (el′o-rēn) trademark for a preparation of tricyclamol, an anticholinergic.

eluate (el′u-āt) the substance separated out by, or the product of, elution or elutriation.

eluent (e-lu′ent) the solution used in elution.

elution (e-loo′shun) in chemistry, separation of material by washing; the process of pulverizing substances and mixing them with water in order to separate the heavier constituents, which settle out in solution, from the lighter.

elutriation (e-loo″tre-a′shun) purification of a substance by dissolving it in a solvent and pouring off the solution, thus separating it from the undissolved foreign material.

Em. emmetropia.

emaciation (e-ma″se-a′shun) excessive leanness; a wasted condition of the body.

emailloid (e-ma′loid) ameloblast.

emanation (em″ah-na′shun) that which is given off, such as a gaseous disintegration product given off from radioactive substances, or an effluvium.

emasculation (e-mas″ku-la′shun) removal of the penis or testes.

embalming (em-bahm′ing) treatment of a dead body to retard decomposition.

embarrass (em-bar′as) to impede the function of; to obstruct.

Embden-Meyerhof pathway (em′den-mi′er-hof) the series of enzymatic reactions in the anaerobic conversion of glucose to lactic acid, resulting in energy in the form of adenosine triphosphate (ATP).

embedding (em-bed′ing) fixation of tissue in a firm medium, in order to keep it intact during cutting of thin sections.

embole (em′bo-le) the reducing of a dislocated limb.

embolectomy (em″bo-lek′to-me) surgical removal of an embolus.

emboli (em′bo-li) plural of *embolus.*

embolic (em-bol′ik) pertaining to embolism or an embolus.

embolism (em′bo-lizm) the sudden blocking of an artery by a clot of foreign material (embolus) that has been brought to its site of lodgment by the blood current. The obstructing material is most often a blood clot, but may be a fat globule, air bubble, piece of tissue, or clump of bacteria.

SYMPTOMS. The symptoms of an embolism usually do not appear until the embolus lodges within a blood vessel and suddenly obstructs the blood flow. Emboli usually lodge at divisions of an artery, where the vessel narrows. The signs of obstruction appear almost immediately with severe pain at the site. If the embolus lodges in an extremity the area becomes pale, numb, and cold to the touch, and normal arterial pulse below the site is absent. Fainting, nausea and vomiting and eventually severe shock may occur if a large vessel is occluded. Unless the obstruction is relieved, gangrene of the adjacent tissues served by the affected vessel develops.

PREVENTION. THROMBOPHLEBITIS AND PHLEBOTHROMBOSIS are the most common predisposing causes of embolism, particularly one which lodges in an extremity. In order to prevent the development of emboli it is necessary to avoid venous stasis in patients who are confined to bed because of surgery, illness, or injury. In addition to physical inactivity, heart failure and pressure on the veins of the legs and pelvis can inhibit blood flow and thus set the stage for inflammation, clot formation, and the possibility of embolism.

Although frequent changing of position, exercise, and early ambulation are necessary to the prevention of thrombosis and embolism, sudden and extreme movements should be avoided. Under no circumstances should the legs be massaged to relieve "muscle cramps," especially when the pain is located in the calf and the patient has not been up and about; pain in the calf may be symptomatic of a thrombosis.

The occurrence of an air embolism can be avoided by careful handling of equipment used for intravenous therapy and correct technique in administering intramuscular injections.

TREATMENT AND PATIENT CARE. Immediate care of the patient with an embolism of an extremity must be prompt, especially if the affected blood vessel is large and gangrene is a real possibility. The purpose of initial treatment is facilitation of blood flow to the part. This is accomplished by lowering the limb to a dependent position and wrapping it to prevent loss of body warmth and combat constriction of the blood vessels. Direct heat is not applied to ischemic tissue because it may further damage the tissues and accelerate the development of gangrene.

Heparin may be given immediately to decrease the possibility of further clot formation. Spasms of the blood vessels may be relieved by an antispasmodic drug or by blocking the sympathetic nerves by local injection of procaine. If conservative measures are not effective, surgery may be necessary to remove the obstructing clot and restore circulation.

Postoperatively the patient's vital signs are monitored and the extremity evaluated frequently to assess circulation. The affected limb should show signs of adequate circulation, that is, warmth, return of color and feeling, and normal PULSE. If these are not present or the limb shows signs of increasing ischemia, the surgeon should be notified. Signs of bleeding at the operative site also should be reported, particularly if the patient has received anticoagulant medication. Exercise of the limb and ambulation are begun only after the surgeon has assessed the patient's status and given permission.

cerebral e., embolism of a cerebral artery, one of the three main causes of CEREBRAL VASCULAR ACCIDENT (stroke).

pulmonary e., obstruction of the pulmonary artery or one of its branches by an embolus. The embolus usually is a blood clot swept into circulation from a large peripheral vein—particularly one in the leg or pelvis. The condition of THROMBOSIS predisposes the patient to pulmonary embolism, as do fracture and other traumas to the lower extremity, surgical and postpartal confinement to bed, and chronic illnesses requiring bed rest. Plugging of a large pulmonary vessel can cause sudden death. Symptoms include sudden onset of chest pain, a cough productive of bright red sputum, tachycardia, and rapid, shallow respirations. Treatment usually consists of administration of oxygen, morphine sulfate to relieve pain, and anticoagulant drugs to aid in removal of the clot.

embololalia (em″bo-lo-la′le-ah) the interpolation of meaningless words or phrases in a spoken sentence.

embolophrasia (em″bo-lo-fra′ze-ah) embololalia.

embolus (em′bo-lus), pl. *em′boli* [Gr.] a clot or other plug, usually part or all of a thrombus, brought by the blood from another vessel and forced into a smaller one, thus obstructing circulation (EMBOLISM).

saddle e., one situated at the bifurcation of a large artery, sometimes blocking both branches.

embryectomy (em″bre-ek′to-me) excision of an extrauterine embryo or fetus.

embryo (em′bre-o) a new organism in the earliest stage of development; the human young from the time of fertilization of the ovum until the beginning of the third month. After the second month the unborn baby is usually referred to as the fetus. adj., **em′bryonal, embryon′ic.**

Immediately after fertilization takes place, cell division begins and progresses at a rapid rate. At approximately 4 weeks the cell mass becomes a recognizable embryo from 7 to 10 mm. long with rudimentary organs. The beginnings of the eyes, ears, and extremities can be seen. By the end of the second month the embryo has grown to a length of 2 to 2.5 cm., and the head is the most prominent part because of the rapid development of the brain; the sex can be distinguished at this stage.

At the time of fertilization the ovum contains the potential beginnings of a human being. As cell division takes place the cells of the blastoderm (embryonic disk) gradually form three layers from which all the body structures develop. The ectoderm (outer layer) gives rise to the epidermis of the skin and its appendages, and to the nervous system. The mesoderm (middle layer) develops into muscle, connective tissue, the circulatory organs, circulating lymph and blood cells, endothelial tissues within the closed vessels and cavities, and the epithelium portion of the urogenital system. From the entoderm (internal layer) are derived those portions not arising from the ectoderm, the liver, pancreas, and the lungs.

embryocardia (em″bre-o-kar′de-ah) a symptom in which the heart sounds resemble those of the fetus, there being very little difference in the quality of the first and second sounds.

embryoctony (em″bre-ok′to-ne) destruction of the living embryo or fetus.

embryologist (em″bre-ol′o-jist) an expert in embryology.

embryology (em″bre-ol′o-je) the science of the development of the individual during the embryonic stage and, by extension, in several or even all preceding and subsequent stages of the life cycle. adj., **embryolog′ic.**

embryoma (em″bre-o′mah) a general term applied to neoplasms thought to be derived from embryonic cells or tissues, including dermoid cysts, teratomas, embryonal carcinomas, etc.

e. of kidney, Wilms' tumor.

embryonization (em-bre″o-nĭ-za′shun) reversion of a tissue or cell to the embryonic form.

embryonoid (em′bre-ŏ-noid″) resembling an embryo.

embryopathy (em″bre-op′ah-the) a morbid condition resulting from interference with normal embryonic development, with consequent congenital anomalies.

rubella e., congenital deformities in an infant due to RUBELLA (German measles) in the mother during early pregnancy; called also rubella syndrome.

embryoplastic (em′bre-o-plas″tik) pertaining to or concerned in formation of an embryo.

embryotomy (em″bre-ot′o-me) dismemberment of the fetus in difficult labor in which a normal delivery is impossible.

embryotoxon (em″bre-o-tok′son) a ringlike opacity at the margin of the cornea.

anterior e., embryotoxon.

posterior e., a developmental anomaly in which there is a ringlike opacity at Schwalbe's ring, with thickening and anterior displacement of the latter.

embryotroph (em′bre-o-trōf″) the total nutriment (histotroph and hemotroph) made available to the embryo.

embryotrophy (em″bre-ot′ro-fe) the nutrition of the early embryo.

embryulcus (em″bre-ul′kus) a blunt hook for removal of the fetus from the uterus.

emedullate (e-med′u-lāt) to remove bone marrow.

emergent (e-mer′jent) 1. coming out from a cavity or other part. 2. coming on suddenly.

emesis (em′ĕ-sis) the act of vomiting. Also used as a word termination, as in *hematemesis.*

emetic (e-met′ik) 1. causing vomiting. 2. an agent that causes vomiting. A strong solution of salt (1 tablespoon to 1 cup of water), mustard water (1 tablespoon to 1 cup of water), and powdered ipecac or ipecac syrup are examples of emetics.

Emetics should not be used when lye or other strong alkalis or acids have been swallowed, since vomiting may rupture the already weakened walls of the esophagus. Among the acids and alkalis for which emetics should not be used are sodium hydroxide (caustic soda), potassium hydroxide (caustic potash), and carbolic acid. Emetics should be avoided also when kerosene, gasoline, nail polish remover, or lacquer thinner has been swallowed, since vomiting of these substances may draw them into the lungs.

emetine (em′ĕ-tēn) an alkaloid derived from ipecac or produced synthetically. Its hydrochloride salt is used as an antiamebic.

emetocathartic (em″ĕ-to-kah-thar′tik) 1. both emetic and cathartic. 2. an emetocathartic agent.

E.M.F. electromotive force.

-emia word element [Gr.], *condition of the blood.*

emigration (em″ĭ-gra′shun) the escape of leukocytes through the walls of small blood vessels; diapedesis.

eminence (em′ĭ-nens) a projection or boss.

eminentia (em″ĭ-nen′she-ah), pl. *eminen′tiae* [L.] eminence.

emiocytosis (e″me-o-si-to′sis) the ejection of material, e.g., insulin granules, from a cell.

emissary (em′ĭ-sār″e) affording an outlet, referring especially to the venous outlets from the dural sinuses through the skull.

emission (e-mish′un) a discharge; specifically an involuntary discharge of semen.

nocturnal e., reflex emission of semen during sleep.

Emivan (em′ĭ-van) trademark for preparations of ethamivan, a respiratory stimulant.

emmenagogue (ĕ-men′ah-gog) an agent or measure that promotes menstruation.

emmenia (ĕ-me′ne-ah) menstruation. adj., **emmen′ic.**

emmenology (em″ĕ-nol′o-je) the sum of knowledge about menstruation and its disorders.

emmetrope (em′ĕ-trōp) a person who has no refractive error of vision.

emmetropia (em″ĕ-tro′pe-ah) the ideal optical condition, parallel rays coming to a focus on the retina. adj., **emmetrop′ic.**

emollient (e-mol′yent) 1. soothing and softening, as an emollient bath given for various skin disorders. 2. an agent that softens or soothes the skin, or soothes an irritated internal surface.

emotion (e-mo′shun) a state of mental excitement characterized by alteration of feeling tone and by physical changes in the body. adj., **emo′tional.** The physical form of emotion may be outward and evident to others, as in crying, laughing, blushing, or a variety of facial expressions. However, emotion is not always reflected in one's appearance and actions even though psychic changes are taking place. Joy, grief, fear, and anger are examples of emotions.

empathize (em′pah-thīz) to experience or feel empathy; to enter into another's feelings.

empathy (em′pah-the) the recognition of and entering into another's feelings. adj., **empath′ic.**

emperipolesis (em-per″ĭ-po-le′sis) lymphocytic penetration of and movement within another cell.

emphysema (em″fĭ-se′mah, em″fi-ze′mah) a pathologic accumulation of air in tissues or organs. The term is generally used to designate chronic pulmonary emphysema, a lung disorder in which the terminal bronchioles become plugged with mucus. Eventually there is a loss of elasticity in the lung tissue so that inspired air becomes trapped in the lungs, making breathing difficult, especially during the expiratory phase.

bullous e., emphysema in which bullae form in areas of lung tissue so that these areas do not contribute to respiration.

chronic pulmonary e., emphysema of the lungs that develops slowly over a period of years and in some persons may gradually lead to serious disability. It is found most frequently in men over 40.

In many cases, it occurs as a result of prolonged respiratory difficulties, such as chronic bronchial ASTHMA, BRONCHITIS, or TUBERCULOSIS, that have caused partial obstruction of the smaller divisions of the bronchi. (See also CHRONIC OBSTRUCTIVE PULMONARY DISEASE.)

Chronic emphysema may also occur without serious preceding respiratory problems. Some authorities suggest that a defect in the elastic tissue of the lungs may make certain persons susceptible to the disease. It is found with some frequency in aged persons whose lungs have lost their natural elasticity.

Chronic emphysema of the lungs kills over 10,000 Americans a year and the number of deaths has been increasing sharply. The reasons for this are not fully known. As with other respiratory ailments, however, one factor may be the increasing pollution of the air that accompanies urbanization, industrialization, and the growing number of automobiles. Another reason may be the increase in tobacco smoking. Although there is no proof that smoking actually causes emphysema, there is a higher proportion of smokers who inhale or smoke heavily among emphysema sufferers than among the general population. It is known that the continuance of smoking seriously aggravates the disease.

SYMPTOMS. As the lungs become less efficient, breathing becomes more difficult for chronic emphysema sufferers. There is often a persistent cough that is moist and wheezing in nature. The patient often develops a barrel-shaped chest and has an anxious facial expression. Cardiac complications, especially enlargement and dilatation of the right ventricle with resultant right heart failure (COR PULMONALE), may develop from pulmonary emphysema.

TREATMENT. See CHRONIC OBSTRUCTIVE PULMONARY DISEASE.

interlobular e., accumulation of air in the septa between lobules of the lungs.

interstitial e., presence of air in the peribronchial and interstitial tissues of the lungs.

intestinal e., a condition marked by accumulation of gas under the tunica serosa of the intestine.

lobar e., emphysema involving less than all the lobes of the affected lung.

lobar e., congenital, lobar e., infantile, a condition characterized by overinflation, commonly affecting one of the upper lobes and causing respiratory distress in early life.

panacinar e., panlobular e., generalized obstructive emphysema affecting all lung segments, with atrophy and dilatation of the alveoli and destruction of the vascular bed.

subcutaneous e., air or gas in the subcutaneous tissues.

surgical e., subcutaneous emphysema following operation.

unilateral e., emphysema affecting only one lung, frequently due to congenital defects in circulation.

vesicular e., panacinar emphysema.

emphysematous (em″fĭ-sem′ah-tus) of the nature of or affected with emphysema.

empiricism (em-pir′ĭ-sizm) skill or knowledge based entirely on experience. adj., **empir′ic.**

Empirin (em′pĭ-rin) trademark for tablets containing acetylsalicylic acid, acetophenetidin, and caffeine, used as an analgesic. One form of Empirin contains codeine and requires a prescription.

emprosthotonos (em″pros-thot′o-nos) tetanic forward flexure of the body.

empty-sella syndrome a clinical syndrome in which the diaphragm of the sella turcica is vestigial, the sella turcica forms an extension of the subarachnoid space and is filled with cerebrospinal fluid, and the pituitary fossa appears to be empty, although the pituitary gland is present in a flattened form.

empyema (em″pi-e′mah) accumulation of pus in a body cavity, particularly the presence of a purulent exudate within the pleural cavity (pyothorax). It occurs as an occasional complication of pleurisy or some other respiratory disease. Symptoms include dyspnea,, coughing, chest pain on one side, malaise, and fever. Thoracentesis may be done to confirm the diagnosis and determine the specific causative organism. The condition is treated with antibiotics, rest, and sedative cough mixtures.

empyesis (em″pi-e′sis) a pustular eruption.

emulgent (e-mul′jent) 1. effecting a straining or purifying process. 2. a renal artery or vein. 3. a medicine that stimulates bile or urine flow.

emulsifier (e-mul″sĭ-fi′er) a substance used to make an emulsion.

emulsion (e-mul′shun) a mixture of two immiscible liquids, one being dispersed throughout the other in small droplets; a colloid system in which both the dispersed phase and the dispersion medium are liquids. Margarine, cold cream, and various medicated ointments are emulsions. In some emulsions the suspended particles tend to join together and settle out; hence the container must be shaken each time the emulsion is used.

emulsoid (e-mul′soid) a colloid system in which the dispersion medium is liquid, usually water, and the disperse phase consists of highly complex organic substances, such as starch or glue, which absorb much water, swell, and become distributed throughout the dispersion medium.

emunctory (e-mungk′to-re) 1. excretory or cleansing. 2. an excretory organ or duct.

emylcamate (e-mil′kah-māt) a tranquilizer.

enamel (e-nam′el) the white, compact, and very hard substance covering and protecting the dentin of the crown of a tooth.

mottled e., defective enamel, with a chalky white appearance or brownish stain, caused by excessive amounts of fluorine in drinking water and food preparations during the period of enamel calcification.

e. organ, a process of epithelium forming a cap over a dental papilla and developing into the enamel.

enanthema (en-an′the-mah) an eruption upon a mucous surface. adj., **enanthem′atous.**

enantiomorph (en-an′te-o-morf″) one of a pair of isomeric substances, the molecular structures of which are mirror opposites of each other.

enarthrosis (en″ar-thro′sis) a joint in which the rounded head of one bone is received into a socket in another, permitting motion in any direction; called also ball-and-socket joint.

encapsulation (en-kap″su-la′shun) enclosure within a capsule.

encephal(o)- word element [Gr.], *brain.*

encephalalgia (en″sef-ah-lal′je-ah) cephalalgia; pain within the head; headache.

encephalatrophy (en″sef-ah-lat′ro-fe) atrophy of the brain.

encephalic (en″sĕ-fal′ik) 1. pertaining to the brain. 2. within the skull.

encephalitis (en′sef-ah-li′tis) inflammation of the brain. adj., **encephalit′ic.**

There are many types of encephalitis, depending on the causative agent and the structures involved. A large percentage of the cases are caused by viruses; some are transmitted from animals to man, as in equine encephalitis, and some from man to man, as in HERPES SIMPLEX encephalitis. Another name for the disease is sleeping sickness. The symptoms may be mild, with headache and a general malaise and muscle ache similar to that associated with influenza. The more acute and serious symptoms may include fever, delirium, convulsions, coma, and, in a significant number of patients, death.

Treatment is essentially symptomatic and is aimed at control of high fever, maintenance of fluid and electrolyte balance, and constant maintenance of respiratory and urinary function as required.

Convalescence from acute cases with serious damage to the central nervous system usually is prolonged and efforts at physical rehabilitation are needed to overcome the neurological and musculoskeletal complications that may develop. In some cases personality changes and emotional disturbances may require extensive treatment.

acute disseminated e., postinfection encephalitis.

cortical e., inflammation involving only the cortex of the brain.

Economo's e., a form of epidemic encephalitis, the original type described by von Economo, marked by increasing languor, apathy, and drowsiness, passing into lethargy; observed in various parts of the world between 1915 and 1926. Called also lethargic encephalitis.

epidemic e., a viral encephalitis occurring epidemically.

equine e., equine encephalomyelitis.

hemorrhagic e., herpes encephalitis in which there is inflammation of the brain with hemorrhagic foci and perivascular exudate.

herpes e., that caused by a herpesvirus, resembling equine encephalomyelitis.

e. hyperplas'tica, an acute nonsuppurating form of encephalitis.

infantile e., inflammation of the brain in children following infections.

Japanese B e., a form of epidemic encephalitis of varying severity occurring in Japan and other Pacific islands, China, U.S.S.R., and probably much of the Far East.

lead e., encephalitis with cerebral edema due to lead poisoning.

lethargic e., a form of epidemic encephalitis characterized by increasing languor, apathy, and drowsiness (see also ECONOMO'S ENCEPHALITIS).

e. neonato'rum, encephalitis of the newborn.

e. periaxia'lis diffu'sa, a subacute or chronic leukoencephalopathy of children and adolescents (see also SCHILDER'S DISEASE).

postinfection e., an acute disease of the central nervous system seen in patients convalescing from infectious, usually viral, diseases.

postvaccinal e., acute encephalitis sometimes occurring after vaccination.

Russian spring-summer e., a form of epidemic encephalitis acquired in forests from infected ticks, but also transmitted in other ways, as by ingestion of the flesh or milk of infected animals. It ranges in severity from mild to fatal, with degenerative changes in organs other than those of the nervous system.

St. Louis e., a viral disease first observed in 1932 in Illinois. It occurs during the late summer and early fall, and is clinically similar to western equine encephalomyelitis. It is usually transmitted by certain mosquitoes.

encephalocele (en-sef'ah-lo-sēl") hernial protrusion of brain substance through a congenital or traumatic opening of the skull.

encephalocystocele (en-sef"ah-lo-sis'to-sēl) hernial protrusion of the brain distended by fluid.

encephalogram (en-sef'ah-lo-gram") the film obtained by encephalography.

encephalography (en-sef"ah-log'rah-fe) radiography of the brain.

encephaloid (en-sef'ah-loid) 1. resembling the brain or brain substance. 2. medullary carcinoma.

encephalolith (en-sef'ah-lo-lith") a brain calculus.

encephalology (en-sef'ah-lol'o-je) the sum of knowledge regarding the brain, its functions, and its diseases.

encephaloma (en-sef"ah-lo'mah) 1. any swelling or tumor of the brain. 2. medullary carcinoma.

encephalomalacia (en-sef"ah-lo-mah-la'she-ah) softening of the brain.

encephalomeningitis (en-sef"ah-lo-men"in-ji'-tis) meningoencephalitis; inflammation of the brain and meninges.

encephalomeningocele (en-sef"ah-lo-mĕ-ning'-go-sĕl) protrusion of the brain and meninges through a defect in the skull.

encephalomeningopathy (en-sef"ah-lo-men"in-gop'ah-the) disease involving the brain and meninges.

encephalomere (en-sef'ah-lo-mēr") one of the segments making up the embryonic brain.

encephalometer (en"sef-ah-lom'ĕ-ter) an instrument used in locating certain of the brain regions.

encephalomyelitis (en-sef"ah-lo-mi"ĕ-li'tis) inflammation of the brain and spinal cord.

acute disseminated e., postinfection encephalitis.

benign myalgic e., a disease usually occurring in epidemics, characterized by headache, fever, myalgia, muscular weakness, and emotional lability.

equine e., eastern, a viral disease similar to western equine encephalomyelitis, but occurring in a region extending from New Hampshire to Texas and as far west as Wisconsin, and in Canada, Mexico, the Carribean, and parts of Central and South America.

equine e., Venezuelan, a viral disease of horses and mules; the infection in man resembles influenza, with little or no indication of nervous system involvement; the causative agent was first isolated in Venezuela.

equine e., western, a viral disease of horses and mules, communicable to man, occurring chiefly as a meningoencephalitis, with little involvement of the medulla oblongata or spinal cord; observed in the United States chiefly west of the Mississippi River.

granulomatous e., a disease marked by granulomas and necrosis of the walls of the cerebral and spinal ventricles.

postvaccinal e., inflammation of the brain and spinal cord following vaccination or infection with vaccinia virus.

encephalomyeloneuropathy (en-sef"ah-lo-mi"-ĕ-lo-nu-rop'ah-the) a disease involving the brain, spinal cord, and nerves.

encephalomyelopathy (en-sef"ah-lo-mi"ĕ-lop'ah-the) a disease involving the brain and spinal cord.

encephalomyeloradiculitis (en-sef"ah-lo-mi"ĕ-lo-rah-dik"u-li'tis) inflammation of the brain, spinal cord, and spinal nerve roots.

encephalomyeloradiculopathy (en-sef"ah-lo-mi"ĕ-lo-rah-dik"u-lop'ah-the) a disease involving the brain, spinal cord, and spinal nerve roots.

encephalomyocarditis (en-sef"ah-lo-mi"o-kar-di'-tis) a viral disease charcterized by degenerative and inflammatory changes in skeletal and cardiac muscle and by lesions of the central nervous system resembling those of poliomyelitis.

encephalon (en-sef'ah-lon) the brain; with the spinal cord (medulla spinalis) constituting the central nervous system.

encephalopathy (en-sef"ah-lop'ah-the) any degenerative disease of the brain.

biliary e., bilirubin e., kernicterus.

boxer's e., traumatic encephalopathy.

hepatic e., a condition, usually occurring secondarily to advanced liver disease, marked by disturbances of consciousness that may progress to deep coma (hepatic coma), psychiatric changes of varying degree, flapping tremor, and fetor hepaticus.

hypernatremic e., a severe hemorrhagic encephalopathy induced by the hyperosmolarity accompanying hypernatremia and dehydration.

lead e., brain disease caused by lead poisoning.

portal-systemic e., hepatic encephalopathy.

progressive subcortical e., Schilder's disease.

traumatic e., general slowing of mental functions, occasional confusion, and scattered memory loss, due to cumulative punishment absorbed in the boxing ring. Called also boxer's encephalopathy.

Wernicke's e., an inflammatory hemorrhagic

form due to thiamine deficiency associated with alcoholism (see also WERNICKE'S ENCEPHALOPATHY).

encephalopuncture (en-sef"ah-lo-pungk'tūr) surgical puncture of the brain.

encephalopyosis (en-sef"ah-lo-pi-o'sis) suppuration or abscess of the brain.

encephalorrhagia (en-sef"ah-lo-ra'je-ah) hemorrhage within or from the brain.

encephalosclerosis (en-sef"ah-lo-sklĕ-ro'sis) hardening of the brain.

encephalosis (en"sef-ah-lo-'sis) any organic brain disease.

encephalotomy (en"sef-ah-lot'o-me) 1. craniotomy (2). 2. dissection or anatomy of the brain.

enchondroma (en"kon-dro'mah) a benign growth of cartilage arising in the metaphysis of a bone. adj., **enchondro'matous.**

enchondromatosis (en-kon"dro-mah-to'sis) a condition characterized by hamartomatous proliferation of cartilage cells within the metaphysis of several bones, causing thinning of the overlying cortex and distortion of the growth in length. Called also dyschondroplasia.

enchondrosarcoma (en-kon"dro-sar-ko'mah) central chondrosarcoma.

enclave (en'klāv) tissue detached from its normal connection and enclosed within another organ.

enclitic (en-klit'ik) having the planes of the fetal head inclined to those of the maternal pelvis.

encopresis (en"ko-pre'sis) incontinence of feces not due to organic defect or illness.

encysted (en-sist'ed) enclosed in a sac, bladder, or cyst.

end(o)- word element [Gr.], *within; inward.*

endadelphos (end"ah-del'fos) a monster in which a parasitic twin is enclosed within the body of the other twin (the autosite).

Endamoeba (en"dah-me'bah) a genus of amebas parasitic in the intestines of invertebrates.

endangiitis (en"dan-je-i'tis) inflammation of the endangium.

endangium (en-dan'je-um) tunica intima (inner coat) of a blood vessel.

endaortitis (en"da-or-ti'tis) inflammation of the membrane lining the aorta.

endarterectomy (en"dar-ter-ek'to-me) excision of thickened atheromatous areas of the innermost coat of an artery.

endarterial (end"ar-te're-al) within an artery.

endarteritis (en"dar-ter-i'tis) inflammation of the innermost coat (tunica intima) of an artery.

e. oblit'erans, a form in which the lumen of the smaller vessels become narrowed or obliterated as a result of proliferation of the tissue of the intimal layer.

end-artery (end-ar'ter-e) an artery that does not anastomose with other arteries.

endbrain (end'brān) telencephalon.

end-bulb (end'bulb) one of the small encapsulated bodies at the end of sensory nerve fibers in skin, mucous membranes, muscles, and other areas. They are called also Krause's bulbs or corpuscles.

endemic (en-dem'ik) 1. present in a community at all times. 2. a disease of low morbidity that is constantly present in a human community, but clinically recognizable in only a few.

endemiology (en-de"me-ol'o-je) the science dealing with all the factors relating to occurrence of endemic disease.

endemoepidemic (en"de-mo-ep"ĭ-dem'ik) endemic, but occasionally becoming epidemic.

endergonic (en"der-gon'ik) characterized or accompanied by the absorption of energy; requiring the input of free energy.

end-feet (end'fēt) button- or knoblike terminal enlargements of naked nerve fibers which end in a synapse with dendrites of another cell.

ending (end'ing) a termination, especially the peripheral termination of a nerve or nerve fiber.

endoaneurysmorrhaphy (en"do-an"u-riz-mor'-ah-fe) opening of an aneurysmal sac and suture of the orifices.

endoangiitis (en"do-an"je-i'tis) endangiitis.

endoappendicitis (en"do-ah-pen"dĭ-si'tis) inflammation of the mucous membrane of the vermiform appendix.

endoarteritis (en"do-ar"ter-i'tis) endarteritis.

endoblast (en'do-blast) entoderm.

endobronchitis (en"do-brong-ki'tis) inflammation of the epithelial lining of the bronchi.

endocardial (en"do-kar'de-al) 1. situated or occurring within the heart. 2. pertaining to the endocardium.

e. cushions, elevations on the atrioventricular canal of the embryonic heart which later help form the interatrial septum.

endocarditis (en"do-kar-di'tis) inflammation of the inner lining of the heart (the endocardium) usually involving the heart valves. adj., **endocardit'ic.** Bacterial endocarditis is an acute or subacute, febrile, systemic disease characterized by bacterial infection of the heart valves or irregular areas on the endocardium, with formation of bacteria-laden vegetations on these areas. Intensive chemotherapy with antibiotic drugs has done much to reduce the seriousness of this disease. The nonbacterial forms include verrucous and rheumatic endocarditis.

atypical verrucous e., see verrucous ENDOCARDITIS.

bacterial e., a febrile systemic disease marked by bacterial or fungal infection of the heart valves, with formation of pathogen-laden vegetations: the acute form has an abrupt onset and a rapidly progressive course, and is caused by virulent organisms—e.g., *Staphylococcus aureus,* gram-negative bacteria, and fungi—capable of invading other tissues; the subacute form has an insidious onset and protracted course, and is due to various bacteria, usually α-hemolytic streptococci. Called also infective endocarditis.

infective e., bacterial endocarditis.

Libman-Sacks e., see verrucous ENDOCARDITIS.

Löffler's e., Löffler's fibroplastic parietal e., endocarditis associated with eosinophilia, marked by fibroplastic thickening of the endocardium, resulting in congestive heart failure, persistent tachycardia, hepatomegaly, splenomegaly, serous effusions into the pleural cavity, and edema of the limbs.

mural e., that affecting the lining of the walls of the heart chambers only.

parietal e., mural endocarditis.

rheumatic e., that associated with rheumatic fever.

rickettsial e., endocarditis caused by invasion of the heart valves with *Coxiella burnetii;* it is a sequela of Q fever, usually occurring in persons who have had rheumatic fever.

syphilitic e., endocarditis resulting from extension of syphilitic infection from the aorta.

tuberculous e., that resulting from extension of a tuberculous infection from the pericardium and myocardium.

valvular e., that affecting the membrane over the heart valves only.

vegetative e., verrucous e., nonbacterial endocarditis with formation of shreds of fibrin on the ulcerated valves, frequently found in association with systemic lupus erythematosus, in which case it is known as Libman-Sacks disease or atypical verrucous endocarditis.

endocardium (en″do-kar-′de-um) the endothelial lining membrane of the heart and the connective tissue bed on which it lies.

endocervicitis (en″do-ser″vĭ-si′tis) inflammation of the endocervix.

endocervix (en″do-ser′viks) 1. the mucous membrane lining the canal of the cervix uteri. 2. the region of the opening of the cervix uteri into the uterine cavity. adj., **endocer′vical.**

endochondral (en″do-kon′dral) situated, formed, or occurring within cartilage.

endocolitis (en″do-ko-li′tis) inflammation of the mucous membrane of the colon.

endocranial (en″do-kra′ne-al) within the cranium.

endocranitis (en″do-kra-ni′tis) inflammation of endocranium.

endocranium (en″do-kra′ne-um) the endosteal layer of the dura mater of the brain.

endocrine (en′do-krin) 1. secreting internally. 2. pertaining to internal secretions; hormonal.

e. glands, glands that regulate body activity by special secretions, the hormones, which are delivered directly into the blood. Each of the glands within the endocrine system has one or more specific functions, but they all are dependent upon the other glands in the system for maintenance of a normal hormonal balance in the body.

The PITUITARY GLAND (hypophysis cerebri), which is about the size of a pea, lies at the base of the brain and is called the master gland because it regulates the functions of other endocrine glands. It also has some vital functions of its own, such as controlling the body's growth through the growth hormone (somatotropin).

Some pituitary hormones that directly affect other glands in the endocrine system are: thyrotropic hormone (thyroid-stimulating hormone, TSH), which stimulates the thyroid gland; adrenocorticotropic hormone (ACTH), which affects the cortex of the adrenal gland; and the gonadotropic hormones (FSH, LH, and LTH), which have a role in the development and proper functioning of the gonads.

The THYROID GLAND is situated in the neck, its two lateral lobes lying on either side of the larynx. It secretes the hormone thyroxine, which controls the metabolic rate, and calcitonin, which lowers plasma calcium and phosphate levels and serves as an antagonist to parathyroid hormone. The PARATHYROID GLANDS are located behind the thyroid and are embedded in its capsule. There are two pairs of parathyroid glands; their secretion, parathyroid hormone, regulates the blood calcium and phosphorus levels.

Small groups of specialized cells, scattered throughout the pancreas, are known as the islands of Langerhans. The beta cells secrete the hormone insulin, which is necessary for proper utilization of carbohydrates. (See also DIABETES MELLITUS.) The alpha cells secrete glucagon, a hormone that stimulates glycogenolysis in the liver.

The ADRENAL GLANDS, one atop each kidney, are each two glands in one, being made up of two parts, the cortex and medulla, with separate hormonal secretions. There are at least 26 hormones produced by the adrenal glands, including epinephrine, corticosterone, and aldosterone. They are vital to the protection of the body during stress and danger, and to the adaptation of the body to changes in its environment.

The GONADS, or sex glands, consist of the TESTES in the male and the OVARIES in the female. Besides producing sperm and ova, respectively, they manufacture the androgens and estrogens, hormones responsible for the special characteristics of the male and female, respectively.

The PINEAL GLAND and the THYMUS are also sometimes included as endocrine glands, although the exact function of each is unknown.

endocrinism (en-dok′rĭ-nizm) endocrinopathy.

endocrinologist (en″do-krĭ-nol′o-jist) an individual skilled in endocrinology, and in the diagnosis and treatment of disorders of the glands of internal secretion, i.e., the endocrine glands.

endocrinology (en″do-krĭ-nol′o-je) study of the endocrine system.

endocrinopathy (en″do-krĭ-nop′ah-the) any disease due to disorder of the endocrine system. adj., **endocrinopath′ic.**

endocrinotherapy (en″do-kri″no-ther′ah-pe) treatment of disease by the administration of endocrine preparations; hormonotherapy.

endocrinous (en-dok′rĭnus) of or pertaining to an internal secretion (hormone) or to a gland producing such a secretion, i.e., to an endocrine gland.

endocystitis (en″do-sis-ti′tis) inflammation of the bladder mucosa.

endocytosis (en″do-si-to′sis) the uptake by a cell of particles that are too large to diffuse through its wall; it includes both phagocytosis and pinocytosis.

endoderm (en′do-derm) entoderm.

Endodermophyton (en″do-der-mof′ĭ-ton) *trichophyton.*

endodontia (en′do-don′she-ah) endodontics.

endodontics (en″do-don′tiks) the branch of dentistry concerned with the etiology, prevention, diagnosis, and treatment of conditions that affect the tooth pulp, root, and periapical tissues.

endodontist (en″do-don′tist) a dentist who specializes in endodontics.

endodontitis (en″do-don-ti′tis) inflammation of the dental pulp; pulpitis.

endodontium (en″do-don′she-um) dental pulp.

endoenteritis (en″do-en″tĕ-ri′tis) inflammation of the intestinal mucosa.

endoenzyme (en″do-en′zīm) an intracellular enzyme; an enzyme that is retained in a cell and does not normally diffuse out of the cell into the surrounding medium.

FUNCTIONS OF ENDOCRINE GLANDS

GLAND	HORMONE	ACTION OF HORMONE
PITUITARY		
Anterior lobe	Thyrotropic hormone	Stimulates thyroid gland
	Somatotropic hormone	Stimulates growth
	Gonadotropic hormones (LH, FSH, LTH)	Affect growth, maturity and functioning of primary and secondary sex organs
	Adrenocorticotropic hormone (ACTH)	Stimulates cortex of adrenal glands
Posterior lobe	Antidiuretic hormone	Decreases production of urine
	Oxytocin	Stimulates uterine contractions
THYROID	Thyroxine Triiodothyronine	Stimulates metabolism (catabolic phase)
	Calcitonin	Inhibits hypercalcemia
PARATHYROID	Parathyroid hormone	Regulates blood calcium level
ADRENAL		
Cortex	Hormones divided into three main groups:	
	Glucocorticoids	Tend to increase amount of sugar in blood
	Mineralocorticoids	Tend to increase amount of blood sodium and decrease amount of potassium in blood
	Androgens (male hormones)	Govern certain secondary sex characteristics All corticoids important for defense against stress or injury to body tissues
Medulla	Epinephrine (Adrenaline); "fight or flight" hormone	Elevates blood pressure; converts glycogen to glucose when needed by muscles for energy; increases heartbeat rate; dilates bronchioles
OVARIES	Estrone and progesterone	Stimulate development of secondary sex characteristics Effect repair of endometrium after menstruation
TESTES	Testosterone	Essential for normal functioning of male reproductive organs Stimulates development of male secondary sex characteristics
ISLANDS OF LANGERHANS OF PANCREAS	Insulin	Promotes metabolism of carbohydrates
	Glucagon	Stimulates glycogenolysis in the liver
THYMUS	Thymosin	Important in establishment of cell-mediated immunity

From Keane, C. B.: Saunders Review for Practical Nurses. 3rd ed. Philadelphia, W. B. Saunders Co., 1977.

endogamy (en-dog′ah-me) 1. fertilization by union of separate cells having the same chromatin ancestry. 2. restriction of marriage to persons within the same community. adj., **endog′amous.**

endogenous (en-doj′ĕ-nus) produced within or caused by factors within the organism.

endointoxication (en″do-in-tok″sĭ-ka′shun) poisoning by an endogenous toxin.

endolaryngeal (en″do-lah-rin′je-al) situated on or occurring within the larynx.

Endolimax (en″do-li′maks) a genus of amebas found in the colon of man, other mammals, birds, amphibians, and cockroaches.

endolymph (en′do-limf) the fluid within the membranous labyrinth of the ear.

endolysin (en-dol′ĭ-sin) a bactericidal substance in cells; acting directly on bacteria.

endometriosis (en″do-me″tre-o′sis) a condition in which tissue more or less perfectly resembling the uterine mucous membrane occurs aberrantly in various locations in the pelvic cavity. adj., **endometriot′ic.** The condition may be characterized by pelvic pain, abnormal uterine or rectal bleeding, dysmenorrhea, and symptoms of pressure within the pelvic cavity. Sterility and dyspareunia also may be present.

Treatment is based on the age of the patient and the extent of the endometrial growth. In young women exogenous hormone therapy is employed, and, whenever feasible, the patient is encouraged to become pregnant since interruption of menstruation is thought to retard the progress of the disease. In older women and in cases of extensive growth, surgical treatment involving complete hysterectomy is indicated. X-ray therapy in doses large enough to produce destruction of the reproductive organs is sometimes employed when there is definite evidence of advanced endometriosis and surgery is contraindicated or refused.

endometritis (en″do-me-tri′tis) inflammation of the endometrium.

puerperal e., endometritis following childbirth.

syncytial e., a benign tumor-like lesion with infiltration of the uterine wall by large syncytial trophoblastic cells.

endometrium (en″do-me′tre-um) the mucous membrane lining the uterus. adj., **endome′trial.**

endomitosis (en″do-mi-to′sis) mitosis taking place without dissolution of the nuclear membrane, and not followed by cytoplasmic division, resulting in doubling of the number of chromosomes within the nucleus. adj., **endomitot′ic.**

endomorph (en′do-morf) an individual having the type of body build in which entodermal tissues predominate: there is relative preponderance of soft roundness throughout the body, with large digestive viscera and fat accumulations, and with large trunk and thighs and tapering extremities.

endomorphy (en′do-mor″fe) the condition of being an endomorph. adj., **endomor′phic.**

endomyocarditis (en″do-mi″o-kar-di′tis) inflammation of the endocardium and myocardium.

endomysium (en″do-mis′e-um) the sheath of delicate reticular fibrils that surrounds each muscle fiber.

endoneuritis (en″do-nu-ri′tis) inflammation of the endoneurium.

endoneurium (en″do-nu′re-um) the interstitial connective tissue in a peripheral nerve, separating individual nerve fibers. adj., **endoneu′rial.**

endonuclease (en″do-nu′kle-ās) a nuclease that cleaves internal bonds of polynucleotides.

endoparasite (en″do-par′ah-sīt) a parasite that lives within the body of the host. adj., **endoparasit′ic.**

endopelvic (en″do-pel′vik) within the pelvis.

endopeptidase (en″do-pep′tĭ-dās) a peptidase capable of acting on any peptide linkage in a peptide chain.

endopericarditis (en″do-per″ĭ-kar-di′tis) inflammation of the endocardium and pericardium.

endoperimyocarditis (en″do-per″ĭ-mi″o-kar-di′-tis) inflammation of the endocardium, pericardium, and myocardium.

endoperitonitis (en″do-per″ĭ-to-ni′tis) inflammation of the serous lining of the peritoneal cavity.

endophlebitis (en″do-flĕ-bi′tis) inflammation of the intima of a vein.

endophthalmitis (en″dof-thal-mi′tis) inflammation of the ocular cavities and their adjacent structures.

endophyte (en′do-fīt) a parasitic plant organism living within its host's body.

endophytic (en″do-fit′ik) 1. pertaining to an endophyte. 2. growing inward; proliferating on the interior of an organ or structure.

endoplasm (en′do-plazm) the more centrally located cytoplasm of a cell. adj., **endoplas′mic.**

endoreduplication (en″do-re-du″plĭ-ka′shun) replication of chromosomes without subsequent cell division.

end organ (end″or′-gan) one of the larger, encapsulated endings of sensory nerves.

endosalpingitis (en″do-sal″pin-ji′tis) inflammation of the endosalpinx.

endosalpingoma (en″do-sal″ping-go′mah) adenomyoma of the uterine tube.

endosalpingosis (en″do-sal″ping-go′sis) 1. endometriosis involving the uterine tube. 2. ovarian endometriosis in which the abnormal mucosa resembles tubal mucosa rather than endometrium.

endosalpinx (en″do-sal′pinks) the mucous membrane lining the oviduct (uterine tube).

endoscope (en′do-skōp) an instrument used for direct visual inspection of hollow organs or body cavities. Specially designed endoscopes are used for such examinations as BRONCHOSCOPY, CYSTOSCOPY, GASTROSCOPY, and PROCTOSCOPY.

Although the design of an endoscope may vary according to its specific use, all endoscopes have similar working elements. The viewing part (scope) may be a hollow metal or fiber tube fitted with a lens system that permits viewing in a variety of directions. The endoscope also has a light source, power cord, and power source. Accessories that might be used with an endoscope for diagnostic or therapeutic purposes include suction tip, tubes, and suction pump; forceps for removal of biopsy tissue or a foreign body; and electrode tip for cauterization.

endoscopy (en-dos′ko-pe) visual examination of interior structures of the body with an endoscope. adj., **endoscop′ic.**

endosepsis (en″do-sep′sis) septicemia originating from causes inside the body.

endoskeleton (en″do-skel′ĕ-ton) the cartilaginous and bony skeleton of the body, exclusive of that part of the skeleton of dermal origin.

endosmosis (en″dos-mo′sis) inward osmosis; inward passage of liquid through a membrane of a cell or cavity, by which one fluid passes through a septum into a cavity that contains fluid of a different density. adj., **endosmot′ic.**

endosome (en′do-sōm) a body thought to consist of deoxyribonucleic acid, observed in the vesicular nucleus of certain protozoa.

endosteal (en-dos′te-al) 1. pertaining to the endosteum. 2. occurring or located within a bone.

endosteitis (en-dos″te-i′tis) inflammation of the endosteum.

endosteoma (en-dos″te-o′mah) a tumor in the medullary cavity of a bone.

endosteum (en-dos′te-um) the tissue lining the medullary cavity of a bone.

endostoma (en″dos-to′mah) endosteoma.

endotendineum (en″do-ten-din′e-um) the delicate connective tissue separating the secondary bundles (fascicles) of a tendon.

endothelia (en″do-the′le-ah) [Gr.] plural of *endothelium.*

endothelial (en″do-the′le-al) pertaining to or made up of endothelium.

endotheliocyte (en″do-the′le-o-sīt″) a large mononuclear phagocytic wandering cell of the circulating blood and tissues. Called also endothelial leukocyte.

endothelioid (en″do-the′le-oid) resembling endothelium.

endotheliolysin (en″do-the″le-ol′ĭ-sin) an antibody that causes the dissolution of endothelial cells. adj., **endotheliolyt′ic.**

endothelioma (en″do-the″le-o′mah) a tumor arising from the endothelial lining of blood vessels.

endotheliosis (en″do-the″le-o′sis) proliferation of endothelial elements.

endotheliotoxin (en″do-the″le-o-tok′sin) a specific toxin that acts on endothelium of capillaries and small veins, producing hemorrhage.

endothelium (en″do-the′le-um), pl. *endothe′lia* [Gr.] the layer of epithelial cells that lines the cavities of the heart and of the blood and lymph vessels, and the serous cavities of the body.

endothermal, endothermic (en″do-ther′mal; en″-do-ther′mik) 1. characterized by the absorption of heat. 2. pertaining to endothermy.

endothermy (en′do-ther″me) production of heat in the tissues by the resistance they offer to the passage of the high-frequency current.

endothrix (en′do-thriks) a dermatophyte whose growth and spore production are confined chiefly within the shaft of a hair.

endotoxemia (en″do-toks-e′me-ah) the presence of endotoxins in the blood.

endotoxic (en″do-tok′sik) pertaining to or possessing endotoxin.

endotoxin (en″do-tok′sin) a heat-stable toxin present in the intact bacterial cell but not in cell-free filtrates of cultures of intact bacteria. They are found primarily in enteric bacilli, in which they are identical with the O antigen, but are also found in certain of the gram-negative cocci and in *Pasteurella* and *Brucella* species. The endotoxins are lipopolysaccharide complexes that occur in the cell wall. They are pyrogenic and increase capillary permeability, the activity being substantially the same regardless of the species of bacteria from which they are derived.

endotracheal (en″do-tra′ke-al) within the trachea.

e. tube, an AIRWAY catheter inserted in the trachea during endotracheal INTUBATION to assure patency of the upper airway by allowing for removal of secretions and maintenance of an adequate air passage. Endotracheal intubation may be accomplished through the mouth using an orotracheal tube, or through the nose using a nasotracheal tube. A variety of endotracheal tubes is available. The tubes are almost always "cuffed" to allow for their use with a mechanical ventilator. The cuff is a rubber balloon-like device that fits over the lower end of the tube. It is attached to a narrow tube that extends outside the body and allows for inflation of the cuff. Once the cuff is inflated there is no flow of air through the trachea other than that going through the endotracheal tube.

Passage of an endotracheal tube during surgery is a well established and long used technique. In recent years the procedure has become a part of medical management of ventilatory failure as an alternative to TRACHEOTOMY. Endotracheal intubation has the advantage of not requiring a surgical procedure as does tracheotomy, removal of the tube (extubation) is less involved, and the procedure can be repeated as necessary.

The endotracheal tube cannot be used for long-term relief of ventilatory failure. After 24 hours the tube can begin to cause extensive and permanent damage to the tissues because of pressure and resultant ischemia. Some conscious patients cannot tolerate the tube because of excessive gagging and local discomfort.

Complications of endotracheal intubation include damage to the vocal cords, erosion, and eventual stricture of the larynx. Pulmonary infections may result from interference with the normal protective mechanisms of the glottis and from the introduction of pathogenic organisms into the respiratory tract and difficulty in their removal by coughing.

PATIENT CARE. After the tube has been inserted by the physician and the cuff inflated, the orotracheal tube is secured to the patient's face. The respiratory apparatus for assisted ventilation must be stabilized on the patient's chest, which is protected by padding. Secure anchoring of the tube and apparatus is necessary to prevent tension on or misplacement of the endotracheal tube.

The inhaled air must be adequately humified and protected from contamination as much as possible. SUCTIONING of secretions via the tube is done with gentleness and according to the basic guidelines established for this procedure. The patient will re-

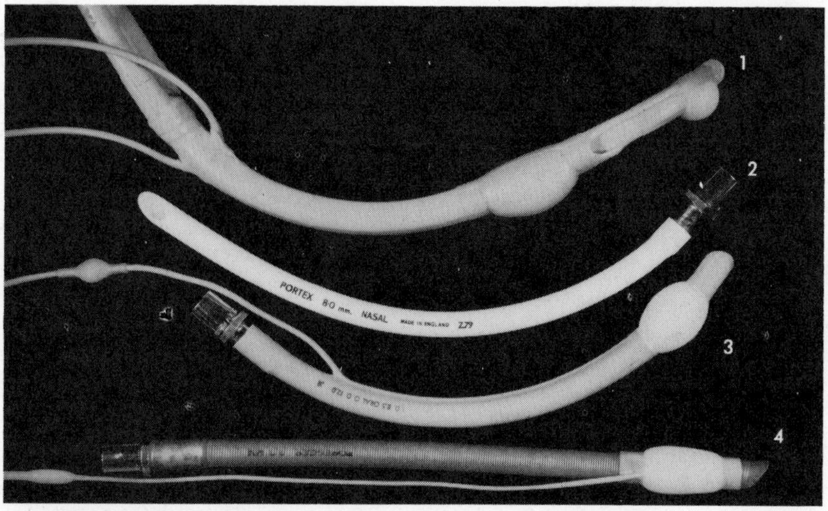

Endotracheal tubes (from top to bottom): (1) The Robert-Shaw double-lumen tube to isolate the flow to each lung. Note the individual inflatable cuffs for the trachea and the left bronchus; (2) The Portex nasotracheal tube, without attached cuff; (3) An orotracheal tube with attached inflatable cuff (very commonly used); and (4) The LA (Latex-Armored) tube.Note the spiral winding to prevent kinking. (From Sanderson, R. G., Ed.: *The Cardiac Patient.* 1972.)

quire mouth care and frequent observation for signs of pressure against the lips and nose. An emergency tracheotomy tray and an extra endotracheal tube are kept at the patient's bedside.

endovasculitis (en″do-vas″ku-li′tis) endangiitis.

Endoxan (en-dok′san) trademark for a preparation of cyclophosphamide, an antineoplastic agent.

end plate (end′plāt) a flattened discoid expansion at the myoneural junction, where a myelinated motor nerve fiber joins a skeletal muscle fiber.

endrin (en′drin) a highly toxic insecticide of the chlorinated hydrocarbon group.

enema (en′ĕ-mah) 1. introduction of fluid into the rectum. 2. a solution introduced into the rectum to promote evacuation of feces or as a means of administering nutrient or medicinal substances, or opaque material in roentgen examination of the lower intestinal tract (see also BARIUM TEST). Unless otherwise ordered, the solution is warmed to 105° F. (40.5° C.), the patient is placed in Sims' left lateral position, and the rectal tube is inserted. The container of fluid is usually held 18 inches above the buttocks.

Fleet e., trademark for an enema containing, in each 100 ml., 16 gm. sodium biphosphate and 6 gm. sodium phosphate, packaged in a plastic squeeze bottle fitted with a 2-inch, prelubricated rectal tube.

energy (en′er-je) power that may be translated into motion, overcoming resistance, or effecting physical change; the ability to do work. Energy assumes several forms; it may be thermal (in the form of heat), electrical, mechanical, chemical, radiant, or kinetic. In doing work, the energy is changed from one form to another or to several forms. In these changes some of the energy is "lost" in the sense that it cannot be recaptured and used again. Usually there is loss in the form of heat, which escapes or is dissipated unused. All energy changes give off a certain amount of the energy as heat.

All activities of the body require energy, and all needs are met by the consumption of food containing energy in chemical form. The human diet comprises three main sources of energy: carbohydrates, proteins, and fats. Of these three, carbohydrates most readily provide the kind of energy needed to activate muscles. Proteins work to build and restore body tissues. The body transforms chemical energy derived from food by the process of METABOLISM, an activity that takes place in the individual cell. Molecules of the food substances providing energy pass through the cell wall. Inside the cell, chemical reactions occur that produce the new forms of energy and yield by-products such as water and waste materials. (See also ADENOSINE.)

free e., the energy equal to the maximum amount of work that can be obtained from a process occurring under conditions of fixed temperature and pressure.

nuclear e., energy that can be liberated by changes in the nucleus of an atom (as by fission of a heavy nucleus or by fusion of light nuclei into heavier ones with accompanying loss of mass).

enervation (en″er-va′shun) 1. lack of nervous energy. 2. removal of a nerve or a section of a nerve.

enflagellation (en-flaj″ĕ-la′shun) the formation of flagella; flagellation.

ENG electronystagmograph.

engagement (en-gāj′ment) the entrance of the fetal head or presenting part into the superior pelvic strait.

engastrius (en-gas′tre-us) a double monster in which one fetus is contained within the abdomen of the other.

engorgement (en-gorj′ment) local congestion; distention with fluids; hyperemia.

engram (en′gram) a lasting mark or trace. The term is applied to the definite and permanent trace left by a stimulus in the protoplasm of a tissue (see ENGRAPHIA). In psychology, it is the lasting trace left in the psyche by anything that has been experienced psychically; a latent memory picture.

engraphia (en-gra′fe-ah) the theory that stimuli leave definite traces (engrams) on the protoplasm,

ENEMAS

TYPE	PREPARATION	PURPOSES
Magnesium, glycerin, and water (one, two, three)	Mix 1 oz. magnesium sulfate, 2 oz. glycerin, and 3 oz. hot water.	To increase intestinal fluids, thereby causing pressure and stimulating peristalsis; glycerin acts as lubricant
Milk and molasses	Mix 180 ml. milk with 180. ml. molasses	Carminative: To relieve distention caused by flatus; to stimulate peristalsis
Oil retention	120 ml. mineral oil or glycerin, heated to 100° F.	To soften feces
Saline	1 tsp. salt to 1 pt. water	To relieve constipation or cleanse the rectal area, especially for removal of mucus
Soapsuds (S.S.)	30 ml. pure castile soap to 500 ml. water	Cleansing of rectal area; soap acts as an irritant to intestinal lining, stimulates peristalsis
Sodium bicarbonate	Add 1 tsp. sodium bicarbonate (baking soda) to 500 ml. water	To soothe mucous membranes and neutralize gastrointestinal acids

which, with repetition, induce a habit that persists after the stimuli have ceased.

enhexymal (en-hek′sĭ-mal) hexobarbital, an ultra-short acting barbiturate.

enkatarrhaphy (en″kah-tar′ah-fe) the operation of burying a structure by suturing together the sides of tissues adjacent to it.

enol (e′nol) one of two tautomeric forms of a substance, the other being the keto form; the enol is formed from the keto by migration of hydrogen from the adjacent carbon atom to the carbonyl group.

enolase (e′no-lās) an enzyme in glycolytic systems that changes phosphoglyceric acid into phosphopyruvic acid.

enophthalmos (en″of-thal′mos) a backward displacement of the eyeball into the orbit.

enostosis (en″os-to′sis) a bony growth within a bone cavity or on the internal surface of the bone cortex.

Enovid (en-o′vid) trademark for preparations of mestranol and norethynodrel, used to inhibit ovulation.

ensiform (en″sĭ-form) sword-shaped; xiphoid.
e. cartilage, the xiphoid process.

ensomphalus (en-som′fah-lus) a double monster with blended bodies, two separate navels, and two umbilical cords.

enstrophe (en′stro-fe) inversion; especially of the margin of the eyelids.

E.N.T. ear, nose, and throat.

entad (en′tad) toward a center; inwardly.

ental (en′tal) inner; central.

entamebiasis (en″tah-me-bi′ah-sis) infection by *Entamoeba.*

Entamoeba (en″tah-me′bah) a genus of amebas parasitic in the intestines of vertebrates.
E. co′li, a nonpathogenic form found in the intestinal tract of man.
E. gingiva′lis, a nonpathogenic species found in the human mouth.
E. histolyt′ica, a species causing AMEBIC DYSENTERY and abscess of the liver.

entasia (en-ta′ze-ah) a constrictive spasm; tonic spasm.

enter(o)- word element [Gr.] *intestine.*

enteral (en′ter-al) within, by way of, or pertaining to the small intestine.

enterectomy (en″ter-ek′to-me) excision of a portion of the intestine.

enterelcosis (en″ter-el-ko′sis) ulceration of the intestine.

enteric (en-ter′ik) pertaining to the small intestine.
e.-coated, designating a special coating applied to tablets or capsules which prevents release and absorption of their contents until they reach the intestine.
e. fever, typhoid fever.

enteritis (en″tĕ-ri′tis) inflammation of the intestine, especially the small intestine, a general condition that can be produced by a variety of causes. Bacteria and certain viruses may irritate the intestinal tract and produce symptoms of abdominal pain, nausea, vomiting, and diarrhea. Similar effects may result from poisonous foods such as mushrooms and berries, or from a harmful chemical present in food or drink. Enteritis may also be the consequence of overeating, alcoholic excesses, or emotional tension.

Rest and bland diet are generally prescribed. In cases of bacterial infection antibiotics may be helpful. Severe dehydration, which may accompany enteritis, is treated with replacement of lost fluids and electrolytes.

choleriform e., an acute cholera-like diarrheal disease with a high fatality rate prevalent in epidemic and endemic forms in the Western Pacific area since 1938.

e. cys′tica chron′ica, a form marked by cystic dilatations of the intestinal glands, due to closure of their openings.

e. gra′vis, an often fatal disease characterized by severe abdominal pain, nausea, vomiting, and bloody diarrhea, with mucosal necrosis and hemorrhage and edema of the submucosa, most prominent in the jejunum and proximal ileum.

membranous e., mucomembranous e., mucous e., mucous colitis.

e. necrot′icans, an inflammation of the intestines due to *Clostridium perfringens* type F, characterized by necrosis.

e. nodula′ris, enteritis with enlargement of the lymph nodes.

phlegmonous e., a condition with symptoms resembling those of peritonitis, which may be secondary to other intestinal diseases, e.g., chronic obstruction, strangulated hernia, carcinoma.

e. polypo′sa, enteritis marked by polypoid growths in the intestine, due to proliferation of the connective tissue.

regional e., a chronic inflammatory disorder of the intestinal tract that may involve any area of the intestine but is characteristically located in the terminal ileum; called also terminal ileitis, regional ileitis, and Crohn's disease.

The cause of the disease is not known. A search for environmental causes has been fruitless, but there is some evidence to suggest that it may be related to viral or other transmissible agents in certain genetically susceptible persons. It most often affects individuals in the 15 to 20 year age bracket and in the 55 to 60 year age range. The incidence of the disease is higher in Jewish persons and, in the United States, is low in Indians and blacks. It occurs more often in urban populations than in rural.

SYMPTOMS. Regional enteritis is primarily a diarrheal disease with frequent loose and watery stools a characteristic symptom. There is a history of malaise, anorexia, abdominal cramps, and a general feeling of ill-health. These symptoms increase in severity and are accompanied by severe weight loss, persistent diarrhea, abdominal pain that is usually felt in the right lower quadrant, and low grade fever. The patient suffers from a fluid and electrolyte imbalance.

Complications of the disease include stricture formation, perforation of the ileum, development of fistulas to the urinary bladder, and hemorrhage. There also may be neurological complications, including tetany and grand mal seizures.

TREATMENT. About half of the cases treated surgically have a recurrence of symptoms. For this reason the treatment of choice is conservative management with supportive measures that include a well-balanced, high caloric, high protein diet to compensate for the poor absorption of food elements from the intestinal tract. There should be some limitation of physical activity to provide rest and to avoid unnecessary expenditure of energy. Medications that may be prescribed include drugs to control diarrhea, antimicrobial agents when indicated, and anti-inflammatory agents such as the adrenal corticosteroids.

enteroanastomosis (en″ter-o-ah-nas″to-mo′sis) enteroenterostomy.

Enterobacteriaceae (en″ter-o-bak-te″re-a′se-e) a family of gram-negative, rod-shaped bacteria (order Eubacteriales) occurring as plant or animal parasites or as saprophytes.

enterobiasis (en″ter-o-bi′ah-sis) infection with nematodes of the genus *Enterobius,* especially E. *vermicularis.*

Enterobius (en″ter-o′be-us) a genus of nematode worms.

E. vermicula′ris, the seatworm or pinworm, a small white worm parasitic in the upper part of the large intestine, and occasionally in the female genitals and bladder. Infection is frequent in children, sometimes causing itching. (See also WORMS.)

enterocele (en′ter-o-sēl″) intestinal hernia.

enterocentesis (en″ter-o-sen-te′sis) surgical puncture of the intestine.

enteroclysis (en″ter-ok′lĭ-sis) the injection of liquids into the intestine.

enterococcus (en″ter-o-kok′us), pl. *enterococ′ci* [Gr.] any streptococcus of the human intestine.

enterocoele (en′ter-o-sēl″) the body cavity formed by outpouchings from the archenteron.

enterocolectomy (en″ter-o-ko-lek′to-me) resection of part of the intestine, including the ileum, cecum, and colon.

enterocolitis (en″ter-o-ko-li′tis) inflammation of the small intestine and colon.

hemorrhagic e., enterocolitis characterized by hemorrhagic breakdown of the intestinal mucosa, with inflammatory cell infiltration.

necrotizing e., pseudomembranous e., an acute, superficial necrosis of the mucosa of the small intestine and colon, with shock and dehydration, and passage per rectum of seromucus, often mixed with blood, and shreds or casts of the bowel wall.

enterocolostomy (en″ter-o-ko-los′to-me) surgical anastomosis of the small intestine to the colon.

enterocrinin (en″ter-ok′rĭ-nin) an extract of the mucosa of the small intestine, said to be a physiological hormone, which stimulates the intestine to secretory activity.

enterocutaneous (en″ter-o-ku-ta′ne-us) pertaining to or communicating with the intestine and the skin, or surface of the body.

enterocyst (en′ter-o-sist″) a cyst proceeding from subperitoneal tissue.

enterocystocele (en″ter-o-sis′to-sēl) hernia of the bladder and intestine.

enterocystoma (en″ter-o-sis-to′mah) vitelline cyst.

enterodynia (en″ter-o-din′e-ah) pain in the intestine.

enteroenterostomy (en″ter-o-en″ter-os′to-me) surgical anastomosis between two segments of the intestine.

enteroepiplocele (en″ter-o-e-pip′lo-sēl) hernia of the intestine and omentum.

enterogastritis (en″ter-o-gas-tri′tis) inflammation of the small intestine and stomach.

enterogastrone (en″ter-o-gas′trōn) a hormone of the duodenum that mediates the humoral inhibition of gastric secretion and motility produced by ingestion of fat. Called also anthelone E.

enterogenous (en″ter-oj′ĕ-nus) 1. arising from the primitive foregut. 2. originating within the small intestine.

enterogram (en′ter-o-gram″) an instrumental tracing of the movements of the intestine.

enterography (en″ter-og′rah-fe) a description of the intestine.

enterohepatitis (en″ter-o-hep″ah-ti′tis) inflammation of the intestine and liver.

enterohepatocele (en″ter-o-hep′ah-to-sēl″) an umbilical hernia containing intestine and liver.

enterohydrocele (en″ter-o-hi′dro-sēl) hernia with hydrocele.

enterokinase (en″ter-o-ki′nās) enteropeptidase.

enterokinesia (en″ter-o-ki″ne′se-ah) peristalsis.

enterokinetic (en″ter-o-ki-net′ik) pertaining to or stimulating peristalsis.

enterokinin (en″ter-o-ki′nin) an extract of the mucosa of the small intestine, said to be a physiological hormone, which stimulates intestinal motility.

enterolith (en′ter-o-lith″) a calculus in the intestine.

enterology (en″ter-ol′o-je) scientific study of the intestine.

enterolysis (en″ter-ol′ĭ-sis) surgical separation of intestinal adhesions.

enteromegaly (en″ter-o-meg′ah-le) enlargement of the intestines.

enteromerocele (en″ter-o-me′ro-sĕl) femoral hernia.

enteromycosis (en″ter-o-mi-ko′sis) fungal disease of the intestine.

enteron (en′ter-on) the gut or alimentary canal; usually used in medicine with specific reference to the small intestine.

enteroparesis (en″ter-o-pah-re′sis) relaxation of the intestine resulting in dilatation.

enteropathogen (en″ter-o-path′o-jen) a microorganism which causes disease of the intestine. adj., **enteropathogen′ic.**

enteropathogenesis (en″ter-o-path″o-jen′ĕ-sis) the production of disease or disorder of the intestine.

enteropathy (en″ter-op′ah-the) any disease of the intestine.

gluten e., celiac disease.

protein-losing e., a nonspecific term referring to conditions, e.g., adult CELIAC DISEASE, associated with excessive loss of enteric plasma proteins.

enteropeptidase (en″ter-o-pep′tĭ-dās) an enzyme of the intestinal juice which activates the proteolytic enzyme of the pancreatic juice by converting trypsinogen into trypsin. Called also enterokinase.

enteropexy (en′ter-o-pek″se) surgical fixation of the intestine to the abdominal wall.

enteroplasty (en′ter-o-plas″te) plastic repair of the intestine.

enteroplegia (en″ter-o-ple′je-ah) adynamic ileus.

enteroptosis (en″ter-op-to′sis) abnormal downward displacement of the intestine. adj., **enteroptot′ic.**

enterorrhagia (en″ter-o-ra′je-ah) intestinal hemorrhage.

enterorrhaphy (en″ter-or′ah-fe) suture of the intestine.

enterorrhexis (en″ter-o-rek′sis) rupture of the intestine.

enteroscope (en′ter-o-skōp″) an instrument for inspecting the inside of the intestine.

enterosepsis (en″ter-o-sep′sis) sepsis developed from the intestinal contents.

enterospasm (en′ter-o-spazm″) intestinal colic.

enterostasis (en″ter-o-sta′sis) intestinal stasis.

enterostenosis (en″ter-o-stĕ-no′sis) narrowing or stricture of the intestine.

enterostomal (en″ter-o-sto′mal) relating to or having undergone an enterostomy.

e. therapist, one who is certified to assist in the specialized care of patients who have undergone enterostomy. Information about local therapists available for consultation can be obtained by writing to The International Association for Enterostomal Therapy, Ravenwood Hospital and Medical Center, 4550 North Windchester, Chicago, Illinois 60640. (See also STOMA.)

enterostomy (en″ter-os′to-me) the artificial formation of a permanent opening into the intestine through the abdominal wall (see also COLOSTOMY and ILEOSTOMY.)

enterotomy (en″ter-ot′o-me) incision of the intestine.

enterotoxemia (en″ter-o-tok-se′me-ah) a condition characterized by the presence in the blood of toxins produced in the intestines.

enterotoxigenic (en″ter-o-tok″sĭ-jen′ik) producing, produced by, or pertaining to production of enterotoxin.

enterotoxin (en″ter-o-tok′sin) 1. a toxin specific for the cells of the intestinal mucosa. 2. a toxin arising in the intestine. 3. an exotoxin that is protein in nature and relatively heat-stable, produced by staplylococci.

enterotoxism (en″ter-o-tok′sizm) autointoxication of enteric origin.

enterotropic (en″ter-o-trop′ik) affecting the intestines.

enterovaginal (en″ter-o-vaj′ĭ-nal) pertaining to or communicating with the intestine and the vagina, as an enterovaginal fistula.

enterovesical (en″ter-o-ves′ĭ-kal) pertaining to or communicating with the intestine and urinary bladder.

Entero-Vioform (en″ter-o-vi′o-form) trademark for a preparation of iodochlorhydroxyquin, a topical anti-infective, used largely for treatment of amebiasis.

enterovirus (en″ter-o-vi′rus) any of a subgroup of picornaviruses infecting the gastrointestinal tract and discharged in the excreta, including the poliovirus, coxsackievirus, and echovirus.

enterozoon (en″ter-o-zo′on) an animal parasite in the intestines. adj., **enterozo′ic.**

enthetobiosis (en-thet″o-bi-o′sis) a term suggested to denote the dependency of an organism on a mechanical device implanted within the body, for example, dependency of a patient on an electronic cardiac pacemaker to regulate the heart beat. The relationship between the organism and the device is critical. Called also epenthetobiosis.

ento- word element [Gr.], *within; inner.*

entoblast (en′to-blast) the entoderm.

entocele (en′to-sēl) an internal hernia.

entochoroidea (en″to-ko-roi′de-ah) the inner layer of the choroid of the eye.

entoderm (en′to-derm) the innermost of the three primitive germ layers of the embryo; from it are derived the epithelium of the pharynx, respiratory tract (except the nose), digestive tract, bladder, and urethra. adj., **entoder′mal, entoder′mic.**

entoectad (en″to-ek′tad) from within outward.

entomere (en″to-mēr) a blastomere normally destined to become entoderm.

entomion (en-to′me-on) the tip of the posteroinferior, or mastoid, angle of the parietal bone.

entomology (en″to-mol′o-je) that branch of biology concerned with the study of insects.

medical e., that concerned with insects that cause disease or serve as vectors of pathogens.

entopic (en-top′ik) occurring in the proper place.

entoptic (en-top′tik) originating within the eye.

entoptoscopy (en″top-tos′ko-pe) inspection of the interior of the eye.

entoretina (en″to-ret′ĭ-nah) the nervous or inner layer of the retina.

entotic (en-tot′ik) situated in or originating within the ear.

entozoon (en″to-zo′on) an internal animal parasite. adj., **entozo′ic.**

entropion (en-tro′pe-on) inversion, or the turning inward, as of the margin of an eyelid.

e. u′veae, inversion of the margin of the pupil.

enucleate (e-nu′kle-āt) to remove whole and clean, as the eye from its socket.

enucleation (e-nu″kle-a′shun) removal of an organ or other mass intact from its supporting tissues, as of the eyeball from the orbit.

enuresis (en″u-re′sis) involuntary discharge of urine, usually referring to involuntary discharge of urine during sleep at night; bed-wetting. adj., **enuret′ic.** It occurs most often in children who are very sound sleepers or who have small bladder capacity. In many cases enuresis is due to emotional rather than physical causes. If it persists after the age of 6, a physical or emotional disorder is likely to be present.

envenomation (en-ven″o-ma′shun) the poisonous effects caused by the bites, stings, or effluvia of insects and other arthropods, or the bites of snakes.

environment (en-vi′ron-ment) the sum total of all the conditions and elements that make up the surroundings and influence the development of an individual.

Enzactin (en-zak′tin) trademark for preparations of triacetin, a local antifungal agent.

enzygotic (en″zi-got′ik) developed from one zygote.

enzymatic (en″zi-mat′ik) of, relating to, caused by, or of the nature of an enzyme.

enzyme (en′zīm) a protein capable of accelerating or producing by catalytic action some change in a substrate for which it is often specific. The substance acted upon by an enzyme is called a substrate. In an enzymatic reaction a portion of one substrate is transferred to another substrate or metabolized. Each enzyme is specific for a certain type of substrate and may catalyze the reaction in either direction.

Enzymes are essential for a number of the life processes and are responsible for functions such as digestion, maintenance of acid-base balance, and energy utilization.

The digestive enzmes are divided into three groups: amylases, or starch splitters; the lipases, or fat splitters; and the proteases, which split proteins.

Enzymes are sensitive to changes in acidity and alkalinity and can act as toxins. If obstruction of the pancreatic duct causes powerful digestive enzymes of the pancreas to be retained and made active in that organ, acute symptoms can occur. A slowing up of the enzymatic action can also cause serious illness or death.

It is thought that improper functioning of enzymes causes some nerve disorders. There has been a growing recognition of a number of hereditary diseases caused by defective enzyme systems. Phenylketonuria (PKU), for example, is caused by the inherited inability of the body to convert the amino acid phenylalanine into tyrosine.

By a number of biochemical tests performed in clinical laboratories the activity levels of many enzymes in body fluids (e.g., serum) can be determined, and variations from previously normal levels can help the physician in diagnosing and following the course of a disease, e.g., MYOCARDIAL INFARCTION and pancreatitis.

activating e., one that activates a given amino acid by attaching it to the corresponding transfer ribonucleic acid.

adaptive e., induced enzyme.

allosteric e., one containing an ALLOSTERIC SITE.

autolytic e., one that produces autolysis of the cell in which it exists.

brancher e., branching e., α-glucan-branching glycosyltransferase: an enzyme involved in conversion of amylose to amylopectin; deficiency of this enzyme causes amylopectinosis.

clotting e., coagulating e., one that catalyzes the conversion of soluble into insoluble proteins.

constitutive e., one produced by a microorganism regardless of the presence or absence of the specific substrate acted upon.

debrancher e., debranching e., dextrin-1,6-glucosidase: an enzyme that acts on glucose residues of the glycogen molecule, and is important in glycogenolysis; deficiency of this enzyme causes Forbes' disease.

digestive e., a substance that catalyzes the process of digestion.

extracellular e., one existing outside of the cell secreting it; called also ectoenzyme.

glycolytic e., one that catalyzes the conversion of sugar to pyruvic acid.

induced e., inducible e., one whose production requires or is stimulated by a specific small molecule, the inducer, which is the substrate of the enzyme or a compound structurally related to it.

inhibitory e., one whose action blocks another reaction or a reaction sequence.

lipolytic e., one that catalyzes the hydrolysis of fat.

mucolytic e., one that catalyzes the hydrolytic depolymerization of mucopolysaccharides.

proteolytic e., one that catalyzes the hydrolysis of proteins and various split products of proteins, the final product being small peptides and amino acids.

redox e., one that catalyzes oxidation-reduction reactions.

repressible e., one whose rate of production is decreased as the concentration of certain metabolites is increased.

respiratory e's, enzymes of the mitochondria, e.g., cytochrome oxidase, which serve as catalysts for cellular oxidations.

splitting e., one that catalyzes the splitting of a fragment from a molecule, e.g., the splitting out of CO_2 from a carboxyl group (decarboxylation).

steatolytic e., lipolytic enzyme.

transferring e., a transferase; one that catalyzes the transference of various radicals between molecules.

uricolytic e., one that catalyzes the conversion of uric acid to urea.

yellow e's, flavoproteins isolated from several sources, which take part in oxidations and reductions.

enzymic (en-zi'mik) enzymatic.

enzymology (en″zi-mol'o-je) the study of enzymes and enzymatic action.

enzymolysis (en″zi-mol'ĭ-sis) disintegration induced by an enzyme.

enzymopathy (en″zi-mop'ah-the) an inborn error of metabolism consisting of defective or absent enzymes, as in the glycogenoses or the mucopolysaccharidoses.

enzymopenia (en-zi″mo-pe'ne-ah) deficiency of an enzyme in the blood. adj., **enzymope'nic.**

enzymuria (en″zi-mu're-ah) the presence of enzymes in the urine.

EOG electro-oculogram.

eonism (e'o-nizm) tranvestism in the male.

eosin (e'o-sin) any of a class of rose-colored stains or dyes, all being bromine derivatives of fluorescein; eosin Y, the sodium salt of tetrabromfluorescein, is much used in histologic and laboratory procedures.

eosinopenia (e″o-sin″o-pe'ne-ah) abnormal deficiency of eosinophils in the blood.

eosinophil (e″o-sin'o-fil) an element readily stained by eosin; specifically, a granular leukocyte with a nucleus that usually has two lobes connected by a thread of chromatin, and cytoplasm containing coarse, round granules of uniform size.

eosinophilia (e″o-sin″o-fil'e-ah) 1. the formation and accumulation of an abnormally large number of eosinophils in the blood. 2. the condition of being readily stained with eosin. adj., **eosinophil'ic.**

tropical e., a disease characterized by anorexia, malaise, cough, leukocytosis, and an increase in eosinophils.

eosinophilic (e″o-sin″o-fil'ik) staining readily with eosin; pertaining to eosinophils or to eosinophilia.

epallobiosis (ep″al-o-bi-o'sis) a term suggested to denote the dependency of an organism on an extracorporal life-support system, as in the use of an artificial kidney or heart-lung machine to perform a vital body function.

epaxial (ep-ak'se-al) situated above or upon an axis.

epencephalon (ep″en-sef'ah-lon) 1. cerebellum. 2. metencephalon.

ependyma (ĕ-pen'dĭ-mah) the membrane lining the cerebral ventricles and the central canal of the spine. adj., **epen'dymal.**

epenthetobiosis (ĕp-en-thĕt″o-bi-o'sis) enthetobiosis.

ephapse (e-faps′) a point of lateral contact (other than a synapse) between nerve fibers across which impulses are conducted directly through the nerve membranes. adj., **ephap′tic.**

ephebiatrics (e-fe″be-at′riks) the branch of medicine that deals especially with the diagnosis and treatment of diseases and problems peculiar to youth.

ephebic (ĕ-fe′bik) pertaining to youth or the period of puberty and adolescence.

ephebogenesis (ef″e-bo-jen′ĕ-sis) the bodily changes occurring at puberty. adj., **ephebogenet′ic.**

ephebology (ef″e-bol′o-je) the study of puberty.

ephedrine (ĕ-fed′rin, ef′ĕ-drin) an adrenergic alkaloid obtained from several species of the shrub *Ephedra* or produced synthetically; used, in the form of ephedrine hydrochloride or ephedrine sulfate, as a bronchodilator.

ephelis (ĕfe′lis), pl. *ephel′ides* [Gr.] a freckle.

Ephynal (ef′ĭ-nal) trademark for a preparation of vitamin E.

epi- word element [Gr.], *upon.*

epiandrosterone (ep″ĭ-an-dros′ter-ōn) an androgenic steroid less active than androsterone and excreted in small amounts in normal human urine.

epiblepharon (ep″ĭ-blef′ah-ron) a developmental anomaly in which a horizontal fold of skin stretches across the border of the eyelid; on the lower lid it may press the lashes against the eyeball.

epibulbar (ep″ĭ-bul′bar) situated upon the eyeball.

epicanthus (ep″ĭ-kan′thus) a vertical fold of skin on either side of the nose, sometimes covering the inner canthus; a normal characteristic in persons of certain races, but anomalous in others. adj., **epican′thal, epican′thic.**

epicardia (ep″ĭ-kar′de-ah) the lower portion of the esophagus, extending from the esophageal hiatus to the cardia, the upper orifice of the stomach.

epicardium (ep″i-kar′de-um) the inner layer of the serous pericardium, which is in contact with the heart.

epichorion (ep″ĭ-ko′re-on) the portion of the uterine mucosa enclosing the implanted conceptus.

epicondyle (ep″ĭ-kon′dīl) an eminence upon a bone, above its condyle.

epicondylitis (ep″ĭ-kon″dĭ-li′tis) inflammation of an epicondyle or of tissues adjoining the humeral epicondyle.

epicranium (ep″ĭ-kra′ne-um) the structures collectively that cover the skull.

epicritic (ep″ĭ-krit′ik) determining accurately; said of cutaneous nerve fibers sensitive to fine variations of touch or temperature.

epicystotomy (ep″ĭ-sis-tot′o-me) cystotomy by the suprapubic method.

epicyte (ep′ĭ-sīt) cell membrane.

epidemic (ep″ĭ-dem′ik) 1. attacking many people in a region at the same time; widely diffused and rapidly spreading. 2. a disease of high morbidity which is only occasionally present in the human community.

epidemicity (ep″ĭ-dĕ-mis′ĭ-te) the quality of being widely diffused and rapidly spreading throughout a community.

epidemiogenesis (ep″ĭ-de″me-o-jen′ĕ-sis) the spread of a communicable disease to epidemic proportions.

epidemiography (ep″ĭ-de″me-og′rah-fe) a treatise upon or an account of epidemics.

epidemiologist (ep″ĭ-de″me-ol′o-jist) an expert in epidemiology.

epidemiology (ep″ĭ-de″me-ol′o-je) 1. the study of the relationships of various factors determining the frequency and distribution of diseases in the human community. 2. the field of medicine dealing with the determination of specific causes of localized outbreaks of infection, toxic poisoning, or other disease of recognized etiology. adj., **epidemiolog′ic.**

epidermis (ep″ĭ-der′mis) the outermost, nonvascular layer of the SKIN, derived from the embryonic ectoderm, varying in thickness from $\frac{1}{200}$ to $\frac{1}{20}$ inch, and composed of, from within outward, five layers: basal layer, prickle-cell layer, granular layer, clear layer, and horny layer. adj. **epider′mal, epider′mic.**

epidermitis (ep″ĭ-der-mi′tis) inflammation of the epidermis.

epidermodysplasia (ep″ĭ-der″mo-dis-pla′ze-ah) faulty development of the epidermis.

e. verrucifor′mis, a skin condition due to a virus identical with or closely related to the virus of common warts, in which the lesions are red or red-violet and widespread and tend to become malignant.

epidermoid (ep″ĭ-der′moid) 1. resembling the epidermis. 2. an intracranial cystlike mass formed by inclusion of epidermal cells.

epidermoidoma (ep″ĭ-der″moi-do′mah) a cerebral or meningeal tumor formed by inclusion of ectodermal elements at the time of closure of the neural groove.

epidermolysis (ep″ĭ-der-mol′ĭ-sis) a loosened state of the epidermis with formation of blebs and bullae either spontaneously or at the site of trauma.

e. bullo′sa, a variety with development of bullae and vesicles, often at the site of trauma; in the hereditary forms, there may be severe scarring after healing, or extensive denuded areas after rupture of the lesions.

epidermomycosis (ep″ĭ-der″mo-mi-ko′sis) dermatophytosis.

epidermophytid (ep″ĭ-der-mof′ĭ-tid) dermatophytid.

epidermophytin (ep″ĭ-der-mof′ĭ-tin) a filtrate of Epidermophyton cultures that induces a hypersensitivity reaction of the tuberculin type; used in treatment of epidermophytosis.

Epidermophyton (ep′ĭ-der-mof′ĭ-ton) a genus of fungi. *E. flocco′sum* attacks both skin and nails but not hair, and is one of the causative organisms of tinea cruris, tinea pedis (athlete's foot), and onychomycosis.

epidermophytosis (ep″ĭ-der″mo-fi-to′sis) a fungal skin infection, especially one due to *Epidermophyton;* dermatophytosis.

epididymectomy (ep″ĭ-did″ĭ-mek′to-me) excision of the epididymis.

epididymis (ep″ĭ-did′ĭ-mis), pl. *epididym′ides* [Gr.] an elongated, cordlike structure along the posterior border of the testis in the ducts of which the sperm are stored. adj., **epidid′ymal.**

epididymitis (ep″ĭ-did″ĭ-mi′tis) inflammation of the epididymis. Nonspecific epididymitis may result from an infection in the urinary tract, especially in the prostate. Rarely it may be traced to an infection elsewhere in the body. Tuberculosis, mumps, and gonorrhea may be complicated by epididymitis. Symptoms include sudden severe pain in the testes followed by scrotal swelling and tenderness. Treatment is usually with antibiotics, rest in bed, and avoidance of alcoholic beverages, spiced foods, sexual excitement, and physical exercise until all symptoms have disappeared.

epididymo-orchitis (ep″ĭ-did″ĭ-mo-or-ki′tis) inflammation of the epididymis and testis.

epididymotomy (ep″ĭ-did″ĭ-mot′o-me) incision of the epididymis.

epididymovasostomy (ep″ĭ-did″ĭ-mo-vas-os′to-me) surgical anastomosis of the epididymis to the ductus deferens.

epidural (ep″ĭ-du′ral) situated upon or outside the dura mater.

epidurography (ep″ĭ-du-rog′rah-fe) radiography of the spine after a radiopaque medium has been injected into the epidural space.

epiestriol (ep″ĭ-es′tre-ol) an estrogenic steroid found in pregnant women.

epigastralgia (ep″ĭ-gas-tral′je-ah) pain in the epigastrium.

epigastrium (ep″ĭ-gas′tre-um) the upper and middle region of the abdomen, located within the sternal angle. adj., **epigas′tric.**

epigenesis (ep″ĭ-jen′ĕ-sis) the development of an organism from an undifferentiated cell, consisting in the successive formation and development of organs and parts that do not preexist in the fertilized egg. adj., **epigenet′ic.**

epiglottis (ep″ĭ-glot′is) the lidlike cartilaginous structure overhanging the entrance to the larynx. adj., **epiglot′tic.** The muscular action of swallowing closes the opening to the trachea by placing the larynx against the epiglottis. This prevents food and drink from entering the larynx and trachea, directing it instead into the esophagus. (See Plates 5 and 6.)

epilation (ep″ĭ-la′shun) the removal of hair by the roots.

epilemma (ep″ĭ-lem′ah) endoneurium.

epilepsy (ep′ĭ-lep″se) paroxysmal transient disturbances of nervous system function resulting from abnormal electrical activity of the brain. It is not a specific disease, but rather a group of symptoms that are manifestations of any of a number of conditions that overstimulate nerve cells of the brain. The estimated incidence of epilepsy is 0.5 per cent of the population, making it a relatively common disease. Over 70 per cent of those having epilepsy experience their first attack before the age of 20, usually while in their teens. It is slightly more prevalent in males.

TYPES. There are several methods for classifying the various types of epilepsy. On the basis of origin, epilepsy is idiopathic (cryptogenic, essential, genetic) or symptomatic (acquired, organic). Symptomatic epilepsy has a physical cause, for example, brain tumor, injury to the brain at birth, a wound or blow to the head, or an endocrine disorder.

On the basis of clinical manifestations and electroencephalographic readings, four types are recognized: (1) grand mal (major epilepsy) with subgroups including generalized, focal (localized), and jacksonian (rolandic), (2) petit mal (minor epilepsy), (3) psychomotor, and (4) autonomic (diencephalic).

SYMPTOMS. The symptoms of epilepsy vary according to amount and type of brain tissue involved. In major seizures, or grand mal, there is a sudden loss of consciousness, frequently preceded by an aura, and immediately followed by generalized convulsions in which there are biting movements and violent shaking of the limbs. The aura can be considered a warning of an impending seizure, although it is probably an early symptom of the attack. The aura, not always experienced by every patient with epilepsy, lasts from a fraction of a second to a few seconds and can include auditory or visual hallucinations, ringing in the ears, unpleasant odors or tastes, illusions that the environment is familiar (déjà vu), and other sensory and perceptual aberrations.

In minor seizures, petit mal, the loss of consciousness lasts only a few seconds. There usually is twitching about the eyes or mouth, the subject remains seated or standing and appears to have had no more than a lapse of attention or a moment of absentmindedness. This form of epilepsy is seen especially in children.

Psychomotor epilepsy, associated with disease of the temporal lobe, is manifested by a very brief clouding of consciousness with some repeated meaningless movement such as hand clapping. It is followed by brief periods of forgetfulness. If the autonomic nervous system is affected, the symptoms may include flushing, pallor, tachycardia, hypertension, perspiration, or other visceral symptoms.

In jacksonian epilepsy the specific portion of the brain controlling certain muscles may be diseased or irritated. The convulsions start in a specific group of muscles, such as those in the hand or leg, and progress to involve other muscles. The involuntary movement may develop into a complete grand mal attack with loss of consciousness.

DIAGNOSIS. Epilepsy is suspected in all persons having recurrent episodes of changes in consciousness and involuntary movements. A complete assessment of the patient's status is necessary, including a complete history, physical and neurological examination, and laboratory studies of the blood and spinal fluid. The latter are especially useful in determining whether an infection is the cause of the seizures. Roentgenographic examination of the skull usually are done. The diagnosis is confirmed by ELECTROENCEPHALOGRAM and ECHOENCEPHALOGRAM, which are helpful in locating the site and possibly the cause of the seizures.

TREATMENT AND PATIENT CARE. Surgical removal of the brain lesion, for example, tumor or scar tissue, is indicated in a limited number of patients. The large majority of cases are treated by medications that prevent disabling effects of the disease. The anticonvulsant drugs that may be prescribed include phenobarbital, diphenylhydantoin (Dilantin), and trimethadione (Tridione).

The patient is instructed in the effects of the drugs prescribed for him, the importance of continuing medications after seizures are controlled and until otherwise instructed by the physician, and the need to report immediately any untoward reactions to his medication. Members of his family should be taught the proper care of a person having a convulsive seizure. (See also CONVULSION.)

The Epilepsy Foundation of America, 733 15th Street, Washington, D.C. 20005, supplies information on all aspects of epilepsy and can refer patients and their families to specialists and clinics in their locality.

One of the major challenges to persons working in the health field and concerned with the care of patients with epilepsy is the dispelling of myths and superstitions about the disease and the propagation of accurate information. Most persons with epilepsy can lead normal lives with few restrictions, but many are subjected to unfair employment practices and social stigma because of prejudices resulting from the general public's ignorance of the effects of epilepsy.

myoclonus e., see MYOCLONUS EPILEPSY.

epileptic (e″ĭ-lep′tik) 1. pertaining to or affected with epilepsy. 2. a person affected with epilepsy.

epileptiform (ep″ĭlep′tĭ-form) 1. resembling epilepsy or its manifestations. 2. occurring in severe or sudden paroxysms.

epileptogenic (ep″ĭ-lep″to-jen′ik) causing an epileptic seizure.

epileptoid (ep″ĭ-lep′toid) epileptiform.

epileptology (ep″ĭ-lep-tol′o-je) the study of epilepsy.

epimenorrhagia (ep″ĭ-men″o-ra′je-ah) too frequent and excessive menstruation.

epimenorrhea (ep″ĭ-men″o-re′ah) abnormally frequent menstruation.

epimer (ep″ĭ-mer) one of two or more isomers which differ only in the position of one carbon atom.

epimerase (ĕ-pim′er-āse) an isomerase that catalyzes the inversion of asymmetric groups in substrates (epimers) having more than one center of asymmetry.

epimere (ep′ĭ-mēr) the dorsal portion of a somite, from which is formed muscles innervated by the dorsal ramus of a spinal nerve.

epimerite (ep″ĭ-mer′īt) an organelle of certain protozoa by which they attach themselves to epithelial cells.

epimerization (e-pim″er-i-za′shun) the changing of one epimeric form of a compound into another, as by enzymatic action.

epimorphosis (ep″ĭ-mor-fo′sis) the regeneration of a piece of an organism by proliferation at the cut surface. adj., **epimor′phic.**

epimysium (ep″ĭ-mis′e-um) the fibrous sheath around an entire skeletal muscle. (See Plate 4.)

epinephrectomy (ep″ĭ-nĕ-frek′to-me) adrenalectomy.

epinephrine (ep″ĭ-nef′rin) a hormone produced by the medulla, or inner core, of the ADRENAL GLANDS; called also adrenaline (Great Britain). Its function is to aid in the regulation of the sympathetic branch of the AUTONOMIC NERVOUS SYSTEM. At times when a person is highly stimulated, as by fear, anger, or some challenging situation, extra amounts of epinephrine are released into the bloodstream, preparing the body for energetic action. The arteries are contracted and blood pressure rises; heartbeat speeds up and so does breathing; the rate at which the blood will clot is increased, and so is the rate of oxygen consumption by the body. Simultaneously, extra sugar is released into the blood from its storage place in the liver for quick conversion into energy. The person has a suddenly increased feeling of muscular strength and aggressiveness.

Some disorders of the adrenal glands, such as Addison's disease, reduce the output of epinephrine below normal. By contrast, excessive activity of the adrenals often seen in highly emotional persons, tends to produce tenseness, palpitation, high blood pressure, perhaps diarrhea, and overaggressiveness. Certain adrenal tumors result in the production of too much epinephrine. Removal of the tumor relieves symptoms.

Epinephrine is also produced synthetically. It can be administered parenterally, topically, or by inhalation, and acts as a vasoconstrictor, antispasmodic, and sympathomimetic. It is used as an emergency heart stimulant and to relieve symptoms in allergic conditions such as urticaria (hives) and asthma. It is the most effective drug for counteracting the lethal effects of anaphylactic shock.

epineural (ep′ĭ-nu′ral) situated upon a neural arch.

epineurium (ep″ĭ-nu′re-um) the sheath of a peripheral nerve. adj., **epineu′rial.**

epinosis (ep″ĭ-no′sis) a psychic or imaginary state of illness secondary to an original illness.

epiphysiolysis (ep″ĭ-fiz″e-ol′ĭ-sis) separation of the epiphysis from the diaphysis of a bone.

epiphysis (e-pif′ĭ-sis), pl. *epiph′yses* [Gr.] 1. the end of a long bone, usually wider than the shaft, and either entirely cartilaginous or separated from the shaft by a cartilaginous disk. 2. part of a bone formed from a secondary center of ossification, commonly found at the ends of long bones, on the margins of flat bones, and at tubercles and processes; during the period of growth epiphyses are separated from the main portion of the bone by cartilage. adj., **epiphys′eal.**

e. cere′bri, pineal body.

epiphysitis (e-pif″ĭ-si′tis) inflammation of an epiphysis or of the cartilage joining the epiphysis to a bone shaft.

epipial (ep″ĭ-pi′al) situated upon the pia mater.

epiplocele (e-pip′lo-sēl) omental hernia.

epiploenterocele (ep″ĭ-plo-en′ter-o-sēl″) a hernia containing intestine and omentum.

epiplomerocele (ep″ĭ-plo-me′ro-sēl) a femoral hernia containing omentum.

epiplomphalocele (ep″ĭ-plom-fal′o-sēl) an umbilical hernia containing omentum.

epiploon (e-pip′lo-on), pl. *epip′loa* [Gr.] the greater omentum. adj., **epiplo′ic.**

episclera (ep″ĭ-skle′rah) the loose connective tissue forming the sclera and the conjunctiva..

episcleral (ep″ĭ-skle′ral) 1. overlying the sclera. 2. pertaining to the episclera.

episcleritis (ep″ĭ-skle-ri′tis) inflammation of the episclera and adjacent tissues.

episioperineoplasty (e-piz″e-o-per″ĭ-ne′o-plas″te) plastic repair of the vulva and perineum.

episioperineorrhaphy (e-piz″e-o-per″ĭ-ne-or′ah-fe) suture of the vulva and perineum.

episioplasty (e-piz′e-o-plas″te) plastic repair of the vulva.

episiorrhaphy (e-piz″e-or′ah-fe) 1. suture of the labia majora. 2. suture of a lacerated perineum.

episiostenosis (e-piz″e-o-stĕ-no′sis) narrowing of the vulvar orifice.

episiotomy (e-piz″e-ot′o-me) incision of the vulva, most often done during the second stage of labor to avoid lacerations of the perineum as the infant is delivered.

episome (ep'ĭ-sōm) in bacterial genetics, any accessory extrachromosomal replicating genetic element that can exist either autonomously or integrated with the chromosome.

epispadias (ep"ĭ-spa'de-as) a congenital malformation with absence of the upper wall of the urethra, occurring in both sexes, but more commonly in the male, the urethral opening being located anywhere on the dorsum of the penis. adj., **epispa'diac, epispa'dial.**

episplenitis (ep"ĭ-sple-ni'tis) inflammation of the capsule of the spleen.

epistaxis (ep"ĭ-stak'sis) hemorrhage from the nose, usually due to rupture of small vessels overlying the anterior part of the cartilaginous nasal septum; nosebleed. A minor nosebleed may be caused by a blow on the nose, irritation from foreign bodies, or vigorous nose-blowing during a cold. Sometimes it occurs in connection with menstruation. If bleeding persists in spite of the following first-aid measures, medical attention is advisable.

The victim should sit up with the head tilted back. The soft portion of the nose is grasped firmly between the thumb and forefinger. If this does not stop the bleeding, small wads of cotton or gauze are gently inserted into the nose and then the nostrils are pressed firmly together again. This often helps a clot to form. If a clot fails to form, cold compresses are applied about the nose, the lips, and the back of the neck. If the bleeding still persists, cauterization of the blood vessel may be necessary.

Sometimes nosebleed has serious underlying causes. Arteriosclerosis is a possible cause in the elderly. Polyps and other fleshy growths in the nose, food allergy, hypertension, vitamin deficiencies, or any disease producing a bleeding tendency may produce nosebleed. Nosebleeds in children are sometimes a sign of rheumatic fever. If the nose bleeds often or profusely or if the bleeding is difficult to stop, a physician should be consulted.

Bleeding from the nose that does not originate in the nose itself is a serious indication that some damage has been done internally, either by injury or disease. Medical attention is necessary to trace the bleeding to its source. The blood probably originates in the stomach, the lungs, within the skull, or in passages related to these parts.

episternal (ep"ĭ-ster'nal) 1. situated on or over the sternum. 2. pertaining to the episternum.

episternum (ep"ĭ-ster'num) the manubrium, or upper piece of the sternum.

epitendineum (ep"ĭ-ten-din'e-um) the fibrous sheath covering a tendon.

epithalamus (ep"ĭ-thal'ah-mus) the part of the thalamencephalon just superior and posterior to the thalamus, comprising the pineal body and adjacent structures; considered by some to include the stria medullaris.

epithelial (ep"ĭ-the'le-al) pertaining to or composed of epithelium.

epithelialization (ep"ĭ-the"le-al-ĭ-za'shun) healing by the growth of epithelium over a denuded surface.

epithelialize (ep"ĭ-the'le-al-īz) to cover with epithelium.

epitheliitis (ep"ĭ-the"le-i'tis) inflammation of the epithelium.

epithelioid (ep"ĭ-the'le-oid) resembling epithelium.

epitheliolysin (ep"ĭ-the"le-ol'ĭ-sin) a cytolysin formed in the serum in response to injection of epithelial cells from a different species; it is capable of destroying epithelial cells of animals of the donor species.

epitheliolysis (ep"ĭ-the"le-ol'ĭ-sis) destruction of epithelial tissue. adj., **epitheliolyt'ic.**

epithelioma (ep"ĭ-the"le-o'mah) any tumor derived from epithelium. adj., **epithelio'matous.**

e. adenoi'des cys'ticum, trichoepithelioma.

epitheliosis (ep"ĭ-the"le-o'sis) proliferation of conjunctival epithelium, forming trachoma-like granules.

epitheliotropic (ep"ĭ-the"le-o-trop'ik) having a special affinity for epithelial cells.

epithelium (ep"ĭ-the'le-um), pl. *epithe'lia* [Gr.] the cellular covering of internal and external surfaces of the body, including the lining of vessels and other small cavities. It consists of cells joined by small amounts of cementing substances. Epithelium is classified into types on the basis of the number of layers deep and the shape of the superficial cells.

ciliated e., epithelium bearing vibratile, hairlike processes (cilia) on its free surface.

columnar e. epithelium whose cells are of much greater height than width.

cuboidal e., epithelium whose cells are of approximately the same height and width, and appear square in transverse section.

germinal e., thickened peritoneal epithelium covering the gonad from earliest development; formerly thought to give rise to germ cells.

glandular e., that composed of secreting cells.

pigmentary e., pigmented e., that made of cells containing granules of pigment.

sense e., sensory e., neuroepithelium (1).

simple e., that composed of a single layer of cells.

squamous e., that composed of flattened platelike cells.

stratified e., epithelium made up of cells arranged in layers.

transitional e., a type characteristically found lining hollow organs, such as the urinary bladder, that are subject to great mechanical change due to contraction and distention, originally thought to represent a transition between stratified squamous and columnar epithelium.

epithelization (ep"ĭ-the"lĭ-za'shun) epithelialization.

epithiazide (ep"ĭ-thi'ah-zīd) an antihypertensive and diuretic.

epitonic (ep"ĭ-ton'ik) abnormally tense or tonic.

epitrichium (ep"ĭ-trik'e-um) periderm.

epitrochlea (ep"ĭ-trok'le-ah) the inner condyle of the humerus.

epitympanum (ep"ĭ-tim'pah-num) the upper part of the tympanum. adj., **epitympan'ic.**

epizoic (ep"ĭ-zo'ik) pertaining to or caused by an epizoon.

epizoon (ep"ĭ-zo'on), pl. *epizo'a* [Gr.] an external animal parasite.

epizootic (ep"ĭ-zo-ot'ik) 1. attacking many animals in any region at the same time; widely diffused and rapidly spreading. 2. a disease of high morbidity which is only occasionally present in an animal community.

eponychium (ep″o-nik′e-um) 1. the narrow band of epidermis extending from the nail wall onto the nail surface; commonly called cuticle. 2. the horny fetal epidermis at the site of the future nail.

eponym (ep′o-nim) a name or phrase formed from or including a person's name, e.g., Hodgkin's disease, Cowper's gland, Schick test. adj., **eponym′ic, epon′ymous.**

epoophoron (ep″o-of′o-ron) a vestigial structure associated with the ovary.

epoxy (ĕ-pok′se) 1. containing one atom of oxygen bound to two different carbon atoms. 2. a resin composed of epoxy polymers and characterized by adhesiveness, flexibility, and resistance to chemical actions.

Eprolin (ep′ro-lin) trademark for a preparation of vitamin E.

epsilon-aminocaproic acid (ep′sĭ-lon am″ĭ-no-kah-pro′ik) see ε-AMINOCAPROIC ACID.

Epsom salt (ep′sum) magnesium sulfate, a cathartic.

Epstein-Barr virus (ep′stīn-bar) a herpesvirus that is the etiologic agent of infectious mononucleosis. It has been isolated from cells cultured from Burkitt's lymphoma, and has been found in certain cases of nasopharyngeal cancer. Called also EB virus.

epulis (ep-u′lis), pl. *epu′lides* [Gr.] any tumor of the gingiva.

epulosis (ep″u-lo′sis) a scarring over; cicatrization. adj., **epulot′ic.**

Equanil (ek′wah-nil) trademark for preparations of meprobamate, a minor tranquilizer.

equation (e-kwa′zhun) an expression of equality between two parts.

Henderson-Hasselbalch e., a formula for calculating the pH of a buffer solution such as blood plasma, $pH = pK' + \log\frac{(BA)}{(HA)}$; (HA) is the concentration of a weak acid; (BA) the concentration of a weak salt of this acid; pK′ the buffer system.

equilibration (e″kwĭ-lĭ-bra′shun) the achievement of a balance between opposing elements or forces.

equilibrium (e″kwĭ-lib′re-um) a state of balance between opposing forces or influences. In the body, equilibrium may be chemical or physical. A state of chemical equilibrium is reached when the body tissues contain the proper proportions of various salts and water. (See also ACID-BASE BALANCE and FLUID BALANCE.) Physical equilibrium, such as the state of balance required for walking, standing, or sitting, is achieved by a very complex interplay of opposing sets of muscles. The labyrinth of the inner ear contains the semicircular canals, or organs of balance, and relays to the brain information about the body's position and also the direction of body motions.

dynamic e., the condition of balance between varying, shifting, and opposing forces that is characteristic of living processes.

equine (e′kwīn) pertaining to, characteristic of, or derived from the horse.

equinovarus (e-kwi″no-va′rus) talipes equinovarus; a foot deformity in which the heel is turned inward and the foot is plantar flexed.

equipotential (e″kwĭ-po-ten′shal) having similar and equal power or capability.

equipotentiality (e″kwĭ-po-ten″she-al′ĭ-te) the quality or state of having similar and equal power; the capacity for developing in the same way and to the same extent.

equivalent (e-kwiv′ah-lent) 1. of equal force, power, value, etc. 2. something that has equivalent properties.

chemical e., that weight in grams of a substance that will produce or react with 1 mole of hydrogen ion or 1 mole of electrons.

epilepsy e., any disturbance, mental or physical, that may take the place of an epileptic seizure.

Joule's e., the mechanical equivalent of heat or the amount of work expended in raising the temperature of a pound of water through 1° F.; 772 foot-pounds. Symbol J.

Er chemical symbol, *erbium.*

erasion (e-ra′zhun) removal by scraping or curettage.

Erb's palsy (erbs) Erb-Duchenne paralysis.

Erb-Duchenne paralysis (erb′du-shen′) paralysis of the upper roots of the brachial plexus due to destruction of the fifth and sixth cervical roots, without involvement of the small muscles of the hand. Called also Duchenne's paralysis and Erb's palsy.

Erb-Goldflam disease (erb gōlt′flahm) myasthenia gravis.

erbium (er′be-um) a chemical element, atomic number 68, atomic weight 167.26, symbol Er. (See table of ELEMENTS.)

erectile (e-rek′tīl) capable of erection.

erection (e-rek′shun) the condition of becoming rigid and elevated, as erectile tissue when filled with blood; applied especially to the swelling and rigidity that occur in the penis as a result of sexual or other types of stimulation. Impulses received by the nervous system stimulate a flow of blood from the arteries leading to the penis, where the erectile tissue fills with blood, and the penis becomes firm and erect. Erection makes possible the transmission of semen into the body of the female (see REPRODUCTION). Erection can also occur to some extent in the clitoris and the nipples of the female.

erector (e-rek′tor) [L.] a structure that erects, as a muscle that holds up or raises a part.

erethism (er′ĕ-thizm) excessive irritability or sensitivity to stimulation. adj., **erethis′mic, erethis′tic.**

erethisophrenia (er″ĕ-thiz″o-fre′ne-ah) exaggerated mental excitability.

erg (erg) a unit of work or energy, equivalent to 2.4 $\times 10^{-8}$ gram (small) calories, or to 0.624 $\times 10^{12}$ electron volts.

ergasia (er-ga′ze-ah) 1. a hypothetical substance that stimulates the activity of body cells. 2. any mentally integrated function, activity, reaction, or attitude of an individual.

ergastic (er-gas′tik) 1. having potential energy. 2. pertaining to ergasia.

ergocalciferol (er″go-kal-sif′er-ol) vitamin D_2; an oil-soluble antirachitic vitamin (see also VITAMIN D and table of the principal VITAMINS).

ergocornine (er″go-kor′nēn) an alkaloid from ergot, once used in peripheral vascular disorders.

ergocristine (er″go-kris′tēn) an alkaloid from ergot, once used in peripheral vascular disorders.

ergocryptine (er″go-krip′tēn) an alkaloid from ergot, once used in peripheral vascular disorders.

ergograph (er′go-graf) an instrument for measuring work done in muscular action.

ergonovine (er″go-no′vin) an alkaloid from ergot or produced synthetically, used as an oxytocic and to relieve migraine.

ergophore (er′go-fōr) in Ehrlich's side-chain theory, the group of atoms in a molecule that brings about the specific activity of the substance.

ergoplasm (er′go-plazm) granular endoplasmic reticulum.

ergosterol (er-gos′ter-ol) a sterol occurring in animal and plant tissues which on ultraviolet irradiation becomes a potent antirachitic substance, vitamin D_2 (ergocalciferol).

ergot (er′got) the dried sclerotium of the fungus *Claviceps purpurea,* which attacks rye plants. Ergot alkaloids are used as oxytocics and in the treatment of migraine. (See also ERGOTISM.)

ergotamine (er-got′ah-min) an alkaloid derived from ergot, used as an oxytocic and in the treatment of migraine.

ergotaminine (er″go-tam′ĭ-nēn) an isomer of ergotamine.

ergotherapy (er″go-ther′ah-pe) treatment of disease by physical effort.

ergotism (er′go-tizm) chronic poisoning produced by ingestion of ergot, marked by cerebrospinal symptoms, spasm, cramps, or by a kind of dry gangrene.

ergotoxine (er″go-tok′sēn) a toxic crystalline alkaloid originally isolated from ergot (*Claviceps purpurea*), consisting of a mixture of ergocornine, ergocristine, and ergocryptine, which exert both oxytocic and adrenergic blocking effects. Because of the variability of these effects, neither ergotoxine nor any of its constituents is currently used in medicine.

Ergotrate (er′go-trāt) trademark for preparations of ergonovine, an ergot alkaloid.

eridodictyon (er″e-o-dik′te-on) the dried leaf of *Eriodictyon californicum,* used in pharmaceutical preparations.

erogenous (ĕ-roj′ĕ-nus) arousing erotic feelings.

e. zones, areas of the body stimulation of which produces erotic desire, e.g., the oral, anal, and genital orifices and the nipples.

erosio (e-ro′ze-o) [L.] erosion.

e. interdigita′lis blastomycet′ica, an eroded lesion occurring between the fingers, almost always between the third and fourth fingers, due to *Candida albicans.*

erosion (e-ro′zhun) an eating or gnawing away; a shallow or superficial ulceration; in dentistry, the wasting away or loss of substance of a tooth by a chemical process that does not involve known bacterial action. adj., **ero′sive.**

cervical e., destruction of the squamous epithelium of the vaginal portion of the cervix, due to irritation; the eroded area is covered by columnar epithelium.

erotic (ĕ-rot′ik) pertaining to sexual love or to lust.

eroticism, erotism (e-rot′ĭ-sizm; er′o-tizm) a sexual instinct or desire; the expression of one's instinctual energy or drive, especially the sex drive.

anal e., fixation of libido at (or regression to) the anal phase of infantile development, producing egotistic, dogmatic, stubborn, miserly character.

genital e., achievement and maintenance of libido at the genital phase of psychosexual development, permitting acceptance of normal adult relationships and responsibilities.

oral e., fixation of libido at (or regression to) the oral phase of infantile development, producing passive, insecure, sensitive character.

erotize (er′o-tīz) to endow with erotic meaning or significance.

erotogenic (ĕ-ro″to-jen′ik) producing erotic feeling.

erotomania (ĕro″to-ma′ne-ah) morbidly exaggerated sexual behavior or reaction; preoccupation with sexuality.

erotopathy (er″o-top′ah-the) any perversion of the sexual impulse.

erotophobia (ĕ-ro″to-fo′be-ah) morbid dread of sexual love.

errhine (er′īn) promoting a nasal discharge; an agent that so acts.

Ertron (er′tron) trademark for preparations of vitamin D_2 (ergocalciferol).

eructation (e″ruk-ta′shun) the oral ejection of gas or air from the stomach; belching.

eruption (e-rup′shun) 1. the act of breaking out, appearing, or becoming visible, as eruption of the teeth. 2. visible efflorescent lesions of the skin due to disease, with redness, prominence, or both; a rash. adj., **erup′tive.**

creeping e., a peculiar eruption that appears to migrate, due to burrowing beneath the skin of certain larvae (see also LARVA MIGRANS).

drug e., dermatitis medicamentosa.

Kaposi's varicelliform e., a generalized and serious vesiculopustular eruption of viral origin, superimposed on preexisting atopic dermatitis; it may be due to the herpes simplex virus (eczema herpeticum) or vaccinia (eczema vaccinatum).

erysipelas (er″ĭ-sip′ĕ-las) a febrile disease characterized by inflammation and redness of the skin and subcutaneous tissues, and due to Group A hemolytic streptococci.

The visible symptoms of erysipelas, a form of cellulitis, are round or oval patches on the skin that promptly enlarge and spread, becoming swollen, tender, and red. The affected skin is hot to the touch, and, occasionally, the adjacent skin blisters. Headache, vomiting, fever, and sometimes complete prostration can occur. Sulfonamide compounds or antibiotics are used in the treatment. Care must be taken to avoid spreading the disease to other areas of the body.

swine e., a contagious and highly fatal disease of pigs, caused by *Erysipelothrix insidiosa.*

erysipelatous (er″ĭ-sĭ-pel′ah-tus) pertaining to or of the nature of erysipelas.

erysipeloid (er″ĭ-sip′ĕ-loid) an infective dermatitis or cellulitis due to infection with *Erysipelothrix insidiosa;* it usually begins in a wound (often the result of a prick by a fish bone) and remains localized, rarely becoming generalized and septicemic.

Erysipelothrix (er″ĭ-sip′ĕ-lo-thriks″) a genus of bacteria containing a single species.

E. insidio′sa, E. rhusiopath′iae, the causative organism of swine erysipelas, which also infects sheep, turkeys, and rats. An erythematous-edematous lesion, commonly on the hand, resulting from contact with infected meat, hides, or bones, represents the usual type of infection in man (see also ERYSIPELOID).

erythema (er″ĭ-the′mah) redness of the skin caused by congestion of the capillaries in the lower layers of the skin. It occurs with any skin injury, infection, or inflammation.

e. ab ig′ne, that due to exposure to radiant heat.

e. indura′tum, a chronic necrotizing vasculitis, usually occurring on the calves of young women (see also BAZIN'S DISEASE).

e. margina′tum, a type of erythema multiforme in which the reddened areas are disk-shaped, with elevated edges.

e. mi′grans, geographic tongue.

e. multifor′me, a symptom complex with highly polymorphic skin lesions, including macular papules, vesicles, and bullae; attacks of the disorder are usually self-limited but recurrences are the rule.

toxic e., e. tox′icum, a generalized erythematous or erythematomacular eruption due to administration of a drug or to bacterial toxins or other toxic substances.

e. feta′lis, e. neonator′um, a blood dyscrasia of the newborn characterized by agglutination and hemolysis of erythrocytes and usually due to incompatibility between the infant's blood and the mother's. In most cases the fetus has Rh-positive blood and its mother has Rh-negative blood (see RH FACTOR). Called also hemolytic disease of the newborn.

In Rh incompatibility the mother builds up immune bodies (antibodies) against the cells of the fetus; these bodies pass through the placenta, entering the fetal circulation. They then proceed to destroy the fetal erythrocytes very rapidly. In order to compensate for this rapid destruction of red blood cells, there is an ever increasing effort on the part of the fetus to avoid anemia. The result of this compensatory action is the release of very immature red blood cells (erythroblasts). Thus an extremely high percentage of the fetal erythrocytes are erythroblasts, and the condition is called erythroblastosis.

SYMPTOMS. If the fetus survives under these circumstances, it is jaundiced and usually anemic at birth. The immune bodies from the mother's blood usually circulate in the baby's blood for 1 to 2 months after birth, continuing their destruction of red blood cells unless an exchange TRANSFUSION is done.

Other symptoms depend on the number of red cells destroyed and the amount of damage done to other tissues of the body, such as the brain and central nervous system.

TREATMENT. The usual treatment for erythroblastosis fetalis is exchange transfusion in which the infant's blood is replaced with Rh-negative blood. The average amount used for transfusion of this kind is 400 ml. This measure stops the destruction of the infant's red cells, and gradually the Rh-negative blood is replaced with the baby's own blood. In about 6 weeks the immune bodies left over from the mother's blood have been destroyed and are no longer a menace to the baby.

Recent developments in the management of erythroblastosis include AMNIOCENTESIS and intrauterine fetal transfusion. The former is puncture of the amniotic sac through the maternal abdomen and is done for the purpose of obtaining a sample of AMNIOTIC FLUID for analysis. This allows for determination of concentration of bilirubin pigments and protein in the amniotic fluid; a high concentration indicates excessive destruction of fetal erythrocytes. If there is a mild hemolysis the mother is watched closely and allowed to deliver at term. In more severe cases, induced labor and premature delivery are usually advised so that further destruction of erythrocytes will not take place and an exchange transfusion can be performed as soon as possible. For cases of very severe hemolysis it has been recommended that an intrauterine transfusion be administered to the fetus. This is a very delicate procedure, not without risks, and advised only if the mother's past history and the present evidence indicate that the infant would not survive or would suffer damage from erythroblastosis. Both amniocentesis and intrauterine transfusion are hazardous procedures that should be performed only by trained personnel in well equipped medical centers.

erythematous (er″ĭ-them′ah-tus) characterized by erythema.

erythr(o)- word element [Gr.], *red; erythrocyte.*

erythrasma (er″ĭ-thraz′mah) a chronic bacterial infection of the major skin folds due to *Corynebacterium minutissimum,* marked by red or brownish patches on the skin.

erythredema polyneuropathy (ĕ-rith″rĕ-de′mah pol″ĭ-nu-rop′ah-the) a disease of infancy and early childhood marked by pain and swelling in, and pink coloration of, the fingers and toes, and by listlessness, irritability, failure to thrive, profuse perspiration, and sometimes scarlet coloration of the cheeks and tip of the nose. Called also acrodynia.

erythremia (er″ĭ-thre′me-ah) polycythemia vera.

erythrism (ĕ-rith′rizm) redness of the hair and beard with a ruddy complexion. adj., **erythris′tic.**

erythritol (ĕ-rith′rĭ-tol) a polyhydric alcohol which is about twice as sweet as sucrose, found in algae, lichens, grasses, and several fungi.

erythrityl (ĕ-rith′rĭ-til) the univalent radical from erythritol.

e. tetranitrate, a vasodilator used in angina pectoris and coronary insufficiency; because of its explosiveness it must be diluted, as with lactose.

erythroblast (ĕ-rith′ro-blast) originally, any nucleated erythrocyte, but now more generally used to designate the nucleated precursor from which an erythrocyte develops.

basophilic e., see under NORMOBLAST.

orthochromatic e., see under NORMOBLAST.

polychromatophilic e., see under NORMOBLAST.

erythroblastemia (ĕ-rith″ro-blas-te′me-ah) the presence in the peripheral blood of abnormally large numbers of nucleated red cells; erythroblastosis.

erythroblastoma (ĕ-rith″ro-blas-to′mah) a tumor-like mass composed of nucleated red cells.

erythroblastomatosis (ĕ-rith″ro-blas″to-mah-to′sis) a condition marked by the formation of erythroblastomas.

erythroblastopenia (ĕ-rith″ro-blas″to-pe′ne-ah) abnormal deficiency of erythroblasts.

erythroblastosis (ĕ-rith″ro-blas-to′sis) the presence of erythroblasts in the circulating blood. adj., **erythroblastot′ic.**

erythrochloropia (ĕ-rith″ro-klo-ro′pe-ah) ability to distinguish only red and green, not blue and yellow.

erythrochromia (ĕ-rith″ro-kro′me-ah) hemorrhagic, red pigmentation of the cerebrospinal fluid.

erythroclasis (er″ĭ-throk′lah-sis) fragmentation of the red blood cells. adj., **erythroclas′tic.**

erythrocuprein (ĕ-rith″ro-koo′prin) a copper-protein compound contained in erythrocytes.

erythrocyanosis (ĕ-rith″ro-si″ah-no′sis) coarsely mottled bluish or red discoloration on the legs and thighs, especially of girls; thought to be a circulatory reaction to exposure to cold.

erythrocyte (ĕ-rith′ro-sīt) a red blood cell, or corpuscle; one of the formed elements in the peripheral blood. For immature forms see NORMOBLAST. Normally, in the human, mature erythrocytes are biconcave disks that have no nuclei and are about 7.7 microns in diameter, consisting mainly of hemoglobin and a supporting framework, called the stroma. Erythrocyte formation (erythropoiesis) takes place in the red bone marrow in the adult, and in the liver, spleen, and bone marrow of the fetus. Erythrocyte formation requires an ample supply of certain dietary elements such as iron, cobalt, and copper, amino acids, and certain vitamins.

The functions of erythrocytes include transportation of oxygen and carbon dioxide. They also are important in the maintenance of a normal ACID-BASE BALANCE, and, since they help determine the viscosity of the blood, they also influence its specific gravity.

The average life span of a red blood cell is 120 days. They are subjected to much wear and tear in circulation and eventually are removed by cells of the RETICULOENDOTHELIAL SYSTEM, particularly in the liver, bone marrow, and spleen. In spite of this constant destruction and production of red cells, the body maintains a fairly constant number of erythrocytes: between 4 and 5 million per cu. mm. of blood in women and 5 to 6 million per cu. mm. in men. A decreased number of erythrocytes constitutes one form of ANEMIA.

Red blood cells are destroyed whenever they are exposed to solutions that are not isotonic to blood plasma. If the erythrocyte is placed in a solution that is more dilute than plasma (distilled water for example) the cell will swell until osmotic pressure bursts the cell membrane. If the erythrocyte is placed in a solution more concentrated than plasma, the cell will lose water and shrivel or crenate. It is for this reason that solutions to be given intravenously must be isotonic to plasma.

e. sedimentation rate, an expression of the extent of settling of erythrocytes in a column of fresh citrated or otherwise treated blood, per unit of time (see also SEDIMENTATION RATE).

erythrocythemia (ĕ-rith″ro-si-the′me-ah) an increase in the number of erythrocytes in the blood, as in erythrocytosis.

erythrocytic (ĕ-rith″ro-sit′ik) of or pertaining to erythrocytes.

erythrocytin (ĕ-rith″ro-si′tin) a substance in red cells thought to function in the first stage of blood clotting.

erythrocytolysin (ĕ-rith″ro-si-tol′ĭ-sin) a substance that produces erythrocytolysis.

erythrocytolysis (ĕ-rith″ro-si-tol′ĭ-sis) dissolution of erythrocytes and escape of hemoglobin.

erythrocytometer (ĕ-rith″ro-si-tom′ĕ-ter) a device for measuring or counting erythrocytes.

erythrocyto-opsonin (ĕ-rith″ro-si″to-op-so′nin) hemopsonin.

erythrocytorrhexis (ĕ-rith″ro-si″to-rek′sis) a morphologic change in erythrocytes, consisting in the escape from the cells of round, shiny granules and splitting off of particles; called also plasmorrhexis.

erythrocytosis (ĕ-rith″ro-si-to′sis) increase in the total red cell mass secondary to any of a number of nonhematogenic systemic disorders in response to a known stimulus (secondary polycythemia), in contrast to primary polycythemia (polycythemia vera.)

stress e., an apparent polycythemia seen in active, anxiety-prone persons, resulting from diminished plasma volume.

erythroderma (ĕ-rith″ro-der′mah) abnormal redness of the skin over widespread areas of the body.

congenital ichthyosiform e., a generalized hereditary dermatitis with scaling, occurring in bullous and nonbullous forms.

e. desquamati′vum, a condition resembling and probably identical with severe seborrheic dermatitis, affecting newborn breast-fed infants, characterized by generalized exfoliative dermatitis and marked erythroderma. Called also Leiner's disease.

lymphomatous e., widespread redness of the skin associated with lymphoma.

maculopapular e., a reddish eruption composed of maculae and papules.

psoriatic e., a generalized psoriasis vulgaris, showing the chemical characteristics of exfoliative dermatitis.

erythrodontia (ĕ-rith″ro-don′she-ah) reddish brown pigmentation of the teeth.

erythrogenesis (ĕ-rith″ro-jen′ĕ-sis) the production of erythrocytes.

e. imperfec′ta, congenital hypoplastic anemia. (1).

erythrogenic (ĕ-rith″ro-jen′ik) 1. producing erythrocytes. 2. producing a sensation of red. 3. producing or causing erythema.

erythrogonium (ĕ-rith″ro-go′ne-um) promegaloblast.

erythroid (er′ĭ-throid) 1. of a red color; reddish. 2. pertaining to the developmental series of cells ending in erythrocytes.

erythrokeratodermia (ĕ-rith″ro-ker″ah-to-der′me-ah) a reddening and hyperkeratosis of the skin.

e. figura′ta varia′bilis, e varia′bilis, a rare hereditary disorder marked by circumscribed erythematous and hyperkeratotic plaques on the skin which vary in size and shape within hours or days; they appear shortly after birth and persist into adolescence or adulthood.

erythrokinetics (ĕ-rith″ro-ki-net′iks) the quantitative, dynamic study of *in vivo* production and destruction of erythrocytes.

erythrolabe (ĕ-rith′ro-lāb) the pigment in retinal cones that is more sensitive to the red range of the spectrum than are the other pigments (chlorolabe and cyanolabe).

erythroleukemia (ĕ-rith″ro-lu-ke′me-ah) a malignant blood dyscrasia, one of the myeloproliferative disorders, with atypical erythroblasts and myeloblasts in the peripheral blood.

erythrolysin (er″ĭ-throl′ĭ-sin) erythrocytolysin.

erythrolysis (er″ĭ-throl′ĭ-sis) erythrocytolysis; dissolution of erythrocytes and escape of hemoglobin.

erythromania (ĕ-rith″ro-ma′ne-ah) uncontrollable blushing.

erythromelalgia (ĕ-rith″ro-mel-al′je-ah) paroxysmal, bilateral vasodilation, particularly of the extremities, with burning pain and increased skin temperature and redness.

erythromycin (ĕ-rith″ro-mi′sin) a broad-spectrum antibiotic produced by a strain of *Streptomyces erythreus.* It is effective against a wide variety of organisms, including gram-negative and gram-positive bacteria. It may be administered orally or parenterally.

erythron (er′ĭ-thron) the circulating erythrocytes in the blood, their precursors, and all the body elements concerned in their production.

erythroneocytosis (ĕ-rith″ro-ne″o-si-to′sis) the presence of immature erythrocytes in the blood.

erythropenia (ĕ-rith″ro-pe′ne-ah) deficiency in the number of erythrocytes.

erythrophage (ĕ-rith′ro-fāj) a phagocyte that ingests erythrocytes.

erythrophagia, erythrophagocytosis (ĕ-rith″ro-fa′je-ah; ĕ-rith″ro-fag″o-si-to′sis) phagocytosis of erythrocytes.

erythropheresis (ĕ-rith″ro-fĕ-re′sis) the reduction of the red cell volume by removal of whole blood and replacement with plasma or albumin.

erythrophil (ĕ-rith′ro-fil) 1. a cell or other element that stains easily with red. 2. erythrophilous.

erythrophilous (er″ĭ-throf′ĭ-lus) easily staining red.

erythrophobia (ĕ-rith″ro-fo′be-ah) 1. a neurotic manifestation marked by blushing at the slightest provocation. 2. morbid aversion to red.

erythrophthisis (ĕ-rith″ro-thi′sis) a condition characterized by severe impairment of the restorative power of the erythrocyte-forming tissues.

erythroplasia (ĕ-rith″ro-pla′ze-ah) a condition of the mucous membranes characterized by erythematous papular lesions.

e. of Queyrat, squamous cell carcinoma *in situ,* manifested as a circumscribed, velvety, erythematous papular lesion on the glans penis, coronal sulcus, or prepuce, leading to scaling and superficial ulceration.

erythropoiesis (ĕ-rith″ro-poi-e′sis) the formation of erythrocytes. adj., **erythropoiet′ic.**

erythropoietin (ĕ-rith″ro-poi′ĕ-tin) the term applied to the substance(s) serving as the humoral regulator of erythropoiesis.

erythroprosopalgia (ĕ-rith″ro-pros″o-pal′je-ah) a nervous disorder marked by redness and pain in the face.

erythropsia (er″ĭ-throp′se-ah) a defect of vision in which objects appear tinged with red.

erythropsin (er″ĭ-throp′sin) rhodopsin, the visual purple.

erythrosis (er″ĭ-thro′sis) 1. reddish or purplish discoloration of the skin and mucous membranes, as in polycythemia vera. 2. hyperplasia of the hematopoietic tissue.

erythrostasis (ĕ-rith″ro-sta′sis) the stoppage of erythrocytes in the capillaries, as in sickle cell anemia.

erythruria (er″ĭ-throo′re-ah) excretion of red urine.

Es chemical symbol, *einsteinium.*

escape (es-kāp) the act of becoming free.

vagal e., the exhaustion of or adaptation to neural chemical mediators in the regulation of systemic arterial pressure.

ventricular e., extrasystole in which a ventricular pacemaker becomes effective before the sinoatrial pacemaker; it usually occurs with slow sinus rates and often, but not necessarily, with increased vagal tone.

eschar (es′kar) 1. a slough produced by a thermal burn, a corrosive application, or by gangrene. 2. tache noire.

escharotic (es-kah-rot′ik) 1. capable of producing an eschar; corrosive. 2. a corrosive or caustic agent.

Escherichia (esh″ĕ-rik′e-ah) a genus of widely distributed gram-negative bacteria (family Enterobacteriaceae), occasionally pathogenic for man.

E. co′li, a species constituting the greater part of the normal intestinal flora of man and other animals; called also colon bacillus. Pathogenic strains are the cause of many cases of urinary tract infections and of epidemic diarrheal diseases, especially in children.

Escherichieae (esh″er-ĭ-ki′e-e) a tribe of bacteria (family Enterobacteriaceae), comprising the coliform bacteria.

eschrolalia (es″kro-la′le-ah) coprolalia.

escorcin (es-kor′sin) a brown powder prepared from a substance extracted from the horse chestnut; used in detecting corneal and conjunctival lesions.

escutcheon (es-kuch′an) the pattern of distribution of the pubic hair.

eserine (es′er-ēn) physostigmine, a cholinesterase inhibitor.

Esidrix (es′ĭ-driks) trademark for a preparation of hydrochlorothiazide, a diuretic.

-esis word element [Gr.], *state; condition.*

Eskabarb (es′kah-barb) trademark for a preparation of phenobarbital, an anticonvulsant, hypnotic, and sedative.

Eskadiazine (es″kah-di′ah-zēn) trademark for a preparation of sulfadiazine; an antibacterial agent.

Esmarch's bandage (es′marks) an India rubber bandage applied upward around (from the distal part to the proximal) a part in order to expel blood from it; the part is often elevated as the elastic pressure is applied.

eso- word element [Gr.], *within.*

esoethmoiditis (es″o-eth″moi-di′tis) inflammation of the ethmoid sinuses.

esogastritis (es″o-gas-tri′tis) inflammation of the gastric mucosa.

esophageal (ĕ-sof″ah-je′al) of or pertaining to the esophagus.

esophagectasia (ĕ-sof″ah-jek-ta′ze-ah) dilatation of the esophagus.

esophagectomy (ĕ-sof″ah-jek′to-me) excision of a portion of the esophagus.

esophagism (ĕ-sof′ah-jism) spasm of the esophagus.

esophagitis (ĕ-sof″ah-ji′tis) inflammation of the esophagus.

peptic e., inflammation of the esophagus due to a reflux of acid and pepsin from the stomach.

esophagobronchial (ĕ-sof″ah-go-brong′ke-al) pertaining to or communicating with the esophagus and a bronchus.

esophagocele (ĕ-sof″ah-go-sēl″) abnormal distention of the esophagus; protrusion of the esophageal mucosa through a rupture in the muscular coat.

esophagodynia (ĕ-sof″ah-go-din′e-ah) pain in the esophagus.

esophagoenterostomy (ĕ-sof″ah-go-en″ter-os′to-me) surgical formation of an anastomosis between the esophagus and the small intestine.

esophagoesophagostomy (ĕ-sof″ah-go-ĕ-sof″ah-gos′to-me) anastomosis between two formerly remote parts of the esophagus.

esophagogastrectomy (ĕ-sof″ah-go-gas-trek′to-me) excision of the esophagus and stomach.

esophagogastric (ĕ-sof″ah-go-gas′trik) pertaining to the esophagus and the stomach.

esophagogastroanastomosis (ĕ-sof″ah-go-gas″-tro-ah-nas″to-mo′sis) esophagogastrostomy.

esophagogastroplasty (ĕ-sof″ah-go-gas′tro-plas″-te) plastic repair of the esophagus and stomach.

esophagogastroscopy (ĕ-sof″ah-go-gas-tros′ko-pe) endoscopic inspection of the esophagus and stomach.

esophagogastrostomy (ĕ-sof″ah-go-gas-tros′to-me) anastomosis of the esophagus to the stomach.

esophagography (ĕ-sof″ah-gog′rah-fe) roentgenography of the esophagus.

esophagojejunostomy (ĕ-sof″ah-go-je″joo-nos′to-me) anastomosis of the esophagus to the jejunum.

esophagomalacia (ĕ-sof″ah-go-mah-la′she-ah) softening of the walls of the esophagus.

esophagometer (ĕ-sof″ah-gom′ĕ-ter) an instrument for measuring the esophagus.

esophagomyotomy (ĕ-sof″ah-go-mi-ot′o-me) incision through the muscular coat of the esophagus.

esophagoplasty (ĕ-sof′ah-go-plas″te) plastic repair of the esophagus.

esophagoplication (ĕ-sof″ah-go-pli-ka′shun) infolding of the wall of an esophageal pouch.

esophagoptosis (ĕ-sof″ah-gop-to′sis) prolapse of the esophagus.

esophagorespiratory (ĕ-sof″ah-go-re-spi′rah-to″-re) pertaining to or communicating with the esophagus and respiratory tract (trachea or a bronchus).

esophagoscope (ĕ-sof′ah-go-skōp″) an endoscope for examination of the esophagus.

esophagoscopy (ĕ-sof″ah-gos′ko-pe) direct visual examination of the esophagus with an esophagoscope. Esophagoscopy usually is done as a diagnostic procedure for the purpose of locating and inspecting a disorder of the esophagus. After the esophagoscope has been inserted it is possible to obtain samples of tissue for microscopic study. In some instances the esophagoscope can be used to remove a foreign object that has become lodged in the esophagus.

PATIENT CARE. Food and liquids are withheld for at least 6 hours prior to the procedure so that the stomach will be empty and there will be no regurgitation during the procedure. An operative permit should be signed before this examination is done. Sedatives are usually given about an hour before the procedure to relax the patient and help him cooperate with the physician. Although the procedure is not painful, it is uncomfortable and difficult for the patient. The newer, more flexible endoscopes have greatly reduced the discomfort of the procedure. The throat is anesthetized with a local anesthetic such as cocaine or tetracaine (Pontocaine) to depress the gag reflex and reduce local reaction to the passage of the instrument. Since there may be some toxic reaction to the local anesthetic the patient should be observed carefully for dyspnea, excitement, dizziness, or headache and an emergency tray containing epinephrine and barbiturates should be readily available.

The patient is placed on his back with his head and shoulders extending over the edge of the treatment table. The patient's head is supported by an attendant and, if it seems likely that he will move about, he is restrained. This is necessary because a sudden movement might cause perforation of the esophagus.

Food and fluids are withheld for several hours after the procedure is completed, and the patient is instructed not to take anything by mouth until the gag reflex has returned. This is necessary because there is danger of aspiration as long as the gag reflex is depressed. Hoarseness and a sore throat usually remain for a few days after the examination.

esophagostenosis (ĕ-sof″ah-go-stĕ-no′sis) stricture of the esophagus.

esophagostomy (ĕ-sof″ah-gos′to-me) the creation of an artificial opening into the esophagus.

esophagotomy (ĕ-sof″ah-got′o-me) incision of the esophagus.

esophagotracheal (ĕ-sof″ah-go-tra′ke-al) pertaining to or communicating with the esophagus and trachea.

esophagus (ĕ-sof′ah-gus) the musculomembranous passage extending from the pharynx to the stomach, consisting of an outer fibrous coat, a muscular layer, a submucous layer, and an inner mucous membrane. The junction between the stomach and esophagus is closed by a muscular ring known as the cardiac sphincter, which opens to allow the passage of food into the stomach. In an adult the esophagus is usually 10 to 12 inches long. (See also DIGESTIVE SYSTEM and Plate 9.)

Disorders of the esophagus often involve either an obstruction or a reflux (backward flow) of food and gastric juices. Foreign bodies, accidentally swallowed and lodged in the esophageal passage, can obstruct the flow of foods and fluids, as can malignant or benign tumors. The term ACHALASIA is used to describe a particular disturbance in motility which leads to obstruction at the level of the cardiac sphincter.

Esophagitis, inflammation of the mucous membrane lining the esophagus, may occur in conjunction with gastroenteritis, or as a result of a backward flow of the gastric contents upward into the esophagus. The symptoms of hiatal hernia are due in large part to this type of reflux. Hiatal hernia is a protrusion of the stomach, colon, or other intestinal organs through the esophageal hiatus, a narrow opening in the diaphragm through which the esophagus normally passes. When the herniation occurs the normal downward passage of food is interrupted.

Esophageal varices are varicose veins of the esophagus and occur most often as a result of obstruction in the portal circulation, especially in portal hypertension. These varices are potentially dangerous since they tend to rupture easily and may result in serious hemorrhage.

Visual examination of the interior lining of the esophagus is accomplished by ESOPHAGOSCOPY.

esophoria (es″o-fo′re-ah) HETEROPHORIA in which there is deviation of the visual axis of one eye toward that of the other eye in the absence of visual fusional stimuli.

esosphenoiditis (es″o-sfe″noi-di′tis) osteomyelitis of the sphenoid bone.

esotropia (es″o-tro′pe-ah) STRABISMUS in which there is deviation of the visual axis of one eye toward that of the other eye, resulting in diplopia. Called also cross-eye and convergent strabismus. adj., **estrop′ic.**

E.S.P. extrasensory perception.

E.S.R. erythrocyte sedimentation rate.

essence (es′ens) 1. the distinctive or individual principle of anything. 2. a mixture of alcohol with a volatile oil.

essential (ĕ-sen′shal) 1. constituting the necessary or inherent part of a thing; giving a substance its peculiar and necessary qualities. 2. indispensable; required in the diet, as essential fatty acids. 3. idiopathic; self-existing; having no obvious external exciting cause.

E.S.T. electroshock therapy.

ester (es′ter) a compound formed from an alcohol and an acid by removal of water.

esterase (es′ter-ās) any enzyme that catalyzes the hydrolysis of esters into its alcohol and acid.

esterification (es-ter″ĭ-fĭ-ka′shun) conversion of an acid into an ester by combination with an alcohol and removal of a molecule of water.

esterify (es-ter′ĭ-fi) to combine with an alcohol with elimination of a molecule of water, forming an ester.

esterolysis (es″ter-ol′ĭ-sis) the hydrolysis of an ester into its alcohol and acid. adj., **esterolyt′ic.**

esthematology (es″them-ah-tol′o-je) esthesiology.

esthesiogenic (es-the″ze-o-jen′ik) producing sensation.

esthesiology (es-the″ze-ol′o-je) the scientific study or description of the sense organs and sensations.

esthesiometer (es-the″ze-om′ĕ-ter) an instrument for measuring tactile sensibility; tactometer.

esthesioneurosis (es-the″ze-o-nu-ro′sis) any disorder of the sensory nerves.

esthesiophysiology (es-the″ze-o-fiz″e-ol′o-je) the physiology of sensation and sense organs.

esthesodic (es″thĕ-zod′ik) conducting or pertaining to conduction of sensory impulses.

esthetics (es-thet′iks) the branch of philosophy dealing with beauty; in dentistry, a philosophy concerned especially with the appearance of a dental restoration, as achieved through its color or form.

Estinyl (es′tĭ-nil) trademark for a preparation of ethinyl estradiol.

estival (es′tĭ-val, ĕ-sti′val) pertaining to or occurring in summer.

estivation (es″tĭ-va′shun) the dormant state in which certain animals pass the summer.

estivoautumnal (es″tĭ-vo-aw-tum′nal) occurring in summer and autumn.

estradiol (es″trah-di′ol, es-tra′de-ol) the most potent naturally occurring ESTROGEN in humans; pharmacologically, it is usually used in the form of its esters (e.g., estradiol benzoate, cyprionate, and valerate), or as a semisynthetic derivative (estinyl estradiol).

estrin (es′trin) estrogen.

estrinization (es″trin-ĭ-za′shun) production of the cellular changes in the vaginal epithelium characteristic of estrus.

estriol (es′tre-ol) a relatively weak human ESTROGEN, being a metabolic product of estradiol and estrone found in high concentration in the urine.

estrogen (es′tro-jen) a generic term for estrus-producing compounds; the female sex hormones, including estradiol, estriol, and estrone.

In humans, the estrogens are formed in the ovary, adrenal cortex, testis, and fetoplacental unit, and are responsible for female secondary sex characteristic development, and during the menstrual cycle, act on the female genitalia to produce an environment suitable for fertilization, implantation, and nutrition of the early embryo.

Estrogen is used as a palliative in post-menopausal cancer of the breast and in prostatic cancer, in oral contraceptives, for relief of menopausal discomforts, etc. There is evidence from controlled studies that estrogen therapy for menopausal symptoms is closely linked to cancer of the endometrium. The degree of risk is closely associated with the dosage and the length of time it is taken.

estrogenic (es″tro-jen′ik) estrus-producing; having the properties of, or properties similar to, an estrogen.

estrone (es′trōn) an ESTROGEN isolated from pregnancy urine, the human placenta, and palm kernel oil, and also prepared synthetically.

estruation (es″troo-a′shun) estrus.

Estrugenone (es″troo-jen′ōn) trademark for a preparation of estrone.

estrum (es′trum) estrus.

estrus (es′trus) the recurrent, restricted period of sexual receptivity in female mammals other than human females, marked by intense sexual urge (see also estrous CYCLE). adj., **es′trual, es′trous.**

e.s.u. electrostatic unit.

Etamon (et′ah-mon) trademark for a preparation of tetraethylammonium, a ganglionic blocking agent.

ethacrynic acid (eth″ah-krin′ik) a powerful diuretic used orally or parenterally, and effective in promoting sodium and chloride excretion.

ethambutol (ĕ-tham′bu-tōl) a tuberculostatic agent.

ethamivan (ĕ-tham′ĭ-van) a compound used as a respiratory stimulant and to hasten recovery from general anesthesia.

ethanol (eth′ah-nol) the major ingredient of alcoholic beverages; called also ethyl alcohol and grain alcohol.

ethanolamine (eth″ah-nol-ah′mēn) a colorless, moderately viscous liquid with an ammonical odor contained in cephalins and phospholipids, and derived metabolically by decarboxylation of serine. The oleate is used as a sclerosing agent in the treatment of varicose veins.

ethaverine (eth″ah-ver′ēn) a compound used as a relaxant for vascular smooth muscle.

ethchlorvynol (eth-klōr′vĭ-nol) a sedative.

ethene (eth′ēn) ethylene.

ether (e′ther) 1. diethyl ether: a colorless, transparent, mobile, very volatile, highly inflammable liquid with a characteristic odor; given by inhalation to produce general ANESTHESIA. 2. any of various volatile liquids mostly containing diethyl ether or resembling it.

nitrofurfuryl methyl e., a compound used as a topical fungicide and sporicide for skin infections.

vinyl e., a clear colorless liquid used as an inhalation anesthetic.

ethereal (e-the're-al) 1. pertaining to, prepared with, containing, or resembling ether. 2. evanescent; delicate.

etherization (e"ther-ĭ-za'shun) induction of anesthesia by means of ether.

ethinamate (ĕ-thin'ah-māt) a short-acting, nonbarbiturate sedative.

ethinyl trichloride (eth'ĭ-nil) trichloroethylene, an anesthetic.

ethionamide (ĕ-thi"on-am'īd) a tuberculostatic agent.

ethionine (ĕ-thi'o-nin) the ethyl homologue of methionine.

ethisterone (ĕ-this'ter-ōn) a synthetic progestational steroid.

ethmocarditis (eth"mo-kar-di'tis) inflammation of the connective tissue of the heart.

ethmoid (eth'moid) 1. sievelike; cribriform. 2. the ethmoid bone.

e. bone, the sievelike bone that forms a roof for the nasal fossae and part of the floor of the anterior cranial fossa (see also table of BONES).

ethmoidal (eth-moi'dal) pertaining to the ethmoid bone.

ethmoidectomy (eth"moi-dek'to-me) excision of the ethmoid cells or of a portion of the ethmoid bone.

ethmoiditis (eth"moi-di'tis) inflammation of the ethmoid bone or ethmoid sinuses.

ethmoidotomy (eth"moi-dot'o-me) incision into the ethmoid sinus.

ethnic (eth'nik) pertaining to a social group who share cultural bonds or physical (racial) characteristics.

ethnobiology (eth"no-bi-ol'o-je) the scientific study of physical characteristics of different races of mankind.

ethnology (eth-nol'o-je) the science dealing with the races of man, their descent, relationship, etc.

ethoheptazine (eth"o-hep'tah-zēn) an analgesic.

ethohexadiol (eth"o-heks-a'de-ol) an insect repellant.

ethologist (ĕ-thol'o-jist) a person skilled in ethology.

ethology (ĕ-thol'o-je) the scientific study of animal behavior, particularly in the natural state. adj., **etholog'ical.**

ethopropazine (eth"o-pro'pah-zēn) a homologue of promethazine, a phenothiazine used as the hydrochloride salt in the treatment of parkinsonism.

ethosuximide (eth"o-suk'sĭ-mīd) an anticonvulsant.

ethotoin (e-tho'to-in) an anticonvulsant used in the treatment of grand mal epilepsy.

ethoxazene (eth-ok'sah-zēn) an azo dye; the hydrochloride salt is used to relieve pain associated with chronic urinary tract infections.

ethoxzolamide (eth"ok-zol'ah-mīd) a diuretic of the carbonic anhydrase inhibitor type, used mainly to reduce intraocular pressure in glaucoma.

ethyl (eth'il) the monovalent radical, C_2H_5.

e. acetate, a flavoring agent and antispasmodic.

e. alcohol, ALCOHOL, the major ingredient of alcoholic beverages; called also ethanol and grain alcohol.

e. biscoumacetate, an anticoagulant.

e. bromide, an inhalation anesthetic.

e. carbamate, urethan.

e. chaulmoograte, a mixture of the ethyl esters of the unsaturated fatty acids of CHAULMOOGRA OIL, which has been used in the treatment of leprosy.

e. chloride, a local anesthetic applied topically to intact skin.

e. oxide, a transparent, colorless liquid used as a pharmaceutical solvent.

e. phenylephrine, ethylphenylephrine.

e. vanillin, a flavoring agent.

ethylcellulose (eth"il-sel'u-lōs) an ethyl ether of cellulose; used as a pharmaceutical tablet binder.

ethylene (eth'ĭ-lēn) a colorless, highly flammable gas with a slightly sweet taste and odor, used as an inhalation anesthetic to induce general ANESTHESIA.

ethylenediamine (eth'ĭ-lēn-di"ah-mēn) a solvent used in pharmaceutical preparations.

ethylmorphine (eth"il-mor'fēn) the ethyl ester of morphine; its hydrochloride salt is used as an antitussive and narcotic, and topically as a chemotic.

ethylnoradrenaline (eth"il-nor-ah-dren'ah-lin) ethylnorepinephrine.

ethylnorepinephrine (eth"il-nor-ep"ĭ-nef'rin) a sympathomimetic agent used as the hydrochloride salt in the treatment of bronchial asthma.

ethylparaben (eth"il-par'ah-ben) an antifungal agent.

ethylphenylephrine (eth"il-fen"il-ef'rin) a sympathomimetic circulatory stimulant; used as the hydrochloride salt.

ethynodiol (ĕ-thi"no-di'ol) a semisynthetic steroid; the diacetate ester is used as an anovulatory progesterone.

ethynyl (eth"ĭ-nil) the group —C≡CH, when it occurs in organic compounds; present in various oral contraceptives.

etiolation (e"te-o-la'shun) 1. blanching or paleness of a plant grown in the dark due to lack of chlorophyll. 2. the process by which the skin becomes pale when deprived of sunlight.

etiology (e"te-ol'o-je) the science dealing with causes of disease. adj., **etiolog'ic, etiolog'ical.**

etioporphyrin (e"te-o-por'fĭ-rin) a porphyrin obtained from hematoporphyrin.

Eu chemical symbol, *europium.*

eu- word element [Gr.], *normal; good; well; easy.*

Eubacteriales (u"bak-te"re-a'lēz) an order of Schizomycetes comprising the true bacteria.

Eubacterium (u"bak-te're-um) a genus of bacteria found in the intestinal tract as parasites, and as saprophytes in soil and water.

eubiotics (u"bi-ot'iks) the science of healthy living.

eucalyptol (u"kah-lip'tol) a colorless liquid obtained from eucalyptus oil and other sources; used as an expectorant, flavoring agent, and local anesthetic.

eucalyptus oil (u″kah-lip′tus) a volatile oil from fresh leaf of species of *Eucalyptus,* the chief constituent of which is eucalyptol.

eucatropine (u-kat′ro-pēn) a mydriatic used as the hydrochloride salt.

euchlorhydria (u″klōr-hi′dre-ah) the presence of the normal amount of hydrochloric acid in the gastric juice.

eucholia (u-ko′le-ah) normal condition of the bile.

euchromatin (u-kro′mah-tin) that state of chromatin in which it stains lightly, is genetically active, and is considered to be partially or fully uncoiled.

euchromatopsy (u-kro′mah-top″se) normal color vision.

eucrasia (u-kra′ze-ah) 1. a state of health; proper balance of different factors constituting a healthy state. 2. a state in which the body reacts normally to ingested or injected drugs, proteins, etc.

eudiemorrhysis (u″di-ĕ-mor′ĭ-sis) the normal flow of blood through the capillaries.

eudiometer (u″de-om′ĕ-ter) an instrument for measuring and analyzing gases.

eudipsia (u-dip′se-ah) ordinary, normal thirst.

euergasia (u″er-ga′ze-ah) normal psychobiologic functioning.

euesthesia (u″es-the′ze-ah) a normal state of the senses.

eugenics (u-jen′iks) the study and control of procreation as a means of improving hereditary characteristics of future generations.

negative e., that concerned with prevention of reproduction by individuals having inferior or undesirable traits.

positive e., that concerned with promotion of optimal mating and reproduction by individuals having desirable or superior traits.

eugenol (u′jĕ-nol) the chief constituent of clove oil, also obtained from other sources, used as a dental topical analgesic and antiseptic.

euglobulin (u-glob′u-lin) one of a class of globulins characterized by being insoluble in water but soluble in saline solutions.

euglycemia (u″gli-se′me-ah) a normal level of glucose in the blood. adj., **euglyce′mic.**

eugonic (u-gon′ik) growing luxuriantly; said of bacterial cultures.

eukaryon (u-kar′e-on) 1. a highly organized nucleus bounded by a nuclear membrane, a characteristic of cells of higher organisms. 2. eukaryote.

eukaryosis (u″kar-e-o′sis) the state of having a true nucleus.

eukaryote (u-kar′e-ōt) an organism whose cells have a true nucleus bounded by a nuclear membrane, and exhibit mitosis.

eukaryotic (u″kar-e-ot′ik) pertaining to a eukaryon or to a eukaryote.

eukinesia (u″ki-ne′ze-ah) normal or proper motor function or activity. adj., **eukinet′ic.**

eulaminate (u-lam′ĭ-nāt) having the normal number of laminae, as certain areas of the cerebral cortex.

Eulenburg's disease (oil′en-burgz) myotonia congenita.

eumetria (u-me′tre-ah) a normal condition of nerve impulse, so that a voluntary movement just reaches the intended goal; the proper range of movement.

eunuch (u′nuk) a male deprived of the testes or external genitals, especially one castrated before puberty (so that male secondary sex characteristics fail to develop).

eunuchoid (u′nŭ-koid) 1. resembling a eunuch. 2. a person who resembles a eunuch.

eunuchoidism (u′nŭ-koi-dizm″) deficiency of the testes or of their secretion, with impaired sexual power and eunuchoid symptoms.

female e., hypogonadism in which the ovaries fail to function at puberty, resulting in infertility, absence of development of secondary sex characteristics, infantile sexual organs, and excessive growth of the long bones.

hypergonadotropic e., that associated with secretion of high levels of gonadotropins, as in Klinefelter's syndrome.

hypogonadotropic e., that due to lack of gonadotropin secretion.

eupancreatism (u-pan′kre-ah-tizm″) normal functioning of the pancreas.

eupepsia (u-pep′se-ah) good digestion; the presence of a normal amount of pepsin in the gastric juice. adj., **eupep′tic.**

euphoretic (u″fo-ret′ik) 1. pertaining to, characterized by, or producing euphoria. 2. an agent that produces eupthoria.

euphoria (u-for′re-ah) bodily comfort; well-being; absence of pain or distress. In psychiatry, abnormal or exaggerated sense of well-being. adj., **euphor′ic.**

euphoriant (u-for′e-ant) euphoretic.

euplastic (u-plas′tik) readily becoming organized; adapted to tissue formation.

euploid (u′ploid) 1. having a balanced set or sets of chromosomes, in any number. 2. a euploid individual or cell.

euploidy (u′ploi-de) the state of being euploid.

eupnea (ūp-ne′ah) normal respiration. adj., **eupne′ic.**

eupraxia (u-prak′se-ah) intactness of reproduction of coordinated movements. adj., **euprac′tic.**

Euraz (u′raks) trademark for preparations of crotamiton, an acaricide.

eurhythmia (u-rith′me-ah) regularity of the pulse.

europium (u-ro′pe-um) a chemical element, atomic number 63, atomic weight 151.96, symbol Eu. (See table of ELEMENTS.)

Eurotium (u-ro′she-um) a genus of fungi or molds.

eury- word element [Gr.], *wide; broad.*

eurycephalic (u″rĭ-sĕ-fal′ik) having a wide head.

euryon (u′re-on) a point on either parietal bone marking either end of the greatest transverse diameter of the skull.

eustachian tube (u-sta′ke-an) the narrow channel that connects the tympanum with the nasopharynx; called also auditory tube. The eustachian tube serves to equalize pressure on either side of the tympanic membrane (eardrum). In children this tube is wider and shorter than in adults, and thus children are especially prone to infections of the middle ear that originate in the pharynx and travel through the tube. (See also Plate 15.)

euthanasia (u″thah-na′ze-ah) 1. an easy or painless death. 2. the deliberate ending of life of a person suffering from an incurable disease; called also mercy killing.

In recent years the term euthanasia has been broadened to include the practice of withholding extraordinary means or "heroic" measures, and thus allowing the patient to die. A distinction is made between positive and negative euthanasia. In positive or active euthanasia there is the deliberate ending of life; an action is taken to cause death in a person. Negative or passive euthanasia is the withholding of life-preserving procedures and treatments that would prolong the life of one who is incurably and terminally ill and could not survive without them.

Many persons feel that they have a "right to die," that the decision is theirs as to whether extraordinary means should be taken to prolong their lives. The Euthanasia Education Council, 250 West 57th St., New York, NY 10019, provides free of charge a copy of the *Living Will*. This simple one-page document states that in a situation in which there is no hope for recovery, the person signing the will does not wish to have his life prolonged by artificial means or heroic measures. The Living Will is not legally binding in most states at the present time; it is simply a statement as to how the person who has signed it chooses to die.

euthenics (u-then′iks) the science of race improvement by regulation of environment.

euthermic (u-ther′mik) characterized by the proper temperatures; promoting warmth.

euthyroid (u-thi′roid) having a normally functioning thyroid gland.

eutocia (u-to′she-ah) normal labor, or childbirth.

Eutrombicula (u″trom-bik′u-lah) a subgenus of *Trombicula* (see also CHIGGER).

E. alfreddugè′si, the common chigger of the United States; called also *Trombicula alfreddugèsi.*

eutrophia (u-tro′fe-ah) a state of normal (good) nutrition.

eutrophication (u″tro-fĭ-ka′shun) the accidental or deliberate promotion of excessive growth (multiplication) of one kind of organism to the disadvantage of other organisms in the same ecosystem.

ev, EV electron volt.

evacuant (e-vak′u-ant) 1. promoting evacuation. 2. an agent that promotes evacuation.

evacuation (e-vak″u-a′shun) 1. an emptying or removal, especially the removal of any material from the body by discharge through a natural or artificial passage. 2. material discharged from the body, especially the discharge from the bowels.

evagination (e-vaj″ĭ-na′shun) an outpouching of a layer or part.

evaluation (e-val″u-a′shun) a critical appraisal or assessment; a judgment of the value, worth, character, or effectiveness of that which is being assessed. In the health care field, this includes assessment of the patient's status on the health/illness continuum, and evaluation of the effectiveness of patient care activities in bringing about a change in his status.

The basic components of evaluation are (1) identifying the parameters of the subject of appraisal, (2) developing criteria specific to the topic within the parameters, (3) data gathering, (4) measuring the data against the criteria, and (5) employing the results of assessment for improvement of the process, status, behavior, or activity evaluated.

Parameters are the exact dimensions or fixed limits that clearly define the area of evaluation. They establish the frame of reference within which the process will take place and are essential to accurate interpretation and meaningful use of the results of the evaluation. Parameters to be considered might include the framework of time within which the data gathering will take place, description of the kinds of data to be obtained, and specification of the patient population selected for evaluation of patient care. In a NURSING AUDIT, for example, the medical records chosen for audit might be those of patients whose admission and discharge dates were within a specific period of time, and whose age range and diagnoses were similar. Since it is a *nursing* audit, the kind of data collected should be limited to information related to the area of nursing activities and the resulting patient care outcomes recorded on the patient's chart.

In the assessment of a patient's status on the health/illness continuum, the parameters might limit the appraisal to respiratory function, neuromuscular function, emotional status, or any of a number of areas that are important to accomplishing the overall goals and objectives of health care for that specific patient.

Parameters may vary widely, then, depending on what is being appraised and the goals and purposes of the evaluation. They focus the attention of the evaluators on specifics rather than generalities and allow for a more analytic and logical approach to the task of evaluation.

A *criterion* is a standard on which a judgment is based; a set of criteria is useful only insofar as it provides a sound basis for decision-making and action. The criteria developed for the purpose of evaluation may be stated in a number of ways, but they must be pertinent to the previously established parameters and objectives. If, for example, the parameters limit an assessment to nursing activities related to adult patients with new colostomies, the objectives would be concerned with the ability of the patient to manage his colostomy and resume his daily life at home and at work. The criteria must be stated within the confines of these parameters and they must be compatible with the objectives. The criteria are written as positive outcomes; that is, they clearly state the specific things the patient has demonstrated an ability to do as a result of the nursing care he has received. It should be noted that, although objectives project future desired ends, and criteria state outcomes in terms of what has been accomplished, both are based on the same concept.

Criteria should be measurable, that is, stated in terms that denote logical and sequential steps in the progression toward a desirable goal. In some instances criteria may be relatively easy to state because they are based on previously and scientifically determined norms and values. In the area of assessment of a patient's physiologic status one could use as criteria the normal range of values for laboratory tests, the acceptable limits of vital sign readings, the normal range of joint motion, or any of the established quantifiable values and standards.

Criteria related to patient care activities also should reflect a systematic and analytic approach. If they are related to patient education, they should be written in behavioral terms that describe the specific units of behavior one would look for to determine whether a change is taking or has taken place. For example, is the patient able to change his colostomy drainage bags without assistance?

Criteria represent the "ideal," but they should not be considered as inflexible and permanently fixed. They may, and often do, require revision after having been tested in the process of evaluation and found to be irrelevant, impractical, or unachievable because of factors that are difficult or impossible to control. They may prove to be invalid because they do not measure what they were intended to measure, or they may be of little use because they do not lead to the detection of deficiencies that need correction. When criteria do fail to serve the function for which they are intended, it may be that those developing the criteria are not sufficiently knowledgeable about the area of assessment and thus need the help of practitioners who are more experienced.

Data gathering involves the collection of information that gives factual and objective evidence about the subject being evaluated. The evidence may be obtained through observation, interview, the review of patient records, and, as in the case of assessment of a patient's health/illness status, through such procedures as laboratory analysis and testing, radiologic studies, and other diagnostic techniques.

The data collected become documented evidence, which is then measured against the established criteria. If the evidence indicates that all of the criteria are being met, there is no indication of a problem in the area of evaluation. If the evidence shows that certain criteria are not met, these deficiencies are identified as the ones needing attention so that there can be progress toward the stated goals.

Evans blue (ev′anz) an odorless green, bluish green, or brown powder dye, used as a diagnostic acid in estimation of blood volume. The dye is injected into the bloodstream and after a sufficient period of time samples of the blood are taken to determine the degree of dilution of the dye.

eventration (e″ven-tra′shun) 1. protrusion of the bowels through the abdomen. 2. removal of the abdominal viscera.

e. of the diaphragm, diaphragmatic e., elevation of the dome of the diaphragm into the thoracic cavity, usually due to phrenic nerve paralysis.

eversion (e-ver′zhun) a turning inside out; a turning outward.

evert (e-vert′) to turn inside out; to turn outward.

Evipal (e′vĭ-pal) trademark for a preparation of hexobarbital, an ultrashort-acting barbiturate.

evisceration (e-vis″er-a′shun) 1. extrusion of the viscera, or internal organs; disembowelment. 2. removal of the contents of the eyeball, leaving the sclera.

evolution (ev″o-lu′shun) the process of development in which an organ or organism becomes more and more complex by the differentiation of its parts; a continuous and progressive change according to certain laws and by means of resident forces.

convergent e., the development, in animals that are only distantly related, of similar structures or functions in adaptation to similar environment.

organic e., the origin and development of species; the theory that existing organisms are the result of descent with modification from those of past times.

evulsion (e-vul′shun) extraction by force.

Ewing's tumor (sarcoma) (u′ingz) a malignant tumor of bone that arises in medullary tissue, occurring more often in cylindrical bones, with pain, fever, and leukocytosis as prominent symptoms.

ex- work element [L.], *away from; without; outside;* sometimes used to denote *completely.*

exacerbation (eg-zas″er-ba′shun) increase in severity of a disease or any of its symptoms.

examination (eg-zam″ĭ-na′shun) inspection or investigation, especially as a means of diagnosing disease, qualified according to the methods used, as physical, cystoscopic, etc.

exanthem (eg-zan′them) 1. any cutaneous eruptive disease or fever. 2. the eruption which characterizes an eruptive fever.

e. sub′itum, an acute viral disease of infants and young children, with continuous or remittent fever, falling by crises, and followed by a rash on the trunk (see also ROSEOLA INFANTUM).

exanthema (eg″zan-the′mah) pl. *exanthem′ata* [Gr.] exanthem.

exanthematous (eg″zan-them′ah-tus) characterized by or of the nature of an eruption or rash.

exarticulation (eks″ar-tik″u-la′shun) amputation at a joint; partial removal of a joint.

excavation (eks″kah-va′shun) 1. the act of hollowing out. 2. a hollowed-out space, or pouchlike cavity.

atrophic e., cupping of the optic disk, due to atrophy of the optic nerve fibers.

e. of optic disk, physiologic e., a normally occurring depression in the center of the optic disk.

rectouterine e., Douglas' cul-de-sac.

rectovesical e., the space between the rectum and bladder in the peritoneal cavity of the male.

vesicouterine e., the space between the bladder and uterus in the peritoneal cavity of the female.

excavator (eks′kah-va″tor) a scoop or gouge for surgical use.

excerebration (ek″ser-ĕ-bra′shun) removal of the brain.

excipient (ek-sip′e-ent) any more or less inert substance added to a drug to give suitable consistency or form to the drug; a vehicle.

excise (ek-sīz′) to remove by cutting.

excision (ek-sizh′un) removal, as of an organ, by cutting.

excitability (ek-sīt″ah-bil′ĭ-te) readiness to respond to a stimulus; irritability.

excitant (ek-sīt′ant) an agent producing excitation of the vital functions, or of those of the brain.

excitation (ek″si-ta′shun) an act of irritation or stimulation; a condition of being excited; the addition of energy, as the excitation of a molecule by absorption of photons.

indirect e., electrostimulation of a muscle by placing the electrode on its nerve.

excitomotor (ek-si″to-mo′tor) tending to produce motion or motor function; an agent that so acts.

excitosecretory (ek-si″to-se-kre′to-re) producing increased secretion.

excitovascular (ek-si″to-vas′ku-lar) causing vascular changes.

exclave (eks′klāv) a detached part of an organ.

exclusion (ek-skloo′zhun) a shutting out or elimination; surgical isolation of a part, as of a segment of intestine, without removal from the body.

excoriation (ek″sko-re-a′shun) any superficial loss

of substance, such as that produced on the skin by scratching.

excrement (ek′skrĕ-ment) fecal matter; matter cast out as waste from the body.

excrementitious (ek″skrĕ-men-tish′us) pertaining to or of the nature of excrement.

excrescence (ek-skres′ens) an abnormal outgrowth; a projection of morbid origin. adj., **excres′cent**.

excreta (ek-skre′tah) excretion products; waste material excreted or eliminated from the body, including FECES, URINE, and PERSPIRATION. Mucus and carbon dioxide also can be considered excreta. The organs of excretion are the intestinal tract, kidneys, lungs, and skin.

excrete (ek-skrēt′) to throw off or eliminate, as waste matter, by a normal discharge.

excretion (ek-skre′shun) 1. the act, process, or function of excreting. 2. material that is excreted. adj., **ex′cretory**. Ordinarily, what is meant by excretion is the evacuation of feces. Technically, excretion can refer to the expulsion of any matter, whether from a single cell or from the entire body, or to the matter excreted.

excursion (ek-skur′zhun) a range of movement regularly repeated in performance of a function, e.g., excursion of the jaws in mastication. adj., **excur′sive**.

excystation (ek″sis-ta′shun) escape from a cyst or envelope, as in that stage in the life cycle of parasites occurring after the cystic form has been swallowed by the host.

exercise (ek′ser-siz) performance of physical exertion for improvement of health or correction of physical deformity.

active e., motion imparted to a part by voluntary contraction and relaxation of its controlling muscles.

active assistive e., voluntary contraction of muscles controlling a part, assisted by a therapist or by some other means.

active resistive e., motion voluntarily imparted to a part against resistance.

Buerger-Allen e's, specific exercises intended to improve circulation to the feet and legs (see also BUERGER-ALLEN EXERCISES).

corrective e., therapeutic exercise.

isometric e., active exercise performed against stable resistance, without change in the length of the muscle.

isotonic e., active exercise without appreciable change in the force of muscular contraction, with shortening of the muscle.

Kegel e's, a program of exercises designed to strengthen the pelvic-vaginal muscles in stress incontinence in women (see also KEGEL EXERCISES).

muscle-setting e., voluntary contraction and relaxation of skeletal muscles without movement of the associated part of the body; called also static exercise.

passive e., motion imparted to a segment of the body by another individual, machine, or other outside force, or produced by voluntary effort of another segment of the patient's own body.

range of motion (ROM) e's, exercises that move each joint through its full range of motion, that is, to the highest degree of motion of which each joint normally is capable.

static e., muscle-setting exercise.

e. testing, a technique for evaluating circulatory response to physical stress; called also stress testing. The procedure involves continuous electrocardiographic monitoring during physical exercise, the objective being to increase the intensity of physical exertion until a target heart rate is reached or signs and symptoms of cardiac ischemia appear.

Clinical exercise testing has become an important tool in screening for and diagnosing early ischemic heart disease that cannot be detected by a standard resting EKG, and in predicting the probability of the development of the condition in later years. The technique cannot determine the location of the lesion causing cardiac ischemia and therefore must be supplemented with angiocardiography when coronary occlusion is detected.

Three basic forms of exercise are used: the treadmill, step climbing, and the bicycle ergometer. The procedure must be performed in a clinical setting where medical personnel are available in the event symptoms of dyspnea, vertigo, extreme fatigue, severe arrhythmias, and other abnormal EKG readings develop during the exercise.

Exercise testing also may be used to assess the pulmonary status of a patient with a respiratory disease. As the patient performs specific exercises, blood samples are drawn for BLOOD GAS ANALYSIS, and ventilatory function tests such a tidal volume, total lung capacity, and vital capacity are conducted. An example of the kind of exercise test that may be used is the *step test*, in which the patient steps up and down on a 20-cm.-high platform 30 times a minute.

therapeutic e., the scientific use of bodily movement to restore normal function in diseased or injured tissues or to maintain a state of well-being. Called also corrective exercise. As with any type of therapy, a therapeutic exercise program is designed to correct specific disabilities of the individual patient. The program is evaluated periodically and modified as indicated by the progress of the patient and his response to the prescribed regimen. Exercises affect the body locally and systemically, and bring about changes in the nervous, circulatory, and endocrine systems as well as the musculoskeletal system.

Among the types of therapeutic exercise are those that (1) increase or maintain mobility of the joints and surrounding soft tissues, (2) develop coordination through control of individual muscles, (3) increase muscular strength and endurance, and (4) promote relaxation and relief of tension.

JOINT MOBILITY. In the absence of a disability that prohibits mobility, the regular day-to-day activities of living maintain the normal movements of the joints. If, however, motion is restricted for any reason, the soft tissues become dense and hard and adaptive shortening of the connective tissues takes place. These changes begin to develop within four days after a joint has been immobilized and are evident even in a normal joint that has been rendered immobile. It is for this reason that therapeutic exercises to prevent loss of joint motion are so important and should be begun as soon as possible after an injury has occurred or a disease process has begun.

Prevention of the loss of joint motion is much less costly and time-consuming than correction of tissue changes that seriously impair joint mobility. It is recommended that each joint should be put through its full range of motion three times at least twice daily. If the patient is not able to carry out these exercises, he is assisted by a therapist or member of his family who has been instructed in the exercises. Inflammation of the joint, as in arthritis, may cause some pain on motion, and so passive exercises are done slowly and gently with the joint as relaxed as possible. Procedures that stretch tight muscles to increase joint motion should be done only by a skilled therapist who understands the hazards of fracture and bleeding within the joint, which can occur if the exercises are done improperly or too strenuously.

MUSCLE TRAINING. Exercises of this type are taught to the patient who has lost some control over a major skeletal muscle. By learning precise and conscious control over a specific muscle, the patient is able to strengthen and coordinate its movement with normal motor patterns and thus enhance his mobility. Muscle training or neuromuscular re-education demands full cooperation of the patient. He must be capable of understanding the purpose of the exercises and able to follow directions and give his full attention to the muscle isolated for retraining. The training sessions are held in a quiet, comfortable atmosphere in which the patient is able to concentrate on the task of controlling the activity of the specific muscle.

The development of conscious control over individual muscles is useful in the rehabilitation of patients with a variety of disorders, including physical trauma, diseases such as poliomyelitis that affect the motor neurons, and congenital disorders such as cerebral palsy. It demands full concentration and mental awareness on the part of the patient and involves a systematic program of sequential activities carried out under the direction of a therapist who is knowledgeable in the technique. Although it requires much effort on the part of the patient and the therapist, the attainment of muscle control and coordination is a very satisfying reward.

MUSCLE STRENGTH AND ENDURANCE. Improvement of muscle strength and endurance is particularly important in the rehabilitation of patients whose goal is to return to an active and productive life after a debilitating illness or disabling injury. The exercises are prescribed according to the individual needs of the patient and usually involve more than one group of muscles. Endurance exercises, usually of the low-resistance type, demand repetition and persistence beyond the point of fatigue. When developing a program of this type it is necessary to take into account the patient's need for motivation and the pitfalls of boredom from monotony. The various activities included in occupational therapy can be useful in maintaining the patient's interest and cooperation.

RELIEF OF TENSION. Exercises that promote relaxation of the muscles and provide relief from the effects of tension are useful in a wide variety of disorders ranging from mild tension headache to insomnia. Patients who are especially tense may require several sessions of instruction in relaxation before they can learn the technique.

exeresis (ek-ser′ĕ-sis) surgical removal, or excision.

exergonic (ek″ser-gon′ik) accompanied by the release of free energy.

exflagellation (eks-flaj″ĕ-la′shun) the protrusion or formation of flagelliform microgametes from a microgametocyte in malarial parasites and some related sporozoa.

exfoliation (eks-fo″le-a′shun) a falling off in scales or layers, adj., **exfo′liative.**

lamellar e. of newborn, a congenital hereditary disorder in which the infant is born completely covered with a collodion- or parchment-like membrane that peels off within 24 hours, after which there may be complete healing, or the scales may re-form and the process repeated. In the more severe form, the infant (harlequin fetus) is completely covered with thick, horny, armor-like scales, and is usually stillborn or dies shortly after birth. Called also ichthyosis congenita, ichthyosis fetalis, and lamellar ichthyosis of newborn.

exhalation (eks″hah-la′shun) 1. the giving off of watery or other vapor, or of an effluvium. 2. a vapor or other substance exhaled or given off. 3. the act of breathing out.

exhaustion (eg-zawst′yun) 1. privation of energy with consequent inability to respond to stimuli; lassitude. 2. withdrawal. 3. a condition of emptiness caused by withdrawal. 4. emptying by a process of withdrawal.

heat e., an effect of excessive exposure to heat (see also HEAT EXHAUSTION).

exhibitionism (ek″sĭ-bish′ĕ-nizm) a sexual deviation in which pleasure is gained by exposure of the genitals to persons of the opposite sex in socially unacceptable circumstances. It is more common in men than in women, and in adults it is difficult to correct. It may be resorted to by an individual who is unable for physical or psychologic reasons to gain sexual gratification by normal means. A common cause is a feeling of sexual inadequacy; for this the exposure is a compensation. Exhibitionism may also be a form of masochism in which a feeling of guilt drives the person to behavior for which he knows he will be punished. Psychotherapy is necessary to deal with this type of sexual deviation.

exhibitionist (ek″sĭ-bish′ĕ-nist) a person who indulges in exhibitionism.

exo- word element [Gr.], *outside of; outward.*

exobiology (ek″so-bi-ol′o-je) the science concerned with study of life on planets other than the earth.

exocardia (ek″so-kar′de-ah) congenital displacement of the heart; ectocardia.

exocardial (ek″so-kar′de-al) situated, occurring, or developed outside the heart.

exocolitis (ek″so-ko-li′tis) inflammation of the outer coat of the colon.

exocrine (ek′so-krin) 1. secreting externally via a duct. 2. denoting such a gland or its secretion.

exocytosis (ek″so-si-to′sis) 1. the discharge from a cell of particles that are too large to diffuse through the wall; the opposite of endocytosis. 2. the aggregation of migrating leukocytes in the epidermis as part of the inflammatory response.

exodeviation (ek″so-de″ve-a′shun) a turning outward; in ophthalmology, exotropia.

exodontics (ek″so-don′tiks) that branch of dentistry dealing with extraction of teeth.

exoenzyme (ek″so-en′zīm) an enzyme that acts outside the cell that secretes it.

exoerythrocytic (ek″so-ĕ-rith″ro-sit′ik) occurring or situated outside the red blood cells (erythrocytes), a term applied to a stage in the development of malarial parasites that takes place in cells other than erythrocytes.

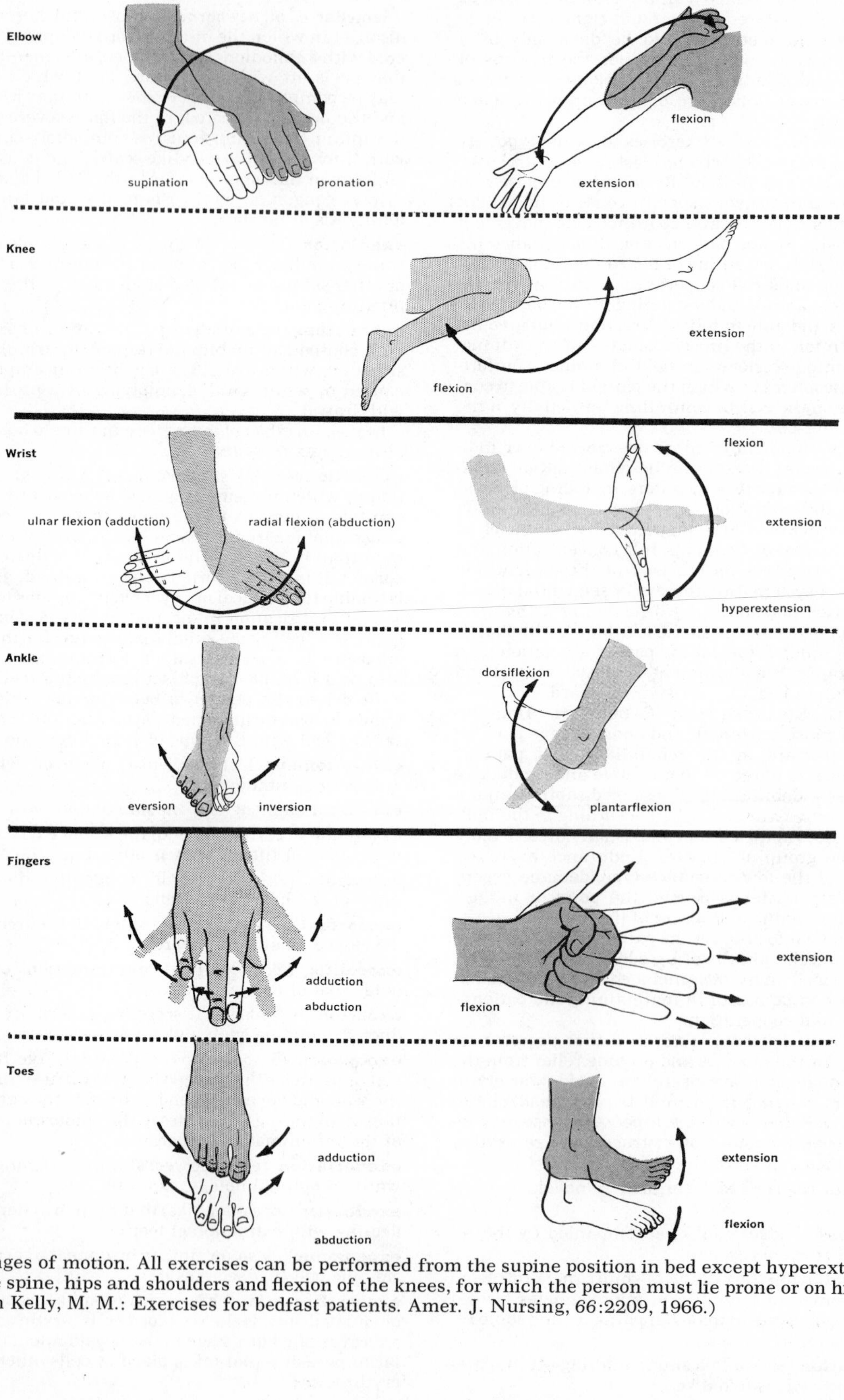

Ranges of motion. All exercises can be performed from the supine position in bed except hyperextension of the spine, hips and shoulders and flexion of the knees, for which the person must lie prone or on his side. (From Kelly, M. M.: Exercises for bedfast patients. Amer. J. Nursing, *66*:2209, 1966.)

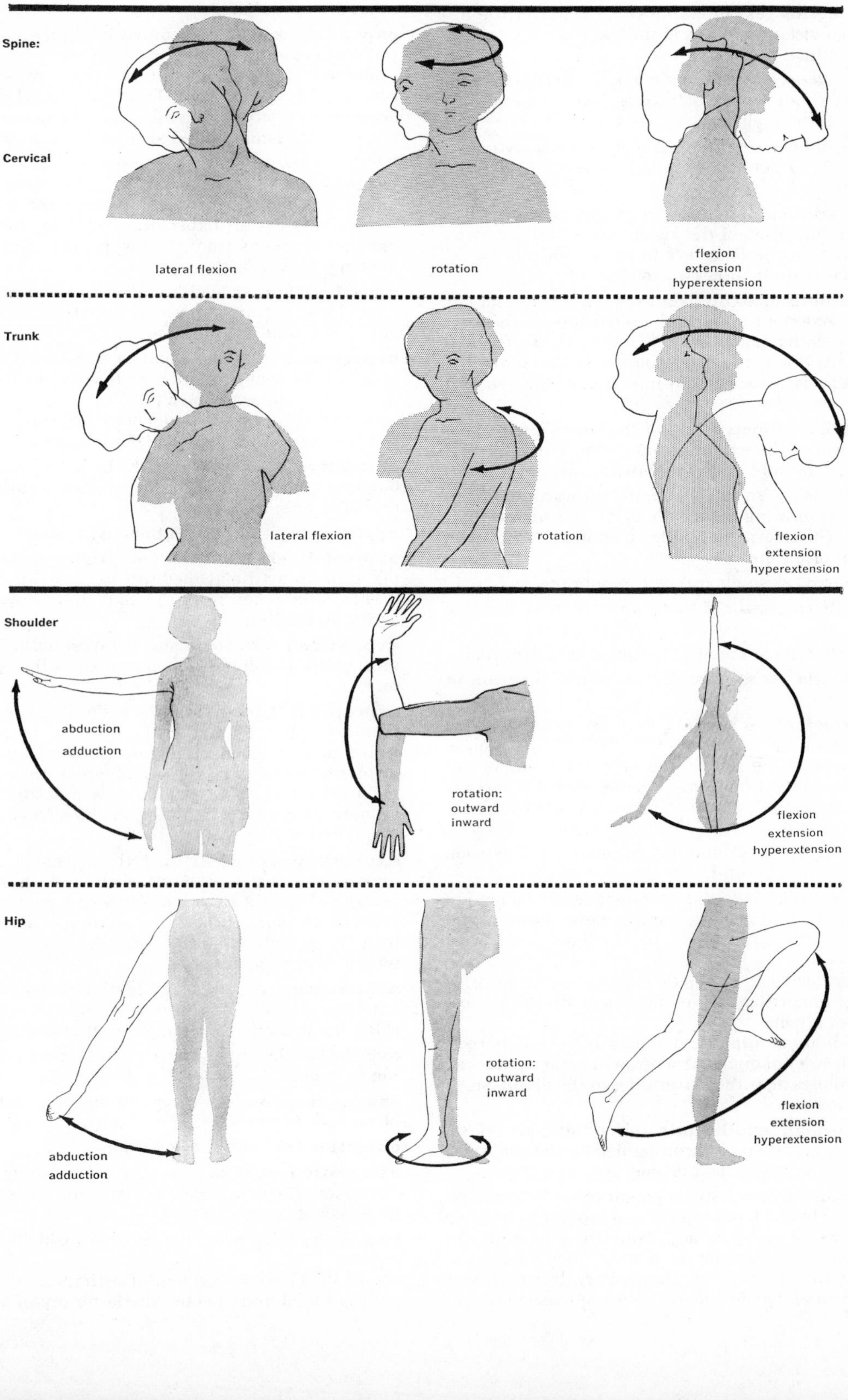
Spine:
Cervical
lateral flexion
rotation
flexion
extension
hyperextension
Trunk
lateral flexion
rotation
flexion
extension
hyperextension
Shoulder
abduction
adduction
rotation:
outward
inward
flexion
extension
hyperextension
Hip
rotation:
outward
inward
flexion
extension
hyperextension
abduction
adduction

exogamy (ek-sog'ah-me) 1. protozoan fertilization by union of elements that are not derived from the same cell. 2. marriage outside a particular group.

exogenous (ek-soj'ĕ-nus) originating outside or caused by factors outside the organism.

exomphalus (eks-om'fah-los) 1. hernia of the abdominal viscera into the umbilical cord. 2. congenital umbilical hernia.

exonuclease (ek"so-nu'kle-ās) a nuclease that cleaves single mononucleotides from the end of a polynucleotide chain.

exopeptidase (ek"so-pep'tĭ-dās) a proteolytic enzyme whose action is limited to terminal peptide linkages.

exophoria (ek"so-fo're-ah) HETEROPHORIA in which there is deviation of the visual axis of an eye away from that of the other eye in the absence of visual fusional stimuli. adj., **exopho'ric.**

exophthalmia, exophthalmos (ek"sof-thal'me-ah; ek"sof-thal'mos) abnormal protrusion of the eye. adj., **exophthal'mic.** It results in a marked stare and is usually due to HYPERTHYROIDISM. Occasionally the condition is caused by an infection of the eye or a tumor behind the eye.

exophthalmometry (ek"sof-thal-mom'ĕ-tre) measurement of the extent of protrusion of the eyeball in exophthalmos. adj., **exophthalmomet'ric.**

exophytic (ek"so-fit'ik) growing outward; in oncology, proliferating externally or on the surface epithelium of an organ or other structure in which the growth originated.

exoplasm (ek'so-plazm) cell membrane.

exorbitism (ek-sor'bĭ-tizm) protrusion of the eyeball.

exormia (ek-sor'me-ah) a papular skin eruption.

exoserosis (ek"so-se-ro'sis) an oozing of serum or exudate.

exoskeleton (ek"so-skel'ĕ-ton) an external hard framework, as a crustacean's shell, that supports and protects the soft tissues of lower animals, derived from the ectoderm. In vertebrates the term is sometimes applied to structures produced by the epidermis, as hair, nails, hoofs, teeth, etc.

exosmosis (ek"sos-mo'sis) osmosis or diffusion from within outward.

exostosis (ek"sos-to'sis), pl. *exosto'ses* [Gr.] a benign new growth projecting from a bone surface and characteristically capped by cartilage. adj., **exostot'ic.**

e. cartilagin'ea, a variety of osteoma consisting of a layer of cartilage developing beneath the periosteum of a bone.

hereditary multiple e., a generally benign, hereditary disorder of enchondral growth of bone, marked by exostoses near the extremities of the diaphysis of long bones.

exothermal, exothermic (ek"so-ther'mal; ek"so-ther'mik) marked or accompanied by the evolution of heat; liberating heat or energy.

exotoxin (ek"so-tok'sin) a potent toxin formed and excreted by the bacterial cell, and found free in the surrounding medium. adj., **exotox'ic.** Exotoxins are heat labile, and protein in nature. They are detoxified with retention of antigenicity by treatment with formaldehyde and are the most poisonous substances known to man. Bacteria of the genus *Clostridium* are the most frequent producers of exotoxins; diptheria, botulism, and tetanus are all caused by bacterial toxins.

exotropia (ek"so-tro'pe-ah) STRABISMUS in which there is permanent deviation of the visual axis of one eye away from that of the other, resulting in diplopia. Called also divergent strabismus and walleye. adj., **exotro'pic.**

expander (ek-span'der) something that enlarges or prolongs; extender.

plasma volume e., a substance that can be transfused to maintain fluid volume of the blood in event of great necessity, supplemental to the use of whole blood and plasma. Called also artificial plasma extender and plasma volume extender.

expectorant (ek-spek'to-rant) 1. promoting expectoration. 2. an agent that promotes expectoration.

liquefying e., an expectorant that promotes the ejection of mucus from the respiratory tract by decreasing its viscosity.

expectoration (ek-spek"to-ra'shun) 1. the coughing up and spitting out of material from the lungs, bronchi, and trachea. 2. sputum.

experiment (ek-sper'ĭ-ment) a procedure done in order to discover or demonstrate some fact or general truth. adj., **experimen'tal.**

control e., one made under standard conditions, to test the correctness of other observations.

expiration (ek"spĭ-ra'shun) 1. the act of breathing out, or expelling air from the lungs. 2. termination, or death. adj., **expi'ratory.**

expire (ek-spīr) 1. to breathe out. 2. to die.

explant 1. (eks-plant') to take from the body and place in an artificial medium for growth. 2. (eks'plant) tissue taken from the body and grown in an artificial medium.

exploration (eks"plo-ra'shun) investigation or examination for diagnostic purposes. adj., **explo'ratory.**

exposure (eks-po'zhur) 1. the act of laying open, as surgical exposure. 2. the condition of being subjected to something, as to infectious agents or extremes of weather or radiation, which may have a harmful effect. 3. in radiology, a measure of the amount of ionizing radiation at the surface of the irradiated object, e.g., the body.

expression (eks-presh'un) 1. the aspect or appearance of the face as determined by the physical or emotional state. 2. the act of squeezing out or evacuating by pressure. 3. the manifestation of a heritable trait in an individual carrying the gene or genes which determine it.

expressivity (eks"pres-siv'ĭ-te) the extent to which a heritable trait is manifested by an individual carrying the principal gene or genes that determine it.

expulsive (eks-pul'siv) driving or forcing out; tending to expel.

exsanguination (eks-sang"gwĭ-na'shun) extensive blood loss due to internal or external hemorrhage.

exsection (ek-sek'shun) excision.

exsiccation (ek"sĭ-ka'shun) the act of drying out; in chemistry, the deprival of a crystalline substance of its water of crystallization.

exstrophy (ek'stro-fe) the turning inside out of an organ.

e. of the bladder, congenital deficiency of the abdominal wall and bladder, the latter organ appearing to be turned inside out, with the internal surface of the posterior wall showing through the opening in the anterior wall.

ext. external; extract.

extender (ek-sten′der) something that enlarges or prolongs; expander.

artificial plasma e., plasma volume e., plasma volume expander.

extension (ek-sten′shun) 1. the movement by which the two ends of any jointed part are drawn away from each other. 2. a movement bringing the members of a limb into or toward a straight condition.

Buck's e., extension of a fractured leg by weights, the foot of the bed being raised so that the body makes counterextension.

Codivilla's e., extension for fractures made by a weight pulling on calipers or a nail passed through the lower end of the bone.

nail e., Steinmann e., extension exerted on the distal fragment of a fractured bone by means of a nail or pin (Steinmann pin) driven into the fragment.

extensor (ek-sten′sor) [L.] any muscle that extends a joint.

exteriorize (eks-te′re-or-īz) 1. to form a correct mental reference of the image of an object seen. 2. in psychiatry, to turn one's interest outward. 3. to transpose an internal organ to the exterior of the body.

extern (eks′tern) a medical student or graduate in medicine who assists in patient care in the hospital but does not reside there.

external (eks-ter′nal) situated or occurring on the outside. In anatomy, situated toward or near the outside; lateral.

externalize (eks-ter′nah-līz) to direct outwardly an internal conflict.

externus (ek-ster′nus) external; in anatomy, denoting a structure farther from the center of an organ or cavity.

exteroception (ek″ster-o-sep′shun) the perception of stimuli originating outside or at a distance from the body.

exteroceptor (ek″ster-o-sep′tor) a sensory nerve ending stimulated by the immediate external environment, such as those in the skin and mucous membranes. adj., **exterocep′tive.**

exterofective (ek″ster-o-fek′tiv) responding to external stimuli; a term applied to the cerebrospinal nervous system.

extima (ek′stĭ-mah) outermost; the outermost coat of a blood vessel; the adventitia.

extinction (eks-ting′shun) in psychology, the disappearance of a conditioned response as a result of nonreinforcement; also, the process by which the disappearance is accomplished. (See also CONDITIONING.)

extirpation (ek″ster-pa′shun) complete removal or eradication of an organ or tissue.

extorsion (eks-tor′shun) tilting of the upper part of the vertical meridian of the eye away from the midline of the face.

extra- word element [L.], *outside; beyond the scope of; in addition.*

extra-articular (ek″strah-ar-tik′u-lar) situated or occurring outside a joint.

extracapsular (ek″strah-kap′su-lar) situated or occurring outside a capsule.

extracellular (ek″strah-sel′u-lar) situated or occurring outside a cell or cells.

extracorporeal (ek″strah-kor-po′re-al) situated or occurring outside the body.

e. circulation, the circulation of blood outside of the body, as through an ARTIFICIAL KIDNEY for removal of substances usually excreted in the urine, or through a HEART-LUNG MACHINE for carbon dioxide-oxygen exchange.

extracorticospinal (ek″strah-kor″tĭ-ko-spi′nal) outside the corticospinal tract.

extract (ek′strakt) a concentrated preparation of a vegetable or animal drug.

allergenic e., an extract of the protein of any substance to which a person may be sensitive.

cell-free e., the solution obtained by rupturing cells and removing all particulate matter.

chondodendron tomentosum e., an alcoholic extract from curare obtained from the South American shrub *Chondodendron tomentosum;* used as a skeletal muscle relaxant.

liver e., a brownish, somewhat hygroscopic powder prepared from mammalian livers; used as a hematopoietic.

malt e., a product containing dextrin, maltose, a small amount of glucose, and amylolytic enzymes; used as a nutritive and emulsifying agent.

ox bile e., one prepared from the fresh bile of the ox; used as a choleretic.

extraction (ek-strak′shun) 1. the process or act of pulling or drawing out. 2. the preparation of an extract.

breech e., extraction of an infant from the uterus in cases of breech presentation.

flap e., removal of a cataract by making a flap in the cornea.

serial e., the selective extraction of deciduous teeth during an extended period of time to allow autonomous adjustment.

vacuum e., delivery of a fetus by application of a vacuum.

extractive (ek-strak′tiv) any substance present in an organized tissue, or in a mixture in a small quantity, and requiring extraction by a special method.

extractor (ek-strak′tor) an instrument for removing a calculus or foreign body.

extradural (ek″strah-du′ral) situated or occurring outside the dura mater.

extraembryonic (ek″strah-em″bre-on′ik) not occurring as a part of the embryo proper; applied specifically to the fetal membranes.

extramarginal (ek″strah-mar′jĭ-nal) below the limit of consciousness.

extramastoiditis (ek″strah-mas″toi-di′tis) inflammation of tissues adjoining the mastoid process.

extramural (eks″trah-mu′ral) situated or occurring outside the wall of an organ or structure.

extraplacental (eks″trah-plah-sen′tal) independent of the placenta.

extrapulmonary (eks″trah-pul′mo-na″re) not connected with the lungs.

extrapyramidal (eks″trah-pĭ-ram′ĭ-dal) outside the pyramidal tracts.

e. disease, e. syndrome, any of a group of clinical disorders marked by abnormal involuntary movements, alterations in muscle tone, and postural disturbances; the group includes parkinsonism, chorea, athetosis, etc.

e. system, e. tract, a functional, rather than anatomical, unit comprising the nuclei and fibers (excluding those of the pyramidal tract) involved in motor activities; they control and coordinate especially the postural, static, supporting, and locomotor mechanisms. It includes the corpus striatum, subthalamic nucleus, substantia nigra, and red nucleus, along with their interconnections with the reticular formation, cerebellum, and cerebrum; some authorities include the cerebellum and vestibular nuclei.

extrasensory perception (ek″strah-sen′so-re) knowledge of, or response to, an external thought or objective event not achieved as the result of stimulation of the sense organs; abbreviated E.S.P.

extrasystole (ek″strah-sis′to-le) a premature cardiac contraction that is independent of the normal rhythm and arises in response to an impulse outside the sinoatrial node.

atrial e., one in which the stimulus is thought to arise in the atrium elsewhere than at the sinoatrial node.

atrioventricular e., one in which the stimulus is thought to arise in the atrioventricular node.

interpolated e., a contraction taking place between two normal heartbeats.

nodal e., atrioventricular extrasystole.

retrograde e., a premature ventricular contraction followed by a premature atrial contraction, due to transmission of the stimulus backward, usually over the bundle of His.

ventricular e., one in which either a pacemaker or a re-entry site is in the ventricular structure.

extratubal (ek′strah-tu′bal) situated or occurring outside a tube.

extrauterine (ek″strah-u′ter-in) situated or occurring outside the uterus.

e. pregnancy, ectopic pregnancy.

extravasation (eks-trav″ah-za′shun) 1. a discharge or escape, as of blood, from a vessel into the tissues; blood or other substance so discharged. 2. the process of being extravasated.

extravascular (ek″strah-vas′ku-lar) situated or occurring outside a vessel or the vessels.

extraversion (ek″strah-ver′zhun) extroversion.

extravert (ek″strah-vert) extrovert.

extremitas (ek-strem′ĭ-tas), pl. *extremita′tes* [L.] extremity.

extremity (ek-strem′ĭ-te) 1. the distal or terminal portion of elongated or pointed structures. 2. the arm or leg.

extrinsic (ek-strin′sik) of external origin.

e. factor, a hematopoietic vitamin that combines with intrinsic factor for absorption and is needed for erythrocyte maturation; called also VITAMIN B_{12} and CYANOCOBALAMIN.

extroversion (eks″tro-ver′zhun) 1. a turning inside out; exstrophy. 2. direction of one's energies and attention outward from the self.

extrovert (ek′stro-vert) a person whose interest is turned outward.

extrude (ek-strood′) 1. to force out, or to occupy a position distal to that normally occupied. 2. in dentistry, to occupy a position occlusal to that normally occupied.

extrusion (ek-stroo′zhun) 1. a pushing out. 2. in dentistry, the condition of a tooth pushed too far forward from the line of occlusion.

extubation (eks″tu-ba′shun) removal of a tube used in intubation.

exuberant (eg-zu′ber-ant) copious or excessive in production; showing excessive proliferation.

exudate (eks′u-dāt) a fluid with a high content of protein and cellular debris which has escaped from blood vessels and has been deposited in tissues or on tissue surfaces, usually as a result of inflammation.

exudation (eks″u-da′shun) 1. the escape of fluid, cells, or cellular debris from blood vessels and deposition in or on the tissue. 2. exudate.

exudative (eks-oo′dah-tiv) of or pertaining to a process of exudation.

exumbilication (eks″um-bil″ĭ-ka′shun) 1. marked protrusion of the navel. 2. umbilical hernia.

eye (i) the organ of vision. (See Plate 15.) In the embryo the eye develops as a direct extension of the brain, and thus is a very delicate organ. To protect the eye the bones of the skull are shaped so that an orbital cavity protects the dorsal aspect of each eyeball. In addition, the conjunctival sac covers the front of the eyeball and lines the upper and lower eyelids. Tears from the lacrimal duct constantly wash the eye to remove foreign objects, and the lids and eyelashes aid in protecting the front of the eye.

STRUCTURE. The eyeball has three coats. The cornea is the clear transparent layer on the front of the eyeball. It is a continuation of the sclera (the white of the eye), the tough outer coat that helps protect the delicate mechanism of the eye. The choroid is the middle layer and contains blood vessels. The third layer, the retina, contains rods and cones, which are specialized cells that are sensitive to light. Behind the cornea and in front of the lens is the iris, the circular pigmented band around the pupil. The iris works much like the diaphragm in a camera, widening or narrowing the pupil to adjust to different light conditions.

FUNCTION. The refraction or bending of light rays so that they focus on the retina and can thus be transmitted to the optic nerve is accomplished by three structures: the aqueous humor, a watery substance between the cornea and lens; the lens, a crystalline structure just behind the iris; and the vitreous humor, a jelly-like substance filling the space between the lens and the retina. Unlike the lens of a camera, the lens of the eye focuses by a process called accommodation. This means that when the eye sees something in the distance, muscles pull the lens, stretching it until it is thin and almost flat, so that the light rays are only slightly bent as they pass through it. When the object is close, the muscles relax and the elastic lens becomes thicker, bending the light rays and focusing them on the retina.

Because the eye must function under many different circumstances, there are two different sets of nerve cells in the retina, the cone-shaped and the rod-shaped cells. They cover the full range of adaptation to light, the cones being sensitive in bright light, and the rods in dim light. The cones are responsible for color vision. It is now believed that there are three types of cones, each containing a substance that reacts to light of a different color—one set for red, one for green, and the third for violet. These are the primary colors in light, which, when mixed together, give white. White light stimulates all three sets of color cells; any other color stimulates one or two. Lack of a set of color cells causes COLOR BLINDNESS, which usually affects either the red or the green cells.

The optic nerve, which transmits the nerve impulses from the retina to the visual center of the brain, contains nerve fibers from the many nerve cells in the retina. The small spot where it leaves the retina does not have any light-sensitive cells, and is called the blind spot.

The eyes are situated in the front of the head in such a way that human beings have stereoscopic vision, the ability to judge distances. Because the eyes are set apart, each eye sees farther around an object on its own side than does the other. The brain superimposes the two slightly different images and judges distances from the composite image. (See also VISION.)

DISORDERS OF THE EYE. If the eyeball is too short or too long, the lens focuses the image not on the retina, but behind or in front of it. The former condition is called hyperopia, or farsightedness, and the latter myopia, or nearsightedness. An irregularity in the curvature of the cornea or lens can cause the impaired vision of ASTIGMATISM.

STRABISMUS, or squint, or crossed eyes, is usually caused by weakness in some of the muscles that control movement of the eyeball.

CONJUNCTIVITIS is an inflammation of the membrane that covers the front of the eyeball and lines the eyelids.

When small pieces of the retina become detached from the underlying layers, the result is DETACHMENT OF THE RETINA. Repair by surgery can usually prevent blindness produced by retinal detachment.

PRESBYOPIA (usually taking the form of hyperopia) occurs in older persons and develops as the lens loses its elasticity with the passing years. Correction is easily made with properly prescribed eyeglasses.

The three major disorders causing blindness in the United States are CATARACT, GLAUCOMA, and TRACHOMA.

Foreign bodies in the eyes are common occurences. Cinders, grit, or other foreign bodies are best removed by lifting the eyelid by the lashes. The foreign body will usually remain on the surface of the lid, and can easily be removed. Particles embedded in the eyeball must be removed by a physician.

Eyestrain is fatigue of the eyes caused by improper use, uncorrected defects in the vision, or an eye disorder. Symptoms may include aching or pains in the eyes, or a hot, scratchy feeling in the eyelids. Headache, blurring or dimness of vision, and sometimes dizziness or nausea may also occur.

artificial e., a prosthetic organ inserted in the eye socket to replace the eyeball. It may be made of glass or plastic and most are designed to be worn day and night. When a patient becomes weak and debilitated and unable to care for the prosthesis, he must depend on members of the health care team to give proper care according to the routine that has been established and preferred by the patient.

Cleaning of an artificial eye is similar in principle to care of dentures; both are handled with care to avoid damage and are cleansed according to the dictates of good hygienic principles. The prosthesis is removed while the patient is lying down so that the eye falls into the hand and is not likely to be dropped and broken. The prosthesis is removed by depressing the lower eyelid and allowing the artificial eye to slide out and down.

Mild soap and water are most often used for cleansing the artificial eye. Alcohol or other chemicals can damage prostheses made of plastic. If the eye is not replaced in the eye socket immediately after cleansing, it is stored in water or contact lens soaking solution.

The prosthesis is inserted by lifting the upper eyelid with the thumb or forefinger and placing the notched edge of the eye toward the nose. The prosthesis is placed as far as possible under the upper lid and then the lower lid is depressed to allow the eye to slip into place. Insertion of the eye can be made easier by moistening it with water before insertion.

The hands are washed thoroughly before removal and insertion of the prosthesis. If it is necessary to wipe the eye of the patient wearing a prosthesis, one should gently wipe toward the nose to avoid dislodging it.

cross e., esotropia.

pink e., pinkeye.

wall e., exotropia.

eyeball (i'bawl) the ball or globe of the eye.

eye bank an institution or agency whose primary purpose is to collect, prepare, and supply to ophthalmologists eye tissue for transplantation. Those institutions equipped with special laboratory facilities also conduct research and store eye tissue. The Eye Bank Association of America (E.B.A.A.) coordinates eye banks in the United States and establishes medical ethical standards for the various collecting and distributing agencies throughout the country. Individuals wishing to donate their eyes may make arrangements to do so prior to their death, or the legal next-of-kin may give permission for the donation at the time of death. At the present time, the demand for usable eyes is far greater than the available supply.

eyebrow (i'brow) 1. supercilium; the transverse elevation at the junction of the forehead and the upper eyelid. 2. supercilia; the hairs growing on this elevation.

eyecup (i'kup) a small vessel for application of cleansing or medicated solution to the exposed area of the eyeball. 2. physiologic cup.

eyeglass (i'glas) a lens for aiding the sight.

eyeground (i'grownd) the fundus of the eye as seen with an ophthalmoscope.

eyelash (i'lash) cilium; one of the hairs growing on the edge of an eyelid.

eyelid (i'lid) either of two movable folds (upper and lower) protecting the anterior surface of the eyeball.

eyepiece (i'pēs) the lens or system of lenses of a microscope (or telescope) nearest the user's eye, serving to further magnify the image produced by the objective.

eyestrain (i'strān) eye fatigue caused by overuse of the eye or by an uncorrected defect in focus of the eye.

F

F chemical symbol, *fluorine.*

F. Fahrenheit; field of vision; formula; French (catheter size).

F_1 first filial generation, a term used in genetics.

F_2 second filial generation, a term used in genetics.

fabella (fah-bel'ah), pl. *fabel'lae* [L.] a sesamoid fibrocartilage in the gastrocnemius muscle. (See table of BONES.)

fabism (fa'bizm) favism.

Fabry's disease (syndrome) (fah-brēz') a hereditary disorder of phospholipid metabolism (see also ANGIOKERATOMA CORPORIS DIFFUSUM).

face (fās) 1. the anterior, or ventral, aspect of the head from the forehead to the chin, inclusive. 2. any presenting aspect or surface. adj. **fa'cial.**

moon f., the peculiar rounded face seen in various conditions, such as in Cushing's syndrome, or after administration of adrenal corticoids.

facet (fas'et) a small, plane surface on a hard body, such as a bone.

facetectomy (fas"ĕ-tek'to-me) excision of the articular facet of a vertebra.

faci(o)- word element [L.], *face.*

facial (fa'shal) of or pertaining to the face.

f. nerve, the seventh cranial nerve; its motor fibers supply the muscles of facial expression. These are a complex group of cutaneous muscles that move the eyebrows, skin of the forehead, corners of the mouth, and other parts of the face concerned with frowning, smiling, achieving a look of surprise, or any of the many and varied expressions of emotion. The sensory fibers of the facial nerve provide a sense of taste in the forward two-thirds of the tongue, and also supply the submaxillary, sublingual, and lacrimal glands for secretion.

Irritation of the facial nerve can produce a paralysis known as BELL'S PALSY. Usually the paralysis involves only one side of the face with a resulting distortion of facial expression, inability to close the mouth on one side, and difficulty in closing the eye on the affected side.

facies (fa'she-ēz), pl. *fa'cies* [L.] 1. the face. 2. a specific surface of a body structure, part, or organ. 3. the expression or appearance of the face.

adenoid f., the dull expression with open mouth, in children with adenoid growths.

f. hepat'ica, a thin face with sunken eyeballs, sallow complexion, and yellow conjunctivae, characteristic of certain chronic liver disorders.

f. hippocrat'ica, a drawn, pinched, and livid appearance indicative of approaching death.

f. leonti'na, a peculiar, deeply furrowed, lion-like appearance of the face seen in certain cases of advanced lepromatous leprosy.

Parkinson's f., parkinsonian f., a stolid masklike expression of the face, with infrequent blinking, which is pathognomonic of PARKINSON'S DISEASE.

facilitation (fah-sil"ĭ-ta'shun) hastening or assistance of a natural process; the increased excitability of a neuron after stimulation by a subthreshold presynaptic impulse. The resistance is diminished so that second application of the stimulus evokes the reaction more easily.

faciobrachial (fa"she-o-bra'ke-al) pertaining to the face and arm.

faciocervical (fa"she-o-ser'vĭ-kal) pertaining to the face and neck.

faciolingual (fa"she-o-ling'gwal) pertaining to the face and tongue.

facioplasty (fa'she-o-plas"te) restorative or plastic surgery of the face.

facioplegia (fa"she-o-ple'je-ah) facial paralysis. adj., **faciople'gic.**

facioscapulohumeral (fa"she-o-skap"u-lo-hu'meral) pertaining to the face, scapula, and arm.

F.A.C.O.G. Fellow of the American College of Obstetricians and Gynecologists.

F.A.C.P. Fellow of American College of Physicians.

F.A.C.S. Fellow of American College of Surgeons.

F.A.C.S.M. Fellow of the American College of Sports Medicine.

factitial (fak-tish'al) artifically produced; produced unintentionally.

factitious (fak-tish'us) artificial; not natural.

factor (fak'tor) an agent or element that contributes to the production of a result.

accelerator f., factor V, one of the CLOTTING factors.

antianemia f., extrinsic factor (see CYANOCOBALAMIN and VITAMIN B_{12}).

antihemophilic f., AHF, factor VIII, one of the CLOTTING factors.

antihemorrhagic f., vitamin K.

antinuclear f. (ANF), an autoantibody against constituents of cell nuclei, present in the sera in systemic lupus erythematosus and occasionally in rheumatoid arthritis and other collagen diseases.

antipernicious anemia f., cyanocobalamin.

antirachitic f., vitamin D.

antiscorbutic f., ascorbic acid.

antisterility f., vitamin E.

citrovorum f., folinic acid, a factor necessary for the growth of *Leuconostoc citrovorum.*

clotting f's, coagulation f's, factors essential to normal blood clotting, whose absence, diminution, or excess may lead to abnormality of the clotting mechanism; 12 factors, commonly designated by Roman numerals (I to V and VII to XIII) have been described (factor VI is no longer considered to have a clotting function). PLATELET FACTORS, designated by Arabic numerals, also play a role in clotting (see also CLOTTING).

extrinsic f., a hematopoietic vitamin that combines with intrinsic factor for absorption from the intestine and is needed for erythrocyte maturation; called also CYANOCOBALAMIN and VITAMIN B_{12}.

F f., fertility f., the episome that determines the mating type of conjugating bacteria, being present in the donor (male) bacterium and absent in the recipient (female).

fibrin stabilizing f., factor XIII, one of the CLOTTING factors.

Hageman f., factor XII, one of the CLOTTING factors.

intrinsic f., a glycoprotein secreted by gastric glands, necessary for the absorption of VITAMIN B_{12} (cyanocobalamin, extrinsic factor). Its absence results in pernicious anemia.

LE f., an immunoglobulin (a 7S antibody) that reacts with leukocyte nuclei, found in the serum in systemic lupus erythematosus.

modifying f's, multiple factors which affect the degree of expressivity of another gene.

multiple f's, two or more genes that cooperate, blend, or cumulate to produce a certain characteristic.

platelet f's, factors important in hemostasis that are contained in or attached to the platelets (see also PLATELET FACTORS).

R f., resistance f., the bacterial plasmid (R plasmid) responsible for resistance to antibiotics; it is transmitted to other bacterial cells by conjugation, as well as to the progeny of any cell containing it.

Rh f., Rhesus f., genetically determined antigens present on the surface of erythrocytes; incompatibility for these antigens between mother and offspring is responsible for ERYTHROBLASTOSIS FETALIS (see also RH FACTOR).

rheumatoid f., a protein of high molecular weight in the serum of most patients with rheumatoid arthritis, detectable by serologic tests.

spreading f., hyaluronidase.

Stuart f., Stuart-Prower f., factor X, one of the CLOTTING factors.

transfer f. (TF), a factor occurring in sensitized lymphocytes that has the capacity to transfer delayed hypersensitivity to a normal (nonreactive) individual.

facultative (fak'ul-ta″tiv) not obligatory; pertaining to or characterized by the ability to adjust to particular circumstances or to assume a particular role.

f. anaerobe, a microorganism that can live and grow with or without molecular oxygen.

faculty (fak'ul-te) 1. a normal power or function, especially of the mind. 2. the teaching staff of an institute of learning.

FAD flavin-adenine dinucleotide.

fae- for words beginning thus, see those beginning *fe-*.

Fahr-Volhard disease (far fōl'hart) the malignant form of arteriolar nephrosclerosis.

Fahrenheit scale (far'en-hīt) a temperature scale with the ice point at 32 and the normal boiling point of water at 212 degrees (212° F.). (For equivalents of Fahrenheit and Celsius temperatures, see Appendix.)

Fahrenheit thermometer (far'en-hīt) a thermometer employing the Fahrenheit scale. The abbreviation 100° F. should be read "one hundred degrees Fahrenheit."

failure (fāl'yer) inability to perform or to function properly.

heart f., inability of the heart to maintain a circulation sufficient to meet the body's needs (see also HEART FAILURE).

kidney f., renal f., inability of the kidney to excrete metabolites at normal plasma levels under normal loading, or inability to retain electrolytes when intake is normal; in the acute form, marked by uremia and usually by oliguria, with hyperkalemia and pulmonary edema.

respiratory f., ventilatory f., a life-threatening condition in which respiratory function is inadequate to maintain the body's needs for oxygen supply and carbon dioxide removal while at rest (see also RESPIRATORY FAILURE).

faint (fānt) temporary loss of consciousness due to generalized cerebral ischemia; syncope. This may be due to a nervous reaction stemming from such causes as fear, hunger, pain, or any emotional or physical shock. Although fainting may be considered a very mild form of shock, it is not as serious and usually is not accompanied by the rapid, weak pulse and cold, clammy skin characteristic of true shock.

The person who is about to faint should be made to lie down with the legs somewhat elevated, and collar and clothing loosened. If this is not feasible, he should lower his head between his knees for about 5 minutes.

If a person has lost consciousness, he should be kept lying down with the feet and legs slightly elevated. Tight clothing should be loosened. Smelling salts (ammonium carbonate) or aromatic spirits of ammonia may be held under the victim's nose until he revives. Prolonged loss of consciousness indicates a condition more serious than simple fainting and should be treated by a physician.

falcial (fal'shal) pertaining to a falx.

falciform (fal'sĭ-form) sickle-shaped.

f. ligament, a sickle-shaped sagittal fold of peritoneum that helps to attach the liver to the diaphragm and separates the right and left lobes of the liver.

falcular (fal'ku-lar) falciform.

fallopian tube (fah-lo'pe-an) uterine tube.

Fallot's tetralogy (fal-ōz' tĕ-tral'o-je) a combination of congenital cardiac defects, namely, pulmonary stenosis, ventricular septal defects, dextroposition of the aorta, so that it overrides the interventricular septum and receives venous as well as arterial blood, and right ventricular hypertrophy (see also TETRALOGY OF FALLOT).

fallout (fawl'owt) the settling to the earth's surface of radioactive fission products from the atmosphere after a nuclear explosion.

falx (falks), pl. *fal'ces* [L.] a sickle-shaped structure.

f. cerebel'li, the fold of dura mater separating the cerebellar hemispheres.

f. cer'ebri, a sickle-shaped fold of dura mater in the longitudinal fissure, which separates the two cerebral hemispheres.

F.A.M.A. Fellow of American Medical Association.

familial (fah-mil'e-al) occurring in or affecting members of a family more than would be expected by chance.

family (fam'ĭ-le) 1. a group descended from a common ancestor. 2. a taxonomic category subordinate to an order (or suborder) and superior to a tribe (or subfamily).

Fanconi's syndrome (disease) (fan-kōn'ēz) 1. a hereditary disorder marked by pancytopenia, hypoplasia of bone marrow, patchy brown skin discoloration due to melanin deposition, and multiple musculoskeletal and genitourinary anomalies. 2. a hereditary disorder marked by aminoaciduria, glycosuria, hyperphosphaturia, deposition of cystine throughout the body, and by rickets, osteomalacia, and short stature.

Fannia (fan'e-ah) a genus of flies whose larvae

have caused both intestinal and urinary infestation in man.

fantasy (fan'tah-se) an imagined sequence of events or mental images that serves to satisfy unconscious wishes or to express unconscious conflicts.

farad (far'ad) the unit of electric capacity; capacity to hold 1 coulomb with a potential of 1 volt.

faradism (far'ah-dizm) 1. faradization. 2. induced current.

faradization (far"ah-dĭ-za'shun) therapeutic use of interrupted current.

farcy (far'se) the more chronic and constitutional form of GLANDERS.

farsightedness (far-sīt'ed-nes) a condition in which vision for distant objects is better than for near objects; called also HYPEROPIA.

fascia (fash'e-ah), pl. *fas'ciae* [L.] a sheet or band of fibrous tissue such as lies deep to the skin or invests muscles and various body organs. adj., **fas'cial.**

aponeurotic f., a dense, firm, fibrous membrane investing the trunk and limbs and giving off sheaths to the various muscles.

f. cribro'sa, the superficial fascia of the thigh covering the saphenous opening.

crural f., the investing fascia of the leg.

deep f., aponeurotic fascia.

endothoracic f., that beneath the serous lining of the thoracic cavity.

extrapleural f., a prolongation of the endothoracic fascia sometimes found at the root of the neck, important as possibly modifying the auscultatory sounds at the apex of the lung.

f. la'ta, the external investing fascia of the thigh.

Scarpa's f., the deep, membranous layer of the subcutaneous abdominal fascia.

superficial f., 1. a fascial sheet lying directly beneath the skin. 2. subcutaneous tissue.

thyrolaryngeal f., the fascia covering the thyroid gland and attached to the cricoid cartilage.

transverse f., that between the transversalis muscle and the peritoneum.

fascicle (fas'ĭ-k'l) a small bundle or cluster, especially of nerve or muscle fibers.

fascicular (fah-sik'u-lar) clustered together; pertaining to or arranged in bundles or clusters; pertaining to a fascicle.

fasciculated (fah-sik'u-lāt-ed) clustered together or occurring in bundles, or fasciculi.

fasciculation (fah-sik"u-la'shun) 1. the formation of fasicles. 2. a small local involuntary muscular contraction visible under the skin, representing spontaneous discharge of a number of fibers innervated by a single motor nerve filament.

fasciculus (fah-sik'u-lus), pl. *fascic'uli* [L.] fascicle.

f. cuneatus of medulla oblongata, the continuation into the medulla oblongata of the fasciculus cuneatus of the spinal cord.

f. cuneatus of spinal cord, the lateral portion of the posterior funiculus of the spinal cord, composed of ascending fibers that end in the nucleus cuneatus.

f. gracilis of medulla oblongata, the continuation into the medulla oblongata of the fasciculus gracilis of the spinal cord.

f. gracilis of spinal cord, the median portion of the posterior funiculus of the spinal cord, composed of ascending fibers that end in the nucleus gracilis.

fasciectomy (fas"e-ek'to-me) excision of fascia.

fasciitis (fas"e-i'tis) inflammation of a fascia.

nodular f., proliferative f., a benign, reactive proliferation of fibroblasts in the subcutaneous tissues and commonly associated with the deep fascia.

pseudosarcomatous f., a benign soft tissue tumor occurring subcutaneously and sometimes arising from deep muscle and fascia.

fasciodesis (fas"e-od'ĕ-sis) suture of a fascia to skeletal attachment.

Fasciola (fah-si'o-lah) a genus of flukes.

F. hepat'ica, the common liver fluke of herbivores, occasionally found in the human liver.

fasciola (fah-si'o-lah), pl. *fasci'olae* [L.] 1. a small band or striplike structure. 2. a small bandage. adj., **fasi'olar.**

fascioliasis (fas"e-o-li'ah-sis) infection with *Fasciola.*

fasciolopsiasis (fas"e-o-lop-si"ah-sis) infection with *Fasciolopsis.*

Fasciolopsis (fas"e-o-lop'sis) a genus of trematodes.

F. bus'ki, the largest of the intestinal flukes, found in the small intestines of residents throughout Asia.

fascioplasty (fas'e-o-plas"te) plastic repair of a fascia.

fasciorrhaphy (fas"e-or'ah-fe) repair of a lacerated fascia.

fasciotomy (fas"e-ot'o-me) incision of a fascia.

fast (fast) 1. immovable, or unchangeable; resistant to the action of a specific drug, stain, or destaining agent. 2. abstention from food.

fastigium (fas-tij'e-um) [L.] 1. the highest point in the roof of the fourth ventricle of the brain. 2. the acme, or highest point. adj., **fastig'ial.**

fat (fat) 1. the adipose or fatty tissue of the body. 2. an oily substance consisting of glycerin (a form of alcohol called also glycerol) and a group of fatty acids, chiefly palmitic, stearic, and oleic acids, combined as glycerin esters. Fats consist of carbon, hydrogen, and oxygen in various chemical combinations. They occur in most foods, especially in meats and dairy products. Fats may be solid such as butter, or liquid, such as olive oil.

The fat-soluble vitamins, A, D, and K, are found in fats. Between 15 and 35 per cent of the average human diet is fat, and about 95 per cent of the fat we eat is absorbed and utilized or stored in the body. In addition, fat is produced by the body from carbohydrates and some from proteins. Fat accounts for some 15 per cent of the average person's body weight.

Digestion of fat is accomplished in the intestines. The products of fat digestion are absorbed through the intestinal walls and distributed by the blood to various storage regions in the body. Some fat is used for tissue building but most of it is stored for future energy needs. These reserves are continuously being converted into carbohydrates for the body's work, and are continuously being replaced by new reserves.

When the intake of food exceeds the energy needs of the body, the food stored as fat accumulates in layers under the skin. Such fat layers provide insulation for the body against low temperatures. The insulating effect is due to the fact that there are few blood vessels in fatty tissue, and hence the heat of circulating blood is lost slowly from the body.

OBESITY. Although people vary in their tendency to put on fat, OBESITY is almost invariably the result of eating more than one needs. Obesity is a definite hazard to health. It places an unnatural burden on the heart and for this reason is a common cause of CORONARY OCCLUSION (heart attack). DIABETES MELLITUS and ARTERIOSCLEROSIS are major and serious diseases associated with obesity.

SATURATED AND UNSATURATED FATS. Fats are composed of FATTY ACIDS in various combinations with glycerin. These fatty acids (and the fats they form) can be classified as saturated or unsaturated. The molecules of saturated fatty acids are constructed with single bonds between the carbon and hydrogen atoms so that they contain all the hydrogen possible; i.e., they are "saturated" with hydrogen. Unsaturated fatty acids contain double bonds so that they can take on more hydrogen under certain conditions. All of the common unsaturated fatty acids are liquid at room temperature. Through the process of hydrogenation, hydrogen can be incorporated into certain unsaturated fatty acids so that they are converted into solid fats for cooking purposes. Margarine is an example of the hydrogenation of unsaturated fatty acids into a solid substance.

Research has indicated that the unsaturated fats (called also polyunsaturates) are less likely than saturated fats to be used by the body in ways injurious to health. The theory supporting this claim is that the body's normal supply of cholesterol and its concentration in serum are increased by saturated fats, which are found mainly in animal fats, such as meat, butter, and eggs. The unsaturated fats, found in large quantities in vegetable oils such as corn oil and safflower oil, are thought to help reduce the amount of cholesterol in the blood. Some researchers hold that eating foods rich in cholesterol itself, such as the animal fats, will also increase the amount of cholesterol in the blood.

Although the body's own normal production of cholesterol is essential to the functioning of body systems, it is known that the formation of fatty deposits in the arteries, a condition called ATHEROSCLEROSIS, can impede the flow of blood and cause damage to the coronary arteries of the heart and other arteries. Cholesterol is recognized as an important factor in these conditions, although its exact contribution is still not clear (see also CHOLESTEROL).

fatal (fa'tal) causing death; deadly; mortal; lethal.

fatigability (fat″ĭ-gah-bil′ĭ-te) easy susceptibility to fatigue.

fatigue (fah-tēg′) a state of increased discomfort and decreased efficiency resulting from prolonged exertion; a generalized feeling of tiredness or exhaustion; loss of power or capacity to respond to stimulation. Fatigue is a normal reaction to intense physical exertion, emotional strain, or lack of rest. It is the body's way of saying that one ought to slow down, relax, and get more rest and sleep. Fatigue that is not relieved by rest may have a more serious origin. It may be a symptom of generally poor physical condition, of specific disease, or of severe emotional stress.

Poor living habits, including improper diet, lack of sleep, and insufficient fresh air and exercise, are a common cause of fatigue. Often, however, fatigue signals an oncoming illness. Fatigue is associated with a wide variety of diseases, including tuberculosis, anemia, thyroid disorders, heart ailments, diabetes mellitus, and cancer.

Sometimes fatigue is psychologic in origin. Tiredness and a loss of interest in one's work may actually result from boredom with the daily routine. If one is certain that there is nothing wrong physically, steps should be taken to vary the daily round, to seek new and more active ways to spend leisure time, perhaps to revive old interests that have been neglected.

Sometimes the demands made upon a person's nervous system are excessive and nervous exhaustion, or nervous prostration, occurs. This state of abnormal fatigue is usually brought on by the inability to cope emotionally with long periods of trouble. Insomnia combines with deep discouragement, and the person is mentally and physically exhausted. The resulting symptoms are sometimes grouped together under the descriptive term, neurasthenia, or nerve weakness. They include poor memory, irritability, aches and pains, lack of appetite, heart palpitations, and dizziness. Occasionally because of his emotional state, the person has difficulty with a particular organ and may suffer from an imaginary ailment. A cardiac neurosis, in which the individual is convinced he has heart disease, is fairly common. The combat fatigue suffered by soldiers in battle is a type of neurosis.

fatty (fat'e) pertaining to or characterized by fat.

f. acid, an organic compound of carbon, hydrogen, and oxygen that combines with glycerin to form fat. All fats are esters of fatty acids and glycerin, the fatty acids accounting for 90 percent of the molecule of most natural fats. Fatty acids may be saturated or unsaturated, depending on their content of hydrogen. Saturated fatty acids contain all the hydrogen atoms possible in the molecule. They are solid at room temperature and are the components of the common animal fats, such as butter and lard. Unsaturated fatty acids contain one or more free bonds which allow for taking on more hydrogen atoms under certain conditions; in other words, they are not "saturated" with hydrogen atoms. The unsaturated fatty acids are liquid at room temperaure and are found in oils such as olive oil and linseed oil.

From a nutritional standpoint, some fatty acids are essential for proper growth and metabolism, and a deficiency of these fatty acids can lead to eczema and other skin disorders. Such deficiencies are rare, however, because the fatty acids occur in abundance in many foods, such as butter, whole milk, egg yolk, nuts, and vegetables.

f. degeneration, deposit of fat globules in a tissue.

fauces (faw′sēz) the passage from the mouth to the pharynx. adj., **fau′cial.**

faucitis (faw-si′tis) inflammation of the fauces.

faveolate (fah-ve′o-lāt) honeycombed; alveolate.

faveolus (fah-ve′o-lus) foveola.

favism (fa′vizm) an acute hemolytic anemia caused by ingestion of fava beans or inhalation of the pollen of the plant, usually occurring in certain individuals as a result of a genetic abnormality with a deficiency in an enzyme, glucose-6-phosphate dehydrogenase, in the erythrocytes. Called also fabism.

favus (fa′vus) a type of tinea capitis, with formation of prominent honeycomb-like masses, due to *Trichophyton schoenleini.*

F-Cortef (ef-kor′tef) trademark for a preparation of fludrocortisone, a synthetic corticoid.

F.D. fatal (lethal) dose; focal distance.

F.D.A. Food and Drug Administration.

Fe chemical symbol, *iron* (L. *ferrum.*)

fear (fēr) a normal emotional response, in contrast to anxiety and phobia, to consciously recognized external sources of danger; it is manifested by alarm, apprehension, or disquiet.

febricide (feb′rĭ-sīd) lowering bodily temperature; an agent that so acts.

febrifacient (feb″rĭ-fa′shent) producing fever.

febrifuge (feb″rĭ-fūj) an agent that reduces body temperature in fever; antipyretic.

febrile (feb′ril) pertaining to fever; feverish.

fecal (fe′kal) pertaining to or of the nature of feces.

f. impaction, accumulation of putty-like or hardened feces in the rectum or sigmoid. The condition often occurs in patients with long-standing bowel problems and chronic constipation. It also may develop when barium is introduced into the intestinal tract and not completely removed.

Symptoms include painful defecation, feeling of fullness in the rectum, and constipation or a diarrheic stool. Rectal examination reveals a hard or putty-like mass. The condition can be prevented in most cases by adequate removal of barium after radiologic studies, and by careful monitoring of the bowel movements of elderly patients with bowel problems.

Fecal impaction usually requires digital removal with a gloved finger to break up the mass. Prior to removal the patient is given an oil retention ENEMA to help soften the mass. An injection of 30 to 60 ml. of hydrogen peroxide may help break up the fecal mass through foaming action.

fecalith (fe′kah-lith) an intestinal concretion formed around a center of fecal material.

fecaloid (fe′kal-oid) resembling feces.

fecaloma (fe″kal-o′mah) a tumor-like accumulation of feces in the rectum; stercoroma.

fecaluria (fe″kal-u′re-ah) the presence of fecal matter in the urine.

feces (fe′sēz), pl. of faex [L.] body waste discharged from the intestine; called also stool, excreta, or excrement. The feces are formed in the colon and pass down into the rectum by the process of peristalsis. When the rectum is sufficiently distended, nerve endings in its wall signal a need for evacuation, which is made possible by a voluntary relaxation of the sphincter muscles around the outer part of the anus.

The frequency of bowel movements varies according to the individual body make-up, type of intestine, eating habits, physical activity, and custom. Although one bowel movement a day is the average, a movement every 2 or 3 days may be considered normal. A balanced diet and an established routine can promote regular bowel movements.

CHARACTERISTICS. Normally the stool is soft and formed and brownish in color. An abnormality in color, odor, or consistency usually indicates a disorder of the intestinal tract or of the accessory organs of the digestive system. Black, tarry stools may indicate intestinal bleeding, especially in the upper portion of the tract. Some drugs, such as those containing iron or bismuth, can produce tarry stools. Bright red blood in the feces can indicate a wide variety of disorders ranging from HEMORRHOIDS to a malignancy of the rectum. Clay-colored stools result from an absence or deficiency of BILE in the intestinal tract, and indicate obstruction of the biliary tract or decreased production of bile by the liver. Greenish-colored feces often accompany diarrhea, especially in infants, and may be caused by growth of certain bacteria.

Bulky, fatty stools, having a foul odor, are characteristic of CYSTIC FIBROSIS. Other causes of fatty feces include GALLBLADDER disease, pancreatic disorders, SPRUE, and excessive intake of fat in the diet. Feces containing large amounts of mucus often occur in COLITIS and other irritations of the intestinal tract.

The stool of a newborn, full-term infant is called meconium. It is a dark greenish brown color, smooth and semisolid in consistency.

DISINFECTION. In many types of communicable diseases it is necessary to decontaminate the feces before they are flushed into the sewage system. Chlorinated lime, Lysol, or formalin may be used for this purpose. The contents of the bedpan used by the patient should be thoroughly covered with the disinfectant and allowed to stand for several hours. The contents are then disposed of in a hopper or commode, and the bedpan is rinsed and sterilized, preferably with live steam or by autoclave.

OBSERVATIONS. Because the characteristics of the feces can be of help in the diagnosis of various diseases, it is important to inspect the stool for color, consistency, odor, and number of stools per day. Abnormalities should be noted on the patient's chart or reported to the physician.

SPECIMENS. A sample of the feces (stool specimen) may be required as a diagnostic aid. The specimen should be collected in a sterile bedpan and transferred into a sterile container, using a wooden spatula or tongue blade for this purpose. In order for certain types of intestinal parasites to be discovered in the feces, the specimen must be fresh and kept warm until examined in the laboratory. Microorganisms that may be detected include the typhoid and paratyphoid bacilli, the anthrax bacilli, and *Entomoeba histolytica,* which causes AMEBIC DYSENTERY.

Specimens of the feces may be examined for occult (hidden) blood. This test is indicated when intestinal bleeding is suspected but the stools do not appear to contain blood when examined by gross inspection.

feculent (fek′u-lent) 1. having dregs or sediment. 2. excrementitious.

fecundation (fe″kun-da′shun) fertilization; impregnation.

fecundity (fe-kun′dĭ-te) the ability to produce offspring frequently and in large numbers. In demography, the physiological ability to reproduce, as opposed to fertility.

feeblemindedness (fe″b′l-mīnd′ed-nes) former name for MENTAL RETARDATION.

feedback (fēd′bak) the return of some of the output of a system as input so as to exert some control in the process; feedback is negative when the return exerts an inhibitory control; positive when it exerts a stimulatory effect.

feeding (fēd′ing) the taking or giving of food.

artificial f., feeding of a baby with food other than mother's milk.

breast f., the feeding of an infant at the breast (see also BREAST FEEDING).

forced f., administration of food by force to those who cannot or will not receive it.

intravenous f., administration of nutrient fluids through a vein (see also INTRAVENOUS INFUSION).

sham f., feeding in which the food is chewed and swallowed but does not enter the stomach, because of diversion to the exterior by an esophageal fistula or other device.

tube f., feeding of liquids and semisolid foods through a nasogastric tube (see also TUBE FEEDING).

Feer's disease (fārz) erythredema polyneuropathy.

Fehling's solution (fa'lingz) (1) 34.66 gm. cupric sulfate in water to make 500 ml.; (2) 173 gm. crystallized potassium and sodium tartrate and 50 gm. sodium hydroxide in water to make 500 ml.; mix equal volumes of (1) and (2) at time of use.

Feingold diet (fīn'gōld) a special diet used in the control of HYPERACTIVITY in children. The dietary program requires avoiding all foods containing artificial color and flavoring, and limiting the intake of fruits and vegetables in which salicylates occur naturally. Among these are apples, apricots, blackberries, cucumbers, grapes, oranges, peaches, plums, raspberries, tea, and tomatoes.

fellatio (fĕ-la'she-o) oral stimulation or manipulation of the penis.

felon (fel'on) a purulent infection involving the pulp of the distal phalanx of a finger.

feltwork (felt'werk) a complex of closely interwoven fibers, as of nerve fibers.

Felty's syndrome (fel'tēz) chronic (rheumatoid) arthritis, splenomegaly, leukopenia, pigmented spots on the skin of the legs, and other inconsistent evidence of hypersplenism, namely, anemia and thrombocytopenia.

female (fe'māl) 1. an individual of the sex that produces ova or bears young. 2. feminine.

feminine (fem'ĭ-nin) pertaining to the female sex, or having qualities normally characteristic of the female.

feminism (fem'ĭ-nizm) the appearance or existence of female secondary sex characters in the male.

feminization (fem"ĭ-nĭ-za'shun) 1. the normal induction or development of female sex characters. 2. the induction or development of female secondary sex characters in the male.

testicular f., a condition in which the subject is phenotypically female, but lacks nuclear sex chromatin and is of XY chromosomal sex.

femoral (fem'o-ral) pertaining to the femur or to the thigh.

f. artery, the chief artery of the thigh (see table of ARTERIES).

f. canal, the medial part of the femoral sheath lateral to the base of the lacunar ligament.

f. nerve, the largest branch of the lumbar plexus (see table of NERVES).

f. triangle, the area formed superiorly by the inguinal ligament, laterally by the sartorius muscle, and medially by the adductor longus muscle. Called also Scarpa's triangle.

f. vein, the chief vein of the thigh (see table of VEINS).

femorocele (fem'o-ro-sēl") femoral hernia.

femorotibial (fem"o-ro"tib'e-al) pertaining to the femur and tibia.

femto- (fem'to) a combining form used in naming units of measurement to indicate one-quadrillionth (10^{-15}) of the unit designated by the root with which it is combined.

femur (fe'mur), pl. *fem'ora* [L.] 1. the thigh bone, extending from the pelvis to the knee; the longest and strongest bone in the body. Its proximal end articulates with the acetabulum, a cup-like cavity in the pelvic girdle. The greater and lesser trochanters are the two processes (prominences) at the proximal end of the femur. 2. the thigh.

fenestra (fĕ-nes'trah), pl. *fenes'trae* [L.] a window-like opening.

f. coch'leae, a round opening in the inner wall of the middle ear covered by the secondary tympanic membrane; called also round window.

f. vestib'uli, an oval opening in the inner wall of the middle ear, which is closed by the stapes; called also oval window.

fenestrate (fen'es-trāt) to pierce with one or more openings.

fenestration (fen"es-tra'shun) 1. the act of perforating or the condition of being perforated. 2. the surgical creation of a new opening in the labyrinth of the ear for the restoration of hearing in otosclerosis.

aortopulmonary f., aortic septal defect.

fenfluramine (fen-flōōr'ah-mēn) an anorectic that seems to depress rather than stimulate the central nervous system, as do the amphetamines; used as the hydrochloride salt.

fentanyl (fen'tah-nil) a piperidine derivative; the citrate salt is used as a narcotic analgesic, and in combination with droperidol as a neuroleptanalgesic.

Feosol (fe'o-sol) trademark for preparations of ferrous sulfate, an iron preparation.

Fergon (fer'gon) trademark for preparations of ferrous gluconate, an iron preparation.

ferment (fer'ment) 1. to undergo fermentation. 2. any substance that causes fermentation.

fermentation (fer"men-ta'shun) enzymatic decomposition, especially of carbohydrates; the anaerobic conversion of foodstuffs to particular products, as opposed to aerobic conversion (oxidation).

fermium (fer'me-um) a chemical element, atomic number 100, atomic weight 253, symbol Fm. (See table of ELEMENTS.)

ferning (fern'ing) the appearance of a fernlike pattern in a dried specimen of cervical mucus, an indication of the presence of estrogen.

-ferous word element [L.], *bearing; producing.*

ferredoxin (fer"ĕ-dok'sin) a nonheme iron-containing protein, also having a high sulfide content, which serves as an acceptor molecule in electron transport from chlorophyll during the formation of NADPH in photosynthesis.

ferric (fer'ik) containing iron in its plus-three oxidation state, Fe(III) (sometimes designated Fe^{3+}).

f. chloride, $FeCl_3$, used as a reagent and topically as an astringent and antiseptic.

ferritin (fer'ĭ-tin) the iron-apoferritin complex, one of the forms in which iron is stored in the body.

ferrocholinate (fer"o-ko'lin-āt) a compound of ferric hydroxide and choline dihydrogen citrate, used orally in iron-deficiency anemia.

ferrokinetics (fer"o-ki-net'iks) the turnover or rate of change of iron in the body.

Ferrolip (fer'o-lip) trademark for preparations of ferrocholinate, a hematinic.

ferroprotein (fer"o-pro'te-in) a protein combined

with an iron-containing radical; ferroproteins are respiratory carriers.

ferrotherapy (fer″o-ther′ah-pe) therapeutic use of iron and iron compounds.

ferrous (fer′us) containing iron in its plus-two oxidation state, Fe(II) (sometimes designated Fe^{2+}).

f. carbonate, $FeCO_3$; a hematinic useful in treatment of iron deficiency anemia but extremely irritating to the gastric and intestinal mucosa.

f. fumarate, the anhydrous salt of a combination of ferrous iron and fumaric acid; used as a hematinic.

f. gluconate, a hematinic that is less irritating to the gastrointestinal tract than other hematinics, and generally used as a substitute when ferrous sulfate cannot be tolerated.

f. sulfate, the most widely used hematinic for the treatment of iron deficiency anemia. It is believed to be less irritating then equivalent amounts of ferric salts and is more effective.

All iron preparations should be administered after meals, never on an empty stomach. The patient should be warned that the drugs cause stools to turn dark green or black. Overdosage may cause severe systemic reactions.

ferrum (fer′um) [L.] iron (symbol Fe).

fertility (fer-til′ĭ-te) the capacity to conceive or to induce conception. adj., **fer′tile.** Many factors, including poor diet, general ill health, and emotional stress, may lessen fertility. Sterility, or a complete inability to conceive children, is fairly rare. Most childless couples can be helped to have children with medical assistance in determining and correcting the conditions which lessen their fertility.

FERTILITY IN WOMEN. Any disturbance of the endocrine glands may lessen fertility. These glands influence every stage of the sexual cycle, from the maturing of the ovum in the ovary to its implantation in the uterus. Thus, an imbalance in the endocrine system may affect fertility in several different ways. The ovum may fail to mature, or may be sterile, or the fertilized ovum may not come to rest properly in the uterus. Many types of endocrine disturbance can now be corrected by administration of hormones.

Any deformation of the reproductive organs may affect fertility. In a few cases, the uterus may be undeveloped. More common, however, is retroverted uterus, which was thought for some years to be a cause of infertility. In those cases in which the retroverted uterus does contribute to infertility, exercises or a mechanical support may often be sufficient to correct the condition.

If the uterine tubes are blocked, the ovum and sperm will be prevented from uniting. This condition can be detected by passing a gas, such as carbon dioxide, into the uterus under controlled pressure. The gas goes into the tubes and, if the tubes are open, escapes into the abdomen, from which it is harmlessly discharged. In some cases, it is thought that the gas may unblock stopped-up tubes, as well as detect them. Similar information is obtained by instilling a radiopaque material into the uterus and tubes and obtaining x-rays. In the rare instances in which a portion of the tube is completely blocked, surgery may be advised. As long as one tube and one ovary continue to function normally, however, the woman continues to be fertile to some degree, even if the tube and the ovary are on opposite sides of the uterus.

Painful intercourse (dyspareunia) may result in infertility by diminishing the frequency of intercourse. This is an abnormal condition and should have medical attention. Pain during intercourse may be a result of a malfunction of the glands that lubricate the vagina. Often the difficulty is psychologic in origin, the result of sexual fears or inhibitions. Most serious of this type of condition is vaginismus, in which the muscles in the vagina contract, blocking the entry of the penis and making intercourse impossible.

Among other conditions that can cause infertility or sterility in women is salpingitis, an inflammation of the uterine tubes, a principal complication of gonorrhea, although it may also result from tuberculosis and other infections. Eventually the tubes become closed at both ends and pus accumulates within them, a condition known as pyosalpinx. Another cause of sterility is chronic cervicitis, resulting in production of mucus harmful to the migration of the sperm into the uterus.

Proper nutrition may be an important factor in fertility. A healthy diet is a necessary part of any treatment designed to remedy infertility. Vitamin supplements are occasionally suggested.

Weight control is another factor in treatment for infertility, since both overweight and underweight women are found to have less than normal fertility.

Emotional stress may directly or indirectly lessen fertility. Repressed hostilities or fears of pregnancy may cause muscle spasms which reduce the chance of pregnancy. Although the effects of emotional factors are still somewhat mysterious, it appears that these factors may affect fertility in other ways as well. Often a couple adopt a child after giving up hope, and unexpectedly have a child of their own shortly afterward, possibly because of the decrease in anxiety. In many cases, psychologic counseling is an important part of treatment for infertility, particularly if the doctor can find no organic reason for it.

FERTILITY IN MEN. At one time, a couple's inability to have children was almost always ascribed to infertility in the wife. It is now recognized that in about 40 per cent of all childless couples, the husband is lacking in fertility. This is not related to virility, which is the ability to perform intercourse, but to the quantity and vitality of the sperm cells in the sexual emission. There is no disturbance of the sexual act.

Impotence in the male is inability to maintain an erection or to achieve orgasm, making coitus impossible. It has no direct relationship with fertility, except that in preventing completion of the sexual act it also prevents conception. An impotent man may be very fertile, because his testes produce many sperm cells, while one who is virile may suffer from decreased fertility. A great many cases of impotence are the result of emotional disturbances, and can often be successfully treated.

The only way of discovering low fertility in the male is by laboratory examination of the semen. To determine the fertility of the male, the physician examines a sample of the semen under the microscope. Infertility may result from too few sperm cells, or from a high proportion of malformed cells, or from a low level of vitality of the sperm. Also, an obstruction in the passages from the testes may block or prevent the exit of the sperm.

Treatment for male infertility varies with the

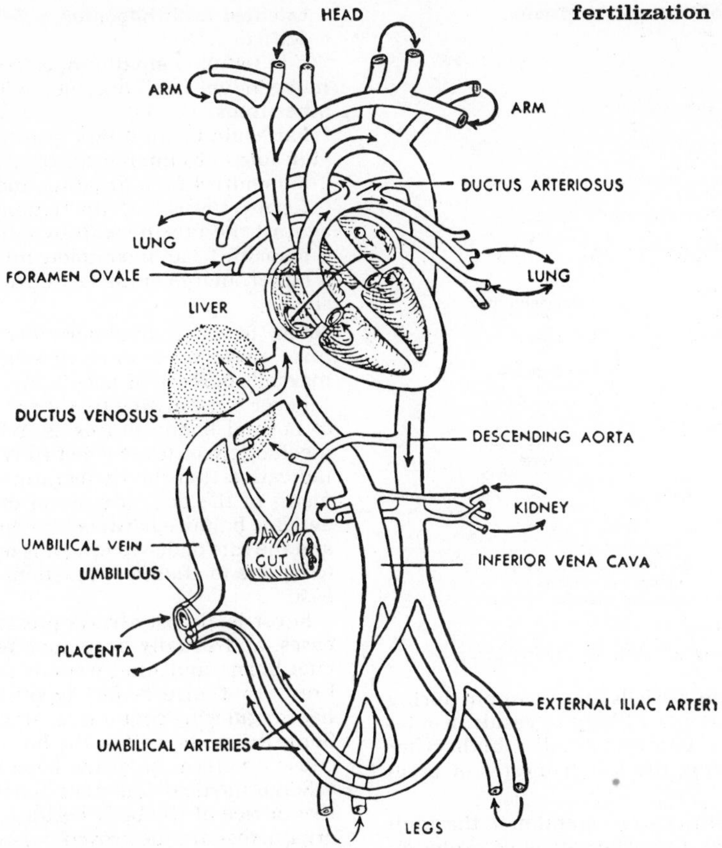

Fetal circulation. (From King, B. G., and Showers, M. J.: Human Anatomy and Physiology. 6th ed. Philadelphia, W. B. Saunders Co., 1969.)

cause of the infertility. In some cases, increased rest and a better diet may be sufficient to raise the level of effective sperm cells. When several factors are involved, medical treatment or psychotherapy may be necessary. In a few cases, the man may be wholly sterile, as may happen as a result of mumps suffered in adolescence or adulthood. Gonorrhea and tuberculosis may also cause sterility.

fertilization (fer″tĭ-lĭ-za′shun) in human reproduction, the process by which the male's sperm unites with the female's ovum. By this event, also called conception, a new life is created and the sex and other biologic traits of the new individual are determined. These traits are determined by the combined genes and chromosomes that exist in the sperm and ovum.

After injection into the vagina, the sperm cells—millions of them—make use of their whiplike tails to swim through the cervix toward the uterus. Most are destroyed along the way by secretions in the vagina, but some reach the uterus and a few may enter the UTERINE TUBES. A very small number may survive as long as 48 hours. If during this period only one sperm succeeds in entering a uterine tube and meeting there an ovum ready to be fertilized, conception can occur. This event is possible only during a period of about 4 days of the month. After the sperm lodges in the ovum, the tail disappears, but the head unites with the ovum to form the embryo. (See also REPRODUCTION.)

fervescence (fer-ves′ens) increase of fever or body temperature.

fester (fes′ter) to suppurate superficially.

festinant (fes′tĭ-nant) accelerating.

festination (fes″tĭ-na′shun) an involuntary tendency to take short accelerating steps in walking.

fetal (fe′tal) of or pertaining to a fetus or to the period of its development.

f. circulation, the circulation of blood through the body of the fetus and to and from the placenta through the umbilical cord. Oxygenated blood from the placenta is carried to the embryo by the umbilical vein. The blood from the embryo is returned to the placenta by two umbilical arteries. Oxygenation of the fetal blood and disposal of its waste products is carried on through the placenta. When the lungs begin to function at birth some of the fetal vessels, such as the ductus arteriosus, and the fetal passages, such as the foramen ovale, begin to fall into disuse. This is a gradual process of fibrosis that takes place in the period after birth.

f. alcohol syndrome, a group of symptoms characterized by mental and physical abnormalities of the infant and linked to the maternal intake of alcohol during pregnancy.

Clinical manifestations, which can be present in varying degrees, include mental retardation, hyperactivity, cardiac and genital abnormalities, a small head with low-set ears, small eyes, flat nose with upturned nostrils, poorly developed extremities, and webbed fingers and toes.

The risk and extent of abnormalities appear to be dose related and are most likely to be increased when the daily intake of pure alcohol exceeds

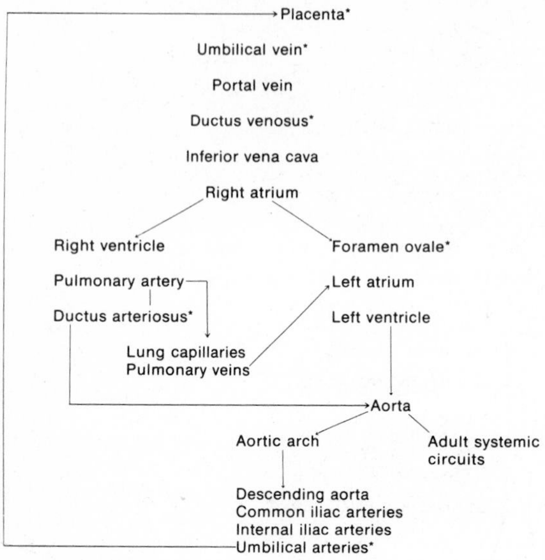

*Cease function at birth or shortly after.

one-half ounce. The periods of gestation during which the alcohol is most likely to result in fetal damage are three to four-and-a-half months after conception and during the last trimester of pregnancy.

fetalization (fe″tal-ĭ-za′shun) retention in the adult of characters that at an earlier stage of evolution were only infantile and were rapidly lost as the organism attained maturity.

fetation (fe-ta′shun) 1. development of the fetus. 2. pregnancy.

feticide (fēt′ĭ-sīd) destruction of the fetus.

fetid (fet′id) having a rank, disagreeable smell.

fetish (fet′ish, fe′tish) an object symbolically endowed with special meaning; e.g., an object or body part with special erotic interest.

fetoglobulin (fe′to-glob′u-lin) fetoprotein.

fetography (fe-tog′rah-fe) roentgenography of the fetus *in utero.*

fetology (fe-tol′o-je) that branch of medicine dealing with the fetus *in utero.*

fetometry (fe-tom′ĕ-tre) measurement of the fetus, especially of its head.

fetoplacental (fe″to-plah-sen′tal) pertaining to the fetus and placenta.

fetoprotein (fe″to-pro′tēn) a fetal antigen that also occurs in adults in certain diseases; α-fetoprotein appears in the serum of patients with hepatoma and embryonal adenocarcinoma; γ-fetoprotein in that of patients with a variety of neoplasms, including sarcomas and leukemias; and β-fetoprotein (found to be identical with normal liver ferritin) in the fetal liver and in adults with a variety of liver diseases.

fetor (fe′tor) stench or offensive odor.

hepatic f., f. hepat′icus, the peculiar odor of the breath characteristic of hepatic disease.

f. o′ris, halitosis.

fetus (fe′tus) [L.] the developing young in the uterus, specifically the unborn offspring in the postembryonic (see also EMBRYO) period, in man from seven or eight weeks after fertilization until birth. adj., **fe′tal.**

calcified f., lithopedion; a fetus that has become calcified.

f. in fet′tu, a small, imperfect fetus, incapable of independent life, contained within the body of another fetus.

harlequin f., an infant affected with the more severe form of lamellar EXFOLIATION of the newborn.

mummified f., a dried-up and shriveled fetus.

f. papyra′ceus, a fetus flattened by being pressed against the uterine wall by a living twin.

parasitic f., an incomplete minor fetus attached to a larger, more completely developed fetus, or autosite.

fever (fe′ver) 1. an abnormally high body temperature; pyrexia. 2. any disease characterized by marked increase of body temperature.

Fever is a warning that there is some disturbance of normal bodily processes. While the physiologic mechanism of fever is not fully understood, it is an indication that the temperature-regulating mechanisms of the body are out of order, and the body's delicate balance between the rate of producing heat and the rate of dissipating it is upset. This is thought to be due to chemical reactions resulting from disease.

Fever is almost always present in infectious diseases, and usually accompanies seriously infected cuts, burns, and other wounds. Abnormalities in the brain that affect the hypothalamus, where the heat-regulating center is located, can produce fever. Some drugs, as well as the hormone thyroxine, can cause an elevation of the body temperature.

Some medical scientists consider fever a protective device of the body because certain pathogenic organisms are destroyed when the temperature rises well above normal. It is also believed that the increased metabolic rate accompanying fever allows the cells to increase their production of immune substances that defend the body against bacterial invasion. Fever brings discomfort, weakness or fatigue, and sometimes pain, causing the patient to rest and in this way conserving his energy for battle against the disease. Sometimes fever itself is destructive, as in SUNSTROKE. Prolonged or very high fever usually must be controlled.

NORMAL AND ABNORMAL TEMPERATURE. Although fever is defined as abnormal temperature increase, it is not always easy to determine when an increase in temperature is abnormal. This is especially true of the lower temperature readings. If the temperature is 37.7° C. (100° F.) by mouth or 38.3° C. (101° F.) or above by rectum, fever is almost decidedly present. However, a mouth temperature of 37.2° C. (99° F.) may or may not indicate fever even though the reading is above the manufacturer's 37° C. (98.6° F.) arrow on the thermometer scale. This arrow indicates normal temperature on the basis of a statistical average, and is by no means the normal temperature for everyone. Normal temperature varies somewhat from person to person. Also, in each person there are slight temperature variations throughout the day.

Since it is sometimes important to judge whether or not fever is present by interpreting readings under the 37.7° C. (100° F.) mark, it is recommended that a person determine his own particular normal, or basal, temperature. This is done by averaging a number of readings taken over a period of time. Once the basal temperature is determined, it can be assumed that when there is an increase of a degree or two above that figure (and in all cases when the reading is over 37.7° C. [100° F.]), fever is present.

There are a few exceptions to this rule. Children often have a slightly raised temperature after lively activity, and adults have a considerably raised temperature while engaged in strenuous sports. This rise is of course temporary and disappears with rest. During and soon after emotional excitement there may also be a rise in temperature. In women there is a slight increase in temperature at the time of ovulation.

EFFECTS OF FEVER. The feverish person feels weak. Often there is a sensation of soreness in muscles and bones, and there may also be chills, headache, thirst, loss of appetite, constipation, a coated tongue, and dry skin. In children a sudden onset of high fever may bring on CONVULSIONS and DELIRIUM although the illness itself may not be serious.

In fever the pulse rate is likely to increase at the rate of about eight to ten beats per minute for each degree of temperature rise. The metabolic rate—the speed of chemical reactions in the body—also increases.

TREATMENT. The treatment of fever includes detection and elimination of the primary cause whenever possible, and the relief of symptoms. Fluids are given orally or intravenously as necessary to prevent dehydration. Frequent, small feedings of high-calorie, high-protein liquids are recommended to combat fatigue and the debility brought about by an increased metabolic rate. Vitamin supplements may be prescribed in prolonged, low-grade fevers.

Antipyretic drugs such as aspirin and sodium salicylate are used when the body temperature rises to a dangerous level. In cases of extreme fever, as in sunstroke, it is sometimes advisable to cool the patient quickly in a bath of cold water. Other measures to reduce body temperature are discussed under PATIENT CARE.

PATIENT CARE. The feverish patient's temperature, pulse, and respiration should be taken and recorded at least every 4 hours, and more frequently if the temperature rises above 38.8° C. (102° F.) or if the patient has chills or signs of delirium. The shivering accompanying a fever is a reaction of the body to the cold of its environment. The patient feels cold because his body temperature is much higher in relation to the surrounding air than it normally is. In response to the stimulus of cold the muscles begin a rhythmic contraction in an effort to produce more heat. When this occurs warmth should be provided the patient in the form of extra blankets and the application of a hot water bottle filled with warm, *not hot,* water. At the same time efforts should be made to bring the body temperature down to the normal range if the physician has left a written order to this effect. Because fever is considered beneficial in some cases, it is important to know the wishes of the physician in regard to the use of nursing measures to reduce fever.

Sponging alternate parts of the body and extremities with cool water or a mixture of alcohol and water is an effective means of reducing fever. The purpose of the sponging is to increase evaporation of moisture and thereby increase heat loss from the body surface. The part being sponged should be left exposed to the air until it is almost dry, and then lightly covered while another part of the body is being sponged. Alcohol is often used with the cool bath water because it evaporates more quickly than water. An ice cap or cold compress to the forehead helps to reduce the fever and relieve headache and delirium. In some instances the physician may order a cool water enema.

During the sponging procedure the patient's temperature is taken every 30 minutes. A sudden reduction in temperature is not desirable, and should the patient's temperature appear to be dropping too quickly the sponge bath is discontinued. After the procedure is completed the bed linens and patient's gown should be changed as necessary to leave him dry and comfortable.

A prolonged or extremely high fever is likely to produce severe dehydration. For this reason the patient is observed for symptoms of fluid depletion, the fluid intake and output are measured and recorded, and the urine is observed for color and concentration. If delirium or convulsions are likely to accompany the fever, side rails should be applied to the bed and someone should be in constant attendance to prevent the patient from injuring himself.

For specific types of fevers, see the eponymic or descriptive name, as TYPHOID FEVER.

f. blister, an itching or stinging sore on the skin or mucous membrane, due to infection with the virus of HERPES SIMPLEX. It often accompanies fever, and is most commonly seen about the lips or nose. Called also herpes febrilis.

continued f., continuous f., persistently elevated body temperature, showing no or little variation and never falling to normal during any 24-hour period.

intermittent f., an attack of MALARIA or other fever, with recurring paroxysms of elevated temperature separated by intervals during which the temperature is normal.

periodic f., a hereditary condition characterized by repetitive febrile episodes and anatomic disturbances, occurring in precise or irregular cycles of days, weeks, or months.

remittent f., elevated body temperature showing fluctuation each day, but never falling to normal.

fiber (fi'ber) an elongated threadlike structure.

A f's, myelinated fibers of the somatic nervous system having a diameter of 1μ to 22μ and a conduction velocity of 5 to 120 meters per second.

accelerating f's, accelerator f's, adrenergic fibers that transmit the impulses which accelerate the heart beat.

adrenergic f's, nerve fibers that liberate epinephrine-like substances at the time of passage of nerve impulses across a synapse.

alpha f's, motor and proprioceptive fibers of the A type having conduction velocities of 70–120 meters per second and ranging from 13μ to 22μ in diameter.

arcuate f's, any of the bow-shaped fibers in the brain, such as those connecting adjacent gyri in the cerebral cortex, or the external or internal arcuate fibers of the medulla oblongata.

association f's, nerve fibers that interconnect portions of the cerebral cortex within a hemisphere. Short association fibers interconnect neighboring gyri; long fibers interconnect more widely separated gyri and are arranged into bundles or fasciculi.

B f's, myelinated preganglionic autonomic axons having a fiber diameter of $\leq 3\mu$ and a conduction velocity of 3 to 15 meters per second.

beta f's, touch and temperature fibers of the A type having conduction velocities of 30–70 meters per second and ranging from 8μ to 13μ in diameter.

C f's, unmyelinated postganglionic fibers of the autonomic nervous system; also, the unmyelinated fibers at the dorsal roots, having a diameter of 0.3μ

to 1.3μ and a conduction velocity of 0.6 to 2.3 meters per second.

cholinergic f's, nerve fibers that liberate acetylcholine at the synapse.

collagenous f., a soft, flexible, white fiber, the most characteristic constituent of all types of connective tissues.

Corti's f's, Corti's rods.

dark f's, muscle fibers rich in sarcoplasm and having a dark appearance.

depressor f's, nerve fibers which, when stimulated reflexly, cause a diminished vasomotor tone and thereby a decrease in arterial pressure.

elastic f's, yellowish fibers of elastic quality traversing the intercellular substance of connective tissue.

gamma f's, A fibers that conduct touch and pressure impulses and innervate the intrafusal fibers of the muscle spindle; they conduct at velocities of 15–40 meters per second and range from 3μ to 7μ in diameter.

gray f's, unmyelinated nerve fibers found largely in the sympathetic nerves.

intrafusal f's, modified muscle fibers which, surrounded by fluid and enclosed in a connective tissue envelope, compose the muscle spindle.

lattice f's, reticular fibers.

light f's, muscle fibers poor in sarcoplasm and more transparent than dark fibers.

medullated f's, myelinated fibers.

motor f's, nerve fibers transmitting motor impulses to a muscle fiber.

muscle f., any of the cells comprising the contractile elements of muscular tissue. (See also Plate 4.)

myelinated f's, grayish white nerve fibers encased in a myelin sheath.

nerve f., a slender process of a neuron, especially the prolonged axon that conducts nerve impulses. (See also Plate 12.)

nonmedullated f's, unmyelinated fibers.

osteogenetic f's, osteogenic f's, precollagenous fibers formed by osteoclasts and becoming the fibrous component of bone matrix.

postganglionic f's, nerve fibers passing to involuntary muscle and gland cells, the cell bodies of which lie in the autonomic ganglia.

preganglionic f's, nerve fibers passing to the autonomic ganglia, the cell bodies of which lie in the brain or spinal cord.

pressor f's, nerve fibers which, when stimulated reflexly, cause or increase vasomotor tone.

projection f's, bundles of axons that connect the cerebral cortex with the subcortical centers, brain stem, and spinal cord.

Purkinje's f's, modified cardiac muscle fibers in the subendothelial tissue concerned with conducting impulses in the heart.

radicular f's, fibers in the roots of the spinal nerves.

reticular f's, immature connective tissue fibers, staining with silver, forming the reticular framework of lymphoid and myeloid tissue, and occurring in interstitial tissue of glandular organs, the papillary layer of the skin, and elsewhere.

Sharpey's f's, those that pass from the periosteum and embed in the periosteal lamellae.

spindle f's, achromatic filaments extending between the poles of a dividing cell and making a spindle-shaped configuration.

T f., a fiber given off at right angles from the axon of a nerve cell.

unmyelinated f's, nerve fibers that lack a myelin sheath.

fibercolonoscope (fi″ber-ko-lōn′o-skōp) a fiberscope for viewing the colon.

fibergastroscope (fi″ber-gas′tro-skōp) a fiberscope for viewing the stomach.

fiber-illuminated (fi′ber-il-loo″min-a′ted) transmitting light by means of bundles of glass or plastic fibers, utilizing a lens system to transmit the image; said of endoscopes of such design.

fiberoptic (fi″ber-op-tik) pertaining to fiberoptics; coated with flexible glass or plastic fibers having special optical properties and orientation.

fiberoptics (fi″ber-op′tiks) the transmission of an image along flexible bundles of glass or plastic fibers having special optical properties and orientation.

fiberscope (fi′ber-skōp) a flexible endoscope whose lumen is coated with fiberoptic glass or plastic fibers having special optical properties.

fibr(o)- word element [L.], *fiber; fibrous.*

fibra (fi′brah), pl. *fi′brae* [L.] fiber.

fibril (fi′bril) a minute fiber or filament. adj., **fibril′lar, fib′rillary.**

fibrillation (fi″brĭ-la′shun) 1. a small, local, involuntary, muscular contraction, due to spontaneous activation of single muscle cells or muscle fibers. 2. the quality of being made up of fibrils. 3. the initial degenerative changes in osteoarthritis, marked by softening of the articular cartilage and development of vertical clefts between groups of cartilage cells.

atrial f., a cardiac arrhythmia marked by rapid randomized contractions of the atrial myocardium, causing a totally irregular, often rapid, ventricular rate.

ventricular f., a cardiac arrhythmia marked by fibrillary contractions of the ventricular muscle due to rapid repetitive excitation of myocardial fibers without coordinated ventricular contraction. Ventricular fibrillation is a frequent cause of CARDIAC ARREST. An apparatus called a defibrillator sometimes is used to alleviate fibrillation. The defibrillator delivers an electric shock to the heart muscle, depolarizing the muscle and ending the irregular contractions. The heart is then able to resume normal, regular contractions.

fibrillogenesis (fi-bril″o-jen′ĕ-sis) the formation and development of fibrils.

fibrin (fi′brin) an insoluble protein that is essential to CLOTTING of blood, formed from fibrinogen by action of thrombin.

fibrinocellular (fi″brĭ-no-sel′u-lar) made up of fibrin and cells.

fibrinogen (fi-brin′o-jen) a high-molecular-weight protein in the blood plasma that by the action of thrombin is converted into fibrin; called also clotting factor I. In the CLOTTING mechanism, fibrin threads form a meshwork for the basis of a blood clot. Most of the fibrinogen in the circulating blood is formed in the liver. Normal quantities of fibrinogen in the plasma vary from 100 to 700 mg. per 100 ml. of plasma.

Commercial preparations of human fibrinogen are used to restore blood fibrinogen levels to normal after extensive surgery, or to treat diseases and hemorrhagic conditions that are complicated by AFIBRINOGENEMIA.

fibrinogenemia (fi-brin″o-jĕ-ne′me-ah) hyperfibrinogenemia.

fibrinogenolysis (fi-brin″o-jĕ-nol′ĭ-sis) the proteolytic destruction of fibrinogen in the circulating blood. adj., **fibrinogenolyt′ic.**

fibrinogenopenia (fi-brin″o-jen″o-pe′ne-ah) decreased fibrinogen in the blood.

fibrinoid (fi′brĭ-noid) 1. resembling fibrin. 2. a homogeneous, eosinophilic, relatively acellular refractile substance with some of the staining properties of fibrin.

fibrinokinase (fi″brĭ-no-ki′nās) a non–water-soluble plasminogen activator derived from animal tissues.

fibrinolysin (fi″brĭ-nol′ĭ-sin) 1. plasmin. 2. a preparation of proteolytic enzyme formed from profibrinolysin (plasminogen) by action of physical agents or by specific bacterial kinases; used to promote dissolution of thrombi.

fibrinolysis (fi″brĭ-nol′ĭ-sis) the dissolution of fibrin by enzymatic action. adj. **fibrinolyt′ic.**

fibrinopenia (fi″brĭ-no-pe′ne-ah) deficiency of fibrinogen in the blood.

fibrinopeptide (fi″brĭ-no-pep′tīd) either of two peptides (A and B) split off from fibrinogen during blood CLOTTING by the action of thrombin.

fibrinoscopy (fi″brĭ-nos′ko-pe) inoscopy.

fibrinous (fi′brĭ-nus) pertaining to or of the nature of fibrin.

fibrinuria (fi″brĭ-nu′re-ah) discharge of fibrin in the urine.

fibroadenoma (fi″bro-ad″ĕ-no′mah) adenoma containing fibrous elements.

fibroadipose (fi″bro-ad′ĭ-pōs) both fibrous and fatty.

fibroangioma (fi″bro-an″je-o′mah) an angioma containing much fibrous tissue.

fibroareolar (fi″bro-ah-re′o-lar) both fibrous and areolar.

fibroblast (fi′bro-blast) an immature fiber-producing cell of connective tissue capable of differentiating into a chondroblast, collagenoblast, or osteoblast. Called also fibrocyte. adj., **fibroblas′tic.**

fibroblastoma (fi″bro-blas-to′mah) any tumor arising from fibroblasts, now classified as fibromas and or fibrosarcomas.

fibrocalcific (fi″bro-kal-sif′ik) pertaining to or characterized by partially calcified fibrous tissue.

fibrocarcinoma (fi″bro-kar″sĭ-no′mah) scirrhous carcinoma.

fibrocartilage (fi″bro-kar′tĭ-lij) cartilage made up of parallel, thick, compact collagenous bundles, separated by narrow clefts containing the typical cartilage cells (chondrocytes).

fibrochondritis (fi″bro-kon-dri′tis) inflammation of fibrocartilage.

fibrochondroma (fi″bro-kon-dro′mah) chondroma containing areas of fibrosis.

fibrocyst (fi′bro-sist) cystic fibroma.

fibrocystic (fi″bro-sis′tik) characterized by an overgrowth of fibrous tissue and the development of cystic spaces, especially in a gland.

f. disease of pancreas, cystic fibrosis.

fibrocystoma (fi″bro-sis-to′mah) cystic fibroma.

fibrocyte (fi′bro-sīt) a cell that produces fibrous tissue; called also FIBROBLAST.

fibrodysplasia (fi″bro-dis-pla′ze-ah) fibrous dysplasia.

fibroelastic (fi″bro-e-las′tik) both fibrous and elastic.

fibroelastosis (fi″bro-e″las-to′sis) overgrowth of fibroelastic elements.

endocardial f., a condition characterized by left ventricular hypertrophy and conversion of the endocardium into a thick fibroelastic coat, with ventricular capacity sometimes reduced, but often increased.

fibroenchondroma (fi″bro-en″kon-dro′mah) enchondroma containing fibrous elements.

fibroepithelioma (fi″bro-ep″ĭ-the″le-o′mah) a tumor composed of both fibrous and epithelial elements.

fibroglia (fi-brog′le-ah) border fibrils in close relation to the surface of fibroblasts.

fibroglioma (fi″bro-gli-o′mah) a glioma containing excessive fibrous tissue.

fibroid (fi′broid) 1. having a fibrous structure; resembling a fibroma. 2. fibroma. 3. LEIOMYOMA; *fibroids* is a colloquial term for leiomyoma of the UTERUS.

f. tumor, fibroma.

fibroidectomy (fi″broi-dek′to-me) excision of a uterine fibroma (leiomyoma).

fibrolipoma (fi″bro-lĭ-po′mah) a lipoma containing excessive fibrous tissue. adj., **fibrolipo′matous.**

fibroma (fi-bro′mah) a tumor composed mainly of fibrous or fully developed connective tissue.

ameloblastic f., an odontogenic fibroma, marked by simultaneous proliferation of both epithelial and mesenchymal tissue, without formation of enamel or dentin.

cementifying f., cementoblastoma; a tumor usually occurring in the mandible of older persons and consisting of fibroblastic tissue containing masses of cementum-like tissue.

chondromyxoid f. of bone, a benign neoplasm apparently derived from cartilage-forming connective tissue.

cystic f., one that has undergone cystic degeneration.

f. myxomato′des, myxofibroma; a fibroma containing myxomatous tissue.

nonosteogenic f., a degenerative and proliferative lesion of the medullary and cortical tissues of bone.

odontogenic f., a benign tumor of the jaw arising from the embryonic portion of the tooth germ, the dental papilla, or dental follicle, or later from the periodontal membrane.

ossifying f., ossifying f. of bone, a benign, relatively slow-growing, central bone tumor, usually of the jaws, especially the mandible, which is composed of fibrous connective tissue within which bone is formed.

fibromatoid (fi-bro′mah-toid) resembling fibroma; fibroma-like.

fibromatosis (fi″bro-mah-to′sis) 1. the presence of multiple fibromas. 2. the formation of a fibrous, tumor-like nodule arising from the deep fascia, with a tendency to local recurrence.

f. gingi′vae, a diffuse fibroma of the gingivae and palate, manifested as a dense, smooth or nodular overgrowth of the tissues.

palmar f., fibromatosis involving the palmar fascia, and resulting in Dupuytren's contracture.

plantar f., fibromatosis involving the plantar fascia manifested as single or multiple nodular swellings, sometimes accompanied by pain but usually unassociated with contractures.

fibromatous (fi-bro'mah-tus) pertaining to or of the nature of fibroma.

fibromuscular (fi"bro-mus'ku-lar) both fibrous and muscular.

fibromyitis (fi"bro-mi-i'tis) inflammation of muscle with fibrous degeneration.

fibromyoma (fi"bro-mi-o'mah) a myoma containing fibrous elements, a leiomyoma.

fibromyomectomy (fi"bro-mi"o-mek'to-me) excision of a fibromyoma (leiomyoma).

fibromyositis (fi"bro-mi"o-si'tis) inflammation of fibromuscular tissue.

fibromyxoma (fi"bro-mik-so'mah) a fibroma containing myxomatous tissue; myxofibroma.

fibromyxosarcoma (fi"bro-mik"so-sar-ko'mah) a sarcoma containing fibrous and mucous elements.

fibroneuroma (fi"bro-nu-ro'mah) neurofibroma.

fibropapilloma (fi"bro-pap"ĭ-lo'mah) a papilloma containing much fibrous tissue.

fibroplasia (fi"bro-pla'ze-ah) the formation of fibrous tissue, as in the healing of a wound. adj., **fibroplas'tic**.

retrolental f., a condition characterized by retinal vascular proliferation and tortuosity and by the presence of fibrous tissue behind the lens, leading to detachment of the retina and arrest of growth of the eye, generally attributed to use of excessively high concentrations of oxygen in the care of premature infants.

fibrosarcoma (fi"bro-sar-ko'mah) a sarcoma arising from collagen-producing fibroblasts.

odontogenic f., a malignant tumor of the jaws, originating from one of the mesenchymal components of the tooth or tooth germ.

fibroserous (fi"bro-se'rus) composed of both fibrous and serous elements.

fibrosis (fi-bro'sis) formation of fibrous tissue; fibroid degeneration. adj., **fibrot'ic.**

cystic f., cystic f. of pancreas, a generalized hereditary disorder with widespread dysfunction of exocrine glands, chronic pulmonary disease, pancreatic deficiency, high levels of electrolytes in sweat, and sometimes biliary cirrhosis. (See also CYSTIC FIBROSIS.)

diffuse interstitial pulmonary f., progressive fibrosis of the pulmonary alveolar walls, with steadily progressive dypsnea, resulting in death from oxygen lack or right heart failure.

endomyocardial f., idiopathic myocardiopathy occurring endemically in various regions of Africa and rarely in other areas, characterized by cardiomegaly, by marked thickening of the endocardium with dense, white fibrous tissue that frequently extends to involve the inner third or half of the myocardium, and by congestive heart failure.

mediastinal f., development of whitish, hard fibrous tissue in the upper portion of the mediastinum, sometimes obstructing the air passages and large blood vessels.

periureteric f., progressive development of fibrous tissue spreading from the great midline vessels and causing strangulation of one or both ureters.

postfibrinous f., that occurring in tissues in which fibrin has been deposited.

proliferative f., that in which the fibrous elements continue to proliferate after the original causative factor has ceased to operate.

pulmonary f., diffuse interstitial pulmonary fibrosis.

retroperitoneal f., deposition of fibrous tissue in the retroperitoneal space, producing vague abdominal discomfort, and often causing blockage of the ureters, with resultant hydronephrosis and impaired renal function, which may result in renal failure. Called also Ormond's disease.

f. u'teri, a morbid condition characterized by overgrowth of the smooth muscle and increase in the collagenous fibrous tissue of the uterus, producing a thickened, coarse, tough myometrium.

fibrositis (fi"bro-si'tis) inflammatory hyperplasia of the white fibrous tissue, especially of the muscle sheaths and fascial layers of the locomotor system, causing pain and stiffness; called also muscular rheumatism.

fibrothorax (fi"bro-tho'raks) adhesion of the two pleural layers, the lung being covered by thick non-expansible fibrous tissue.

fibrous (fi'brus) composed of or containing fibers.

f. dysplasia, localized overgrowth of fibrous tissue in bone (see also fibrous DYSPLASIA).

fibula (fib'u-lah) the lateral and smaller of the two bones of the leg. (see also table of BONES). adj. **fib'u-lar.**

ficin (fi'sin) a highly active, crystallizable protein-ase from the sap of fig trees, which catalyzes the hydrolysis of many proteins at acid (4.1) pH, the clotting of milk, and "digestion" of some living worms, e.g., whipworms. It also shows esterase activity.

F.I.C.S. Fellow of the International College of Surgeons.

field (fēld) 1. an area or open space, as an operative field or visual field. 2. a range of specialization in knowledge, study, or occupation. 3. in embryology, the developing region within a range of modifying factors.

auditory f., the space or range within which stimuli will be perceived as sound.

high-power f., the area of a slide visible under the high magnification system of a microscope.

individuation f., a region in which an organizer influences adjacent tissue to become a part of a total embryo.

low-power f., the area of a slide visible under the low magnification system of a microscope.

morphogenetic f., an embryonic region out of which definite structures normally develop.

visual f., the area within which stimuli will produce the sensation of sight with the eye in a straight-ahead position.

fila (fi'lah) [L.] plural of *filum.*

filaceous (fi-la'shus) composed of filaments.

filament (fil'ah-ment) a delicate fiber or thread.

filamentous (fil"ah-men'tus) composed of long, threadlike structures.

Filaria (fĭ-la're-ah) a former generic name for members of the superfamily Filarioidea.

F. bancrof'ti, *Wuchereria bancrofti.*

F. medinen'sis, *Dracunculus medinensis.*

filaria (fĭ-la're-ah,), pl. *fila'riae* [L.] a nematode worm of the superfamily Filarioidea. adj., **fila'rial.**

filariasis (fil"ah-ri'ah-sis) infection with filariae. The organism causing the most common form of filariasis is *Wuchereria bancrofti.* Most often encountered in central Africa, the southwest Pacific, and eastern Asia, the disease also occurs in the West Indies and in tropical South and Central America. It is transmitted by the *Culex* mosquito or by mites or flies. The larvae invade lymphoid tissues and then grow to adult worms an inch or two long. The resulting obstruction of the lymphatic circulation causes swelling, inflammation, and pain. Repeated infections over many years, with impaired circulation and formation of excess connective tissue, may cause enlargement of the affected part, usually the arm, leg, or scrotum. In cases of extreme enlargement, known as ELEPHANTIASIS, the affected part may grow to many times its normal size.

The larvae can be killed by treatment with diethylcarbamazine, but there is as yet no effective way of treating the adult worms. Edema of the legs can be reduced by rest and by the use of pressure bandages. The prognosis is favorable for all but the most severe cases.

filaricide (fĭ-lăr'ĭ-sīd) an agent that destroys filariae. adj., **filaricid'al.**

filariform (fĭ-lăr'ĭ-form) resembling filariae; threadlike.

Filarioidea (fĭ-la"re-oi'de-ah) a superfamily of nematode parasites (filariae), the adults of which are threadlike worms that invade the tissues and body cavities, where the female deposits microfilariae (prelarvae). These microfilariae are ingested by bloodsucking insects in whom they pass their developmental stage and are returned to man by the bites of such insects (see also FILARIASIS).

filiform (fil'ĭ-form, fi'lĭ-form) 1. threadlike. 2. an extremely slender bougie.

filipin (fil'ĭ-pin) an antifungal antibiotic.

fillet (fil'et) 1. a loop, as of cord or tape, for making traction. 2. in the nervous system, a long band of nerve fibers.

film (film) 1. a thin layer or coating. 2. a thin sheet of material (e.g., gelatin, cellulose acetate) specially treated for use in photography or radiography; used also to designate the sheet after exposure to the energy to which it is sensitive.

bite-wing f., an x-ray film for radiography of oral structures, with a protruding tab to be held between the upper and lower teeth.

gelatin f., absorbable, a sterile, nonantigenic, absorbable, water-insoluble coating used as an aid in surgical closure and repair of defects in the dura mater and pleura.

spot f., a radiograph of a small anatomic area obtained (1) by rapid exposure during fluoroscopy to provide a permanent record of a transiently observed abnormality, or (2) by limitation of radiation passing through the area to improve definition and detail of the image produced.

x-ray f., film sensitized to roentgen (x-) rays, either before or after exposure.

film badge (film baj) a pack of radiographic film or films worn as a badge, used for the detection and approximate measurement of radiation exposure of personnel.

filopressure (fi"lo-presh'ur) compression of a blood vessel by a thread.

filter (fil'ter) a device for eliminating certain elements, as (1) particles of certain size from a solution, or (2) rays of certain wavelength from a stream of radiant energy.

Berkefeld's f., one composed of diatomaceous earth, impermeable to ordinary bacteria.

Millipore f., trademark for a device used to filter nutrient solutions as they are administered intravenously.

Pasteur-Chamberland f., a hollow column of unglazed porcelain through which liquids are forced by pressure or by vacuum exhaustion.

Wood's f., a nickel-oxide filter that holds back all but a few violet rays and passes ultraviolet rays of about 365 nm. (see also WOOD'S LIGHT).

filterable, filtrable (fil'ter-ah-b'l; fil'trah-b'l) capable of passing through the pores of a filter.

filtrate (fil'trāt) a liquid that has passed through a filter.

filtration (fil-tra'shun) passage through a filter or through a material that prevents passage of certain molecules.

filum (fi'lum), pl. *fi'la* [L.] a threadlike structure or part.

f. termina'le, a slender, threadlike prolongation of the spinal cord from the conus medullaris to the back of the coccyx.

fimbria (fim'bre-ah,), pl. *fim'briae* [L.] 1. a fringe, border, or edge; a fringelike structure. 2. one of the minute filamentous appendages of certain bacteria, associated with antigenic properties of the cell surface.

f. hippocam'pi, the band of white matter along the median edge of the ventricular surface of the hippocampus.

fimbriae of uterine tube, the numerous divergent fringelike processes on the distal part of the infundibulum of the uterine tube.

fimbriate (fim'bre-āt) fringed.

finger (fing'ger) one of the five digits of the hand.

baseball f., partial permanent flexion of the terminal phalanx of a finger caused by a ball or other object striking the end or back of the finger, resulting in rupture of the attachment of the extensor tendon.

clubbed f., one with enlargement of the terminal phalanx with constant osseous changes.

hammer f., mallet f., permanent flexion of the distal phalanx of a finger.

webbed f's, fingers more or less united by strands of tissue; syndactyly.

fingerprint (fing'ger-print) 1. an impression of the cutaneous ridges of the fleshy distal portion of a finger. 2. in biochemistry, the characteristic pattern of a peptide after subjection to an analytical technique.

Finney's pyloroplasty (fin'ēz) enlargement of the pyloric canal by establishment of an inverted U-shaped anastomosis between the stomach and duodenum after longitudinal incision.

Finsen's lamp (fin'senz) a carbon arc lamp operating at 50 volts and 50 amperes, so constructed that radiation is concentrated on an area 1 inch square; a water-cooled quartz system is used to remove caloric radiation and a compression quartz piece to dehematize the skin.

Finsen's light (fin'senz) light consisting mainly of violet and ultraviolet rays given off by Finsen's lamp; used in treatment of lupus and similar diseases.

first aid (ferst ād) emergency care and treatment of an injured person before complete medical and surgical treatment can be secured.

Fishberg concentration test (fish'berg) determination of the ability of the kidneys to maintain excretion of solids under conditions of reduced water intake and a high protein diet, in which urine samples are collected and tested for specific gravity. The patient is given a high-protein dinner (unless he is azotemic) with not more than 200 ml. of fluid, and nothing thereafter until the test is completed. Urine voided during the night is discarded. The morning urine is saved and the urine of one hour later and two hours later is saved. If the specific gravity of any of these three specimens is less than 1.022 there is impairment of renal function.

fission (fish'un) 1. the act of splitting. 2. asexual reproduction in which the cell divides into two (binary fission) or more (multiple fission) daughter parts, each of which becomes an individual organism. 3. nuclear fission; the splitting of the atomic nucleus, with release of energy.

fissiparous (fĭ-sip'ah-rus) propagated by fission.

fissula (fis'u-lah), pl. *fis'sulae* [L.] a small cleft.

fissura (fis-ur'rah,), pl. *fissu'rae* [L.] fissure.

fissure (fish'er) a narrow slit or cleft, especially one of the deeper or more constant furrows separating the gyri of the brain.

abdominal f., a congenital cleft in the abdominal wall.

anal f., f. in ano, a painful lineal ulcer at the margin of the anus.

anterior median f., a longitudinal furrow along the midline of the ventral surface of the spinal cord and medulla oblongata.

f. of Bichat, transverse fissure (2).

branchial f., branchial cleft.

central f., fissure of Rolando.

collateral f., a longitudinal fissure on the inferior surface of the cerebral hemisphere between the fusiform gyrus and the hippocampal gyrus.

Henle's f's, spaces filled with connective tissue between the muscular fibers of the heart.

hippocampal f., one extending from the splenium of the corpus callosum almost to the tip of the temporal lobe; called also hippocampal sulcus.

longitudinal f., the deep fissure between the cerebral hemispheres.

palpebral f., the longitudinal opening between the eyelids.

portal f., porta hepatis.

posterior median f., 1. a shallow vertical groove in the closed part of the medulla oblongata, continuous with the posterior median sulcus of the spinal cord. 2. a shallow vertical groove dividing the spinal cord throughout its whole length in the midline posteriorly. Called also posterior median sulcus.

presylvian f., the anterior branch of the fissure of Sylvius.

Rolando's f., f. of Rolando, a groove running obliquely across the superolateral surface of the cerebral hemisphere, separating the frontal from the parietal lobe. Called also central fissure and central sulcus.

f. of round ligament, one on the visceral surface of the liver, lodging the round ligament in the adult.

sylvian f., f. of Sylvius, one extending laterally between the temporal and frontal lobes, and turning posteriorly between the temporal and parietal lobes.

transverse f., 1. porta hepatis. 2. the transverse cerebral fissure between the diencephalon and the cerebral hemispheres; called also fissure of Bichat.

zygal f., a cerebral fissure consisting of two branches connected by a stem.

fistula (fis'tu-lah) any abnormal, tubelike passage within body tissue, usually between two internal organs, or leading from an internal organ to the body surface. Some fistulas are created surgically, for diagnostic or therapeutic purposes; others occur as a result of injury or as congenital abnormalities. Among the many kinds of fistulas, the anal type (fistula in ano) is one of the most common. This generally develops as a result of a break, or fissure, in the wall of the anal canal or rectum, or an abscess here. Treatment is by surgery.

In women, difficult labor in childbirth may result in the formation of a vesicovaginal fistula, between the bladder and the vagina, with resulting leakage of urine into the vagina. In a vesicointestinal fistula, there is leakage of urine from the bladder into the intestine. In rectovaginal fistula, feces escape through the wall of the anal canal or rectum into the vagina. The latter condition, formerly a serious hazard of childbirth, is now rare; also, like other kinds of fistulas, it can be corrected by surgery.

With the types of fistulas described here, typical symptoms are pain in the affected region and an abnormal discharge through the skin near the anus or through the vagina. Fistulas at different places of the body may be caused by tuberculosis, actinomycosis (a fungus infection), the presence of diverticula, or some other serious disease, and the fistula itself may be a site of infection and discomfort.

arteriovenous f., a fistula between an artery and a vein.

blind f., one open at one end only, opening on the skin (external blind fistula) or on an internal surface (internal blind fistula).

branchial f., a persisting branchial cleft.

complete f., one extending from the skin to an internal body cavity.

craniosinus f., one between the cerebral space and one of the sinuses, permitting escape of cerebrospinal fluid into the nose.

Eck's f., an artificial communication made between the portal vein and the vena cava.

fecal f., a colonic fistula opening on the external surface of the body and discharging feces.

gastric f., an abnormal passage communicating with the stomach; often applied to an artificially created opening, through the abdominal wall, into the stomach.

horseshoe f., a semicircular fistulous tract about the anus, with both openings on the skin.

incomplete f., blind fistula.

pulmonary arteriovenous f., congenital, a congenital anomalous communication between the pulmonary arterial and venous systems, allowing unoxygenated blood to enter the systemic circulation.

umbilical f., an abnormal passage communicating with the gut or the urachus at the umbilicus.

fistulectomy (fis″tu-lek'to-me) excision of a fistula.

fistulization (fis″tu-lĭ-za'shun) 1. the process of becoming fistulous. 2. surgical creation of a fistula.

fistulotomy (fis″tu-lot'o-me) incision of a fistula.

fistulous (fis'tu-lus) pertaining to or of the nature of a fistula.

fixation (fik-sa′shun) 1. the act or operation of holding, suturing, or fastening in a fixed position. 2. the condition of being held in a fixed position. 3. in psychiatry, the cessation of the development of personality at a stage short of complete maturity. 4. in microscopy, the treatment of material so that its structure can be examined in greater detail with minimal alteration of the normal state, and also to provide information concerning the chemical properties (as of cell constituents) by interpretation of fixation reactions. 5. in chemistry, the process whereby a substance is removed from the gaseous or solution phase and localized. 6. in ophthalmology, direction of the gaze so that the visual image of the object falls on the fovea centralis. 7. in film processing, the chemical removal of all undeveloped salts of the film emulsion, as on x-ray films.

complement f., f. of complement, the combining of complement with the antigen-antibody complex, rendering the complement inactive, or fixed. (See also COMPLEMENT FIXATION.)

fixative (fik′sah-tiv) an agent used in preserving a histologic or pathologic specimen so as to maintain the normal structure of its constituent elements.

flaccid (flak′sid) weak, lax, soft; applied especially to muscles.

flagellar (flah-jel′ar) of or pertaining to a flagellum.

flagellate (flaj′ĕ-lāt) 1. any microorganism having flagella. 2. any protozoon of the subphylum Mastigophora. 3. having flagella.

flagellation (flaj″el-la′shun) 1. massage by tapping the part with the fingers. 2. whipping or being whipped to achieve erotic pleasure. 3. exflagellation.

flagelliform (flah-jel′ĭ-form) shaped like a flagellum or lash.

flagellosis (flaj″ĕ-lo′sis) infection with flagellate protozoa.

flagellum (flah-jel′um), pl. *flagel′la* [L.] a mobile, whiplike process, such as the coiled, filamentous appendage, originating in the cell wall or outer layers of cytoplasm of rod-shaped bacteria, certain protozoa, etc., and serving as an organ of locomotion.

flail (flāl) exhibiting abnormal or pathologic mobility, as flail chest or flail joint.

f. chest, a loss of stability of the chest wall due to multiple rib fractures or detachment of the sternum from the ribs as a result of a severe crushing chest injury. The loose chest segment moves in a direction which is the reverse of normal; that is, the segment moves inward during inspiration and outward during expiration (PARADOXICAL RESPIRATION). Other manifestations of flail chest include shortness of breath, cyanosis, and extreme pain in the area of trauma.

Emergency treatment is aimed at stabilizing the loose chest segment to reduce ineffective and exhausting chest movement, and to provide for adequate ventilation of the lungs. The segment may be immobilized by application of a weighted object, such as a sandbag, or by splinting the area using a bulky dressing and tape. The patient is transported lying on the affected side to further stabilize the chest wall. Positive pressure resuscitation is administered, using a bag-mask or the mouth-to-mouth technique.

f. joint, an unusually movable joint.

flame (flām) 1. the luminous, irregular appearance usually accompanying combustion, or an appearance resembling it. 2. to render sterile by exposure to a flame.

flank (flangk) the side of the body between the ribs and ilium.

flap (flap) 1. a mass of tissue for GRAFTING, usually including skin, only partially removed from one part of the body so that it retains its own blood supply during transfer to another site. (See also GRAFT.) 2. an uncontrolled movement.

island f., a flap consisting of skin and subcutaneous tissue, with a pedicle made up of only the nutrient vessels.

jump f., one cut from the abdomen and attached to a flap of the same size on the forearm. The forearm flap is transferred later to some other part of the body to fill a defect there.

pedicle f., pedicle graft.

rope f., one made by elevating a long strip of tissue from its bed except at its two ends, the cut edges then being sutured together to form a tube.

skin f., a full-thickness mass or flap of tissue containing epidermis, dermis, and subcutaneous tissue.

sliding f., a flap carried to its new position by a sliding technique.

tube f., tunnel f., rope flap.

flare (flār) a diffuse area of redness on the skin around the point of application of an irritant, due to vasomotor reaction.

flask (flask) a laboratory vessel, usually of glass and with a constricted neck.

flatfoot (flat′foot) a condition in which one or more arches of the foot have flattened out.

flatness (flat′nes) a peculiar sound lacking resonance, heard on percussing an abnormally solid part.

flatulence (flat′u-lens) excessive formation of gases in the stomach or intestine.

flatulent (flat′u-lent) characterized by flatulence; distended with gas.

flatus (fla′tus) 1. gas or air in the gastrointestinal tract. 2. gas or air expelled through the anus.

flatworm (flat′werm) an individual organism of the phylum Platyhelminthes (see also WORMS).

flav(o)- word element [L.], *yellow.*

flavanone (fla′vah-nōn) flavonoid compounds formed by reduction of the 2:3 double bond of a flavone.

flavin (fla′vin) any of a group of water-soluble yellow pigments widely distributed in animals and plants, including riboflavin and yellow enzymes.

f. adenine dinucleotide (FAD), a coenzyme that is a condensation product of riboflavin phosphate and adenylic acid; it forms the prosthetic group of certain enzymes, including D-amino acid oxidase and xanthine oxidase, and is important in electron transport in mitochondria.

f. mononucleotide (FMN), a derivative of riboflavin that serves as a coenzyme for a number of oxidative enzymes.

flavivirus (fla″ve-vi′rus) one of a subcategory of togaviruses; the type species is the yellow fever virus.

Flavobacterium (fla″vo-bak-te′re-um) a genus of bacteria (family Achromobacteraceae) characteristically producing yellow, orange, red, or yellow-brown pigmentation, found in soil and water; some species are said to be pathogenic.

flavone (fla′vōn) a substance, $C_{15}H_{10}O_2$, the basis of several yellow dyes.

flavonoid (fla′vo-noid) a generic term for a group of compounds widely distributed in higher plants; one subgroup (anthocyanins) accounts for most of the yellow, red, and blue pigmentation, while another (bioflavonoids) are concerned in maintenance of a normal state of capillary walls.

flavonol (fla′vo-nol) a yellow crystalline flavonoid, formed by introduction of an OH group at C-3 of a flavone.

flavoprotein (fla″vo-pro′te-in) a conjugated protein containing flavin.

flavoxate (fla-voks′āt) a smooth muscle relaxant; the hydrochloride salt is used in treatment of spasms of the urinary tract.

flaxseed (flak′sēd) linseed; used as a topical demulcent and as an emollient.

fl.dr. fluid dram.

flea (fle) a small, wingless, bloodsucking insect. Many fleas are ectoparasites and may act as disease carriers; they act as vectors of such diseases as plague, tularemia, and brucellosis.

Fleet enema (flēt) trademark for an enema containing, in each 100 ml., 16 gm. sodium biphosphate and 6 gm. sodium phosphate, packaged in a plastic squeeze bottle fitted with a 2-inch, prelubricated rectal tube.

Fleming (flem′ing) Sir Alexander (1881–1955). Scottish bacteriologist and discoverer of PENICILLIN. He was born at Lochfield in Scotland and served as a captain in the army medical corps during World War I. The first result of his search for an antibacterial substance that would not be toxic to human tissue was the discovery of lysozyme, but his epochal discovery was of penicillin in 1938. In 1943 he was made fellow of the Royal Society, was knighted and given the John Scott medal in 1944, and was awarded the Nobel prize in 1945.

flesh (flesh) the soft muscular tissue of the animal body.

goose f., cutis anserina; erection of the papillae of the skin, as from cold or shock.

proud f., exuberant amounts of soft, edematous, unhealthy-looking granulation tissue developing during healing of large surface wounds.

flex (fleks) to bend or put in a state of flexion.

flexibilitas (flek″sĭ-bil′ĭ-tas) [L.] flexibility.

f. ce′rea, a cataleptic state in which the limbs retain any position in which they are placed; called also waxy flexibility.

flexibility (flek″sĭ-bil′ĭ-te) the state of being unusually pliant.

waxy f., flexibilitas cerea.

flexion (flek′shun) the act of bending or the condition of being bent.

flexor (flek′sor) any muscle that flexes a joint (see table of MUSCLES).

flexura (flek-shu′rah), pl. *flexu′rae* [L.] flexure.

flexure (flek′sher) a bend or fold; a curvation.

caudal f., the bend at the aboral end of the embryo.

cephalic f., the curve in the mid-brain of the embryo.

cervical f., a bend in the neural tube of the embryo at the junction of the brain and spinal cord.

colic f., left, the angular junction of the transverse and descending colon.

colic f., right, the angular junction of the ascending and transverse colon.

dorsal f., one of the flexures in the mid-dorsal region of the embryo.

duodenojejunal f., the bend at the junction of duodenum and jejunum.

hepatic f., right colic flexure.

lumbar f., the ventral curvature in the lumbar region of the back.

mesencephalic f., a bend in the neural tube of the embryo at the level of the mesencephalon, or mid-brain.

pontine f., a flexure of the hindbrain in the embryo.

sacral f., caudal flexure.

sigmoid f., sigmoid colon.

splenic f., left colic flexure.

flint disease (flint) chalicosis.

floating kidney excessive mobility of the kidney; called also hypermobile kidney. NEPHROPTOSIS refers to a dropping of the kidney from its normal position. Surgical correction, by NEPHROPEXY, is necessary when the condition interferes with normal kidney function.

floccillation (flok″sĭ-la′shun) carphology; involuntary picking at the bedclothes, seen in grave fevers and in conditions of great exhaustion.

floccose (flok′ōs) wooly; said of bacterial growth composed of short, curved chains variously oriented.

flocculation (flok″u-la′shun) a colloid phenomenon in which the disperse phase separates in discrete, usually visible, particles rather than in a continuous mass, as in coagulation.

flocculent (flok′u-lent) containing downy or flaky shreds.

flocculus (flok′u-lus), pl. *floc′uli* [L.] 1. a small tuft or mass, as of wool or other fibrous material. 2. a small mass on the lower side of each cerebral hemisphere, continuous with the nodule of the vermis. adj., **floc′cular.**

flora (flo′rah) the collective plant organisms of a given locality.

intestinal f., the bacteria normally residing within the lumen of the intestine.

Floraquin (flōr′ah-kwin) trademark for a preparation of diiodohydroxyquin, an antiamebic.

Florinef (flōr′ĭ-nef) trademark for preparations of fludrocortisone, a synthetic adrenal corticoid.

Floropryl (flōr′o-pril) trademark for preparations of isoflurophate, an anticholinesterase inhibitor used topically as a miotic in glaucoma.

flowmeter (flo′me-ter) an apparatus for measuring the rate of flow of liquids or gases.

floxuridine (floks-ūr′ĭ-den) a derivative of fluouracil used as an antiviral and antineoplastic agent; abbreviated FUDR.

fl.oz. fluid ounce.

flu (floo) popular name for INFLUENZA.

intestinal f., a popular name for what may be any of several disorders of the stomach and intestinal tract (see also INTESTINAL FLU).

fluctuation (fluk″tu-a′shun) a variation, as about a fixed variation or mass; a wavelike motion.

fludrocortisone (floo″dro-kor′tĭ-sōn) a synthetic adrenal corticoid with effects similar to those of hydrocortisone and desoxycorticosterone.

fluid (floo′id) 1. a liquid or gas; any liquid of the body. 2. composed of molecules which freely change their relative positions without separation of the mass.

allantoic f., the fluid contained within the allantosis.

amniotic f., the fluid within the amnion that bathes the developing fetus and protects it from mechanical injury (see also AMNIOTIC FLUID).

body f's, the fluids within the body, composed of water, electrolytes, and nonelectrolytes. The volume and distribution of body fluids vary with age, sex, and amount of adipose tissue. Throughout life there is a slow decline in the volume of body fluids; obesity decreases the relative amount of water in the body.

Although the body fluids are continuously in motion, moving in and out of the cells, tissue spaces, and vascular system, physiologists consider them to be "compartmentalized." Fluid within the cell membranes is called *intracellular* fluid and comprises about two-thirds of the total body fluids. The remaining one-third is outside the cell and is called *extracellular* fluid. The extracellular fluid can be further divided into tissue fluid (*interstitial* fluid), which is found in the spaces between the blood vessels and surrounding cells, and intravascular fluid, which is the fluid component of blood.

Intracellular fluid serves as a medium for the basic materials needed by cells for growth, repair, and performance of their various functions. Extracellular fluid circulates in the spaces between the cells and brings to them the nutrients and other substances needed for cell function.

The composition of intracellular fluid differs from that of extracellular fluid, and the difference in these components is important to the normal functioning of the cells. For example, extracellular fluid contains large amounts of the positively charged sodium ions and relatively small amounts of similarly charged potassium ions, whereas intracellular fluid contains these ions in inverse concentrations. The gain and loss of sodium is particularly important in the maintenance of FLUID BALANCE because of the ability of sodium to retain water.

The movement of body fluids and their components from one compartment to another is essential for the maintenance of constant internal conditions (HOMEOSTASIS) that allow for nutrition of the cell, excretion of waste products, and the production of energy and other specific functions of the cells. The substances passing through the cell membranes are transported by DIFFUSION and active transport. These processes are dependent on differences in the concentrations of the intracellular and extracellular fluids, the permeability of the membranes, and the effect of the positively and negatively charged ions in the fluids. The concentrations of the body fluids, particularly in regard to the amount of osmotically active particles in proportion to the amount of water (OSMOLALITY), are important to the movement of fluids in and out of their compartments. As we know from the principles of OSMOSIS, the concentration of the fluids on either side of the cell membrane directly affects the rate at which water moves in and out of the cell.

The maintenance of a proper balance between the intracellular and extracellular fluid volumes is essential to health. In patients with HEART FAILURE

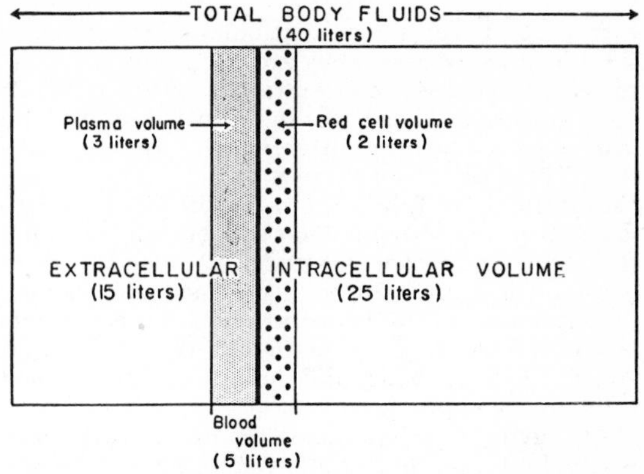

Diagrammatic representation of the body fluids, showing the extracellular fluid volume, intracellular fluid volume, blood volume and total body fluids. (From Guyton, A. C.: Textbook of Medical Physiology. 5th ed. Philadelphia, W. B. Saunders Co., 1976.)

and renal failure the balance becomes upset, producing either localized or generalized EDEMA. Excessive fluid loss produces DEHYDRATION of the cells and impaired cellular function.

cerebrospinal f., the fluid contained within the ventricles of the brain, the subarachnoid space, and the central canal of the spinal cord (see also CEREBROSPINAL FLUID).

f. dram, a unit of liquid measure of the apothecaries' system, containing 60 minims, and equivalent to 3.697 ml. (See also Table of Weights and Measures in the Appendix.)

interstitial f., the extracellular fluid bathing most tissues, excluding the fluid within the lymph and blood vessels.

f. ounce, a unit of liquid measure of the apothecaries' system, being 8 fluid drams, or the equivalent of 29.57 ml. (See also Table of Weights and Measures in the Appendix.)

seminal f., semen.

spinal f., the fluid within the spinal canal.

synovial f., synovia.

fluid balance a state in which the volume of body water and its solutes (electrolytes and nonelectrolytes) is within normal limits and there is normal distribution of fluids within the intracellular and extracellular compartments. The total volume of body fluids should be about 60 per cent of the body weight, and it should be distributed so that one-third is extracellular fluid and two-thirds intracellular fluid. Although this distribution remains constant in a healthy individual, there is continuous movement of fluid into and out of the various compartments.

Most organs are concerned in some way with the maintenance of fluid balance within the body; however, the KIDNEYS play a major role in regulating most of the constituents of the fluids. It is in the renal tubules that water is reabsorbed into the blood stream or allowed to enter the urine for excretion. The antidiuretic hormone (ADH) controls this process. It is also in the distal tubules of the kidneys that sodium reabsorption takes place and this process is influenced by the hormone aldosterone.

Water and sodium are particularly important in fluid balance because they are the components directly affecting the concentration (OSMOLALITY) of the fluids and, therefore, their distribution. The body does not tolerate differences in osmotic pressure. Thus, whenever there is an imbalance in the concentration of fluids, there is shifting of the fluids, with water moving from the less concentrated fluid to the more concentrated until an equilibrium is established. In addition to these osmotic factors, the movement of fluids in and out of compartments is affected by capillary permeability, arterial and venous blood pressure, and the rate of flow of bood through the capillaries.

The adaptive mechanisms for maintaining normal volume and distribution of fluids inside and outside the cells function only as long as there is adequate and equal intake and output of water and electrolytes. When either gains or losses of these components of body fluids are excessive and prolonged, a fluid imbalance exists. If the condition persists, the result is circulatory collapse and death.

A deficit of body fluids is manifested by either intracellular or extracellular dehydration, or both. The result is an insufficient volume of fluid to meet the needs of the cells. The deficit can be made up by oral or parenteral administration of fluids. It is essential, however, that in making up the deficit overenthusiastic use of intravenous fluids does not produce an excess of water and an imbalance in the other direction.

An excess of water can be manifested as water intoxication, circulatory overload (vascular hypervolemia), and increased volume of water within the cell or interstitial spaces (EDEMA).

A fluid balance record is kept on each patient who is susceptible to or already suffering from a disturbance in the balance of body fluids. This record, also called the record of intake and output, shows the amount of fluid entering the body and the amount lost from the body. Intake includes *all* routes by which water enters the body: by mouth, by rectum, via irrigation tubes, and parenterally. Output consists of all fluids lost via the urinary tract and the intestinal tract, whether by suction, vomiting and diarrhea, or by drainage from wounds and from fistulas. An accurate measuring and recording of fluid intake and output can be a valuable aid in detecting imbalances and in determining the amount needed for fluid replacement.

In addition to measurement and recording of intake and output and evaluation of the clinical signs of fluid imbalance, certain laboratory tests are helpful in the accurate assessment of a patient's hydration status. Among these are OSMOLALITY, SERUM SODIUM, and BLOOD UREA NITROGEN. The serum osmolality expresses the status of the concentration of dissolved particles in the serum. When the body is dehydrated by excessive fluid loss or inadequate intake, the serum is less dilute or more concentrated than it normally would be and the serum osmolality is increased. Conversely, overhydration of the body would be reflected in a less concentrated serum and a decrease in serum osmolality. Because of osmotic pressure, a state of equilibrium exists between the osmolality of serum and that of the fluid within the cells. Water moves freely across the cell membrane to maintain that equilibrium. It is possible, therefore, to determine the state of hydration within the cells by determining the osmolality of the serum. It is for this reason that serum osmolality reflects total body hydration.

Measurement of serum sodium is of value in determining the body's state of hydration because of the ability of sodium to retain water. Serum sodium concentration is not an index of sodium deficit or excess, but rather an index of water deficit or excess. An elevated level of sodium in the blood (hypernatremia) would indicate that the loss of water from the body has exceeded the loss of sodium, as might occur, for example, in the administration of osmotic diuretics, uncontrolled diabetes insipidus, gastroenteritis, and extensive burns.

An elevated blood urea nitrogen (BUN) can be caused by dehydration and is indicative of an imbalance between the rate of urea synthesis and its excretion by the kidneys. If the kidneys are functioning normally, the elevated BUN resulting from dehydration can be relieved by an increased fluid intake. Dehydration also plays a major role in the development of HYPERGLYCEMIC HYPEROSMOLAR NONKETOTIC COMA.

fluidextract (floo″id-ek′strakt) a liquid preparation of a vegetable drug, containing alcohol as a solvent or preservative, or both, of such strength that each milliliter contains the therapeutic constituents of 1 gm. of the standard drug it represents.

fluidrachm (floo′ĭ-dram) fluid dram.

fluke (flo͞ok) an organism of the class TREMATODA (phylum Platyhelminthes), characterized by a body that is usually flat and often leaflike. Trematodes can infect the blood, liver, intestines, and lungs. (See also WORM.)

flumen (floo′men), *flu′mina* [L.] a stream.

flu′mina pilo′rum, the lines along which the hairs of the body are arranged.

flumethasone (floo-meth′ah-sōn) an anti-inflammatory glucocorticoid used topically in the treatment of certain dermatoses.

flumethiazide (floo″mĕ-thi′ah-zīd) a sulfonamide compound used as a diuretic and antihypertensive.

fluocinolone acetonide (floo″o-sin′o-lōn) an anti-inflammatory glucocorticoid used topically in eczematous dermatoses.

fluocortolone (floo″o-kor′to-lōn) an anti-inflammatory glucocorticoid.

fluorescein (floo″o-res′e-in) a fluorescing dye; the sodium salt is used in solution to reveal corneal lesions and as a test of circulation in the retina and extremities.

fluorescence (floo″o-res′ens) the property of emitting light while exposed to light, the wavelength of the emitted light being longer than that of the absorbed light. adj., **fluores′cent.**

fluoridation (floo″or-ĭ-da′shun) treatment with fluorides; the addition of fluorides to drinking water as a measure to reduce the incidence of dental caries.

Minute traces of fluoride are found in almost all food, but the quantity apparently is too small to meet the requirements of the body in building tooth enamel that resists cavities. Drinking water containing one part fluoride to one million parts of water does meet this need. It has been found to reduce tooth decay in children by as much as 40 to 60 per cent. Since few natural water supplies contain the necessary amount of fluoride, it usually must be added if protection against tooth decay is desired. Recent evidence suggests that the fluoridation of water has little direct effect in reducing tooth decay in adults. But children raised on fluoridated water develop a resistance to tooth decay that carries over into their adult lives.

In spite of all the evidence in favor of fluoridation, some communities have hesitated to add the chemical to their water. Where this is true, it is possible to obtain other means of fluoride protection. Dentists may apply fluoride solutions directly to a child's teeth, beginning as soon as the first teeth appear, and repeat this treatment every 3 or 4 years until the child is 13. This has been found to reduce caries by about 40 per cent.

Fluoridated water can be bought by the bottle or prepared at home, but both methods require special care and are far more costly to the individual than is the fluoridation of a public water supply. The dentist or physician may prescribe sodium fluoride drops to be added to milk, water, or juice. The use of these drops must be carefully supervised, since a slight excess of fluoride causes mottling of teeth (dental FLUOROSIS) and since, like most medicines, fluoride in large amounts is a poison. A dentifrice containing fluoride may also prove effective. The physician or dentist should be consulted before any fluoride preparation is used.

fluoride (floo′ō-rīd) any binary compound of fluorine.

fluoridization (floo″or-ĭ-dĭ-za′shun) 1. application of fluoride solution to the teeth. 2. fluoridation.

fluorine (floo′or-ēn) a chemical element, atomic number 9, atomic weight 18.998, symbol F. (See table of ELEMENTS.)

fluorochrome (floo′or-o-krōm) a fluorescent compound, as a dye, used to mark protein with a fluorescent label.

fluorography (floo″or-og′rah-fe) fluororoentgenography.

Fluoromar (flo′or-o-mar) trademark for a preparation of fluroxene, a general anesthetic.

fluorometholone (flo″or-o-meth′o-lōn) an anti-inflammatory glucocorticoid used topically in dermatoses that have an allergic or inflammatory basis and are associated with pruritus.

fluorophosphate (floo″or-o-fos′fāt) an organic compound containing fluorine and phosphorus.

diisopropyl f., isoflurophate.

fluororoentgenography (floo″or-o-rent″gen-og′rah-fe) the photographic recording of fluoroscopic images on small films, using a fast lens; a procedure used in mass roentgenography of the chest. Called also fluorography and photofluorography.

fluoroscope (floo′or-o-skōp″) an instrument for visual observation of the form and motion of the deep structures of the body by means of x-ray. The patient is put into position so that the part to be viewed is placed between an x-ray tube and a fluorescent screen. X-rays from the tube pass through the body and project the bones and organs as shadowy images on the screen. Examination by this method is called fluoroscopy.

The advantage of the fluoroscope is that the action of joints, organs, and entire systems of the body can be observed directly. The use of radiopaque media aids in this process. (See also BARIUM TEST.)

fluoroscopy (floo″or-os′ko-pe) examination by means of the fluoroscope.

fluorosis (floo″o-ro′sis) a condition due to ingestion of excessive amounts of fluorine. (See also FLUORIDATION.)

dental f., a mottled discoloration of the enamel of the teeth occurring in chronic endemic fluorosis.

endemic f., chronic, that due to unusually high concentrations of fluorine in the natural drinking water supply, typically causing dental fluorosis but also combined osteosclerosis and osteomalacia.

fluorouracil (floo″or-o-ūr′ah-sil) an antimetabolite used as a antineoplastic agent.

Fluothane (floo′o-thān) trademark for a preparation of halothane, a general anesthetic.

fluoxymesterone (floo-ok″se-mes′ter-ōn) an anabolic androgenic steroid used in the palliative treatment of certain cancers.

fluphenazine (floo-fen′ah-zēn) a major tranquilizer, used as the enanthate ester and hydrochloride salt.

fluprednisolone (floo″pred-nis′o-lōn) an anti-inflammatory glucocorticoid used in the treatment of joint diseases and allergic disorders.

flurandrenolide, flurandrenolone (floo″an-dren′o-līd; floo″an-dren′o-lōn) a glucocorticoid used topically in the treatment of certain skin diseases.

flurazepam (floor-az′ĕ-pam) a hypnotic, used as the hydrochloride salt.

flurogestone (floor″o-jes′tōn) a progestin, used as the acetate ester.

flurothyl (floor′o-thil) a volatile liquid used as a convulsant; administered by inhalation for therapy of psychiatric disorders for which convulsive therapy is usually employed.

fluroxene (floor-oks′ēn) a volatile liquid administered by inhalation to produce general anesthesia.

flush (flush) redness, usually transient, of the face and neck.

hectic f., a persistent or chronic flush associated with chronic debilitating disease, usually febrile.

malar f., hectic flush at the malar eminence.

flutter (flut′er) a rapid vibration or pulsation.

atrial f., cardiac arrhythmia in which the atrial contractions are rapid (200–320 per minute), but regular.

diaphragmatic f., peculiar wavelike fibrillations of the diaphragm of unknown cause.

impure f., atrial flutter in which the atrial rhythm is irregular.

mediastinal f., abnormal mobility of the mediastinum during respiration.

pure f., atrial flutter in which the atrial rhythm is regular.

ventricular f., a possible transition stage between ventricular tachycardia and ventricular fibrillation, the electrocardiogram showing rapid, uniform, and virtually regular oscillations, 250 or more per minute.

flutter-fibrillation (flut′er-fi-brĭ-la′shun) impure flutters that vary from moment to moment in their resemblance to flutter or fibrillation, respectively.

flux (fluks) 1. an excessive flow or discharge. 2. matter discharged.

bloody f., dysentery.

fly (flī) a dipterous, or two-winged insect, which is often the vector of organisms causing disease.

Fm chemical symbol, *fermium.*

FMN flavin mononucleotide.

focus (fo′kus), pl. *fo′ci* [L.] 1. the point of convergence of light rays or sound waves. 2. the chief center of a morbid process. adj., **fo′cal.**

foe- for words beginning thus, see those beginning *fe-*

fog (fog) a colloid system in which the dispersion medium is a gas and the dispersed particles are liquid.

fogging (fog′ing) in ophthalmology, a method of determining refractive error in astigmatism, the patient being first made artifically myopic by means of plus spheres, in order to relax all accommodation before using cylinders.

fold (fōld) plica; a thin, recurved margin, or doubling.

amniotic f., the folded edge of the amnion where it rises over and finally encloses the embryo.

aryepiglottic f., a fold of mucous membrane extending on each side between the lateral border of the epiglottis and the summit of the arytenoid cartilage.

circular f's, the permanent transverse folds of the luminal surface of the small intestine.

costocolic f., a fold of peritoneum passing from the left colic flexure to the adjacent part of the diaphragm. Called also phrenicocolic ligament.

Douglas f., a crescentic line marking the termination of the posterior layer of the sheath of the rectus abdominis muscle just below the level of the iliac crest.

gastric f's, the series of folds in the mucous membrane of the stomach.

gluteal f., the crease separating the buttocks from the thigh.

head f., a fold of blastoderm at the cephalic end of the developing embryo.

lacrimal f., a fold of mucous membrane at the lower opening of the nasolacrimal duct.

mucosal f., mucous f., a fold of mucous membrane.

nail f., the fold of palmar skin around the base and sides of the nail of a finger or toe.

neural f., one of the paired folds lying on either side of the neural plate that form the neural tube.

palmate f's, folds on the anterior and posterior walls of the cervical canal.

semilunar f. of conjunctiva, a mucous fold at the medial angle of the eye.

spiral f., a spirally arranged elevation in the mucosa of the first part of the cystic duct.

tail f., a fold of the blastoderm at the caudal end of the developing embryo.

transverse f's three permanent transverse folds in the rectum.

ventricular f., vestibular f., a false vocal cord.

vestigial f., a pericardial fold enclosing the remnant of the embryonic left anterior cardinal vein.

vocal f., a fold of mucous membrane in the larynx, forming the inferior boundary of the ventricle of the larynx, the vocal muscle being situated deep to it; called also true vocal cord.

folic acid (fo′lik) one of the VITAMINS of the B complex. Folic acid is an essential growth factor and is necessary to the proper formation of blood in the body, and a deficiency of this vitamin typically produces anemia. Green vegetables, liver, and yeast are major sources of folic acid in the diet. It is also produced synthetically. Folic acid deficiency may result from the inability of the body to utilize the vitamin.

f. a. antagonist, a compound, such as aminopterin, that neutralizes the action of folic acid, thus producing folic acid deficiency; used particularly in treatment of leukemias and Hodgkin's disease.

folie (fo-le′) [Fr.] psychosis; insanity.

f. à deux (ah duh′) the occurrence of identical psychoses simultaneously in two closely associated persons.

f. circulaire (ser″ku-lair′) the circular form of manic-depressive psychosis.

f. du doute (du doot) pathologic inability to make even the most trifling decisions.

f. du pourquoi (du poor-kwah′) psychopathologic constant questioning.

f. gémellaire (zha″mĕ-lair′) psychosis occurring simultaneously in twins.

f. musculaire (mus″ku-lār′) severe chorea.

f. raisonnante (rez″un-nahnt′) the delusional form of any psychosis.

folinic acid (fo-lin′ik) a folic acid derivative necessary for the growth of *Leuconostoc citrovorum;* used in treating megaloblastic anemias not due to vitamin B_{12} deficiency and in folic acid deficiency, and as an antidote to toxic effects of folic acid antagonists. Called also citrovorum factor.

folium (fo′le-um), pl. *fo′lia* [L.] a leaflike structure, especially one of the leaflike subdivisions of the cerebellar cortex.

follicle (fol′ĭ-k′l) a sac or pouchlike depression or cavity. adj., **follic′ular.**

atretic f., a graafian follicle that has involuted.

dental f., the structure within the substance of the jaws enclosing a tooth before its eruption; the dental sac and its contents.

gastric f's, lymphoid masses in the gastric mucosa.

graafian f., a maturing ovarian follicle among whose cells fluid has begun to accumulate, leading to the formation of a single cavity and leaving the ovum located in the cumulus oophorus; called also vesicular ovarian follicle.

hair f., one of the tubular invaginations of the epidermis enclosing the hairs, and from which the hairs grow.

lymph f., lymphatic f., 1. a small collection of actively proliferating lymphocytes in the cortex of a lymph node. 2. a small collection of lymphoid tissue in the mucous membrane of the gastrointestinal tract; such collections may occur singly (solitary lymphatic follicle) or closely packed together (aggregated lymphatic follicles).

Naboth's f's, nabothian f's, Naboth's cysts.

ovarian f., the ovum and its encasing cells, at any stage of its development.

ovarian f., primary, an immature ovarian follicle consisting of an immature ovum and the few specialized epithelial cells surrounding it.

primordial f., an ovarian follicle consisting of an ovum enclosed by a single layer of cells.

sebaceous f., a hair follicle with a relatively large sebaceous gland, producing a relatively insignificant hair.

solitary f's, 1. areas of concentrated lymphatic tissue in the mucosa of the colon. 2. small lymph follicles scattered throughout the mucosa and submucosa of the small intestine. Called also solitary glands.

thyroid f's, discrete cystlike units filled with a colloid substance, constituting the lobules of the thyroid gland.

vesicular f., graafian follicle.

follicle-stimulating hormone FSH; one of the gonadotropic hormones of the anterior lobe of the PITUITARY GLAND that stimulates the growth and maturation of graafian follicles in the ovary, and stimulates spermatogenesis in the testis.

folliculitis (fŏ-lik″u-li′tis) inflammation of a follicle(s); used ordinarily in reference to hair follicles, but sometimes in relation to follicles of other kinds.

f. bar′bae, a papulopustular folliculitis of the beard; called also barber's itch or SYCOSIS BARBAE.

Folliculitis barbae is caused by staphylococci. It is marked by pustules in the hair follicles, intense itching, and pain when the hairs are touched or moved as in shaving. The disease can be stubborn and last for months or even years. Occasionally it leads to skin abscess. The condition is treated with bland hot compresses, antibiotics locally and systemically, and epilation of the infected hair.

keloid f., infection of hair follicles of the back of the neck and scalp, occuring chiefly in men, producing large, irregular keloid plaques and scarring.

folliculoma (fŏ-lik″u-lo′mah) granulosa-theca cell tumor.

folliculus (fŏ-lik′u-lus), pl. *follic′uli* [L.] follicle.

Follutein (fŏ-lu′te-in) trademark for a preparation of chorionic gonadotropin.

Folvite (fōl′vīt) trademark for preparations of folic acid.

fomentation (fo″men-ta′shun) treatment by warm, moist applications; also, the substance thus applied.

fomes (fo′mēz), pl. *fo′mites* [L.] an inanimate object or material on which disease-producing agents may be conveyed.

fontanel, fontanelle (fon″tah-nel′) a soft spot; one of the membrane-covered spaces remaining at the junction of the sutures in the incompletely ossified skull of the fetus or infant. Actually there are two soft spots close together, representing gaps in the bone structure which will be filled in by bone during the normal process of growth. The anterior fontanel is diamond shaped and lies at the junction of the frontal and parietal bones. This fontanel usually fills in and closes between the eighth and fifteenth months of life. The posterior fontanel lies at the junction of the occipital and parietal bones, is triangular in shape and usually closes by the third or fourth month of life. Though these "soft spots" may appear very vulnerable, they may be touched gently without harm. Care should be exercised that they be protected from strong pressure or direct injury.

food (fo͞od) anything which, when taken into the body, serves to nourish or build up the tissues or to supply body heat.

f. poisoning, a group of acute illnesses due to ingestion of contaminated food. It may result from allergy; toxemia from foods, such as those inherently poisonous or those contaminated by poisons; foods containing poisons formed by bacteria or foodborne infections. Food poisoning usually causes inflammation of the gastrointestinal tract (gastroenteritis). This may occur quite suddenly, soon after the poisonous food has been eaten. The symptoms are acute, and include tenderness, pain or cramps in the abdomen, nausea, vomiting, diarrhea, weakness, and dizziness.

Food poisoning is often falsely attributed to ptomaines, substances that are formed when protein foods "spoil," or decompose. Because ptomaines produce toxic reactions when injected into experimental animals, "ptomaine poisoning" was formerly believed to be responsible for food-poisoning symptoms in human beings. It is now known that the human digestive system is well able to cope with these substances. Although they should be avoided, spoiled foods are not necessarily harmful. When they are, it is because foods in the process of decomposition frequently harbor disease-causing bacteria.

Bacterial food poisoning may be staphylococcal in origin or it may result from other microorganisms, as in BOTULISM or salmonella infections.

Staphylococcal poisoning is the most common form of food poisoning in the United States. If a food handler is afflicted with a staphylococcal infection, or if he is a carrier, one of the rare persons who carries the disease without suffering infection, he may pass the bacteria on to food. In some foods, the bacteria will multiply very quickly, especially if the food is not refrigerated. Staphylococci are toxin-producing bacteria which do not harm the body directly but produce poisonous substances in the body, causing disease symptoms. The symptoms of staphylococcal poisoning result from the effects of the toxins which have built up in the staphylococci-harboring food. The condition does not spread throughout the body and is not contagious.

Custard-filled pastry is the food most liable to contain staphylococci. Other susceptible foods are cream, milk, cheddar cheese, potato salad, many kinds of sauces, and processed meats, especially ham. These foods should always be purchased from reliable dealers and be kept refrigerated.

Staphylococcal poisoning is characterized by a sudden, sometimes violent onset of nausea, vomiting, and weakness. There may be severe diarrhea. It is rarely serious, except for young children, the elderly, and persons who are weakened by other illness. Symptoms may appear as soon as a half hour or as late as 4 hours after the contaminated food is eaten.

There are a number of poisonous berries and over 80 kinds of poisonous mushrooms. Every year people die or become seriously ill because they have decided that one of these looks good enough to eat. Children are frequently tempted by poisonous holly berries or the berries that grow on privet (the shrub often used for hedges). Adults often place their faith in some incorrect notion, such as the old superstition that you can tell mushrooms from toadstools by cooking a silver coin with them; the coin is supposed to tarnish if the variety is poisonous. These mistaken notions cause a number of deaths every year. Although it is possible to learn to identify poisonous mushrooms and berries, it is much wiser to play safe. Children should be trained not to eat things they find in the woods or fields.

Mushroom poisoning causes a sudden reduction in the concentration of sugar in the blood. There may be convulsions, severe abdominal pain, intense thirst, nausea, vomiting, diarrhea, dimness of vision, and symptoms resembling those of alcoholic intoxication. Symptoms appear 6 to 15 hours after eating.

Mussels and clams may grow in beds, contaminated by the typhoid bacillus (*Salmonella typhi*) and other pathogens. Mussels, clams, and certain other shellfish are dangerous during some seasons of the year. They become poisonous as a result of feeding on microorganisms that appear in the ocean during the warm months, particularly in the Pacific. Shellfish poisoning is characterized by paralysis of the respiratory tract. The symptoms vary. There may be trembling about the lips or loss of power in the muscles of the neck. Symptoms develop within 5 to 30 minutes after eating.

FIRST AID FOR FOOD POISONING

1. Give the patient weak tea and, when he can tolerate them, soft foods.

2. Keep the patient warm and apply heat to the abdomen by means of an electric pad or hot water bottle.

3. The patient should be seen by a physician as soon as possible.

Botulism and Poisoning from Mushrooms, Berries, or Shellfish. If the patient has difficulty seeing, swallowing, or breathing; or if his eyes are sunken; or if his breath has a sweet, fruity odor, his condition is serious and a physician should be called immediately.

Food and Drug Administration an agency of the Department of Health, Education and Welfare whose principal purpose is to enforce the Federal Food, Drug and Cosmetic Act. The agency insures that foods for sale in the United States are safe, pure, and wholesome; that drugs and therapeutic devices are safe and effective; that cosmetics are harmless; and that all these products are correctly labeled and packaged. The F.D.A. is also responsible for enforcing the federal act that requires informative labels on any household product that is toxic, corrosive, irritant, inflammable, or generates pressure through decomposition or heat.

If a product in interstate commerce is proved to be faulty, the F.D.A. is authorized to bring court action or seize the adulterated or incorrectly labeled merchandise and to prosecute the responsible person or company.

foot (foot) the distal part of the primate leg, upon which the individual stands and walks.

athlete's f., a chronic, superficial fungal infection of the skin of the foot (see also ATHLETE'S FOOT).

dangle f., drop f., a condition in which the foot hangs in a plantar-flexed position, due to lesion of the peroneal nerve.

flat f., flatfoot.

immersion f., a condition resembling trench foot occurring in persons who have spent long periods in water.

Madura f., maduromycosis of the foot.

march f., painful swelling of the foot, usually with fracture of a metatarsal bone, after excessive foot strain.

trench f., a condition of the feet resembling FROSTBITE, due to the prolonged action of water on the skin combined with circulatory disturbance due to cold and inaction.

footboard (foot'bōrd) a device placed at the foot of the bed and situated so that the feet rest firmly against it and are at right angles to the legs. It is used to relieve the weight of the bedclothes and to maintain proper positioning of the feet while a patient is confined to bed. Its purpose is to prevent the development of footdrop. It also helps maintain good posture because it prevents the patient from slipping down in bed.

A footboard can be made from wood or improvised from a cardboard box. When the patient is a child and immobilization of the foot, as well as correct positioning, is desired, rubber-soled tennis shoes can be nailed to the footboard and the child's feet laced into the shoes.

footdrop (foot'drop) dropping of the foot from paralysis of the anterior muscles of the leg.

foot-pound (foot'pownd) the amount of energy necessary to raise 1 pound of mass a distance of 1 foot.

foramen (fo-ra'men), pl. *foram'ina* [L.] a natural opening or passage, especially one into or through a bone.

apical f., an opening at or near the apex of the root of a tooth.

auditory f., external, the external acoustic meatus.

auditory f., internal, the passage for the auditory (vestibulocochlear) and facial nerves in the pars petrosa of the temporal bone.

cecal f., f. ce'cum, 1. a blind opening between the frontal crest and the crista galli. 2. a depression on the dorsum of the tongue at the median sulcus.

condyloid f., anterior, hypoglossal canal.

condyloid f., posterior, condylar canal.

epiploic f., an opening connecting the two sacs of the peritoneum, situated below and behind the porta hepatis.

ethmoidal foramina, foram'ina ethmoida'lis, small openings in the ethmoid bone at the junction of the medial wall with the roof of the orbit, the anterior transmitting the nasal branch of the ophthalmic nerve and the anterior ethmoid vessels, the posterior transmitting the posterior ethmoid vessels.

incisive f., one of the openings of the incisive canals into the incisive fossa of the hard palate.

interventricular f., a passage from the third to the lateral ventricle of the brain.

intervertebral f., a passage for a spinal nerve and vessels formed by notches on the pedicles of adjacent vertebrae.

jugular f., an opening formed by the jugular notches of the temporal and occipital bones.

f. mag'num, a large opening in the anterior inferior part of the occipital bone, between the cranial cavity and spinal canal.

mastoid f., an opening in the temporal bone behind the mastoid process.

f. of Monro, interventricular foramen.

obturator f., the large opening between the pubic bone and the ischium.

optic f., optic canal.

f. ova'le, 1. the septal opening in the fetal heart that provides a communication between the atria. The opening closes at birth; failure to close results in atrial septal defect (see also CONGENITAL HEART DEFECT). 2. an aperture in the great wing of the sphenoid for vessels and nerves.

palatine f., anterior, incisive foramen.

f. rotun'dum, a round opening in the great wing of the sphenoid for the maxillary branch of the trigeminal nerve.

sacral foramina, anterior, eight passages (four on each side) on the pelvic surface of the sacrum for the anterior branches of the sacral nerves.

sacral foramina, posterior, eight passages (four on each side) on the dorsal surface of the sacrum for the posterior branches of the sacral nerves.

Scarpa's f., an opening behind the upper medial incisor, for the nasopalatine nerve.

sciatic f., either of two foramina, the greater and the smaller sciatic foramina, formed by the sacrotuberal and sacrospinal ligaments in the sciatic notch of the hip bone.

sphenopalatine f., a space between the orbital and sphenoidal processes of the palatine bone, opening into the nasal cavity and transmitting the sphenopalatine artery and the nasal nerves.

spinous f., a hole in the great wing of the sphenoid for the middle meningeal artery.

supraorbital f., passage in the frontal bone for the supraorbital vessels and nerve; often present as a notch bridged only by fibrous tissue.

thebesian foramina, minute openings in the walls of the right atrium through which the smallest cardiac veins (thebesian veins) empty into the heart.

transverse f., the passage in either transverse process of a cervical vertebra that, in the upper six vertebrae, transmits the vertebral vessels.

vena cava f., an opening in the diaphragm for the inferior vena cava and some branches of the right vagus nerve.

vertebral f., 1. the large opening in a vertebra formed by its body and its arch. 2. transverse foramen.

f. of Vesalius, an occasional opening medial to the foramen ovale of the sphenoid, for passage of a vein from the cavernous sinus.

Weitbrecht's f., a foramen in the capsule of the shoulder joint.

f. of Winslow, epiploic foramen.

Forbes' disease (forbz) glycogenosis (type III) in which a deficiency of the debrancher enzyme dextrin-1,6-glucosidase affects the heart and liver, with hepatomegaly, hypoglycemia, acidosis, stunted growth, and doll facies. Called also Cori's disease and limit dextrinosis.

force (fōrs) energy or power; that which originates or arrests motion or other activity.

catabolic f., energy derived from the metabolism of food.

electromotive f., the force that, by reason of differences in potential, causes a flow of electricity from one place to another, giving rise to an electric current.

reserve f., energy above that required for normal functioning. In the heart it is the power that will take care of the additional circulatory burden imposed by bodily exertion.

Van der Waals f's, the relatively weak, short-range forces of attraction existing between atoms and molecules, which results in the attraction of nonpolar organic compounds to each other (hydrophobic bonding).

forceps (fōr′seps), pl. *for′cipes* [L.] a two-bladed instrument with a handle for compressing or grasping tissues in surgical operations, and for handling sterile dressings, etc.

alligator f., strong toothed forceps having a double clamp.

bayonet f., a forceps whose blades are offset from the axis of the handle.

capsule f., a forceps for removing the lens capsule in cataract.

Chamberlen f., the original form of obstetric forceps.

clamp f., a forceps-like clamp with an automatic lock, for compressing arteries, etc.

dressing f., forceps with scissor-like handles for grasping lint, drainage tubes, etc., in dressing wounds.

obstetric f., forceps for extracting the fetal head from the maternal passages.

rongeur f., a forceps designed for use in cutting bone.

Fordyce's disease (fōr′dīs-ez) a developmental anomaly marked by enlarged and ectopic sebaceous glands that appear as minute yellowish papules on the oral mucosa.

forearm (fōr′arm) the part of the arm between the elbow and wrist; antebrachium.

forebrain (fōr′brān) prosencephalon: 1. the portion of the brain developed from the anterior of the three primary brain vesicles in the early embryo, and comprising the diencephalon and telencephalon. 2. the most anterior of the primary brain vesicles.

foreconscious (fōr′kon-shus) preconscious; material not ordinarily in consciousness, but subject to voluntary recall.

forefinger (fōr′fing-ger) the first or index finger.

forefoot (fōr′foot) the front part of the foot.

foregut (fōr′gut) the endodermal canal of the embryo cephalic to the junction of the yolk stalk, giving rise to the pharynx, lung, esophagus, stomach, liver, and most of the small intestine.

forehead (fōr′ed) the part of the face above the eyes; the anterior portion of the cranium. Called also frons.

foreskin (fōr′skin) prepuce; a loose fold of skin that covers the glans penis. It is a continuation of the loose skin that covers the entire penis and scrotum.

forewaters (fōr′wat-erz) the part of the amniotic sac that pouches into the uterine cervix in front of the presenting part of the fetus.

fork (fork) a pronged instrument.

tuning f., a device that produces harmonic vibration when its two prongs are struck; used to test hearing and bone conduction.

formaldehyde (fōr-mal′dĕ-hīd) a gaseous compound with strongly disinfectant properties. It is used in solution (formol) for disinfection of excreta and utensils and also in the preparation of toxoids from toxins.

formalin (fōr′mah-lin) a 37 per cent solution of gaseous formaldhyde used as a fixative.

formamidase (form-am′ĭ-dās) an enzyme that catalyzes the hydrolysis of formylkynurenine to kynurenine and formate in tryptophan metabolism.

formatio (fōr-ma′she-o), pl. *formatio′nes* [L.] formation.

formation (fōr-ma′shun) 1. the process of giving shape or form; the creation of an entity, or of a structure of definite shape. 2. a structure of definite shape.

reaction f., the development of mental mechanisms which hold in check and repress the components of forbidden wishes.

formic acid (fōr′mik) a colorless, pungent liquid with vesicant properties, from nettles and ants and other insects; derivable from oxalic acid and from glycerin and from the oxidation of formaldehyde.

formication (fōr″mĭ-ka′shun) a sensation as if small insects were crawling on the body.

formiciasis (fōr″mĭ-si′ah-sis) a morbid condition caused by ant bites.

formilase (fōr′mĭ-lās) an enzyme that changes acetic acid into unstable formic acid.

formiminoglutamic acid (fōrm-im″ĭ-no-gloo-tam′-ik) a product in the metabolism of histidine, which accumulates in the urine of humans and rats deficient in folic acid.

formol (fōr′mol) formaldehyde solution.

formula (fōr′mu-lah), pl. *for′mulae, for′mulas* [L.] 1. an expression, using numbers or symbols, of the composition of, or of directions for preparing, a compound, such as a medicine, or of a procedure to follow to obtain a desired result, or of a single concept. 2. a milk mixture for feeding an infant, composed of milk and other ingredients—usually sugar and water—in proportions prescribed by the pediatrician (see also INFANT).

chemical f., a combination of symbols used to express the chemical components of a substance.

empirical f., a chemical formula that expresses the proportions of the elements present in a substance.

molecular f., a chemical formula expressing the number of each element present in a substance, without indicating how they are linked.

official f., one officially established by a pharmacopeia or other recognized authority.

rational f., structural formula.

spatial f., stereochemical f., a chemical formula giving the numbers of atoms of each element present in a molecule of a substance, which atom is linked to which, the types of linkages involved, and the relative positions of the atoms in space.

structural f., a chemical formula showing the spatial arrangement of the atoms and the linkage of every atom.

formulary (fōr′mu-ler″e) a collection of formulae.

National F., a book of standards for certain pharmaceuticals and preparations not included in the U.S.P; revised every 5 years, and recognized as a book of official standards by the Pure Food and Drug Act of 1906. Abbreviated N.F.

formyl (fōr′mil) the radical, HCO or H·C:O—, of formic acid.

fornix (fōr′niks), pl. *for′nices* [L.] 1. an archlike structure or the vaultlike space created by such a structure. 2. fornix of cerebrum; either of a pair of arched fiber tracts that unite under the corpus callosum, so that together they comprise two columns, a body, and two crura.

Foroblique (fōr-o-blēk′) trademark for an obliquely forward visual telescopic system used in certain cystoscopes.

Fort Bragg fever pretibial fever.

Forthane (fōr′thān) trademark for a preparation of methylhexaneamine, a sympathomimetic used as a nasal decongestant.

fossa (fos′ah), pl. *fos′sae* [L.] a trench or channel; in anatomy, a hollow or depressed area.

amygdaloid f., the depression in which the tonsil is lodged.

cerebral f., any of the depressions on the floor of the cranial cavity.

condylar f., condyloid f., either of two pits on the lateral portion of the occipital bone.

coronoid f., a depression in the humerus for the coronoid process of the ulna.

cranial f., any one of the three hollows (anterior, middle, and posterior) in the base of the cranium for the lobes of the brain.

digastric f., a depression on the inner surface of the mandible, giving attachment to the anterior belly of the digastric muscle.

epigastric f., 1. one in the epigastric region. 2. urachal fossa.

ethmoid f., the groove in the cribriform plate of the ethmoid bones, for the olfactory bulb.

glenoid f., mandibular fossa.

hyaloid f., a depression in the front of the vitreous body, lodging the lens.

hypophyseal f., a depression in the sphenoid lodging the pituitary gland; called also pituitary fossa.

iliac f., a concave area occupying much of the inner surface of the ala of the ilium, especially anteriorly; from it arises the iliac muscle.

incisive f., a slight depression on the anterior surface of the maxilla above the incisor teeth.

infratemporal f., an irregularly shaped cavity medial or deep to the zygomatic arch.

interpeduncular f., a depression on the inferior surface of the midbrain, between the two cerebral peduncles, the floor of which is the posterior perforated substance.

ischiorectal f., a potential space between the pelvic diaphragm and the skin below it; an anterior recess extends a variable distance between the pelvic and urogenital diaphragms.

mandibular f., a depression in the inferior surface of the pars squamosa of the temporal bone at the base of the zygomatic process, in which the condyle of the mandible rests; called also glenoid fossa.

mastoid f., a small triangular area between the posterior wall of the external acoustic meatus and the posterior root of the zygomatic process of the temporal bone.

nasal f., the portion of the nasal cavity anterior to the middle meatus.

navicular f., 1. the vaginal vestibule between the vaginal orifice and the frenulum of the pudendal labia. 2. the lateral expansion of the urethra of the glans penis; called also lacuna majus. 3. a depression on the internal pterygoid process of the sphenoid, giving attachment to the tensor veli palatini muscle.

f. ova′lis cor′dis, a fossa in the right atrium of the heart; the remains of the fetal foramen ovale.

ovarian f., a shallow pouch on the posterior surface of the broad ligament of the uterus in which the ovary is located.

pituitary f., hypophyseal fossa.

subarcuate f., a depression in the posterior inner surface of the pars petrosa of the temporal bone.

subpyramidal f., a depression on the internal wall of the middle ear.

subsigmoid f., a fossa between the mesentery of the sigmoid flexure and that of the descending colon.

supraspinous f., a depression above the spine of the scapula.

temporal f., an area on the side of the cranium bounded posteriorly and superiorly by the temporal lines, anteriorly by the frontal and zygomatic bones, and laterally by the zygomatic arch, lodging the temporal muscle.

tibiofemoral f., a space between the articular surfaces of the tibia and femur mesial or lateral to the inferior pole of the patella.

urachal f., one on the inner abdominal wall, between the urachus and the hypogastric artery.

fossette (fŏ-set′) 1. a small depression. 2. a small, deep corneal ulcer.

fossula (fos′u-lah), pl. *fos′ulae* [L.] a small fossa.

Fothergill's disease (foth′er-gilz) 1. scarlatina anginosa. 2. tic douloureux.

Fothergill's neuralgia (foth′er-gilz) tic douloureux.

foulage (foo-lahzh′) [Fr.] kneading and pressing of the muscles in massage.

fourchette (foor-shet′) [Fr.] the posterior junction of the labia minora.

fovea (fo′ve-ah), pl. *fo′veae* [L.] a small pit or depression.

f. centra′lis ret′inae, a small pit in the center of the macula lutea, composed of slim, elongated cones; it is the area of clearest vision, because here the layers of the retina are spread aside, permitting light to fall directly on the cones.

foveate (fo′ve-āt) pitted.

foveation (fo″ve-a′shun) formation of pits on a surface, as on the skin; a pitted condition.

foveola (fo-ve′o-lah), pl. *fove′olae* [L.] a minute pit or depression.

Fowler's positon (fow′lerz) the head of the patient's bed is raised 18 to 20 inches above the level, with the knees also elevated.

Fowler's solution (fow′lerz) potassium arsenite solution, composed of arsenic trioxide, potassium bicarbonate, and water; has been used as an antileukemic agent.

Fox-Fordyce disease (foks for′dīs) a condition of unknown causation characterized by plugging of the pores of the apocrine sweat glands and vesiculation of the epidermis.

foxglove (foks′gluv) *Digitalis purpurea,* the source of digitalis.

Fr chemical symbol, *francium.*

fracture (frak′chur) 1. the breaking of a part, especially a bone. 2. a break in the continuity of bone. Fractures may be caused by trauma, by twisting due to muscle spasm, or indirect loss of leverage or by disease that results in decalcification of the bone.

TREATMENT. Immediate first aid consists in splinting the bone. No attempt should be made to set the bone; it should be splinted "as it lies"; i.e., it should be supported in such a way that the injured part will remain steady and will resist jarring if the victim is moved.

A fracture is treated by reduction, which means that the broken ends are pulled into alignment and the continuity of the bone is established so that healing can take place and the bone is "made whole" again. Closed reduction is performed by manual manipulation of the fractured bone so that the fragments are brought into proper alignment; no surgical incision is made. Open reduction is done only when it is necessary to débride and cleanse the area, as in an open fracture. A fracture may also require internal fixation with pins, nails, metal plates, or screws to stabilize the alignment.

Once reduction is accomplished the bone is immobilized by application of a CAST or by an apparatus exerting TRACTION on the distal end of the bone.

avulsion f., separation of a small fragment of bone cortex at the site of attachment of a ligament or tendon.

Barton's f., fracture of the distal end of the radius into the wrist joint.

Bennett's f., fracture of the base of the first metacarpal bone, running into the carpometacarpal joint, complicated by subluxation.

blow-out f., fracture of the orbital floor caused by a sudden increase of intraorbital pressure due to traumatic force; the orbital contents herniate into the maxillary sinus so that the inferior rectus or inferior oblique muscle may become incarcerated in the fracture site, producing diplopia on looking up.

capillary f., one that appears on a roentgenogram as a fine, hairlike line, the segments of bone not being separated; sometimes seen in fractures of the skull.

closed f., one that does not produce an open wound.

Colles' f., fracture of the lower end of the radius, the distal fragment being displaced backward; if the lower fragment is displaced forward, it is a reversed Colles' fracture.

comminuted f., one in which the bone is splintered or crushed (see illustration).

complete f., one involving the entire cross section of the bone.

compound f., open fracture.

compression f., one produced by compression.

depressed f., fracture of the skull in which a fragment is depressed.

direct f., one at the site of injury.

dislocation f., fracture of a bone near an articulation with concomitant dislocation of that joint.

double f., fracture of a bone in two places.

Dupuytren's f., Pott's fracture.

Duverney's f., fracture of the ilium just below the anterior inferior spine.

fissure f., a crack extending from a surface into, but not through, a long bone.

greenstick f., one in which one side of a bone is broken, the other being bent (see illustration).

impacted f., fracture in which one fragment is firmly driven into the other (see illustration).

incomplete f., one that does not involve the complete cross section of the bone.

indirect f., one at a point distant from the site of injury.

interperiosteal f., greenstick or incomplete fracture.

intrauterine f., fracture of a fetal bone incurred in utero.

lead pipe f., one in which the bone cortex is slightly compressed and bulged on one side with a slight crack on the other side of the bone.

Le Fort's f., bilateral horizontal fracture of the maxilla. Le Fort fractures are classified as follows: *Le Fort I fracture,* a horizontal segmented fracture of the alveolar process of the maxilla, in which the teeth are usually contained in the detached portion of the bone. *Le Fort II fracture,* unilateral or bilateral fracture of the maxilla, in which the body of the maxilla is separated from the facial skeleton and the separated portion is pyramidal in shape; the fracture may extend through the body of the maxilla down the midline of the hard palate, through the floor of the orbit, and into the nasal cavity. *Le Fort III fracture,* a fracture in which the entire maxilla and one or more facial bones are completely separated from the craniofacial skeleton; such fractures are almost always accompanied by multiple fractures of the facial bones.

Monteggia's f., one in the proximal half of the shaft of the ulna, with dislocation of the head of the radius (see illustration).

open f., one in which a wound through the adjacent or overlying soft tissues communicates with the site of the break; called also compound fracture (see illustration).

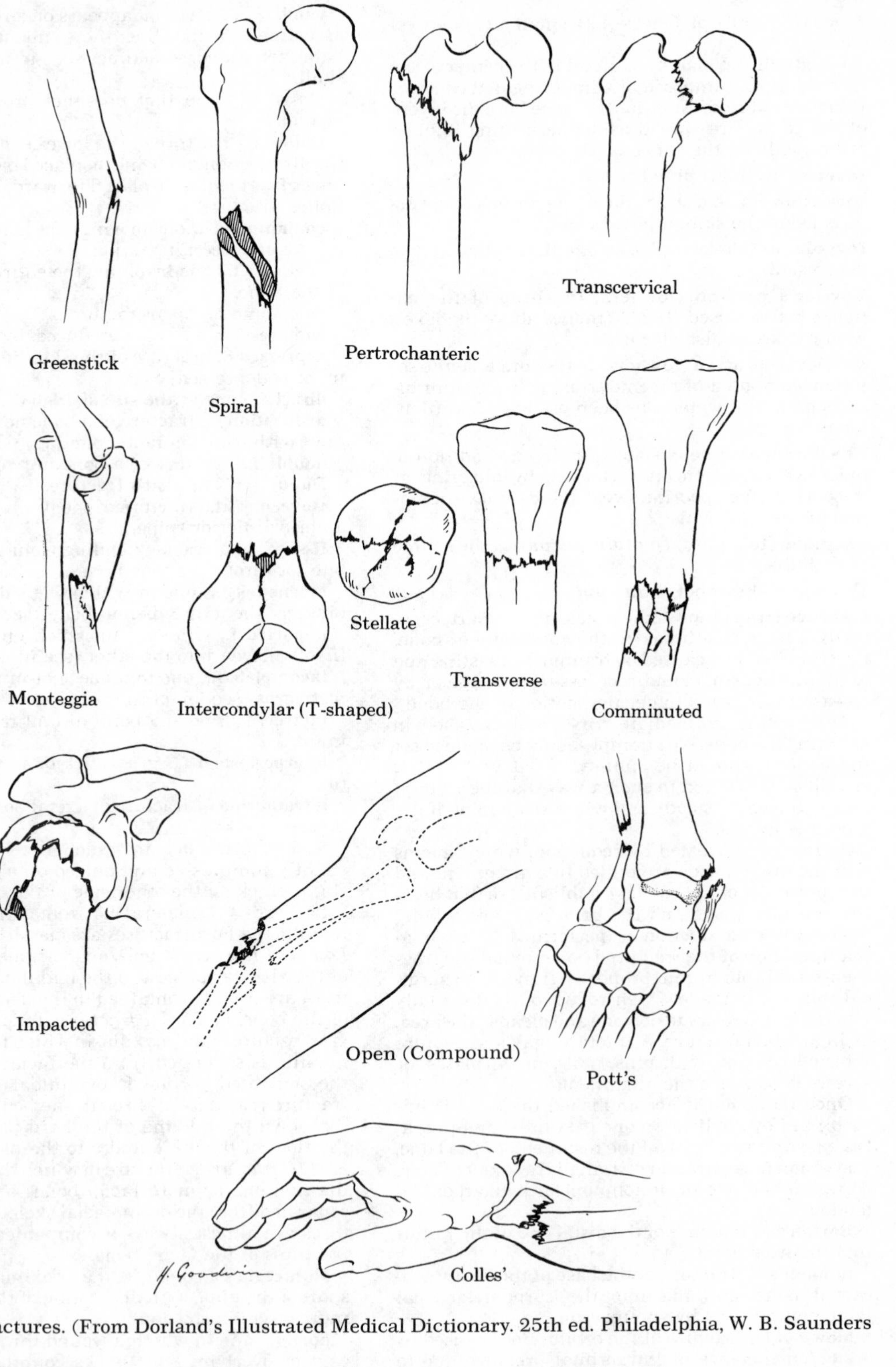

Types of fractures. (From Dorland's Illustrated Medical Dictionary. 25th ed. Philadelphia, W. B. Saunders Co., 1974.)

pathologic f., one occurring in diseased bone with only slight or no trauma.

pertrochanteric f., fracture of the femur passing through the greater trochanter (see illustration).

ping-pong f., an indented fracture of the skull, resembling the indentation that can be produced with the finger in a ping-pong ball; when elevated it resumes and retains its normal position.

Pott's f., fracture of lower part of fibula with serious injury of the lower tibial articulation.

simple f., closed fracture.

Smith's f., reversed Colles' fracture.

spiral f., one in which the bone has been twisted apart (see illustration).

spontaneous f., pathologic fracture.

sprain f., the separation of a tendon from its insertion, taking with it a piece of bone.

stellate f., one with a central point of injury, from which radiate numerous fissures (see illustration).

Stieda's f., a fracture of the internal condyle of the femur.

transcervical f., one through the neck of the femur (see illustration).

transverse f., one at right angles to the axis of the bone (see illustration).

trophic f., one due to a nutritional (trophic) disturbance.

fracture-dislocation (frak′chur-dis″lo-ka′shun) a fracture of a bone near a joint, also involving dislocation.

frae- for words beginning thus, see those beginning *fre-*.

fragilitas (frah-jil′ĭ-tas) [L.] fragility.

f. crin′ium, a brittleness of the hair.

f. os′sium congen′ita, osteogenesis imperfecta.

fragility (frah-jil′ĭ-te) susceptibility, or lack of resistance, to influences capable of causing disruption of continuity or integrity.

f. of blood, erythrocyte fragility.

capillary f., abnormal susceptibility of capillary walls to rupture.

erythrocyte f., susceptibility of erythrocytes to hemolysis when subjected to mechanical trauma (mechanical fragility) or when exposed to increasingly hypotonic saline solutions (osmotic fragility). A test of erythrocyte osmotic fragility is used in diagnosing hemolytic anemia. Called also fragility of blood.

fragmentation (frag″men-ta′shun) division into small pieces.

frambesia (fram-be′ze-ah) yaws.

frambesioma (fram-be″ze-o′mah) mother yaw; the initial cutaneous lesion of YAWS.

frame (frām) a rigid supporting structure or a structure for immobilizing a part.

Balkan f., an apparatus for continuous extension in treatment of fractures of the femur, consisting of an overhead bar, with pulleys attached, by which the leg is supported in a sling.

Bradford f., a rectangular structure of gas pipe across which are stretched two strips of canvas, used as a bed frame for patients with fractures or disease of the hip or spine.

quadriplegic standing f., a device for supporting in the upright position a patient whose four limbs are paralyzed.

Stryker f., one consisting of canvas stretched on anterior and posterior frames, on which the patient can be rotated around his longitudinal axis (see also STRYKER FRAME).

Franceschetti's syndrome see mandibulofacial DYSOSTOSIS.

Francisella (fran″sĭ-sel′ah) a genus of bacteria.

f. tularen′sis, the etiologic agent of tularemia; called also PASTEURELLA TULARENSIS.

francium (fran′se-um) a chemical element, atomic number 87, atomic weight 223, symbol Fr. (See table of ELEMENTS.)

Frankenhaüser's ganglion (frang′ken-hoy″zerz) a ganglion near the cervix uteri; called also cervical, or cervicouterine, ganglion.

F.R.C.P. Fellow of the Royal College of Physicians.

F.R.C.S. Fellow of the Royal College of Surgeons.

freckle (frek″l) a pigmented spot on the skin due to accumulation of melanin resulting from exposure to sunlight (see also LENTIGO).

melanotic f. of Hutchinson, a noninvasive malignant melanoma occurring most often on the face of women during the fourth decade; called also lentigo maligna.

freeze-drying (frēz-dri′ing) a method of tissue preparation in which the tissue specimen is frozen and then dehydrated at low temperature in a high vacuum.

freeze-etching (frēz-ech′ing) a method used to study unfixed cells by electron microscopy, in which the object to be studied is placed in 20 per cent glycerol, frozen at −100° C., and then mounted on a chilled holder.

freezing point (fre′zing) the temperature at which a liquid begins to freeze; for water, 0° C., or 32° F.

Frei's disease (frīz) lymphogranuloma venereum.

Frei's test (frīz) intracutaneous injection of antigen derived from infected chick embryos, used in the diagnosis of lymphogranuloma venereum.

Freiberg's disease (fri′bergz) osteochondrosis of the head of the second metatarsal bone.

fremitus (frem′ĭ-tus) a vibration perceptible on palpation or auscultation.

tactile f., a vibration, as in the chest wall, felt on the thorax while the patient is speaking.

tussive f., one felt on the chest while the patient coughs.

vocal f., one caused by speaking, perceived on auscultation.

French scale (french) a scale used for denoting size of catheters, sounds, and other tubular instruments, each unit being roughly equivalent to 0.33 mm. in diameter.

frenectomy (fre-nek′to-me) excision of a frenum (frenulum).

frenoplasty (fre′no-plas″te) the correction of an abnormally attached frenum by surgically repositioning it.

frenotomy (fre-not′o-me) the cutting of a frenum (frenulum).

frenulum (fren′u-lum,), pl. *fren′ula* [L.] a small fold of integument or mucous membrane that limits the movements of an organ or part.

f. of clitoris, a fold formed by union of the labia minora with the clitoris.

f. of ileocecal valve, a fold formed by the joined extremities of the ileocecal valve, partially encircling the lumen of the colon.

f. labio′rum puden′di, fourchette.

f. lin'guae, the midline fold connecting the under surface of the tongue and floor of the mouth; called also frenulum of tongue.

f. of lip, a median fold of mucous membrane connecting the inside of each lip to the corresponding gum.

f. of prepuce of penis, a fold under the penis connecting it with the prepuce.

f. of superior medullary velum, a band lying in the superior medullary velum at its attachment to the inferior colliculi.

f. of tongue, the vertical fold of mucous membrane under the tongue, attaching it to the floor of the mouth.

frenum (fre'num,), pl. *fre'na* [L.] a restraining structure or part; see FRENULUM.

frequency (fre'kwen-se) in statistics, the number of occurrences of a determinable entity per unit of time or population, e.g., cases of disease per 100,000 population.

Freud (froid) Sigmund (1856–1939). Clinical neurologist and founder of psychoanalysis. Born in Freiberg in Moravia, and educated at the University of Vienna, he studied in Paris in 1885 under the neurologist J. M. Charcot, who encouraged him to investigate hysteria from a psychologic point of view. Freud stressed the existence of an unconscious that exerts a dynamic influence on consciousness, and was led to develop his method of "free association" in order to discover these buried memories. He emphasized the role of sexuality in the development of neurotic conditions, and published *Interpretation of Dreams* (1900), *Psychopathology of Everyday Life* (1901), and many more works. He was also director of the *International Journal of Psychology.* Fleeing the Nazi regime in Vienna in 1938, he died in London.

freudian (froi'de-an) pertaining to Sigmund Freud, the founder of PSYCHOANALYSIS, and to his doctrines regarding the causes and treatment of neuroses and psychoses (see also NEUROSIS and PSYCHOSIS).

friable (fri'ah-b'l) easily pulverized or crumbled.

friction (frik'shun) the act of rubbing.

friction rub an auscultatory sound caused by the rubbing together of two serous surfaces.

Fried's rule (frēds) the dose of a drug for an infant less than 2 years old is obtained by multiplying the child's age in months by the adult dose and dividing the result by 150.

Friedländer's disease (frēd'len-derz) endarteritis obliterans.

Friedländer's pneumonia (frēd'len-derz) a form characterized by massive mucoid inflammatory exudates in a lobe of the lung, due to *Klebsiella pneumoniae.*

Friedman's test (frēd'manz) a test for pregnancy, based on the effects on ovaries of a mature, non-pregnant female rabbit, produced by injection of the patient's urine (see also PREGNANCY TESTS).

Friedreich's ataxia (frēd'rīks) hereditary sclerosis of the dorsal and lateral columns of the spinal cord, usually beginning in childhood or youth. It is attended by ataxia, speech impairment, scoliosis, and peculiar swaying and irregular movements, with paralysis of the muscles, especially of the lower extremities.

Friedreich's disease (frēd'rīks) 1. paramyoclonus multiplex. 2. Friedreich's ataxia.

frigidity (frĭ-jid'ĭ-te) coldness; especially, sexual unresponsiveness of the female to physical stimulation.

frigorific (frig"o-rif'ik) producing coldness.

Fröhlich's syndrome (fra'liks) a condition associated with lesions of the hypothalamus and pituitary gland, marked by obesity and sexual infantilism; called also adiposogenital dystrophy. It is treated with pituitary extract.

frolement (frōl-maw') [Fr.] 1. a rustling sound heard on auscultation in pericardial disease. 2. a brushing movement in massage.

frons (fronz) [L.] the forehead.

frontad (frun'tad) toward a front, or frontal aspect.

frontal (frun'tal) 1. pertaining to the forehead. 2. denoting a longitudinal plane passing through the body from side to side, and dividing it into front and back parts.

f. bone, the unpaired bone constituting the anterior part of the skull (see also table of BONES).

f. lobe, the rostral (anterior) portion of the cerebral hemisphere.

frontalis (fron-ta'lis) [L.] frontal.

frost (frost) a deposit resembling frozen dew or vapor.

urea f., the appearance on the skin of salt crystals left by evaporation of the sweat in urhidrosis.

frostbite (frost'bīt) injury to tissues due to exposure to cold. Usually the first areas of the body to freeze are the nose, ears, fingers, and toes. The flesh feels cold to the touch, and frozen parts become pale and feel numb. There may also be some prickly or itchy sensation. A person suffering from frostbite may feel no warning pain.

In mild cases of frostbite proper treatment can rather quickly restore normal circulation of blood. In more serious cases the area may become painfully inflamed, and blistering may follow. Especially severe frostbite can cause death of the injured tissues and gangrene may result.

TREATMENT. The frozen parts should be gradually and gently rewarmed. Hot water bottles or other applications of heat are contraindicated, as is rubbing or massaging, which may further damage the injured tissues. Cool or lukewarm water may be used to rewarm the frozen parts. If water is not available, the part may be rewarmed by covering it with warm clothing or by placing it in contact with any other part of the body that is warm. Contrary to a common theory, frostbite should *never* be treated by rubbing the affected area with snow or by the application of snow or ice.

frottage (fro-tahzh') [Fr.] 1. a rubbing movement in massage. 2. sexual gratification by rubbing against a person of the opposite sex.

frotteur (fro-tur') one who practices frottage (2).

frozen section (fro'zen) a specimen of tissue that has been quick-frozen, cut by microtome, and stained immediately for rapid diagnosis of possible malignant lesions. A specimen processed in this manner is not satisfactory for detailed study of the cells, but it is valuable because it is quick and gives the surgeon immediate information regarding the malignancy of a piece of tissue.

fructofuranose (fruk"to-fu'rah-nōs) the combining and more reactive form of fructose.

β-fructofuranosidase (fruk"to-fu"rah-no'sĭ-dās) an

enzyme occurring in yeasts and other organisms that catalyzes the hydrolysis of sugars with a terminal unsubstituted β-D-fructofuranosyl residue.

fructokinase (fruk″to-ki′nās) an enzyme that catalyzes the transfer of a high-energy phosphate group to D-fructose.

fructose (fruk′tōs) a sugar found in honey and many sweet fruits; called also levulose and fruit sugar. It is used in solution as a fluid and nutrient replenisher.

fructosemia (fruk″to-se′me-ah) the presence of fructose in the blood, as in fructose intolerance.

fructoside (fruk′to-sīd) a compound that bears the same relation to fructose as a glucoside does to glucose.

fructosuria (fruk″to-su′re-ah) the presence of fructose in the urine.

essential f., a benign hereditary disorder of carbohydrate metabolism due to a defect in fructokinase and manifested only by fructose in the blood and urine.

fructosyl (fruk′to-sil) a radical of fructose.

fruit (fro͞ot) the matured ovary of a plant, including the seed and its envelopes.

frustration (frus-tra′shun) increased emotional tension due to failure to achieve sought gratifications or satisfactions.

FSH follicle-stimulating hormone.

Fuadin (fu′ah-din) trademark for a preparation of stibophen, used as an antischistosomal and in the treatment of granuloma inguinale.

fuchsin (fook′sin) any of several red to purple dyes.

acid f., a mixture of sulfonated fuchsins; used in various complex stains.

basic f., a histologic stain, a mixture of pararosaniline, rosaniline, and magenta II. Also, a mixture of rosaniline and pararosaniline hydrochlorides used as a local anti-infective.

fucose (fu′kōs) a monosaccharide occurring as L-fucose in a number of mucopolysaccharides and mucoproteins.

fucosidase (fu-ko′sĭ-dās) an enzyme occurring in two forms that catalyzes the hydrolysis of fucoside to an alcohol and fucose.

fucoside (fu′ko-sīd) an acetal derivative of fucose.

fucosidosis (fu″ko-sĭ-do′sis) a hereditary neurovisceral disease due to deficient enzymatic activity of fucosidase and resulting in accumulation of fucose in all tissues; it is marked by progressive cerebral degeneration, muscle weakness with eventual spasticity, emaciation, cardiomegaly, thick skin, and excessive sweating.

FUDR floxuridine.

-fugal word element [L.], *driving away; fleeing from; repelling.*

fugue (fūg) a dissociative reaction in which amnesia is accompanied by physical flight from customary surroundings.

fulgurate (ful′gu-rāt) 1. to come and go like a flash of lightning. 2. to destroy by contact with electric sparks generated by a high-frequency current.

fulguration (ful″gu-ra′shun) destruction of living tissue by electric sparks generated by a high-frequency current.

fulminate (ful′mĭ-nāt) to occur suddenly with great intensity. adj., **ful′minant.**

Fulvicin (ful′vĭ-sin) trademark for a preparation of griseofulvin, an antibiotic used as a fungistatic in dermatophytoses.

fumagillin (fu″mah-jil′in) an antibiotic elaborated by strains of *Aspergillus fumigatus;* used as an antimicrobial.

fumarase (fu′mah-rās) an enzyme that catalyzes the interconversion of fumarate and malate.

fumarate (fu′mar-āt) a salt of fumaric acid.

ferrous f., the anhydrous salt of a combination of ferrous iron and fumaric acid; used as a hematinic.

fumaric acid (fu′mar-ik) an unsaturated dibasic acid; it is the *trans*-isomer of maleic acid and an intermediate in the tricarboxylic acid cycle.

fumigation (fu″mĭ-ga′shun) exposure to disinfecting fumes.

Fumiron (fūm′i-ron) trademark for a preparation of ferrous fumarate; a hematinic.

function (fungk′shun) the special, normal, or proper action of any part or organ.

functional (fungk′shun-al) pertaining to or fulfilling a function; affecting the function but not the structure.

f. disease, a disease involving body functions but without detectable tissue damage.

fundament (fun′dah-ment) 1. a base or foundation, as the breech or rump. 2. the anus and parts adjacent to it.

fundectomy (fun-dek′to-me) excision of the fundus of an organ, as of the stomach.

fundiform (fun′dĭ-form) shaped like a loop or sling.

fundoplication (fun″do-pli-ka′shun) mobilization of the lower end of the esophagus and plication of the fundus of the stomach up around it, in the treatment of hiatal hernia.

fundus (fun′dus), pl. *fun′di* [L.] the bottom or base of anything; used in anatomic nomenclature as a general term to designate the bottom or base of an organ, or the part of a hollow organ farthest from its mouth. adj., **fun′dal, fun′dic.**

f. of bladder, the base or posterior surface of the urinary bladder.

f. of eye, the back portion of the interior of the eyeball, visible through the pupil by use of the ophthalmoscope.

f. of gallbladder, the inferior, dilated portion of the gallbladder.

f. of stomach, the part of the stomach to the left and above the level of the opening between the stomach and esophagus.

f. tym′pani, the floor of the tympanic cavity.

f. u′teri, f. of uterus, the part of the uterus above the orifices of the uterine tubes.

funduscope (fun′dus-skōp) ophthalmoscope. adj., **funduscop′ic.**

fundusectomy (fun″dŭ-sek′to-me) excision of the fundus of the stomach.

fungal (fun′gal) pertaining to or caused by a fungus.

fungate (fun′gāt) to produce fungus-like growths; to grow rapidly, like a fungus.

fungemia (fun-je′me-ah) the presence of fungi in the blood stream.

fungi (fun′ji) [L.] plural of *fungus.*

fungicide (fun′jĭ-sīd) an agent that destroys fungi. adj., **fungici′dal.**

fungicidin (fun″jĭ-si′din) nystatin, an antifungal antibiotic.

fungiform (fun′jĭ-form) shaped like a fungus, or mushroom.

fungistasis (fun″jĭ-sta′sis) inhibition of the growth of fungi. adj., **fungistat′ic.**

fungistat (fun′jĭ-stat) a substance that checks the growth of fungi.

fungitoxic (fun″jĭ-tok′sik) exerting a toxic effect upon fungi.

Fungizone (fun′jĭ-zōn) trademark for a preparation of amphotericin B, an antibiotic used in cryptococcal meningitis and systemic fungal infections.

fungoid (fun′goid) resembling a fungus.

chignon f., a nodular growth on the hair.

fungosity (fun-gos′ĭ-te) a fungoid growth or excrescence.

fungous (fun′gus) of the nature of, caused by, or resembling a fungus.

fungus (fun′gus), pl. *fun′gi* [L.] a general term for a group of eukaryotic protists (mushrooms, yeasts, molds, etc.) marked by the absence of chlorophyll and the presence of a rigid cell wall. Fungi are present in the soil, air, and water, but only a few species can cause disease. Among the fungal diseases (mycoses) are HISTOPLASMOSIS, COCCIDIOIDOMYCOSIS, RINGWORM, ATHLETE'S FOOT, and THRUSH. Although the fungal diseases develop slowly, are difficult to diagnose, and are resistant to treatment, they are rarely fatal.

funicle (fu′nĭ-k'l) funiculus.

funiculitis (fu-nik″u-li′tis) 1. inflammation of the spermatic cord. 2. inflammation of that portion of a spinal nerve root which lies within the intervertebral canal.

funiculus (fu-nik′u-lus), pl. *funic′uli* [L.] a cord; a cordlike structure or part, especially one of the large bundles of nerve tracts making up the white matter of the spinal cord. adj., **funic′ular.**

anterior f., the white substance of the spinal cord lying on either side between the anterior median fissure and the ventral root.

lateral f., f. latera′lis, the lateral mass of fibers on either side of the spinal cord, between the anterolateral and posterolateral sulci.

posterior f., the white substance of the spinal cord lying on either side between the posterior median sulcus and the dorsal root.

f. spermat′icus, the spermatic cord.

funiform (fu′nĭ-form) resembling a rope or cord.

funnel chest (fun′el) a congenital abnormality of the anterior chest wall in which the sternum is depressed; called also PECTUS EXCAVATUM.

Furacin (fu′rah-sin) trademark for preparations of nitrofurazone, an antibacterial agent.

Furadantin (fūr″ah-dan′tin) trademark for preparations of nitrofurantoin, an antibacterial used in urinary tract infections.

Furaspor (fūr′ah-spōr) trademark for a preparation of nitrofurfuryl methyl ether, used as a topical fungicide and sporicide for skin infections.

furazolidone (fu″rah-zol′ĭ-dōn) a yellow, odorless, crystalline powder, used as a local antibacterial and antiprotozoal.

furcal (fur′kal) forked.

furfuraceous (fur″fu-ra′shus) fine and loose; said of scales resembling dandruff or bran.

furosemide (fur-o′sĕ-mīd) an oral diuretic.

Furoxone (fur-ok′sōn) trademark for preparations of furazolidone, an antibacterial and antiprotozoal.

furrow (fur′o) a groove or trench.

atrioventricular f., the transverse groove marking off the atria of the heart from the ventricles.

digital f., any one of the transverse folds across the joints on the palmar surface of a finger.

gluteal f., the furrow that separates the buttocks.

furuncle (fu′rung-k'l) a focal suppurative inflammation of the skin and subcutaneous tissues, enclosing a central slough or "core"; called also BOIL. It is caused by staphylococci, which enter through the hair follicles, and its formation is favored by constitutional or digestive derangement and local irritation.

furunculoid (fu-rung′ku-loid) resembling a furuncle or boil.

furunculosis (fu-rung″ku-lo′sis) 1. the persistent sequential occurrence of furuncles over a period of weeks or months. 2. the simultaneous occurrence of a number of furuncles.

Fusarium (fu-sa′re-um) a genus of fungi; some species are plant pathogens and some are opportunistic infectious agents of man and animals.

fuscin (fus′in) a brown pigment of the retinal epithelium.

fusible (fu′zĭ-b'l) capable of being melted.

fusiform (fu′zĭ-form) spindle-shaped.

fusimotor (fu″sĭ-mo′tor) denoting motor nerve fibers (of gamma motoneurons) that innervate intrafusal fibers of the muscle spindle.

fusion (fu′zhun) 1. the act or process of melting. 2. the abnormal coherence of adjacent parts or bodies. 3. the coordination of separate images of the same object in the two eyes into one. 4. the operative formation of an ankylosis or arthrosis.

diaphyseal-epiphyseal f., operative establishment of bony union between the epiphysis and diaphysis of a bone.

nerve f., nerve anastomosis done to induce regeneration for resupplying empty tracts of a nerve with new growth of fibers.

nuclear f., the fusion of two atomic nuclei to form a single heavier nucleus, resulting in the release of enormous amounts of energy.

spinal f., surgical creation of ankylosis between contiguous vertebrae; spondylosyndesis.

fusional (fu′zhun-al) marked by fusion.

Fusobacterium (fu″zo-bak-te′re-um) a genus of anaerobic gram-negative bacteria found as normal flora in the mouth and large bowel, and often in necrotic tissue, probably as secondary invaders.

F. plau′tivincen′ti, a species found in necrotizing ulcerative gingivitis (trench mouth) and in necrotizing ulcerative stomatitis.

fusocellular (fu″zo-sel′u-lar) having spindle-shaped cells.

fusospirillosis (fu″zo-spi″rĭ-lo′sis) trench mouth.

fusospirochetal (fu″zo-spi″ro-ke′tal) of or caused by fusiform bacilli and spirochetes.

fusospirochetosis (fu″zo-spi″ro-ke-to′sis) trench mouth.

G

G. gram (or grams); gingival; glucose; gonidial.

g gravity; the unit of force exerted upon a body during acceleration and deceleration.

g. gram (or grams).

Ga chemical symbol, *gallium.*

gadolinium (gad″o-lin′e-um) a chemical element, atomic number 64, atomic weight 157.25, symbol Gd. (See table of ELEMENTS.)

gag (gag) 1. a surgical device for holding the mouth open. 2. to retch, or strive to vomit.

g. reflex, elevation of the soft palate and retching elicited by touching the back of the tongue or the wall of the pharynx; called also pharyngeal reflex.

gait (gāt) the manner or style of walking.

g. analysis, evaluation of the manner or style of walking, usually done by observing the individual as he walks naturally in a straight line. The normal forward step consists of two phases: the *stance phase,* during which one leg and foot are bearing most or all of the body weight, and the *swing phase,* during which the foot is not touching the walking surface and the body weight is borne by the other leg and foot. In a complete two-step cycle both feet are in contact with the floor at the same time for about 25 percent of the time. This part of the cycle is called the *double-support phase.*

An analysis of each component of the three phases of ambulation is an essential part of the diagnosis of various neurologic disorders and the assessment of patient progress during rehabilitation and recovery from the effects of a neurologic disease, a musculoskeletal injury or disease process, or amputation of a lower extremity.

antalgic g., the limp characteristics of cured cases of coxalgia, marked by avoidance of weight-bearing on the affected side.

ataxic g., an unsteady, uncoordinated walk, employing a wide base.

double-step g., a gait in which there is a noticeable difference in the length and/or timing of alternate steps.

drag-to g., a gait in which the feet are dragged (rather than lifted) toward the CRUTCHES.

equine g., a walk accomplished mainly by flexing the hip joint; seen in crossed-leg palsy.

festinating g., one in which the patient involuntarily moves with short, accelerating steps, often on tiptoe, as seen in Parkinson's disease; festination.

four-point g., a gait in forward motion using CRUTCHES.

gluteal g., the gait characteristic of paralysis of the gluteus medius muscle, marked by a listing of the trunk toward the affected side at each step.

helicopod g., a gait in which the feet describe half circles, as in some hysterical disorders.

hemiplegic g., a gait involving flexion of the hip because of footdrop and circumduction of the leg.

intermittent double-step g., a hemiplegic gait in which there is a pause after the short step of the normal foot, or in some cases after the step of the affected foot.

Oppenheim's g., a gait marked by irregular oscillation of the head, limbs, and body; seen in some cases of multiple sclerosis.

spastic g., a walk in which the legs are held together and move in a stiff manner, the toes seeming to drag and catch.

steppage g., the gait in footdrop in which the advancing leg is lifted high in order that the toes may clear the ground. It is due to paralysis of the anterior tibial and peroneal muscles, and is seen in lesions of the lower motor neuron, such as multiple neuritis, lesions of the anterior motor horn cells, and lesions of the cauda equina.

swing-through g., that in which the CRUTCHES are advanced and then the legs are swung past them.

swing-to g., that in which the CRUTCHES are advanced and the legs are swung to the same point.

tabetic g., an ataxic gait in which the feet slap the ground; in daylight the patient can avoid some unsteadiness by watching his feet.

three-point g., that in which both CRUTCHES and the affected leg are advanced together and then the normal leg is moved forward.

two-point g., that in which the right foot and left CRUTCH or cane are advanced together, and then the left foot and right crutch.

waddling g., exaggerated alternation of lateral trunk movements with an exaggerated elevation of the hip, suggesting the gait of a duck; characteristic of progressive muscular dystrophy.

galact(o)- word element [Gr.], *milk.*

galactacrasia (gah-lak″tah-kra′ze-ah) an abnormal state of the breast milk.

galactagogue (gah-lak′tah-gog) 1. promoting the flow of milk. 2. an agent that promotes the flow of milk.

galactan (gah-lak′tan) a carbohydrate that yields galactose upon hydrolysis.

galactemia (gal″ak-te′me-ah) the presence of milk in the blood.

galactic (gah-lak′tik) 1. pertaining to milk. 2. galactagogue.

galactin (gah-lak′tin) a hormone of the anterior pituitary gland (see also PROLACTIN).

galactischia (gal″ak-tisk′e-ah) suppression of milk secretion.

galactoblast (gah-lak′to-blast) a colostrum corpuscle in the acini of the mammary gland.

galactobolic (gah-lak″to-bol′ik) of or relating to the action of neurohypophyseal peptides which contract the mammary myoepithelium and cause ejection of milk.

galactocele (gah-lak′to-sēl) 1. a milk-containing, cystic enlargement of the mammary gland. 2. hydrocele filled with milky fluid.

galactolipid, galactolipin (gah-lak″to-lip′id; gah-lak″to-lip′in) a cerebroside which yields galactose on hydrolysis.

galactoma (gal″ak-to′mah) galactocele (1).

galactometer (gal″ak-tom′ĕ-ter) an instrument for measuring the specific gravity of milk; lactometer.

galactophore (gah-lak′to-fōr) 1. galactophorous. 2. a milk duct.

galactophoritis (gah-lak″to-fo-ri′tis) inflammation of the milk ducts.

galactophorous (gal″ak-tof′o-rus) conveying milk.

galactophygous (gal″ak-tof′ĭ-gus) arresting the flow of milk.

galactoplania (gah-lak″to-pla′ne-ah) secretion of milk in some abnormal part.

galactopoiesis (gah-lak″to-poi-e′sis) the production of milk by the mammary glands.

galactopoietic (gah-lak″to-poi-et′ik) 1. pertaining to, marked by, or promoting milk production. 2. an agent that promotes milk flow.

galactopyra (gah-lak″to-pi′rah) milk fever.

galactorrhea (gah-lak″to-re′ah) excessive or spontaneous milk flow; persistent secretion of milk irrespective of nursing; lactorrhea.

galactosamine (gah-lak″to-sam′in) an amino derivative of galactose.

galactoscope (gah-lak′to-skōp) a device for showing the proportion of cream in milk.

galactose (gah-lak′tōs) a monosaccharide derived from lactose. D-galactose is found in lactose, cerebrosides of the brain, raffinose of the sugar beet, and in many gums and seaweeds; L-galactose is found in flaxseed mucilage.

g. tolerance test, a laboratory test done to determine the liver's ability to convert the sugar galactose into glycogen. Two methods may be used. The oral method requires about 5 hours to complete, and the intravenous method, which is more accurate, requires about 2 hours. With the oral method, elimination of more than 3 gm. of galactose in the urine during a 5-hour period indicates liver damage. With the intravenous method, all galactose should have been eliminated from the blood 45 minutes after its injection.

galactosemia (gah-lak″to-se′me-ah) a genetically determined biochemical disorder in which there is a lack of the enzyme necessary for proper metabolism of galactose. Normally the sugar derived from lactose in milk is changed by enzymatic action into glucose. In galactosemia the enzyme glactose-1-phosphate uridyl transferase is absent. This means that normal conversion of galactose to glucose does not take place and the galactose accumulates in the tissues and blood.

The disorder becomes manifest soon after birth and is characterized by feeding problems, vomiting and diarrhea, abdominal distention, enlargement of the liver, mental retardation, and elevated blood and urine galactose levels. Cataracts also may develop.

The disorder can be detected by a sensitivity test so that early diagnosis and treatment are possible. If the disease is detected early, before there is damage to the central nervous system, the symptoms of the disorder can be prevented.

Treatment consists of exclusion from the diet of milk and all foods containing galactose or lactose. Milk substitutes are used and the diet is planned to substitute necessary nutrients normally obtained from products containing lactose or galactose.

galactosidase (gah-lak″to-si′dās) an enzyme that catalyzes the conversion of galactoside to galactose; it occurs in two forms: α-galactosidase (melibiase) and β-galactosidase (lactase).

galactoside (gah-lak′to-sīd) a glycoside containing galactose.

galactosis (gal″ak-to′sis) the formation of milk by the lacteal glands.

galactostasis (gal″ak-tos′tah-sis) 1. cessation of milk secretion. 2. abnormal collection of milk in the mammary glands.

galactosuria (gah-lak″to-su′re-ah) the presence of galactose in the urine.

galactotherapy (gah-lak″to-ther′ah-pe) treatment of a nursing infant by medication given the mother or wet nurse.

galactotoxin (gah-lak″to-tok′sin) a basic substance formed in milk.

galactozymase (gah-lak″to-zi′mās) a starch-liquefying enzyme.

galacturia (gal″ak-tu′re-ah) chyluria; the discharge of urine with a milky appearance.

galea (ga′le-ah), pl. *ga′leae* [L.] a helmet-shaped structure.

g. aponeurot′ica, aponeurosis connecting the frontal and occipital bellies of the occipitofrontal muscle.

Galen (ga′len) [Claudius Galenus] (A.D. 130–200). The celebrated Greek physician to the Roman Emperor Marcus Aurelius. Although he did not dissect the human cadaver, he made many valuable anatomic and physiologic observations on animals (and applied many of them inaccurately to man), and his writings on these and other subjects were extensive. His influence on medicine was profound for many

GALACTOSEMIA: FOOD PLAN FOR ALL THE FAMILY MEMBERS

Food Group	Servings During One Day		
	Preschool	*School Age*	*Adults*
Milk (Nutramigen for child with galactosemia)[1]	3 to 4 cups	4 or more cups	2 cups
Fruits[2] and vegetables[3]	4 or more small servings	4 or more	4 or more
Meats, fish, eggs, poultry[4]	2 or more small servings	2 or more	2 or more
Breads and cereals (milk free for child with galactosemia)	4 or more	4 or more	4 or more

From "Parent's Guide for the Galactose-free Diet," published by the California State Department of Health, 2151 Berkeley Way, Berkeley, California.

[1]If Nutramigen is not drunk in these amounts, calcium and vitamin D should be given as supplements.

[2]Include every day a serving of one of these: citrus, tomato, melon, strawberries, broccoli, raw cabbage, green peppers.

[3]Include a deep yellow or dark green, leafy vegetable at least every other day. Omit beets, peas, and lima beans for the child with galactosemia.

[4]Nuts, peanuts, and peanut butter are also included in this group.

centuries—his teleology ("nature does nothing in vain") being particularly attractive to the medieval mind, although it was stultifying as regards advances in medical thought and practice.

galenicals, galenics (gah-len′ĭ-kals; gah-len′iks) medicines prepared according to the formulae of Galen. The term is now used to denote standard preparations containing one or several organic ingredients, as contrasted with pure chemical substances.

galeophobia (ga″le-o-fo′be-ah) morbid fear of cats; ailurophobia.

gall (gawl) the bile.

gallamine triethiodide (gal′ah-min tri″eth-i′o-dīd) a skeletal muscle relaxant.

gallbladder (gawl′blad-er) the pear-shaped organ located below the liver. It serves as a storage place for bile. The gallbladder may be subject to such disorders as inflammation and the formation of GALLSTONES.

Acute inflammation of the gallbladder (CHOLECYSTITIS) causes severe pain and tenderness in the right upper abdomen, accompanied by fever, nausea, prostration, and sometimes jaundice. If the inflammation does not subside quickly, the gallbladder must be removed before it becomes gangrenous and ruptures.

Chronic inflammation of the gallbladder may cause habitual indigestion, accompanied by flatulence and nausea. The indigestion is most evident after heavy meals or meals of fatty foods. There also may be repeated attacks of pain in the right upper abdomen; these may be very brief or may last as long as several hours. Gallstones are often present. The condition may respond to conservative treatment with diet and medications or it may require surgical removal of the gallbladder, especially if there are gallstones.

Diagnosis of disorders of the gallbladder is aided by CHOLECYSTOGRAPHY; x-ray films are made after a contrast medium has been administered so that the gallbladder and bile ducts are clearly silhouetted. Studies may be done to determine the presence of gallstones or obstructions to the flow of bile in the biliary tract.

SURGERY OF THE GALLBLADDER. The two surgical procedures most commonly performed on the gallbladder are cholecystectomy and cholecystostomy. In cholecystectomy the gallbladder is removed; in cholecystostomy an incision is made into the gallbladder for the purpose of drainage. Surgical procedures involving the common bile duct are sometimes done in the treatment of various disorders of the gallbladder and biliary tract and may entail a surgical incision into the common bile duct (choledochotomy) which is usually done for removal of gallstones (choledocholithotomy).

Patient Care. During the preoperative period the patient usually receives a thorough physical examination as well as specific tests for liver function and x-ray studies of the gallbladder and bile ducts. Since nausea and flatulence are common occurrences in these patients both before and after surgery, a nasogastric tube is usually inserted prior to surgery.

When the patient returns from the operating room a careful check should be made for drainage tubes, which may have been inserted during surgery. Most drains are devised so that bile and serous fluid from the operative site drain directly onto the dressings applied over the wound. Other drains or tubes, such as the T tube or Y tube, should be opened immediately and attached to a drainage apparatus so that the bile is collected in a bottle and can be measured periodically. In either case dressings over the wound are checked frequently for signs of hemorrhage or abnormalities in the drainage. When bile leakage is excessive the dressings will need frequent reinforcing and the outer layers will require frequent changing to keep the patient dry and comfortable and to avoid irritation of the skin around the incision.

It is especially important to observe the patient for signs of jaundice, bile pigment in the urine, and light-colored stools during the postoperative period. Any of these conditions may indicate improper drainage of bile from the gallbladder and resultant accumulation of bile pigments in the blood. If the patient complains of severe abdominal pain before or after removal of drains or tubes, this situation should be reported to the physician at once.

Galli Mainini test (gal′e mi-ne′ne) a test for pregnancy; sperm are found in the urine of male frogs 1 to 4 hours after injection of urine from a pregnant woman (see also PREGNANCY TESTS).

gallium (gal′e-um) a chemical element, atomic number 31, atomic weight 69.72, symbol Ga. (See table of ELEMENTS.)

gallon (gal′on) a unit of liquid measure (4 quarts, or 3.785 liters, or 3785 ml.).

gallop (gal′op) a disordered rhythm of the heart. (See also gallop RHYTHM.)

gallstone (gawl′stōn) a stonelike mass, called a calculus, that forms in the gallbladder. The presence of gallstones is known medically as cholelithiasis. Their cause is unknown, although there is evidence of a connection between gallstones and obesity. They are most common in women after pregnancy, and in men and women past 35.

Gallstones may be present for years without causing trouble. The usual symptoms, however, are vague discomfort and pain in the upper abdomen. There may be indigestion and nausea, especially after eating fatty foods. X-rays will generally reveal the presence of gallstones, either directly or by use of a dye introduced into the gallbladder (CHOLECYSTOGRAPHY).

The most common complication of gallstones occurs when one of the stones escapes from the gallbladder and travels along the common bile duct, where it may lodge, blocking the flow of bile to the intestine and causing obstructive jaundice. This condition should be corrected by surgery before the liver is damaged.

When a gallstone travels through or obstructs a bile duct it can cause severe biliary colic, probably the most severe pain that can be experienced. The pain is located in the upper right quadrant of the abdomen, and radiates through to the scapula. Morphine is usually not given to relieve the pain because it increases spasm of the biliary sphincters. Other drugs such as papaverine hydrochloride and atropine may be given to promote relaxation and thereby relieve the pain. Treatment may also include insertion of a nasogastric tube for the purpose of gastric suction to relieve distention in the upper gastrointestinal tract.

Surgery is the preferred method of treatment and is performed as soon as the patient is able to withstand it. In most cases the gallbladder is removed and a tube is inserted to establish drainage of bile that has been dammed up by the stone. (See also surgery of the GALLBLADDER.)

galvanic current (gal-van′ik) a steady direct electric current.

galvanism (gal′vah-nizm) 1. unidirectional electric current derived from a chemical battery. 2. galvanotherapy.

galvanization (gal″vah-nĭ-za′shun) galvanotherapy.

galvanocautery (gal″vah-no-kaw′ter-e) cautery by a wire heated by galvanic current.

galvanocontractility (gal″vah-no-kon″trak-til′ĭ-te) contractility in response to stimulation by galvanic current.

galvanometer (gal″vah-nom′ĕ-ter) an instrument for measuring current by electromagnetic action.

galvanopalpation (gal″vah-no-pal-pa′shun) testing of nerves of the skin by means of galvanic current.

galvanosurgery (gal″vah-no-ser′jer-e) the use of galvanocautery in surgery.

galvanotaxis (gal″vah-no-tak′sis) the tendency of an organism to arrange itself in a medium so that its axis bears a certain relation to the direction of the current in the medium.

galvanotherapy (gal″vah-no-ther′ah-pe) the therapeutic use of galvanic current.

galvanotropism (gal″vah-not′ro-pizm) the tendency of an organism to turn or move under the action of electric current.

gamete (gam′ēt) 1. one of two cells, male (spermatozoon) and female (ovum), whose union is necessary in sexual reproduction to initiate the development of a new individual. 2. the malarial parasite in its sexual form in a mosquito's stomach, either male (microgamete) or female (macrogamete); the latter is fertilized by the former to develop into an ookinete. adj., **gamet′ic.**

gametocide (gam′ĕ-to-sīd″) an agent that destroys gametes or gametocytes. adj., **gametoci′dal.**

gametocyte (gah-met′o-sīt) that sexual stage of the malarial parasite in the blood which may produce gametes when taken into the mosquito host; it may be male (microgametocyte) or female (macrogametocyte).

gametogenesis (gam″ĕ-to-jen′ĕ-sis) the development of the male and female sex cells (gametes). adj, **gametogen′ic.**

gametogony (gam″ĕ-tog′o-ne) the development of merozoites into male and female gametes, which later fuse to form a zygote.

gamma (gam′ah) the third letter of the Greek alphabet, γ; used in names of chemical compounds to distinguish one of three or more isomers or to indicate the position of substituting atoms or groups.

g. globulin, a plasma protein developed in the lymphoid tissues and reticuloendothelial system in response to invasion by harmful agents such as bacteria, viruses, and toxins. There are three types of plasma proteins: albumin, globulins, and fibrinogen. Fibrinogen and albumin are manufactured by the liver; fibrinogen plays a vital role in the process of clotting. Gamma globulins are specific protein molecules that react chemically with the invading agent and are capable of destroying it; thus they play an important role in providing IMMUNITY. (See also IMMUNOGLOBULIN.) Almost all ANTIBODIES produced in defense of the body are gamma globulin molecules.

Commercial preparations of gamma globulin are derived from blood serum and are used for prevention, modification, and treatment of various infectious diseases. This type of gamma globulin, which is an immune serum, contains almost all the known antibodies circulating in the blood. It provides a passive immunity, usually for about 6 weeks. Certain specific types of gamma globulin may be used to raise the body's resistance to measles, mumps, and poliomyelitis.

The production of gamma globulin may be increased in the body by the invasion of harmful microorganisms. An abnormal amount of gamma globulin in the blood, a condition known as hypergammaglobulinemia, may be indicative of a chronic infection or certain malignant blood diseases.

There is also a rare condition, AGAMMAGLOBULINEMIA, in which the body is unable to produce gamma globulin; patients suffering from this condition are extremely susceptible to infection and must be given frequent injections of gamma globulin serum. (See also Disorders of the IMMUNE RESPONSE.)

g. rays, γ-rays, electromagnetic emissions from radioactive substances. Gamma rays are similar to and have the same general properties as x-rays, except that they are produced through the disintegration of certain radioactive elements. They consist of high energy photons, have short wavelengths, and have no mass and no electric charge.

Radium, uranium, and thorium are examples of radioactive metals that emit three types of rays: alpha, beta, and gamma rays. Of these three forms of radiation, the gamma rays are the most penetrating and therefore are sometimes used in the treatment of deep-seated malignancies (see also RADIOTHERAPY).

gamma benzene hexachloride (gam′ah ben′zēn hek″sah-klōr′īd) lindane, a pediculicide and scabicide.

gammacism (gam′ah-sizm) imperfect utterance of *g* and *k* sounds.

gammaglobulinopathy (gam″ah-glob″u-lin-op′ah-the) gammopathy.

gammopathy (gam-mop′ah-the) abnormal proliferation of the lymphoid cells producing immunoglobulins; the gammopathies include multiple myeloma, macroglobulinemia, and Hodgkin's disease. Called also gammaglobulinopathy.

Gamna's disease (gam′naz) splenomegaly with thickening of the splenic capsule and the presence of small brownish areas (Gamna's nodules), iron-containing pigment being deposited in the splenic pulp.

Gamna's nodules (gam′naz) brown or yellow pigmented nodules seen in the spleen in certain cases of enlargement, as in Gamna's disease and siderotic splenomegaly.

gamogenesis (gam″o-jen′ĕ-sis) sexual reproduction.

gangli(o)- word element [Gr.], *ganglion.*

ganglial (gang′gle-al) pertaining to a ganglion.

gangliated (gang′gle-āt″ed) provided with ganglia; ganglionated.

gangliectomy (gang″gle-ek′to-me) excision of a ganglion; ganglionectomy.

gangliform (gang′glĭ-form) having the form of a ganglion.

gangliitis (gang″gle-i′tis) inflammation of a ganglion; ganglionitis.

ganglioblast (gang′gle-o-blast″) an embryonic cell of the cerebrospinal ganglia.

gangliocyte (gang′gle-o-sīt) a ganglion cell.

gangliocytoma (gang″gle-o-si-to′mah) ganglioneuroma.

ganglioform (gang′gle-o-form″) gangliform.

ganglioglioma (gang″gle-o-gli-o′mah) a glioma rich in mature neurons or ganglion cells.

ganglioglioneuroma (gang″gle-o-gli″o-nu-ro′mah) ganglioneuroma.

ganglioma (gang″gle-o′mah) ganglioneuroma.

ganglion (gang′gle-on), pl. *gan′glia, ganglions* [Gr.] 1. a knot or knotlike mass; used in anatomic nomenclature as a general term to designate a group of nerve cell bodies, located outside the central nervous system. Occasionally applied to certain nuclear groups within the brain or spinal cord, e.g., basal ganglia. 2. a form of cystic tumor occurring on an aponeurosis or tendon, as the wrist. adj., **gan′glial, ganglion′ic.**

Arnold's g., otic ganglion.

autonomic ganglia, aggregations of cell bodies of neurons of the autonomic nervous system; the parasympathetic and the sympathetic ganglia combined.

basal ganglia, masses of gray matter centrally embedded with the thalamus in the cerebral hemisphere, comprising the corpus striatum (caudate and lentiform nuclei), amygdaloid body, and claustrum. Sometimes the thalamus is considered as part of the basal ganglia; the tuber cinereum, corpora geniculata, and even the corpora quadrigemina have also been included. Called also basal nuclei.

cardiac ganglia, ganglia of the superficial cardiac plexus under the arch of the aorta.

carotid g., an occasional small enlargement in the internal carotid plexus.

celiac ganglia, two irregularly shaped ganglia, one on each crus of the diaphragm within the celiac plexus.

cephalic ganglia, parasympathetic ganglia in the head, consisting of the ciliary, otic, pterygopalatine, and submandibular ganglia.

cerebrospinal ganglia, those associated with the cranial and spinal nerves.

cervical g., 1. any of the three ganglia (inferior, middle, and superior) of the sympathetic trunk in the neck region. 2. one near the cervix uteri.

cervicothoracic g., a ganglion on the sympathetic trunk anterior to the lowest cervical or first thoracic vertebra. It is formed by a union of the seventh and eighth cervical and first thoracic ganglia. Called also stellate ganglion.

cervicouterine g., one near the cervix uteri.

ciliary g., a parasympathetic ganglion in the posterior part of the orbit.

coccygeal g., glomus coccygeum.

Corti's g., spiral ganglion.

dorsal root g., spinal ganglion.

false g., an enlargement on a nerve that does not have a true ganglionic structure.

Frankenhäuser's g., cervical ganglion (2).

gasserian g., trigeminal ganglion.

geniculate g., the sensory ganglion of the facial nerve, on the geniculum of the facial nerve.

g. im′par, the ganglion commonly found in front of the coccyx, where the sympathetic trunks of the two sides unite.

inferior g., the lower of two ganglia of the glossopharyngeal nerve as it passes through the jugular foramen. 2. the lower of two ganglia of the vagus nerve as it passes through the jugular foramen.

jugular g., superior ganglion (1 and 2).

Ludwig's g., a ganglion near the right atrium of the heart, connected with the cardiac plexus.

lumbar ganglia, the ganglia on the sympathetic trunk, usually four or five on either side.

lymphatic g., a lymph node.

otic g., a parasympathetic ganglion next to the medial surface of the mandibular division of the trigeminal nerve, just inferior to the foramen ovale. Its postganglionic fibers supply the parotid gland. Called also Arnold's ganglion.

parasympathetic ganglia, aggregations of cell bodies of cholinergic neurons of the parasympathetic nervous system; these ganglia are located near to or within the wall of the organs being innervated. See also Plate 14.

petrous g., inferior ganglion (1).

pterygopalatine g., a parasympathetic ganglion in a fossa in the sphenoid bone, formed by postganglionic cell bodies that synapse with preganglionic fibers from the fascial nerve via the nerve of the pterygopalatine canal. Called also sphenopalatine ganglion.

sacral ganglia, those of the sacral part of the sympathetic trunk, usually three or four on either side.

Scarpa's g., vestibular ganglion.

semilunar g., 1. trigeminal ganglion. 2. [pl.] celiac ganglia.

sensory g., any of the ganglia of the peripheral nervous system that transmit sensory impulses; also, the collective masses of nerve cell bodies in the brain subserving sensory functions.

simple g., a cystic tumor in a tendon sheath.

sphenopalatine g., pterygopalatine ganglion.

spinal ganglia, ganglia on the posterior root of each spinal nerve.

spiral g., the ganglion on the cochlear nerve, located within the modiolus, sending fibers peripherally to the organ of Corti and centrally to the cochlear nuclei of the brain stem. Called also Corti's ganglion.

stellate g., cervicothoracic ganglion.

submandibular g., submaxillary g., a parasympathetic ganglion located superior to the deep part of the submandibular gland, on the lateral surface of the hyoglossal muscle; its postganglionic fibers supply the sublingual and submandibular glands.

superior g., 1. the upper of two ganglia on the glossopharyngeal nerve as it passes through the jugular foramen. 2. the upper of two ganglia of the vagus nerve just as it passes through the jugular foramen. Called also jugular ganglion.

sympathetic ganglia, aggregations of cell bodies of adrenergic neurons of the sympathetic nervous system; these ganglia are arranged in chainlike fashion on either side of the spinal cord.

thoracic ganglia, the ganglia on the thoracic portion of the sympathetic trunk, 11 or 12 on either side.

trigeminal g., a ganglion on the sensory root of the fifth cranial nerve, situated in a cleft within the dura mater on the anterior surface of the pars petrosa of the temporal bone, and giving off the ophthalmic and maxillary and part of the mandibular nerve. Called also gasserian ganglion and semilunar ganglion.

tympanic g., an enlargement on the tympanic branch of the glossopharyngeal nerve.

vestibular g., the sensory ganglion of the vestibular part of the eighth cranial nerve, located in the upper part of the lateral end of the internal acoustic meatus. Called also Scarpa's ganglion.

Walther's g., glomus coccygeum.

Wrisberg's ganglia, cardiac ganglia.

wrist g., cystic enlargement of a tendon sheath on the back of the wrist.

ganglionated (gang′gle-o-nāt″ed) provided with ganglia; gangliated.

ganglionectomy (gang″gle-o-nek′to-me) excision of a ganglion; gangliectomy.

ganglioneuroma (gang″gle-o-nu-ro′mah) a benign neoplasm composed of nerve fibers and mature ganglion cells; called also gangliocytoma, ganglioglioneuroma, and ganglioma.

ganglionic (gang″gle-on′ik) pertaining to a ganglion.

g. blockade, inhibition by drugs of nerve impulse transmission at autonomic ganglionic synapses.

ganglionitis (gang″gle-o-ni′tis) inflammation of a ganglion; gangliitis.

ganglionostomy (gang″gle-o-nos′to-me) surgical creation of an opening into a cystic tumor on a tendon sheath or aponeurosis.

ganglioplegic (gang″gle-o-ple′jik) 1. blocking transmission of impulses through the sympathetic and parasympathetic ganglia. 2. an agent that so acts.

ganglioside (gang′gle-o-sīd) a class of galactose-containing cerebrosides found in central nervous system tissues; they are glycolipids of the basic composition ceramide-glucose-galactose-N-acetyl neuraminic acid. The form GM_1 accumulates in tissues in generalized gangliosidosis, the form GM_2 in Tay-Sachs disease.

gangliosidosis (gang″gle-o-si-do′sis) a lipid storage disorder marked by accumulation of gangliosides in tissues due to an enzyme defect. In generalized gangliosidosis, a hereditary defect in β-galactosidase causes accumulation of galactoside GM_1, resulting in mental retardation, hepatomegaly, skeletal deformities, and, often, a cherry-red spot. In TAY-SACHS DISEASE, a defect of hexosaminidase A results in accumulation of ganglioside GM_2.

gangosa (gang-go′sah) one of the late lesions of yaws, manifested as a destructive ulceration of the nose, nasopharynx, and hard palate.

gangrene (gang′grēn) the death of body tissue, generally in considerable mass, usually associated with loss of vascular (nutritive) supply, and followed by bacterial invasion and putrefaction. Although it usually affects the extremities, gangrene sometimes may involve the internal organs. Symptoms depend on the site and include fever, pain, darkening of the skin, and an unpleasant odor. If the condition involves an internal organ, it is generally attended by pain and collapse. Treatment includes correcting the causes and is frequently successful with modern medications and surgery.

TYPES OF GANGRENE. The three major types of gangrene are moist, dry, and gas gangrene. Moist and dry gangrene result from loss of blood circulation due to various causes; gas gangrene occurs in wounds infected by anaerobic bacteria, among which are various species of *Clostridium,* which break down tissue by gas production and by toxins.

Moist gangrene is caused by sudden stoppage of blood, resulting from burning by heat or acid, severe freezing, physical accident that destroys the tissue, a tourniquet that has been left on too long, or a clot or other embolism. At first, tissue affected by moist gangrene has the color of a bad bruise, is swollen, and often blistered. The gangrene is likely to spread with great speed. Toxins are formed in the affected tissues and absorbed.

Dry gangrene occurs gradually and results from slow reduction of the blood flow in the arteries. There is no subsequent bacterial decomposition; the tissues become dry and shriveled. It occurs only in the extremities, and can occur with ARTERIOSCLEROSIS, in old age, or in advanced stages of DIABETES MELLITUS. BUERGER'S DISEASE can also sometimes cause dry gangrene. Symptoms include gradual shrinking of the tissue, which becomes cold and lacking in pulse, and turns first brown and then black. Usually a line of demarcation is formed where the gangrene stops, owing to the fact that the tissue above this line continues to receive an adequate supply of blood.

Gas gangrene results from dirty lacerated wounds infected by anaerobic bacteria, especially species of *Clostridium.* It is an acute, severe, painful condition in which muscles and subcutaneous tissues become filled with gas and a serosanguineous exudate.

INTERNAL GANGRENE. In strangulated HERNIA, a loop of intestine is caught in the bulge and its blood supply is cut off; gangrene may occur in that section of tissue. In acute APPENDICITIS, areas of gangrene may occur in the walls of the appendix with consequent rupture through a gangrenous area. In severe cases of CHOLECYSTITIS, which is usually associated with GALLSTONES, gangrene may develop where the stones compress the mucous membrane. Thrombosis of the mesenteric artery may result in gangrene. Gangrene can be a rare complication of LUNG abscess in pneumonia; a symptom is brown sputum with a foul smell.

PREVENTION. To prevent gangrene in an open wound, the wound should be kept as clean as possible. If a tourniquet is applied, it must be loosened for about 1 minute in every 10 minutes to keep fresh blood in the tissue. Burned skin requires careful and antiseptic handling (see also BURN). FROSTBITE is especially dangerous, for the freezing impedes circulation and skin becomes tender and easily broken.

gangrenous (gang′grĕ-nus) pertaining to, marked by, or of the nature of gangrene.

Ganser's syndrome (gan′serz) amnesia, disturbance of consciousness, and hallucinations, associated with senseless answers to questions, and absurd acts.

Gantrisin (gan′trĭ-sin) trademark for preparations of sulfisoxazole, an antibacterial sulfonamide.

Garamycin (gar″ah-mi′sin) trademark for a preparation of gentamicin, an antibiotic.

Gardner's syndrome (gahrd′nerz) familial polyposis of the colon associated with osseous and soft tissue tumors.

gargle (gar′g′l) 1. a solution for rinsing the mouth and throat. 2. to rinse the mouth and throat by holding a solution in the open mouth and agitating it by expulsion of air from the lungs.

gargoylism (gar'goil-izm) HURLER'S SYNDROME, the prototypical form of mucopolysaccharidosis.

Garré's osteomyelitis (gar-āz') sclerosing nonsuppurative osteomyelitis.

gas (gas) any elastic aeriform fluid in which the molecules are widely separated from each other and so have free paths.

coal g., a gas produced by the destructive distillation of coal and used for domestic cooking. It is poisonous because it contains carbon monoxide.

g. gangrene, a condition often resulting from dirty, lacerated wounds in which the muscles and subcutaneous tissue become filled with gas and a serosanguineous exudate. It is due to species of *Clostridium* that break down tissue by gas production and by toxins.

laughing g., nitrous oxide.

marsh g., methane.

g. pains, pains caused by distention of the stomach or intestines by accumulations of air or other gases. The presence of gas is indicated by the distention of the abdomen and by belching or the discharge of gas by rectum. Gas-forming foods include highly flavored vegetables such as onions, cabbage, and turnips, and members of the bean family. Melons and raw apples are gas-forming fruits. Seasonings and other chemical irritants are also likely to produce gas in the intestinal tract.

sewer g., the mixture of gases and vapors from a sewer; often dangerous from the contained materials resulting from the decay of organic matter.

tear g., a gas that produces severe lacrimation by irritating the conjunctivae.

gaster (gas'ter) [Gr.] stomach.

Gasterophilus (gas"ter-of'ĭ-lus) a genus of flies, the horse botflies, the larvae of which develop in the gastrointestinal tract of horses and may sometimes infect man.

gastr(o)- word element [Gr.], *stomach.*

gastradenitis (gas"trad-ĕ-ni'tis) inflammation of the gastric glands.

gastralgia (gas-tral'je-ah) pain in the stomach; gastric colic.

gastramine (gas'trah-min) an analogue of histamine used in place of it in gastric function tests to stimulate gastric secretion (see also BETAZOLE).

gastrectomy (gas-trek'to-me) excision of the stomach (total gastrectomy) or a portion of it (partial or subtotal gastrectomy). Indications for surgical removal of part or all of the stomach include malignant tumors and gastric ULCER that does not respond to medical management or is complicated by perforation or hemorrhage. (See also surgery of the STOMACH.)

gastric (gas'trik) pertaining to, affecting, or originating in the stomach.

g. analysis, analysis of the stomach contents by microscopy and tests to determine the amount of acid present. The tests performed are of value in diagnosing peptic ulcer, cancer of the stomach, and pernicious anemia. They include tests for free and total acid, for occult blood, and for lactic acid. Hyperacidity frequently is associated with benign ulcers; free acid is decreased in malignant tumors. Achlorhydria, or total absence of free hydrochloric acid, is characteristic of untreated pernicious anemia.

Procedures for a gastric analysis vary according to the type of test meal or stimulating substance given to increase the flow of gastric juices. Alcohol, caffeine, or histamine may be used as a stimulant. All gastric analyses require that the patient be in a fasting state, that he refrain from smoking, and that he remain calm and undisturbed prior to withdrawal of the stomach's contents. Measures must be taken to make the passage of the stomach tube as easy as possible for the patient under the circumstances. Once the stomach tube is in place specimens are obtained at varying intervals, depending on the stimulant administered.

One type of gastric analysis does not require the passage of a stomach tube. This is the DIAGNEX BLUE test, sometimes called a "tubeless gastric analysis." This test determines free hydrochloric acid by qualitative means; though it is of value as a screening device, it cannot be used as conclusive evidence in those cases in which hydrochloric acid is not excreted.

g. juice, the secretion of glands in the walls of the stomach for use in digestion. Its essential ingredients are pepsin, an enzyme that breaks down proteins in food, and hydrochloric acid, which destroys bacteria and is of assistance in the digestive process.

At the sight and smell of food, the stomach increases its output of gastric juice. When the food reaches the stomach, it is thoroughly mixed with the juice, the breakdown of the proteins is begun and the food then passes on to the duodenum for the next stage of digestion.

Normally the hydrochloric acid in gastric juice does not irritate or injure the delicate stomach tissues. However, in certain persons the stomach produces too much gastric juice, especially between meals when it is not needed, and the gastric secretions presumably erode the stomach lining, producing a peptic ULCER, and also hinder its healing once an ulcer has formed.

g. ulcer, an ULCER of the inner wall of the stomach. It is one of the two most common types of peptic ulcer, the other type being duodenal ulcer.

gastricism (gas'trĭ-sizm) gastric disorder.

gastricsin (gas-trik'sin) a proteolytic enzyme isolated from gastric juice; its precursor is pepsinogen but differs from pepsin in molecular weight and in the amino acid content at the N terminal.

gastrin (gas'trin) a polypeptide hormone secreted by certain cells of the pyloric glands, which strongly stimulates secretion of gastric acid and pepsin, and weakly stimulates secretion of pancreatic enzymes and gallbladder contraction.

gastrinoma (gas"trin-o'mah) a gastrin-secreting, non-beta islet cell tumor of the pancreas, associated with Zollinger-Ellison syndrome.

gastritis (gas-tri'tis) inflammation of the lining of the stomach. Gastritis is one of the most common stomach disorders, and occurs in acute, chronic, and toxic forms.

acute g., severe gastritis caused by food poisoning, overeating, excessive intake of alcoholic beverages, or bacterial or viral infection, and often accompanied by enteritis. The outstanding symptom of acute gastritis is abdominal pain. There is a feeling of distention, with loss of appetite, nausea, and headache. There may be a slight fever and vomiting.

The substance causing the irritation can often be identified and it should of course be avoided. A bland diet of liquids and easily digested food should be followed for 2 or 3 days. Simply prepared solid foods in small quantities can then be added.

chronic g., an inflammation of the stomach that may occur repeatedly or continue over a period of time. Pain, especially after eating, and symptoms associated with indigestion occur in chronic gastritis. Among its possible causes are vitamin deficiencies, abnormalities of the gastric juice, ulcers, hiatus hernia, excessive use of alcohol, chronic emotional tension, or a combination of any of these factors.

Chronic gastritis is treated with a bland diet. Food should be taken frequently, in small amounts. Antacids may also be used in moderation to minimize stomach acidity. A tranquilizer or mild sedative may help relieve tension and thus speed the healing process.

giant hypertrophic g., Menetrier's disease.

toxic g., gastritis resulting from ingestion of a corrosive substance such as a strong acid or poison. There is acute burning and cramping stomach pain, accompanied by diarrhea and vomiting. The vomitus may be bloody. The victim may collapse.

This condition is an emergency and immediate measures must be taken to prevent serious damage to the tissues of the stomach. First-aid measures are begun at once to flush out and neutralize the POISON.

gastroanastomosis (gas″tro-ah-nas″to-mo′sis) gastrogastrostomy.

gastrocamera (gas″tro-kam′er-ah) a small camera which can be passed down the esophagus to photograph the inside of the stomach.

gastrocardiac (gas″tro-kar′de-ak) pertaining to the stomach and the heart.

gastrocele (gas′tro-sēl) hernial protrusion of the stomach or of a gastric pouch.

gastrocolic (gas″tro-kol′ik) pertaining to or communicating with the stomach and colon.

gastrocolitis (gas″tro-ko-li′tis) inflammation of the stomach and colon.

gastrocolostomy (gas″tro-ko-los′to-me) surgical anastomosis of the stomach to the colon.

gastrocolotomy (gas″tro-ko-lot′o-me) incision into the stomach and colon.

gastrocutaneous (gas″tro-ku-ta′ne-us) pertaining to the stomach and skin, or communicating with the stomach and the cutaneous surface of the body, as a gastrocutaneous fistula.

gastrodiaphany (gas″tro-di-af′ah-ne) examination of the stomach by transillumination of its walls with a small electric lamp passed down the esophagus.

gastrodidymus (gas″tro-did′ĭ-mus) symmetrical conjoined twins joined in the abdominal region.

Gastrodiscoides (gas″tro-dis-koi′dēz) a genus of trematodes parasitic in the intestinal tract.

gastroduodenal (gas″tro-du″o-de′nal) pertaining to the stomach and duodenum.

gastroduodenitis (gas″tro-du″o-dĕ-ni′tis) inflammation of the stomach and duodenum.

gastroduodenoscopy (gas″tro-du″o-dĕ-nos′ko-pe) endoscopic examination of the stomach and duodenum.

gastroduodenostomy (gas″tro-du″o-dĕ-nos′to-me) anastomosis of the stomach to a formerly remote part of the duodenum.

gastrodynia (gas″tro-din′e-ah) pain in the stomach.

gastroenteralgia (gas″tro-en″ter-al′je-ah) pain in the stomach and intestines.

gastroenteric (gas″tro-en-ter′ik) pertaining to the stomach and intestines.

gastroenteritis (gas″tro-en″tĕ-ri′tis) inflammation of the lining of the stomach and intestine. Psychologic causes of gastroenteritis include fear, anger, and other forms of emotional upset. Allergic reactions to certain foods can cause gastroenteritis, as can irritation by excessive use of alcohol. Severe gastroenteritis, with such symptoms as headache, nausea, vomiting, weakness, diarrhea, and gas pains, may result from various infectious and contagious diseases, such as TYPHOID FEVER, INFLUENZA, and FOOD POISONING.

gastroenteroanastomosis (gas″tro-en″ter-o-ah-nas″to-mo′sis) surgical anastomosis of the stomach to the small intestine.

gastroenterocolitis (gas″tro-en″ter-o-ko-li′tis) inflammation of the stomach, small intestine,, and colon.

gastroenterologist (gas″tro-en″ter-ol′o-jist) a physician specializing in gastroenterology.

gastroenterology (gas″tro-en″ter-ol′o-je) the study of the stomach and intestine and their diseases.

gastroenteropathy (gas″tro-en″ter-op′ah-the) any disease of the stomach and intestine.

gastroenteroptosis (gas″tro-en″ter-op-to′sis) downward displacement or prolapse of the stomach and intestine.

gastroenterostomy (gas″tro-en″ter-os′to-me) surgical anastomosis of the stomach to the intestine.

gastroenterotomy (gas″tro-en″ter-ot′o-me) incision into the stomach and intestine.

gastroesophageal (gas″tro-ĕ-sof″ah-je′al) pertaining to the stomach and esophagus.

gastroesophagitis (gas″tro-e-sof″ah-ji′tis) inflammation of the stomach and esophagus.

gastroesophagostomy (gas″tro-e-sof″ah-gos′to-me) surgical anastomosis between the stomach and esophagus.

gastrofiberscope (gas″tro-fi′ber-skōp) a fiberscope for viewing the stomach.

gastrogastrostomy (gas″tro-gas-tros′to-me) surgical creation of an anastomosis of two previously remote portions of the stomach, such as anastomosis between the pyloric and cardiac ends of the stomach, performed for hourglass contraction of the stomach, a condition in which the organ contracts at the middle.

gastrogavage (gas″tro-gah-vahzh′) artificial feeding through a tube passed into the stomach.

gastrogenic (gas″tro-jen′ik) originating in the stomach.

Gastrografin (gas″tro-gra′fin) trademark for a preparation of meglumine diatrizoate, a diagnostic radiopaque medium.

gastrograph (gas′tro-graf) an instrument for registering motions of the stomach.

gastrohepatic (gas″tro-hĕ-pat′ik) pertaining to the stomach and liver.

gastrohepatitis (gas″tro-hep″ah-ti′tis) inflammation of the stomach and liver.

gastroileac (gas″tro-il′e-ak) pertaining to the stomach and ileum.

gastroileitis (gas″tro-il″e-i′tis) inflammation of the stomach and ileum.

gastroileostomy (gas″tro-il″e-os′to-me) surgical anastomosis of the stomach to the ileum.

gastrointestinal (gas″tro-in-tes′tĭ-nal) pertaining to the stomach and intestine.

g. series, G.I. series, an examination of the upper gastrointestinal tract using barium as the contrast medium for a series of x-ray films. Called also a barium meal (see BARIUM TEST).

g. tract, the stomach and intestines in continuity (see also DIGESTIVE SYSTEM).

gastrojejunocolic (gas″tro-je-joo″no-kol′ik) pertaining to the stomach, jejunum, and colon.

gastrojejunostomy (gas″tro-je-joo-nos′to-me) surgical anastomosis of the stomach to the jejunum.

gastrolienal (gas″tro-li-e′nal) pertaining to the stomach and spleen; gastrosplenic.

gastrolith (gas′tro-lith) a calculus in the stomach.

gastrolithiasis (gas″tro-lĭ-thi′ah-sis) the presence or formation of gastroliths.

gastrology (gas-trol′o-je) study of the stomach and its diseases.

gastrolysis (gas-trol′ĭ-sis) surgical division of perigastric adhesions to mobilize the stomach.

gastromalacia (gas″tro-mah-la′she-ah) softening of the wall of the stomach.

gastromegaly (gas″tro-meg′ah-le) enlargement of the stomach.

gastromycosis (gas″tro-mi-ko′sis) fungal infection of the stomach.

gastromyxorrhea (gas″tro-mik″so-re′ah) excessive secretion of mucus by the stomach.

gastrone (gas′trōn) a reputed hormonal inhibitor of gastric acid secretion, extracted from gastric mucus.

gastroparalysis (gas″tro-pah-ral′ĭ-sis) paralysis of the stomach; gastroplegia.

gastropathy (gas-trop′ah-the) any disease of the stomach.

gastropexy (gas′tro-pek″se) surgical fixation of the stomach.

Gastrophilus (gas-trof′ĭ-lus) *Gasterophilus.*

gastrophrenic (gas″tro-fren′ik) pertaining to the stomach and diaphragm.

gastroplasty (gas′tro-plas″te) plastic repair of the stomach.

gastroplegia (gas″tro-ple′je-ah) gastroparalysis.

gastroplication (gas″tro-pli-ka′shun) treatment of gastric dilatation by stitching a fold in the stomach wall.

gastroptosis (gas″trop-to′sis) downward displacement of the stomach.

gastropulmonary (gas″tro-pul′mo-ner″e) pertaining to the stomach and lungs.

gastropylorectomy (gas″tro-pi″lo-rek′to-me) excision of the pyloric part of the stomach.

gastropyloric (gas″tro-pi-lor′ik) pertaining to the stomach and pylorus.

gastrorrhagia (gas″tro-ra′je-ah) hemorrhage from the stomach.

gastrorrhaphy (gas-tror′ah-fe) suture of the stomach.

gastrorrhea (gas″tro-re′ah) excessive secretion by the glands of the stomach.

gastroschisis (gas-tros′kĭ-sis) a congenital fissure of the abdominal wall.

gastroscope (gas′tro-skōp) an endoscope especially designed for passage into the stomach to permit examination of its interior. The gastroscope is a hollow, cylindrical tube fitted with special lenses and

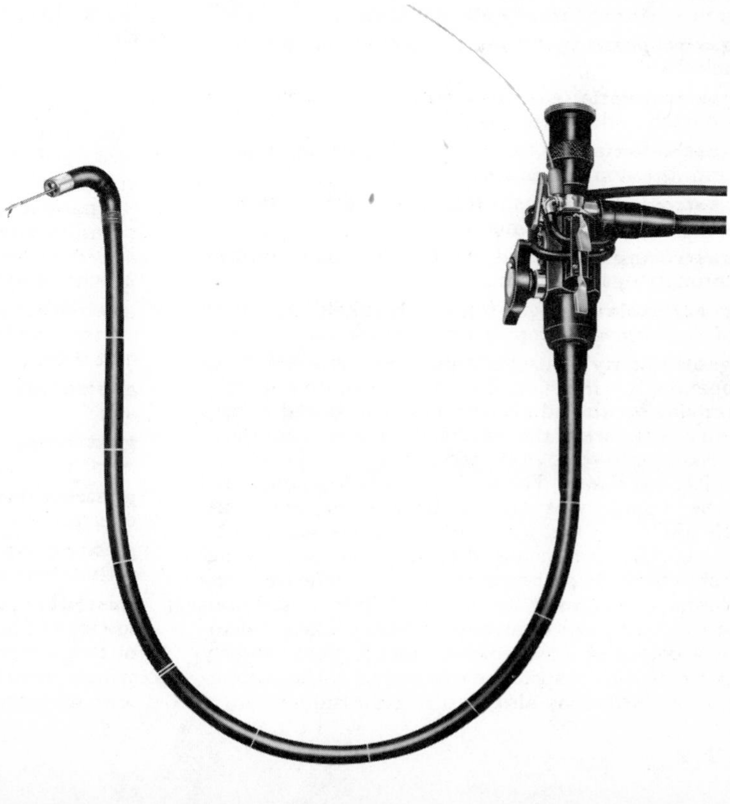

Fiberoptic gastroscope. (Courtesy of American Cystoscope Makers, Inc.)

lights. The newer types of gastroscope are made of glass fiber (fiberscope) which is more flexible. Each glass fiber reflects light and creates a mirror effect, making it possible to "go around corners," and facilitating visualization of the curvature of the stomach.

gastroscopy (gas-tros′ko-pe) inspection of the interior of the stomach with a gastroscope.

PATIENT CARE. For 6 to 8 hours prior to the examination the patient is not allowed to take any food or liquids by mouth. The stomach should be empty during the procedure to facilitate inspection of its lining and to avoid vomiting and aspiration of liquids into the lungs.

A sedative, usually a barbiturate, and an analgesic such as meperidine (Demerol) are given 30 minutes to 1 hour before the examination. The patient is awake during the procedure, which is not painful but is uncomfortable and exhausting. The sedatives help relieve apprehension and fear so that the patient can be more cooperative during the examination.

A local anesthetic such as cocaine or tetracaine (Pontocaine) is sprayed on the posterior pharynx to depress the gag reflex and reduce local reaction to the passage of the gastroscope. The patient is watched for toxic reaction to these drugs, and an emergency tray containing barbiturates and adrenalin must be readily available.

For passage of the conventional metal gastroscope the patient should be lying on his back. He may sit on the side of the bed or lie on his side facing the physician if a fiberscope is passed. If it seems likely that the patient will not be able to lie still he should be restrained, as there is danger that a sudden movement may cause the endoscope to perforate the esophagus or stomach.

After the procedure is completed the patient should be provided with rest and an opportunity to sleep. Foods and liquids are withheld until the gag reflex returns (usually about 4 hours).

gastrospasm (gas′tro-spazm) spasm of the stomach.

gastrosplenic (gas″tro-splen′ik) pertaining to the stomach and spleen; gastrolienal.

gastrostaxis (gas″tro-stak′sis) the oozing of blood from the stomach mucosa.

gastrostenosis (gas″tro-stĕ-no′sis) contraction or shrinkage of the stomach.

gastrostogavage (gas-tros″to-gah-vahzh′) feeding through a gastric fistula.

gastrostolavage (gas-tros″to-lah-vahzh′) irrigation of the stomach through a gastric fistula.

gastrostomy (gas-tros′to-me) the creation of an opening into the stomach. This procedure is done to provide for the administration of food and liquids when stricture of the esophagus or other conditions make swallowing impossible.

PATIENT CARE. The patient who is to undergo this type of surgery usually has been ill for some time. He often has nutritional deficiencies brought on by a steadily increasing difficulty in swallowing. Sometimes the patient is a small child who has accidentally swallowed lye or some other caustic substance, or he may be an adult who has taken a corrosive poison in an attempted suicide. Some elderly patients with obstructive carcinoma of the esophagus or throat may also require gastrostomy.

A primary consideration in the care of these patients is the patient's acceptance of the gastrostomy as a substitute for eating. There are many social and emotional factors associated with eating and sharing a meal with others. The hospital staff must be sensitive to the problems the patient will encounter in his adjustment to the changes a gastrostomy may bring to his life. Whenever possible the patient should be taught to feed himself and care for his gastrostomy. It is important that he have privacy while doing this and that he be encouraged to ask questions and seek assistance from the members of the health care team.

The skin around the opening must be protected from irritation by the gastric juices, which may leak from the opening and act as a corrosive on the skin. In some cases the gastrostomy tube can be removed after each feeding. A device called the Barnes-Redo prosthesis is available for use by patients with a permanent gastrostomy. This device is designed so that a cap can be fitted over a nylon tube permanently installed in the opening. When food or liquids are to be given the cap is unscrewed and a catheter is passed into the nylon tube. After feeding is completed the catheter is removed and the cap is screwed tightly over the nylon tube.

Feedings for a gastrostomy patient are gradually increased according to his tolerance. At first, water and glucose are given at regular intervals. If there is no leakage and the patient has no difficulty with these liquids, other liquids and puréed foods are gradually added until a full meal can be tolerated.

In order to stimulate gastric secretions and aid digestion, the patient should see, smell, and taste small amounts of food before each feeding. It is recommended that he be allowed to chew small bits of food even though he cannot swallow them. This allows for proper stimulation of the gums and teeth and helps promote the health of the mouth and teeth.

Feedings should be warmed before they are given through the tube. Although commercially prepared liquid feedings are more convenient, they often cause diarrhea and are not as nutritionally adequate as regular meals. The foods to be given through the tube should be cooked until they are soft and then puréed in an electric blender. They can be diluted with the water in which they have been cooked, so that no vitamins are lost. The hospital or clinic dietician usually must work very closely with the patient and his family, instructing them in the planning and preparation of the patient's meals and offering suggestions for a variety of foods that will provide a well balanced diet.

gastrothoracopagus (gas″tro-thor″ah-kop′ah-gus) symmetrical conjoined twins joined at the abdomen and thorax.

gastrotomy (gas-trot′o-me) incision into the stomach.

gastrotonometer (gas″tro-to-nom′ĕ-ter) an instrument for measuring intragastric pressure.

gastrotropic (gas″tro-trop′ik) having affinity for or exerting a special effect on the stomach.

gastrotympanites (gas″tro-tim″pah-ni′tēz) tympanitic distension of the stomach.

gastrula (gas′troo-lah) an embryo in the stage following the blastula stage; the simplest type consists of two layers of cells, the ectoderm and entoderm, which have invaginated to form the archenteron and an opening, the blastopore.

gastrulation (gas″troo-la′shun) the formation of a gastrula.

Gatch bed (gach) a bed fitted with jointed springs, which may be adjusted to various back rest and knee rest positions.

Gaucher's cells (go′shāz) a large cell characteristic of Gaucher's disease, with eccentrically placed nuclei and fine wavy fibrils parallel to the long axis of the cell.

Gaucher's disease (go-shāz′) a hereditary disorder of glucocerebroside metabolism, marked by the presence of Gaucher's cells in the marrow, and by hepatosplenomegaly and erosion of the cortices of long bones and pelvis. The adult form is associated with moderate anemia and thrombocytopenia, and yellowish pigmentation of the skin; in the infantile form there is, in addition, marked central nervous system impairment; in the juvenile form there are rapidly progressive systemic manifestations but moderate central nervous system involvement.

gauntlet (gawnt′let) a bandage covering the hand and fingers like a glove.

gauze (gawz) a light, open-meshed fabric of muslin or similar material.

absorbent g., white cotton cloth of various thread counts and weights, supplied in various lengths and widths and in different forms (rolls or folds).

petrolatum g., a sterile material produced by saturation of sterile absorbent gauze with sterile white petrolatum.

gavage (gah-vahzh′) [Fr.] 1. forced feeding, especially through a tube passed into the stomach (see also TUBE feeding). 2. superalimentation.

Gay's gland (gāz) specialized sweat and sebaceous glands around the anus; called also circumanal glands.

g-cal. gram calorie (small calorie).

Gd chemical symbol, *gadolinium.*

Ge chemical symbol, *germanium.*

Gee's disease, Gee-Herter disease, Gee-Herter-Heubner disease (gēz; ge-her′ter; ge-her′ter-hoib′ner) the infantile form of CELIAC DISEASE.

Gee-Thaysen (ge-thi′sen) the adult form of CELIAC DISEASE.

gegenhalten (ga″gen-halt′en) [Ger.] an involuntary resistance to passive movement as may occur in cerebral cortical disorders.

Geiger counter, Geiger-Müller counter (gi′ger; gi′ger-mil′er) an amplifying device that indicates the presence of ionizing particles emitted by a substance; used as a means of determining the presence of radioactivity.

Geissler's tube (gīs′lerz) an x-ray tube containing a highly rarified gas.

gel (jel) a colloid that is firm in consistency, although containing much liquid; a colloid in a gelatinous form.

gelatin (jel′ah-tin) a substance obtained by partial hydrolysis of collagen derived from skin, white connective tissue, and bones of animals; used as a suspending agent for various drugs or in manufacture of capsules and suppositories; suggested for intravenous use as a plasma substitute, and has been used as an adjuvant protein food. In absorbable film and sponge, it is used in surgical procedures.

zinc g., a preparation of zinc oxide, gelatin, glycerin, and purified water, applied topically as a protective.

gelatinase (jĕ-lat′ĭ-nās) an enzyme that liquefies gelatin, but does not affect fibrin and egg albumin; occurs among bacteria, molds, and yeasts.

gelatinize (jĕ-lat′ĭ-nīz) to convert into a jelly, or to become converted into gelatin.

gelatinoid (jĕ-lat′ĭ-noid) resembling gelatin.

gelatinolytic (jĕ-lat″ĭ-no-lit′ik) dissolving or splitting up gelatin.

gelatinous (jĕ-lat′ĭ-nus) like jelly or softened gelatin.

gelation (jĕ-la′shun) conversion of a sol into a gel.

Gelfilm (jel′film) trademark for absorbable gelatin film, used as an aid in surgical closure and repair of defects in the dura mater and pleura.

Gelfoam (jel′fōm) trademark for preparations of absorbable gelatin sponge, used as a local hemostatic.

gelose (jel′ōs) agar.

gelosis (je-lo′sis) a hard, swollen lump in a tissue, especially in muscle.

gemellology (jem″el-ol′o-je) the scientific study of twins and twinning.

geminate (jem′ĭ-nāt) paired; occurring in twos.

gemistocyte (jem-is′to-sīt) an astrocyte in which the cell body swells considerably, the nucleus is in an eccentric position, and the cytoplasm is clearly visible. adj., **gemistocyt′ic.**

gemmation (jĕ-ma′shun) development of a new organism from a protuberance on the cell body of the parent, a form of asexual reproduction; called also budding.

gemmule (jem′ūl) 1. a reproductive bud; the immediate product of gemmation. 2. any one of the many little excrescences upon the protoplasmic process of a nerve cell.

Gemonil (jem′o-nil) trademark for a preparation of metharbital, an anticonvulsant barbiturate.

-gen word element [Gr.], *an agent that produces.*

genal (je′nal) pertaining to the cheek; buccal.

gender (jen′der) sex; the category to which an individual is assigned on the basis of sex.

gene (jēn) one of the biologic units of heredity, self-reproducing, and located at a definite position (locus) on a particular chromosome. Genes make up segments of the complex DEOXYRIBONUCLEIC ACID (DNA) molecule that controls cellular reproduction and function. There are thousands of genes in the chromosomes of each cell nucleus; they play an important role in heredity because they control the individual physical, biochemical, and physiologic traits inherited by offspring from their parents. Through the genetic code of DNA they also control the day-to-day functions and reproduction of all cells in the body. For example, the genes control the synthesis of structural proteins and also the enzymes that regulate various chemical reactions that take place in a cell.

The gene is capable of replication. When a cell multiplies by mitosis each daughter cell carries a set of genes that is an exact replica of that of the parent cell. This characteristic of replication explains how genes can carry hereditary traits through successive generations without change.

allelic g's, genes situated at corresponding loci in a pair of chromosomes.

complementary g's, two independent pairs of nonallelic genes, neither of which will produce its effect in the absence of the other.

dominant g., one that produces an effect (the phenotype) in the organism regardless of the state of the corresponding allele. An example of a trait determined by a dominant gene is brown eye color.

histocompatibility g., one that determines the specificity of tissue antigenicity and thus the compatibility of donor and recipient in tissue transplantation and blood transfusion.

holandric g's, genes located on the Y chromosome and appearing only in male offspring.

leaky g., one in which a switch in the sequence of bases in a nucleotide results in the production of a mutant protein that, because of a single amino acid replacement, has only partial enzymatic activity; a hypomorph.

lethal g., one whose presence brings about the death of the organism or permits survival only under certain conditions.

mutant g., one that has undergone a detectable mutation.

operator g., one serving as a starting point for reading the genetic code, and which, through interaction with a repressor, controls the activity of structural genes associated with it in the operon.

recessive g., one that produces an effect in the organism only when it is transmitted by both parents, i.e., only when the individual is homozygous.

regulator g., repressor g., one that synthesizes repressor, a substance which, through interaction with the operator gene, switches off the activity of the structural genes associated with it in the operon.

sex-linked g., one that is carried on a sex chromosome, especially an X chromosome.

structural g., one that forms templates for messenger RNA and is thereby responsible for the amino acid sequence of specific polypeptides.

supplementary g's, two independent pairs of genes that interact in such a way that one dominant will produce its effect even in the absence of the other, but the second requires the presence of the first to be effective.

genera (jen'er-ah) [L.] plural of *genus.*

generation (jen"ĕ-ra'shun) 1. the process of reproduction. 2. a class composed of all individuals removed by the same number of successive ancestors from a common predecessor, or occupying positions on the same level in a genealogical (pedigree) chart.

alternate g., reproduction by alternate asexual and sexual means in an animal or plant species.

asexual g., direct g., production of a new organism not originating from union of gametes.

filial g., first, the first-generation offspring of two parents; symbol F_1.

filial g., second, all of the offspring produced by two individuals of the first filial generation; symbol F_2.

parental g., the generation with which a particular genetic study is begun; symbol P_1.

sexual g., production of a new organism from the zygote formed by the union of gametes.

spontaneous g., the discredited concept of continuous generation of living organisms from nonliving matter.

generative (jen'ĕ-ra"tiv) pertaining to reproduction.

generic (jĕ-ner'ik) 1. pertaining to a genus. 2. nonproprietary; denoting a drug name not protected by a trademark, usually descriptive of the drug's chemical structure.

genesiology (jĕ-ne"ze-ol'o-je) the sum of what is known concerning generation.

genesis (jen'ĕ-sis) creation; origination; used as a word termination joined to an element indicating the thing created, e.g., carcinogenesis.

genetic (jĕ-net'ik) 1. pertaining to reproduction or to birth or origin. 2. inherited.

g. code, the arrangement of nucleotides in the polynucleotide chain of a chromosome that governs the transmission of genetic information to proteins, i.e., determines the sequence of amino acids in the polypeptide chain making up each protein synthesized by the cell. Genetic information is coded in DNA by means of four bases (two purines: adenine and guanine; and two pyrimidines: thymine and cystosine). Each adjacent sequence of three bases (a codon) determines the insertion of a specific amino acid. In RNA, uracil replaces thymine.

geneticist (jĕ-net'ĭ-sist) a specialist in genetics.

genetics (jĕ-net'iks) the branch of biology dealing with the phenomena of heredity and the laws governing it.

biochemical g., the science concerned with the chemical and physical nature of genes and the mechanism by which they control the development and maintenance of the organism.

The field of biochemical genetics is relatively new and recently it has become the study of the cause of many specific diseases that are now known to be inherited. These diseases include those resulting from the improper synthesis of hemoglobins and protein, such as SICKLE CELL ANEMIA and THALASSEMIA, both of which are hereditary anemias; some 200 inborn errors of metabolism, such as PHENYLKETONURIA and GALACTOSEMIA, in which lack or alteration of a specific enzyme prohibits proper metabolism of carbohydrates, proteins, or fats and thus produces pathologic symptoms; and genetically determined variations in response to certain drugs, for example, isoniazid.

clinical g., the study of the possible genetic factors influencing the occurrence of a pathologic condition. In addition to the diseases mentioned under biochemical genetics, other aspects of clinical genetics include the study of chromosomal aberrations, such as those that cause mental retardation and DOWN'S SYNDROME (mongolism), and immunogenetics, or the genetic aspects of the IMMUNE RESPONSE and the transmission of genetic factors from generation to generation.

genetotrophic (jĕ-net"o-trōf'ik) pertaining to genetics and nutrition; relating to problems of nutrition that are hereditary in nature, or transmitted through the genes.

genetous (jen'ĕ-tus) dating from fetal life.

Geneva Convention (jĕ-ne'vah) an international agreement of 1864, whereby, among other pledges, the signatory nations pledged themselves to treat the wounded and the army medical and nursing staff as neutrals on the field of battle.

genial (je'ne-al) pertaining to the chin.

genic (jen'ik) pertaining to or caused by the genes.

-genic word element [Gr.], *giving rise to; causing.*

genicular (jĕ-nik'u-lar) pertaining to the knee.

geniculate (jĕ-nik'u-lāt) bent, like a knee.

geniculum (jĕ-nik′u-lum), pl. *genic′ula* [L.] a little knee; used in anatomic nomenclature to designate a sharp kneelike bend in a small structure or organ.

genioplasty (je′ne-o-plas″te) plastic surgery of the chin.

genital (jen′ĭ-tal) 1. pertaining to reproduction, or the reproductive organs. 2. [pl.] the REPRODUCTIVE ORGANS.

genitalia (jen″ĭ-ta′le-ah) the REPRODUCTIVE ORGANS; called also the genitals.

The internal female reproductive organs consist of the ovaries, uterine tubes, uterus, and vagina. The external genitalia, referred to collectively as the vulva, consist of the mons pubis, labia majora, labia minora, clitoris, vestibule of the vagina, vulvovaginal glands, and the bulb of the vestibule. (See Plate 11.)

The male genitalia consist of the testes, seminiferous (semen-carrying) tubules, epididymides, ductus deferentes, ejaculatory ducts, seminal vesicles, prostate, bulbourethral glands, and glans penis. (See Plate 11.)

genitaloid (jen′ĭ-tal-oid″) pertaining to the primordial germ cells, before future sexuality is distinguishable.

genito- word element [L.], relating to the organs of reproduction.

genitocrural (jen″ĭ-to-kroo′ral) pertaining to the genitalia and the thigh.

genitofemoral (jen″ĭ-to-fem′o-ral) genitocrural.

genitoplasty (jen′ĭ-to-plas″te) plastic surgery on the reproductive (genital) organs.

genitourinary (jen′ĭ-to-u′rĭ-ner″e) pertaining to the genitalia and urinary apparatus; urogenital.

g. system, the organs of reproduction, together with the organs concerned with production and excretion of urine; called also urogenital system. (See Plate 11.)

genoblast (jen′o-blast) 1. the nucleus of the impregnated ovum. 2. a mature germ cell.

genocopy (jen′o-kop″e) an individual whose phenotype mimics that of another genotype but whose character is determined by a distinct assortment of genes.

genodermatosis (je″no-der″mah-to′sis) a genetic disorder of the skin, usually generalized.

genome (je′nōm) the complete set of hereditary factors contained in the haploid set of chromosomes. adj., **genom′ic.**

genotype (jen″o-tīp) 1. the entire genetic constitution of an individual; also, the alleles present at one or more specific loci. 2. the type species of a genus. adj., **genotyp′ic.**

-genous word element [Gr.], *arising or resulting from; produced by.*

gentamicin (jen″tah-mi′sin) an antibiotic elaborated by fungi of the genus *Micromonospora,* effective against *Pseudomonas* and certain other gram-negative bacilli; the sulfate salt is prepared as a cream and ointment for topical application.

gentian (jen′shan) the dried rhizome and roots of *Gentiana lutea;* has been used as a bitter tonic.

g. violet, a dye derived from triphenylmethane, used as a topical anti-infective, stain, and internal anthelmintic; called also methylrosaniline chloride.

gentianophilic (jen″shan-o-fil′ik) staining readily with gentian violet.

gentianophobic (jen″shan-o-fo′bik) not staining with gentian violet.

genu (je′nu), pl. *gen′ua* [L.] the knee.

g. extror′sum, bowleg.

g. intror′sum, knock-knee.

g. recurva′tum, hyperextensibility of the knee joint.

g. val′gum, knock-knee.

g. va′rum, bowleg.

genus (je′nus), pl. *gen′era* [L.] a taxonomic category (taxon) subordinate to a tribe (or subtribe) and superior to a species (or subgenus).

geo- word element [Gr.], *the earth; the soil.*

geobiology (je″o-bi-ol′o-je) the biology of terrestrial life.

geode (je′ōd) a dilated lymph space.

geomedicine (je″o-med′ĭ-sin) the branch of medicine dealing with the influence of climatic and environmental conditions on health.

geophagia, geophagism (je″o-fa′je-ah; je-of′ah-jizm) the habit of eating clay or earth (soil); chthonophagia.

geotaxis (je″o-tak′sis) geotropism.

geotrichosis (je″o-trĭ-ko′sis) a candidiasis-like infection due to *Geotrichum candidum,* which may attack the bronchi, lungs, mouth, or intestinal tract.

Geotrichum (je-ot′rĭ-kum) a genus of yeastlike fungi.

G. can′didum, a species found in the feces and dairy products.

geotropism (je-ot′ro-pizm) a tendency of growth or movement toward or away from the earth; the influence of gravity on growth.

ger-, gero-, geronto- word element [Gr.], *old age; the aged.*

geratic (jĕ-rat′ik) pertaining to old age.

geratology, gereology (jer″ah-tol′o-je; jer″e-ol′o-je) the science dealing with old age.

geriatrics (jer″e-at′riks) the branch of medicine dealing with the problems of aging and diseases of the elderly. It is related to the science of gerontology, which is the study of the aging process in all its aspects, social as well as biologic. Geriatrics grows increasingly important as modern medicine and a rising standard of living lengthen life expectancy and increase the proportion of aged persons in society.

An important part of geriatrics is concerned with helping older persons to live happy and satisfying lives. Geriatric specialists encourage their patients to follow useful and interesting pursuits and to adopt a sound mental attitude toward aging itself. The prevention of disease is also important in geriatrics, and stress is placed on suitable exercise, rest, and nutrition, and on maintenance of proper body weight. Regular and thorough medical examinations are another essential factor in the control of illness.

There are few illnesses, if any, that affect only elderly persons. Certain disorders, however, tend to be characteristic problems of advancing age. These include decline of vision and hearing and deterioration of the teeth. The wear and tear of living may also produce increasing stiffness and other disorders of the joints, and the bones may become somewhat brittle and tend to break more easily.

Among the diseases that often affect older persons are ARTERIOSCLEROSIS and heart disease. Other disorders that may often occur in the aged are HERNIA, CATARACT, enlargement of the prostate in men, CANCER, and prolapse of the rectum or uterus. Advances in modern surgery have made it possible to treat these conditions in elderly patients with excellent results.

In geriatrics, increasing emphasis is also being given to the older person's psychologic welfare—his social contacts, economic security, interest in living, work opportunities after retirement, and a continuing sense of belonging to society. Geriatrics recognizes that health of mind is essential to the health of the body. (See also AGED.)

germ (jerm) 1. a pathogenic microorganism. 2. living substance capable of developing into an organ, part, or organism as a whole; a primordium.

wheat g., the embryo of wheat, which contains tocopherol, thiamine, riboflavin, and other vitamins.

German measles (jer′man me′zelz) a contagious, mild viral infection, most common in children between the ages of 3 and 12 years; called also RUBELLA or 3-day measles. The disease is usually mild in children, but it has been found to cause various developmental abnormalities in fetuses of mothers who contract it during pregnancy.

germanium (jer-ma′ne-um) a chemical element, atomic number 32, atomic weight 72.59, symbol Ge. (See table of ELEMENTS.)

germicidal (jer″mĭ-si′dal) destructive to pathogenic microorganisms.

germicide (jer′mĭ-sīd) an agent that destroys pathogenic microorganisms.

germinal (jer′mĭ-nal) pertaining to or of the nature of a germ cell or the primitive stage of development.

germination (jer″mĭ-na′shun) the sprouting of a seed or spore or of a plant embryo.

germinative (jer′mĭ-na″tiv) pertaining to germination or to a germ cell.

germinoma (jer″mĭ-no′mah) a neoplasm of germ tissue (testis or ovum), e.g., a seminoma.

gerocomia (jer″o-ko′me-ah) the care of old men; the hygiene of old age.

geroderma, gerodermia (jer″o-der′mah; jer″o-der′me-ah) dystrophy of the skin and genitals, giving the appearance of old age.

gerodontics (jer″o-don′tiks) dentistry dealing with the dental problems of older people. adj., **gerodon′tic.**

gerodontist (jer″o-don′tist) a dentist specializing in gerodontics.

gerodontology (jer″o-don-tol′o-je) study of the dentition and dental problems in the aged and aging.

geromarasmus (jer″o-mah-raz′mus) the emaciation sometimes characteristic of old age.

geromorphism (jer″o-mor′fizm) premature senility.

gerontal (jĕ-ron′tal) pertaining to old age.

gerontologist (jer″on-tol′o-jist) a physician specializing in gerontology.

gerontology (jer″on-tol′o-je) the scientific study of the problems of aging in all its aspects.

gerontopia (jer″on-to′pe-ah) second sight; improvement of vision, especially near vision, in the aged, a sign of incipient cataract. Called also senopia.

gerontotherapeutics (je-ron″to-ther″ah-pu′tiks) the science of retarding and preventing the development of many of the aspects of senescence.

gerontoxon (jer″on-tok′son) arcus senilis.

gestagen (jes′tah-jen) any hormone with progestational activity.

gestalt (ges-tawlt′) a whole perceptual configuration.

gestaltism (gĕ-stawl′tizm) the theory in psychology that the objects of mind, as immediately presented to direct experience, come as complete unanalyzable wholes or forms (Gestalten) that cannot be split up into parts.

gestation (jes-ta′shun) the period of development of the young in viviparous animals, from the time of fertilization of the ovum to birth. (See also PREGNANCY.)

g. period, the duration of pregnancy, in the human female about 266 days.

gestosis (jes-to′sis) any toxemic manifestation in pregnancy.

GFR glomerular filtration rate.

G.I. gastrointestinal; globin (zinc) insulin.

Giannuzzi's crescents (jah-noot′zēz) crescent-shaped patches surrounding the mucous tubercles in mixed glands.

giant cell tumor 1. a bone tumor, ranging from benign to frankly malignant, composed of cellular spindle cell stroma containing multinucleated giant cells resembling osteoclasts. 2. a benign, small, yellow, tumor-like nodule of tendon sheath origin, most often of the wrist and fingers or ankle and toes, laden with lipophages and containing multinucleated giant cells.

giantism (ji′an-tizm) 1. gigantism. 2. excessive size, as of cells or nuclei.

Giardia (je-ar′de-ah) a genus of flagellate protozoa parasitic in the intestines of man and animals, which may cause protracted, intermittent diarrhea with symptoms suggesting malabsorption.

G. intestina′lis, G. lam′blia, a species parasitic in the intestines of man.

giardiasis (je″ar-di′ah-sis) infection with *Giardia.*

gibbosity (gĭ-bos′ĭ-te) the condition of being humped; kyphosis.

gibbous (gib′us) humped; protuberant.

gibbus (gib′us) a hump.

Gibney boot (gib′ne) an adhesive tape support used in the treatment of sprains and other painful conditions of the ankle, the tape being applied in a basket-weave fashion with strips placed alternately under the sole of the foot and around the back of the leg.

Gibraltar fever (jĭ-brawl′ter) brucellosis.

Gibson murmur (gib′sun) a long rumbling sound occupying most of systole and diastole, usually localized in the second left interspace near the sternum, and usually indicative of patent ductus arteriosus.

Giemsa stain (gēm′sah) a solution containing azure II-eosin, azure II, glycerin, and methanol; used for staining protozoan parasites, *Leptospira, Borrelia,* viral inclusion bodies, and *Rickettsia.*

Gierke's disease (gēr′kez) glycogenosis (type I) in which deficiency of the hepatic enzyme glucose-

6-phosphatase results in liver and kidney involvement, with hepatomegaly, hypoglycemia, hyperuricemia, and gout. Called also von Gierke's disease and hepatorenal glycogenosis.

giga- (gi'gah) word element [Gr.], *huge;* used in naming units of measurement to designate an amount 10^9 (one billion) times the size of the unit to which it is joined, e.g., gigameter (10^9 meters); symbol G.

gigantism (ji-gan'tizm, ji'gan-tizm) abnormal overgrowth of the body or a part; excessive size and stature. Generally applied to a rare abnormality of the PITUITARY GLAND that causes excessive growth in a child so that he becomes an unusually tall adult. If the abnormality is extreme, he may reach a height of 8 feet or more, although the body proportions usually are normal.

The condition is brought on by overproduction of growth hormone occurring before the growing ends of bone have closed. The opposite condition, DWARFISM, is caused by underproduction of the same hormone. (Overproduction of growth hormone in adults causes ACROMEGALY.) Gigantism can be corrected only by early diagnosis in childhood and removal by surgery of part of the pituitary gland or by x-ray treatment.

cerebral g., gigantism in the absence of increased levels of growth hormone, attributed to a cerebral defect; infants are large, and accelerated growth continues for the first 4 or 5 years, the rate being normal thereafter. The hands and feet are large, the head large and dolichocephalic, the eyes have an antimongoloid slant, with hypertelorism. The child is clumsy, and mental retardation of varying degree is usually present.

gigantomastia (ji-gan"to-mas'te-ah) extreme hypertrophy of the breast.

Gilbert's disease (zhēl-bārz') benign hereditary hyperbilirubinemia marked by mild intermittent jaundice and often by fatigue, weakness, and abdominal pain.

Gilles de la Tourette's syndrome (disease) (zhēl"dĕ-lah-toor-etz') facial and vocal tics with onset in childhood, progressing to generalized jerking movements in any body part, with echolalia and coprolalia.

Gimbernat's ligament (him-ber-nāts') a membrane with its base just medial to the femoral ring, one side attached to the inguinal ligament and the other to the pectineal line of the pubis. Called also lacunar ligament.

gingiva (jin-ji'vah; jin'jĭ-vah), pl. *gingi'vae* [L.] covering the tooth-bearing border of the jaw; the gum. adj., **gingi'val.**

alveolar g., the portion overlying the alveolar process and firmly attached to it.

areolar g., the portion attached to the alveolar process by loose areolar connective tissue.

free g., the portion covering part of the crowns of the teeth, but not attached to them.

gingivalgia (jin"jĭ-val'je-ah) pain in the gingiva.

gingivectomy (jin"jĭ-vek'to-me) surgical excision of all loose infected and diseased gingival tissue to eradicate periodontal infection and reduce the depth of the gingival sulcus.

gingivitis (jin"jĭ-vi'tis) a general term for inflammation of the gums, of which bleeding is one of the primary symptoms. Other symptoms include swelling, redness, pain, and difficulty in chewing. There are numerous causes for this condition, and it can lead to a more serious disorder, PERIODONTITIS.

One of the most common causes of gingivitis is the accumulation of food particles in the crevices between the gums and the teeth. Other causes are general poor health, irregular teeth, badly fitting fillings or dentures that irritate the gums, and infections such as VINCENT'S ANGINA and TRENCH MOUTH.

Gingivitis is best prevented by correct brushing of the teeth and proper gum care. A good diet containing the necessary minerals and vitamins is also important. Vitamin deficiencies and anemia and other blood dyscrasias are often accompanied by gingivitis.

necrotizing ulcerative g., TRENCH MOUTH; a gingival infection marked by redness and swelling, necrosis, pain, hemorrhage, a necrotic odor, and often a pseudomembrane. Extension to the oral mucosa is called necrotizing ulcerative gingivostomatitis.

gingivo- word element [L.], *gingival.*

gingivoglossitis (jin"jĭ-vo-glŏ-si'tis) inflammation of the gingiva and tongue.

gingivolabial (jin"jĭ-vo-la'be-al) pertaining to the gingivae and lips.

gingivoplasty (jin'jĭ-vo-plas"te) surgical remodeling of the gingiva.

gingivosis (jin"jĭ-vo'sis) a chronic, diffuse inflammation of the gums, with desquamation of the papillary epithelium and mucous membrane.

gingivostomatitis (jin"jĭ-vo-sto"mah-ti'tis) inflammation of the gingiva and oral mucosa.

herpetic g., that due to infection with herpes simplex virus, with redness of the oral tissues, formation of multiple vesicles and painful ulcers, and fever.

necrotizing ulcerative g., that due to extension to the oral mucosa of necrotizing ulcerative gingivitis (TRENCH MOUTH) (see also VINCENT'S ANGINA).

ginglymus (jing'glĭ-mus) a joint that allows movement in but one plane, forward and backward, as does a door hinge; called also hinge joint.

girdle (ger'd'l) an encircling or confining structure.

pectoral g., shoulder girdle.

pelvic g., the encircling bony structure supporting the lower limbs.

shoulder g., thoracic g., the encircling bony structure supporting the upper limbs.

Gitaligin (jĭ-tal'ĭ-jin) trademark for a preparation of gitalin, a cardiotonic.

gitalin (jit'ah-lin) amorphous gitalin; a mixture of digitalis glycosides used as a cardiotonic in congestive heart failure and cardiac arrhythmias.

glabella (glah-bel'ah) the area on the frontal bone above the nasion and between the eyebrows.

glabrous (gla'brus) smooth and bare.

gladiolus (glah-di'o-lus) the main portion or body of the sternum.

glairy (glār'e) resembling white of an egg.

gland (gland) an aggregation of cells specialized to secrete or excrete materials not related to their ordinary metabolic needs. Glands are divided into two main groups, endocrine and exocrine. adj., **glan'dular.**

The ENDOCRINE GLANDS, or ductless glands, discharge their secretions (hormones) directly into the blood; they include the adrenal, pituitary, thyroid, and parathyroid glands, the islands of Langerhans in the pancreas, the gonads, the thymus, and the pineal body.

The exocrine glands, which discharge through ducts opening on an external or internal surface of the body, include the salivary, sebaceous, and sweat glands, the liver, the gastric glands, the pancreas, the intestinal, mammary, and lacrimal glands, and the prostate.

The organs sometimes called lymph glands are more accurately called lymph nodes; they are not glands in the usual sense.

acinous g., one made up of one or more oval or spherical sacs (acini).

adrenal g., a flattened body above either kidney, an endocrine gland consisting of a cortex and medulla, the former elaborating steroid hormones, and the latter epinephrine and norepinephrine; called also suprarenal gland. (See also ADRENAL GLAND.)

apocrine g., one whose discharged secretion contains part of the secreting cells.

areolar g's, Montgomery's glands.

axillary g's, lymph nodes situated in the axilla.

Bartholin g's, vulvovaginal glands, two minute glands, one on each side of the vagina, their ducts opening on the vulva (see also BARTHOLIN GLANDS).

Bowman's g's, olfactory glands.

bronchial g's, seromucous glands in the mucosa and submucosa of the bronchial walls.

Brunner's g's, glands in the duodenum secreting intestinal juice.

buccal g's, seromucous glands on the inner surface of the cheeks; called also genal glands.

bulbocavernous g's, bulbourethral g's, two glands embedded in the substance of the sphincter of the male urethra, posterior to the membranous part of the urethra; their secretion lubricates the urethra; called also Cowper's glands.

cardiac g's, mucus-secreting glands of the cardiac part (cardia) of the stomach.

celiac g's, lymph nodes anterior to the abdominal aorta.

ceruminous g's, cerumin-secreting glands in the skin of the external auditory canal.

cervical g's, 1. the lymph nodes of the neck. 2. compound clefts in the wall of the uterine cervix.

ciliary g's, sweat glands that have become arrested in their development, situated at the edges of the eyelids; called also Moll's glands.

circumanal g's, specialized sweat and sebaceous glands around the anus; called also Gay's glands.

Cobelli's g's, mucous glands in the esophageal mucosa just above the cardia.

coccygeal g., glomus coccygeum.

compound g., one made up of a number of smaller units whose excretory ducts combine to form ducts of progressively higher order.

conglobate g., a lymph node.

Cowper's g's, bulbourethral glands.

ductless g's, endocrine g's.

duodenal g's Brunner's glands.

Ebner's g's, serous glands at the back of the tongue near the taste buds.

eccrine g., one of the ordinary, or simple, sweat glands, which are of the merocrine type.

fundic g's, fundus g's, very numerous, tubular glands in the mucosa of the fundus and body of the stomach that contain the cells which produce acid and pepsin.

gastric g's, the secreting glands of the stomach, including the fundic, cardiac, and pyloric glands.

Gay g's, circumanal glands.

genal g's, buccal glands.

glossopalatine g's, mucous glands at the posterior end of the smaller sublingual glands.

haversian g's, folds on synovial surfaces regarded as secretors of synovia.

hematopoietic g's, glandlike bodies, e.g., the spleen, that take a part in blood formation.

hemolymph g's, minute nodes resembling small lymph nodes but red or brown in color and containing blood sinuses instead of or alongside lymph spaces. They occur especially in the retroperitoneal tissue near the origin of the superior mesenteric and renal arteries, but are also found elsewhere. They are believed to take part in blood destruction and formation. Two varieties are distinguished—splenolymph glands and marrow-lymph glands.

holocrine g., one whose discharged secretion contains the entire secreting cells.

intestinal g's, straight tubular glands in the mucous membrane of the intestines, opening, in the small intestine, between the bases of the villi, and containing argentaffin cells. Called also crypts, or glands, of Lieberkühn.

jugular g., a lymph node behind the clavicular insertion of the sternocleidomastoid muscle.

Krause's g., an accessory lacrimal gland deep in the conjunctival connective tissue, mainly near the upper fornix.

lacrimal g's, the glands that secrete tears (see also LACRIMAL APPARATUS).

g's of Lieberkühn, intestinal glands.

lingual g's, the seromucous glands on the surface of the tongue.

lingual g's, anterior, seromucous glands near the apex of the tongue.

Littre's g's, 1. preputial glands. 2. the male urethral glands.

lymph g., lymph node.

mammary g., the milk-secreting organ of female mammals, existing also in a rudimentary state in the male (see also BREAST and MAMMARY GLAND).

marrow-lymph g's, hemolymph glands having a marrow-like tissue.

meibomian g's, sebaceous follicles between the cartilage and conjunctiva of the eyelids.

merocrine g., one whose discharged secretion contains no part of the secreting cells.

mixed g's, 1. seromucous glands. 2. glands that have both exocrine and endocrine portions.

Moll's g's, ciliary glands.

Montgomery's g's, sebaceous glands in the mammary areola; called also areolar glands.

mucous g's, glands that secrete mucus.

olfactory g's, small mucous glands in the olfactory mucosa; called also Bowman's glands.

parathyroid g's, small bodies in the region of the thyroid glands, developed from the entoderm of the brachial clefts, occurring in a variable number of pairs, commonly two; they secrete parathyroid hormone and are concerned chiefly with the metabolism of calcium and phosphorus (see also PARATHYROID GLANDS).

parotid g., the large salivary gland located in front of the ear (see also PAROTID GLAND).

peptic g's, gastric glands that secrete pepsin.

pineal g., a small, conical structure attached by a stalk to the posterior wall of the third ventricle of the cerebrum (see also PINEAL BODY).

pituitary g., the hypophysis; the epithelial body of

dual origin at the base of the brain in the sella turcica, attached by a stalk to the hypothalamus; it consists of two main lobes, the anterior lobe, secreting several important hormones which regulate the proper functioning of the thyroid, gonads, adrenal cortex, and other endocrine organs, and the posterior lobe, whose cells serve as a reservoir for hormones having antidiuretic and oxytocic action, releasing them as needed. (See also PITUITARY GLAND.)

preputial g's, small sebaceous glands of the corona of the penis and the inner surface of the prepuce, which secrete smegma; called also Littre's glands and Tyson's glands.

prostate g., prostate.

pyloric g's, the mucin-secreting glands of the pyloric part of the stomach.

salivary g's, glands of the oral cavity whose combined secretion constitutes the saliva (see also SALIVARY GLANDS).

sebaceous g., holocrine glands of the corium that secrete an oily material (sebum) into the hair follicles.

sentinel g., an enlarged lymph node, considered to be pathognomonic of some pathologic condition elsewhere.

seromucous g's, glands that are both serous and mucous.

serous g., a gland that secretes a watery albuminous material, commonly but not always containing enzymes.

sex g's, sexual g's, gonads (see OVARY and TESTIS).

simple g., one with a nonbranching duct.

Skene's g's, the largest of the female urethral glands, which open into the urethral orifice; they are regarded as homologous with the prostate. Called also paraurethral ducts.

solitary g's, solitary follicles.

splenolymph g's, hemolymph glands having more of the splenic type of tissue.

sublingual g., a salivary gland on either side under the tongue.

submandibular g., submaxillary g., a salivary gland on the inner side of each ramus of the lower jaw.

sudoriferous g's, sudoriparous g's, sweat glands.

suprarenal g., adrenal gland.

sweat g's, glands that secrete sweat, situated in the corium or subcutaneous tissue, opening by a duct on the body surface; they promote cooling of the body by evaporation of the secretion (see also SWEAT GLANDS).

target g., one specifically affected by a pituitary hormone.

thymus g., a ductless glandlike body in the anterior mediastinal cavity, which is involved in cell-mediated immunity (see also THYMUS).

thyroid g., an endocrine gland consisting of two lobes, one on each side of the trachea, joined by a narrow isthmus, producing hormones (thyroxine and triiodothyronine), which require iodine for their elaboration and which are concerned in regulating metabolic rate; it also secretes calcitonin (see also THYROID GLAND).

tubular g., any gland made up of or containing a tubule or tubules.

Tyson's g's, preputial glands.

urethral g's, mucous glands in the wall of the urethra; in the male, called also Littre's glands.

vulvovaginal g's, two minute glands, one on either side of the vaginal orifice, their ducts opening on the vulva (see also BARTHOLIN GLANDS).

Waldeyer's g's, glands in the attached edge of the eyelid.

Weber's g's, the tubular mucous glands of the tongue.

glanders (glan′derz) a disease of horses communicable to man, and caused by the glanders bacillus, *Pseudomonas mallei.* It is marked by a purulent inflammation of the mucous membranes and an eruption of nodules on the skin that coalesce and break down, forming deep ulcers, which may end in necrosis of cartilage and bones. The more chronic and constitutional form is known as farcy.

glandilemma (glan″dĭ-lem′ah) the capsule or outer envelope of a gland.

glandula (glan′du-lah), pl. *glan′dulae* [L.] gland.

glandular (glan′du-lar) 1. pertaining to or of the nature of a gland. 2. pertaining to the glans penis.

g. fever, an acute infectious disease caused by the Epstein-Barr virus (see also infectious MONONUCLEOSIS).

glandule (glan′dūl) a small gland.

glans (glanz), pl. *glan′des* [L.] a small, rounded mass or glandlike body.

g. clitor′idis, the erectile tissue on the free end of the clitoris.

g. pe′nis, the cap-shaped expansion of the corpus spongiosum at the end of the penis.

Glanzmann's disease, thrombasthenia (glanz′-manz) thrombasthenia.

glass (glas) 1. a hard, brittle, often transparent material, usually consisting of the fused amorphous silicates of potassium or sodium, and of calcium, with silica in excess. 2. a container, usually cylindrical, made from glass. 3. (pl.) lenses worn to aid or improve vision (see also GLASSES and LENS).

Wood's g., Wood's filter.

glasses (glas′ez) spectacles; LENSES arranged in a frame holding them in the proper position before the eyes, as an aid to vision.

bifocal g., glasses with lenses having two different refracting powers, one for distant and one for near vision.

trifocal g., lenses that have three different refracting powers, one for distant, one for intermediate, and one for near vision.

glaucarubin (glaw″kah-ru′bin) a crystalline glycoside obtained from the fruit of *Simaruba glauca;* used as an amebicide.

glaucoma (glaw-ko′mah) a group of diseases of the eye characterized by increased intraocular pressure, resulting in pathological changes in the optic disk and typical visual field defects, and eventually blindness if it is not treated successfully. adj., **glauco′matous.** Glaucoma is responsible for almost half of all cases of adult blindness, and strikes more than 2 per cent of all those over 40 years of age in the United States. It rarely occurs in anyone under 40. There is evidence that it is much more common in patients with diabetes mellitus. The cause is unknown, but proper treatment, given early enough, can halt its disabling effects.

The normal eye is filled with aqueous humor in an amount carefully regulated to maintain the shape of the eyeball. In glaucoma, the balance of this fluid is disturbed; fluid is formed more rapidly than it leaves the eye, and pressure builds up. The increased pressure damages the retina and disturbs the vision, for example, by the loss of side vision. If not relieved by proper treatment, the pressure will eventually damage the optic nerve, interrupting the flow of impulses and causing blindness.

There are two principal forms of glaucoma. The acute form may cause a sudden dimming of the vision, often with severe pain in the eye. Chronic glaucoma, which is more common, does not usually cause pain, and affects the vision very gradually. The patient frequently does not notice the effects of chronic glaucoma until after he has already suffered some loss of vision.

SYMPTOMS AND DIAGNOSIS. The symptoms of glaucoma are loss of side vision, so that the patient seems to be "looking down a rifle barrel," blurred or fogged vision, and the appearance of colored rings or halos around bright objects. These symptoms do not necessarily indicate glaucoma, but anyone over 40 who experiences any of them should consult an opthalmologist immediately.

Glaucoma is diagnosed with the help of a tonometer, which measures the pressure inside the eyeball.

TREATMENT. Treatment for glaucoma varies with the type and severity of the case. If it is detected early, it can generally be treated satisfactorily with miotics and other drugs that help reduce the pressure inside the eye. In some advanced cases, relatively simple surgery may be necessary to provide the fluid with a new outflow channel.

The effects of untreated glaucoma cannot be remedied. If the condition is neglected until partial or total blindness sets in, the retina and optic nerve cannot be repaired to restore sight.

congenital g., that due to defective development of the structures in and around the anterior chamber of the eye, and resulting in impairment of the aqueous humor.

infantile g., congenital glaucoma that may be fully developed at birth with enlarged eyes and hazy corneas, or may develop at any time up to two or three years of age.

juvenile g., congenital glaucoma differing from the infantile form in that it occurs in older children and young adults, and there is no gross enlargement of the eyeball.

narrow-angle g., a form of primary glaucoma in an eye characterized by a shallow anterior chamber and a narrow angle, in which filtration is compromised as a result of the iris blocking the angle.

open-angle g., a form of primary glaucoma in an eye in which the angle of the anterior chamber remains open, but filtration is gradually diminished because of the tissues of the angle.

primary g., increased intraocular pressure occurring in an eye without previous disease.

secondary g., increased intraocular pressure due to disease or injury to the eye.

g. sim′plex, glaucoma without pronounced symptoms, but attended with progressive loss of vision.

gleet (glēt) 1. chronic gonorrheal urethritis. 2. a urethral discharge, especially one that is mucous or purulent.

glenoid (gle′noid) resembling a pit or socket.

g. cavity, a depression in the lateral angle of the scapula for articulation with the humerus.

g. fossa, a depression in the temporal bone in which the condyle of the lower jaw rests; called also mandibular fossa.

g. lip, a ring of fibrocartilage joined to the rim of the glenoid cavity.

glia (gli′ah) neuroglia; the supporting structure of nervous tissue, consisting, in the central nervous system, of astrocytes, oligodendrocytes, and microglia.

gliacyte (gli′ah-sīt) a cell of the glia or neuroglia.

gliadin (gli′ah-din) an alcohol-soluble protein from wheat.

glial (gli′al) of or pertaining to glia or neuroglia.

glioblastoma (gli″o-blas-to′mah) any malignant astrocytoma.

g. multifor′me, astrocytoma Grade III or IV; a rapidly growing tumor, usually of the cerebral hemispheres, composed of spongioblasts, astroblasts, and astrocytes.

gliococcus (gli″o-kok′us) a micrococcus forming gelatinous matter.

gliocyte (gli′o-sīt) gliacyte.

gliocytoma (gli″o-si-to′mah) glioma.

gliogenous (gli-oj′ĕnus) produced or formed by neuroglia.

glioma (gli-o′mah) a tumor composed of neuroglia in any of its states of development; sometimes extended to include all intrinsic neoplasms of the brain and spinal cord, as astrocytomas, ependymomas, etc.

g. ret′inae, retinoblastoma.

gliomatosis (gli″o-mah-to′sis) excessive development of the neuroglia, especially of the spinal cord, in certain cases of syringomylia.

gliomatous (gli-o′mah-tus) pertaining to or of the nature of glioma.

glioneuroma (gli″o-nu-ro′mah) glioma combined with neuroma.

gliosarcoma (gli″o-sar-ko′mah) glioma combined with sarcoma.

gliosis (gli-o′sis) an excess of astroglia in damaged areas of the central nervous system.

gliosome (gli′o-sōm) one of the small cytoplasmic processes of neuroglial cells.

Glisson's capsule (glis′unz) a sheath of connective tissue enclosing the hepatic artery, hepatic duct, and portal vein.

Glisson's disease (glis′unz) rickets.

glissonitis (glis″o-ni′tis) inflammation of Glisson's capsule.

globi (glo′bi) 1. plural of *globus*. 2. encapsulated globular masses containing bacilli; seen in smears of lepromatous leprosy lesions.

globin (glo′bin) the protein constituent of hemoglobin; also, any member of a group of proteins similar to the typical globin.

globinometer (glo″bĭ-nom′ĕ-ter) an instrument for determining the proportion of oxyhemoglobin in the blood.

globoside (glob′o-sīd) a sphingoglycolipid containing acetylated amino sugars and simple hexoses, occurring in human serum, spleen, liver, and erythrocytes, and accumulating in tissues in Sandhoff's disease.

globule (glob′ūl) a small spherical mass; a little globe or pellet, as of medicine. adj., **glob′ular.**

globulin (glob′u-lin) a class of proteins which are insoluble in water, but soluble in saline solutions (euglobulins), or water-soluble proteins (pseudoglobulins) whose other physical properties resemble those of true globulins. The plasma proteins are divided into three main types: fibrinogen, globulins, and albumin. Globulins are further divided into three groups: alpha, beta, and gamma globulins. The alpha and beta globulins perform various functions in the circulation, such as transporting other proteins to various parts of the body, combining with other substances so they can be transported and chemically reacting with other substances. The GAMMA GLOBULINS are essential to the establishment of immunity because nearly all ANTIBODIES are gamma globulin molecules (see also IMMUNOGLOBULINS).

accelerator g., a substance present in plasma, but not in serum, that functions in the formation of intrinsic and extrinsic thromboplastin; called also CLOTTING factor V.

antihemophilic g., AHG, CLOTTING factor VIII.

antilymphocyte g., ALG, a substance used as an immunosuppressive agent in organ transplantation, usually in combination with immunosuppressive drugs; it is the gamma globulin fraction of antilymphocyte serum.

immune g., 1. immunoglobulin. 2. a serum globulin that has been modified in response to infection or to injection of certain materials and contains antibodies to the antigens eliciting their production; used as a passive immunizing agent against measles or tetanus and in prophylaxis or treatment of whooping cough.

serum g., the fraction of proteins precipitated from blood serum by half saturation with ammonium sulfate; the principal groups include the α-, β-, and γ-globulins.

globulinuria (glob″u-lin-u′re-ah) the presence of globulins in the urine.

globus (glo′bus), pl. *glo′bi* [L.] 1. a sphere or ball; a spherical mass. 2. a subjective sensation as of a lump or mass.

g. hyster′icus, the subjective sensation of a lump in the throat.

g. pal′lidus, the smaller and more medial part of the lentiform nucleus of the brain.

glomangioma (glo-man″je-o′mah) a benign, often painful tumor derived from a glomus, usually occurring on the distal portion of the fingers or toes, in the skin, or in deeper structures.

glomectomy (glo-mek′to-me) excision of a glomus.

glomera (glom′er-ah) plural of *glomus.*

glomerular (glo-mer′u-lar) pertaining to or of the nature of a glomerulus, especially a renal glomerulus.

glomeruli (glo-mer′u-li) plural of *glomerulus.*

glomerulitis (glo-mer″u-li′tis) inflammation of the glomeruli of the kidney.

glomerulonephritis (glo-mer″u-lo-nĕ-fri′tis) a variety of NEPHRITIS characterized by inflammation of the capillary loops in the glomeruli of the kidney. It occurs in acute, subacute, and chronic forms and is usually secondary to an infection, especially with the hemolytic streptococcus.

lobular g., a form in which all glomeruli are affected, with accentuation of the lobulation of the glomerular tufts; it is marked by constant proteinuria and microscopic hematuria.

glomerulopathy (glo-mer″u-lop′ah-the) any disease, especially any noninflammatory disease, of the renal glomeruli.

diabetic g., intercapillary glomerulosclerosis.

glomerulosclerosis (glo-mer″u-lo-sklĕ-ro′sis) arteriolar nephrosclerosis.

intercapillary g., Kimmelstiel-Wilson syndrome, a degenerative complication of DIABETES MELLITUS, manifested as albuminuria, edema, hypertension, renal insufficiency, and retinopathy.

glomerulus (glo-mer′u-lus), pl. *glomer′uli* [L.] a small tuft or cluster; a small convoluted mass of capillaries, especially a network of vascular tufts encased in the malpighian capsule of the kidney. adj., **glomer′ular.**

The glomerulus is an integral part of the NEPHRON, the basic unit of the KIDNEY. Each nephron is capable of forming urine by itself, and each kidney has approximately a million nephrons. The specific function of each glomerulus is to bring blood (and the waste products it carries) to the nephron. As the blood flows through the glomerulus, about one-fifth of the plasma passes through the glomerular membrane, collects in the malpighian capsule, and then flows through the renal tubules. Much of this fluid passes back into the blood via the small capillaries around the tubules (peritubular capillaries). The continuous filtration of fluid from the glomeruli and its reabsorption into the peritubular capillaries is made possible by a high pressure in the glomerular capillary bed and a low pressure in the peritubular bed.

Any disease of the glomeruli, such as acute or chronic glomerulonephritis, must be considered serious because it interferes with the basic functions of the kidneys, that is, filtration of liquids and excretion of certain end products of metabolism and excess sodium, potassium, and chloride ions that may accumulate in the blood.

glomoid (glo′moid) resembling a glomus.

glomus (glo′mus), pl. *glom′era* [L.] a small histologically recognizable body composed primarily of fine arterioles connecting directly with veins, and having a rich nerve supply.

g. carot′icum, carotid body.

g. choroi′deum, an enlargement of the choroid plexus of the lateral ventricle.

coccygeal g., g. coccyg′eum, a collection of arteriovenous anastomoses formed, close to the tip of the coccyx, by the median sacral artery.

gloss(o)- word element [Gr.], *tongue.*

glossal (glos′al) pertaining to the tongue.

glossalgia (glŏ-sal′je-ah) pain in the tongue.

glossectomy (glŏ-sek′to-me) excision of all or a portion of the tongue.

Glossina (glŏ-si′nah) a genus of biting flies, including the tsetse flies, which serve as vectors of trypanosomes causing various forms of TRYPANOSOMIASIS in man and animals.

glossitis (glŏ-si′tis) inflammation of the tongue.

rhomboid g., median, a congenital anomaly of the tongue, with a flat or slightly raised reddish patch or plaque on the midline of the dorsal surface.

glossocele (glos′o-sēl) swelling and protrusion of the tongue.

glossodynia (glos″o-din′e-ah) pain in the tongue.

glossograph (glos′o-graf) an apparatus for registering tongue movements in speech.

glossolalia (glos″o-la′le-ah) unintelligible speech.

glossology (glŏ-sol′o-je) 1. the sum of knowledge regarding the tongue. 2. a treatise on nomenclature.

glossopathy (glŏ-sop′ah-the) any disease of the tongue.

glossopharyngeal (glos″o-fah-rin′je-al) pertaining to the tongue and pharynx.

g. nerve, the ninth cranial nerve; it supplies the carotid sinus, mucous membrane, and muscles of the pharynx, soft palate, and posterior third of the tongue, and the taste buds in the posterior third of the tongue. By serving the carotid sinus, the glossopharyngeal nerve provides for reflex control of the heart. It is also responsible for the swallowing reflex, for stimulating secretions of the parotid glands, and for the sense of taste in the posterior third of the tongue. (See also table of NERVES.)

glossoplasty (glos′o-plas′te) plastic surgery of the tongue.

glossorrhaphy (glŏ-sōr′ah-fe) suture of the tongue.

glossospasm (glos′o-spazm) spasm of the tongue.

glossotomy (glŏ-sot′o-me) incision of the tongue.

glossotrichia (glos″o-trik′e-ah) hairy tongue.

glottic (glot′ik) pertaining to the glottis or to the tongue.

glottis (glot′is), pl. *glot′tides* [Gr.] the vocal apparatus of the larynx, consisting of the true vocal cords (vocal folds) and the opening between them.

gluc(o)- word element [Gr.], *sweetness; glucose.* See also words beginning *glyco-*.

glucagon (gloo′kah-gon) a polypeptide hormone secreted by the pancreatic alpha cells that increases blood glucose concentration. The commercial preparation, glucagon hydrochloride, is used to relieve hypoglycemic coma from any cause, especially hyperinsulinism.

glucagonoma (gloo″kah-gon-o′mah) a malignant glucagon-secreting tumor of the alpha cells of the pancreas.

glucinium (gloo-sin′e-um) beryllium.

glucocerebroside (gloo″ko-ser′ĕ-bro-sid) a cerebroside containing a glucose sugar; it accumulates in the tissues in Gaucher's disease.

glucocorticoid (gloo″ko-kor′tĭ-koid) any corticoid substance that increases gluconeogenesis, raising the concentration of liver glycogen and blood sugar, i.e., cortisol (hydrocortisone), cortisone, and corticosterone. These hormones influence protein, fat, and carbohydrate metabolism. They promote mobilization of fat from fat stores and transport of amino acids into the extracellular compartment. By increasing the concentration of amino acids in the blood the glucocorticoids provide the liver with the chemical needed to convert proteins and fats into glucose (gluconeogenesis). The amino acids in the blood are also used by the body in times of stress to repair cellular damage and to build tissue resistance to trauma (see also ALARM REACTION). The various glucocorticoids are used therapeutically for their anti-inflammatory effects.

glucofuranose (gloo″ko-fu′rah-nōs) a form of glucose in which carbon atoms 1 and 4 are bridged by an oxygen atom.

glucogenic (gloo″ko-jen′ik) giving rise to or producing sugar.

glucokinase (gloo″ko-ki′nās) an enzyme that in the presence of ATP catalyzes glucose to glucose-6-phosphate.

glucokinetic (gloo″ko-ki-net′ik) activating sugar so as to maintain the sugar level of the body.

glucokinin (gloo″ko-kin′in) a substance obtained from vegetable tissues and yeast; when injected into animals, it produces hyperglycemia, and in depancreatized dogs has an insulin-like effect.

gluconate (gloo′ko-nāt) a salt of gluconic acid.

ferrous g., a compound used in the treatment of iron deficiency anemia (see also FERROUS GLUCONATE).

gluconeogenesis (gloo″ko-ne″o-jen′ĕ-sis) the synthesis of glucose from noncarbohydrate sources, such as amino and fatty acids. Called also glyconeogenesis.

gluconic acid (gloo-kon′ik) an intermediate product formed in the biosynthesis of pentoses.

glucophore (gloo′ko-fōr) the group of atoms in a molecule that gives the compound a sweet taste.

glucoprotein (gloo″ko-pro′te-in) glycoprotein.

glucopyranose (gloo″ko-pi′rah-nōs) a form of glucose in which carbon atoms 1 and 5 are bridged by an oxygen atom.

glucosamine (gloo″ko-sam′in) an α-amino derivative of dextrose (δ-glucose), obtained from mucin and chitin by hydrolysis.

glucosan (gloo′ko-san) an anhydro-polymer yielding a hexose on hydrolysis.

glucose (gloo′kōs) 1. D-glucose; a simple sugar, a monosaccharide in certain foodstuffs, especially fruit, and in normal blood; the chief source of energy for living organisms. (See also DEXTROSE.) 2. liquid glucose.

Glucose, whose molecular formula is $C_6H_{12}O_6$, is the end product of carbohydrate digestion; very soon after digestion the other monosaccharides (fructose and galactose) are converted into glucose. Because of this conversion, glucose is the only monosaccharide present in significant amounts in the body fluids. The metabolism of glucose produces energy for the body cells; the rate of metabolism is controlled by insulin. Glucose that is not needed for energy is stored in the form of glycogen as a source of potential energy, readily available when needed. Most of the glycogen is stored in the liver and muscle cells. When these and other body cells are saturated with glycogen, the excess glucose is converted into fat and stored as adipose tissue.

The normal fasting level for glucose in the blood is between 70 and 90 mg. per 100 ml. Unusually high levels of glucose in the blood (hyperglycemia) may indicate such diseases as DIABETES MELLITUS, HYPERTHYROIDISM, or hyperpituitarism. Levels of blood sugar below 40 mg. per 100 ml. (HYPOGLYCEMIA) may be caused by diseases of the kidneys or liver, hypopituitarism, and hyperinsulinism, an uncommon condition in which too much insulin is produced. A GLUCOSE TOLERANCE TEST is done to assess the ability of the body to metabolize glucose.

liquid g., a thick syrupy, sweet liquid, consisting chiefly of dextrose, with dextrins, maltose, and water, obtained by incomplete hydrolysis of starch; used as a flavoring agent, as a food, and in the treatment of dehydration.

g.-1-phosphate, an intermediate in carbohydrate metabolism.

g.-6-phosphate, an intermediate in carbohydrate metabolism.

g. tolerance test, a test of the body's ability to utilize carbohydrates. It is often used to detect abnormalities of carbohydrate metabolism such as occur in diabetes mellitus, hypoglycemia, and liver and adrenocortical dysfunction.

There are two types of glucose tolerance tests. In the standard test, which is used most often, the patient is given a single dose of 100 gm. of glucose, and blood and urine specimens are collected periodically for up to 6 hours. The Exton and Rose test is also useful for the diagnosis of diabetes mellitus and is completed in 1 hour.

In the standard test the patient must be in a fasting state when the test is begun, and a blood sample is taken for measurement of fasting glucose before the test dose is given. Glucose is given dissolved in water and flavored with lemon juice, or commercial preparations in the form of a carbonated drink or gelatin, which are more palatable and provide exactly 100 gm. of glucose, may be used.

One-half hour after the glucose is ingested a blood sample and urine specimen are obtained. The specimens are collected at hourly intervals for the next 4 or 5 hours as indicated. Each specimen must be labeled with the exact time it was collected. The patient may be allowed to drink water during the testing period but he may not drink anything else or eat or smoke until the test is completed.

Usually the patient experiences some weakness and perspires excessively, and he may faint during the test. These are normal reactions to a fall in the blood glucose level as insulin is secreted in response to the presence of glucose.

In both the standard test and in the Exton and Rose test the patient is usually fed a high-carbohydrate diet for 3 days before the test. In the Exton and Rose test the patient is given 50 gm. of glucose, and blood and urine samples are obtained 30 minutes later. Immediately after these specimens are collected he is given a second dose of 50 gm. of glucose. Half an hour later specimens of blood and urine are obtained.

NORMAL VALUES. *Standard test* (results given in milligrams per 100 ml. of blood): fasting—80 mg.; 30 min.—150 mg.; 60 min.—135 mg.; 2 hours—100 mg.; 2½ hours—80 mg. *Exton and Rose test* (results given in milligrams per 100 ml. of blood): Fasting—80 mg., urine neg.; 30 min.—150 mg., urine neg.; 1 hour—160 mg., urine neg.

glucosidase (gloo-ko'sĭ-dās) an enzyme of the hydrolase class that splits glucoside, occurring as α-, β-, and α-1,3-glucosidase; α-glucosidase (maltase) occurs in intestinal juice, and β-glucosidase (cellobiase) in the kidney, liver, and intestinal mucosa.

glucosin (gloo'ko-sin) a group of bases derived from glucose by the action of ammonia; some are highly toxic.

glucosulfone (gloo″ko-sul'fōn) a dapsone derivative; the sodium salt is used as a leprostatic and tuberculostatic.

glucosuria (gloo″ko-su're-ah) 1. the presence of glucose in the urine. 2. dextrosuria.

glucuronic acid (gloo″ku-ron'ik) an acid formed by oxidation of glucose in animal metabolism and found in urine combined with camphor, chloroform, chloral, and other aromatic bodies.

β-glucuronidase (gloo″ku-ron'ĭ-dās) an enzyme that attacks glycosidic linkages in natural and synthetic glucuronides and has been implicated in estrogen metabolism and cell division; occurs in the spleen, liver, and endocrine glands.

glucuronide (gloo-ku'ron-īd) any compound with glucuronic acid.

glutamate (gloo'tah-māt) a salt of glutamic acid; in biochemistry, the term is often used interchangeably with glutamic acid.

glutamic acid (gloo-tam'ik) a crystalline dibasic nonessential amino acid, widely distributed in proteins; its hydrochloride salt is used as a gastric acidifier. The monosodium salt of L-glutamic acid (sodium glutamate) is used in treating encephalopathies associated with hepatic disease, and to enhance the flavor of foods and tobacco.

glutamic-oxaloacetic transaminase (gloo-tam'ik ok″sah-lo-ah-se'tik trans-am'ĭ-nās) GOT, an enzyme normally present in serum (SGOT) and various tissues, especially the heart and liver; it is released into the serum as a result of tissue injury and is present in increased concentration in myocardial infarction or acute damage to liver cells. (See also SERUM GLUTAMIC-OXALOACETIC TRANSAMINASE.)

glutamic-pyruvic transaminase (gloo-tam'ik pi-roo'vik trans-am'ĭ-nās) GPT, an enzyme normally present in the serum (SGPT) and body tissues, especially the liver; it is released into the serum as a result of tissue injury and is present in increased concentration in acute damage to liver cells. (See also SERUM GLUTAMIC-PYRUVIC TRANSAMINASE.)

glutaminase (gloo-tam'ĭ-nās) an enzyme that catalyzes the splitting of glutamine into glutamic acid and ammonia.

glutamine (gloo'tah-min) an amide of glutamic acid, occurring in the juices of many plants and in some animal tissues; it is an important carrier of urinary ammonia and is broken down in the kidney by glutaminase.

Glutan H-C-L (gloo'tan) trademark for capsules containing glutamic acid hydrochloride, a gastric acidifier.

glutaraldehyde (gloo″tahr-al'dĕ-hīd) a compound used as a tissue fixative for light and electron microscopy because of its preservation of fine structural detail and localization of enzyme activity.

glutathione (gloo″tah-thi'ōn) a tripeptide in animal and plant tissues composed of glutamic acid, cysteine, and aminoacetic acid; it acts as a respiratory carrier of oxygen.

oxidized g., the precursor of reduced glutathione.

reduced g., a tripeptide present in red blood cells, deficiency of which probably predisposes erythrocytes to the oxidant and hemolytic effects of certain drugs.

gluteal (gloo'te-al) pertaining to the buttocks.

g. muscles, three muscles, the greatest, middle, and least, which extend, abduct, and rotate the thigh; called also gluteus maximus, medius, and minimus muscles. (See also table of MUSCLES.)

g. nerves, nerves that innervate the gluteal muscles (see also table of NERVES.)

glutelin (gloo'tĕ-lin) a simple protein from the seeds of cereals.

gluten (gloo'ten) the protein of wheat and other grains that gives dough its tough elastic character; avoidance of this substance will alleviate CELIAC DISEASE (nontropical sprue) in certain persons.

g. enteropathy, celiac disease.

glutethimide (gloo-teth'ĭ-mīd) a hypnotic and sedative.

glutin (gloo'tin) 1. a viscid substance from the glutelin of wheat. 2. gelatin in its soft or dissolved state.

glutinous (gloo'tĭ-nus) adhesive; sticky.

glutitis (gloo-ti'tis) inflammation of the gluteal muscles.

glycemia (gli-se'me-ah) the presence of glucose in the blood.

glyceraldehyde (glis"er-al'dĕ-hīd) a compound, glyceric aldehyde, formed by the oxidation of glycerol.

glyceric acid (glĭ-ser'ik) an intermediate product in the transformation in the body of carbohydrate to lactic acid formed by oxidation of glycerin.

glyceride (glis'er-īd) an organic acid ester of glycerin, designated, according to the number of ester linkages, as a mono-, di-, or triglyceride.

glycerin (glis'er-in) a clear, colorless, syrupy liquid, used as a humectant and as a solvent for drugs; it is a trihydric sugar alcohol, being the alcoholic component of fats. Called also glycerol.

glycerite (glis'er-īt) a preparation of a medicinal substance in glycerin.

glycerol (glis'er-ol) glycerin.

glycerophosphate (glis"er-o-fos'fāt) a combination of a base with glycerin and phosphoric acid.

glycerose (glis'er-ōs) a sugar formed by oxidizing glycerin; there are two glyceroses, glyceraldehyde and dihydroxyacetone.

glyceryl (glis'er-il) the trivalent radical of glycerin.

g. monostearate, an emulsifying agent.

g. triacetate, triacetin, a topical antifungal agent.

g. trinitrate, a colorless or yellowish, oily liquid; a vasodilator used principally in ANGINA PECTORIS; called also NITROGLYCERIN.

glycine (gli'sēn) a nonessential amino acid occurring as a constituent of many proteins. It has been synthesized and is used as a gastric antacid and dietary supplement. Called also aminoacetic acid and glycocoll.

glycobiarsol (gli"ko-bi-ar'sol) an intestinal amebicide.

glycocalyx (gli"ko-kal'iks) the glycoprotein-polysaccharide covering that surrounds many cells.

glycocholate (gli"ko-ko'lāt) a salt of glycocholic acid.

glycocholic acid (gli"ko-ko'lik) a conjugated form of one of the bile acids that yields glycine and cholic acid on hydrolysis.

glycocoll (gli'ko-kol) glycine.

glycogen (gli'ko-jen) a polysaccharide that is the chief carbohydrate storage material in animals. It is formed by and largely stored in the liver, and to a lesser extent in muscles; it is depolymerized to glucose and liberated as needed. Called also animal starch.

g. disease, g. storage disease, glycogenosis.

glycogenase (gli'ko-jĕ-nās) an enzyme that splits glycogen into dextrin and maltose.

glycogenesis (gli"ko-jen'ĕ-sis) the conversion of glucose to glycogen for storage in the liver. adj., **glycogenet'ic.**

glycogenic (gli"ko-jen'ik) pertaining to, characterized by, or promoting glycogenesis; pertaining to glycogen.

glycogenolysis (gli"ko-jĕ-nol'ĭ-sis) the splitting up of glycogen in the liver, yielding glucose.

glycogenosis (gli"ko-jĕ-no'sis), pl. *glycogeno'ses.* a group of genetically determined disorders of glycogen metabolism, marked by abnormal storage of glycogen in the tissues of the body. Called also glycogen disease or glycogen storage disease. See GIERKE'S DISEASE (glycogenosis, type I), POMPE'S DISEASE (type II), FORBES' DISEASE (type III), AMYLOPECTINOSIS (type IV), McARDLE'S DISEASE (type V), and HERS' DISEASE (type IV).

generalized g., Pompe's disease.

hepatorenal g., Gierke's disease.

myophosphorylase deficiency g., McArdle's disease.

glycogeusia (gli"ko-gu'se-ah) a sweet taste in the mouth.

glycol (gli'kol) any one of a group of aliphatic dihydric alcohols, having marked hygroscopic properties and useful as solvents and plasticizers.

glycolic acid (gli-kol'ik) an intermediate product in the transformation in the body of serine to glycine.

glycolipid (gli"ko-lip'id) a lipid containing carbohydrate groups, usually galactose but also glucose, inositol, or others; the glycolipids include the cerebrosides.

glycolysis (gli-kol'ĭ-sis) the breaking down of sugars into simpler compounds, chiefly pyruvate or lactate. adj., **glycolyt'ic.**

glyconeogenesis (gli"ko-ne"o-jen'ĕ-sis) gluconeogenesis.

glyconucleoprotein (gli"ko-nu"kle-o-pro'te-in) nucleoprotein bearing carbohydrate groups.

glycopenia (gli"ko-pe'ne-ah) a deficiency of sugar in the tissues.

glycopexis (gli"ko-pek'sis) fixation or storing of sugar or glycogen. adj., **glycopec'tic.**

glycophilia (gli"ko-fil'e-ah) a condition in which a small amount of glucose produces hyperglycemia.

glycoprotein (gli"ko-pro'te-in) any of a class of conjugated proteins consisting of a compound of protein with a carbohydrate group.

glycoptyalism (gli"ko-ti'ah-lizm) glycosialia.

glycopyrrolate (gli"ko-pir'o-lāt) an anticholinergic used to reduce gastric acid secretion and hypermotility.

glycorrachia (gli"ko-ra'ke-ah) the presence of sugar in the cerebrospinal fluid.

glycorrhea (gli"ko-re'ah) any sugary discharge from the body.

glycosamine (gli"ko-sam'in) glucosamine.

glycosecretory (gli"ko-se-kre'to-re) concerned in secretion of glycogen.

glycosemia (gli"ko-se'me-ah) glycemia.

glycosialia (gli"ko-si-a'le-ah) glucose in the saliva; glycoptyalism.

glycosialorrhea (gli"ko-si"ah-lo-re'ah) excessive flow of saliva containing sugar.

glycosidase (gli'ko-sĭ-dās) any of a large group of hydrolytic enzymes acting on glycosyl compounds.

glycoside (gli'ko-sīd) any compound containing a carbohydrate molecule (sugar), particularly any such natural product in plants, convertible, by hydrolytic cleavage, into a sugar and a nonsugar component (aglycone), and named specifically for the sugar contained, as glucoside (glucose), pentoside (pentose), fructoside (fructose), etc.

cardiac g., any one of a group of glycosides occurring in certain plants (*Digitalis*, etc.), having a characteristic action on the heart.

glycosometer (gli″ko-som′ĕ-ter) an instrument for determining the proportion of glucose in urine.

glycosphingolipid (gli″ko-sfing″o-lip′id) a sphingolipid containing the sugar glucose or galactose.

glycostatic (gli″ko-stat′ik) tending to maintain a constant sugar level.

glycosuria (gli″ko-su′re-ah) abnormally high sugar content in the urine.

renal g., glycosuria due to an inherited inability of the renal tubules to reabsorb glucose completely.

glycosyl (gli′ko-sil) a radical derived from a carbohydrate.

glycotropic (gli″ko-trop′ik) having an affinity for sugar; causing hyperglycemia.

glycuresis (gli″ku-re′sis) the normal increase in the glucose content of the urine that follows an ordinary carbohydrate meal.

glycyrrhiza (glis″ĭ-ri′zah) the dried roots and rhizome of the legume *Glycyrrhiza glabra,* or licorice; used as a flavored vehicle for drugs.

glyoxylic acid (gli″ok-sil′ik) an acid formed in the oxidative deamination of glycine.

Glytheonate (gli-the′o-nāt) trademark for a preparation of theophylline sodium glycinate, a smooth muscle relaxant, myocardial stimulant, and diuretic.

gm. gram.

gnath(o)- word element [Gr.], *jaw.*

gnathic (nath′ik) pertaining to the jaw or cheeks.

gnathion (na′the-on) the most outward and everted point on the profile curvature of the chin.

gnathitis (nah-thi′tis) inflammation of the jaw.

gnathocephalus (na″tho-sef′ah-lus) a headless monster with jaws.

gnathodynamometer (na″tho-di″nah-mom′ĕ-ter) an instrument for measuring the force exerted in closing the jaws.

gnathology (nah-thol′o-je) the science dealing with the masticatory apparatus as a whole.

gnathoplasty (na′tho-plas″te) plastic repair of the jaw or cheek.

gnathoschisis (nah-thos′kĭ-sis) congenital cleft of the upper jaw, as in cleft palate.

gnosia (no′se-ah) the faculty of perceiving and recognizing. adj., **gnos′tic.**

goiter (goi′ter) enlargement of the thyroid gland, causing a swelling in the front part of the neck. adj., **goit′rous.** Simple endemic goiter is usually caused by lack of iodine in the diet. Although the administration of iodine will not cure simple goiter, it will prevent it or stop an existing goiter from enlarging. If there is evidence of pressure against the throat, or the possibility of a malignancy, the goiter may be removed surgically.

Exophthalmic, or toxic, goiter (known also as Graves′ disease) is accompanied by excessive concentrations of thyroid hormones in the blood, which produce the symptoms of HYPERTHYROIDISM. There is protrusion of the eyeballs (exophthalmos) and there may be other ocular changes. Treatment of this type of goiter may include surgical removal of the thyroid or medical management with administration of iodine compounds and other antithyroid drugs. Depending on the age and sex of the patient, therapeutic doses of radioactive iodine may also be used.

aberrant g., goiter of an supernumerary thyroid gland.

adenomatous g., that caused by adenoma or multiple colloid nodules of the thyroid gland.

Basedow g., a colloid goiter which has become hyperfunctioning after administration of iodine.

colloid g., a large, soft thyroid gland with distended spaces filled with colloid.

cystic g., one with cysts formed by mucoid or colloid degeneration.

endemic g., see GOITER.

exophthalmic g., enlargement of the thyroid with protrusion of the eyeballs; see GOITER.

fibrous g., goiter in which the capsule and the stroma of the thyroid gland are hyperplastic.

follicular g., parenchymatous goiter.

intrathoracic g., one in which a portion of the enlarged gland is in the thoracic cavity.

nodular g., goiter with circumscribed nodules within the gland.

parenchymatous g., goiter marked by increase in follicles and proliferation of epithelium.

perivascular g., one that surrounds a large blood vessel.

retrovascular g., goiter with a process or processes behind an important blood vessel.

substernal g., goiter in which a portion of the enlarged gland is beneath the sterum.

suffocative g., one that causes dyspnea by pressure.

toxic g., exophthalmic goiter.

vascular g., one due chiefly to dilatation of the blood vessels.

goitrogen (goi′tro-jen) a goiter-producing agent.

goitrogenic (goi-tro-jen′ik) producing goiter.

goitrogenicity (goi″tro-jĕ-nis′ĭ-te) the tendency to produce goiter.

gold (gōld) a chemical element, atomic number 79, atomic weight 196.967, symbol Au. (See table of ELEMENTS.) Gold and many of its compounds are used in medicine, especially in treating rheumatoid arthritis. Gold salts are among the most toxic of therapeutic agents and must be given only under strict medical supervision. Toxic reactions may vary from mild to severe kidney or liver damage and blood dyscrasias.

radioactive g., a RADIOISOTOPE of gold; used in treating certain types of cancer (see also RADIOGOLD).

g. sodium thiomalate, an odorless, fine, white to yellowish powder with a metallic taste; used in treatment of rheumatoid arthritis and nondisseminated lupus erythematosus.

g. sodium thiosulfate, used in treatment of rheumatoid arthritis.

g. thioglucose, aurothioglucose, used in treating rheumatoid arthritis.

Goldblatt kidney (gōld′blat) a kidney with obstruction of its blood flow, resulting in renal hypertension.

Goldflam's disease (gōlt′flahmz) myasthenia gravis.

Goldflam-Erb disease (gōlt′flahm-erb) myasthenia gravis.

Golgi apparatus (complex) (gol′je) a complex of membranes and vesicles in a cell, seen in stained preparations as an irregular network of blackened canals or solid strands; it plays a role in the secretory activity of the cell.

Golgi neurons (cells) (gol′je) 1. (*type I*): pyramidal cells with long axons, which leave the gray matter of the central nervous system, traverse the white matter, and terminate in the periphery. 2. (*type II*): stellate neurons with short axons in the cerebral and cerebellar cortices and in the retina.

Golgi tendon organ (gol′je) any of the mechanoreceptors arranged in series with muscle in the tendons of mammalian muscles, being the receptor for stimuli responsible for the lengthening reaction.

gomitoli (go-mit′o-li) a network of capillaries in the upper infundibular stem (of the hypothalamus), which surround terminal arterioles of the superior hypophyseal arteries and that lead into the portal veins to the adenohypophysis.

gomphosis (gom-fo′sis) a type of fibrous joint in which a conical process is inserted into a socket-like portion.

gonad (go′nad, gon′ad) a sex gland; a gamete-producing gland; the OVARY in the female and the TESTIS in the male. adj., **gonad′al, gonad′ial.** The ovary produces the ovum and the testis produces the spermatozoon. In addition, the gonads secrete hormones that influence the development of the reproductive organs at puberty, and they control other physical traits that differentiate men from women, such as pitch of the voice and body form and size (the secondary sex characters). The hormones produced by the ovary include ESTROGEN and PROGESTERONE. The principal hormone produced by the testis is called TESTOSTERONE.

gonadectomy (go″nah-dek′to-me) removal of a gonad.

gonadopathy (go″nah-dop′ah-the) any disease of the gonads.

gonadotherapy (go-nad″o-ther′ah-pe) treatment with gonadal hormones.

gonadotrophic (go-nad″o-trōf′ik) gonadotropic.

gonadotrophin (go-nad″o-trōf′in) gonadotropin.

gonadotropic (go-nad″o-trop′ik) stimulating the gonads; applied to hormones of the anterior PITUITARY GLAND which influence the gonads.

g. hormone, one that has influence on the gonads.

gonadotropin (go-nad″o-trōp′in) a substance that has a stimulating effect upon the gonads, especially the hormone secreted by the anterior PITUITARY GLAND.

chorionic g., a gonad-stimulating principle from human pregnancy urine or from the serum of pregnant mares; used in treatment of underdevelopment of the gonads (see also CHORIONIC GONADOTROPIN).

gonaduct (go′nah-dukt) the duct of a gonad; an oviduct or seminal duct.

gonagra (go-nag′rah) gout in the knee.

gonalgia (go-nal′je-ah) pain in the knee.

gonangiectomy (go-nan″je-ek′to-me) vasectomy.

gonarthritis (gon″ar-thri′tis) inflammation of the knee joint.

gonarthrocace (gon″ar-throk′ah-se) tuberculous arthritis of the knee joint.

gonarthrotomy (gon″ar-throt′o-me) incision into the knee joint.

gonecystis (gon″ĕ-sis′tis) a seminal vesicle.

gonecystitis (gon″ĕ-sis-ti′tis) inflammation of a seminal vesicle.

gonecystolith (gon″ĕ-sis′to-lith) a concretion in a seminal vesicle.

gonecystopyosis (gon″ĕ-sis″to-pi-o′sis) suppuration of a seminal vesicle.

gonidium (go-nid′e-um), pl. *gonid′ia* [Gr.] 1. the algal component of the thallus of a lichen. 2. a motile reproductive unit of certain nitrogen-fixing bacteria. adj., **gonid′ial.**

goniometer (go″ne-om′ĕ-ter) an instrument for measuring angles; the instrument used in GONIOMETRY.

finger g., one for measuring the limits of flexion and extension of the joints between the phalanges of the fingers.

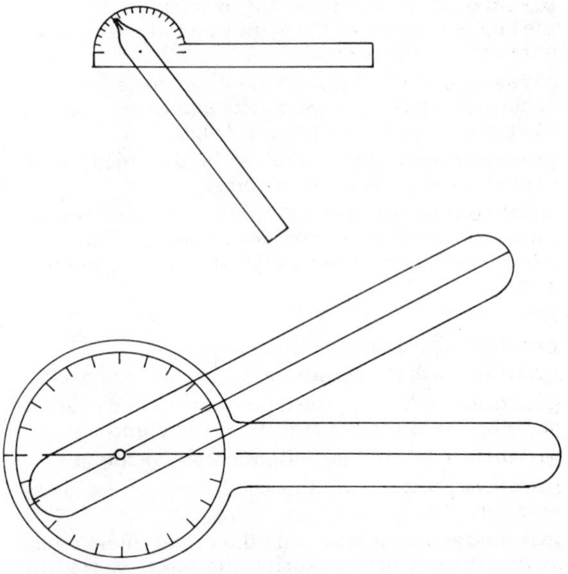

Two examples of universal goniometers commonly used by the clinician. (From Krusen, F. H., Kottke, F. J., and Ellwood, P. M., Jr.: Physical Medicine and Rehabilitation. 2nd ed. Philadelphia, W. B. Saunders Co., 1971.)

goniometry (go″ne-om′ĕ-tre) the measurement of range of motion in a joint. The technique may be used as a diagnostic or therapeutic measure to determine the functional status of a patient with a musculoskeletal or neurological disability. There is a variety of tools and techniques by which joint motion can be measured, but for most clinical purposes the simple universal goniometer is an adequate instrument. The system for recording measurements of range of motion may be somewhat complex or it may be based upon the simple technique of relating the degree of joint motion to a full circle (360 degrees).

In this system of measurement the axis of the goniometer is placed in alignment with the axis of rotation of the joint, and the 0° position of the circle is assigned in terms of one of the bones of the joint in alignment with a point above the head of the patient. In the sagittal plane, which divides the body into right and left halves, motion that rotates the distal member of the joint toward the 0° position is flexion, and motion which rotates it away from the 0° position is extension. In the frontal plane, which

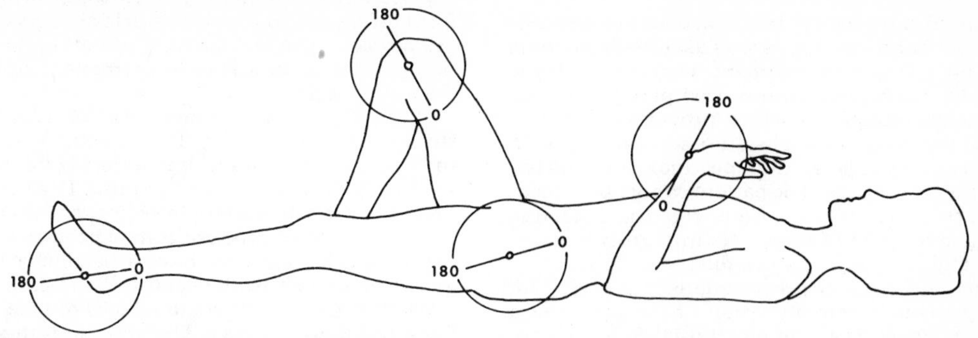

The full circle or 360° system of goniometry applied to several joints of the body, illustrating the locations of the zero degree (0°) position. (From Krusen, F. H., Kottke, F. J., and Ellwood, P. M., Jr.: Physical Medicine and Rehabilitation. 2nd ed. Philadelphia, W. B. Saunders Co., 1971.)

divides the body into ventral and dorsal portions, motion toward the 0° position is abduction (that is, toward the midline of the body), and motion away from the 0° position is adduction.

The 360° system for measurement of joint motion is relatively simple and easily understood by members of the health care team. For this reason it is frequently used. It is especially important, however, that all persons using this or any other system for joint measurement communicate with one another and come to a mutual understanding of the terms to be used and the purposes for which goniometry is being utilized.

gonion (go′ne-on), pl. *go′nia* [Gr.] the most inferior, posterior, and lateral point on the angle of the mandible. adj., **go′nial.**

goniopuncture (go″ne-o-pungk′cher) insertion of a knife blade through the clear cornea, just within the limbus, across the anterior chamber of the eye and through the opposite corneoscleral wall, in treatment of glaucoma.

gonioscope (go′ne-o-skōp″) an optical instrument for examining the angle of the anterior chamber of the eye and for demonstrating ocular motility and rotation.

gonioscopy (go″ne-os′ko-pe) examination of the angle of the anterior chamber of the eye with a gonioscope.

goniotomy (go″ne-ot′o-me) an operation for glaucoma; it consists in opening Schlemm's canal under direct vision.

gono- word element [Gr.], *seed; semen.*

gonococcemia (gon″o-kok-se′me-ah) the presence of gonococci in the blood.

gonococcide (gon″o-kok′sīd) an agent destructive to gonococci.

gonococcus (gon″o-kok′us), pl. *gonococ′ci* [L.] an individual of the species *Neisseria gonorrhoeae,* the etiologic agent of GONORRHEA. adj., **gonococ′cal.**

gonocyte (gon′o-sīt) the primitive reproductive cell of the embryo.

gonophore (gon′o-fōr) an accessory reproductive organ, such as the oviduct.

gonorrhea (gon″o-re′ah) a highly contagious bacterial infection of the genitourinary system. adj., **gonorrhe′al.** It is the most common veneral disease.

CAUSE. Gonorrhea is caused by the bacterial organism *Neisseria gonorrhoeae,* or gonococcus. Characteristically, the gonococcus attacks the mucous membranes of the genital and urinary organs, producing inflammation and pus. In adults the disease is almost always contracted by coitus with an infected person.

Occasionally the gonococci may attack the membranes of the eye, resulting in blindness if untreated. This is not common in adults. The eyes of babies, however, may be infected at birth during passage through the birth canal of an infected mother. The condition that results is called ophthalmia neonatorum, and in the past it was a major cause of blindness in babies. Today it is routine, and required by law in some states, for all newborn infants to receive eye drops (penicillin or silver nitrate) at birth as a protection against gonorrheal infection.

SYMPTOMS. The first symptoms of gonorrhea usually appear within a week after exposure to the gonococcus, but they may take as long as 3 weeks to develop. In men the inflammation generally causes a painful burning sensation during urination, and the infected penis discharges a whitish fluid, or pus. If the condition remains untreated, the discharge increases and continues for 2 or 3 months. As the infection spreads to other membranes, complications such as inflammation of the prostate and the testes may result and may cause sterility.

A woman infected with gonorrhea may feel no pain and notice no early symptoms. She may, however, experience pain in the lower abdomen, with or without a burning sensation during urination or a whitish discharge from the vagina. If the infection is allowed to reach other organs of her reproductive system, the ovaries and the uterine tubes may become inflamed and sterility may result.

If uncontrolled, the gonococcal infection may continue to spread and affect other parts of the body such as the bladder, kidneys, and rectum. The disease can also cause inflammation of the joints, resulting in painful arthritis. As the infection spreads it can lead to meningitis or to peritonitis, and may even cause death if the gonococci enter the blood and lodge in the valves of the heart, causing endocarditis.

DIAGNOSIS AND TREATMENT. Diagnosis is confirmed by the presence of gonococci in the discharge from the penis or vagina or in fluid from any affected area. Gonorrhea can be cured with comparative speed, particularly in its early stages. Penicillin and other antibiotics, as well as the sulfonamide drugs, are effective in treatment. The drug of choice is usually penicillin, administered in a single dose of the long-acting form, which provides concentrations of the drug in the blood for several weeks. In cases of allergy to penicillin, spectinomycin and tetracycline can be used. The patient cannot be considered cured until cultures taken from the discharge are negative for 3 to 4 weeks. No immunity is established and reinfection is possible.

PATIENT CARE. The greatest danger in caring for these patients is contamination of the eyes and a resulting gonorrheal conjunctivitis. Special care must be taken with bed linens, urinals, and bedpans since these can be grossly contaminated with vaginal or urethral discharge. While administering care the hands should be covered with rubber gloves and then washed thoroughly for a full minute after the gloves are removed. It is best to wear a protective gown such as that worn during isolation technique whenever personal care is given the patient. Although gonorrhea is contracted by coitus, the gonococci can infect the eyes or an open wound or break in the skin.

Gonyaulax (gon″e-aw′laks) a genus of dinoflagellates found in fresh, salt, or brackish waters, having yellow to brown chromatophores.

G. catanel′la, a poisonous species which helps to form the destructive red tide in the ocean; see also under POISON.

gonycampsis (gon″ĭ-kamp′sis) abnormal curvature of the knee.

gonyocele (gon′e-o-sel″) synovitis or tuberculous arthritis of the knee.

gonyoncus (gon″e-ong′kus) tumor of the knee.

Goodell's sign (good′elz) softening of the cervix uteri and vagina; a sign of pregnancy.

Goodpasture's syndrome (good-pas′churz) glomerulonephritis associated with hemoptysis, an uncommmon, rapidly progressive, usually fatal condition affecting chiefly young men.

GOT glutamic-oxaloacetic transaminase, an enzyme normally present in serum (SGOT) and various body tissues, especially the heart and liver.

gouge (gowj) a hollow chisel for cutting and removing bone.

goundou (go͞on′doo) a sequel of yaws, seen in natives of Central and South America, with headache, purulent nasal discharge, and formation of bony exostoses at the side of the nose.

gout (gowt) a hereditary form of arthritis in which uric acid appears in excessive quantities in the blood and may be deposited in the joints and other tissues. During an acute attack of gout there is swelling, inflammation, and extreme pain in a joint, frequently that of the big toe. After several years of attacks, the chronic form of the disease may set in, permanently damaging and deforming joints and destroying cells of the kidney. About 95 per cent of all cases occur in men and the first attack rarely occurs before the age of 30.

CAUSES. The causes of gout are not fully understood. It is a disorder of the metabolism of purines. These nitrogenous substances are found in high-protein foods and the net product of their metabolism is uric acid. For unknown reasons, the uric acid, normally expelled in the urine, is retained in the blood in excess amounts. Uric acid crystals are deposited in the joints and in cartilage, where they form lumps called tophi. The uric acid crystals also predispose to the formation of calculi in the kidney (kidney stones) and lead to permanent damage of the kidney cells.

ACUTE GOUT. The acute form of gout usually strikes without warning. The affected joint, which in 70 per cent of cases is that of the big toe, becomes swollen, inflamed, and very painful. The first attack may follow an operation, infection, or minor irritation such as tight shoes, or it may have no apparent cause. The patient may have a headache or fever, and often cannot walk because of the pain.

Without treatment, acute attacks of gout usually last a few days or weeks. The symptoms then disappear completely until the next attack. As the disease progresses, the attacks tend to last longer and the intervals between attacks become shorter.

Treatment. An acute attack of gout can be treated successfully with any of several medicines. Colchicine has long been used to treat gout. In most cases, colchicine relieves the pain and swelling in 72 hours or less, although it does not affect the high concentration of uric acid. In very severe attacks, or for patients who are not helped by colchicine, phenylbutazone or oxyphenbutazone may be used instead. Corticotropin or the cortisones may be combined with one of these medicines. Indomethacin has also been effective in acute cases.

The patient should be kept in bed, with the affected joint protected, throughout the attack and for 24 hours after it subsides. Walking too soon after the attack may set off another one.

CHRONIC GOUT. After a number of acute attacks of gout, the patient who goes without medical treatment may develop the symptoms of chronic gout. This seldom occurs less than 10 years after the first acute attack.

The joints affected by chronic gout degenerate in the same way as joints affected by RHEUMATOID ARTHRITIS, and they may eventually lose their ability to move. In 10 to 20 per cent of those with chronic gout, damage to the renal tubules occurs as the result of the formation of kidney stones.

Treatment. Chronic gout is treated with probenecid or other medicines which promote the urinary excretion of uric acid. Other treatment may also be necessary if the kidney is involved. Sometimes surgery to remove the tophi and correct deformities may be helpful.

MANAGEMENT BETWEEN ATTACKS. If acute gout is recognized at an early stage and treated correctly, the development of the chronic form can generally be prevented.

Since uric acid is the end product of purine metabolism, the patient is usually put on a diet limiting the amount of foods of a high purine content, such as sweetbreads, kidney, liver, sardines, anchovies, and meat extracts and gravies. He also should keep his weight within normal limits and is instructed to increase his daily intake of liquids to encourage the production of urine. Medications such as probenecid, which prevents the retention or uric acid in the body and the formation of tophi, may be prescribed. Another drug, allopurinol, which prevents the formation of uric acid by blocking an enzyme step, has been used successfully in the long-term treatment of gout.

G.P. general practitioner; general paresis (see DEMENTIA PARALYTICA).

G6PD glucose-6-phosphate dehydrogenase.

GPT glutamic-pyruvic transaminase, an enzyme normally present in serum (SGPT) and body tissues, especially the liver.

gr. grain.

graafian follicle (graf'e-an) a small sac, embedded in the OVARY, that encloses an ovum. At puberty each ovary has a large number of immature follicles, each of which contains an undeveloped egg cell. These structures are called primordial, or primitive, graafian follicles. About every 28 days between puberty and the onset of menopause, one of these follicles develops to maturity, or ripens.

As the follicle ripens, it increases in size. The ovum within becomes larger, the follicular wall becomes thicker, and fluid collects in the follicle and surrounds the egg. At this point, it is also known as a vesicular ovarian follicle. The follicle also secretes estradiol, the hormone that prepares the endometrium to receive a fertilized egg. As the follicle matures, it moves to the surface of the ovary and forms a projection. When fully mature, the graafian follicle breaks open and releases the ovum, which passes into the UTERINE TUBES. This release of the ovum is called OVULATION; it occurs midway in the menstrual cycle, generally about 14 days after the commencement of the menstrual flow.

The released ovum travels down the tube to the uterus, a process that takes about 3 days. Meanwhile, the empty graafian follicle in the ovary becomes filled with cells containing a yellow substance, the corpus luteum, or yellow body. The corpus luteum secretes progesterone, a hormone that causes further change in the endometrium, allowing it to provide a good milieu in which a fertilized ovum can grow through the stages of gestation to become a fetus.

gracile (gras'il) slender; delicate.

Gradenigo's syndrome (grah-dě-ne'gōz) sixth nerve palsy and unilateral headache in suppurative disease of the middle ear, due to involvement of the abducens and trigeminal nerves by direct spread of the infection.

gradient (gra'de-ent) rate of increase or decrease of a variable value, or its representative curve.

graduate (grad'u-āt) 1. person who has received a degree from a university or college. 2. a measuring vessel marked by a series of lines.

graduated (grad'u-āt"ed) marked by a succession of lines, steps, or degrees.

graft (graft) 1. any tissue or organ for implantation or transplantation. 2. to implant or transplant such tissue. (See also FLAP and GRAFTING.)

autodermic g., autoepidermic g., a skin graft taken from the patient's own body.

autologous g., autoplastic g., a graft taken from another area of the patient's own body; an autograft.

avascular g., a graft of tissue in which not even transient vascularization is achieved.

bone g., a piece of bone used to take the place of a removed bone or bony defect.

cable g., a nerve graft made up of several sections of nerve in the manner of a cable.

cutis g., dermal graft.

delayed g., a skin graft that is sutured back into its bed and subsequently shifted to a new recipient.

dermal g., dermic g., skin from which epidermis and subcutaneous fat have been removed, used instead of fascia in various plastic procedures.

epidermic g., a piece of epidermis implanted on a raw surface.

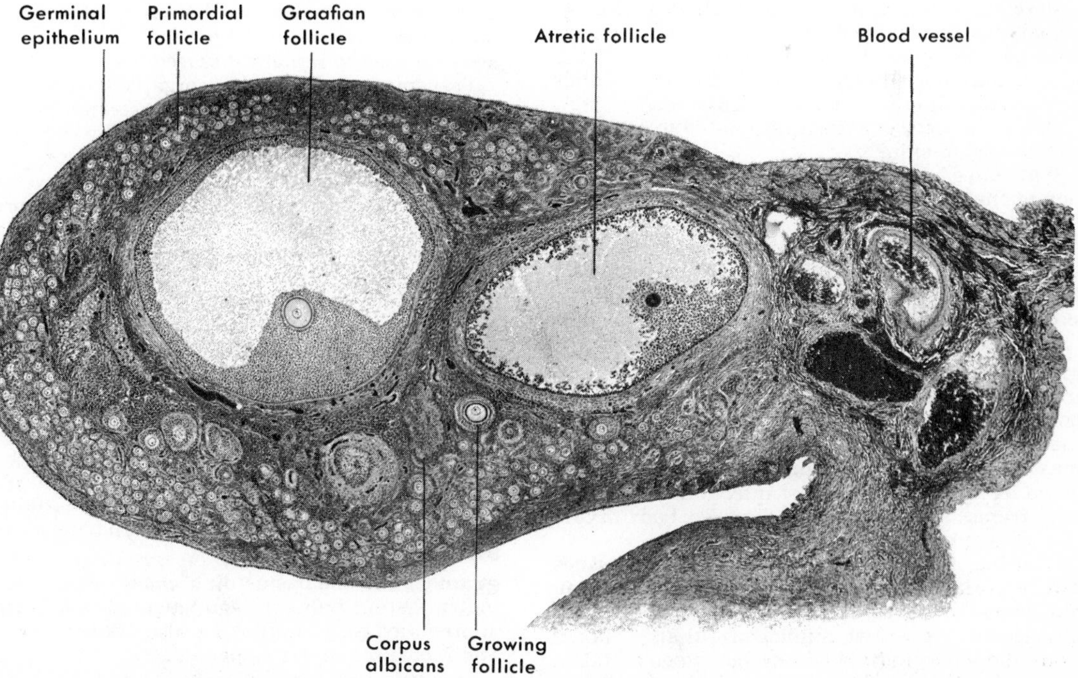

Retouched photomicrograph of transection of ovary of *Macacus rhesus*. (From Bloom, W., and Fawcett, D. W.: A Textbook of Histology. 10th ed. Philadelphia, W. B. Saunders Co., 1975.)

fascia g., a graft of tissue taken from the external investing fascia of the leg (fascia lata).

fascicular g., a nerve graft in which bundles of nerve fibers are approximated and sutured separately.

free g., a graft of tissue completely freed from its bed, in contrast to a flap.

full-thickness g., a skin graft consisting of the full thickness of the skin, with little or none of the subcutaneous tissue.

heterodermic g., a skin graft taken from a donor of another species.

heterologous g., heteroplastic g., a graft of tissue transplanted between animals of different species; a heterograft or xenograft.

homologous g., a graft of tissue obtained from the body of another animal of the same species but with a genotype differing from that of the recipient; a homograft or allograft.

isologous g., isoplastic g., a graft of tissue transplanted between genetically identical individuals; an isograft.

lamellar g., replacement of the superficial layers of an opaque cornea by a thin layer of clear cornea from a donor eye.

Ollier-Thiersch g., a very thin skin graft in which long, broad strips of skin, consisting of the epidermis, rete, and part of the corium, are used.

omental g's, free or attached segments of omentum used to cover suture lines following gastrointestinal or colonic surgery.

pedicle g., see pedicle FLAP.

penetrating g., a full-thickness corneal transplant.

periosteal g., a piece of periosteum to cover a denuded bone.

pinch g., a piece of skin graft about ¼ inch in diameter, obtained by elevating the skin with a needle and slicing it off with a knife.

rope g., rope flap.

sieve g., a skin graft from which tiny circular islands of skin are removed so that a larger denuded area can be covered, the sievelike portion being placed over one area, and the individual islands over surrounding or other denuded areas.

skin g., a piece of skin transplanted to replace a lost portion of skin.

split-skin g., a skin graft consisting of only a portion of the skin thickness.

sponge g., a bit of sponge inserted into a wound to promote the formation of granulations.

thick-split g., a skin graft cut in pieces, often including about two thirds of the full thickness of the skin.

Thiersch g., Ollier-Thiersch graft.

grafting (graf′ting) the implanting or transplanting of skin or other tissue from another part of the body or from another person to serve as replacement for damaged or missing tissue. The purpose may be to encourage healing, to improve function, to act as a safeguard against infection, to improve appearance, or to replace a diseased body organ. (See also TRANSPLANTATION.)

Grafting of skin is most common, but other tissues can be grafted, such as bone, cartilage, muscle, fat, blood vessels, nerves, and certain body organs. Usually, grafts are either autologous—that is, taken from the same individual—or homologous, taken from another individual. The autologous graft (autograft) is the most commonly used and the most successful. A graft from a genetically identical individual, e.g., an identical twin, is an isologous graft (isograft), and a graft in which the donor and recipient are of different species is a heterologous graft (heterograft or xenograft).

SKIN GRAFTING. The most important function of skin grafting is to promote the healing of large surfaces that have been burned or wounded, or that have become ulcerated or cancerous.

The skin to be grafted is cut usually from the chest, thigh, or abdomen, from the lower part of the neck, or from behind the ear. It may be removed in very thin strips or as a thin layer of superficial skin, and it must be placed in its new location without delay. If delay is unavoidable, it is placed in a saline solution or refrigerated.

In this kind of so-called free graft, in which the skin is cut entirely away from the body before transplantation, the skin is sewed into place and a pressure dressing is applied or a tissue glue is used. The skin must then depend for its nourishment on the surrounding tissue in the new location.

If a large thick area of skin containing much underlying tissue is to be moved, it is usually done by means of a pedicle graft—that is, the skin is not completely removed but is left partially attached to the body so that it continues to receive nourishment from its original site while it is beginning to grow in its new site. For example, an injured hand that needs the transplant may be strapped against the abdominal wall to receive a pedicle graft of skin from the abdomen. (See also PLASTIC SURGERY.)

OTHER GRAFTS. Eye surgeons have developed one of the most dramatic and useful grafting procedures, called keratoplasty, in which part or all of a diseased cornea that has become opaque is removed and replaced by healthy corneal tissue from an eye bank.

Cartilage and bone are other tissue that can be successfully transplanted from one individual to another. Cartilage lends itself particularly well to various shapes and is widely used in reconstructive surgery. Bone grafts are sometimes used instead of metal plates in operations to repair fractures. They are also used to replace diseased bone.

Transplanting of an entire organ from one person to another has been done, and transplants from animal to human have been attempted. There has been success in some instances of kidney transplants, especially when the donor and recipient have been identical twins. The major problem in this procedure is the rejection phenomena. Heart transplants have also been performed in humans. Surgical and scientific ingenuity are now tending toward the construction of artificial organs, substituting for the heart, kidney, or other organs (see ARTIFICIAL ORGAN). Arteries of plastic tubing have been used in surgical procedures.

Graham's law (gra′amz) the rate of diffusion of a gas through porous membranes varies inversely with the square root of its density.

grain (grān) 1. a seed, especially of a cereal plant. 2. the twentieth part of a scruple: 0.065 gm.; abbreviated gr. (See also Table of Weights and Measures in the Appendix.)

gram (gram) the basic unit of mass (weight) of the metric system, being the equivalent of 15.432 grains; abbreviated G., g., or gm. (See also Table of Weights and Measures in the Appendix.)

g. calorie, see small CALORIE.

-gram word element [Gr.], *written; recorded.*

Gram's stain (gramz) a staining procedure in which bacteria are stained with crystal violet, treated with strong iodine solution, decolorized with ethanol or ethanol-acetone, and counterstained with a contrasting dye; those retaining the stain are gram-positive, and those losing the stain but staining with the counterstain are gram-negative.

gramicidin (gram″ĭ-si′din) an antibacterial substance produced by the growth of *Bacillus brevis,* one of the two principal components of tyrothricin; called also gramicidin D. Gramicidin S is a closely related substance produced by a thermophilic strain of *B. brevis.*

gram-molecule (gram-mol′ĕ-kūl) a quantity in grams numerically equal to the molecular weight of the substance.

gram-negative (gram-neg′ah-tiv) not staining with GRAM'S STAIN, a primary characteristic of certain microorganisms.

gram-positive (gram-poz′ĭ-tiv) staining with GRAM'S STAIN, a primary characteristic of certain microorganisms.

grand mal (grahn mahl) [Fr.] a major epileptic seizure attended by loss of consciousness and convulsive movements, as distinguished from petit mal, a minor seizure (see also EPILEPSY).

granular (gran′u-lar) made up of or marked by the presence of granules or grains.

g. cell tumor, a benign, circumscribed, tumor-like lesion of soft tissue, particularly of the tongue, skin, and muscle, composed of large cells with prominent granular cytoplasm; considered by some to arise from myoblasts (myoblastoma) and by others from neurogenic elements (granular cell schwannoma); still others regard it as a manifestation of lipid storage cell disease.

g. reticulum, rough-surfaced endoplasmic reticulum.

granulatio (gran″u-la′she-o), pl. *granulatio′nes* [L.] a granule, or granular mass.

granulation (gran″u-la′shun) 1. the division of a hard substance into small particles. 2. the formation in wounds of small, rounded masses of tissue during healing; also the mass so formed.

arachnoid g's, enlarged arachnoid villi projecting into the venous sinuses and creating slight depressions on the inner surface of the cranium.

exuberant g's, excessive proliferation of granulation tissue in the healing of a wound.

g. tissue, the new tissue formed in repair of wounds of soft tissue, consisting of connective tissue cells and ingrowing young vessels. It ultimately forms the cicatrix.

granule (gran′ūl) 1. a small particle or grain. 2. a small pill made of sucrose.

acidophil g's, granules staining with acid dyes.

albuminous g's, granules seen in the cytoplasm of many normal cells, which disappear on the addition of acetic acid, but are not affected by ether or chloroform.

aleuronoid g's, colorless myeloid colloidal bodies found in the base of pigment cells.

alpha g's, 1. coarse, highly refractive, eosinophil granules of leukocytes, composed of albuminous matter. 2. the acidophil granules in the cells of the pituitary gland.

amphophil g's, beta granules.

azur g's, azurophil g's, granules that stain easily with azure dyes; they are coarse, reddish granules and are seen in many lymphocytes.

Babès-Ernst g's, metachromatic granules.

basophil g's, granules staining with basic dyes.

beta g's, presecretion granules found in the pituitary gland and islands of Langerhans of the pancreas.

carbohydrate g's, particles of carbohydrate matter in body fluids in the course of being assimilated.

chromatic g's, chromophilic g's, Nissl bodies.

cone g's, the nuclei of the visual cells in the outer nuclear layer of the retina which are connected with the cones.

delta g's, fine basophil granules in the lymphocytes.

eosinophil g's, those staining with eosin (see also alpha granules [1]).

epsilon g's, neutrophil granules.

fuchsinophil g's, those staining with fuchsin.

gamma g's, basophil granules found in the blood, bone marrow, and tissues.

Grawitz's g's, minute granules seen in the erythrocytes in the basophilia of lead poisoning.

hyperchromatin g's, azur granules.

iodophil g's, granules staining brown with iodine, seen in polymorphonuclear leukocytes in various acute infectious diseases.

juxtaglomerular g's, osmophilic secretory granules present in the juxtaglomerular cells, closely resembling zymogen granules.

Kölliker's interstitial g's, granules seen in the sarcoplasm of muscle fibers.

metachromatic g's, granules present in many bacterial cells, having an avidity for basic dyes and causing irregular staining of the cell.

Much's g's, granules and rods found in tuberculous sputum which do not stain by the usual processes for acid-fast bacilli but do stain with Gram's stain.

Neusser's g's, basophil granules seen about the nuclei of leukocytes.

neutrophil g's, neutrophilic granules from the protoplasm of polymorphonuclear leukocytes; called also epsilon granules.

Nissl's g's, Nissl bodies.

oxyphil g's, alpha granules (1).

pigment g's, small masses of coloring matter in pigment cells.

protein g's, minute particles of various proteins, some anabolic and others catabolic.

rod g's, the nuclei of the visual cells in the outer nuclear layer of the retina which are connected with the rods.

Schüffner's g's, small granules seen in erythrocytes infected with the malarial parasite *Plasmodium vivax* when stained by certain methods; called also Schüffner's dots.

seminal g's, the small granular bodies in the semen.

thread g's, mitochondria.

zymogen g's, secretory granules in certain cells, containing enzyme precursors that become active after they have left the cell.

granuloadipose (gran″u-lo-ad′ĭ-pōs) showing fatty degeneration containing granules of fat.

granuloblast (gran′u-lo-blast″) an immature granulocyte.

granulocyte (gran′u-lo-sīt″) any cell containing granules, especially a granular leukocyte.

band-form g., band cell.

granulocytopenia (gran″u-lo-si″to-pe′ne-ah) agranulocytosis.

granulocytopoiesis (gran″u-lo-si″to-poi-e′sis) the production of granulocytes. adj., **granulocytopoiet′ic.**

granulocytosis (gran″u-lo-si-to′sis) an excess of granulocytes in the blood.

granuloma (gran″u-lo′mah) a circumscribed mass consisting mainly of histiocytes, occurring in reaction to the presence of a living agent (infectious granuloma) or a nonliving foreign body, or sometimes idiopathically.

apical g., modified granulation tissue containing elements of chronic inflammation located adjacent to the root apex of a tooth with infected necrotic pulp.

benign g. of thyroid, chronic inflammation of the thyroid gland, converting it into a bulky tumor that later becomes extremely hard.

coccidioidal g., the secondary, progressive, chronic (granulomatous) stage of coccidioidomycosis.

dental g., one usually surrounded by a fibrous sac continuous with the periodontal ligament and attached to the root apex of a tooth.

eosinophilic g., a form of xanthomatosis characterized by the presence of rarefactions or cysts in one or more bones, sometimes associated with eosinophilia.

g. fissura′tum, a firm, whitish, fissured, fibrotic granuloma of the gum and buccal mucosa, occurring on an edentulous alveolar ridge and between the ridge and the cheek.

foreign body g., a localized histiocytic reaction to a foreign body in the tissue.

g. inguina′le, a granulomatous disease that is associated with uncleanliness, and is caused by the microorganism *Donovania granulomatis,* sometimes, called Donovan body. Although granuloma inguinale is generally considered to be a venereal disease, there is no absolute proof that it is transmitted by sexual contact. It is possible that natural resistance to the disease is very high, so that only a few of the persons exposed are affected.

Generally, 10 days to 3 months elapse after exposure before the first symptoms appear. Small painless ulcers that bleed easily may occur first. Swelling in the groin may then follow. A new ulcer or ulcers may appear as the old one heals, so that granuloma inguinale may eventually cover the reproductive organs, buttocks, and lower abdomen. The extensive sores give off a foul odor. As persons who have the disease seem to develop little immunity to it, granuloma inguinale may be present for many years.

In recent years, both streptomycin and tetracyclines have been successfully employed to treat the disease. Excellent results have been obtained with troleandomycin. There is no known preventive for granuloma inguinale, although the disease is rare where sanitary living conditions prevail.

lethal midline g., a rare, destructive necrotizing granuloma that results in destruction of the midface and invariably in death. It is always preceded by longstanding nonspecific inflammation of the nose or nasal sinuses, with purulent, often bloody discharge.

lipoid g., a granuloma containing lipoid cells; xanthoma.

lipophagic g., a granuloma attended by the loss of subcutaneous fat.

Majocchi's g., trichophytic granuloma.

paracoccidioidal g., paracoccidioidomycosis.

peripheral giant cell reparative g., a pedunculated or sessile lesion of the gingivae or alveolar ridge, apparently arising from the periodontal or mucoperiosteum, and usually due to trauma.

g. pyogen′icum, septic g., a fungating pedunculated growth in which the granulations consist of masses of pyogenic organisms.

swimming pool g., a granulomatous lesion at the site of a swimming pool injury, attributed to *Mycobacterium balnei;* it tends to heal spontaneously in a few months or years.

g. telangiectat′icum, a form characterized by numerous dilated blood vessels.

trichophytic g., a form of tinea corporis, occurring chiefly on the lower legs, due to *Trichophyton* infecting the hairs at the site of involvement, marked by raised, circumscribed, rather boggy granulomas, disseminated or arranged in chains; the lesions are slowly absorbed, or undergo necrosis, leaving depressed scars. Called also Majocchi's granuloma.

g. trop′icum, yaws.

ulcerating g. of pudenda, venereal g., g. vene′reum granuloma inguinale.

granulomatosis (gran″u-lo″mah-to′sis) the formation of multiple granulomas.

g. siderot′ica, a condition in which brownish nodules are seen in the enlarged spleen.

Wegener's g., a progressive disease, with granulomatous lesions of the respiratory tract, focal necrotizing arteriolitis with mainly glomerular renal involvement, and, finally, widespread inflammation of all organs of the body.

granulomatous (gran″u-lo′mah-tus) composed of granulomas.

granulomere (gran′u-lo-mēr″) the center portion of a platelet in a dry, stained blood smear, apparently filled with fine, purplish red granules.

granulopenia (gran″u-lo-pe′ne-ah) agranulocytosis.

granuloplastic (gran′u-lo-plas″tik) forming granules.

granulopoiesis (gran″u-lo-poi-e′sis) the formation and development of granulocytes. adj., **granulopoiet′ic.**

granulosa cell tumor (gran″u-lo′sah) an ovarian tumor originating in the solid mass of cells (granulosa cells) that surrounds the ovum in a developing graafian follicle. It may be associated with excessive production of estrogen, inducing endometrial hyperplasia with menorrhagia.

granulosa-theca cell tumor an ovarian tumor predominantly composed of either granulosa cells (follicular cells) or theca cells, and often associated with excessive production of estrogen, with hyperplasia of the breast and endometrium and carcinoma of the endometrium. When luteinized, i.e., having cells resembling those of the corpus luteum, it is known as luteoma.

granulose (gran′u-lōs) amylose (2).

granulosis (gran″u-lo′sis) the formation of granules.

g. ru′bra na′si, redness and marked sweating confined to the nose and surrounding area of the face, with red papules and sometimes many small vesicles, seen most often in children, and usually clearing up at puberty.

granum (gra′num) [L.] grain.

graph (graf) a diagram or curve representing varying relationships between sets of data. Often used as a word ending denoting a recording instrument.

graphorrhea (graf″o-re′ah) in psychiatry, the writing of a meaningless flow of words.

graphospasm (graf′o-spazm) writer's cramp.

-graphy word element [Gr.], *writing or recording; a method of recording.* adj., **graph′ic.**

grattage (grah-tahzh′) [Fr.] removal of granulations by scraping.

gravedo (grah-ve′do) head cold; nasal catarrh.

gravel (grav′el) calculus occurring in small particles.

Graves' disease (grāvz) an association of hyperthyroidism, goiter, and exophthalmos, with accelerated pulse rate, profuse sweating, nervous symptoms, psychic disturbances, emaciation, and elevated basal metabolism. Called also exophthalmic GOITER.

gravid (grav′id) pregnant; containing developing young.

gravida (grav′ĭ-dah) a pregnant woman; called gravida I (primigravida) during the first pregnancy, gravida II (secundigravida) during the second, and so on.

gravidic (grah-vid′ik) occurring in pregnancy.

gravidocardiac (grav″ĭ-do-kar′de-ak) pertaining to heart disease in pregnancy.

gravimetric (grav″ĭ-met′rik) pertaining to measurement by weight; performed by weight, as the gravimetric method of drug assay.

gravity (grav′ĭ-te) weight; tendency toward the center of the earth.

specific g., the weight of a substance compared with that of another taken as a standard (see also SPECIFIC GRAVITY).

Gravlee Jet Washer (grav′le) a diagnostic instrument consisting of a cannula, an adjustable rubber flange, a saline reservoir, and a 30 ml. syringe, and employed to obtain endometrial cells for cytologic and histologic examination. The procedure of endometrial washing for which the Gravlee Jet Washer is used, provides a relatively quick and easy means of screening for endometrial carcinoma in its early stages.

Grawitz's granules (grah′vits-ez) minute granules seen in the erythrocytes in the basophilia of lead poisoning.

gray matter, gray substance gray areas of the nervous system, so called because the nerve fibers in these areas are not enveloped in a white fatty material called the MYELIN sheath. These fibers are described as unmyelinated, or nonmedullated. White matter or substance is the term used to describe the tissues composed of myelinated, or medullated, fibers.

The bodies of the nerve cells are centered in the gray matter. The cerebral cortex is composed of gray matter and there are some deep-seated masses of gray matter within the cerebellum. In the spinal cord there is a central core of gray matter surrounded by white matter. On a cross section of the spinal cord the gray matter follows the general pattern of the letter H.

green (grēn) 1. the color of grass or of an emerald. 2. a green dye.

benzaldehyde g., malachite green.

brilliant g., a basic dye having powerful bacteriostatic properties for gram-positive organisms; used topically as an anesthetic.

indocyanine g., a dye used as a diagnostic aid in the determination of blood volume, cardiac output, and hepatic function.

malachite g., a triphenylmethane dye used as a stain for bacteria and as an antiseptic for wounds.

Paris g., Schweinfurt g., an emerald green compound of copper and arsenic, used as an insecticide on plants.

Greenfield's disease (grēn′fēldz) the infantile form of metachromatic LEUKODYSTROPHY.

grenz rays (grenz) very soft electromagnetic radiation of wavelengths about 2 angstroms.

grid (grid) 1. a grating; in radiology, a device consisting essentially of a series of narrow lead strips closely spaced on their edges and separated by spacers of low density material; used to reduce the amount of scattered radiation reaching the x-ray film. 2. a chart with horizontal and perpendicular lines for plotting curves.

baby g., a direct-reading chart on infant growth.

Wetzel g., a direct-reading chart for evaluating physical fitness in terms of body build, developmental level, and basal metabolism.

grip (grip) 1. influenza. 2. a grasping or clasping.

devil's g., epidemic pleurodynia.

grippe (grip) influenza.

griseofulvin (gris″e-o-ful′vin) an antibiotic used orally for treatment of fungal infections of the skin, nails, and scalp. Treatment usually must be prolonged and patient must be watched for signs of leukopenia, which often occurs when drug is administered over a long period of time.

groin (groin) the junctional region between the abdomen and thigh.

groove (gro͞ov) a narrow, linear hollow or depression.

branchial g., an external furrow lined with ectoderm, occurring in the embryo between two branchial arches.

Harrison's g., a horizontal groove along the lower border of the thorax corresponding to the costal insertion of the diaphragm; seen in rickets.

medullary g., neural g., that formed by the beginning invagination of the neural plate of the embryo to form the neural tube.

gross (grōs) coarse or large; visible to the naked eye.

ground substance (ground) the gel-like material in which connective tissue cells and fibers are imbedded.

group (gro͞op) 1. an assemblage of objects having certain things in common. 2. a number of atoms forming a recognizable and usually transferable portion of a molecule.

alcohol g., an organic radical consisting of one atom each of carbon and oxygen with three atoms of hydrogen (primary alcohol group), with two atoms of hydrogen (secondary alcohol group), or with only one atom of hydrogen (tertiary alcohol group).

azo g., the bivalent radical, —N=N—.

blood g's, categories into which blood can be classified on the basis of agglutinogens (see also BLOOD GROUP).

coli-aerogenes g., a group of microorganisms including *Escherichia coli, Aerobacter aerogenes,* and a variety of intermediate forms; called also coliform bacilli or coliform bacteria.

colon-typhoid-dysentery g., collectively, bacteria of the genera *Escherichia, Salmonella,* and *Shigella.*

peptide g., the bivalent radical, —CO·NH—, formed by reaction between the NH_2 and COOH groups of adjacent amino acids.

prosthetic g., the non–amino acid portion of a conjugated protein.

saccharide g., a combination of carbon, hydrogen, and oxygen atoms in a hypothetical molecule, $C_6H_{10}O_5$, the number of which in the compound determines the specific name of the polysaccharide.

group-transfer (gro͞op″trans′fer) denoting a chemical reaction (excluding oxidation and reduction) in which molecules exchange functional groups, a process catalyzed by enzymes called transferases.

growing pains (gro′ing) recurrent quasirheumatic limb pains peculiar to early youth, once believed to be caused by the growing process. It is now recognized that growth does not cause pain and that these pains can be a symptom of many different disorders.

growth (grōth) 1. the progressive development of a living thing, especially the process by which the body reaches its point of complete physical development. 2. an abnormal formation of tissue, such as a tumor.

HUMAN GROWTH. Human growth from infancy to maturity involves great changes in body size and appearance, including the development of the sexual characteristics. The growth process is not a steady one: at some times growth occurs rapidly, at others slowly. Individual patterns of growth vary widely because of differences in heredity and environment. Children tend to have physiques similar to those of their parents or of earlier forebears; however, environment may modify this tendency. Living conditions, including nutrition and hygiene, have considerable influence on growth.

Glands and Growth. The regulators of growth are the ENDOCRINE GLANDS, which are themselves subject to hereditary influence. The PITUITARY GLAND secretes growth hormone, which controls general body growth, particularly the growth of the skeleton, and also influences METABOLISM.

In addition to influencing growth directly, the pituitary gland has a central role in regulating the other endocrine glands. These other glands in turn control many body functions, and they secrete the various hormones that directly regulate metabolism.

Variations in Growth Rates. The growth of different individuals varies a great deal. It should be remembered that the rate of growth we call "normal" is really only an average rate. There is a wide range of growth rates, almost all of them quite normal. Of the children of a given sex and age, only about two-thirds will have physical measurements that fall close to the average.

Periods of Rapid Growth. Children in general have two periods of noticeably rapid growth. One occurs after birth, the other near puberty. In the first year of life the average baby grows about 50 per cent in height and about triples his weight. Thereafter his development proceeds more slowly until he reaches the rapid growth associated with puberty, which generally takes place between the ninth and thirteenth years in girls and between the eleventh and fifteenth years in boys.

During the pubertal period of rapid growth the sexual differences become evident. The girl begins to assume the characteristics of a woman's physique, with full breasts, rounded hips, and soft deposits of fatty tissue, and she begins MENSTRUATION. The boy likewise undergoes changes associated with masculinity: enlargement of the testes, broadening of shoulders, deepening of the voice, and appearance of facial hair. In both sexes the appearance of pubic hair accompanies these developments. The average girl may attain her adult size by the age of 17, the average boy by 18 or 19.

GROWTH DISORDERS. Disorders in growth are usually traceable to excess or shortage of pituitary secretions, and may arise from hereditary defects or from glandular abnormalities. Abnormally large secretions of growth hormone can produce GIGANTISM. Failure of the pituitary gland to develop sufficiently or to secrete adequate amounts of growth hormone may result in DWARFISM. In adulthood, overproduction of growth hormone may lead to ACROMEGALY, a disorder characterized by abnormal growth of the hands and feet and coarse thickening of the facial features. In certain cases, such hormonal imbalance or deficiency may be relieved by surgery or by giving hormone substitutes. These growth disorders are uncommon, however.

g. hormone, a substance that stimulates growth, especially a secretion of the anterior lobe of the PITUITARY GLAND that directly influences protein, carbohydrate, and lipid metabolism and controls the rate of skeletal and visceral growth.

grumous (groo′mus) lumpy or clotted.

gryposis (grĭ-po′sis) abnormal curvature, as of the nails.

GSH reduced glutathione.

G6PD glucose-6-phosphate dehydrogenase.

GSSG oxidized glutathione.

GU genitourinary.

guanase (gwan′ās) guanine deaminase (see DEAMINASE).

guanethidine (gwan-eth′i-den) an adrenergic-blocking agent; the sulfate salt is used as an antihypertensive.

guanidoacetic acid (gwan″ĭ-do-ah-se′tik) an intermediate product in the synthesis of creatine.

guanine (gwan′ēn) a purine base, one of the fundamental components of nucleic acids (DNA and RNA).

guanosine (gwan′o-sēn) a nucleoside, guanine riboside, one of the major constituents of RNA.

g. triphosphate, an energy-rich compound involved in several metabolic reactions.

guaranine (gwah-rah′nin) caffeine.

Guillain-Barré syndrome (ge-yan′bar-ra′) a relatively rare disease affecting the nerves; called also acute idiopathic polyneuritis, postinfectious polyneuritis, and Landry's paralysis.

The cause of the disease is unknown; however, it usually follows a febrile illness within 10 to 21 days and is believed by some to be related to an autoimmune mechanism. Because it is characterized by a flaccid paralysis, it is sometimes mistaken for poliomyelitis.

The early symptoms are fever, malaise, nausea, or prostration. Muscular weakness usually starts in the lower extemities and tends to go upward through the body, but it may affect the facial muscles and arms first and then move downward. The paralysis is not accompanied by loss of sensation, but rather by abnormal sensations of tingling and numbness. The classic cerebrospinal fluid findings are of an elevated protein level without an increase in the number of leukocytes. The cerebrospinal fluid pressure is within normal limits.

The progression of the paralysis may stop at any point. Once the weakness reaches its maximum, the paralysis remains unchanged for days or weeks. Improvement begins spontaneously and continues for weeks, or rarely, months. The prognosis for full recovery is good.

Guillain-Barré syndrome affects primarily the ventral roots of the spinal cord, hence the motor disturbances. The sensory counterpart of this syndrome affects the dorsal roots and is usually called Guillain-Barré-Strohl syndrome. The symptoms of this disease include severe stabbing pains at first, followed by abnormally exaggerated response to painful stimuli.

There is no specific treatment for the disease. It must run its course and for this reason skilled patient care is imperative, particularly in the acute phase, when respiratory failure is a very real possibility. All measures needed to prevent complications in the patient who cannot move about in bed are required for these patients. The experience of paralysis and sensory disturbances is an ordeal for the patient. He will need continued physical and psychological support throughout all stages of recovery, which may last for weeks or months, depending on the individual patient.

guillotine (gil′o-tēn) a surgical instrument with a sliding blade for excising a tonsil or the uvula.

Gull's disease (gulz) atrophy of the thyroid gland with myxedema.

gullet (gul′et) the passage to the stomach, including both the esophagus and pharynx.

Gullstrand's slit lamp (gul′strandz) an apparatus for projecting a narrow flat beam of intense light into the eye (see also Gullstrand's slit LAMP).

gum (gum) 1. a mucilaginous excretion of various plants. 2. gingiva.

karaya g., sterculia g., the dried gummy exudate from *Sterculia urens* and other *Sterculia* species; used as a bulk cathartic. It has adhesive properties and is used as a dental adhesive and in fitting ileostomy appliances.

gumma (gum′ah) a soft, gummy tumor, such as that occurring in tertiary syphilis.

gummatous (gum′ah-tus) of the nature of gumma.

gummy (gum′e) resembling gum or gumma.

Gunn's dots (gunz) white dots seen about the macula lutea on oblique illumination.

Günther's disease (gin′terz) congenital erythropoietic porphyria.

gurney (ger′ne) a wheeled cot used in hospitals.

gustation (gus-ta′shun) the act of tasting or the sense of taste. adj., **gus′tatory.**

gut (gut) 1. the bowel or intestine. 2. the primitive digestive tube, consisting of the fore-, mid-, and hindgut. 3. catgut.

gutta (gut′ah), pl. *gut′tae* [L.] a drop.

gutta-percha (gut″ah-per′chah) the coagulated latex of a number of tropical trees of the family Sapotaceae; used as a dental cement and in splints.

guttat. [L.] *gutta′tim* (drop by drop).

guttate (gut′āt) resembling a drop.

guttatim (gŭ-ta′tim) [L.] drop by drop.

guttering (gut′er-ing) the cutting of a gutter-like excision in bone.

guttural (gut′er-al) pertaining to the throat.

gymnocyte (jim′no-sīt) a cell with no cell wall.

Gymnodinium (jim″no-din′e-um) a genus of dinoflagellates, most species of which have many colored chromatophores, found in fresh, salt, and brackish waters; when present in great numbers, they help to form the destructive red tide in the ocean.

gymnospore (jim′no-spōr) a spore without a protective envelope.

gyn-, gyne-, gyneco-, gyno- word element [Gr.], *woman.*

gynaeco- for words beginning thus, see those beginning *gyneco-.*

gynandrism (jĭ-nan′drizm) 1. hermaphroditism. 2. female pseudohermaphroditism.

gynandroblastoma (jĭ-nan″dro-blas-to′mah) an ovarian tumor containing elements of both arrhenoblastoma and granulosa cell tumor; it produces both androgenic and estrogenic effects.

gynandroid (jĭ-nan′droid) a hermaphrodite or a female pseudohermaphrodite.

gynandromorph (jĭ-nan′dro-morf) an organism exhibiting gynandromorphism.

gynandromorphism (jĭ-nan″dro-mor′fizm) the presence of chromosomes of both sexes in different tissues of the body, producing a mosaic of male and female sex characteristics. adj., **gynandromorph′ous.**

gynecic (jĭ-ne′sik) pertaining to women.

gynecogenic (jin″ĕ-ko-jen′ik) producing female characteristics.

gynecography (jin″ĕ-kog′rah-fe) roentgenography of the female reproductive organs.

gynecoid (jin′ĕ-koid) woman-like.

gynecologist (gi″nĕ-kol′o-jist, jin″ĕ-kol′o-jist) a specialist in gynecology.

gynecology (gi″nĕ-kol′o-je, jin″ĕ-kol′o-je) the branch of medicine dealing with diseases of the genital tract in women. adj., **gynecolog′ic.**

gynecomania (jin″ĕ-ko-ma′ne-ah) satyriasis.

gynecomastia (jin″ĕ-co-mas′te-ah) excessive development of mammary glands in the male, even to the functional state.

gynecopathy (jin″ĕ-kop′ah-the) any disease peculiar to women.

gynephobia (jin″ĕ-fo′be-ah) morbid aversion to women.

Gynergen (jin′er-jen) trademark for a preparation of ergotamine, an alkaloid of ergot used also to treat migraine.

gynogenesis (jin″o-jen′ĕ-sis) development of an egg that is stimulated by a sperm in the absence of any participation of the sperm nucleus.

gynomerogon (jin″o-mer′o-gon) an organism produced by gynomerogony and containing only the maternal set of chromosomes.

gynomerogony (jin″o-mer-og′o-ne) development of a portion of a fertilized ovum containing only the female pronucleus.

gynopathic (jin″o-path′ik) pertaining to disease of women.

gynoplastics (jin′o-plas″tiks) plastic or reconstructive surgery of female reproductive organs. adj., **gynoplas′tic.**

gypsum (jip′sum) native calcium sulfate, which, when calcined, becomes plaster of Paris.

gyrate (ji′rāt) convoluted; ring- or spiral-shaped.

gyration (ji-ra′shun) revolution about a fixed center.

gyre (jīr) gyrus.

gyrectomy (ji-rek′to-me) excision or resection of a cerebral gyrus, or a portion of the cerebral cortex.

Gyrencephala (ji″ren-sef′ah-lah) a group of higher mammals, including man, having a brain marked by convolutions.

gyrencephalic (ji″ren-sĕ-fal′ik) pertaining to the Gyrencephala; having a brain marked by convolutions.

gyrospasm (ji′ro-spazm) rotatory spasm of the head.

gyrus (ji′rus), pl. *gy′ri* [L.] one of the many convolutions of the surface of the brain caused by infolding of the cortex (gy′ri cere′bri), separated by fissures or sulci.

angular g., one continuous anteriorly with the supramarginal gyrus.

annectent gyri, various small folds on the cerebral surface that are too inconstant to bear specific names; called also gyri transitivi.

Broca's g., inferior frontal gyrus.

central g., anterior, precentral gyrus.

central g., posterior, postcentral gyrus.

cerebral gyri, the tortuous elevations (convolutions) on the surface of the cerebral hemisphere, caused by infolding of the cortex and separated by fissures or sulci.

cingulate g., an arch-shaped convolution situated just above the corpus callosum.

frontal g., any of the three (inferior, middle, and superior) gyri of the frontal lobe.

fusiform g., one on the inferior surface of the hemisphere between the inferior temporal and parahippocampal gyri, consisting of a lateral (lateral occipitotemporal gyrus) and a medial (medial occipitotemporal gyrus) part.

hippocampal g., g. hippocam′pi, one on the inferior surface of each cerebral hemisphere, lying between the hippocampal and collateral fissures; called also parahippocampal gyrus.

infracalcarine g., lingual g., one on the occipital lobe forming the inferior lip of the calcarine sulcus and, with the cuneus, the visual cortex.

marginal g., the middle frontal gyrus.

occipital g., any of the three (superior, middle, and inferior) gyri of the occipital lobe.

occipitotemporal g., lateral, the lateral portion of the fusiform gyrus.

occipitotemporal g., median, the medial portion of the fusiform gyrus.

orbital gyri, irregular gyri on the orbital surface of the frontal lobe.

parahippocampal g., hippocampal gyrus.

paraterminal g., a thin sheet of gray matter in front of and ventral to the genu of the corpus callosum.

postcentral g., the convolution of the frontal lobe immediately behind the central sulcus; the primary sensory area of the cerebral cortex. Called also posterior central gyrus.

precentral g., the convolution of the frontal lobe immediately in front of the central sulcus; the primary motor area of the cerebral cortex. Called also anterior central gyrus.

g. rec′tus, a cerebral convolution on the orbital aspect of the frontal lobe.

supracallosal g., indusium griseum.

supramarginal g., that part of the inferior parietal convolution which curves around the upper end of the fissure of Sylvius.

temporal g., any of the gyri of the temporal lobe, including inferior, middle, superior, and transverse temporal gyri; the more prominent of the latter (anterior transverse temporal gyrus) represents the cortical center for hearing.

gy′ri transiti′vi, annectant gyri.

uncinate g., the uncus.

H

H chemical symbol, *hydrogen.*

H. (*ho'ra*) [L.] (hour).

H$^+$ symbol, *hydrogen ion.*

Ha chemical symbol, *hahnium.*

habena (hah-be'nah) the peduncle of the pineal body.

habenula (hah-ben'u-lah), pl. *haben'ulae* [L.] 1. any frenulum, especially one of a series of structures in the cochlea. 2. a triangular area in the dorsomedial aspect of the thalamus rostral to the pineal gland.

habit (hab'it) 1. an action that has become automatic or characteristic by repetition. 2. predisposition; bodily temperament.

habituation (hah-bich"u-a'shun) 1. the gradual adaptation to a stimulus or to the environment. 2. a condition due to repeated consumption of a drug, with a desire to continue its use, but with little or no tendency to increase the dose. (See also DRUG ABUSE.)

habitus (hab'ĭ-tus) [L.] habit; body conformation.

h. enteroptot'icus, the body conformation seen in enteroptosis, marked by a long, narrow abdomen.

h. phthis'icus, a body conformation predisposing to pulmonary tuberculosis, marked by pallor, emaciation, poor muscular development, and small bones.

hachement (ahsh-maw') [Fr.] a hacking or chopping stroke in massage.

hae- for words beginning thus, see also those beginning *he-*.

Haemadipsa (he"mah-dip'sah) a genus of leeches.

Haemaphysalis (hem"ah-fis'ah-lis) a genus of ticks, several species of which are important as vectors of disease.

Haemophilus (he-mof'ĭ-lus) *Hemophilus.*

hafnium (haf'ne-um) a chemical element, atomic number 72, atomic weight 178.49, symbol Hf. (See table of ELEMENTS.)

Hagedorn's needle (hahg'ĕ-dornz) a form of flat suture needle.

Hageman factor (hāg'ĕ-man) clotting factor XII.

hahnium (hah'ne-um) a chemical element, atomic number 105, atomic weight 260, symbol Ha. (See table of ELEMENTS.)

Hailey-Hailey disease (ha'le-ha'le) benign familial pemphigus.

hair (hār) a threadlike structure, especially the specialized epidermal structure developing from a papilla sunk in the corium, produced only by mammals and characteristic of that group of animals. Also, the aggregate of such hairs.

auditory h's, hairlike attachments of the epithelial cells of the inner ear.

bamboo h., trichorrhexis nodosa.

beaded h., hair marked with alternate swellings and constrictions; seen in monilethrix.

h. bulb, the bulbous expansion at the lower end of a hair root.

burrowing h., one that grows horizontally in the skin.

club h., a hair whose root is surrounded by a bulbous enlargement composed of keratinized cells, preliminary to normal loss of the hair from the follicle.

h. follicle, a pouchlike depression in the skin in which a hair develops from the matrix at its base and grows to emerge from its opening on the body surface.

Frey's h's, stiff hairs mounted in a handle; used for testing the sensitiveness of pressure points of the skin.

ingrown h., one that has curved and reentered the skin.

lanugo h., the fine hair on the body of the fetus.

moniliform h., beaded hair.

pubic h., the hair on the external genitalia; called also pubes.

sensory h's, hairlike projections on the surface of sensory epithelial cells.

tactile h's, hairs sensitive to touch.

taste h's, short hairlike processes projecting freely into the lumen of the pit of a taste bud from the peripheral ends of the taste cells.

terminal h., the coarse hair on various areas of the body during adult years.

twisted h., pilus tortus; a hair which at spaced intervals is twisted through an axis of 180 degrees, being abnormally flattened at the site of twisting.

hairball (hār'bawl) trichobezoar; a concretion of hair sometimes found in the stomach or intestines of man or other animals.

halation (hah-la'shun) indistinctness of the visual image caused by strong illumination coming from the same direction as the object being viewed.

halazone (hal'ah-zōn) a white, crystalline powder used as a disinfectant for water supplies.

halcinonide (hal-sin'o-nīd) a topical corticosteroid used in the treatment of acute and chronic dermatoses.

Haldol (hal'dol) trademark for a preparation of haloperidol, an antipsychotic agent.

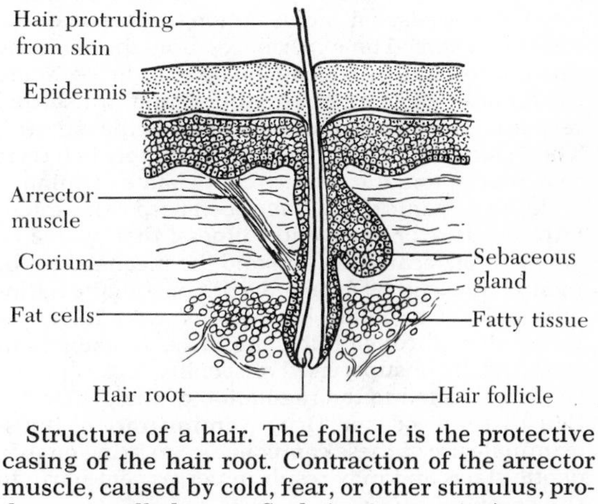

Structure of a hair. The follicle is the protective casing of the hair root. Contraction of the arrector muscle, caused by cold, fear, or other stimulus, produces so-called goose flesh (cutis anserina).

Haldrone (hal'drōn) trademark for a preparation of paramethasone acetate, a corticosteroid.

half-life (haf'līf) the time in which the radioactivity usually associated with a particular isotope is reduced by half through radioactive decay.

half-value layer (haf-val'u) that thickness of a given substance (a filter) which will reduce the intensity of an x-ray beam by half.

halibut liver oil (hal'ĭ-but) a fixed oil from fresh or suitably preserved livers of halibut species; used as a source of vitamins A and D.

halide (hal'īd) a compound of a halogen with an element or radical.

halisteresis (hah-lis"ter-e'sis) deficiency of mineral salts (calcium) in a part, as in osteomalacia.

halitosis (hal"ĭ-to'sis) offensive odor of the breath.

halitus (hal'ĭ-tus) an expired breath.

Hallervorden-Spatz syndrome (hal'er-for"den spatz) a hereditary disorder involving marked reduction in the number of myelin sheaths of the globus pallidus and substantia nigra, with accumulations of iron pigment, progressive rigidity beginning in the legs, choreoathetoid movements, dysarthria, and progressive mental deterioration.

hallucination (hah-lu"sĭ-na'shun) a sensory impression (sight, touch, sound, smell, or taste) that has no basis in external stimulation. Hallucinations can have psychologic causes, as in mental illness, or they can result from drugs, alcohol, organic illnesses, such as brain tumor or senility, or exhaustion. When hallucinations have a psychologic origin, they usually represent a disguised form of a repressed conflict.

auditory h., a hallucination of hearing; the most common type.

gustatory h., a hallucination of taste.

haptic h., tactile hallucination.

hypnagogic h., a hallucination occurring between sleeping and awakening.

olfactory h., a hallucination of smell.

tactile h., a hallucination of touch.

visual h., a hallucination of sight.

hallucinogen (hah-lu'sĭ-no-jen") an agent capable of producing hallucinations or false sensory perceptions. adj., **hallucinogen'ic.** Drugs that have hallucinogenic properties include mescaline, LSD (lysergic acid diethylamide), and psilocybin. Certain mushrooms and seeds and cactus button (peyote) are also hallucinogenic. The experiences brought about by the use of hallucinogens involve a more acute "awareness" of one's environment and a distorted response to visual, auditory, and tactile stimuli. They can also cause a person to exhibit behavior that is symptomatic of a psychotic state of mind.

Hallucinogenic drugs have been used experimentally in research on mental illness; their value in determining brain function and the mechanisms of mental illness is yet to be proved. Abuse of the hallucinogenic compounds by persons who have obtained them through illicit channels, or taken them in medically unsupervised or socially unacceptable settings, has led to the regulation of their distribution by the Food and Drug Administration. Indiscriminate use of these compounds can bring on psychotic states and may result in permanent harm to the psyche.

hallucinogenesis (hah-lu"sĭ-no-jen'ĕ-sis) the production of hallucinations.

hallucinosis (hah-lu"sĭ-no'sis) the experiencing of more or less constant hallucinations.

acute h., alcoholic h., alcoholic psychosis marked by auditory hallucinations and delusions of persecution.

hallux (hal'uks) the great toe.

h. doloro'sa, a painful disease of the great toe, usually associated with flatfoot.

h. flex'us, hallux rigidus.

h. mal'leus, hammer toe affecting the great toe.

h. rig'idus, painful flexion deformity of the great toe with limitation of motion at the metatarsophalangeal joint.

h. val'gus, angulation of the great toe toward the other toes of the foot.

h. va'rus, angulation of the great toe away from the other toes of the foot.

halmatogenesis (hal"mah-to-jen'ĕ-sis) a sudden alteration of type from one generation to another.

halo (ha'lo) a circular structure, such as a luminous circle seen surrounding an object or light.

Fick's h., a colored circle appearing around a light, experienced by wearers of contact lenses.

h. glaucomato'sus, glaucomatous h., a narrow light zone surrounding the optic disk in glaucoma.

senile h., a zone of variable width around the optic disk, due to exposure of various elements of the choroid as a result of senile atrophy of the pigmented epithelium.

halogen (hal'o-jen) an element of a closely related chemical family, all of which form similar (saltlike) compounds in combination with sodium. The halogens are bromine, chlorine, fluorine, and iodine.

halometer (hah-lom'ĕ-ter) 1. an instrument for measuring ocular halos. 2. an instrument for estimating the size of erythrocytes by measuring the diffraction halos they produce.

haloperidol (hal"o-per'ĭ-dol) an antipsychotic drug of the butyrophenone series.

halophil (hal'o-fil) a halophilic microorganism.

halophilic (hal"o-fil'ik) pertaining to or characterized by an affinity for salt; requiring a high concentration of salt for optimal growth.

Halotestin (hal"o-tes'tin) trademark for a preparation of fluoxymesterone, an androgen used in the palliative treatment of certain cancers and in replacement therapy in primary hypogonadism and testicular hypofunction.

halothane (hal'o-thān) a colorless, mobile, nonflammable, heavy liquid used by inhalation to produce ANESTHESIA.

Ham test one for paroxysmal nocturnal hemoglobinuria, performed by incubating red cells in an acid environment; a positive test may be obtained in other forms of anemia.

hamartia (ham-ar'she-ah) a defect of tissue combination in development.

hamartoblastoma (ham-ar"to-blas-to'mah) a tumor developing from a hamartoma.

hamartoma (ham"ar-to'mah) a benign tumor-like nodule composed of an overgrowth of mature cells and tissues normally present in the affected part, but often with one element predominating.

hamartomatous (ham"ar-to'mah-tus) pertaining to a disturbance in growth of a tissue in which the cells of a circumscribed area outstrip those of the surrounding areas.

hamate (ham′āt) hooked, as the hamate bone.

Hamman's disease (ham′anz) interstitial emphysema of the lungs due to spontaneous rupture of the alveoli.

Hamman-Rich syndrome (ham′an rich) diffuse interstitial pulmonary fibrosis.

hammer (ham′er) the malleus, the largest of the three bones of the ear.

h. toe, a condition in which the proximal phalanx of the toe—most often that of the second toe—is extended and the second and distal phalanges are flexed, causing a clawlike appearance.

hamstring (ham′string) one of the tendons that laterally and medially bound the depression in the posterior region of the knee (popliteal space).

inner h's, the tendons of the gracilis, sartorius, and two other muscles of the leg.

outer h., the tendon of the biceps muscle of the thigh.

hamulus (ham′u-lus), pl. *ham′uli* [L.] any hook-shaped process.

hand (hand) the terminal part of an arm, or of the upper (anterior) extremity of a primate.

ape h., one with the thumb permanently extended.

cleft h., a malformation in which the division between the fingers extends into the metacarpus; also, a hand with the middle digits absent.

claw h., see CLAWHAND.

drop h., wristdrop.

lobster-claw h., cleft hand.

obstetrician's h., the contraction of the hand in tetany; the hand is flexed at the wrist, the fingers at the metacarpophalangeal joints but extended at the interphalangeal joints, the thumb being strongly flexed into the palm.

writing h., in Parkinson's disease, assumption of the position by which a pen is commonly held.

hand-foot-and-mouth disease a mild, highly infectious virus disease of children, with vesicular lesions in the mouth and on the hands and feet.

Hand-Schüller-Christian disease (hand shil′er kris′chan) chronic idiopathic histiocytosis with multifocal histiocytic lipogranulomas of bone and of the skin, the histiocytes containing abundant cholesterol. It affects chiefly children and young adults. Called also Hand's disease, Schüller's disease, Schüller-Christian disease, and chronic idiopathic xanthomatosis.

The three classic symptoms of the syndrome are softened areas of the skull and other flat, membranous bones, exophthalmos, and diabetes insipidus. However, all three symptoms are rarely found in one patient. Otitis frequently accompanies the disease. Skin lesions resembling those of seborrheic dermatitis may appear, as may xanthomas.

There is no specific treatment. X-ray therapy is sometimes helpful in treating specific local lesions and corticosteroids have been used with success in some cases. Complete recovery does occur, but about 40 per cent of the cases terminate fatally.

H and E hematoxylin and eosin (stain).

handedness (hand′ed-nes) the preferential use of the hand of one side in all voluntary motor acts.

handicap (han′de-kap) any physical or mental defect or characteristic that prevents a person from taking part freely in the activities appropriate for his age. A handicap may be the result of an accident or a disease, or it may be congenital. It may be obvious—blindness, paralysis, or disfiguring scars—or unnoticeable—a heart defect, slight mental retardation, or a chronic disease such as hemophilia.

Hanger's test (hang′erz) a test for liver cell disease based on the flocculation of a cephalin-cholesterol emulsion by the patient's serum (see also CEPHALIN-CHOLESTEROL FLOCCULATION TEST).

hangnail (hang′nāl) a shred of eponychium at one side of a nail. Hangnail is prevented by gently pushing the cuticle instead of cutting it, and it is treated by clipping off the shred of skin and applying antiseptic to the area to prevent infection.

Hanot's disease (an-ōz′) biliary cirrhosis.

Hansen's bacillus (han′sunz) *Mycobacterium leprae,* the causative agent of leprosy.

Hansen's disease (han′sunz) leprosy.

haphalgesia (haf″al-je′ze-ah) pain on touching objects.

haploid (hap′loid) having half the number of chromosomes characteristically found in the somatic (diploid) cells of an organism; typical of the gametes of a species whose union restores the diploid number.

haploidy (hap′loi-de) the state of being haploid.

haploscope (hap′lo-skōp) a stereoscope for testing the visual axis. adj., **haploscop′ic.**

haplotype (hap′lo-tīp) the group of alleles of linked genes contributed by either parent; the haploid genetic constitution contributed by either parent.

Hapsburg jaw (haps′berg) a mandibular prognathous jaw, often accompanied by Hapsburg lip.

Hapsburg lip (haps′berg) a thick, overdeveloped lower lip that often accompanies Hapsburg jaw.

hapten, haptene (hap′ten; hap′tēn) the portion of an antigenic molecule or complex that determines its immunologic specificity. adj. **hapten′ic.**

haptic (hap′tik) tactile.

haptics (hap′tiks) the science of the sense of touch.

haptoglobin (hap″to-glo′bin) a group of serum alpha-2 globulin glycoproteins that bind free hemoglobin; the different types, genetically determined, are distinguished electrophoretically.

haptophore (hap′to-fōr) in Ehrlich's side-chain theory, the specific group of the molecule of toxins, agglutinins, precipitins, opsonins, and lysins by which they become attached to their antibodies, antigens, or the receptors of cells, thus making possible their specific activity.

Harada's syndrome a syndrome, possibly caused by a virus, consisting of uveomeningitis associated with retinochoroidal detachment, temporary or permanent deafness and blindness, and sometimes, though often transiently, alopecia, vitiligo, and poliosis.

harelip (hār′lip) congenitally cleft lip (see also CLEFT LIP).

Harmonyl (har′mo-nil) trademark for preparations of deserpidine, a tranquilizer.

Harrison antinarcotic act (har′ĭ-sun) a federal law, enacted March 1, 1915, that regulates the possession, sale, purchase, and prescription of opium and coca and all their preparations, natural and synthetic derivatives and salts. These include the drugs cocaine, morphine, codeine, and papaverine. Laws patterned after the Harrison antinarcotic act in some states prohibit the possession or sale of derivatives of barbituric acid except under proper licenses, so that they may not be dispensed without a prescription.

Harrison's groove (har′ĭ-sunz) a horizontal groove along the lower border of the thorax corresponding to the costal insertion of the diaphragm; seen in rickets.

Hartmann's solution (hart′manz) a solution containing sodium chloride, sodium lactate, and phosphates of calcium and potassium; used intravenously as a systemic alkalizer and as a fluid and electrolyte replenisher.

Hartnup disease (hart′nup) a genetically determined disorder of intestinal and renal transport of neutral alpha-amino acids, with pellagra-like skin lesions, transient cerebellar ataxia, constant renal aminoaciduria and other biochemical abnormalities.

harvest fever spirochetosis affecting harvest workers, due to *Leptospira grippotyphosa,* with fever, diarrhea, conjunctivitis, stupor, and vomiting.

Harvey (har′ve) William (1578–1657). English physician and physiologist. Born at Folkestone in Kent, he attended the universities of Cambridge and Padua, and announced in 1628 his discovery of the circulation of blood, which was a model of accurate experimentation and inductive proof, and the first application of quantitative demonstration in any biologic investigation. His *De generatione animalium* is important in the history of embryology, for in it Harvey rejected the doctrine of preformation of the fetus and stated that almost all animals, and man himself, are produced from eggs.

Hashimoto's disease (hash″ĭ-mo′tōz) a progressive disease of the thyroid gland with degeneration of its epithelial elements and replacement by lymphoid and fibrous tissue; called also struma lymphomatosis.

hashish (hash-ēsh′) a preparation of the unadulterated resin scraped from the flowering tops of female hemp plants (*Cannabis sativa*), smoked or chewed for its intoxicating effects. It is far more potent than marihuana.

haustration (hos-tra′shun) 1. the formation of a haustrum. 2. a haustrum.

haustrum (hos′trum), pl. *haus′tra* [L.] one of the pouches of the colon, produced by adaptation of its length to the tenia coli, or by collection of circular muscle fibers at 1 or 2 cm. distances, and responsible for the sacculated appearance.

Haverhill fever (ha′ver-il) a form of RATBITE FEVER, an acute febrile disease caused by *Streptobacillus moniliformis,* transmitted by the bite of an infected rat, and characterized by an erythematous eruption and more or less generalized arthritis, with adenitis, headache, and vomiting; first described in Haverhill, Mass., in 1926.

haversian (ha-ver′shan) named for the English physician and anatomist Clopton Havers, 1650–1702.

h. canal, any of the anastomosing channels of the harversian system in compact bone, containing blood and lymph vessels, and nerves.

h. glands, synovial villi.

h. system, a haversian canal and its concentrically arranged lamellae, constituting the basic unit of structure in compact bone (osteon).

hay fever a seasonal allergy characterized by sneezing, itchy and watery eyes, running nose, and burning palate and throat.

Like all allergies, hay fever is caused by sensitivity to certain substances—most commonly pollens and the spores of molds. Pollen is the fertilizing element of flowering plants. It is a fine dust, easily airborne, that enters the body by inhalation. Ragweed pollen is a particular nuisance to persons subject to hay fever. Mold is a fungus that grows on animal and vegetable matter. The spores of molds are dustlike reproductive units that are also present in the air we breathe.

The amount of pollen in the air varies with the season and geographic area. East of the Rocky Mountains, the peak of the regional hay fever season occurs between mid-August and mid-September, when the air is heavy with the pollen of the ragweed plant. An appreciable number of hay fever sufferers are also reactive to the spring pollens from grasses and trees. Mold-bearing plants such as wheat, barley, and corn are prevalent in the agricultural areas of the Midwest, and attacks of hay fever caused by mold spores are common there as these crops ripen.

Hay fever deserves to be recognized as more than a mere nuisance. By causing lack of sleep and loss of appetite, it can lower the body's resistance to disease. It can cause inflammation of the ears, sinuses, throat, and bronchi. A number of hay fever sufferers develop ASTHMA.

Hay fever can be relieved, although not cured, by antihistamines and sympathomimetic drugs such as ephedrine and phenylpropanolamine hydrochloride. Sedatives, may be prescribed for nervous or tense persons. A series of preventive injections (desensitization) may be recommended in advance of the hay fever season. This consists of administering controlled and gradually increasing amounts of the offending substance in order to develop a certain amount of immunity. In some cases it may be helpful to avoid part of the hay fever season by taking a vacation in an area that is relatively free of the annoying pollen. Air conditioning may also help give relief by filtering much of the pollen from the air. (See also ALLERGY.)

nonseasonal h. f., perennial h. f., nonseasonal allergic rhinitis.

Haygarth's nodes (ha′garths) joint swellings in rheumatoid arthritis.

Hb hemoglobin.

HCG human chorionic gonadotropin.

HCl hydrochloric acid.

H disease Hartnup disease.

H & E hematoxylin and eosin (stain).

He chemical symbol, *helium.*

head (hed) the anterior or superior part of a structure or organism, in vertebrates containing the brain and the organs of special sense.

articular h., an eminence on a bone by which it articulates with another bone.

h. injury, traumatic injury to the head resulting from a fall or violent blow. Such an injury may be open or closed and may involve a brain CONCUSSION, skull fracture, or contusions of the brain. All head injuries are potentially dangerous because there may be a slow leakage of blood from damaged blood vessels into the brain, or the formation of a blood clot which gradually increases pressure against brain tissue (see cranial HEMATOMA). One of the most common complications of head injury is subdural hematoma, resulting from the oozing of blood from the cortical veins and the small blood vessels that lie between the arachnoid and the dura mater. A less common but more serious complication that constitutes an extreme surgical emergency is epidural hematoma, a collection of blood in the space between the skull and the dura mater. The leaking of blood into the epidural space progresses rapidly and therefore requires immediate treatment. A third complication that may occur following head injury is herniation of either the brain stem or a part of the cerebellum through the tentorial hiatus (*transtentorial herniation*). This is an extreme emergency demanding immediate relief of pressure against the blood vessels serving the brain stem and cerebellum.

Long-term effects of head injury may include chronic headache, disturbances in mental and motor function, and a host of other symptoms that may or may not be psychogenic. Organic brain damage and posttraumatic epilepsy resulting from scar formation are possible sequels to head injury.

TREATMENT. The method of treatment will depend on the kind and amount of damage inflicted on the brain and surrounding membranes. Surgical procedures to relieve intracranial pressure may include the drilling of burr holes in the skull to aspirate accumulated blood, and intracranial surgery to remove hematomas. Edema of brain tissue may be reduced by the intravenous administration of mannitol. Dexamethasone (Decadron), an anti-inflammatory steroid that has little salt-retaining action, is often used. If no immediate surgery is indicated, the physician may choose to treat the head injury conservatively, with rest and quiet and the careful monitoring of the patient for signs of change in the neurologic status.

PATIENT CARE. Continuous monitoring of the vital signs and assessment of the patient's neurologic status are essential to the care of the patient with a head injury. His intake and output is measured and recorded and fluid intake limited according to the degree of edema present. Intravenous fluids must be given with caution and oral liquids allowed as soon as the patient is able to swallow. An excessively large urinary output is reported immediately, as this may indicate damage to the hypothalamus and suppression of antidiuretic hormone.

Any one of the following symptoms should be reported to the physician: (1) changes in the patient's blood pressure, pulse, or respiratory rate, especially slowing of the pulse with a rising blood pressure; (2) extreme restlessness or excitability following a period of comparative calm; (3) deepening stupor or loss of consciousness; (4) headache that increases in intensity; (5) vomiting, especially persistent, projectile vomiting; (6) unequal size of pupils; (7) inability to move one or more extremity; (8) leakage of spinal fluid (clear yellow or pink-tinged) from the nose or ear.

When leakage of spinal fluid is suspected, this can be verified by using a Clinistix test for sugar. If it is positive, the leaking fluid is spinal fluid rather than mucus. When there is leakage of spinal fluid through the nose, the patient must be warned not to blow his nose. Leakage of spinal fluid from the nose or the ear demands absolute bed rest with the head elevated 30 degrees to maintain neutral intracranial pressure and promote healing.

Patients who are unconscious must be watched closely for respiratory difficulty or inability to swallow. If the patient cannot swallow, his head must be turned to the side and his mouth and trachea suctioned as necessary to prevent aspiration of mucus into the lungs. A TRACHEOSTOMY set and VENTILATOR should be readily at hand in case severe respiratory embarrassment occurs.

Side rails are applied and the head board of the bed is padded with pillows or a blanket if the patient is delirious or if convulsions are anticipated. An accurate record of the patient's intake and output is kept and the patient is observed for signs of retention of urine, incontinence, or abdominal distention.

nerve h., the optic disk.

headache (hed'āk) a pain or ache in the head. One of the most common ailments of man, it is a symptom rather than a disorder in itself. It accompanies many diseases and conditions, including emotional distress. (See also MIGRAINE.)

Although recurring headache may be an early sign of serious organic disease relatively few headaches are caused by disease-induced structural changes. Most result from vasodilation of blood vessels in tissues surrounding the brain, or from tension in the neck and scalp muscles.

Treatment of headache varies according to its severity and its tendency to recur. A mild transient headache can be relieved by the administration of an analgesic such as aspirin; however, aspirin and other drugs should not be taken habitually. It is best to determine the primary cause of the headache. A tranquilizer may be useful when stress and tension are shown to be responsible for recurring headaches. If the cause is found to be a vascular disturbance, the physician may prescribe vasoconstricting drugs such as ergotamine or ergotamine plus caffeine.

cluster h., a migraine-like disorder marked by attacks of unilateral intense pain over the eye and forehead, with flushing and watering of the eyes and nose; attacks last about an hour and occur in clusters.

histamine h., cluster headache.

tension h., a type due to prolonged overwork or emotional strain, or both, affecting especially the occipital region.

healing (hēl'ing) the restoration of structure and function of injured or diseased tissues. The healing processes include blood clotting, tissue mending, scarring, and bone healing.

INFLAMMATION. When an injury occurs, the body's first-aid mechanisms automatically begin to operate. The blood vessels in the neighborhood of the injury dilate to provide an increased blood supply. At the same time the pores in the thin walls of the capillaries also widen, letting more plasma than usual flow through to the injured tissues. The immediate result is twofold: the increased flow of blood and plasma brings the body's repair materials to the spot in large quantities, and the increase in fluid at the spot distends tissues, presses on nerves, and raises the local temperature. This whole process is called INFLAMMATION. It is one of the body's protective devices. Inflammation causes, pain, which impairs the function of the injured part.

BLOOD CLOTTING. If the skin is broken and there is bleeding, another mechanism, blood CLOTTING, goes into operation at the site of the injury. Twelve essential clotting substances, or factors, have been recognized. Of the four chief ones, only three are ordinarily present in the blood; the fourth is locked in the tissues. Not until tissue is damaged, and the fourth substance is liberated, is the blood clotting, or coagulating, mechanism put to work.

In the BLOOD there are fragments of protoplasm known as platelets. Even though no more than a few drops of blood may flow from a cut, platelets by the tens of thousands come in contact with the rough edge of injured tissue, and they disintegrate. Thus they liberate thromboplastin, the fourth substance essential for clotting, at the spot where it is needed. The thromboplastin acts upon one of the constituents of the blood, prothrombin, and in the presence of calcium, also a normal constituent of the blood, the prothrombin changes to a similar but active material, thrombin. Now the newly formed thrombin reacts with another chemical in the blood, fibrinogen, to form fibrin. This substance, the end product of the series of chemical reactions, is insoluble and spongelike and has the property of being able to contract. It forms a network of threads that enmesh the erythrocytes; it pulls them together, as it contracts, into a tough mass called a clot, which acts like a cork to stop up the opening.

The platelets help to stop the flow of blood in two additional ways. They release a chemical that stimulates the muscle walls of nearby blood vessels to contract, narrowing the channels along which blood is flowing to the cut and also narrowing the cut end that needs to be plugged. And the platelets themselves, being sticky, act as a natural adhesive, helping to seal up the cut. They are both chemical and mechanical agents.

THE MENDING PROCESS. The same materials that arrest bleeding prepare the site for mending. The fibrin threads contract and pull together the edges of the wound under the natural adhesive patch of the clot, and the repair cells go to work. These repair cells are a variety of connective tissue, long and spindle-shaped, with fibrous branches; they bind the edges of the wound neatly together. This done, their work is ended; their remnants and the remnants of cells damaged in the injury are cleared away by scavenger cells (phagocytes), cellular sanitation squads that keep all kinds of microscopic debris from cluttering the body tissues.

SCAR FORMATION. When a cut is relatively clean and small, the edges of tissue are brought together in a neat seam and there is no visible evidence of the repair. The repair cells have acted as basting stitches, and they are disposed of when the tissues themselves effect a permanent juncture with their own cells. A clean, dry surgical incision in which there is practically no loss of tissue heals in much the same way.

When a wound is extensive, with uneven edges, the repair cells are unable to pull the edges together. Instead, they build a bridge across the gap. These cells of connective tissue, the fibroblasts, are not skin and cannot change into skin. They harden into tough, contracting, white scar tissue (granulation tissue).

In the type of wound just described, the physician stitches the edges of the damaged tissues together, giving the body the conditions under which it can do its own repair work. But when so much tissue has been lost that the wound must be left open or gaping, as in an abscess or ulcer, this cannot be done, and the fibroblasts must fill in the wound from the depth and sides before it can be covered over. In addition to being unsightly, the scars from extensive wounds may interfere with nerves, blood vessels, and muscles. In such cases, PLASTIC SURGERY may be necessary or advisable to restore function or for cosmetic reasons.

BONE HEALING. When a bone is broken, the healing process works on similar principles; but the task requires different material, as strong as the original

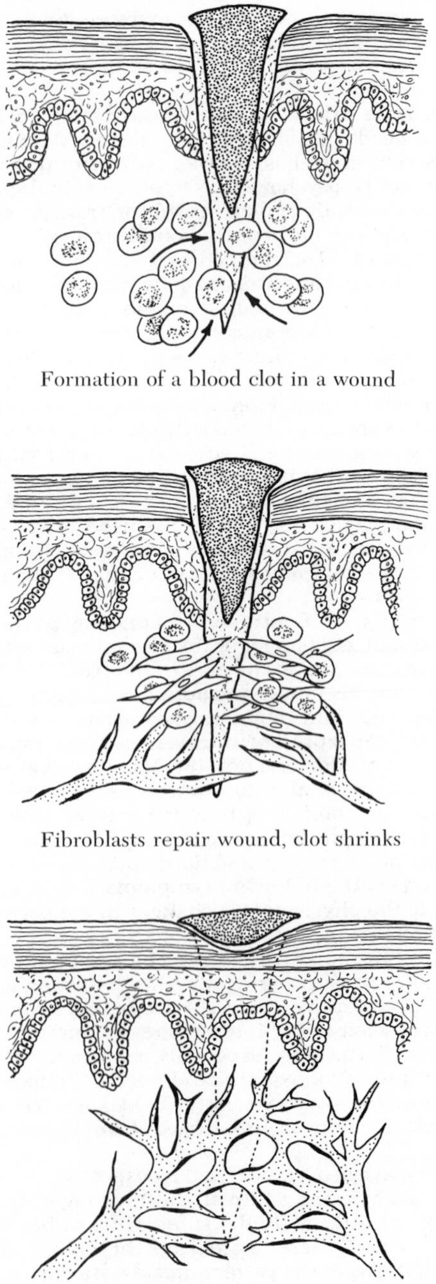

Formation of a blood clot in a wound

Fibroblasts repair wound, clot shrinks

Normal blood supply returns to healing wound

Wound healing.

bone and capable of hardening rapidly. The first repair cells bind the broken ends of bone together, and along these bonds, the osteoblasts, bone-forming cells, begin at once to grow. Callus, a tough binding material, holds the break firm until the new bone is properly hardened, and eventually it also turns into true bone. When the task is done, bone-scavenger cells (osteoclasts) clear away excess repair cells and trim the mended area to nearly its original size. When the break is jagged and the ends are out of alignment, the body's repair mechanisms fill in with their mending materials, but often not adequately. The physician helps the natural process by setting the fracture and giving the body the necessary start for a good bone repair job.

There are various factors that favorably influence the healing process. The chief ones are youth (healing is slow in elderly people), rest of the injured part, adequate nutrition, with plenty of protein and vitamins, and warmth.

h. by first intention, union of accurately coapted edges of a wound, with an irreducible minimum of granulation tissue.

h. by second intention, union by adhesion of granulating surfaces.

health (helth) a state of physical, mental, and social well-being.

public h., the field of medicine that is concerned with safeguarding and improving the health of the community as a whole.

Health Maintenance Organization (HMO) a broad term encompassing a variety of health care delivery systems utilizing group practice and providing alternatives to the fee-for-service private practice of medicine and other allied health professions.

Although there may be wide variation in organizational pattern and in the membership and ownership of the organization, the major goal of any HMO is to allow for investment in and incentives to use a prepaid and organized comprehensive health care system that serves a defined population. The enrolled population enters into a contract with the organization, agreeing to pay, or have paid on their behalf, a fixed sum, in return for which the HMO makes available the health care personnel, facilities, and services that the population may require. The services are available on a 24 hour a day, 7 day a week basis. Some HMO's may provide directly the entire range of health services, including rehabilitation, dental, and mental health care. Others may agree to provide directly or arrange to pay only for physicians' services, in-hospital care, and outpatient emergency and preventive medical services. The kinds of services available are stipulated in the contract between the organization and its enrolled population. The emphasis of a health maintenance organization is on preventive rather than crisis-oriented medical care. Additional information can be obtained by writing to the U.S. Department of Health, Education and Welfare, Health Services Administration, 5600 Fisher Lane, Rockville, MD 20852.

Health Systems Agency (HSA) a regional health care planning agency created by enactment of the National Health Planning and Resources Development Act of 1974 (Public Law 93-641). Some 211 such agencies have been established to serve designated geographic regions throughout the United States. These regions are known as *health service areas.*

FUNCTIONS. As stated in the law, functions of the HSA include: (1) improving the health of residents of a health service area, (2) increasing the accessibility, acceptability, continuity, and quality of the health services provided, (3) restraining increases in the cost of health services, and (4) preventing unnecessary duplication of health resources.

STAFF. The staff of an HSA provides the agency with expertise in at least the following: "(i) administration, (ii) the gathering and analysis of data, (iii) health planning, and (iv) development and use of health resources."

GOVERNING BODY. The governing body of an HSA is responsible for the internal affairs of the agency, including matters related to the staff of the agency, the agency's budget, and procedures and criteria. Responsibilities of the governing body (and Executive Committee if any) other than those related to internal affairs include "the establishment of the health systems plan and annual implementation plan, approval of grants and contracts entered into, issuing of an annual report of the activities of the agency, and conduct of its business meetings in public."

Requirements for *membership* of the governing body are: "(1) a majority (but not more than 60%) of the members shall be residents of the health service area served by the entity who are not providers of health care and who are broadly representative of the social, economic, linguistic, and racial populations, geographic areas of the HSA, and major purchasers of health care; (2) residents of the health service area who represent (a) physicians, dentists, nurses, and other health professionals, (b) health care institutions (particularly hospitals, long-term care facilities, and health maintenance organizations), (c) health care insurers, (d) health professional schools, and (e) the allied health professionals."

The law further stipulates that members of the governing body who are direct providers of health care shall constitute not less than one-third of the membership of the governing body or executive committee of a health systems agency. The membership also should include "public elected officials and other representatives of governmental authorities in the agency's health service area and representatives of public and private agencies in the area concerned with health."

SHPDA. In addition to the creation of HSAs throughout the country, Public Law 93-641 also provides for the formation of STATE HEALTH PLANNING AND DEVELOPMENT AGENCIES (SHPDAs), which are designated by each state's Governor and approved by the Secretary of HEW. The SHPDA conducts reviews of existing health services of an area and considers health system changes proposed by HSAs, certifying the need for services and programs recommended by the HSAs.

healthy (helth′e) pertaining to, characterized by, or promoting health.

hearing (hēr′ing) the sense by which sounds are perceived, by conversion of sound waves into nerves impulses, which are then interpreted by the brain. Also, the capacity to perceive sound. The organ of hearing is the EAR, which is divided into three sections, the outer, middle, and inner ear. Each plays a special role in hearing. Connecting the middle ear with the nasopharynx is the eustachian tube, through which air enters to equalize the pressure on both sides of the TYMPANIC MEMBRANE (eardrum). See also Plate 15.

THE MECHANICS OF HEARING. When sound waves strike the tympanic membrane, they start it vibrating. Most of the sound waves simply bounce off; what remains may be a very tiny vibration of the drum. To be useful, the ear must be able to record very light sound, and yet survive a violent sound such as a thunderclap.

The problem of protecting the tympanic membrane is handled by two tiny muscles that damp the vibrations in the eardrum and ossicles. The main problem, that of hearing, is solved by the ear's transmitting chain of membrane-ossicles-cochlea, a mechanical transformer that converts the large-amplitude sound waves striking the drum into smaller, more concentrated vibrations.

The ossicles act as a series of levers, each one amplifying the minute movement of the eardrum as it passes it along. By the time the stirrup taps the window of the cochlea, it has 22 times the pressure of the original vibration. The thin oval window membrane vibrates in turn, setting the fluid in the cochlea in motion along its spiral course. The constricted channel of the cochlea multiplies the pressure still further, until the original vibrations reach the nerve ends in the form of powerful sideways motions rubbing against the sensitive hairlike cells of the organ of Corti. The vibrations are transformed into impulses that pass along the vestibulocochlear nerve to the brain, and the waves of pressure in the cochlea are released by way of another membrane-covered window, the round window, at the other end of the cochlea.

It is still not certain how the organ of Corti transforms the vibrations into nerve impulses. There are two major theories. One, the Helmholtz theory, points out that the organ of Corti is shaped much like a piano or harp, with long strands at one end and short ones at the other. Perhaps these strands vibrate sympathetically, each strand for a different note, just as the strings of a harp or piano will vibrate when another instrument is played nearby. The second theory, the telephone theory, holds that the frequency of notes is transmitted to the brain by nerve impulses of the same frequency. This is the principle on which the telephone is based.

There are technical objections to both theories. It is possible that the organ of Corti operates on both principles—for example, like the telephone for low notes and according to the Helmholtz theory for high notes, with the two systems overlapping in the middle range, where the ear is more sensitive.

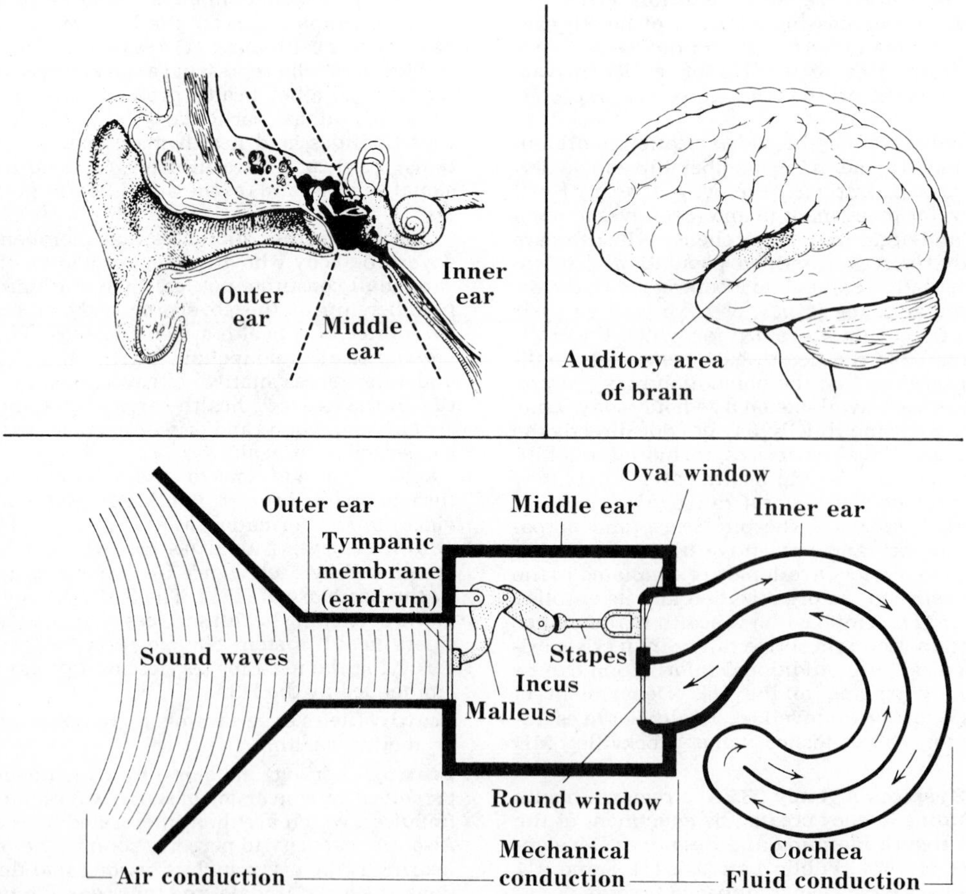

As sound is conducted from the external ear to the inner ear, the sound waves undergo considerable transformation. The tympanic membrane (eardrum), ossicles and cochlea act as a mechanical transformer to concentrate the sound waves so that they can be picked up by nerve endings in the inner ear and transmitted to the brain.

Whatever system the ear uses, it is a remarkably versatile organ. The human ear can distinguish more than 1500 separate musical tones, can recognize thousands of different sounds and can hear clearly from the softest whisper to the roar of a factory or a battleship's guns. See also DEAFNESS for discussion of hearing loss.

h. aid, an instrument to amplify sounds for the hard of hearing. There are two types of electronic hearing aids: the air-conduction type, which is worn in the external acoustic meatus, and the bone-conduction type, which is worn in back of the ear over the mastoid process.

Those who have conductive DEAFNESS can often use any one of the better aids with good results. Patients with OTOSCLEROSIS will probably need the bone-conduction type of instrument. Those with sensorineural deafness, caused by injury to the vestibulocochlear nerve, or mixed deafness may have more trouble selecting a suitable hearing aid, and may get less satisfactory results.

Those wearing a hearing aid for the first time should have special training in its proper use. A hearing aid picks up and amplifies all the sounds in the vicinity. Often a person whose hearing has declined gradually will have lost the facility to ignore background noises. When he first tries a hearing aid, his ears will be assaulted by the sounds of passing cars, of doors slamming, of telephones ringing. Training in how to filter out these noises and concentrate on the essential is necessary if the person is to get good results from his hearing aid. For best results, this should be combined with lessons in lip-reading.

heart (hart) the hollow muscular organ lying slightly to the left of the midline of the chest. The heart serves as a pump controlling the blood flow in two circuits, the pulmonary and the systemic (see also CIRCULATORY SYSTEM).

DIVISIONS OF THE HEART. The septum, a thick muscular wall, divides the heart into right and left halves. Each half is again divided into upper and lower quarters or chambers. The lower chambers are called ventricles; the upper chambers are called atria. The right side of the heart, consisting of the right atrium and right ventricle, sends blood into the pulmonary circuit. The left side, consisting of the left atrium and left ventricle, sends blood into the systemic circuit.

VALVES OF THE HEART. Between the right atrium and right ventricle is the tricuspid valve. Similarly, the left atrium and left ventricle are connected by the mitral, or bicuspid, valve. In addition to the valves between the atrium and ventricle on each side of the heart, there are valves at the blood's exit points: the pulmonary valve opening from the right ventricle into the pulmonary artery, and the aortic valve opening from the left ventricle into the aorta. These valves, both within the heart and leading out of it, open and shut in such a way as to keep the blood flowing in one direction through the heart's two separate pairs of chambers: from atrium to ventricle and out through its appropriate artery.

LAYERS OF THE HEART. The heart wall is composed of three layers of tissues. Its chambers are lined by a delicate membrane, the endocardium. The thick muscular wall essential to normal pumping action of the heart is called the myocardium. The thin but sturdy membranous sac surrounding the exterior of the heart is called the pericardium.

THE HEART'S PACEMAKER. The heart is made up of special muscle tissue, capable of continuous rhythmic contraction without tiring. The impulse that starts the heartbeat has its origin in an area of the right atrium called the sinoatrial node; it is this special tissue that acts as a pacemaker for the heart. It transmits the impulse in a fraction of a second through the atria to another group of similarly sensitive fibers called the atrioventricular node, which conducts the stimulus into the ventricular walls, resulting in contraction of the ventricles. (See also PACEMAKER.)

PUMPING ACTION. Although the right and left sides of the heart serve two separate branches of the circulation, each with its distinct function, they are coordinated so that the heart efficiently serves both sides with a single pumping action. The valve action on both sides is also coordinated with the two phases of the pumping action. Thus during diastole, the relaxation phase, oxygen-poor blood returning from the systemic circulation and accumulated in the right atrium pours into the right ventricle. At the same time, the oxygen-rich blood that has accumulated in the left atrium returning from the pulmonary circulation pours into the left ventricle. The walls of both atria contract to press blood into the relaxed ventricles. In the next contraction phase (systole) the valve between the atrium and ventricle on each side closes, and the muscular walls contract the ventricles and force the blood through the pulmonary artery and the aorta. At the end of the contraction the pulmonary and aortic valves snap shut, preventing any backward surge of the blood into the ventricles. The diastole follows, the ventricles again filling with the flow from their separate atria, and the cycle is repeated. (See also Plate 5).

DISORDERS OF THE HEART. The heart is subject to a variety of disorders. Among them are CONGENITAL HEART DEFECTS, which begin or exist at the time of birth. Disorders of this nature may interfere with the flow of the blood from the heart to the lungs. TETRALOGY OF FALLOT and PATENT DUCTUS ARTERIOSUS are examples of congentital heart defects.

In syphilitic heart disease, there is damage to the aorta or the aortic valve, interfering with the proper functioning of the valve, so that the blood may flow backward into the heart as well as forward from the ventricle.

Another heart ailment is rheumatic heart disease, associated with RHEUMATIC FEVER. The disease can injure the endocardium, the valves, or the muscle fibers. The valves may lose their original efficiency, so that passage of the blood is hindered.

Coronary insufficiency is a condition in which the coronary arteries are unable to transport an adequate supply of oxygenated blood to nourish the heart muscle itself. One form of coronary insufficiency, manifested as ANGINA PECTORIS, may be precipitated by hampered circulation of the blood caused by arteriosclerotic narrowing of the coronary artery, combined with a stepped-up demand for oxygen during exercise or some other form of exertion.

A "heart attack" is the common description for the condition in which the formation of a blood clot within a coronary artery may shut off, or occlude, the blood flow to a section of the heart muscle. This is called a CORONARY OCCLUSION or THROMBOSIS, and can damage or cause permanent injury to the affected area of myocardium (MYOCARDIAL INFARCTION).

HEART FAILURE is the inability of the heart to perform its function of pumping sufficient blood to assure a normal flow through the circulation. The heart is unable to pump out the blood returned to it from the veins. In the condition known as congestive heart failure, one or more chambers of the heart do not empty adequately during contraction of the heart muscle. This results in shortness of breath, edema, and abnormal retention of sodium and water in body tissues.

Cardiac arrhythmias are disturbances in the normal rate and rhythm of the heartbeat. Electrical impulses that affect the rate and rhythm of the heartbeat are generated in the heart's pacemaker—the sinoatrial node—and distributed to the heart muscle by the heart's conduction system. The sinoatrial node is subject to the influence of the autonomic nervous system and it also responds to chemical changes in the blood and to certain drugs. Tissue necrosis such as that in myocardial infarction or resulting from arteriosclerotic coronary artery disease also can block the passage of electrical impulses. When there is a disturbance in any part of the heart's conduction system or electric generating function, the patient may experience a heartbeat that is speeded up (tachycardia) or slowed down (bradycardia). The various forms of arrhythmia are sinus arrhythmia, extrasystole, heart block, atrial fibrillation, atrial flutter, and paroxysmal tachycardia.

HEART SURGERY. Many heart disorders can be corrected by surgery of the heart. Since the 1950's, special techniques in heart surgery have become possible, primarily because of several new developments. One was the introduction of antibiotics to aid in controlling infection. Another was the technique of induced HYPOTHERMIA, which allows for removal of the body's supply of oxygenated blood for as long as 8 to 10 minutes without causing damage to body tissues. Thus hypothermia permits surgeons to drain the heart in order to repair defects.

A third development was the invention of the HEART-LUNG MACHINE, or pump-oxygenator. This machine, when connected to the patient's circulatory system, relieves the heart and lungs of their tasks of pumping and oxygenating blood, by providing for extracorporeal circulation.

Among the severe congenital defects which in many cases may be treated surgically are patent ductus arteriosus, coarctation of the aorta, and atrial and ventricular septal defect. Another congenital (sometimes acquired) heart defect that may be treated surgically is pulmonary stenosis.

Acquired heart defects that may in certain cases be treated by surgery include stenosis, or narrowing of the mitral or aortic valves, constrictive pericarditis, and aneurysm of the aorta or of the heart wall itself.

Patient Care. Prior to surgery the patient is given instructions in coughing and deep breathing so that he can perform these procedures after surgery. They are necessary to provide complete expansion of the lungs and to prevent pulmonary complications postoperatively. He is also told what to expect postoperatively; for example, he can expect a tight feeling in his chest, there may be a tube inserted in the chest cavity, and his blood pressure, pulse, and respiration rate will be taken and recorded frequently. To allay his fears of choking or suffocating and to familiarize him with some of the machinery that may be used after surgery, some physicians wish to have the patient acquainted with the suction machine and the respirator, which are kept available in case of need.

During the preoperative period it is important to observe the patient carefully so as to become familiar with his individual characteristics, such as rate and volume of pulse, depth and rate of respiration, tolerance to physical activity, and tolerance to pain or discomfort. Later, these preoperative observations are used as a basis for comparison with the patient's postoperative condition.

Preparation of the patient's unit for postoperative care should include assembling a suction apparatus for removing mucus from the mouth and throat, poles for holding infusion bottles, and equipment for taking and recording blood pressure. An oxygen

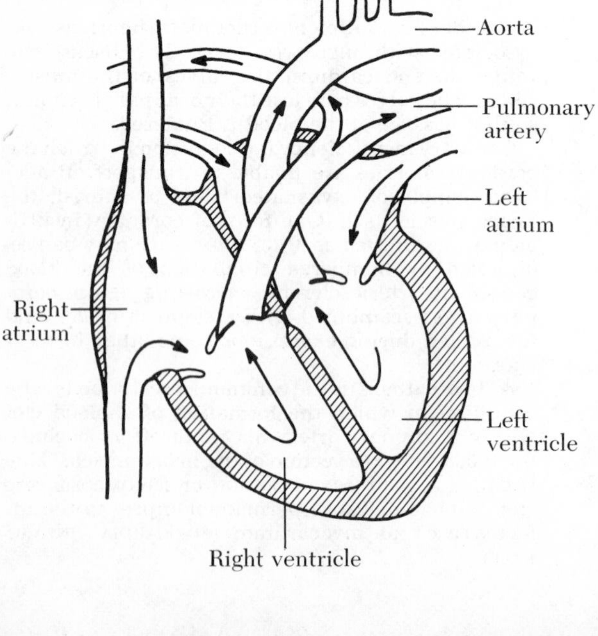

Blood enters the right atrium from the body and then passes into the right ventricle, where it is pumped into the lungs. It returns from the lungs into the left atrium. It enters the left ventricle and then is pumped to the body via the aorta.

tank may be set up, and if a mucolytic agent such as Alevaire is to be administered, this equipment should also be on hand. To avoid delay in an emergency, a cardiac arrest tray containing scalpel, hemostats, and rib spreaders should be readily available in the event CARDIAC MASSAGE is necessary. One should also be prepared for assisting with a THORACENTESIS should the accumulation of fluid in the chest require this procedure. If hypothermia has been used during surgery, it will be necessary to have equipment available for keeping the body at lowered temperatures and also for applying external heat when hypothermia is discontinued.

Immediately after surgery the radial pulse, respiration, and blood pressure are observed for character and rate as often as every 5 minutes until they become stabilized. Use of monitoring instruments allows for continued observation of these variables. Any change in blood pressure, variance in the volume or rhythm of pulse or respiratory changes must be reported at once. Generalized cyanosis is reported to the physician, as is blanching or mottling of the lower extremities, which may indicate the presence of an embolism. Surgical dressings are checked carefully and at frequent intervals for signs of hemorrhage or restriction of chest expansion. All drainage tubes, such as urinary catheter or nasogastric tube, must be attached to the proper apparatus for drainage. The amount and type of drainage obtained is carefully observed and recorded. The CHEST TUBE is attached to closed drainage or to chest suction apparatus (see THORACIC SURGERY). After the patient has recovered from anesthesia he usually is put in Fowler's position. The surgeon may allow him to lie on his back or on the operative side.

Maintenance of a patent AIRWAY is most important in these patients because retention of secretions in the respiratory tract is common. Coughing is encouraged. In some cases suctioning, bronchoscopy, or tracheostomy may be required to open the airway and remove mucous plugs and secretions. Oxygen is administered as needed. Positioning of the patient should be done only according to the specific wishes of the surgeon, since improper positioning may produce thrombosis or other complications in certain types of surgery.

heartbeat (hart'bēt) the cycle of contraction of the heart muscle, during which the chambers of the heart contract. The beat begins with a rhythmic impulse in the sinoatrial node, which serves as a pacemaker for the heart. (See also HEART.)

heart block impairment of conduction in heart excitation; often applied specifically to atrioventricular heart block.

When isolated impulses from the atria fail to reach the ventricles, heartbeats are missed and the block is called incomplete. When no impulses reach the ventricles from the atria the heart block is complete, with the result that the atria and the ventricles beat at separate rates. In this case the beats remain regular but the rate of the ventricular beats is greatly slowed down.

Heart block can occur with various forms of heart disease, and as a result of excessive dosage of digitalis. A particularly severe instance of heart block can be complicated by the Stokes-Adams disease, in which a sudden attack of unconsciousness results from the slowed heartbeat. It may be accompanied by convulsions.

The treatment for heart block caused by digitalis overdosage is to stop the medication temporarily and give reduced amounts thereafter. When heart block results from a form of heart disease, treatment is given for the underlying cause. An artificial PACEMAKER may be used in the treatment of complete heart block and Stokes-Adams disease.

atrioventricular (A-V) h. b., a form in which the blocking is at the atrioventricular junction. It is *first degree* when A-V conduction time is prolonged; *second degree* (partial heart block) when some but not all atrial impulses reach the ventricle; *third degree* (complete heart block) when no atrial impulses at all reach the ventricle, and the atria and ventricles act independently of each other.

bundle-branch h. b., a form in which one ventricle is excited before the other because of absence of conduction in one of the branches of the bundle of His.

complete h. b., see atrioventricular heart block.

interventricular h. b., bundle-branch heart block.

Mobitz type I h. b., second degree A-V heart block in which the P-R interval increases progressively until an atrial impulse is blocked.

Mobitz type II h. b., second degree A-V heart block in which the P-R interval is fixed, with periodic blocking of an atrial impulse.

sinoatrial h. b., partial or complete impairment of conduction from the sinoatrial node to the atria, resulting in delay or absence of an atrial beat.

heartburn (hart'burn) pyrosis; a burning sensation in the esophagus, or below the sternum in the region of the heart. It is one of the common symptoms of indigestion.

Heartburn often occurs when there is distention of a part of the esophagus, particularly the lower part. This may happen when the stomach regurgitates part of its contents, forcing them upward into the esophagus. Since this matter is acid, it acts as an irritant, producing discomfort or pain.

Excessive acidity (hyperacidity) is thought to be a cause of heartburn, occurring when the stomach secretes an excessive amount of hydrochloric acid. Recent evidence, however, indicates that hyperacidity in itself may not be the actual cause, and that heartburn results from excessive gastric secretions only when there is improper eating or emotional disturbance.

There is no doubt that emotional disturbance, excitement, and nervous tension are frequent causes of heartburn. The functions of the stomach, both those of motion and secretion, are controlled by the VAGUS NERVE, one of the cranial nerves. Emotional stress can stimulate this nerve, which in turn starts the churning of the stomach and the flow of the various gastric juices; it can also cause contraction and spasm of the pylorus. If some of the stomach contents are displaced into the esophagus during this nervous activity, heartburn may result.

Treatment of heartburn is aimed at determining its underlying cause. Antacids may be used to relieve the symptoms but they will not cure heartburn and should not be used indiscriminately.

heart failure (hart'fāl-ūr) inability of the heart to maintain a circulation sufficient to meet the body's needs; most often applied to myocardial failure affecting the right or left ventricle.

backward h. f., a concept of heart failure emphasizing the contribution of passive engorgement of the systemic venous system as a cause.

congestive h. f., that marked by breathlessness and abnormal retention of sodium and water, resulting in edema, with congestion of the lungs or peripheral circulation, or both.

TREATMENT. Treatment for heart failure includes rest to reduce the oxygen requirements of the body, medications such as digitalis to strengthen the heart action and diuretics to control the edema, along with dietary measures.

PATIENT CARE. The patient with acute congestive failure is usually placed on complete bed rest with severe limitation of activities as long as the symptoms of edema, dyspnea, ascites, and venous engorgement are present. He must be fed, bathed, dressed, and otherwise cared for as though he could not lift a finger to help himself. For some patients this is extremely difficult and depressing. Care should be taken not to give the patient the impression that he is causing any difficulties for those assigned to his care.

In addition to measuring the patient's intake and output it is usually necessary to record his weight daily. This information is used as a guide to the response to medication and treatment and the amount of fluid being retained in the tissues.

Oxygen is administered as needed to relieve dyspnea and cyanosis (see also OXYGEN THERAPY). The position of the patient in bed may also help relieve these symptoms. If the patient tires easily while sitting up in Fowler's position, he may rest more comfortably if he is allowed to lay his arms and head on an overbed table that has been padded with pillows (orthopneic position). Since edematous tissue breaks down more readily and is thus more susceptible to ulceration than normal tissue, routine skin care is extremely important.

Dietary restrictions, such as limiting the intake of sodium to reduce edema, should be explained thoroughly to the patient and his family. If fluids by mouth also are restricted, care should be taken to regulate the amount taken at any given period so that the total amount allowed is evenly distributed over a 24-hour period.

Chronic congestive failure does not always require hospitalization. Medications such as digitalis and a diuretic are used to control the condition and may keep the patient free of symptoms unless complications develop.

forward h. f., a concept of heart failure emphasizing the inadequacy of cardiac output as the primary cause and considering venous distention to be secondary.

high output h. f., that in which cardiac output remains high, associated with hyperthyroidism, anemia, emphysema, etc.

left-sided h. f., left ventricular h. f., failure of the left ventricle to maintain a normal output of blood. Since the left ventricle does not empty completely, it cannot accept blood returning from the lungs via the pulmonary veins. The pulmonary veins become engorged and fluid seeps out through the veins and collects in the pleural cavity. Pulmonary edema and pleural effusion result. In many cases heart failure begins on the left side and eventually involves both sides of the heart.

low-output h. f., that in which cardiac output is diminished, associated with cardiovascular diseases.

right-sided h. f., right ventricular h. f., failure of proper functioning of the right ventricle, with subsequent engorgement of the systemic veins, producing pitting edema, enlargement of the liver, and ascites.

heart-lung machine a mechanical device that temporarily takes over the functions of the heart and lungs; called also a pump-oxygenator. It is used as an aid to surgery.

The "heart" of the machine is a pump that draws blood from the patient's vessels before it reaches the heart. The blood is routed through a "lung" chamber (usually made of plastic), where it receives oxygen. The oxygenated blood is then returned to the patient's vessels and pumped through his circulatory system. This method of circulating the blood outside the patient's body is known as extracorporeal circulation.

heart murmur any sound in the heart region other than normal heart sounds (see also MURMUR). A murmur may be caused by several different factors, including changes in the valves of the heart or blood leaking through a disease-scarred valve that does not close properly.

RHEUMATIC FEVER is a common cause of heart murmur. A murmur may also indicate other types of heart disease. In many cases, however, the murmur may be of the innocent or "functional" type, which does not indicate any heart damage at all and causes no trouble. Such murmurs vary from time to time, and often go away completely.

heart rate the number of contractions of the cardiac ventricles per unit of time.

heart sounds the sounds heard on the surface of

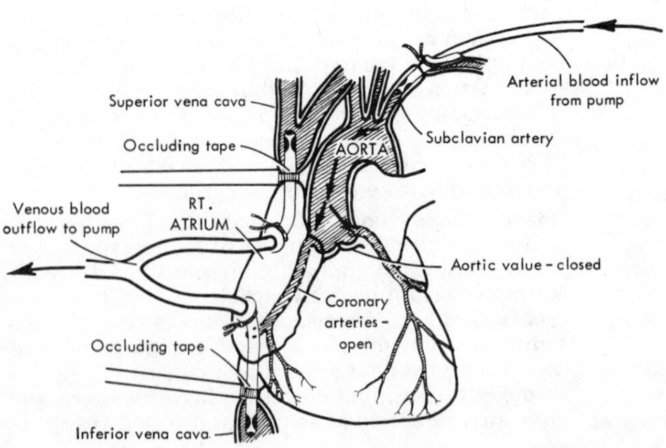

Extracorporeal circulation, illustrating flow of blood from the body and return. The coronary arteries are filled, but no blood enters the cardiac chambers (except coronary venous return). (From Storer, E. H., Pate, J. W., and Sherman, R. T.: The Science of Surgery. New York, McGraw-Hill Book Co., 1964.)

the chest in the heart region. They are amplified by and heard more distinctly through a stethoscope. These sounds are caused by the vibrations of the normal cardiac cycle. They may be produced by muscular action, valvular actions, motion of the heart, and blood as it passes through the heart.

The first heart sound is heard as a firm but not sharp "lubb" sound. It consists of four components: a low-frequency, indistinct vibration caused by ventricular contraction; a louder sound of higher frequency caused by closure of the mitral and tricuspid valves; a vibration caused by opening of the semilunar valves and early ejection of blood from the ventricles; and a low-pitched vibration produced by rapid ejection.

The second heart sound is shorter and higher pitched than the first, is heard as a "dupp" and is produced by closure of the aortic and pulmonary valves.

The third heart sound is very faint and is caused by blood rushing into the ventricles. It can be heard in most normal persons between the ages of 10 and 20 years.

The fourth heart sound is rarely audible in a normal heart but can be demonstrated on graphic records. It is short and of low frequency and intensity, and is caused by atrial contraction. The vibrations arise from atrial muscle and from blood flow into, and distention of, the ventricles.

ABNORMALITIES IN HEART SOUNDS. Failure of the heart muscle to contract is characterized by a gallop or triple rhythm. Accentuation of the third heart sound (protodiastolic gallop) is caused by the filling of a large flabby ventricle with blood under high venous pressure. A presystolic gallop is an accentuated fourth heart sound and is also caused by blood filling a dilated and inert ventricle. Merging of the third and fourth heart sounds is called a mesodiastolic or summation gallop. A very rare abnormality in which four heart sounds are heard distinctly is called a "locomotive" rhythm.

HEART MURMURS are sounds other than the normal heart sounds emanating from the heart region. They are often heard as blowing or hissing sounds as blood leaks through diseased and malfunctioning valves.

HEAT human erythrocyte agglutination test.

heat (hēt) energy that raises the temperature of a body or substance; also, the rise of the temperature itself. Heat is associated with molecular motion, and generated in various ways, including combustion, friction, chemical action, and radiation. The total absence of heat is absolute zero, at which all molecular activity ceases.

BODY HEAT. *Heat Production.* Body heat is the by-product of the metabolic processes of the body. The hormones thyroxine and epinephrine increase metabolism and consequently increase body heat. Muscular activity also produces body heat. At complete rest (basal metabolism) the amount of heat produced from muscular activity may be as low as 25 per cent of the total body heat. During exercise or shivering the percentage may rise to 60 per cent.

Body temperature is regulated by the thermostatic center in the HYPOTHALAMUS. A body temperature above the normal range is called FEVER.

Heat Loss. Loss of body heat occurs in three ways: by radiation (heat waves), by conduction to air or objects in contact with the body, and by evaporation of perspiration. Some body heat is lost in expiration of air and in elimination of urine and feces.

APPLICATIONS OF EXTERNAL HEAT. *Purposes.* Local applications of heat may be used to provide warmth and promote comfort, rest, and relaxation. Heat is also applied locally to promote suppuration and drainage from an infected area by hastening the inflammatory process; to relieve congestion and swelling by dilating the blood vessels, thereby increasing circulation; and to improve repair of diseased or injured tissues by increasing local metabolism.

Effects. Factors that determine the physiologic action of heat include the type of heat used, length of time it is applied, age and general condition of the patient, and area of body surface to which the heat is applied. Moist heat is more penetrating than dry heat. Prolonged applications of heat produce an increase in skin secretions, resulting in a softening of the skin and a lowering of its resistance. Extreme heat produces constriction of the blood vessels; moderate heat produces vascular dilation. Repeated applications of heat will result in an increased tolerance to heat so that the individual may be burned without his being aware of it. Elderly persons and infants are more susceptible to burns from high temperatures.

Heat applied to an infected area can localize the infection; for this reason, external heat should not be applied to the abdomen when appendicitis is suspected, because it may lead to rupture of the inflamed appendix.

Methods. In general, applications of heat are dry or wet. Dry heat may be applied to the superficial tissues in the form of hot water bottles, electric heating pads, or an electric incandescent bulb with a

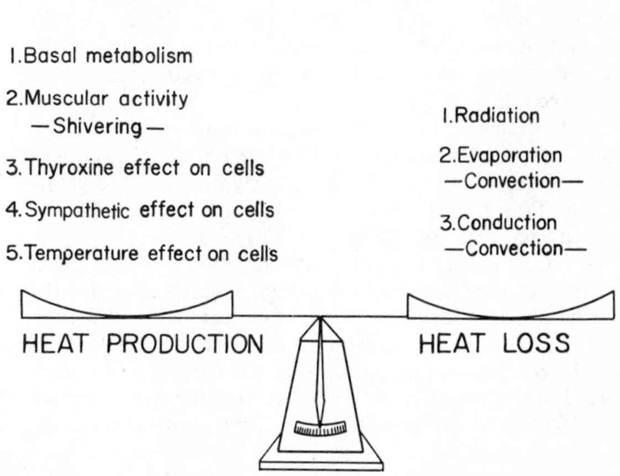

Balance of heat production versus heat loss. (From Guyton, A. C.: Textbook of Medical Physiology. 5th ed. Philadelphia, W. B. Saunders Co., 1976.)

heat cradle. Three modes of heat application to deeper tissues are shortwave, ultrasound, and microwave DIATHERMY.

Hot water bottles should be filled with water not exceeding 125° F. (52° C.), and should be about half full; the air is expelled before the bottle is sealed. The hot water bottle is covered with a flannel or cotton covering before it is applied and this covering should remain dry at all times, unless the hot water bottle is used over moist dressings to keep them warm. The hot water bottle should be refilled at least every 2 hours.

Electric heating pads are never used over wet dressings or in other areas where moisture may come in contact with the electricity. Those used in hospitals should have an automatic control and the thermostat should be turned to low or medium.

Heat lamps may generate heat through ultraviolet or infrared radiation. Ultraviolet rays are more penetrating than infrared rays. Moderate radiation from ultraviolet rays produces local vasodilation and stimulates growth of tissue cells. It must be used with caution because of the danger of producing deep burns.

Infrared rays provide surface heat but penetrate to a depth of only 10 mm. Prolonged and intense application can lead to burning and blistering of the skin. Before being exposed to infrared rays, the skin should be cleansed and all ointments or other medicinal preparations removed.

The heat cradle employs an ordinary bed cradle to support the top bed covers and an electric light bulb to generate heat. This type of apparatus is often used for patients with circulatory disturbances of the extremities.

Moist or wet heat can be applied in a variety of ways, including baths, hot packs, HYDROCOLLATOR, soaks, and compresses (see also HYDROTHERAPY).

Uses. Local applications of heat are used for a variety of disorders. Perineal lacerations and surgical incisions heal more readily when dry heat is applied. Circulatory disturbances of the extremities, and the ulcers they sometimes cause, are amenable to applications of heat. Moderate heat is used to relax the muscles and reduce spasm that often accompanies muscle strain (see also DIATHERMY).

Heat, applied by boiling, autoclaving, flaming, or burning, is a commonly used physical antiseptic.

h. exhaustion, a disorder resulting from overexposure to heat or to the sun; called also heat prostration. Long exposure to extreme heat or too much activity under a hot sun causes excessive sweating, which removes large quantities of salt and fluid from the body. When the amount of salt and fluid in the body falls too far below normal, heat exhaustion may result.

SYMPTOMS. The early symptoms of heat exhaustion are headache and a feeling of weakness and dizziness, usually accompanied by nausea and vomiting. There may also be cramps in the muscles of the arms, legs, or abdomen. These first symptoms are similar to the early signs of SUNSTROKE, or heat stroke, but the disorders are not the same and should be treated differently. In heat exhaustion, the person turns pale and perspires profusely. His skin is cool and moist, his pulse and breathing are rapid. His body temperature remains at a normal level or slightly below, whereas in sunstroke the body temperature may be dangerously elevated. He may seem confused and may find it difficult to coordinate his body movements. Ordinarily he remains conscious.

TREATMENT. In cases of heat exhaustion, a physician should be called and the victim should lie quietly in a cool place. He should be given half a teaspoonful of salt dissolved in tomato juice or in half a glass of water every 15 minutes for 2 hours if he tolerates it. After he has taken the salt, hot tea or coffee may be given.

If the condition is accompanied by cramps, the pain may be relieved by gentle massage of the painful area or by firm hand pressure. In cases of severe heat exhaustion and cramps, it may be necessary to keep the victim at rest in bed for a day or more.

PREVENTION. Heat exhaustion and other heat disorders may be prevented by avoiding long exposure to sun or heat. When the weather is very hot, or when working in an extremely hot place, it is essential to drink plenty of water. Salt tablets should be taken if the stomach tolerates them, or a half to one teaspoonful of salt can be added to each quart of drinking water. Regular breaks from work are necessary, and in the event of weakness or dizziness, the victim should stop working at once and rest in a cool place.

latent h., the heat that a body may absorb without changing its temperature.

molecular h., the product of the molecular weight of a substance multiplied by its specific heat.

prickly h., h. rash, miliaria; inflammation of the skin, due to retention of sweat, occurring during hot, humid weather.

sensible h., the heat that, when absorbed by a body, produces a rise in temperature.

specific h., the number of calories required to raise the temperature of 1 gm. of a particular substance one degree centigrade.

h. stroke, a severe life-threatening condition resulting from prolonged exposure to heat. See SUNSTROKE.

heavy-chain disease a monoclonal gammopathy in which there is elaboration of immunoglobulin of class IgG that lacks certain antigenic determinants. The resultant globulin fragment (molecular weight, 53,000), resembling the Fc fragment, is found in both serum and urine. Symptoms include recurring bacterial infections, anemia, enlargement of lymphoid organs, and edema of the palate. Histologically there is lymphoma, ranging from Hodgkin's disease to reticulum cell sarcoma. Heavy-chain disease involving the IgA and IgM systems has also been reported.

hebephrenia (heb″ĕ-fre′ne-ah) a clinical form of SCHIZOPHRENIA coming on soon after the onset of puberty and marked by rapid deterioration, hallucinations, absurd delusions, senseless laughter and silly mannerisms. Called also hebephrenic schizophrenia. adj., **hebephren′ic.**

Heberden's nodes (he′ber-denz) small, hard nodules, formed usually at the distal interphalangeal joints of the fingers in osteoarthritis.

hebetic (hĕ-bet-′ik) pertaining to puberty.

hebetude (heb′ĕ-tūd) mental dullness; apathy.

hebosteotomy, hebotomy (he-bos″te-ot′o-me; he-bot′o-me) pubiotomy.

hecatomeric (hek″ah-to-mer′ik) having processes

that divide in two, one going to each side of the spinal cord; said of certain neurons.

hecto- (hek'to) word element [Fr.], *hundred;* used in naming units of measurement to designate an amount 100 times (10^2) the size of the unit to which it is joined, e.g., hectoliter (100 liters); symbol h.

hectogram (hek'to-gram) one hundred grams; 3.53 ounces.

hectoliter (hek'to-le"ter) one hundred liters; 26.42 gallons.

hectometer (hek'to-me"ter) one hundred meters; 109.36 yards.

hedonism (he'don-izm) excessive devotion to pleasure.

Hedulin (hed'u-lin) trademark for a preparation of phenindione, an anticoagulant.

heel (hēl) the hindmost part of the foot; called also calx. By extension, a part comparable to the heel of the foot, or the hindmost portion of an elongate structure.

Thomas h., a shoe correction consisting of a heel $\frac{1}{2}$ inch longer and $\frac{1}{6}$ to $\frac{1}{8}$ inch higher on the inside; used to bring the heel of the foot into varus and to prevent depression in the region of the head of the talus.

Heerfordt's disease (hār'forts) uveoparotid fever.

Hegar's sign (ha'garz) compressibility and softening of the lower uterine segment, an indication of pregnancy.

Heimlich maneuver (hīm'lik) a technique for removing foreign matter from the trachea of a choking victim. The maneuver is also recommended as a preliminary step in the emergency treatment of accident victims in need of artificial ventilation. Before administering mouth-to-mouth respiration the maneuver is carried out to clear material that may prevent adequate ventilation of the lungs. The technique may be carried out with the victim in a standing position or lying down.

STANDING POSITION. The rescuer stands behind the victim and wraps his arms around the victim's waist, allowing the victim's head, arms, and upper torso to hang forward. A fist is made with one hand and held with the other. The fist is then placed against the victim's abdomen at a point slightly above the umbilicus and below the rib cage. The rescuer's fist is then pressed into the victim's abdomen with a forceful upward thrust. The maneuver may be repeated if necessary to clear the air passages.

SUPINE POSITION. The victim is placed on his back with his head turned to one side. The rescuer kneels astride the victim's hips and places both hands on his abdomen, one hand upon the other. The heel of the lower hand is placed slightly above the umbilicus and below the rib cage. Pressure is applied to the victim's abdomen with a forceful upward thrust. The maneuver may be repeated if necessary to clear the air passages.

Heine-Medin disease (hi'nĕ-ma'din) the major form of POLIOMYELITIS.

Heineke-Mikulicz pyloroplasty (hi'nĕ-kĕ mik'-u-lich) enlargement of a pyloric stricture by incising the pylorus longitudinally and suturing the incision transversely.

HeLa cells (he'lah) cells of the first continuously cultured carcinoma strain, descended from a human cervical carcinoma; used in the study of life processes, including viruses, at the cell level.

helcoid (hel'koid) like an ulcer.

heli(o)- (he'le-o) word element [Gr.], *sun.*

helianthin (he"le-an'thin) methyl orange; an orange-yellow aniline dye used as a pH indicator.

helical (hel'ĭ-kal) shaped like a helix.

helicine (hel'ĭ-sin) spiral.

helicoid (hel'ĭ-koid) coiled; spiral.

helicopodia (hel"ĭ-ko-po'de-ah) helicopod gait.

helicotrema (hel"ĭ-ko-tre'mah) the passage that connects the scala tympani and the scala vestibuli at the apex of the cochlea.

heliotaxis (he"le-o-tak'sis) the motile response of an organism to the stimulus of light; phototaxis.

heliotherapy (he"le-o-ther'ah-pe) treatment of disease by exposing the body to the sun's rays; therapeutic use of the sun bath.

heliotropism (he"le-ot'ro-pizm) phototropism; the tendency of an organism to orient itself in relation to the stimulus of light.

helium (he'le-um) a chemical element, atomic number 2, atomic weight 4.003, symbol He. (See table of ELEMENTS.)

Helium is a chemically inert element that is odorless, tasteless, and noncombustible. Because of its low density it is easily moved through the air passages and therefore requires little effort in breathing on the part of the patient who is in respiratory distress. Although helium itself has no chemical therapeutic value, when combined with oxygen it facilitates the delivery of this gas to the lungs. The administration of helium-oxygen combination usually is employed as an initial measure to relieve diffuse airway obstruction and to prevent exhaustion of the patient who is having difficulty breathing through restricted air passages. Once the bronchial passages have been opened, conventional oxygen therapy is continued to relieve hypoxia.

It should be noted that helium causes the voice to be high-pitched and the spoken word difficult to understand. This should be explained to the patient with the assurance that the effect is harmless and temporary.

helix (he'liks) 1. a coiled structure. 2. the superior and posterior free margin of the pinna of the ear.

double h., Watson-Crick h., a representation of the structure of DEOXYRIBONUCLEIC ACID (DNA), consisting of two coiled chains, each of which contains information completely specifying the other chain.

Hellin's law (hel'inz) one in about 89 pregnancies ends in the birth of twins; one in 89^2, or 7921, of triplets; one in 89^3, or 704,969, of quadruplets.

helminth (hel'minth) a parasitic worm; a nematode or trematode.

helminthagogue (hel-min'thah-gog) anthelmintic; vermifuge; an agent that expels worms or intestinal animal parasites.

helminthemesis (hel"min-them'ĕ-sis) the vomiting of worms.

helminthiasis (hel"min-thi'ah-sis) an infection with worms.

helminthology (hel"min-thol'o-je) the scientific study of parasitic worms.

helminthoma (hel"min-tho'mah) a tumor caused by a parasitic worm.

heloma (he-lo'mah) a corn.

h. du'rum, hard corn, the usual type occurring over joints of the toes.

h. mol'le, a soft corn.

helotomy (he-lot'o-me) excision or paring of a corn or callus.

hemabarometer (hem"ah-bah-rom'ĕ-ter) an instrument for ascertaining the specific gravity of blood.

hemacytometer (he"mah-si-tom'ĕ-ter) hemocytometer.

hemadsorption (hem"ad-sorp'shun) the adherence of red cells to other cells. adj., **hemadsor'bent.**

hemadynamometer (he"mah-di"nah-mom'ĕ-ter) an instrument for measuring blood pressure.

hemadynamometry (he"mah-di"nah-mom'ĕ-tre) measurement of blood pressure.

hemagglutination (he"mah-gloo"tĭ-na'shun) agglutination of erythrocytes.

hemagglutinin (he"mah-gloo'tĭ-nin) an antibody that causes agglutination of erythrocytes.

cold h., one that acts only at temperatures near 4° C.

warm h., one that acts only at temperatures near 37° C.

hemal (he'mal) pertaining to blood.

hemanalysis (he"mah-nal'ĭ-sis) analysis of the blood.

hemangiectasis (he-man"je-ek'tah-sis) dilatation of blood vessels.

hemangioameloblastoma (he-man"je-o-ah-mel"-o-blas-to'mah) a highly vascular ameloblastoma.

hemangioblast (he-man'je-o-blast") a mesodermal cell that gives rise to both vascular endothelium and hemocytoblasts.

hemangioblastoma (he-man"je-o-blas-to'mah) a capillary hemangioma of the brain consisting of proliferated blood vessel cells or angioblasts.

hemangioendothelioblastoma (he-man"je-o-en"do-the"le-o-blas-to'mah) a tumor of mesenchymal origin of which the cells tend to form endothelial cells and line blood vessels.

hemangioendothelioma (he-man"je-o-en"do-the"le-o'mah) a hemangioma in which endothelial cells are the predominant component.

hemangiofibroma (he-man"je-o-fi-bro'mah) a hemangioma containing fibrous tissue.

hemangioma (he-man"je-o'mah) a benign tumor made up of newly formed blood vessels, clustered together. Hemangioma may be present at birth in various parts of the body, including the liver and bones. In the majority of cases, however, it appears as a network of small blood-filled capillaries near the surface of the skin, forming a reddish or purplish birthmark. These marks are not malignant.

Types of hemangiomas include "strawberry" or "raspberry" marks, port-wine stains, and cavernous hemangiomas; the latter is a less common type in which the birthmark has a soft, spongy consistency. With the exception of port-wine stains, superficial hemangiomas often disappear of their own accord as the person grows older. Cavernous hemangiomas should be treated early, since the lesions tend to grow and there is the possibility of severe hemorrhage should the lesion be injured and start to bleed. Treatment is by irradiation, injection of a sclerosing agent, or surgery.

hemangiomatosis (he-man"je-o-mah-to'sis) the presence of multiple hemangiomas.

hemangiopericytoma (he-man"je-o-per"ĭ-si-to'-mah) a tumor composed of spindle cells with a rich vascular network, which apparently arises from pericytes.

hemangiosarcoma (he-man"je-o-sar-ko'mah) a malignant tumor of vascular tissue; called also angiosarcoma.

hemaphein (hem"ah-fe'in) a brown coloring matter of the blood and urine. adj., **hemaphe'ic.**

hemarthros, hemarthrosis (hem-ar'thros; hem"-ar-thro'sis) blood in a joint cavity.

hemat(o)- word element [Gr.], *blood.* See also words beginning *hem-* and *hemo-*.

hematein (hem"ah-te'in) a compound occurring in reddish brown plates with a metallic luster; the coloring principle of hematoxylin.

hematemesis (hem"ah-tem'ĕ-sis) the vomiting of blood. The appearance of the vomitus depends on the amount and character of the gastric contents at the time blood is vomited and on the length of time the blood has been in the stomach. Gastric acids change bright red blood to a brownish color and the vomitus is often described as "coffee-ground" in color. Bright red blood in the vomitus indicates a fresh hemorrhage and little contact of the blood with gastric juices.

The most common causes of hematemesis are PEPTIC ULCER, gastritis, esophageal lesions or varices, and cancer of the stomach. Benign tumors, traumatic postoperative bleeding, and swallowed blood from points in the nose, mouth, and throat can also produce hematemesis.

hematencephalon (hem"at-en-sef'ah-lon) effusion of blood into the brain.

hemathermous (hem"ah-ther'mus) warm-blooded; hematothermal.

hematic (he-mat'ik) 1. pertaining to the blood. 2. hematinic.

hematidrosis (hem"ah-tĭ-dro'sis) excretion of bloody sweat.

hematimeter (hem"ah-tim'ĕ-ter) device for counting blood corpuscles; a hemocytometer.

hematin (hem'ah-tin) a compound formed by the oxidation of heme from the ferrous Fe (II) to the ferric Fe (III) state; it does not combine with oxygen.

hematinemia (hem"ah-tĭ-ne'me-ah) the presence of heme in the blood.

hematinic (hem"ah-tin'ik) 1. improving the quality of the blood. 2. an agent that improves the quality of the blood, increasing the hemoglobin level and the number of erythrocytes; examples are iron preparations, liver extract, and the B complex vitamins.

hematinometer (hem"ah-tĭ-nom'ĕ-ter) an instrument for measuring the hemoglobin of the blood; hemoglobinometer.

hematinuria (hem"ah-tin-u're-ah) the presence of heme in the urine.

hematobilia (hem"ah-to-bil'e-ah) bleeding into the biliary passages.

hematoblast (hem'ah-to-blast") hemocytoblast.

hematocele (hem'ah-to-sēl") an effusion of blood into a cavity, especially into the tunica vaginalis testis.

hematochezia (hem″ah-to-ke′ze-ah) blood in the feces.

hematochromatosis (hem″ah-to-kro″mah-to′sis) hemochromatosis.

hematochyluria (hem″ah-to-ki-lu′re-ah) the discharge of blood and chyle in the urine.

hematocolpometra (hem″ah-to-kol″po-me′trah) accumulation of menstrual blood in the vagina and uterus.

hematocolpos (hem″ah-to-kol′pos) accumulation of menstrual blood in the vagina.

hematocrit (he-mat′o-krit) the volume percentage of erythrocytes in whole blood; also, the apparatus or procedures used in its determination. The hematocrit (which means, literally, "to separate blood") is determined by centrifuging a blood sample to separate the cellular elements from the plasma; the results of the test indicate the ratio of cell volume to plasma volume and are expressed as milliliters of packed cells per 100 ml. of blood, or in volumes per 100 ml. Normal range is 40 to 54 volumes per 100 ml. for males, and 37 to 47 volumes per 100 ml. for females. The hematocrit, in conjunction with other hematologic tests, provides information about the size, functioning capacity, and number of erythrocytes.

hematocryal (hem″ah-to-kri′al) poikilothermic.

hematocrystallin (hem″ah-to-kris′tah-lin) hemoglobin.

hematocyanin (hem″ah-to-si′ah-nin) a chromoprotein occurring in the blood of mollusks and arthropods. It is a blue respiratory pigment and contains 0.17 to 0.38 per cent of copper.

hematocyst (hem′ah-to-sist″) effusion of blood into the bladder or in a cyst.

hematocyturia (hem″ah-to-si-tu′re-ah) the presence of erythrocytes in the urine.

hematogenic (hem″ah-to-jen′ik) 1. hematopoietic. 2. hematogenous.

hematogenous (hem″ah-toj′ĕ-nus) produced by or derived from the blood; disseminated through the bloodstream or by the circulation.

hematoid (hem′ah-toid) like blood.

hematoidin (hem″ah-toi′din) a substance apparently chemically identical with bilirubin but formed in the tissues from hemoglobin, particularly under conditions of reduced oxygen tension.

hematologist (he″mah-tol′o-jist) a specialist in hematology.

hematology (he″mah-tol′o-je) the science dealing with the morphology of blood and blood-forming tissues, and with their physiology and pathology. adj., **hematolog′ic.**

hematolymphangioma (hem″ah-to-lim-fan″je-o′mah) a tumor composed of blood and lymph vessels.

hematolysis (hem″ah-tol′ĭ-sis) hemolysis.

hematoma (he″mah-to′mah) a localized collection of extravasated blood, usually clotted, in an organ, space, or tissue. Contusions (bruises) and black eyes are familiar forms of hematoma that are seldom serious. Hematomas can occur almost anywhere on the body; they are almost always present with a fracture and are especially serious when they occur inside the skull, where they may produce local pressure on the brain. In minor injuries the blood is absorbed unless infection develops.

CRANIAL HEMATOMA. The two most common kinds of cranial hematomas are extradural (epidural) and subdural. The word dural refers to the dura mater. *Extradural hematoma* occurs above the dura mater, between it and the skull. It is most often caused by a heavy blow to the head that damages the upper surface of the dura mater. Blood seeps into the surrounding tissue, forming a tumor-like mass or hematoma. Since the skull is rigid, the hematoma presses inward against the brain. If the pressure continues, the brain can be affected. An extradural hematoma can involve rupture of an artery, with hemorrhage, causing severe pressure that can be quickly fatal.

Subdural hematoma occurs beneath the dura mater, between the tough casing and the more delicate membranes covering the tissue of the brain, the pia-arachnoid. This kind of injury is more often caused by the head's striking an immovable object, such as the floor, than by a blow from a moving object. There may be no severe head injury or fracture. A blow to the head can cause the brain to move violently, tearing blood vessels and forming a swelling that may include fluid from the brain tissue. A chronic subdural hematoma may remain and increase in size. (See also HEAD INJURY.)

Symptoms. The most common symptoms of extradural hematoma occur within a few hours after injury. There can be a sudden or gradual loss of consciousness, partial or full paralysis on the side opposite the injury, and dilation of the pupil of the eye on the same side as the injury.

The symptoms of chronic subdural hematoma are similar to those of a brain tumor, and may come and go. Diagnosis is difficult, particularly in older people. There may be subtle personality changes, or the patient may become confused, weak in various parts of the body, vague and drowsy.

Subdural hematoma may occasionally occur in babies as a result of birth injury. Unless the injury is discovered and treated at an early stage, the child's mental and physical development may be retarded, and spastic paralysis can occur. Early surgery is usually successful in preventing permanent symptoms and disabilities.

Treatment. Prompt surgery is the only treatment for extradural hematoma. The clotted blood is removed by a combination of suction and irrigation methods through openings made in the skull, and the bleeding is controlled. The same surgery is used for subdural hematomas.

SEPTAL HEMATOMA. Injury to the nose sometimes causes hematoma of the nasal septum. Its symptoms include nasal obstruction and headache. The condition may be treated by incision and drainage or may clear up spontaneously in a few weeks. If the hematoma becomes infected, an abscess may result, requiring drainage and treatment with antibiotics.

hematomediastinum (hem″ah-to-me″de-ah-sti′num) effusion of blood into the mediastinum.

hematometra (hem″ah-to-me′trah) an accumulation of menstrual blood in the uterus.

hematometry (he″mah-tom′ĕ-tre) measurement of hemoglobin and estimation of the percentage of various cells of the blood.

hematomphalocele (hem″at-om-fal′o-sēl) an umbilical hernia containing blood.

hematomyelia (hem″ah-to-mi-e′le-ah) hemorrhage into the substance of the spinal cord.

hematomyelitis (hem″ah-to-mi″ĕ-li′tis) acute myelitis with bloody effusion into the spinal cord.

hematomyelopore (hem″ah-to-mi′ĕ-lo-pōr″) formation of canals in the spinal cord due to hemorrhage.

hematonephrosis (hem″ah-to-nĕ-fro′sis) the presence of blood in the renal pelvis.

hematopathology (hem″ah-to-pah-thol′o-je) the study of diseases of the blood; hemopathology.

hematophagous (hem″ah-tof′ah-gus) subsisting on blood.

hematophilia (hem″ah-to-fil′e-ah) hemophilia.

hematopoiesis (hem″ah-to-poi-e′sis) the formation and development of blood cells, usually taking place in the bone marrow.

extramedullary h., the formation of and development of blood cells outside the bone marrow, as in the spleen, liver, and lymph nodes.

hematopoietic (hem″ah-to-poi-et′ik) 1. pertaining to or affecting the formation of blood cells. 2. an agent that promotes the formation of blood cells.

hematoporphyria (hem″ah-to-por-fēr′e-ah) a constitutional state marked by abnormal quantity of porphyrin (uroporphyrin and coproporphyrin) in the tissues and secreted in the urine, pigmentation of the face (and later of the bones), sensitivity of the skin to light, vomiting, and intestinal disturbance; see PORPHYRIA.

hematoporphyrin (hem″ah-to-por′fĭ-rin) an iron-free derivative of heme, a product of the decomposition of hemoglobin.

hematoporphyrinemia (hem″ah-to-por″fĭ-rĭ-ne′me-ah) hematoporphyrin in the blood.

hematoporphyrinuria (hem″ah-to-por″fĭ-rĭ-nu′re-ah) hematoporphyrin in the urine.

hematorrhachis (hem″ah-tor′ah-kis) hemorrhage into the vertebral canal.

hematorrhea (hem″ah-to-re′ah) copious hemorrhage.

hematosalpinx (hem″ah-to-sal′pinks) an accumulation of blood in the uterine tube.

hematoscheocele (hem″ah-tos′ke-o-sēl″) an accumulation of blood within the scrotum.

hematoscope (hem′ah-to-skōp″) an instrument for the optical or spectroscopic examination of blood.

hematoscopy (hem″ah-tos′ko-pe) analysis of blood with the hematoscope.

hematospectroscopy (hem″ah-to-spek-tros′ko-pe) spectroscopic examination of blood.

hematospermatocele (hem″ah-to-sper-mat′o-sēl) a spermatocele containing blood.

hematospermia (hem″ah-to-sper′me-ah) blood in the semen.

hematosteon (hem″ah-tos′te-on) hemorrhage into the medullary cavity of a bone.

hematothermal (hem″ah-to-ther′mal) homoiothermic.

hematotoxic (hem″ah-to-tok′sik) 1. pertaining to blood poisoning. 2. poisonous to the blood and hematopoietic system.

hematotrachelos (hem″ah-to-trah-ke′los) distention of the cervix uteri with blood.

hematotropic (hem″ah-to-trop′ik) having a special affinity for or exerting a specific effect on the blood or blood cells.

hematotympanum (hem″ah-to-tim′pah-num) hemorrhage into the middle ear.

hematoxylin (hem″ah-tok′sĭ-lin) an acid coloring matter obtained from the wood of a tree (*Haematoxylon campechianum*); used as a stain for histologic specimens and as an indicator.

hematuria (hem″ah-tu′re-ah) the discharge of blood in the urine. The urine may be slightly blood tinged, grossly bloody, or a smoky brown color.

Hematuria is symptomatic of disease or injury to a part of the urinary system. Tumors of the bladder, cystitis, urethritis, and small kidney stones passing along the ureter can cause blood in the urine. Vascular diseases and some types of kidney disorders produce hematuria. Traumatic injury to the kidney is usually but not always accompanied by hematuria.

PATIENT CARE. When hematuria is suspected because of the outward appearance of the urine, a specimen should be saved and sent to the laboratory for microscopic analysis. An accurate record of the patient's intake and output of fluids is kept and the characteristics of the urine should be noted on the patient's chart. If hematuria occurs suddenly and unexpectedly this should be reported immediately to the physician in charge.

heme (hēm) the nonprotein, insoluble, iron protoporphyrin constituent of hemoglobin, of various other respiratory pigments, and of many cells, both animal and vegetable. It is an iron compound of protoporphyrin and so constitutes the pigment portion or protein-free part of the hemoglobin molecule, and is responsible for its oxygen-carrying properties.

hemeralopia (hem″er-al-o′pe-ah) day blindness; defective vision in a bright light.

hemi- (hem′ĭ) word element [Gr.], *half.*

hemiacardius (hem″e-ah-kar′de-us) an unequal twin in which the heart is rudimentary, its circulation being assisted by the other twin.

hemiachromatopsia (hem″e-ah-kro″mah-top′se-ah) loss of the normal perception of color in half, or in corresponding halves, of the visual field.

hemialbumose (hem″e-al′bu-mōs) a digestion product of certain proteins; normally found in bone marrow, and occurring in the urine in osteomalacia and diphtheria.

hemialbumosuria (hem″e-al″bu-mo-su′re-ah) hemialbumose in the urine.

hemiamyosthenia (hem″e-ah-mi″os-the′ne-ah) lack of muscular power on one side of the body.

hemianacusia (hem″e-an″ah-koo′ze-ah) loss of hearing in one ear.

hemianalgesia (hem″e-an″al-je′ze-ah) analgesia on one side of the body.

hemianencephaly (hem″e-an″en-sef′ah-le) congenital absence of one side of the brain.

hemianesthesia (hem″e-an″es-the′ze-ah) anesthesia of one side of the body.

crossed h., h. crucia′ta, loss of sensation on one side of the face and loss of pain and temperature sense on the opposite side of the body.

hemianopia, hemianopsia (hem″e-ah-no′pe-ah; hem″e-ah-nop′se-ah) defective vision or blindness in half of the visual field; usually applied to bilateral defects caused by a single lesion. adj., **hemianop′ic, hemianop′tic.**

hemianosmia (hem″e-an-oz′me-ah) absence of the sense of smell in one nostril.

hemiapraxia (hem″e-ah-prak′se-ah) inability to perform coordinated movements on one side of the body.

hemiataxia (hem″e-ah-tak′se-ah) ataxia on one side of the body.

hemiathetosis (hem″e-ath″ĕ-to′sis) athetosis of one side of the body.

hemiatrophy (hem″e-at′ro-fe) atrophy of one side of the body or one half of an organ of part.

hemiballism, hemiballismus (hem″ĭ-bal′izm; hem″ĭ-bah-liz′mus) violent motor restlessness of half of the body, most marked in the upper extremity.

hemic (he′mik, hem′ik) pertaining to blood.

hemicardia (hem″ĭ-kar′de-ah) the presence of only one side of a four-chambered heart.

hemicellulose (hem″ĭ-sel′u-lōs) general name for a group of high molecular weight carbohydrates resembling cellulose but more soluble and more easily decomposed.

hemicephalia (hem″ĭ-sĕ-fa′le-ah) congenital absence of the cerebrum.

hemicephalus (hem″ĭ-sef′ah-lus) a fetus exhibiting hemicephalia.

hemichorea (hem″e-ko-re′ah) chorea affecting only one side of the body.

hemichromatopsia (hem″ĭ-kro″mah-top′se-ah) defective perception of color in half of the visual field.

hemicolectomy (hem″ĭ-ko-lek′to-me) excision of approximately half of the colon.

hemicorporectomy (hem″ĭ-kor″po-rek′to-me) surgical removal of the lower part of the body, including the bony pelvis, external genitalia, and the lower part of the rectum and anus.

hemicrania (hem″ĭ-kra′ne-ah) 1. headache on one side of the head. 2. a developmental anomaly with absence of half of the cranium.

hemicraniosis (hem″ĭ-kra″ne-o′sis) hyperostosis of one side of the cranium and face.

hemidiaphoresis (hem″ĭ-di″ah-fo-re′sis) sweating on one side of the body only.

hemidysesthesia (hem″ĭ-dis″es-the′ze-ah) a disorder of sensation affecting only one side of the body.

hemidystrophy (hem″ĭ-dis′tro-fe) unequal development of the two sides of the body.

hemiectromelia (hem″e-ek″tro-me′le-ah) a developmental anomaly with imperfect limbs on one side of the body.

hemiepilepsy (hem″e-ep′ĭ-lep″se) epilepsy affecting one side of the body.

hemifacial (hem″ĭ-fa′shal) affecting one side of the face.

hemigastrectomy (hem″ĭ-gas-trek′to-me) excision of half of the stomach.

hemigeusia (hem″ĭ-gu′ze-ah) absence of the sense of taste on one side of the tongue.

hemiglossectomy (hem″ĭ-glŏ-sek′to-me) excision of part of the tongue.

hemiglossitis (hem″ĭ-glŏ-si′tis) inflammation of half of the tongue.

hemignathia (hem″ĭ-na′the-ah) a developmental anomaly characterized by partial or complete lack of the lower jaw on one side.

hemihidrosis (hem″ĭ-hĭ-dro′sis) sweating on one side of the body only.

hemihypalgesia (hem″ĭ-hi″pal-je′ze-ah) diminished sensitivity to pain on one side of the body.

hemihyperesthesia (hem″ĭ-hi″per-es-the′ze-ah) increased sensitivity of one side of the body.

hemihyperhidrosis (hem″ĭ-hi″per-hĭ-dro′sis) excessive sweating on one side of the body.

hemihyperplasia (hem″ĭ-hi″per-pla′ze-ah) overdevelopment of one side of the body or of half of an organ or part.

hemihypertonia (hem″ĭ-hi″per-to′ne-ah) increased muscle tone on one side of the body.

hemihypertrophy (hem″ĭ-hi-per′tro-fe) overgrowth of one side of the body or of a part.

hemihypesthesia (hem″ĭ-hi″pes-the′ze-ah) diminished sensitivity on one side of the body.

hemihypoplasia (hem″ĭ-hi″po-pla′ze-ah) underdevelopment of one side of the body or of half of an organ or part.

hemihypotonia (hem″ĭ-hi″po-to′ne-ah) diminished muscle tone on one side of the body.

hemilaminectomy (hem″ĭ-lam″ĭ-nek′to-me) excision of part of a vertebral lamina.

hemilaryngectomy (hem″ĭ-lar″in-jek′to-me) excision of part of the larynx.

hemilateral (hem″ĭ-lat′er-al) affecting one side of the body only.

hemilesion (hem″ĭ-le′zhun) a lesion on one side of the spinal cord.

hemimelia (hem″ĭ-me′le-ah) congenital absence of all or part of the distal half of a limb.

hemimelus (hem-im′ĕ-lus) an individual exhibiting hemimelia.

hemin (he′min) the crystalline chloride of heme.

heminephrectomy (hem″ĭ-nĕ-frek′to-me) excision of part (half) of a kidney.

hemiopia (hem″e-o′pe-ah) hemianopia.

hemipagus (hem-ip′ah-gus) twin fetuses joined laterally at the thorax.

hemiparalysis (hem″ĭ-pah-ral′ĭ-sis) paralysis of one side of the body.

hemiparanesthesia (hem″ĭ-par″an-es-the′ze-ah) anesthesia of the lower half of one side.

hemiparaplegia (hem″ĭ-par″ah-ple′je-ah) paralysis of the lower half of one side.

hemiparesis (hem″ĭ-pah-re′sis) paresis affecting one side of the body.

hemiparesthesia (hem″ĭ-par″es-the′ze-ah) perverted sensation on one side.

hemipeptone (hem″ĭ-pep′tōn) a form of peptone obtained from pepsin digestion.

hemiplegia (hem″ĭ-ple′je-ah) paralysis of one side of the body; usually caused by a brain lesion, such as a tumor, or by a cerebral vascular accident. adj., **hemiple′gic.** The paralysis occurs on the side opposite the brain disorder. This is explained by the fact that motor axons from the cerebral cortex enter the medulla oblongata and form two well defined bands known at the pyramidal tracts. The majority of the fibers in these tracts cross to the opposite side; therefore damage to the right hemisphere of the brain affects motor control of the left half of the body. (See also CEREBRAL VASCULAR ACCIDENT for symptoms and care of the patient with hemiplegia.)

Hemiptera (hem-ip′ter-ah) an order of arthropods (class Insecta) characterized usually by the presence of two pairs of wings; including some 30,000 species, known as the true bugs, and characterized by having mouth parts adapted to piercing or sucking.

hemipyocyanin (hem″ĭ-pi″o-si′ah-nin) an antibiotic produced by the growth of *Pseudomonas aeruginosa,* which is active against certain fungi.

hemirachischisis (hem″ĭ-rah-kis′kĭ-sis) fissure of the vertebral column without prolapse of the spinal cord.

hemisacralization (hem″ĭ-sa″kral-ĭ-za′shun) fusion of the fifth lumbar vertebra to the first segment of the sacrum on only one side.

hemisection (hem″ĭ-sek′shun) division into two equal parts; bisection.

hemispasm (hem′ĭ-spazm) spasm affecting only one side.

hemisphere (hem′ĭ-sfēr) half of a spherical or roughly spherical structure or organ.

cerebral h., one of the paired structures constituting the largest part of the brain, which together comprise the extensive cerebral cortex, centrum semiovale, basal ganglia, and rhinencephalon, and contain the lateral ventricle. See also BRAIN.

dominant h., that cerebral hemisphere which is more concerned than the other in the integration of sensations and the control of many functions.

hemispherium (hem″ĭ-sfe′re-um), pl. *hemisphe′ria* [L.] hemisphere.

hemithorax (hem″ĭ-tho′raks) one side of the chest; the cavity lateral to the mediastinum.

hemithyroidectomy (hem″ĭ-thi″roi-dek′to-me) excision of one lobe of the thyroid.

hemivertebra (hem″ĭ-ver′tĕ-brah) a developmental anomaly in which one side of a vertebra is incompletely developed.

hemizygosity (hem″ĭ-zi-gos′ĭ-te) the state of having only one of a pair of alleles transmitting a specific character. adj., **hemizy′gous.**

hemizygote (hem″ĭ-zi′got) an individual exhibiting hemizygosity.

hemo- word element [Gr.], *blood.* See also words beginning *hem-* and *hemato-.*

hemoalkalimeter (he″mo-al″kah-lim′ĕ-ter) an apparatus for estimating the alkalinity of the blood.

hemobilia (he″mo-bil′e-ah) hematobilia.

hemoblast (he′mo-blast) hemocytoblast.

hemoblastosis (he″mo-blas-to′sis) a general term for proliferative disorders of the blood-forming tissues.

hemocatheresis (he″mo-kah-ther′ĕ-sis) the destruction of erythrocytes.

hemochorial (he″mo-ko′re-al) denoting a type of placenta in which maternal blood comes in direct contact with the chorion.

hemochromatosis (he″mo-kro″mah-to′sis) a disorder of iron metabolism with excess deposition of iron in the tissues, bronze skin pigmentation, cirrhosis of the liver, and diabetes mellitus. Called also bronze diabetes and iron storage disease. adj., **hemochromotot′ic.**

hemochrome (he′mo-krōm) an oxygen-carrying pigment of the blood.

hemochromogen (he″mo-kro′mo-jen) any compound formed by the combination of heme with a nitrogenous compound.

hemochromometer (he″mo-kro-mom′ĕ-ter) an instrument for making color tests of the blood to determine the proportion of hemoglobin.

hemochromoprotein (he″mo-kro″mo-pro′te-in) a colored, conjugated protein with respiratory functions, found in the blood of animals.

hemoclasis (he-mok′lah-sis) destruction of erythrocytes. adj., **hemoclas′tic.**

hemoconcentration (he″mo-kon″sen-tra′shun) increase in the proportion of formed elements in the blood, as a result of a decrease in its fluid content.

hemoconia (he″mo-ko′ne-ah), pl. *hemoco′niae* [L.] small, round or dumbbell-shaped bodies exhibiting brownian movement, observed in blood platelets in darkfield microscopy of a wet film of blood.

hemoconiosis (he″mo-ko″ne-o′sis) presence in blood of excessive amounts of hemoconia.

hemocryoscopy (he″mo-kris-os′ko-pe) the ascertaining of the freezing point of blood.

hemocrystallin (he″mo-kris′tah-lin) hemoglobin.

hemocuprein (he″mo-koo′prin) a copper and protein compound isolated from erythrocytes.

hemocyanin (he″mo-si′ah-nin) hematocyanin.

hemocyte (he′mo-sīt) a blood cell.

hemocytoblast (he″mo-si′to-blast) the free stem cell from which, according to some theorists, all other blood cells are derived.

hemocytoblastoma (he″mo-si″to-blas-to′mah) a tumor containing all the cells typical of bone marrow.

hemocytocatheresis (he″mo-si″to-kah-ther′ĕ-sis) destruction of erythrocytes.

hemocytogenesis (he″mo-si″to-jen′ĕ-sis) formation of blood cells; hematopoiesis.

hemocytology (he″mo-si-tol′o-je) the study of blood cells.

hemocytolysis (he″mo-si-tol′ĭ-sis) hemolysis.

hemocytometer (he″mo-si-tom′ĕ-ter) an instrument used in counting blood cells, commonly applied to a combination of counting chambers with coverglasses and pipets for erythrocytes and leukocytes, all meeting established specifications.

hemocytotripsis (he″mo-si″to-trip′sis) disintegration of blood cells by pressure.

hemodiagnosis (he″mo-di″ag-no′sis) diagnosis by examination of the blood.

hemodialysis (he″mo-di-al′ĭ-sis) removal of certain elements from the blood by virtue of difference in rates of their diffusion through a semipermeable membrane while the blood is being circulated outside the body. (See also KIDNEY.)

hemodialyzer (he″mo-di′ah-līz″er) an apparatus for performing hemodialysis. Popularly called artificial KIDNEY.

hemodiastase (he″mo-di′as-tās) an amylolytic enzyme found in the blood.

hemodilution (he″mo-di-lu′shun) increase in the fluid content of blood, resulting in diminution of the concentration of formed elements.

hemodynamics (he″mo-di-nam′iks) the study of

the movements of the blood and the forces concerned therein. adj., **hemodynam'ic.**

hemoendothelial (he″mo-en-do-the'le-al) denoting a type of placenta in which maternal blood comes in contact with the endothelium of chorionic vessels.

hemoferrum (he″mo-fer'um) oxyhemoglobin.

hemoflagellate (he″mo-flaj'ĕ-lāt) any flagellate protozoan parasitic in the blood.

hemofuscin (he″mo-fūs'in) a brownish-yellow pigment resulting from hemoglobin decomposition; it gives urine a deep ruddy color.

hemogenesis (he″mo-jen'ĕ-sis) the formation of blood; hematogenesis.

hemogenic (he″mo-jen'ik) pertaining to production of blood.

hemoglobin (he″mo-glo'bin) the oxygen-carrying pigment of the blood, the principal protein in the erythrocyte; it makes up approximately 33 per cent of the cell and averages between 14 and 16 gm. per 100 ml. of whole blood. The pigment in hemoglobin gives blood its red color. Symbol Hb.

Hemoglobin is a chromoprotein, that is, a protein combined with a colored compound. The protein is globin; the pigment is heme, which is red. When erythrocytes are broken down, degradation of hemoglobin releases the pigment bilirubin, which is converted into pigments responsible for the characteristic color of bile. Heme is a complex molecule containing iron.

Hemoglobin has the property of combining chemically with certain gases to form various substances; one of the most important is oxyhemoglobin, formed by the combination of oxygen and hemoglobin. This function of hemoglobin is important in respiration because it provides a means of transporting oxygen from the lungs to the tissues. The oxygen combined with hemoglobin in arterial blood is responsible for its bright red color; venous blood has a darker color because of its lower oxygen content.

Hemoglobin also combines readily with carbon monoxide; this is what happens in carbon monoxide poisoning.

Hemoglobin has been classified according to various types. For example, adult hemoglobin, fetal hemoglobin, and hemoglobin in sickle cell anemia are called hemoglobin A, F, and S, respectively. Homozygosity for hemoglobin S results in sickle cell anemia; heterozygosity in sickle cell trait. Hemoglobins C, D, E, F, I, and J are found in persons with certain blood abnormalities.

Hemoglobin determinations are often used as aids in diagnosing different types of anemias. The amount of hemoglobin may be expressed in grams per 100 ml. of blood or in percentages of normalcy. A value as low as 80 per cent may be considered within the normal range. The results reported in grams are considered more accurate. The normal range expressed in these terms is 14.0 to 18.0 gm. per 100 ml. of blood for men, and 12.0 to 16.0 gm. per 100 ml. of blood for women.

hemoglobinemia (he″mo-glo″bĭ-ne'me-ah) presence of excessive hemoglobin in the blood plasma.

hemoglobinolysis (he″mo-glo″bĭ-nol'ĭ-sis) the splitting up of hemoglobin.

hemoglobinometer (he″mo-glo″bĭ-nom'ĕ-ter) a laboratory instrument for colorimetric determination of the hemoglobin content of the blood.

hemoglobinopathy (he″mo-glo″bĭ-nop'ah-the) any hematologic disorder due to alteration in the genetically determined molecular structure of hemoglobin, with characteristic clinical and laboratory abnormalities and often overt anemia.

hemoglobinous (he″mo-glo'bĭ-nus) containing hemoglobin.

hemoglobinuria (he″mo-glo″bĭ-nu're-ah) the presence of free hemoglobin in the urine. adj., **hemoglobinu'ric.**

epidemic h., hemoglobinuria of young infants, with cyanosis, jaundice, hemorrhage, and polyuria.

intermittent h., that occurring in isolated episodes, e.g., after exposure to cold (paroxysmal cold hemoglobinuria), or idiopathically, usually during the night, with hemosiderinuria, increased amounts of plasma hemoglobin, a positive acid-serum or sucrose-hemolysis test, and often leukopenia or thrombocytopenia (paroxysmal nocturnal hemoglobinuria).

malarial h., blackwater fever.

march h., a rare form following prolonged exercise.

paroxysmal h., intermittent hemoglobinuria.

toxic h., that which is consequent upon the ingestion of various poisons.

hemogram (he'mo-gram) a graphic representation of the differential blood count.

hemohistioblast (he″mo-his'te-o-blast″) the hypothetical stem cell from which all blood cells are derived.

hemoid (he'moid) resembling blood.

hemokinesis (he″mo-ki-ne'sis) the flow of blood in the body. adj., **hemokinet'ic.**

hemolith (he'mo-lith) a concretion in the walls of a blood vessel.

hemolymph (he'mo-limf) 1. blood and lymph. 2. the blood of invertebrates having open blood-vascular systems.

hemolymphangioma (he″mo-lim-fan″je-o'mah) hematolymphangioma.

hemolysate (he-mol'ĭ-sāt) the product resulting from hemolysis.

hemolysin (he-mol'ĭ-sin) a substance that liberates hemoglobin from erythrocytes by interrupting their structural integrity.

hemolysis (he-mol'ĭ-sis) rupture of erythrocytes with release of hemoglobin into the plasma.

Some microbes form substances called hemolysins that have the specific action of destroying red blood corpuscles; the beta-hemolytic streptococcus is an example.

Intravenous administration of a hypotonic solution or plain distilled water will cause the red cells to fill with fluid until their membranes rupture and the cells are destroyed.

In a transfusion reaction or in ERYTHROBLASTOSIS FETALIS, incompatibility causes the red blood cells to clump together. The agglutinated cells become trapped in the smaller vessels and eventually disintegrate, releasing hemoglobin into the plasma. Kidney damage may result as the hemoglobin crystallizes and obstructs the renal tubules, producing renal shutdown and uremia.

Snake venoms and certain vegetable poisons, e.g., mushrooms, may cause hemolysis. A great variety of chemical agents can lead to destruction of erythrocytes if there is exposure to a sufficiently high concentration of the substance. These chemical hemolytics include arsenic, lead, benzene, acetanilid, nitrites, and potassium chlorate.

hemolysoid (he-mol′ĭ-soid) a hemolysin so altered that it still combines with erythrocytes but does not cause hemolysis.

hemolytic (he″mo-lit′ik) pertaining to, characterized by, or producing hemolysis.

h. anemia, anemia caused by the increased destruction of erythrocytes. It may result from Rh incompatibility (see RH FACTOR and ERYTHROBLASTOSIS FETALIS); from mismatched blood transfusions; from industrial poisons such as benzene, trinitrotoluene (TNT) or aniline; and from hypersensitivity to certain antibiotics and tranquilizers. Hemolytic anemia may occur as a result of a disorder of the IMMUNE RESPONSE in which B-cell–produced antibodies fail to recognize erythrocytes that are "self" and directly attack and destroy them. Hemolytic anemia may also appear in the course of other diseases such as widespread cancer, leukemia, Hodgkin's disease, acute alcoholism, and liver diseases. In addition to the usual symptoms of anemia, the patient may exhibit JAUNDICE.

Severe hemolytic anemia may be very quickly fatal. Victims must be hospitalized immediately so that transfusions can be given and other treatment begun. If the cause of the condition can be located, and if it can be successfully treated, there is a good chance of recovery. In some cases, surgery to remove the SPLEEN may bring about great improvement. (See also ANEMIA for a discussion of patient care.)

h. disease of newborn, a condition marked by excessive blood destruction in newborn infants; caused by transplacental transfer of antibodies produced by the mother in response to passage of incompatible blood from the fetal to the maternal circulation and usually the result of incompatibility of the Rh factor. (See also ERYTHROBLASTOSIS FETALIS.)

h. jaundice, a rare, chronic, and generally hereditary disease characterized by periods of excessive hemolysis due to abnormal fragility of the erythrocytes, which are small and spheroidal. It is accompanied by enlargement of the spleen and by jaundice. The hereditary or congenital form is known as congenital familial icterus and familial acholuric jaundice; the acquired form is known as acquired hemolytic jaundice.

hemolyze (he′mo-līz) to subject to or to undergo hemolysis.

hemomediastinum (he″mo-me″de-ah-sti′num) an effusion of blood into the mediastinum.

hemometer (he-mom′ĕ-ter) hemoglobinometer.

hemometra (he″mo-me′trah) hematometra.

hemonephrosis (he″mo-nĕ-fro′sis) effused blood in the renal pelvis; hematonephrosis.

hemopathology (he″mo-pah-thol′o-je) the study of diseases of the blood.

hemopathy (he-mop′ah-the) any disease of the blood. adj., **hemopath′ic.**

hemopericardium (he″mo-per″ĭ-kar′de-um) an effusion of blood in the pericardial cavity.

hemoperitoneum (he″mo-per″ĭ-to-ne′um) an effusion of blood in the peritoneal cavity.

hemopexin (he″mo-pek′sin) a heme-binding serum protein.

hemopexis (he″mo-pek′sis) coagulation of blood.

hemophagocyte (he″mo-fag′o-sīt) a cell that destroys blood corpuscles.

hemophil (he′mo-fil) 1. thriving on blood. 2. a microorganism that grows best in media containing hemoglobin.

hemophilia (he″mo-fil′e-ah) a condition characterized by impaired coagulability of the blood, and a strong tendency to bleed. The *classic disease* is hereditary, and limited to males, being transmitted always through the female to the second generation, but many similar conditions attributable to the absence of different factors from the blood are now recognized.

SYMPTOMS. In addition to excessive bleeding from minor wounds, a hemophiliac may be subject to spontaneous hemorrhages under the skin and in the gums, gastrointestinal tract, joints, and muscles. Hemarthrosis may cause the joints to stiffen and may result in permanent crippling if it is permitted to go untreated.

TREATMENT. General treatment is directed toward raising the level of clotting factor VIII (AHF, or antihemophilic factor) in the patient's blood. Serious occurrences of bleeding require transfusion of fresh whole blood or of blood plasma to replace lost blood and to increase temporarily the clotting power of the hemophiliac. The patient must learn to avoid trauma and to obtain prompt medical attention for any bleeding, no matter how slight it may seem. Before any surgery or dental treatment the patient must be given an infusion of special plasma. Also, arrangements should be made for blood donors so that there will be sufficient blood available for transfusion if it is needed. Whenever these patients must receive injections, a small needle is used, pressure is applied at the site after the needle is withdrawn and the area should be inspected frequently for bleeding until the danger of hemorrhage is past.

h. A, classical hemophilia, due to deficiency of clotting factor VIII, transmitted by the female to the male as a sex-linked recessive abnormality.

h. B, a form similar to classical hemophilia but due to a deficiency of clotting factor IX; called also Christmas disease.

h. C, an autosomal dominant form due to deficiency of clotting factor XI.

vascular h., angiohemophilia.

hemophiliac (he″mo-fil′e-ak) a person affected with hemophilia.

hemophilic (he″mo-fil′ik) 1. pertaining to hemophilia. 2. living or growing especially well in blood.

hemophilioid (he″mo-fil′e-oid) resembling classical hemophilia clinically, but not due solely to clotting factor VIII deficiency.

Hemophilus (he-mof′ĭ-lus) a genus of gram-negative bacteria, most species of which have a nutritional requirement for the constituents of fresh blood.

H. aegyp′tius, an organism closely related to *H. influenzae,* which is the cause of pinkeye (acute contagious conjunctivitis).

H. ducrey′i, the causative agent of chancroid.

H. influen′zae, a species once thought to be the cause of epidemic influenza; it produces a highly fatal form of meningitis, especially in infants.

H. vagina′lis, a hemophilic bacterium associated, possibly causally, with human vaginitis.

hemophoric (he″mo-for′ik) conveying blood.

hemophthalmia (he″mof-thal′me-ah) extravasation of blood inside the eye.

hemopleura (he″mo-ploo′rah) hemothorax.

hemopneumopericardium (he″mo-nu″mo-per″ĭ-kar′de-um) effused blood and air in the pericardium.

hemopneumothorax (he″mo-nu″mo-tho′raks) an accumulation of blood and air in the pleural cavity.

hemopoiesis (he″mo-poi-e′sis) hematopoiesis. adj., **hemopoiet′ic.**

hemoprecipitin (he″mo-pre-sip′ĭ-tin) a precipitin specific for blood.

hemoprotein (he″mo-pro′te-in) a conjugated protein whose nonprotein portion is heme.

hemopsonin (he″mop-so′nin) an opsonin that renders erythrocytes more liable to phagocytosis. Called also erythrocyto-opsonin.

hemoptysis (he-mop′tĭ-sis) coughing and spitting of blood as a result of bleeding from any part of the respiratory tract. In true hemoptysis the sputum is bright red and frothy with air bubbles; it must not be confused with the dark red or black color of hematemesis.

Although recent developments in drug therapy have reduced the incidence of serious bleeding in tuberculous patients, tuberculosis remains a common cause of hemoptysis. Other causes may be bronchiectasis, lung abscess, or malignancy. In acute pneumonia the sputum may be bright red or it may contain old blood which gives it a characteristic rusty appearance. Vascular disorders such as congestive heart failure, pulmonary infarction, and aortic aneurysm can also cause hemoptysis.

Treatment is aimed at the primary cause of the symptom. The patient with severe hemorrhage is more likely to die from drowning in his own blood than from blood loss. Emergency measures for severe hemoptysis include application of an ice pack to the neck and chest, administration of a sedative, and absolute bed rest with the head of the bed elevated slightly. The patient may be given codeine to depress the cough reflex, and he should be instructed to cough with the glottis open, without straining.

parasitic h., a disease due to infection of the lungs with lung flukes of the genus *Paragonimus,* with cough and spitting of blood and gradual deterioration of health.

hemorrhage (hem′ŏ-rij) the escape of blood from a ruptured vessel. Hemorrhage can be external, internal, or into the skin or other tissues. Blood from an artery is bright red in color and comes in spurts; that from a vein is dark red and comes in a steady flow.

SYMPTOMS. Aside from the obvious flow of blood from a wound or body orifice, massive hemorrhage can be detected by other signs, such as restlessness, cold and clammy skin, thirst, increased and thready pulse, rapid and shallow respirations, and a drop in blood pressure. If the hemorrhage continues unchecked, the patient may complain of visual disturbances, ringing in the ears, or extreme weakness.

FIRST AID

From Severe wound

1. Apply direct pressure on the wound with a thick compress of gauze or any other available clean cloth. If necessary, use bare hands or fingers.

2. When bleeding has been controlled, bind the compress firmly in place with strips of cloth.

3. If direct pressure does not control bleeding, apply digital pressure at the appropriate pressure point.

Internal Bleeding

1. Following injury, blood flowing from the mouth, nose, or ears may indicate fracture of the skull or serious internal injury. Do *not* move the patient. Summon medical help immediately.

2. Until help arrives, the patient should be covered with a blanket or coat. If possible, keep the head and chest a little lower than the body and elevate the legs.

Further treatment consists of measures to stop the flow of blood, to combat shock and circulatory collapse, and to replace lost blood by transfusion.

capillary h., oozing of blood from minute vessels.

cerebral h., a hemorrhage into the cerebrum; one of the three main causes of CEREBRAL VASCULAR ACCIDENT (stroke).

concealed h., internal hemorrhage.

fibrinolytic h., that due to abnormalities in the fibrinolytic system and not dependent on hypofibrinogenemia.

internal h., that in which the extravasated blood remains within the body.

intracranial h., bleeding within the cranium, which may be extradural, subdural, subarachnoid, or cerebral.

petechial h., subcutaneous hemorrhage occurring in minute spots.

postpartum h., that which follows soon after labor.

primary h., that which soon follows an injury.

secondary h., that which follows an injury after a considerable lapse of time.

hemorrhagenic (hem″o-rah-jen′ik) causing hemorrhage.

hemorrhagic (hem″o-raj′ik) pertaining to or characterized by hemorrhage.

h. disease of newborn, a self-limited hemorrhagic disorder of the first days of life, caused by deficiency of vitamin K–dependent blood clotting factors II, VII, IX, and X.

epidemic h. fever, an acute infectious disease characterized by fever, purpura, peripheral vascular collapse, and acute renal failure, caused by a filterable agent thought to be transmitted to man by mites or chiggers.

h. fevers, a group of viral diseases of diverse etiology but having many similar clinical characteristics: increased capillary permeability, leukopenia, and thrombocytopenia are common to all. They are manifested by sudden onset, fever, headache, generalized myalgia, backache, conjunctivitis, and severe prostration, followed by various hemorrhagic symptoms, which result in focal inflammatory reaction and necrosis, with mild leukocytosis.

hemorrhea (hem″o-re′ah) hematorrhea.

hemorrheology (he″mo-re-ol′o-je) the scientific study of the deformation and flow properties of cellular and plasmatic components of blood in macroscopic, microscopic, and submicroscopic dimensions and the rheologic properties of vessel structure with which the blood comes in direct contact.

hemorrhoid (hem′ŏ-roid) an enlarged (varicose) vein in the mucous membrane inside or just outside the rectum that causes pain, itching, discomfort, and bleeding.

Hemorrhoids (called also piles) are usually caused by straining to evacuate hard, dry stools.

They sometimes occur in pregnancy because of pressure on the veins from the enlarged uterus. They may result from pressure on the veins caused by a disorder of the liver or the heart or may be symptomatic of a tumor or growth that causes pressure against the veins.

Temporary relief from hemorrhoids can usually be obtained by cold compresses, sitz baths, fecal softeners, or an analgesic ointment. Treatment of the condition is by surgical removal of the hemorrhoids by ligation and excision (HEMORRHOIDECTOMY) or by Barron ligation.

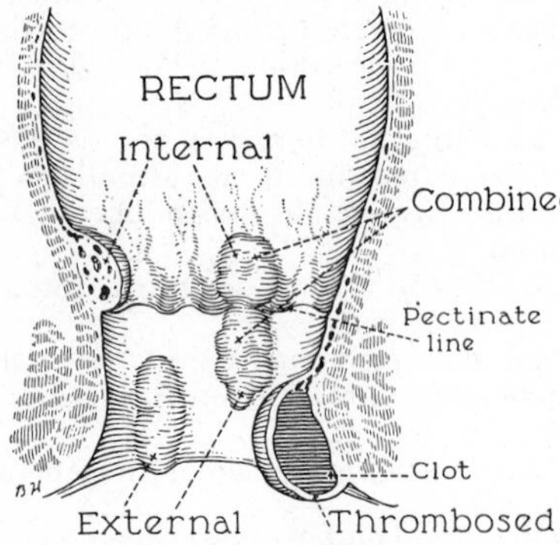

Types of hemorrhoids.

external h., one distal to the pectinate line.

internal h., one originating above the pectinate line and covered by mucous membrane.

prolapsed h., an internal hemorrhoid that has descended below the pectinate line and protruded outside the anal sphincter.

strangulated h., an internal hemorrhoid that has prolapsed sufficiently and for long enough time for its blood supply to become occluded by the constricting action of the anal sphincter.

hemorrhoidectomy (hem″ŏ-roi-dek′to-me) surgical excision of hemorrhoids. Although the operation is considered minor and dressings may not be needed, the patient may experience much discomfort and require analgesic drugs and frequent nursing measures to relieve discomfort.

PATIENT CARE. Postoperatively the patient must be watched for signs of hemorrhage, an uncommon occurrence but one that can develop quickly. The patient may be placed on his abdomen to relieve pressure on the operative site, or he may lie on his back with a rubber air ring under the buttocks for support. Warm stiz baths are usually begun the day after surgery to relieve disomfort. Compresses of witch hazel or some other astringent agent may be applied to reduce swelling and promote healing. Difficulty in evacuating often occurs during the immediate postoperative period. Sitz baths are quite helpful in relieving this situation.

hemosiderin (he″mo-sid′er-in) an insoluble form of storage iron, visible microscopically both with and without the use of special stains.

hemosiderinuria (hem″o-sid″er-in-u′re-ah) the presence of hemosiderin in the urine.

hemosiderosis (he″mo-sid″ĕ-ro′sis) a focal or general increase in tissue iron stores without associated tissue damage.

hemospermia (he″mo-sper′me-ah) the presence of blood in the semen.

hemostasis (he″mo-sta′sis, he-mos′tah-sis) arrest of the escape of blood by either natural (clot formation or vessel spasm) or artificial (compression or ligation) means, or the interruption of blood flow to a part.

hemostat (he′mo-stat) 1. a small surgical clamp for constricting blood vessels. 2. an antihemorrhagic agent.

hemostatic (he″mo-stat′ik) 1. checking blood flow. 2. an agent that checks the flow of blood.

hemostyptic (he″mo-stip′tik) hemostatic.

hemotherapy (he″mo-ther′ah-pe) the use of blood in treating disease.

hemothorax (he″mo-tho′raks) collection of blood in the pleural cavity.

hemotoxic (he″mo-tok′sik) hematotoxic.

hemotoxin (he″mo-tok′sin) an exotoxin characterized by hemolytic activity.

hemotroph (he′mo-trōf) the sum total of the nutritive material from the circulating blood of the maternal body, utilized by the early embryo. adj., **hemotroph′ic.**

henbane (hen′bān) hyoscyamus.

Henle's fissure (hen′lēz) spaces filled with connective tissue between the muscular fibers of the heart.

Henle's layer (hen′lēz) the outermost layer of the inner root sheath of the hair follicle.

Henle's ligament (hen′lēz) a lateral expansion of the lateral edge of the rectus abdominis which attaches to the pubic bone.

Henle's loop (hen′lēz) the U-shaped loop of the uriniferous tubule of the kidney.

Henle's membrane (hen′lēz) fenestrated membrane.

Henle's sheath (hen′lēz) the endoneurium, especially the delicate continuation around terminal branches of nerve fibers; called also connective tissue sheath of Key and Retzius.

Henle's tubules (hen′lēz) the straight ascending and descending portions of a renal tubule forming Henle's loop.

Henoch's chorea (hen′ōks) chronic progressive electric chorea.

Henoch's disease (purpura) (hen′ōks) Schönlein-Henoch purpura in which abdominal symptoms predominate.

Henry's law (hen′rēz) the solubility of a gas in a liquid solution is proportionate to the partial pressure of the gas.

hepar (he′par) [L.] liver.

heparin (hep′ah-rin) an anticoagulant mucopolysaccharide acid occurring in tissues, most abundantly in the liver, or a mixture of active principles from the livers or lungs of domestic animals (sodium heparin) which renders the blood incoagulable; used in the prevention and treatment of thrombosis, in bacterial endocarditis, in postoperative pulmonary embolism, and frostbite, and in repair of vascular injury. Heparin is an ANTICOAGULANT and a patient receiving this drug must be watched for signs of spontaneous bleeding.

heparinize (hep′er-ĭ-nīz″) to treat with heparin.

hepat(o)- (hep′ah-to) word element [Gr.], *liver.*

hepatalgia (hep″ah-tal′je-ah) pain in the liver.

hepatatrophia (hep″ah-tah-tro′fe-ah) atrophy of the liver.

hepatectomize (hep″ah-tek′to-mīz) to deprive of the liver by surgical removal.

hepatectomy (hep″ah-tek′to-me) surgical excision of liver tissue.

hepatic (hĕ-pat′ik) pertaining to the liver.

h. duct, the excretory duct of the liver, or one of its branches in the lobes of the liver (see also BILE DUCTS).

hapatic(o)- (hĕ-pat′ĭ-ko) word element [Gr.], *hepatic duct.*

hepaticoduodenostomy (hĕ-pat″ĭ-ko-du″o-dĕ-nos′to-me) anastomosis of the hepatic duct to the duodenum.

hepaticoenterostomy (hĕ-pat″ĭ-ko-en″ter-os′to-me) anastomosis of the hepatic duct to the intestine (duodenum or jejunum).

hepaticogastrostomy (hĕ-pat″ĭ-ko-gas-tros′to-me) anastomosis of the hepatic duct to the stomach.

hepaticojejunostomy (hĕ-pat″ĭ-ko-je″joo-nos′to-me) anastomosis of the hepatic duct to the jejunum.

hepaticolithotomy (hĕ-pat″ĭ-ko-lĭ-thot′o-me) incision of the hepatic duct with removal of calculi.

hepaticolithotripsy (hĕ-pat″ĭ-ko-lith′o-trip″se) the crushing of a calculus in the hepatic duct.

hepaticostomy (hĕ-pat″ĭ-kos′to-me) fistulization of the hepatic duct.

hepaticotomy (hĕ-pat″ĭ-kot′o-me) incision of the hepatic duct.

hepatin (hep′ah-tin) glycogen.

hepatitis (hep″ah-ti′tis) inflammation of the liver. It may be secondary to other disorders such as AMEBIC DYSENTERY, CIRRHOSIS, or infectious MONONUCLEOSIS, it may be drug-induced, or it may be due to a viral infection. The virus can be transmitted by the fecal-oral route through contaminated foods or liquids (most often, hepatitis A). In serum hepatitis (most often, hepatitis B) the virus is present in the serum of a blood donor and is transmitted by administration of infected blood or blood products. Improved sterilization techniques for disinfecting needles, syringes, intravenous equipment, and other articles that might be contaminated with the virus, and the use of disposable equipment, have largely erased this source of infection.

The only immunization generally available is passive protection by immune serum globulin. Research is being conducted to develop active and passive specific prevention of hepatitis B.

SYMPTOMS. The symptoms of hepatitis include loss of appetite, nausea, fever, local tenderness in the region of the liver, and enlargement of the liver. As the disease progresses, jaundice becomes evident and there is rapid loss of weight and strength.

TREATMENT. Bed rest is prescribed and continued until the patient is free of symptoms. During the convalescent period physical activities are limited, sometimes for as long as 2 to 3 months, to prevent permanent damage to the liver. The diet is planned to provide an adequate intake of protein to repair damaged tissue cells, and a high intake of carbohydrates, which are thought to have a protective effect on the liver cells. There are no specific drugs used in the treatment of hepatitis.

PATIENT CARE. During the acute phase of the disease the patient with infectious hepatitis is cared for under "enteric precautions" (see ISOLATION TECHNIQUE). Special care must be used in the handling of all articles and equipment contaminated by bodily excretions from the patient. The patient must be encouraged to rest as much as possible and to eat all of the meals and between-meal feedings offered to him. If nausea or other conditions interfere with adequate intake of the prescribed diet, the situation should be reported to the physician so that supplemental feedings may be administered intravenously.

h. A, infectious hepatitis; an acute viral (hepatitis virus A) illness, usually transmitted by oral ingestion of infected material, but also by blood transfusion (see hepatitis B), usually beginning with fever, malaise, and nonspecific gastrointestinal symptoms, followed by jaundice, pruritus, dark urine, pale stools, and hepatomegaly with tenderness. The incubation period is short (one to six weeks).

anicteric h., a mild hepatitis without jaundice, usually seen in young children. May be confused with gastrointestinal "flu."

h. B, serum hepatitis; an acute viral (hepatitis virus B) illness once considered to be transmitted only by parenteral exposure (contaminated needles and administration of blood or blood products) but now known to be transmitted also by oral ingestion of contaminated material. The incubation period is relatively long (4 to 24 weeks) and the acute illness tends to be more prolonged than that of hepatitis A.

infectious h., hepatitis A.

serum h., hepatitis B.

transfusion h., hepatitis B.

viral h., hepatitis A and hepatitis B.

hepatization (hep″ah-tĭ-za′shun) transformation into a liver-like mass, especially the solidified state of the lung in lobar pneumonia. The early stage, in which the pulmonary exudate is blood stained, is called red hepatization. The later stage, in which the red cells disintegrate and a fibrinosuppurative exudate persists, is called gray hepatization.

hepatoblastoma (hep″ah-to-blas-to′mah) a malignant intrahepatic tumor consisting chiefly of embryonic tissue, occurring in infants and young children.

hepatocarcinoma (hep″ah-to-kar″sĭ-no′mah) carcinoma derived from the parenchymal cells of the liver (hepatocytes).

hepatocele (hep′ah-to-sēl″) hernia of the liver.

hepatocellular (hep″ah-to-sel′u-lar) pertaining to or affecting liver cells.

hepatocholangitis (hep″ah-to-ko″lan-ji′tis) inflammation of the liver and bile ducts.

hepatocirrhosis (hep″ah-to-sĭ-ro′sis) cirrhosis of the liver.

hepatocuprein (hep″ah-to-koo′prin) a copper protein present in liver tissue.

hepatocystic (hep″ah-to-sis′tik) pertaining to the liver and gallbladder.

hepatocyte (hep′ah-to-sīt″) a parenchymal liver cell.

hepatodynia (hep″ah-to-din′e-ah) pain in the liver.

hepatogastric (hep″ah-to-gas′trik) pertaining to the liver and stomach.

hepatogenic (hep″ah-to-jen′ik) 1. giving rise to or forming liver tissue. 2. hepatogenous.

hepatogenous (hep″ah-toj′ĕ-nus) 1. originating in or caused by the liver. 2. hepatogenic.

hepatogram (hep′ah-to-gram″) 1. a tracing of the liver pulse in the sphygmogram. 2. a roentgenogram of the liver.

hepatography (hep″ah-tog′rah-fe) 1. a treatise on the liver. 2. roentgenography of the liver. 3. the recording of the liver pulse.

hepatojugular (hep″ah-to-jug′u-lar) pertaining to the liver and jugular vein.

h. reflux, distention of the jugular vein induced by manual pressure over the liver; it suggests insufficiency of the right heart.

hepatolenticular degeneration (hep″ah-to-len-tik′u-lar) a hereditary disorder of copper metabolism, marked by a pigmented ring at the outer margin of the cornea, degenerative changes in the brain, cirrhosis of the liver, splenomegaly, tremor, rigidity, contractures, psychic disturbances, dysphagia, and increasing weakness and emaciation. Commonly called Wilson's disease.

hepatolienography (hep″ah-to-li″ĕ-nog′rah-fe) roentgenography of the liver and spleen.

hepatolith (hep′ah-to-lith″) a calculus in the liver.

hepatolithectomy (hep″ah-to-lĭ-thek′to-me) removal of a calculus from the liver.

hepatolithiasis (hep″ah-to-lĭ-thi′ah-sis) the presence of calculi in the biliary ducts of the liver.

hepatology (hep″ah-tol′o-je) the scientific study of the liver and its diseases.

hepatolysin (hep″ah-tol′ĭ-sin) a cytolysin destructive to liver cells.

hepatolysis (hep″ah-tol′ĭ-sis) destruction of the liver cells. adj., **hepatolyt′ic.**

hepatoma (hep″ah-to′mah) 1. any tumor of the liver. 2. a malignant hepatic tumor whose cells resemble parenchymal liver cells.

hepatomalacia (hep″ah-to-mah-la′she-ah) softening of the liver.

hepatomegaly (hep″ah-to-meg′ah-le) enlargement of the liver.

hepatomelanosis (hep″ah-to-mel″ah-no′sis) melanosis of the liver.

hepatomphalocele (hep″ah-tom′fah-lo-sēl″) umbilical hernia with liver involvement in the hernial sac.

hepatonephric (hep″ah-to-nef′rik) pertaining to the liver and kidney.

hepatopathy (hep″ah-top′ah-the) any disease of the liver.

hepatopexy (hep′ah-to-pek″se) surgical fixation of a displaced liver to the abdominal wall.

hepatopleural (hep″ah-to-ploo′ral) pertaining to the liver and pleura or pleural cavity.

hepatopneumonic (hep″ah-to-nu-mon′ik) pertaining to, affecting, or communicating with the liver and lungs.

hepatoportal (hep″ah-to-por′tal) pertaining to the portal system of the liver.

hepatopulmonary (hep″ah-to-pul′mo-ner″e) hepatopneumonic.

hepatorenal (hep″ah-to-re′nal) pertaining to the liver and kidneys.

hepatorrhaphy (hep″ah-tor′ah-fe) suture of the liver.

hepatorrhexis (hep″ah-to-rek′sis) rupture of the liver.

hepatoscan (hep′ah-to-skan″) a surface scintiscan of the liver.

hepatoscopy (hep″ah-tos′ko-pe) examination of the liver.

hepatosis (hep″ah-to′sis) any functional disorder of the liver.

serous h., veno-occlusive disease of the liver.

hepatosplenitis (hep″ah-to-sple-ni′tis) inflammation of the liver and spleen.

hepatosplenography (hep″ah-to-sple-nog′rah-fe) roentgenography of the liver and spleen.

hepatosplenomegaly (hep″ah-to-sple″no-meg′ah-le) enlargement of the liver and spleen.

hepatotherapy (hep″ah-to-ther′ah-pe) administration of liver or liver extract.

hepatotomy (hep″ah-tot′o-me) incision of the liver.

hepatotoxemia (hep″ah-to-tok-se′me-ah) septicemia originating in the liver.

hepatotoxin (hep″ah-to-tok′sin) a toxin that destroys liver cells. adj., **hepatotox′ic.**

hepta- (hep′tah) word element [Gr.], *seven.*

heptabarbital (hep″tah-bar′bĭ-tal) a short-acting barbiturate used as a hypnotic and sedative.

heptachromic (hep″tah-kro′mik) 1. pertaining to or exhibiting seven colors. 2. having vision for all seven colors of the spectrum.

heptapeptide (hep″tah-pep′tīd) a polypeptide containing seven amino acids.

heptaploidy (hep′tah-ploi″de) the state of having seven sets of chromosomes. adj., **hep′taploid.**

heptose (hep′tōs) a sugar whose molecule contains seven carbon atoms.

hereditary (hĕ-red′ĭ-ter″e) transmissible or transmitted from parent to offspring; genetically determined.

heredity (hĕ-red′ĭ-te) the genetic transmission of traits from parents to offspring. The hereditary material is contained in the ovum and sperm, so that the child's heredity is determined at the moment of conception.

CHROMOSOMES AND GENES. Inside the nucleus of each germ cell are structures called *chromosomes.* A chromosome is composed of DEOXYRIBONUCLEIC ACID (DNA) on a framework of protein. Genes are segments of the DNA molecule; there are thousands of GENES in each cell. Each gene carries a specific hereditary trait. These traits are physical, biochemical, and physiologic. Thus genes affect not only the physical appearance of an individual but also his physiologic makeup, his tendency to develop certain diseases, and the daily activities of all the cells of his body.

The human ovum contains 23 chromosomes. The sperm also contains 23 chromosomes, and aside from the pair determining the sex, each one is similar in shape and size to one in the ovum. When the sperm penetrates the ovum, the fertilized ovum thus contains 23 pairs of chromosomes, or 46 chromosomes in all.

The fertilized ovum then begins to reproduce itself by dividing (mitosis). The original cell divides and forms two cells, each of these divides and forms a total of four cells and so on until a many-celled embryo begins to take form.

In the process of cell division, the chromosomes in the nucleus have the ability to make duplicates of themselves. They do not split in two, but instead each one produces another chromosome exactly like itself. When the two cells are formed from one, the chromosomes are divided so that each cell contains the same number and kind of chromosomes as the original. For this reason, all the cells in the developing embryo and in the human body, except the ovum and sperm, contain identical sets of 46 chromosomes.

The ovum and the sperm are formed by a special process of cell division (meiosis) in which each sperm or ovum receives only one member of each chromosome pair. If this were not true, and sperm or ova contained the full complement of 46 chromosomes, the cells of the offspring would have 92 chromosomes, their offspring would have 184 and so on. As it is, the amount of hereditary material in the body cells remains constant from generation to generation.

In the formation of the germ cells, it is a matter of chance which member of each pair of chromosomes goes to a given ovum or sperm. It is also purely a matter of chance which sperm fertilizes an ovum. Incredible as it seems, there are, all in all, about 70 trillion possible combinations of chromosomes that a child can inherit.

INHERITED TRAITS. Although many of the details of human heredity are not known, in general we can say that the child receives a set of genes from his parents. These genes, or hereditary determinants, develop into characteristics which reflect those of his parents, grandparents, and other ancestors. Before birth these inherited traits are influenced by conditions within the mother's body. After birth they are shaped in various ways by environmental influences such as diet, training, and education.

Some specific aspects of human heredity are well understood, for example, the inheritance of eye color. Remember that one member of a chromosome pair is contributed by one parent and the other by the other parent. A gene in one chromosome acts on the same trait as a gene in the same position on the other chromosome.

It has been found that one gene may be more powerful in its influence than the other gene that acts on the same trait. The more powerful gene is then said to be dominant, and the other gene is said to be recessive. A gene that produces blue eyes, for example is recessive to a gene that produces brown eyes.

SEX DETERMINATION. Of the 23 pairs of chromosomes in each of the body cells, one pair is distinctly different from the others. The members of this pair are the sex chromosomes, and they determine the sex of offspring. In the female, they look alike and are termed X chromosomes. But in the male, one sex chromosome is an X chromosome and the other is a smaller, Y chromosome. Thus each germ cell produced by the male contains either an X or a Y chromosome. If a sperm containing a Y chromosome fertilizes an egg, the child will be male. If the sperm has an X chromosome, the child will be female.

In the development of the male embryo it is essential that fetal male hormones (androgens) be released at a certain time during early gestation. Otherwise, the infant will be born with external female genitalia even though he has the chromosomal sex pattern of a male and has no internal female reproductive organs.

SEX-LINKED TRAITS. Certain hereditary traits are known as sex-linked because they are carried on the X chromosome. Color blindness is an example. This condition, in which colors appear as varying shades of gray, is rare in females but appears in about 8 per cent of the male population. The genes for color vision are located on the X chromosomes, and the gene for normal vision is dominant to that for color blindness. A female having one gene for normal vision on one X chromosome and one for color blindness on the other will have normal vision, since the color blindness gene is recessive. A male, however, having only one X chromosome, will be color blind if that chromosome has the recessive gene, since there is no corresponding dominant gene to suppress it.

It is possible for a female to be color blind, if she has two of the recessive genes, but it is quite rare that these two genes come together in one person.

Another characteristic associated with sex is baldness. The gene for baldness is dominant in males and recessive in females. Thus a male need have only one gene for baldness for the trait to be expressed, but a female must have two.

HEREDITARY DISEASES. Hereditary diseases should be distinguished from congenital birth defects. A congenital defect is one that the infant is born with, such as a cleft lip, a birthmark, or congenital syphilis, but the defect can arise during conception or pregnancy and not be related to heredity. Hereditary diseases, on the other hand, are passed from generation to generation by genes. Some diseases, such as cystic fibrosis, are transmitted by recessive genes.

Classic HEMOPHILIA is a hereditary disease transmitted by a sex-linked gene. A recessive gene carried on the X chromosome is responsible for it, and it is transmitted in the same way as color blindness. In the extremely rare cases of a female carrying two recessive genes for the trait, the victim usually dies at the onset of menstruation.

Medical scientists believe that although certain diseases are not inherited directly, the tendency to contract them may be inherited. Epilepsy, for example, occurs more frequently in some families than in others. The tendency to develop allergy, asthma, and bronchitis also seems to run in families. Whether these conditions actually develop in a person with such a tendency depends on environmental circumstances. Strong evidence indicates that nearsightedness, farsightedness, and night blindness have a hereditary basis.

Certain mental disorders are known to be hereditary. It has been dicovered in recent years that there is an abnormality in the chromosomes in children afflicted with DOWN'S SYNDROME (mongolism). This condition is classified as a trisomy, which refers to the state of having an extra chromosome per cell. Inborn errors of metabolism such as PHENYLKETONURIA and GALACTOSEMIA are inherited.

ROLE OF MUTATION. Mutation is the term used for a spontaneous change in a chromosome or gene. Normally chromosomes duplicate themselves exactly during cell division. Occasionally, however, the new cells contain an altered gene or chromosome. If the mutation occurs in an ovum or sperm involved in reproduction, the new trait will be expressed in the offspring.

Many mutations are so minor that they have no visible effect. A mutation that is very harmful will usually result in the death of the fetus and spontaneous abortion. Occasionally a mutation is beneficial. Favorable mutations gradually tend to spread through a population. The accumulation of mutations over millions of years has contributed to evolution.

heredofamilial (her″ĕ-do-fah-mil′e-al) occurring in certain families under circumstances that implicate a hereditary basis.

Hering's theory color perception depends on a visual substance in the retina which is variously modified by anabolism for black, green, and blue, and by catabolism for white, red, and yellow.

Hering-Breuer reflexes inflation and deflation reflexes that help regulate the rhythmic ventilation of the lungs, thereby preventing overdistention and extreme deflation. These reflexes arise outside the respiratory center in the brain; that is, the receptor sites are located in the respiratory tract, mainly in the bronchi and bronchioles. They are activated by either a stretching or a non-stretching and compression of the lung; the impulses are transmitted from the receptor sites through the vagus nerve to the brain stem and thence to the respiratory center.

The *inflation* reflex acts to inhibit inspiration and thereby prevents further inflation. When the lung tissue is stretched by inflation, the stretch receptors respond by sending impulses to the respiratory center, which in turn slows down inspiration. As the expiratory phase begins, the receptors are no longer stretched, impulses are no longer sent, and inspiration can begin again. This is called the Hering-Breuer *deflation* reflex. It is also believed that in addition to the cessation of impulses from the stretch receptors, there may be an activation of compression receptors which transmit impulses that inhibit expiration, thus allowing inspiration to begin.

hermaphrodism (her-maf′ro-dizm) hermaphroditism.

hermaphrodite (her-maf′ro-dīt) an individual whose body contains tissue of both male and female gonads. The ovaries and testes may be present as separate organs, or ovarian and testicular tissue may be combined in the same organ (ovotestis). See also HERMAPHRODITISM.

hermaphroditism (her-maf′ro-di-tizm″) a state characterized by the presence of both ovarian and testicular tissue and of ambiguous morphologic criteria of sex, a rare condition in human beings. Hermaphroditism is not to be confused with pseudohermaphroditism, in which an individual with only one kind of gonad possesses reproductive organs that reflect some characteristics of the opposite sex, owing to improper balance of male and female hormones or other endocrine disorder.

bilateral h., that in which gonadal tissue typical of both sexes occurs on each side of the body.

false h., pseudohermaphroditism.

lateral h., presence of gonadal tissue typical of one sex on one side of the body and tissue typical of the other sex on the opposite side.

transverse h., that in which the external genital organs are typical of one sex and the gonads typical of the other sex.

true h., coexistence in the same person of both ovarian and testicular tissue, with somatic characters typical of both sexes.

unilateral h., presence of gonadal tissue typical of both sexes on one side and of only an ovary or a testis on the other.

hermetic (her-met′ik) impervious to the air.

hernia (her′ne-ah) the abnormal protrusion of part of an organ or tissue through the structures normally containing it. adj., **her′nial.** In this condition, a weak spot or other abnormal opening in a body wall permits part of the organ to bulge through. A hernia may develop in various parts of the body; it occurs most commonly in the region of the abdomen.

A layman's term for hernia is rupture. The word rupture is misleading, because it suggests tearing and nothing is torn in a hernia. A hernia is either acquired or congenital.

Although various supports and trusses can be tried in an effort to contain the hernia, the best treatment of this condition is surgical repair of the weakness in the muscle wall through which the hernia protrudes. This procedure is called HERNIORRHAPHY.

h. cer′ebri, protrusion of brain substance through the skull.

crural h., femoral hernia.

diaphragmatic h., protrusion of some of the contents of the abdomen through an opening in the diaphragm into the chest cavity. The condition may be congenital or acquired, in some cases as a result of severe injury. Hiatal hernia is one type of diaphragmatic hernia. Symptoms, which are noted especially when the stomach is full after a meal, include heartburn, indigestion, difficulty in breathing, and pain that may in some instances extend to the neck and arms. Some cases require surgical treatment. In less severe cases, treatment includes small meals of bland, easily digested food, moderate exercise, and sleeping with the upper part of the body in a raised position.

fat h., hernial protrusion of peritoneal fat through the abdominal wall.

femoral h., protrusion of a loop of intestine into the femoral canal, a tubular passageway that carries nerves and blood vessels to the thigh; this type occurs more often in women than in men.

hiatal h., hiatus h, protrusion of a structure, often a portion of the stomach, through the esophageal hiatus of the diaphragm.

Holthouse's h., an inguinal hernia that has turned outward into the groin.

incarcerated h., one that cannot be readily reduced, but without obstruction or strangulation; sometimes applied to an irreducible hernia with intestinal obstruction but no strangulation.

incisional h., hernia after operation at the site of the surgical incision, owing to improper healing or to excessive strain on the healing tissue; such strain may be caused by excessive muscular effort, such as that involved in lifting or severe coughing, or by obesity, which creates additional pressure on the weakened area.

inguinal h., hernia occurring in the groin, or inguen, where the abdominal folds of flesh meet the thighs. It is often the result of increased pressure within the abdomen, whether due to lifting, coughing, straining, or accident. Inguinal hernia accounts for about 75 per cent of all hernias.

A sac formed from the peritoneum and containing a portion of the intestine or omentum, or both, pushes either directly outward through the weakest point in the abdominal wall (direct hernia) or downward at an angle into the inguinal canal (indirect hernia). Indirect inguinal hernia (the common form) occurs more often in males because it follows the tract that develops when the testes descend into the scrotum before birth, and the hernia itself may descend into the scrotum. In the female, the hernia follows the course of the round ligament of the uterus.

Inguinal hernia begins usually as a small breakthrough. It may be hardly noticeable, appearing as a soft lump under the skin, no larger than a marble, and there may be little pain. As time passes, the pressure of the contents of the abdomen against the weak abdominal wall may increase the size of the opening and, accordingly, the size of the lump formed by the hernia. In the early stages, an inguinal hernia is usually reducible—it can be pushed gently back into its normal place.

irreducible h., one that cannot be restored by manipulation.

reducible h., one that can be returned by manipulation.

scrotal h., inguinal hernia which has passed into the scrotum.

strangulated h., one that is tightly constricted. As any hernia progresses and bulges out through the weak point in its containing wall, the opening in the wall tends to close behind it, forming a narrow neck. If this neck is pinched tight enough to cut off the blood supply, the hernia will quickly swell and become strangulated. This is a very dangerous condition that can appear suddenly and requires immediate medical attention. Unless the blood supply is restored promptly, gangrene can set in and may cause death.

If a hernia suddenly grows larger, becomes tense and will not go back into place, and there is pain and nausea, the hernia is strangulated. Occasionally, especially in the elderly, there is no pain or tenderness when a hernia is strangulated.

umbilical h., protrusion of part of the intestine at the umbilicus, occurring most frequently in infants (see also UMBILICAL HERNIA).

vaginal h., hernia into the vagina; called also colpocele.

vaginal h., posterior, downward protrusion of the pouch of Douglas with its intestinal contents, between the posterior vaginal wall and the rectum; called also enterocele.

herniation (her″ne-a′shun) abnormal protrusion of an organ or other body structure through a defect or natural opening in a covering membrane, muscle or bone.

h. of nucleus pulposus, rupture or prolapse of the nucleus pulposus into the spinal canal, or against the spinal cord (see also slipped DISK).

tonsillar h., protrusion of the cerebellar tonsils through the foramen magnum.

transtentorial h., downward displacement (caudal transtentorial herniation; uncal herniation) of the medial brain structures through the tentorial notch by a supratentorial mass, exerting pressure on the underlying structures, including the brain stem.

uncal h., transtentorial herniation.

hernioid (her′ne-oid) resembling hernia.

herniology (her″ne-ol′o-je) the study of hernia.

hernioplasty (her′ne-o-plas″te) surgical repair of hernia, with reconstruction of the abdominal wall.

herniorrhaphy (her″ne-or′ah-fe) surgical repair of HERNIA, with suture of the abdominal wall. When the weakened area is very large, hernioplasty is done and some type of strong synthetic material is sewn over the defect to reinforce the area.

Postoperative care is similar to that for any type of abdominal surgery. The patient is protected from respiratory infections which may cause coughing and undue strain on the suture line. Ambulation is usually not restricted, and the physician instructs the patient in activities he may resume when discharged from the hospital.

heroin (her′o-in) a highly addictive narcotic derived from morphine; also called diacetylmorphine. Its sale is prohibited in the United States and in many other countries of the world.

heroinism (her′o-in-izm″) addiction to heroin.

herpangina (her″pan-ji′nah) an infectious febrile disease of children due to a coxsackievirus, marked by vesicular or ulcerated lesions on the fauces or soft palate.

herpes (her′pēz) any inflammatory skin disease caused by a herpesvirus and characterized by the formation of small vesicles in clusters. When used alone the term may refer to *herpes simlex* or to *herpes zoster*.

h. cor′nea, herpetic inflammation involving the cornea.

h. febri′lis, herpes simplex occurring as a concomitant of fever, commonly about the lips and nares; called also *fever blisters* and *cold sores*. Treatment is neither specific nor very satisfactory.

h. genita′lis, herpes simplex of the genitals. The incidence of active genital herpes is difficult to determine because many cases present very mild symptoms or none at all and the disease is frequently misdiagnosed. Genital herpes is currently the most common cause of vesiculoulcerative lesions of the genitalia in women seen in venereal disease clinics, and often is associated with gonorrhea, trichomoniasis, and condyloma acuminata. The disease usually is transmitted by sexual contact, but this is not the only mode of transmission, as man is extremely susceptible to infection by *Herpesvirus hominis* and there is the likelihood that overcrowded conditions could allow for other modes of transmission, particularly via the hands.

SYMPTOMS. In the male the vesicles usually are found on the glans penis or the prepuce. The disease often is self-limiting and the lesions of a primary infection frequently heal in about a week, or they can serve as a portal of entry for other infectious agents.

In the female the symptoms are more severe in a primary infection than in recurrent episodes. The primary infection is most likely to occur during the teens or young adulthood. The vesicular eruptions typical of herpesvirus infection involve the vulva, perineum, and buttocks. Lesions of the cervix may vary from small superficial ulcers with diffuse inflammation to a single, large, necrotic ulcer. Other symptoms include malaise, fever, and anorexia. There also may be involvement of neural structures and neurologic symptoms.

Diagnosis can be readily established by cytologic examination of scrapings from the base of the lesion (TZANCK'S TEST).

COMPLICATIONS. As stated above, a primary herpetic infection usually is self-limiting and, barring secondary infection, immediate complications are rare. In some instances the infection can be complicated by urethral stricture, meningoencephalitis, labial fusion, and lymphatic suppuration.

Herpetic infection of the female genital tract can be extremely hazardous to infants born of infected mothers. The risk of spontaneous abortion is significantly high when the infection occurs during the first 20 weeks of pregnancy. When infection occurs after 32 weeks, there is a strong possibility that the infant will develop neonatal herpes, which appears within a few days after birth and is almost always fatal. Prevention may be accomplished by cesarean section. Congenital anomalies associated with maternal herpes include microcephaly, retinal dysplasia. diffuse brain damage, and mental retardation.

Although there is at present no conclusive evidence that type II herpesvirus infection can lead to cervical carcinoma, there is evidence of a strong link between the two diseases.

TREATMENT. Unfortunately, there presently is no effective antiviral therapy for genital herpes; hence treatment must be symptomatic. Local and systemic analgesic may be prescribed and mild antiseptic compresses applied to reduce the risk of a secondary bacterial infection. It is recommended that soaps and other chemicals that may cause irritation should be avoided. Photodynamic inactivation of the herpes simplex virus has been found to present the hazard of increasing the potential for malignancy.

h. labia'lis, herpes febrilis.

ocular h., herpes of the eye and its adnexa.

h. progenitalis, herpes genitalis.

h. sim'plex, an acute viral disease marked by groups of vesicles, each about 3 to 6 mm. in diameter, on the skin, often on the borders of the lips or the nares (*h. labialis, cold sores*), or on the genitals (*h. genitalis*). It often accompanies fever (*fever blisters*), although there are other precipitating factors, such as the common cold, sunburn, skin abrasions, and emotional disturbances. Often called herpes. (See also HERPESVIRUS.) Treatment is neither specific nor very satisfactory. Tincture of benzoin and camphorated lip ice may help dry the lesions. In some cases smallpox vaccination reduces the occurrence of the lesions.

traumatic h., a self-limiting cutaneous herpesvirus infection following trauma, the virus entering through burns or other wounds; the temperature rises moderately, and vesicles appear around the wound. Called also wrestler's herpes.

h. zoster, an acute viral disease characterized by inflammation of spinal ganglia and by a vesicular eruption along the area of distribution of a sensory nerve, caused by the virus of chickenpox; called also shingles and zoster.

The disease may appear in persons who have been exposed to chickenpox, and it sometimes accompanies other diseases such as pneumonia, tuberculosis, and lymphoma or is triggered by trauma or injection of certain drugs. In some cases it appears without any apparent reason for activation.

Treatment is symptomatic and is aimed at relieving the pain and itching of the blisters. Local applications of calamine lotion or other lotions to dry the blisters may help. Herpes zoster is a very exhausting disease, especially for elderly people, because the constant itching and pain are difficult to control, even with systemic analgesics in some cases.

Herpes zoster affecting the eye causes severe conjunctivitis and possible ulceration and scarring of the cornea if not treated successfully.

h. zos'ter o'ticus, herpes zoster of the ear due to involvement of the geniculate ganglion, with motor impairment, pain that may be excruciating, and herpetic lesions of the auricle, auditory canal, and tympanic membrane; called also herpes zoster auricularis and Ramsay Hunt syndrome.

herpesvirus (her'pēz-vi'rus) any of a large group of DNA viruses found in many animal species, with a nucleocapsid of about 100 mμ in diameter, composed of 162 capsomers, and sometimes enclosed in a loose membrane. The viruses mature in the nucleus of the infected cell, where they induce the formation of a characteristic inclusion body; some also induce formation of a cytoplasmic inclusion body.

The various strains of herpes simplex virus affecting man (*Herpesvirus hominis*) fall into two major types. *Type I* infections are primarily nongenital, for example, *herpes labialis* or "cold sores" and ocular herpes. *Type II* infections are primarily genital, affecting the mucocutaneous border of the genitalia in females and males. Exceptions are the neonate with a cutaneous infection caused by type II and contracted during birth, or possibly transplacentally, and renal transplant recipients with a type II cutaneous herpes.

Other herpesvirus infections include varicella (CHICKENPOX) and HERPES ZOSTER (which are different manifestations of infection by the same virus), as well as cytomegalic inclusion disease and INFECTIOUS MONONUCLEOSIS. Herpesviruses can also cause benign aseptic meningitis and encephalitis with a mortality rate as high as 70%.

Infection with *Herpesvirus hominis* is almost universal in Western countries. By early adulthood neutralizing antibodies are present in 90 percent of the population; however, the majority of individuals with a *primary* infection present no symptoms and the disease goes undiagnosed. The primary infection is almost always a self-limited disease, but recurrent reactivation of the infection can present severe clinical manifestations that are difficult to treat.

After the primary infection is healed, the virus remains in the body, a virus-host balance is established, and the disease enters a quiescent or latent stage during which no active lesions are apparent. Despite the presence of circulating antibody, the quiescent stage can be interrupted by reactivation of the disease. During the active phase the local lesions usually reappear at the site of the primary infection. The factors that precipitate recurrent episodes are not fully understood, but it is known that in institutions and in other conditions of overcrowding minor epidemics do occur, and such conditions do enhance predisposition to overt disease. (See also HERPES SIMPLEX and HERPES GENITALIS.)

herpetic (her-pet'ik) pertaining to or of the nature of herpes; relating to or caused by herpesviruses.

herpetiform (her-pet'ĭ-form) resembling herpes.

Hers' disease (herz) glycogenosis (type VI) in which a deficiency in liver phosphorylase affects the liver and leukocytes, with hepatomegaly, mild hypoglycemia, mild acidosis, and growth retardation.

hersage (ār-sahzh') [Fr.] surgical separation of the fibers of a peripheral nerve.

hertz (herts) a unit of frequency, equal to one cycle per second; symbol, Hz.

hesperidin (hes-per'ĭ-din) a bioflavonoid used to reduce capillary fragility.

heter(o)- word element [Gr.], *other; dissimilar.*

heteradelphus (het″er-ah-del′fus) a twin monster with one fetus more developed than the other.

heterecious (het″er-e′shus) requiring different hosts in different stages of development; a characteristic of certain parasites.

heteresthesia (het″er-es-the′ze-ah) variation of cutaneous sensibility on adjoining areas.

heteroagglutination (het″er-o-ah-gloo″tĭ-na′shun) agglutination of particulate antigens of one species by agglutinins derived from another species.

heteroagglutinin (het″er-o-ah-gloo′tin-in) an agglutinin that is capable of heteroagglutination.

heteroantibody (het″er-o-an″tĭ-bod′e) an antibody combining with antigens originating from a species foreign to the antibody producer.

heteroantigen (het″er-o-an′tĭ-jen) an antigen originating from a species foreign to the antibody producer.

heteroblastic (het″er-o-blas′tik) originating in a different kind of tissue.

heterocellular (het″er-o-sel′u-lar) composed of cells of different kinds.

heterocephalus (het″er-o-sef′ah-lus) a monster with two unequal heads.

heterochromatin (het″er-o-kro′mah-tin) that state of chromatin in which it is dark-staining, genetically inactive, and tightly coiled.

heterochromia (het″er-o-kro′me-ah) diversity of color in a part normally of one color.

h. i′ridis, difference in color of the iris in the two eyes, or in different areas in the same iris.

heterochronia (het″er-o-kro′ne-ah) irregularity in time; occurrence at abnormal times.

heterochronic (het″er-o-kron′ik) 1. pertaining to or characterized by heterochronia. 2. existing for different periods of time; showing a difference in ages.

heterochthonous (het″er-ok′tho-nus) originating in an area other than that in which it is found.

heterocyclic (het″er-o-si′klik) having or pertaining to a closed chain or ring formation that includes atoms of different elements.

heterocytotropic (het″er-o-si″to-trop′ik) having an affinity for cells from different species.

heterodermic (het″er-o-der′mik) denoting a skin graft from an individual of another species.

heterodont (het′er-o-dont″) having teeth of different shapes, as molars, incisors, etc.

heterodromous (het″er-od′ro-mus) moving or acting in other than the usual or forward direction.

heteroerotism (het″er-o-er′o-tizm) sexual feeling directed toward another person.

heterogamety (het″er-o-gam′ĕ-te) production by an individual of one sex (as the human male) of unlike gametes with respect to the sex chromosomes. adj., **heterogamet′ic.**

heterogamy (het″er-og′ah-me) the conjugation of gametes differing in size and structure, to form the zygote from which the new organism develops.

heterogeneity (het″er-o-jĕ-ne′ĭ-te) the state of being heterogeneous.

heterogeneous (het″er-o-je′ne-us) not of uniform composition, quality, or structure.

heterogenesis (het″er-o-jen′ĕ-sis) 1. alternation of generations; reproduction differing in character in successive generations. 2. asexual generation.

heterogenote (het′er-o-je″nōt) a cell that has an additional genetic fragment, different from its intact genotype; usually resulting from transduction.

heterogenous (het″er-oj′ĕ-nus) of other origin; not originating in the body.

heterogony (het″er-og′o-ne) heterogenesis.

heterograft (het′er-o-graft″) a graft of tissue transplanted between individuals of different species; a xenograft.

heterography (het″er-og′rah-fe) writing of other than the intended words.

heterohemagglutination (het″er-o-he″mah-gloo″tĭ-na′shun) agglutination of erythrocytes by a hemagglutinin derived from an individual of a different species.

heterohemagglutinin (het″er-o-he″mah-gloo′tĭ-nin) a hemagglutinin that agglutinates erythrocytes of organisms of other species.

heterohemolysin (het″er-o-he-mol′ĭ-sin) a hemolysin that destroys erythrocytes of animals of other species than that of the animal in which it is formed.

heteroimmunity (het″er-o-im-mu′nĭ-te) 1. an immune state induced in an individual by immunization with cells of an animal of another species. 2. a state in which an immune response to exogenous antigen (e.g., drugs or pathogens) results in immunopathological changes. adj., **heteroimmune′.**

heterokeratoplasty (het″er-o-ker′ah-to-plas″te) grafting of corneal tissue taken from an individual of another species.

heterokinesis (het″er-o-ki-ne′sis) the differential distribution of the sex chromosomes in the developing gametes of a heterogametic organism.

heterolalia (het″er-o-la′le-ah) utterance of inappropriate or meaningless words instead of those intended.

heterolateral (het″er-o-lat′er-al) relating to the opposite side; contralateral.

heterologous (het″er-ol′o-gus) 1. made up of tissue not normal to the part. 2. derived from an individual of a different species.

heterolysin (het″er-ol′ĭ-sin) an antibody that lyzes cells of species other than the one in which it is formed.

heterolysis (het″er-ol′ĭ-sis) destruction of cells of one species by lysin from another species. adj., **heterolyt′ic.**

heteromeric (het″er-o-mer′ik) sending processes through one of the commissures to the white matter of the opposite side of the spinal cord.

heterometaplasia (het″er-o-met″ah-pla′ze-ah) formation of tissue foreign to the part where it is formed.

heterometropia (het″er-o-mĕ-tro′pe-ah) the state in which the refraction in the two eyes differs.

heteromorphosis (het″er-o-mor-fo′sis) the development, in regeneration, of an organ or structure different from the one that was lost.

heteromorphous (het″er-o-mor′fus) of abnormal shape or structure.

heteronomous (het″er-on′ŏ-mus) subject to different laws; in biology, subject to different laws of growth or specialized along different lines. In psychology, subject to another's will.

hetero-osteoplasty (het″er-o-os′te-o-plas″te) osteoplasty with bone taken from an individual of another species.

heteropagus (het″er-op′ah-gus) a conjoined twin monster consisting of inequally developed components.

heteropathy (het″er-op′ah-the) abnormal or morbid sensibility to stimuli.

heterophasia, heterophemia (het″er-o-fa′ze-ah; het″er-o-fe′me-ah) the utterance of words other than those intended by the speaker.

heterophil (het″er-o-fil″) 1. a finely granular polymorphonuclear leukocyte represented by neutrophils in man, but characterized in other mammals by granules that have variable sizes and staining characteristics. 2. heterophilic.

heterophilic (het″er-o-fil′ik) 1. having affinity for other antigens or antibodies besides the one for which it is specific. 2. staining with a type of stain other than the usual one.

heterophonia (het″er-o-fo′ne-ah) any abnormality of the voice.

heterophoria (het″er-o-fo′re-ah) failure of the visual axes to remain parallel after the visual fusional stimuli have been eliminated. The various forms of heterophoria are spoken of as phorias, their direction being indicated by the appropriate prefix, as *cyclo*phoria, *eso*phoria, *exo*phoria, *hyper*phoria, and *hypo*phoria. adj., **heterophor′ic.**

heterophthalmia (het″er-of-thal′me-ah) difference in the direction of the axes, or in the color, of the two eyes.

heteroplasia (het″er-o-pla′ze-ah) replacement of normal by abnormal tissues; malposition of normal cells. adj., **heteroplas′tic.**

heteroplasty (het′er-o-plas″te) plastic repair with tissue derived from an individual of a different species.

heteroploid (het′er-o-ploid″) 1. characterized by heteroploidy. 2. an individual or cell with an abnormal number of chromosomes.

heteroploidy (het′er-o-ploi″de) the state of having an abnormal number of chromosomes.

heteropsia (het″er-op′se-ah) unequal vision in the two eyes.

heteropyknosis (het″er-o-pik-no′sis) 1. the quality of showing variations in density throughout. 2. a state of differential condensation observed in different chromosomes, or in different regions of the same chromosome; it may be attenuated (negative heteropyknosis) or accentuated (positive heteropyknosis). adj., **heteropyknot′ic.**

heterosexual (het″er-o-seks′u-al) 1. pertaining to, characteristic of, or directed toward the opposite sex. 2. a person with erotic interests directed toward the opposite sex.

heterosexuality (het″er-o-seks″u-al′ĭ-te) sexual attraction to persons of the opposite sex.

heterosis (het″er-o′sis) the existence, in the first generation hybrid, of greater vigor than is shown by either parent.

heterostimulation (het″er-o-stim″u-la′shun) stimulation of an animal with antigenic material originating in another species.

heterotaxia (het″er-o-tak′se-ah) abnormal position of viscera.

heterotherm (het′er-o-therm″) an organism characterized by heterothermy.

heterothermy (het′er-o-ther″me) exhibition of widely different body temperatures at different times or under different conditions. adj., **heterother′mic.**

heterotonia (het″er-o-to′ne-ah) a state characterized by variations in tension or tone. adj., **heteroton′ic.**

heterotopia (het″er-o-to′pe-ah) displacement or misplacement of parts. adj., **heterotop′ic.**

heterotoxin (het″er-o-tok′sin) a toxin formed outside the body.

heterotransplant (het″er-o-trans′plant) tissue taken from one individual and transplanted into one of a different species; a xenograft.

heterotrichosis (het″er-o-trĭ-ko′sis) growth of hairs of different colors on the body.

heterotroph (het′er-o-trōf″) a heterotrophic organism.

heterotrophic (het″er-o-trof′ik) unable to synthesize metabolic products from inorganic materials; requiring complex organic substances (growth factors) for nutrition.

heterotropia (het″er-o-tro′pe-ah) failure of the visual axes to remain parallel when fusion is possible (see also STRABISMUS).

heterotypic (het″er-o-tip′ik) pertaining to, characteristic of, or belonging to a different type. adj., **heterotyp′ical.**

heteroxenous (het″er-ok′sĕ-nus) requiring more than one host to complete the life cycle.

heterozygosity (het″er-o-zi-gos′ĭ-te) the state of having different alleles in regard to a given character. adj., **heterozy′gous.**

heterozygote (het″er-o-zi′gōt) an individual exhibiting heterozygosity.

HETP hexaethyltetraphosphate.

Hetrazan (het′rah-zan) trademark for preparations of diethylcarbamazine, a compound used in combating filarial infections.

Heubner-Herter disease (hoib′ner her′ter) celiac disease of infants.

heuristic (hu-ris′tik) encouraging or promoting investigation; conducive to discovery.

hex(a)- (hek′sah) word element [Gr.], *six.*

Hexa-Betalin (hek″sah-ba′tah-lin) trademark for preparations of pyridoxine hydrochloride, a form of vitamin B_6.

hexachlorophene (hek″sah-klo′ro-fēn) a detergent and germicidal compound commonly incorporated in soaps and dermatologic agents.

hexachromic (hek″sah-kro′mik) 1. pertaining to or exhibiting six colors. 2. able to distinguish only six of the seven colors of the spectrum.

hexad (hek′sad) 1. a group or combination of six similar or related entities. 2. an element with a valence of six.

hexadimethrine (hek″sah-di-meth′rēn) a compound used to neutralize the anticoagulant action of heparin.

hexaethyltetraphosphate (hek″sah-eth″il-tet″-

rah-fos′fāt) a powerful anticholinesterase that has been tried in the treatment of myasthenia gravis; also used as an insecticide.

hexamethonium (hek″sah-mĕ-tho′ne-um) a ganglion-blocking ammonium compound used as an antihypertensive.

hexamine (hek′sah-min) methenamine, a urinary antiseptic.

hexaploidy (hek′sah-ploi″de) the state of having six sets of chromosomes (6n).

hexavalent (hek″sah-va′lent) having a valence of six.

Hexavibex (hek″sah-vi′beks) trademark for a preparation of pyridoxine, a form of vitamin B_6.

hexavitamin (hek″sah-vi′tah-min) a preparation of vitamin A, vitamin D, ascorbic acid, thiamine hydrochloride, riboflavin, and niacinamide.

hexestrol (hek-ses′trol) a synthetic estrogenic hormone.

hexethal (hek′sĕ-thal) a short- to intermediate-acting barbiturate.

hexetidine (hek-set′ĭ-dēn) a compound used as an antifungal.

hexobarbital (hek″so-bar′bĭ-tal) an ultrashort-acting sedative and hypnotic; also used as the sodium salt to induce general anesthesia.

hexobarbitone (hek″so-bar′bĭ-tōn) hexobarbital.

hexocyclium methylsulfate (hek″so-si′kle-um) an anticholinergic having antisecretory and antispasmodic activities; used in the management of peptic ulcer and other gastrointestinal disorders accompanied by hyperacidity, hypermotility, and spasm.

hexokinase (hek″so-ki′nās) an enzyme that catalyzes the transfer of a high-energy phosphate group of a donor to D-glucose, producing D-glucose-6-phosphate.

hexosamine (hek′sōs-am″in) a nitrogenous sugar in which an amino group replaces a hydroxyl group.

hexose (hek′sōs) a monosaccharide containing six carbon atoms in a molecule.

hexosephosphate (hek″sōs-fos′fāt) an ester of glucose with phosphoric acid that aids in the absorption of sugars and is important in carbohydrate metabolism.

hexuronic acid (hek″su-ron′ik) ascorbic acid.

hexylcaine (hek′sil-kān) a local anesthetic, used as the hydrochloride salt.

hexylresorcinol (hek″sil-rĕ-zor′sĭ-nol) an anthelmintic for intestinal roundworms and trematodes.

h. pill, one containing hexylresorcinol, with a rupture-resistant coating which disintegrates in the digestive tract.

HF Hageman factor, or clotting factor XII.

Hf chemical symbol, *hafnium.*

Hg chemical symbol, *mercury* (L. *hydrargyrum*).

Hgb hemoglobin.

HGF hyperglycemic-glycogenolytic factor (glucagon).

HGH human growth hormone.

HHNK hyperglycemic hyperosmolar nonketonic coma.

hiatus (hi-a′tus), pl. *hia′tus* [L.] a gap, cleft, or opening. adj., **hia′tal.**

aortic h., h. aor′ticus, the opening in the diaphragm through which the aorta and thoracic duct pass.

esophageal h., h. esophage′us, the opening in the diaphragm for the passage of the esophagus and the vagus nerves.

h. hernia, protrusion of any structure through the esophageal hiatus of the diaphragm.

hibernation (hi″ber-na′shun) the dormant state in which certain animals pass the winter, marked by narcosis and by sharp reduction in body temperature and metabolism.

artificial h., a state of reduced metabolism, muscle relaxation, and a twilight sleep resembling narcosis, produced by controlled inhibition of the sympathetic nervous system and causing attenuation of the homeostatic reactions of the organism.

hibernoma (hi″ber-no′mah) a rare benign tumor made up of large polyhedral cells with a coarsely granular cytoplasm, occurring on the back or around the hips.

hiccough, hiccup (hik′up) spasmodic involuntary contraction of the diaphragm that results in uncontrolled breathing in of air; called also singultus. The peculiar noise of hiccups is produced by a beginning inspiration that is suddenly checked by closure of the glottis.

Hiccups may be due to a variety of causes, such as rapid eating or irritation in the digestive system or the respiratory system, or of the diaphragm muscle itself. Hiccups sometimes occur as a complication following some kinds of surgery, and in serious diseases such as uremia and epidemic encephalitis. They may also have emotional causes. Hiccups are serious only when they persist for a long time; usually they stop after a few minutes.

Standard home remedies for hiccups include holding the breath, swallowing sugar or a bread crust, pulling the tongue forward, applications of cold to the back of the neck, simply sipping water slowly, and breathing into a paper bag. The paper bag device has the effect of cutting off the normal exchange of air with the surrounding atmosphere. The air in the bag, after a few breaths, will have an increasingly high carbon dioxide content, and so will the air in the lungs, and finally the blood. As a consequence, the automatic respiratory centers in the brain call for stronger and deeper breathing to get rid of the carbon dioxide. This frequently makes the contractions of the diaphragm more regular and eliminates the hiccups.

In extreme cases of prolonged hiccups sedative drugs or tranquilizers may be necessary.

Hicks contractions (hiks) Braxton Hicks contractions.

hidr(o)- (hid′ro) word element [Gr.], *sweat.*

hidradenitis (hi″drad-ĕ-ni′tis) inflammation of the sweat glands.

h. suppurati′va, a severe, chronic, recurrent suppurative infection of the apocrine sweat glands.

hidradenoma (hi″drad-ĕ-no′mah) a general term for tumors of the skin, the components of which resemble epithelial elements of sweat glands; they may be nodular (solid) or papillary.

hidrocystoma (hid″ro-sis-to′mah) a retention cyst of a sweat gland.

hidropoiesis (hid″ro-poi-e′sis) the formation of sweat. adj., **hidropoiet′ic.**

hidrorrhea (hid″ro-re′ah) profuse perspiration.

hidroschesis (hĭ-dros′kĕ-sis) suppression of perspiration.

hidrotic (hĭ-drot′ik, hi-drot′ik) pertaining to, characterized by, or causing sweating.

hieralgia (hi″er-al′je-ah) pain in the sacrum.

hierolisthesis (hi″er-o-lis-the′sis) displacement of the sacrum.

high blood pressure a disorder of the circulatory system marked by persistently excessive pressure of the blood against the walls of the arteries (see also HYPERTENSION).

hilitis (hi-li′tis) inflammation of a hilus.

hillock (hil′ok) a small prominence or elevation.

hilum (hi′lum) hilus.

hilus (hi′lus), p., *hi′li* [L.] a depression or pit on an organ, giving entrance and exit to vessels and nerves. adj., **hi′lar.**

hindbrain (hīnd′brān) the rhombencephalon, the portion of the brain developed from the most caudal of the three primary brain vesicles of the early embryo, comprising the metencephalon and myelencephalon.

hindfoot (hīnd′foot) the posterior portion of the foot, comprising the region of the talus and calcaneus.

hindgut (hīnd′gut) a pocket formed beneath the caudal portion of the developing embryo, which develops into the distal portion of the small intestine, the colon and the rectum.

Hinton test (hin′ton) a serologic test for syphilis.

hip (hip) 1. the region of the body at the articulation of the femur and the hip at the base of the lower trunk. These bones meet at the hip joint. Called also coxa. 2. loosely, the hip joint.

At each hip joint, the smooth, rounded head of the femur fits into the deeply recessed socket (the acetabulum) in the hip bone, which comprises the ilium, ischium, and pubis. The joint is covered by a tough, flexible protective capsule and is heavily reinforced by strong ligaments that stretch across the joint.

As in most joints, the ends of the bones, where they meet at the hip joint, are covered with a layer of cartilage that reduces friction and absorbs shock. The synovial membrane lines the socket and lubricates the joint with synovia. Cushioning is provided by small fluid-filled sacs, or bursae.

FRACTURE AND DISLOCATION. The hip is much more susceptible to fracture than to dislocation. The hip joint is very stable and possesses great strength; severe injury is necessary to dislocate it and it will often fracture first. Hip fractures usually involve the neck or the base of the neck of the femur. A fracture usually causes the leg to appear shortened, with the foot pointing outward; usually the victim is unable to raise his leg and there is pain, swelling, and discoloration around the joint. The diagnosis is confirmed by x-ray examination.

A wrench of considerable force, such as may occur in an automobile accident, in skiing, or in football, may dislocate the hip. Dislocation usually tears the capsule and ligaments that bind the joint together, and fragments may be torn from the rim of the hip socket.

First-aid measures are the same for a fractured hip as for a dislocated hip. In either case the injured person will probably not be able to lift his heel while lying on his back. If the victim must be moved, his

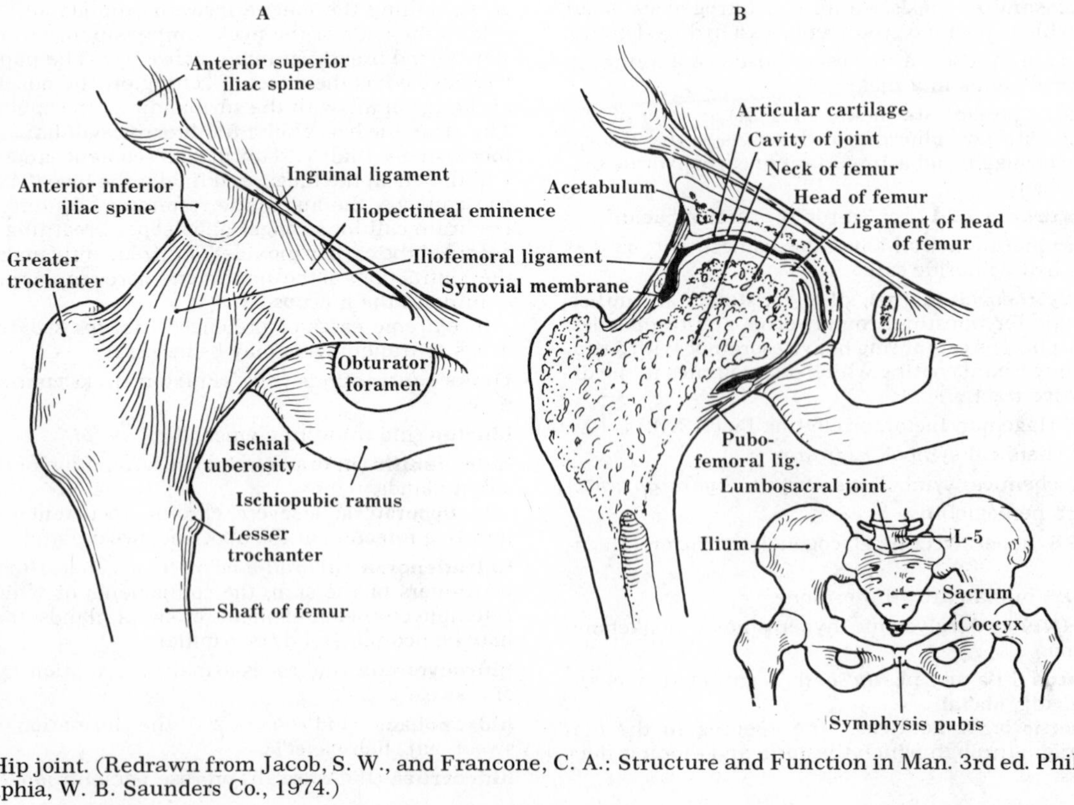

Hip joint. (Redrawn from Jacob, S. W., and Francone, C. A.: Structure and Function in Man. 3rd ed. Philadelphia, W. B. Saunders Co., 1974.)

legs should be gently brought together and tied at the thigh and ankle; the uninjured leg is used as a splint. If possible, a stretcher should be improvised for carrying him.

CONGENITAL DISLOCATION. Congenital dislocation of the hip occurs more frequently in females than in males. It may not be evident until the child starts to walk, when it causes limping or waddling. It is important that the condition be recognized before the child does much walking on the weakened joint. Early treatment can cure the condition, but neglect for a year or two may make reconstruction of the hip joint necessary.

OTHER HIP DISORDERS. Like most joints, the hip may be affected by ARTHRITIS and by BURSITIS, or inflammation of the bursae.

A condition known as slipped capital femoral epiphysis occasionally occurs in growing children. The epiphysis is a cartilaginous disk found at the heads of long bones throughout the body; it is the site at which bone growth takes place and it becomes permanently united to the bone only when growth has finished. There is an epiphyseal line at the top of the femur where the head of the bone joins its neck. Injury to the femur of a child, or its subjection to unusual pressure, may cause the epiphysis to slip out of alignment. This produces shortening of the leg, limitation of movement of the hip, and pain. If the condition is diagnosed early enough it may be corrected with splints and plaster casts.

h. bone, os coxae, which comprises the ilium, ischium, and pubis (see also table of BONES).

h. joint, the ball and socket joint formed between the head of the femur and the acetabulum of the hip bone.

h.-joint disease, tuberculosis of the hip joint; called also coxalgia.

Hippel's disease (hip'elz) angiomatosis confined chiefly to the retina.

hippocampus (hip″o-kam'pus), pl. *hippocam'pi* [L.] a curved elevation on the floor of the inferior horn of the lateral ventricle; it is an important functional component of the limbic system.

h. ma'jor, hippocampus.

h. mi'nor, the lower of two medial elevations in the lateral cerebral ventricle (see also CALCAR AVIS).

Hippocrates (hĭ-pok'rah-tēz) (late 5th century B.C.). "Father of Medicine." Son of a priest-physician, he was born on the island of Cos. By stressing that there is a natural cause for disease he did much to dissociate the care of the sick from the influence of magic and superstition. His carefully kept records of treatment and solicitous observation of the ill provided a foundation for clinical medicine in the case report; and by reporting also unsuccessful methods of treatment he anticipated the modern scientific attitude. The way for the professional nurse was prepared by his emphasis on the importance of skilled bedside care, and his bedside example demonstrated the value of clinical instruction. A moral code for medicine has been established by his ideals of ethical conduct and practice as embodied in the Hippocratic Oath.

"I swear by Apollo the physician, by Æsculapius, Hygeia, and Panacea, and I take to witness all the gods, all the goddesses, to keep according to my ability and my judgment the following Oath:

"To consider dear to me as my parents him who taught me this art; to live in common with him and if necessary to share my goods with him; to look upon his children as my own brothers, to teach them this art if they so desire without fee or written promise; to impart to my sons and the sons of the master who taught me and the disciples who have enrolled themselves and have agreed to the rules of the profession, but to these alone, the precepts and the instruction. I will prescribe regimen for the good of my patients according to my ability and my judgment and never do harm to anyone. To please no one will I prescribe a deadly drug, nor give advice which may cause his death. Nor will I give a woman a pessary to procure abortion. But I will preserve the purity of my life and my art. I will not cut for stone, even for patients in whom the disease is manifest; I will leave this operation for practitioners (specialists in this art). In every house where I come I will enter only for the good of my patients, keeping myself far from all intentional ill-doing and all seduction, and especially from the pleasures of love with women or with men, be they free or slaves. All that may come to my knowledge in the exercise of my profession or outside my profession or in daily commerce with men, which ought not to be spread abroad, I will keep secret and will never reveal. If I keep this oath faithfully, may I enjoy my life and practice my art, respected by all men and in all times; but if I swerve from it or violate it, may the reverse be my lot."

Hippocratic (hip″o-krat'ik) relating to HIPPOCRATES.

hippuria (hĭ-pu're-ah) an excess of hippuric acid in urine.

hippuric acid (hĭ-pu'rik) a compound formed by conjugation of benzoic acid and glycine; it occurs in the urine of herbivorous animals, rarely in human urine.

hippus (hip'us) abnormal exaggeration of the rhythmic contraction and dilation of the pupil, independent of changes in illumination or in fixation of the eyes.

hirci (her'si), sing. *hir'cus* [L.] the hairs growing in the axilla.

hircus (her'kus), pl. *hir'ci* [L.] one of the hairs growing in the axilla.

Hirschsprung's disease (hirsh'sproongz) congenital absence of the parasympathetic nerve ganglia in the anorectum or proximal rectum, resulting in massive enlargement of the colon, constipation, and obstruction. Severe cases may require surgery in early infancy; less severe cases can be treated with enemas and laxatives but surgery often is required eventually. Called also aganglionic megacolon and congenital megacolon.

hirsute (her'sūt) shaggy; hairy.

hirsuties, hirsutism (her-su'she-ēz; her'sūt-izm) abnormal hairiness, especially in women.

hirudicide (hĭ-roo'dĭ-sīd) an agent that is destructive to leeches.

hirudin (hĭ-roo'din) the active principle of the buccal secretion of leeches; it prevents clotting of the blood.

His's bundle (his'ez) a band of atypical cardiac muscle fibers connecting the atria with the ventricles of the heart; called also atrioventricular bundle.

His's disease (his'ez) trench fever; called also His-Werner disease.

hist(io)(o)- word element [Gr.], *tissue.*

Histadyl (his'tah-dil) trademark for preparations of methapyrilene, an antihistamine.

Histalog (his'tah-log) trademark for a preparation of betazole, an analogue of histamine, used as a substitute for histamine in gastric function tests.

histaminase (his-tam′ĭ-nās) an enzyme that inactivates histamine.

histamine (his′tah-min) an amine produced by the breakdown of histidine, a common amino acid derived from protein that occurs naturally in the body. Histamine is found in all tissues of the body. adj., **histamin′ic.**

Although histamine was discovered in 1909, its role is still not fully understood. Histamine normally functions as a stimulant to the production of gastric juice. It also dilates the small blood vessels, as part of the regular adaptation of the body to changing inner and exterior conditions. An excess of histamine can dilate blood vessels to the extent that extravasation occurs. This appears as the reddening and swelling known as inflammation. Continued extravasation causes edema. Histamine also constricts bronchial smooth muscle.

In certain people, histamine may bring on a severe form of headache, known medically as histaminic cephalalgia. It usually occurs during sleep, and is caused by release of histamine into the system. It is treated by desensitizing the patient to histamine.

An excess of histamine apparently is released when the body comes in contact with certain substances to which it is sensitive. This excess histamine is believed to be the final cause of hay fever, urticaria (hives), and most other allergies, as well as certain stomach upsets and some headaches. It is possible that histamine also causes vomiting, diarrhea, and muscular spasm, since these reactions are seen in animals injected with histamine. The fact that a person suffering from shock has large amounts of histamine in the blood suggests that histamine also plays a role in this condition, but its presence may be an incidental side effect.

Substances that block some of the effects of histamine, the ANTIHISTAMINES, have proved useful in preventing some types of vomiting, and they are the main medications for relieving allergies.

h. phosphate, a compound used in tests of gastric function and to reduce sensitivity to histamine.

histaminemia (his″tah-min-e′me-ah) histamine in the blood.

histidase (his′tĭ-dās) an enzyme of the liver that converts histidine to urocanic acid.

histidine (his′tĭ-din) a naturally occurring amino acid, essential for optimal growth of infants; its decarboxylation results in formation of histamine.

histidinemia (his″tĭ-dĭ-ne′me-ah) a hereditary metabolic defect marked by excessive histidine in the blood and urine due to deficient histidase activity; many affected persons show mild mental retardation and disordered speech development.

histidinuria (his″tĭ-dĭ-nu′re-ah) an excess of histidine in the urine. (See also HISTIDINEMIA).

histiocyte (his′te-o-sīt″) a large phagocytic interstitial cell of the reticuloendothelial system; a macrophage. adj. **histiocyt′ic.**

histiocytoma (his″te-o-si-to′mah) a tumor containing histiocytes.

histiocytosis (his″te-o-si-to′sis) a condition marked by the abnormal appearance of histiocytes in the blood.

lipid h., Niemann-Pick disease.

h. X, a generic term embracing eosinophilic granuloma, Letterer-Siwe disease, and Hand-Schüller-Christian disease.

histiogenic (his″te-o-jen′ik) formed by the tissues.

histioid (his′te-oid) histoid.

histoblast (his′to-blast) a tissue-forming cell.

histochemistry (his″to-kem′is-tre) that branch of histology that deals with the identification of chemical components in cells and tissues.

histocompatibility (his″to-kom-pat″ĭ-bil′ĭ-te) the quality of a cellular or tissue graft enabling it to be accepted and functional when transplanted to another organism. adj., **histocompat′ible.**

h. genes, genes that determine the specificity of tissue antigenicity and thus the compatibility of donor and recipient in tissue transplantation.

histodialysis (his″to-di-al′ĭ-sis) disintegration or breaking down of tissue.

histodifferentiation (his″to-dif″er-en″she-a′shun) the acquisition of tissue characteristics by cell groups during development.

histogenesis (his″to-jen′ĕ-sis) differentiation of cells into the specialized tissues forming the various organs and parts of the body.

histogram (his′to-gram) a graph in which values found in a statistical study are represented by lines or symbols placed horizontally or vertically, to indicate frequency distribution.

histoid (his′toid) 1. developed from one kind of tissue. 2. resembling one of the tissues of the body.

histoincompatibility (his″to-in″kom-pat″ĭ-bil′ĭ-te) the quality of a cellular or tissue graft preventing its acceptance or functioning when transplanted to another organism; said of the relationship between the genotypes (histocompatibility genes) of donor and host in which a graft generally will be rejected. adj., **histoincompat′ible.**

histokinesis (his″to-ki-ne′sis) movement in the tissues of the body.

histologist (his-tol′o-jist) one who specializes in histology.

histology (his-tol′o-je) that department of anatomy dealing with the minute structure, composition, and function of tissues. adj. **histolog′ic, histolog′ical.**

pathologic h., the science of diseased tissues.

histolysis (his-tol′ĭ-sis) breaking down of tissues. adj., **histolyt′ic.**

histoma (his-to′mah) any tissue tumor.

histone (his′tōn) a simple protein, soluble in water and insoluble in dilute ammonia, found combined as salts with acidic substances, such as nucleic acids or the globin of hemoglobin.

histonomy (his-ton′o-me) the scientific study of tissues based on the translation into biologic terms of quantitative laws derived from histologic measurement.

histonuria (his″to-nu′re-ah) histone in the urine.

histopathology (his″to-pah-thol′o-je) pathologic histology.

histophysiology (his″to-fiz″e-ol′o-je) the correlation of function with the microscopic structures of cells and tissues.

Histoplasma (his″to-plaz′mah) a genus of fungi.

H. capsula′tum, a species of pathogenic fungi that cause infection (histoplasmosis) in man.

histoplasmin (his″to-plaz′min) a preparation of growth products of *Histoplasma capsulatum,* injected intracutaneously as a test for histoplasmosis.

histoplasmosis (his"to-plaz-mo'sis) a systemic fungal disease caused by inhalation of dust contaminated by *Histoplasma capsulatum.* Histoplasmosis is particularly common in the rural Midwest, but is worldwide in distribution and has been seen in most sections of the United States, including urban areas. It is not transmitted from one person to another. The disease begins in the lungs and may spread to other organs. Infection is usually asymptomatic, but may cause acute pneumonia, or disseminated reticuloendothelial hyperplasia with hepatosplenomegaly and anemia, or an influenza-like illness with joint effusion and erythema nodosum. Reactivated infection involves the lungs, meninges, heart, peritoneum, and adrenals in that order of frequency. On x-ray the lungs may resemble tuberculous lungs.

The specific drug used in the treatment of histoplasmosis is amphotericin B, an antifungal antibiotic. In extreme cases surgery may be necessary to remove the affected portions of the lung.

historrhexis (his"to-rek'sis) the breaking up of tissue.

histotherapy (his"to-ther'ah-pe) treatment by administration of animal tissues.

histothrombin (his"to-throm'bin) thrombin derived from connective tissue.

histotome (his'to-tōm) a cutting instrument used in microtomy; microtome.

histotomy (his-tot'o-me) dissection of tissues; microtomy.

histotoxic (his"to-tok'sik) poisonous to tissue.

histotroph (his'to-trōf) the sum total of nutritive material derived from maternal tissue other than the blood, utilized by the early embryo.

histotrophic (his"to-trof'ik) 1. encouraging formation of tissue. 2. pertaining to histotroph.

histotropic (his"to-trop'ik) having affinity for tissue cells.

histrionism (his'tre-o-nizm") a morbid or hysterical adoption of an exaggerated manner and gestures. adj., **histrion'ic.**

hives (hīvz) a vascular reaction characterized by sudden outbreaks of itching and burning swellings on the skin; called also URTICARIA.

Hl latent hyperopia.

Hm manifest hyperopia.

HMO health maintenance organization.

HNO_2 nitrous acid.

HNO_3 nitric acid.

Ho chemical symbol, *holmium.*

H_2O water.

H_2O_2 hydrogen peroxide.

hoarseness (hōrs'nes) a rough quality of the voice.

Hodgkin's disease (hoj'kinz) a primary lymph node neoplastic disease characterized by painless, progressive enlargement of the lymph nodes, spleen, and lymphoid tissues generally, which often begins in a cervical node on the side of the neck and spreads through the body. Called also malignant granuloma and lymphogranuloma. The disease accounts for only 1% of all malignancies in the United States, but because it primarily affects young persons, it accounts for 10% of malignancies in the 15 to 30 year range. It is almost twice as common among males as among females and is more often fatal in men. With early diagnosis and treatment, 90 percent of patients with localized Hodgkin's disease can have a 10 year survival rate without recurrence. The overall prognosis is less favorable in patients who are diagnosed after the disease has spread through the body.

Symptoms. The first sign of the disease usually is an enlargement of a cervical node. Occasionally there may be swelling of nodes on both sides of the neck or enlargement of nodes elsewhere in the body. Severe itching is often an early sign of the disorder.

As Hodgkin's disease progresses, it is usually marked by sweating, weakness, fever, and loss of weight and appetite. It spreads through the lymphatic system, involving other lymph nodes elsewhere in the body as well as the spleen, liver, and bone marrow. The lymph nodes and the spleen and liver may swell, and by obstructing other organs may cause coughing, breathlessness, or enlargement of the abdomen. The patient often becomes anemic, and because of blood changes the body becomes less able to combat infections.

The disease is classified according to stages of development of the malignancy. These stages are helpful in establishing the prognosis and prescribing treatment. In stage I only one localized lymph node region is involved. Stage IE indicates involvement of a single extralymphatic organ. Stage II indicates two or more involved nodes on the same side of the diaphragm. Stage IIE indicates involvement of an extralymphatic organ and one or more nodes on the same side of the diaphragm. IIS designates splenic involvement with localization below the diaphragm. In Stage III there is disease on both sides of the diaphragm, sometimes with splenic involvement (IIIS) or extralymphatic organ involvement (IIIE), or both. In Stage IV there is diffuse involvement of one or more extralymphatic organs or tissues with or without associated lymph node involvement.

Diagnosis and Treatment. The diagnosis is established on the basis of four histologic patterns associated with the disease: predominance of lymphocytes, mixed cellularity, lymphocyte depletion, and nodular sclerosis. The presence of giant Reed-Sternberg cells is presumptive evidence of Hodgkin's disease; however, these or similar cells have also been found in patients in infectious mononucleosis and thus their presence alone is not clearly indicative of Hodgkin's Disease.

Treatment is by large doses of radiation of the affected nodes using a cobalt machine or a linear accelerator capable of delivering a high dosage of radiation deep into the tissues. Patients with systemic involvement usually are treated by chemotherapy alone or in conjunction with radiotherapy. The drugs (see also ANTINEOPLASTICS) are administered in combination; for example, the treatment known as COPP includes cyclophosphamide (Cytoxan), vincristine sulfate (Oncovin), procarbazine, and prednisone. Another combination known as MOPP substitutes mechlorethamine (Mustargen) for Cytoxan. The dosage pattern is individualized according to patient response and tolerance. The basic pattern is to give the drugs for two weeks and then withhold them for two weeks to allow for bone marrow recovery. The pattern is repeated for six courses, after which it may be changed to accommodate the patient's needs.

Hodgson's disease (hoj'sonz) aneurysmal dilatation of the proximal part of the aorta.

hodoneuromere (ho"do-nu'ro-mēr) a segment of

the embryonic trunk with its pair of nerves and their branches.

Hoffmann's sign (hof′manz) 1. increased mechanical irritability of the sensory nerves in tetany; the ulnar nerve is usually tested. 2. a sudden nipping of the nail of the index, middle, or ring finger produces flexion of the terminal phalanx of the thumb and of the second and third phalanx of some other finger; called also digital reflex.

hol(o)- word element [Gr.], *entire; whole.*

holandric (hol-an′drik) inherited exclusively through the male descent; transmitted through genes located on the Y chromosome.

holarthritis (hol″ar-thri′tis) inflammation of all the joints.

holergasia (hol″er-ga′ze-ah) a psychiatric disorder involving the entire personality. adj., **holargas′tic.**

holistic (ho-lis′tik) pertaining to totality, or to the whole.

Hollenhorst plaques atheromatous emboli containing cholesterol crystals in the retinal arterioles, a sign of impending serious cardiovascular disease.

Holmgren test (holm′gren) one for detection of imperfect perception of color, based on matching various strands of yarn.

holmium (hol′me-um) a chemical element, atomic number 67, atomic weight 164.930, symbol Ho. (See table of ELEMENTS.)

holoacardois (hol″o-ah-kar′de-us) an unequal twin fetus in which the heart is entirely absent.

holoblastic (hol″o-blas′tik) undergoing cleavage in which the entire ovum participates; completely dividing.

Holocaine (ho′lo-kān) trademark for a preparation of phenacaine, a local anesthetic.

holocrine (hol′o-krin) wholly secretory: noting that type of glandular secretion in which the entire secreting cell, along with its accumulated secretion, forms the secreted matter of the gland, as in the sebaceous glands; cf. apocrine and merocrine.

holodiastolic (hol″o-di″ah-stol′ik) pertaining to the entire diastole.

holoendemic (hol″o-en-dem′ik) affecting practically all the residents of a particular region.

holoenzyme (hol″o-en′zim) the active compound formed by combination of a coenzyme and an apoenzyme.

hologynic (hol″o-jin′ik) inherited exclusively through the female descent; transmitted through genes located on attached X chromosomes.

holoprosencephaly (hol″o-pros″en-sef′ah-le) developmental failure of cleavage of the prosencephalon with a deficit in midline facial development and with cyclopia in the severe form; sometimes due to trisomy 13–15.

holorachischisis (hol″o-rah-kis′kĭ-sis) fissure of the entire vertebral column with prolapse of the spinal cord.

holosystolic (hol″o-sis-tol′ik) pertaining to the entire systole.

homaluria (hom″ah-lu′re-ah) production and excretion of urine at a normal, even rate.

Homan's sign (ho′manz) discomfort behind the knee on forced dorsiflexion of the foot; a sign of thrombosis in the leg.

homatropine (ho-mat′ro-pin) an anticholinergic alkaloid obtained by the condensation of tropine and mandelic acid; used to produce parasympathetic blockade and as a mydriatric.

h. hydrobromide, a compound used topically in the eye as a cycloplegic and mydriatic.

h. methylbromide, a compound used as an inhibitor of gastric spasm and secretion.

homeo- word element [Gr.], *similar; same; unchanging.*

homeomorphous (ho″me-o-mor′fus) of like form and structure.

homeopathy (ho″me-op′ah-the) a system of therapeutics founded by Samuel Hahnemann (1755–1843) in which diseases are treated by drugs that are capable of producing in healthy persons symptoms like those of the disease to be treated, the drug being administered in minute doses. adj., **homeopath′ic.**

homeoplasia (ho″me-o-pla′ze-ah) formation of new tissue like that normal to the part. adj., **homeoplas′tic.**

homeostasis (ho″me-o-sta′sis) a tendency of biological systems to maintain stability while continually adjusting to conditions that are optimal for survival. adj., **homeostat′ic.** Homeostatic mechanisms are necessary for the body to regain its balance when disease or injury occurs and to maintain that balance if it is to remain healthy. Many of the medications and treatments prescribed during illness are given to help preserve this dynamic equilibrium within the body. Without successful physiological homeostasis, in which relatively constant conditions are maintained in the internal environment, the body cannot survive.

It is through homeostatic mechanisms that body temperature is kept within normal range, the osmotic pressure of the blood and its hydrogen ion concentration (pH) is kept within strict limits, nutrients are supplied to cells as needed, and waste products are removed before they accumulate and reach toxic levels of concentration. These are but a few examples of the thousands of homeostatic control systems within the body. Some of these systems operate within the cell and others operate within an aggregate of cells (organs) to control the complex interrelationships among the various organs.

The changes that occur in homeostasis are a result of *negative feedback.* The term negative feedback is used because whenever a factor approaches either of the two extremes in a normal range, the condition acts as a stimulus to produce a negative or opposing effect. We know that cellular function, especially normal function, can continue in the human body only when certain conditions are held within a narrow range, the "normal" range that sustains life. When particular factors go beyond the normal range, a corrective action takes place to compensate for the extreme and return the system to a normal balance. For example, an abnormally high level of carbon dioxide in the blood acts as a stimulus, and through negative feedback triggers HYPERVENTILATION, which in turn causes a loss of carbon dioxide and a return to normal concentration.

Homeostatic feedback mechanisms tend to be slower than voluntary responses and so there is always a lag between stimulus and response in homeostasis. The nerve fibers reserved for the processes of homeostasis have a considerably slower rate of transmission than do voluntary nerve fibers, and many of the messages of homeostasis are carried by such chemical messengers as hormones and carbon dioxide in the blood.

Because of the lag, the adjustments made through homeostatic mechanisms are not always perfect. If the lag becomes too great, the compensating mechanisms may be too extreme or occur out of phase, and produce "overshoots" of increasing magnitude each time the input enters and goes through the circuit of stimulus–response–effect. This situation can bring about collapse of the system.

Positive feedback leads to instability which can produce serious and even fatal results. In this situation the initiating stimulus produces a condition similar to the one already existing. In this way the mechanism enters a vicious and sometimes deadly cycle. A mild degree of positive feedback can be overcome by the normal negative feedback control systems of the body. If these systems fail, however, death will ensue. In some instances positive feedback and overshoots can result in overproduction of a normal body chemical and bring about such conditions as allergies, epilepsy, cirrhosis of the liver, and nephritis. In a malignancy the homeostatic mechanism has gone awry and inhibitors of cell division do not function at the point at which cell division should cease; thus the cells continue to divide and produce new growth.

homeotherapy (ho″me-o-ther′ah-pe) treatment with a substance similar to the causative agent of the disease.

homeothermal (ho″me-o-ther′mal) homoiothermic.

homeotypical (ho″me-o-tip′ĭ-kal) resembling the normal or usual type.

homo- (ho′mo) 1. word element [Gr.], *same; similar.* 2. chemical prefix indicating addition of one CH_2 group to the main compound.

homoarterenol (ho″mo-ar″tĕ-re′nol) nordefrin, a sympathomimetic agent.

homobiotin (ho″mo-bi′o-tin) a homologue of biotin having an additional CH_2 group in the side chain and acting as a biotin antagonist.

homocystine (ho″mo-sis′tēn) a homologue of cystine which results from demethylation of methionine.

homocystinuria (ho″mo-sis″tin-u′re-ah) an inborn error of sulfur amino acid metabolism due to lack of the enzyme cystathionine synthase; it is characterized by homocystine in the urine and by mental retardation, hepatomegaly, ectopia lentis, and cardiovascular and skeletal disorders.

homocytotropic (ho″mo-si″to-trop′ik) having an affinity for cells of individuals of the same species.

homodromous (ho-mod′ro-mus) moving or acting in the same or in the usual direction.

homogametic (ho″mo-gah-met′ik) having only one kind of gamete with respect to the sex chromosomes, as in the human female.

homogenate (ho-moj′ĕ-nāt) material obtained by homogenization.

homogeneity (ho″mo-jĕ-ne′ĭ-te) the state of being homogeneous.

homogeneous (ho″mo-je′ne-us) of uniform quality, composition, or structure.

homogenesis (ho″mo-jen′ĕ-sis) reproduction by the same process in each generation.

homogenic (ho″mo-jen′ik) homozygous.

homogenicity (ho″mo-jĕ-nis′ĭ-te) homogeneity.

homogenize (ho-moj′ĕ-nīz) to convert into material that is of uniform quality or consistency throughout; to render homogeneous.

homogentisic acid (ho″mo-jen-tis′ik) 2,5-dihydroxyphenyl acetic acid, an intermediate product in the metabolism of tyrosine and phenylalanine, excreted in the urine in an inborn error of metabolism (PHENYLKETONURIA).

homograft (ho′mo-graft) a graft of tissue transplanted between individuals of the same species, but of a different genotype; an allograft.

homoiotherm (ho-moi′o-therm) an animal that exhibits homoiothermy; a so-called warm-blooded animal.

homoiothermy (ho-moi′o-ther″me) maintenance of a constant body temperature despite variation in environmental temperature. adj., **homoiother′mic.**

homolateral (ho″mo-lat′er-al) ipsilateral; pertaining to or situated on the same side.

homologous (ho-mol′ŏ-gus) 1. corresponding in structure, position, origin, etc. 2. derived from an animal of the same species but of different genotype; allogeneic.

homologue (hom′ŏ-log) 1. any homologous organ or part. 2. in chemistry, one of a series of compounds distinguished by addition of a CH_2 group in successive members.

homology (ho-mol′ŏ-je) the state of being homologous.

homolysin (ho-mol′ĭ-sin) a lysin produced by injection into the body of an antigen derived from an individual of the same species.

homonomous (ho-mon′ŏ-mus) subject to the same laws; in biology, subject to the same laws of growth or developed along the same line.

homonymous (ho-mon′ĭ-mus) 1. having the same or corresponding sound or name. 2. standing in the same relation.

homophilic (ho″mo-fil′ik) reacting only with specific antigen.

homoplastic (ho″mo-plas′tik) denoting a transplantation or grafting of tissue taken from another individual of the same species.

homoplasty (ho′mo-plas″te) 1. operative replacement of lost parts or tissues by similar parts from another individual of the same species. 2. similarity between organs or their parts not due to common ancestry.

homorganic (hom″or-gan′ik) produced by the same or by homologous organs.

homosexual (ho″mo-seks′u-al) 1. sexually oriented toward persons of the same sex. 2. a homosexual individual.

homosexuality (ho″mo-seks″u-al′ĭ-te) sexual orientation toward persons of the same sex.

homotherm (ho′mo-therm) homoiotherm.

homotopic (ho″mo-top′ik) occurring at the same place upon the body.

homotype (ho′mo-tīp) a part having reversed symmetry with its mate, as the hand. adj., **homotyp′ic.**

homozygosis (ho″mo-zi-go′sis) the formation of a zygote by the union of gametes that have one or more identical alleles.

homozygosity (ho″mo-zi-gos′ĭ-te) the state of having identical alleles in regard to a given character or characters. adj., **homozy′gous.**

homozygote (ho″mo-zi′gōt) an individual exhibiting homozygosity.

homunculus (ho-mung′ku-lus) a dwarf without deformity or disproportion of parts.

hookworm (hook′werm) a parasitic roundworm, found mostly in the southeastern part of the United States, that enters the human body through the skin and migrates to the intestines, where it attaches itself to the intestinal wall and sucks blood from it for nourishment. Once fairly common, hookworm disease is now largely confined to poor, rural areas where modern sanitation is lacking.

The kind of hookworm most common in the United States and Central America is *Necator americanus,* which literally means "American killer." This hookworm is about half an inch long, with sharp hooklike teeth and a muscular gullet used in sucking blood. The female, slightly larger than the male, can lay more than 10,000 eggs a day, any one of which can hatch into a larva and invade the human body. Another common hookworm is *Ancylostoma duodenale.*

The larval hookworms enter the body by burrowing through the skin, usually that of the sole of the foot. The first sign of the disease may appear on the skin as small eruptions that develop into pus-filled blisters; this condition is sometimes called "ground itch."

Meanwhile the hookworms enter blood vessels and are carried by the blood into the lungs. They leave the lungs, propel themselves up the trachea, are swallowed and washed through the stomach and end up in the intestines. Here, if left alone, they will make a permanent home, using their host's body as a source of nourishment.

By the time they reach the intestines, about 6 weeks after they enter the body as larvae, the worms are full-grown adults. Each worm now attaches itself by its hooked teeth to the intestinal wall, where it sucks its host's blood by contraction and expansion of its gullet. If large numbers of worms are present, they can cause considerable loss of blood and severe anemia. The symptoms include pallor and loss of energy; the appetite may increase.

The thousands of eggs laid every day by each female worm pass out of the body in the stool, in which they can easily be seen. If the stool is not properly disposed of, the larvae that hatch from the eggs may infect other persons.

TREATMENT AND PREVENTION. A nutritious, high-protein diet supplemented by iron is given to relieve anemia and improve the health. Specific drugs include the anthelmintics mebendazole, bephenium hydroxynaphthoate, tetrachloroethylene, and chenopodium oil. When left untreated, hookworm can cause not only anemia but also bronchial inflammation and, occasionally, stunting of growth, retardation of mental development, and even death.

Hookworm infection can be prevented by installation of sanitary toilets or, if that is not possible, by disposal of human feces in deep holes so that the soil with which the human foot comes in contact is not contaminated. Shoes should be worn out of doors to protect the feet from infection.

hordeolum (hōr-de′o-lum) inflammation of one or more sebaceous glands of the eyelid; called also STY.

horizon (hŏ-ri′zon) a specific anatomic stage of embryonic development, of which 23 have been defined, beginning with the unicellular fertilized egg and ending 7 to 9 weeks later, with the beginning of the fetal stage.

hormesis (hōr-me′sis) stimulation by a subinhibitory concentration of a toxic substance.

hormonagogue (hōr-mōn′ah-gog) an agent that increases the production of hormones.

hormone (hōr′mon) a chemical transmitter substance produced by cells of the body and transported by the bloodstream to the cells and organs on which it has a specific regulatory effect. adj. **hormo′nal.** Hormones act as chemical messengers to body organs, stimulating certain life processes and retarding others. Growth, reproduction, sexual attributes, and even mental conditions and personality traits are dependent on hormones.

Hormones are produced by various organs and body tissues, but mainly by the ENDOCRINE GLANDS, such as the pituitary, thyroid, and gonads (testes and ovaries). Each gland apparently manufactures several kinds of hormones; the adrenal glands alone produce more than 25 varieties. The total number of hormones is still unknown, but each has its unique function and its own chemical formula. After a hormone is discharged by its parent gland into the capillaries or the lymph, it may travel a circuitous path through the bloodstream to exert influence on cells, tissues, and organs (target organs) far removed from its site of origin.

One of the best-known hormones is INSULIN, a protein manufactured by the beta cells of the islands of Langerhans in the pancreas that is important in carbohydrate metabolism. Other important hormones are THYROXINE, an iodine-carrying amino acid produced by the thyroid gland; CORTISONE, a member of the steroid family from the adrenal glands; and the sex hormones, ESTROGEN from the ovaries and ANDROGEN from the testes.

Certain hormone substances can be synthesized in the laboratory for treatment of human disease. Animal hormones can also be used, as endocrine hormones are to some extent interchangeable among species. Extracts from the pancreas of cattle, for example, enabled diabetes sufferers to live normal lives even before the chemistry of insulin was fully understood.

We now know that any significant imbalance in the kind and number of hormones produced by the glands must be corrected if the body and mind are to function properly. Extreme imbalances account for such forms of abnormal development as DWARFISM and CRETINISM. Hormonal imbalance can also cause changes in personality such as excessive excitability, lethargy, or fatigue. Thanks to modern endocrinology, hormone and glandular disorders are yielding more and more to the physician's treatment.

adaptive h., one that is secreted during adaptation to unusual circumstances.

adrenocortical h., one of the steroids produced by the adrenal cortex (see also CORTICOSTEROID).

adrenocorticotropic h., a hormone elaborated by the anterior lobe of the PITUITARY GLAND that stimulates the action of the ADRENAL CORTEX (see also ACTH).

adrenomedullary h's, substances secreted by the adrenal medulla, including epinephrine and norepinephrine.

androgenic h's, the masculinizing hormones, androsterone and testosterone.

antidiuretic h., ADH, one from the posterior lobe of the pituitary gland that suppresses the secretion of urine; VASOPRESSIN.

corpus luteum h., progesterone.

cortical h., corticosteroid.

estrogenic h's, substances capable of producing certain biological effects, the most characteristic of which are the changes which occur in mammals at estrus; the naturally occurring estrogenic hormones are β-estradiol, estrone, and estriol.

follicle-stimulating h. (FSH), one of the gonadotropic hormones of the anterior lobe of the pituitary gland that stimulates follicular growth in the ovary and spermatogenesis in the testis.

gonadotropic h., one that has an influence on the gonads.

growth h., a substance that stimulates growth, especially a secretion of the anterior lobe of the PITUITARY GLAND that directly influences protein, carbohydrate, and lipid metabolism and controls the rate of skeletal and visceral growth. Called also somatotropin.

interstitial cell-stimulating h., luteinizing hormone.

lactation h., lactogenic h., prolactin.

luteinizing h., a gonadotropic hormone of the anterior pituitary gland, acting with follicle-stimulating hormone to cause ovulation of mature follicles and secretion of estrogen by thecal and granulosa cells of the ovary; it is also concerned with corpus luteum formation. In the male, it stimulates development of the interstitial cells of the testes and their secretion of testosterone. Called also interstitial cell-stimulating hormone.

luteotropic h., prolactin.

melanocyte-stimulating h. (MSH), a substance from the anterior pituitary that influences the formation or deposition of melanin in the body.

parathyroid h., a polypeptide hormone secreted by the parathyroid glands that influences calcium and phosphorus metabolism and bone formation.

placental h., one secreted by the placenta, including chorionic gonadotropin, relaxin, and other substances having estrogenic, progestational, or adrenocorticoid activity.

progestational h's, substances, including PROGESTERONE, that are concerned mainly with preparing the endometrium for nidation of the fertilized ovum if conception has occurred.

sex h's, hormones having estrogenic (female sex hormones) or androgenic (male sex hormones) activity.

somatotrophic h., somatotropic h., growth hormone.

thymic h., thymosin.

thyrotropic h., a hormone of the anterior lobe of the pituitary gland that exerts a stimulating influence on the thyroid gland; called also thyrotropin and thyroid-stimulating hormone (TSH).

hormonopoiesis (hōr-mo″no-poi-e′sis) the production of hormones. adj., **hormonopoiet′ic.**

hormonotherapy (hōr-mo″no-ther′ah-pe) treatment by the use of hormones; endocrinotherapy.

horn (hōrn) a pointed projection such as the paired processes on the head of various animals, or other structure resembling them in shape.

anterior h. of spinal cord, the horn-shaped structure seen in transverse section of the spinal cord, formed by the anterior column of the cord.

cicatricial h., a hard, dry outgrowth from a cicatrix, commonly scaly and rarely osseous.

posterior h. of spinal cord, the horn-shaped structure seen in transverse section of the spinal cord, formed by the posterior column of the cord.

sebaceous h., a hard outgrowth of the contents of a sebaceous cyst.

warty h., a hard, pointed outgrowth of a wart.

Horner's syndrome (hōr′nerz) sinking in of the eyeball, ptosis of the upper eyelid, slight elevation of the lower lid, constriction of the pupil, narrowing of the palpebral fissure, and anhidrosis caused by paralysis of the cervical sympathetic nerve supply.

horopter (hōr-op′ter) the sum of all points seen in binocular vision with the eyes fixed.

hospital (hos′pit'l) an institution for the care and treatment of the sick and injured.

hospitalization (hos″pit'l-i-za′shun) 1. the placing of a patient in a hospital. 2. the period of confinement in a hospital.

host (hōst) 1. an animal or plant that harbors and provides sustenance for another organism (the parasite). 2. the recipient of an organ or other tissue derived from another organism (the donor).

accidental h., one that accidentally harbors an organism that is not ordinarily parasitic in the particular species.

alternate h., intermediate host.

definitive h., final h., the organism in which a parasite passes its adult and sexual existence.

intermediate h., the organism in which a parasite passes its larval or nonsexual existence.

paratenic h., an animal acting as a substitute intermediate host of a parasite, usually having acquired the parasite by ingestion of the original host.

h. of predilection, the host preferred by a parasite.

primary h., definitive host.

reservoir h., one that serves as a host for a pathogenic parasite and may serve as the source from which the parasite is transmitted to other species.

secondary h., intermediate host.

transfer h., one that is used until the appropriate definitive host is reached, but is not necessary to completion of the life cycle of the parasite.

housemaid's knee a swelling at the front of the knee, caused by enlargement of a bursa in front of the patella (kneecap), with accumulation of fluid within it.

The condition is so called because it was formerly supposed to be common among domestic workers who injured the knee by frequent kneeling.

The knee swells, is tender to the touch, and hurts when bent; if the bursa continues to be aggravated, these symptoms become acute. The injury may result in BURSITIS. Infection is possible if the knee is cut or scratched.

The condition can be treated by withdrawal of the fluid with a hollow needle and syringe. Sometimes the bursa must be removed altogether to prevent a chronic or recurrent condition.

Howell-Jolly bodies (how′el zho-le′) small, round or oval bodies, probably nuclear remnants, seen in erythrocytes when stains are added to fresh blood and found in various anemias and after splenectomy or splenic atrophy.

Hp haptoglobin, a serum protein that binds free hemoglobin.

HPG human pituitary gonadotropin.

HPL human placental lactogen.

HPO hyperbaric (high-pressure) oxygenation.

hr. hour.

HSA human serum albumin.

5-HT serotonin (5-hydroxytryptamine).

ht. height.

Hubbard tank (hub'ard) a tank designed for full immersion of the body for the purpose of employing HYDROTHERAPY. A narrow section at the middle of the tank allows the therapist to reach the patient, and wider sections at each end permit full abduction of the patient's legs and arms. The tank is fitted with an aerator that agitates the water and provides gentle massage and débridement of wounds. An overhead crane facilitates transfer of the patient to and from the tank. The Hubbard tank is especially useful in the treatment of patients with extensive burns and those with chronic arthritic disorders in which there is involvement of several joints.

Huhner test (hoon'er) determination of the number and condition of spermatozoa in mucus aspirated from the canal of the cervix uteri within 2 hours after coitus.

hum (hum) a low, steady, prolonged sound.

venous h., a continuous blowing or singing sound heard on ausculation at the base of the neck with the patient in upright position; due to increased venous flow, it is exaggerated in anemia and fever.

human erythrocyte agglutination test an adaptation of the sheep cell agglutination test; human Rh-positive cells coated with incomplete anti-Rh antibody are used instead of the sheep red blood cells sensitized with rabbit gamma globulin. The sera of some patients with rheumatoid arthritis will agglutinate these cells. The agglutination may be inhibited by some normal sera, and not others, and this test is the basis for the determination of the inherited gamma globulin groups (Gm system). Abbreviated HEAT.

Humatin (hu'mah-tin) trademark for preparations of paromomycin sulfate, an antibiotic.

humectant (hu-mek'tant) 1. moistening. 2. a moistening or diluent medicine.

humeral (hu'mer-al) of or pertaining to the humerus.

humeroradial (hu"mer-o-ra'de-al) pertaining to the humerus and radius.

humeroscapular (hu"mer-o-skap'u-lar) pertaining to the humerus and scapula.

humeroulnar (hu"mer-o-ul'nar) pertaining to the humerus and ulna.

humerus (hu'mer-us) the bone of the upper arm, extending from shoulder to elbow. It consists of a shaft and two enlarged extremities. The proximal end has a smooth round head that articulates with the scapula to form the shoulder joint. Just below the head are two rounded processes called the greater and lesser tubercles. Just below the tubercles is the "surgical neck," so named because of its liability to fracture. The distal end of the humerus has two articulating surfaces: the trochlea, which articulates with the ulna, and the capitulum, which articulates with the radius, at the elbow.

humidifier (hu-mid'ĭ-fi"er) an apparatus for controlling humidity by adding moisture to the air.

humidity (hu-mid'ĭ-te) the degree of moisture in the air.

h. therapy, the therapeutic use of water to prevent or correct a moisture deficit in the respiratory tract. Under normal conditions the respiratory tract is kept moist by humidifying mechanisms that allow for evaporation of water from the respiratory mucosa. If these mechanisms fail to work, are bypassed as in ENDOTRACHEAL INTUBATION, or are inadequate to overcome the drying and irritating effects of therapeutic gases and mucosal crusting, some form of humidification must be provided.

The principal reasons for employing humidity therapy are: (1) to prevent drying and irritation of the respiratory mucosa, (2) to facilitate ventilation and diffusion of oxygen and other therapeutic gases being administered, and (3) to aid in the removal of thick and viscous secretions that obstruct the air passages. Another important use of water aerosol therapy is to aid in obtaining an induced sputum specimen.

Humidity therapy may be delivered in a variety of ways. Humidifiers and vaporizers increase the water content of an environment and are limited to the treatment of upper respiratory disorders because they produce particles that are too large to penetrate deeply into the lungs. Nebulizers generate clouds or mists of particles that are extremely small and thus capable of penetrating more deeply into the bronchioles and small structures of the lower respiratory tract. Examples of these include jet instruments and ultrasonic nebulizers.

humor (hu'mor), pl. *humo'res, humors* [L.] any fluid or semifluid in the body, adj., **hu'moral.**

aqueous h., the fluid produced in the eye and filling the spaces (anterior and posterior chambers) in front of the lens and its attachments.

ocular h., either of the humors of the eye—aqueous or vitreous.

vitreous h., the fluid portion of the vitreous body; often used to designate the entire vitreous body.

Humorsol (hu'mor-sol) trademark for a solution of demecarium bromide, used in the treatment of glaucoma.

hunchback (hunch'bak) a rounded deformity, or hump, of the back, or a person with such a deformity. The condition is called also KYPHOSIS and is the result of an abnormal backward curvature of the spine.

hunger (hung'ger) a craving, as for food.

air h., dyspnea affecting both inspiration and expiration, characteristic of diabetic acidosis and coma. Called also Kussmaul's respiration.

Hunner's ulcer (hun'erz) an ulcer involving all layers of the bladder wall, occurring in chronic interstitial cystitis.

Hunt's neuralgia (huntz) neuralgia involving the geniculate ganglion, the pain being limited to the middle ear and external acoustic meatus; called also geniculate neuralgia.

Hunter (hun'ter) John (1728–1793). "Founder of scientific surgery." Born in England, he learned dissection from his brother William and then acquired extensive knowledge of gunshot wounds in the army, of which he was later appointed surgeon-general. Upon retiring from the army, he practiced surgery and lectured on anatomy and surgery. His merit rests with the sound pathologic reasons upon which his surgical procedures were based. Hunter was also the first to study teeth scientifically. In 1783 he was elected a member of the Royal Society of Medicine and of the Royal Academy of Surgery at Paris.

Hunter's canal (hun'terz) a fascial tunnel in the middle third of the medial part of the thigh, containing the femoral vessels and saphenous nerve. Called also adductor canal.

Huntington's chorea (hunt'ing-tunz) a rare hereditary disease characterized by quick involuntary movements, speech disturbances, and mental deterioration due to degenerative changes in the cerebral cortex and basal ganglia; called also chronic or hereditary chorea.

The disease appears in adulthood, usually between the ages of 30 to 45, and the patient's condition deteriorates over a period of 15 years or so, progressing to total incapacitation and death. There is no treatment as yet that is successful in curing this disorder. Sedatives and tranquilizers may be used to relieve the symptoms.

Hurler's syndrome (hoor'lerz) the prototypical form of MUCOPOLYSACCHARIDOSIS, with gargoyle-like facies, dwarfism, severe somatic and skeletal changes, severe mental retardation, cloudy corneas, deafness, cardiovascular defects, hepatosplenomegaly, and joint contractures. Called also gargoylism.

Hürthle cells (her'tel) large eosinophilic cells sometimes found in the thyroid gland (see also HÜRTHLE CELL TUMOR).

Hürthle cell tumor (her'tel) a new growth of the thyroid gland composed wholly or predominantly of large cells (Hürthle cells) having abundant granular, eosinophilic cytoplasm. Such tumors are usually benign (Hürthle cell adenoma) but on occasion may be locally invasive or may rarely metastasize (Hürthle cell carcinoma, or malignant Hürthle cell tumor).

Hutchinson's pupil (huch'in-sunz) a pupil that is dilated while the pupil of the other eye is not.

Hutchinson's triad (huch'in-sunz) diffuse interstitial keratitis, labyrinthine disease, and Hutchinson's teeth, seen in congenital syphilis.

Hutchinson-Gilford disease (huch'in-sun-gil'ford) progeria.

HVL half-value layer.

hyal(o)- word element [Gr.], *glassy.*

hyalin (hi'ah-lin) a translucent albuminoid substance obtainable from the products of amyloid degeneration.

hyaline (hi'ah-līn) glassy; pellucid.

h. cartilage, cartilage with a glassy, translucent appearance, the matrix and embedded collagenous fibers having the same index of refraction.

h. membrane disease, a disorder of newborn infants, usually premature, characterized by the formation of a hyalin-like membrane lining the terminal respiratory passages. Infants with this disease do not secrete adequate quantities of a substance called surfactant, which is secreted by the epithelium of the alveoli and decreases the surface tension of the fluids lining the alveoli and bronchioles. When the surface tension is kept low, air can pass through the fluids and into the alveoli. If the surface tension is not decreased by adequate supplies of surfactant, the alveoli cannot fill with air and there is partial or complete collapse of the lung (atelectasis). Thus the infant with hyaline membrane disease suffers from respiratory embarrassment with severe DYSPNEA and cyanosis. (See also RESPIRATORY DISTRESS SYNDROME OF NEWBORN.)

The cause of hyaline membrane disease is not known, but it seldom occurs in full-term infants, and may develop in infants whose mothers are diabetic or in infants delivered by cesarean section.

There is no cure for hyaline membrane disease. The infant is given oxygen and positive pressure breathing with a VENTILATOR, and usually is fed through a stomach tube to avoid aspiration of liquids into the lungs. As a safeguard against pneumonia, which frequently accompanies this disease, antibiotics may be prescribed. Infants who are able to survive the first few days usually recover very quickly.

hyalinization (hi"ah-lin"ĭ-za'shun) conversion into a substance resembling glass.

hyalinosis (hi"ah-lĭ-no'sis) hyaline degeneration.

hyalinuria (hi"ah-lĭ-nu're-ah) hyalin in the urine.

hyalitis (hi"ah-li'tis) inflammation of the vitreous body.

asteroid h., hyalitis marked by spherical or star-shaped bodies in the vitreous (see also BENSON'S DISEASE).

h. puncta'ta, a form marked by small opacities.

h. suppurati'va, purulent inflammation of the vitreous body.

hyalogen (hi-al'o-jen) an albuminous substance occurring in cartilage, vitreous humor, etc., and convertible into hyalin.

hyaloid (hi'ah-loid) pellucid; like glass.

hyalomere (hi'ah-lo-mēr") the pale, homogeneous portion of a blood platelet.

Hyalomma (hi"ah-lom'ah) a genus of ticks occurring only in Africa, Asia, and Europe; ectoparasites of animals and man, they may transmit disease and cause serious injury by their bite.

hyalomucoid (hi"ah-lo-mu'koid) the mucoid of the vitreous body.

hyalonyxis (hi"ah-lo-nik'sis) the act of puncturing the vitreous body.

hyalophagia (hi"ah-lo-fa'je-ah) the eating of glass.

hyaloplasm (hi'ah-lo-plazm") 1. the more fluid portion of the cytoplasm of a cell, in which the other elements are dispersed. Called also cytochylema and paraplasm. 2. axoplasm.

nuclear h., karyolymph.

hyaloserositis (hi"ah-lo-se"ro-si'tis) inflammation of serous membranes marked by conversion of the serous exudate into a pearly coating of the affected organ.

hyalosis (hi"ah-lo'sis) degenerative changes in the vitreous humor.

asteroid h., the presence of spherical or star-shaped opacities in the vitreous humor.

hyalosome (hi-al'o-sōm) a structure resembling the nucleolus of a cell, but staining only slightly.

hyaluronic acid (hi"ah-lu-ron'ik) a sulfate-free mucopolysaccharide in the intercellular substance of various tissues, especially the skin; also isolated from the vitreous humor, synovial fluid, umbilical cord, etc.

hyaluronidase (hi"ah-lu-ron'ĭ-dās) an enzyme that catalyzes the hydrolysis of hyaluronic acid, the "cement material" of connective tissues; it is found in leeches, snake and spider venom, in testes, and is produced by various pathogenic bacteria, enabling them to spread through tissue. A preparation from mammalian testes is used to promote absorption and diffusion of solutions injected subcutaneously. When hyaluronidase is mixed with fluids administered subcutaneously, absorption is more rapid and less uncomfortable. This is especially valuable when large amounts of fluid must be given by hypodermoclysis instead of intravenously. The drug should be dissolved just before it is used and usually is injected with the first portion of the fluid to be given. Hyaluronidase should not be given in areas where there is infection. Since it hastens absorption, it must be given with caution when administered with toxic drugs, as the toxic reaction can occur very rapidly.

Hyazyme (hi′ah-zīm) trademark for a preparation of hyaluronidase for injection.

hybrid (hi′brid) an offspring of parents of different species.

hybridization (hi″brid-ĭ-za′shun) the production of hybrids.

hydantoin (hi-dan′to-in) a crystalline base, glycolyl urea, derivable from allantoin.

hydatid (hi′dah-tid) 1. a hydatid cyst. 2. any cystlike structure.

h. cyst, the larval stage of the tapeworm *Echinococcus granulosis* or *E. multilocularis,* containing daughter cysts, each of which has many scolices; it is the cause of hydatid disease. Called also echinococcus cyst and hydatid.

h. disease, an infection, usually of the liver, caused by larval forms (hydatid cysts) of TAPEWORMS of the genus *Echinococcus,* and characterized by the development of expanding cysts. In the infection caused by *E. granulosis,* single or multiple cysts that are unilocular in character are formed, and in that caused by *E. multilocularis,* the host's tissues are invaded and destroyed as the cyst(s) enlarge by peripheral budding. Called also echinococcosis.

h. mole, hydatidiform mole.

h. or Morgagni, a cystlike remnant of the müllerian duct attached to a testis or to the oviduct.

sessile h., the hydatid of Morgagni connected with a testis.

stalked h., the hydatid of Morgagni connected with an oviduct.

hydatidiform (hi″dah-tid′ĭ-form) resembling a hydatid.

h. mole, an abnormal pregnancy resulting from a pathologic ovum, with proliferation of the epithelial covering of the chorionic villi and dissolution and cystic cavitation of the avascular stroma of the villi. It results in a mass of cysts resembling a bunch of grapes. Called also hydatid mole.

hydatidocele (hi″dah-tid′o-sēl) a tumor of the scrotum containing hydatids.

hydatidoma (hi″dah-tĭ-do′mah) a tumor containing hydatids.

hydatidosis (hi″dah-tĭ-do′sis) hydatid disease.

hydatidostomy (hi″dah-tĭ-dos′to-me) incision and drainage of a hydatid cyst.

hydatiduria (hi″dah-tĭ-du′re-ah) excretion of hydatid cysts in the urine.

Hydeltra (hi-del′trah) trademark for preparations of prednisolone, a compound used as a glucocorticoid.

hydr(o)- word element [Gr.], *hydrogen; water.*

hydracetin (hi-dras′ĕ-tin) acetylphenylhydrazine, an erythrocyte depressant.

hydraeroperitoneum (hi-dra″er-o-per″ĭ-to-ne′um) water and gas in the peritoneal cavity.

hydragogue (hi″drah-gog) 1. increasing the fluid content of the feces. 2. a purgative that causes evacuation of watery stools.

hydralazine hydrochloride (hi-dral′ah-zēn) an antihypertensive and vasodilator; used in peripheral vascular disease, essential and early malignant hypertension, thrombophlebitis, and other conditions in which dilation of the blood vessels of the extremities is desired.

The drug may be administered orally, intramuscularly, or intravenously. Dosage is adjusted to the individual patient's response. The blood pressure should be checked frequently, especially during parenteral administration of the drug. Side effects are rare with therapeutic doses, but the drug must be administered with caution to patients with coronary artery disease, advanced kidney damage, and existing or incipient cerebral vascular accident.

hydramnios (hi-dram′ne-os) excess of amniotic fluid.

hydranencephaly (hi″dran-en-sef′ah-le) absence of the cerebral hemispheres, their normal site being occupied by cerebrospinal fluid.

hydrargyria (hi″drar-jir′e-ah) chronic poisoning from mercury.

hydrargyrum (hi-drar′jĭ-rum) [L.] mercury (symbol Hg).

hydrarthrosis (hi″drar-thro′sis) an accumulation of watery fluid in the cavity of a joint. adj., **hydrarthro′dial.**

hydrase, hydratase (hi′drās; hi′drah-tās) any enzyme that catalyzes the hydration-dehydration of C — O linkages.

hydrate (hi′drāt) 1. a compound of water with a radical. 2. a salt or other compound that contains water of crystallization.

hydration (hi-dra′shun) the absorption of or combination with water.

hydraulics (hi-draw′liks) the science dealing with the mechanics of liquids.

hydrazine (hi′drah-zin) a gaseous diamine, H_4N_2, or any of its substitution derivatives.

hydremia (hi-dre′me-ah) excess of water in the blood.

hydrencephalocele (hi″dren-sef′ah-lo-sēl″) hernial protrusion of brain tissue containing fluid.

hydrencephalomeningocele (hi″dren-sef″ah-lo-mĕ-ning′go-sēl) hernial protrusion, through a cranial defect, of meninges containing cerebrospinal fluid and brain substance.

hydroa (hi-dro′ah) a vesicular eruption, with intense itching and burning, occurring on skin surfaces exposed to sunlight.

hydroappendix (hi″dro-ah-pen′diks) distention of the vermiform appendix with watery fluid.

hydrobilirubin (hi″dro-bil″ĭ-roo′bin) a bile pigment.

hydrocalycosis (hi″dro-kal″ĭ-ko′sis) distention of a single calix of the kidney with accumulated urine.

hydrocarbon (hi″dro-kar′bon) an organic compound that contains carbon and hydrogen only.

alicyclic h., one that has cyclic structure and aliphatic properties.

aliphatic h., a compound in which the carbons are

attached in a chain with no ring form.

aromatic h., one that has cyclic structure and a closed conjugated system of double bonds.

cyclic h., one of a series of hydrocarbons having the general formula C_nH_{2n}, the carbon atoms being thought of as having a closed ring structure.

saturated h., one that has the maximum number of hydrogen atoms for a given carbon structure.

unsaturated h., an aliphatic or alicyclic hydrocarbon that has less than the maximum number of hydrogen atoms for a given carbon structure.

hydrocele (hi′dro-sēl) a painless swelling of the scrotum caused by a collection of fluid in the tunica vaginalis testis, the outermost covering of the testes. It can be removed by withdrawing the fluid by tapping through the outer layer of tissue, or by cutting away the outer layer of tissue. The latter operation makes it impossible for the hydrocele to recur.

hydrocelectomy (hi″dro-se-lek′to-me) excision of a hydrocele.

hydrocephalocele (hi″dro-sef′ah-lo-sēl″) hydrencephalocele.

hydrocephaloid (hi″dro-sef′ah-loid) resembling hydrocephalus.

h. disease, a condition resembling hydrocephalus, but with depressed fontanels, following severe diarrhea.

hydrocephalus (hi″dro-sef′ah-lus) a condition characterized by enlargement of the cranium caused by abnormal accumulation of cerebrospinal fluid; called also water on the brain. adj., **hydroceph-al′ic.** Although hydrocephalus occurs occasionally in adults, it is usually associated with a congenital defect in infants. When the regular flow or absorption of the CEREBROSPINAL FLUID is impaired by a congenital malformation of the ventricular system, the fluid accumulates in the brain and enlarges the ventricles.

There is no known effective treatment for hydrocephalus other than surgery. The procedures most often used employ the SHUNT technique, so called because it shunts the fluid away from the cranial cavity and into the jugular vein, where it is absorbed into the bloodstream. The shunt technique is not the final answer to all problems of hydrocephalus, and research continues on possible alternative methods.

PATIENT CARE. The child with hydrocephalus requires frequent changing of position of the head as well as of the body. Decubitus ulcers (pressure sores) on the head are a constant threat because of the weight and size of the head and the child's inability to move it. The child should be picked up and held frequently, especially during feeding periods. Care must be taken that the head is well supported while the child is being held.

hydrochloric acid (hi″dro-klōr′ik) HCl, a normal constituent of gastric juice in man and other animals. The absence of free hydrochloric acid in the stomach, called achlorhydria, may be found with chronic gastritis, gastric carcinoma, pernicious anemia, pellagra, and alcoholism. This condition is also referred to as gastric anacidity.

Hyperacidity of the gastric juice is often associated with emotional stress and tension and is believed to be a factor in the development of peptic ULCER.

Dilute hydrochloric acid may be administered to aid digestion in achlorhydria. The preparation should be given well diluted and the patient is instructed to take the solution through a straw to avoid damage to the teeth. It is administered 30 minutes before each meal.

hydrochloride (hi″dro-klōr′īd) an addition salt of hydrochloric acid with an organic base.

hydrochlorothiazide (hi″dro-klōr″o-thi′ah-zīd) a white, crystalline compound used as a diuretic and antihypertensive agent.

hydrocholecystis (hi″dro-ko″le-sis′tis) distention of gallbladder with watery fluid.

hydrocholeresis (hi″dro-ko″lĕ-re′sis) secretion of bile relatively low in specific gravity, viscosity, and total solid content.

hydrocholeretic (hi″dro-ko″ler-et′ik) 1. pertaining to or producing hydrocholeresis. 2. an agent that stimulates an increased output of bile of low specific gravity.

hydrocirsocele (hi″dro-sir′so-sēl) hydrocele with variocele.

hydrocodone (hi″dro-ko′dōn) a synthetic analgesic used in the form of the bitartrate salt as an antitussive. Continued use may cause addiction. Called also dihydrocodeinone.

Hydrocollator (hi-drok″o-la′tor) trademark for a canvas-enclosed pack of silica gel that is immersed in water and heated to 140° to 160° F. and applied to a body part for the purpose of applying local HEAT. The pack has the advantage of maintaining heat for 20 to 30 minutes and therefore requires no replacement during a treatment prescribed for this period of time. The pack is heavier than electric heating pads and hot water bottles, but should not be placed under the part being treated so that body weight presses against it. Several layers of terry cloth are placed between the pack and the patient's skin to avoid burning. The packs are stored in special containers which maintain the moisture and do not allow the packs to become completely dry. These same containers are used in heating the Hydrocollator pack.

hydrocolloid (hi″dro-kol′oid) a colloid in which water is the dispersion medium.

hydrocolpos (hi″dro-kol′pos) collection of watery fluid in the vagina.

hydrocortamate (hi″dro-kor′tah-māt) a synthetic glucocorticoid used in the topical treatment of dermatoses.

hydrocortisone (hi″dro-kor′tĭ-sōn) the pharmaceutical term for cortisol, the principal GLUCOCORTICOID secreted by the adrenal gland; it is used for its anti-inflammatory action.

Hydrocortone (hi″dro-kor′tōn) trademark for preparations of hydrocortisone, a corticosteroid.

hydrocyanic acid (hi″dro-si-an′ik) a volatile liquid that is extremely poisonous because it checks the oxidation process in protoplasm.

hydrocyst (hi′dro-sist) a cyst with watery contents.

HydroDiuril (hi″dro-di′u-ril) trademark for a preparation of hydrochlorothiazide, a diuretic and antihypertensive.

hydroflumethiazide (hi″dro-floo″mĕ-thi′ah-zīd) an antihypertensive and diuretic.

hydrogel (hi′dro-jel) a gel that contains water.

hydrogen (hi′dro-jen) a chemical element, atomic number 1, atomic weight 1.00797, symbol H. (See table of ELEMENTS.) It exists as the mass 1 isotope (protium, or light or ordinary hydrogen), mass 2 isotope (deuterium, heavy hydrogen), and mass 3 isotope (tritium).

heavy h., hydrogen having double the mass of ordinary hydrogen; deuterium.

h. ion concentration, the degree of concentration of hydrogen ions (the acid element) in a solution. Its symbol is pH, and expresses the degree to which a solution is acidic or alkaline. The pH range extends from 0 to 14, pH 7 being neutral. A pH of less than 7 indicates acidity, above 7 indicates alkalinity. See also ACID-BASE BALANCE.

h. monoxide, water, H_2O.

h. peroxide, H_2O_2, used in solution as an anti-bacterial agent. A 3 per cent solution foams on touching skin or mucous membrane and appears to have a mechanical cleansing action.

h. sulfide, an ill-smelling, colorless, poisonous gas, H_2S; much used as a chemical reagent. Called also hydrosulfuric acid.

hydrogenase (hi′dro-jen-ās″) an enzyme that catalyzes the reduction of various substances by combining them with molecular hydrogen.

hydrogenate (hi′dro-jen-āt″) to cause to combine with hydrogen; to reduce with hydrogen.

hydrogymnastics (hi″dro-jim-nas′tiks) therapeutic exercise performed in water.

hydrokinetic (hi″dro-ki-net′ik) relating to movement of water or other fluid, as in a whirlpool bath.

hydrokinetics (hi″dro-ki-net′iks) the science dealing with fluids in motion.

hydrolase (hi′dro-lās) one of the six main classes of enzymes, comprising those that catalyze the hydrolysis of a compound.

hydrology (hi-drol′o-je) the study of water and its uses.

Hydrolose (hi′dro-lōs) trademark for a preparation of methylcellulose, a laxative.

hydro-lyase (hi″dro-jen-li′ās) an adaptive enzyme formed by *Escherichia coli,* which catalyzes the breakdown of formic acid to carbon dioxide and hydrogen.

hydrolymph (hi′dro-limf) the thin blood of certain animals.

hydrolysate (hi-drol′ĭ-zat) any compound produced by hydrolysis.

protein h., a mixture of amino acids prepared by splitting a protein with acid, alkali, or enzyme. Such preparations provide the nutritive equivalent of the original material in the form of its constituent amino acids and are used in special diets or for patients unable to take the ordinary food proteins.

hydrolysis (hi-drol′ĭ-sis) the cleavage of a compound by the addition of water, the hydroxyl group being incorporated in one fragment and the hydrogen atom in the other. adj., **hydrolyt′ic.**

hydroma (hi-dro′mah) hygroma.

hydromeningitis (hi″dro-men″in-ji′tis) meningitis with serous effusion.

hydromeningocele (hi″dro-mĕ-ning′go-sēl) protrusion of the meninges, containing fluid, through a defect in the skull or vertebral column.

hydrometer (hi-drom′ĕ-ter) an instrument for determining the specific gravity of a fluid.

hydrometra (hi″dro-me′trah) collection of watery fluid in the uterus.

hydrometrocolpos (hi″dro-me″tro-kol′pos) collection of watery fluid in the uterus and vagina.

hydrometry (hi-drom′ĕ-tre) measurement of specific gravity with a hydrometer.

hydromicrocephaly (hi″dro-mi″kro-sef′ah-le) smallness of the head with an abnormal amount of cerebrospinal fluid.

hydromorphone (hi″dro-mor′fōn) a hydrogenated ketone of morphine used as an analgesic. Called also dihydromorphinone.

h. hydrochloride, the crystalline compound used as a narcotic analgesic.

hydromphalus (hi-drom′fah-lus) a cystic accumulation of watery fluid at the umbilicus.

hydromyelia (hi″dro-mi-e′le-ah) dilatation of the central canal of the spinal cord with an abnormal accumulation of fluid.

hydromyelomeningocele (hi″dro-mi″ĕ-lo-mĕ-ning′go-sēl) a defect of the spine marked by protrusion of the membranes and tissue of the spinal cord, forming a fluid-filled sac.

hydromyoma (hi″dro-mi-o′mah) a leiomyoma with cystic degeneration.

hydronephrosis (hi″dro-nĕ-fro′sis) distention of the renal pelvis and calices with urine. adj., **hydronephrot′ic.** If it is allowed to progress, the functioning units of the kidney are destroyed. The collecting tubules dilate and the muscular walls of the renal pelvis and calices stretch, are replaced by fibrous tissue, and eventually form a large, fluid-filled, functionless sac.

The cause of hydronephrosis is obstruction or atrophy of the urinary tract. Mechanical obstruction may result from ureteral tumors, calculi, NEPHROPTOSIS, benign or malignant hyperplasia of the prostate, or carcinoma of the bladder, urethra, or glans penis. Inflammatory obstruction is the outcome of a urinary tract infection that produces edema and narrowing of the ureters or urethra. Rarely there occurs during pregnancy a loss of muscle tone in the urinary tract. The atony is thought to be induced by placental hormones.

SYMPTOMS. The patient usually complains of recurrent attacks of pain in the kidney region. The pain may be described as dull and nagging, or sharp. Examination of the urine often reveals the presence of pus and blood; there is fever if infection develops. If both kidneys are involved, uremia develops as the functional units of the kidneys are destroyed.

Diagnosis is established by extensive urologic examination with detailed PYELOGRAPHY, which usually reveals the cause of the obstruction and accumulation of fluid in the pelvis.

TREATMENT. The urinary tract must be drained by whatever means necessary; this may involve a simple dilatation of the ureter or urethra or it may require surgery of the affected kidney. When urinary tract infection is present as a cause or result of the hydronephrosis, urinary antiseptics and antibiotics are administered until the urine becomes sterile.

hydropericarditis (hi″dro-per″ĭ-kar-di′tis) pericarditis with watery effusion.

hydropericardium (hi″dro-per″ĭ-kar′de-um) an excess of transudate in the pericardial cavity.

hydroperitoneum (hi″dro-per″ĭ-to-ne′um) a collection of fluid in the peritoneal cavity; ASCITES.

hydrophilia (hi″dro-fil′e-ah) the property of absorbing water; having a strong affinity for water. adj., **hydrophil′ic.**

hydrophobia (hi″dro-fo′be-ah) rabies.

hydrophobic (hi″dro-fo′bik) 1. pertaining to hydrophobia (RABIES). 2. repelling water; insoluble in water.

hydrophthalmus (hi″drof-thal′mos) distention of the eyeball in infantile glaucoma.

hydrophysometra (hi″dro-fi″so-me′trah) collection of fluid and gas in the uterus.

hydropic (hi-drop′ik) affected with dropsy, or hydrops.

hydropneumatosis (hi″dro-nu″mah-to′sis) collection of fluid and gas in the tissues.

hydropneumogony (hi″dro-nu-mo′go-ne) injection of air into a joint to detect the presence of effusion.

hydropneumopericardium (hi″dro-nu″mo-per″ĭ-kar′de-um) fluid and gas in the pericardium.

hydropneumoperitoneum (hi″dro-nu″mo-per″ĭ-to-ne′um) fluid and gas in the peritoneal cavity.

hydropneumothorax (hi″dro-nu″mo-tho′raks) a collection of fluid and gas within the pleural cavity.

hydrops (hi′drops) [L.] abnormal accumulation of serous fluid in the tissues or in a body cavity; called also dropsy.

fetal h., h. feta′lis, accumulation of fluid in the entire body of the newborn infant, in erythroblastosis fetalis.

hydropyonephrosis (hi″dro-pi″o-nĕ-fro′sis) urine and pus in the renal pelvis.

hydroquinone (hi″dro-kwin′ōn) a topical skin-depigmenting agent.

hydrorrhea (hi″dro-re′ah) a copious watery discharge.

h. gravida′rum, watery discharge from the gravid uterus.

hydrosalpinx (hi″dro-sal′pinks) accumulation of watery fluid in a uterine tube.

hydrosarcocele (hi″dro-sar′ko-sēl) hydrocele and sarcocele together.

hydroscheocele (hi-dros′ke-o-sēl″) a scrotal hernia containing fluid.

hydrosol (hi′dro-sol) a colloid in which the dispersion medium is a liquid.

hydrospirometer (hi″dro-spi-rom′ĕ-ter) a spirometer in which a column of water serves as an index.

hydrostat (hi′dro-stat) a device for regulating the height of a fluid in a column or reservoir.

hydrostatic (hi″dro-stat′ik) pertaining to a liquid in a state of equilibrium.

hydrostatics (hi″dro-stat′iks) the science of equilibrium of fluids.

hydrosulfuric acid (hi″dro-sul-fu′rik) hydrogen sulfide.

hydrosyringomyelia (hi″dro-sĭ-ring″go-mi-e′le-ah) distention of the central canal of the spinal cord, with the formation of cavities and degeneration.

hydrotaxis (hi″dro-tak′sis) an orientation movement of motile organisms or cells in response to the influence of water or moisture.

hydrotherapy (hi″dro-ther′ah-pe) the external use of water in the treatment of disease and injury. adj., **hydrotherapeu′tic.** Because of its physical properties related to the conduction of heat, buoyancy, and cleansing action, water is an ideal agent for applications of HEAT and COLD to obtain desired physiological effects, débridement of wounds that are extensive and not easily cleansed by other methods, and the implementation of programs of therapeutic EXERCISE.

Applications of moist heat and warm water help relieve pain and improve circulation, promote relaxation and reduce muscle tightness, and serve to localize infections. Examples of hydrotherapeutic measures of this type include warm baths, HYDROCOLLATOR packs, and compresses of toweling, wool, and other cloth materials. Special equipment such as the HUBBARD TANK and whirlpool baths are fitted with devices that mechanically agitate the water, thereby providing gentle massage and a cleansing action in addition to the therapeutic effects of heat.

Applications of cold water include cold packs, ice compresses, cold baths on all or part of the body, and cold showers. The cold water decreases body temperature, reduces swelling and constricts blood vessels, thereby reducing blood flow to the treated part. Brief applications of cold water increase the pulse and respiration rates and produce a rise in blood pressure. Removal from the cold water to a warmer environment induces relaxation and brings about a decrease in the vital signs.

The special properties of buoyancy, cohesion, and viscosity make water a particularly useful medium in which exercises may be carried out. For patients who cannot tolerate weight bearing on the joints, walking exercises under water are of great value. The buoyant effect of the water in an exercise pool allows for a wider range of motion and permits fuller use of the muscles with less discomfort. This is especially important in exercising painful arthritic joints. The cohesion and viscosity of water account for its resistance to objects moving through it. This resistance can be used to good advantage in the progressive improvement of muscle strength and endurance by exercise. An additional benefit of underwater exercising is its psychological impact on the patient who has impaired mobility. In the water he has a feeling of movement accomplished with relatively more ease than outside the water and thus has a good "body image" of mobility.

Water under pressure may be applied in a spray or jet stream to all or a part of the body for the purpose of providing stimulation and massage, depending on the amount of pressure used. This procedure, called a douche, may also be used to provide a cleansing action to the part being treated.

hydrothermal, hydrothermic (hi″dro-ther′mal; hi″dro-ther′mik) relating to the temperature effects of water, as in hot baths.

hydrothionemia (hi″dro-thi″o-ne′me-ah) hydrogen sulfide in the blood.

hydrothionuria (hi″dro-thi″o-nu′re-ah) hydrogen sulfide in the urine.

hydrothorax (hi″dro-tho′raks) the presence of noninflammatory serous fluid within the pleural cavity.

hydrotropism (hi-drot′ro-pizm) a growth response of a nonmotile organism to the presence of water or moisture.

hydrotympanum (hi″dro-tim′pah-num) a collection of serous fluid in the middle ear.

hydroureter (hi″dro-u-re′ter) distention of the ureter with fluid.

hydrous (hi′drus) containing water.

hydrovarium (hi″dro-va′re-um) a collection of serous fluid in an ovary.

hydroxide (hi-drok′sīd) any compound of hydroxyl with another radical.

hydroxocobalamin (hi-drok″so-ko-bal′ah-min) an analogue of cyanocobalamin (vitamin B_{12}) having exceptionally long-acting hematopoietic activity; used in the treatment of pernicious anemia and other macrocytic anemias.

hydroxy- a chemical prefix indicating presence of the univalent radical OH.

hydroxyamphetamine (hi-drok″se-am-fet′ah-mēn) a compound used as a sympathomimetic nasal decongestant, pressor, and mydriatic.

hydroxyapatite (hi-drok″se-ap′ah-tīt) an inorganic constituent of bone matrix and teeth, imparting rigidity to these structures.

hydroxybenzene (hi-drok″sĭ-ben′zēn) phenol.

hydroxybutyric acid (hi-drok″sĭ-bu-tir′ik) a poisonous acid sometimes occurring in the urine in diabetes (ketoacidosis).

hydroxychloroquine (hi-drok″sĭ-klo′ro-kwin) a drug used as the sulfate salt in the treatment of malaria, lupus erythematosus, rheumatoid arthritis, and symptomatic giardiasis.

25-hydroxycholecalciferol (hi-drok″sĭ-ko″le-kal-sif′er-ol) a metabolically activated form of cholecalciferol synthesized in the liver.

hydroxycorticosterone (hi-drok″sĭ-kor″tĭ-ko-stēr′ōn) cortisol, a corticosteroid.

hydroxydione (hi-drok″sĭ-di′ōn) a steroid preparation used as the sodium salt to produce basal anesthesia.

hydroxyl (hi-drok′sil) the univalent radical OH.

hydroxylase (hi-drok′sĭ-lās) any enzyme that brings about the coupled oxidation of two donors, with incorporation of oxygen into one of them.

hydroxylysine (hi-drok″sĭ-li′sēn) a naturally occurring amino acid.

hydroxyphenamate (hi-drok″sĭ-fen′ah-māt) a minor tranquilizer.

hydroxyprogesterone (hi-drok″sĭ-pro-jes′ter-ōn) a long-acting progesterone used as the caproate ester in the treatment of corpus luteum deficiency.

hydroxyproline (hi-drok″sĭ-pro′lēn) an amino acid produced in the digestion of hydrolytic decomposition of proteins, especially of collagens.

hydroxystilbamidine (hi-drok″sĭ-stil-bam′ĭ-dēn) a compound used in treatment of leishmaniasis and blastomycosis.

hydroxytetracycline (hi-drok″sĭ-tĕ″trah-si′klēn) oxytetracycline, a broad-spectrum antibiotic.

5-hydroxytryptamine (hi-drok″sĭ-trip′tah-mēn) serotonin.

hydroxyzine (hi-drok′sĭ-zēn) a central nervous system depressant having antispasmodic, antihistaminic, and antifibrillatory actions; used as the hydrochloride or pamoate salt.

hydruria (hi-droo′re-ah) excretion of urine of low specific gravity.

hygiene (hi′jēn) 1. the science of health and its preservation. 2. a condition or practice, such as cleanliness, that is conducive to preservation of health. adj., **hygien′ic.**

mental h., the science dealing with development of healthy mental and emotional reactions and habits.

oral h., the proper care of the mouth and teeth.

social h., the science dealing with prevention and cure of venereal disease.

hygienics (hi″je-en′iks) a system of principles for promoting health.

hygienist (hi′je-en″ist) a specialist in hygiene.

dental h., a dental health specialist whose primary concern is maintenance of dental health and prevention of oral disease (see also under DENTAL).

hygro- (hi′gro) word element [Gr.], *moisture.*

hygroma (hi-gro′mah) an accumulation of fluid in a sac, cyst, or bursa. adj., **hygrom′atous.**

cystic h., h. cys′ticum, an endothelium-lined, fluid-containing lesion of lymphatic origin, encountered most often in infants and children and occurring in various regions of the body, most commonly in the posterior triangle of the neck, behind the sternocleidomastoid muscle (hygroma colli cysticum).

Fleischmann's h., enlargement of a bursa in the floor of the mouth, to the outer side of the genioglossus muscle.

hygrometer (hi-grom′ĕ-ter) an instrument for measuring atmospheric moisture.

hygroscope (hi′gro-skōp) an instrument for showing variation in atmospheric moisture.

hygroscopic (hi″gro-skop′ik) readily absorbing moisture.

Hygroton (hi′gro-ton) trademark for a preparation of chlorthalidone, a diuretic.

hymen (hi′men) the membranous fold partly or completely closing the vaginal orifice. adj., **hy′menal.**

hymenectomy (hi″men-ek′to-me) excision of the hymen.

hymenitis (hi″men-i′tis) inflammation of the hymen.

hymenolepiasis (hi″men-o-lep-i′ah-sis) infection due to organisms of species of *Hymenolepis.*

Hymenolepis (hi″men-ol′ĕ-pis) a genus of TAPEWORMS; three species, *H. diminu′ta, H. lanceola′ta,* and *H. na′na,* have been found in man.

hymenology (hi″men-ol′o-je) the science of the membranes.

hymenotomy (hi″men-ot′o-me) incision of the hymen.

hyoepiglottidean (hi″o-ep″ĭ-glŏ-tid′e-an) pertaining to the hyoid bone and epiglottis.

hyoglossal (hi″o-glos′al) pertaining to the hyoid bone and tongue or to the hyoglossal muscle.

hyoid (hi′oid) 1. shaped like Greek letter upsilon (υ). 2. pertaining to the hyoid bone.

h. bone, a horseshoe-shaped bone situated at the base of the tongue, just below the thyroid cartilage. (See also table of BONES.)

hyoscine (hi′o-sin) scopolamine.

hyoscyamine (hi″o-si′ah-mēn) an anticholinergic alkaloid usually obtained from species of the plant *Hyoscyamus* or other genera of the family Solanaceae. The hydrobromide and sulfate salts are used to produce parasympathetic blockage.

hyoscyamus (hi″o-si′ah-mus) the dried leaf of *Hyoscyamus niger,* which contains hyoscyamine and scopolamine; used in tincture or extract to produce parasympathetic blockade.

hyp- see HYPO-.

hypacusia (hi″pah-ku′ze-ah) slightly diminished acuteness of the sense of hearing.

hypalbuminosis (hi″pal-bu″mĭ-no′sis) hypoalbuminosis.

hypalgesia (hi″pal-je′ze-ah) diminished sensibility to pain. adj. **hypalge′sic.**

hypamnios (hi-pam′ne-os) deficiency of amniotic fluid.

hypanakinesia (hi″pan-ah-ki-ne′se-ah) hypokinesia.

hypaxial (hi-pak′se-al) beneath an axis, as the axis of the vertebral column.

hyper- word element [Gr.], *abnormally increased; excessive.*

hyperacid (hi″per-as′id) abnormally or excessively acid.

hyperacidity (hi″per-ah-sid′ĭ-te) excessive acidity.

hyperactive (hi″per-ak′tiv) exhibiting hyperactivity.

hyperactivity (hi″per-ak-tiv′ĭ-te) abnormally increased activity. Developmental hyperactivity of children (*hyperkinesia*) is characterized by constant motion and fidgetiness, excitability and impulsiveness, distractibility and short attention span, low tolerance for frustration, and poor muscle coordination. Although they exhibit a normal to high IQ, these children do not do well in school and have learning difficulties.

Patterns of behavior vary in individual children and even in the same child from day to day, at times from hour to hour. The condition usually abates during adolescence.

A small percentage of cases of hyperactivity result from brain damage and psychoses; however, the specific cause or causes of most cases have not been determined. Recent research has shown some correlation between the intake of synthetic colors and flavors in food and the incidence of hyperactivity. Some success in relief of the behavioral pattern of hyperactivity has been achieved through the use of the Feingold diet. This diet restricts the intake of these artificial substances and limits foods which contain natural salicylates, including apples, apricots, blackberries, cucumbers, grapes, oranges, peaches, plums, raspberries, tea, and tomatoes.

Medications that have been tried with varying degrees of success are stimulants and antidepressants, which have the paradoxical effect of calming the child, and tranquilizers. This form of drug therapy is highly controversial and is only a palliative measure that is not without risks.

hyperacusia, hyperacusis (hi″per-ah-ku′ze-ah; hi″per-ah-ku′sis) abnormal acuteness of the sense of hearing.

hyperacute (hi″per-ah-kūt′) extremely acute.

hyperadenosis (hy″per-ad″ĕ-no′sis) enlargement of glands.

hyperadiposis (hi″per-ad″ĭ-po′sis) extreme fatness.

hyperadrenalemia (hi″per-ah-dre″nah-le′me-ah) increased amount of adrenal secretion in the blood.

hyperadrenalism, hyperadrenia (hi″per-ah-dren′al-izm; hi″per-ah-dre′ne-ah) overactivity of the adrenal glands.

hyperadrenocorticalism, hyperadrenocorticism (hi″per-ah-dre″no-kor′tĭ-kal-izm″; hi″per-ah-dre″no-kor′tĭ-sizm) hypersecretion of the adrenal cortex; CUSHING'S SYNDROME.

hyperaffectivity (hi″per-ah″fek-tiv′ĭ-te) abnormally increased sensibility to mild stimuli; abnormally heightened emotional reactivity.

hyperalbuminemia (hi″per-al-bu″mĭ-ne′me-ah) excessive albumin content of the blood.

hyperaldosteronemia (hi″per-al-dos″ter-o-ne′me-ah) excess of aldosterone in the blood.

hyperaldosteronism (hi″per-al-dos′ter-ōn-izm″) an abnormality of electrolyte metabolism produced by excessive secretion of aldosterone, it may be primary (called Conn's syndrome) or occur secondarily in response to extra-adrenal disease. There may be hypertension, hypokalemia, alkalosis, muscular weakness, polyuria, and polydipsia. Called also aldosteronism.

hyperaldosteronuria (hi″per-al-dos″ter-o-nu′re-ah) excess of aldosterone in the urine.

hyperalgesia (hi″per-al-je′ze-ah) excessive sensitiveness to pain. adj., **hyperalge′sic.**

hyperalimentation (hi″per-al″ĭ-men-ta′shun) a program of parenteral administration of all nutrients for patients with gastrointestinal dysfunction; also called total parenteral alimentation (TPA) and total parenteral nutrition (TPN).

The procedure originated as an emergency life-saving technique following surgery for severe and massive trauma of the gastrointestinal tract. It has recently become a relatively common means of providing bowel rest and nutrition in spite of inherent risks. Although primarily employed as a short-term temporary measure until either surgical or medical treatment corrects the gastrointestinal dysfunction, it has been used with some success as long-term therapy for selected patients on an outpatient basis.

Hyperalimentation may be employed in the following conditions: malnutrition from such acute and chronic inflammatory bowel diseases as regional ILEITIS (Crohn's disease) and ULCERATIVE COLITIS, partial or total obstruction of the gastrointestinal tract that cannot be relieved immediately by surgery, congenital anomalies in the newborn prior to surgery, massive burns that produce critical protein loss, and other disorders in which malnutrition is a threat to the life of the patient who cannot receive nutrients via the digestive tract.

The nutrient mix is tailored to the individual needs and tolerance of the patient. There is not complete agreement among the experts as to the ideal mix, especially of amino acids. The primary goal is to provide sufficient food elements, calories, vitamins, minerals, electrolytes, and other nutrients to allow growth and repair of tissues and normal cellular function.

Administration of the nutrients is accomplished via a CENTRAL VENOUS CATHETER, usually inserted in the superior vena cava. The route of administration, constant rate of flow required, and potential patient sensitivity to the elements administered, all contribute to the potential complications of hyperalimentation.

Of the many complications that may develop, the most common are febrile reactions arising from patient intolerance to the required rate of flow, reactions due to individual sensitivity to some of the elements in the nutrient mix, and infection from contamination of either the site of insertion of the catheter or the apparatus used to administer the nutrients. Other complications that may develop include phlebitis and thrombosis of the vena cava, electrolyte imbalance, hyperglycemia, cardiac overload, dehydration, metabolic acidosis, and mechanical trauma to the heart.

PATIENT CARE. The patient receiving hyperalimentation requires almost continuous monitoring and assessment of his status by skilled members of the health care team who are fully aware of the hazards of the procedure. The physician, nurse, and pharmacist are essential members of that team, working cooperatively to meet the needs of the patient and avoid complications. During the first 24 hours the patient is watched closely for signs of pneumothorax, hemothorax, internal bleeding, and cardiac complications.

Principles of strict aseptic technique must be followed in the daily changing of dressings and in handling the nutrient solution and the administration equipment. The catheter through which the nutrients are administered should not be used for administration of medication, blood, or any other substance that may induce clotting in the vein.

Vital signs are checked frequently and any indication of a developing infection is attended to immediately. The urine is checked regularly throughout the day for sugar and acetone as a means of assessing the body's ability to utilize available carbohydrate. Daily blood sugar tests are done for the same reason. (See also HYPERGLYCEMIC HYPEROSMOLAR NONKETOTIC COMA.)

The rate of flow is checked regularly every half-hour to assure that the rate is constant. If, for any reason, the rate falls behind, no effort is made to increase the rate to catch up. If the nutrient mix is used up before a fresh supply is available, 5% dextrose may be given to keep the catheter and vein patent. Any unused nutrient remaining after a 24-hour period is discarded to reduce the danger of contamination.

hyperalkalinity (hi″per-al″kah-lin′ĭ-te) excessive alkalinity.

hyperammoniemia (hi″per-ah-mo″ne-e′me-ah) excess of ammonia in the blood.

hyperammoniuria (hi″per-ah-mo″ne-u′re-ah) excess of ammonia in the urine.

hyperamylasemia (hi″per-am″il-a-se′me-ah) abnormally high levels of amylase in the blood serum.

hyperanakinesia (hi″per-an″ah-ki-ne′ze-ah) excessive motor activity.

hyperaphia (hi″per-a′fe-ah) abnormal acuteness of the sense of touch. adj., **hyperaph′ic.**

hyperazotemia (hi″per-az″o-te′me-ah) excess of nitrogenous matter in the blood.

hyperazoturia (hi″per-az″o-tu′re-ah) excess of nitrogenous matter in the urine.

hyperbaric (hi″per-bār′ik) characterized by greater than normal pressure or weight; applied to gases under greater than atmospheric pressure, or to a solution of greater specific gravity than another taken as a standard of reference.

h. oxygenation, exposure to oxygen under conditions of greatly increased pressure; abbreviated HPO, for high-pressure oxygenation. This treatment is given to patients who, for various reasons, need more oxygen than they can take in by breathing while in the ordinary atmosphere, or even in an oxygen tent.

The patient is placed in a sealed enclosure, called a hyperbaric chamber. Compressed air is introduced to raise the atmospheric pressure to several times normal. At the same time the patient is given pure oxygen through a face mask. The increase in atmospheric pressure forces enough air into the patient so that the pressure within his body equals the pressure outside. Thus all his tissues become flooded with more than the usual supply of oxygen. While the patient is in the chamber, pressure changes are controlled with extreme care to avoid injury to his lungs or other tissues.

USE OF HYPERBARIC OXYGENATION. This form of treatment may be administered in many types of disorders in which oxygen supply is deficient. If, because of injury or disease, the lungs or heart are unable to maintain good circulation, the increase in oxygen can temporarily compensate for the reduction in circulation. If injury or disease has caused the breaking or blocking of arteries, an extra supply of oxygen in the vessels that are still functioning will help.

Hyperbaric oxygenation has been used with apparent success in some cases of heart surgery and other operations during which a forced supply of oxygen to the patient is vital. During such operations, the surgeon and his assistants must work within the chamber. Since the high pressure could cause the physical and mental disturbances of BENDS, as sometimes happens with deep-sea divers, it must be carefully controlled. All persons must be decompressed after leaving the chamber.

Patients suffering from tetanus and gas gangrene, infections caused by bacteria that are resistant to antibiotics but vulnerable to oxygen, are helped by hyperbaric oxygenation. The technique is apparently also useful in radiotherapy for cancer. When full of oxygen, cancer cells seem more vulnerable to radiation.

Carbon monoxide poisoning can be treated by hyperbaric oxygenation. Carbon monoxide molecules, displacing the oxygen in the erythrocytes, usually cause asphyxiation, but hyerbaric oxygenation can often keep the patient alive until the carbon monoxide has been eliminated from his system.

hyperbarism (hi″per-bar′izm) a condition due to exposure to ambient gas pressure or atmospheric pressures exceeding the pressure within the body.

hyperbetalipoproteinemia (hi″per-ba″tah-lip″o-pro″te-in-e′me-ah) hyperlipoproteinemia (type II).

hyperbilirubinemia (hi″per-bil″i-roo″bĭ-ne′me-ah) excess of bilirubin in the blood.

hyperbrachycephalic (hi″per-brak″e-sĕ-fal′ik) having a very short, wide head, with a cephalic index of 85.5 or more.

hyperbulia (hi″per-bu′le-ah) excessive willfulness.

hypercalcemia (hi″per-kal-se′me-ah) excess of calcium in the blood; calcemia.

idiopathic h., a condition of infants, associated with vitamin D intoxication, characterized by elevated serum calcium levels, increased density of the skeleton, mental deterioration, and nephrocalcinosis.

hypercalciuria (hi″per-kal″se-u′re-ah) excess of calcium in the urine.

hypercapnia, hypercarbia (hi″per-kap′ne-ah; hi″-per-kar′be-ah) excess of carbon dioxide in the blood, indicated by an elevated P_{CO_2} as determined by BLOOD GAS ANALYSIS, and resulting in respiratory ACIDOSIS. adj., **hypercap′nic.**

hypercatharsis (hi″per-kah-thar′sis) excessive purgation.

hypercellularity (hi″per-sel″u-lar′ĭ-te) abnormal increase in the number of cells present, as in bone marrow. adj., **hypercell′ular.**

hyperchloremia (hi″per-klo-re′me-ah) excess of chlorides in the blood. adj., **hyperchlore′mic.**

hyperchlorhydria (hi″per-klōr-hi′dre-ah) excess of HYDROCHLORIC ACID in the gastric juice.

hypercholesteremia, hypercholesterolemia (hi″per-ko-les″ter-e′me-ah; hi″per-ko-les″ter-ol-e′me-ah) excess of cholesterol in the blood.

familial h., hyperlipoproteinemia (type II).

hypercholia (hi″per-ko′le-ah) excessive secretion of bile.

hyperchromatism (hi″per-kro′mah-tizm) 1. excessive pigmentation. 2. degeneration of cell nuclei, which become filled with particles of pigment, or chromatin. 3. increased staining capacity. adj., **hyperchromat′ic.**

hyperchromatosis (hi″per-kro″mah-to′sis) hyperchromatism.

hyperchromemia (hi″per-kro-me′me-ah) a high color index of the blood.

hyperchromia (hi″per-kro′me-ah) 1. hyperchromatism. 2. abnormal increase in the hemoglobin content of erythrocytes. adj., **hyperchro′mic.**

hyperchylia (hi″per-ki′le-ah) excessive secretion of gastric juice.

hyperchylomicronemia (hi″per-ki″lo-mi″kro-ne′me-ah) the presence in the blood of an excessive number of particles of fat (chylomicrons).

hypercoagulability (hi″per-ko-ag″u-lah-bil′ĭ-te) abnormally increased coagulability of the blood.

hypercorticism (hi″per-kor′tĭ-sizm) hyperadrenocorticism.

hypercryalgesia, hypercryesthesia (hi″per-kri″al-je′ze-ah; hi″per-kri″es-the′ze-ah) excessive sensitiveness to cold.

hypercupriuria (hi″per-ku″pre-u′re-ah) an excess of copper in the blood.

hypercyanotic (hi″per-si″ah-not′ik) extremely cyanotic.

hypercythemia (hi″per-si-the′me-ah) excess of erythrocytes in the blood.

hypercytosis (hi″per-si-to′sis) an abnormally increased number of cells, especially of leukocytes.

hyperdactyly (hi″per-dak′tĭ-le) the presence of supernumerary digits on the hand or foot.

hyperdicrotic (hi″per-di-krot′ik) markedly dicrotic.

hyperdistention (hi″per-dis-ten′shun) excessive distention.

hyperdiuresis (hi″per-di″u-re′sis) excessive secretion of urine.

hyperdontia (hi″per-don′she-ah) a condition characterized by the presence of supernumerary teeth.

hyperdynamia (hi″per-di-na′me-ah) excessive muscular activity. adj., **hyperdynam′ic.**

hyperemesis (hi″per-em′ĕ-sis) excessive vomiting. adj., **hyperemet′ic.**

h. gravida′rum, excessive and pernicious vomiting of pregnancy, usually in the first trimester. The condition is more serious than simple MORNING SICKNESS, a common discomfort during the first 3 months of pregnancy. The exact cause of hyperemesis gravidarum is not known; however, psychologic factors are thought to play an important role in its development and control.

SYMPTOMS. The patient complains of uncontrollable nausea, persistent retching and vomiting, inability to take any food by mouth, and exhaustion

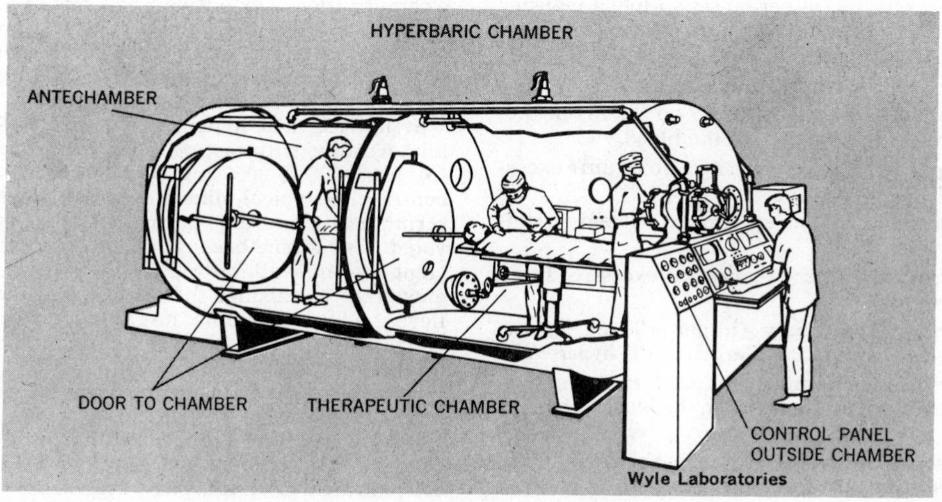

Hyperbaric chamber. (Courtesy of Wyle Laboratories.)

due to restlessness and lack of sleep. As the condition persists the patient becomes severely dehydrated, develops a fever, and may show signs of peripheral nerve involvement and jaundice. The urine may contain blood, bile, albumin, and ketone bodies as starvation develops. Although hyperemesis gravidarum is rarely fatal, these latter symptoms indicate a grave illness that demands prompt treatment.

TREATMENT. The physical symptoms of the patient are relieved by intravenous administration of fluids and nutrients and mild sedation to promote rest and relaxation. There is some controversy as to the value of psychotherapy; however, it is generally agreed that the patient will need help in overcoming emotional problems and nervous tension if they contribute to the occurrence of the disorder.

Dietary treatment may include limiting the intake of liquids, eating a snack of crackers or dry toast before arising, and avoiding excessive fat in the diet.

PATIENT CARE. The hospitalized patient should be placed in a quiet, well ventilated room that is free from odors or sights that may cause nausea. She should be encouraged to talk about her fears and anxieties if she indicates a desire to do so. The nursing staff should be alert to signs of depression or fears of pregnancy, labor, or the responsibilities of motherhood. Recovery is much more likely if the patient is able to vocalize her fears and seek aid in solving the mental conflicts that may be an underlying cause of her illness. Those who care for her should be sympathetic, optimistic, and reassuring in discussing her condition with her.

h. lacten'tium, the vomiting of nursing babies.

hyperemia (hi"per-e'me-ah) an excess of blood in a part. adj., **hypere'mic.**

active h., arterial h., that due to local or general relaxation of arterioles.

leptomeningeal h., congestion of the pia-arachnoid.

passive h., that due to obstruction to flow of blood from the area.

reactive h., that due to increase in blood flow after its temporary interruption.

venous h., passive hyperemia.

hyperencephalus (hi"per-en-sef'ah-lus) a monster with the cranial vault absent and the brain exposed.

hypereosinophilia (hi"per-e"o-sin"o-fil'e-ah) an extreme degree of eosinophilia.

hyperepinephrinemia (hi"per-ep"ĭ-nef"rĭ-ne'me-ah) excessive epinephrine in the blood.

hyperequilibrium (hi"per-e"kwĭ-lib're-um) excessive tendency to vertigo.

hypererethism (hi"per-er'ĕ-thizm) extreme irritability.

hyperergasia, (hi"per-er-ga'ze-ah) excessive functional activity.

hyperergia, hyperergy (hi"per-er'je-ah; hi"per-er'je) hypersensitivity to allergens. adj., **hyperer'gic.**

hypererythrocythemia (hi"per-ĕ-rith"ro-si-the'-me-ah) excess of erythrocytes in the blood; hypercythemia.

hyperesophoria (hi"per-es"o-fo're-ah) deviation of the visual axes upward and inward.

hyperesthesia (hi"per-es-the'ze-ah) a state of abnormally increased sensitivity to stimuli. adj., **hyperesthet'ic.**

hyperexophoria (hi"per-ek"so-fo're-ah) deviation of the visual axes upward and outward.

hyperextension (hi"per-ek-sten'shun) extension of a limb or part beyond the normal limit.

hyperferremia (hi"per-fĕ-re'me-ah) excess of iron in the blood. adj., **hyperferre'mic.**

hyperfibrinogenemia (hi"per-fi-brin"o-jĕ-ne'me-ah) excessive fibrinogen in the blood; fibrinogenemia.

hyperflexion (hi"per-flek'shun) flexion of a limb or part beyond the normal limit.

hyperfunction (hi"per-fungk'shun) excessive functioning of a part or organ.

hypergalactia, hypergalactosis (hi"per-gah-lak'she-ah; hi"per-gal"ak-to'sis) excessive secretion of milk.

hypergammaglobulinemia (hi"per-gam"ah-glob"u-lin-e'me-ah) increased gamma globulins in the blood. adj., **hypergammaglobuline'mic.**

hypergenesis (hi"per-jen'ĕ-sis) excessive development.

hypergenitalism (hi"per-jen'ĭ-tal-izm") hypergonadism.

hypergeusesthesia, hypergeusia (hi"per-gu"-zes-the'ze-ah; hi"per-gu'ze-ah) abnormal acuteness of the sense of taste.

hypergia (hi-per'je-ah) diminished sensitivity to allergens.

hyperglandular (hi"per-glan'du-lar) marked by excessive glandular activity.

hyperglobulia (hi"per-glo-bu'le-ah) excess of erythrocytes; erythrocytosis; polycythemia.

hyperglobulinemia (hi"per-glob"u-lin-e'me-ah) excess of globulin in the blood.

hyperglycemia (hi"per-gli-se'me-ah) excess of glucose in the blood.

hyperglycemic (hi"per-gli-se'mik) characterized by or causing hyperglycemia.

h. hyperosmolar nonketotic coma (HHNK), a metabolic derangement in which there is an abnormally high serum glucose level without ketoacidosis. It can occur as a complication of borderline and unrecognized DIABETES MELLITUS, in pancreatic disorders that interfere with the production of insulin, as a complication of extensive burns, and in conditions marked by an excess of steroids, as in steroid therapy or acute stress conditions. The condition also may develop during HYPERALIMENTATION, HEMODIALYSIS, and PERITONEAL DIALYSIS.

SYMPTOMS. The hyperglycemia of HHNK is usually extreme, with fasting blood sugar levels ranging from 600 to 3000 mg. per 100 ml. of blood. In contrast to typical diabetic coma, however, the serum acetone level is normal or only slightly elevated. This occurs because, although there is sufficient insulin available to avoid ketosis, there is not enough to metabolize the glucose and thereby relieve the hyperglycemia. It is also believed that the glucocorticoids and dehydration inhibit the production of ketone bodies.

Hyperosmolality, resulting from the extremely high concentration of sugar in the blood, causes a shift of water from the intracellular fluid (the less concentrated solution) into the blood (the higher concentrated solution). This results in cellular dehydration. Another symptom of HHNK, polyuria, occurs because the high plasma osmolality prevents the normal osmotic return of water to the blood by the renal tubules, and it is excreted in the urine. This leads to a decreased blood volume, which severely hampers the kidney's excretion of glucose and a vicious cycle is begun.

TREATMENT. It is essential that HHNK be recognized early and treatment begun immediately to break the chain of metabolic aberrations that are occurring. It is estimated that the mortality rate of HHNK is 60% to 70%, and the probable reason for this high mortality rate is failure to recognize the condition and institute prompt corrective measures.

Insulin is administered in small doses, the amount and frequency depending on periodic assessment of blood glucose levels. The objective is to avoid the extremes of hyperglycemia and insulin shock. Intravenous fluids are administered cautiously, so that the sodium and water deficits can be corrected without producing extreme shifts of water from the blood into the intracellular compartment and thus failing to correct the hyperosmolar condition of the blood. Electrolytes other than the sodium lost through diuresis also must be replaced as indicated by laboratory findings.

Dehydration plays a major role in the development of severe HHNK; thus patient care is concerned with careful monitoring of those patients susceptible to its development, especially the elderly, the debilitated, and the mild or unsuspected diabetic. Maintenance of an adequate fluid balance can do much to prevent the hyperosmolar condition and the development of a chain of events that can rapidly lead to coma and death.

hyperglyceridemia (hi″per-glis″er-ĭ-de′me-ah) excess of glycerides in the blood.

hyperglycinemia (hi″per-gli″sĭ-ne′me-ah) a hereditary metabolic disorder involving excessive glycine in the blood and urine. One form is characterized by episodic vomiting, lethargy, dehydration, ketosis, and increased susceptibility to infection; a second form by generalized hypotonia, lethargy, absence of reflexes, and periodic myoclonic jerks.

hyperglycinuria (hi″per-gli″sin-u′re-ah) an excess of glycine in the urine (see also HYPERGLYCINEMIA).

hyperglycogenolysis (hi″per-gli″ko-jĕ-nol′ĭ-sis) excessive splitting up of glycogen (glycogenolysis).

hyperglycorrachia (hi″per-gli″ko-ra′ke-ah) excessive sugar in the cerebrospinal fluid.

hyperglycosuria (hi″per-gli″ko-su′re-ah) extreme glycosuria.

hypergnosia (hi″per-no′se-ah) a paranoic condition marked by distortion of perception with a tendency to project psychic conflicts to the environment.

hypergonadism (hi″per-go′nad-izm) abnormally increased functional activity of the gonads, with excessive growth and precocious sexual development.

hyperhedonia (hi″per-he-do′ne-ah) morbid increase of pleasure in agreeable acts.

hyperhemoglobinemia (hi″per-he″mo-glo″bĭ-ne′me-ah) an excess of hemoglobin in the blood.

hyperhidrosis (hi″per-hĭ-dro′sis) excessive perspiration. adj., **hyperhidrot′ic.**

hyperhydration (hi″per-hi-dra′shun) abnormally increased water content of the body.

hyperidrosis (hi″per-ĭ-dro′sis) hyperhidrosis.

hyperimmune (hi″per-im-mūn′) possessing very large quantities of specific antibodies in the serum.

hyperinflation (hi″per-in-fla′shun) excessive inflation or expansion, as of the lungs; overinflation.

hyperinsulinism (hi″per-in′su-lin-izm″) 1. excessive secretion of insulin by the pancreas, resulting in hypoglycemia. 2. insulin shock from overdosage of insulin.

hyperinvolution (hi″per-in″vo-lu′shun) superinvolution.

hyperirritability (hi″per-ir″ĭ-tah-bil′ĭ-te) pathological responsiveness to slight stimuli.

hyperisotonic (hi″per-i″so-ton′ik) denoting a solution containing more than 0.45 per cent salt, in which erythrocytes become crenated as a result of exosmosis.

hyperkalemia (hi″per-kah-le′me-ah) excess of potassium in the blood. adj., **hyperkale′mic.** Symptoms may include hyperactivity of the gastrointestinal tract producing diarrhea and nausea; muscle weakness, usually beginning in the extremities and extending inward to the trunk; tingling of the hands, feet, and tongue; and slow irregular pulse. As the amount of potassium continues to increase, a flaccid paralysis of the muscles of respiration develops; eventually the cardiac muscle may fail, bringing about cardiac arrest.

hyperkeratinization (hi″per-ker″ah-tin-ĭ-za′shun) excessive development of keratin in the epidermis.

hyperkeratosis (hi″per-ker″ah-to′sis) 1. hypertrophy of the horny layer of the skin, or any disease characterized by it. 2. hypertrophy of the cornea. adj., **hyperkeratot′ic.**

epidermolytic h., a hereditary disease, with hyperkeratosis, blisters, and erythema; at birth, the skin is entirely covered with thick, horny, armor-like plates that are soon shed, leaving a raw surface on which the scales re-form.

hyperketonemia (hi″per-ke″to-ne′me-ah) abnormally increased concentration of ketone bodies in the blood.

hyperketonuria (hi″per-ke″to-nu′re-ah) excessive ketone in the urine.

hyperketosis (hi″per-ke-to′sis) excessive formation of ketone.

hyperkinemia (hi″per-ki-ne′me-ah) abnormally high cardiac output.

hyperkinesia (hi″per-ki-ne′ze-ah) abnormally increased motor function or activity. See also HYPERACTIVITY.

hyperkinetic (hi″per-ki-net′ik) pertaining to or marked by hyperkinesia.

h. syndrome, a disorder of childhood, usually abating during adolescence, marked by overactivity, distractibility, restlessness, and low tolerance for frustration. (See also HYPERACTIVITY.)

hyperlactation (hi″per-lak-ta′shun) lactation in greater than normal amount or for a longer than normal period.

hyperleukocytosis (hi″per-lu″ko-si-to′sis) excess of leukocytes in the blood.

hyperlipemia (hi″per-li-pe′me-ah) an excess of lipids in the blood.

carbohydrate-induced h., hyperlipoproteinemia (type IV).

fat-induced h., hyperlipoproteinemia (type I).

hyperlipoproteinemia (hi″per-lip″o-pro″te-in-e′-

me-ah) an excess of lipoproteins in the blood. The familial type occurs in five forms, distinguished chemically by the ratio of plasma levels of cholesterol and triglycerides, characterized clinically as follows. *Type I:* repeated bouts of abdominal colic, xanthoma of the skin and eyes, and hepatosplenomegaly. *Type II:* tendinous xanthoma, tuberous xanthoma, and accelerated atherosclerosis. *Type III:* planar xanthoma and, less often, tendinous xanthoma and atherosclerosis. *Type IV:* early coronary atherosclerosis and sometimes the symptoms of type I. *Type V:* the symptoms of type I.

hyperliposis (hi″per-lĭ-po′sis) excess of fat in the blood serum or tissues.

hyperlithuria (hi″per-lĭ-thu′re-ah) excess of uric (lithic) acid in the urine.

hypermastia (hi″per-mas′te-ah) 1. excessive size of mammary glands. 2. the presence of one or more supernumerary mammary glands; polymastia.

hypermenorrhea (hi″per-men″o-re′ah) excessive uterine bleeding occurring at regular intervals, the period of flow being of usual duration.

hypermetabolism (hi″per-mĕ-tab′o-lizm) increased metabolism.

extrathyroidal m., abnormally elevated basal metabolism unassociated with thyroid disease.

hypermetria (hi″per-me′tre-ah) ataxia in which movements overreach the intended goal.

hypermetrope (hi″per-met′rōp) hyperope.

hypermetropia (hi″per-mĕ-tro′pe-ah) farsightedness; hyperopia.

hypermnesia (hi″perm-ne′ze-ah) extreme retentiveness of memory.

hypermorph (hi′per-morf) 1. a person who is tall, but of low sitting height. 2. in genetics, a hypermorphic mutant gene, i.e., one exaggerating or increasing normal activity. adj., **hypermor′phic.**

hypermotility (hi″per-mo-til′ĭ-te) excessive or abnormally increased motility, as of the gastrointestinal tract.

hypermyotonia (hi″per-mi″o-to′ne-ah) excessive muscular tonicity.

hypermyotrophy (hi″per-mi-ot′ro-fe) excessive development of muscular tissue.

hypernatremia (hi″per-na-tre′me-ah) an excess of sodium in the blood, indicative of water loss exceeding the sodium loss. adj., **hypernatre′mic.**

hyperneocytosis (hi″per-ne″o-si-to′sis) leukocytosis with an excessive number of immature forms of leukocytes.

hypernephroma (hi″per-nĕ-fro′mah) carcinoma of the kidney whose cells resemble those from the adrenal cortex.

hypernoia (hi″per-noi′ah) excessive mental activity.

hypernutrition (hi″per-nu-trish′un) overfeeding and its ill effects.

hyperonychia (hi″per-o-nik′e-ah) hypertrophy of the nails.

hyperope (hi′per-ōp) a person with hyperopia.

hyperopia (hi″per-o′pe-ah) farsightedness; a visual defect in which parallel light rays reaching the eye come to focus behind the retina, vision being better for distant objects than for near. (See also VISION.)

Most children are born with some degree of farsightedness. As the child grows the condition decreases and usually disappears by the age of 8 years. If the child is excessively farsighted, however, the constant effort to focus may cause headaches and fatigue.

The eyeglasses used to correct hyperopia are convex; that is, they bend the light rays toward the center, helping the lens of the eye to focus them on the retina.

hyperorchidism (hi″per-or′kĭ-dizm) abnormally increased functional activity of the testes.

hyperorexia (hi″per-o-rek′se-ah) excessive appetite.

hyperorthocytosis (hi″per-or″tho-si-to′sis) leukocytosis with a normal proportion of the various forms of leukocytes.

hyperosmia (hi″per-oz′me-ah) abnormal acuteness of the sense of smell.

hyperosmolarity (hi″per-oz″mo-lar′ĭ-te) abnormally increased osmotic concentration of a solution.

hyperostosis (hi″per-os-to′sis) excessive growth of bony tissue. adj., **hyperostot′ic.**

frontal internal h., h. fronta′lis intern′a, a new formation of bone tissue protruding in patches on the internal surface of the cranial bones in the frontal region.

infantile cortical h., a disease of young infants characterized by soft tissue swellings over the affected bones, fever, and irritability, and marked by periods of remission and exacerbation.

Morgagni's h., frontal internal hyperostosis.

hyperoxaluria (hi″per-ok″sah-lu′re-ah) an excess of oxalate in the urine.

primary h., a genetic disorder characterized by urinary excretion of oxalate, with nephrolithiasis, nephrocalcinosis, early onset of renal failure, and often a generalized deposit of calcium oxalate.

hyperoxemia (hi″per-ok-se′me-ah) excessive acidity of the blood.

hyperoxia (hi″per-ok′se-ah) an abnormally increased supply or concentration of oxygen.

hyperparasite (hi″per-par′ah-sīt) a parasite that preys on a parasite. adj., **hyperparasit′ic.**

hyperparathyroidism (hi″per-par″ah-thi′roi-dizm) abnormally increased activity of the parathyroid glands, causing loss of calcium from the bones and excessive secretion of calcium and phosphorus by the kidney. Among the symptoms are kidney stones, back pain, joint pains, thirst, nausea, and vomiting. The condition also makes bones more subject to fracture.

About 90 per cent of cases of primary hyperparathyroidism are caused by a benign tumor. Secondary hyperparathyroidism is usually associated with hyperplasia of the parathyroid glands. It is most commonly found in chronic kidney disease, but is also found in childhood rickets and osteomalacia.

If a parathyroid tumor is present, it is removed surgically. If there is hyperplasia of all of the parathyroids, three of the glands and part of the fourth must be removed surgically.

The outlook for the patient is directly related to the extent of kidney damage. Damaged bones, despite deformity, fracture, and cysts, will heal completely if the tumor is removed. Once significant kidney damage has occurred, however, it may continue to progress.

hyperpepsinia (hi″per-pep-sin′e-ah) excessive secretion of pepsin in the stomach.

hyperperistalsis (hi″per-per″ĭ-stal′sis) excessively active peristalsis.

hyperphalangism (hi″per-fal′an-jizm) the presence of a supernumerary phalanx on a finger or toe.

hyperphasia (hi″per-fa′ze-ah) excessive talkativeness.

hyperphenylalaninemia (hi″per-fen″il-al″ah-nĭ-ne′me-ah) an excess of phenylalanine in the blood, as in phenylketonuria.

hyperphonesis (hi″per-fo-ne′sis) intensification of the sound in auscultation or percussion.

hyperphoria (hi″per-fo′re-ah) HETEROPHORIA in which there is permanent upward deviation of the visual axis of an eye in the absence of visual fusional stimuli.

hyperphosphatasia (hi″per-fos″fah-ta′ze-ah) excess of phosphatase in the body.

hyperphosphatemia (hi″per-fos″fah-te′me-ah) an excess of phosphates in the blood.

hyperphosphaturia (hi″per-fos″fah-tu′re-ah) an excess of phosphates in the urine.

hyperphrenia (hi″per-fre′ne-ah) 1. extreme mental excitement. 2. accelerated mental activity.

hyperpigmentation (hi″per-pig″men-ta′shun) abnormally increased pigmentation.

hyperpituitarism (hi″per-pĭ-tu′ĭ-tar-izm″) a condition due to pathologically increased activity of the PITUITARY GLAND, especially increased secretion of growth hormone, resulting in acromegaly or gigantism.

hyperplasia (hi″per-pla′ze-ah) abnormal increase in volume of a tissue or organ caused by the formation and growth of new normal cells. adj., **hyperplas′tic.**

hyperplasmia (hi″per-plaz′me-ah) 1. excess in the proportion of blood plasma to corpuscles. 2. increase in size of erythrocytes through absorption of plasma.

hyperploid (hi′per-ploid) 1. characterized by hyperploidy. 2. a hyperploid individual or cell.

hyperploidy (hi′per-ploi″de) the state of having more than the typical number of chromosomes in unbalanced sets, as in Down's syndrome.

hyperpnea (hi″perp-ne′ah) abnormal increase in depth and rate of respiration. adj., **hyperpne′ic.**

hyperponesis (hi″per-po-ne′sis) excessive action-potential output from the motor and premotor areas of the cortex. adj., **hyperponet′ic.**

hyperposia (hi″per-po′ze-ah) abnormally increased ingestion of fluids for relatively brief periods.

hyperpotassemia (hi″per-pot″ah-se′me-ah) hyperkalemia; excess of potassium in the blood.

hyperpragic (hi″per-praj′ik) characterized by excessive activity.

hyperpraxia (hi″per-prak′se-ah) abnormal activity; restlessness.

hyperprolinemia (hi″per-pro″lĭ-ne′me-ah) a disorder of amino acid metabolism marked by excessive proline in the blood.

hyperprosexia (hi″per-pro-sek′se-ah) preoccupation with one idea to the exclusion of all others.

hyperproteinemia (hi″per-pro″te-ĭ-ne′me-ah) an excess of protein in the blood.

hyperproteosis (hi″per-pro″te-o′sis) a condition due to excess of protein in the diet.

hyperpselaphesia (hi″perp-sel″ah-fe′ze-ah) increased tactile sensitiveness.

hyperpsychosis (hi″per-si-ko′sis) exaggeration of the function of thought.

hyperptyalism (hi″per-ti′ah-lizm) abnormally increased secretion of saliva.

hyperpyrexia (hi″per-pi-rek′se-ah) excessively high fever. adj., **hyperpyrex′ial, hyperpyrex′ic.**

malignant h., malignant hyperthermia.

hyperreactive (hi″per-re-ak′tiv) showing a greater than normal response to stimuli.

hyperreflexia (hi″per-re-flek′se-ah) exaggeration of reflexes.

hyperresonance (hi″per-rez′o-nans) exaggerated resonance on percussion.

hypersalemia (hi″per-sah-le′me-ah) abnormally increased content of salt in the blood.

hypersalivation (hi″per-sal″ĭ-va-shun) abnormally increased secretion of saliva.

hypersecretion (hi″per-se-kre′shun) excessive secretion.

hypersensitivity (hi″per-sen″sĭ-tiv′ĭ-te) a state of altered reactivity in which the body reacts with an exaggerated immune response to a foreign agent; anaphylaxis and allergy are forms of hypersensitivity. adj., **hypersen′sitive.**

delayed h., a slowly developing increase in cell-mediated immune response to a specific antigen, as occurs in graft rejection, autoimmune disease, etc.

immediate h., antibody-mediated hypersensitivity characterized by lesions resulting from release of histamine and other vasoactive substances, as occurs in anaphylaxis.

hypersensitization (hi″per-sen″sĭ-ti-za′shun) the induction of hypersensitivity.

hypersialosis (hi″per-si″ah-lo′sis) excessive secretion of the salivary glands.

hypersomnia (hi″per-som′ne-ah) pathologically excessive sleep or drowsiness.

hypersplenism (hi″per-splen′izm) a condition characterized by exaggeration of the hemolytic function of the spleen, resulting in deficiency of peripheral blood elements, and by hypercellularity of the bone marrow and splenomegaly.

hypersthenia (hi″per-sthe′ne-ah) increased strength or tonicity. adj., **hypersthen′ic.**

hypertelorism (hi″per-te′lo-rizm) abnormally increased distance between two organs or parts.

ocular h., orbital h., increase in the interocular distance, often associated with cleidocranial or craniofacial dysostosis and sometimes with mental deficiency.

Hypertensin (hy″per-ten′sin) trademark for a preparation of angiotensin amide, a vasoconstrictor substance.

hypertensinogen (hi″per-ten-sin′o-jen) angiotensinogen.

hypertension (hi″per-ten′shun) persistently high pressure of the blood against the arterial walls; diagnosis is based on at least three consecutive daily or weekly blood pressure readings. A *mild* or borderline case of hypertension is characterized by a systolic blood pressure that consistently falls in the 140–159 mm. Hg range and a diastolic blood pressure that consistently falls in the 90–95 mm. Hg range. *Moderate* to *severe* hypertensive patients are those whose systolic blood pressure consistently measures 160 mm. Hg or higher or whose diastolic blood pressure consistently measures above 95 mm. Hg, or both. These criteria, used by the Department of Health, Education and Welfare, are not the only ones employed to diagnose hypertension in some individuals. In many cases severe hypertension is relative to age, sex, race, and medical history. If there is damage to the heart, kidneys, or liver, any elevation of blood pressure may be considered dangerous.

It is estimated that one in ten Americans are hypertensive, and undiagnosed cases could double that number. The condition occurs most frequently in men over 35 years of age and in women over 45 years; however, in recent years screening clinics have detected it in increasing numbers of teenagers. Hypertension is more severe and more prevalent in blacks than in whites. Since 1950 improvement in diagnosis and treatment of hypertension has brought about a 65 percent decrease in the death rate.

TYPES AND CAUSES. Hypertension may be classified as primary or secondary. In 85 to 90 percent of the cases the causes of hypertension cannot be determined. Such cases are classified as *primary* or *essential* hypertension. Factors contributing to the development of this disease include heredity, obesity, excessive intake of salt, smoking, and an aggressive, hyperactive personality. A stressful environment also may produce a tendency toward hypertension. It is known that there is a direct relationship between hypertension and ATHEROSCLEROSIS. Elevated blood pressure levels speed up the atherosclerotic process, and the complications of essential hypertension are directly related to this accelerated process.

The remaining 5 to 10 percent of cases, classified as *secondary* hypertension, can be traced to a specific disease such as tumor of the adrenal gland (PHEOCHROMOCYTOMA) and stricture of the renal artery (renal hypertension).

Malignant hypertension occurs most often in persons in their twenties or thirties and differs from other types of hypertension in that it progresses rapidly and may prove fatal if not treated immediately after symptoms develop, before damage is done to the blood vessels. Especially affected are the blood vessels in the eye, resulting in damage to the retina. The kidneys or heart may fail, or the cerebral blood vessels may rupture, resulting in a CEREBRAL VASCULAR ACCIDENT. With proper care malignant hypertension can be kept under control for years. Without adequate treatment the disease can be fatal within two years.

PATIENT CARE. The major goal in the treatment and control of hypertension is prevention of complications. These include stroke from cerebral hemorrhage or thrombosis, congestive heart failure, heart attack, and kidney damage.

Success of treatment depends on close supervision of the patient and his cooperation with his prescribed regimen of drug therapy and moderation in his life style. Unfortunately, many patients have difficulty following the prescribed treatment, and through lack of understanding and misinformation, fail to take their medications. Recent studies show that 40 to 70 percent of hypertensive patients stop taking their medication, usually because they begin to feel better and do not see the need to continue taking the drugs, or because they have unpleasant side effects and do not realize that other medications can be substituted to keep their blood pressure under control.

Patient supervision and education are a constant challenge to the members of the health team striving to prevent the complications of hypertension. The patient must understand that he has a condition that will persist throughout his life and that, although there are means of controlling his hypertension, these are effective only insofar as he is willing and able to accept responsibility for carrying out the regimen prescribed for him.

The patient should be informed of factors contributing to his hypertension, the purpose of the special diet, exercises, and medications prescribed, and the need to consult with his physician or other health care practitioner should any difficulties arise from the medications he is taking.

Drugs that may be prescribed include the DIURETICS, which are usually the first medication used when diet and weight reduction do not effectively control the blood pressure. These drugs act to prevent sodium and water reabsorption by the kidneys and are thought to bring about a combined effect of reducing the plasma volume and causing dilatation of the smooth muscles of the blood vessels. If the diuretics alone are not effective, the physician will add an adrenergic blocking agent, for example, reserpine (Serpasil), methyldopa (Aldomet), and guanethidine (Ismelin). Other antihypertensive agents thay may be used are hydralazine (Apresoline) and mecamylamine (Inversine).

The drugs used in the treatment of hypertension are often used in combination which allows for decrease in the dosage of a single medication that may be producing side effects, and also provides for drug interactions that can produce additive or potentiating effects. The kinds of drugs used and the combinations of drugs are determined by the response of the individual patient, and this demands continued supervision and assessment of the patient's status.

portal h., abnormally increased pressure in the portal circulation.

hypertensive (hi″per-ten′siv) 1. characterized by or causing increased tension or pressure, as abnormally high blood pressure. 2. a person with hypertension.

hypertensor (hi″per-ten′sor) a substance that raises the blood pressure.

hyperthecosis (hi″per-the-ko′sis) hyperplasia and excessive luteinization of the cells of the inner stromal layer of the ovary.

hyperthelia (hi″per-the′le-ah) the presence of supernumerary nipples.

hyperthermalgesia (hi″per-ther″mal-je′ze-ah) abnormal sensitiveness to heat.

hyperthermesthesia (hi″per-therm″es-the′ze-ah) increased sensibility for heat.

hyperthermia (hi″per-ther′me-ah) greatly increased temperature. adj., **hyperther′mal, hyperther′mic.**

malignant h., a syndrome affecting patients undergoing general anesthesia, marked by rapid rise in body temperature, signs of increased muscle metabolism, and, usually, rigidity.

hyperthrombinemia (hi″per-throm″bĭ-ne′me-ah) an excess of thrombin in the blood.

hyperthymia (hi″per-thi′me-ah) excessive emotionalism.

hyperthymism (hi″per-thi′mizm) excessive thymus activity.

hyperthyroidism (hi″per-thi′roi-dizm) excessive functional activity of the thyroid gland. adj. **hyperthy′roid.** It is predominantly a disease of adult women, with peak incidence between 30 and 50 years of age. The clinical state of hyperthyroidism is also called *thyrotoxicosis.* It most commonly occurs as part of a syndrome which may include goiter, exophthalmos, and MYXEDEMA and is known as *Graves' disease* or *Basedow's disease.*

The cause of hyperthyroidism is unknown. There is much evidence to indicate a strong hereditary factor in the development of Graves' disease and myxedema. Some theorists consider it to be an AUTOIMMUNE DISEASE, while others believe it to be precipitated by an emotionally traumatic event in the patient's life. Graves' disease sometimes occurs after the intake of desiccated thyroid for weight reduction. It appears after the medication is no longer taken and is, perhaps, a "rebound" effect.

SYMPTOMS. The manifestations of hyperthyroidism may vary from mild symptoms of weakness, insomnia, weight loss, and tremulousness to extreme tachycardia, palpitations, exertional dyspnea, and ankle edema. The patient with Graves' disease also exhibits an enlarged thyroid (goiter) and abnormal protrusion of the eyes (exophthalmia).

The hyperthyroid patient's metabolic rate is greatly accelerated, producing a speeding up of all the bodily processes and an emotional upheaval in response to the increased physical activity. The patient often experiences episodes of emotional extremes with episodes of crying and depression followed by intense physical activity and mental euphoria and hysteria.

TREATMENT AND PATIENT CARE. General measures of support for the patient suffering from hyperthyroidism include physical and emotional rest and a high caloric, nutritional diet supplemented with vitamins and calcium. A sedative such as phenobarbital may be prescribed to promote rest. Adrenergic blocking agents are prescribed to control the symptoms of tremor, restlessness, and tachycardia. These drugs include reserpine, guanethidine, and propranolol. The choice of additional drugs and surgical intervention will depend on the age of the patient, the size of the goiter, and the patient's response to selected therapies.

It is important that the patient and his family understand the course of the disease, the patient's helplessness in controlling his emotions without medication and support from those around him, and the need to follow conscientiously the regimen prescribed. The patient's environment should be as calm and nonstimulating as possible, both at home and in the hospital.

Radioactive Iodine. The drug of choice for middle aged persons and nonpregnant women usually is radioactive iodine (^{131}I). Its main disadvantage is the possibility of the development of hypothyroidism resulting from "overeffective" treatment. This may occur immediately after treatment is begun or long after treatment is completed. The dosage depends on the size of the gland and the thyroid's sensitivity to radiation. The radioactive iodine is administered orally, usually in one small dose, and the patient is allowed to return home.

Patients receiving larger doses are placed in isolation for eight days, the half-life of ^{131}I. Radioactive iodine is excreted by the kidneys and circulates in the blood; hence, precautions are necessary with the handling of needles and syringes used on the patient, and with bedpans and specimen bottles used for the collection of urine.

All patients receiving ^{131}I must be observed for signs of THYROID CRISIS resulting from radiation-induced thyroiditis. Patients receiving small doses of radioactive iodine may require two and sometimes three doses. They also require adjunctive therapy in the form of potassium iodide therapy or the antithyroid drugs, or both, if hyperthyroidism is not controlled within two or three months.

It should be remembered that the objective of treatment with radioactive iodine and the antithyroid drugs is reduction of thyroid activity to normal levels. This is not easily accomplished, and so the patient must be evaluated frequently for signs of ineffective treatment with persistence of symptoms, and for overeffective treatment which can bring about symptoms of hypothyroidism.

Antithyroid Drugs. The antithyroid drugs, especially propylthiouracil, are prescribed as initial treatment for children, young adults, and pregnant women. The prime candidates for this therapy are patients with small goiters, recent onset of the disease, and mild symptoms. Iodine preparations such as propylthiouracil and saturated solution of potassium iodide (SSKI) have only a temporary effect. They require that the patient take the medication at the prescribed time and strictly according to schedule. These drugs also produce agranulocytosis, which can develop rather quickly. For this reason patients receiving these drugs must be instructed to report to the physician any sore throat, fever, or rash, so that WBC tests can be done and the patient's condition evaluated.

The iodine preparations often are given routinely for a period of 10 to 14 days prior to surgery to reduce the vascularity of the thyroid. Another principal use of the antithyroid drugs is in the treatment of THYROID CRISIS.

Surgery. Subtotal THYROIDECTOMY is the treatment of choice in children who fail to respond to or have an adverse reaction to antithyroid drugs, in adults who cannot or are not willing to follow prolonged drug therapy, and in patients with greatly enlarged thyroids or whose glands are likely to develop carcinoma.

hyperthyroxinemia (hi″per-thi-rok″sin-e′me-ah) an excess of thyroxine in the blood.

hypertonia (hi″per-to′ne-ah) abnormally increased tonicity or strength.

h. oc′uli, high intraocular pressure; glaucoma.

hypertonic (hi″per-ton′ik) 1. pertaining to or characterized by an increased tonicity or tension. 2. having an osmotic pressure greater than that of the solution with which it is compared.

hypertonicity (hi″per-to-nis′ĭ-te) the state or quality of being hypertonic.

hypertrichiasis, hypertrichosis (hi″per-trĭ-ki′-ah-sis; hi″per-trĭ-ko′sis) excessive hairiness.

hypertriglyceridemia (hi″per-tri-glis″er-ĭ-de′me-ah) an excess of triglycerides in the blood; a familial form occurs in hyperlipoproteinemia types I and IV.

hypertrophy (hi-per′tro-fe) increase in volume of a

tissue or organ produced entirely by enlargement of existing cells. adj., **hypertroph'ic.**

ventricular h., hypertrophy of the myocardium of a ventricle, causing undue deviation of the axis of the electrocardiogram.

hypertropia (hi"per-tro'pe-ah) STRABISMUS in which there is permanent upward deviation of the visual axis of one eye.

hyperuricemia (hi"per-u"rĭ-se'me-ah) an excess of uric acid in the blood. adj., **hyperurice'mic.**

hypervalinemia (hi"per-val"ĭ-ne'me-ah) an inborn error of metabolism characterized by elevated levels of serum valine, valinuria, and failure to thrive.

hypervascular (hi"per-vas'ku-lar) extremely vascular.

hyperventilation (hi"per-ven"tĭ-la'shun) 1. increase of air in the lungs above the normal amount. 2. abnormally prolonged and deep breathing, usually associated with acute anxiety or emotional tension. It is most commonly seen in nervous, anxious females who have other functional disturbances related to emotional problems. A transient, respiratory ALKALOSIS commonly results from hyperventilation. More prolonged hyperventilation may be caused by disorders of the central nervous system, or by drugs, such as high concentrations of salicylate, that increase the sensitivity of the respiratory centers.

Symptoms of hyperventilation include "faintness" or impaired consciousness without actual loss of consciousness. At the outset the patient may have felt a tightness of the chest, a sensation of smothering, and some degree of apprehension. Other symptoms may be related to the heart and digestive tract, for example, palpitation or pounding of the heart, fullness in the throat, and pain over the stomach region. In prolonged attacks the patient may exhibit tetany with muscular spasm of the hands and feet.

Immediate treatment consists of having the patient rebreathe in a paper bag, to replace the carbon dioxide he has been "blowing off" during hyperventilation. He may need to be convinced that there is nothing seriously wrong with him in the organic sense and that he can control the "attack" by using the paper bag for rebreathing. Treatment of the underlying emotional disturbance is recommended.

hyperviscosity (hi"per-vis-kos'ĭ-te) excessive viscosity.

hypervitaminosis (hi"per-vi"tah-mĭ-no'sis) a condition produced by ingestion of excessive amounts of vitamins; symptom complexes are associated with excessive intake of vitamins A and D.

hypervolemia (hi"per-vo-le'me-ah) abnormal increase in the volume of circulating fluid (plasma) in the body.

hypesthesia (hi"pes-the'ze-ah) abnormally diminished sensitiveness; hypoesthesia.

hypha (hi'fah), pl. *hy'phae* [L.] one of the filaments composing the mycelium of a fungus. adj., **hy'phal.**

hyphedonia (hīp"he-do'ne-ah) diminution of power of enjoyment.

hyphema (hi-fe'mah) hemorrhage into the anterior chamber of the eye.

hyphemia (hi-fe'me-ah) 1. oligemia, or deficiency of blood. 2. hyphema.

hyphidrosis (hīp"hĭ-dro'sis) too scanty perspiration.

Hyphomycetes (hi"fo-mi-se'tēz) the mycelial (hyphal) fungi, i.e., the molds.

hypn(o)- word element [Gr.], *sleep; hypnosis.*

hypnagogic (hip"nah-goj'ik) 1. producing sleep. 2. occurring just before sleep; said of dreams.

hypnagogue (hip'nah-gog) 1. hypnotic; inducing sleep. 2. an agent that produces sleep.

hypnalgia (hip-nal'je-ah) pain during sleep.

hypnoanalysis (hip"no-ah-nal'ĭ-sis) psychoanalysis with use of hypnosis to help uncover unconscious material.

hypnoanesthesia (hip"no-an"es-the'ze-ah) reduction of sensitivity to pain by hypnosis.

hypnodontics (hip"no-don'tiks) the application of hypnosis and controlled suggestion in the practice of dentistry.

hypnogenic (hip"no-jen'ik) inducing sleep or a hypnotic state.

hypnoid (hip'noid) resembling hypnosis.

hypnolepsy (hip'no-lep"se) narcolepsy.

hypnology (hip-nol'o-je) the scientific study of sleep or of hypnotism.

hypnonarcosis (hip"no-nar-ko'sis) light hypnosis combined with narcosis.

hypnosis (hip-no'sis) an artificially induced passive state in which there is increased amenability and responsiveness to suggestions and commands. In hypnosis, a drowsy phase is followed by a sleep that is light or deep, depending on the cooperation of the sleeper. Although this sleep seems normal, a part of the sleeper remains aware of the outside world and of the wishes of the hypnotist.

STATE OF HYPNOSIS. The nature of hypnosis and the way it works are still largely unknown. One widely accepted theory is that the person's ego—that is, the part of his mind that consciously restrains his instincts—is temporarily weakened under hypnosis at his own wish. How deeply he responds depends on many psychologic and biologic factors. The ability to respond to hypnosis varies from person to person; it tends to increase after successive experiences.

It is not true that a hypnotized person will do absolutely anything he is asked. Most subjects, for instance, will not respond to any suggestions they would consider immoral or illegal if they were awake.

USE OF HYPNOSIS. A common medical use of hypnosis is in treating mental illness. Historically, Sigmund Freud developed his theory of the unconscious as a result of his experiments with a hypnotized patient. Out of this theory came some of the techniques of PSYCHOANALYSIS. By lessening the mind's unconscious defenses, hypnosis can make some patients able to recall and even reexperience important childhood events that have long been forgotten or repressed by the conscious mind.

In certain cases when the use of anesthetics is not advisable, hypnosis has been used successfully during dental treatment, setting of fractures, and childbirth, usually in addition to pain-killing medicines.

hypnotherapy (hip"no-ther'ah-pe) the therapeutic use of hypnotism.

hypnotic (hip-not'ik) 1. pertaining to or inducing hypnosis or sleep. 2. an agent that induces sleep.

hypnotism (hip′no-tizm) the method or practice of inducing hypnosis.

hypnotize (hip′no-tīz) to put into a condition of hypnosis.

hypnotoxin (hip″no-tok′sin) a hypothetical toxin that is supposed to accumulate during the waking hours until it is sufficient to inhibit the activity of the cortical cells and induce sleep.

hypo (hi′po) 1. a colloquial abbreviation of hypodermic. 2. sodium thiosulfate, used as a photographic fixing agent.

hypo- word element [Gr.], *abnormally decreased; deficient; beneath; under.*

hypoacidity (hi″po-ah-sid′ĭ-te) decreased acidity.

hypoacusia, hypoacusis (hi″po-ah-ku′ze-ah; hi″po-ah-ku′sis) slightly diminished auditory sensitivity.

hypoadrenalism (hi″po-ah-dren′al-izm) deficiency of adrenal activity, as in Addison's disease.

hypoadrenocorticism (hi″po-ah-dre″no-kor′tĭ-sizm) diminished activity of the adrenal cortex; Addison's disease.

hypoaffectivity (hi″po-ah″fek-tiv′ĭ-te) abnormally diminished sensitivity to superficial stimuli; abnormally decreased emotional reactivity.

hypoalbuminemia (hi″po-al-bu″mĭ-ne′me-ah) abnormally low levels of albumin in the blood.

hypoalbuminosis (hi″po-al-bu-mĭ-no′sis) abnormally low level of albumin.

hypoaldosteronism (hi″po-al-dos′ter-ōn-izm″) deficiency of aldosterone in the body.

hypoalimentation (hi″po-al″ĭ-men-ta′shun) insufficient nourishment.

hypoazoturia (hi″po-az″o-tu′re-ah) diminished nitrogenous material in the urine.

hypobaric (hi″po-bār′ik) characterized by less than normal pressure or weight; applied to gases under less than atmospheric pressure, or to solutions of lower specific gravity than another taken as a standard of reference.

hypobaropathy (hi″po-bār-op′ah-the) the disturbances experienced at high altitudes due to reduced air pressure and lack of oxygen; altitude sickness.

hypoblast (hi′po-blast) the entoderm. adj., **hypoblas′tic.**

hypocalcemia (hi″po-kal-se′me-ah) diminished calcium in the blood.

hypocalciuria (hi″po-kal″se-u′re-ah) an abnormally diminished amount of calcium in the urine.

hypocapnia (hi″po-kap′ne-ah) diminished carbon dioxide in the blood. adj., **hypocap′nic.**

hypocarbia (hi″po-kar′be-ah) hypocapnia.

hypocellularity (hi″po-sel″u-lar′ĭ-te) abnormal decrease in the number of cells present, as in bone marrow.

hypochloremia (hi″po-klo-re′me-ah) diminished chlorides in the blood. adj., **hypochlore′mic.**

hypochlorhydria (hi″po-klōr-hi′dre-ah) deficiency of hydrochloric acid in the gastric juice.

hypochlorization (hi″po-klōr″ĭ-za′shun) reduction of sodium chloride in the diet.

hypochlorous acid (hi″po-klōr′us) an unstable compound used as a disinfectant and bleaching agent.

hypochloruria (hi″po-klo-ru′re-ah) diminished chloride content in the urine.

hypocholesteremia, hypocholesterolemia (hi″po-ko-les″ter-e′me-ah; hi″po-ko-les″ter-ol-e′me-ah) low level of cholesterol in the blood.

hypochondria (hi″po-kon′dre-ah) hypochondriasis.

hypochondriac (hi″po-kon′dre-ak) 1. pertaining to the hypochondrium. 2. a person affected with hypochondriasis.

hypochondriasis (hi″po-kon-dri′ah-sis) abnormal concern about one's health. The hypochondriac exaggerates trivial symptoms and often believes that he is suffering from some serious ailment.

True hypochondriasis is a type of neurosis caused by an unresolved conflict in the patient's unconscious mind. His fears are usually related to a specific organ, such as the heart, eyes, or lungs. This organ often has a deep symbolic connection with the inner conflict causing the neurosis. In many cases, the relationship between the patient's mind and the organ on which his fears center is so strong that he develops real symptoms, even though there is no physical disorder to explain them.

The treatment of hypochondriasis is usually difficult and of long duration. Psychotherapy is the most effective means of dealing with this disorder.

hypochondrium (hi″po-kon′dre-um) the upper abdominal region on either side, just below the thorax. adj., **hypochon′drial.**

hypochromasia (hi″po-kro-ma′ze-ah) 1. staining less intensely than normal. 2. decrease of hemoglobin in erythrocytes so that they are abnormally pale. adj. **hypochromat′ic.**

hypochromatism (hi″po-kro′mah-tizm) abnormally deficient pigmentation, especially deficiency of chromatin in a cell nucleus.

hypochromatosis (hi″po-kro″mah-to′sis) the gradual fading and disappearance of the nucleus (the chromatin) of a cell.

hypochromemia (hi″po-kro-me′me-ah) abnormally low color index of the blood.

hypochromia (hi″po-kro′me-ah) 1. hypochromatism. 2. decrease of hemoglobin in the erythrocytes so that they are abnormally pale. adj., **hypochro′mic.**

hypochylia (hi″po-ki′le-ah) deficiency of chyle.

hypocomplementemia (hi″po-kom′plĕ-men-te′me-ah) diminution of complement levels in the blood.

hypocorticism (hi″po-kor′tĭ-sizm) hypoadrenocorticism.

hypocrinism (hi″po-krin′izm) a state due to deficient secretion of an endocrine gland.

hypocupremia (hi″po-ku-pre′me-ah) abnormally diminished concentration of copper in the blood.

hypocyclosis (hi″po-si-klo′sis) insufficient accommodation in the eye.

hypocythemia (hi″po-si-the′me-ah) deficiency in the number of erythrocytes in the blood.

hypodactyly (hi″po-dak′tĭ-le) less than the usual number of digits on the hand or foot.

Hypoderma (hi″po-der′mah) a genus of ox-warble or heel flies, whose larvae cause warbles in cattle and a form of larva migrans in man.

hypodermiasis (hi″po-der-mi′ah-sis) a creeping eruption of the skin in man and cattle caused by the larvae of *Hypoderma.*

hypodermic (hi″po-der′mik) 1. beneath the skin; injected into subcutaneous tissues. 2. a hypodermic, or subcutaneous, injection; a hypodermic syringe.

hypodermoclysis (hi″po-der-mok′lĭ-sis) the introduction into the subcutaneous tissues of fluids, especially physiologic sodium chloride solution, in large quantity; particularly useful in the administration of fluids to small children and elderly persons not suited to intravenous infusion. The most common sites for insertion of the needles for hypodermoclysis are the anterior aspect of the thighs and the loose tissue below each breast. Two needles are used to deliver the fluid; one in each thigh or on each side of the chest. This method of introducing fluids into the body is contraindicated in cases of edema, and it may be complicated by abscess formation, puncture of a large blood vessel, and necrosis and sloughing of the tissues due to poor absorption. The enzyme hyaluronidase (Alidase, Wydase) is injected into the tubing at each injection site at the start of clysis, and sometimes an additional 1 ml. is added to the solution to facilitate absorption. Called also subcutaneous infusion.

hypodipsia (hi″po-dip′se-ah) abnormally diminished thirst.

hypodynamia (hi″po-di-na′me-ah) abnormally diminished power. adj., **hypodynam′ic.**

hypoeccrisia (hi″po-e-kriz′e-ah) abnormally diminished excretion. adj., **hypoeccrit′ic.**

hypoendocrinism (hi″po-en-dok′rĭ-nizm) insufficiency of endocrine gland activity.

hypoergasia (hi″po-er-ga′ze-ah) abnormally decreased functional activity.

hypoergia (hi″po-er′je-ah) 1. hypoergasia. 2. hyposensitivity to allergens.

hypoergic (hi″po-er′jik) 1. less energetic than normal. 2. pertaining to or characterized by hypoergy.

hypoergy (hi″po-er′je) abnormally diminished reactivity; hyposensitivity.

hypoesophoria (hi″po-es″o-fo′re-ah) deviation of the visual axes downward and inward.

hypoesthesia (hi″po-es-the′ze-ah) a state of abnormally decreased sensitivity to stimuli. adj., **hypoesthet′ic.**

hypoexophoria (hi″po-ek″so-fo′re-ah) deviation of the visual axes downward and laterally.

hypoferremia (hi″po-fĕ-re′me-ah) deficiency of iron in the blood.

hypofibrinogenemia (hi″po-fi-brin″o-jĕ-ne′me-ah) deficiency of fibrinogen in the blood.

hypofunction (hi″po-fungk′shun) diminished functioning.

hypogalactia (hi″po-gah-lak′she-ah) deficiency of milk secretion. adj., **hypogalac′tous.**

hypogammaglobulinemia (hi″po-gam″ah-glob″u-lin-e′me-ah) an immunological deficiency state marked by abnormally low levels of generally all classes of serum gamma globulins, with heightened susceptibility to infectious diseases. It may be congenital or secondary, or it may be physiological, which occurs in normal infants and which, when prolonged, is called transient hypogammaglobulinemia. (See also AGAMMAGLOBULINEMIA.)

acquired h., hypogammaglobulinemia that becomes manifest after early childhood; the condition may be primary (that is, without discoverable underlying cause) or secondary (that is, associated with such conditions as multiple myeloma, lymphoma, and chronic lymphoid leukemia, in which there is failure of gamma globulin synthesis).

congenital h., hypogammaglobulinemia in which the manifestations of immunologic inadequacy appear shortly after birth.

hypogastric (hi″po-gas′trik) pertaining to the hypogastrium.

hypogastrium (hi″po-gas′tre-um) the lowest middle abdominal region.

hypogenesis (hi″po-jen′ĕ-sis) defective development.

hypogenitalism (hi″po-jen′ĭ-tal-izm″) lack of sexual development because of deficient activity of the gonads; hypogonadism.

hypogeusesthesia, hypogeusia (hi″po-gu″zes-the′ze-ah; hi″po-gu′ze-ah) abnormally diminished acuteness of the sense of taste.

hypoglossal (hi″po-glos′al) situated beneath the tongue, as the hypoglossal nerve.

hypoglottis (hi″po-glot′is) 1. the under side of the tongue. 2. ranula.

hypoglycemia (hi″po-gli-se′me-ah) an abnormally low level of sugar (glucose) in the blood. The condition may result from an excessive rate of removal of glucose from the blood or from decreased secretion of glucose into the blood. Overproduction of insulin from the islands of Langerhans or an overdose of exogenous insulin can lead to increased utilization of glucose, so that glucose is removed from the blood at an accelerated rate. Some large tumors of the retroperitoneal area and tumors of the islands of Langerhans can increase the production of insulin and result in rapid removal of glucose from the blood. Because the liver is the source of most of the glucose entering the blood while a person is fasting, damage to the liver cells can result in impaired ability to convert glycogen into glucose. If secretion of the adrenocortical hormones, especially the GLUCOCORTICOIDS, is deficient, the protein precursors of glucose are not available and the blood glucose level drops as the liver's glycogen supply is depleted.

SYMPTOMS. Hypoglycemia may be tolerated by normal persons for brief periods of time without symptoms; however, if the blood sugar level remains very low for a prolonged period of time, symptoms of cerebral dysfunction develop. These include mental confusion, hallucinations, convulsions, and eventually deep coma as the nervous system is deprived of the glucose needed for its normal metabolic activities. Other symptoms are a result of a greatly increased secretion of epinephrine, a normal response to hypoglycemia. The patient then experiences increased pulse rate, tachycardia, a rise in blood pressure, sweating, and anxiety. (See also INSULIN SHOCK.)

TREATMENT. An acute episode of hypoglycemia demands emergency treatment with intravenous injections of glucose. If the patient can swallow and no facilities for intravenous therapy are available, sugar, candy, sweetened fruit juice, or honey may be given by mouth.

Specific treatment depends on the primary cause of hypoglycemia. If hyperinsulinism is due to a tumor or hyperplasia of the islands of Langerhans, surgical intervention is necessary to remove this cause of hypoglycemia. The large sarcomas of the retroperitoneal or mediastinal areas that cause hyperinsulinism also must be treated surgically.

When the cause of hypoglycemia is an endocrine or liver disease that results in decreased secretion of glucose, treatment includes dietary changes that are aimed at avoiding extremes in blood glucose level and maintaining an adequate level of glucose in the blood at all times. The diet is high in protein and fat and low in carbohydrate content and is given in frequent, small feedings during the day and before retiring. This regimen avoids extreme fluctuations in blood glucose concentration by restricting carbohydrate intake, and supplies adequate precursors of glycogen through the protein intake.

hypoglycemic (hi″po-gli-se′mik) pertaining to, characterized by, or producing hypoglycemia.

h. drugs, drugs that lower the blood sugar level. The hormone INSULIN lowers the blood sugar by increasing the metabolism of sugar. Some synthetic hypoglycemic agents such as chlorpropamide and tolbutamide have been used in the treatment of older diabetics. However, the Food and Drug Administration has warned that these drugs may cause heart disease. Because of their toxicity and questionable effectiveness, most physicians prefer to control the diabetes of older patients with diet alone.

hypoglycogenolysis (hi″po-gli″ko-jĕ-nol′ĭ-sis) defective splitting up of glycogen in the body.

hypoglycorrachia (hi″po-gli″ko-ra′ke-ah) abnormally low sugar content in the cerebrospinal fluid.

hypogonadism (hi″po-go′nad-izm) decreased functional activity of the gonads, with retardation of growth and sexual development.

hypogonadotropic (hi″po-gon″ah-do-trōp′ik) relating to or caused by deficiency of gonadotropin.

hypohidrosis (hi″po-hĭ-dro′sis) abnormally diminished secretion of sweat. adj., **hypohidrot′ic.**

hypokalemia (hi″po-kah-le′me-ah) abnormally low potassium levels in the blood, which may lead to neuromuscular and renal disorders and to electrocardiographic abnormalities.

hypokalemic (hi″po-kah-le′mik) 1. pertaining to or characterized by hypokalemia. 2. an agent that lowers blood potassium levels.

hypokinesia (hi″po-ki-ne′ze-ah) abnormally diminished motor activity. adj., **hypokinet′ic.**

hypoleydigism (hi″po-li′dig-izm) abnormally diminished secretion of androgens by Leydig's cells.

hypolipidemic (hi″po-lip″ĭ-de′mik) promoting the reduction of lipid concentrations in the serum.

hypomagnesemia (hi″po-mag″nĕ-se′me-ah) abnormally low magnesium content of the blood, manifested chiefly by neuromuscular hyperirritability.

hypomania (hi″po-ma′ne-ah) mania of a mild type. adj., **hypoman′ic.**

hypomastia (hi″po-mas′te-ah) abnormal smallness of mammary glands.

hypomenorrhea (hi″po-men″o-re′ah) diminution of menstrual flow or duration.

hypomere (hi′po-mēr) 1. one of the ventrolateral portions of the fusing myotomes in embryonic development, forming muscles innervated by the ventral rami of the spinal nerves. 2. the lateral plate of mesoderm that develops into the walls of the body cavities.

hypometabolism (hi″po-mĕ-tab′o-lizm) decreased metabolism; low metabolic rate.

hypometria (hi″po-me′tre-ah) ataxia in which movements fall short of the intended goal.

hypomnesia (hi″pom-ne′ze-ah) defective memory.

hypomorph (hi′po-morf) 1. a person short in standing height as compared to his sitting height. 2. in genetics, a hypomorphic mutant gene, i.e., showing only a slight reduction of the activity it influences. adj., **hypomor′phic.**

hypomotility (hi″po-mo-til′ĭ-te) deficient power of movement in any part.

hypomyotonia (hi″po-mi″o-to′ne-ah) deficient muscular tonicity.

hypomyxia (hi″po-mik′se-ah) decreased secretion of mucus.

hyponatremia (hi″po-na-tre′me-ah) deficiency of sodium in the blood; salt depletion.

hyponeocytosis (hi″po-ne″o-si-to′sis) leukopenia with the presence of immature leukocytes in the blood.

hyponoia (hi″po-noi′ah) sluggish mental activity.

hyponychium (hi″po-nik′e-um) the thickened epidermis beneath the free distal end of the nail of a digit. adj., **hyponych′ial.**

hypo-orthocytosis (hi″po-or″tho-si-to′sis) leukopenia with a normal proportion of the various forms of leukocytes.

hypopancreatism (hi″po-pan′kre-ah-tizm″) diminished activity of the pancreas.

hypoparathyroidism (hi″po-par″ah-thi′roi-dizm) a disorder caused by underproduction of the parathyroid hormone. It most often occurs as a result of accidental removal of, or damage to, one or all of the parathyroids during thyroid surgery. Insufficiency of parathyroid hormone causes lowering of the calcium content of the blood and may result in TETANY, of which the most obvious sign is spasm of the muscles, especially those of the fingers and toes.

Treatment consists of raising the lowered calcium content of the blood. There are various forms in which calcium can be administered, and calcium injections will bring immediate improvement. However, if there is complete absence of parathyroid function the patient will have to continue to take oral preparations of calcium indefinitely. Transplantation of parathyroid glands has been attempted as substitution therapy.

hypophalangism (hi″po-fal′an-jizm) absence of a phalanx on a finger or toe.

hypopharynx (hi″po-far′ingks) laryngopharynx.

hypophonesis (hi″po-fo-ne′sis) diminution of the sound in auscultation or percussion.

hypophonia (hi″po-fo-ne′ah) a weak voice due to incoordination of the vocal muscles.

hypophoria (hi″po-fo′re-ah) HETEROPHORIA in which there is permanent downward deviation of the visual axis of an eye in the absence of visual fusional stimuli.

hypophosphatasia (hi″po-fos″fah-ta′ze-ah) an inborn error of metabolism marked by abnormally low serum alkaline phosphatase activity and excretion of phosphoethanolamine in the urine. It is manifested by rickets in infants and children and by osteomalacia in adults. It is most severe in babies under six months of age.

hypophosphatemia (hi″po-fos″fah-te′me-ah) deficiency of phosphates in the blood. See also HYPOPHOSPHATASIA. adj., **hypophosphate′mic.**

hypophosphaturia (hi″po-fos″fah-tu′re-ah) abnormally decreased levels of urinary phosphate.

hypophrenia (hi″po-fre′ne-ah) mental retardation.

hypophrenic (hi″po-fren′ik) 1. below the diaphragm. 2. mentally retarded.

hypophysectomy (hi-pof″ĭ-sek′to-me) excision of the hypophysis, or pituitary gland.

hypophyseal, hypophysial (hi″po-fiz′e-al) pertaining to the hypophysis (PITUITARY GLAND).

hypophyseoportal (hi″po-fiz″e-o-por′tal) denoting the portal system of the pituitary gland, in which hypothalamic venules connect with capillaries of the anterior pituitary.

hypophysioprivic (hi″po-fiz″e-o-priv′ik) due to deficiency of hormonal secretion of the hypophysis.

hypophysis (hi-pof′ĭ-sis), pl. *hypoph′yses* [Gr.] an epithelial body of dual origin at the base of the brain in the sella turcica, attached by a stalk to the hypothalamus; called also PITUITARY GLAND. It is composed of two main lobes, the anterior lobe (adenohypophysis, anterior pituitary), secreting several important hormones that regulate the proper functioning of the thyroids, gonads, adrenal cortex, and other endocrine glands, and the posterior lobe (neurohypophysis, posterior pituitary), whose cells serve as a reservoir for hormones having antidiuretic and oxytocic action, releasing them as needed.
h. cer′ebri, hypophysis.
h. sic′ca, posterior pituitary.

hypopiesis (hi″po-pi-e′sis) abnormally low pressure, in particular, low blood pressure.

hypopigmentation (hi″po-pig″men-ta′shun) abnormally decreased pigmentation.

hypopituitarism (hi″po-pĭ-tu′ĭ-tar-izm″) the condition resulting from diminution or cessation of hormonal secretion by the pituitary gland, especially the anterior pituitary. Symptoms vary with the degree of dysfunction.

hypoplasia, hypoplasty (hi″po-pla′ze-ah; hi′po-plas″te) incomplete development of an organ or tissue. adj., **hypoplas′tic.**

hypopnea (hi-pop′ne-ah) abnormal decrease in depth and rate of respiration. adj., **hypopne′ic.**

hypoporosis (hi″po-po-ro′sis) deficient callus formation after bone fracture.

hypoposia (hi″po-po′ze-ah) abnormally diminished ingestion of fluids.

hypopotassemia (hi″po-pot″ah-se′me-ah) hypokalemia.

hypopraxia (hi″po-prak′se-ah) abnormally diminished activity.

hypoprosody (hi″po-pros′o-de) diminution of the normal variation of stress, pitch, and rhythm of speech.

hypoproteinemia (hi″po-pro″te-ĭ-ne′me-ah) deficiency of protein in the blood.

hypoprothrombinemia (hi″po-pro-throm″bĭ-ne′-me-ah) deficiency of prothrombin in the blood.

hypopselaphesia (hi″pop-sel″ah-fe′ze-ah) dullness of tactile sensitiveness.

hypopsychosis (hi″po-si-ko′sis) diminution of the function of thought.

hypoptyalism (hi″po-ti′ah-lizm) abnormally decreased secretion of saliva.

hypopyon (hi-po′pe-on) pus in the anterior chamber of the eye.

hyporeactive (hi″po-re-ak′tiv) showing less than normal response to stimuli.

hyporeflexia (hi″po-re-flek′se-ah) diminution or weakening of reflexes.

hyposalemia (hi″po-sah-le′me-ah) diminution of salt levels in the blood.

hyposalivation (hi″po-sal″ĭ-va′shun) hypoptyalism.

hyposcleral (hi″po-skle′rol) beneath the sclera.

hyposecretion (hi″po-se-kre′shun) diminished secretion.

hyposensitivity (hi″po-sen″sĭ-tiv′ĭ-te) 1. abnormally decreased sensitivity. 2. the state of being less sensitive to a specific allergen after repeated and gradually increasing doses of the offending substance. adj., **hyposen′sitive.**

hyposensitization (hi″po-sen″sĭ-tĭ-za′shun) the act or process of inducing hyposensitivity.

hyposmia (hi-poz′me-ah) diminished acuteness of the sense of smell.

hyposmolarity (hi-poz″mo-lar′ĭ-te) abnormally decreased osmolar concentration of a solution.

hyposomnia (hi″po-som′ne-ah) pathologically diminished sleep; insomnia.

hypospadiac (hi″po-spa′de-ak) 1. pertaining to hypospadias. 2. a person affected with hypospadias.

hypospadias (hi″po-spa′de-as) a developmental anomaly in the male in which the urethra opens on the under side of the penis or on the perineum.
female h., a developmental anomaly in the female in which the urethra opens into the vagina.

hypostasis (hi-pos′tah-sis) poor or stagnant circulation in a dependent part of the body or an organ.

hypostatic (hi″po-stat′ik) 1. pertaining to, due to, or associated with hypostasis. 2. abnormally static; said of certain inherited traits that are liable to be suppressed by other traits.

hyposthenia (hi″pos-the′ne-ah) diminished strength or tonicity. adj., **hyposthen′ic.**

hyposthenuria (hi″pos-thĕ-nu′re-ah) excretion of urine of low specific gravity.

hypostomia (hi″po-sto′me-ah) a developmental anomaly characterized by abnormal smallness of the mouth, the slit being vertical instead of horizontal.

hypostypsis (hi″po-stip′sis) moderate astringency. adj., **hypostyp′tic.**

hyposynergia (hi″po-sĭ-ner′je-ah) defective coordination.

hypotelorism (hi″po-te′lo-rizm) abnormally decreased distance between two organs or parts.
ocular h., orbital h., abnormal decrease in the intraocular distance.

hypotension (hi″po-ten′shun) diminished tension; lowered blood pressure. A consistently low blood pressure with a systolic pressure less than 100 mm. of mercury is no cause for concern. In fact, low blood pressure often is associated with long life and an old age free of illness. An extremely low blood pressure is occasionally a symptom of a serious condition. In shock there is a disproportion between the blood volume and the capacity of the circulatory system, resulting in greatly reduced blood pressure.

Hypotension may be associted with Addison's disease and inadequate thyroid function, but in both cases the primary disease produces so many other symptoms that the hypotension is considered comparatively unimportant.

orthostatic h., postural h., a form of low blood presure that occurs on assumption of the erect position.

hypotensive (hi″po-ten′siv) 1. characterized by or causing diminished tension or pressure, as abnormally low blood pressure. 2. a person with abnormally low blood pressure.

hypotensor (hi″po-ten′sor) a substance that lowers the blood pressure.

hypothalamus (hi″po-thal′ah-mus) a portion of the brain, lying beneath the thalamus at the base of the cerebrum, and forming the floor and part of the walls of the third ventricle. Anatomically, it includes the optic chiasm, mammilary bodies, tuber cinereum, infundibulum, and pituitary gland, but for physiological purposes, the pituitary gland is considered a distinct structure. adj., **hypothalam′ic.**

Some cells in the hypothalamus control heat production and others control heat loss; thus the hypothalamus is said to contain the temperature-regulating center of the body. It also contains the mechanism for regulating functional activity of the posterior lobe of the PITUITARY GLAND, and the secretory activity of the anterior lobe of the pituitary. Because of its influence in the production of pituitary hormones, the hypothalamus indirectly plays an important role in the regulation of fat and carbohydrate metabolism, in body fluid balance and electrolyte content and in internal secretion of other endocrine glands.

The hypothalamus is a coordinating center for the autonomic nervous system and therefore influences many involuntary actions such as gastrointestinal motility and secretion, sweating, changes in arterial pressure and urinary output. Behaviorial functions associated with the hypothalamus include sleep, wakefulness, alertness, and reactions to pain and pleasure.

hypothenar (hi-poth′ĕ-nar) 1. the fleshy eminence on the palm along the ulnar margin. 2. relating to this eminence.

hypothermia (hi″po-ther′me-ah) low temperature. adj., **hypother′mal, hypother′mic.** Hypothermia may be symptomatic of a disease or disorder of the temperature-regulating mechanism of the body, or it may be induced for certain surgical procedures or as a therapeutic measure.

induced h., deliberate reduction of the temperature of all or part of the body; sometimes used as an adjunct to anesthesia in surgical procedures involving a limb, and as a protective measure in cardiac and neurologic surgery. The hypothermia may be continued only for the duration of the operation or it may be prolonged for as long as 5 days, depending on the reason for its use.

LOCAL HYPOTHERMIA. This is a type of refrigeration anesthesia restricted to a part of the body, such as a limb. It usually is used to produce surgical anesthesia immediately before amputation. The advantages of this type of anesthesia include minimal risk of shock, lowering of cell metabolism, and elimination of the need for inhalation anesthesia in patients who are poor surgical risks.

The part to be anesthetized is packed in ice or wrapped in a special refrigeration unit consisting of coiled tubes. Tourniquets are applied to the limb to inhibit circulation and avoid general chilling of the patient. The limb is chilled for 3 to 5 hours before amputation.

GENERAL HYPOTHERMIA. Generalized lowering of the body temperature decreases the metabolism of tissues and thereby the need for oxygen; it is used in various surgical procedures, especially on the heart. The body temperature is maintained between 89° F. (32° C.) and 78° F. (26° C.).

To induce general hypothermia, the patient may be immersed in ice water, packed in crushed ice or ice packs, or wrapped in a cooling blanket containing coils through which cold water or an antifreeze, or both, are circulated. The fastest method for achieving hypothermia is extracorporeal cooling of the blood; the patient's blood is removed through a cannula inserted in a large vessel, circulated through refrigerated coils and returned via another cannulated vessel.

Rewarming of the patient is accomplished simply by removing the ice packs or cooling blankets and allowing the temperature to rise gradually and naturally. In most cases regular blankets are used to maintain body warmth. External heat in the form of hot water bottles or warm tub baths, if used at all, must be applied with extreme caution to avoid burning the patient.

PATIENT CARE. During hypothermia and the rewarming process the patient's temperature, pulse, respiration, and blood pressure must be checked frequently. Special electronic thermometers are often used so that the body temperature can be monitored at all times. In prolonged hypothermia, cardiac irregularities or respiratory difficulties may develop quickly; the patient must be watched constantly for changes in the vital signs, and any changes must be reported immediately. The skin also should be observed for signs of developing decubitus ulcers, edema, or marked discoloration.

The patient should be turned every 2 hours, with special attention to proper positioning and good body alignment. Decreased secretion of saliva and mouth-breathing demand frequent mouth care. The eyes may need to be irrigated frequently and covered with compresses moistened with physiologic saline solution if the corneal reflex is diminished and eye secretions are reduced.

Intake and output are measured and recorded. An indwelling catheter is inserted prior to induction of hypothermia and is left in place until normal body temperature is established. This is necessary because urinary output is diminished during hypothermia. Fluids are given intravenously and the oral intake of food and liquids is prohibited because of depression of the gag reflex.

Shivering during prolonged hypothermia must be avoided as it tends to elevate the body temperature and increase metabolic needs, thereby defeating the purpose of hypothermia. Chlorpromazine may be ordered as a precaution against shivering.

During the rewarming process the patient must be observed for signs of increased tendency to bleed and of gastric distention; these are common complications. After the body temperature returns to normal and becomes stabilized, the patient is allowed to progress to a normal diet and physical activities.

symtomatic h., pathologic reduction of body temperature as a result of decreased heat production or increased heat loss. Hypothyroidism, severe blood loss with circulatory failure, and damage to the heat-producing cells of the hypothalamus can lead to decreased heat production. Prolonged exposure to cold, overdosage of antipyretic drugs, such as aspirin, and profuse sweating (diaphoresis) are some causes of increased heat loss and resultant hypothermia.

hypothesis (hi-poth'ĕ-sis) a supposition that appears to explain a group of phenomena and is assumed as a basis of reasoning and experimentation.

hypothrombinemia (hi"po-throm"bĭ-ne'me-ah) deficiency of thrombin in the blood, resulting in a tendency to bleed.

hypothymia (hi"po-thi'me-ah) abnormally diminished emotionalism.

hypothymism (hi"po-thi'mizm) diminished thymus activity.

hypothyroidism (hi"po-thi'roi-dizm) deficiency of THYROID GLAND activity, with underproduction of thyroxine, or the condition resulting from it. adj., **hypothy'roid.** In its severe form it is called MYXEDEMA and is characterized by physical and mental sluggishness, obesity, loss of hair, enlargement of the tongue, and thickening of the skin. In children the condition is known as CRETINISM.

hypotonia (hi"po-to'ne-ah) abnormally decreased tonicity or strength.

hypotonic (hi"po-ton'ik) 1. having an abnormally reduced tonicity or tension. 2. having an osmotic pressure lower than that of the solution with which it is compared.

hypotoxicity (hi"po-tok-sis'ĭte) abnormally reduced toxic quality.

hypotransferrinemia (hi"po-trans-fer"ĭ-ne'me-ah) deficiency of transferrin in the blood.

hypotrichosis (hi"po-trĭ-ko'sis) presence of less than the normal amount of hair.

hypotrophy (hi-pot'ro-fe) abiotrophy.

hypotropia (hi"po-tro'pe-ah) STRABISMUS in which there is permanent downward deviation of the visual axis of one eye.

hypotympanotomy (hi"po-tim"pah-not'o-me) surgical opening of the hypotympanum.

hypotympanum (hi"po-tim'pah-num) the lower part of the cavity of the middle ear, in the temporal bone.

hypoventilation (hi"po-ven"tĭ-la'shun) reduction in the amount of air entering the pulmonary alveoli.

hypovitaminosis (hi"po-vi"tah-mĭ-no'sis) a condition produced by lack of an essential vitamin.

hypovolemia (hi"po-vo-le'me-ah) abnormally decreased volume of circulating fluid (plasma) in the body. adj., **hypovole'mic.**

hypovolia (hi"po-vo'le-ah) diminished water content or volume, as of extracellular fluid.

hypoxanthine (hi"po-zan'thēn) an intermediate product of uric acid synthesis, formed from adenylic acid and itself a precursor of xanthine.

hypoxemia (hi"pok-se'me-ah) deficient oxygenation of the blood. The most reliable method for measuring the degree of hypoxemia is BLOOD GAS ANALYSIS to determine the partial pressure of oxygen in the arterial blood. Insufficient oxygenation of the blood eventually leads to HYPOXIA.

hypoxia (hi-pok'se-ah) a broad term meaning diminished availability of oxygen to the body tissues. adj., **hypox'ic.** Its causes are many and varied. There may be a deficiency of oxygen in the atmosphere, as in ALTITUDE SICKNESS, or a pulmonary disorder that interferes with adequate ventilation of the lungs. Anemia or circulatory deficiencies can lead to inadequate transport and delivery of oxygen to the tissues. Finally, edema or other abnormal conditions of the tissues themselves may impair the exchange of oxygen and carbon dioxide between the capillaries and the tissues.

SYMPTOMS. Signs and symptoms of hypoxia vary according to its cause. Generally they include dyspnea, rapid pulse, syncope, and mental disturbances such as delirium or euphoria. Cyanosis is not always present and in some cases is not evident until the hypoxia is far advanced. The localized pain of ANGINA PECTORIS due to hypoxia occurs because of impaired oxygenation of the myocardium. Discoloration of the skin and eventual ulceration that sometimes accompany varicose veins are a result of hypoxia of the involved tissues.

TREATMENT. The treatment of hypoxia depends on the primary cause. Administration of oxygen by inhalation may be useful in some cases and of no help in others. For example, in situations in which there is difficulty with the transport of oxygen from the lungs to other parts of the body, increasing the intake of oxygen will do little to correct the problem of distribution (see OXYGEN THERAPY). In some vascular diseases the administration of vasodilators may help increase circulation, hence oxygen supply, to the tissues.

hyps(o)- word element [Gr.], *height.*

hypsarhythmia (hip"sah-rith'me-ah) a term for an electroencephalographic abnormality sometimes observed in infants, with random high-voltage slow waves and spikes arising from multiple foci and spreading to all cortical areas; the disorder is characterized by spasms or quivering spells, and is commonly associated with mental retardation.

hypsokinesis (hip"so-ki-ne'sis) a backward swaying or falling in erect posture, seen in paralysis agitans and other neurologic disorders.

hyster(o)- word element [Gr.], *uterus; hysteria.*

hysteralgia (his"tĕ-ral'je-ah) pain in the uterus.

hysteratresia (his"ter-ah-tre'ze-ah) atresia of the uterus.

hysterectomy (his"tĕ-reck'to-me) surgical removal of the UTERUS.

abdominal h., that performed through the abdominal wall.

cesarean h., cesarean section followed by removal of the uterus.

radical h., excision of the uterus, upper vagina, and parametrium.

subtotal h., that in which the cervix is left in place.

total h., that in which the uterus and cervix are completely excised.

vaginal h., that performed through the vagina.

hysteresis (his-tĕ-re'sis) the failure of coincidence of two associated phenomena, such as that exhibited in the differing temperatures of gelation and of liquefaction of a reversible colloid.

hystereurynter (his"ter-u-rin'ter) an instrument for dilating the ostium uteri.

hystereurysis (his"ter-u'rĭ-sis) dilation of the ostium uteri.

hysteria (his-te're-ah) a form of psychoneurosis in which the individual converts anxiety created by emotional conflict into physical symptoms that have no organic basis; called also conversion reaction or conversion hysteria. The term hysteria is also used to describe a state of tension or excitement in which there is a temporary loss of control over the emotions. adj., **hyster′ical.**

The patient with conversion hysteria is mentally ill. He converts his mental distress into physical symptoms in an effort to escape severe emotional conflict. The physical symptoms may include blindness, deafness, mutism, or paralysis of an arm or leg. In most cases the symptom can be related to some aspect of the conflict. For example, a college student interested in creative writing, but majoring in music because her parents want her to, may attempt to solve the problem by developing a loss of hearing. She then has an excuse for not continuing with the music and can at the same time satisfy her own desires without openly defying her parents. The patient who employs such methods is unaware that he is using the physical symptom to solve his emotional problem. Treatment is by PSYCHOTHERAPY in which the patient is helped to resolve the emotional conflict in a more normal manner.

The milder form of hysteria that is characterized by such symptoms as crying, pointless laughter, shouting, aimless walking about, or a temper tantrum usually results from an incident in which a person is pushed beyond his normal endurance. It might be provoked by danger, severe fright, or the reception of bad news.

hysterics (his-ter′iks) popular term for an uncontrollable emotional outburst.

hysterocatalesy (his″ter-o-kat′ah-lep″se) hysteria with cataleptic symptoms.

hysterocele (his′ter-o-sēl″) hernia of the uterus.

hysterocleisis (his″ter-o-kli′sis) surgical closure of the ostium uteri.

hysterodynia (his″ter-o-din′e-ah) pain in the uterus.

hysteroepilepsy (his″ter-o-ep′ĭ-lep″se) severe hysteria with epileptic convulsions.

hysterogenic (his″ter-o-jen′ik) causing hysterical phenomena or symptoms.

hysterography (his″tĕ-rog′rah-fe) 1. the graphic recording of the strength of uterine contractions in labor. 2. radiography of the uterus after instillation of a contrast medium.

hysteroid (his″ter-oid) resembling hysteria.

hysterolith (his′ter-o-lith″) a uterine calculus.

hysterolysis (his″tĕ-rol′ĭ-sis) freeing of the uterus from adhesions.

hysterometer (his″tĕ-rom′ĕ-ter) an instrument for measuring the uterus.

hysterometry (his″tĕ-rom′ĕ-tre) measurement of the uterus.

hysteromyoma (his″ter-o-mi-o′mah) leiomyoma of the uterus.

hysteromyomectomy (his″ter-o-mi″o-mek′to-me) local excision of a leiomyoma of the uterus.

hysteromyotomy (his″ter-o-mi-ot′o-me) incision of the uterus for removal of a solid tumor.

hysteropathy (his″tĕ-rop′ah-the) any uterine disease; metropathy.

hysteropexy (his′ter-o-pek″se) fixation of a displaced uterus by surgery.

hysteropia (his″tĕ-ro′pe-ah) a hysterical disorder of vision.

hysteroptosis (his″ter-op-to′sis) prolapse of the uterus.

hysterorrhaphy (his″tĕ-ror′ah-fe) 1. suture of the uterus. 2. hysteropexy.

hysterorrhexis (his″ter-o-rek′sis) rupture of the uterus.

hysterosalpingectomy (his″ter-o-sal″pin-jek′to-me) excision of the uterus and uterine tubes.

hysterosalpingography (his″ter-o-sal″ping-gog′rah-fe) roentgenography of the uterus and uterine tubes.

hysterosalpingo-oophorectomy (his″ter-o-sal-ping″go-o″of-o-rek′to-me) excision of the uterus, uterine tubes, and ovaries.

hysterosalpingostomy (his″ter-o-sal″ping-gos′to-me) anastomosis of a uterine tube and the uterus.

hysteroscope (his′ter-o-skōp″) an endoscope used in direct visual examination of the canal of the uterine cervix and the cavity of the uterus.

hysterospasm (his′ter-o-spazm″) spasm of the uterus.

hysterotomy (his″tĕ-rot′o-me) incision of the uterus.

hysterotrachelorrhaphy (his″ter-o-tra″kĕ-lor′ah-fe) suture of the uterus and uterine cervix.

hysterotrachelotomy (his″ter-o-tra″kĕ-lot′o-me) incision of the uterus and uterine cervix.

hysterotraumatism (his″ter-o-traw′mah-tizm) hysterical symptoms following injury.

hysterotubography (his″ter-o-tu-bog′rah-fe) hysterosalpingography.

Hytakerol (hi-tak′er-ol) trademark for preparations of dihydrotachysterol, used to increase the blood calcium level.

Hz hertz (cycles per second).

I

I chemical symbol, *iodine.*

^{131}I, I 131 symbol for the radioactive isotope of iodine of atomic mass 131, half-life, 8.07 days; also written I^{131}.

-ia (e′ah) word element, *state; condition.*

-iasis word element [Gr.], *condition; state.*

iatr(o)- word element [Gr.], *medicine; physician.*

iatric (i-at′rik) pertaining to medicine or to a physician.

iatrochemistry (i-at″ro-kem′is-tre) the name of a school of medicine of the 17th century, which espoused the theory that all phenomena of life and disease were based on chemical action.

iatrogenic (i-at″ro-jen′ik) resulting from the activity of a physician; said of any adverse condition in a patient resulting from treatment by a physician or surgeon.

iatrophysics (i-at″ro-fiz′iks) 1. treatment of disease by physical or mechanical means. 2. medical physics. 3. the early theory that all vital phenomena are controlled by the laws of physics.

ibuprofen (i-bu′pro-fen) a nonsteroidal anti-inflammatory agent indicated in symptomatic relief of rheumatoid arthritis and osteoarthritis. It is similar in action to aspirin but less apt to cause gastrointestinal side effects.

ICD intrauterine contraceptive device.

Iceland disease benign myalgic encephalomyelitis.

ichor (i′kor) a watery discharge from wounds or sores. adj., **i′chorous.**

ichorrhea (i″ko-re′ah) copious discharge of ichor.

ichthammol (ik-tham′ol) an ammoniated coal tar product, used in ointment form for certain skin diseases.

ichthyismus (ik″the-iz′mus) ichthyotoxism.

ichthyoid (ik′the-oid) fishlike.

Ichthyol (ik′the-ol) trademark for a preparation of ichthammol.

ichthyology (ik″the-ol′o-je) the study of fishes.

ichthyophagous (ik″the-of′ah-gus) eating or subsisting on fish.

ichthyosarcotoxin (ik″the-o-sar″ko-tok′sin) a toxin found in the flesh of poisonous fishes.

ichthyosarcotoxism (ik″the-o-sar″ko-tok′sizm) poisoning due to ingestion of poisonous fish, marked by various gastrointestinal and neurological disturbances.

ichthyosis (ik″the-o′sis) 1. any of several generalized skin disorders marked by dryness, roughness, and scaliness, due to hypertrophy of the horny layer, resulting from excessive production or retention of keratin, or a molecular defect in the keratin. 2. ichthyosis vulgaris. adj., **ichthyot′ic.**

i. congen′ita, lamellar exfoliation of the newborn.

i. feta′lis, lamellar exfoliation of the newborn.

i. hys′trix, a rare form of epidermolytic hyperkeratosis marked by generalized, dark brown, linear verrucoid ridges somewhat like porcupine skin.

lamellar i. of newborn, see LAMELLAR EXFOLIATION OF THE NEWBORN.

ichthyotoxin (ik″the-o-tok′sin) any toxic substance derived from fish.

ichthyotoxism (ik″the-o-tok′sizm) any intoxication due to an ichthyotoxin.

I.C.N. International Council of Nurses.

I.C.S. International College of Surgeons.

ICSH interstitial cell-stimulating hormone (luteinizing hormone).

ictal (ik′tal) pertaining to, characterized by, or due to a stroke or an acute epileptic seizure.

icteric (ik-ter′ik) pertaining to or affected with jaundice.

i. index, a rough determination of the concentration of bilirubin in the blood; it is indicative of liver function. The color intensity of the blood is measured and reported in units. Preparation of the patient includes fasting because chyle can render the sample of blood unsatisfactory. Normal range for the icteric index is 4 to 8 units.

icterogenic (ik″ter-o-jen′ik) causing jaundice.

icterohepatitis (ik″ter-o-hep″ah-ti′tis) inflammation of the liver with marked jaundice.

icteroid (ik′ter-oid) resembling jaundice.

icterus (ik′ter-us) jaundice.

i. gra′vis, acute yellow atrophy of the liver.

i. gra′vis neonato′rum, severe jaundice in the newborn, usually a form of isoimmunization with Rh factor. (See also KERNICTERUS.)

i. neonato′rum, jaundice in newborn infants.

ictus (ik′tus) a seizure, stroke, blow, or sudden attack. adj., **ic′tal.**

ICU intensive care unit.

I.D. infective dose.

I.D.$_{50}$ median infective dose.

id (id) 1. a freudian term used to describe that part of the personality which harbors the unconscious, instinctive impulses that lead to immediate gratification of primitive needs such as hunger, the need for air, the need to move about and relieve body tension, and the need to eliminate. Id impulses are physiologic and body processes, as opposed to the EGO and SUPEREGO, which are psychologic and social processes. The id is dominated by the pleasure principle and some gratification of the id impulses is necessary for survival of a person's personality. 2. a rash associated with but remote from the main lesion of the disease; considered to be an allergic reaction to the causative agent of the disease; often used as a suffix of a root representing the causative factor, as syphilid.

-id [Gr.] 1. a suffix meaning having the shape of, or resembling. 2. see ID (2).

-ide (īd) suffix indicating a binary compound.

idea (i-de′ah) a mental impression or conception.

autochthonous i., a strange idea that comes into the mind in some unaccountable way, but is not a hallucination.

compulsive i., an idea that persists despite reason

and will and that drives one to action, usually inappropriate.

dominant i., a morbid or other impression that controls or colors every action and thought.

fixed i., a persistent morbid impression or belief that cannot be changed by reason.

i. of reference, the incorrect idea that the words and actions of others refer to one's self, or the projection of the causes of one's own imaginary difficulties upon someone else.

ideal (i-de'al) a pattern or concept of perfection.

ego i., the standard of perfection unconsciously created by a person for himself.

ideation (i″de-a'shun) the formation of ideas or images. adj., **idea'tional.**

idée fixe (e-da' fēks') fixed idea.

identification (i-den″tĭ-fĭ-ka'shun) a defense mechanism by which an individual unconsciously takes as his own the characteristics, postures, achievements, or other identifying traits of other persons or groups. Identification plays a major role in the development of the SUPEREGO and of awareness and acceptance of the standards and rules accepted by society. However, as a person matures emotionally, his own self-identity should become clearer as he relates more to his own personal achievements and less to the accomplishments and successes of others with whom he identifies.

Identification is not to be confused with imitation, which is a conscious process. It should be pointed out also that overuse of identification as a defense mechanism denies one the opportunity of enjoying the benefits and self-satisfaction derived from his own accomplishments.

ideogenetic, ideogenous (i″de-o-jĕ-net'ik; i″de-oj'ĕ-nus) induced by or related to vague sense impressions rather than organized images.

ideology (i″de-ol'o-je, id″e-ol'o-je) 1. the science of the development of ideas. 2. the body of ideas characteristic of an individual or of a social unit.

ideomotion (i″de-o-mo'shun) muscular action induced by a dominant idea.

idio- word element [Gr.], *self; peculiar to a substance or organism.*

idiocy (id'e-o-se) severe MENTAL RETARDATION.

amaurotic familial i., a group of hereditary disorders due to an inborn defect of lipid metabolism, in which sphingolipids accumulate in the brain (see also AMAUROTIC FAMILIAL IDIOCY).

mongolian i., former name for Down's syndrome.

idioglossia (id″e-o-glos'e-ah) imperfect articulation, with utterance of meaningless vocal sounds. adj., **idioglot'tic.**

idiogram (id'e-o-gram) a drawing or photograph of the chromosomes of a particular cell.

idiopathic (id″e-o-path'ik) self-originated; occurring without known cause.

idiopathy (id″e-op'ah-the) a morbid state arising without known cause.

idiosome (id'e-o-sōm″) the centrosome of a spermatocyte, together with the surrounding Golgi apparatus and mitochondria.

idiosyncrasy (id″e-o-sing'krah-se) 1. a habit or quality of body or mind peculiar to any individual. 2. an abnormal susceptibility to an agent (e.g., a drug) that is peculiar to the individual. adj., **idiosyncrat'ic.**

idiot (id'e-ot) a person afflicted with severe MENTAL RETARDATION.

mongolian i., former name for a person afflicted with Down's syndrome.

i.-savant, a person who is generally mentally retarded, yet has a particular mental faculty developed to an unusually high degree, as for mathematics, music, etc.

idiotrophic (id″e-o-trof'ik) capable of selecting its own nourishment.

idioventricular (id″e-o-ven-trik'u-lar) pertaining to the cardiac ventricle alone.

idoxuridine (i″doks-ūr'ĭ-den) a pyrimidine analogue that prevents replication of DNA viruses; used topically in herpes simplex keratitis.

IDU idoxuridine.

Ig immunoglobulin of any of the five classes: IgA, IgD, IgE, IgG, and IgM.

ignipuncture (ig″nĭ-pungk'tūr) therapeutic puncture with hot needles.

ignis (ig'nis) [L.] fire.

i. sa'cer, 1. ergotism. 2. herpes zoster.

ile(o)- word element [L.], *ileum.*

ileac (il'e-ak) 1. of the nature of ileus. 2. pertaining to the ileum.

ileal (il'e-al) pertaining to the ileum.

i. conduit, use of a segment of the ileum for the diversion of urinary flow from the ureters. The segment is resected from the intestine with nerves and blood supply intact. The proximal end of the segment is closed, forming a pouch, and the ends of the ureters are sutured to it. The distal end is brought to the outside of the abdominal wall and effaced to form a stoma. The remaining ends of the small intestine are anastomosed to reestablish bowel continuity, the ileal loop no longer being a part of the intestinal tract. Called also urinary ileostomy and the Bricker procedure.

Indications for an ileal conduit include surgical removal of the bladder for severe trauma or malignancy, congenital defect of the urinary tract, and neurogenic nonfunctioning bladder in which other devices to maintain urinary flow are unsatisfactory.

Prior to surgery, the placement of the stoma is determined by a thorough examination of the abdomen while the patient assumes various body positions. The site is selected so that old scar tissue, skin folds, bony prominences, and the umbilicus are avoided. Paraplegics or others wearing braces for ambulation must have the stoma placed so that there is no pressure on it from the appliance.

PATIENT CARE. The diversion of urinary flow to a collection pouch outside the body presents a very real challenge to the patient and those responsible for helping him develop a positive attitude about himself and his ability to achieve the goal of independence and rehabilitation. Psychologically he must adjust to a new body image, and he must deal with the most personal and intimate problems associated with the collection and disposal of urine. He will be concerned with the physical, social, and recreational limitations imposed by the stoma and with his acceptance socially. He will fear embarrassment from odors and leakage of urine, with his appearance and mode of dress, and with the amount of time involved in emptying and caring for the collection apparatus. With adequate instruction and continued support and reassurance, each of his concerns can be dealt with in a positive and helpful manner.

Because there is continuous drainage of urine down the ureters from the kidneys, the appliance for collection of urine must be worn at all times. In most cases the appliance must be emptied every 3 to 4 hours, depending on the amount of fluid intake and whether a leg bag is also used. These pouches are reusable for a short period of time and are discarded at the patient's discretion. They are cleaned with soap and water and may be rinsed in white vinegar to help eliminate odor. Commercial deodorizers are also available.

Skin irritation and infection around the stoma is always a danger because the moisture that collects under the faceplate of the appliance provides an ideal environment for the development of fungus (yeast or mold) infections. Soap and water are used to clean the area, which is then thoroughly dried and treated with such topical medications as Mycostatin powder and Kenalog spray to protect the skin.

It is especially important that the patient receive coordinated care from all available members of the health care team. The certified ostomy care specialist is an invaluable source of help and guidance for the patient and his family. In many communities there is an ostomy club whose members have some type of stoma and who meet regularly to share their experiences and to learn about self-care. Information about these and other local resources can be obtained by contacting the United Ostomy Association, Inc., and the International Association for Enterostomal Therapy. (See also STOMA.)

ileectomy (il″e-ek′to-me) excision of the ileum.

ileitis (il″e-i′tis) inflammation of the ileum, or distal portion of the small intestine. It may result from infection, obstruction, severe irritation, or faulty absorption of material through the intestinal walls.

A specific type of inflammation of unknown cause involving the small and large intestines is known as regional ileitis, REGIONAL ENTERITIS or Crohn's disease. The advanced stage is marked by hardening, thickening, and ulceration of parts of the bowel lining. An obstruction may cause the development of a fistula.

A common symptom of ileitis is pain in the lower right quadrant of the abdomen or around the umbilicus. Other symptoms include loss of appetite, loss of weight, anemia, and diarrhea, which may alternate with periods of constipation. Treatment may require medication to remove any source of infection, special diet or surgery if there is obstruction.

ileocecal (il″e-o-se′kal) pertaining to the ileum and cecum.

i. valve, the valve guarding the opening between the ileum and cecum; called also ileocolic valve.

ileocecostomy (il″e-o-se-kos′to-me) surgical anastomosis of the ileum to the cecum.

ileocolic (il″e-o-kol′ik) pertaining to the ileum and colon.

i. valve, ileocecal valve.

ileocolitis (il″e-o-ko-li′tis) inflammation of the ileum and colon.

i. ulcero′sa chron′ica, chronic ileocolitis with fever, rapid pulse, anemia, diarrhea, and right iliac pain.

ileocolostomy (il″e-o-ko-los′to-me) surgical anastomosis of the ileum to the colon.

ileocolotomy (il″e-o-ko-lot′o-me) incision of the ileum and colon.

ileocystoplasty (il″e-o-sis′to-plas″te) repair of the wall of the urinary bladder with an isolated segment of the wall of the ileum.

ileocystostomy (il″e-o-sis-tos′to-me) use of an isolated segment of ileum to create a passage from the urinary bladder to an opening in the abdominal wall.

ileoileostomy (il″e-o-il″e-os′to-me) surgical anastomosis between two parts of the ileum.

ileorectal (il″e-o-rek′tal) pertaining to or communicating with the ileum and rectum.

ileorrhaphy (il″e-or′ah-fe) suture of the ileum.

ileosigmoidostomy (il″e-o-sig″moi-dos′to-me) surgical anastomosis of the ileum to the sigmoid colon.

ileostomy (il″e-os′to-me) an artificial opening (stoma) created in the small intestine (ileum) and brought to the surface of the abdomen for the purpose of evacuating feces. Ileostomy may be done in the treatment of ULCERATIVE COLITIS, REGIONAL ILEITIS (Crohn's disease), congenital defects of the bowel, CANCER, trauma, and other conditions requiring bypass of the colon.

An ileostomy may be temporary or permanent. When the ileostomy is done in conjunction with partial or complete removal of the colon and anus, it is always permanent. The stoma created by ileostomy usually is located in the right lower quadrant of the abdomen.

PATIENT CARE. The patient with an ileostomy requires care similar to that of the patient with a COLOSTOMY. Attention must be paid to the physical and psychological adjustments demanded of the patient as he works through his problems and strives to lead a normal and productive life.

The appliance for collection of feces must be worn continuously and emptied every 4 to 5 hours because there is continuous flow of feces through the ileostomy. The pouch should be changed at least once every week and more often if skin irritation, leakage, or persistent odor becomes a problem. The patient's main concerns will be obstruction and diarrhea. He must be taught the signs of developing obstruction and the technique for gentle irrigation and massage around the stoma to remove material obstructing the movement of intestinal contents. If either irrigation or massage will not relieve the obstruction, he is instructed to report to his physician.

Diarrhea is a more frequent problem in a patient with an ileostomy and is more likely to result in serious difficulties arising from fluid and electrolyte loss and an upset in the ACID-BASE BALANCE. The patient must be aware of the early signs and symptoms of these difficulties and report to his physician should they occur.

The patient's diet need not be severely restricted, but he should be warned to avoid foods that produce gas and those likely to lead to obstruction, for example popcorn, nuts, and seeds. He is instructed to chew all of his food thoroughly in order to facilitate digestion of the food before it passes through the ileostomy.

Skin irritations are a constant threat, as are topical fungus (yeast and mold) infections that may develop around the stoma. Because of the liquidity of the feces there is always danger of leakage around the pouch where it fits over the stoma. The skin must be cleansed frequently and protected with a skin barrier such as Kenalog spray and karaya gum.

The patient requires continued support as he

learns to care for and live with his ileostomy. Fortunately, there are many sources of assistance for him, his family, and members of the health care team responsible for his care and rehabilitation. (See also STOMA.)

urinary i., use of a segment of the ileum as a stoma for the diversion of urinary flow from the ureters (see also ILEAL CONDUIT).

ileotomy (il″e-ot′o-me) incision of the ileum.

Iletin (il′ĕ-tin) trademark for preparations of insulin for injection.

ileum (il′e-um) the distal portion of the small intestine, extending from the jejunum to the cecum.

duplex i., congenital duplication of the ileum.

ileus (il′e-us) intestinal obstruction, especially failure of peristalsis. The condition frequently accompanies peritonitis and usually results from disturbances in neural stimulation of the bowel. It also may occur in many painful conditions involving the thoracolumbar region, for example, the colicky pains of GALLSTONES or KIDNEY stones and spinal injuries.

SYMPTOMS. The principal symptoms of ileus are abdominal pain and distention, vomiting (the vomitus may contain fecal material), and constipation. If the intestinal obstruction is not relieved, the circulation in the wall of the intestine is impaired and the patient appears extremely ill with symptoms of SHOCK and DEHYDRATION.

TREATMENT. Distention of the abdomen is relieved by decompression, which involves INTUBATION with a long, balloon-tipped tube (e.g., MILLER-ABBOTT TUBE) that extends to the site of the obstruction, and use of constant suction. Because of the disruption in absorption of fluids and nutrients from the intestinal tract, fluids, electrolytes, and glucose are given intravenously. Surgical intervention to remove the cause of ileus is usually necessary when the obstruction is complete or the bowel is likely to become gangrenous. The type of surgical procedure will depend on the condition of the bowel and the cause of the obstruction. In some cases ILEOSTOMY or COLOSTOMY, either temporary or permanent, may be necessary. (See also INTESTINAL OBSTRUCTION.)

adynamic i., ileus resulting from inhibition of bowel motility, which may be produced by various causes, most frequently peritonitis.

dynamic i., hyperdynamic i., spastic ileus.

mechanical i., that due to mechanical causes, such as hernia, adhesions, volvulus, etc.

meconium i., ileus in the newborn due to blocking of the bowel with thick meconium.

paralytic i., adynamic ileus.

spastic i., that due to persistent contracture of a bowel segment.

i. subpar′ta, ileus due to pressure of the gravid uterus on the pelvic colon.

ili(o)- word element [L.], *ilium.*

iliac (il′e-ak) pertaining to the ilium.

iliadelphus (il″e-ah-del′fus) symmetrical conjoined twins united in the iliac region; iliopagus.

Ilidar (il′ĭ-dar) trademark for a preparation of azepetine, an adrenergic blocking agent used to dilate peripheral blood vessels.

iliofemoral (il″e-o-fem′o-ral) pertaining to the ilium and femur.

ilioinguinal (il″e-o-ing′gwĭ-nal) pertaining to the iliac and inguinal regions.

iliolumbar (il″e-o-lum′bar) pertaining to the iliac and lumbar regions.

iliopagus (il″e-op′ah-gus) symmetrical conjoined twins united in the iliac region.

iliopectineal (il″e-o-pek-tin′e-al) pertaining to the ilium and pubes.

iliotrochanteric (il″e-o-tro″kan-ter′ik) pertaining to the ilium and femoral trochanter.

ilium (il′e-um), pl. *il′ia* [L.] the lateral, flaring portion of the hip bone. adj., **il′iac.** (See also table of BONES.)

illness (il′nes) a condition marked by pronounced deviation from the normal healthy state; sickness.

illumination (ĭ-lu″mĭ-na′shun) the lighting up of a part, cavity, organ, or object for inspection.

axial i., light transmitted or reflected along the axis of a microscope.

darkfield i., dark-ground i., the casting of peripheral light rays upon a microscopical object from the side, the center rays being blocked out; the object appears bright on a dark background.

direct i., light thrown from above or from the direction of observation.

focal i., light thrown upon the focus of a lens or mirror.

oblique i., light from a source at one side of the object.

through i., light from a source behind and shining through the object.

illuminator (ĭ-lu′mĭ-na″tor) the source of light for viewing an object.

illusion (ĭ-lu′zhun) a mental impression derived from misinterpretation of an actual sensory stimulus. adj., **illu′sional.**

Ilotycin (i″lo-ti′sin) trademark for preparations of erythromycin, an antibiotic.

im- 1. a prefix, replacing *in-* before words beginning *b, m,* and *p.* 2. a chemical prefix indicating the bivalent group $>$NH.

I.M. intramuscularly.

I.M.A. Industrial Medical Association.

image (im′ij) a picture or concept with more or less likeness to an objective reality.

body i., the three-dimensional concept of one's self, recorded in the cortex by the perception of ever changing postures of the body, and constantly changing with them.

mirror i., 1. the image of light made visible by the reflecting surface of the cornea and lens when illuminated through the slit lamp. 2. an image with right and left relations reversed, as in the reflection of an object in a mirror.

motor i., the organized cerebral model of the possible movements of the body.

imago (ĭ-ma′go), pl. *ima′goes* or *imag′ines* [L.] 1. the adult or definitive form of an insect. 2. in psychoanalysis, a childhood memory or fantasy of a loved person that persists in adult life.

imbalance (im-bal′ans) lack of balance; especially lack of balance between muscles, as in insufficiency of ocular muscles.

autonomic i., defective coordination between the sympathetic and parasympathetic nervous systems, especially with respect to vasomotor activities.

sympathetic i., vagotonia.

vasomotor i., autonomic imbalance.

imbecile (im′bĕ-sil) defective mentally; a person exhibiting imbecility.

imbecility (im″bĕ-sil′ĭ-te) MENTAL RETARDATION less severe than idiocy but more severe than moronity.

imbibition (im″bĭ-bish′un) absorption of a liquid.

imbricated (im′brĭ-kāt″ed) overlapping like shingles.

imidazole (im″id-az′ōl) a base found combined with alanine in histidine.

imide (im′īd) any compound containing the bivalent group, >NH, to which are attached only acid radicals.

iminazole (im″in-az′ōl) imidazole.

imipramine (ĭ-mip′rah-mēn) an antidepressant, used as the hydrochloride salt.

immature (im″ah-tūr) unripe or not fully developed.

immersion (ĭ-mer′zhun) 1. the plunging of a body into a liquid. 2. the use of the microscope with the object and object glass both covered with a liquid.

i. foot, a condition resembling trench foot occurring in persons who have spent long periods in water.

immiscible (ĭ-mis′ĭ-b′l) not susceptible of being mixed.

immobilization (ĭ-mo″bĭ-lĭ-za′shun) the rendering of a part incapable of being moved.

immobilize (im-mo′bil-īz) to render incapable of being moved, as by a cast.

immune (ĭ-mūn′) 1. being highly resistant to a disease because of the formation of humoral antibodies or the development of immunologically competent cells, or both, or as a result of some other mechanism, as interferon activities in viral infections. 2. characterized by the development of humoral antibodies or cellular IMMUNITY, or both, following antigenic challenge. 3. produced in response to antigenic challenge, as immune serum globulin.

i. reaction, 1. immune response. 2. formation of a papule and areola without development of a vesicle following smallpox vaccination.

i. response, the reaction to and interaction with substances interpreted by the body as not-self, the result being humoral and cellular IMMUNITY. Called also immune reaction. The immune response depends on a functioning THYMUS and the conversion of stem cells to B- and T-lymphocytes. These B- and T-cells contribute to ANTIBODY production, cellular immunity, and immunologic memory.

DISORDERS OF THE IMMUNE RESPONSE. Pathologic conditions associated with an abnormal immune reponse (immunopathy) may result from: (1) immunodepression, that is, an absence or deficient supply of the components of either humoral or cellular immunity, or both; (2) excessive production of gamma globulins; (3) overreaction to antigens of extrinsic origin, that is, antigens from outside the body; and (4) abnormal response of the body to its own cells and tissues.

Those conditions arising from immunosuppression include agammaglobulinemia (the absence of gamma globulins) and hypogammaglobulinemia (a decrease of circulating antibodies). Factors that may cause or contribute to suppression of the immune response include: (1) congenital absence of the thymus or of the stem cells that are precursors of B- and T-lymphocytes; (2) malnutrition, in which there is a deficiency of the specific nutrients essential to the life of antibody-synthesizing cells; (3) cancer, viral infections, and extensive burns, all of which overburden the immune response mechanisms and rapidly deplete the supply of antigen-specific antibody; (4) certain drugs, including alcohol and heroin, some antibiotics, antipsychotics, and the ANTINEOPLASTICS used in the treatment of CANCER.

Overproduction of gamma globulins is manifested by an excessive proliferation of plasma cells (multiple myeloma).

Hypersensitivity is the result of an overreaction to substances entering the body. Examples of this kind of inappropriate immune response include HAY FEVER, drug and food ALLERGIES, extrinsic ASTHMA, serum sickness, and ANAPHYLAXIS.

AUTOIMMUNE DISEASES are manifestations of the body's abnormal response to and inability to tolerate its own cells and tissues. For reasons not yet fully understood, the body fails to interpret its own cells as *self* and, as it would with other foreign (*not-self*) substances, utilizes antibodies and immunologically competent cells to destroy and contain them.

immunifacient (ĭ-mu″nĭ-fa′shent) producing immunity.

immunity (ĭ-mu′nĭ-te) 1. the condition of being immune; security against a particular disease; nonsusceptibility to the invasive or pathogenic effects of foreign microorganisms or to the toxic effect of antigenic substances. Called also functional or protective immunity. 2. heightened responsiveness to antigenic challenge that leads to more rapid binding or elimination of antigen than in the nonimmune state; it includes both humoral and cell-mediated immunity (see below). 3. the capacity to distinguish foreign material from *self,* and to neutralize, eliminate, or metabolize that which is foreign (*not-self*) by the physiologic mechanisms of the IMMUNE RESPONSE.

The mechanisms of immunity are essentially concerned with the body's ability to recognize and dispose of substances which it interprets as foreign and harmful to its well-being. When such a substance enters the body, complex chemical and mechanical activities are set into motion to defend and protect the body's cells and tissues. The foreign substance, usually a protein, is called an ANTIGEN, that is, one which generates the production of an antagonist. The most common response to the antigen is the production of ANTIBODY. The antigen-antibody reaction is an essential component of the overall immune response. A second type of activity, cellular response, is also an essential component.

The various and complex mechanisms of immunity are basic to the body's ability to protect itself against specific infectious agents and parasites, to accept or reject cells and tissues from other individuals, as in blood transfusions and organ transplants, and to protect against cancer, as when the immune system recognizes malignant cells as not-self and destroys them.

In recent years there has been extensive research into the body's ability to differentiate between cells, organisms, and other substances that are self, and therefore not alien to the body, and those which are not self and therefore must be eliminated. A major motivating force behind these research efforts has been the need for more information about rejection of transplanted tissues, the growth and proliferation of malignant cells, the inability of certain individuals to develop normal immunological responses, as in immune deficient diseases, and the failure of the body to recognize its own tissues, as in AUTOIMMUNE DISEASE.

IMMUNOLOGICAL RESPONSES. Immunological responses in humans can be divided into two broad categories: humoral immunity, which takes place in the body fluids (humors) and is concerned with antibody and complement activities; and cell-mediated or cellular immunity, which involves a variety of activities designed to destroy or at least contain cells that are recognized by the body as alien and harmful. Both types of responses are instigated by lymphocytes that originate in the bone marrow as stem cells and later are converted into mature cells having specific properties and functions.

The two kinds of lymphocytes that are important to establishment of immunity are T-lymphocytes (T-cells) and B-lymphocytes (B-cells). The T-lymphocytes are converted by the THYMUS and are therefore called thymus-dependent. Lymphocytes of this type eventually become sensitized so that they are able to recognize and dispose of such foreign substances as microbes, tissues from other individuals, and other kinds of antigens. They are involved in cellular immunity.

The B-lymphocytes are bursa-dependent or "bursa-equivalent" cells, so named because they were first identified during research studies that centered around the immunologic activity of the bursa of Fabricius, a lymphoid organ in the chicken. Although humans have no discrete bursa and the exact site of B-lymphocyte production in humans has not been established, the name B-cell has been retained. B-lymphocytes mature into plasma cells that are primarily responsible for forming antibodies, thereby providing humoral immunity.

Humoral Immunity. At the time that a substance enters the body and is interpreted as foreign, antibodies are released from plasma cells and enter the body fluids where they can react with the specific antigens for which they were formed. This release of antibodies is stimulated by antigen-specific groups (clones) of B-lymphocytes. Each B-lymphocyte has IMMUNOGLOBULIN M (IgM) receptors which play a major role in capturing its specific antigen and in launching production of the immunoglobulins (which are antibodies) that are capable of neutralizing and destroying that particular type of antigen.

Most of the B-lymphocytes activated by the presence of their specific antigen become plasma cells, which then synthesize and export antibodies. The activated B-lymphocytes that do not become plasma cells continue to reside as "memory" cells in the lymphoid tissue, where they stand ready for future encounters with antigens that may enter the body. It is these memory cells that provide continued immunity after initial exposure to the antigens.

There are two types of humoral immune response: primary and secondary. The primary response begins immediately after the initial contact with an antigen; the resulting antibody appears 48 to 72 hours later. The antibodies produced during this primary response are predominantly of the IgM class of immunoglobulins.

A secondary response occurs within 24 to 48 hours. This reaction produces large quantities of immunoglobulins that are predominantly of the IgG class. The secondary response persists much longer than the primary response and is the result of repeated contact with the antigens. This phenomenon is the basic principle underlying consecutive IMMUNIZATIONS.

The ability of the antibody to bind with or "stick to" antigen renders it capable of destroying the antigen in a number of ways; for example, agglutination and opsinization. Antibody also "fixes" or activates COMPLEMENT, which is the second component of the humoral immune system. Complement is the name given a complex series of enzymatic proteins which are present but inactive in normal serum. When complement fixation takes place, the antigen, antibody, and complement become bound together. The cell membrane of the antigen (which usually is a bacterial cell) then ruptures, resulting in dissolution of the antigen cell and a leakage of its substance

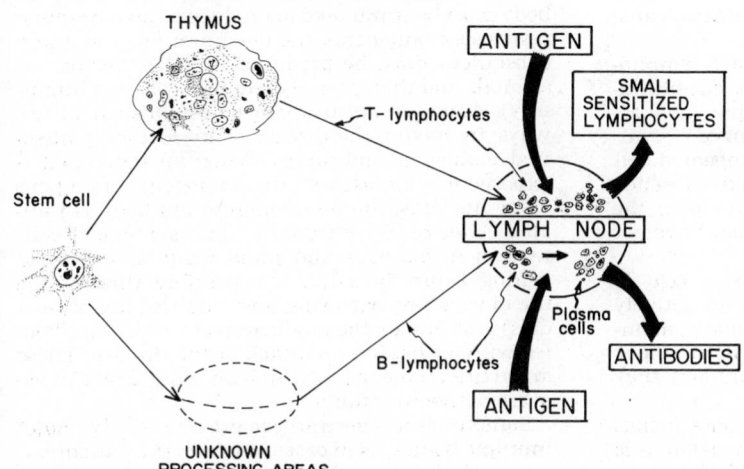

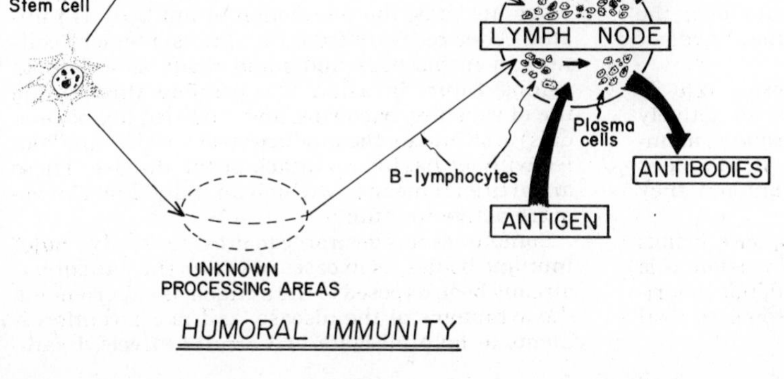

Formation of antibodies and sensitized lymphocytes by a lymph node in response to antigens. This figure also shows the origin of *thymic* ("T") and *bursal* ("B") lymphocytes that are responsible for the cellular and humoral immune processes of the lymph nodes. (From Guyton, A. C.: Textbook of Medical Physiology. 5th ed. Philadelphia, W. B. Saunders Co., 1976.)

into the body fluids. This destructive process is called lysis.

Cellular Immunity. This type of immune response is dependent upon T-lymphocytes, which are primarily concerned with a delayed type of immune response. Examples of this type of response include the rejection of transplanted organs, defense against slowly developing bacterial diseases that result from intracellular infections, and recognition and rejection of self cells undergoing alteration, for example, those infected with viruses, and cancer cells that have tumor-specific antigens on their surfaces. These responses are called cell-mediated immune (CMI) responses.

The T-lymphocyte becomes sensitized by its first contact with a specific antigen. Subsequent exposure to the antigen stimulates a host of chemical and mechanical activities, all designed to either destroy or inactivate the offending antigen. Some of the sensitized T-lymphocytes combine with the antigen to deactivate it, while others set about to destroy the invading organism by direct invasion or the release of chemical factors. These chemical factors, through their influence on macrophages and unsensitized lymphocytes, enhance the effectiveness of the immune response.

Among the more active chemical factors are lymphokines, which are potent and biologically active proteins. The names of the lymphokines are somewhat descriptive of their functions. Factors that directly affect the macrophages are: the macrophage chemotactic factor (MCF), which attracts macrophages to the invasion site; macrophage migration inhibiting factor (MIF), which causes macrophages to remain at the invasion site; and macrophage activating factor (MAF), which stimulates the metabolic activities of these large cells, thereby improving their ability to ingest the foreign invaders.

Another factor, a protein called INTERFERON, is produced by the body cells, especially T-lymphocytes, following viral infection or in response to a wide variety of inducers, such as certain nonviral infectious agents and synthetic polymers.

A portion of the population of T-lymphocytes is transformed into "killer cells" by the lymphocyte transforming factor (LTF). These activated lymphocytes produce a lymphotoxin or cytotoxin, which damages the cell membranes of the antigens, causing them to rupture.

In order to ensure an ample supply of T-lymphocytes, two additional factors are at work. The blastogenic factor stimulates lymphocytes that have already undergone conversion to sensitized T-lymphocytes to increase their number by repeated cell division and the formation of clones. In the absence of antigens, TRANSFER FACTOR (TF) takes over the task of sensitizing those lymphocytes that have not been exposed to antigen.

Lymphocytes that have been converted into T-cells or B-cells but are not used either to actively engage in the immune response or to reside as memory cells, can return to the blast stage. If, at a later time they are needed to interact with antigen, they can become sensitized again.

It is apparent that the immune response brings about intensive activity at the site of invasion; it is not only the pathogen that is destroyed, but invariably, there is death and damage to some normal tissues.

Interactions Between the Two Systems. There are several areas in which the cellular and humoral systems interact and thereby improve the efficiency of the overall immune response. For example, a by-product of the enzymatic activity of the complement system acts as a chemotactic factor, attracting T-lymphocytes and macrophages to the invasion site. In another example, although T-lymphocytes are not required for the production of antibody, there is optimal antibody production after interaction between T-cells and B-cells.

Future research is expected to shed more light on all aspects of the immune response and the ways in which the various components function independently and interact with each other. One theory of immunity postulates that an interaction between the B-lymphocytes and T-lymphocytes at the surface of a macrophage causes the release of an RNA or an RNA-antigen complex. It is believed that the length of time that an uncommitted lymphocyte is exposed to this complex determines its fate, that is, whether it will become a B-cell or a T-cell. If the exposure is lengthy, the lymphoblast will develop into a plasma cell capable of producing antibody. Hence, it is postulated that the RNA-antigen complex determines whether the immune response will be humoral or cellular.

Abnormalities of the immune response system are discussed under Disorders of the IMMUNE RESPONSE.

TYPES OF IMMUNITY. An individual may be naturally immune to certain pathological conditions, or he may acquire immunity through either active or passive means.

Natural immunity is a genetic characteristic of an individual and is due to the particular species and race to which he belongs, to his sex, and to his individual ability to produce immune bodies. All humans are immune to certain diseases that affect animals of the lower species; males are more resistant to some disorders than are females, and vice versa. Persons of one race are more susceptible to some diseases than those of another race that has had exposure to the infectious agents through successive generations. One's individual ability to produce immune bodies, and thereby ward off pathogens, is influenced by his state of physical health, his nutritional status, and his emotional response to stress.

In order for an individual to acquire immunity his body must be stimulated to produce its own immune response components (active immunity) or these substances must be produced by other persons or animals and then passed on to him (passive immunity). *Active immunity* can be established in two ways: by having the disease or by receiving modified pathogens and toxins. When an individual is exposed to a disease and the pathogenic organisms enter his body, the production of antibody is initiated. After recovery from the illness, memory cells remain in his body and stand ready as a defense against future invasion. It is possible, through the use of vaccines, bacterins, and modified toxins (toxoids) to stimulate the production of specific antibodies without having an attack of the disease. These are artificial means by which an individual can acquire active immunity.

Sometimes it is desirable to provide "ready-made" immune bodies, as in cases in which the patient has already been exposed to the antigen, is experiencing the symptoms of the disease, and needs reinforcements to help mitigate its harmful effects. Examples of conditions for which an individual may be given such *passive immunity* include tetanus, diphtheria, and a venomous snake bite. The patient is given immune serum, which contains antibodies (including antitoxin) produced by the animal from which the serum was taken, or *gamma globulin.*

It is not always necessary that the patient actually suffer from the disease and exhibit its symptoms before passive immunity is provided. In some instances in which exposure to an infectious agent is suspected, immune bodies may be given to ward off a full-blown attack or at least to lessen its severity.

Another way in which immunity can be passively acquired is across the placental barrier from fetus to mother. The maternal antibody thus acquired serves as protection for the newborn until he can actively establish immunity on his own. Although humoral immunity can be acquired in this way, cellular immunity cannot.

immunization (im″u-nĭ-za′shun) the process of rendering a subject immune, or of becoming immune. Called also inoculation and vaccination; the word vaccine originally referred to the substance used to immunize against SMALLPOX, the first immunization developed. Now, however, the term is used for any preparation used in active immunization.

active i., inoculation, usually by injection, with a specific antigen to promote antibody formation in the body. The antigenic substance may be in one of four forms: (1) dead disease bacteria, as in TYPHOID FEVER immunization; (2) dead viruses, as in the Salk POLIOMYELITIS injection; (3) live attenuated virus, e.g., smallpox vaccine and Sabin polio vaccine (taken orally); and (4) toxoids, altered forms of toxins produced by bacteria, as in immunization against TETANUS and DIPHTHERIA.

Since active immunization induces the body to produce its own antibodies and to go on producing them, protection against disease will last several years, in some cases for life.

passive i., transient immunization produced by the introduction into the system of serum (antiserum) or antitoxin that already contains antibodies. The person immunized is protected only as long as these antibodies remain in his blood and are active—usually from 4 to 6 weeks.

immunize (im′u-nīz) to render immune.

immunoassay (im″u-no-as′sa) the measurement of antigen-antibody interaction, as by immunofluorescent techniques, radioimmunoassay, etc.

immunobiology (im″u-no-bi-ol′o-je) that branch of biology dealing with immunologic effects on such phenomena as infectious disease, growth and development, recognition phenomena, hypersensitivity, heredity, aging, cancer, and transplantation.

immunochemistry (im″u-no-kem′is-tre) the study of the chemical basis of immune phenomena and their interactions.

immunocompetence (im′u-no-kom′pĕ-tens) the capacity to develop an immune response following antigenic challenge. adj., **immunocom′petent.**

immunocyte (im′u-no-sīt) any cell of the lymphoid series which can react with antigen to produce antibody or to participate in cell-mediated reactions.

immunodeficiency (im″mu-no-dĕ-fish′en-se) a deficiency of the immune response due to hypoactivity or decreased numbers of lymphoid cells. adj., **immunodefi′cient.**

immunodiffusion (im″mu-no-dĭ-fu′zhun) the diffusion of antigen and antibody from separate reservoirs to form decreasing concentration gradients in hydrophilic gels.

immunoelectrophoresis (im″u-no-e-lek″tro-fo-re′sis) a method of distinguishing proteins and other materials on the basis of their electrophoretic mobility and antigenic specificities.

immunoferritin (im″mu-no-fer′ĭ-tin) an antibody labeled with ferritin.

immunofiltration (im″mu-no-fil-tra′shun) the extraction of antibodies in pure form by subjection of serum to insoluble specific antigen, the antigen then being removed from the antibody by treatment with soluble carriers.

immunofluorescence (im″mu-no-floo″o-res′ens) a method of determining the location of antigen (or antibody) in a tissue section or smear by the pattern of fluorescence resulting when the specimen is exposed to the specific antibody (or antigen) labeled with a fluorochrome.

immunogen (im′u-no-jen) any substance capable of eliciting an immune response.

immunogenetics (im″u-no-jĕ-net′iks) the study of the genetic factors controlling the individual's immune response and the transmission of those fac-

REVISED SCHEDULE FOR ACTIVE IMMUNIZATION AND TUBERCULIN TESTING OF NORMAL INFANTS AND CHILDREN IN THE UNITED STATES*

2 mo.	DTP[1]	TOPV[2]
4 mo.	DTP	TOPV
6 mo.	DTP	TOPV
1 yr.	Measles[3]	Tuberculin Test[4]
1–12 yr.	Rubella[3]	Mumps[3]
1½ yr.	DTP	TOPV
4–6 yr.	DTP	TOPV
14–16 yr.	Td[5]	and thereafter every 10 years

[1]DTP – diphtheria and tetanus toxoids combined with pertussis vaccine.

[2]TOPV – trivalent oral polio virus vaccine. The above recommendation is suitable for breast-fed as well as bottle-fed infants.

[3]May be given at one year as measles-rubella or measles-mumps-rubella combined vaccines.

[4]Frequency of repeated tuberculin tests depends on risk of exposure of the child and on the prevalence of tuberculosis in the population group.

[5]Td – combined tetanus and diphtheria toxoids (adult type) for those over six years of age in contrast to diphtheria and tetanus (DT) containing a larger amount of diphtheria antigen.

Tetanus toxoid at time of injury: For clean, minor wounds, no booster dose is needed by a fully immunized child unless more than 10 years have elapsed since the last dose.

For contaminated wounds, a booster dose should be given if more than five years have elapsed since the last dose.

Routine smallpox vaccination is no longer recommended.

*Approved by the Committee on Infectious Diseases, October 17, 1971, American Academy of Pediatrics

tors from generation to generation. adj., **immunogenet'ic.**

immunogenic (im"u-no-jen'ik) producing immunity; evoking an immune response.

immunogenicity (im"u-no-jĕ-nis'ĭ-te) the ability of a substance to provoke an immune response. adj., **immuogen'ic.**

immunoglobulin (im"u-no-glob'u-lin) a protein of animal origin with known ANTIBODY activity. Immunoglobulins are major components of what is called the humoral IMMUNE RESPONSE system. They are synthesized by lymphocytes and plasma cells and found in the serum and in other body fluids and tissues, including the urine, spinal fluid, lymph nodes, and spleen. (See also IMMUNITY.)

Each immunoglobulin molecule consists of four polypeptide chains: two heavy chains (H-chains) and two light chains (L-chains). There are five antigenically different kinds of H-chains, and this difference is the basis for the classification of immunoglobulins. Each class varies in its chemical structure and in its number of antigen-binding sites and adheres to and reacts only with the specific antigen for which it was produced.

The five classes of immunoglobulins (Ig) are: IgA, IgD, IgE, IgG, and IgM. Two types of IgA have been identified. They are serum IgA and secretory IgA (sIgA). They are both known to have antiviral properties; their production is stimulated by oral vaccines and aerosol immunizations.

IgD is found in trace quantities in the serum. Its function is not yet clear.

IgE is called the reaginic antibody and is generally present in increased levels in persons with allergy. When IgE attaches itself to cells within the body, for example, those of the mucous membrane and skin, the cells become sensitized to allergens, causing them to release histamine and histamine-like substances when they come in contact with the allergen. Such allergic reactions as hives, hay fever, asthma, and anaphylactic shock are thought to be manifestations of IgE-mediated reactions.

IgG is the most abundant of the five classes of immunoglobulins. It is the major antibody in the secondary humoral response of immunity, serves to activate the complement system, and is frequently involved in opsonization. IgG is the only immunoglobulin that can cross the placental barrier.

IgM is principally concerned with the primary antibody response, appearing soon after initial invasion by an antigen and capable of destroying the antigen when it is first introduced. Like the IgG, IgM activates the complement system and together these two classes of immunoglobulins serve as specific antitoxins against the toxins of diphtheria, tetanus, botulism, and anthrax microorganisms, and snake venoms.

immunologist (im"u-nol'o-jist) a specialist in immunology.

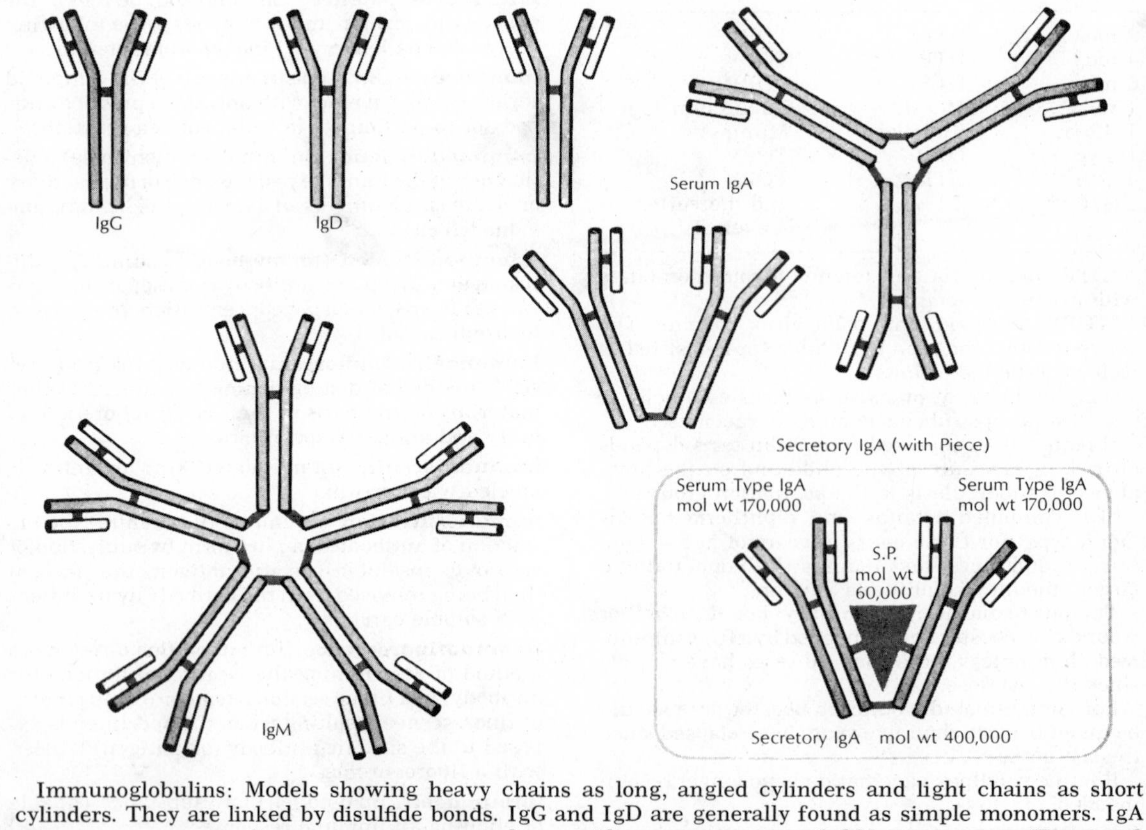

Immunoglobulins: Models showing heavy chains as long, angled cylinders and light chains as short cylinders. They are linked by disulfide bonds. IgG and IgD are generally found as simple monomers. IgA exists as a monomer, dimer, or trimer, or as a dimer with a secretory piece. IgM is a pentamer. (Reprinted with permission from Tomasi, T. B.: The Gamma Globulins: First Line of Defense. *Hospital Practice,* Vol. 2, No. 7 and from *Immunobiology,* R. A. Good and D. W. Fisher, Eds. Sinauer Associates, Inc., Sunderland, Mass., 1971.)

immunology (im″u-nol′o-je) the scientific study of all aspects of immunity, including allergy, hypersensitivity, etc. adj., **immunolog′ic.**

immunopathology (im″u-no-pah-thol′o-je) that branch of biomedical science concerned with immune reactions associated with disease, whether the reactions be beneficial, without effect, or harmful. adj., **immunopatholog′ic.**

immunoprecipitation (im″u-no-pre-sip″ĭ-ta′shun) precipitation resulting from interaction of specific antibody and antigen.

immunoproliferative (im″u-no-pro-lif′er-ah-tiv) characterized by the proliferation of the lymphoid cells producing immunoglobulins, as in the gammopathies.

immunosorbent (im″u-no-sor′bent) an insoluble support for antigen, used to absorb homologous antibodies from a mixture.

immunosuppressant (im″u-no-su-pres′ant) immunosuppressive.

immunosuppression (im″u-no-sŭ-presh′un) inhibition of the formation of antibodies to antigens that may be present; used in transplantation procedures to prevent rejection of the transplanted organ or tissue.

immunosuppressive (im″u-no-sŭ-pres′iv) 1. pertaining to or inducing immunosuppression. 2. an agent that induces immunosuppression.

immunosurveillance (im″u-no-ser-va′lens) the monitoring function of the immune system whereby it recognizes and reacts against aberrant cells arising within the body.

immunotherapy (im″u-no-ther′ah-pe) the production of passive immunity.

immunotoxin (im″u-no-tok′sin) an antitoxin.

immunotransfusion (im″u-no-trans-fu′zhun) transfusion of blood from a donor previously rendered immune to the disease affecting the patient.

impacted (im-pak′ted) being wedged in firmly. In obstetrics, denoting twins so situated during delivery that the pressure of one against the other prevents complete engagement of either.

impaction (im-pak′shun) the condition of being wedged in firmly.

fecal i., a collection of putty-like or hardened feces in the rectum or sigmoid (see also FECAL IMPACTION).

impalpable (im-pal′pah-b′l) not detectable by touch.

impar (im′par) not even; unequal; unpaired.

impatent (im-pa′tent) not open; closed.

impedance (im-ped′dans) obstruction or opposition to passage or flow, as of an electric current or other form of energy.

acoustic i., an expression of the opposition to passage of sound waves, being the product of the density of a substance and the velocity of sound in it.

imperforate (im-per′fo-rāt) not open; abnormally closed.

impermeable (im-per′me-ah-b′l) not permitting passage, as for fluid.

impetigo (im″pĕ-ti′go) a streptococcal or staphylococcal skin infection marked by vesicles or bullae that become pustular, rupture, and form yellow crusts, called also impetigo contagiosa or impetigo vulgaris. The disease occurs most frequently in children, especially in very young infants because of their low resistance. It is spread by direct contact with the moist discharges of the lesions. If not properly treated, it can be serious or even fatal to newborn infants.

Treatment consists of cleansing the lesions with soap and water and then wiping the surrounding skin with alcohol. Care should be taken to avoid spreading the infection and the patient should be isolated. The lesions should be kept dry and open to the air as much as possible. Local applications of an antibiotic ointment may clear up the lesions; however, systemic administration of antibiotics usually is recommended.

implant 1. (im-plant′) to insert or to graft (tissue or radioactive material) into intact tissues or a body cavity. 2. (im′plant) any material inserted or grafted into the body.

implantation (im″plan-ta′shun) 1. the insertion of an organ or tissue in a new site in the body. 2. the attachment and embedding of the fertilized ovum in the endometrium. 3. the insertion or grafting into the body of biological, living, inert, or radioactive material.

impotence (im′po-tens) inability of the male to achieve or maintain an erection of sufficient rigidity to perform sexual intercourse successfully. adj., **im′potent.**

There is no direct relationship between impotence and FERTILITY, except that in preventing coitus it also prevents conception. An impotent man may be very fertile, because his testes produce many spermatozoa. Many cases of impotence are the result of emotional disturbances, and can be treated successfully.

impregnation (im″preg-na′shun) 1. the act of fertilizing or rendering pregnant. 2. saturation.

impressio (im-pres′e-o), pl. *impressio′nes* [L.] impression (1).

impression (im-presh′un) 1. a slight indentation or depression, as one produced in the surface of one organ by pressure exerted by another. 2. a negative imprint of an object made in some plastic material that later solidifies. 3. an effect produced upon the mind, body, or senses by some external stimulus or agent.

imprinting (im′print-ing) a species-specific, rapid kind of learning during a critical period of early life in which social attachment and identification are established.

impulse (im′puls) 1. a sudden pushing force. 2. a sudden uncontrollable act. 3. nerve impulse.

cardiac i., movement of the chest wall caused by the heart beat.

nerve i., the electrochemical process propagated along nerve fibers.

impulsion (im-pul′shun) an abnormal impulse to perform certain acts, usually of a disagreeable nature.

In chemical symbol, *indium.*

in- 1. a prefix, *in, within,* or *into.* 2. an intensive prefix. 3. a negative or privative prefix.

inactivation (in-ak″tĭ-va′shun) the destruction of activity, as of a virus, by the action of heat or other agent.

inanimate (in-an′ĭ-mat) 1. without life. 2. lacking in animation.

inanition (in″ah-nish′un) the exhausted state due to prolonged undernutrition; starvation.

inappetence (in-ap′ĕ-tens) lack of appetite or desire.

inarticulate (in″ar-tik′u-lāt) 1. not having joints; disjointed. 2. uttered so as to be unintelligible; incapable of articulate speech.

inassimilable (in″ah-sim′ĭ-lah-b'l) not susceptible of being utilized as nutriment.

inborn (in′born) inherited; formed or implanted during fetal life.

inbreeding (in′brēd-ing) the mating of closely related individuals or of individuals having closely similar genetic constitutions.

incarceration (in-kar″sĕ-ra′shun) unnatural retention or confinement of a part.

incest (in′sest) sexual activity between persons so closely related that marriage between them is legally or culturally prohibited.

incidence (in′sĭ-dens) the rate at which a certain event occurs, as the number of new cases of a specific disease occurring during a certain period.

incident (in-sĭ-dent) impinging upon, as incident radiation.

incineration (in-sin″ĕ-ra′shun) the act of burning to ashes.

incipient (in-sip′e-ent) beginning to exist; coming into existence.

incision (in-sizh′un) 1. a cut or a wound made by a sharp instrument. 2. the act of cutting.

incisive (in-si′siv) 1. having the power of cutting; sharp. 2. pertaining to the incisor teeth.

i. bone, the portion of the maxilla bearing the incisors; developmentally, it is the premaxilla, which in humans later fuses with the maxilla, but in most other vertebrates persists as a separate bone.

incisor (in-si′zor) 1. adapted for cutting. 2. any one of the four front teeth of either jaw.

incisure (in-si′zher) a cut, notch, or incision.

Rivinus i., tympanic notch; a defect in the upper tympanic part of the temporal bone, filled by the upper portion of the tympanic membrane.

inclination (in″klĭ-na′shun) a sloping or leaning; the angle of deviation from a particular line or plane of reference.

i. of the pelvis, the angle between the plane of the pelvic inlet and the horizontal plane.

inclusion (in-kloo′zhun) 1. the act of enclosing or the condition of being enclosed. 2. anything that is enclosed; a cell inclusion.

i. bodies, round, oval, or irregular shaped bodies in the cytoplasm and nuclei of cells, as in diseases due to viral infection, such as rabies, smallpox, etc.

cell i., a usually lifeless, often temporary, constituent in the cytoplasm of a cell.

i. conjunctivitis, conjunctivitis affecting primarily newborn infants, caused by a strain of *Chlamydia trachomatis,* beginning as an acute purulent conjunctivitis and leading to papillary hypertrophy of the palpebral conjunctiva.

incoagulability (in″ko-ag″u-lah-bil′ĭ-te) the state of being incapable of coagulation. adj., **incoag′ulable.**

incompatible (in″kom-pat′ĭ-b'l) not suitable for combination, simultaneous administration, or transplantation; mutually repellent.

incompatibility (in″kom-pat″ĭ-bil′ĭ-te) the quality of being incompatible.

incompetence (in-kom′pĕ-tens) 1. inability to function properly. 2. the legal status of an incompetent.

incompetent (in-kom′pĕ-tent) 1. not able to function properly. 2. a person determined by the courts to be unable to manage his own affairs.

incontinence (in-kon′tĭ-nens) 1. inability to control excretory functions. 2. immoderation or excess. adj., **incon′tinent.**

Fecal incontinence may result from disorders of the nervous system or weakening of the anal sphincters in elderly persons. Anal or rectal surgery and anal tears resulting from childbirth also may impair control.

Urinary incontinence has many possible causes. Stress, anger, or anxiety can increase the urge to urinate. Incontinence sometimes occurs after surgery or in connection with irritation of the urinary tract by inflammation or injury. In some instances incontinence is due to an obstruction that prevents normal emptying of the urinary bladder, resulting in constant dribbling of the overflow. An uncontrolled flow can result from spasm of the bladder, or from the development of a fistula between the bladder and urethra, vagina, or rectum. Damage to the spinal cord or brain by injury or disease also hinders bladder control.

PATIENT CARE. The ultimate goal in the care of an incontinent patient is to keep him dry, comfortable, and odor-free, and to help him achieve some degree of independence and social acceptability. Loss of control of urine and feces can be a devastating blow emotionally and can present multiple problems because of complications that can develop.

Management of the problems begins with a thorough assessment of the situation. How much control can the patient be expected to accomplish in view of the level of neural and muscular function he has to work with? Has he had an opportunity to participate in planning the program and in setting realistic goals for himself? Is he mentally competent to participate in planning and carrying out a bowel and bladder training program? (See also BLADDER TRAINING and BOWEL TRAINING.) If the patient cannot take part in setting goals and planning a program for their achievement, has he at least been made aware of them and has he been given an explanation of the purpose of each technique employed? Is there a member of the family who can give a satisfactory history of the patient's former eating and elimination habits?

Once the program is planned it is best to get the patient out of bed to go to the bathroom or to a commode chair. If he must be confined to bed he should be offered the bedpan on a regular schedule designed according to his needs. If he is incontinent at night, the time should be noted and a bedpan or urinal offered at the time he usually voids in bed. Regularity is also important in the eating of meals and snacks. An accurate record is kept of his intake and output, and certain foods and fluids known to cause difficulties are limited.

For those patients who cannot for one reason or another achieve control it is necessary to employ some techniques other than a training program for the collection of urine and feces. Penile clamps for males may be helpful in cases of urinary incontinence. URETEROSTOMY and ILEAL CONDUIT are alternatives that may be considered for certain patients having problems with control of urinary flow. Indwelling CATHETERS must be used with restraint because of the dangers of infection. And in some cases there is no other choice but to use some type of protective pants that can be worn over an absorbent pad.

Finding a way to keep the incontinent patient clean and dry can be a very real challenge. It requires knowing the patient as a person and making no assumptions about his ability to cooperate and achieve control until an effort has been made to involve him in a plan for control. It demands ingenuity, perseverance, and patience and a very real desire to help the patient cope with his problem.

stress i., involuntary escape of urine due to strain on the orifice of the bladder, as in coughing or sneezing.

incoordination (in″ko-or″dĭ-na′shun) lack of normal adjustment of muscular motions; failure to work harmoniously.

incorporation (in-kor″po-ra′shun) 1. the union of one substance with another, or with others, in a composite mass. 2. an unconscious mental mechanism in which a person figuratively ingests the psychic representation of another person, or parts of him.

increment (in′krĕ-ment) an increase or addition; the amount by which a value or quantity is increased. adj., **incremen′tal.**

incrustation (in″krus-ta′shun) 1. the formation of a crust. 2. a crust, scab, or scale.

incubate (in′ku-bāt) 1. to subject to or to undergo incubation. 2. material that has undergone incubation.

incubation (in″ku-ba′shun) 1. the provision of proper conditions for growth and development, as for bacterial or tissue cultures. 2. the development of an infectious disease from time of the entrance of the pathogen to the appearance of clinical symptoms. 3. the development of the embryo in the egg of oviparous animals. 4. the maintenance of an artificial environment for an infant, especially a premature infant.

i. period, the interval of time required for development; especially the time between invasion of the body by a pathogenic organism and appearance of the first symptoms of disease. Incubation periods vary from a few days to several months, depending on the causative organism and type of disease.

incubator (in′ku-ba″ter) an apparatus for maintaining optimal conditions (temperature, humidity, etc.) for growth and development, especially one used in the early care of premature infants, or one used for cultures, The primary purpose of the incubator used for premature infants is to surround the infant with some of the environmental conditions normally provided in the uterus and necessary until he reaches approximately the level of development of a full-term infant.

The temperature within the incubator is regulated so that the infant's temperature is maintained between 96° and 98° F. (35.5° to 36.6° C.). Humidity is kept at 50 to 60 per cent unless there is respiratory difficulty, in which case the humidity may be raised as high as 85 to 100 per cent. Oxygen is added in concentrations not exceeding 30 to 40 per cent only as long as the infant is cyanotic because of the dan-

INCUBATION PERIODS OF COMMUNICABLE DISEASES

Usually about 0–7 days

Disease	Incubation Period Avg.	Incubation Period Range	Isolation	Immunization
Anthrax	1–4	(1–7)	"Clean" technique	
Bacillary dysentery	2–4	(1–7)	Till stool negative	
Chancroid	3–5	(1–12)	From sexual contact	
Cholera	3	(1–5)	Till stool negative (quarantine)	
Dengue	5–6	(3–15)	Screen	
Diphtheria	2–5		Till nose and throat negative	Toxoid/antitoxin
Epidemic diarrhea of newborn	6–7	(2–21)	Yes (quarantine)	
Erysipelas	0–2		"Clean" technique	
Food poisoning				
staphylococcus	2–4	(1–6) hr.	From food handling	Antitoxin
salmonella	12	(6–48) hr.	From food handling	Antitoxin
botulism	18–24	(2–48) hr.	From food handling	Antitoxin
Gonorrhea	3–5	(1–14)	From sexual contact and children	
Impetigo contagiosa	5		From child contacts	
Infectious keratoconjunctivitis	5–7			
Influenza	1–3		Acute stage	Formalin-virus
Meningitis, meningococcic	7	(2–10)	24 hr., if treated	
Paratyphoid	1–10		Till stool and urine negative	Vaccine
Plague	3–6		Till well	Formalin-vaccine
Pneumonia, bacterial	1–3		Respiratory precautions	
Puerperal infection	1–3		Till well	
Relapsing fever (tick)	3–6	(2–12)		
Rocky Mountain spotted fever	3–10			Yolk-sac vaccine
Scabies	1–2		From school	
Scarlet fever	2–5		Respiratory precautions	
Tularemia	3	(1–10)		
Yellow fever	3–6		Screen	Modified-virus

Continued on page 514.

ger of retrolental FIBROPLASIA with high concentrations of oxygen.

incubus (in′ku-bus) 1. nightmare. 2. a heavy mental burden.

incudal (ing′ku-dal) pertaining to the incus.

incudectomy (ing″ku-dek′to-me) excision of the incus.

incudiform (ing-ku′dĭ-form) anvil-shaped.

incudomalleal (ing″ku-do-mal′e-al) pertaining to the incus and malleus.

incudostapedial (ing″ku-do-stah-pe′de-al) pertaining to the incus and stapes.

incurable (in-kūr′ah-b′l) 1. not susceptible of being cured. 2. a person with a disease that cannot be cured.

incus (ing′kus) the middle of the three ossicles of the ear; called also anvil (see also table of BONES).

Indecidua (in″dĕ-sid′u-ah) a division of the class Mammalia comprising the mammals without a decidua, including whales and ungulates.

index (in′deks), pl. *indexes* or *in′dices* [L.] 1. the second digit of the hand, the forefinger. 2. the numerical ratio of measurement of any part in comparison with a fixed standard.

alveolar i., gnathic index.

cephalic i., 100 times the maximum breadth of the skull divided by its maximum length.

cerebral i., the ratio of the greatest transverse to the greatest anteroposterior diameter of the cranial cavity.

color i., the relative amount of hemoglobin in an erythrocyte compared with that of a normal individual of the same age and sex. The percentage of hemoglobin is divided by the percentage of erythrocytes.

gnathic i., the degree of prominence of the jaws; the distance from the basion to the front of the jaw expressed as a percentage of the distance from the

INCUBATION PERIODS OF COMMUNICABLE DISEASES (*Concluded*)

Usually about 7–14 days

Disease	Incubation Period Avg.	Range	Isolation	Immunization
Coccidioidomycosis	10–15	(7–21)	Till sputum negative	
Equine encephalitis	5–15			
Infectious mononucleosis	11	(7–15)	Respiratory precautions	
Leptospirosis	9–10	(4–19)		
Lymphocytic choriomeningitis	8–13			
Measles	9–14		Till 5 days after rash	Immune globulin
Pertussis	5–9	(2–21)	From school and susceptibles	Vaccine
Poliomyelitis	7–14	(3–35)	First 2 weeks	Vaccine
Primary atypical pneumonia	11	(7–21)	Respiratory precautions	
Psittacosis	6–15		Till afebrile	
Relapsing fever (louse)	7	(5–12)	To delouse	
Scrub typhus	7–10	(7–14)		
Smallpox	12	(7–21)	Till scabs off (quarantine)	Vaccinia
Trichinosis	9	(2–28)		
Typhoid fever	7–14	(3–38)	Till stool and urine negative	Vaccine
Typhus fever	12	(6–15)	To delouse (quarantine)	Vaccine

Usually over 14 days

Disease	Incubation Period Avg.	Range	Isolation	Immunization
Amebic dysentery	21–28	(8–90)	From food handling	
Brucellosis	14	(6–30+)		
Chickenpox	14	(12–21)	Till skin clear	
German measles	16–18	(10–21)	First week	
Granuloma inguinale	10–90		From sexual contact	
Hepatitis, infectious	25	(15–35)	Stool disinfection for 3 weeks	Immune globulin
Hepatitis, serum	80–100	(60–180)		
Lymphogranuloma venereum	7–28		From sexual contact	
Malaria	10–17	(to 35+)	Screen	
Mumps	18	(12–26)	Till glands down	
Q fever	14–21			Vaccine
Rabies	14–42	(10–180)	Aseptic technique	Attenuated vaccine
Rickettsialpox	10–24			
Syphilis	21	(10–90)	From sexual contact and children	
Tetanus	4–21			Toxoid
Tuberculosis	Variable		"Open" cases	BCG vaccine
Yaws	30–90		Desirable till treated	

From The SK&F Pocket Book of Medical Tables. 15th ed. Philadelphia, Smith Kline & French Laboratories, 1966.

basion to the midpoint of the nasal suture.

hemolytic i., a formula for calculating increased erythrocyte destruction.

icteric i., a rough determination of bilirubin in the blood (see also ICTERIC INDEX).

length-breadth i., cephalic index.

length-height i., vertical index.

leukopenic i., a fall of 1000 or more in the total leukocyte count within $1\frac{1}{2}$ hours after ingestion of food; it indicates allergic hypersensitivity to that food.

nasal i., 100 times the width of the nose, divided by its length.

opsonic i., a measure of opsonic activity determined by the ratio of the number of microorganisms phagocytized by normal leukocytes in the presence of serum from an individual infected by the microorganism, to the number phagocytized in serum from a normal individual.

orbital i. (of Broca), 100 times the height of the opening of the orbit divided by its width.

phagocytic i., the average number of bacteria ingested per leukocyte of the patient's blood.

refractive i., the refractive power of a medium compared with that of air (assumed to be 1).

sacral i., 100 times the breadth of the sacrum divided by the length.

thoracic i., the ratio of the anteroposterior diameter of the thorax to the transverse diameter.

vertical i., 100 times the height of the skull divided by its length.

vital i., the ratio of births to deaths within a given time in a population.

volume i., the index indicating the size of the erythrocytes as compared to the normal.

indican (in'dĭ-kan) 1. a substance formed by decomposition of tryptophan in the intestines and excreted in the urine. 2. a yellow indoxyl glycoside from indigo plants.

indicanuria (in"dĭ-kan-u're-ah) an excess of indican in the urine.

indication (in"dĭ-ka'shun) a sign or circumstance that points to or shows the cause, treatment, etc., of a disease.

indicator (in'dĭ-ka"ter) 1. the index finger, or the extensor muscle of the index finger. 2. any substance that indicates the appearance or disappearance of a chemical by a color change or attainment of a certain pH.

indigestion (in"dĭ-jes'chun) lack or failure of digestive function; commonly used to denote vague abdominal discomfort after meals. Among the symptoms of indigestion are heartburn, nausea, flatulence, cramps, a disagreeable taste in the mouth, belching, and sometimes vomiting or diarrhea. Ordinary indigestion can result from eating too much or too fast; from eating when tense, tired, or emotionally upset; from food that is too fatty or spicy; and from heavy food or food that has been badly cooked or processed.

Indigestion and its symptoms may also accompany other disorders such as allergy, migraine, influenza, typhoid fever, food poisoning, peptic ulcer, inflammation of the gallbladder (chronic cholecystitis), appendicitis, and coronary occlusion ("heart attack").

indigitation (in-dij"ĭ-ta'shun) intussusception (1).

indigo (in'dĭ-go) a blue dyeing material from various leguminous and other plants, being the aglycone of indican; also made synthetically; sometimes found in the sweat and urine.

indium (in'de-um) a chemical element, atomic number 49, atomic weight 114.82, symbol In. (See table of ELEMENTS.)

individuation (in"dĭ-vid"u-a'shun) 1. the process of developing individual characteristics. 2. differential regional activity in the embryo occurring in response to organizer influence.

indocyanine green (in"do-si'ah-nēn) a dye used intravenously as a diagnostic aid in the determination of blood volume, cardiac output, and hepatic function.

indole (in'dōl) a compound obtained from coal tar and indigo and produced by decomposition of tryptophan in the intestine, where it contributes to the peculiar odor of feces. It is excreted in the urine in the form of indican.

indolent (in'do-lent) causing little pain; slow growing.

indomethacin (in"do-meth'ah-sin) an anti-inflammatory, analgesic, and antipyretic agent, used in arthritic disorders and degenerative joint disease.

indoxyl (in-dok'sil) an oxidation product of indole formed in tryptophan decomposition, and excreted in the urine as indican.

indoxyluria (in-dok"sil-u're-ah) an excess of indoxyl in the urine.

inducer (in-dūs'er) in biosynthesis, a compound that induces synthesis of a specific enzyme or sequence of enzymes, by antagonizing the corresponding repressor, or by some other mechanism.

induction (in-duk'shun) 1. the process or act of inducing, or causing to occur, especially the production of a specific morphogenetic effect in the embryo through evocators or organizers, or the production of anesthesia or unconsciousness by use of appropriate agents. 2. the generation of an electric current or magnetic properties in a body because of its proximity to an electrified or magnetized object.

inductor (in-duk'tor) a tissue elaborating a chemical substance that acts to determine the growth and differentiation of embryonic parts.

indulin (in'du-lin) a coal tar dye used as a histologic stain.

indurated (in'du-rāt"ed) hardened; abnormally hard.

induration (in"du-ra'shun) the quality of being hard; the process of hardening; an abnormally hard spot or place. adj., **indura'tive.**

black i., the hardening and pigmentation of the lung tissue, as in pneumonia.

brown i., 1. a deposit of altered blood pigment in the lung in pneumonia. 2. increase of the pulmonary connective tissue and excessive pigmentation, due to chronic congestion from valvular heart disease, or to anthracosis.

cyanotic i., hardening of an organ from chronic venous congestion.

granular i., cirrhosis.

gray i., induration of lung tissue in or after pneumonia, without pigmentation.

red i., interstitial pneumonia in which the lung is red and congested.

indusium griseum (in-du'ze-um gris'e-um) [L.] a thin layer of gray matter on the dorsal surface of the corpus callosum.

inebriant (ĭ-ne′bre-ant) 1. causing drunkenness. 2. an agent that causes drunkenness.

inelastic (in″e-las′tik) lacking elasticity.

inert (in-ert′) inactive.

inertia (in-er′she-ah) [L.] inactivity; inability to move spontaneously.

colonic i., weak muscular activity of the colon, leading to distention of the organ and constipation.

i. time, the time required to overcome the inertia of a muscle after reception of a stimulus from a nerve.

uterine i., sluggishness of uterine contractions in labor.

in extremis (in ek-stre′mis) [L.] at the point of death.

infancy (in′fan-se) the first 2 years of life.

infant (in′fant) a young child from birth to 2 years of age.

NEEDS OF THE INFANT. Emotional and physical needs include love and security, a sense of trust, warmth and comfort, feeding and sucking pleasure.

GROWTH AND DEVELOPMENT. Development is a continuous process, and each child progresses at his own rate. There is a developmental sequence, which means that the changes leading to maturity are specific and orderly. The various types of growth and development and the accompanying changes in appearance and behavior are interrelated; that is, physical, emotional, social, and spiritual developments affect one another in the progress toward maturity.

Development of muscular control proceeds from the head downward (cephalocaudal development). The infant controls the head first and gradually acquires the ability to control the neck, then the arms, and finally the legs and feet. Movements are general and random at first, beginning with use of the larger muscles and progressing to specific smaller muscles, such as those needed to handle small objects.

Factors that influence growth and development are: hereditary traits, sex, environment, nationality and race, and physical makeup.

INFANT CARE. A plan of care should be designed within the framework of the natural rhythms of a normal infant. The plan should be sensible, taking into account the family's needs as well as the needs of the infant.

Bathing. A sponge bath is usually advised during the first 2 weeks of life. After that, the tub bath provides not only cleanliness but also an opportunity for exercise as the infant kicks and splashes in the water. There is no definite time at which the bath should be given, but it is best to plan the bath before a feeding.

The room should be warm (about 75° to 80° F. [23.8° to 26.6° C.]) and free from drafts. The temperature of the bath water should be about 90° to 100° F. (32.2° to 37.7° C.), or comfortably warm to the inner arm. The scalp should be washed with soap and water once or twice a week, or daily if the baby has CRADLE CAP. Special attention should be given to the folds and creases of the arms, legs, and genitalia. A lotion may be applied after the bath but it usually is not necessary; talcum, if used at all, should be applied sparingly to avoid caking and accumulations in the folds of the skin which may harbor bacteria.

Clothing. The infant's garments should be loose so that he can move about freely. He should be kept comfortably warm, but not overheated because this leads to prickly heat. The number of gowns, shirts, diapers, or other articles of clothing needed will depend on laundry facilities and the taste and wishes of the family. Diapers require special laundering to remove all traces of soap and stains and to destroy bacteria. Ideally, diapers should be boiled for 5 minutes in soapy water and then washed and rinsed thoroughly, with several rinses to remove the soap. If possible they should be hung outdoors to dry.

Fresh Air. A daily outing for fresh air and sunshine is recommended if the temperature is above freezing and if there is no strong wind. Sunburn, overheating, and glare in the infant's eyes should be avoided.

Sleep. The average infant spends a large part of his time sleeping. Needs of individual infants vary, but at 3 months most infants sleep about 16 hours out of the 24. This length of time will gradually decrease as he grows older.

ARTIFICIAL FEEDING. The advantages and disadvantages of breast feeding as opposed to artificial feeding are discussed under BREAST FEEDING. In artificial feeding the infant is fed from a bottle until he learns to drink from a cup. A formula prescribed by the pediatrician is given; when the baby is about 2 to 4 weeks of age, cereal and pureed foods are added to the diet. Vitamins A, D, and C (usually in the form of orange juice) are given every day. At about 4 months boiled egg yolk may be given and soup may also be tried. When an infant is first given solid foods he may make a sucking action with his tongue and then push the food out of his mouth. This does not indicate a dislike for the taste; the infant is simply learning how to handle solid foods in his mouth. At 5 months custards and simple puddings may be given for variety. At 6 months a variety of food can be offered and the infant may be weaned from the breast or bottle to a cup. By 12 months the infant should be able to handle most simple foods but his interest in eating may dwindle as he begins to notice other things that distract his attention.

Preparation of Formula. The type of milk and sugar to be used in the formula depends on the pediatrician's orders and the infant's tolerance. Evaporated milk, condensed milk, homogenized milk, or dried milk can be used. The sugar included in the formula may be sucrose (cane sugar), dextrose or a mixture of dextrose and maltose. There are several proprietary milk products available; some are said to closely resemble breast milk in composition. They have the advantages of convenience, sterility, and compactness and usually require only the addition of boiled water for preparation.

Generally there are two methods for sterilizing the formula: the terminal method and the aseptic method. In the terminal method the formula is prepared and poured into bottles and filled bottles are sterilized by heat. In the aseptic method the formula and bottles are sterilized separately and then the bottles are filled and capped under aseptic conditions.

Enough formula for 24 hours should be prepared at one time and poured into 8-oz. bottles. The bottles of formula are kept refrigerated until one is needed for feeding; it is then reheated to a tepid temperature. (Recent evidence, however, shows that infants tolerate cold formula as well as that which has been warmed.) Any formula left in the bottle after feeding should be poured out and the bottle and nipple immediately rinsed with cold water to remove the milk.

Average Achievement Levels of Infants, 1 Month to 1 Year

1 Month

Physical

Weight: 8 pounds. Gains about 5 to 7 ounces weekly during first 6 months of life
Height: Gains approximately 1 inch a month for the first 6 months
Pulse: 120–150
Respirations: 30–60

Motor Control

Head sags when supported. May lift head from time to time when he is held against his mother's shoulder
Makes crawling movements when prone on a flat surface
Lifts head intermittently, though unsteadily, when in prone position. Cervical curve begins to develop as the infant learns to hold his head erect
Can turn his head to the side when prone
Can push with feet against a hard surface to move himself forward
Has "dance" reflex when held upright with feet touching the bed or examining table
Shows a well developed tonic neck reflex (head turned to one side, the arm extended on the same side, and the other arm flexed to his shoulder)
Holds hands in fists. Does not reach with hands. Can grasp an object placed in his hand, but drops it immediately

Vision

Stares indefinitely at his surroundings and apparently notices faces and bright objects, but only if they are in his line of vision. Activity diminishes when he regards a human face
Can follow an object to the midline of vision

Vocalization and Socialization

Utters small throaty sounds
Smiles indefinitely
Shows a vague and indirect regard of faces and bright objects
Cries when hungry or uncomfortable

2 Months

Physical

Posterior fontanel closed

Motor Control

Can hold head erect in midposition. Can lift head and chest a short distance above bed or table when lying on his abdomen
Tonic neck and Moro reflexes are fading
Can turn from side to back
Can hold a rattle for a brief time

Vision

Can follow a moving light or object with his eyes

Vocalization and Socialization

Shows a "social smile" in response to another's smile. This is the beginning of social behavior. It may not appear until the third month
Has learned that by crying he will get attention. His crying becomes differentiated; the sound of his crying varies with the reason for crying, e.g., hunger, sleepiness, or pain
Pays attention to the speaking voice

3 Months

Physical

Weight: 12–13 pounds

Motor Control

Holds his hands up in front of him and stares at them
Plays with hands and fingers
Reaches for shiny objects but misses them
Can carry hand or object to mouth at will
Holds head erect and steady. Raises chest, usually supported on forearms
Has lost the walking or dancing reflex
Grasping reflex has weakened
Sits, back rounded, knees flexed when supported

Vision

Shows binocular coordination (vertical and horizontal vision) when an object is moved from right to left and up and down in front of his face
Turns eyes to an object in his marginal field of vision
Voluntarily winks at objects which threaten his eyes

Vocalization and Socialization

Laughs aloud and shows pleasure in making sounds
Cries less
Smiles in response to mother's face

AVERAGE ACHIEVEMENT LEVELS OF INFANTS, 1 MONTH TO 1 YEAR (*Continued*)

4 MONTHS

Physical

Weight: Between 13 and 14 pounds

Drools between 3 and 4 months of age. This indicates the appearance of saliva. He does not know how to swallow saliva, which therefore runs from his mouth

Motor Control

Symmetrical body postures predominate

Holds head steady when in sitting position

Lifts head and shoulders at a 90-degree angle when on abdomen and looks around

Tries to roll over. Can turn from back to side

Thumb apposition in grasping occurs between third and fourth months

Holds hands predominantly open. Activates arms at sight of proferred toy

Sits with adequate support and enjoys being propped up

Tonic neck reflex has disappeared

Sustains portion of own weight

Vision

Recognizes familiar objects

Stares at rattle placed in his hand and takes it to his mouth

Follows moving objects well. Even the most difficult types of eye movements are present

Arms are activated on sight of dangling toy

Vocalization and Socialization

Laughs aloud and smiles in response to smiles of others

Initiates social play by smiling

Vocalizes socially; i.e., he coos and gurgles when talked to

He does not cry when scolded. He is very "talkative"

"Talking" and crying follow each other quickly

Shows evidence of wanting social attention and of increasing interest in other members of the family

Enjoys having people with him

5 MONTHS

Physical

Weight: Twice the birth weight (15–16 pounds)

Motor Control

Sits with slight support. Holds back straight when pulled to sitting position

Can use thumb in partial apposition to fingers more skillfully

Can balance head well

Reaches for objects which are beyond his grasp. Grasps objects independently of direct stimulation of the palm of the hand (partial grasp). Grasps with the whole hand. Accepts an object handed to him

Has completely lost the Moro reflex

Vocalization and Socialization

Vocalizes his displeasure when a desired object is taken from him

6 MONTHS

Physical

Gains about 3 to 5 ounces weekly during the second 6 months of life

Grows about 1/2 inch a month

May be teething

Motor Control

Sits momentarily without support if placed in a favorable leaning position

Grasps with simultaneous flexion of fingers

Retains transient hold on 2 blocks, one in either hand

Pulls himself up to a sitting position

Completely turns over from stomach to stomach with rest periods during the complete turn. This ability is important in protecting him from falling out of bed

Springs up and down when sitting

Bangs with object held in his hand, rattle or spoon

Hitches. Hitching is locomotion backward when in a sitting position. Movement of the body is aided by use of his arms and hands. This ability is usually present by the sixth month

Vocalization and Socialization

Babbles from the third to the eighth month

Vocalizes several well defined syllables. Actively vocalizes pleasure with crowing or cooing. Babbling is not linked with specific objects, people, or situations

Cries easily on slight provocation (change of position or withdrawal of a toy)

Thrashes arms and legs when frustrated

Begins to recognize strangers (fifth to sixth month)

Average Achievement Levels of Infants, 1 Month to 1 Year (*Continued*)

7 Months

Motor Control

When lying down, lifts head as if he were trying to sit up
Sits briefly, leaning forward on his hands. Control of trunk is more advanced
Plays with his feet and puts them in his mouth
Bounces actively when held in a standing position
Can approach a toy and grasp it with one hand
Can transfer a toy from one hand to the other with varying degrees of success
Rolls more easily from back to stomach

Vocalization and Socialization

Vocalizes his eagerness
Vocalizes "m-m-m" when crying
Makes polysyllabic vowel sounds
Emotional development, 7 to 8 months: Shows fear of strangers
Emotional instability shown by easy and quick changes from crying to laughing

8 Months

Motor Control

Sits alone steadily
Complete thumb apposition
Hand-eye coordination is perfected to the point that random reaching and grasping no longer persist

Vocalization and Socialization

Greets strangers with coy or bashful behavior, turning away, hanging his head, crying or even screaming, and refuses to play with strangers or even accept toys from them
Shows nervousness with strangers
Emotional development: "Eight months' anxiety," to be distinguished from anaclitic depression, occurs between the sixth and eighth months as a result of the child's increased capacity for discriminating between friend and stranger
Affection or love of family group appears
Emotional instability still shown by easy changes from laughing to crying
Stretches arm to loved adult as in invitation to come

9 Months

Motor Control

Shows good coordination and sits alone
Holds his bottle with good hand-mouth coordination. Can put the nipple in and out of his mouth at will
Preference for the use of one hand is marked
Crawls instead of hitching. Crawling may be seen as early as the fourth month; the average age is about nine months. In crawling the infant is prone, his abdomen touching the floor, his head and shoulders supported with the weight borne on the elbows. The body is pulled along by the movement of the arms while the legs drag. The leg movements may resemble swimming or kicking movements
Creeps. This is a more advanced type of locomotion than crawling. The trunk is carried above the floor, but parallel to it. The infant uses both his hands and knees in propelling himself forward. Not all infants follow this pattern of hitching, crawling, and creeping. Different children stress different means of locomotion and may even skip a stage. (This is particularly likely if an infant is sick or for some other reason is unable to practice moving about)
Raises himself to a sitting position. Requires help to pull self to feet

Vocalization and Socialization

Shows the beginning of imitative expression. Sounds stand for things to him. Says "Da-da" or some such expression
Responds to adult anger. Cries when scolded

10 Months

Motor Control

Sits steadily for an indefinite time. Does not enjoy lying down unless he is sleepy
Makes early stepping movements when held
Pulls himself to his feet, holding to the crib rail or similar support. (This is a good time to begin use of the play pen or yard)
Creeps and cruises about very well. (Cruising is walking sideways while holding on to a supporting object with both hands)
Can pick up objects fairly well and pokes them with his fingers
Feeds himself a cracker or some such food which he can hold in his hand
Is able crudely to release a toy
Can bring his hands together

Vocalization and Socialization

Says one or two words and imitates an adult's inflection
Pays attention to his name
Plays simple games as bye-bye and pat-a-cake (motor control is such that he can bring his hands together) and peek-a-boo

Feeding the Infant. The infant should be picked up and held during the feeding. This provides him with physical contact that conveys a sense of warmth and security, and also avoids the dangers of strangulation or aspiration of the formula and prevents the possibility of the infant sucking air from a half-empty bottle. He should be positioned so that his head and shoulders are elevated and well supported.

The opening in the nipple may be a cross-cut or a group of small holes. The nipples should be firm and the opening small enough so that some sucking effort is required and the formula is not taken too rapidly.

During the feeding the infant's position should be changed so that he can eliminate bubbles of air that may have accumulated in his stomach. The position for "burping" or "bubbling" the infant is not important as long as his head and shoulders are higher than the rest of his body. He may be turned on his abdomen for burping. Holding the infant in a sitting position in one's lap is less likely to contaminate the infant than is the shoulder method. After the feeding is completed the infant should be placed in bed on his side or abdomen to facilitate the removal of air from the stomach and reduce the danger of aspiration if he regurgitates some of the formula.

floppy i., floppy i. syndrome, a congenital myopathy of infants, marked clinically by myotonia and muscle weakness.

immature i., one weighing between 17 oz. and $2\frac{1}{5}$ lb. (500 to 999 gm.) at birth, with little chance of survival.

mature i., one weighing $5\frac{1}{2}$ lb. (2500 gm.) or more at birth, with optimal chance of survival.

newborn i., the human young during the first 2 to 4 weeks after birth.

postmature i., one carried for more than 294 days from the beginning of the last menstrual period or 280 days from the date of conception.

premature i., one weighing between $2\frac{1}{5}$ and $5\frac{1}{2}$ lb. (1000 to 2499 gm.) at birth, with poor to good chance of survival (see also PREMATURE INFANT).

infantile (in'fan-tīl) relating to infancy; having features or traits characteristic of early childhood.

i. paralysis, poliomyelitis.

infantilism (in-fan'tĭ-lizm, in'fan-tĭ-lizm) persistence of the characters of childhood into adult life, marked by mental retardation, underdevelopment of the reproductive organs, and often dwarfism.

infarct (in'farkt) a localized area of ischemic necrosis produced by occlusion of the arterial supply or the venous drainage of the part.

anemic i., one due to sudden interruption of flow of arterial blood to the area.

bland i., an uninfected infarct.

hemorrhagic i., one that is red owing to oozing of erythrocytes into the injured area.

pale i., anemic infarct.

red i., hemorrhagic infarct.

septic i., one in which the tissues have been invaded by pathogenic organisms.

white i., anemic infarct.

infarction (in-fark'shun) 1. the formation of an infarct. 2. an infarct.

cardiac i., myocardial infarction.

cerebral i., an ischemic condition of the brain, causing a persistent focal neurologic deficit in the area affected.

AVERAGE ACHIEVEMENT LEVELS OF INFANTS, 1 MONTH TO 1 YEAR (*Concluded*)

11 MONTHS

Motor Control

Stands erect with the help of his mother's hand or supporting himself by holding on to some object as the side of his play yard

12 MONTHS

Physical

Weight: Three times his birth weight (21–22 pounds)
Height: 29 inches
Head and chest are equal in circumference
Has 6 teeth
Pulse: 100–140 per minute.
Respirations: 20–40 per minute

Motor Control

Stands for a moment alone, or possibly longer
Walks with help. Cruises, walking sideways around chairs or from chair to chair, holding on with one hand
Lumbar curve and the compensating dorsal curve develop as he learns to walk
Can sit down from standing position without help
Holds a crayon adaptively to make a stroke and can mark on a piece of paper
Can pick up small bits of food and transfer them to his mouth. Can drink from a cup and eat from a spoon, but requires help. He likes to eat with his fingers
Cooperates in dressing; e.g., he can put his arm through a sleeve. Can take off his socks

Vocalization and Socialization

Can say 2 words besides "Mama" and "Dada"
Slow vocabulary growth, as a rule, owing to his interest in walking
Knows his own name
Uses expressive jargon. Communicates with himself and those around him
Inhibits simple acts on command. Recognizes the meaning of "No, no"
Shows jealousy, affection, anger, and other emotions. He may cry for affection. He loves an audience, and will repeat a performance which brings a response. Crying is more often associated with irritation or frustration than it formerly was. Stiffens in resistance
Loves rhythms
Still egocentric, concerned only with himself

From Marlow, D. R.: Textbook of Pediatric Nursing. 3rd ed. Philadelphia, W. B. Saunders Co., 1969.

myocardial i., gross necrosis of the myocardium, due to interruption of the blood supply to the area (see also CORONARY OCCLUSION).

pulmonary i., localized necrosis of lung tissue, due to obstruction of the arterial blood supply.

infection (in-fek′shun) 1. invasion and multiplication of microorganisms in body tissues, especially that causing local cellular injury due to competitive metabolism, toxins, intracellular replication, or antigen-antibody response. 2. an infectious disease.

The infectious process is similar to a circular chain with each link representing one of the factors involved in the process. An infectious disease occurs only if each link is present and in proper sequence. These links are: (1) the causative agent, which must be of sufficient number and virulence or capable of destroying normal tissue; (2) reservoirs in which the organism can thrive and reproduce; for example, body tissues and the wastes of humans, animals, and insects, and contaminated food and water; (3) a portal through which the pathogen can leave the host; for example, via the respiratory tract and intestinal tract; (4) a mode of transfer, that is, the hands, air currents, vectors, fomites, or other means by which the pathogens can be moved from one place or person to another; and (5) a portal of entry through which the pathogens can enter the body of a (6) susceptible host. Open wounds, the respiratory, intestinal, and reproductive tracts are examples of portals of entry. The host must be susceptible to the disease, not having any immunity to it, or lacking adequate resistance to overcome the invasion by the pathogens.

The body responds to the invasion of causative organisms by the formation of ANTIBODIES and by a series of physiologic changes known as INFLAMMATION.

The spectrum of infectious agents changes with the passage of time and the introduction of drugs and chemicals designed to destroy them. The advent of antibiotics and the resultant development of resistant strains of bacteria have introduced new types of pathogens little known or not previously thought to be significantly dangerous to man. The gram-positive organisms were the most common infectious agents 25 years ago. Today the gram-negative microorganisms, and *Proteus, Pseudomonas,* and *Serratia* are particularly troublesome, especially in the development of hospital-acquired infections. It can safely be predicted that within the next two or three decades other lesser known pathogens and new strains of bacteria will emerge as the most common causes of infections.

The development of resistant strains of pathogens can be limited by the judicious use of antibiotics. This requires culturing and sensitivity testing for a specific antibiotic to which the identified causative organism has been found to be sensitive. If the patient has been receiving a broad-spectrum antibiotic prior to culture and sensitivity testing, this should be discontinued as soon as the specific antibiotic for the organism has been found. It would be helpful, too, if the general public understood that antibiotics are not cure-alls and that there is danger in using them indiscriminately. In some instances an antibiotic can upset the normal flora of the body, thus compromising the body's natural resistance and making it more susceptible to a second infection. (See also SUPERINFECTION.)

Although antibacterials have greatly reduced mortality and morbidity rates for many infectious diseases, the ultimate outcome of an infectious process depends on the effectiveness of the host's IMMUNE RESPONSES. The antibacterial drugs provide a holding action, keeping the growth and reproduction of the infectious agent in check until the interaction between the organism and the immune bodies of the host can subdue the invaders.

Intracellular infectious agents include viruses, mycobacteria, *Brucella, Salmonella,* and many others. Infections of this type are overcome primarily by T-lymphocytes and their products, which are the components of cell-mediated IMMUNITY. Extracellular infectious agents live outside the cell; these include pneumococcus, streptococcus, and hemophilus. These microorganisms have a carbohydrate capsule that acts as an antigen to stimulate the production of antibody, an essential component of humoral IMMUNITY.

Infection may be transmitted by direct contact, by indirect contact, or by vectors. Direct contact may be with body excreta such as urine, feces, or mucus, or with drainage from an open sore, ulcer, or wound. Indirect contact refers to transmission via inanimate objects such as bed linens, bedpans, drinking glasses, or eating utensils. Vectors are flies, mosquitoes, or other insects capable of harboring and spreading the infectious agent.

airborne i., infection by inhalation of organisms suspended in air on water droplets or dust particles.

cross i., infection transmitted between patients infected with different pathogenic microorganisms.

droplet i., infection due to inhalation of respiratory pathogens suspended on liquid particles exhaled by someone already infected.

dustborne i., infection by inhalation of pathogens that have become affixed to particles of dust.

endogenous i., that due to reactivation of organisms present in a dormant focus, as occurs in tuberculosis, etc.

exogenous i., that caused by organisms not normally present in the body but which have gained entrance from the environment.

mixed i., infection with more than one kind of organism at the same time.

pyogenic i., infection by pus-producing organisms.

secondary i., infection by a pathogen following an infection by a pathogen of another kind.

terminal i., an acute infection occurring near the end of a disease and often causing death.

waterborne i., infection by microorganisms transmitted in water.

infectious (in-fek′shus) caused by or capable of being communicated by infection.

i. disease, one due to organisms ranging in size from viruses to parasitic worms; it may be contagious in origin, result from nosocomial organisms, or be due to endogenous microflora from the nose and throat, skin, or bowel (see also COMMUNICABLE DISEASE).

infective (in-fek′tiv) infectious, capable of producing infection; pertaining to or characterized by the presence of pathogens.

inferior (in-fēr′e-or) situated below, or directed downward; in anatomy, used in reference to the lower surface of a structure, or to the lower of two (or more) similar structures.

infertility (in″fer-til′ĭ-te) diminution or absence of the ability to produce offspring. adj., **infer′tile.** (See also FERTILITY.)

infestation (in″fes-ta′shun) parasitic attack or subsistence on the skin and/or its appendages, as by insects, mites, or ticks; sometimes used to denote parasitic invasion of the organs and tissues, as by helminths.

infiltrate (in-fil′trāt) 1. to penetrate the interstices of a tissue or substance. 2. material deposited by infiltration.

infiltration (in″fil-tra′shun) the diffusion or accumulation in a tissue or cells of substances not normal to it or in amounts in excess of the normal; also, the material so accumulated.

adipose i., fatty infiltration.

calcareous i., deposit of lime and magnesium salts in the tissues.

cellular i., the migration and accumulation of cells within the tissues.

fatty i., 1. a deposit of fat in tissues, especially between cells. 2. the presence of fat vacuoles in the cell cytoplasm.

urinous i., the extravasation of urine into a tissue.

infirm (in-ferm′) weak; feeble, as from disease or old age.

infirmary (in-fir′mah-re) a hospital or place where the sick or infirm are maintained or treated.

inflammation (in″flah-ma′shun) a localized protective response elicited by injury or destruction of tissues, which serves to destroy, dilute, or wall off both the injurious agent and the injured tissue. adj., **inflam′matory.** The injury may be caused by a physical blow, or by exposure to an excessive amount of radiation from sunlight, x-rays, or an ultraviolet lamp; or it may be caused by corrosive chemicals, burns, extreme heat or cold, or foreign objects. Inflammation is also the usual response to a bacterial infection.

The physiologic changes that take place during the inflammatory process include vascular dilatation, leukocytosis, and fluid exudation. The vascular changes occur at the site of the injury to the tissues. The damaged cells liberate a toxic substance (necrosin), in response to which the capillaries and arteries dilate so that there is an increased flow of fluid and protein to the area. The speed of circulation is decreased with the result that leukocytes leave the blood vessels and enter the tissue spaces. The vascular changes are responsible for the redness that accompanies inflammation.

Leukocytosis means an increase in the number of white blood cells. The injured tissues release chemicals that attract the leukocytes to the site of injury. There they ingest, or surround and destroy, the cause of the inflammation.

Body fluids also collect at the site. This increase of fluids is called exudation. The exudate brings immune bodies (antibodies) and special enzymes, and also helps in the removal of dead bacteria, destroyed tissue cells, and blood cells.

The four classic symptoms of inflammation are redness (rubor), swelling (tumor), heat (calor), and pain (dolor). Loss of function of the part may also occur.

TREATMENT. Treatment of inflammation depends on the cause. Heat can sometimes be applied to an inflammation to promote the circulation of blood through the area. On the other hand application of cold initially may reduce swelling and thus reduce pain. If the inflammation results from a wound, the wound should be cleaned and painted with a mild antiseptic.

The treatment of advanced or widespread conditions of inflammation caused by a bacterial infection is intended to destroy the bacteria, increase the patient's resistance to any possible infection, and eliminate from the body any toxins formed by the bacteria. Treatment therefore consists of medicines such as the sulfonamides and antibiotics, vitamins to help increase the patient's resistance to infection, and antitoxins to help eliminate any toxins. Surgery may be required to remove foreign bodies, drain pus, and otherwise promote healing.

acute i., inflammation, usually of sudden onset, marked by the classical signs of heat, redness, swelling, pain and loss of function, and in which vascular and exudative processes predominate.

catarrhal i., a form affecting mainly a mucous surface, marked by a copious discharge of mucus and epithelial debris.

chronic i., prolonged and persistent inflammation marked chiefly by new connective tissue formation; it may be a continuation of an acute form or a prolonged low-grade form.

exudative i., one in which the prominent feature is an exudate.

fibrinous i., one marked by an exudate of coagulated fibrin.

granulomatous i., a form, usually chronic, attended by formation of granulomas.

interstitial i., inflammation affecting chiefly the stroma of an organ.

parenchymatous i., inflammation affecting chiefly the essential tissue elements of an organ.

productive i., proliferative i., one leading to the production of new connective tissue fibers.

pseudomembranous i., an acute inflammatory response to a powerful necrotizing toxin, e.g., diphtheria toxin, characterized by formation on a mucosal surface of a false membrane composed of precipitated fibrin, necrotic epithelium, and inflammatory leukocytes.

purulent i., suppurative inflammation.

serous i., one producing a serous exudate.

specific i., one due to a particular microorganism.

subacute i., a condition intermediate between chronic and acute inflammation, exhibiting some of the characteristics of each.

suppurative i., one marked by pus formation.

toxic i., one due to a poison, e.g., a bacterial product.

traumatic i., one that follows a wound or injury.

ulcerative i., that in which necrosis on or near the surface leads to loss of tissue and creation of a local defect (ulcer).

inflation (in-fla′shun) distention or the act of distending, with air, gas, or fluid.

inflection, inflexion (in′flek-shun) the act of bending inward, or the state of being bent inward.

influenza (in″floo-en′zah) an acute viral infection of the respiratory tract, occurring in isolated cases, epidemics, and pandemics. Called also grippe (or grip) and flu. adj., **influen′zal.** Three main types of the virus have been recognized, labeled by researchers as types A (with many subgroups, labeled A_1, A_2, etc.), B, and C. The A_2 virus is a comparatively new strain that first emerged in 1957. The disease it produces is often called Asian flu.

SYMPTOMS. Influenza has a brief incubation period. The symptoms appear suddenly and though the virus enters the respiratory tract it soon affects the entire body. The symptoms include fever, chills, headache, sore throat, cough, gastrointestinal disturbances, muscular pain, and neuralgia.

TREATMENT. There is no drug that will cure influenza. An antibiotic may be prescribed to ward off complications of secondary bacterial infections such as pneumonia and bronchitis. Bed rest, increasing the intake of fluids, and aspirin to relieve aches and discomfort and help control fever are prescribed.

PREVENTION. A vaccine is available, although it does not always provide complete immunity against all forms of influenza viruses that may be present. The vaccine is strongly advised for people over 65, pregnant women and all who have chronic heart, lung, or kidney disease. Other precautions include avoiding contact with others who have influenza, avoiding crowded places when there is a local epidemic, and observing good personal hygiene to increase the body's resistance.

infra- word element [L.], *beneath.*

infra-axillary (in″frah-ak′sĭ-ler″e) below the axilla.

infraclavicular (in″frah-klah-vik′u-lar) below the clavicle.

infraclusion (in″frah-kloo′zhun) a condition in which the occluding surface of a tooth does not reach the normal occlusal plane and is out of contact with the opposing tooth.

infracostal (in″frah-kos′tal) below a rib.

infraction (in-frak′shun) incomplete bone fracture without displacement.

infrahyoid (in″frah-hi′oid) below the hyoid bone.

inframaxillary (in″frah-mak′sĭ-ler″e) beneath the maxilla.

infranuclear (in″frah-nu′kle-ar) below a nucleus.

infraorbital (in″frah-or′bĭ-tal) lying under or on the floor of the orbit.

infrapatellar (in″frah-pah-tel′ar) beneath the patella.

infrared (in″frah-red′) denoting elctromagnetic radiation of wavelength greater than that of the red end of the spectrum, having wavelengths of 0.75–1000 μm. Infrared rays are sometimes subdivided into long-wave or far infrared (about 3.0–1000 μm.) and short-wave or near infrared (about 0.75–3.0 μm.). They are capable of penetrating body tissues to a depth of 10 mm. Sources of infrared rays include heat lamps, hot water bottles, steam radiators, and incandescent light bulbs.

Infrared rays are used therapeutically to promote muscle relaxation, to speed up the inflammatory process, and to increase circulation to a part of the body. (See also HEAT.)

infrascapular (in″frah-skap′u-lar) below the scapula.

infrasonic (in″frah-son′ik) below the frequency range of sound waves.

infraspinous (in″frah-spi′nus) beneath the spine of the scapula.

infrasternal (in″frah-ster′nal) beneath the sternum.

infratrochlear (in″frah-trok′le-ar) beneath the trochlea.

infraversion (in″frah-ver′zhun) 1. downward deviation of the eye. 2. infraclusion.

infundibuliform (in″fun-dib′u-lĭ-form) shaped like a funnel.

infundibulum (in″fun-dib′u-lum), pl. *infundib′ula* [L.] 1. any funnel-shaped passage. 2. conus arteriosus, the anterosuperior portion of the right ventricle of the heart. adj., **infundib′ular.**

ethmoidal i., 1. a passage connecting the nasal cavity with the anterior ethmoidal cells and frontal sinus. 2. a sinuous passage connecting the middle meatus of the nose with the anterior ethmoidal cells and often with the frontal sinus.

i. of hypothalamus, a hollow, funnel-shaped mass in front of the tuber cinereum, extending to the posterior lobe of the pituitary gland.

i. of uterine tube, the distal, funnel-shaped portion of the uterine tube.

infusion (in-fu′zhun) 1. the steeping of a substance in water to obtain its soluble principles. 2. the product obtained by this process. 3. the slow therapeutic introduction of fluid other than blood into a vein (see also INTRAVENOUS INFUSION). Note—An *infusion* flows in by gravity, an *injection* is forced in by a syringe, an *instillation* is dropped in, an *insufflation* is blown in, and an *infection* slips in unnoticed.

subcutaneous i., administration of fluids directly into subcutaneous tissues for the purpose of providing hydration. (See also HYPODERMOCLYSIS.)

ingesta (in-jes′tah) material taken into the body by mouth.

ingestant (in-jes′tant) a substance that is or may be taken into the body by mouth or through the digestive system.

ingestion (in-jes′chun) the taking of food, drugs, etc., into the body by mouth.

ingravescent (in″grah-ves′ent) gradually becoming more severe.

ingrown nail (in′grōn) aberrant growth of a toenail, with one or both lateral margins pushing deeply into adjacent soft tissue, causing pain, inflammation, and possible infection. The condition occurs most frequently in the great toe, and is often caused by pressure from tight-fitting shoes. Another common cause is improper cutting of the toenails, which should be cut straight across or with a curved toenail scissors so that the sides are a little longer than the middle.

inguen (ing′gwen), pl. *in′guina* [L.] the groin.

inguinal (ing′gwĭ-nal) pertaining to the groin.

i. canal, the oblique passage in the lower anterior abdominal wall, through which passes the round ligament of the uterus in the female, and the spermatic cord in the male.

i. hernia, hernia occurring in the groin; protrusion of intestine or omentum, or both, either directly through a weak point in the abdominal wall (direct inguinal hernia) or downward into the inguinal canal (indirect inguinal hernia). (See also inguinal HERNIA.)

INH trademark for preparations of isoniazid, a tuberculostatic.

inhalant (in-ha′lant) a substance that is or may be taken into the body by way of the nose and trachea (through the respiratory system).

inhalation (in″hah-la′shun) 1. the act of breathing in. 2. an agent to be inhaled as a vapor.

inhaler (in-ha′ler) an apparatus for administering vaporized or volatilized agents by inhalation, or for protecting the lungs from harmful substances in the air.

inheritance (in-her′ĭ-tans) 1. the acquisition of

characters or qualities by transmission from parent to offspring. 2. that which is transmitted from parent to offspring. (See also GENE, DEOXYRIBONUCLEIC ACID, and HEREDITY.)

maternal i., the transmission of characters that are dependent on peculiarities of the egg cytoplasm produced, in turn, by nuclear genes.

inhibition (in″ĭ-bish′un, in″hĭ-bish′un) arrest or restraint of a process; in psychiatry, the unconscious restraining of an instinctual drive. adj., **inhib′itory.**

competitive i., inhibition of enzyme activity by an inhibitor (a substrate analogue) that competes with the substrate for binding sites on the enzymes.

contact i., inhibition of cell division in normal animal cells when in close contact with each other.

noncompetitive i., inhibition of enzyme activity by substances that combine with the enzyme at a site other than that utilized by the substrate.

inhibitor (in-hib′ĭ-tor) 1. any substance that interferes with a chemical reaction, growth, or other biologic activity. 2. a chemical substance that inhibits or checks the action of a tissue organizer or the growth of microorganisms.

inion (in′e-on) the external occipital protuberance. adj., **in′ial.**

iniopagus (in″e-op′ah-gus) a twin monster joined at the occiput.

initis (ĭ-ni′tis) inflammation of the substance of a muscle.

injected (in-jek′ted) 1. introduced by injection. 2. congested.

injection (in-jek′shun) 1. the forcing of a liquid into a part, as into the subcutaneous tissues, the vascular tree, or an organ. 2. a substance so forced or administered; in pharmacy, a solution of a medicament suitable for injection. 3. congestion.

Immunizing substances, or inoculations, are generally given by injection. When a patient is unconscious, injection may be the only means of administering medication, and in some cases nourishment. Some medicines cannot be given by mouth because chemical action of the digestive juices would change or reduce their effectiveness, or because they would be removed from the body too quickly to have any effect. Certain potent medicines must be injected because they would irritate body tissues if administered any other way. Occasionally a medication is injected so that it will act more quickly.

In addition to the most common types of injections described below, injections are sometimes made into arteries, bone marrow, the spine, the sternum, the pleural space of the chest region, the peritoneal cavity, and joint spaces. In sudden heart failure, heart-stimulating drugs may be injected directly into the heart (intracardiac injection).

hypodermic i., subcutaneous injection.

intracutaneous i., intradermal i., injection of small amounts of material into the corium or substance of the skin. This method is used in diagnostic procedures and in administration of regional anesthetics, as well as in treatment procedures. In certain allergy tests, the allergen is injected intracutaneously. These injections are given in an area where the skin and hair are sparse, usually on the inner part of the forearm. A 25-gauge needle, $\frac{3}{8}$ or $\frac{1}{2}$ inch long, is recommended. The needle is inserted at a 10- to 15-degree angle to the skin.

intramuscular i., injection into the substance of a muscle, usually the muscle of the upper arm, thigh, or buttock. Intramuscular injections are given when the substance is to be absorbed quickly. They should be given with extreme care, especially in the buttock, because the sciatic nerve may be injured or a large blood vessel may be entered if the injection is not made correctly into the upper, outer quadrant of the buttock. The deltoid muscle at the shoulder is also used, but less commonly than the gluteus muscle of the buttock; care must be taken to insert the needle in the center, 2 cm. below the acromion.

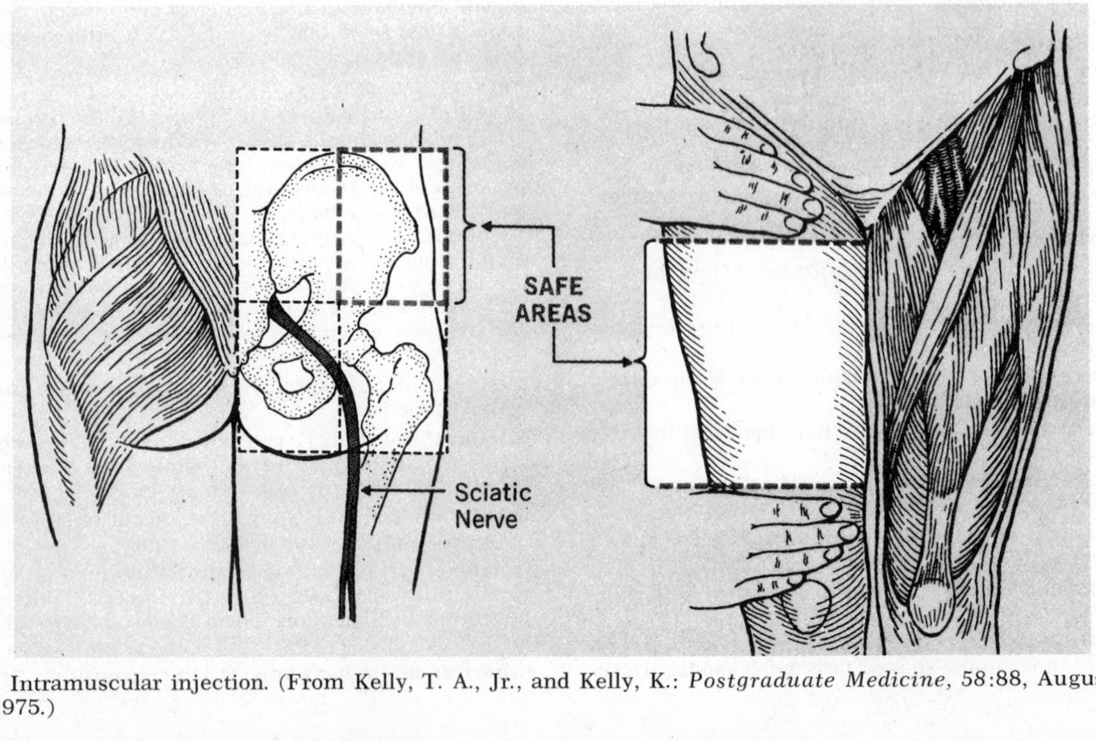

Intramuscular injection. (From Kelly, T. A., Jr., and Kelly, K.: *Postgraduate Medicine*, 58:88, August 1975.)

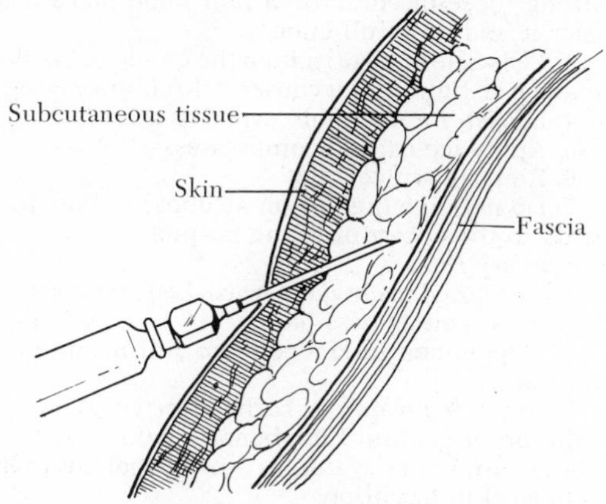

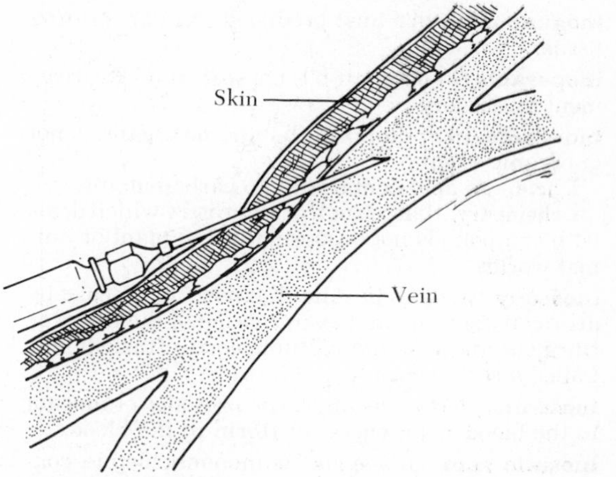

Left: subcutaneous, or hypodermic, injection, in which fluid medicines are introduced into the body through a hypodermic needle that pierces only the skin and the tissue beneath it. Right: intravenous injection, in which the needle is inserted into a vein. Only occasionally are injections made into arteries.

Injections into the anterolateral aspect of the thigh are considered the safest because there is less danger of damage to a major blood vessel or nerve. The area permits multiple injections, is more accessible, and easier to stabilize, particularly in pediatric patients or others who are restless and uncooperative. The vastus lateralis muscle is located by identifying the trochanter and the side of the knee cap and then drawing a visual line between the two. The distance is then divided into thirds and the needle inserted into the area identified as the middle third.

The needle should be at least $1\frac{1}{2}$ inches long so that the liquid is injected deep into the muscle tissue. The gauge of the needle depends on the viscosity of the fluid being injected. As a general rule, not more than 5 ml. is given in an intramuscular injection. The needle is inserted at a 90-degree angle to the skin. When the gluteus maximus muscle is the site chosen for the injection, the patient should be in a prone position with the toes turned in if possible. This position relaxes the muscle and makes the injection less painful.

intravenous i., an injection made into a vein. Intravenous injections are used when rapid absorption is called for, when fluid cannot be taken by mouth, or when the substance to be administered is too irritating to be injected into the skin or muscles. In certain diagnostic tests and x-ray examinations a drug or dye may be administered intravenously. Blood transfusions also are given by this route. (See also INTRAVENOUS INFUSION.)

subcutaneous i., injection made into the subcutaneous tissues; called also hypodermic injection. Although usually fluid medications are injected, occasionally solid materials, such as steroid hormones, are administered subcutaneously in small, slowly absorbed pellets to prolong their effect. Subcutaneous injections may be given wherever there is subcutaneous tissue, usually in the upper, outer arm or thigh. A 25-gauge needle $\frac{3}{4}$ inch long is usually used, and the amount injected should not exceed 2 ml. The needle is held at a 45-degree angle to the skin.

injury (in′ju-re) harm or hurt; a wound or maim; usually applied to damage inflicted on the body by an external force.

inlay (in′la) material laid into a defect in tissue; in dentistry, a filling made outside the tooth to correspond with the cavity form and then cemented into the cavity.

inlet (in′let) a means or route of entrance.

pelvic i., the upper limit of the pelvic cavity.

I.N.N. International Nonproprietary Names, the designations recommended by the World Health Organization for pharmaceuticals.

innate (ĭ-nāt′, in′āt) inborn; hereditary; congenital.

innervation (in″er-va′shun) 1. the distribution or supply of nerves to a part. 2. the supply of nervous energy or of nerve stimulation sent to a part.

innidiation (ĭ-nid″e-a′shun) development of cells in a part to which they have been carried by metastasis.

innocent (in′o-sent) not malignant; benign.

innocuous (ĭ-nok′u-us) harmless.

innominate (ĭ-nom′ĭ-nāt) nameless.

i. artery, brachiocephalic trunk, the first branch of the arch of the aorta.

i. bone, the hip bone.

i. veins, the brachiocephalic veins, which unite to form the superior vena cava.

inochondritis (in″o-kon-dri′tis) inflammation of a fibrocartilage.

inoculability (ĭ-nok″u-lah-bil′ĭ-te) the state of being inoculable.

inoculable (ĭ-nok′u-lah-b′l) 1. susceptible of being inoculated; transmissible by inoculation. 2. not immune against a transmissible disease.

inoculation (ĭ-nok″u-la′shun) 1. introduction of pathogenic microorganisms, injective material, serum, or other substances into tissues of living organisms or into culture media; introduction of a disease agent into a healthy individual to produce a mild form of the disease, followed by IMMUNITY.

inoculum (ĭ-nok′u-lum) material used in inoculation.

inocyte (in′o-sīt) a cell of fibrous tissue.

inogenesis (in″o-jen′ĕ-sis) the formation of fibrous tissue.

inogenous (in-oj'ĕ-nus) produced from or forming tissue.

inoperable (in-op'er-ah-b'l) not susceptible to treatment by surgery.

inorganic (in"or-gan'ik) 1. having no organs. 2. not of organic origin.

i. acid, an acid containing no carbon atoms.

i. chemistry, that branch of chemistry which deals with compounds not occurring in the plant or animal worlds.

inoscopy (in-os'ko-pe) the diagnosis of disease by artificial digestion and examination of the fibers or fibrinous matter of the sputum, blood, effusions, etc. Called also fibrinoscopy.

inosemia (in"o-se'me-ah) 1. the presence of inositol in the blood. 2. an excess of fibrin in the blood.

inosinic acid (in"o-sin'ik) a mononucleotide constituent of muscle, made up of hypoxanthine, ribose, and phosphoric acid.

inositol (in-o'sĭ-tol) a sugar-like vitamin of the B complex found in many animal and plant tissues; it is concerned in the growth of yeast and certain bacteria, and has been shown to have lipotropic action on fatty liver in rats and to be curative of mouse alopecia.

inosituria (in"o-si-tu're-ah) the presence of inositol in the urine.

inotropic (in'o-trop"ik) affecting the force of muscular contractions.

inquest (in'kwest) a legal inquiry before a coroner or medical examiner, and usually a jury, into the manner of death.

insalubrious (in"sah-lu'bre-us) injurious to health.

insanity (in-san'ĭ-te) a legal term for mental illness, roughly equivalent to PSYCHOSIS and implying inability to be responsible for one's acts. adj., **insane'**.

inscriptio (in-skrip'she-o), pl. *inscriptio'nes* [L.] inscription.

i. tendin'ea, intersectio tendinea.

inscription (in-skrip'shun) 1. a mark or line. 2. that part of a prescription containing the names and amounts of the ingredients.

insect (in'sekt) any individual of the class Insecta.

i. bites and stings, injuries caused by the mouth parts and venom of insects and of certain related creatures, known as arachnids—spiders, scorpions, ticks—but popularly classified with insects. Bites and stings can be the cause of much discomfort. Usually there is no real danger, although a local infection can develop from scratching. Some insects, however, establish themselves on the skin as parasites, others inject poison, and still others transmit disease. A knowledge of first-aid measures for bites and stings can do much to relieve discomfort, to prevent infection and, in some cases, even to save a life.

FIRST AID FOR INSECT BITES AND STINGS

Stings of Bees, Wasps, Hornets, Yellow Jackets

1. For bee sting, scrape stinger out with fingernail or remove with tweezers, holding tweezers flat against skin to avoid squeezing more venom into wound.

2. To relieve itching, apply (a) paste of sodium bicarbonate (baking soda) and water, or (b) a paste of water and unseasoned meat tenderizer.

In Case of Allergic Reaction to Bee or Wasp Stings

1. Call a physician immediately.

2. If the sting is on a limb, apply a constricting bandage above the sting as follows: Use a wide, strong piece of cloth; tie a half knot; place a stick over it and tie a full knot.

3. Twist the stick to tighten the bandage but do not make it so tight that it causes a throbbing sensation.

4. Loosen for 1 minute every 10 minutes.

5. Apply ice or cold compresses.

6. Remove stinger.

7. Do not give the person alcohol or allow him to walk to the doctor or to the hospital.

Chigger Bites

1. If exposed to chiggers, wash body with soap and water as soon as possible.

2. Apply denatured alcohol or sulfur ointment to the skin.

3. Apply ice water, or bathe affected parts with a solution of sodium bicarbonate (baking soda) and water, ammonia water, or an alcohol solution, to relieve skin irritation.

Ticks

1. To remove ticks, dab kerosene, gasoline, or some kind of oil on skin where ticks are embedded. If ticks do not drop off in half an hour, remove them carefully with tweezers or in some other way, being careful not to use bare hands.

2. Wash the bite and paint with antiseptic.

Stings of Poisonous Scorpions, Spiders, Centipedes

1. Call a physician immediately.

2. Have patient lie down.

3. If sting is on a limb, apply a constricting bandage above the sting as follows: Use a wide, strong piece of cloth; tie a half knot; place a stick over it and tie a full knot.

4. Twist the stick to tighten the bandage but do not make it so tight that it causes a throbbing sensation.

5. Loosen for 1 minute every 10 minutes.

6. Apply ice to the sting.

7. Do not give the person alcohol or allow him to walk to the doctor or to the hospital.

Insecta (in-sek'tah) a class of arthropods whose members are characterized by division of the body into three distinct regions: head, thorax, and abdomen.

insecticide (in-sek'tĭ-sīd) an agent that kills insects. adj., **insec'ticidal.**

Insectivora (in"sek-tiv'o-rah) an order of small, terrestrial and nocturnal mammals, including moles, shrews, etc., which feed primarily on insects.

insectivore (in-sek'tĭ-vōr) any individual of the order Insectivora. adj., **insec'tivorous.**

insemination (in-sem"ĭ-na'shun) the deposit of seminal fluid within the vagina or cervix.

artificial i., that done by artificial means.

insensible (in-sen'sĭ-b'l) 1. devoid of sensibility or consciousness. 2. not perceptible to the senses.

insertion (in-ser'shun) 1. the act of implanting, or condition of being implanted. 2. the site of attachment, as of a muscle to the bone that it moves.

velamentous i., attachment of the umbilical cord to the fetal membranes.

insidious (in-sid'e-us) coming on stealthily; of gradual and subtle development.

insight (in'sīt) self-understanding; in psychiatry, referring to the extent to which the patient is aware of his illness and understands its nature.

in situ (in si'tu) [L.] in its normal place; confined to the site of origin.

insoluble (in-sol′u-b′l) not susceptible of being dissolved.

insomnia (in-som′ne-ah) abnormal wakefulness; an inability to fall asleep easily or to remain asleep throughout the night. The frequency of persistent insomnia is high.

The causes of insomnia may be physical or psychologic or, most often, a combination of both. Some persons are more sensitive to conditions around them than others, and may be kept awake by slight noises, light, or sharing their bed. Beverages that contain caffeine, such as coffee, tea, and cola drinks, keep some people awake. A heavy meal shortly before bedtime may prevent sleep. Drinking large quantities of fluids may cause an uncomfortable feeling of distention of the bladder.

The type of bedding may be a cause of insomnia. Changing to a firmer or softer mattress, doing without a pillow, or making other changes in the bedding may help. Those who are bothered by the weight of blankets may sleep better under lightweight blankets, or with a device that supports the bedclothes at the foot of the bed.

Personal problems and worries about job, finances, or family matters may cause wakefulness, and the inability to sleep disappears when the problems are solved. More difficult to deal with are the deeper psychologic problems such as anxiety, irrational fears, and tensions or frequent nightmares that produce resistance to sleep.

insomniac (in-som′ne-ak) a person suffering from insomnia.

insorption (in-sorp′shun) movement of a substance into the blood, especially from the gastrointestinal tract into the circulating blood.

inspection (in-spek′shun) visual examination for detection of features or qualities perceptible to the eye.

inspersion (in-sper′zhun) sprinkling, as with powder.

inspiration (in″spĭ-ra′shun) the drawing of air into the lungs. adj., **inspi′ratory.**

inspissated (in-spis′āt-ed) being thickened, dried, or made less fluid by evaporation.

instep (in′step) the dorsal part of the arch of the foot.

instillation (in″stĭ-la′shun) administration of a liquid drop by drop.

instinct (in′stinkt) a complex of unlearned responses characteristic of a species. adj., **instinc′tive.**

death i., in psychoanalysis, the latent instinctive impulse toward death.

herd i., the instinct or urge to be one of a group and to conform to its standards of conduct and opinion.

instrumentarium (in″stroo-men-ta′re-um) the equipment or instruments required for any particular operation or purpose; the physical adjuncts with which a physician combats disease.

insufficiency (in″sŭ-fish′en-se) inability to perform properly an allotted function.

adrenal i., hypoadrenalism.

aortic i., inadequacy of the aortic valve, permitting blood to flow back into the left ventricle of the heart.

cardiac i., inability of the heart to perform its function properly; heart failure.

coronary i., decrease in flow of blood through the coronary blood vessels.

ileocecal i., inability of the ileocecal valve to prevent backflow of contents from the cecum into the ileum.

pulmonary i., insufficiency of the pulmonary valve, permitting blood to flow into the right ventricle of the heart.

respiratory i., a condition in which respiratory function is inadequate to meet the body's needs when increased physical activity places extra demands on it (see also RESPIRATORY INSUFFICIENCY).

thyroid i., hypothyroidism.

valvular i., failure of a cardiac valve to close perfectly, causing the blood to flow back through the orifice (valvular regurgitation); named, according to the valve affected, aortic, mitral, pulmonary, or tricuspid insufficiency.

velopharyngeal i., failure of velopharyngeal closure due to cleft palate, muscular dysfunction, etc., resulting in defective speech.

venous i., inadequacy of the venous valves with impairment of venous drainage, resulting in edema.

insufflation (in″sŭ-fla′shun) the blowing of a powder, vapor, or gas into a body cavity.

perirenal i., injection of air around the kidney for roentgen examination of the adrenal glands.

tubal i., insufflation of carbon dioxide gas through the uterus into the uterine tubes as a test of their patency. Called also Rubin's test.

insufflator (in′sŭ-fla″tor) an instrument used in insufflation.

insula (in′su-lah), pl. *in′sulae* [L.] a triangular area of the cerebral cortex that forms the floor of the lateral cerebral fossa; called also island of Reil.

insular (in′su-lar) pertaining to the insula or to an island, as the islands of Langerhans.

insulation (in″sŭ-la′shun) 1. the surrounding of a space or body with material designed to prevent the entrance or escape of radiant energy. 2. the material so used.

insulin (in′su-lin) a protein hormone, the active antidiabetic principle formed by the beta cells of the islands of Langerhans of the pancreas and secreted into the blood, where it regulates carbohydrate, lipid, and amino acid metabolism; also, a preparation of the active principle of the pancreas, used therapeutically in DIABETES MELLITUS and sometimes in other conditions.

Types of insulin vary in the rapidity of action and the duration of effectiveness. Regular insulin is effective almost immediately after injection and reaches its peak of action within 2 hours. It is used most often in diabetic emergencies and in regulating dosage for a patient when diabetes is first diagnosed. Crystalline insulin is made of zinc-insulin crystals and is usually given to patients who are allergic to regular insulin. Other types of insulin developed in recent years contain substances that prolong the action of insulin. Protamine zinc insulin (PZI), isophane insulin (NPH), globin zinc insulin, and insulin lente are examples of long-acting preparations of insulin.

ADMINISTRATION OF INSULIN. Protamine zinc, isophane, and lente insulin are all cloudy and milky in appearance and must be thoroughly mixed by gently rolling the bottle between the palms before the drug is withdrawn from the ampule. Vigorous shaking is avoided because it produces air bubbles that may alter the dosage measured in the syringe.

When regular insulin and NPH insulin are to be given in a single injection it is necessary to mix the

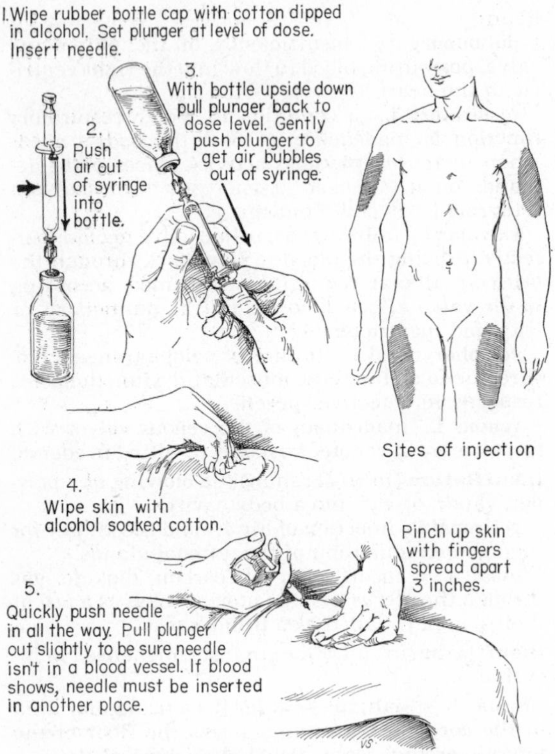
1. Wipe rubber bottle cap with cotton dipped in alcohol. Set plunger at level of dose. Insert needle.
2. Push air out of syringe into bottle.
3. With bottle upside down pull plunger back to dose level. Gently push plunger to get air bubbles out of syringe.
Sites of injection
4. Wipe skin with alcohol soaked cotton.
Pinch up skin with fingers spread apart 3 inches.
5. Quickly push needle in all the way. Pull plunger out slightly to be sure needle isn't in a blood vessel. If blood shows, needle must be inserted in another place.

Injection of insulin. (From Dowling, H. F., and Jones, T.: That the Patient May Know. Philadelphia, W. B. Saunders Co., 1959.)

preparations in the following manner: (1) inject air into the NPH vial; (2) inject air into the regular insulin vial and then withdraw the required dosage; (3) withdraw NPH insulin dosage; (4) put an air bubble in the syringe and mix the two types of insulin.

Insulin is administered at room temperature. It is stored in the refrigerator (never frozen) and removed about one hour prior to administration. The vial should be left in its cardboard container to reduce the danger of contamination and to prevent light from damaging the insulin.

Insulin is measured in units, and is available in varying strengths, for example, U40, U80, and U100. The term U100 means that there are 100 units per milliliter of insulin. When measuring the drug in an insulin syringe, one must *be careful to use the calibrations on the syringe that correspond with the strength of insulin being used.* If the insulin is marked U80, then the measurements on the syringe must be for U80 insulin. Some insulin syringes have calibrations for U40 insulin on one side and for U80 insulin on the other. Others have calibrations for U40 or U80 or U100 only.

Insulin is injected deep into the subcutaneous tissue of the upper arm or thigh. Because of the frequency with which the injections are given, the sites should be rotated to avoid the formation of excessive amounts of scar tissue and to provide ample time for healing before the site is used again. The anterior surface of the abdomen may also be used as a site of injection.

HYPOGLYCEMIA and INSULIN SHOCK result when the level of insulin in the body is too high, because of overdose, failure to eat a full meal at the expected time, more than the usual amount of exercise, an emotional or physical upset, or some change in the body chemistry, as in infection, surgical operation, etc.

i. shock, a condition of circulatory insufficiency caused by an overdose of insulin or decreased food intake with the usual dose. Insulin shock is an ever present danger against which those who take insulin for diabetes mellitus must learn to protect themselves.

DIFFERENCES BETWEEN INSULIN SHOCK AND DIABETIC ACIDOSIS

	INSULIN SHOCK	DIABETIC ACIDOSIS
Cause	Too much insulin	Too little insulin
Symptoms		
Onset	Sudden	Gradual
Breathing	Shallow	Noisy and deep
Skin	Moist	Dry
Hunger, thirst	Extreme hunger	Extreme thirst
Urine	Little or no sugar	Much sugar
Treatment	Sugar is eaten	Insulin is injected

SYMPTOMS. The first reaction to an overdose of insulin is usually tremors, cold sweating, and extreme hunger. The symptoms may differ in some cases, and can include nausea, dizziness, headache, and marked drowsiness. If the urine is tested at this time, it will show no sugar or a trace at most. The blood sugar content likewise is drastically lowered. The patient suddenly becomes weaker and has a quickened pulse and perhaps muscular spasms, such emotional reactions as excessive laughing or crying and convulsions.

The ultimate stage of insulin shock is unconsciousness. This is a serious emergency requiring the services of a physician. Death seldom occurs, but an undue delay can result in permanent harm.

Insulin shock, produced intentionally, has been used in the treatment of affective psychoses (see also SHOCK THERAPY).

TREATMENT. Insulin shock occurs most often when meals are delayed or irregular, and sometimes after unusual physical exertion. Diabetics should recognize the symptoms of insulin shock and immediately take some form of sugar at the first sign of such an attack, either sugar by the lump or spoonful, or a glass of orange juice with sugar added. (See also DIABETES MELLITUS.)

First Aid for Insulin Shock

1. If the person is conscious, immediately give him sugar or a food rich in sugar, such as candy or orange juice.

2. If the patient is semiconscious or unconscious, don't force food or liquid. Call a physician, or take the patient to a hospital.

insulinemia (in″su-lin-e′me-ah) the presence of insulin in the blood.

insulinogenesis (in″su-lin″o-jen′ĕ-sis) the formation and release of insulin by the islands of Langerhans.

insulinogenic (in″su-lin″o-jen′ik) relating to insulinogenesis.

insulinoma (in″su-lin-o′mah) a tumor of the beta cells of the islands of Langerhans; although usually benign, it is one of the chief causes of hypoglycemia.

insulitis (in″su-li′tis) cellular infiltration of the islands of Langerhans, possibly in response to invasion by an infectious agent.

insuloma (in″su-lo′mah) insulinoma.

insusceptibility (in″sŭ-sep″tĭ-bil′ĭ-te) the state of being unaffected or uninfluenced; immunity.

intake (in′tāk) the substances, or the quantities thereof, taken in and utilized by the body. The record of intake and output is called FLUID BALANCE record.

integration (in″tĕ-gra′shun) harmonious assimilation into a common body or activity; anabolic activity.

integument (in-teg′u-ment) a covering or investment; the skin.

integumentary (in-teg″u-men′tar-e) 1. pertaining to or composed of skin. 2. serving as a covering.

integumentum (in-teg″u-men′tum) [L.] integument.

in tela (in te′lah) [L.] in tissue; relating especially to stained histologic preparations.

intellect (in′tĕ-lekt) the mind, thinking faculty, or understanding.

intellectualization (in″tĕ-lek″chu-al-ĭ-za′shun) the mental process in which reasoning is used as a defense against confronting unconscious conflict and its stressful emotions.

intelligence (in-tel′ĭ-jens) the ability to comprehend or understand. It is basically a combination of reasoning, memory, imagination, and judgment. Each of these faculties relies upon the others.

The brain may store up many memories, but they are useful only when brought to surface consciousness at the right time and in the right connection. Imagination is the faculty of associating several memories—they may be of facts, images, or sensations—to produce another fact or image. In general, the more efficiently the brain combines memories in an orderly fashion, the greater the intelligence. Imagination, however, must be governed by reason and judgment. Reason is the ability to draw logical conclusions by relating memories and observations. Judgment relies on experience to choose between different forms of reasoning. All these factors are controlled by the cerebral cortex (see also BRAIN).

In speaking of general intelligence, authorities often distinguish between a number of different kinds of basic mental ability. One of these is verbal aptitude, the ability to understand the meaning of words and to use them effectively in writing or speaking. Another is skill with numbers, the ability to add, subtract, multiply, and divide and to use these skills in problems. The capacity to work with spatial relationships, that is, with visualizing how objects take up space, is still another (for example, how two triangles can fit together to make a square). Perception, memory, and reasoning may also be considered different basic abilities. Often a person is more proficient in some of these areas than he is in others. Commonly, for example, a child may excel in using words but have some difficulty with arithmetic, or the opposite may be true.

In the United States, schoolgirls often achieve verbal skills more quickly than boys, while boys are often more skillful in spatial relations and number work. As a person grows older and as his interests and needs develop and change, his aptitudes may change as well.

These abilities are the ones that are usually examined by intelligence tests. There are others, however, that may be as important or more important. Determination and perseverance make intelligence effective and useful. Artistic talent, such as proficiency in art or music, and creativity, the ability to use thought and imagination to produce original ideas, are difficult to measure but are certainly part of intelligence.

i. quotient, I.Q., a numerical expression of intellectual capacity obtained by multiplying the mental age of the subject, ascertained by testing, by 100 and dividing by his chronologic age.

intensimeter (in″ten-sim′ĕ-ter) a device for measuring intensity of roentgen rays.

intention (in-ten′shun) a manner of HEALING.

inter- word element [L.], *between.*

interarticular (in″ter-ar-tik′u-lar) between articulating surfaces.

interatrial (in″ter-a′tre-al) between the atria of the heart.

interbrain (in′ter-brān) 1. thalamencephalon. 2. diencephalon.

intercalary (in-ter′kah-ler″e) inserted between; interposed.

intercalated (in-ter′kah-la″ted) inserted between.

intercartilaginous (in″ter-kar″tĭ-laj′ĭ-nus) between, or connecting, cartilages.

intercellular (in″ter-sel′u-lar) between the cells.

interchondral (in″ter-kon′dral) intercartilaginous.

intercilium (in″ter-sil′e-um) the space between the eyebrows.

interclavicular (in″ter-klah-vik′u-lar) between the clavicles.

intercondylar (in″ter-kon′dĭ-lar) between two condyles.

intercostal (in″ter-kos′tal) between two ribs.

intercourse (in′ter-kōrs) mutual exchange.

sexual i., coitus.

intercricothyrotomy (in″ter-kri″ko-thi-rot′o-me) incision of the larynx through the lower part of the fibroelastic membrane of the larynx (cricothyroid membrane); inferior laryngotomy.

intercurrent (in″ter-kur′ent) occurring during the course of, as a disease occurring during the course of an already existing disease.

interdigital (in″ter-dij′ĭ-tal) between two digits (fingers or toes).

interdigitation (in″ter-dij″ĭ-ta′shun) 1. an interlocking of parts by finger-like processes. 2. one of a set of finger-like processes.

interface (in′ter-fās) in chemistry, the boundry between two systems or phases.

interfascicular (in″ter-fah-sik′u-lar) between adjacent fascicles.

interfemoral (in″ter-fem′o-ral) between the thighs.

interferon (in″ter-fēr′on) a class of small soluble proteins released by cells invaded by virus, which induces in noninfected cells the formation of an antiviral protein that inhibits viral multiplication. The production of interferon is not restricted to viral infections; it may be released in response to a wide variety of inducers, such as certain nonviral and infectious agents, e.g., rickettsiae, bacteria, and synthetic polymers.

interfibrillar (in″ter-fi′bril-ar) between fibrils.

interfilar (in″ter-fi′lar) between or among the fibrils of a reticulum.

interictal (in″ter-ik′tal) occurring between attacks or paroxysms.

interkinesis (in″ter-ki-ne′sis) the period between the first and second divisions in meiosis.

interlobar (in″ter-lo′bar) between lobes.

interlobitis (in″ter-lo-bi′tis) inflammation of the pleura between lobes of the lung; called also interlobular pleurisy.

interlobular (in″ter-lob′u-lar) between lobules.

intermaxillary (in″ter-mak′sĭ-ler″e) between the maxillae.

intermediate (in″ter-me′de-at) 1. between; intervening; resembling, in part, each of two extremes. 2. a substance formed in a chemical process that is essential to formation of the end product of the process.

intermedin (in″ter-me′din) melanocyte-stimulating hormone.

intermedius (in″ter-me′de-us) [L.] intermediate; in anatomy, denoting a structure lying between a lateral and a medial structure.

intermeningeal (in″ter-mě-nin′je-al) between the meninges.

intermittent (in″ter-mit′ent) marked by alternating periods of activity and inactivity.

i. positive-pressure breathing (IPPB), a form of respiratory therapy utilizing a VENTILATOR for the treatment of patients with inadequate breathing. As the name implies, the treatment involves application of pressure only during the inspiratory phase, its purpose being to assist the patient to breathe more deeply. Among the types of ventilators used in IPPB therapy are the Bird Mark VII, the Bennett PR-2, and the RETIC automatic respirator. The RETIC is an example of the newer, more simply designed units that are generally smaller in size and are portable.

IPPB may be prescribed for a patient who is unable to cough effectively (as during the postoperative period), and for one who is suffering from a chronic obstructive or restrictive pulmonary disease and whose breathing is further impaired by either infection or trauma. IPPB is frequently used as a means of providing deep pulmonary AEROSOL therapy, in the relief of bronchospasms and in the removal of bronchial secretions.

Overenthusiastic use of IPPB at the time ventilators made their debut on the medical scene has led some to question the superiority of this treatment over such less expensive and more conservative measures as POSTURAL DRAINAGE and instruction of the patient in effective deep breathing and coughing techniques. It is now generally agreed that IPPB offers an acceptable alternative to these techniques when the patient is unable or unwilling to make the necessary effort to ventilate his lungs adequately. There remain, however, inherent risks in IPPB and no one should attempt to administer assisted ventilation without extensive knowledge and operational skill in the use of a ventilator.

intermural (in″ter-mu′ral) between the walls of an organ or organs.

intermuscular (in″ter-mus′ku-lar) between muscles.

intern (in′tern) a medical graduate serving and residing in a hospital preparatory to being licensed to practice medicine.

internal (in-ter′nal) situated or occurring within or on the inside; in anatomy, many structures formerly called internal are now termed medial.

internalization (in-ter″nal-ĭ-za′shun) a mental mechanism whereby certain external attributes, attitudes, or standards are unconsciously taken as one's own.

internatal (in″ter-na′tal) between the nates, or buttocks.

interneuron (in″ter-nu′ron) a neuron between the primary afferent neuron and the final motor neuron (motoneuron).

internist (in-ter′nist) a specialist in internal medicine.

internode (in′ter-nōd) a space between two nodes.

internship (in′tern-ship) the position of an intern in a hospital, or the term of service.

internuclear (in″ter-nu′kle-ar) situated between nuclei or between nuclear layers of the retina.

internuncial (in″ter-nun′shal) transmitting impulses between two different parts.

internus (in-ter′nus) [L.] internal; in anatomy, denoting a structure nearer to the center of an organ or part.

interoceptor (in″ter-o-sep′tor) a sensory nerve terminal located in and transmitting impulses from the viscera. adj., **interocep′tive.**

interofective (in″ter-o-fek′tiv) affecting the interior of the organism—a term applied to the autonomic nervous system.

interolivary (in″ter-ol′ĭ-ver″e) between the olivary bodies.

interorbital (in″ter-or′bĭ-tal) between the orbits.

interosseous (in″ter-os′e-us) between two bones.

interpalpebral (in″ter-pal′pě-bral) between the eyelids.

interparietal (in″ter-pah-ri′ě-tal) 1. intermural. 2. between the parietal bones.

interparoxysmal (in″ter-par″ok-siz′mal) between paroxysms.

interphalangeal (in″ter-fah-lan′je-al) situated between two contiguous phalanges.

interphase (in′ter-fāz) the interval between two successive cell divisions, during which the chromosomes are not individually distinguishable.

interplant (in′ter-plant) an embryonic part isolated by transference to an indifferent environment provided by another embryo.

interpolation (in-ter″po-la′shun) 1. surgical transplantation of tissue. 2. the determination of intermediate values in a series on the basis of observed values.

interproximal (in″ter-prok′sĭ-mal) between two adjoining surfaces.

interpubic (in″ter-pu′bik) between the pubic bones.

interpupillary (in″ter-pu′pĭ-ler″e) between the pupils.

interscapular (in″ter-skap′u-lar) between the scapulae.

intersectio (in″ter-sek′she-o), pl. *intersectio′nes* [L.] intersection.

i. tendin'ea, a fibrous band traversing the belly of a muscle, dividing it into two parts; called also inscriptio tendinea.

intersection (in"ter-sek'shun) a site at which one structure crosses another.

intersex (in'ter-seks) 1. intersexuality. 2. an individual who exhibits intersexuality.

female i., a female pseudohermaphrodite.

male i., a male pseudohermaphrodite.

true i., a true hermaphrodite.

intersexuality (in"ter-seks"u-al'ĭ-te) an intermingling, in varying degrees, of the characters of each sex, including physical form, reproductive tissue, and sexual behavior, in one individual, as a result of some flaw in embryonic development (see also HERMAPHRODITISM and PSEUDOHERMAPHRODITISM). adj., **intersex'ual.**

interspace (in'ter-spās) a space between similar structures.

interspinal (in"ter-spi'nal) between two spinous processes.

interstice (in-ter'stis) an interval, space, or gap in a tissue or structure.

interstitial (in"ter-stish'al) pertaining to or situated betweeen parts or in the interspaces of a tissue.

i. cell-stimulating hormone, luteinizing hormone.

i. cells, the cells of the connective tissue of the ovary or the testis (Leydig's cells), which furnish the internal secretion of those structures.

i. fluid, the extracellular fluid bathing most tissues, excluding the fluid within the lymph and blood vessels.

i. plasma cell pneumonia, a form affecting infants and debilitated persons, including those receiving certain drugs, in which cellular detritus containing plasma cells appears in lung tissue; it is caused by *Pneumocystis carinii.*

i. tissue, connective tissue between the cellular elements of a structure.

interstitium (in"ter-stish'ĭ-um) 1. interstice. 2. interstitial tissue.

intertransverse (in"ter-trans-vers') situated between or connecting the transverse processes of the vertebrae.

intertrigo (in"ter-tri'go) an erythematous skin eruption occurring on apposed surfaces of the skin, as the creases of the neck, folds of the groin and armpit, and beneath pendulous breasts. It is caused by moisture, warmth, friction, sweat retention, and infectious agents. Symptoms include burning, itching, moistness, redness, maceration, and sometimes erosions, fissures, and exudations. It is most likely to occur in obese persons, and particularly in those with diabetes mellitus. Intertrigo is most prevalent in hot and humid regions.

In treatment of intertrigo, the apposing body surfaces should be thoroughly cleansed and dried, and then sprinkled with talcum powder containing zinc oxide. Sometimes gauze strips between the adjacent skin surfaces will keep the area dry and exposed to air.

intertubular (in"ter-tu'bu-lar) between tubules.

interureteral, interureteric (in"ter-u-re'ter-al; in"ter-u"rĕ-ter'ik) between the ureters.

intervaginal (in"ter-vaj'ĭ-nal) between sheaths.

interval (in'ter-val) the space between two objects or parts; the lapse of time between two events.

atrioventricular i., A–V i., P–R i.

c.-a. i., cardioarterial i., the time between the apex beat and arterial pulsation.

lucid i., a brief period of remission of symptoms in a psychosis.

postsphygmic i., the short period (0.08 second) of ventricular diastole, after the sphygmic period, and lasting until the atrioventricular valves open. Called also postsphygmic period.

P–R i., in electrocardiography, the time between the onset of the P wave (atrial activity) and the QRS complex (ventricular activity).

presphygmic i., the first phase of ventricular systole, being the period (0.04–0.06 sec.) immediately after closure of the atrioventricular valves and lasting until the semilunar valves open. Called also presphygmic period.

QRST i., Q–T i., the duration of ventricular electrical activity.

intervalvular (in"ter-val'vu-lar) between valves.

intervascular (in"ter-vas'ku-lar) between blood vessels.

interventricular (in"ter-ven-trik'u-lar) between the ventricles of the heart.

intervertebral (in"ter-ver'tĕ-bral) between two vertebrae.

i. disk, the layer of fibrocartilage between the bodies of adjoining vertebrae (see also slipped DISK).

intervillous (in"ter-vil'us) between or among villi.

intestinal (in-tes'tĭ-nal) pertaining to the intestine.

i. bypass, a surgical procedure in which all but a few inches of the proximal jejunum and terminal ileum are bypassed in order to bring about malabsorption of digested food. The procedure is done for the purpose of correcting obesity. Also called jejunoileal bypass or shunt. Patients having this type of surgery must be meticulously managed so that severe nutritional CIRRHOSIS and serious loss of water and electrolytes are avoided.

i. flu, a popular term for what may be any of several disorders of the stomach and intestinal tract. The symptoms are nausea, diarrhea, abdominal cramps, and fever.

During the acute stage all foods should be avoided. Carbonated soft drinks such as ginger ale or cola can be taken in moderation to relieve the nausea. Cola is also useful in offsetting the effects of the diarrhea.

When the symptoms subside, the diet should at first be confined to liquids and soft, bland foods. Milk and dairy products, butter, and fats generally, fruits and greens should be avoided completely until the patient is free of all symptoms. If the symptoms persist a physician should be consulted.

i. obstruction, any hindrance to the passage of the intestinal contents. Causes may be mechanical or neural or both. Some of the more common mechanical causes are HERNIA, ADHESIONS of the peritoneum, VOLVULUS, INTUSSUSCEPTION, malignant or benign tumor, congenital defect, and local inflammation. Failure of peristalsis (adynamic ILEUS) is frequently associated with PERITONITIS; it also may occur with GALLSTONES, uremia, heavy metal poisoning, infection, and spinal injury.

SYMPTOMS. The most characteristic symptoms are abdominal pain, vomiting, and distention. The symptoms may be mild at first and in its early stages the condition can be confused with less serious disorders of the intestinal tract. Under no circumstances should the patient be given a laxative or purgative because it will aggravate the situation. If the obstruction continues the patient suffers from dehydration and shock because of inadequate absorption of fluids, electrolytes, and nutrients from the intestinal tract. If the bowel becomes strangulated and circulation to the bowel wall is obstructed, the patient shows signs of peritonitis with extreme tenderness and rigidity of the abdomen.

TREATMENT. The basic steps of treatment are decompression of the intestine, replacement of fluids and electrolytes, and removal of the cause of the obstruction.

Decompression is accomplished by INTUBATION with a special tube (usually the MILLER-ABBOTT TUBE) designed to reach past the pyloric sphincter and into the intestine. Constant suction is then applied to remove accumulations of gas and liquids.

Fluids, sodium chloride, and glucose are administered intravenously at a specific rate as ordered by the physician. Transfusions of whole blood plasma may be given as necessary to restore normal blood values.

Surgical removal of the cause of obstruction is usually necessary in cases of complete obstruction. If there is no evidence of strangulation of the bowel, the surgeon may choose to postpone surgery until dehydration and shock have been overcome and a normal electrolyte balance is restored. The type of surgical procedure performed depends on the cause of the obstruction and whether or not the intestine is gangrenous. In some cases a COLOSTOMY may be necessary before the damaged portion of the bowel is removed. A surgical incision into the cecum with insertion of a drainage tube (cecostomy) may be done when intestinal intubation is not successful in relieving distention.

PATIENT CARE. Observations of the patient with intestinal obstruction include location and character of abdominal pain, degree of distention, and occurrence or absence of bowel movements or passing of flatus. Should defecation occur a specimen is saved for examination and laboratory analysis. If there is vomiting, the amount and special characteristics of the vomitus should be noted and recorded. In severe cases of obstruction of the small bowel the vomitus may contain fecal material because of the reversal of peristalsis and forcing of the intestinal contents backward into the stomach.

Foods and fluids by mouth are restricted. If a Miller-Abbott tube has been inserted it should be irrigated as necessary to keep the lumen open so that intestinal decompression by suction siphonage is achieved. Frequent mouth care is necessary to relieve the dryness and foul taste that accompanies intestinal obstruction and vomiting.

Urinary output is measured and recorded because there is a possibility that pressure on the bladder will produce urinary retention. In some cases catheterization may be necessary.

Preoperative Care. If conservative measures fail to relieve the obstruction, or if the bowel has become strangulated, surgery is indicated. Before the operation the surgeon may order a low enema. The entire abdomen is shaved. Suction siphonage is continued and the intestinal tube is left in place when the patient goes to the operating room.

Postoperative Care. Routine postoperative care of the patient with abdominal surgery is indicated. Specific measures depend on the type of surgical procedure done. Suction siphonage is usually continued until peristalsis resumes. The passing of flatus or feces should be noted on the patient's chart because it indicates a return of normal peristaltic movements of the bowel. In some cases a cecostomy tube or rectal tube is inserted during surgery; the tube is attached to a drainage bottle and the amount and type of material collected in the bottle are recorded. If there is evidence that the tube has become obstructed the surgeon should be notified, because he may wish to order saline irrigations to keep the tube open and draining freely. The skin around the site of insertion of a cecostomy tube should be protected with gauze impregnated with petrolatum. The area must be washed frequently to avoid erosion of the skin by intestinal contents leaking around the tube.

See also COLOSTOMY for patient care after that procedure.

i. tract, the small and large intestines in continuity. The long, coiled tube of the intestine is the part of the digestive system where most of the digestion of food takes place.

The small intestine has three parts: the duodenum (connected to the stomach), the jejunum, and the ileum. The small intestine is small only in diameter; in length it is about 20 feet.

The large intestine, just below the ileum of the small intestine, is about 5 feet long. It is made up of the cecum (to which the appendix is attached), the colon (comprising the ascending, transverse, and descending colon and the sigmoid), and the rectum.

The digestion of food is completed in the small intestine. The digested food is absorbed through the walls of the small intestine into the blood (see also DIGESTIVE SYSTEM).

Indigestible parts of the food pass into the large intestine. Here the liquid from the wastes is gradually absorbed back into the body through the intestinal walls. The waste itself is formed into fairly solid feces and pushed down into the rectum for evacuation.

Among the disorders of the intestinal tract are the disturbances of function, such as DIARRHEA, CONSTIPATION, and COLITIS; the organic diseases, ULCERATIVE COLITIS, APPENDICITIS, and ILEITIS; and communicable diseases, such as DYSENTERY. Colitis is characterized by constipation, sometimes alternating with diarrhea. Ulcerative colitis is a disorder in which ulcers may appear in the wall of the large intestine. Ileitis is a disorder of the ileum, or lower portion of the small intestine. A symptom of both is diarrhea. Dysentery, which is characterized by diarrhea, is the result of infection by bacteria, viruses, or various parasites.

intestine (in-tes′tin) the part of the alimentary tract extending from the pyloric opening of the stomach to the anus. It is a membranous tube, comprising the small intestine and large intestine; called also bowel and gut (see also INTESTINAL TRACT, and see Plates 9 and 10).

intestinum (in″tes-ti′num), pl. *intesti′na* [L.] intestine.

intima (in′tĭ-mah) the innermost coat of a blood vessel; called also tunica intima. adj., **in′timal.**

intimitis (in″tĭ-mi′tis) endarteritis; inflammation of the innermost coat of an artery.

Intocostrin (in″to-kos′trin) trademark for a preparation of tubocurarine, a curare derivative used as a skeletal muscle relaxant.

intolerance (in-tol′er-ans) inability to withstand or

consume; inability to absorb or metabolize nutrients.

intorsion (in-tor′shun) tilting of the upper part of the vertical meridian of the eye toward the midline of the face.

intoxication (in-tok″sĭ-ka′shun) 1. poisoning; the state of being poisoned. 2. the condition produced by excessive use of alcohol.

Intoxication in the sense of poisoning can be caused by carbon monoxide, lead, or other toxic agents. Some medications can be poisonous in excessive doses. Intoxication can also occur in persons who have an allergy to medications such as penicillin, to various serums, and to other substances. Any type of drug addiction is medically recognized as a state of intoxication. In addition to those mentioned there are the commonly recognized types of poisoning, such as those caused by chemicals and food contaminants.

Acid intoxication and alkaline intoxication are ACIDOSIS and ALKALOSIS, respectively, of a severe grade.

Intoxication in the sense of drunkenness occurs when the concentration of alcohol in the blood reaches about one-tenth of 1 per cent. (See also ALCOHOLISM.)

intra- word element [L.], *inside of; within.*

intra-abdominal (in″trah-ab-dom′ĭ-nal) within the abdomen.

intra-arterial (in″trah-ar-te′re-al) within an artery.

intra-articular (in″trah-ar-tik′u-lar) within a joint.

intracanalicular (in″trah-kan″ah-lik′u-lar) within canaliculi.

intracapsular (in″trah-kap′su-lar) within a capsule.

intracardiac (in″trah-kar′de-ak) within the heart.

intracartilaginous (in″trah-kar″tĭ-laj′ĭ-nus) within a cartilage.

intracellular (in″trah-sel′u-lar) within a cell or cells.

intracervical (in″trah-ser′vĭ-kal) within the canal of the cervix uteri.

intracisternal (in″trah-sis-ter′nal) within a subarachnoid cistern.

intracranial (in″trah-kra′ne-al) within the cranium.

i. pressure screw, a device for measuring the degree of pressure being exerted within the subarachnoid space. Monitoring can be done on a continuous or an intermittent basis. The screw is inserted through a burr hole in the frontal area of the skull just behind the hairline and a capped 3-way stop cock is attached to the pressure screw. High-pressure tubing joined to the screw leads to a manometer on which pressure changes can be directly visualized, or to equipment which displays the information on an oscilloscope or graph. Readings on changes in intracranial pressure can thus be obtained by watching the manometer or by monitoring the oscilloscope or graphic display. When the manometer is used, point zero is established after positioning the patient with the head of the bed elevated 30 degrees.

Through the use of the intracranial pressure screw, elevations in intracranial pressure can be detected before changes in the vital signs and other symptoms of increased pressure become apparent. In this way measures can be taken to reduce the pressure before irreversible damage is done to the brain tissue.

The major risks of the intracranial pressure screw are infection and leakage of cerebrospinal fluid, either of which necessitates removal of the screw.

intracutaneous (in″trah-ku-ta′ne-us) within the substance of the skin.

i. injection, an injection into the corium or substance of the skin; called also intradermal injection (see also intracutaneous INJECTION).

intracystic (in″trah-sis′tik) within the bladder or a cyst.

intradermal (in″trah-der′mal) within the dermis.

i. injection, intracutaneous injection.

intraductal (in″trah-duk′tal) within a duct.

intradural (in″trah-du′ral) within or beneath the dura mater.

intrafusal (in″trah-fu′zal) pertaining to the striated fibers within a muscle spindle.

intrahepatic (in″trah-hĕ-pat′ik) within the liver.

intralesional (in″trah-le′zhun-al) occurring in or introduced directly into a localized lesion.

intralobar (in′trah-lo′bar) within a lobe.

intralocular (in″trah-lok′u-lar) within the loculi of a structure.

intraluminal (in″trah-lu′mĭ-nal) within the lumen of a tubular structure.

intramedullary (in″trah-med′u-lār″e) within (1) the spinal cord, (2) the medulla oblongata, or (3) the marrow cavity of a bone.

intramural (in″trah-mu′ral) within the wall of an organ.

intramuscular (in″trah-mus′ku-lar) within the muscular substance.

i. injection, an injection made into the substance of a muscle (see also intramuscular INJECTION).

intraocular (in″trah-ok′u-lar) within the eye.

intraoperative (in″trah-op′er-a″tiv) occurring during a surgical operation.

intraoral (in″trah-o′ral) within the mouth.

intraorbital (in″trah-or′bĭ-tal) within the orbit.

intraparietal (in″trah-pah-ri′ĕ-tal) 1. intramural. 2. within the parietal region of the brain.

intrapartum (in″trah-par′tum) occurring during childbirth or during delivery.

intraperitoneal (in″trah-per″ĭ-to-ne′al) within the peritoneal cavity.

intrapleural (in″trah-ploo′ral) within the pleura.

intrapsychic (in″trah-si′kik) taking place within the mind.

intrapulmonary (in″trah-pul′mo-ner″e) within the substance of the lung.

intraspinal (in″trah-spi′nal) within the substance of the spinal column.

intrasternal (in″trah-ster′nal) within the sternum.

intrathecal (in″trah-the′kal) within a sheath; through the theca of the spinal cord into the subarachnoid space.

intrathoracic (in″trah-tho-ras′ik) within the thorax.

intratracheal (in″trah-tra′ke-al) endotracheal.

intratubal (in″trah-tu′bal) within a tube.

intratympanic (in″trah-tim-pan′ik) within the tympanic cavity.

intrauterine (in″trah-u′ter-in) within the uterus.

i. contraceptive device, IUD, a mechanical device inserted into the uterine cavity for the purpose of contraception. These devices are made of metallic, plastic, or other substances and are manufactured in various sizes and shapes. Examples include the Hall-Stone ring, Lippes loop, Brinberg bow, and Margulies coil. Their exact effect is not known but it is believed that they increase mobility of the ovum through the uterine tube and interfere with implantation of the fertilized ovum.

After the IUD has been inserted, the patient is instructed to have yearly follow-up examinations. Contraindications to insertion include recent pelvic infection, suspected pregnancy, cervical stenosis, myoma of the uterus, and abnormal uterine bleeding. They are not recommended for women who have never been pregnant because of the severe pain and bleeding that they produce in the majority of these patients.

intravasation (in-trav″ah-za′shun) the entrance of foreign material into vessels.

intravascular (in″trah-vas′ku-lar) within a vessel or vessels.

intravenous (in″trah-ve′nus) within a vein.

i. infusion, administration of fluids through a vein; called also phleboclysis, venoclysis, and intravenous feeding. This method of feeding is used most often when a patient is suffering from severe dehydration and is unable to drink fluids because he is unconscious, recovering from an operation, unable to swallow normally, or vomiting persistently. Medications are also given directly into the veins when necessary (see also intravenous INJECTION).

The fluid to be infused is prescribed by the physician. Within the past decade intravenous therapy has progressed rapidly and is no longer limited to replacement of body fluids and electrolyte supplements. Many medications are now administered by intravenous infusion, and the danger of drug incompatibility is a very real hazard. Incompatibility charts are not entirely reliable as sources of information about chemical interaction of drug additives combined in an intravenous infusion. For this reason admixing should be done by a clinical pharmacologist. Intravenous antibiotics should be mixed only with electrolytes. Because of their local irritating effects on the vein, concentrated doses of potassium chloride and dextrose solutions with a concentration higher than 10 per cent should not be given through a peripheral vein. (See also HYPERALIMENTATION.)

The rate of flow is regulated by a control clip on the tubing close to the container and there is a glass or plastic drip regulator in the line through which the rate at which the fluid is flowing from the container can be observed. It is extremely important that the intravenous solution is administered at the proper rate of flow; otherwise the patient may become overhydrated or underhydrated. (See also FLUID BALANCE.)

PATIENT CARE. Before the intravenous infusion is begun the patient's arm or leg is immobilized in a comfortable position, preferably with a special board designed for this purpose. The tape, gauze or canvas straps used to hold the limb stationary are applied snugly, but not so tight as to impede circulation. The label of each container of fluid or medication is very carefully checked against the physician's orders before it is connected to the infusion apparatus. Fluids should be checked for precipitation and cloudiness and discarded if either of these is detected. If there is no vacuum in the bottle, it should be discarded because of the likelihood of contamination.

The size of the needle or catheter is chosen so that it is neither too large nor too small for insertion into the vein selected for the infusion. Local preparation of the site of the venipuncture is important in the prevention of infection. Alcohol swabs are being replaced with antiseptics that have a providone-iodine base. The cleansed area must be completely dry before the needle is inserted.

After the vein has been entered, the needle or catheter should be secured with tape and the tubing coiled and taped along the leg or arm so that tension on the needle is avoided. The bottle and tubing should be changed every 24 hours and an indwelling intravenous catheter is replaced at least every 72 hours.

The site of venipuncture is closely watched for signs of infiltration. If swelling occurs or the patient complains of severe pain in the area the needle should be removed. If the flow of solution stops, this may indicate pressure on the tip of the needle and may be relieved by gentle manipulation of the needle. The area also is watched for signs of phlebitis. These include redness, swelling, heat, and induration around the site. When these signs appear the catheter is removed and a new site is chosen.

Following completion of the intravenous infusion the tubing is clamped off and the needle or catheter is quickly withdrawn. Before attempting to remove the needle, it is necessary to remove all tape from the needle or the catheter. Immediately after the needle is removed a dry, sterile gauze sponge is gently pressed down on the site to control leakage of blood and prevent the formation of a hematoma. A small sterile bandage is then placed over the site to prevent infection.

The amount and type of solution, time the infusion was started and completed, and any untoward reaction of the patient are recorded on the patient's chart.

intraventricular (in″trah-ven-trik′u-lar) within a ventricle.

intravital (in″trah-vi′tal) occurring during life.

intra vitam (in′trah vi′tam) [L.] during life.

intrinsic (in-trin′sik) situated entirely within, or pertaining exclusively to, a part.

i. factor, a glycoprotein secreted by the gastric glands, which is necessary for the assimilation and absorption of cyanocobalamin (extrinsic factor, vitamin B_{12}) contained in food, an essential for the production of the antianemia factor. It is absent in PERNICIOUS ANEMIA.

introitus (in-tro′ĭ-tus), pl. *intro′itus* [L.] the entrance to a cavity or space.

introjection (in″tro-jek′shun) a mental mechanism in which loved or hated external objects are unconsciously and symbolically taken within oneself.

intromission (in″tro-mish′un) the entrance of one part or object into another.

introspection (in″tro-spek′shun) contemplation or observation of one's thoughts and feelings; self-analysis. adj., **introspec′tive.**

introsusception (in″tro-sŭ-sep′shun) intussusception.

introversion (in″tro-ver′zhun) 1. the turning outside in, more or less completely, of an organ. 2. preoccupation with oneself, with reduction of interest in the outside world.

introvert (in′tro-vert) a person whose interests are turned inward upon himself.

intubate (in′tu-bāt) to perform intubation.

intubation (in″tu-ba′shun) the insertion of a tube, as into the larynx. The purpose of intubation varies with the location and type of tube inserted; generally the procedure is done to allow for drainage, to maintain an open airway, or for the administration of anesthetics or OXYGEN.

Intubation into the stomach or intestine is done to remove gastric or intestinal contents for the relief or prevention of distention, or to obtain a specimen for analysis. A rubber or plastic nasogastric tube is introduced through the nose and into the stomach. The shorter tubes designed for intubation into the stomach include Levin tubes and Salem sumps. Longer tubes include the Harris, Cantor, MILLER-ABBOTT, and Abbott-Rawson tubes, all of which are designed to pass through the stomach and into the small intestine. The tubes usually are attached to a suction apparatus so that gas and liquids can be removed. A nasogastric tube also may be inserted for the purpose of providing nourishment (see also TUBE FEEDING).

The SENGSTAKEN-BLAKEMORE TUBE is a triple-lumen tube with an esophageal balloon, a gastric balloon, and gastric tubes with sucking ports at its tip. It is used to stop hemorrhage from gastric and esophageal varices.

A tube may be inserted in the common bile duct to allow for drainage of bile from the ducts that drain the liver after surgery on the gallbladder or the common bile duct.

Endotracheal intubation can be achieved by insertion of an ENDOTRACHEAL TUBE via the mouth or

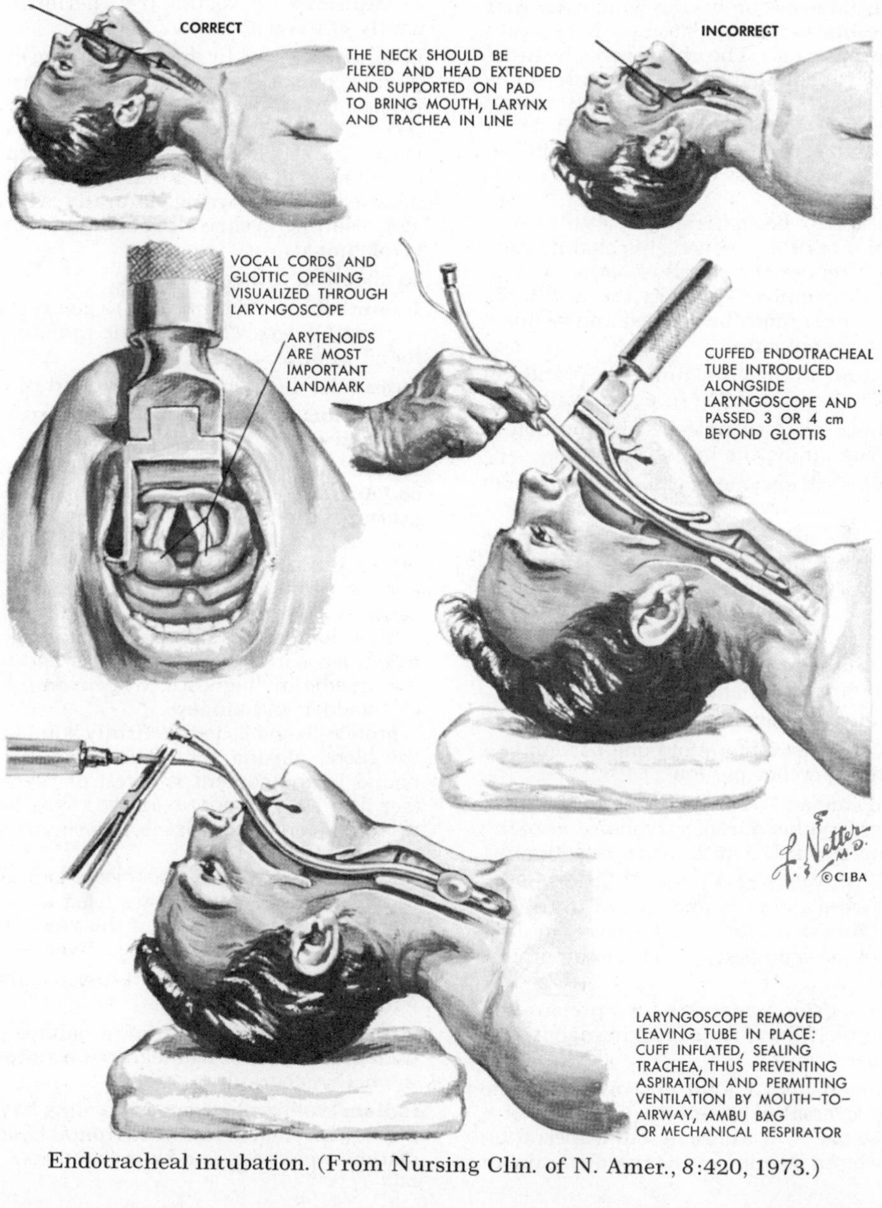
CORRECT
THE NECK SHOULD BE FLEXED AND HEAD EXTENDED AND SUPPORTED ON PAD TO BRING MOUTH, LARYNX AND TRACHEA IN LINE
INCORRECT
VOCAL CORDS AND GLOTTIC OPENING VISUALIZED THROUGH LARYNGOSCOPE
ARYTENOIDS ARE MOST IMPORTANT LANDMARK
CUFFED ENDOTRACHEAL TUBE INTRODUCED ALONGSIDE LARYNGOSCOPE AND PASSED 3 OR 4 cm BEYOND GLOTTIS
F. Netter M.D.
©CIBA
LARYNGOSCOPE REMOVED LEAVING TUBE IN PLACE: CUFF INFLATED, SEALING TRACHEA, THUS PREVENTING ASPIRATION AND PERMITTING VENTILATION BY MOUTH–TO–AIRWAY, AMBU BAG OR MECHANICAL RESPIRATOR

Endotracheal intubation. (From Nursing Clin. of N. Amer., 8:420, 1973.)

nose. It is done for the purpose of assuring patency of the upper airway. The tube is inserted (usually after a laryngoscope has been introduced to serve as a guide) between the vocal cords, through the larynx, and far enough into the trachea that the cuff is beyond the larynx. TRACHEOSTOMY is also a form of endotracheal intubation.

intumescence (in″tu-mes′ens) 1. a swelling, normal or abnormal. 2. the process of swelling. adj., **intumes′cent.**

intussusception (in″tŭ-sŭ-sep′shun) 1. prolapse of one part of the intestine into the lumen of an immediately adjacent part, causing INTESTINAL OBSTRUCTION. 2. the reception into an organism of matter, such as food, and its transformation into new protoplasm.

Intussusception is a rather rare disorder. Most cases occur in children during the first year of life, and some cases occur in the second year, but very few thereafter. The condition may be caused by a growth in the intestine or by any condition that causes the intestine to contract strongly. Frequently there is no obvious cause. The child seems healthy, yet paroxysms of abdominal pain begin, with vomiting and restlessness. Within 12 to 24 hours bloody mucus is passed by rectum. On the second day a high fever may appear. Death can occur within 2 to 4 days after the onset unless the condition is remedied by surgery.

The diagnosis may be confirmed by BARIUM TEST in the form of a barium enema. This examination will frequently reduce the intussusception and in some cases will completely correct the condition. Treatment by surgery may be advised and ordinarily gives a permanent cure.

intussusceptum (in″tŭ-sŭ-sep′tum) the portion of intestine that has prolapsed in intussusception.

intussuscipiens (in″tŭ-sŭ-sip′e-ens) the portion of the intestine containing the intussusceptum.

inulase (in′u-lās) an enzyme that converts inulin to fructose.

inulin (in′u-lin) a starch occurring in the rhizome of certain plants, which on hydrolysis yields fructose. It is used as a measure of glomerular function in tests of renal function.

inunction (in-ungk′shun) 1. the act of anointing or applying an ointment by friction. 2. an ointment made with lanolin as a menstruum.

in utero (in u′ter-o) [L.] within the uterus.

invaginate (in-vaj′ĭ-nāt) to infold one portion of a structure within another portion.

invagination (in-vag″ĭ-na′shun) 1. the infolding of one part within another part of a structure, as of the blastula during gastrulation. 2. intussusception.

invasiveness (in-va′siv-nes) 1. the ability of microorganisms to enter the body and spread in the tissues. 2. the ability to infiltrate and actively destroy surrounding tissue, a property of malignant tumors. adj., **inva′sive.**

Inversine (in-ver′sēn) trademark for a preparation of mecamylamine, a ganglionic blocking agent used as an antihypertensive.

inversion (in-ver′zhun) 1. a turning inward, inside out, or other reversal of the normal relation of a part. 2. homosexuality. 3. a chromosomal aberration due to the inverted reunion of the middle segment after breakage of a chromosome at two points, resulting in a change in sequence of genes or nucleotides.

carbohydrate i., the hydrolysis of disaccharides or polysaccharides to monosaccharides.

invert (in′vert) a homosexual.

invertase (in-ver′tās) β- fructofuranosidase.

invertebrate (in-ver′tĕ-brāt) 1. having no vertebral column. 2. any animal that has no vertebral column.

invertin (in-ver′tin) β-fructofuranosidase.

investment (in-vest′ment) material in which a denture, tooth, crown, or model for a dental restoration is enclosed for curing, soldering, or casting, or the process of such enclosure.

inveterate (in-vet′er-it) confirmed and chronic; long-established and difficult to cure.

in vitro (in ve′tro) [L.] within a glass; observable in a test tube; in an artificial environment.

in vivo (in ve′vo) [L.] within the living body.

involucrum (in″vo-lu′krum), pl. *involu′cra* [L.] a covering or sheath, as of a sequestrum.

involuntary (in-vol′un-tār″e) performed independently of the will.

involution (in″vo-lu′shun) 1. a rolling or turning inward. 2. one of the movements involved in the gastrulation of many animals. 3. a retrograde change of the entire body or in a particular organ, as the retrograde changes in the female genital organs that result in normal size after delivery. 4. the progressive degeneration occurring naturally with advancing age, resulting in shriveling of organs or tissues. adj., **involu′tional.**

Io chemical symbol, *ionium.*

Iodamoeba (i-o″dah-me′bah) a genus of amebas, including *I. buetsch′lii,* parasitic in man, and *I. su′is,* found in pigs.

iodide (i′o-dīd) a binary compound of iodine.

iodination (i″o-dĭ-na′shun) the incorporation or addition of iodine in a compound.

iodine (i′o-dīn) a chemical element, atomic number 53, atomic weight 126.904, symbol I. (See table of ELEMENTS.) Iodine is essential in nutrition, being especially prevalent in the colloid of the THYROID GLAND. It is used in the treatment of HYPOTHYROIDISM and as a topical antiseptic. Iodine is a frequent cause of poisoning (see also IODISM).

Since iodine salts are opaque to x-rays, they can be combined with other compounds and used as contrast media in diagnostic x-ray examinations of the gallbladder and kidneys.

protein-bound i., iodine firmly bound to protein in the blood plasma. The determination of protein-bound iodine content is a test of thyroid function (see also PROTEIN-BOUND IODINE TEST). Iodine makes up 65 per cent of thyroxine, a hormone produced by the thyroid gland.

radioactive i., a RADIOISOTOPE of iodine; called also radioiodine. ^{131}I and ^{125}I are used in the diagnosis and treatment of disease of the THYROID GLAND and is scintiscanning of the lungs, liver, etc.

iodinophilous (i″o-din-of′ĭ-lus) easily stainable with iodine.

iodipamide (i″o-dip′ah-mīd) a radiopaque medium used in the form of its meglumine and sodium salts in cholecystography.

iodism (i′o-dizm) chronic poisoning by iodine or iodides, with coryza, ptyalism, frontal headache, emaciation, weakness, and skin eruptions.

iodoalphionic acid (i″o-do-al″fe-on′ik) a white or yellowish compound used as a contrast medium in cholecystography.

iodobrassid (i-o″do-bras′id) a compound used in iodide therapy and as a radiopaque medium.

iodochlorhydroxyquin (i″o-do-klōr″hi-drok′sĭ-kwin) a spongy yellowish powder used as a topical anti-infective in the treatment of amebiasis, *Trichomonas vaginalis* infection, and eczema.

iododerma (i″o-do-der′mah) any skin lesion resulting from iodism.

iodoform (i-o′do-form) a topical anti-infective.

iodoglobulin (i″o-do-glob′u-lin) an iodine-containing globulin (protein).

iodomethamate (i-o″do-meth′ah-māt) an acid compound; the sodium salt is used as a radiopaque medium for urography.

iodophilia (i″o-do-fil′e-ah) a reaction shown by leukocytes in certain pathologic conditions, as in toxemia and severe anemia, in which the polymorphonuclears show diffuse brownish coloration when treated with iodine or iodides.

iodophthalein (i″o-do-thal′ēn) an iodine-containing compound; the sodium salt is used as a radiopaque medium in cholecystography.

iodopyracet (i-o″do-pi′rah-set) a radiopaque medium used in urography.

iodotherapy (i″o-do-ther′ah-pe) treatment with iodine or iodides.

iodum (i-o′dum) [L.] iodine.

ion (i′on) an atom or group of atoms having a charge of positive (cation) or negative (anion) electricity by virtue of having gained or lost an electron, and forming one of the elements of an ELECTROLYTE. adj., **ion′ic.**

dipolar i., zwitterion.

hydrogen i., the positively charged hydrogen atom (H^+), which is the positive ion of all acids.

hydroxyl i., the negatively charged group, OH^-, present to excess in alkaline solutions.

ion-exchange resin a high-molecular-weight, insoluble polymer of simple organic compounds with the ability to exchange its attached ions for other ions in the surrounding medium. They are classified as cation- or anion-exchange resins, depending on which ions the resin exchanges. Cation-exchange resins are used to restrict sodium absorption in edematous states; anion-exchange resins are used as antacids in the treatment of ulcers. Ion-exchange resins may also be classified as carboxylic, sulfonic, etc., depending on the nature of the active groups.

ionium (i-o′ne-um) a radioactive isotope of thorium, which emits both alpha and gamma rays; symbol, Io.

ionization (i″on-i-za′shun) 1. the dissociation of a substance in solution into ions. 2. iontophoresis.

i. chamber, an enclosure containing two or more electrodes between which an electric current may be passed when the enclosed gas is ionized by radiation; used for determining the intensity of x-rays and other rays.

ionogen (i-on′o-jen) a substance that may be ionized.

ionometer (i″o-nom′ĕ-ter) an instrument for measuring the intensity or quantity of radiation from an ionizing radiation source.

ionophose (i′o-no-fōz″) a violet phose.

ionotherapy (i″o-no-ther′ah-pe) 1. iontophoresis. 2. treatment with ultraviolet rays.

iontophoresis (i-on″to-fo-re′sis) the introduction of ions of soluble salts into the body by an electric current.

iopanoic acid (i″o-pah-no′ik) an acid used as a radiopaque medium in cholecystography.

iophendylate (i″o-fen′dĭ-lāt) a radiopaque medium used in myelography.

iophenoxic acid (i″o-fen-oks′ik) an acid used as a radiopaque medium in cholecystography.

iothalamate (i″o-thal′ah-māt) a radiopaque medium used in angiography and urography.

iothiouracil (i″o-thi″o-u′rah-sil) a drug that inhibits thyroid activity.

ipecac (ip′ĕ-kak) the dried rhizome and roots of *Cephaelis ipecacuanha* or *Cephaelis acuminata;* used as an emetic or expectorant.

ipomea (i″po-me′ah) the dried root of *Ipomaea orizabensis;* used as a cathartic.

IPPB INTERMITTENT POSITIVE-PRESSURE BREATHING, a principle used in the operation of certain types of VENTILATORS.

Ipral (ip′ral) trademark for preparations of probarbital, an intermediate-acting barbiturate.

iproniazid (i″pro-ni′ah-zid) a monoamine oxidase inhibitor used as a psychic stimulant.

ipsi- word element [L.], *same; self.*

ipsilateral (ip″sĭ-lat′er-al) situated on or affecting the same side.

I.Q. intelligence quotient (see also INTELLIGENCE).

Ir chemical symbol, *iridium.*

Ircon (ir′kon) trademark for a preparation of ferrous fumarate, used as a hematinic.

irid(o)- word element [Gr.], *iris of the eye; a colored circle.*

iridal (i′rĭ-dal) pertaining to the iris.

iridalgia (i″rĭ-dal′je-ah) pain in the iris.

iridauxesis (ir″id-awk-se′sis) thickening of the iris.

iridectomesodialysis (ir″ĭ-dek″to-me″so-di-al′ĭ-sis) excision and separation of adhesions around the inner edge of the iris.

iridectomy (ir″ĭ-dek′to-me) excision of part of the iris.

iridectropium (ir″ĭ-dek-tro′pe-um) eversion of the iris.

iridemia (ir″ĭ-de′me-ah) hemorrhage from the iris.

iridencleisis (ir″ĭ-den-kli′sis) surgical incarceration of a slip of the iris within a corneal or limbal incision to act as a wick for aqueous drainage in glaucoma.

irideremia (ir″ĭ-der-e′me-ah) congenital absence of the iris.

irides (ir′ĭ-dēz) [Gr.] plural of *iris.*

iridescence (ir″ĭ-des′ens) the condition of gleaming with bright and changing colors. adj., **irides′cent.**

iridesis (i-rid′ĕ-sis) repositioning of the pupil by fixation of a sector of iris in a corneal or limbal incision.

iridic (i-rid′ik) pertaining to the iris.

iridium (ĭ-rid′e-um, ī-rid′e-um) a chemical element, atomic number 77, atomic weight 192.2, symbol Ir. (See table of ELEMENTS.)

iridoavulsion (ir″ĭ-do-ah-vul′shun) complete tearing away of the iris from its periphery.

iridocapsulitis (ir″ĭ-do-kap″su-li′tis) inflammation of the iris and lens capsule.

iridocele (i-rid′o-sēl) hernial protrusion of part of the iris through the cornea.

iridochoroiditis (ir″ĭ-do-ko″roi-di′tis) inflammation of the iris and choroid.

iridocoloboma (ir″ĭ-do-kol″o-bo′mah) congenital fissure or coloboma of the iris.

iridoconstrictor (ir″ĭ-do-kon-strik′tor) a muscle element or an agent that acts to constrict the pupil of the eye.

iridocyclectomy (ir″ĭ-do-si-klek′to-me) excision of part of the iris and of the ciliary body.

iridocyclitis (ir″ĭ-do-si-kli′tis) inflammation of the iris and ciliary body.

heterochromic i., a unilateral low-grade form leading to depigmentation of the iris of the affected eye; called also heterochromic uveitis.

iridocyclochoroiditis (ir″ĭ-do-si″klo-ko″roi-di′tis) inflammation of the iris, ciliary body, and choroid.

iridocystectomy (ir″ĭ-do-sis-tek′-to-me) excision of part of the iris to form an artificial pupil.

iridodesis (ir″ĭ-dod′ĕ-sis) iredesis.

iridodialysis (ir″ĭ-do-di-al′ĭ-sis) separation or loosening of the iris from its attachments.

iridodilator (ir″ĭ-do-di-la′tor) a muscle element or an agent that acts to dilate the pupil of the eye.

iridodonesis (ir″ĭ-do-do-ne′sis) tremulousness of the iris on movement of the eye, occurring in subluxation of the lens.

iridokeratitis (ir″ĭ-do-ker″ah-ti′tis) inflammation of the iris and cornea.

iridokinesia, iridokinesis (ir″ĭ-do-ki-ne′ze-ah; ir″ĭ-do-ki-ne′sis) contraction and expansion of the iris. adj., **iridokinet′ic.**

iridoleptynsis (ir″ĭ-do-lep-tin′sis) thinning or atrophy of the iris.

iridology (ir″ĭ-dol′o-je) the study of the iris as associated with disease.

iridomalacia (ir″ĭ-do-mah-la′she-ah) softening of the iris.

iridomesodialysis (ir″ĭ-do-me″so-di-al′ĭ-sis) surgical loosening of adhesions around the inner edge of the iris.

iridomotor (ir″ĭ-do-mo′tor) pertaining to movements of the iris.

iridoncus (ir″ĭ-dong′kus) tumor or swelling of the iris.

iridoparalysis (ir″ĭ-do-pah-ral′ĭ-sis) iridoplegia.

iridoperiphakitis (ir″ĭ-do-per″ĭ-fah-ki′tis) inflammation of the lens capsule.

iridoplegia (ir″ĭ-do-ple′je-ah) paralysis of the sphincter of the iris, with lack of contraction or dilation of the pupil; called also iridoparalysis.

iridoptosis (ir″ĭ-dop-to′sis) prolapse of the iris.

iridopupillary (ir″ĭ-do-pu′pĭ-ler′e) pertaining to the iris and pupil.

iridorhexis (ir″ĭ-do-rek′sis) 1. rupture of iris. 2. the tearing away of the iris.

iridoschisis (ir″ĭ-dos′kĭ-sis) splitting of the mesodermal stroma of the iris into two layers, with fibrils of the anterior layer floating in the aqueous.

iridosclerotomy (ir″ĭ-do-sklĕ-rot′o-me) incision of the sclera and of the edge of the iris in glaucoma.

iridosteresis (ir″ĭ-do-stĕ-re′sis) removal of all or part of the iris.

iridotasis (ir″ĭ-dot′ah-sis) stretching of the iris in treatment of glaucoma.

iridotomy (ir″ĭ-dot′o-me) incision of the iris.

iris (i′ris), pl. *ir′ides* [Gr.] the circular pigmented membrane behind the cornea, perforated by the pupil; the most anterior portion of the vascular tunic of the eye, it is made up of a flat bar of circular muscular fibers surrounding the pupil, a thin layer of plain muscle fibers by which the pupil is dilated, and, posteriorly, of two layers of pigmented epithelial cells. (See also Plate 15.)

iritis (i-ri′tis) inflammation of the iris. adj., **irit′ic.** The condition may be acute, occurring suddenly with pronounced symptoms, or chronic, with less severe but longer-lasting symptoms.

CAUSE. The cause of iritis is often obscure. Frequently the condition is associated with rheumatic diseases, particularly rheumatoid arthritis, and with diabetes mellitus, syphilis, diseased teeth, tonsillitis, and other infections. It may also be caused by trauma.

SYMPTOMS. Iritis is characterized by severe pain, usually radiating to the forehead and becoming worse at night. The eye is usually red and the pupil contracts and may be irregular in shape; there is extreme sensitivity to light, together with blurring of vision and tenderness of the eyeball. The iris becomes swollen and discolored. If not treated promptly, iritis can be dangerous because of scarring and adhesions that may cause impaired vision and possibly blindness.

TREATMENT. Caring for iritis calls for treatment of the underlying cause and then dilation of the pupil with atropine drops to prevent scarring or adhesions. Certain steroid drugs may be used to reduce the inflammation quickly. Warm compresses may also help to lessen the inflammation and pain. A protective covering allows the eye to rest.

With proper treatment, acute iritis usually clears up fairly quickly, although it may recur. For permanent relief, elimination or control of the underlying cause is necessary.

serous i., iritis with a serous exudate.

iritoectomy (ir″ĭ-to-ek′to-me) iridectomy.

iritomy (i-rit′o-me) iridotomy.

irium (ir′e-um) sodium lauryl sulfate.

iron (i′ern) a chemical element, atomic number 26, atomic weight 55.847, symbol Fe. (See table of ELEMENTS.) Iron is chiefly important to the human body because it is the main constituent of hemoglobin, cytochrome, and other components of respiratory enzyme systems. A constant although small intake of iron in food is needed to replace erythrocytes that are destroyed in the body processes.

Most iron reaches the body in food, where it occurs naturally in the form of iron compounds. These are converted for use in the body by the action of the hydrochloric acid produced in the stomach. This acid separates the iron from the food and combines with it in a form that is readily assimilable by the body. Vitamin C enhances the absorption of food iron. The administration of alkalis hampers iron absorption.

IRON DEFICIENCIES. The amount of new iron needed every day by the adult body is about 15 mg. A child needs a bit more in proportion to his weight. Although these amounts are very small, iron deficiencies may cause serious disorders.

The most common form of anemia results from iron deficiency. A great loss of blood, such as may result from bleeding ulcers, hemorrhoids, or injury, may cause a deficiency of iron. Women who lose much blood in menstruation may have to supplement their diet with iron-rich food. Iron deficiency sometimes occurs in pregnancy as a result of increased demands on the mother's blood. Iron deficiency may also occur in infants, since milk contains little iron. Although babies are born with an extra supply of hemoglobin, by the age of 2 or 3 months they need iron-rich food to supplement milk.

Iron preparations, such as ferrous sulfate, may be necessary in the treatment of iron deficiency anemia; they should be administered after meals, never on an empty stomach. The patient should be warned that the drugs cause stools to turn dark green or black. Overdosage may cause severe systemic reactions.

FOOD SOURCES OF IRON. Liver is the richest source of iron, containing enough in 6 oz. for a whole day's supply for an adult. Other iron-rich foods include lean meat, oysters, kidney beans, whole-wheat bread, kale, spinach, egg yolk, turnip tops, beet greens, carrots, apricots, and raisins.

i. lung, a popular name for a type of VENTILATOR that provides controlled, automatic breathing for a patient whose respiratory muscles are paralyzed; it consists of a metal tank, enclosing the patient's body with his head outside, and within which artificial respiration is maintained by alternating negative and positive pressure. Called also Drinker respirator.

radioactive i., a RADIOISOTOPE of iron; a mixture of ^{55}Fe and ^{59}Fe has been used in blood studies. Called also radioiron.

i. storage disease, hemochromatosis.

Ironate (i′ron-āt) trademark for a preparation of ferrous sulfate, used in iron deficiency anemia.

Irosul (i′ro-sul) trademark for preparations of ferrous sulfate, used in iron deficiency anemia.

irotomy (i-rot′o-me) iridotomy.

irradiate (ĭ-ra′de-āt) to treat with radiant energy.

irradiation (ĭ-ra″de-a′shun) exposure to radiant energy (heat, roentgen rays, etc.) for therapeutic or diagnostic purposes (see also RADIATION).

There are many kinds of rays, all traveling at the speed of light. Every living thing is subject to some irradiation by cosmic rays, ultraviolet rays in sunlight, and other natural radiation in the environment. Such radiation is usually slight and harmless. In large amounts, certain kinds of radiation—those rays with a greater frequency and producing more energy—cause direct harm to living cells.

USES. Irradiation of certain foods, including milk, kills harmful bacteria and prevents spoilage. X-ray photography is used in industrial research and in diagnosis of disorders within the body.

Radiation therapy (see also RADIOTHERAPY) usually refers to treatment by x-rays and gamma rays. X-rays are produced by bombarding a tungsten target with high-speed electrons in a vacuum tube; gamma rays are emitted by radium and other radioactive substances, including RADIOISOTOPES of iodine, gold, phosphorus, and cobalt. X-rays may be employed to kill organisms causing skin diseases, for example, or to destroy the abnormal cells that form tumors. Gonads, blood cells, and cancer cells are especially sensitive to radiation, particularly to x-rays and gamma rays. These rays are used principally for the treatment of cancer, and the radiotherapist attempts to destroy diseased cells without producing other ill effects.

Other rays are also used medically. Infrared rays produce a radiant heat used for the treatment of sprains and bursitis; tissues such as muscles and joints are relaxed and soothed by the penetration of these rays. Ultraviolet rays are used in sun lamps to treat skin diseases, such as acne and psoriasis.

PROTECTION AGAINST HARMFUL EFFECTS. Excessive radiation can cause RADIATION SICKNESS in the person exposed; sterility or genetic mutations in offspring are other possible results of excessive exposure to radiation. Hence the great danger from the blasts of nuclear or thermonuclear explosions and from the radioactive materials (fallout) scattered by these blasts.

The harmful effects of radiation are determined by both the degree of exposure and the type of radiation. Prevention must take into account time, distance, and shielding of both areas and people. Persons who are employed in nuclear power plants or other places where radioactive materials are accumulated must be properly shielded, and should wear or carry a dosimeter on which the amount of radiation received is recorded. Proper shielding is necessary also for radiologists, nurses, and others who spend much time near radiation emitted from either machinery or materials. (See also RADIATION PROTECTION.)

Since radiation effects, such as those of x-rays, build up in the body, a person should not be exposed to any more radiation during his lifetime than is necessary, and all radiotherapy must be under the control of a competent medical practitioner. In many states, all radiation-producing equipment must be registered.

Radiologists reduce harmful effects by limiting the field of exposure, by means of fast films, filters, and other technical devices. This shortens measurably the length of exposure of patients receiving medical and dental x-rays.

irreducible (ir″rĕ-doo′sĭ-b′l) not susceptible to reduction, as a fracture, hernia, or chemical substance.

irrigation (ir″ĭ-ga′shun) washing of a body cavity or wound by a stream of water or other fluid.

GENERAL PRINCIPLES. A steady, gentle stream is used in irrigation. The pressure should be sufficient to reach the desired area, but not enough to force the fluid beyond the area to be irrigated. The greater the height of the container of solution, the greater will be the pressure exerted by the stream of solution. Return flow of solution must always be allowed for. Directions about the type of solution to be used, the strength desired, and correct temperature should be followed carefully. Aseptic technique must be observed if sterile irrigation is ordered.

BLADDER. The purpose is to cleanse the bladder or to apply medication to the bladder lining. Aseptic technique must be used. The amount and type of solution will be ordered by the physician. A syringe and basin are used for single irrigations; other apparatus may be used for continuous or intermittent irrigations.

Ear. The stream is kept flowing steadily but with very low pressure; excessive pressure is painful and may spread infection to the middle ear. The patient usually is seated for this procedure, but he may lie on his side, with the ear to be irrigated uppermost while the solution is entering the ear. The head is turned to allow for return flow. The output flow of solution must never be obstructed.

Eye (Conjunctival Sac). The patient's head is turned to the side so that the eye to be irrigated is lower than the other eye. The solution is allowed to run over the eyelids to cleanse them and to accustom the patient to the flow of the solution. The flow of solution is directed from the inner to outer corner of the eye. The eyelids are separated by exerting pressure on the facial bones, not on the eyeball.

Perineum. The purpose of the procedure is to cleanse the vulva. The type of solution is specified by the physician. Flow of the solution is from front to back. The patient is instructed to wipe from the front to back to avoid contamination from the anal region.

Throat (Oral Pharynx). This type of irrigation reaches a more extensive area than does gargling. The temperature of the solution may be slightly higher than for other irrigations because the mouth and throat are more accustomed to hot liquids. The patient may be more comfortable sitting, with his head bent forward slightly. The patient is instructed to hold his breath while the solution is flowing.

irritability (ir″ĭ-tah-bil′ĭ-te) 1. ability of an organism or a specific tissue to react to the environment. 2. the state of being abnormally responsive to slight stimuli, or unduly sensitive.

myotatic i., the ability of a muscle to contract in response to stretching.

irritable (ir′ĭ-tah-b'l) 1. capable of reacting to a stimulus. 2. abnormally sensitive to stimuli.

irritant (ir′ĭ-tant) 1. causing irritation. 2. an agent that causes irritation.

irritation (ir″ĭ-ta′shun) 1. the act of stimulating. 2. a state of overexcitation and undue sensitivity. adj., **ir′ritative.**

ischemia (is-ke′me-ah) deficiency of blood in a part, due to functional constriction or actual obstruction of a blood vessel. adj., **ische′mic.**

myocardial i., deficiency of blood supply to the heart muscle, due to obstruction or constriction of the coronary arteries (see also CORONARY INSUFFICIENCY).

ischi(o)- word element [Gr.], *ischium.*

ischiadic, ischial (is″ke-ad′ik; is′ke-al) ischiatic.

ischialgia (is″ke-al′je-ah) pain in the ischium.

ischiatic (is″ke-at′ik) pertaining to the ischium.

ischidrosis (is″kĭ-dro′sis) anhidrosis.

ischiobulbar (is″ke-o-bul′bar) pertaining to the ischium and the bulb of the urethra.

ischiocapsular (is″ke-o-kap′su-lar) pertaining to the ischium and the capsular ligament of the hip joint.

ischiocele (is′ke-o-sēl″) hernia through the sacrosciatic notch.

ischiococcygeal (is″ke-o-kok-sij′e-al) pertaining to the ischium and coccyx.

ischiodidymus (is″ke-o-did′ĭ-mus) conjoined twins united at the pelvis.

ischiodynia (is″ke-o-din′e-ah) pain in the ischium.

ischiofemoral (is″ke-o-fem′o-ral) pertaining to the ischium and femur.

ischiohebotomy (is″ke-o-he-bot′o-me) surgical division of the ischiopubic ramus and ascending ramus of the pubes.

ischioneuralgia (is″ke-o-nu-ral′je-ah) sciatica.

ischiopagus (is″ke-op′ah-gus) conjoined twins fused at the ischial region.

ischiopubic (is″ke-o-pu′bik) pertaining to the ischium and pubes.

ischiorectal (is″ke-o-rek′tal) pertaining to the ischium and rectum.

ischium (is′ke-um) the inferior, dorsal portion of the hip bone (see also table of BONES).

ischuria (is-ku′re-ah) retention of suppression of the urine. adj., **ischuret′ic.**

iseikonia (i″si-ko′ne-ah) iso-iconic. adj., **iseikon′ic.**

island (i′land) a cluster of cells or an isolated piece of tissue.

blood i's, aggregations of mesenchymal cells in the angioblast of the embryo, developing into vascular endothelium and blood cells.

i's of Langerhans, irregular microscopic structures scattered throughout the pancreas, composed of alpha cells, which secrete glucagon and beta cells, which secrete insulin (see also DIABETES MELLITUS).

i. of Reil, insula.

islet (i′let) an island.

i's of Langerhans, islands of Langerhans.

Walthard's i's, microscopic inclusions of the ovarian germinal epithelium, which have been implicated in the development of Brenner tumors.

Ismelin (is′me-lin) trademark for a preparation of guanethidine, an antihypertensive.

iso- word element [Gr.], *equal; alike; same.*

isoagglutinin (i″so-ah-gloo′tĭ-nin) an isoantigen that acts as an agglutinin.

isoalloxazine (i″so-ah-lok′sah-zēn) an isomer of alloxazine from which riboflavin and other flavins are derived.

isoamyl nitrite (i″so-am′il) amyl nitrite, a vasodilator.

isoanaphylaxis (i″so-an″ah-fi-lak′sis) anaphylaxis produced by serum from an individual of the same species.

isoantibody (i″so-an′tĭ-bod″e) an antibody produced by one individual that reacts with isoantigens of another individual of the same species.

isoantigen (i″so-an′tĭ-jen) an antigen existing in alternative (allelic) forms in a species, thus inducing an immune response when one form is transferred to members of the species who lack it; typical isoantigens are the blood group antigens.

isobar (i′so-bahr) 1. one of two or more chemical species with the same atomic weight but different atomic numbers. 2. a line on a map or chart depicting the boundries of an area of constant atmospheric pressure.

isobornyl thiocyanoacetate (i″so-bor′nil thi″o-si″ah-no-as′ĕ-tāt) a pediculicide.

isobucaine (i″so-bu′kān) a local anesthetic, used as the hydrochloride salt.

isocaloric (i″so-kah-lo′rik) providing the same number of calories.

isocarboxazid (i″so-kar-bok′sah-zid) a monoamine oxidase inhibitor used as an antidepressant.

isocellular (i″so-sel′u-lar) made up of identical cells.

isochromatic (i″so-kro-mat′ik) of the same color throughout.

isochromatophil (i″so-kro-mat′o-fil) staining equally with the same stain.

isochromosome (i″so-kro′mo-sōm) an abnormal chromosome having a median centromere and two identical arms, formed by transverse, rather than normal longitudinal, splitting of a replicating chromosome.

isochronic, isochronous (i″so-kron′ik; i-sok′ro-nus) performed in equal times; said of motions and vibrations occurring at the same time and being equal in duration.

isocoria (i″so-ko′re-ah) equality of size of the pupils of the two eyes.

isocortex (i″so-kor′teks) neopallium.

isocytolysin (i″so-si-tol′ĭ-sin) an isoantigen that acts as a cytolysin.

isocytosis (i″so-si-to′sis) equality in size of cells, especially of erythrocytes.

isodactylism (i″so-dak′tĭ-lizm) relatively even length of the fingers.

isodiametric (i″so-di″ah-met′rik) measuring the same in all diameters.

isodontic (i″so-don′tik) having all the teeth alike.

isodose (i′so-dōs) a radiation dose of equal intensity to more than one body area.

isoelectric (i″so-e-lek′trik) showing no variation in electric potential.

i. period, the moment in muscular contraction when no deflection of the galvanometer is produced.

isoenzyme (i″so-en′zīm) one of the many forms in which a protein catalyst may exist in a single species, the various forms differing chemically, physically, and/or immunologically, but catalyzing the same reaction.

isoflurophate (i″so-floo′ro-fāt) an anticholinesterase inhibitor used as a miotic in glaucoma.

isogamety (i″so-gam′ĕ-te) production by an individual of one sex of gametes identical with respect to the sex chromosome. adj., **isogamet′ic.**

isogamy (i-sog′ah-me) reproduction resulting from union of two gametes identical in size and structure, as in protozoa. adj., **isog′amous.**

isogeneic (i″so-jĕ-ne′ik) having the same genetic constitution; syngeneic.

isogeneric (i″so-jĕ-ner′ik) of the same kind; belonging to the same species.

isogenesis (i″so-jen′ĕ-sis) similarity in the processes of development.

isograft (i′so-graft) a graft between genetically identical individuals.

isohemagglutination (i″so-he″mah-gloo″tĭ-na′shun) agglutination of erythrocytes caused by an isohemagglutinin.

isohemagglutinin (i″so-he″mah-gloo′tĭ-nin) an isoantigen that agglutinates erythrocytes.

isohemolysin (i″so-he-mol′ĭ-sin) an isoantigen that causes hemolysis.

isohemolysis (i″so-he-mol′ĭ-sis) hemolysis produced by isohemolysin. adj., **isohemolyt′ic.**

isohypercytosis (i″so-hi″per-si-to′sis) increase in the number of leukocytes, with normal proportions of neutrophil cells.

isohypocytosis (i″so-hi″po-si-to′sis) decrease in the number of leukocytes with normal relation between the number of various forms.

iso-iconia (i″so-i-ko′ne-ah) a condition in which the image of an object is the same in both eyes. adj., **iso-icon′ic.**

isoimmunization (i″so-im″u-nĭ-za′shun) development of antibodies in response to isoantigens.

isolate (i′so-lāt) 1. to separate from others, or set apart. 2. a group of individuals prevented by geographic, genetic, ecologic, or social barriers from interbreeding with others of their kind.

isolation (i″so-la′shun) the act of isolating or state of being isolated, such as (*a*) the physiologic separation of a part, as by tissue culture or by interposition of inert material; (*b*) the segregation of patients with a communicable disease; (*c*) the successive propagation of a growth of microorganisms until a pure culture is obtained; (*d*) the chemical extraction of an unknown substance in pure form from a tissue; (*e*) the defensive failure to connect behavior with motives, or contradictory attitudes and behavior with each other.

i. technique, special precautionary measures and procedures used in the care of a patient with a COMMUNICABLE DISEASE. In recent years the Center for Disease Control (CDC) in Atlanta, Georgia, has identified five general types of isolation procedures. These techniques take into account the site of infection and the mode of transmission, eliminating the need for strictly isolating every patient and thus sparing many patients from the psychological trauma of total separation and ostracism. A manual explaining each of the types, special precautions to be taken, and a set of cards giving concise information about isolation procedures for specific communicable diseases can be obtained by writing to the Superintendant of Documents, U.S. Government Printing Office, Washington, D.C. 20402, and asking for Publication 2054. Additional cards for posting on the patients' doors also can be obtained from this address.

The five types of isolation identified by the CDC are described as follows. *Strict isolation* is recommended for patients with diseases that are highly infectious or that can be transmitted by both direct contact and airborne routes. This type of isolation requires a private room, gowns, masks, and proper handwashing. Diseases requiring strict isolation include staphylococcal and streptococcal pneumonia, extensive burns infected with *Staphylococcus aureus* or Group A streptococcus, and rubella, smallpox, and diphtheria. Personnel caring for these patients should have up-to-date immunization against the diseases for which vaccines are available.

Respiratory isolation requires a private room, handwashing on entering and leaving the room, and masks for all susceptible persons who must enter the room. If possible, those who are susceptible should be excluded from the patient area. Examples of diseases requiring respiratory isolation are chickenpox, German measles, pertussis (whooping cough), meningococcal meningitis, and sputum-positive tuberculosis.

Enteric precautions require a private room for children only. Masks are not necessary but gowns and gloves are worn by all persons having contact with the patient or with articles contaminated with fecal material. All such contaminated articles must be disinfected or discarded. Examples of diseases requiring this type of isolation are cholera, viral hepatitis (infectious and serum), and salmonellosis (including typhoid fever).

Wound and skin precautions are recommended for infected wounds and for impetigo. A private room is desirable and all persons having direct contact with the patient should wear gowns. Gloves are worn when direct contact with the infected area is necessary, and masks are worn during dressing changes. Special precautions are necessary for the handling and disinfection of instruments, dressings, and bed linens.

Protective (reverse) isolation is required in the care of all patients who have seriously impaired resistance to infectious diseases, for example, patients with certain lymphomas and leukemia, those receiving immunosuppressive therapy, and those with agranulocytosis. This type of isolation requires a private room that is under slightly positive pressure to prevent contaminated air from flowing into the room. Gowns, masks, and gloves must be worn by all persons entering the room and having direct contact with the patient. Under some circumstances caps and shoe booties are worn. (See also PROTECTIVE ISOLATION.)

GENERAL PRINCIPLES OF PATIENT CARE. In addition to the specific measures taken to prevent the spread of certain types of infectious diseases, there are general principles that are basic to the care of any patient who is a source of infection to others or likely to become infected by those who are in contact with him. The factors most important in preventing the spread of infection are proper disinfection techniques and conscientious handwashing. The hands are used for many tasks in patient care and are therefore likely to be an excellent source of infection if they are not washed properly before and after each contact with the patient or with articles in his environment.

Disinfection can be concurrent or terminal. *Concurrent disinfection* refers to immediate destruction of infectious agents as they leave the body, or after they have contaminated linen, eating utensils, hospital equipment, and other objects that have come in contact with the patient, his excreta, or discharge from wounds. Concurrent disinfection is a continuous process in the daily care of the patient.

Terminal disinfection refers to destruction of pathogenic microorganisms remaining in the patient's environment after he is no longer considered to be a source of infection.

The spread of microorganisms can be kept at a minimum if it is always kept in mind that one must touch only "clean" to "clean" and "contaminated" to "contaminated." Once a clean article comes in contact with a contaminated article, both must be considered contaminated. In this context the word "clean" does not mean unsoiled; it means that an object is free from the organisms causing the patient's illness. Unsoiled linen, for example, might be contaminated with infectious agents and therefore could not be considered clean.

While carrying out the multitude of special procedures and precautionary measures necessary in isolation technique, one must not forget their psychologic impact on the patient. He should be told the reason for the precautions with special emphasis on concern for his well-being as well as for the protection of others. Unless he is very seriously ill some provision should be made for diversional activities that will help relieve the loneliness and boredom that result from isolation from other human beings.

Visitors are limited to a very few persons and they should be instructed in the ways in which the patient's disease can be spread and the precautions necessary to prevent infection of others. If the patient is a child and his parents are allowed to stay with him, they should wear gowns, masks, and head coverings while they are in the patient's unit. Toys, books, and other items brought into the unit for the child's amusement must be of the type that can be thoroughly disinfected; otherwise it will be necessary to dispose of them when he is no longer ill.

SETTING UP THE ISOLATION UNIT. Specific steps in setting up the unit will depend on hospital policy and the patient's disease. When the patient is being cared for in the home it is necessary to improvise with the facilities available. Ideally the patient should be in a room with an adjoining bath, both rooms being considered as the unit and as contaminated areas. When a bathroom is available, there is running water for handwashing and for obtaining and disposing of bath water. When running water is not available in the unit, basins and a pitcher are needed for proper handwashing.

If the patient has not entered the unit before it is set up, upholstered furniture, rugs, and other articles that would be difficult or impossible to disinfect should be removed. The usual items included in a hospital unit such as wash basin, water pitcher and glass, soap and soap dish, bedpan and urinal are kept in their usual places, cleansed daily and disinfected terminally. Supplies of extra linen and isolated gowns and masks are kept in an area away from the immediate surroundings of the patient. Paper or plastic bags are used to line the inside of the wastebasket in the patient's room and also the container for discarded paper towels. Small paper bags are used at the bedside for disposal of paper tissues used by the patient. Most hospitals use large, sturdy paper bags for contaminated linen; however, some may use laundry bags marked "isolation." The linen may require special handling and often is autoclaved before laundering so that all microorganisms are destroyed. In the home the linen should be soaked in a disinfectant before laundering.

Hospital equipment such as thermometer tray, stethoscope, and sphygmomanometer are kept in the patient's unit for his individual use and are disinfected terminally. Disposable needles and syringes, intravenous equipment, catheters, and drainage tubes are discarded in a lined container set aside for this purpose.

Rubber gloves, catheter trays, and other equipment that is not disposable must be soaked in Lysol solution for 30 minutes before it is cleaned, dried, and returned to the hospital supply room.

The patient's bathroom should contain antibacterial soap, paper towels, a nail brush, and Lysol or other disinfectant for soaking articles. If the patient's excreta is to be disinfected before it is flushed into the sewage system, chlorinated lime or Lysol may be used for this purpose (see also FECES).

SPECIFIC ISOLATION PROCEDURES. *Handwashing.*

Proper washing of the hands is necessary each time the patient receives care, or the hands are grossly contaminated. Running water is much preferred to the use of a basin and pitcher of water. When running water is not available a second person must assist by pouring water from a pitcher over the hands being washed.

Friction between the hands during the handwashing is very important in removal of microorganisms from the lines and crevices in the skin. A clean nail brush is used to clean beneath the fingernails. The wrists and arms usually can be considered uncontaminated; therefore the hands are kept below the level of the elbows during the handwashing procedure. If bar soap is used, it is kept in the hands during the entire procedure until the hands are rinsed for the last time. The hands should be washed for one full minute.

When foot pedals are not used to control the flow of water, the faucet handles are to be considered contaminated and a paper towel must be used to turn off the water after the hands have been cleaned.

Gown Technique. If the gown is disposable, it is discarded in a lined container in the patient's room or anteroom. If it is the type that is worn more than once, a hat rack or other device is placed inside the patient's unit and is used to hold a gown that has been worn, and is therefore contaminated on the outside, but is not soiled and can be worn again. The outside of the gown is contaminated and so the gown is hung with the contaminated side out. The inside of the gown and the neck band are considered clean because they are not touched by the hands after they have been contaminated. When the gown is put on, it is removed from the hook by grasping the inside of the neckband. Then the arms are slid into the sleeves, keeping the hand inside one sleeve as the other sleeve is adjusted. The back edges of the gown are brought together away from the body and then folded over and tied.

When removing the gown the back ties are loosened first. The cuff of the left sleeve is pulled over the hand, and with the left hand inside the sleeve the right sleeve is pulled down over the right hand. The gown is then shrugged off the shoulders and the hands removed from the sleeves. If the gown is to be discarded it is rolled with the inside out. If it is to be worn again it is hung on the hook with the contaminated side to the outside. Immediately after the gown is removed the hands must be washed.

Face Mask. The mask is worn for protection against contamination by droplet infection. Sneezing or coughing by the patient may release infectious organisms from his respiratory tract. A mask should fit snugly and cover both the nose and mouth. It should not be worn for more than 1 hour at a time. If it is necessary to stay in the patient's immediate environment for a longer period than this, the mask is discarded and replaced by a fresh one.

Gloves. Gloves are worn if there are dressings to be changed, or if there is the possibility of gross contamination of the hands from excreta. The gloves are removed by grasping the cuff on the outside and turning the glove wrong side out. The ungloved hand is then slipped under the cuff of the other glove so that it is removed by turning it wrong side out. The gloves are then placed in a basin of Lysol solution or other disinfectant and soaked for 30 minutes. The hands are washed immediately after removal of the gloves.

Cap. Some types of isolation require that a cap be worn. A clean cap is worn each time one enters the patient's unit and is discarded before leaving the unit. When removing the cap, care must be taken to avoid contamination of the hands if they have already been washed.

Feeding the Patient. Disposable plates, cups, and food trays are preferred. The meal can be prepared in the kitchen and brought to the patient's unit. Silverware is usually kept in the patient's unit, washed after use and wrapped in a paper towel until it is needed again. Uneaten food is wrapped in a paper bag or newspaper and placed in a lined container. If a bathroom is available, some of the food may be flushed down the toilet. Milk and other liquids can be disposed of in the same manner.

TERMINAL DISINFECTION. If the patient is to continue to stay in the hospital and the isolation is discontinued, he should be given a bath and shampoo, dressed in clean clothes, and placed in a clean room while disinfection is carried out. If he is to be discharged, the bath, shampoo, and change of clothes are done immediately before he leaves the hospital and he is placed in another room until he is discharged.

All equipment must be decontaminated or wrapped and prepared for discard before it is removed from the unit. A special technique called "fogging" is used in some hospitals when decontamination is desired, although the Center for Disease Control does not recognize it as an effective method of decontamination.

In the home the furniture in the room is washed with Lysol solution and the windows are opened so that the room is exposed to fresh air for several hours. The mattress and bed covers should be exposed to direct sunlight for 8 hours if possible.

isolecithal (i″so-les′ĭ-thal) having a small amount of yolk evenly distributed throughout the cytoplasm of the ovum.

isoleucine (i″so-lu′sēn) an amino acid produced by hydrolysis of fibrin and other proteins; essential for optimal infant growth and for nitrogen equilibrium in adults.

isologous (i-sol′o-gus) characterized by an identical genotype.

isolysin (i-sol′ĭ-sin) a lysin acting on cells of animals of the same species as that from which it is derived.

isolysis (i-sol′ĭ-sis) lysis of cells by isolysins. adj., **isolyt′ic.**

isomer (i′so-mer) any compound exhibiting, or capable of exhibiting isomerism. adj., **isomer′ic.**

isomerase (i-som′er-ās) a major class of enzymes comprising those that catalyze the process of isomerization, such as the interconversion of aldoses and ketoses.

isomerism (i-som′ĕ-rizm) the possession by two or more distinct compounds of the same molecular formula, each molecule having the same number of atoms of each element, but in different arrangement.

isomerization (i-som″ĕ-rĭ-za′shun) the process whereby any isomer is converted into another isomer, usually requiring special conditions of temperature, pressure, or catalysts.

isometheptene (i″so-meth′ep-tēn) a sympathomimetic used as a vasoconstrictor and antispasmodic.

isometric (i″so-met′rik) maintaining, or pertaining to, the same measure, or length; of equal dimensions.

i. contraction, muscle contraction without appreciable shortening or change in distance between its origin and insertion.

i. exercise, active exercise performed against stable resistance, without change in the length of the muscle.

isometropia (i″so-mĕ-tro′pe-ah) equality in refraction of the two eyes.

isomorphism (i″so-mor′fizm) identity in form; in genetics, referring to genotypes of polypoid organisms that produce similar gametes even though containing genes in different combinations on homologous chromosomes. adj., **isomor′phic.**

isoniazid (i″so-ni′ah-zid) an antibacterial compound used in treatment of tuberculosis.

isonicotinoylhydrazine (i″so-nik″o-tin″o-il-hi′-drah-zēn) isoniazid.

isopathy (i-sop′ah-the) the treatment of disease by means of products of the disease or with material from the affected organ. adj. **isopath′ic.**

isophoria (i″so-fo′re-ah) correspondence of the visual axes of the two eyes; equality in the tension of the vertical muscles of the two eyes.

Isophrin (i′so-frin) trademark for a preparation of phenylephrine, a local vasoconstrictor.

isoprecipitin (i″so-pre-sip′ĭ-tin) an isoantigen that acts as a precipitin.

isopregnenone (i″so-preg′ne-nōn) dydrogesterone.

isoprenaline (i″so-pren′ah-lēn) isoproterenol.

isopropamide (i″so-pro′pah-mīd) an anticholinergic used in the form of the iodide to suppress gastric secretion and motility in the management of peptic ulcer and other intestinal ailments.

isopropanol (i″so-pro′pah-nol) isopropyl alcohol, used as a solvent and as a rubefacient.

isoproterenol (i″so-pro″tĕ-re′nol) a sympathomimetic used chiefly in the form of the hydrochloride and sulfate salts, as a bronchodilator.

isopter (i-sop′ter) a curve representing areas of equal visual acuity in the field of vision.

isopyknosis (i″so-pik-no′sis) the quality of showing uniform density throughout, especially the uniformity of condensation observed in comparison of different chromosomes or in different areas of the same chromosome. adj., **isopyknot′ic.**

Isordil (i′sor-dil) trademark for a preparation of isosorbide, a coronary vasodilator.

isorrhea (i″so-re′ah) an equilibrium between the intake and output, by the body, of water and/or solutes. adj., **isorrhe′ic.**

isosexual (i″so-seks′u-al) pertaining to or characteristic of the same sex.

isosmotic (i″soz-mot′ik) having the same osmotic pressure.

isosorbide (i″so-sor′bīd) an osmotic diuretic; the dinitrate of isosorbide is used as a coronary vasodilator in treatment of coronary insufficiency and angina pectoris.

Isospora (i-sos′po-rah) a genus of sporozoan parasites (order Coccidia), found in birds, amphibians, reptiles, and various mammals, including man; *I. bel′li* and *I. hom′inis* cause coccidiosis in man.

isospore (i′so-spōr) 1. an isogamete of organisms that reproduce by spores. 2. an asexual spore produced by a homosporous organism.

isosthenuria (i″sos-thĕ-nu′re-ah) maintenance of a constant osmolality of the urine, regardless of changes in osmotic pressure of the blood.

isotherapy (i″so-ther′ah-pe) isopathy.

isotherm (i′so-therm) a line on a map or chart depicting the boundaries of an area in which the temperature is the same.

isothermal, isothermic (i″so-ther′mal; i″so-ther′-mik) having the same temperature.

isotone (i′so-tōn) one of several nuclides having the same number of neutrons, but differing in number of protons in their nuclei.

isotonia (i″so-to′ne-ah) 1. a condition of equal tone, tension, or activity. 2. equality of osmotic pressure between two elements of a solution or between two different solutions.

isotonic (i″so-ton′ik) 1. of equal tension. 2. denoting a solution in which body cells can be bathed without net flow of water across the semipermeable cell membrane; also, denoting a solution having the same tonicity as another solution with which it is compared.

i. contraction, muscle contraction without appreciable change in the force of contraction; the distance between the muscle's origin and insertion becomes lessened.

i. exercise, active exercise without appreciable change in the force of muscular contraction, with shortening of the muscle.

isotope (i′so-tōp) a chemical element having the same atomic number as another (i.e., the same number of nuclear protons), but having a different atomic mass (i.e., a different number of nuclear neutrons).

radioactive i., one having an unstable nucleus and which emits characteristic radiation during its decay to a stable form. (See also RADIOISOTOPE.)

stable i., one that does not transmute into another element with emission of corpuscular or electromagnetic radiations.

isotropic (i″so-trop′ik) 1. having like properties in all directions, as in a cubic crystal or a piece of glass. 2. being singly refractive.

isotropy (i-sot′ro-pe) the quality or condition of being isotropic.

isotypical (i″so-tip′ĭ-kal) of the same kind.

isoxsuprine (i-sok′su-prēn) a vasodilator used as the hydrochloride salt.

isozyme (i′so-zīm) isoenzyme.

issue (ish′ū) a discharge of pus, blood, or other matter; a suppurating lesion emitting such a discharge.

isthmectomy (is-mek′to-me) excision of an isthmus, especially of the isthmus of the thyroid.

isthmoparalysis, isthmoplegia (is″mo-pah-ral′ĭ-sis; is″mo-ple′je-ah) paralysis of the isthmus faucium.

isthmus (is′mus) a narrow connection between two larger bodies or parts. adj., **isth′mian.**

i. of auditory tube, i. of eustachian tube, the narrowest part of the eustachian tube at the junction of its bony and cartilaginous parts.

i. of fauces, i. fau′cium, the constricted aperture

between the cavity of the mouth and the pharynx.

i. of rhombencephalon, the narrow segment of the fetal brain, forming the plane of separation between the rhombencephalon and cerebrum.

i. of thyroid, the band of tissue joining the lobes of the thyroid.

i. of uterine tube, the narrower, thicker-walled portion of the uterine tube closest to the uterus.

i. of uterus, the constricted part of the uterus between the cervix and the body of the uterus.

Isuprel (i′su-prel) trademark for a preparation of isoproterenol, a sympathomimetic bronchodilator.

isuria (i-su′re-ah) excretion of urine at a uniform rate.

itch (ich) a skin disease attended with itching.

bakers' i., any of several inflammatory dermatoses of the hands, especially chronic candidal paronychia, seen with special frequency in bakers.

barber's i., infection and irritation of the hair follicles of the beard region (see also SYCOSIS BARBAE).

dhobie i., allergic contact dermatitis, caused by catechols in the marking fluid used on laundry by native washermen (dhobie) in India.

grain i., itching dermatitis due to a mite, *Pyemotes ventricosus,* which preys on certain insect larvae which live on straw, grain, and other plants.

grocers' i., a vesicular dermatitis caused by certain mites found in stored hides, dried fruits, grain, copra, and cheese.

ground i., the itching eruption caused by the entrance into the skin of the larvae of the hookworm *Ancylostoma duodenale* or *Necator americanus* (see also HOOKWORM DISEASE).

seven-year i., scabies.

swimmers' i., an itching dermatitis due to penetration into the skin of larval forms (cercaria) of schistosomes, occurring in bathers in waters infested with these organisms.

winter i., itching of the skin in cold weather, unassociated with structural lesions.

itching (ich′ing) pruritus; an unpleasant cutaneous sensation, provoking the desire to scratch or rub the skin.

iteroparity (it″er-o-par′ĭ-te) the state, in an individual organism, of reproducing repeatedly, or more than once in a lifetime.

-itis, pl. *-it′ides.* Word element [Gr.], *inflammation.*

ITP idiopathic thrombocytopenic purpura.

Itrumil (it′roo-mil) trademark for a preparation of iothiouracil, a drug that inhibits thyroid activity.

I.U. immunizing unit; International unit.

IUCD intrauterine contraceptive device (see also CONTRACEPTION).

IUD intrauterine contraceptive device (see also CONTRACEPTION).

I.V. intravenously.

I.V.T. intravenous transfusion.

Ixodes (ik-so′dēz) a genus of hard-bodied ticks (family Ixodidae); some species are vectors of disease.

ixodiasis (ik″so-di′ah-sis) any disease or lesion due to tick bites; infestation with ticks.

ixodic (ik-sod′ik) pertaining to, or caused by, ticks.

Ixodidae (iks-od′ĭ-de) a family of ticks (superfamily Ixodoidea), comprising the hard-bodied ticks.

Ixodides (iks-od′ĭ-dēz) the ticks, a suborder of Acarina, including the superfamily Ixodoidea.

Ixodoidea (iks″o-doi′de-ah) a superfamily of arthropods (suborder Ixodides), comprising both the hard- and soft-bodied ticks.

J

J symbol, *Joule's equivalent; joule.*

jacket (jak'et) an encasement or covering for the trunk, especially the thorax.

plaster-of-Paris j., a casing of plaster of Paris enveloping the body, for the purpose of giving support or correcting deformities (see also CAST).

Sayre's j., a plaster-of-Paris jacket used as a support for the vertebral column.

strait j., straitjacket.

jacksonian epilepsy (jak-so'ne-an) a form of EPILEPSY marked by clonic movements that start in one muscle group and spread systematically to adjacent groups.

jactitation (jak"tĭ-ta'shun) restless tossing to and fro in acute illness.

janiceps (jan'ĭ-seps) a double monster with one head and two opposite faces.

jaundice (jawn'dis) yellowness of skin, sclerae, and excretions due hyperbilirubinemia and deposition of BILE pigments. Called also icterus. It is usually first noticeable in the eyes, although it may come on so gradually that it is not immediately noticed by those in daily contact with the jaundiced person.

Jaundice is not a disease. It is a symptom of one of a number of different diseases and disorders of the LIVER, GALLBLADDER, and blood. One such disorder is the presence of a gallstone in the common bile duct, which carries bile from the liver to the intestine. This may obstruct the flow of bile, causing it to accumulate and enter the bloodstream. The obstruction of bile flow may cause bile to enter the urine, making it dark in color, and also decrease the bile in the stool, making it light and clay-colored. This condition requires surgery to remove the gallstone before it causes serious liver injury.

Jaundice may also be a symptom of infectious (viral) HEPATITIS. This very infectious disease may result in damage to the liver if not treated.

Certain diseases of the blood, such as hemolytic anemia, increase the amount of yellow pigment in the bile, causing jaundice.

The pigment causing jaundice is called BILIRUBIN. It is derived from hemoglobin that is released when erythrocytes are hemolyzed and therefore is constantly being formed and introduced into the blood as worn-out or defective erythrocytes are destroyed by the body. Normally the liver cells absorb the bilirubin and secrete it along with other bile constituents. If the liver is diseased, or if the flow of bile is obstructed, or if destruction of erythrocytes is excessive, the bilirubin accumulates in the blood and eventually will produce jaundice. A diagnostic test for determination of the level of bilirubin in the blood, called the VAN DEN BERGH TEST, is of value in detecting elevated bilirubin levels at the earliest stages before jaundice appears, when liver disease or hemolytic anemia is suspected.

acholuric j., jaundice without bilirubinemia, associated with elevated unconjugated bilirubin that is not excreted by the kidney.

acute febrile j., acute infectious j., infectious hepatitis.

cholestatic j., that resulting from abnormality of bile flow in the liver.

hematogenous j., hemolytic jaundice.

hemolytic j., jaundice associated with HEMOLYTIC ANEMIA.

hemorrhagic j., leptospiral jaundice.

hepatocellular j., jaundice caused by injury to or disease of the liver cells.

homologous serum j., serum hepatitis.

infectious j., infective j., 1. infectious hepatitis. 2. leptospiral jaundice.

leptospiral j., severe leptospirosis with fever, jaundice, myalgia, and occasionally with nephritis and meningitis. The symptoms last from 10 days to 2 weeks and recovery is usually uneventful. Called also Weil's disease.

nonhemolytic j., that due to an abnormality in bilirubin metabolism.

obstructive j., that due to blockage of the flow of bile.

physiologic j., mild icterus neonatorum during the first few days after birth.

jaw (jaw) either of the two opposing bony structures (maxilla and mandible) of the mouth of vertebrates; they bear the teeth and are used for seizing prey, for biting, or for masticating food.

j. bone, the mandible or maxilla, especially the mandible.

Hapsburg j., a mandibular prognathous jaw, often accompanied by Hapsburg lip.

phossy j., phosphonecrosis.

jaw-winking (jaw-wingk'ing) elevation of a congenitally ptotic eyelid when the mouth is opened, giving the appearance of constant winking.

Jeanselme's nodules (zhah-selmz') gummata of tertiary syphilis and of nonvenereal treponemal diseases, located on joint capsules, bursae, or tendon sheaths.

jejunectomy (jĕ"joo-nek'to-me) excision of the jejunum.

jejunitis (jĕ"joo-ni'tis) inflammation of the jejunum.

jejunocecostomy (jĕ-joo"no-se-kos'to-me) anastomosis of the jejunum to the cecum.

jejunocolostomy (jĕ-joo"no-ko-los'to-me) anastomosis of the jejunum to the colon.

jejunoileitis (jĕ-joo"no-il"e-i'tis) inflammation of the jejunum and ileum.

jejunoileostomy (jĕ-joo"no-il"e-os'to-me) anastomosis of the jejunum to the ileum.

jejunojejunostomy (jĕ-joo"no-je"joo-nos'to-me) surgical anastomosis between two portions of the jejunum.

jejunorrhaphy (jĕ-joo-nor'ah-fe) operative repair of the jejunum.

jejunostomy (jĕ"joo-nos'to-me) surgical creation of a permanent opening between the jejunum and the surface of the abdominal wall.

jejunotomy (jĕ"joo-not'o-me) incision of the jejunum.

jejunum (jĕ-joo'num) that part of the small intestine extending from the duodenum to the ileum. adj., **jeju'nal.**

jelly (jel'e) a soft, coherent, resilient substance; generally, a colloidal semisolid mass.

cardiac j., a jelly present between the endothelium and myocardium of the embryonic heart that transforms into the connective tissue of the endocardium.

contraceptive j., a nongreasy jelly used in the vagina for prevention of conception.

petroleum j., a purified mixture of semisolid hydrocarbons obtained from petroleum (see also PETROLATUM).

Wharton's j., the soft, jelly-like intracellular substance of the umbilical cord.

Jenner (jen'er) Edward (1749–1823). English physician. Born at Berkeley, Gloucestershire, he discovered the principle of smallpox vaccination in 1796. By experimental demonstration, Jenner turned a local country tradition that dairymaids who had contracted cowpox did not acquire smallpox into a permanent working principle in science.

jennerian (jĕ-ne're-an) relating to Edward Jenner, who developed vaccination.

jerk (jerk) a sudden reflex or involuntary movement.

Achilles j., ankle j., plantar extension of the foot elicited by a tap on the Achilles tendon, preferably while the patient kneels on a bed or chair, the feet hanging free over the edge; called also Achilles reflex, and triceps surae jerk or reflex.

biceps j., biceps reflex.

elbow j., involuntary flexion of the elbow on striking the tendon of the biceps or triceps muscle.

jaw j., jaw-jerk reflex.

knee j., contraction of the quadriceps muscle and extension of the leg elicited by tapping the patellar ligament when the leg hangs loosely flexed at a right angle (see also KNEE JERK).

tendon j., tendon reflex.

triceps surae j., ankle jerk.

joint (joint) the site of the junction or union of two or more bones of the body. The primary function of a joint is to provide motion and flexibility to the human frame.

Some joints are immovable, such as certain fixed joints where segments of bone are fused together in the skull. Other joints, such as those between the vertebrae, have extremely limited motion. However, most joints allow considerable motion.

Many joints have an extremely complex internal structure. They are composed not merely of ends of bones but also of ligaments, which are tough whitish fibers binding the bones together; cartilage, which is connective tissue, covering and cushioning the bone ends; the articular capsule, a fibrous tissue that encloses the ends of the bones; the synovial membrane, which lines the capsule and secretes a lubricating fluid (synovia); and sometimes bursae, which are fluid-filled sacs that cushion the movements of muscles and tendons.

Joints are classified by variations in structure that make different kinds of movement possible. The movable joints are usually subdivided into hinge, pivot, gliding, ball-and-socket, condyloid, and saddle joints.

DISEASES AND DISORDERS. Joints are often subject to great stress in day-to-day living; likewise they are exposed daily to injuries of all kinds because of their prominent location on the body. Wrenches and SPRAINS are fairly common. DISLOCATIONS are only slightly less frequent and they may be the aftermath of disease as well as accident.

Joints are also subject to inflammation (ARTHRITIS). The two most prevalent types are OSTEOARTHRITIS, a degenerative joint disorder common to elderly people, and RHEUMATOID ARTHRITIS, which may occur in even the very young and the cause of which is largely unknown. BURSITIS is inflammation of one or more bursae. It may cause pain and partial or complete immobility of the adjacent joint; it may be either acute or chronic. Synovitis, painful inflammation of the lining of the synovial membrane, may be caused by external injury or by disease, for exam-

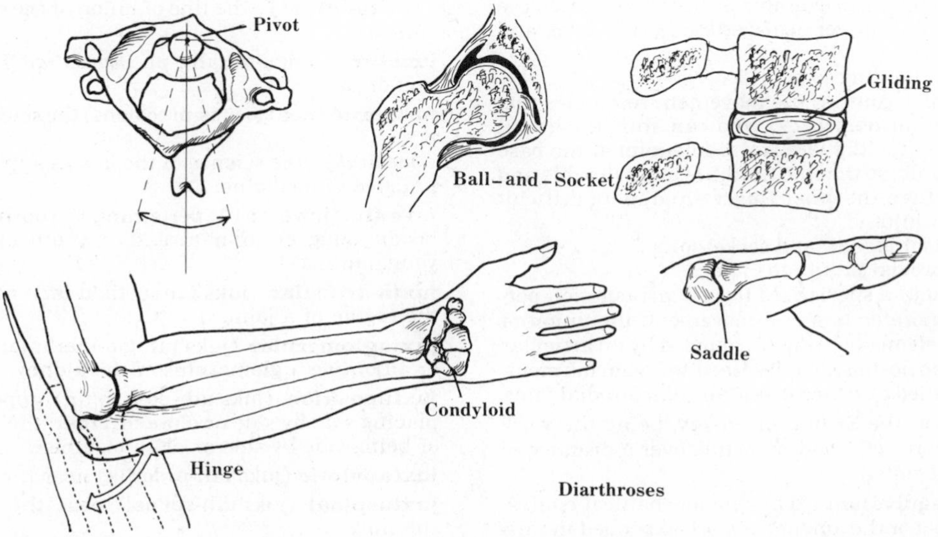

Joints.

ple, tuberculosis or syphilis. ANKYLOSIS is immobility and solidification of a joint.

arthrodial j., gliding joint.

ball-and-socket j., a synovial joint in which the rounded or spheroidal surface of one bone ("ball") moves within a cup-shaped depression ("socket") on another bone, allowing greater freedom of movement than any other type of joint. Called also spheroidal joint.

cartilaginous j., one in which the bones are united by cartilage, providing slight flexible movement; it includes symphysis and synchondrosis.

condyloid j., one in which an ovoid head of one bone moves in an elliptical cavity of another, permitting all movements except axial rotation. Such a joint is found at the wrist, connecting the radius and carpal bones, and at the base of the index finger.

diarthrodial j., synovial joint.

fibrous j., one in which the bones are connected by fibrous tissue and no or very little motion is possible; it includes suture, syndesmosis, and gomphosis. Called also synarthrodial joint.

flail j., an unusually mobile joint.

gliding j., a synovial joint in which the opposed surfaces are flat or only slightly curved, so that the bones slide against each other in a simple and limited way. The intervertebral joints are gliding joints, and many of the small bones of the wrist and ankle meet in gliding joints. Called also arthrodial joint and plane joint.

hinge j., a synovial joint that allows movement in only one plane, foreward and backward. Examples are the elbow and the interphalangeal joints of the fingers. The jaw is primarily a hinge joint but it can also move somewhat from side to side. The knee and ankle joints are hinge joints that also allow some rotary movement. Called also ginglymus.

hip j., the joint formed at the head of the femur and the acetabulum of the hip bone; loosely called hip.

knee j., the compound joint between the femur, patella, and tibia.

pivot j., a joint in which one bone pivots within a bony or an osseoligamentous ring, allowing only rotary movement; an example is the joint between the first and second cervical vertebrae (the atlas and axis).

plane j., gliding joint.

saddle j., a joint whose movement resembles that of a rider on horseback, who can shift in several directions at will; there is a saddle joint at the base of the thumb, so that the thumb is more flexible and complex than the other fingers, and more difficult to treat if injured.

spheroidal j., ball-and-socket joint.

synarthrodial j., fibrous joint.

synovial j., a specialized form of articulation permitting more or less free movement, the union of the bony elements being surrounded by an articular capsule enclosing a cavity lined by synovial membrane. Called also diarthrosis and diarthrodial joint.

joule (jo͞ol) the SI unit of energy, being the work done by force of 1 newton acting over a distance of 1 meter. Symbol J.

Joule's equivalent (jo͞olz) the mechanical equivalent of heat or the amount of work expended in raising the temperature of a pound of water through 1° F.; 772 foot-pounds. Symbol J.

jugal (joo'gal) pertaining to the cheek or zygomatic (cheek) bone.

j. point, the point at the angle formed by the masseteric and maxillary edges of the zygomatic bone. Called also jugale.

jugale (joo-ga'le) jugal point.

jugular (jug'u-lar) 1. pertaining to the neck. 2. one of the jugular veins.

j. veins, large veins that return blood to the heart from the head and neck. (See also table of VEINS and Plate 7.)

Each side of the neck has two sets of jugular veins, external and internal. The external jugular carries blood from the face, neck, and scalp and has two branches, posterior and anterior. The internal jugular vein receives blood from the brain, the deeper tissues of the neck and the interior of the skull. The external jugular vein empties into the subclavian vein, and the internal jugular vein joins it to form the brachiocephalic vein, which carries the blood to the superior vena cava, where it continues to the heart.

If one of these veins is severed, rapid loss of blood will result and air bubbles may enter the circulatory system unless preventive measures are taken. If such an event should occur, a compress should be applied to the wound with pressure. Under no circumstance is a tourniquet used.

jugum (joo'gum), pl. *ju'ga* [L.] a depression or ridge connecting two structures.

j. pe'nis, a forceps for compressing the penis.

juice (jo͞os) any fluid from animal or plant tissue.

gastric j., the liquid secretion of the gastric glands (see also GASTRIC JUICE).

intestinal j., the liquid secretion of glands in the intestinal lining.

pancreatic j., the enzyme-containing secretion of the pancreas, conducted through its ducts to the duodenum.

prostatic j., the liquid secretion of the prostate, which contributes to semen formation.

junction (jungk'shun) the place of meeting or coming together. adj., **junc'tional.**

myoneural j., the point of junction of a nerve fiber with the muscle that it innervates.

sclerocorneal j., the line of union of the sclera and cornea.

junctura (jungk-tu'rah), pl. *junctu'rae* [L.] a junction or joint.

jurisprudence (joor"is-proo'dens) the science of the law.

medical j., the science of the law as applied to the practice of medicine.

juvenile (ju'vĕ-nīl) 1. pertaining to youth or childhood; young or immature. 2. a youth or child; a young animal.

juxta-articular (juks"tah-ar-tik'u-lar) near or in the region of a joint.

juxtaglomerular (juks"tah-glo-mer'u-lar) near to or adjoining a glomerulus of the kidney.

juxtaposition (juks"tah-po-zish'un) apposition; a placing side by side or close together; the condition of being side by side or close together.

juxtapyloric (juks"tah-pi-lor'ik) near the pylorus.

juxtaspinal (juks"tah-spi'nal) near the vertebral column.

K

K chemical symbol, *potassium* (L. *kalium*).

K. cathode; Kelvin (scale).

Ka (*Kathode*) cathode.

Kahler's disease (kah'lerz) multiple myeloma.

Kahn test (kahn) a serologic (precipitation) test for the diagnosis of syphilis.

kak- for words beginning thus, see also those beginning *cac-*.

kakosmia (kak-oz'me-ah) cacosmia.

kala-azar (kah"lah-ah-zar') a highly fatal infectious disease endemic in the tropics and subtropics, caused by the protozoon *Leishmania donovani.* Sandflies of the genus *Phlebotomus* are the vectors. Called also visceral leishmaniasis.

SYMPTOMS. Symptoms are usually vague, resembling those of incipient pulmonary tuberculosis. The disease is often confused with malaria. There may be fever, chills, malaise, cough, anorexia, anemia, and wasting. The *Leishmania* organisms multiply in the cells of the reticuloendothelial system, eventually causing hyperplasia of the cells, especially those of the liver and spleen. Diagnosis is confirmed by demonstration of the parasite.

TREATMENT. Two groups of compounds are recommended: pentavalent organic antimonials, such as sodium antimony gluconate, and aromatic diamidines, such as pentamidine.

Bed rest is prescribed for patients debilitated by anemia. A decrease in white cell count (leukopenia) often accompanies the disease, and therefore the patient's resistance to secondary infections is lowered. In some cases transfusion may be necessary to bring blood values back to normal. The patient is given a well balanced diet and liberal amounts of fluids. Special mouth care and attention to the skin are necessary to avoid complications.

kalemia, kaliemia (kah-le'me-ah; ka"le-e'me-ah) the presence of potassium in the blood.

kaligenous (kah-lij'ĕ-nus) producing potash.

kaliopenia (ka-"le-o-pe'ne-ah) hypokalemia.

kalium (ka'le-um) [L.] potassium (symbol K).

kaliuresis (ka"le-u-re'sis) excretion of potassium in the urine.

kaliuretic (ka"le-u-ret'ik) 1. pertaining to or promoting kaliuresis. 2. an agent that promotes kaliuresis.

kallidin (kal'ĭ-din) kinin liberated by the action of kallikrein on a globulin of blood plasma. Kallidin I is the same as bradykinin; kallidin II is composed of bradykinin with a lysine added at the N-terminal.

kallikrein (kal"ĭ-kre'in) any of a group of enzymes present in various glands, lymph, urine, blood plasma, etc., the major action of which is the liberation of kinins from α-2-globulins, and hence have vasodilator and whealing actions.

kallikreinogen (kal"ĭ-kri'no-jen) the inactive precursor of kallikrein which is normally present in blood.

kanamycin (kan"ah-mi'sin) a broad-spectrum antibiotic derived from *Streptomyces kanamyceticus.*

Kantrex (kan'treks) trademark for preparations of kanamycin, an antibiotic.

kaolin (ka'o-lin) native hydrated aluminum silicate, powdered and freed from gritty particles by elutriation; used externally as an absorbent and protective and internally as a gastrointestinal adsorbent and demulcent in mild diarrhea.

kaolinosis (ka"o-lin-o'sis) pneumoconiosis from inhaling particles of kaolin.

Kaposi's sarcoma (kap'o-sēz) a multifocal, metastasizing, malignant reticulosis with angiosarcoma-like features, involving chiefly the skin.

Kaposi's varicelliform eruption (kap'o-sēz) a generalized and serious vesiculopustular eruption of viral origin, superimposed on preexisting atopic dermatitis; it may be due to the herpes simplex virus (eczema herpticum) or the vaccinia virus (eczema vaccinatum).

Kappadione (kap"ah-di'ōn) trademark for preparations of menadiol sodium diphosphate, used as a prothrombinogenic vitamin.

karaya gum (kar'a-ah) the dried gummy exudation from *Sterculia urens* or other species of *Sterculia,* which becomes gelatinous when moisture is added. It is available in rings that can be molded into any desired shape. Products containing karaya gum are often used as protective skin barriers in the care of COLOSTOMY and other conditions in which there is a STOMA. Called also sterculia gum.

Karell diet (kah'rel) the diet used in the KARELL TREATMENT.

Karell treatment (kah'rel) treatment of heart and kidney disease by keeping the patient in bed and giving only 800 ml. of milk daily for 4 or 5 days, the diet then being gradually increased until, on the thirteenth day the regular diet is resumed.

Kartagener's syndrome (kar-tag'ĕ-nerz) a hereditary syndrome consisting of dextrocardia, bronchiectasis, and sinusitis.

karyo- word element [Gr.], *nucleus.*

karyoclasis (kar"e-ok'lah-sis) karyoklasis.

karyocyte (kar'e-o-sīt") a nucleated cell.

karyogamy (kar"e-og'ah-me) cell conjugation with union of nuclei.

karyogenesis (kar"e-o-jen'ĕ-sis) the formation of a cell nucleus. adj., **karyogen'ic.**

karyokinesis (kar"e-o-ki-ne'sis) division of the nucleus, usually an early stage in the process of cell division, or mitosis. adj., **karyokinet'ic.**

karyoklasis (kar"e-ok'lah-sis) the breaking down of the cell nucleus or nuclear membrane. adj., **karyoklas'tic.**

karyolymph (kar'e-o-limf") the fluid portion of the nucleus of a cell, in which the other elements are dispersed.

karyolysis (kar"e-ol'ĭ-sis) the dissolution of the nucleus of a cell. adj., **karyolyt'ic.**

karyomegaly (kar"e-o-meg'ah-le) abnormal enlargement of the nucleus of a cell.

karyomere (kar'e-o-mēr") 1. chromomere (1). 2. a

vesicle containing only a small portion of the typical nucleus, usually after abnormal mitosis.

karyomitome (kar″e-om′ĭ-tōm) the nuclear chromatin network.

karyomitosis (kar″e-o-mi-to′sis) division of the cell nucleus preceding mitosis.

karyomorphism (kar″e-o-mor′fizm) the shape of a cell nucleus.

karyon (kar′e-on) the nucleus of a cell.

karyophage (kar′e-o-fāj″) a protozoon that phagocytizes the nucleus of the cell it infects.

karyoplasm (kar′e-o-plazm″) nucleoplasm.

karyopyknosis (kar″e-o-pik-no′sis) shrinkage of a cell nucleus, with condensation of the chromatin. adj., **karyopyknot′ic.**

karyorrhexis (kar″e-o-rek′sis) rupture of the cell nucleus in which the chromatin disintegrates into formless granules that are extruded from the cell. adj., **karyorrhec′tic.**

karyosome (kar′e-o-sōm″) any of the condensed irregular clumps of chromatin dispersed in the chromatin network of a cell nucleus.

karyostasis (kar″e-os′tah-sis) the so-called resting stage of the nucleus between mitotic divisions.

karyotheca (kar″e-o-the′kah) the nuclear membrane.

karyotype (kar′e-o-tīp) the chromosomal constitution of the cell nucleus; by extension, the photomicrograph of chromosomes arranged according to the DENVER CLASSIFICATION (see also illustration accompanying CHROMOSOME).

Kashin-Beck disease (kash′in bek) a disabling degenerative disease of the peripheral joints and spine, endemic in eastern Siberia, northern China, and Korea; believed to be caused by ingestion of cereal grains infected with the fungus *Fusarium sporotrichiella.*

kat(a)- word element [Gr.], *down; against.* See also words beginning *cat(a)-.*

katathermometer (kat″ah-ther-mom′ĕ-ter) a thermometer with a wet bulb and a dry bulb, for detecting cooling rates.

Kayser-Fleischer ring (ki′zer flĭsh′er) a gray-green to red-gold pigmented ring at the outer margin of the cornea, seen in progressive lenticular degeneration and pseudosclerosis.

kc. kilocycle.

kc.p.s. kilocycles per second.

Keflex (kef′lex) trademark for preparations of cephalexin, an oral cephalosporin.

Keflin (kef′lin) trademark for a preparation of cephalothin, an analogue of cephalosporin C.

Kegel exercises (ke′gul) specific exercises named after Dr. Arnold H. Kegel, a gynecologist who first developed the exercises to strengthen the pelvic-vaginal muscles as a means of controlling stress incontinence in women. He later learned from patients who had been performing the exercises that strengthening of the pubococcygeus muscle, a sphincteric muscle that surrounds the vagina, also improved feminine sexual response and contributed to the attainment of orgasm. Reasearch has since demonstrated that this muscle contains specialized nerve endings which contribute to a satisfactory sexual experience.

A third area in which the Kegel exercises are important is in NATURAL CHILDBIRTH. The exercises strengthen the pelvic floor and therefore are helpful in reducing discomfort and congestion during pregnancy and in providing support for the pelvic organs before and after birth. During delivery the mother who has developed good tone and conscious control over the pubococcygeus muscle is able to release the muscle and thereby facilitate the passage of the infant through the birth canal. After delivery the exercises maintain the strength of the muscle and greatly diminish the possibility of rectocele and cystocele, dyspareunia, and other aftereffects of delivery.

Most patients must be taught an awareness of the muscle and how to control it. This usually can be done by having the woman shut off urine flow while sitting with the knees widely separated. After a few trials the sensation of control is recognized and the patient is able to perform the exercise on her own. Usually the exercises are begun with five or ten contractions before arising in the morning and also during each voiding of urine. Gradually the number of sessions and the number of contractions are increased until ultimately a pattern of three hundred daily contractions is reached. The exercises require concentration but a small expenditure of energy. Once the muscle has been strengthened it tends to maintain its strength and state of partial contraction at all times. Sexual activity helps preserve the muscle tone.

Keith's bundle (kēths) a bundle of fibers in the wall of the right atrium between the openings of the venae cavae; called also sinoatrial bundle.

Keith's node (kēths) sinoatrial node.

Keith-Flack node (kēth-flak) sinoatrial node.

Keith-Wagener-Barker classification (kēth-wag′en-er-bar′ker) a classification of hypertension and arteriolosclerosis based on retinal changes.

keloid (ke′loid) a sharply elevated, irregularly shaped, progressively enlarging scar, due to excessive collagen formation in the corium during connective tissue repair. adj., **keloid′al.** A keloid is a benign tumor that has its origin usually in a scar from surgery or a burn or other injury. Keloids are generally considered harmless and noncancerous, although they may produce contractures. Ordinarily they cause no trouble beyond an occasional itching sensation.

Surgical removal is not usually effective because it results in a high rate of recurrence. However, intralesional injection of steroids, cryotherapy, and x-ray therapy often are of substantial help. When x-ray therapy is employed, care must be taken not to destroy the surrounding healthy tissue.

Kelvin scale (kel′vin) an absolute scale on which the unit of measurement corresponds to that of the CELSIUS (centigrade) SCALE, but the ice point is at 273.15 degrees (273.15° K.).

Kelvin thermometer (kel′vin) a thermometer employing the KELVIN SCALE.

Kemadrin (kem′ah-drin) trademark for a preparation of procyclidine, an antiparkinsonism drug.

Kempner rice diet (kemp′ner) a special diet restricted to 10 oz. of rice daily, supplemented only by liberal quantities of sugar and fresh or preserved fruits, prescribed for hypertensive vascular disease and kidney disease.

Kenacort (ken′ah-kort) trademark for preparations of triamcinolone, a corticosteroid.

Kenalog (ken′ah-log) trademark for preparations of triamcinolone acetonide, a corticosteroid.

Kenny treatment (ken′e) treatment of poliomyelitis by wrapping the patient in woolen cloths wrung out of hot water and re-educating muscles by passive exercises after pain has subsided.

keno- word element [Gr.], *empty.*

kenotoxin (ke″no-tok′sin) the toxin of fatigue, thought to be produced by muscular contraction.

kerasin (ker′ah-sin) a cerebroside from brain tissue, yielding galactose, sphingosine, and lignoceric acid on hydrolysis.

kerat(o)- word element [Gr.], *horny tissue; cornea.*

keratalgia (ker″ah-tal′je-ah) pain in the cornea.

keratectasia (ker″ah-tek-ta′ze-ah) protrusion of a thin, scarred cornea.

keratectomy (ker″ah-tek′to-me) excision of a portion of the cornea; kerectomy.

keratic (kĕ-rat′ik) 1. pertaining to keratin. 2. pertaining to the cornea.

keratin (ker′ah-tin) a scleroprotein that is the principal constituent of epidermis, hair, nails, horny tissues, and the organic matrix of the enamel of the teeth. Its solution is sometimes used in coating pills when the latter are desired to pass through the stomach unchanged.

keratinase (ker′ah-tin-ās″) a proteolytic enzyme that hydrolyzes keratin.

keratinization (ker″ah-tin″ĭ-za′shun) the development of or conversion into keratin.

keratinocyte (kĕ-rat′ĭ-no-sīt″) the cell of the epidermis that synthesizes keratin, known in its successive stages in the various layers of the skin as basal cell, prickle cell, and granular cell.

keratinous (kĕ-rat′ĭ-nus) containing or of the nature of keratin.

keratitis (ker″ah-ti′tis) inflammation of the cornea. Keratitis may be deep, when the infection causing it is carried in the blood or spreads to the cornea from other parts of the eye, or superficial, caused by bacterial or viral infection or by allergic reaction. Microorganisms causing the inflammation can be introduced into the cornea during the removal of foreign bodies from the eye. All infections of the eye are potentially serious because opaque fibrous tissue or scar tissue may form on the cornea during the healing process and cause partial or total loss of vision.

CAUSES. There are several kinds of keratitis. Dendritic keratitis is a viral form caused by the herpes simplex virus; it usually affects only one eye. A bacterial form, acute serpiginous keratitis, may result from infection by pneumococci, streptococci, or staphylococci. Some kinds of keratitis—dendritic keratitis, for example—may follow symptoms of upper respiratory tract infection, such as fever.

Burns of the cornea, such as those produced by chemicals or ultraviolet rays, also give rise to a form of keratitis. In TRACHOMA, a contagious disease of the conjunctiva, the eyes become inflamed, and small, gritty particles develop on the cornea. Herpetic keratitis may accompany HERPES ZOSTER.

Interstitial keratitis is often caused by congenital syphilis, although occasionally it may also result from acquired SYPHILIS. When caused by congenital syphilis, the disease usually appears when the child is between the ages of 5 and 15. In rare cases, interstitial keratitis may also stem from tuberculosis or rheumatic infection in other parts of the body.

SYMPTOMS. Symptoms vary somewhat among the different forms of keratitis, but pain, which may be severe, and inability to tolerate light (photophobia) are usual. There may also be considerable effusion of tears and a conjunctival discharge.

TREATMENT. Antibiotics are the usual treatment for keratitis caused by an infectious organism. Cortisone is used for other forms, but may be dangerous in some patients. Antiviral agents, such as idoxuridine, have been used to treat herpes simplex (dendritic) keratitis. In cases of syphilitic interstitial keratitis, the syphilis is treated. Congenital interstitial keratitis can be prevented if syphilis is detected early in pregnancy by means of blood tests, and the mother is treated.

keratoacanthoma (ker″ah-to-ak″an-tho′mah) a rapidly growing, benign papular lesion, with a superficial crater filled with a keratin plug, usually on the face; it resolves spontaneously.

keratocele (ker′ah-to-sēl″) hernial protrusion of Descemet's membrane.

keratocentesis (ker″ah-to-sen-te′sis) puncture of the cornea, keratonyxis.

keratoconjunctivitis (ker″ah-to-kon-junk″tĭ-vi′-tis) inflammation of the cornea and conjunctiva.

epidemic k., a highly infectious form, commonly with regional lymph node involvement, occurring in epidemics; an adenovirus has been repeatedly isolated from affected patients.

phlyctenular k., a form marked by formation of a small, gray, circumscribed lesion at the corneal limbus.

k. sic′ca, a condition marked by hyperemia of the conjunctiva, thickening and drying of the corneal epithelium, and itching and burning of the eye.

keratoconus (ker″ah-to-ko′nus) conical protrusion of the central part of the cornea, resulting in an irregular astigmatism.

keratoderma (ker″ah-to-der′mah) hypertrophy of the horny layer of the skin.

k. blennorha′gica, pustular psoriasis associated with gonorrhea.

k. climacter′icum, endocrine k., circumscribed hyperkeratosis of palms and soles, occurring in menopausal women.

keratodermia (ker″ah-to-der′me-ah) keratoderma.

keratogenous (ker″ah-toj′ĕ-nus) giving rise to a growth of horny material.

keratoglobus (ker″ah-to-glo′bus) a bilateral anomaly in which the cornea is enlarged and globular in shape.

keratohelcosis (ker″ah-to-hel-ko′sis) ulceration of the cornea.

keratohemia (ker″ah-to-he′me-ah) deposition of blood in the cornea.

keratohyalin (ker″ah-to-hi′ah-lin) granules in the stratum granulosum of the epidermis. adj., **keratohy′aline.**

keratoid (ker′ah-toid) resembling horn or corneal tissue.

keratoiridoscope (ker″ah-to-i-rid′o-skōp) a compound microscope for examining the eye.

keratoiritis (ker″ah-to-i-ri′tis) inflammation of the cornea and iris, corneoiritis.

keratoleptynsis (ker″ah-to-lep-tin′sis) removal of the anterior portion of the cornea and replacement with bulbar conjunctiva.

keratoleukoma (ker″ah-to-lu-ko′mah) a white opacity of the cornea.

keratolysis (ker″ah-tol′ĭ-sis) loosening or separation of the horny layer of the epidermis.

pitted k., k. planta′re sulca′tum, a tropical disease marked by thickening and deep fissuring of the skin of the soles, occurring during the rainy season.

keratolytic (ker″ah-to-lit′ik) 1. pertaining to or promoting keratolysis. 2. an agent that promotes keratolysis.

keratoma (ker″ah-to′mah) keratosis.

keratomalacia (ker″ah-to-mah-la′she-ah) softening and necrosis of the cornea associated with vitamin A deficiency.

keratome (ker′ah-tōm) a knife for incising the cornea.

keratometer (ker″ah-tom′ĕ-ter) an instrument for measuring the curves of the cornea.

keratometry (ker″ah-tom′ĕ-tre) measurement of corneal curves. adj., **keratomet′ric.**

keratomycosis (ker″ah-to-mi-ko′sis) fungal disease of the cornea.

keratonyxis (ker″ah-to-nik′sis) puncture of the cornea; keratocentesis.

keratopathy (ker″ah-top′ah-the) noninflammatory disease of the cornea.

band k., a condition characterized by an abnormal gray circumcorneal band.

keratoplasty (ker′ah-to-plas″te) plastic surgery of the cornea; corneal grafting.

optic k., transplantation of corneal material to replace scar tissue that interferes with vision.

tectonic k., transplantation of corneal material to replace tissue that has been lost.

keratorhexis (ker″ah-to-rek′sis) rupture of the cornea.

keratoscleritis (ker″ah-to-sklĕ-ri′tis) inflammation of cornea and sclera.

keratoscope (ker′ah-to-skōp″) an instrument for examining the cornea.

keratoscopy (ker″ah-tos′ko-pe) inspection of the cornea.

keratosis (ker″ah-to′sis) any horny growth, such as a wart or callosity.

actinic k., a sharply outlined verrucous or keratotic growth, which may develop into a cutaneous horn, and may become malignant; it usually occurs in the middle aged or elderly and is due to excessive exposure to the sun. Called also senile, or solar, keratosis.

k. follicula′ris, a rare hereditary condition manifested by areas of crusting, verrucous papular growths, usually occurring symmetrically on the trunk, axillae, neck, face, scalp, and retroauricular areas. Called also Darier's disease.

k. palma′ris et planta′ris, congenital, hereditary thickening of the skin of the palms and soles, sometimes with painful lesions resulting from fissuring; often associated with other anomalies.

k. pharyn′gea, horny projections from the tonsils and pharyngeal walls.

k. pila′ris, hyperkeratosis limited to the hair follicles.

k. puncta′ta, a hereditary hyperkeratosis in which the lesions are localized in multiple points on the palms and soles.

seborrheic k., k. seborrhe′ica, a benign, noninvasive tumor of epidermal origin, marked by numerous yellow or brown, sharply marginated, oval, raised lesions.

k. seni′lis, solar k., actinic keratosis.

keratotomy (ker″ah-tot′o-me) incision of the cornea.

kerectomy (kĕ-rek′to-me) keratectomy.

kerion (ke′re-on) a boggy, exudative tumefaction covered with pustules, as may occur in tinea infections.

kernicterus (ker-nik′ter-us) a condition in the newborn marked by severe neural symptoms, associated with high levels of bilirubin in the blood; it is commonly a sequela of icterus gravis neonatorum.

Kernig's sign (ker′nigz) in the supine position the patient can easily and completely extend the leg; in the sitting posture or when lying with the thigh flexed upon the abdomen the leg cannot be completely extended; it is a sign of meningitis.

keto- word element, *ketone group.*

keto acids (ke′to) compounds containing the groups CO (carbonyl) and COOH (carboxyl).

ketoacidosis (ke″to-ah″sĭ-do′sis) acidosis due to accumulation of ketone bodies.

Keto-Diastix trademark for a reagent strip for detection of ketones and glucose in the urine.

ketogenesis (ke″to-jen′ĕ-sis) the production of ketone bodies. adj., **ketogenet′ic.**

ketogenic (ke″to-jen′ik) forming or capable of being converted into ketone bodies.

k. diet, one containing large amounts of fat, with minimal amounts of protein and carbohydrate. The object of such a diet being to produce KETOSIS; it is occasionally used in the treatment of certain types of epilepsy in young children.

ketolysis (ke-tol′ĭ-sis) the splitting up of ketone bodies. adj., **ketolyt′ic.**

ketone (ke′tōn) any compound containing the carbonyl group, CO, and having hydrocarbon groups attached to the carbonyl carbon.

k. bodies, the substances acetone, acetoacetic acid, and β-hydroxybutyric acid; except for acetone (which may arise spontaneously from acetoacetic acid), they are normal metabolic products of lipid within the liver, and are oxidized by muscles; excessive production leads to urinary secretion of these bodies, as in diabetes mellitus. Called also acetone bodies.

Initially, the combustion of fatty acids produces ketones, which eventually are broken down into carbon dioxide and water by the liver and other tissues of the body. Under abnormal conditions, such as uncontrolled DIABETES MELLITUS, starvation, or the intake of a diet composed almost entirely of fat, the breakdown of fatty acids may be halted at the ketone stage, causing increasing levels of ketone bodies in the blood. This condition is called KETOSIS and is directly related to improper utilization or inadequate supplies of carbohydrates, which are necessary for proper combustion of fats.

ketonemia (ke″to-ne′me-ah) an excess of ketone bodies in the blood.

ketonuria (ke″to-nu′re-ah) an excess of ketone bodies in the urine.

ketose (ke'tōs) any sugar that contains a ketone group.

ketosis (ke"to'sis) the accumulation of excessive quantities of ketone bodies in the body tissues and fluids. adj., **ketot'ic.** Ketosis is the result of incomplete combustion of fatty acids, which in turn is the result of improper utilization of, or lack of availability of, carbohydrates. When carbohydrates cannot be used as the source of energy, the body draws on its supply of fats. Deficiency of carbohydrates triggers several hormonal responses and greatly increases the removal of fatty acids from fatty tissues. As a result, large quantities of fatty acids must be oxidized, more in fact than the body cells can handle; thus their oxidation is incomplete and ketones accumulate in the blood and tissues.

Ketosis may result in severe ACIDOSIS because the ketone bodies beta-oxybutyric acid and acetoacetic acid decrease the blood pH and, more important, because when the keto acids are excreted in the urine they take with them large quantities of sodium. The result is a depletion of the alkaline part of the body's buffer system, so that the ACID-BASE BALANCE is upset in favor of acidosis.

Ketosis occurs in uncontrolled DIABETES MELLITUS because carbohydrates are not properly utilized, and in starvation because carbohydrates simply are not available for utilization. Ketosis is sometimes produced intentionally in the treatment of certain types of epilepsy in young children by means of the ketogenic diet, which contains large amounts of fat and little carbohydrate and protein.

The patient with ketosis often has a sweet or "fruity" odor to his breath. This is produced by acetone, a ketone body that is highly volatile and is blown off in small amounts with air expired from the lungs. Although ketosis can give rise to acidosis, acidosis can occur without any corresponding ketosis.

It is also possible to have an extremely high blood sugar without ketoacidosis (HYPERGLYCEMIC HYPEROSMOLAR NONKETOTIC COMA).

ketosteroid (ke"to-ste'roid) a steroid having ketone groups on functional carbon atoms.

17-k's, steroids found in normal urine and in excess in certain tumors, which have a ketone group on the 17th carbon atom, and include certain androgenic and adrenocortical hormones.

Ketostix (ke'to-sticks) trademark for a reagent strip for detection of ketone bodies in the urine.

ketosuria (ke"to-su're-ah) ketose in the urine.

kev kilo (1000) electron volts (3.82×10^{-17} gram-(small) calories, or 1.6×10^{-9} ergs).

Kew Gardens spotted fever rickettsialpox.

kg. kilogram.

kg.-m. kilogram-meter.

khellin (kel'in) an active principle of the fruit of the plant *Ammi visnaga,* used as a coronary vasodilator and bronchodilator.

kHz kilohertz.

kidney (kid'ne) either of the two bean-shaped organs in the lumbar region that filter the blood, excreting the end-products of body metabolism in the form of urine, and regulating the concentrations of hydrogen, sodium, potassium, phosphate, and other ions in the extracellular fluid.

PHYSIOLOGY. In an average adult each kidney is about 4 inches long, 2 inches wide and 1 inch thick, and weighs 4 to 6 oz. In this small area the kidney contains over a million microscopic filtering units, the NEPHRONS. Blood arrives at the kidney by way of the renal artery, and is distributed through arterioles into many millions of capillaries which lead into the nephrons. Fluids and dissolved salts in the blood pass through the walls of the capillaries and are collected within the central capsule of each nephron, the malpighian capsule. The glomerulus, a tuft of capillaries within the capsule, acts as a semipermeable membrane permitting a protein-free ultrafiltrate of plasma to pass through. This filtrate is forced into hairpin-shaped collecting channels in the nephrons, called tubules. Capillaries in the walls of the tubules reabsorb the water and the salts required by the body and deliver them to a system of small kidney veins which, in turn, carry them into the renal vein and return them to the general circulation. Excess water and other waste materials remain in the tubules as urine. The urine contains, besides water, a quantity of urea, uric acid, yellow pigments, amino acids, and trace metals. The urine moves through a system of ducts into a collecting funnel (renal pelvis) in each kidney, whence it is led into the two ureters.

Filtering Capacity. About $1\frac{1}{2}$ quarts (1500 ml.) of urine are excreted daily by the average adult. The efficiency of the normal kidney is one of the most remarkable aspects of the body. It has a filtering capacity of a quart of blood per minute—that is, 15 gallons per hour, or 360 gallons per day. Ordinarily it draws off from the blood about 180 quarts of fluid daily, and returns usually 98 to 99 per cent of the water plus the useful dissolved salts, according to the body's changing needs.

Maintaining Salt and Water Balance. The development of kidneys was an essential step in the evolution of species that could live in fresh water and eventually on dry land. The kidneys still preserve a salt-water environment inside the body, maintaining the proper balance between the salts (ELECTROLYTES) and water. If the water becomes excessive, salt will continue to be returned to the blood while more of the water is excreted in the urine. The opposite happens if there is an excess of salts. Simi-

KIDNEY
(partly in hemisection)

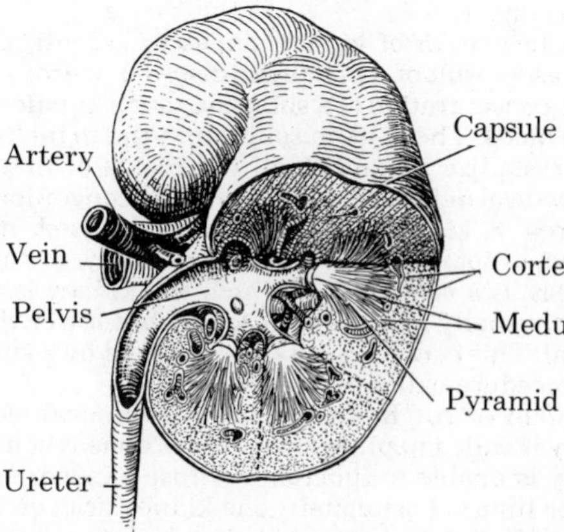

Kidney. (From Dorland's Illustrated Medical Dictionary, 25th ed. Philadelphia, W. B. Saunders Co., 1974.)

larly, the kidneys regulate the amount of potassium in the blood. These functions of the kidneys are controlled by hormones.

Maintaining Acid-Base Balance. The kidneys help control the body's acidity by converting some of the amino acids into ammonia, an alkaline chemical. The kidneys also manufacture enzymes that aid in this conversion.

DISORDERS OF THE KIDNEYS. Disorders of the kidney include inflammation, infection, obstruction, structural defects, injuries, calculus formation, and tumors.

PYELITIS is an inflammation of the renal pelvis. When the inflammation reaches deeper portions of the kidneys, it is called pyelonephritis.

NEPHRITIS is widespread inflammation of the kidney, usually affecting the inner mesh of capillaries (glomeruli). It appears to be caused in certain cases by an allergic reaction to certain varieties of streptococci. NEPHROSIS (called also the nephrotic syndrome) is a noninflammatory condition in which the kidneys lose their control over the water content of the blood, producing widespread edema.

When the kidneys are so badly damaged that they can no longer remove urea and other waste products from the blood, a condition called UREMIA develops. It has many causes, such as severe trauma to the kidney, nephritis, chronic pyelonephritis, hypertension, severe gout, renal calculi with infection, overdose of vitamin D, and diabetes mellitus.

Kidney infection is potentially serious. Many disorders can be completely cured if treated early. Unchecked infection can destroy the organs and lead to uremia. Failure of both kidneys may result in death, because no other organ can eliminate waste products of the blood. Fortunately, one kidney or even less than half a kidney is capable of performing the task of purification. Hence a diseased kidney can be removed, and the other will carry on the function. If both must be removed—a rare circumstance—or if both are destroyed by disease, the only hope is the use of an artifical kidney (see also artificial KIDNEY) or a kidney transplant (see also TRANSPLANTATION).

Antibiotics and other medicines are prescribed for many kidney diseases caused by infection. In a kidney disorder stemming from such diseases as tuberculosis or diabetes mellitus, the underlying disease must also be treated. The kidneys are also subject to cancer.

The formation of kidney stones or calculi, may occur as a result of a metabolic disorder or from the excess concentration of a substance such as calcium in the blood. The salts in solution in the urine may also crystallize around small fragments of matter.

Structural defects in kidneys may be congenital or acquired. A kidney may be displaced, fused, malformed, or totally absent. Floating kidney, or NEPHROPTOSIS, is a condition in which the kidney is displaced, usually to a position somewhat lower than normal. This condition may be corrected by a surgical procedure called NEPHROPEXY.

SURGERY OF THE KIDNEY. Surgical removal of the kidney is called nephrectomy, and is done when the kidney is unable to function because of severe disease or injury. Fortunately, one kidney or even less than half a kidney is capable of performing the necessary task of eliminating waste products of the blood.

When obstruction prevents an adequate flow of urine from the kidney, nephrostomy may be performed. This procedure involves a surgical incision into the pelvis of the kidney and usually includes the insertion of a tube or catheter so that drainage can be established. Removal of large kidney stones may entail a "splitting" of the kidney; that is, an incision is made from one end of the kidney to the other. Removal of a calculus from the pelvis of the kidney is known as a pyelolithotomy. If the stone is located in the upper ureter it is removed by a procedure known as a ureterolithotomy. This operation involves an abdominal incision but the kidney is not incised.

Patient Care. The site of the incision for surgery of the kidney creates special problems. The incision is referred to as a flank incision and, because it is directly below the diaphragm, deep breathing, coughing, and other measures necessary to prevent pulmonary complications are extremely painful and difficult for the patient. Narcotic drugs that relieve pain are usually ordered to be given every 4 hours so that coughing and deep breathing can be done. In addition to these measures, the patient should be turned from side to side and encouraged to get out of bed as soon as ordered by the physician.

If a nephrostomy tube has been inserted, care must be taken that it does not kink while the patient is lying in bed. When he moves about there should be enough slack in the connecting tubes so that there is no tension exerted on the nephrostomy tube. It should be remembered that any type of CATHETER or drainage tube inserted during surgery of the kidney or ureters has been left in place for the purpose of drainage. Those responsible for the postoperative care of the patient must constantly be alert to the possibility of obstruction of catheters or tubes, or their accidental removal. In either case the surgeon should be notified immediately so that steps can be taken to reestablish drainage and prevent serious damage to the kidney.

In most cases when a nephrectomy has been done, a Penrose drain is left in place to facilitate removal of serous material collecting in the space left by the kidney. There will, of course, be no urine in this drainage. It may be blood tinged at first, but should not continue to be bright red in color; if it does, it may indicate hemorrhage and should be reported immediately. The amount, color, consistency, and odor of drainage should be noted and recorded on the patient's chart. Dressings may be changed or reinforced as necessary to keep the patient dry and comfortable. A sterile safety pin may be attached to the end of the drain to keep it in place. The drain must not be compressed by the weight of the patient's body. Small pillows are used to support the area around the drain when the patient is lying on the operative side.

Abdominal distention frequently occurs after renal surgery. Fluids by mouth should be given slowly at first until there is evidence that peristalsis is normal. Warm fluids are preferred to iced drinks. Citrus fruit juices and milk are usually contraindicated. A rectal tube and medications to stimulate peristalsis are often ordered to facilitate the passage of flatus.

Hemorrhage is likely to occur after kidney surgery, especially when the highly vascular parenchyma has been incised. The times at which hemorrhage is most likely to occur are the day of surgery and 8 to 12 days after surgery when there is sloughing of tissue during the healing process. Dressings should be observed frequently and any undue drainage of bright red blood must be reported immediately.

amyloid k., one marked by deposition of amyloid; called also waxy kidney.

artificial k., an extracorporeal device used as a substitute for nonfunctioning kidneys to remove endogenous metabolites from the blood, or as an emergency measure to remove exogenous poisons such as bromides or barbiturates. Called also hemodialyzer. Originally the artificial kidney was used only as a temporary substitute until the kidneys could recover and resume normal function. With the development of a type of cannula that is a semipermanent appliance inserted in the patient's arm, it became possible to treat patients with chronic renal failure.

There are several types of artificial kidneys available but all require the same basic components and all employ the principle of a semipermeable membrane through which dialysis takes place. The artificial kidney utilizes a cellophane membrane, the patient's blood, and a wash or dialyzing solution. The blood usually is removed from the brachial or radial artery and continuously recirculated through the dialyzing tube, which is immersed in the dialyzing solution. This solution is of lower concentration than the patient's blood, and so the solutes in the blood pass through the membrane into the dialyzing solution, until an equilibrium is achieved. Thus are waste products or toxins, or both, removed from the patient's blood.

This procedure is sometimes called hemodialysis because the dialysis takes place between the patient's blood and the dialyzing solution. Another method is PERITONEAL DIALYSIS, in which the dialyzing membrane is the membrane lining the peritoneal cavity, and the dialyzing solution is introduced into the peritoneal cavity.

Patients treated by the artificial kidney are given heparin before treatment is begun so that there will be no clotting of blood during the procedure. In peritoneal dialysis no anticoagulation is necessary.

cake k., a solid, irregularly lobed organ of bizarre shape, formed by fusion of the two renal anlagen. Called also lump kidney.

cicatricial k., a shriveled, irregular, and scarred kidney due to suppurative pyelonephritis.

contracted k., an atrophic kidney that may be scarred and granular.

fatty k., one affected with fatty degeneration.

flea-bitten k., one with small, randomly scattered petechiae on its surface.

floating k., one that is freely movable; called also hypermobile kidney (see also NEPHROPTOSIS).

fused k., a single anomalous organ developed as a result of fusion of the renal anlagen.

Goldblatt k., one with obstruction of its blood flow, resulting in renal hypertension.

horseshoe k., an anomalous organ resulting from fusion of the corresponding poles of the renal anlagen.

hypermobile k., one that is freely movable; called also floating kidney (see also NEPHROPTOSIS).

lump k., cake kidney.

polycystic k., a hereditary congenital condition marked by bilateral multiple renal cysts.

sponge k., a congenital condition in which multiple small cystic dilatations of the collecting tubules of the medullary portion of the renal pyramids give the organ a spongy, porous feeling and appearance.

wandering k., floating or hypermobile kidney (see also NEPHROPTOSIS).

waxy k., amyloid kidney.

kidney failure inability of the kidney to excrete metabolites at normal plasma levels under normal loading, or inability to retain electrolytes when intake is normal; in the acute form, marked by uremia and usually by oliguria, with hyperkalemia and pulmonary edema.

Kienböck's disease (kēn′beks) 1. slowly progressive osteochondrosis of the lunate bone; it may affect other wrist bones. 2. traumatic cavitation of the spinal cord.

Kienböck's unit (kēn′beks) a unit of x-ray exposure equal to 0.1 erythema dose; symbol X.

kilo- word element [Gr.], *one thousand;* used in naming units of measurement to designate an amount 10^3 times the size of the unit to which it is joined.

kilocalorie (kil′o-kal″o-re) large calorie.

kilocycle (kil′o-si′k′l) a unit of 1000 (10^3) cycles; e.g., 1000 cycles per second; applied to the frequency of electromagnetic waves.

kilogram (kil′o-gram) a unit of mass (weight) of the metric system, 1000 grams; equivalent to 15,432 grains, or 2.205 pounds (avoirdupois) or 2.679 pounds (apothecaries' weight); abbreviated kg.

k. calorie, large calorie.

kilogram-meter (kil′o-gram-me″ter) a unit of work, representing the energy required to raise 1 kg. of weight 1 meter vertically against gravitational force, equivalent to 7.2 foot-pounds and to 1000 gram-meters.

kilohertz (kil′o-hertz) one thousand (10^3) hertz; abbreviated kHz.

kiloliter (kil′o-le″ter) 1000 liters; 264 gallons; abbreviated kl.

kilometer (kil′o-me″ter) 1000 meters; 3280.83 feet; five-eighths of a mile; abbreviated km.

kilounit (kil″o-u′nit) a quantity equivalent to one thousand (10^3) units.

kilovolt (kil′o-volt) 1000 volts; abbreviated kv.

k. peak, the maximal amount of voltage that an x-ray machine is using; abbreviated kvp.

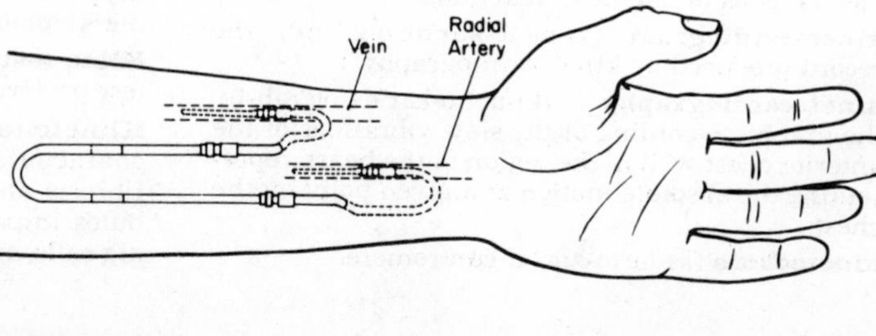

Artificial kidney: schematic drawing showing the tips of the cannula within the vein and artery. (From Fellows, B. J.: The role of the nurse in a chronic dialysis unit. Nursing Clin. N. Amer., *1*:577, 1966.)

Kimmelstiel-Wilson syndrome (kim′el-stēl wil′son) a degenerative complication of DIABETES MELLITUS, with albuminuria, edema, hypertension, renal insufficiency, and retinopathy. Called also intercapillary glomerulosclerosis.

kinanesthesia (kin″an-es-the′ze-ah) loss of the power of perceiving sensations of movement.

kinase (ki′nās) 1. a subclass of the transferases, comprising the enzymes that catalyze the transfer of a high-energy group from a donor (usually ATP) to an acceptor, and named, according to the acceptor, as creatine kinase, fructokinase, etc. 2. an enzyme that activates a zymogen, and named, according to its source, as enterokinase, streptokinase, etc.

kine- word element [Gr.], *movement.* See also words beginning *cine-*.

kinematics (kin″ĕ-mat′iks) that phase of mechanics which deals with the possible motions of a material body.

kinematograph (kin″ĕ-mat′o-graf) an instrument for showing pictures of objects in motion.

kineplasty (kin′ĕ-plas″te) plastic amputation; amputation in which the stump is so formed as to be utilized for producing motion of the prosthesis.

kinesalgia (kin″ĕ-sal′je-ah) pain on muscular exertion.

kinescope (kin′ĕ-skōp) an instrument for ascertaining ocular refraction.

kinesi(o)- word element [Gr.], *movement.*

kinesia (ki-ne′ze-ah) motion sickness.

kinesialgia (ki-ne″se-al′je-ah) kinesalgia.

kinesiatrics (ki-ne″se-at′riks) kinesitherapy.

kinesimeter (kin″ĕ-sim′ĕ-ter) 1. an instrument for quantitative measurement of motions. 2. an instrument for exploring the body surface to test cutaneous sensibility.

kinesiology (ki-ne″se-ol′o-je) scientific study of movement of body parts.

-kinesis word element [Gr.], *movement.*

kinesitherapy (ki-ne″sĭ-ther′ah-pe) treatment of disease by movements or exercise.

kinesthesia (kin″es-the′ze-ah) the sense by which position, weight, and movement are perceived. adj., **kinesthet′ic.**

kinesthesiometer (kin″es-the″ze-om′ĕ-ter) an apparatus for testing kinesthesia.

kinesthesis (kin″es-the′sis) kinesthesia.

kinetic (ki-net′ik) pertaining to or producing motion.

kineticist (ki-net′i-sist) a specialist in kinetics.

kinetics (kĭ-net′iks; ki-net′iks) the scientific study of the turnover, or rate of change, of a specific factor in the body, commonly expressed as units of amount per unit time.

chemical k., the scientific study of the rates and mechanisms of chemical reactions.

kinetocardiogram (ki-ne″to-kar′de-o-gram″) the record produced by kinetocardiography.

kinetocardiography (ki-ne″to-kar″de-og′rah-fe) the graphic recording of the slow vibrations of the anterior chest wall in the region of the heart, representing the absolute motion at a given point on the chest.

kinetochore (ki-ne′to-kōr) a centromere.

kinetogenic (ki-ne″to-jen′ik) causing or producing movement.

kinetoplasm (ki-ne′to-plazm) the most highly contractile portion of the cytoplasm of a cell; applied to the chromatophilic elements in the nervous system.

kinetoplast (ki-ne′to-plast) an accessory body found in many protozoa, primarily the Mastigophora, consisting of the blepharoplast and parabasal body, united by a delicate membrane; loosely called MICRONUCLEUS.

kinetosis (ki″ne-to′sis) any disorder due to unaccustomed motion (see also MOTION SICKNESS).

kinetotherapy (ki-ne″to-ther′ah-pe) kinesitherapy.

kingdom (king′dum) one of the three major categories into which natural objects are usually classified: the animal (including all animals), plant (including all plants), and mineral (including all substance and objects without life). A fourth, the Protista, includes all single-celled organisms.

kinin (ki′nin) any of a group of endogenous peptides that acts on blood vessels, smooth muscles, and nociceptive nerve endings.

venom k., a peptide found in the venom of insects.

kinocilium (ki″no-sil′e-um), pl. *kinocil′ia.* a motile, protoplasmic filament on the free surface of a cell.

kinotoxin (ki″no-tok′sin) a fatigue toxin; kenotoxin.

kinship (kin′ship) a group of individuals of varying degrees of descent from a common ancestor.

Kirschner wire (kērsh′ner) a steel wire for skeletal transfixing of fractured bones and for obtaining skeletal traction in fractures. It is inserted through the soft parts and the bone and is held tight in a clamp.

kl. kiloliter.

Klebs-Löffler bacillus (klebz lef′ler) the diphtheria bacillus, *Corynebacterium diphtheriae.*

Klebsiella (kleb″se-el′ah) a genus of gram-negative bacteria (tribe Escherichieae).

K. friedlän′deri, K. pneumo′niae, the etiologic agent of Friedländer's pneumonia and other respiratory infections.

K. rhinoscleroma′tis, a species isolated from the nasal secretions of patients with rhinoscleroma.

kleptomania (klep″to-ma′ne-ah) an abnormal, uncontrollable desire to steal. This should not be confused with the stage children naturally go through before they understand the concept of ownership. Repeated stealing by an older child may be done simply for the sake of adventure, or it may be an indication of emotional disturbance.

In an adult, the uncontrollable impulse to steal arises from a serious psychologic problem, or neurosis. Since the impulse is an irrational one rooted in subconscious needs of which the person who steals is not aware, he often does not actually covet the object he steals. Sometimes the impulse is expressed by ostensibly borrowing an object and not returning it.

kleptomaniac (klep″to-ma′ne-ak) a person exhibiting kleptomania.

Kline test (klīn) a microscopic slide precipitation test performed for the diagnosis of syphilis.

Klinefelter's syndrome (klīn fel-terz) a condition characterized by the presence of small testes, with fibrosis and hyalinization of the seminiferous tubules, impairment of function and clumping of Leydig cells, and an increase in urinary gonadotropins, associated with an abnormality of the sex chromosomes.

Klippel's disease (klĭ-pelz′) arthritic general pseudoparalysis.

Klippel-Feil syndrome (klĭ-pel′-fīl) shortness of the neck due to reduction in the number of cervical vertebrae or the fusion of multiple hemivertebrae into one osseous mass, with limitation of neck motion and low hairline.

Klumpke's paralysis (kloomp′kez) atrophic paralysis of the lower arm and hand; due to lesion of the eighth cervical and first dorsal nerves. Called also Klumpke-Dejerine paralysis.

Klumpke-Dejerine paralysis (kloomp′kĕ-dezh″-er-ēn′) Klumpke's paralysis.

km. kilometer.

kMc.p.s. kilomegacycles per second.

knee (ne) a complex hinge joint, one of the largest joints of the body, and one that sustains great pressure. The knee is formed by the head of the tibia, the lower end of the femur, and the patella, or kneecap. The bones are jointed by ligaments, and the patella is secured to the adjacent bones by powerful tendons. The fibula is attached at the side of the knee to the tibia. Crescent-shaped pads of cartilage lying on top of the tibia cushion it from the femur and form the gliding surfaces of the joint in motion.

Further cushioning is supplied by bursae, which are located around the main joint, between it and the patella and on the outside of the patella. A capsule of ligaments binds the whole assembly together. The capsule is lined with synovial membrane, which secretes a lubricating fluid (synovia) that makes possible a smooth, gliding motion.

DISORDERS OF THE KNEE. Twists and wrenches of the knee may result from a blow or from pressure. If the injury is followed by swelling and soreness, rest and heat are usually helpful. An elastic bandage may be helpful to bolster the knee against further stress and strain. If symptoms are severe or persistent, they should be reported to a physician.

HOUSEMAID'S KNEE results from frequent kneeling on hard surfaces, causing injury to the front of the knee and inflammation of the bursa in front of the patella, with fluid accumulating within it.

Water on the knee is an excessive accumulation of synovia within the knee joint. The condition may follow a knee injury or result from an infection or acute arthritis. The patella is raised or "floats" on the accumulated fluid, and there is general swelling around the knee. In most cases, the effusion subsides if the joint is rested.

The knee is subject to many joint inflammations that come under the general heading of ARTHRITIS. When the knee is severely inflamed, the patient is confined to bed, and the knee is bound and splinted to rest the joint.

The knee is subject to bone and joint injuries, including DISLOCATION, SPRAIN, and FRACTURE. A fractured patella without wide separation of the parts is often treated by immobilization of the leg for several weeks with a cast or splint, so that the parts can grow together. The surgeon extracts with a needle or syringe the excess blood or fluid that has accumulated in the knee. If the injury is a complicated one, with wide separation of the parts, the parts may be bound together surgically with fine steel wire or similar material. Torn soft tissues are sewed together, and the knee is immobilized in a plaster cast for 4 or 5 weeks.

Recently developed techniques in the surgical restoration of a joint now permit total or partial replacement of the knee. Surgery of this kind is indicated when there has been severe joint damage due to rheumatoid and dejenerative arthritis or a severely traumatic fracture.

Trick knee is a colloquial term referring to a knee that is highly susceptible to injury and that may constantly or intermittently give trouble. It often occurs in athletes, who initially suffer a twist or blow that is sufficiently violent to tear ligaments or to weaken or displace other internal components of the knee. Thereafter, under the stress of athletic competition, the knee may unexpectedly give way or "lock." Upon manipulation the knee often snaps back to normal position. Wearing an elastic bandage during strenuous activity may help keep such a weakened knee in position.

Another condition that interferes with free knee movement may be caused by loose fragments in the knee resulting from tuberculosis of the bone, arthritis, or inflammation of the synovial membrane that lines the knee joint.

KNOCK-KNEE, an inward curving of the knees, is usually caused by irregular bone growth or by weak ligaments; formerly rickets was a common cause.

k. jerk, k. reflex, a kick reflex produced by sharply tapping the patellar liagment. To test this reflex, the

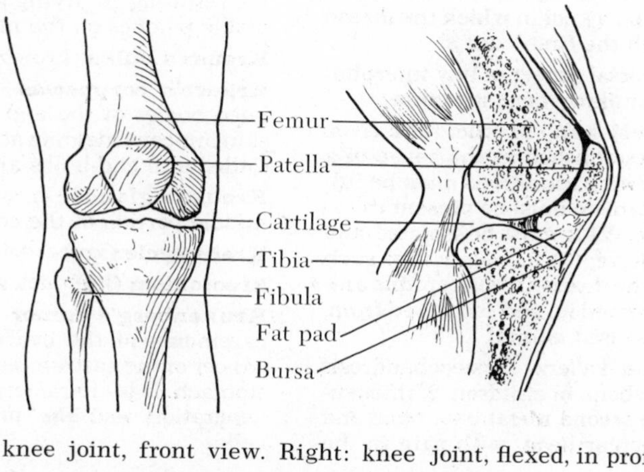

Left: knee joint, front view. Right: knee joint, flexed, in profile.

lower part of the leg is allowed to hang relaxed, usually by crossing the legs at the knees. The physician taps the ligament below the patella with a small rubber hammer. The normal reaction is contraction of the quadriceps muscle, causing involuntary extension of the lower leg. Called also patellar reflex and quadriceps reflex.

The knee jerk is a stretch reflex; striking the patellar ligament stretches the quadriceps muscle at the front of the thigh and causes it to contract. Two nerves are involved; one receives the stimulus and transmits the impulse to the spinal cord, and the other, a motor nerve, receives the impulse and relays it to the quadriceps muscle.

Inadequate response to the knee jerk test may mean that the reflex mechanism involved is in some way impaired. In some people the knee jerk is normally so light that it is nearly imperceptible, and the physician makes other tests to check the reflex mechanism.

kneecap (ne′kap) patella.

knock-knee (nok′ne) a childhood deformity, developing gradually, in which the knees rub together or "knock" in walking and the ankles are far apart; called also genu valgum. At one time, knock-knee and bowleg were common symptoms of rickets. Knock-knee is now more often caused by an irregularity in the growth of the leg bones, sometimes stemming from injury to the bone ends at the knee, or by weak ligaments. The weight of the body, which is not supported properly, turns the knees in and the weak lower legs buckle until the ankles are spread far apart.

Knock-knee in young children varies in seriousness. Milder cases frequently disappear after early childhood as bones, ligaments, and muscles strengthen and coordination improves. More serious cases can often be corrected by strengthening exercises and by proper manipulation of the joints. Sometimes braces are used to ensure the proper alignment of growing legs.

In a very young child, knock-knee involves only the soft bone ends where the bone grows. If allowed to continue for a number of years, the condition can lead to abnormal developments in body structure. The sooner corrective measures are taken, the more effective the treatment is likely to be.

knot (not) 1. an intertwining of the ends or parts of one or more threads, sutures, or strip of cloth. 2. in anatomy, a knoblike swelling or protuberance.

surgeon's k., surgical k., a knot in which the thread is passed twice through the first loop.

knuckle (nuk″l) the dorsal aspect of any interphalangeal joint, or any similarly bent structure.

Koch's law (postulates) (kōks) in order for a given microorganism to be established as the cause of a given disease, the following conditions must be fulfilled: (1) the microorganism must be present in every case of the disease; (2) it must be isolated and cultivated in pure culture; (3) inoculation of such culture must produce the disease in susceptible animals; (4) it must be observed in, and recovered from, the experimentally diseased animal.

Köhler's bone disease (ka′lerz) 1. osteochondrosis of the tarsal navicular bone in children. 2. thickening of the shaft of the second metatarsal bone and changes about its articular head, with pain in the second metatarsophalangeal joint on walking or standing.

koilo- word element [Gr.], *hollowed; concave.*

koilonychia (koi″lo-nik′e-ah) dystrophy of the nails in which they are abnormally thin and concave from side to side, with the edges turned up.

koilorrhachic (koi″lo-rak′ik) having a vertebral column in which the lumbar curvature is anteriorly concave.

koilosternia (koi″lo-ster′ne-ah) pectus excavatum (funnel chest).

Kölliker's interstitial granules (kel′ĭ-kerz) granules seen in the sarcoplasm of muscle fibers.

Kolmer test (kōl′mer) 1. a modification of the Wassermann test for syphilis. 2. a specific complement-fixation test for various bacterial diseases.

kolp- for words beginning thus, see those beginning *colp-*.

kolypeptic (ko″lĕ-pep′tik) hindering or checking digestion.

Konakion (kon″ah-ki′on) trademark for a preparation of phytonadione (vitamin K_1), used as a prothrombinogenic agent.

konometer (ko-nom′ĕ-ter) an apparatus for counting the dust particles in the air.

Koplik's spots (kop′liks) small, irregular, bright red spots on the buccal and lingual mucosa, with a minute bluish white speck in the center of each; they are pathognomonic of beginning measles.

Korsakoff's syndrome (psychosis) (kor-sak′ofs) a psychosis associated with chronic alcoholism and caused by vitamin B_1 (thiamine) deficiency; characteristics include disturbances of orientation, memory defect, susceptibility to external stimulation and suggestion, hallucinations, and, usually, the signs of polyneuritis (wristdrop, etc.). There is irreversible brain damage; confinement to an institution is a frequent outcome of this condition.

Kr chemical symbol, *krypton.*

Krabbe's disease (krab′ēz) a familial form of leukoencephalopathy beginning in infancy, marked pathologically by cerebral demyelination and by the presence of large globoid bodies in the white substance.

Kraepelin's classification (kra′pa-linz) a classification of manic-depressive and schizophrenic groups of mental disease.

kraurosis (kraw-ro′sis) a dried, shriveled condition.

k. vul′vae, atrophy of the female external genitalia, resulting in drying and shriveling, with leukoplakic patches on the mucosa and intense itching.

Krause's bulbs (krow′zez) Krause's corpuscles.

Krause's corpuscles (krow′zez) small encapsulated bodies at the end of sensory nerve fibers in skin, mucous membranes, muscles, and other areas. Called also end-bulbs and Krause's bulbs.

Krause's glands (krow′zez) mucous glands in the middle portion of the conjunctiva.

Krebs cycle (krebz) tricarboxylic acid cycle.

kreotoxism (kre″o-tok′sizm) poisoning by meat.

Krukenberg's tumor (kroo′ken-bergz) a type of carcinoma of the ovary, usually metastatic from cancer of the gastrointestinal tract, especially of the stomach. It is characterized by areas of mucoid degeneration and the presence of signet-ring–like cells.

krypton (krip′ton) a chemical element, atomic number 36, atomic weight 83.80, symbol Kr. (See table of ELEMENTS.)

Kufs' disease (ko͞ofs) the late juvenile, or adult, form of AMAUROTIC FAMILIAL IDIOCY, occurring between 15 and 26 years of age, differing from the infantile form (TAY-SACHS DISEASE) in that it shows no racial predilection, and from the infantile, late infantile (BIELSCHOWSKY'S DISEASE), and juvenile (SPIELMEYER-VOGT DISEASE) forms in that ocular lesions are absent; clinical findings are those of cerebellar or basal ganglia disorders.

Kugelberg-Welander disease a hereditary juvenile form of muscular atrophy, due to lesions of the anterior horns of the spinal cord, with onset principally between 2 and 17 years of age; it is marked by atrophy and weakness of the proximal muscles of the lower extremities and pelvic girdle, followed by involvement of the distal muscles and muscular twitchings.

Kümmell's disease (spondylitis) (kim′elz) compression fracture of vertebra, with symptoms occurring a few weeks after injury, including spinal pain, intercostal neuralgia, motor disturbances of the legs, and kyphosis that is painful on pressure and easily reduced by extension. Called also post-traumatic spondylitis.

Kupffer's cells (ko͞op′ferz) large, stellate or pyramidal, intensely phagocytic cells lining the walls of the hepatic sinusoids and forming part of the reticuloendothelial system.

kuru (koo′roo) a chronic, progressive, uniformly fatal central nervous system disorder due to a virus and transmissible to subhuman primates; seen only in the Fore and neighboring peoples of New Guinea.

Kussmaul's disease (ko͞os′mowlz) an inflammatory disease of the coats of the small and medium-sized arteries, marked by a variety of systemic symptoms (see also COLLAGEN DISEASES). Called also periarteritis nodosa.

Kussmaul's respiration (ko͞os′mowlz) a distressing dyspnea occurring in paroxysms, characteristic of diabetic acidosis and coma. Called also air hunger.

kv. kilovolt.

kvp. kilovolt peak.

kwashiorkor (kwash″e-or′kor) a syndrome occurring in infants and young children soon after weaning. It is due to severe protein deficiency, and the symptoms include edema, pigmentation changes of skin and hair, impaired growth and development, distention of the abdomen (pot belly), and pathologic liver changes.

Kwell (kwel) trademark for preparations of gamma benzene hexachloride, a pediculicide and scabicide.

Kyasanur Forest disease (kyah′sah-nor for′est) a highly fatal virus disease of monkeys in the Kyasanur Forest of India, communicable to man, in whom it produces hemorrhagic symptoms.

kyestein (ki-es′te-in) a film that sometimes floats on stale urine.

kymatism (ki′mah-tizm) myokymia; quivering of muscles.

kymogram (ki′mo-gram) the graphic record (tracing or film) produced by the kymograph.

kymograph (ki′mo-graf) an instrument for recording variations or undulations, arterial or other.

kymography (ki-mog′rah-fe) the use of the kymograph.

Kynex (ki′neks) trademark for preparations of sulfamethoxypyridazine, an antibacterial used in urinary tract and other infections.

kynocephalus (ki″no-sef′ah-lus) a monster with a head like that of a dog.

kynurenine (kin″u-re′nin) a metabolite of tryptophan found in microorganisms and in the urine of normal animals; it is a precursor of kynurenic acid and an intermediate in the conversion of tryptophan to niacin.

kyphos (ki′fos) the hump in the spine in kyphosis.

kyphoscoliosis (ki″fo-sko″le-o′sis) backward (kyphosis) and lateral (scoliosis) curvature of the spine, in vertebral osteochondrosis (Scheuermann's disease).

kyphosis (ki-fo′sis) abnormally increased convexity in the curvature of the thoracic spine as viewed from the side; called also hunchback. adj., **kyphot′ic.** The condition may be the result of an acquired disease, an injury, or a congenital disorder or disease. It never develops from poor posture.

This spinal deformity usually is caused by vertebral tuberculosis (POTT'S DISEASE), or by some other destructive inflammation of the vertebrae (spondylitis). Kyphosis sometimes occurs with certain forms of poliomyelitis and with diseases that cause bone destruction, as happens in osteitis deformans (Paget's disease). An injury, such as a fracture of the spine, treated improperly or not at all, may also result in hunchback. There are some rare cases of kyphosis caused by congenital deformities and diseases. One example, achondroplasia, or fetal rickets, is a congenital bone disorder that affects growth and bone formation.

There are no specific symptoms of kyphosis besides back pain and increasing immobility of the spine. Symptoms vary with the cause, and any back pain or injury should be investigated.

kyrtorrhachic (kir″to-rak′ik) having a vertebral column in which the lumbar curvature is anteriorly convex.

kyto- for words beginning thus, see those beginning *cyto-*.

L

L. Latin; left; length; libra (*pound, balance*); licentiate; light sense; limes (*boundary*); liter, lumbar; coefficient of induction.

L_0 Ehrlich's symbol for a toxin-antitoxin mixture that is completely neutralized and will not kill an animal.

L+ Ehrlich's symbol for a toxin-antitoxin mixture that contains one fatal dose in excess and will kill the experimental animal.

L- chemical prefix (written as small capital) that specifies that the substance corresponds in chemical configuration to the standard substance L-glyceraldehyde. Carbohydrates are named by this method to distinguish them by their chemical composition. The opposite prefix is D-.

l. liter

l- chemical abbreviation, *levo-* (i.e., left or counterclockwise).

λ lambda, the eleventh letter of the Greek alphabet; symbol for *decay constant.*

La chemical symbol, *lanthanum.*

L & A light and accommodation (reaction of the pupils).

labia (la′be-ah) [L.] plural of *labium.*

labial (la′be-al) pertaining to a lip, or labium.

labialism (la′be-ah-lizm″) defective speech with use of labial sounds.

labile (la′bil) 1. gliding; moving from point to point over the surface; unstable. 2. chemically unstable.

lability (lah-bil′ĭ-te) the quality of being labile. In psychiatry, emotional instability; a tendency to show alternating states of gaiety and somberness.

labio- word element [L.], *lip.*

labioglossolaryngeal (la″be-o-glos″o-lah-rin′je-al) pertaining to the lips, tongue, and larynx.

labioglossopharyngeal (la″be-o-glos″o-fah-rin′je-al) pertaining to the lips, tongue, and pharynx.

labiograph (la′be-o-graf″) an instrument for recording movements of the lips in speaking.

labiomental (la″be-o-men′tal) pertaining to the lips and chin.

labionasal (la″be-o-na′zal) pertaining to the lip and nose.

labiopalatine (la″be-o-pal′ah-tin) pertaining to the lips and palate.

labioplasty (la′be-o-plas″te) plastic repair of a lip; cheiloplasty.

labium (la′be-um), pl. *la′bia* [L.] a fleshy border or edge; a lip. adj., **la′bial.**

l. ma′jus (pl. *la′bia majo′ra*), an elongated fold in the female, one on either side of the rima pudendi.

l. mi′nus (pl. *la′bia mino′ra*), the small fold of skin on either side, between the labia majora and the opening of the vagina.

la′bia o′ris, the lips of the mouth.

labor (la′bor) the function of the female organism by which the product of conception is expelled from the uterus through the vagina to the outside world. The process of labor takes place in three stages: (1) opening or dilation of the cervix uteri; (2) passage of the fetus through the birth canal, or vagina; and (3) separation and expulsion of the placenta. (See below.)

Labor is believed to be triggered by the release of oxytocin after a fall in the levels of other hormones. Normally at the end of pregnancy oxytocin, which is stored in the posterior lobe of the pituitary gland, is released and stimulates contraction of the uterine muscles.

First Stage of Labor. The beginning of labor is usually indicated by one or more of the following signs: (1) Show: passage from the vagina of small quantities of blood-tinged mucus. (2) Breaking the "bag of waters": normal rupture of membranes that is indicated by a gush or slow leakage of amniotic fluid from the vagina. (3) True labor contractions.

The first two of these signs are almost always unmistakable. The contractions, however, can be confusing. BRAXTON-HICKS CONTRACTIONS, or "false" labor pains, can be distinguished from true labor contractions by the irregular time intervals between them and by their tendency to disappear when the patient changes position or gets up and walks about. True labor contractions are regularly spaced and usually start in the small of the back, or as a feeling of tightness in the abdomen, or of pressure in the pelvis. The contractions recur at increasingly shorter intervals, every three to five minutes, and become progressively stronger and longer-lasting. The increase in the strength of contractions usually is accompanied by an increase in the amount of show because of rupture of capillaries in the dilating cervix.

This first stage of childbirth is known as the dilation period. The uterus is like a large rubber bottle with a half-inch long neck that is almost closed. As the uterine muscles contract, the cervix becomes thinner (effacement) and more open (dilated) so that the neck of the uterus eventually resembles that of a jar more than that of a bottle.

The length of the first stage of labor varies with each individual patient. It is related to the strength and effectiveness of the contractions and is a period when the mother is instructed to relax as much as possible and let the uterus do the work. Pushing or bearing down is not effective during this stage and is harmful in that it may cause a tearing of the cervix and will only serve to exhaust the mother. She is encouraged to rest and possibly to nap between contractions.

The second stage of labor may be heralded by symptoms of nausea, vomiting, irritability, the urge to bear down, or periods of feeling hot and then cold. These are signs of the period of transition from the first to the second stage of labor.

Second Stage of Labor. This second period, called the expulsion stage, usually is characterized by intense contractions that last for about one full minute and occur at 2 to 3 minute intervals. The cervix is fully dilated and the mother is able to help with this process by bearing down with each uterine contraction, using her abdominal muscles to help expel the infant.

Third Stage of Labor. In this final stage the

placenta detaches itself from the uterine wall and is expelled. The process takes about 15 minutes, and is painless.

PATIENT CARE. Once labor has begun the patient should have someone in constant attendance. She will derive much emotional support from one who is warm, kind, and understanding, and displays a genuine interest in her welfare and that of her infant. It is best to have the same person care for her through the entire labor and birth process.

During labor the strength, frequency, and duration of contractions are noted and recorded. It is expected that the contractions will increase in all three characteristics, but a sudden change in any one should be reported to the physician immediately. The rate, regularity, and volume of the fetal heart tones are checked and recorded periodically. Some apprehensive patients may be helped by allowing them to listen to the infant's heartbeat.

Food and fluids are withheld during active labor, but thirst may cause some discomfort and may be lessened by allowing the patient to moisten her lips with a gauze sponge dipped in ice water. Frequent bathing of the face with a cool washcloth often helps relieve the flushed feeling brought about by the actual hard work being done by the mother. Frequent changing of the patient's gown and the quilted pad protecting the bed linens may be necessary to keep her clean, dry, and comfortable.

If hospital policy allows the husband to remain with his wife during labor, he should be instructed in ways in which he can help his wife and at the same time feel that he is making some contribution in this very important event in their lives. He may wish to participate in keeping a record of the contractions or he might appreciate the opportunity to listen to the fetal heart tones occasionally. If the patient feels that sacral support during each contraction helps mitigate the pain, the husband can be shown how to do this. Some fathers have attended classes for expectant parents and are prepared for their role during labor and delivery. Both husband and wife should be informed of the progress being made during labor so they can feel that something is being accomplished by their efforts.

The mother should be instructed to relax between contractions so as to conserve her strength. She should not bear down until the cervix is dilated, since this effort will only serve to exhaust her and may cause lacerations of the cervix. After the cervix is fully dilated she can speed the birth process by holding her breath and contracting her abdominal muscles. Controlled breathing exercises learned in classes for expectant parents promote relaxation and aid labor. (See also NATURAL CHILDBIRTH.)

Although serious complications rarely develop during labor, they can occur and must be watched for. Observations to report immediately include hyperactivity of the fetus; vaginal bleeding in excess of a heavy show; a rapid and irregular pulse and drop in blood pressure; sudden rise in blood pressure; headache, visual disturbances, extreme restlessness, or rapidly developing edema. A sudden cessation of contractions or a contraction that does not relax may indicate a serious disturbance in the labor process. The appearance of meconium in the vaginal discharge may indicate fetal distress unless the infant is in a breech position.

artificial l., induced labor.

dry l., that in which the amniotic fluid escapes before contraction of the uterus begins.

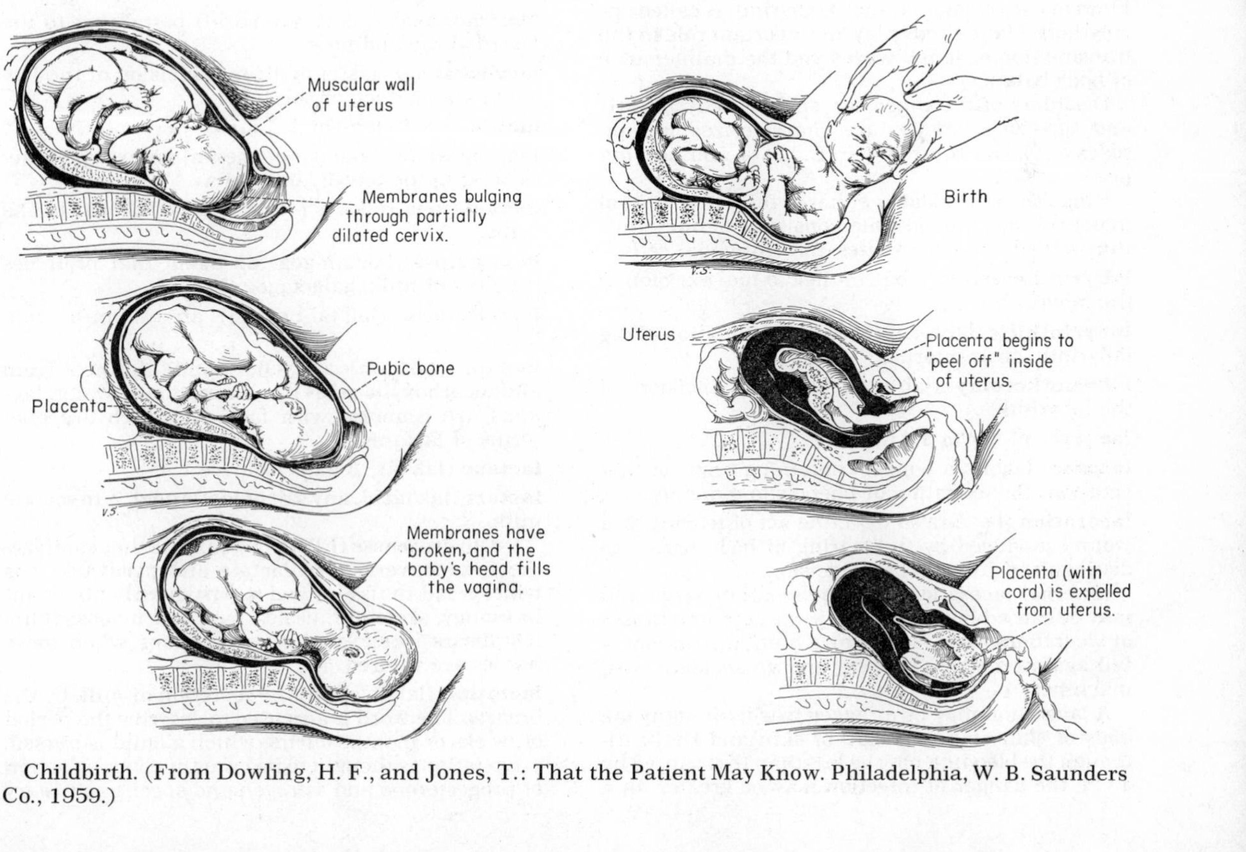
Muscular wall of uterus
Membranes bulging through partially dilated cervix.
Pubic bone
Placenta
Membranes have broken, and the baby's head fills the vagina.
Birth
Uterus
Placenta begins to "peel off" inside of uterus.
Placenta (with cord) is expelled from uterus.

Childbirth. (From Dowling, H. F., and Jones, T.: That the Patient May Know. Philadelphia, W. B. Saunders Co., 1959.)

false l., ineffective pains resembling labor pains, not accompanied by cervical dilation; called also false pains. (See also BRAXTON-HICKS CONTRACTIONS.)

induced l., that which is brought on by extraneous means, e.g., by the use of drugs that cause uterine contractions; called also artificial labor.

instrumental l., delivery facilitated by the use of instruments, particularly forceps.

missed l., that in which contractions begin and then cease, the fetus being retained for weeks or months.

precipitate l., delivery accomplished with undue speed.

premature l., expulsion of a viable infant before the normal end of gestation; usually applied to interruption of pregnancy between the twenty-eighth and thirty-seventh weeks.

spontaneous l., delivery occurring without artificial aid.

laboratory (lab′o-rah-tor″e) a place equipped for making tests or doing experimental work.

labrum (la′brum), pl. *la′bra* [L.] an edge, rim, or lip.

labyrinth (lab′ĭ-rinth) the internal ear, consisting of the vestibule, cochlea, and SEMICIRCULAR CANALS. (See also Plate 15.) adj., **labyrin′thine.** The cochlea is concerned with hearing, and the vestibule and semicircular canals with equilibrium (sense of balance).

The bony portion of the labyrinth (osseous labyrinth) is composed of a series of canals tunneled out of the temporal bone. Inside the osseous labyrinth is the membranous labyrinth, which conforms to the general shape of the osseous labyrinth but is much smaller. A fluid called perilymph fills the space between the osseous and membranous labyrinths. Fluid inside the membranous labyrinth is called endolymph. These fluids play an important role in the transmission of sound waves and the maintenance of body balance.

Disorders of the inner ear, such as labyrinthitis and MENIÈRE'S DISEASE, are characterized by episodes of dizziness, ringing in the ears, and hearing loss.

ethmoid l., ethmoidal l., either of the paired lateral masses of the ethmoid bone, consisting of numerous thin-walled cellular cavities, the ethmoidal cells.

labyrinthectomy (lab′ĭ-rin-thek′to-me) excision of the labyrinth.

labyrinthitis (lab″ĭ-rin-thi′tis) inflammation of the labyrinth; otitis interna.

labyrinthotomy (lab″ĭ-rin-thot′o-me) incision of the labyrinth.

lac (lak), pl. *lac′ta* [L.] milk.

laccase (lak′ās) a copper-containing enzyme that catalyzes the oxidation of phenols to quinones.

laceration (las″ĕ-ra′shun) 1. the act of tearing. 2. a wound produced by the tearing of body tissue, as distinguishd from a cut or incision.

External lacerations may be small or large and may be caused in many ways. Some common causes of lacerations are a blow from a blunt instrument, a fall against a rough surface, and an accident with machinery.

A laceration may be a ragged tear with many tag ends of skin or a torn flap of skin and flesh. Although the bleeding may be less than that caused by a cut, the danger of infection may be greater. In a laceration there is likely to be more damage to surrounding tissue, with a greater area exposed.

Because of the danger of infection, cleaning the laceration is the first and most important step in treatment. If the wound is not extensive or deep, the cleaning is simply done with soap and water. The wound is then covered with dry sterile gauze. If parts of the wound are deep, medical attention should be sought and immunity against tetanus established.

Lacerations within the body occur when an organ is compressed or moved out of place by an external or internal force. This kind of laceration may result from a blow that does not penetrate the skin. Surgical repair is usually necessary for internal lacerations.

lacertus (lah-ser′tus), pl. *lacer′ti* [L.] a name given certain fibrous attachments of muscles.

lacrimal (lak′rĭ-mal) pertaining to tears.

l. apparatus, a group of organs concerned with the production and drainage of tears (see also Plate 15); it is a protective device that helps keep the eye moist and free of dust and other irritating particles.

The lacrimal gland, which secretes tears, lies over the upper, outer corner of the eye; its excretory ducts branch downward toward the eyeball. A constant stream of tears washes down over the front of the eye and is drained off through two small openings located in the inner corner of the eye. Through these openings the tears pass into the lacrimal canaliculus, then through the lacrimal sac into the nasolacrimal duct and finally into the nasal cavity.

lacrimation (lak″rĭ-ma′shun) secretion and discharge of tears.

lacrimator (lak′rĭ-ma″tor) an agent, as a gas, that induces the flow of tears.

lacrimatory (lak′rĭ-mah-to″re) causing a flow of tears.

lacrimonasal (lak″rĭ-mo-na′zal) pertaining to the lacrimal sac and nose.

lacrimotomy (lak″rĭ-mot′o-me) incision of the lacrimal gland, duct, or sac.

lact(o)- word element [L.], *milk.*

lactacidemia (lak-tas″ĭ-de′me-ah) an excess of lactic acid in the blood; lacticemia.

lactaciduria (lak-tas″ĭ-du′re-ah) lactic acid in the urine.

lactagogue (lak′tah-gog) an agent that promotes the flow of milk; galactagogue.

lactalbumin (lak″tal-bu′min) an albumin from milk.

lactam (lak′tam) a cyclic amide formed from aminocarboxylic acids by elimination of water; lactams are isomeric with lactims, which are enol forms of lactams.

lactase (lak′tās) β-galactosidase.

lactate (lak′tāt) 1. any salt of lactic acid. 2. to secrete milk.

l. dehydrogenase (LDH), an enzyme that catalyzes the interconversion of lactate and pyruvate. It is widespread in tissues and is particularly abundant in kidney, skeletal muscle, liver, and myocardium. It appears in elevated concentrations when these tissues are injured.

lactation (lak-ta′shun) the secretion of milk by the breasts. The word is also used to describe the period of weeks or months during which a child is nursed.

Lactation is thought to be brought about by action of progesterone and estrogen and specific pituitary hormones, such as lactogenic hormone (prolactin). Lactation does not begin until at least 3 days after the birth of the baby. Before that, and immediately after birth, the breast secretes colostrum, a fluid containing substances valuable to the baby until milk is formed.

l. hormone, lactogenic hormone, or prolactin.

lacteal (lak′te-al) 1. pertaining to milk. 2. any of the intestinal lymphatics that transport chyle.

lactescence (lak-tes′ens) resemblance to milk.

lactic (lak′tik) pertaining to milk.

l. acid, a compound formed in the body in anaerobic metabolism of carbohydrate, and also produced by bacterial action on milk. The sodium salt of racemic or inactive lactic (sodium lactate) acid is used as an electrolyte and fluid replenisher.

lacticemia (lak″tĭ-se′me-ah) an excess of lactic acid in the blood; lactacidemia.

lactiferous (lak-tif′er-us) conveying milk.

lactifuge (lak′tĭ-fūj) checking or stopping milk secretion; an agent that so acts.

lactigenous (lak-tij′ĕ-nus) producing milk.

lactigerous (lak-tij′er-us) lactiferous.

lactim (lak′tim) see LACTAM.

lactivorous (lak-tiv′o-rus) feeding or subsisting upon milk.

Lactobacillus (lak″to-bah-sil′us) a genus of bacteria, some of which are considered to be etiologically related to dental caries, but are otherwise nonpathogenic. They produce lactic acid by fermentation.

lactobacillus (lak″to-bah-sil′us), pl. *lactobacil′li.* any individual organism of the genus *Lactobacillus.*

lactocele (lak′to-sēl) galactocele.

lactogen (lak′to-jen) any substance that enhances lactation.

human placental l., a hormone secreted by the placenta; it has lactogenic, luteotropic, and growth-promoting activity, and inhibits maternal insulin activity.

lactogenic (lak″to-jen′ik) stimulating the production of milk.

l. hormone, one of the gonadotropic hormones of the anterior pituitary; it stimulates and sustains lactation in postpartum animals, and shows luteotropic activity in certain mammals. Called also prolactin.

lactoglobulin (lak″to-glob′u-lin) a globulin occurring in milk.

immune l's, antibodies (immunoglobulins) occurring in the colostrum of mammals.

lactolase (lak′to-lās) an enzyme that produces lactic acid.

lactometer (lak-tom′ĕ-ter) an instrument for measuring the specific gravity of milk; galactometer.

lactone (lak′tōn) 1. an aromatic liquid from lactic acid. 2. a cyclic organic compound in which the chain is closed by ester formation between a carboxyl and a hydroxyl group in the same molecule.

lactophosphate (lak″to-fos′fāt) any salt of lactic and phosphoric acids.

lactoprotein (lak″to-pro′te-in) a protein derived from milk.

lactorrhea (lak″to-re′ah) excessive or spontaneous milk flow; persistent secretion of milk irrespective of nursing; galactorrhea.

lactose (lak′tōs) a sugar derived from milk, which on hydrolysis yields glucose and galactose.

lactosuria (lak″to-su′re-ah) lactose in the urine.

lactotherapy (lak″to-ther′ah-pe) treatment by milk diet.

lactovegetarian (lak″to-vej″ĕ-ta′re-an) 1. a person who subsists on a diet of milk or milk products and vegetables. 2. pertaining to such a diet.

lactulose (lak′tu-lōs) a synthetic disaccharide used as a cathartic.

lacuna (lah-ku′nah), pl. *lacu′nae* [L.] 1. a small pit or hollow cavity. 2. a defect or gap, as in the field of vision (scotoma). adj., **lacu′nar.**

absorption l., a pit or groove in developing bone that is undergoing resorption; frequently found to contain osteoclasts.

intervillous l., one of the blood spaces of the placenta in which the fetal villi are found.

l. mag′na, the lateral expansion of the urethra of the glans penis; called also navicular fossa.

l. pharyn′gis, a depression of the pharyngeal end of the eustachian tube.

lacunule (lah-ku′nūl) a minute lacuna.

lacus (la′kus), pl. *la′cus* [L.] lake.

l. lacrima′lis, lacrimal lake.

lae- for words beginning thus, see those beginning *le-*.

Laënnec (la-nek′) René Théophile Hyacinthe (1781–1826). French physician. He is known for the invention of the stethoscope in 1819 and his *De l'auscultation médiate,* from which much of our knowledge of chest diseases is derived.

Laënnec's cirrhosis (la-neks′) cirrhosis of the liver associated with alcohol abuse.

Laënnec's pearls (la-neks′) soft casts of the smaller bronchial tubes expectorated in bronchial asthma.

Laetrile (la′ĕ-tril) trademark for a substance derived from apricot pits, alleged to have antineoplastic activity.

Lafora's bodies (lah-fo′rahz) intracytoplasmic inclusions consisting of a complex of glycoprotein and acid mucopolysaccharide; widespread deposits are found in myoclonus epilepsy.

Lafora's disease (lah-fo′rahz) myoclonus epilepsy.

lag (lag) 1. the time elapsing between application of a stimulus and the resulting reaction. 2. the early period after inoculation of bacteria into a culture medium, in which the growth or cell division is slow.

lagena (lah-je′nah) the curved, flask-shaped organ of hearing in vertebrates lower than mammals, corresponding to the cochlear duct.

lageniform (lah-jen′ĭ-form) flask-shaped.

lagophthalmos (lag″of-thal′mos) inability to shut the eyes completely.

lake (lāk) 1. to undergo separation of hemoglobin from erythrocytes. 2. a circumscribed collection of fluid in a hollow or depressed cavity. (See also LACUNA.)

lacrimal l., the triangular space at the medial angle of the eye, where the tears collect. (See also LACRIMAL APPARATUS.)

lal(o)- word element [Gr.], *speech; babbling.*

LaLeche League (la-lesh′) an organization formed in 1957 for the purpose of helping women to breast-feed their infants. Information about the organization and the services it provides can be obtained from local groups or from the LaLeche

League International, Franklin Park, Illinois 60131.

laliatry (lal-i′ah-tre) the study and treatment of disorders of speech.

lallation (lah-la′shun) a babbling, infantile form of speech.

lalognosis (lal″og-no′sis) the understanding of speech.

lalopathology (lal″o-pah-thol′o-je) the branch of medicine dealing with disorders of speech.

lalopathy (lah-lop′ah-the) any speech disorder.

laloplegia (lal″o-ple′je-ah) paralysis of the organs of speech.

lalorrhea (lal″o-re′ah) excessive flow of words.

Lamarck's theory (lah-marks′) the theory that acquired characteristics may be transmitted.

Lamaze method (lah-māz′) a method of preparations for NATURAL CHILDBIRTH developed by the French obstetrician Fernand Lamaze, and based on the Russian psychoprophylactic technique of training the mind and body for the purpose of modifying the perception of pain during labor and delivery. The Lamaze method of prepared childbirth involves class sessions for both parents in which they learn about the birth process and the mechanisms of labor, are taught what to except and what is expected of them during the birth of their child, and are trained in special exercises that develop neuromuscular control, promote physical conditioning, and eliminate or reduce the need for drugs and instruments during delivery. Advocates of the Lamaze method do not claim complete absence of pain during labor and delivery in every case, but they do feel that the method enriches the lives of the parents in many ways and provides for them a means of sharing the birth experience that is denied to them in the more conventional method of hospital deliveries.

lambda (lam′dah) the point of union of the lambdoid and sagittal sutures.

lambdacism (lam′dah-sizm) inability to utter the *l* sound.

lambdoid (lam′doid) shaped like the Greek letter lambda, Λ or λ.

lame (lām) incapable of normal locomotion; deviation from the normal gait.

lamella (lah-mel′ah), pl. *lamel′lae* [L.] 1. a thin scale or plate, as of bone. 2. a medicated disk or wafer to be inserted under the eyelid. adj., **lamel′lar.**

circumferential l., one of the bony plates that underlie the periosteum and endosteum.

concentric l., haversian lamella.

endosteal l., one of the bony plates lying beneath the endosteum.

ground l., interstitial lamella.

haversian l., one of the concentric bony plates surrounding a haversian canal.

intermediate l., interstitial l., one of the bony plates that fill in between the haversian systems.

lamina (lam′ĭ-nah), pl. *lam′inae* [L.] a thin, flat plate or layer; used in anatomic nomenclature to designate such a structure, or a layer of a composite structure.

l. basila′ris, the posterior wall of the cochlear duct, separating it from the scala tympani.

l. choroidocapilla′ris, the inner layer of the choroid, composed of a single-layered network of small capillaries.

l. cribro′sa, 1. fascia cribrosa. 2. (of ethmoid bone) the horizontal plate of ethmoid bone forming the roof of the nasal cavity, and perforated by many foramina for passage of olfactory nerves. 3. (of sclera) the perforated part of the sclera through which pass the axons of the retinal ganglion cells.

epithelial l., the layer of ependymal cells covering the choroid plexus.

l. fus′ca, the pigmentary layer of the sclera.

l. pro′pria, 1. the connective tissue layer of mucous membrane. 2. the middle fibrous layer of the tympanic membrane.

spiral l., l. spira′lis, 1. a double plate of bone winding spirally around the modiolus, dividing the spiral canal of the cochlea into the scala tympani and scali vestibuli. 2. a bony projection on the outer wall of the cochlea in the lower part of the first turn.

terminal l. of hypothalamus, the thin plate derived from the telencephalon, forming the anterior wall of the third ventricle of the cerebrum.

vertebral l., one of the paired dorsal parts of the vertebral arch connected to the pedicles of the vertebra.

laminagraphy (lam″ĭ-nag′rah-fe) a special technique of body-section ROENTGENOGRAPHY.

laminar (lam′ĭ-nar) made up of laminae or layers; pertaining to a lamina.

Laminaria (lam″ĭ-na′re-ah) a genus of seaweeds, the kelps. Its dried stems are used to dilate the uterine cervix in induced ABORTION.

laminated (lam′ĭ-nāt″ed) made up of laminae or thin layers.

lamination (lam″ĭ-na′shun) a laminar structure or arrangement.

laminectomy (lam″ĭ-nek′to-me) surgical excision of the posterior arch of a vertebra. The procedure is most often performed to relieve the symptoms of a ruptured intervertebral disk (slipped DISK). When several disks are involved, spinal fusion may be done so that the vertebrae in the affected area will remain in a fixed position. Bone grafts, usually taken from the iliac crest, are applied to fuse the affected vertebrae permanently, resulting in limitation of movement of this portion of the spine. Laminectomy is also performed for the removal of an intervertebral or spinal cord tumor.

PATIENT CARE. Before surgery the patient will receive treatment for slipped disk. It should be remembered that when the patient is transported to other departments for various preoperative diagnostic tests, special care must be taken to keep the spine in good alignment.

Postoperatively the patient is placed in a bed with bed boards and a firm mattress. His position is changed by "log-rolling" to prevent motion of the vertebral column. In addition he is observed for signs of hemorrhage or leakage of cerebrospinal fluid on the surgical dressing. Should such signs appear, the surgeon should be notified at once. If necessary the dressing may be reinforced until inspected by the physician, but great care must be exercised in the handling of the operative area lest an infection develop and lead to meningitis.

Pain usually persists for some time after surgery, until the local edema and muscle spasms subside. Analgesic medications are given as ordered. Special "bicycle" exercises for the legs may be ordered by the physician to relieve muscle pains of the legs. Early ambulation depends on the desires of the surgeon. If the patient is confined to bed, his position must be changed often to avoid respiratory and pulmonary complications.

laminography (lam″ĭ-nog′rah-fe) a special technique of body-section ROENTGENOGRAPHY.

laminotomy (lam″ĭ-not′o-me) transection of a vertebral lamina.

lamp (lamp) an apparatus for furnishing heat or light.

Finsen's l., a carbon arc lamp operating at 50 volts and 50 amperes and so constructed that radiation is concentrated on an area 1 inch square; a water-cooled quartz system is used to remove caloric radiation and a compression quartz piece to dehematize the skin.

slit l., one embodying a diaphragm containing a slitlike opening, by means of which a narrow, flat beam of intense light may be projected into the eye. It gives intense illumination so that microscopic study may be made of the conjunctiva, cornea, iris, lens, and vitreous, the special feature being that it illuminates a section through the substance of these structures.

sun l., ultraviolet lamp.

ultraviolet l., an electric light bulb that transmits ultraviolet rays; used as a therapeutic device and as a means of obtaining an artificial suntan. (See also ULTRAVIOLET THERAPY.)

Lamperone (lam′per-ōn) trademark for preparations of clofazimine, a tuberculostatic and leprostatic.

lamprophonia (lam″pro-fo′ne-ah) clearness of voice.

lanatoside C (lah-nat′o-sīd) a glycoside obtained from *Digitalis lanata,* used as a cardiotonic where digitalis is recommended.

lance (lans) 1. lancet. 2. to cut or incise with a lancet.

Lancefield classification (lans′fēld) the classification of hemolytic streptococci into groups on the basis of serologic action.

lancet (lan′set) a small, pointed, two-edged surgical knife.

lancinating (lan″sĭ-nāt″ing) tearing, darting, or sharply cutting; used to describe pain.

Landouzy-Déjerine dystrophy (lan-doo′ze-deh″zher-ēn′) a type of MUSCULAR DYSTROPHY.

Landry's paralysis (lan-drēz′) Guillain-Barré syndrome.

Landsteiner's classification (land′sti-nerz) a classification of blood types in which they are designated O, A, B, and AB, depending on the presence or absence of agglutinogens A and B in the erythrocytes; called also International classification.

Langerhans' islands (islets) (lahng′er-hanz) irregular microscopic structures scattered throughout the pancreas, composed of alpha cells, which secrete glucagon; beta cells, which secrete insulin; and delta cells, which secrete gastrin.

lanolin (lan′o-lin) wool fat or wool grease that is refined and incorporated into many commercial preparations. Lanolin is a by-product of the process that accompanies the removal of sheeps' wool from the pelt. In its crude form it is a greasy yellow wax of unpleasant odor. This odor disappears when the lanolin is emulsified and made into salves, creams, ointments, and cosmetics. Although lanolin is slightly antiseptic, it has no other medicinal benefits and is valuable principally because of the ease with which it penetrates the skin, and because it does not turn rancid.

Lanoxin (lah-nok′sin) trademark for preparations of digoxin, a cardiotonic.

lanthanum (lan′thah-num) a chemical element, atomic number 57, atomic weight 138.91, symbol La. (See table of ELEMENTS.)

lanugo (lah-nu′go) the fine hair that covers the body of the fetus.

laparo- word element [Gr.], *loin* or *flank; abdomen.*

laparorrhaphy (lap″ah-ror′ah-fe) suture of the abdominal wall.

laparoscope (lap′ah-ro-skōp″) an endoscope for examining the peritoneal cavity.

laparoscopy (lap″ah-ros′ko-pe) examination by means of the laparoscope. adj., **laparoscop′ic.**

laparotomy (lap″ah-rot′o-me) incision through the flank or, more generally, through any part of the abdominal wall.

laparotrachelotomy (lap″ah-ro-tra″kĕ-lot′o-me) low cervical cesarean section, in which the lower uterine segment is incised.

lapinization (lap″in-i-za′shun) serial passage of a virus or vaccine through rabbits to modify its characteristics.

lapinize (lap″in-īz) to attenuate (as a virus or vaccine) by serial passage through rabbits.

lard (lard) purified internal fat of the abdomen of the hog.

benzoinated l., a preparation of lard containing 1 per cent benzoin; used as a vehicle for drugs and in ointments.

lardacein (lar-da′se-in) a protein found in tissues affected with amyloid degeneration.

lardaceous (lar-da′shus) 1. resembling lard. 2. containing lardacein.

larva (lar′vah), pl. *lar′vae* [L.] an independent, immature stage in the life cycle of an animal, in which it is markedly unlike the parent and must undergo changes in form and size to reach the adult stage.

l. cur′rens, a variant of larva migrans caused by *Strongyloides stercoralis,* in which the progression of the linear lesions is much more rapid.

l. mi′grans, creeping eruption; a convoluted threadlike skin eruption that appears to migrate, caused by the burrowing beneath the skin of roundworm larvae, particularly *Ancylostoma* larvae. Similar lesions are caused by the larvae of botflies.

l. mi′grans, visceral, a condition due to prolonged migration of larvae of animal nematodes in human tissue other than skin.

larval (lar′val) 1. pertaining to larvae. 2. larvate.

larvate (lar′vāt) masked; concealed: said of a disease or of a symptom of a disease.

larvicide (lar′vĭ-sīd) an agent that kills insect larvae.

laryng(o)- word element [Gr.], *larynx.*

laryngalgia (lar″in-gal′je-ah) pain in the larynx.

laryngeal (lah-rin′je-al) pertaining to the larynx.

laryngectomee (lar″in-jek′to-me) a person whose larynx has been removed.

laryngectomy (lar″in-jek′to-me) partial or total removal of the larynx by surgery. It is usually performed as treatment for cancer of the larynx. The patient learns afterward to speak without his voice box.

Instruction in the new method of speaking begins as soon as the operative site has healed. At first, patients have difficulty in forming the sounds of speech, but with continued practice, they can learn to speak well.

There are three methods of speaking without use of the larynx. Esophageal speech, the simplest method, is usually the first one the patient learns. He is taught to belch and then to form simple sounds and words while "burping." With careful instruction and persistent practice, he can make sustained belches that cause a column of air to vibrate in his throat and the walls and roof of his pharynx. This air column substitutes for vocal cords as he forms words with his mouth. Esophageal speech is not smooth, and once the patient has mastered it he begins to learn the smoother, more advanced pharyngeal method.

In pharyngeal speech, a person uses only the limited amount of air that enters the nose and mouth when he breathes through the tracheostomy tube. Sound is generated by blocking this air with quick tongue actions, forcing it to vibrate against the roof of the pharynx at the rear of the mouth. The patient's skill in doing this is developed through diligent practice. By controlling the air and expelling it slowly, it is possible to approach the rhythm and phrasing of normal, fluent speech. As he grows in skill and confidence, the pharyngeal speaker sounds like a person with an ordinary, slightly hoarse voice.

The third method is use of an electronic voice box, which connects the opening of the trachea in the neck to the mouth. It can be removed when the patient desires. Experts discourage use of these devices, however, unless the patient cannot or will not learn pharyngeal speech. They are generally awkward to use and very expensive.

A relatively new surgical procedure that originated in Italy and is now in limited use in the United States involves utilization of muscle tissue remaining after laryngectomy. The soft flaccid folds of tissue are stretched across the air passage to serve as the vibrating mechanism for the production of speech sounds. The tissue also serves as a cover over the larynx to avoid aspiration of food and liquid during eating. This technique must be done at the time of the laryngectomy. It is not done in patients who have been larygectomees for some time.

It is believed that patients having the newer type of surgery can develop better speech than those using esophageal speech.

Patient Care. Because of the physical and emotional adjustments that the patient and his family must make to the surgical procedure and its aftermath, it is especially important that they receive instruction and counseling prior to surgery. They will need help in coping with their fears and anxieties about the patient's ability to communicate after surgery, and they must know that the members of the health care team are available to listen to them uncritically and answer their questions honestly. The patient should be given an explanation about the type of equipment to be used in the immediate postoperative period and the purpose of each procedure. He should be assured that a pencil and paper or other means of communicating by writing will be at his bedside at all times after surgery and that he will not be left without some means of summoning help. It is understandable that one of the greatest fears of these patients is that, since they will be unable to cry out or speak, they will be left alone and might suffocate.

There is some justification for the patient's fear of suffocation; this is the major hazard during the immediate postoperative period. Suctioning is usually ordered every hour and whenever necessary to keep the airway open. Should this not relieve the symptoms of extreme dyspnea and tachycardia, the inner *and outer* cannula may be removed to relieve obstruction. The stoma will not collapse as it might in a tracheostomy patient because the stoma is sutured open. An extra laryngectomy tube is kept at the bedside in case an emergency arises and for daily changing of the outer tube if the surgeon so chooses. It usually is possible to remove the tube permanently after the third or fourth postoperative day. At this time the patient will also be able to swallow liquids.

In preparation for his return home, the patient is taught self-care of his laryngectomy. He is warned against aspirating water into the lungs during bathing or showering. Although a dressing is not necessary for covering the tracheal opening in the neck, the patient may wish to conceal it with a small square of cotton material or wear a collar or scarf of porous material to hide the wound. These types of covering are useful in that they act as filters and remove dust and other irritants from the air being inhaled through the stoma.

Printed material about self-care is available from the local Cancer Society and many communities have a laryngectomee club which offers much moral support and information that are valuable to the patient as he adjusts to his new way of life. Information regarding these laryngectomee clubs and other aspects of postlaryngectomy rehabilitation can be obtained by writing to the American Speech and Hearing Association, 1001 Connecticut Ave., Washington, D.C. 20036.

laryngemphraxis (lar″in-jem-frak′sis) obstruction or closure of the larynx.

laryngismus (lar″in-jiz′mus) spasm of the larynx. adj., **laryngis′mal.**

l. strid′ulus, sudden laryngeal spasm with crowing inspiration.

laryngitis (lar″in-ji′tis) inflammation of the mucous membrane of the larynx, affecting the voice and breathing. Laryngitis may be acute or chronic, or may occur in other forms.

Acute Laryngitis. Acute laryngitis may be caused by overuse of the voice, allergies, irritating dust or smoke, hot or corrosive liquids, or even violent weeping. It also occurs in viral or bacterial infections, and is frequently associated with other diseases of the respiratory tract.

In adults, a mild case of acute laryngitis begins with a dry, tickling sensation in the larynx, followed quickly by partial or complete loss of the voice. There may be a slight fever, minor discomfort, and poor appetite, with recovery after a few days. Other and more uncomfortable symptoms can include a feeling of heat and pain in the throat, difficulty in swallowing, and dry cough followed by expectoration; the voice may be either painful to use or absent. Swelling of the larynx and epiglottis may impair breathing. Increasing difficulty in breathing may be a sign of edematous laryngitis, or croup.

Treatment for acute laryngitis requires that the

patient rest in bed and refrain from talking. The room temperature should be even and warm. The air is kept moist with a humidifier or vaporizer. An ice bag on the throat often is soothing. In some cases, antibiotics may be necessary.

Children are especially vulnerable to laryngitis because of the smallness of their air passages. Most cases in children subside within a few days, but if inflammation and swelling continue to increase, severe dyspnea occurs.

CHRONIC LARYNGITIS. After repeated attacks of the acute type, chronic laryngitis may develop. This is caused mostly by continual irritation from overuse of the voice, tobacco smoke, dust, or chemical vapors, or by a chronic nasal or sinus disorder. Often the moist mucous membrane lining the larynx becomes granulated. The granulation can proceed to thickening and hardening of the mucous membrane, which changes the voice or makes it hoarse. There is little or no pain, though there may be tickling in the throat and a slight cough.

Chronic laryngitis that has persisted for a number of years may result in chronic hypertrophic laryngitis, a condition in which there is a permanent change in the voice because of hypertrophy of the membrane lining the larynx.

Treatment for chronic laryngitis is the same as for the acute form, with elimination of all sources of irritation and reinfection. Hoarseness that lasts longer than 2 weeks may be a warning of tumor or cancer of the larynx, or of a tumor in the thorax that presses on the recurrent laryngeal nerve, which controls the larynx.

OTHER FORMS OF LARYNGITIS. Paroxysmal laryngitis is a nervous disorder affecting infants that seems to be associated with enlarged adenoids and rickets. It consists of unexplained spasms in which the larynx closes, cutting off the air passage, and then suddenly opens. Sometimes the condition may be fatal. Treatment of this form of laryngitis calls for removal of adenoids.

Other types include diphtheritic laryngitis, tuberculous laryngitis, traumatic laryngitis, and allergic laryngitis. Treatment of diphtheritic laryngitis often involves intubation or tracheostomy in order to admit air. Traumatic laryngitis also often requires tracheostomy. Allergic laryngitis, often caused by smoking or other irritants, is treated in the same way as other allergies.

laryngocele (lah-ring′go-sēl) a congenital anomalous air sac communicating with a cavity of the larynx; it may produce a tumor-like lesion visible on the outside of the neck.

laryngocentesis (lah-ring″go-sen-te′sis) surgical puncture of the larynx, with aspiration.

laryngofissure (lah-ring″go-fish′er) median laryngotomy.

laryngogram (lah-ring′go-gram) a roentgenogram of the larynx.

laryngography (lar″ing-gog′rah-fe) roentgenography of the larynx.

laryngology (lar″ing-gol′o-je) that branch of medicine which has to do with the throat, pharynx, larynx, nasopharynx, and tracheobronchial tree.

laryngopathy (lar″ing-gop′ah-the) any disorder of the larynx.

laryngophantom (lah-ring″go-fan′tom) an artificial model of the larynx.

laryngopharyngeal (lah-ring″go-fah-rin′je-al) pertaining to the larynx and pharynx.

laryngopharyngectomy (lah-ring″go-far″in-jek′to-me) excision of the larynx and pharynx.

laryngopharyngitis (lah-ring″go-far″in-ji′tis) inflammation of the larynx and pharynx.

laryngopharynx (lah-ring″go-far′ingks) the portion of the pharynx below the upper edge of the epiglottis, opening into the larynx and esophagus.

laryngophony (lar″ing-gof′o-ne) the vocal sound heard in auscultating the larynx.

laryngoplasty (lah-ring′go-plas″te) plastic repair of the larynx.

laryngoplegia (lah-ring″go-ple′je-ah) paralysis of the larynx.

laryngoptosis (lah-ring″go-to′sis) a lowering and mobilization of the larynx, as sometimes seen in the aged.

laryngorhinology (lah-ring″go-ri-nol′o-je) the branch of medicine that deals with the larynx and nose.

laryngoscleroma (lah-ring″go-skle-ro′mah) scleroma of the larynx.

laryngoscope (lah-ring′go-skōp) an endoscope equipped with a light and mirrors for illumination and examination of the larynx.

laryngoscopy (lar″ing-gos′ko-pe) direct visual examination of the larynx with a laryngoscope. adj., **laryngoscop′ic.**

Before direct examination the patient is given a mild sedative to promote relaxation during the procedure which, though not uncomfortable, may be frightening and exhausting for the patient. Immediately before the laryngoscope is passed, the throat is anesthetized locally with cocaine spray. The patient lies on his back on the examining table with his head extending over the edge. An attendant stands at his head, holding it in position and supporting its weight.

Following the laryngoscopy, fluids and foods are withheld until the effects of the local anesthetic have worn off and the gag reflex has returned.

Indirect laryngoscopy is examination of the larynx by observation of the reflection of it in a laryngeal mirror.

laryngospasm (lah-ring′go-spazm) spasmodic closure of the larynx.

laryngostenosis (lah-ring″go-stě-no′sis) narrowing or stricture of the larynx.

laryngostomy (lar″ing-gos′to-me) surgical creation of an artificial opening into the larynx.

laryngotomy (lar″ing-got′o-me) incision of the larynx.

inferior l., incision of the larynx through the lower part of the fibroelastic membrane of the larynx (cricothyroid membrane).

median l., incision of the larynx through the thyroid cartilage.

subhyoid l., superior l., incision of the larynx through the fibroelastic membrane attached to the hyoid bone and the thyroid cartilage (thyrohyoid membrane).

laryngotracheal (lah-ring″go-tra′ke-al) pertaining to the larynx and trachea.

laryngotracheitis (lah-ring″go-tra″ke-i′tis) inflammation of the larynx and trachea.

laryngotracheotomy (lah-ring″go-tra″ke-ot′o-me) incision of the larynx and trachea.

laryngoxerosis (lah-ring″go-ze-ro′sis) dryness of the larynx.

larynx (lar′ingks) the muscular and cartilaginous structure, lined with mucous membrane, situated at the top of the trachea and below the root of the tongue and the hyoid bone. The larynx contains the vocal cords, and is the source of the sound heard in speech; it is called also the voice box. It is part of the respiratory system, and air passes through the larynx as it travels from the pharynx to the trachea and back again on its way to and from the lungs.

The larynx is composed of nine cartilages (thyroid, cricoid, and epiglottis and the paired arytenoid, corniculate, and cuneiform) held together by muscles and ligaments. (See also Plates 5 and 6.) The largest of these cartilages, the thyroid cartilage, forms the Adam's apple, which protrudes in the front of the neck. Two flexible vocal cords reach from the back to the front wall of the larynx and are manipulated by small muscles to produce sound. The epiglottis, a flap or lid at the base of the tongue, closes the larynx as it is lifted up during swallowing and so prevents passage of food or drink into the larynx and trachea.

DISORDERS OF THE LARYNX. Hoarseness is often the result of inflammation of the mucous membrane of the larynx, or LARYNGITIS. Persistent hoarseness or a change of voice without apparent cause may, however, be a warning signal, an indication of tuberculosis, syphilis, or a tumor.

In cancer of the larynx the first symptom may be persistent hoarseness or the feeling of a lump in the throat, although this feeling, like other laryngeal symptoms, may be caused by emotional stress. Early diagnosis of laryngeal cancer is essential to effective treatment.

Lasègue's sign (lah-sāgz′) in sciatica, aggravation of pain in the back and leg elicited by passive raising of the heel from the bed with the knee straight; no pain is produced when the knee is flexed.

laser (la′zer) a device that transfers light of various frequencies into an extremely intense, small, and nearly nondivergent beam of monochromatic radiation in the visible region, with all the waves in phase; capable of mobilizing immense heat and power when focused at close range, it is used as a tool in surgery, in diagnosis, and in physiologic studies.

Lassa fever (las′ah) a highly fatal, acute, febrile disease caused by an extremely virulent virus, occurring in West Africa, and characterized by progressively increasing prostration, sore throat, ulcerations of the mouth or throat, rash, and general aches and pains.

lassitude (las′ĭ-tūd) weakness; exhaustion.

latency (la′ten-se) a state of being latent.

l. period, 1. latent period. 2. the period from the ages of five to seven years to adolescence, when there is cessation of psychosexual development.

latent (la′tent) dormant or concealed; not manifest; potential.

l. period, a seemingly inactive period, as that between exposure of tissue to an injurious agent and the manifestations of response, or that between the instant of stimulation and the beginning of response.

laterad (lat′er-ad) toward the lateral aspect.

lateral (lat′er-al) 1. denoting a position farther from the median plane or midline of the body or a structure. 2. pertaining to a side.

lateralis (lat″er-a′lis) [L.] lateral.

laterality (lat″er-al′ĭ-te) a tendency to use preferentially the organs (hand, foot, ear, eye) of the same side in voluntary motor acts.

crossed l., the preferential use of contralateral members of the different pairs of organs in voluntary motor acts, e.g., right eye and left hand.

dominant l., the preferential use of ipsilateral members of the different pairs of organs in voluntary motor acts, e.g., right (dextrality) or left (sinistrality) ear, eye, hand, and leg.

lateroduction (lat″er-o-duk′shun) movement of an eye to either side.

lateroflexion (lat″er-o-flek′shun) flexion to one side.

laterotorsion (lat″er-o-tor′shun) twisting of the vertical meridian of the eye to either side.

lateroversion (lat″er-o-ver′zhun) abnormal turning to one side.

latex (la′teks) a viscid, milky juice secreted by some seed plants.

lathyrism (lath′ĭ-rizm) a morbid condition marked by spastic paraplegia, pain, hyperesthesia, and paresthesia, due to ingestion of the seeds of leguminous plants of the genus *Lathyrus*, which includes many kinds of peas. adj., **lathyrit′ic.**

latissimus (lah-tis′ĭ-mus) [L.] widest; in anatomy, denoting a broad structure.

latrodectism (lat″ro-dek′tizm) intoxication due to venom of spiders of the genus *Latrodectus.*

Latrodectus (lat″ro-dek′tus) a genus of poisonous spiders.

L. mac′tans, a species found in the United States; commonly known as the black widow. Its bite may cause severe symptoms or even death. (For first aid, see INSECT BITES AND STINGS.)

LATS long-acting thyroid stimulator.

latus (la′tus) [L.] 1. broad, wide. 2. the side or flank.

laughing gas nitrous oxide.

Laurence-Moon-Biedl syndrome (law′rens mo͞on be′del) a syndrome consisting of obesity, hypogenitalism, retinitis pigmentosa, mental retardation, skull defects, and sometimes syndactyly.

Lauron (law′ron) trademark for a preparation of aurothioglycanide, a gold preparation used in treatment of rheumatoid arthritis.

lavage (lah-vahzh′) 1. irrigation or washing out of an organ or cavity, as of the stomach or intestine. 2. to wash out, or irrigate.

Gastric lavage, or irrigation of the stomach, is usually done to remove ingested poisons. It also may be employed as an emergency procedure if there is danger of vomiting and aspiration during anesthesia, or in cases of persistent vomiting. The solutions used for gastric lavage are physiologic saline, 1 per cent sodium bicarbonate, plain water or a specific antidote for a poison. A nasogastric tube is passed and then the irrigating fluid is funneled into the tube. It is allowed to flow into the stomach by gravity. The solution is removed by siphonage; when the funnel is lowered, the fluid flows out, bringing with it the contents of the stomach.

Lavema (lah-ve′mah) trademark for preparations of oxyphenisatin, a cathartic.

Lavoisier (lah-vwah-zya′) Antoine Laurent (1743–1794). French chemist, born in Paris and later guillotined by the French Revolutionists. Lavoisier demolished the phlogiston theory (a theory of combustion) and explained the true nature of respiration by his introduction of quantitative relations in chemistry. He was secretary and treasurer of a committee seeking the uniformity of weights and measures in France, which led to the establishment of the metric system.

law (law) a uniform or constant fact or principle. For specific laws, see specific names, as MENDEL'S LAW.

l. of independent assortment, the members of gene pairs segregate independently during meiosis (see also MENDEL'S LAW).

l. of segregation, in each generation the ratio of (*a*) pure dominants, (*b*) dominants giving descendants in the proportion of three dominants to one recessive, and (*c*) pure recessives is 1:2:1. This ratio follows from the fact that the two alleles of a gene cannot be a part of a single gamete, but must segregate to different gametes (see also MENDEL'S LAW).

lawrencium (law-ren′se-um) a chemical element, atomic number 103, atomic weight 257, symbol Lw. (See table of ELEMENTS .)

laxative (lak′sah-tiv) a medicine that loosens the bowel contents and encourages evacuation. A laxative with a mild or gentle effect on the bowels is also known as an aperient; one with a strong effect is referred to as a cathartic or a purgative.

Bland laxatives may be used temporarily in the treatment of CONSTIPATION along with other measures. Mineral oil, or liquid petrolatum, and olive oil act as lubricants. Sometimes mineral oil is used in combination with agar, which is bulk-producing. Cascara sagrada aromatic fluid extract and milk of magnesia are two other mild laxatives. Psyllium hydrophilic mucilloid, which is prepared from a plant seed, helps elimination by encouraging the peristaltic movements.

Saline purges, such as sodium phosphate and magnesium sulfate (Epsom salts), flush the intestinal tract. They do this by preventing the intestines from absorbing water; evacuation takes place as soon as water accumulates.

Castor oil is a strong cathartic that effects complete evacuation of the bowels. Its administration is followed by temporary constipation.

DANGERS OF LAXATIVES. Laxatives should be employed only with the advice of a physician. Constipation may be a symptom of serious organic illness as well as the result of improper diet and habits. Also, laxatives taken regularly tend to deprive the colon of its natural muscle tone. In this way laxatives can be the cause of chronic constipation rather than its cure.

Mineral oil taken regularly tends to dilute certain vitamins derived from the food one eats. It can also seep into the lungs, causing a reaction resembling PNEUMONIA, especially in older people.

Purgative salts can produce DEHYDRATION. Laxatives that produce bulk may cause stonelike balls (bezoars) to develop.

A strong cathartic, such as castor oil, can have fatal results if used when there is nausea, vomiting, abdominal pain, or other symptoms of APPENDICITIS. It is also dangerous to use during pregnancy.

Children, in particular, cannot use the same dosage or the strong laxatives taken by adults.

laxator (lak-sa′tor) that which slackens or relaxes.

laxoin (lak′so-in) phenolphthalein, a cathartic.

layer (la′er) stratum; a sheetlike mass of tissue of nearly uniform thickness, several of which may be superimposed, one above the other, as in the epidermis.

ameloblastic l., the inner layer of cells of the enamel organ, which forms the enamel prisms of the teeth.

bacillary l., layer of rods and cones.

basal l., the deepest layer of the epidermis. 2. the deepest layer of the uterine mucosa.

blastodermic l., germ layer.

clear l., stratum lucidum; the clear translucent layer of the epidermis, just beneath the horny layer.

columnar l., 1. layer of rods and cones. 2. mantle layer.

enamel l., the outermost layer of cells of the enamel organ.

ganglionic l. of cerebellum, the thin middle gray layer of the cortex of the cerebellum, consisting of a single layer of Purkinje cells.

germ l., any of the three primary layers of cells formed in the early development of the embryo (ectoderm, entoderm, and mesoderm), from which the organs and tissues develop.

germinative l., 1. malpighian layer. 2. the lower layer of the nail, from which the nail grows.

granular l., 1. the layer of epidermis between the clear and prickle-cell layers; called also stratum granulosum. 2. the deep layer of the cortex of the cerebellum. 3. the layer of follicle cells lining the theca of the vesicular ovarian follicle.

half-value l., the thickness of a given substance which, when introduced in the path of a given beam of rays, will reduce its intensity by one half.

Henle's l., the outermost layer of the inner root sheath of the hair follicle.

horny l., 1. stratum corneum; the outermost layer of the epidermis, consisting of dead and desquamating cells. 2. the outer, compact layer of the nail.

malpighian l., the basal layer and the prickle-cell layer considered together.

mantle l., the middle layer of the wall of the primitive neural tube, containing primitive nerve cells and later forming the gray matter of the central nervous system.

nervous l., all of the retina except the pigment layer; the inner layer of the optic cup.

odontoblastic l., the epithelioid layer of odontoblasts in contact with the dentin of teeth.

Ollier's l., osteogenetic l., the innermost layer of the periosteum.

prickle-cell l., stratum spinosum; the layer of the epidermis between the granular and basal layers, marked by the presence of prickle cells.

l. of rods and cones, a layer of the retina immediately beneath the pigment epithelium, between it and the external limiting membrane, containing the rods and cones.

spinous l., prickle-cell layer.

subendocardial l., the layer of loose fibrous tissue uniting the endocardium and myocardium.

zonal l. of thalamus, a layer of myelinated fibers covering the dorsal surface of the thalamus.

lb. [L.] *li′bra* (pound).

L.D. lethal dose.

L.D.$_{50}$ median lethal dose.

LDH lacate dehydrogenase.

L-dopa (el-do′pah) the naturally occurring form of DOPA, used in the treatment of Parkinson's disease.

L.E. lupus erythematosus.

L.E. cell, a mature neutrophilic polymorphonuclear leukocyte, which has phagocytized a spherical, homogeneous-appearing inclusion, itself derived from another neutrophil; a characteristic of lupus erythematosus, but also found in analogous connective tissue disorders.

L.E. phenomenon, L.E. test, the formation of L.E. cells on incubation of normal neutrophils with the serum of patients with lupus erythematosus.

lead[1] (led) a chemical element, atomic number 82, atomic weight 207.19, symbol Pb. (See table of ELEMENTS.)

l. acetate, a compound used as a reagent and astringent.

l. monoxide, PbO; used as a reagent.

l. poisoning, a form of poisoning caused by the presence of lead or lead salts in the body. Lead poisoning affects the brain, nervous system, blood, and digestive system. It can be either chronic or acute.

Chronic lead poisoning (plumbism) was once fairly common among painters, and was called "painter's colic." It became less frequent as paints composed of other chemicals were substituted for lead-based paints and as plastic toys replaced lead ones. The disease is still seen among children with pica (a craving for unnatural articles of food) who may eat lead paint or coatings.

Symptoms include weight loss, anemia, stomach cramp (lead colic), a bluish black line at the edge of the gums, and constipation. Other symptoms may be mental depression and, in children, irritability and convulsions. In addition to the poisoning, the anemia and weight loss must also be treated, usually by providing an adequate diet. In serious cases, EDTA (calcium disodium edetate) may be prescribed.

Acute lead poisoning, which is rare, can be caused in two ways. Lead may accumulate in the bones, liver, kidneys, brain, and muscles and then be released suddenly to produce an acute condition; or large amounts of lead may be inhaled or ingested at one time. Symptoms are a metallic taste in the mouth, vomiting, bloody or black diarrhea, and muscle cramps. Diagnosis is made by examination of the blood and urine. Treatment consists of immediate removal of unabsorbed lead in the intestinal tract through the administration of mild saline cathartics and enemas. EDTA is given and in most cases measures must be taken to reduce the increased intracranial pressure that accompanies acute lead poisoning.

PREVENTION. An awareness of the prevalence of lead poisoning among children of preschool age who live in poorly maintained housing has led to neighborhood screening surveys in high-risk areas. Blood samples are drawn, and children with lead levels between 40 and 60 mcg./100 ml. receive periodic blood-lead checks. Those with levels between 60 and 80 mcg./100 ml. are treated on an outpatient basis, and those with higher levels usually require hospitalization.

An important aspect of prevention of lead poisoning is determination of sources of lead in the environment and efforts to remove them. Sources include peeling paint from window sills, walls, floors, and bannisters, and from soil around old houses that have shed exterior paint through the years. A vital factor in coping with the problem of lead contamination is public education and development of a community awareness of possible sources and of the need for elimination of these hazards from the environment.

lead[2] (lēd) a specific array (pair) of electrodes used in recording changes in electric potential, created by activity of an organ, such as the heart (electrocardiography) or brain (electroencephalography); applied also to the particular segment of the tracing produced by the potential registered through the specific electrodes; in electrocardiography, lead I records the potential differences between the two arms, lead II between the right arm and left leg, lead III between the left arm and left leg, and lead V from various sites over the heart.

bipolar l., an array involving two electrodes placed at different body sites.

esophageal l., one attached to an electrode inserted in the esophagus.

limb l's, electrodes placed on the arms and left leg.

precordial l's, leads recording electric potential from various sites over the heart, designated V with a subscript numeral indicating the exact site: V_1, fourth intercostal space immediately to the right of the sternum; V_2, fourth intercostal space immediately to the left of the sternum; V_3, midway between V_2 and V_4; V_4, fifth intercostal space in the midclavicular line (the imaginary vertical line on the anterior surface of the body), passing through the center of the nipple; V_5, at the same horizontal level as V_4, in the left anterior axillary line (the imaginary vertical line passing through the middle of the axilla); V_6, left midaxillary line at the same horizontal level as V_4 and V_5.

unipolar l., an array of two electrodes, only one of which transmits potential variations.

Leber's optic atrophy (la-berz′) hereditary bilateral atrophy of the optic nerve affecting postpubertal males; there is rapid loss of vision resulting in permanent central scotoma. Called also Leber's disease.

lecithal (les′ĭ-thal) having a yolk; used especially as a word termination (*isolecithal*, etc.).

lecithin (les′ĭ-thin) any of a group of phospholipids found in animal tissues, especially nerve tissue, the liver, semen, and egg yolk, consisting of esters of glycerol with two molecules of long-chain aliphatic acids and one of phosphoric acid, the latter being esterified with the alcohol group of choline.

lecithinase (les′ĭ-thin-ās″) an enzyme that splits up lecithin (see also PHOSPHOLIPASE).

lecithin-sphingomyelin ratio (L/S ratio), the ratio of lecithin to sphingomyelin in amniotic fluid, the determination of which is helpful in establishing the maturity of the fetus and its susceptibility to *hyaline membrane disease* after birth.

lecitho- word element [Gr.], ***the yolk of an egg*** or ***ovum.***

lecithoblast (les′ĭ-tho-blast″) the primitive entoderm of a two-layered blastodisc.

lecithoprotein (les″ĭ-tho-pro′te-in) a conjugated protein having lecithin as the prosthetic group.

lectin (lek′tin) a term applied to hemagglutinating substances present in saline extracts of certain plant seeds, which specifically agglutinate erythrocytes of certain blood groups.

Ledercillin (led″er-sil′in) trademark for preparations of procaine penicillin G.

leech (lēch) any of the annelids of the class Hirudinea, especially *Hirudo medicinalis;* some species are bloodsuckers, and were formerly used for drawing blood.

Leeuwenhoek (la′ven-hŏŏk) Antonj van (1632–1723). Dutch microscopist. Born in Delft, Holland, he made many interesting discoveries through his careful observations even though his work was not conducted on a definite scientific plan. He gave the first accurate description of the red blood corpuscles in 1674, and in 1677 he described and illustrated the spermatozoa in animals, although he had been anticipated in this discovery by several months. He investigated the structure of muscle, the crystalline lens, and teeth, and was the first to see protozoa and bacteria under the microscope.

Le Fort fracture (lĕ-fort′) bilateral horizontal fracture of the maxilla (see also Le Fort FRACTURE).

leg (leg) the lower limb, especially the part between the knee and foot.

bayonet l., ankylosis of the knee after backward displacement of the tibia and fibula.

bow l., genu varum.

milk l., phlebitis of the femoral vein, with swelling of the leg (see also PHLEGMASIA ALBA DOLENS).

restless l's, a disagreeable, creeping, irritating sensation in the legs, usually the lower legs, relieved only by walking or keeping the legs moving.

Legg's disease, Legg-Calvé disease, Legg-Calvé-Perthes disease, Legg-Calvé-Waldenström disease (legz; leg-kal-va′; leg-kal-va′-per′tēz; leg-kal-va′-vahl′den-strem) osteochrondrosis of the epiphysis of the head of the femur.

legume (leg′ūm) the pod or fruit of a leguminninous plant, such as peas and beans.

legumin (lĕ-gu′min) a globulin characteristically found in the seeds of leguminous plants.

Leiner's disease (li′nerz) erythroderma desquamativum.

leiodermia (li″o-der′me-ah) abnormal smoothness and glossiness of the skin.

leiomyofibroma (li″o-mi-o-fi-bro′mah) epithelioid leiomyoma.

leiomyoma (li″o-mi-o′mah) a benign tumor derived from smooth muscle, most often of the uterus (leiomyoma uteri).

epithelioid l., leiomyoma, usually of the stomach, in which the cells are polygonal rather than spindle shaped.

l. u′teri, leiomyoma of the UTERUS; called also myoma uteri and, colloquially, fibroids. It is the most common of all tumors found in women. It may occur in any part of the uterus, although it is most frequently in the body of the organ.

Leiomyomas usually occur during the third and fourth decades, and are often multiple, although a single tumor may occur. They are usually small but may grow quite large and occupy most of the uterine wall; after menopause, growth usually ceases. Symptoms vary according to the location and size of the tumors. As they grow they may cause pressure on neighboring organs, painful menstruation, profuse and irregular menstrual bleeding, vaginal discharge, or frequent urination, as well as enlargement of the uterus.

In pregnancy, the tumors may interfere with natural enlargement of the uterus with the growing fetus. They may also cause spontaneous abortion and death of the fetus.

Small leiomyomas are usually left undisturbed and are checked at frequent intervals. Larger tumors may be removed surgically. In some instances, hysterectomy is performed.

leiomyosarcoma (li″o-mi″o-sar-ko′mah) a sarcoma containing cells of smooth muscle.

Leishman-Donovan bodies (lēsh′man don′o-van) round or oval bodies found in the reticuloendothelial cells, especially those of the spleen and liver, in kala-azar; they are nonflagellate intracellular forms of *Leishmania donovani.* The term is also used to designate similar forms of *L. tropica* found in macrophages in lesions of cutaneous leishmaniasis.

Leishmania (lēsh-ma′ne-ah) a genus of parasitic protozoa, including *L. brazilien′sis,* the cause of mucocutaneous leishmaniasis; *L. brazilien′sis pifa′noi,* the cause of leishmaniasis tegmentaria diffusa; *L. donova′ni,* the cause of kala-azar; and *L. trop′ica,* the cause of cutaneous leishmaniasis.

leishmaniasis (lēsh″mah-ni′ah-sis) any disease due to infection with *Leishmania.*

American l., mucocutaneous leishmaniasis.

cutaneous l., chronic ulcerative granuloma caused by *Leishmania tropica* and transmitted by the sandfly. It is endemic in the tropics and subtropics, and has various names such as Aleppo boil, Delhi sore, Baghdad sore, and oriental sore. Treatment consists of injections of pentavalent antimonial compounds. Antibiotics are employed to combat secondary infection. Simple lesions may be cleaned, curetted, and left to heal.

mucocutaneous l., a disease endemic in South and Central America caused by *Leishmania braziliensis,* marked by ulceration of the mucous membranes of the nose and throat; widespread destruction of soft tissues in nasal and oral regions may occur. Called also American leishmaniasis. Treatment consists of injections of pentavalent antimonial compounds.

l. tegmenta′ria diffu′sa, a generalized cutaneous disease endemic in South America and Mexico, caused by *Leishmania braziliensis pifanoi,* in which the lesions resemble those of nodular leprosy or of keloid. Pentavalent antimonial compounds are useful in some forms, while others are antimony-resistant. The prognosis for a complete cure is not good; relapses are common.

visceral l., kala-azar.

lemmoblastic (lem″o-blas′tik) forming or developing into a neurolemma cell.

lemmocyte (lem′o-sit) a cell that develops into a neurolemma cell.

lemniscus (lem-nis′kus), pl. *lemnis′ci* [L.] a ribbon or band; in anatomy, a band or bundle of nerve fibers in the central nervous system.

length (length) an expression of the longest dimension of an object, or of the measurement between its two ends.

basialveolar l., the distance from the basion to the lower end of the intermaxillary suture.

basinasal l., the distance from the basion to the center of the suture between the frontal and nasal bones.

crown-heel l., the distance from the crown of the head to the heel in embryos, fetuses, and infants; the equivalent of standing height in older persons.

crown-rump l., the distance from the crown of the head to the breech in embryos, fetuses, and infants; the equivalent of sitting height in older subjects.

focal l., the distance between a lens and an object from which all rays of light are brought to a focus.

wave l., see WAVELENGTH.

lens (lenz) 1. a piece of glass or other transparent material so shaped as to converge or scatter light rays. (See also GLASSES.) 2. crystalline lens; the transparent, biconvex body separating the posterior chamber and the vitreous body of the eye (see also Plate 15). The crystalline lens refracts (bends) light rays so that they are focused on the RETINA. In order for the eye to see objects close at hand, light rays from the objects must be bent more sharply to bring them to focus on the retina; light rays from distant objects require much less refraction. It is the function of the lens to "accommodate" or make some adjustment for viewing near objects and objects at a distance. To accomplish this the lens must be highly elastic so that its shape can be changed and made more or less convex. The more convex the lens, the greater the refraction. Small ciliary muscles create tension on the lens, making it less convex; as the tension is relaxed the lens become more spherical in shape and hence more convex.

With increasing age the lenses lose their elasticity; thus their ability to focus light rays in the retina becomes impaired. This condition is called PRESBYOPIA. In farsightedness (HYPEROPIA) the image is focused behind the retina because the refractive power of the lens is too weak or the eyeball axis is too short. Nearsightedness (MYOPIA) occurs when the refractive power of the lens is too strong or the eyeball is too long, so that the image is focused in front of the retina.

achromatic l., a lens corrected for chromatic aberration.

apochromatic l., one corrected for chromatic and spheric aberration.

biconcave l., one concave on both faces.

biconvex l., one convex on both faces.

bifocal l., one made up of two segments, the upper for far vision and the lower for near vision.

concave l., one with one or both (biconvex) faces curved like a section of the interior of a hollow sphere; it disperses light rays. Called also dispersing lens.

contact l., a thin, curved shell of glass or plastic that is applied directly to the cornea to correct refractive errors (see also CONTACT LENSES).

converging l., **convex l.**, one curved like the exterior of a hollow sphere; it brings light to a focus.

convexoconcave l., one that has one convex and one concave face.

crystalline l., see LENS (2).

cylindrical l., one that is a section of a cylinder cut parallel to its axis, with one surface plane and the other concave or convex.

dispersing l., concave lens.

omnifocal l., a lens whose power increases continuously and regularly in a downward direction, avoiding the discontinuity in field and power inherent in bifocal and trifocal lenses.

orthoscopic l., one that gives a flat and undistorted field of vision.

spherical l., one that has a surface that is the segment of a sphere.

Stokes's l's, an apparatus used in the diagnosis of astigmatism.

trial l's, lenses used in determining visual acuity.

trifocal l., one made up of three segments, the upper for distant, the middle for intermediate, and the lower for near vision (see also GLASSES).

lentectomy (len-tek′to-me) excision of the lens of the eye.

lenticonus (len″tĭ-ko′nus) a congenital conical bulging, anteriorly or posteriorly, of the lens of the eye.

lenticular (len-tik′u-lar) 1. pertaining to or shaped like a lens. 2. pertaining to the lens of the eye. 3. pertaining to the lenticular nucleus.

lenticulostriate (len-tik″u-lo-stri′āt) pertaining to the lenticular nucleus and corpus striatum.

lenticulothalamic (len-tik″u-lo-thah-lam′ik) relating to the lenticular nucleus and the thalamus.

lentiform (len′tĭ-form) lens-shaped.

lentiglobus (len″tĭ-glo′bus) exaggerated curvature of the lens of the eye, producing an anterior spherical bulging.

lentigo (len-ti′go), pl. *lentig′ines* [L.] a flat, brownish pigmented spot on the skin due to increased deposition of melanin and an increased number of melanocytes; a freckle.

l. malig′na, malignant l., melanotic freckle of Hutchinson.

leontiasis (le″on-ti′ah-sis) the leonine facies of lepromatous leprosy, due to nodular invasion of the subcutaneous tissue.

leper (lep′er) a person with leprosy; a term now in disfavor.

lepidic (lĕ-pid′ik) pertaining to scales.

lepidosis (lep″ĭ-do′sis) a scaly eruption.

lepothrix (lep′o-thriks) infection of the axillary and sometimes the pubic hairs, with development of clumps of bacteria on the hairs (see also TRICHOMYCOSIS AXILLARIS).

lepra (lep′rah) leprosy; prior to about 1850, psoriasis.

leprechaunism (lep′rĕ-kon″izm) a lethal familial congenital condition in which the infant is small and has elfin facies and severe endocrine disorders, as indicated in females by an enlarged clitoris.

leprid (lep′rid) the cutaneous lesion or lesions of tuberculoid leprosy: hypopigmented or erythematous maculae or plaques, lacking bacilli.

leproma (lep-ro′mah) a superficial granulomatous nodule, rich in bacilli, the characteristic lesion of lepromatous leprosy. adj., **lepro′matous.**

lepromin (lep′ro-min) a repeatedly boiled, autoclaved, gauze-filtered suspension of finely ground lepromatous tissue and leprosy bacilli, used in the skin test for tissue resistance to leprosy.

leprosarium (lep″ro-sa′re-um) a hospital or colony for treatment and isolation of patients with leprosy.

leprostatic (lep″ro-stat′ik) 1. inhibiting the growth of the leprosy bacillus, *Mycobaterium leprae.* 2. a leprostatic agent.

leprosy (lep′ro-se) inflammatory disease caused by *Mycobacterium leprae* (Hansen's bacillus), and manifested in various ways, depending on the host's ability to develop cell-mediated IMMUNITY. It is a chronic communicable disease characterized by the production of granulomatous lesions of the skin, mucous membranes, and peripheral nervous system. Called also Hansen's disease. Not readily contagious, it often results in severe disability but is rarely fatal. adj., **lep'rous.**

FREQUENCY AND TRANSMISSION. Leprosy is essentially a tropical disease, although it has occurred in every country. It is now rare in the United States and in Europe except for the Mediterranean countries. It is still fairly common in Africa, Asia, and many of the Pacific islands, as well as in the West Indies and Central and South America. About half of the estimated 3 to 4 million cases in the world are in India and China. Leprosy is most prevalent where economic levels and sanitation standards are low.

Leprosy is not inherited, but the actual means of transmission of the disease have not yet been established. It is known that the source of infection is the discharge from lesions of persons with active cases. It is believed that the bacillus enters the body through the skin or through the mucous membranes of the nose and throat. Leprosy is considered one of the least contagious of infectious diseases; only 3 to 5 per cent of those exposed to it ever contract it.

SYMPTOMS. The incubation period of leprosy is often 5 years or more. Early symptoms consist of the development of red or brown patches on the skin, often with pale white centers appearing later. Along with these, there may be loss of sensation in parts of the body. Nodules appear on the body, often with an accompanying fever. Body hair tends to fall out. There may be neuritis and iritis.

In the lepromatous type, open sores later appear on the face, ear lobes, and forehead. Tests show the presence of large numbers of the bacillus in the discharge from these lesions. If the progress of the disease is not checked by treatment, the fingers and toes disintegrate and there may be other disfiguration. Death may occur in extreme cases of this type, but more often it is due to a secondary infection, such as tuberculosis or pneumonia.

In the tuberculoid type, there is loss of sensation on sections of the skin and atrophy of muscles. This often results in the contraction of the hand into a claw.

TREATMENT. Leprosy is most effectively treated with sulfone medications, such as dapsone, developed around 1950. In cases of sulfone resistance, the drug clofazimine (Lamprone) may be prescribed. A semisynthetic antibacterial, rifampin, is very effective in killing leprosy bacilli rapidly, so that patients receiving it may be considered minimal public health risks within a few days after treatment is begun. It often is given in combination with thiambutosine, a second-line drug, with excellent results.

Treatment continues for several years at least, and sometimes indefinitely. In addition to specific medical therapy, adequate rest, diet, and exercise are provided. Physical therapy is employed to retrain affected muscles. Psychiatric help, not only for leprosy patients but for their close contacts and those who only imagine they have been exposed, is invaluable in relieving the anxieties arising from the age-old misconceptions about the disease.

PREVENTION. Measures taken to prevent leprosy include separating infants from leprous parents at birth, and the establishment of clinics and hospitals for diagnosis and treatment. Infected persons are isolated during the contagious period. Many patients return to their homes completely free of symptoms and are able to resume normal living. Cure has been most successful in cases that were diagnosed and treated at an early stage. Especially among the young.

Among the public health measures used to prevent leprosy are the laws in most countries requiring that all cases be reported to the local authorities and that all discharged leprous patients be examined at 6-month intervals. Most countries also refuse entry to immigrants known to be infected.

leptazol (lep″tah-zol) pentylenetetrazol, a convulsant analeptic.

lepto- word element [Gr.], *slender; delicate.*

leptocephalus (lep″to-sef′ah-lus) a person with an abnormally tall, narrow skull.

leptochromatic (lep″to-kro-mat′ik) having a fine chromatin network.

leptocyte (lep′to-sīt) an erythrocyte characterized by a hemoglobinated border surrounding a clear area containing a center of pigment.

leptocytosis (lep″to-si-to′sis) leptocytes in the blood.

leptodactyly (lep″to-dak′tĭ-le) abnormal slenderness of the digits. adj., **leptodac′tylous.**

leptomeninges (lep″to-mĕ-nin′jēz) (plural of *leptomeninx*). the two more delicate components of the meninges: the pia mater and arachnoid considered together. adj., **leptomenin′geal.**

leptomeningitis (lep″to-men″in-ji′tis) inflammation of the leptomeninges.

leptomeningopathy (lep″to-men″ing-gop′ah-the) any disease of the leptomeninges.

leptomonad (lep″to-mo′nad) 1. of or pertaining to *Leptomonas,* a genus of protozoa parasitic in the digestive tract of insects. 2. denoting the leptomonad form; see *promastigote.* 3. a protozoon exhibiting the leptomonad (promastigote) form.

leptopellic (lep″to-pel′ik) having a narrow pelvis.

leptophonia (lep″to-fo′ne-ah) weakness or feebleness of the voice. adj., **leptophon′ic.**

leptoscope (lep′to-skōp) an optical apparatus for measuring the thickness of cell membranes.

Leptospira (lep″to-spi′rah) a genus of bacteria (family Treponemataceae) certain serotypes of which cause leptospirosis.

leptospirosis (lep″to-spi-ro′sis) any of a group of infectious diseases due to certain serotypes of *Leptospira.* The best known is Weil's disease, or leptospiral jaundice; others are mud fever, autumn fever, and swineherd's disease.

The etiologic agent is a spiral organism that infects the kidneys of cattle, swine, dogs, cats, rats, and other animals. The organisms are spread through the animals' urine.

Usually they are inhaled with the air or taken in food or drink by mouth. The disease is most common among people who handle infected animals or the kidneys and other infected tissues of such animals.

SYMPTOMS. Leptospirosis is usually a short illness which produces a variety of symptoms. It begins with fever, acute headache, chills, and sometimes nausea and vomiting. Later, other symptoms may be caused by the effects of the disease upon the kidneys, liver, skin, blood, and other organs. These symptoms can include jaundice, skin rashes, hemorrhages of the skin and mucous membranes, inflammation of the eye, hematuria, and oliguria.

Diagnosis is often difficult because the symptoms resemble those of several other diseases. Jaundice is a key symptom that, when present, aids in diagnosis.

Most cases are mild, consisting only of the early symptoms and having a duration of 1 to 2 weeks. In a few cases, a severe infection may cause damage to the kidneys, liver, or heart. Only rarely is the disease fatal.

TREATMENT AND PREVENTION. Treatment is basically symptomatic. Penicillin or other antibiotics may be prescribed.

Sanitation measures can reduce the spread of the disease in both man and animals. Vaccines for animals are available, but provide only partial immunity to the disease. At the present time there are no vaccines of established value for human beings.

leptotene (lep′to-tēn) the stage of meiosis in which the chromosomes are threadlike in shape.

leptothricosis (lep″to-thrĭ-ko′sis) leptotrichosis.

Leptothrix (lep′to-thriks) a genus of bacteria (family Chlamydobacteriaceae), widely distributed and usually found in fresh water. Some species are found in the human mouth.

leptotrichosis (lep″to-trĭ-ko′sis) any infection due to *Leptothrix.*

l. conjuncti′vae, Parinaud's oculoglandular syndrome caused by *Leptothrix.*

Léri's pleonosteosis (la′rēz) a hereditary syndrome of premature and excessive ossification of the epiphyses of long bones, with short stature, limitation of movement, broadening and deformity of digits, and mongolian facies.

Leriche's syndrome (lĕ-rēsh′ez) fatigue in the hips, thighs, or calves on exercising, absence of pulsation in femoral arteries, impotence, and often pallor and coldness of the legs, usually affecting males and due to obstruction of the terminal aorta.

Leritine (ler′ĭ-tīn) trademark for preparations of anileridine, a narcotic analgesic.

lesbian (lez′be-an) 1. pertaining to lesbianism. 2. a female homosexual.

lesbianism (lez′be-ah-nizm″) homosexuality between women.

Lesch-Nyhan syndrome a hereditary disorder of purine metabolism with physical and mental retardation, compulsive self-mutilation of fingers and lips by biting, choreoathetosis, spastic cerebral palsy, and impaired renal function.

lesion (le′zhun) any pathological or traumatic discontinuity of tissue or loss of function of a part. Lesion is a broad term, including wounds, sores, ulcers, tumors, cataracts, and any other tissue damage. They range from the skin sores associated with eczema to the changes in lung tissue that occur in tuberculosis.

lethal (le′thal) deadly; fatal.

lethargy (leth′ar-je) a condition of drowsiness or indifference. adj., **lethar′gic.**

African l., African trypanosomiasis.

Letterer-Siwe disease (let′er-er si′we) a nonlipid reticuloendotheliosis of early childhood, marked by a hemorrhagic tendency, eczematoid skin eruption, hepatosplenomegaly with lymph node involvement, and progressive anemia.

leucine (lu′sēn) a naturally occurring amino acid, essential for growth in infants and for nitrogen equilibrium in adults.

leuco- for words beginning thus, see also those beginning *leuko-.*

Leuconostoc (loo″ko-nos′tok) a genus of slime-forming saprophytic bacteria (tribe Streptococceae) found in milk and fruit juices, including *L. citro′vorum, L. dextran′icum,* and *L. mesenteroi′des.*

leucovorin (loo″ko-vo′rin) folinic acid.

leuk(o)- word element [Gr.], *white; leukocyte.*

leukapheresis (loo″kah-fĕ-re′sis) the selective removal of leukocytes from withdrawn blood, which is then retransfused in the patient.

leukemia (loo-ke′me-ah) a progressive, malignant disease of the blood-forming organs, marked by distorted proliferation and development of leukocytes and their precursors in the blood and bone marrow. It is accompanied by a reduced number of erythrocytes and blood platelets, resulting in anemia and increased susceptibility to infection and hemorrhage. Other typical symptoms include fever, pain in the joints and bones, and swelling of the lymph nodes, spleen, and liver. adj., **leuke′mic.**

TYPES OF LEUKEMIA. Leukemia is classified clinically on the basis of (1) the duration and character of the disease—acute or chronic; (2) the type of cell involved—myelocytic (myeloid, myelogenous), lymphoid (lymphogenous), or monocytic; and (3) increase or nonincrease in the number of abnormal cells in the blood—leukemic or aleukemic (subleukemic).

In acute leukemia the white cells resemble precursor, or immature, cells. They are larger than normal cells, and they accumulate much more rapidly than in chronic leukemia. They are incapable of performing their normal function of combating infection. In chronic leukemia the white cells are more mature, resembling normal cells and having some limited capacity to oppose invading organisms.

Different types of leukemia dominate in various age groups. Acute lymphoid leukemia occurs in young children, particularly those 3 and 4 years of age. Acute myelocytic leukemia affects principally young adults. Chronic lymphoid leukemia is found chiefly in persons 50 to 70 years old, and chronic myelocytic leukemia in those 30 to 50 years old. Leukemia ranks high among causes of death in children between 4 and 14 years of age in the United States.

The incidence of the disease is growing, and the increase is only partially explained by increased efficiency of detection.

CAUSE. The precise cause of leukemia is unknown. Much research has been directed toward exploring the possibility of a virus or a genetic defect as the cause. Experiments have produced findings that support viral origin in animals. Evidence of possible viral origin in humans is inconclusive.

That radiation is a factor in myelocytic leukemia has been established. When the radiation dose exceeds a certain point, there is a statistical correlation between the size of the dose and the occurrence of leukemia.

It is also known that heredity plays a role in some types of the disease. Leukemia frequency is high among those with Down's syndrome, or mongolism, and the possibility of its development is noticeably greater in a person who has an identical twin with leukemia.

TREATMENT. There is no existing treatment that

can permanently control or cure leukemia. Transfusion and replacement of blood cells relieve the symptoms, and various ANTINEOPLASTIC agents temporarily destroy the leukemic cells, prolonging the life of many patients.

Often no treatment is necessary for chronic lymphoid leukemia, except for irradiation to reduce the larger lymph nodes or spleen. The patient may live a normal life.

Treatment of acute leukemia consists of transfusion, antibiotics, steroids, and antineoplastic chemicals. Still experimental are the use of massive x-ray treatments and grafting of bone marrow from another person.

PATIENT CARE. Most of the patient care problems presented by leukemia result from decrease in the numbers of erythrocytes and platelets, producing a severe anemia and a tendency toward hemorrhage. The patient's energy is conserved by rest in bed and avoidance of activities that produce fatigue. Dyspnea and palpitation occur as the body attempts to compensate for the lack of oxygen supply to the tissue cells. These symptoms may be alarming to the patient and can increase his anxiety. An explanation of the cause of these symptoms may help relieve the anxiety. Rest is also helpful in avoiding symptoms.

Because of constriction of the peripheral blood vessels the patient may experience a continuous feeling of chilliness. Additional warmth should be provided by using warmer clothing or adding an extra lightweight blanket to the bed. Hot water bottles and heating pads are forbidden in most cases because they produce local dilatation of the blood vessels and deprive the vital organs of an adequate blood supply. Decreased sensitivity to heat and cold also present the likelihood of burning the patient without his being aware of it.

The tendency to bleed is common to most leukemia patients and demands careful observation of the patient for signs of hemorrhage. Abnormalities of the urine or stool should be reported. Care must be exercised to avoid trauma that might initiate hemorrhage; for example, if the gums and mouth show a tendency to bleed, brushing of the teeth is discontinued and special mouth care substituted.

Since the patient has a lowered resistance to infection he must be protected from pathogenic microorganisms as much as possible. This may include careful screening of visitors and strict observance of the rules of good personal hygiene.

aleukemic l., leukemia in which the leukocyte count is normal or below normal.

basophilic l., basophilocytic l., leukemia in which basophilic granulocytes predominate.

l. cu′tis, leukemia with leukocytic invasion of the skin marked by pink, reddish brown, or purple macules, papules, and tumors.

embryonal l., stem cell leukemia.

eosinophilic l., leukemia in which eosinophils are the predominating cells.

granulocytic l., myelocytic leukemia.

leukopenic l., aleukemic leukemia.

lymphatic l., lymphoblastic l., lymphocytic l., lymphogenous l., lymphoid l., leukemia associated with hyperplasia and overactivity of the lymphoid tissue, in which the leukocytes are lymphocytes or lymphoblasts.

lymphosarcoma cell l., a form marked by large numbers of lymphosarcoma cells in the peripheral blood; depending on the degree of bone marrow involvement, it may be a variant of lymphosarcoma.

mast cell l., a form marked by overwhelming numbers of tissue mast cells in the peripheral blood.

megakaryocytic l., hemorrhagic thrombocythemia.

micromyeloblastic l., a form marked by the presence of large numbers of micromyeloblasts.

monocytic l., leukemia in which the predominating leukocytes are monocytes.

myeloblastic l., leukemia in which myeloblasts predominate.

myelocytic l., myelogenous l., myeloid l., a form arising from myeloid tissue in which the granular polymorphonuclear leukocytes and their precursors predominate.

plasma cell l., plasmacyte l., a form in which the predominating cell in the peripheral blood is the plasma cell.

promyelocytic l., a form in which the predominant cells are promyeloblasts, rather than myeloblasts, often associated with abnormal bleeding secondary to thrombocytopenia, hypofibrinogenemia, and decreased levels of clotting factor V.

Rieder cell l., myeloblastic leukemia in which the blood contains asynchronously developed cells with immature cytoplasm and a lobulated, relatively more mature nucleus.

stem cell l., leukemia in which the predominating cell is so immature and primitive that its classification is difficult.

subleukemic l., aleukemic leukemia.

leukemid (loo-ke′mid) any of the polymorphic skin eruptions associated with leukemia; clinically, they may be nonspecific, i.e., papular, macular, purpuric, etc., but histopathologically they may represent true leukemic infiltrations.

leukemogen (loo-ke′mo-jen) any substance that produces leukemia. adj., **leukemogen′ic.**

leukemogenesis (loo-ke″mo-jen′ĕ-sis) the induction or development of leukemia.

leukemoid (loo-ke′moid) exhibiting blood and sometimes clinical findings resembling those of true leukemia, but due to some other cause.

leukin (loo′kin) a bactericidal substance from leukocyte extract.

leukoagglutinin (loo″ko-ah-gloo′tĭ-nin) an agglutinin that acts upon leukocytes.

leukoblast (loo′ko-blast) an immature granular leukocyte.

granular l., promyelocyte.

leukoblastosis (loo″ko-blas-to′sis) a general term for proliferation of leukocytes.

leukocidin (loo″ko-si′din) a substance produced by some pathogenic bacteria that is toxic to polymorphonuclear leukocytes (neutrophils).

leukocyte (loo′ko-sīt) a colorless blood corpuscle capable of ameboid movement, whose chief function is to protect the body against microorganisms causing disease and which may be classified in two main groups: granular (basophils, eosinophils, neutrophils) and nongranular (lymphocytes, monocytes). adj., **leukocyt′ic.**

The leukocytes act by moving through blood vessel walls in order to reach a site of injury. Foreign particles such as bacteria may be engulfed or phagocytosed by the leukocytes, especially the neutrophils and monocytes. It is this process that causes the increase in the number of leukocytes in the

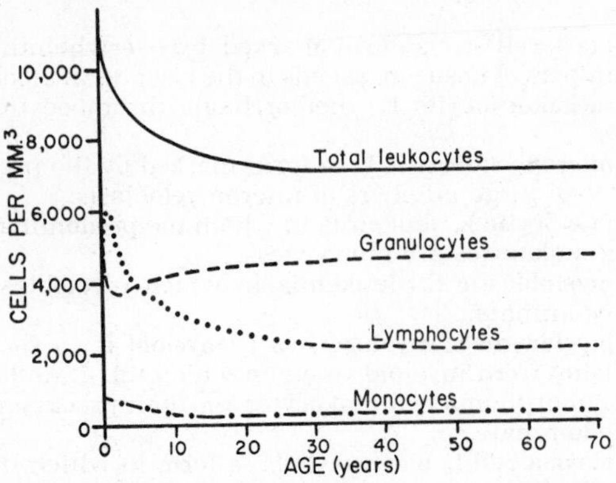

Relative proportions of the different white blood cells at different ages. (From Guyton, A. C.: Textbook of Medical Physiology. 5th ed. Philadelphia, W. B. Saunders Co., 1976.)

blood during infection, and one of the laboratory determinations to diagnose infectious states is based on it. The leukocytes also play some role in the repair of injured tissue, removing debris and preparing the inflammatory site for healing, though their function here is not clear.

agranular l's, nongranular leukocytes.

endothelial l., endotheliocyte.

granular l's, granulocytes; leukocytes containing abundant granules in their cytoplasm, including neutrophils, eosinophils, and basophils.

hyaline l., monocyte.

lymphoid l., nongranular leukocytes.

nongranular l's., leukocytes without specific granules in their cytoplasm, including lymphocytes and monocytes; called also agranulocytes, agranular leukocytes, and lymphoid leukocytes.

polymorphonuclear l., neutrophil (1).

leukocythemia (loo″ko-si-the′me-ah) leukemia.

leukocytoblast (loo″ko-si′to-blast) leukoblast.

leukocytogenesis (loo″ko-si″to-jen′ĕ-sis) the formation of leukocytes.

leukocytolysin (loo″ko-si-tol′ĭ-sin) a lysin that leads to disruption of leukocytes.

leukocytolysis (loo″ko-si-tol′ĭ-sis) disintegration of leukocytes. adj., **leukocytolyt′ic.**

leukocytoma (loo″ko-si-to′mah) a tumor-like mass of leukocytes.

leukocytometer (loo″ko-si-tom′ĕ-ter) an instrument for counting leukocytes.

leukocytopenia (loo″ko-si″to-pe′ne-ah) leukopenia.

leukocytoplania (loo″ko-si″to-pla′ne-ah) wandering of leukocytes; passage of leukocytes through a membrane.

mendelian law (men-de′le-an) Mendel's law.

leukocytopoiesis (loo″ko-si″to-poi-e′sis) the production of leukocytes; leukopoiesis.

leukocytosis (loo″ko-si-to′sis) a transient increase in the number of leukocytes in the blood, due to various causes.

basophilic l., basophilia (2).

mononuclear l., mononucleosis.

pathologic l., that due to some morbid reaction, e.g., infection or trauma.

leukocytotaxis (loo″ko-si″to-tak′sis) leukotaxis.

leukocytotoxin (loo″ko-si″to-tok′sin) a toxin that destroys leukocytes.

leukocyturia (loo″ko-si-tu′re-ah) leukocytes in the urine.

leukoderma (loo″ko-der′mah) an acquired condition with localized loss of pigmentation of the skin.

l. acquisi′tum centrif′ugum, a pigmented nevus surrounded by a ring of depigmentation (see also halo NEVUS).

syphilitic l., indistinct, coarsely mottled hypopigmentation, usually on the sides of the neck, in late secondary syphilis.

leukodystrophy (loo″ko-dis′tro-fe) disturbance of the white substance of the brain. (See also LEUKOENCEPHALOPATHY.)

metachromatic l., a hereditary leukoencephalopathy, marked by accumulation of a sphingolipid (sulfatide) in tissues, with diffuse loss of myelin in the central nervous system and progressive dementia and paralysis; classified according to age of onset as infantile, juvenile, and adult.

leukoedema (loo″ko-ĕ-de′mah) an abnormality of the buccal mucosa, consisting of an increase in thickness of the epithelium, with intracellular edema of the malpighian layer.

leukoencephalitis (loo″ko-en-sef″ah-li′tis) inflammation of the white substance of the brain.

leukoencephalopathy (loo″ko-en-sef″ah-lop′ah-the) any of a group of diseases affecting the white substance of the brain. The term *leukodystrophy* is used to denote such disorders due to defective formation and maintenance of myelin in infants and children.

leukoerythroblastosis (loo″ko-ĕ-rith″ro-blas-to′sis) an anemic condition associated with space-occupying lesions of the bone marrow, marked by a variable number of immature erythroid and myeloid cells in the circulation.

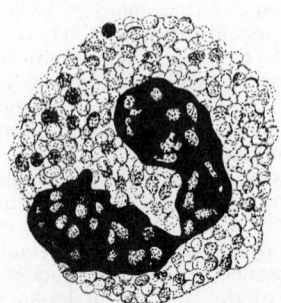

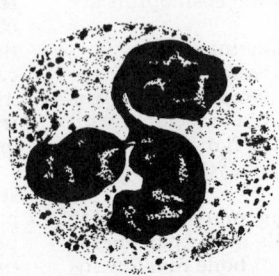

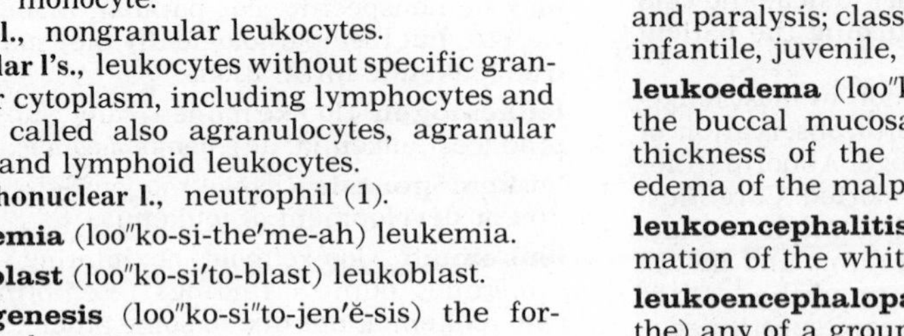

Leukocyte.

leukokeratosis (loo″ko-ker″ah-to′sis) leukoplakia.

leukokoria (loo″ko-ko′re-ah) any condition marked by the appearance of a whitish reflex or mass in the pupillary area behind the lens.

leukolymphosarcoma (loo″ko-lim″fo-sar-ko′mah) lymphosarcoma cell leukemia.

leukolysin (loo-kol′ĭ-sin) leukocytolysin.

leukolysis (loo-kol′ĭ-sis) leukocytolysis.

leukoma (loo-ko′mah) 1. a dense, white corneal opacity. 2. leukoplakia of the buccal mucosa.

l. adhae′rens, a white tumor of the cornea enclosing a prolapsed adherent iris.

leukomyelitis (loo″ko-mi″ĕ-li′tis) inflammation of white matter of the spinal cord.

leukomyelopathy (loo″ko-mi″ĕ-lop′ah-the) disease of the white matter of the spinal cord.

leukonecrosis (loo″ko-nĕ-kro′sis) gangrene with formation of a white slough.

leukonychia (loo″ko-nik′e-ah) abnormal whiteness of the nails, either total or in spots or streaks.

leukopathia (loo″ko-path′e-ah) 1. leukoderma. 2. any disease of the leukocytes.

l. un′guium, leukonychia.

leukopedesis (loo″ko-pĕ-de′sis) diapedesis of leukocytes through blood vessel walls.

leukopenia (loo″ko-pe′ne-ah) reduction of the number of leukocytes in the blood, the count being 5000 or less. adj., **leukope′nic.**

malignant l., pernicious l., agranulocytosis.

leukoplakia (loo″ko-pla′ke-ah) a disease marked by the development on the mucous membranes of the cheeks (leukoplakia buccalis), gums, or tongue (leukoplakia lingualis) of white thickened patches which sometimes show a tendency to fissure and have a pronounced tendency to become malignant. They tend to grow into larger patches, or they may take the form of ulcers. Those in the mouth may in time cause pain during the swallowing of food or in speaking.

Leukoplakia affects mostly elderly or middle-aged men, often as a result of prolonged irritation of the mouth from such varying factors as badly fitting dentures or immoderate use of tobacco.

Treatment is aimed at removing any possible cause of physical or chemical irritation. The patient with leukoplakia should give up tobacco and possibly also alcohol and extremely hot food. Dental attention may be necessary if the patient's teeth are uneven or his dentures do not fit properly. A special mouthwash may be prescribed to be used after each meal.

Surgical removal of the affected area is relatively simple and is frequently the best means of preventing its further development.

l. vul′vae, the presence of hypertrophic grayish-white infiltrated patches on the vulvar mucosa.

leukopoiesis (loo″ko-poi-e′sis) the production of leukocytes; leukocytopoiesis.

leukopsin (loo-kop′sin) visual white; the colorless matter into which rhodopsin is changed by exposure to white light.

leukorrhagia (loo″ko-ra′je-ah) profuse leukorrhea.

leukorrhea (loo″ko-re′ah) a whitish or yellowish, viscid discharge from the vagina or uterine cavity, which may be a symptom of a disorder either in the reproductive organs or elsewhere in the body.

The glands of the vagina and cervix normally secrete a certain amount of mucus-like fluid that moistens the membranes of the vagina. This discharge is frequently increased at the time of ovulation and before a menstrual period. It is also stimulated by sexual excitement, whether or not coitus takes place.

Excessive discharge, however, may indicate an abnormal condition. Yellowish or creamy white discharge, especially if it is thick, often contains pus and provides evidence of an infection. Thinner discharge, and the kinds that seem to be clear mucus, usually indicate that the disorder is chronic, but of less significance.

CAUSES. A frequent cause of leukorrhea is trichomoniasis. The discharge is usually yellowish, has an unpleasant odor and may be accompanied by itching.

Another cause of leukorrhea is infection of the cervix during childbirth. This infection irritates the mucous glands of the cervix, causing them to secrete an excessive amount of mucus. Venereal diseases, especially gonorrhea, are also a common cause of leukorrhea. When the discharge is profuse, thick, and yellowish and there is a burning sensation during urination, gonorrhea should be suspected.

Other bacteria and fungi may be causes of leukorrhea. Infections of the genital tract that cause leukorrhea may originate from foreign bodies, such as tampons, diaphragms, and pessaries, left in the vagina over too long a period.

Leukorrhea sometimes is an early indication of cervical cancer, or of benign conditions, such as polyps or leiomyoma (myoma) of the uterus. It may also be caused by pelvic congestion associated with heart disease, by malnutrition, or by inflammation of the uterine tubes as a result of tuberculosis. In later years, the disorder may be caused by debility.

TREATMENT. Leukorrhea caused by an infection of the reproductive organs is usually treated by douching alone or by douching and medication. The simplest remedy, and usually the first to be prescribed, is a douche of vinegar and water in the proportion of 2 to 4 tablespoonfuls of vinegar to 2 quarts of warm water. If this proves ineffective, a medicated douche may be prescribed, possibly combined with vaginal suppositories. An anti-inflammatory cream or ointment may also be prescribed for irritated external areas.

leukosarcoma (loo″ko-sar-ko′mah) the development of leukemia in patients originally having a well-differentiated, lymphocytic type of malignant lymphoma.

leukosis (loo-ko′sis) proliferation of leukocyte-forming tissue.

leukotaxine (loo″ko-tak′sin) a polypeptide that appears in injured tissue and inflammatory exudates; it promotes leukocytosis and leukotaxis and increases capillary permeability.

leukotaxis (loo″ko-tak′sis) cytotaxis of leukocytes; the tendency of leukocytes to collect in regions of injury and inflammation. adj., **leukotac′tic.**

leukotomy (loo-kot′-o-me) incision of the white matter of the frontal lobe of the brain; called also frontal LOBOTOMY.

leukotoxic (loo″ko-tok′sik) destructive to leukocytes.

leukotoxin (loo″ko-tok′sin) a toxin that destroys leukocytes.

leukotrichia (loo″ko-trik′e-ah) whiteness of the hair.

levallorphan (lev″ah-lor′fan) an antidote to narcotic overdosage; used as the tartrate salt.

levamfetamine, levamphetamine (le″vam-fet′-ah-mēn) the levorotatory form of AMPHETAMINE; used as an anorexic drug in the form of the succinate salt.

levarterenol (lev″ar-tĕ-re′nol) norepinephrine. **l. bitartrate,** a vasopressor.

levator (lĕ-va′tor), pl. *levato′res* [L.] 1. a muscle that elevates an organ or structure. 2. an instrument for raising depressed osseous fragments in fractures.

levigation (lev″ĭ-ga′shun) the grinding to a powder of a moist or hard substance.

Levin tube (lĕ-vin′) a gastroduodenal catheter of sufficiently small caliber to permit transnasal passage.

levo- word element [L.], *left.*

levocardia (le″vo-kar′de-ah) a term denoting normal position of the heart associated with transposition of other viscera (situs inversus).

levoclination (le″vo-kli-na′shun) rotation of the upper poles of the vertical meridians of the two eyes to the left.

levodopa (le″vo-do′pah) a synthetic compound of L-dopa, used as an antiparkinsonian drug. (See also DOPA.)

Levo-Dromoran (le″vo-dro′mo-ran) trademark for preparations of levorphanol, a narcotic analgesic.

levoduction (le″vo-duk′shun) movement of an eye to the left.

levogyration (le″vo-ji-ra′shun) levorotation.

levonordefrin (le″vo-nor′dĕ-frin) a vasoconstrictor.

Levophed (lev′o-fed) trademark for a preparation of levarterenol, a vasopressor.

levopropoxyphene (le″vo-pro-pok′sĭ-fēn) an antitussive; used as the napsylate salt.

levorotation (le″vo-ro-ta′shun) a turning to the left; levogyration.

levorotatory (le″vo-ro′tah-to″re) turning the plane of polarization, or rays of light, to the left.

levorphanol (lēv-or′fah-nol) a narcotic analgesic.

levothyroxine (le″vo-thi-rok′sin) the levorotatory isomer of thyroxine; used as the sodium salt for replacement therapy in hypothyroidism.

levoversion (le″vo-ver′zhun) a turning toward the left.

levulinic acid (lev″u-lin′ik) an acid formed by the action of heat and acid on carbohydrates.

levulose (lev′u-lōs) a sugar from honey and many sweet fruits, used in solution as a fluid and nutrient replenisher; called also fructose and fruit sugar.

levurid (lev′u-rid) an allergic dermatitis ("id") thought to be caused by infection at a remote site by *Candida* or *Cryptococcus.*

Leydig's cells (li′digz) interstitial cells of the testis, which secrete testosterone.

L.F.A. left frontoanterior (position of the fetus).

L.F.P. left frontoposterior (position of the fetus).

L.F.T. left frontotransverse (position of the fetus).

LH luteinizing hormone.

Li chemical symbol, *lithium.*

libido (lĭ-be′do, lĭ-bi′do), pl. *libid′ines* [L.] 1. sexual desire. 2. the energy derived from the primitive impulses. In psychoanalysis the term is applied to the motive power of the sex life; in freudian psychology to psychic energy in general. adj., **libid′inal.**

Libman-Sacks disease (endocarditis) (lib′man-saks) verrucous endocarditis associated with systemic lupus erythematosus; called also atypical verrucous endocarditis.

Librium (lib′re-um) trademark for preparations of chlordiazepoxide, a tranquilizer.

lice (lis) plural of *louse.*

licensure (li′sen-shur) the granting of a permit to perform acts which, without it, would be illegal. The licensure of health care personnel traditionally has been the responsibility of the state licensing boards, governed by licensing statutes enacted by the state.

individual l., the granting of a legal permit that is personal and cannot be transferred to another. The individual seeking the licensure must meet standards for practice as established by the state licensing statutes. In most instances the initial license is granted upon successful completion of an examination administered by the state examining board of the specific profession or vocation, and annual re-registration is required to maintain the license.

institutional l., licensure of an agency providing a particular service to the public. In the health field the licensure of health care agencies, such as hospitals and clinics, has been common practice for many years. Recently, it has been proposed that the term institutional licensure encompass the practice of granting licensure by the employing health agency to individuals employed by the agency. This concept of institutional licensure would transfer from the state to the institution the legal power of determining whether an individual health care practitioner meets the qualifications and standards for practice as determined by the employing agency.

licentiate (li-sen′she-āt) one holding a license from an authorized agency entitling him to practice a particular profession.

lichen (li′ken) 1. any of certain plants formed by the mutualistic combination of an alga and a fungus. 2. any of various papular skin diseases in which the lesions are typically small, firm papules set very close together, the specific kind being indicated by a modifying term.

l. amyloido′sus, a condition characterized by localized cutaneous amyloidosis.

l. chron′icus sim′plex, lichen simplex chronicus.

l. fibromucinoido′sus, l. myxedemato′sus, a condition resembling myxedema but unassociated with hypothyroidism, marked by mucinosis and a widespread eruption of asymptomatic, soft, pale red or yellowish, discrete papules.

l. nit′idus, a skin eruption consisting of many, pinhead-sized, pale, flat, sharply marginated, glistening, discrete papules, scarcely raised above the skin level.

l. pila′ris, lichen spinulosus.

l. planopila′ris, a variant of lichen planus characterized by formation of acuminate horny papules around the hair follicles, in addition to the typical lesions of ordinary lichen planus.

l. pla′nus, an inflammatory skin disease with wide, flat, violaceous, shiny papules in circumscribed patches; it may involve the hair follicles, nails, and buccal mucosa; called also lichen ruber planus.

l. ru'ber monilifor'mis, a variant of lichen simplex chronicus with papules arranged in linear beaded bands.

l. ru'ber pla'nus, lichen planus.

l. sclero'sus et atroph'icus, a chronic atrophic skin disease marked by white papules with an erythematous halo and keratotic plugging. It sometimes affects the vulva (KRAUROSIS VULVAE) or penis (BALANITIS XEROTICA OBLITERANS).

l. scrofuloso'rum, l. scrofulo'sus, any eruption of minute reddish lichenoid follicular papules in children and young adults with tuberculosis.

l. sim'plex chron'icus, a dermatosis of psychogenic origin, marked by a pruritic discrete, or more often, confluent lichenoid papular eruption, usually confined to a localized area. Called also circumscribed or localized neurodermatitis and lichen chronicus simplex. The condition is particularly common in persons of Oriental extraction who live in the United States, and is more common in women over 40 years of age. The lesions may arise from normal skin or they may occur as a complication of other forms of DERMATITIS.

Treatment consists of administration of corticosteroids applied locally as a cream or given by intralesional injection. The area should be protected by light dressings and the patient encouraged to avoid mental stress, emotional upsets, and irritation of the affected area. The application of very hot or very cold compresses may afford temporary relief of the itching.

The condition tends to become chronic with unexplained remissions and reappearance of lesions in a different part of the body.

l. spinulo'sus, a condition in which there is a horn or spine in the center of each hair follicle; called also lichen pilaris.

l. stria'tus, a self-limited condition characterized by a linear lichenoid eruption, usually in children.

l. urtica'tus, papular urticaria.

lichenification (li-ken″ĭ-fĭ-ka'shun) thickening and hardening of the skin, with exaggeration of its normal markings.

lichenoid (li'kĕ-noid) resembling lichen.

Lichtheim's syndrome (likt'hīmz) see subacute combined DEGENERATION of spinal cord.

lidocaine (li'do-kān) a topical anesthetic, used as the hydrochloride salt.

lie (li) the situation of the long axis of the fetus with respect to that of the mother (see also PRESENTATION).

transverse l., the situation during labor when the long axis of the fetus crosses the long axis of the mother. (See also table under POSITION).

lie detector polygraph.

lien (li'en) [L.] spleen. adj., **lie'nal.**

l. accesso'rius, an accessory spleen.

l. mo'bilis, an abnormally movable spleen.

lien(o)- word element [L.], *spleen;* see also words beginning splen(o)-.

lienocele (li-e'no-sēl) hernia of the spleen.

lienography (li″ĕ-nog'rah-fe) roentgenography of the spleen; splenography.

lienomalacia (li-e″no-mah-la'she-ah) abnormal softness of the spleen; splenomalacia.

lienomedullary (li-e″no-med'u-ler″e) pertaining to the spleen and bone marrow; splenomedullary.

lienomyelogenous (li-e″no-mi″ĕ-loj'ĕ-nus) formed in the spleen and bone marrow; splenomyelogenous.

lienomyelomalacia (li-e″no-mi″ĕ-lo-mah-la'she-ah) softening of the spleen and bone marrow; splenomyelomalacia.

lienotoxin (li-e″no-tok'sin) splenotoxin.

lientery (li'en-ter″e) diarrhea with passage of undigested food. adj., **lienter'ic.**

lienunculus (li″en-ung'ku-lus) a detached mass of splenic tissue; an accessory spleen.

ligament (lig'ah-ment) 1. a band of fibrous tissue connecting bones or cartilages, serving to support and strengthen joints. 2. a double layer of peritoneum extending from one visceral organ to another. 3. cordlike remnants of fetal tubular structures that are nonfunctional after birth. adj., **ligament'ous.** The injury suffered when a joint is wrenched with sufficient violence to stretch or tear the ligaments is called a SPRAIN.

accessory l., one that strengthens or supports another.

arcuate l's, the arched ligaments that connect the diaphragm with the lowest ribs and the first lumbar vertebra.

broad l. of uterus, a broad fold of peritoneum supporting the uterus, extending from the side of the uterus to the wall of the pelvis.

capsular l., the fibrous layer of a joint capsule.

conoid l., the posteromedial portion of the coracoclavicular ligament, extending from the coracoid process to the inferior surface of the clavicle.

coracoclavicular l., a band joining the coracoid process of the scapula and the acromial extremity of the clavicle, consisting of two ligaments, the conoid and trapezoid.

costotransverse l., three ligaments (lateral, middle, and superior) that connect the neck of a rib to the transverse process of a vertebra.

cruciate l's of knee, more or less cross-shaped ligaments, one anterior and one posterior, which arise from the femur and pass through the intercondylar space to attach to the tibia.

crural l., inguinal ligament.

deltoid l., medial ligament.

falciform l. of liver, a sickle-shaped sagittal fold of peritoneum that helps to attach the liver to the diaphragm and separates the right and left lobes of the liver. Called also broad ligament of liver.

Gimbernat's l., a membrane with its base just lateral to the femoral ring, one side attached to the inguinal ligament and the other to the pectineal line of the pubis. Called also lacunar ligament.

glenohumeral l's, bands, usually three, on the inner surface of the articular capsule of the humerus, extending from the glenoid lip to the anatomical neck of the humerus.

Henle's l., a lateral expansion of the lateral edge of the rectus abdominis muscle which attaches to the pubic bone.

inguinal l., a fibrous band running from the anterior superior spine of the ilium to the spine of the pubis; called also Poupart's ligament.

lacunar l., Gimbernat's ligament.

Lisfranc's l., a fibrous band extending from the medial cuneiform bone to the second metatarsal.

Lockwood's l., a suspensory sheath supporting the eyeball.

medial l., a large fan-shaped ligament on the medial side of the ankle.

meniscofemoral l's, two small fibrous bands of the knee joint attached to the lateral meniscus, one (the anterior) extending to the anterior cruciate ligament and the other (the posterior) to the medial femoral condyle.

nephrocolic l., fasciculi from the fatty capsule of the kidney passing down on the right side to the posterior wall of the ascending colon and on the left side to the posterior wall of the descending colon.

nuchal l., a broad, fibrous, roughly triangular sagittal septum in the back of the neck, separating the right and left sides.

patellar l., the continuation of the central portion of the tendon of the quadriceps femoris muscle distal to the patella, extending from the patella to the tuberosity of the tibia; called also patellar tendon.

pectineal l., a strong aponeurotic lateral continuation of the lacunar ligament along the pectineal line of the pubis.

periodontal l., the connective tissue structure that surrounds the roots of the teeth and holds them in place in the dental alveoli.

Petit's l., uterosacral ligament.

phrenicocolic l., costocolic fold.

Poupart's l., inguinal ligament.

pulmonary l., a vertical fold extending from the hilus to the base of the lung.

rhomboid l., the ligament connecting the cartilage of the first rib to the undersurface of the clavicle.

round l. of femur, a broad ligament arising from the fatty cushion of the acetabulum and inserted on the head of the femur.

round l. of liver, a fibrous cord from the navel to the anterior border of the liver.

round l. of uterus, a fibromuscular band attached to the uterus near the uterine tube, passing through the abdominal ring, and into the labium majus.

suspensory l. of axilla, a layer ascending from the axillary fascia and ensheathing the smaller pectoral muscle.

suspensory l. of lens, ciliary zonule.

sutural l., a band of fibrous tissue between the opposed bones of a suture or immovable joint.

tendinotrochanteric l., a portion of the capsule of the hip joint.

transverse humeral l., a band of fibers bridging the intertubercular groove of the humerus and holding the tendon in the groove.

trapezoid l., the anterolateral portion of the coracoclavicular ligament, extending from the upper surface of the coracoid process to the trapezoid line of the clavicle.

umbilical l., medial, a fibrous cord, the remains of the obliterated umbilical artery, running cranialward beside the bladder to the umbilicus.

uteropelvic l's, expansions of muscular tissue in the broad ligament of the uterus, radiating from the fascia over the internal obturator muscle to the side of the uterus and the vagina.

uterosacral l., a part of the thickening of the visceral pelvic fascia beside the cervix and vagina; called also Petit's ligament.

ventricular l., vestibular ligament.

vesicouterine l., a ligament that extends from the anterior aspect of the uterus to the bladder.

vestibular l., the membrane extending from the thyroid cartilage in front to the anterolateral surface of the arytenoid cartilage behind; called also ventricular ligament.

vocal l., the elastic tissue membrane extending from the thyroid cartilage in front to the vocal process of the arytenoid cartilage behind.

Weitbrecht's l., a small ligamentous band extending from the ulnar tuberosity to the radius.

ligamentopexy (lig″ah-men′to-pek″se) fixation of the uterus by shortening the round ligament.

ligamentum (lig″ah-men′tum), pl. *ligamen′ta* [L.] ligament.

ligand (li′gand, lig′and) an organic molecule that donates the necessary electrons to form coordinate covalent bonds with metallic ions. Also, an ion or molecule that reacts to form a complex with another molecule.

ligase (li′gās, lig′ās) any of a class of enzymes that catalyze the joining together of two molecules coupled with the breakdown of a pyrophosphate bond in ATP or a similar triphosphate.

ligate (li′gāt) to apply a ligature.

ligation (li-ga′shun) application of a ligature.

ligature (lig′ah-tūr) any material, such as a thread or wire, used in SURGERY to tie off blood vessels to prevent bleeding, or to treat abnormalities in other parts of the body by constricting the tissues.

Ligatures are used both inside and outside the body. If a ligature must be left within the body after an operation, the surgeon will most often use one made of animal tissue that will dissolve or become incorporated in the patient's own body tissue. Ligatures used on the outside of the body for stitches or cuts or incisions can be of any durable material, and are removed after they have served their purpose. Special instruments have been developed for the application of ligatures to parts of the body that are difficult for the surgeon's hands to reach or to work in.

light (līt) electromagnetic radiation with a range of wavelength between 3900 (violet) and 7700 (red) angstroms, capable of stimulating the subjective sensation of sight; sometimes considered to include ultraviolet and infrared radiation as well.

l. adaptation, adaptation of the eye to vision in the sunlight or in bright illumination (photopia), with reduction in the concentration of the photosensitive pigments of the eye.

axial l., central l., light whose rays are parallel to each other and to the optic axis.

cold l., light transmitted through a quartz or plastic structure to dissipate the heat; this lamp may be applied directly to the skin, and used for transillumination of tissues for cancer diagnosis.

diffused l., light whose rays have been scattered by reflection and refraction.

Finsen's l., light consisting mainly of violet and ultraviolet rays given off by FINSEN'S LAMP; used in treatment of lupus and similar diseases.

idioretinal l., intrinsic l., the sensation of light in the complete absence of external stimuli.

Minin l., a lamp for therapeutic administration of violet and ultraviolet light.

oblique l., light falling obliquely on a surface.

polarized l., light of which the vibrations are made over one plane or in circles or ellipses.

reflected l., light whose rays have been turned back from an illuminated surface.

refracted l., light whose rays have been bent out of their original course by passing from one transparent medium to another of different density.

transmitted l., light that passes or has passed through an object.

white l., that produced by a mixture of all wavelengths of electromagnetic energy perceptible as light.

Wood's l., ultraviolet radiation from a mercury vapor source, transmitted through a nickel-oxide filter (Wood's filter or glass), which holds back all but a few violet rays and passes ultraviolet wavelengths of about 365 nm.; used in diagnosis of fungal infections of the scalp and erythrasma, and to reveal the presence of porphyrins and fluorescent minerals.

lightening (līt′en-ing) the sensation of decreased abdominal distention caused by descent of the uterus into the pelvic cavity, 2 or 3 weeks before labor begins.

Lignac-Fanconi disease (lēn-yak′fan-kōn′e) Fanconi syndrome.

lignin (lig′nin) a polysaccharide which along with cellulose forms the cell wall of plants and thus of wood.

lignocaine (lig′no-kān) lidocaine, a topical anesthetic.

lignoceric acid (lig″no-ser′ik) a saturated fatty acid found in wood tar, various cerebrosides, and in small amounts in most natural fats.

limb (lim) 1. one of the paired appendages of the body used in locomotion and grasping; in man, an arm or leg, with all its component parts. 2. a structure or part resembling an arm or leg.

anacrotic l., the ascending portion of an arterial pulse tracing.

catacrotic l., the descending portion of an arterial pulse tracing.

pectoral l., the arm, or a homologous part.

pelvic l., the leg, or a homologous part.

phantom l., sensation, such as paresthesia or pain, subjectively perceived as originating in an absent limb after amputation.

thoracic l., pectoral limb.

limbic (lim′bik) pertaining to a limbus, or margin.

l. system, a group of brain structures common to all mammals, comprising the cortex and related nuclei (see also limbic SYSTEM).

limbus (lim′bus), pl. *lim′bi* [L.] an edge, fringe, or border; used in anatomic nomenclature to designate the edge of the cornea, where it joins the sclera (lim′bus cor′neae), and other margins in the body.

lime (līm) 1. calcium oxide, a corrosively alkaline earth, used for absorbing carbon dioxide from air. 2. the acid fruit of *Citrus aurantifolia.*

l. arsenate, a solution of white arsenic and sodium carbonate in water, used as an insecticide.

chlorinated l., white or grayish granular powder with odor of chlorine; used as a bleaching agent and disinfectant and, formerly, as a topical germicide.

slaked l., calcium hydroxide.

soda l., a mixture of calcium oxide with sodium hydroxide.

sulfurated l., a mixture of calcium sulfide, calcium sulfate, and carbon, used in skin diseases and as a depilatory.

limen (li′men), pl. *lim′ina* [L.] a threshold or boundary.

l. of insula, l. in′sulae, the point at which the cortex of the insula is continuous with the cortex of the frontal lobe.

l. na′si, the upper limit of the vestibule of the nose.

liminal (lim′ĭ-nal) barely perceptible; pertaining to a threshold.

liminometer (lim″ĭ-nom′ĕ-ter) an instrument for measuring the strength of a stimulus that just induces a tendon reflex.

limitans (lim′ĭ-tanz) [L.] limiting.

lincomycin (lin′ko-mi″sin) an antibiotic produced by *Streptomyces lincolnensis;* used as the hydrochloride salt in infections with gram-positive cocci and gram-negative bacilli.

lindane (lin′dān) gamma benzene hexachloride, a powerful insecticide used as a scabicide and pediculicide.

Lindau's disease (lin′dowz) Lindau-von Hippel disease.

Lindau-von Hippel disease (lin′dow von hip′el) a hereditary condition marked by angiomatosis of the retina and cerebellum, which may be associated with similar lesions of the spinal cord and cysts of the viscera; neurologic symptoms, including seizures and mental retardation, may be present. Called also von Hippel-Lindau disease.

line (lin) a stripe, streak, mark, or narrow ridge; often an imaginary line connecting different anatomic landmarks (linea). adj., **lin′ear.**

absorption l's, dark lines in the spectrum due to absorption of light by the substance through which the light has passed.

Beau's l's, transverse furrows on the fingernails, usually a sign of systemic disease but also due to other causes.

blue l., a characteristic line on the gums showing chronic lead poisoning.

cement l., a line visible in microscopic examination of bone in cross section, marking the boundary of an osteon (haversian system).

cleavage l's, linear clefts in the skin indicative of direction of the fibers.

l. of Douglas, a crescentic line marking the termination of the posterior layer of the sheath of the rectus abdominis muscle.

epiphyseal l., one on the surface of an adult long bone, marking the junction of the epiphysis and diaphysis.

gingival l., 1. a line determined by the level to which the gingiva extends on a tooth; called also gum line. 2. any linear mark visible on the surface of the gingiva.

gluteal l., any of the three rough curved lines (anterior, inferior, and posterior) on the gluteal surface of the ala of the ilium.

gum l., gingival line (1).

iliopectineal l., the ridge on the ilium and pubes showing the brim of the true pelvis.

incremental l's, lines supposedly showing the successive layers deposited in a tissue, as in the tooth enamel.

intertrochanteric l., one running obliquely from the greater to the lesser trochanter on the anterior surface of the femur.

lead l., a bluish line at the edge of the gums in lead poisoning.

lip l., a line at the level to which the margin of either lip extends on the teeth.

median l., an imaginary vertical line dividing the body equally into right and left parts.

milk l., the line of thickened epithelium in the embryo along which the mammary glands are developed.

mylohyoid l., a ridge on the inner surface of the lower jaw from the base of the symphysis to the ascending rami behind the last molar tooth.

nuchal l's, three lines (inferior, superior, and highest) on the outer surface of the occipital bone.

pectinate l., one marking the junction of the zone of the anal canal lined with stratified squamous epithelium and the zone lined with columnar epithelium.

semilunar l., a curved line along the lateral border of each rectus abdominis muscle, marking the meeting of the aponeuroses of the internal oblique and transverse abdominal muscles.

Shenton's l., a curved line seen in radiographs of the normal hip, formed by the top of the obturator foramen.

temporal l's, curved ridges, inferior and superior, on the external surface of the parietal bone, continuous with the temporal line of the frontal bone, a ridge that extends upward and backward from the zygomatic process of the frontal bone.

terminal l., one on the inner surface of each pelvic bone, from the sacroiliac joint to the illiopubic eminence anteriorly, separating the false from the true pelvis.

visual l., a line from the point of vision of the retina to the object of vision; called also visual axis.

linea (lin'e-ah), pl. *lin'eae* [L.] a narrow ridge or streak on a surface, as of the body or a bone or other organ; a line.

l. al'ba, white line; the tendinous median line on the anterior abdominal wall between the two rectus muscles.

lin'eae albican'tes, white or colorless lines on the abdomen, breasts, or thighs caused by mechanical stretching of the skin, with weakening of the elastic tissue (see also atrophic STRIAE).

l. as'pera, a rough longitudinal line on the back of the femur for muscle attachments.

lin'eae atroph'icae, atrophic striae.

l. ni'gra, the linea alba when it has become pigmented in pregnancy.

lingua (ling'gwah), pl. *lin'guae* [L.] tongue.

l. geograph'ica, geographic tongue.

l. ni'gra black tongue.

lingual (ling'gwal) pertaining to or near the tongue.

lingula (ling'gu-lah), pl. *lin'gulae* [L.] a small, tonguelike structure, such as the projection from the lower portion of the upper lobe of the left lung (lin'gula pulmo'nis sin'istra), or the bony ridge between the body and great wing of the sphenoid (lin'gula sphenoda'lis). adj., **ling'ular.**

lingulectomy (ling"gu-lek'to-me) excision of the lingula of the left lung.

linguo- word element [L.], *tongue.*

linguopapillitis (ling"gwo-pap"ĭ-li'tis) inflammation or ulceration of the papillae of the edges of the tongue.

liniment (lin'ĭ-ment) a medicinal preparation in an oily, soapy, or alcoholic vehicle, intended to be rubbed on the skin as a counterirritant or anodyne.

camphor l., a preparation of camphor and cottonseed oil used as a local irritant.

camphor and soap l., mixture of green soap, camphor, rosemary oil, alcohol, and purified water, used as a local irritant.

chloroform l., a mixture of chloroform with camphor and soap liniment, used as a local irritant.

medicinal soft soap l., green soap tincture.

linin (li'nin) the substance of the achromatic nuclear reticulum of the cell.

linitis (lĭ-ni'tis) inflammation of gastric cellular tissue.

l. plas'tica, diffuse fibrous proliferation of the submucous connective tissue of the stomach, resulting in thickening and fibrosis so that the organ is constricted, inelastic, and rigid (like a leather bottle). Called also leather bottle stomach.

linkage (lingk'ij) 1. the connection between different atoms in a chemical compound, or the symbol representing it in structural formulas (see also BOND). 2. in genetics, the association of genes having loci on the same chromosome, which results in the tendency of a group of such nonallelic genes to be associated in inheritance.

linseed (lin'sēd) the dried ripe seed of *Linum usitatissimum;* used as a topical demulcent and as an emollient. Called also flaxseed.

lint (lint) an absorbent surgical dressing material.

liothyronine (li"o-thi'ro-nēn) the levorotatory isomer of triiodothyronine; used as the sodium salt in treatment of hypothyroidism.

lip (lip) 1. the upper or lower fleshy margin of the mouth. 2. any liplike part; labium.

cleft l., congenital fissure of the upper lip; harelip (see also CLEFT LIP).

double l., redundancy of the submucous tissue and mucous membrane of the lip on either side of the median line.

glenoid l., a ring of fibrocartilage joined to the rim of the glenoid cavity.

Hapsburg l., a thick, overdeveloped lower lip that often accompanies Hapsburg jaw.

l. reading, understanding of speech through observation of the speaker's lip movements.

lip(o)- word element [Gr.], *fat; lipid.*

lipacidemia (lip"as-ĭ-de'me-ah) an excess of fatty acids in the blood.

lipaciduria (lip"as-ĭ-du're-ah) fatty acid in the urine.

lipase (li'pās, lip'ās) fat-splitting enzyme; any enzyme that catalyzes the splitting of fats into glycerol and fatty acids.

lipectomy (lĭ-pek'to-me) excision of a mass of subcutaneous adipose tissue.

lipedema (lip"ĕ-de'mah) an accumulation of excess fat and fluid in subcutaneous tissues.

lipemia (lĭ-pe'me-ah) an excess of lipids in the blood.

alimentary l., that occurring after ingestion of food.

l. retina'lis, that manifested by a milky appearance of the veins and arteries of the retina.

lipid (lip'id) any of a group of organic substances, including fatty acids, neutral fats, waxes, steroids, and phosphatides, which are insoluble in water, but soluble in alcohol, ether, chloroform, and other fat solvents; lipids are a source of body fuel and an important constituent of cells.

lipidosis (lip"ĭ-do'sis) any disorder of lipid metabolism involving abnormal accumulation of lipids, including Hand-Schüller-Christian disease, Niemann-Pick disease, Tay-Sachs disease, Gaucher's disease, etc.

lipiduria (lip"ĭ-du're-ah) the presence of lipids in the urine.

THE HUMAN BODY

HIGHLIGHTS of STRUCTURE and FUNCTION

SKELETAL SYSTEM

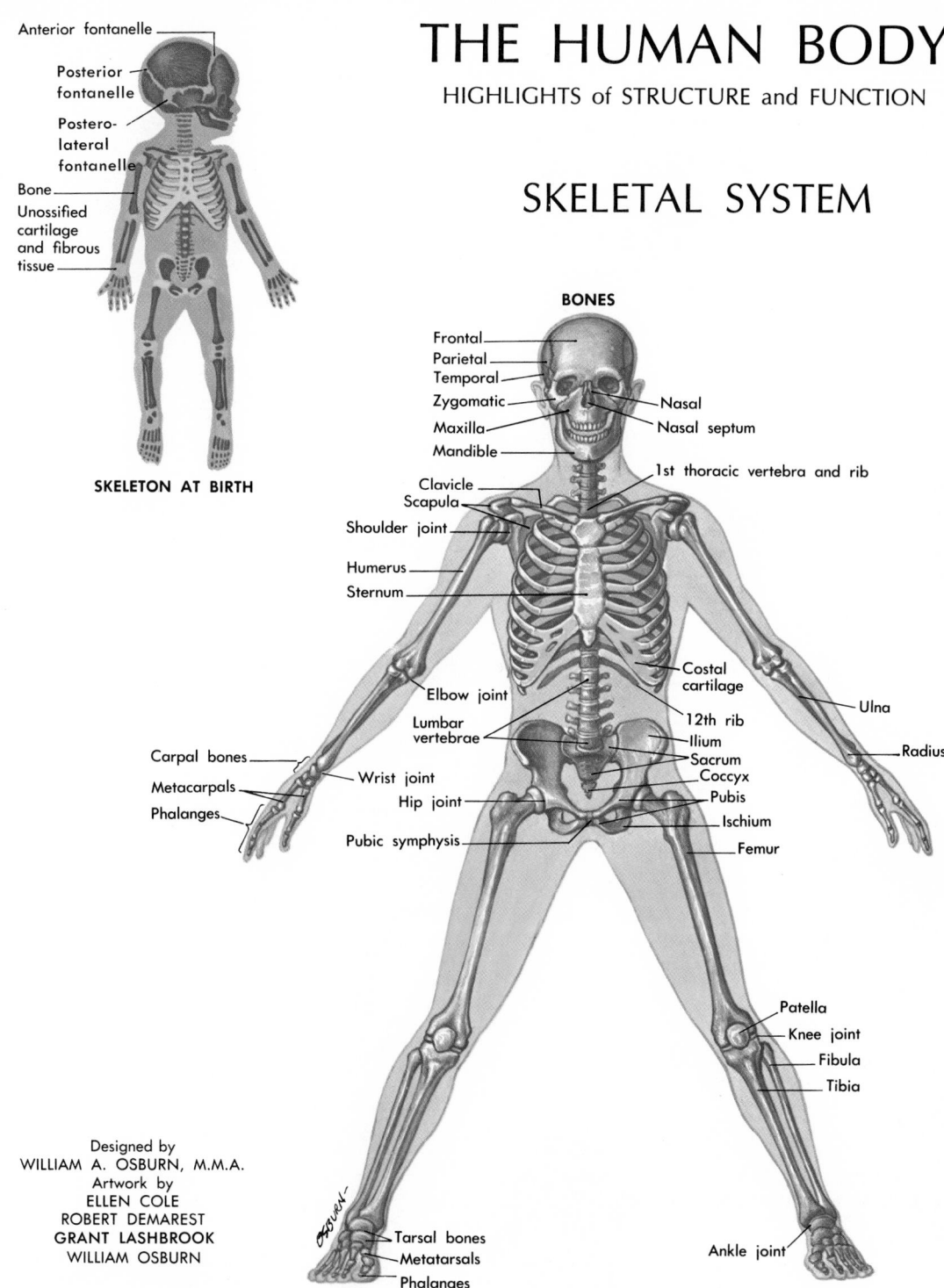

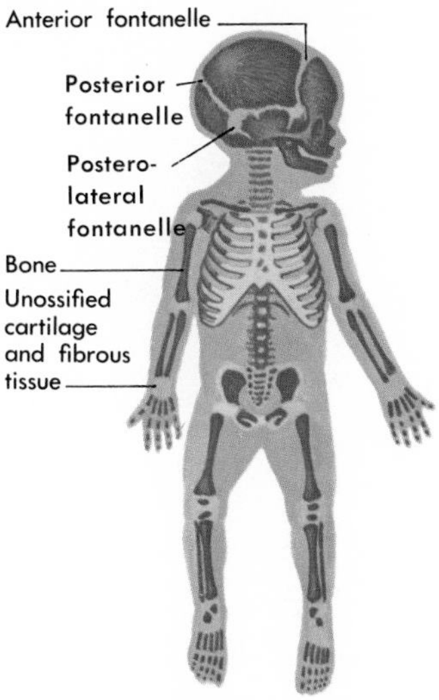

SKELETON AT BIRTH

BONES

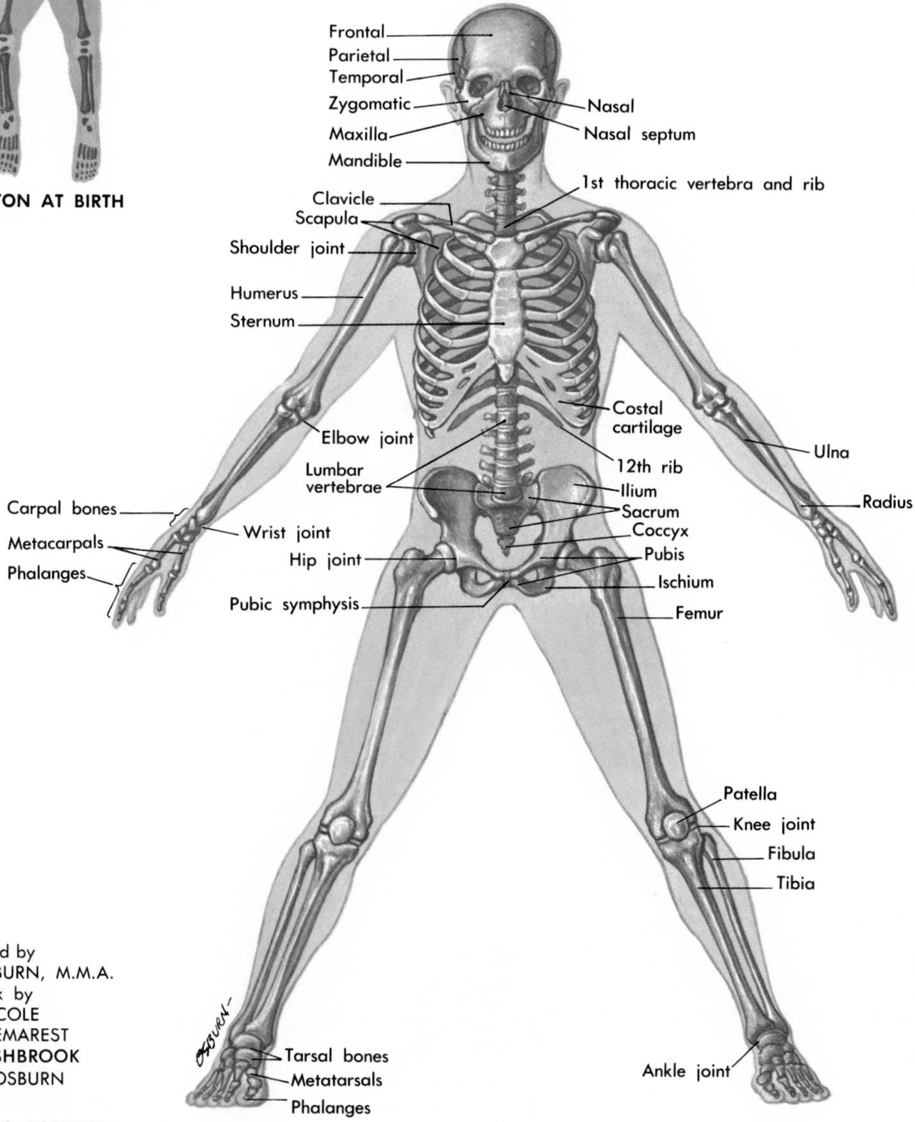

Designed by
WILLIAM A. OSBURN, M.M.A.
Artwork by
ELLEN COLE
ROBERT DEMAREST
GRANT LASHBROOK
WILLIAM OSBURN

W. B. SAUNDERS COMPANY
Philadelphia — London — Toronto

Plate 1

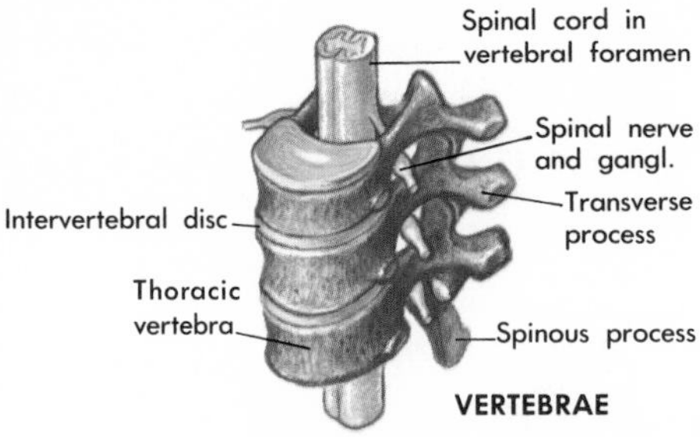

VERTEBRAE

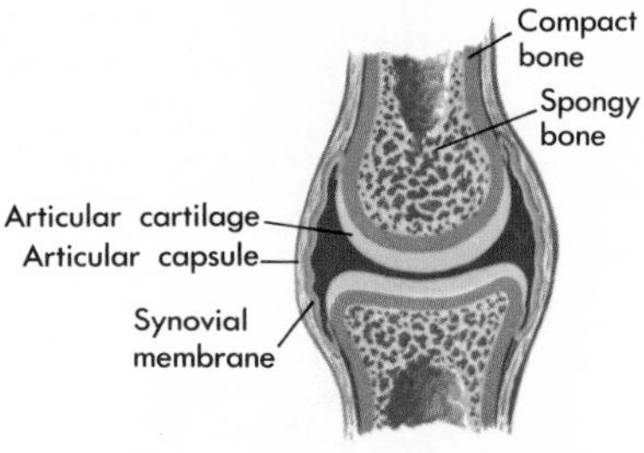

SECTION OF A JOINT

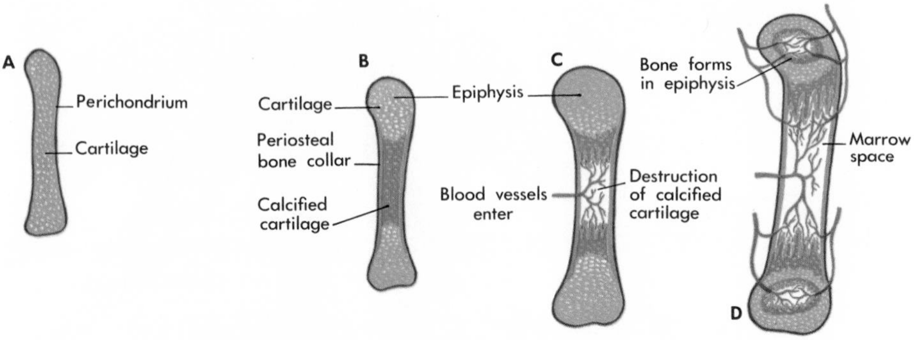

DEVELOPMENT OF BONE

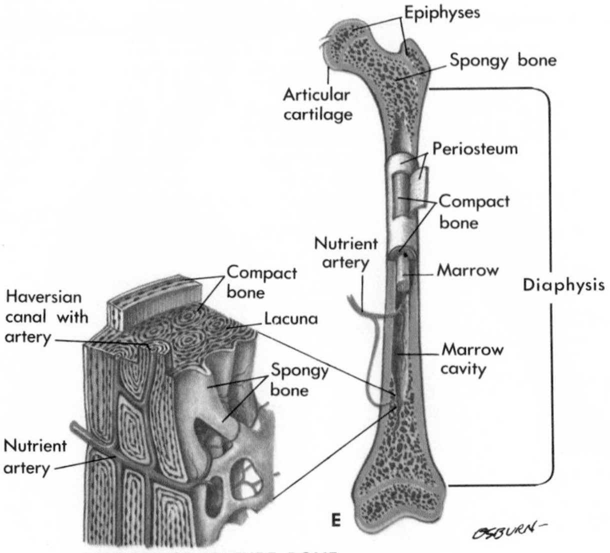

SECTION OF MATURE BONE

Plate 2

SKELETAL MUSCLES

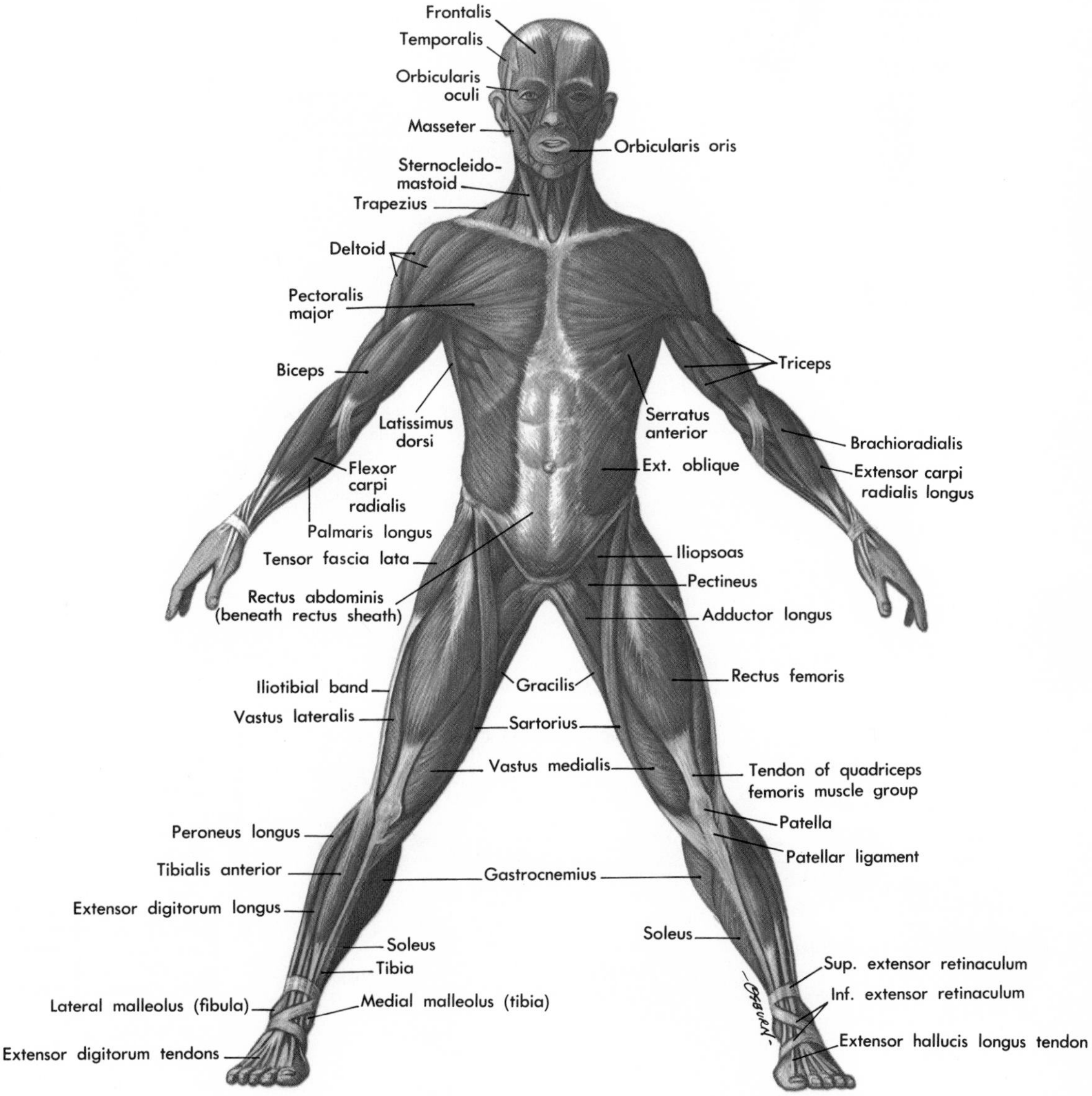
Frontalis
Temporalis
Orbicularis oculi
Masseter
Orbicularis oris
Sternocleido-mastoid
Trapezius
Deltoid
Pectoralis major
Biceps
Triceps
Latissimus dorsi
Serratus anterior
Brachioradialis
Flexor carpi radialis
Ext. oblique
Extensor carpi radialis longus
Palmaris longus
Tensor fascia lata
Iliopsoas
Pectineus
Rectus abdominis (beneath rectus sheath)
Adductor longus
Iliotibial band
Gracilis
Rectus femoris
Vastus lateralis
Sartorius
Vastus medialis
Tendon of quadriceps femoris muscle group
Patella
Peroneus longus
Patellar ligament
Tibialis anterior
Gastrocnemius
Extensor digitorum longus
Soleus
Soleus
Tibia
Sup. extensor retinaculum
Inf. extensor retinaculum
Lateral malleolus (fibula)
Medial malleolus (tibia)
Extensor hallucis longus tendon
Extensor digitorum tendons

Plate 3

HOW A MUSCLE PRODUCES MOVEMENT

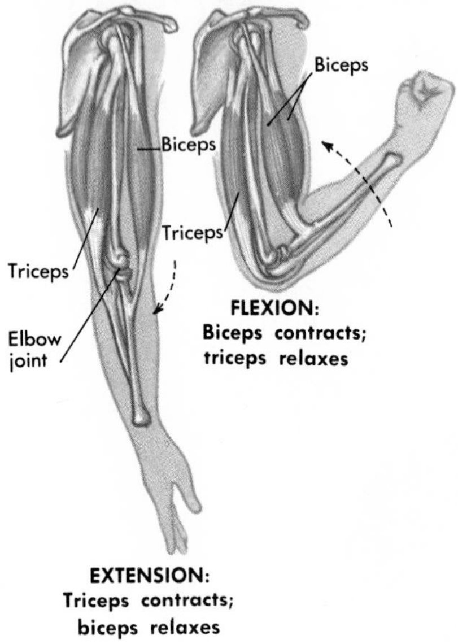

HOW A MUSCLE ATTACHES TO BONE

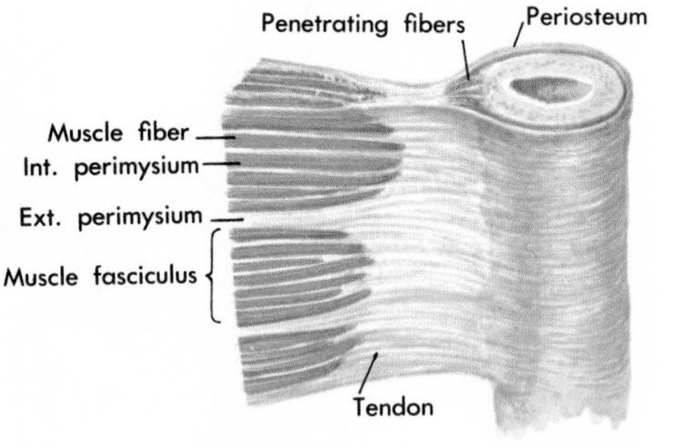

The connective tissue which surrounds the muscle fibers and bundles may (1) form a tendon which fuses with the periosteum, or (2) may fuse directly with the periosteum without forming a tendon.

HOW A MUSCLE CONTRACTS

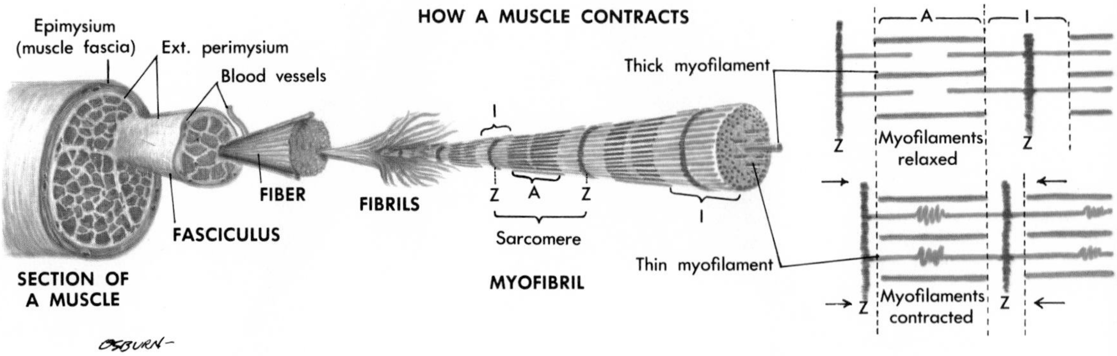

RESPIRATION AND THE HEART

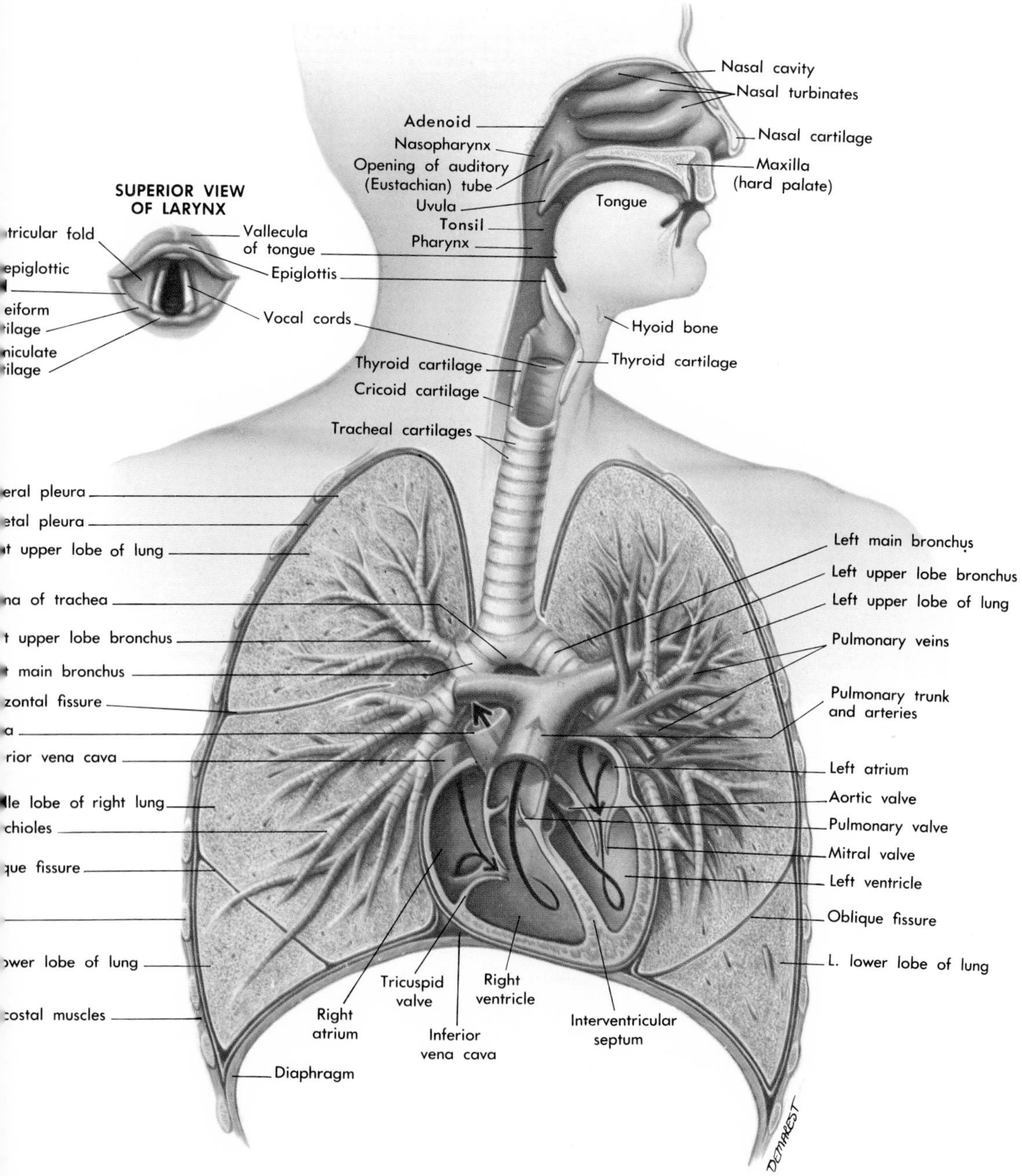

SUPERIOR VIEW OF LARYNX
tricular fold
epiglottic
eiform
ilage
niculate
ilage
Vallecula of tongue
Epiglottis
Vocal cords
Nasal cavity
Nasal turbinates
Nasal cartilage
Maxilla (hard palate)
Adenoid
Nasopharynx
Opening of auditory (Eustachian) tube
Uvula
Tongue
Tonsil
Pharynx
Hyoid bone
Thyroid cartilage
Thyroid cartilage
Cricoid cartilage
Tracheal cartilages
eral pleura
etal pleura
t upper lobe of lung
na of trachea
t upper lobe bronchus
main bronchus
zontal fissure
a
rior vena cava
le lobe of right lung
chioles
que fissure
ower lobe of lung
costal muscles
Left main bronchus
Left upper lobe bronchus
Left upper lobe of lung
Pulmonary veins
Pulmonary trunk and arteries
Left atrium
Aortic valve
Pulmonary valve
Mitral valve
Left ventricle
Oblique fissure
L. lower lobe of lung
Tricuspid valve
Right ventricle
Right atrium
Inferior vena cava
Interventricular septum
Diaphragm
DEMAREST

Plate 5

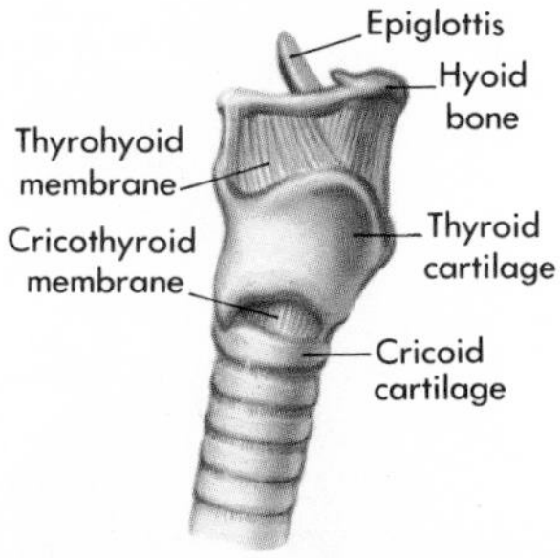

LATERAL VIEW OF THE LARYNX

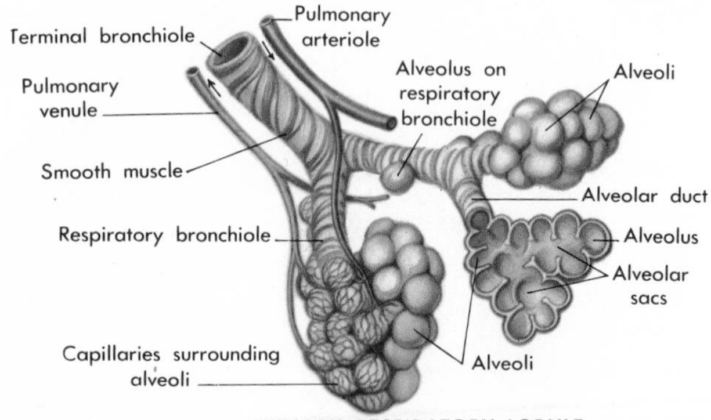

PRIMARY RESPIRATORY LOBULE

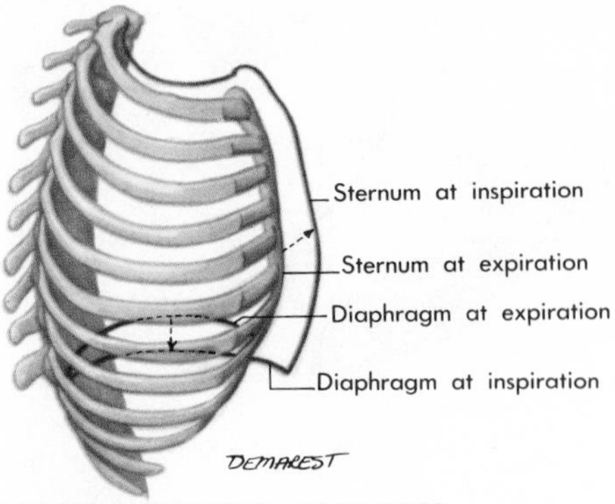

THORACIC RESPIRATORY MOVEMENTS

BLOOD VASCULAR SYSTEM

VEINS

STRUCTURE

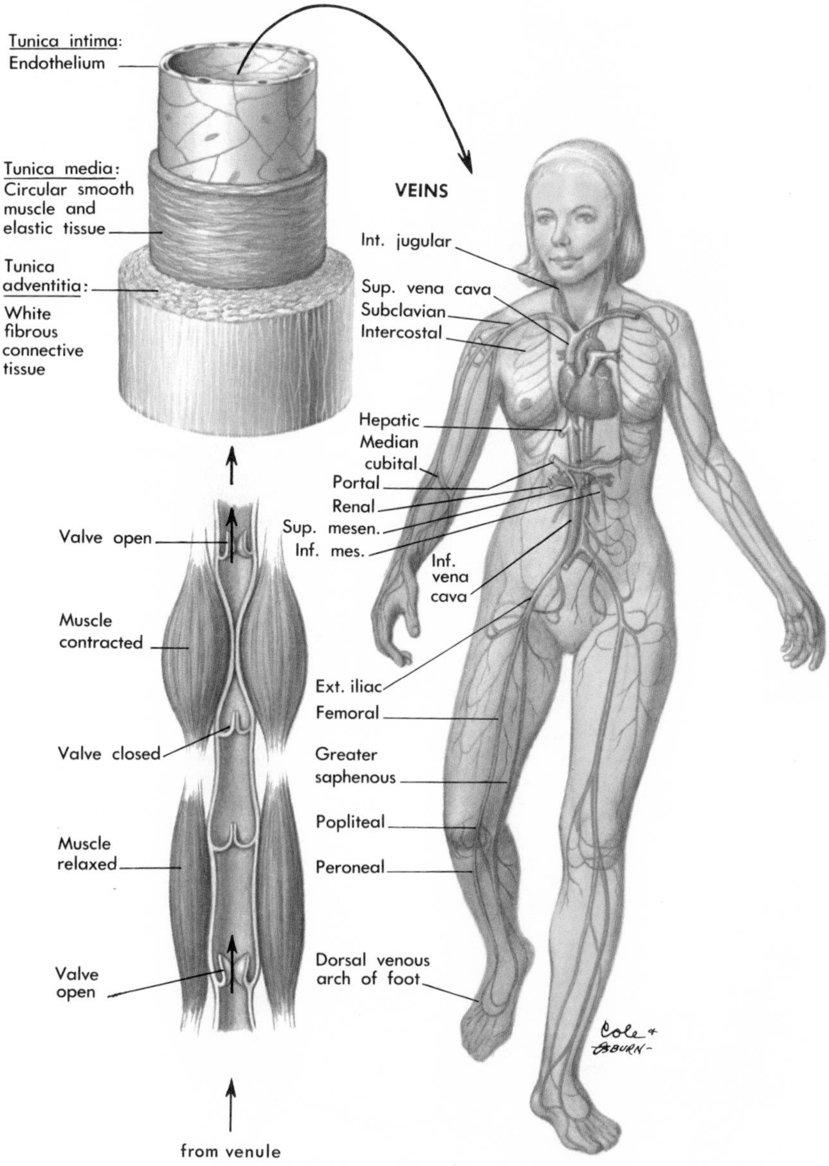

Tunica intima:
Endothelium
Tunica media:
Circular smooth muscle and elastic tissue
Tunica adventitia:
White fibrous connective tissue
Valve open
Muscle contracted
Valve closed
Muscle relaxed
Valve open
from venule
VEINS
Int. jugular
Sup. vena cava
Subclavian
Intercostal
Hepatic
Median cubital
Portal
Renal
Sup. mesen.
Inf. mes.
Inf. vena cava
Ext. iliac
Femoral
Greater saphenous
Popliteal
Peroneal
Dorsal venous arch of foot

ARTERIES

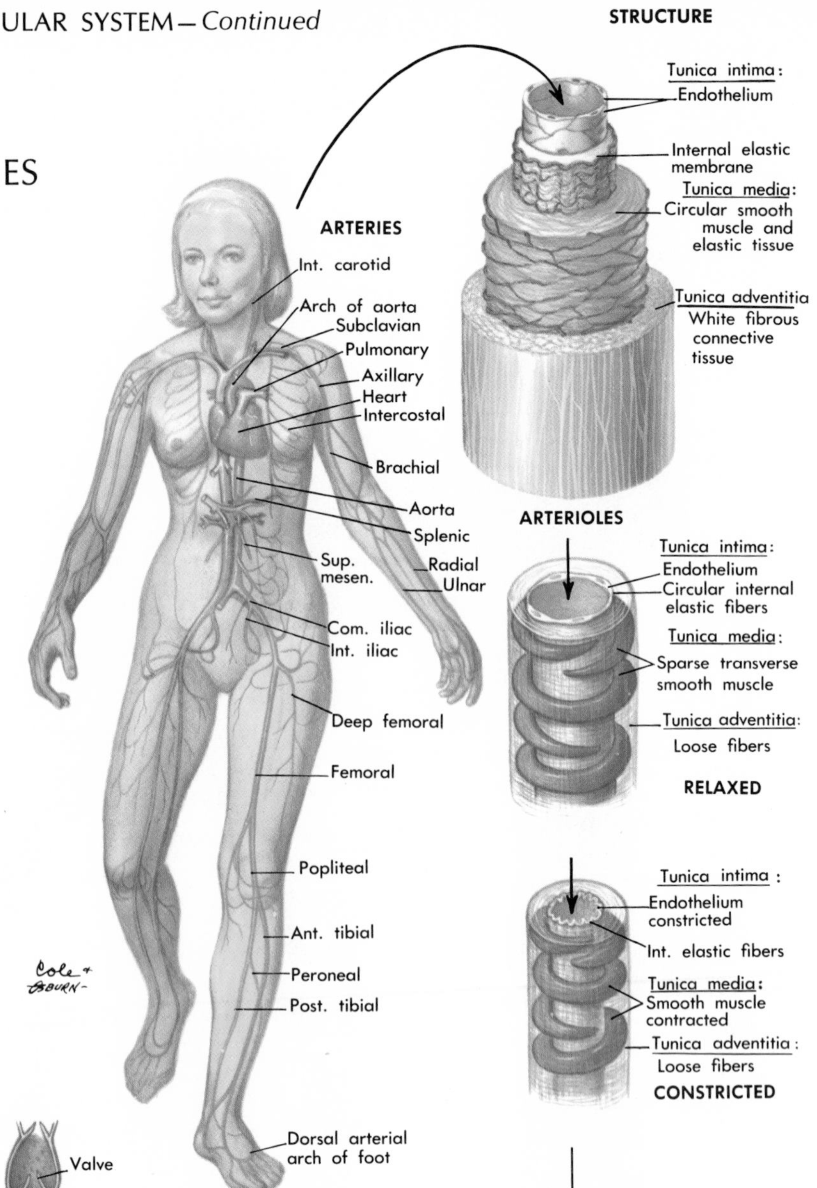
STRUCTURE
Tunica intima:
Endothelium
Internal elastic membrane
Tunica media:
Circular smooth muscle and elastic tissue
Tunica adventitia
White fibrous connective tissue
ARTERIES
Int. carotid
Arch of aorta
Subclavian
Pulmonary
Axillary
Heart
Intercostal
Brachial
Aorta
Splenic
Sup. mesen.
Radial
Ulnar
Com. iliac
Int. iliac
Deep femoral
Femoral
Popliteal
Ant. tibial
Peroneal
Post. tibial
Dorsal arterial arch of foot
Cole + Osburn
ARTERIOLES
Tunica intima:
Endothelium
Circular internal elastic fibers
Tunica media:
Sparse transverse smooth muscle
Tunica adventitia:
Loose fibers
RELAXED
Tunica intima:
Endothelium constricted
Int. elastic fibers
Tunica media:
Smooth muscle contracted
Tunica adventitia:
Loose fibers
CONSTRICTED

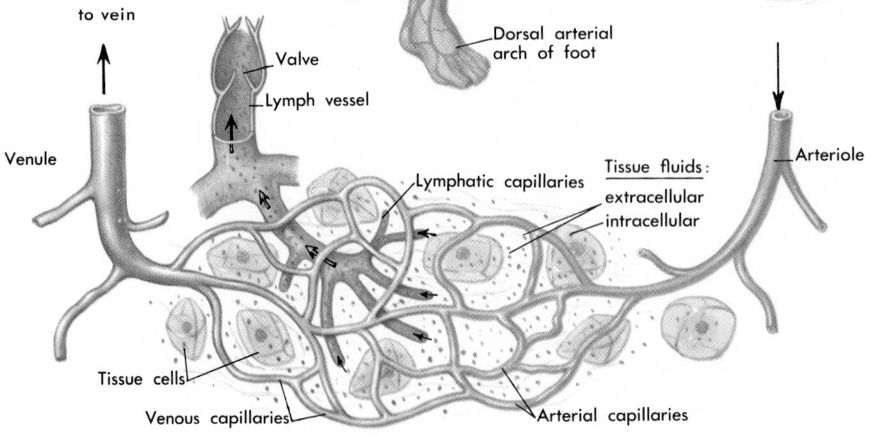
to vein
Venule
Valve
Lymph vessel
Lymphatic capillaries
Tissue fluids:
extracellular
intracellular
Arteriole
Tissue cells
Venous capillaries
Arterial capillaries

A CAPILLARY BED

Plate 8

DIGESTIVE SYSTEM

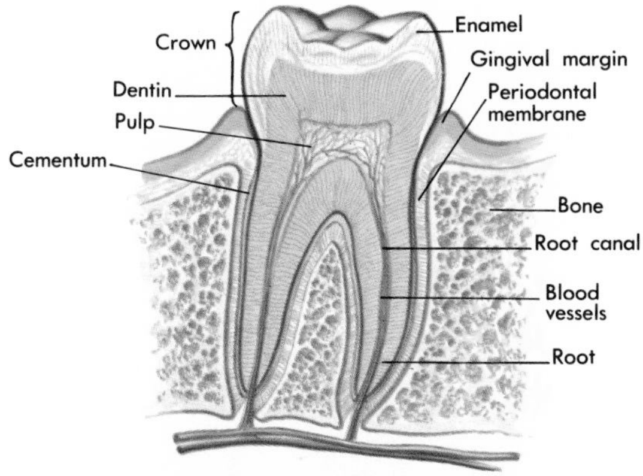
Crown
Dentin
Pulp
Cementum
Enamel
Gingival margin
Periodontal membrane
Bone
Root canal
Blood vessels
Root

SECTION OF A MOLAR TOOTH

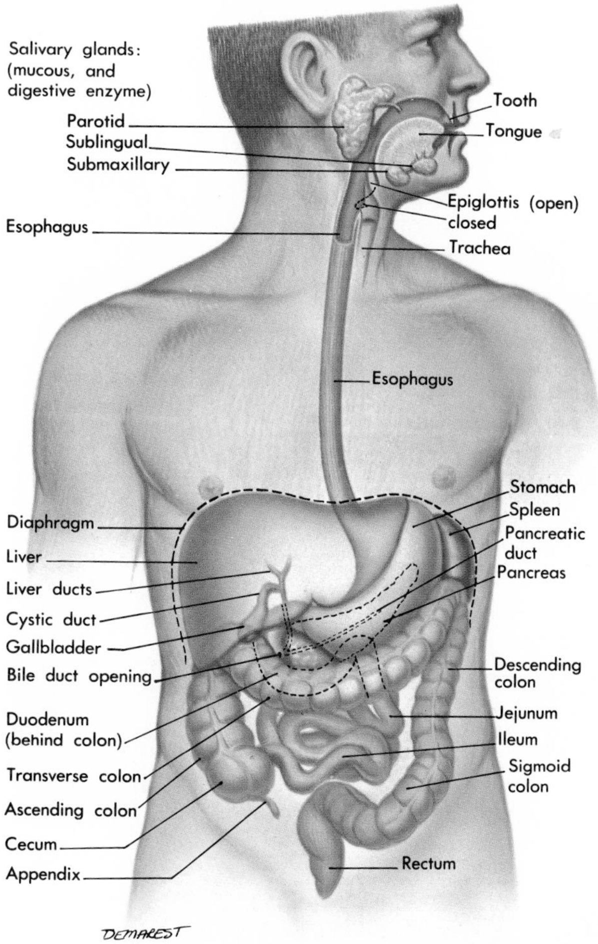
Salivary glands: (mucous, and digestive enzyme)
Parotid
Sublingual
Submaxillary
Esophagus
Tooth
Tongue
Epiglottis (open)
closed
Trachea
Esophagus
Diaphragm
Liver
Liver ducts
Cystic duct
Gallbladder
Bile duct opening
Duodenum (behind colon)
Transverse colon
Ascending colon
Cecum
Appendix
Stomach
Spleen
Pancreatic duct
Pancreas
Descending colon
Jejunum
Ileum
Sigmoid colon
Rectum
DEMAREST

Plate 9

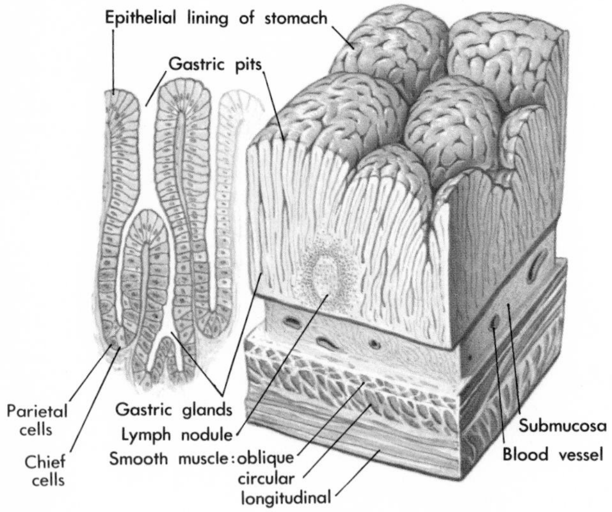

SECTION OF STOMACH WALL

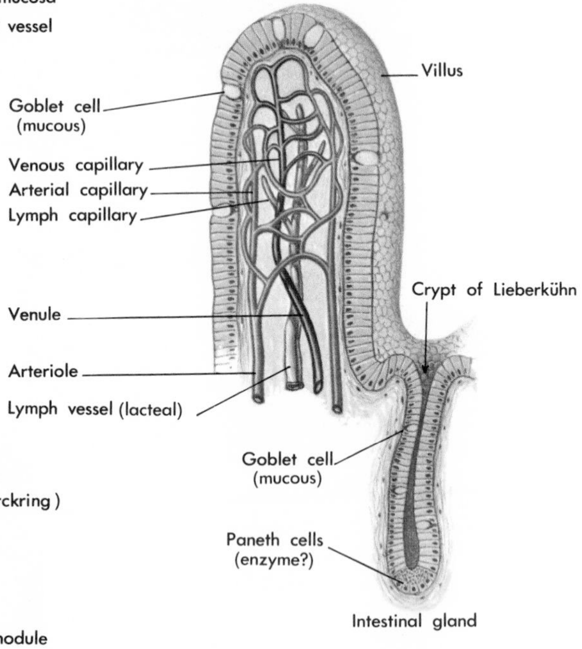

SECTIONS OF SMALL INTESTINE WALL

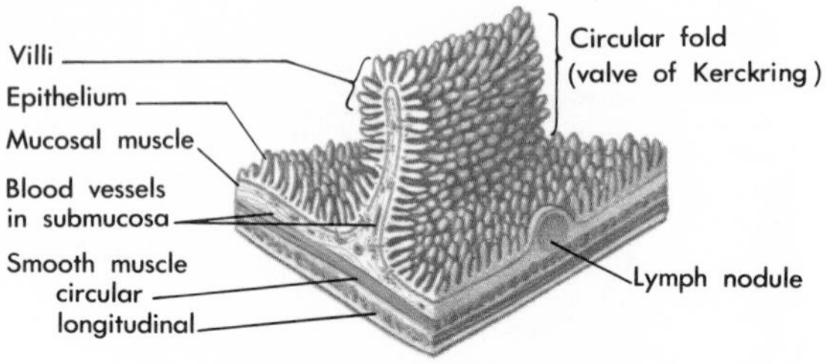

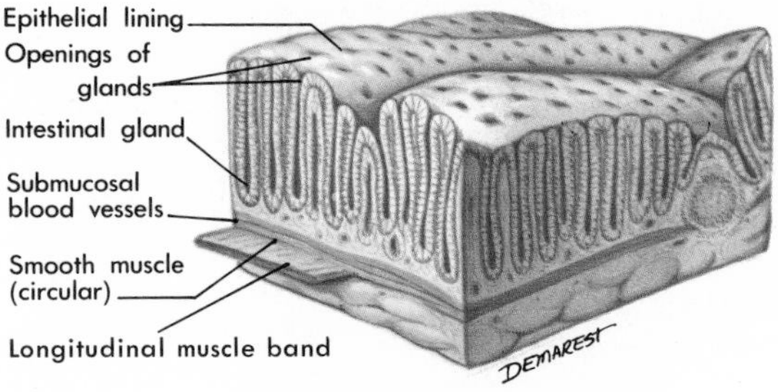

SECTION OF LARGE INTESTINE (COLON)

GENITOURINARY SYSTEM

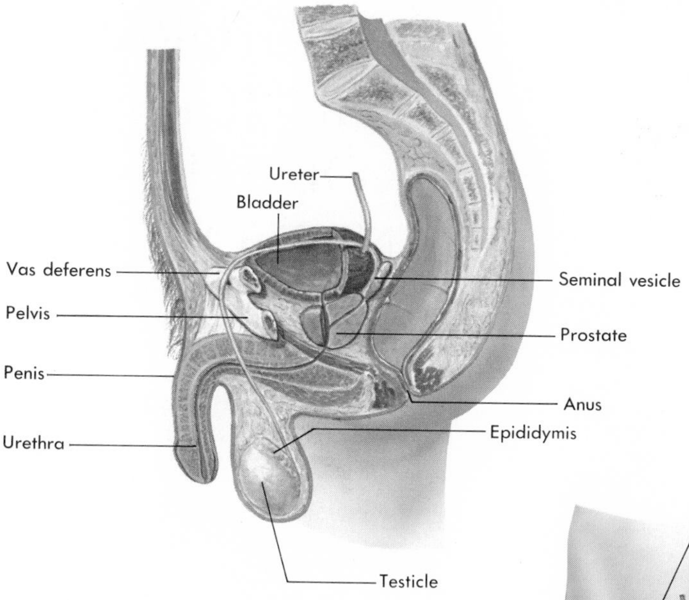

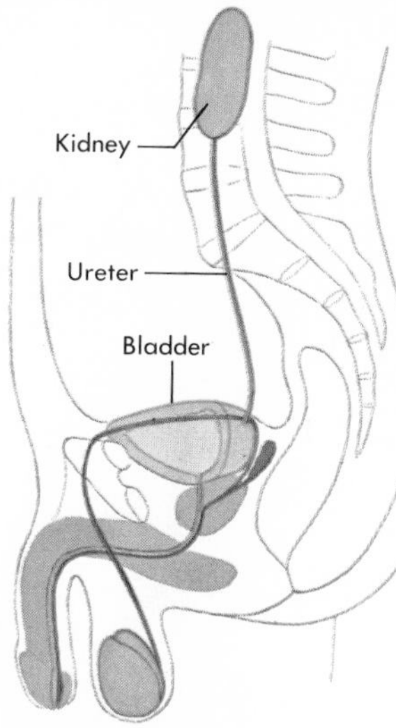

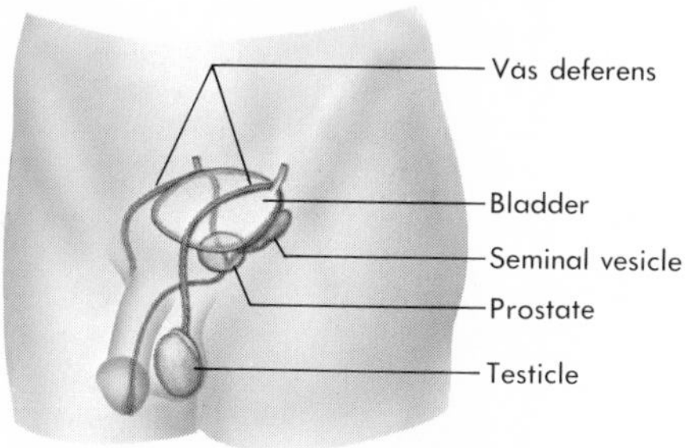

URINARY COMPONENTS

GENITAL COMPONENTS

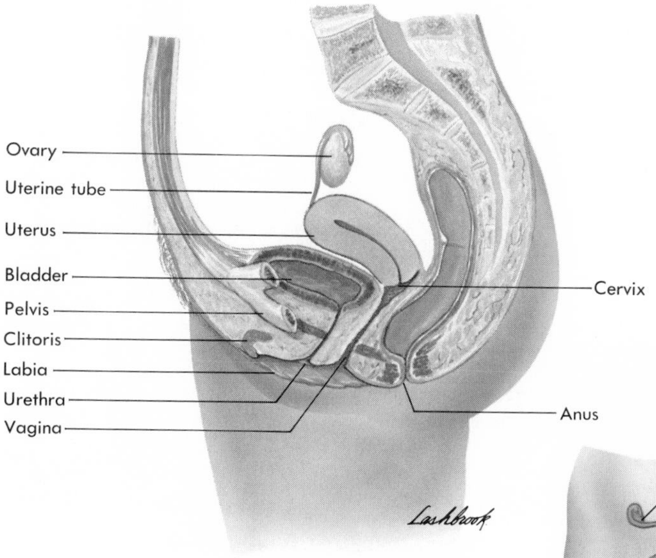

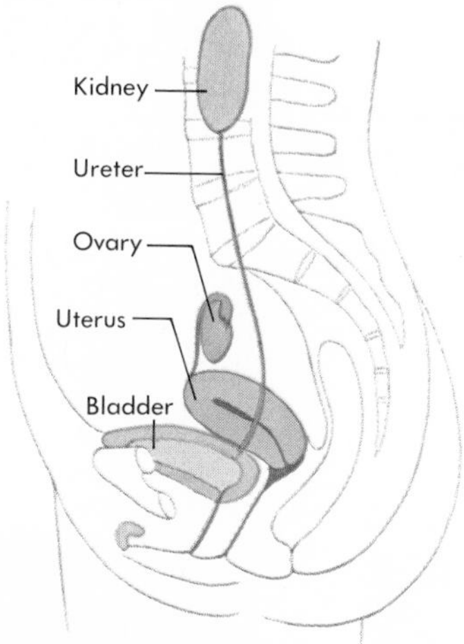

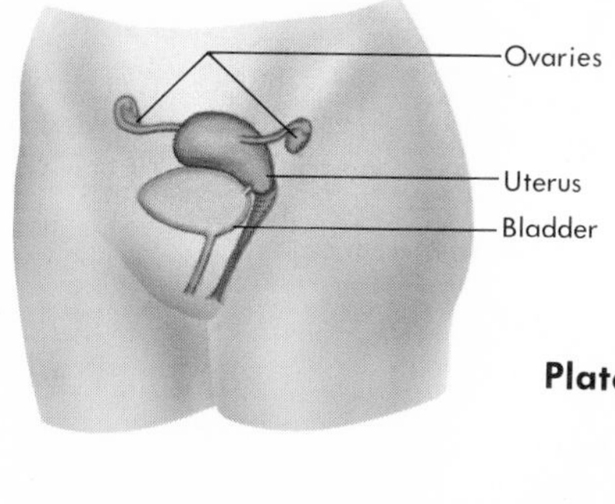

Plate 11

STRUCTURAL HIGHLIGHTS OF THE NERVOUS SYSTEM

GENERAL ARCHITECTURE AND PHYSIOLOGY

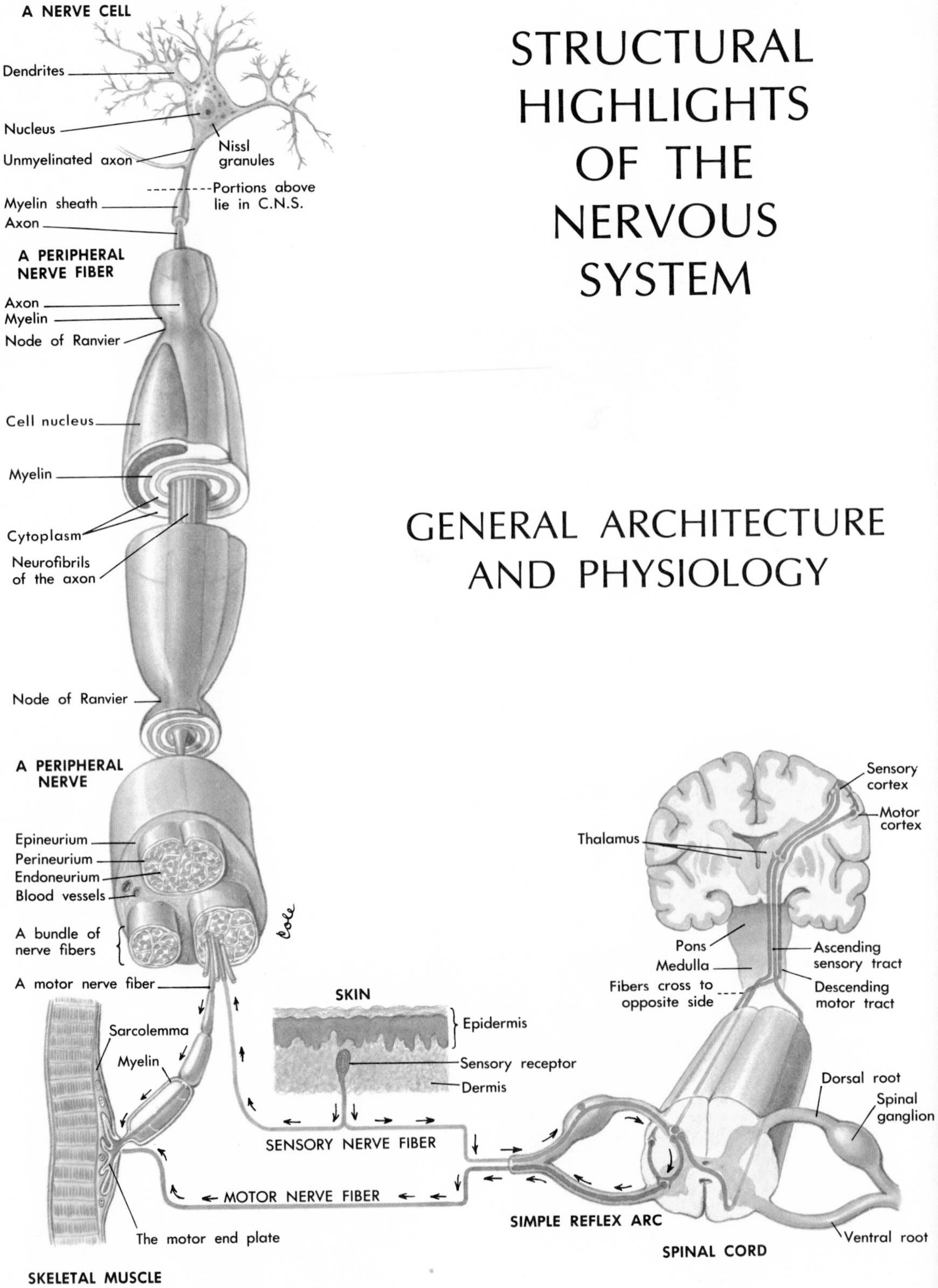

Plate 12

BRAIN AND SPINAL NERVES

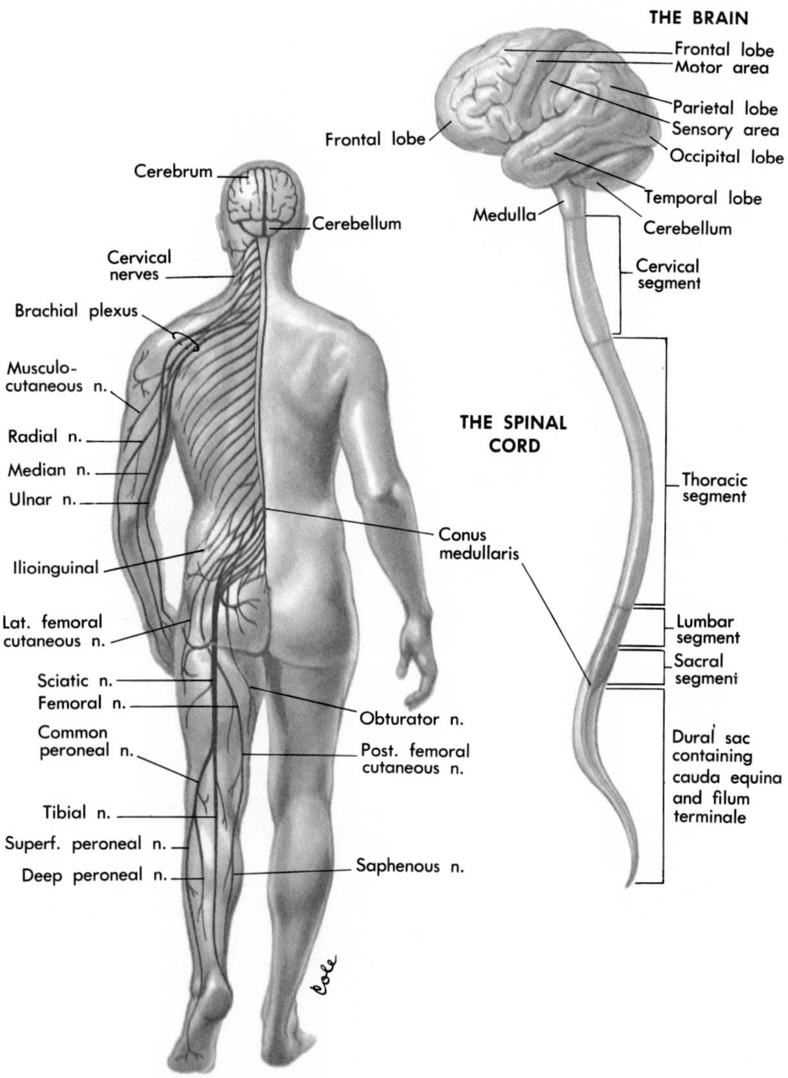

THE BRAIN
Frontal lobe
Motor area
Parietal lobe
Sensory area
Occipital lobe
Temporal lobe
Cerebellum
Frontal lobe
Medulla
Cervical segment
THE SPINAL CORD
Thoracic segment
Lumbar segment
Sacral segment
Dural sac containing cauda equina and filum terminale
Conus medullaris
Cerebrum
Cerebellum
Cervical nerves
Brachial plexus
Musculo-cutaneous n.
Radial n.
Median n.
Ulnar n.
Ilioinguinal
Lat. femoral cutaneous n.
Sciatic n.
Femoral n.
Common peroneal n.
Tibial n.
Superf. peroneal n.
Deep peroneal n.
Obturator n.
Post. femoral cutaneous n.
Saphenous n.
Cole

THE MAJOR SPINAL NERVES

AUTONOMIC NERVES

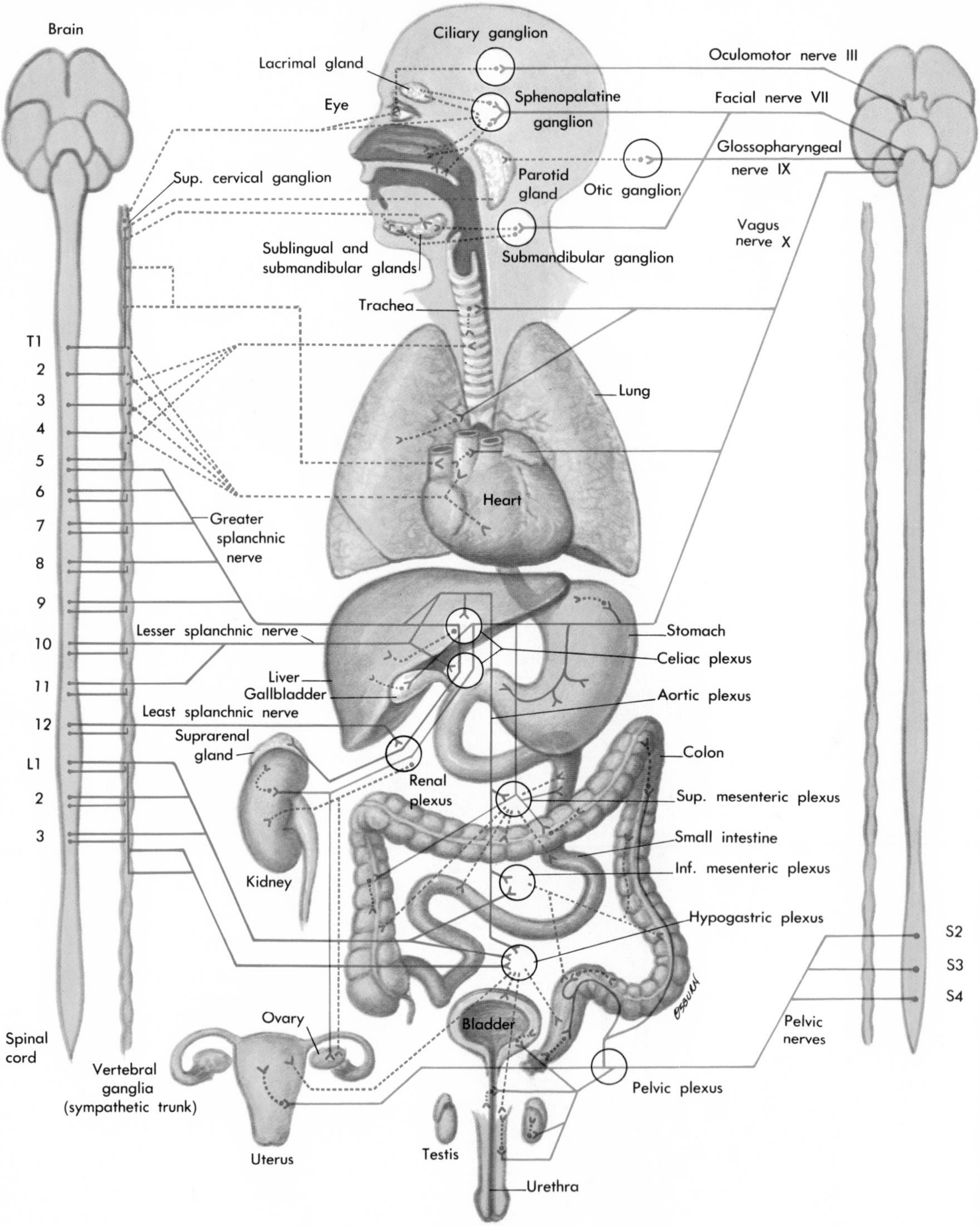

SYMPATHETIC
Thoracolumbar outflow

———	Preganglionic sympathetic fibers
- - - -	Postganglionic sympathetic fibers
———	Preganglionic parasympathetic fibers
- - - -	Postganglionic parasympathetic fibers

PARASYMPATHETIC
Craniosacral outflow

Plate 14

ORGANS OF SPECIAL SENSE

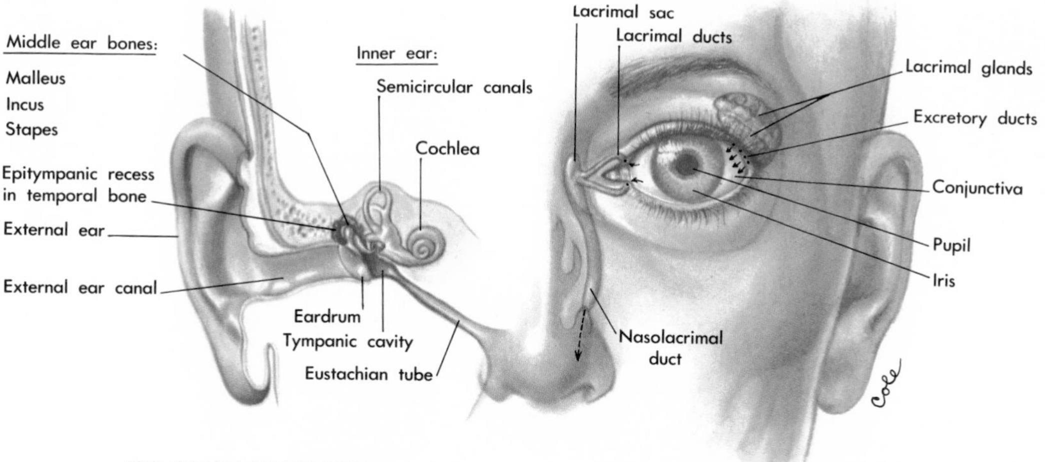

THE ORGAN OF HEARING

THE LACRIMAL APPARATUS AND THE EYE

HORIZONTAL SECTION OF THE EYE

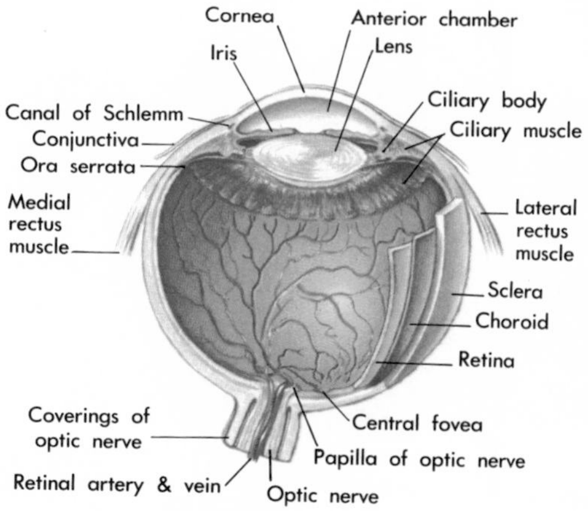

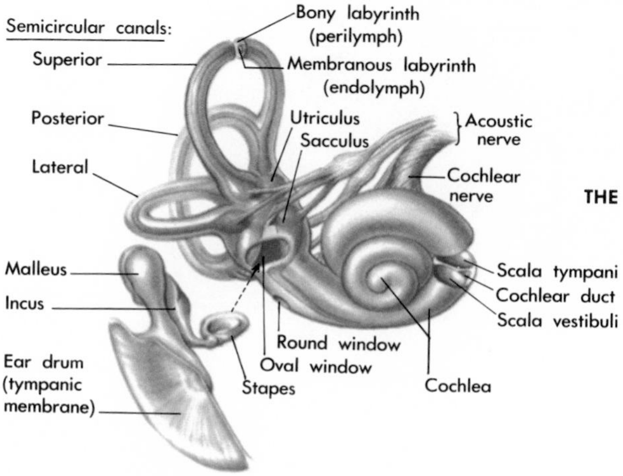

THE MIDDLE EAR AND INNER EAR

Plate 15

PARANASAL SINUSES

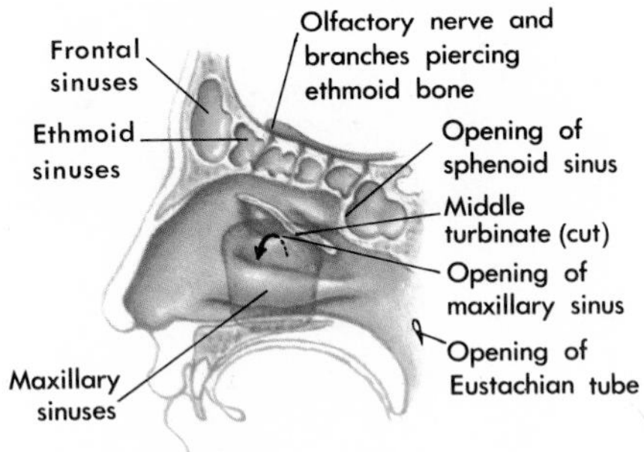

SAGITTAL SECTION OF THE NOSE

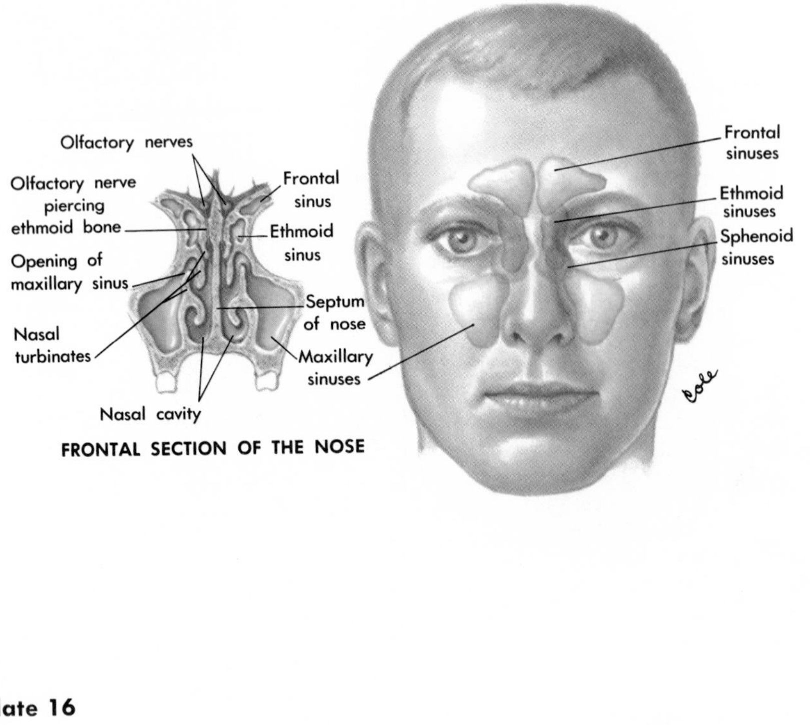

FRONTAL SECTION OF THE NOSE

lipoarthritis (lip″o-ar-thri′tis) inflammation of the fatty tissue of a joint.

lipoatrophy (lip″o-at′ro-fe) atrophy of subcutaneous fatty tissues of the body.

lipoblast (lip′o-blast) a connective tissue cell that develops into a fat cell.

lipocaic (lip″o-ka′ik) a substance extracted from the pancreas that prevents deposit of fat in the liver of animals after experimental pancreatectomy.

lipocardiac (lip″o-kar′de-ak) pertaining to fatty degeneration of the heart.

lipocatabolic (lip″o-kat″ah-bol′ik) pertaining to or effecting catabolism of fat.

lipochondrodystrophy (lip″o-kon″-dro-dis′tro-fe) Hurler's syndrome.

lipochondroma (lip″o-kon-dro′mah) a tumor composed of mature lipomatous and cartilaginous elements.

lipochrome (lip″o-krōm) any one of a group of fat-soluble hydrocarbon pigments, such as carotene, lutein, chromophane, and the natural yellow coloring material of butter, egg yolk, and yellow corn. They are also known as carotenoids.

lipocyte (lip′o-sīt) a fat cell.

lipodystrophy (lip″o-dis′tro-fe) 1. any disturbance of fat metabolism. 2. progressive lipodystrophy.
intestinal l., a malabsorption syndrome marked by diarrhea, steatorrhea, skin pigmentation, arthralgia and arthritis, lymphadenopathy, central nervous system lesions, and infiltration of the intestinal mucosa with macrophages containing PAS-positive material. Called also Whipple's disease.
progressive l., progressive and symmetrical loss of subcutaneous fat from the parts above the pelvis, facial emaciation, and abnormal accumulation of fat about the thighs and buttocks.

lipofibroma (lip″o-fi-bro′mah) a lipoma containing fibrous elements.

lipofuscin (lip″o-fus′in) any of a class of fatty pigments formed by the solution of a pigment in fat.

lipogenesis (lip″o-jen′ĕ-sis) the formation of fat; the transformation of nonfat food materials into body fat. adj., **lipogenet′ic.**

lipogenic (lip″o-jen′ik) producing, forming, or caused by fat.

lipogenous (lĭ-poj′ĕ-nus) producing fatness.

lipogranuloma (lip″o-gran″u-lo′mah) a nodule of lipoid material associated with granulomatous inflammation.

lipogranulomatosis (lip″o-gran″u-lo″mah-to′sis) a condition of faulty lipid metabolism in which yellow nodules of lipoid material are deposited in the skin and mucosae, giving rise to granulomatous reactions.

lipoid (lip′oid) 1. fatlike. 2. lipid.
l. cell tumor, masculinovoblastoma.

lipoidemia (lip″oi-de′me-ah) lipids in the blood; lipemia.

lipoidosis (lip″oi-do′sis) a disturbance of lipid metabolism with abnormal deposit of lipids in the cells.

lipoiduria (lip″oi-du′re-ah) lipids in the urine; lipiduria.

Lipo-Lutin (li″po-lu′tin) trademark for preparations of progesterone, a progestational hormone.

lipolysis (lĭ-pol′ĭ-sis) the splitting up or decomposition of fat. adj., **lipolyt′ic.**

lipoma (lĭ-po′mah) a benign fatty tumor usually composed of mature fat cells.

lipomatosis (lip″o-mah-to′sis) a condition characterized by abnormal localized, or tumor-like, accumulations of fat in the tissues.

lipomatous (lĭpo′mah-tus) affected with, or of the nature of, lipoma.

lipomeria (li″po-me′re-ah) congenital absence of a limb.

lipometabolism (lip″o-mĕ-tab′o-lizm) metabolism of fat. adj., **lipometabol′ic.**

lipomyxoma (lip″o-mik-so′mah) a myxoma containing fatty elements.

lipopenia (lip″o-pe′ne-ah) deficiency of lipids in the body.

lipopeptid (lip″o-pep′tid) any substance composed of amino acids and fatty acids.

lipophage (lip′o-fāj) a cell that absorbs or ingests fat.

lipophagia (lip″o-fa′je-ah) lipophagy.
l. granulomato′sis, intestinal lipodystrophy.

lipophagy (lĭ-pof′ah-je) the absorption of fat; lipolysis. adj., **lipopha′gic.**

lipophilia (lip″o-fil′e-ah) affinity for fat. adj., **lipophil′ic.**

lipopolysaccharide (lip″o-pol″ĕ-sak′ah-rīd) a molecule in which lipids and polysaccharides are linked.

lipoprotein (lip″o-pro′te-in) a combination of a lipid and a protein, having the general properties (e.g., solubility) of proteins. Practically all of the lipids of the plasma are lipoprotein complexes, alpha- and beta-lipoproteins being distinguished by electrophoresis.

liposarcoma (lip″o-sar-ko′mah) a malignant tumor characterized by large anaplastic lipoblasts, sometimes with foci of normal fat cells.

liposis (lĭ-po′sis) lipomatosis.

liposoluble (lip″o-sol′u-b′l) soluble in fats.

lipothymia (li″po-thi′me-ah) syncope.

lipotrophy (lĭ-pot′ro-fe) increase of bodily fat. adj., **lipotroph′ic.**

lipotropic (lip″o-trop′ik) 1. acting on fat metabolism by hastening removal, or decreasing the deposit, of fat in the liver. 2. a lipotropic agent.

lipotropism, lipotropy (lĭ-pot′ro-pizm; lĭ-pot′ro-pe) the condition of being lipotropic.

lipovaccine (lip″o-vak′sēn) a vaccine in a vegetable oil vehicle.

lipoxidase (lĭ-pok′sĭ-dās) lipoxygenase.

lipoxygenase (lĭ-poks′ĭ-jē-nās) an enzyme that catalyzes the oxidation of polyunsaturated fatty acids to form a peroxide of the acid.

Lippes loop (lip′ez) a form of intrauterine contraceptive device.

lipping (lip′ing) 1. a wedge-shaped shadow in the roentgenogram of chondrosarcoma between the cortex and the elevated periosteum. 2. the development of a bony overgrowth in osteoarthritis.

lip reading understanding of speech through observation of the speaker's lip movements; called also speech reading.

lipuria (lĭ-pu′re-ah) lipids in the urine.

Liquaemin (lik′wah-min) trademark for preparations of heparin, an anticoagulant.

Liquamar (lik″wah-mar) trademark for a preparation of phenprocoumon, an anticoagulant.

liquefacient (lik″wĕ-fa′shent) 1. producing or pertaining to liquefaction. 2. an agent that produces liquefaction.

liquefaction (lik″wĕ-fak′shun) conversion into a liquid form.

liquescent (lĭ-kwes′ent) tending to become liquid or fluid.

liquid (lik′wid) 1. a substance that flows readily in its natural state. 2. flowing readily; neither solid nor gaseous.

l. diet, a diet limited to the intake of liquids or foods that can be changed to a liquid state. A liquid diet may be restricted to clear liquids or it may be a full liquid diet (see the table of hospital diets, under DIET).

CLEAR LIQUID DIET. This is a temporary diet of clear liquids without residue. It is not nutritionally adequate, and is used in some acute illnesses and infections, postoperatively (especially after gastrointestinal surgery), and to reduce fecal matter in the colon. Foods allowed include water, tea, coffee, fat-free broth, carbonated beverages, synthetic fruit juices, ginger ale, plain gelatin, and sugar.

FULL LIQUID DIET. This diet can be nutritionally adequate with careful planning. It is used for acute gastritis, as a transition between clear liquid and soft diet, and in conditions in which there is intolerance to solid food. Milk, strained soups, and fruit juices are allowed. Foods that liquefy at body temperature, such as ice cream, flavored gelatin, and soft custards, can be included. Cereal gruels and egg nogs are allowed. When a full liquid diet is used as a TUBE FEEDING it must be of a consistency that will allow easy passage through the tube. Most full liquid diets are given in feedings every 2 to 4 hours.

liquor (lik′er, li′kwor) 1. a liquid, especially an aqueous solution, or a solution not obtained by distillation. 2. a term applied to certain body fluids.

l. am′nii, amniotic fluid.

l. cerebrospina′lis, cerebrospinal fluid.

l. follic′uli, the fluid in the cavity of a developing graafian follicle.

mother l., the liquid remaining after removal of crystals from a solution.

l. san′guinis, blood plasma.

Lisfranc's ligament (lis-frahnks′) a fibrous band extending from the medial cuneiform bone to the second metatarsal.

lissencephaly (lis″en-sef′ah-le) agyria. adj., **lissencephal′ic.**

Lister (lis′ter) Baron Joseph (1827–1912). Founder of modern antiseptic surgery. Born at Upton, Essex, England, Lister set out in a scientific manner to apply Pasteur's discoveries to the prevention of the development of microorganisms in wounds. His research was on the early stages of inflammation and blood coagulation, and in 1865 he successfully used carbolic acid in the treatment of an open fracture. Next he turned his attention to the arrest of hemorrhage in aseptic wounds, which led him to adopt a sulfochromic catgut for tying arteries, a material capable of more speedy absorption than silk or flax, which had long been employed. He wrote articles on amputation and anesthetics. Lister was created a baronet in 1883 and raised to the peerage in 1893, but perhaps the greatest memorial to him is the Lister Institute of Preventive Medicine in London.

Listeria (lis-te′re-ah) a genus of gram-negative bacteria (family Corynebacterium); the single species, *L. monocytog′enes,* is found chiefly in lower animals. In man, it produces upper respiratory disease, septicemia, and encephalitic disease.

listeriosis (lis-tēr″e-o′sis) infection with organisms of the genus *Listeria.*

listerism (lis′ter-izm) the principles and practice of antiseptic and aseptic surgery.

liter (le′ter) the unit of capacity of the metric system, being equal to 1 cubic decimeter; it is equivalent to 1.0567 quarts liquid measure. Abbreviated l.

lith(o)- word element [Gr.], *stone; calculus.*

lithagogue (lith′ah-gog) 1. expelling calculi. 2. an agent that promotes expulsion of calculi.

lithectasy (lĭ-thek′tah-se) extraction of calculi through a mechanically dilated urethra.

lithemia (lĭ-the′me-ah) an excess of uric (lithic) acid in the blood.

lithiasis (lĭ-thi′ah-sis) 1. a condition marked by formation of calculi and concretions. 2. gouty diathesis.

lithic acid (lith′ik) uric acid.

lithium (lith′e-um) a chemical element, atomic number 3, atomic weight 6.939, symbol Li. (See table of ELEMENTS.)

l. carbonate, a psychotropic drug used to treat acute manic attacks and, when given on a maintenance basis, to prevent the recurrence of manic-depressive episodes. Lithium is a safe and effective medication when given under properly controlled conditions, but it has the potential for dangerous side effects.

lithoclast (lith′o-klast) lithotrite.

lithocystotomy (lith″o-sis-tot′o-me) incision of the bladder for removal of stone.

lithodialysis (lith″o-di-al′ĭ-sis) 1. the solution of calculi in the bladder by injected solvents. 2. litholapaxy.

lithogenesis (lith″o-jen′ĕ-sis) formation of calculi, or stones. adj., **lithog′enous.**

litholapaxy (lĭ-thol′ah-pak″se) the crushing of a stone in the bladder and washing out of the fragments.

litholysis (lĭ-thol′ĭ-sis) dissolution of calculi.

lithonephritis (lith″o-nĕ-fri′tis) inflammation of the kidney due to irritation by calculi.

lithonephrotomy (lith″o-nĕ-frot′o-me) excision of a renal calculus.

lithopedion (lith″o-pe′de-on) a calcified fetus.

lithophone (lith′o-fōn) a device for detecting calculi in the bladder by sound.

lithoscope (lith′o-skōp) an instrument for detecting calculi in the bladder.

lithotomy (lĭ-thot′o-me) incision of a duct or organ for removal of calculi.

l. position, the patient lies on his back, legs flexed on the thighs, thighs flexed on the abdomen and abducted. Stirrups may be used to support the feet and legs.

lithotripsy (lith′o-trip″se) the crushing of calculi in the bladder or urethra.

lithotrite (lith′o-trīt) an instrument for crushing calculi; lithoclast.

lithotrity (lĭ-thot′rĭ-te) lithotripsy.

lithous (lith′us) pertaining to or of the nature of a calculus.

lithuresis (lith″u-re′sis) passage of gravel in the urine.

litmus (lit′mus) a blue pigment prepared from *Rocella tinctoria* and other lichens.

l. paper, absorbent paper impregnated with a solution of litmus, dried and cut into strips. It is used to indicate the acidity or alkalinity of solutions. If dipped into alkaline solution it remains blue; acid solution turns it red. It is used to test urine and other body fluids; it has a pH range of 4.5 to 8.3.

Little's disease (lit′elz) congenital spastic stiffness of the limbs, a form of cerebral spastic paralysis due to lack of development of the pyramidal tracts.

Littre's glands (le′trz) 1. small sebaceous glands on the corona of the penis and the inner surface of the prepuce, which secrete smegma; called also preputial glands. 2. mucous glands in the wall of the male urethra.

livedo (lĭ-ve′do) a discolored patch on the skin.

l. annula′ris, l. racemo′sa, l. reticula′ris, reddish blue, netlike mottling of the skin.

liver (liv′er) the large, dark-red gland located in the upper right portion of the abdomen, just beneath the diaphragm (see also Plate 9). its manifold functions include storage and filtration of blood, secretion of bile, conversion of sugars into glycogen, and many other metabolic activities.

STORAGE FUNCTIONS. The liver can store up to 20 per cent of its weight in glycogen and up to 40 percent of its weight in fats. The basic fuel of the body is a simple form of sugar called glucose. This comes to the liver as one of the products of digestion, and is converted into glycogen for storage. It is reconverted to glucose, when necessary, to keep up a steady level of sugar in the blood. This is normally a slow, continuous process, but in emergencies the liver, responding to epinephrine in the blood, releases large quantities of this fuel into the blood for use by the muscles.

As the chief supplier of glucose in the body, the liver is sometimes called on to convert other substances into sugar. The liver cells can make glucose out of protein and fat. This may also work in reverse: the liver cells can convert excess sugar into fat and send it for storage ot other parts of the body.

In addition to these functions, the liver builds many essential proteins and stores up certain necessary vitamins until they are needed by other organs in the body.

PROTECTIVE FUNCTIONS. The liver disposes of worn-out blood cells by breaking them down into their different elements, storing some and sending others to the kidneys for disposal in the urine. It filters and destroys bacteria and also neutralizes poisons.

The liver also helps to maintain the balance of sex hormones in the body. A certain amount of female hormone is normally produced in males, and male hormone in females. When the level of this opposite sex hormone rises above a certain point, the liver takes up the excess and disposes of it.

Finally, the liver polices the proteins that have passed through the digestive system. Some of the amino acids derived from protein metabolism cannot be used by the body; the liver rejects and neutralizes these acids and sends them to the kidneys for disposal.

DISORDERS OF THE LIVER. The liver, with its many complex functions, can be damaged by various disorders and diseases. Often such damage first manifests itself as JAUNDICE. This is a yellowish tinge, best

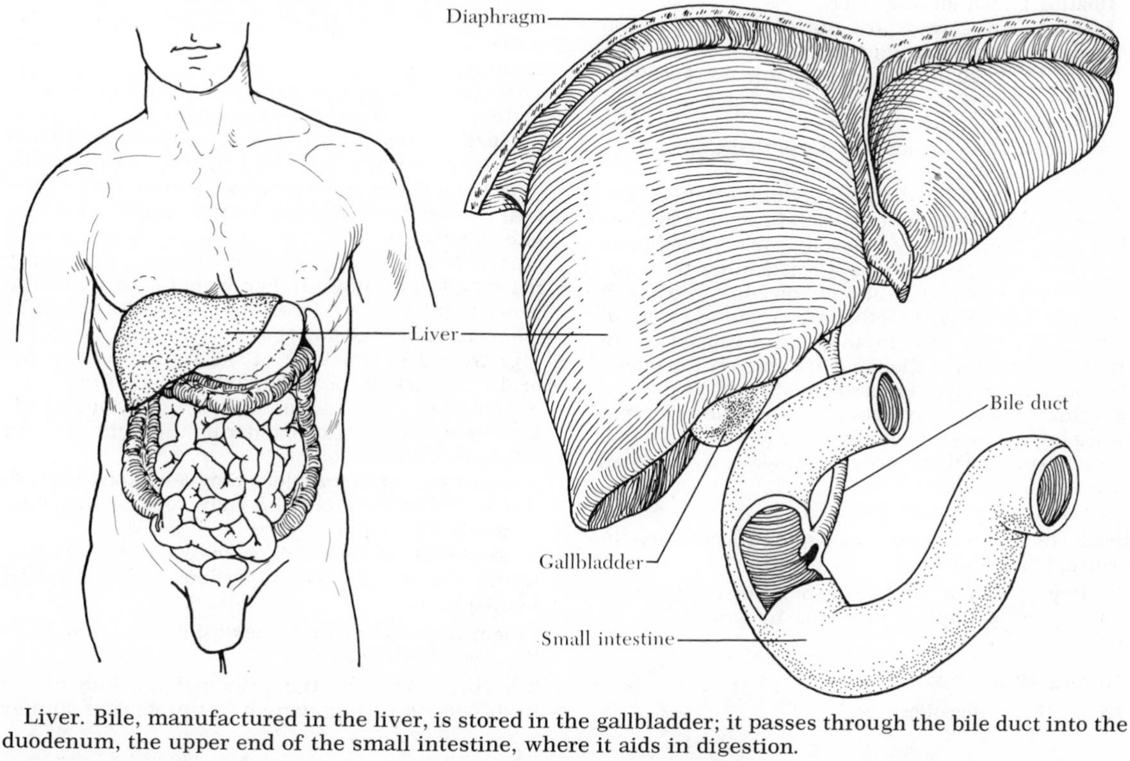

Liver. Bile, manufactured in the liver, is stored in the gallbladder; it passes through the bile duct into the duodenum, the upper end of the small intestine, where it aids in digestion.

seen in the eyes, that is caused by an excess of bile pigment in the blood. Jaundice is not a disease, it is a symptom of any one of a number of liver disorders or blood dyscrasias.

Besides jaundice, other symptoms of liver disease may be a gradual, unexplained swelling of the abdomen, vomiting of blood, and passing of bloody or black tar-like stools.

Infectious, or viral HEPATITIS, is one of the most common diseases of the liver. It is highly contagious and most often affects children and young adults. Its symptoms include jaundice, loss of appetite, fever, and abdominal discomfort.

The liver may be harmed by excessive use of alcohol and by excessive exposure to poisons such as carbon tetrachloride. Certain disorders of the GALLBLADDER also may damage the liver.

CIRRHOSIS of the liver is a chronic inflammation marked by degeneration of the liver cells and thickening of the surrounding tissue; it is the final stage of many kinds of liver damage. The condition often accompanies ALCOHOLISM because of the poor dietary habits of the alcoholic and the toxicity of alcohol. Although alcoholism is the most common cause of cirrhosis, it may also occur as a result of damage from toxins and infections.

Abscess of the liver usually occurs as a complication of peritonitis or abdominal cellulitis, or as an amebic abscess following infection with the *Entamoeba histolytica.*

albuminoid l., amyloid l., one with albuminoid or amyloid degeneration.

biliary cirrhotic l., one in which the bile ducts are clogged and distended, the substance of the organ being inflamed; due to biliary cirrhosis.

l. extract, an extract prepared from mammalian livers; used as a hematopoietic.

fatty l., one affected with fatty infiltration.

floating l., wandering liver.

foamy l., a liver seen post mortem, marked by the presence of numerous gas bubbles.

hobnail l., a liver whose surface is marked with nail-like points from atrophic cirrhosis.

lardaceous l., amyloid liver.

nutmeg l., one presenting a mottled appearance on the cut surface.

sago l., one affected with amyloid degeneration.

l. spots, a lay term for the small brownish patches that appear on the face, neck, or back of the hands of many older people. It is a misleading term because these spots have little or nothing to do with the liver. The spots, smooth, flat, irregularly spaced, and roundish or oval in shape, are caused by an increase in pigmentation and are entirely harmless. Although liver spots are associated with the process of aging, it is actually not age that is the principal cause but many years of exposure to sun and wind.

wandering l., a displaced and movable liver; called also floating liver.

waxy l., albuminoid liver.

livid (liv′id) discolored, as from a contusion or bruise; black and blue.

lividity (lĭ-vid′ĭ-te) the quality of being livid; discoloration, as of dependent parts, by gravitation of blood.

Living Will see EUTHANASIA.

livor (li′vor) discoloration.

l. mor′tis, discoloration on dependent parts of the body after death.

lixiviation (lik-siv″e-a′shun) separation of soluble from insoluble material by use of an appropriate solvent, and drawing off the solution.

L.M. Licentiate in Midwifery.

L.M.A. left mentoanterior (position of the fetus).

L.M.P. left mentoposterior (position of the fetus).

L.M.T. left mentotransverse (position of the fetus).

L.O.A. left occipitoanterior (position of the fetus).

Loa (lo′ah) a genus of filarial nematodes.

L. lo′a, a threadlike worm of West Africa, 1–2 inches long, that inhabits the subcutaneous connective tissue of the body, which it traverses freely. It is seen especially about the orbit and even under the conjunctiva. It causes itching and occasionally edematous swellings (Calabar swellings). The immature forms, or microfilariae, are diurnal, being found in the peripheral circulation in greatest concentrations during the day. Flies of the genus *Chrysops* are the intermediate hosts and vectors.

loading (lōd′ing) administering sufficient quantities of a substance to test a subject's ability to metabolize or absorb it.

loaiasis (lo″ah-i′ah-sis) infection with nematodes of the genus *Loa;* loiasis.

lobar (lo′ber) pertaining to a lobe.

l. atrophy, a progressive atrophy of the cerebral convolutions in a limited area (lobe) of the brain; called also Pick's disease.

l. pneumonia, pneumonia affecting one or more lobes of the lungs (see also PNEUMONIA).

lobate (lo′bāt) divided into lobes.

lobe (lōb) 1. a more or less well defined portion of an organ or gland. 2. one of the main divisions of a tooth crown.

azygos l., a small accessory or anomalous lobe at the apex of the right lung.

caudate l., a small lobe of the liver between the inferior vena cava on the right and the left lobe.

ear l., the lower fleshy, noncartilaginous portion of the external ear.

frontal l., the rostral (anterior) portion of the gray matter of the cerebral hemisphere.

hepatic l., one of the lobes of the liver, designated the right and left and the caudate and quadrate.

occipital l., the most posterior portion of the cerebral hemisphere, forming a small part of its dorsolateral surface.

parietal l., the upper central portion of the gray matter of the cerebral hemisphere, between the frontal and occipital lobes, and above the temporal lobe (see also PARIETAL LOBE).

prefrontal l., the part of the frontal lobe of the brain anterior to the ascending convolution.

quadrate l., 1. precuneus. 2. a small lobe of the liver, between the gallbladder on the right, and the left lobe.

Riedel's l., an anomalous tongue-shaped mass of tissue projecting from the right lobe of the liver.

spigelian l., caudate lobe.

temporal l., a long, tongue-shaped process constituting the lower lateral portion of the cerebral hemisphere.

lobectomy (lo-bek′to-me) excision of a lobe, as of the lung, brain, or liver.

lobeline (lob′ĕ-lin) the principal alkaloid of the herb *Lobelia inflata,* which has properties similar to nicotine; used as a respiratory stimulant and in certain antismoking preparations.

lobitis (lo-bi′tis) inflammation of a lobe, as of the lung.

lobocyte (lo′bo-sīt) a granulocyte with a segmented nucleus.

lobotomy (lo-bot′o-me) cutting of nerve fibers connecting a lobe of the brain with the thalamus. In most cases the affected parts are the prefrontal or frontal lobes, the areas of the brain involved with emotion; thus the operation is referred to as prefrontal, or frontal, lobotomy.

Lobotomy is a form of psychosurgery—a field in which the purpose of the operation is not to remove a growth or repair an injury to the body but to change the patient's mental and emotional state. Today most physicians regard lobotomy as a last resort and use the operation either for certain violent cases when all else has failed or for people with severe and otherwise untreatable anxiety. Although it can make formerly violent and uncontrollable patients calm and docile, it often seems to lead to emotional emptiness.

Furthermore, in recent years, drugs have been developed that have revolutionized the treatment of severe mental illnesses. Among these are the TRANQUILIZERS, which suppress temporarily the violent symptoms of psychosis.

Lobstein's disease (lōb′stīnz) see OSTEOGENESIS IMPERFECTA.

lobulated (lob′u-lāt″ed) made up of lobules.

lobule (lob′ūl) a small segment or lobe, especially one of the smaller divisions making up a lobe. adj., **lob′ular.**

l's of epididymis, the wedge-shaped parts of the head of the epididymis, each comprising an efferent ductule of the testis.

hepatic l., one of the small vascular units comprising the substance of the liver.

l. of lung, one of the smaller subdivisions of the lobes of the lungs (see also BRONCHOPULMONARY SEGMENT).

paracentral l., a lobe on the medial surface of the cerebral hemisphere, continuous with the pre- and postcentral gyri, limited below by the cingulate sulcus.

parietal l., one of two divisions, inferior and superior, of the parietal lobe of the brain.

primary l. of lung, respiratory l., the functional unit of the lung, including a respiratory bronchiole, alveolar ducts and sacs, and alveoli (see also Plate 6).

lobulus (lob′u-lus), pl. *lob′uli* [L.] lobule.

lobus (lo′bus), pl. *lo′bi* [L.] lobe.

local (lo′kal) restricted to or pertaining to one spot or part; not general.

localization (lo″kah-lĭ-za′shun) 1. the determination of a site or place of any process or lesion. 2. restriction to a circumscribed or limited area.

cerebral l., determination of areas of the cortex involved in performance of certain functions.

germinal l., the location on a blastoderm of prospective organs.

lochia (lo′ke-ah) a vaginal discharge occurring during the first week or two after childbirth. adj., **lo′chial.**

l. al′ba, the final vaginal discharge after childbirth, when the amount of blood is decreased and the leukocytes are increased.

l. cruen′ta, lochia rubra.

l. purulen′ta, lochia alba.

l. ru′bra, that occurring immediately after childbirth, consisting almost entirely of blood.

l. sanguinolen′ta, l. sero′sa, the serous vaginal discharge occurring four or five days after childbirth.

lochiocolpos (lo″ke-o-kol′pos) distention of the vagina by retained lochia.

lochiometra (lo″ke-o-me′trah) distention of the uterus by retained lochia.

lochiometritis (lo″ke-o-me-tri′tis) puerperal metritis.

lochiopyra (lo″ke-o-pi′rah) puerperal fever.

lochiorrhagia, lochiorrhea (lo″ke-o-ra′je-ah; lo″ke-o-re′ah) an abnormally profuse lochia.

lochioschesis (lo″ke-os′kĕ-sis) retention of the lochia.

loci (lo′si) [L.] plural of *locus.*

Locke's solution (loks) an aqueous solution of sodium chloride, calcium chloride, potassium chloride, sodium bicarbonate, and dextrose adjusted to pH 7.4; used in physiologic experiments to keep the excised heart beating.

lockjaw (lok′jaw) 1. tetanus. 2. trismus.

Lockwood's ligament (lok′woodz) a suspensory sheath supporting the eyeball.

locomotion (lo″ko-mo′shun) movement, or the ability to move, from one place to another. adj., **locomo′tive.**

locomotor (lo″ko-mo′tor) of or pertaining to locomotion.

l. ataxia, inability to walk properly as a result of damage to the spinal cord by syphilis (see also TABES DORSALIS).

loculus (lok′u-lus), pl. *loc′uli* [L.] 1. a small space or cavity. 2. a local enlargement of the uterus in some mammals, containing an embryo. adj., **loc′ular.**

locus (lo′kus), pl. *lo′ci* [L.] place; site; in genetics, the specific site of a gene on a chromosome.

l. ceru′leus, a pigmented eminence in the superior angle of the floor of the fourth ventricle of the brain.

Löffler's endocarditis (disease) (lef′lerz) endocarditis associated with eosinophilia (see also Löffler's ENDOCARDITIS).

löffleria (lef-le′re-ah) the presence of *Corynebacterium diphtheriae* (diphtheria bacillus) without the ordinary symptoms of diphtheria.

logo(o)- word element [Gr.], *words; speech.*

logadectomy (log″ah-dek′to-me) excision of a portion of the conjunctiva.

logagnosia (log″ag-no′ze-ah) central word defect, as aphasia or alogia.

logagraphia (log″ah-graf′e-ah) inability to express ideas in writing.

logamnesia (log″am-ne′ze-ah) receptive aphasia.

logaphasia (log″ah-fa′ze-ah) expressive aphasia.

logasthenia (log″as-the′ne-ah) disturbance of the mental processes necessary to the comprehension of speech.

logoclonia (log′o-klon″e-ah) spasmodic repetition of the end-syllables of words.

logogram (log′o-gram) the graphic record of the symptoms and signs exhibited by a patient, charted by means of the logoscope.

logokophosis (log″o-ko-fo′sis) word deafness, or auditory aphasia.

logopathy (log-op′ah-the) any disorder of speech due to derangement of the central nervous system.

logopedia, logopedics (log″o-pe′de-ah; log″o-pe′-diks) the study and treatment of speech defects.

logoplegia (log″o-ple′je-ah) paralysis of the speech organs.

logorrhea (log″o-re′ah) excessive or abnormal talkativeness.

logospasm (log′o-spazm) the spasmodic utterance of words.

-logy word element [Gr.], *science; treatise; sum of knowledge in a particular subject.*

loiasis (lo-i′ah-sis) infection with nematodes of the genus *Loa;* loaiasis.

loin (loin) the part of the back between the thorax and pelvis.

Lomotil (lo′mo-til) trademark for preparations of diphenoxylate, an antidiarrheal.

Long (long) Crawford Williamson (1815–1878). American physician, born at Danielsville, Georgia, who in 1842 administered ether to a patient before removing a neck tumor, the first recorded use of an anesthetic in surgery.

long-acting thyroid stimulator (LATS) a substance occurring in the blood in hyperthyroidism, which exerts a stimulating effect on the thyroid of longer duration than does thyrotropin; it is associated with IgG immunoglobulin and may function as an autoantibody.

longissimus (lon-jis′ĭ-mus) [L.] longest.

longitudinalis (lon″jĭ-tu″dĭ-na′lis) lengthwise; in official anatomic nomenclature it designates a structure that is parallel to the long axis of the body or an organ.

longus (long′gus) [L.] long.

loop (lo͞op) a turn or sharp curve in a cordlike structure.

capillary l's, minute endothelial tubes that carry blood in the papillae of the skin.

closed l., a system in which the input to one or more of the subsystems is affected by its own output.

Henle's l., the U-shaped loop of the uriniferous tubule of the kidney.

Lippes l., a form of intrauterine contraceptive device.

L.O.P. left occipitoposterior (position of the fetus).

lophotrichous (lo-fot′rĭ-kus) having two or more flagella at one end (of a bacterial cell).

lordoscoliosis (lor″do-sko″le-o′sis) lordosis complicated with scoliosis.

lordosis (lor-do′sis) forward curvature of the lumbar spine. adj., **lordot′ic.**

Lorfan (lor′fan) trademark for preparations of levallorphan, an antagonist to narcotics.

L.O.T. left occipitotransverse (position of the fetus).

lotio (lo′she-o) [L.] lotion.

l. al′ba, white lotion, an astringent and protectant.

lotion (lo′shun) a liquid suspension or dispersion for external application to the body.

benzyl benzoate l., a preparation of benzyl benzoate, triethanolamine, oleic acid, and water; used as a scabicide.

calamine l., a mixture of calamine, zinc oxide, glycerin, bentonite magma, and calcium hydroxide solution; used as a protectant.

calamine l., phenolated, calamine lotion with liquefied phenol added.

hydrocortisone l., hydrocortisone in an aqueous vehicle for topical application.

white l., a preparation of zinc sulfate and sulfurated potash in purified water; astringent and protectant.

Lotusate (lo′tu-sāt) trademark for a preparation of talbutal, a short- to intermediate-acting barbiturate.

loupe (lo͞op) a magnifying lens.

Louis-Bar syndrome ataxia-telangiectasia.

louse (lows), pl. *lice.* a general name for various parasitic insects, the true lice, which infest mammals and belong to the suborder Anoplura. They are grayish, wingless, and dorsoventrally flattened, and vary in length from one-sixth to one-sixteenth of an inch. Those that are parasitic on man are *Pediculus humanus* var. *capitis,* or head louse, which attaches itself to the hairs of the head; *P. humanus* var. *corporis,* the body or clothes louse; and *Phthirus pubis,* or crab louse, which lives in the pubic hair and in the eyelashes and eyebrows.

Louse infestation is called pediculosis. Lice live on the host's blood, obtained by piercing the skin and sucking the blood through the mouth part. The area bitten itches and may become sore and infected from scratching. Not only are lice an annoyance, but they also transmit some diseases, such as typhus.

TREATMENT. Head lice hatch eggs in silvery oval-shaped envelopes that attach to the shafts of the hairs. The eggs, called nits, can be removed fairly easily with a mild vinegar solution. The hair is combed with a very fine-toothed comb. The lice are effectively destroyed by applications of 1 per cent gamma benzene hexachloride (lindane) in a cream or shampoo.

PREVENTION. Cleanliness, frequent bathing, and frequent changing of clothing are necessary to avoid contracting lice. When infestation is discovered it is necessary to boil or autoclave all clothing and bed linens used by the infected person. Outer clothing that cannot be boiled or autoclaved should be dry cleaned. Dusting with 10 per cent DDT is usually effective in destroying lice on bedclothing, mattresses, and other inanimate objects.

Lowe's disease (lōz) oculocerebrorenal syndrome.

loxapine (loks′ah-pēn) an antipsychotic agent used to control the symptoms of schizophrenia; also used as the succinate salt.

loxoscelism (lok-sos′sĕ-lizm) a morbid condition resulting from the bite of the brown spiders, *Loxosceles reclusa* and *L. laeta,* beginning with a painful erythematous vesicle and progressing to a gangrenous slough of the affected area; first recognized in South America, but a few cases have been diagnosed in North America.

lozenge (loz′enj) troche.

L.P.N. Licensed Practical Nurse.

L.R.C.P. Licentiate of the Royal College of Physicians.

L.R.C.S. Licentiate of the Royal College of Surgeons.

L.S.A. left sacroanterior (position of the fetus).

L.Sc.A. left scapuloanterior (position of the fetus).

L.Sc.P. left scapuloposterior (position of the fetus).

LSD a hallucinogenic compound (lysergic acid diethylamide), derived from lysergic acid, a constituent of ergot alkaloids; called also lysergide. LSD has consciousness-expanding effects and is capable of producing a state of mind in which there is false sense perception (hallucination). (See also HALLUCINOGEN.) The perceptual changes brought about by LSD in normal persons are extremely variable and depend on factors such as age, personality, education, physical make-up, and state of health. The danger of the drug lies in the fact that it loosens control over impulsive behavior and may lead to a full-blown psychosis or less serious mental disorder in persons with latent mental illness. LSD is an experimental drug to be used only under the direct supervision of reliable, authorized scientists. Its distribution is regulated by the Food and Drug Administration of the federal government.

LSD was first developed in 1938 and was believed to be potentially useful in the treatment of mental illness. This theory was based on the belief that the drug could produce a schizophrenic syndrome and that psychiatrists and other persons concerned with mental illness could observe the manifestations of a psychosis under controlled conditions. However, competent investigators have shown that the effect of LSD is more closely related to a toxic psychosis such as that produced by fever, stress, or drugs of many kinds and is of doubtful use in understanding the mechanism of a true psychosis resulting from severe personality disorder. Authorities are hopeful that LSD may eventually prove useful in the investigation of brain function and the mechanism of mental disease but are not in agreement as to how this will come about.

Abuse of LSD by semiscientific investigators and lay persons has led to much publicity, with the result that a black market now operates to make the drug available to those who wish to "increase their awareness" or attain a state of euphoria. Although LSD is not addictive, the greatest number of persons abusing the drug also have been found to be users of marijuana, amphetamines, and barbiturates, and are extremely likely to develop a drug dependence. They apparently use the drug to escape reality rather than for the purpose of helping themselves cope with reality.

The controversy concerning chromosomal damage caused by abuse of LSD is yet to be resolved.

L.S.P. left sacroposterior (position of the fetus).

L.S.T. left sacrotransverse (position of the fetus).

LTH luteotropic hormone (see LUTEOTROPIN).

Lu chemical symbol, *lutetium.*

lubb (lub) a syllable used to represent, or mimic, the first sound of the heart in auscultation (see also LUBB-DUPP).

lubb-dupp (lub′dup) syllables used to represent, or mimic, the combination of the first (lubb) and second (dupp) heart sounds.

lucanthone (loo-kan′thōn) an antischistosomal; used as the hydrochloride salt.

lucidity (loo-sid′ĭ-te) clearness of mind. adj., **lu′cid.**

luciferase (loo-sif′er-ās) an enzyme that catalyzes the bioluminescent reaction in certain animals capable of luminescence.

luciferin (loo-sif′er-in) an organic heat-stable compound that, when acted on by an enzyme (luciferase) in the presence of ATP and molecular oxygen, produces bioluminescence.

lucifugal (loo-sif′u-gal) avoiding, or repelled by, bright light.

lucipetal (loo-sip′ĕ-tal) seeking, or attracted to, bright light.

Ludwig's angina (lo͞od′vigz) diffuse purulent inflammation around the submaxillary gland, beneath the jaw, and about the floor of the mouth, usually due to streptococcal infection.

Ludwig's ganglion (lo͞od′vigz) a ganglion near the right atrium of the heart, connected with the cardiac plexus.

lues (loo′ēz) syphilis. adj., **luet′ic.**

Lugol's solution (loo-golz′) strong iodine solution, each 100 ml. containing 4.5 to 5.5 gm. of iodine and 9.5 to 10.5 gm. of potassium iodide; a source of iodine.

lumb(o)- word element [L.], *loin.*

lumbago (lum-ba′go) pain in the lower part (lumbar region) of the back. Lumbago is a popular term for lower back pain. It embraces a number of illnesses. Such pain may be caused by injury, such as back strain, by arthritis, by abuse of the back muscles (from poor posture, a sagging mattress, or ill fitting shoes, for example), or by a number of other disorders.

lumbar (lum′bar) pertaining to the loins.

l. plexus, one formed by the ventral branches of the second to fifth lumbar nerves in the psoas major muscle (the branches of the first lumbar nerve often are included).

l. puncture, insertion of a hollow needle into the subarachnoid space between the third and fourth lumbar vertebrae; called also SPINAL PUNCTURE. A lumbar puncture may be done to obtain a specimen of CEREBROSPINAL FLUID for examination and to measure the pressure within the cerebrospinal cavities. As a therapeutic measure it is sometimes done to relieve intracranial pressure or to remove blood or pus from the subarachnoid space. A lumbar puncture also is necessary for injection of a spinal anesthetic. For certain x-ray examinations of the skull, such as a pneumoencephalogram, air may be injected via a lumbar puncture. For visualization of the spinal canal and course of the spinal cord a radiopaque dye is injected into the subarachnoid space.

l. vertebrae, the five vertebrae between the thoracic vertebrae and the sacrum.

lumbarization (lum″bar-ĭ-za′shun) nonfusion of the first and second segments of the sacrum so that there is one additional articulated vertebra, the sacrum consisting of only four segments.

lumbocostal (lum″bo-kos′tal) pertaining to the loin and ribs.

lumbodynia (lum″bo-din′e-ah) lumbago.

lumbosacral (lum″bo-sa′kral) pertaining to the lumbar and sacral region, or to the lumbar vertebrae and sacrum.

l. plexus, the lumbar and sacral plexuses considered together, because of their continuous nature.

lumbricoid (lum′brĭ-koid) resembling the earthworm; designating the ascaris, or intestinal roundworms.

lumbricosis (lum″brĭ-ko′sis) infection with lumbrici.

lumbricus (lum′brĭ-kus), pl. *lum′brici* [L.] 1. the earthworm. 2. ascaris.

lumbus (lum′bus) [L.] loin.

lumen (lu′men), pl. *lu′mina* [L.] the cavity or channel within a tube or tubular organ, as a blood vessel or the intestine. adj., **lu′minal.**

luminescence (lu″mĭ-nes′ens) the property of giving off light without a corresponding degree of heat.

luminophore (lu′mĭ-no-fōr″) a chemical group that gives the property of luminescence to organic compounds.

lumirhodopsin (loo″mĭ-ro-dop′sin) an intermediate product of exposure of rhodopsin to light.

lunate (lu′nāt) 1. moon-shaped or crescentic. 2. the lunate bone (see table of BONES).

lung (lung) either of the two main organs of respiration, lying on either side of the heart, within the chest cavity. (See also Plates 5 and 6.) The lungs supply the blood with oxygen inhaled from the outside air, and they dispose of waste carbon dioxide in the exhaled air, as a part of the process known as RESPIRATION.

The lungs are made of elastic tissue filled with interlacing networks of tubes and sacs carrying air, and with blood vessels carrying blood. The bronchi, which bring air to the lungs, branch out within the lungs into many smaller tubes, the bronchioles, which culminate in clusters of tiny air sacs called alveoli, whose total runs into millions. The alveoli are surrounded by a network of capillaries. Through the thin membranes of the capillaries, the air and blood make their exchange of oxygen and carbon dioxide.

The lungs are divided into lobes, the left lung having two lobes and the right lung having three, and are further subdivided into bronchopulmonary segments, of which there are about 20. Protecting each lung is the pleura, a two-layered membrane that envelops the lung and contains lubricating fluid between its inner and outer layers.

MECHANICS OF INFLATION AND DEFLATION. The lungs are inflated by action of the diaphragm and the intercostal muscles. The diaphragm, a large dome-shaped muscle, forms the bottom of the thoracic cage. As it contracts it flattens, increasing the diameter of the thorax and elevating the lower ribs. Both of these actions increase the space for expansion of the lungs.

The external intercostal muscles provide flexibility to the thoracic cage and allow more room for lung expansion by elevating the anterior end of each rib, thereby increasing the anterior-posterior diameter of the chest wall.

Deflation of the lungs is chiefly a passive maneuver. The major muscles involved in expiration are the abdominal muscle group. As these muscles contract, they depress the lower ribs, and, through an increase in abdominal pressure, move the diaphragm upward.

As the lungs are compressed and distended by the respiratory muscles, the pressure within the alveoli (intra-alveolar pressure) rises and falls. During inspiration the pressure becomes slightly negative (–3 mm. Hg) in relation to atmospheric pressure. During expiration the intra-alveolar pressure rises to approximately +3 mm. Hg. The effect of negative pressure within the alveoli is to cause air under atmospheric pressure to flow into the lungs (inspiration). The condition of positive pressure creates the opposite effect, causing air to flow outward (expiration).

The lungs are surrounded by an airtight compartment, the pleural space within the pleural membrane. The intrapleural pressure is less than atmospheric pressure and is expressed as negative pressure. Normally the intrapleural pressure is about –4 mm. Hg. When the lungs are fully expanded this pressure may be as great as –9 mm. Hg. Under normal conditions, however, the intrapleural pressure fluctuates between –4 and –6 mm. Hg.

If anything should penetrate the walls of the pleura, the negative pressure is lost as air rushes into the pleural cavity in response to atmospheric pressure. This condition is called PNEUMOTHORAX. The walls of the alveoli also must remain intact in order to maintain normal intrapleural pressure. If a lesion causes a break in the alveolar membranes, air enters the pleural cavity through the break and produces pneumothorax. Relief of pneumothorax and collapse of the lung from accumulations of either air or fluids may be provided by aspiration of the air or fluid from the thoracic cavity (THORACENTESIS) or by insertion of CHEST TUBES to provide for a gradual reexpansion of the lung. (Specific tests to determine pulmonary volume and capacities are discussed under PULMONARY FUNCTION TESTS.)

DISEASES OF THE LUNGS. The air brought to the lungs is filtered, moistened, and warmed on its way along the respiratory tract but it can nevertheless bring irritants and infectious organisms, and when the body resistance is low for any reason the lungs may suffer diseases of some seriousness. Bacterial PNEUMONIA, once a dangerous disease, is now usually quickly brought under control by antibiotics, but it is still serious and requires prompt medical attention. Viral pneumonia is not effectively treated with antibiotics but is a milder infection than those caused by bacteria.

TUBERCULOSIS of the lungs is a chronic pulmonary infection caused by *Mycobacterium tuberculosis,* usually transmitted by inhalation of infectious material. It was once a widespread and highly fatal disease, but now the prevalence and mortality rate have been reduced drastically because of the improvement in the standard of living and nutrition in many areas, detection of the disease in its earliest stages, and the development of tuberculostatic drugs. There has been some success in inducing specific immunity against tuberculosis by vaccination with BCG (bacille Calmette Guérin) vaccine, a live attenuated strain of bovine tubercle bacilli.

Edema of the lung, or pulmonary EDEMA, is a condition in which the alveoli and interstitial spaces begin to fill with excess fluid. It occurs when the fluid load of the body is too great for the heart, kidneys, or lungs. The condition frequently is a complication of a type of chronic heart disease in which there is weakness of and decreased output from the left ventricle. As the ventricle weakens it becomes less able to accept and remove blood from the pulmonary vascular bed. This produces congestion and engorgement of the pulmonary vessels with escape of fluid into the pulmonary tissues.

Other causes of pulmonary edema include diminished kidney function, which allows for accumulation of body fluids, infections of the lungs which affect the pulmonary capillaries, and a too-rapid administration of intravenous fluids in relation to the ability of the heart and lungs to accommodate an additional fluid load.

PLEURISY is an inflammation of the pleura. Other disorders of the lungs include ASTHMA, BRONCHIECTASIS, ATELECTASIS, EMPHYSEMA, and fungal infections. SILICOSIS and the other PNEUMOCONIOSES are pulmonary diseases caused by inhalation of particulate matter of industrial substances and are often occupation related.

Pulmonary EMBOLISM, while not a primary disease of the lung, does involve an obstruction of the pulmonary artery or one of its branches. The source of obstruction usually is a blood clot that has entered the blood stream from a distant point and been carried to the pulmonary artery. The condition can be fatal if not treated promptly and successfully.

CHRONIC OBSTRUCTIVE PULMONARY DISEASE (COPD) is a classification of lung disease indicating a long-term illness in which there are structural and functional changes in the bronchi and bronchioles, and in the lungs and the blood vessels that serve them. These changes bring about an obstruction of bronchial air flow and loss of elasticity of the lungs. Called also chronic obstructive lung disease (COLD) and diffuse obstructive lung disease (DOLD).

The incidence of COPD is increasing; it is considered the most significant chronic pulmonary disorder in the United States. COPD occurs mainly in association with bronchial ASTHMA, chronic BRONCHITIS, and chronic pulmonary EMPHYSEMA.

Lung Abscess. Lung abscess is an infection of the lung, characterized by a localized accumulation of pus and destruction of tissue. It may be a complication of pneumonia or tuberculosis. A lung abscess may also follow a period of excessive drinking by an alcoholic. Infected matter that has been aspirated may lodge in a bronchiole and produce inflammation. Lung cancer may also be responsible for formation of an abscess.

The first symptoms include a dry cough and chest pain. Later these may be followed by fever, chills, productive cough, headache, perspiration, foul-smelling sputum, and sometimes dyspnea. If the abscess is a complication of pneumonia, the symptoms tend to be moderated to an exaggeration of the pneumonia symptoms.

When a lung abscess forms, it is in the acute stage and treatment with antibiotics usually is effective. POSTURAL DRAINAGE may be prescribed to assist in drainage of exudate from lungs and bronchioles. In most cases, this treatment produces a cure. If the abscess becomes chronic, surgery may be necessary and usually involves removal of the portion of the lung containing the abscess.

Lung Cancer. Malignant growths of the lung are among the most common types of CANCER. Although the exact cause of lung cancer is not known, irritants that are inhaled over a period of time are known to be important predisposing causes. Years ago it was realized that miners of certain ores, men who inhaled the mine dust, developed lung cancer much more often than men in other occupations. Later, other irritants of lung tissue, such as air polluted by fumes from burning fuels or motor exhausts, were singled out as probable causes of the increasing number of cases of the disease in urban and industrial areas. The most obvious irritant, however, and the one most widely encountered, is tobacco smoke, especially cigarette smoke, which is much more frequently and deeply inhaled than the smoke of pipes or cigars.

A study based on autopsies of the lungs of individuals who had died from many varied causes, but whose smoking history was known, showed that unrecognized cancer and precancerous changes in tissue were numerous among smokers and rare among nonsmokers. These findings led the Surgeon General of the United States Public Health Service to appoint a committee to investigate the subject. After an extensive study, the committee issued a report stating that "cigarette smoking is a health hazard of sufficient importance in the United States to warrant appropriate action."

The search for other possible causes of lung cancer has not been neglected. However, no definite findings have been reported thus far.

Since the factors causing lung cancer act slowly and may produce a tumor near the periphery of the lung, early symptoms are vague or may not appear at all, and nearly a third of the cases are in an advanced stage when they are discovered.

The earliest and most common symptom is a cough. Dry at first, this cough later produces sputum which eventually becomes blood-streaked. A wheeze in the chest is frequently a symptom and indicates a partial obstruction in a bronchus. Chest pains, weakness, and loss of weight are later symptoms, as is dyspnea.

Diagnosis depends on a careful physical examination, including a chest x-ray. If a suspicious density is seen on the x-ray, samples of sputum will be examined microscopically for the presence of malignant cells. BRONCHOSCOPY is also done, and at the same time a specimen for biopsy can be obtained or the bronchial secretions can be washed out and the cells stained and examined.

When examination indicates lung cancer, prompt treatment is essential. This may involve the surgical removal of the lobe of the lung containing the cancer or of an entire lung if the malignant cells have spread. A significant number of persons affected by lung cancer can be cured by such operations if the surgery is performed in time. In some cases of widespread involvement surgery is not possible; these patients are treated with x-rays or radium or ANTINEOPLASTIC drugs.

For prevention, regular physical examinations are essential. Chest x-rays should be taken at the first suspicion of trouble and, in any case, should be done annually in people 40 years old or older.

The irritants that can trigger lung cancer must be avoided and, when possible, eliminated. Mine workers should take adequate precautions to avoid inhaling harmful dusts. Public health authorities and industry must act more effectively to control air pollution.

The most important step toward protection against lung cancer is the elimination of cigarette smoking.

State and local units of the American Lung Association (formerly Tuberculosis and Respiratory Disease Association) are excellent sources of information about lung disease and its prevention.

SURGERY OF THE LUNG. Surgical procedures performed on the lung include removal of the entire lung (pneumonectomy), removal of a lobe of the lung (lobectomy), and removal of only a bronchopulmonary segment (segmental resection). The procedure done depends on the size of the area involved and the type of lesion present.

Pneumonectomy is usually necessary for treatment of cancer, multiple abscesses of the lung, or severe bronchiectasis. In this procedure a thoracotomy incision is made and one or two ribs are resected. The large pulmonary vessels (the artery and vein leading to and from the lung) are ligated and cut and the main bronchus serving the lung is closed with sutures. One or more tubes may be inserted to provide for drainage of blood and fluid from the cavity (see also CHEST TUBE).

Cysts, abscesses, or benign tumors that involve only a lobe of the lung are treated by lobectomy. A thoracotomy incision is made and the lung is collapsed before the lobe is removed. The remaining lobes are then reexpanded and chest tubes are inserted for removal of air and fluid.

Some types of lung surgery are aimed at deliberate collapse of the lung for the purpose of permanently or temporarily reducing the size of the thoracic cavity on one side of the chest. Resection of two or more ribs (thoracoplasty) is done primarily for the treatment of tuberculosis; it also may be done following pneumonectomy, in which case its purpose is to partially fill the space left by removal of the lung.

Artificial PNEUMOTHORAX involves injection of a measured amount of air into the pleural cavity. Since the pressure within the pleural cavity is normally lower than atmospheric pressure, the introduction of air will collapse the lung. Because the air is gradually absorbed by the tissues over a period of time, injections of air must be repeated at intervals for as long as collapse of the lung is desired. This procedure is done chiefly as a means of treating tuberculous lesions and allows for immobilization of the lung while healing takes place.

Another method used for collapse of the lung is pneumoperitoneum. As the name implies, this procedure involves injection of air into the peritoneal cavity rather than the thoracic cavity. The injected air causes an upward pressure on the diaphragm which in turn pushes against the lung and hinders its expansion.

If there are adhesions between the lung and the lining of the chest wall they may prevent the collapse of the lung. The cutting of these adhesions is called pneumonolysis.

Patient Care. Before surgery the patient is given an explanation of the procedure to be done and the purpose of the CHEST TUBES, oxygen therapy, and other apparatus to be used postoperatively. Special exercises of the arms, shoulders, and chest muscles are often started before surgery and resumed postoperatively. Their purpose is to strengthen the muscles and provide for continued motion of the shoulder and arm and normal functioning of the remaining lung tissue.

Immediately after surgery the patient's pulse, respirations, and blood pressure are checked and recorded every 15 minutes until they become stabilized. Oxygen is administered by tent, mask, or nasal catheter and the patient is watched closely for signs of respiratory difficulty. Positioning of the patient depends on the specific orders of the surgeon. Generally, the patient is allowed to lie only on his back or the operative side. Lying on the operative side facilitates drainage, and enhances ventilation of the unaffected lung. When turning a patient to the operative side, care must be taken that the tube(s) is not kinked and the patient's weight is adequately supported with pillows so that the tubes are not obstructed. An exception to the turning routine for patients having lung surgery is the pneumonectomy patient. All surgeons recommend that every such patient be placed in the high Fowler position and should not be turned for 24 hours.

Dressings are reinforced but usually they are not changed by the nurse until the drainage tubes have been removed and the incision is closed and healing.

Coughing is encouraged although it may be painful for the patient during the first few postoperative days. Discomfort can be reduced by splinting the chest with the hands or a pillow, or turning the patient onto the operative side during episodes of coughing.

The convalescent period after lung surgery is often long and difficult for the patient. He will need encouragement in continuing his exercises and in other procedures necessary for adequate ventilation and normal function of the remaining lung tissue.

l. calculus, a concretion formed in the bronchi by accretion about an inorganic nucleus, or from calcified portions of lung tissue or adjacent lymph nodes.

l. compliance, a measure of the ability of the lung to distend in response to pressure without disruption; expresses the unit volume of change in the lung per unit of pressure. Compliance or distensibility of the lung is increased in conditions such as emphysema, in which the lung distends more readily, and is decreased in fibrotic conditions in which the lung distends with difficulty.

iron l., a popular name for a type of VENTILATOR that provides controlled, automatic breathing for a patient whose respiratory muscles are paralyzed, consisting of a metal tank, enclosing the patient's body with the head outside, and within which artificial respiration is maintained by alternating negative and positive pressure. Called also Drinker respirator.

l. reflexes, Hering-Breuer reflexes.

lungmotor (lung'mo-tor) an apparatus for forcing air, or air and oxygen, into the lungs.

lungworm (lung'werm) any parasitic worm that invades the lungs, e.g., *Paragonimus westermani* in man.

lunula (loo'nu-lah,), pl. *lu'nulae* [L.] a small, crescentic or moon-shaped area or structure, e.g., the white area at the base of the nail of a finger or toe, or one of the segments of the semilunar valves of the heart.

lupiform (loo'pĭ-form) resembling lupus.

lupoid (loo'poid) 1. pertaining to lupus vulgaris. 2. a variant of sarcoidosis marked by small papular lesions.

lupus (loo'pus) any of a group of skin diseases in which the lesions are characteristically eroded. The term is frequently used alone to refer to lupus vulgaris and sometimes lupus erythematosus, but without a modifier it has no specific meaning.

l. erythemato'sus, an inflammatory disease that takes two forms. One, the systemic or disseminated form, causes deterioration of the connective tissues in various parts of the body. This disease may attack the soft internal organs as well as the bones and muscles, and is often fatal. In its other form, the discoid type, it is a fairly mild skin disorder, in which the lesions typically form a butterfly pattern over the bridge of the nose and cheeks, but other areas may also be involved.

Symptoms of the more serious form vary widely, but may include fever, abdominal pains, and pains in the muscles and joints. Often the symptoms come and go over a long period of time. Diagnosis of the disease is difficult.

The cause is unknown, but the disease is believed not to be infectious and possibly to be related to the allergies. Lupus erythematosus is one of a group of similar disorders known as the COLLAGEN DISEASES. There is no specific treatment, though corticosteroids may be used to control symptoms.

l. vulga'ris, tuberculosis of the skin marked by formation of brownish nodules in the corium, chronic ulceration, and severe scarring.

luteal (loo'te-al) pertaining to or having the properties of the corpus luteum or its active principle.

lutein (loo'te-in) 1. a lipochrome from the corpus luteum, fat cells, and egg yolk. 2. any lipochrome.

luteinic (loo"te-in'ik) pertaining to the corpus luteum, to lutein, or to luteinization.

luteinization (loo"te-in"ĭ-za'shun) the process taking place in the follicle cells of graafian follicles that have matured and discharged their egg: the cells become hypertrophied and there is vascularization and lipid accumulation, (the latter in some species giving a yellow color), the follicles becoming corpora lutea.

luteinizing hormone (loo'te-in-īz"ing) a gonadotropic hormone of the anterior pituitary gland acting, with follicle-stimulating hormone, to cause ovulation of mature follicles and secretion of estrogen by thecal and granulosa cells of the ovary; it is also concerned with corpus luteum formation. In the male, it stimulates development of the interstitial cells of the testes and their secretion of testosterone.

Lutembacher's syndrome (loo'tem-bak"erz) mitral stenosis (usually rheumatic) associated with atrial septal defect.

luteohormone (loo"te-o-hōr'mōn) progesterone.

luteoma (loo"te-o'mah) 1. a luteinized granulosa-theca cell tumor. 2. nodular hyperplasia of ovarian lutein cells sometimes occurring in the last trimester of pregnancy.

luteotropic (loo"te-o-trop'ik) stimulating formation of the corpus luteum.

l. hormone, luteotropin.

luteotropin (loo"te-o-trōp'in) a hormone of the anterior pituitary which stimulates formation of the corpus luteum; identical with prolactin. Called also luteotropic hormone (LTH).

lutetium (loo-te'she-um) a chemical element, atomic number 71, atomic weight 174.97, symbol Lu. (See table of ELEMENTS.)

Lutocylol (loo"to-si'lol) trademark for preparations of ethisterone, a progestational steroid.

Lutrexin (loo-trek'sin) trademark for a preparation of lututrin, a uterine relaxant.

Lutromone (loo'tro-mōn) trademark for a preparation of progesterone, a progestational hormone.

lututrin (loo'tu-trin) a protein or polypeptide substance from the corpus luteum of sow ovaries; used as a uterine relaxant in treatment of functional dysmenorrhea.

Lutz-Splendore-Almeida disease paracoccidioidomycosis.

lux (luks) the unit of illumination, being one lumen per square meter.

luxation (luk-sa'shun) dislocation.

luxus (luk'sus) [L.] excess.

L.V.N. licensed vocational nurse.

Lw chemical symbol, *lawrencium.*

lyase (li'ās) any of a class of enzymes that remove groups from their substrates (other than by hydrolysis), leaving double bonds, or that conversely add groups to double bonds.

lycanthropy, lycomania (li-kan'thro-pe; li"ko-ma'ne-ah) a delusion in which the patient believes himself a wolf.

lycopene (li'ko-pēn) the red carotenoid pigment of tomatoes and various berries and fruits.

lycoperdonosis (li"ko-per"do-no'sis) a respiratory disease due to inhalation of spores of the puffball fungus, *Lycoperdon.*

lye (li) an alkaline percolate from wood ashes; household lye is a crude mixture of sodium hydroxide with some sodium carbonate.

lying-in (li'ing-in) 1. puerperal. 2. puerperium.

lymph (limf) a transparent, usually slightly yellow, often opalescent liquid found within the lymphatic vessels, and collected from tissues in all parts of the body and returned to the blood via the lymphatic system. It is about 95 per cent water; the remainder consists of plasma proteins and other chemical substances contained in the blood plasma, but in slightly smaller percentage than in plasma. Its cellular component consists chiefly of lymphocytes.

The body contains three main kinds of fluid: blood, tissue fluid, and lymph. The blood consists of the blood cells and platelets, the plasma, or fluid portion, and a variety of chemical substances dissolved in the plasma. When the plasma, without its solid particles and some of its dissolved substances, seeps through the capillary walls and circulates among the body tissues, it is known as tissue fluid. When this fluid is drained from the tissues and collected by the lymphatic system, it is called lymph. The LYMPHATIC SYSTEM eventually returns the lymph to the blood, where it again becomes plasma. This movement of fluid through the body is described under CIRCULATORY SYSTEM.

l. node, any of the accumulations of lymphoid tissue organized as definite lymphoid organs along the course of lymphatic vessels, consisting of an outer cortical and an inner medullary part; they are the main source of lymphocytes of the peripheral blood and, as part of the reticuloendothelial system, serve as a defense mechanism by removing noxious agents, e.g., bacteria and toxins, and probably play a role in antibody formation. Sometimes called, incorrectly, lymph glands.

vaccine l., material containing vaccinia virus collected from vaccinial vesicles of calves; used for active immunization against smallpox.

lympha (lim'fah) [L.] lymph.

lymphadenectasis (lim-fad"ĕ-nek'tah-sis) enlargement of a lymph node.

lymphadenectomy (lim-fad"ĕ-nek'to-me) excision of one or more lymph nodes.

lymphadenia (lim"fah-de'ne-ah) hypertrophy of lymph nodes.

lymphadenitis (lim-fad"ĕ-ni'tis) inflammation of lymph nodes.

lymphadenocele (lim-fad'ĕ-no-sēl) a cyst of a lymph node.

lymphadenogram (lim-fad'ĕ-no-gram") the film produced by lymphadenography.

lymphadenography (lim"fad-ĕ-nog'rah-fe) roentgenography of lymph nodes after injection of a contrast medium in a lymphatic vessel.

lymphadenoid (lim-fad′ĕ-noid) resembling the tissues of the lymph nodes. Lymphadenoid tissue includes the spleen, bone marrow, tonsils, and the lymphoid tissues of the organs and mucous membranes.

lymphadenoma (lim-fad″ĕ-no′mah) lymphoma.

lymphadenopathy (lim-fad″ĕ-nop′ah-the) disease of the lymph nodes.

dermatopathic l., regional lymph node enlargement associated with melanoderma and other dermatoses marked by chronic erythroderma.

giant follicular l., nodular well-differentiated lymphocytic malignant lymphoma, microscopically characterized by multiple, proliferative, follicle-like nodules which disturb the normal architecture of the lymph nodes. Called also Brill-Symmers disease and giant follicular lymphoma.

lymphadenosis (lim-fad″ĕ-no′sis) hypertrophy or proliferation of lymphoid tissue.

l. benig′na cu′tis, a benign inflammatory hyperplasia of lymphocytes in the skin, principally on the face or ears, in the form of solitary or disseminated yellowish brown to bluish red nodules that usually involute spontaneously.

lymphadenotomy (lim-fad″ĕ-not′o-me) incision of a lymph node.

lymphagogue (lim′fah-gog) an agent promoting the production of lymph.

lymphangial (lim-fan′je-al) pertaining to a lymphatic vessel.

lymphangiectasia, **lymphangiectasis** (lim-fan″je-ek-ta′se-ah; lim-fan″je-ek′tah-sis) dilatation of the lymphatic vessels. adj., **lymphangiectat′ic.**

lymphangiectomy (lim-fan″je-ek′to-me) excision of one or more lymphatic vessels.

lymphangiitis (lim-fan″je-i′tis) lymphangitis.

lymphangioendothelioma (lim-fan″je-o-en″do-the″le-o′mah) lymphangioma in which endothelial cells are the main component.

lymphangiofibroma (lim-fan″je-o-fi-bro′mah) a fibrosing lymphangioma.

lymphangiogram (lim-fan′je-o-gram″) the film produced by lymphangiography.

lymphangiography (lim-fan″je-og′rah-fe) roentgenography of lymphatic channels after introduction of a contrast medium.

lymphangiology (lim-fan″je-ol′o-je) the scientific study of the lymphatic system.

lymphangioma (lim-fan″je-o′mah) a tumor composed of new-formed lymph spaces and channels. adj., **lymphangio′matous.**

cavernous l., dilation of the lymphatic vessels, resulting in cavities filled with lymph.

cystic l., l. cys′ticum, a cystic growth usually found in the neck or groin, thought to originate from a developmental anomaly of the primitive lymphatic spaces; symptoms are largely due to compression of adjoining structures by the mass.

lymphangiophlebitis (lim-fan″je-o-flĕ-bi′tis) inflammation of lymphatic vessels and veins.

lymphangioplasty (lim-fan′je-o-plas″te) surgical restoration of lymphatic channels.

lymphangiosarcoma (lim-fan″je-o-sar-ko′mah) a malignant tumor of lymphatic vessels, usually arising in a limb that is the site of chronic lymphedema.

lymphangiotomy (lim-fan″je-ot′o-me) incision of a lymphatic vessel.

lymphangitis (lim″fan-ji′tis) inflammation of a lymphatic vessel.

lymphatic (lim-fat′ik) 1. pertaining to lymph or to a lymphatic vessel. 2. a lymphatic vessel.

l. ducts, the two larger vessels into which all lymphatic vessels converge. The right lymphatic duct joins the venous system at the junction of the right internal jugular and subclavian veins and carries lymph from the upper right side of the body. The left lymphatic duct, or thoracic duct, enters the circulatory system at the junction of the left internal jugular and subclavian veins; it returns lymph from the upper left side of the body and from below the diaphragm.

l. system, the lymphatic vessels and lymphoid tissue, considered collectively. (See also CIRCULATORY SYSTEM.)

DISORDERS OF THE LYMPHATIC SYSTEM. Several diseases affect the lymphatic system. LYMPHOGRANULOMA VENEREUM is a viral disease that attacks lymph nodes in the groin and usually is transmitted by sexual contact.

Lymphadenitis is an inflammation of the lymph nodes, particularly in the neck; swollen tonsils is an example. Generalized lymphadenitis can be a symptom of the secondary stage of syphilis.

Cancer attacks the lymphatic system, as it does other systems of the body. A tumor of the lymphoid tissue is known as a lymphoma. The general term lymphosarcoma refers to malignant neoplastic disorders of lymphoid tissue.

l. vessels, the capillaries, collecting vessels, and trunks that collect lymph from the tissues and carry it to the blood stream; called also lymphatics.

lymphaticostomy (lim-fat″ĭ-kos′to-me) surgical creation of a permanent opening into a lymphatic duct, usually the thoracic duct.

lymphatism (lim′fah-tizm) a morbid state due to excessive production or growth of lymphoid tissues, resulting in impaired development and lowered vitality.

lymphatolysis (lim″fah-tol′ĭ-sis) destruction of lymphoid tissue. adj., **lymphatolyt′ic.**

lymphectasia (lim′fek-ta′ze-ah) distention with lymph.

lymphedema (lim″fĕ-de′mah) chronic swelling of a part due to accumulation of interstitial fluid (edema) secondary to obstruction of lymphatic vessels or lymph nodes.

congenital l., Milroy's disease.

lymphemia (lim-fe′me-ah) the presence of an undue number of lymphocytes or their precursors in the blood.

lymphenteritis (lim″fen-ter-i′tis) enteritis with serous infiltration.

lymphnoditis (limf″no-di′tis) inflammation of a lymph node.

lymphoblast (lim′fo-blast) the immature, nucleolated precursor of the mature lymphocyte. adj., **lymphoblas′tic.**

lymphoblastic (lim″fo-blas′tik) pertaining to a lymphoblast; producing lymphocytes.

lymphoblastoma (lim″fo-blas-to′mah) poorly-differentiated lymphocytic malignant LYMPHOMA.

lymphoblastomatosis (lim″fo-blas″to-mah-to′sis) the condition produced by the presence of lymphoblastomas.

lymphoblastosis (lim″fo-blas-to′sis) an excess of lymphoblasts in the blood.

lymphocyte (lim′fo-sīt) a mononuclear, nongranular leukocyte having a deeply staining nucleus containing dense chromatin and a pale-blue–staining cytoplasm. Chiefly a product of lymphoid tissue, it participates in IMMUNITY. adj., **lymphocyt′ic.**

B-l's, bursa-equivalent lymphocytes, i.e., lymphocytes that are thymus-independent, migrating to the tissues without passing through or being influenced by the thymus; they are analogous to the avian leukocytes derived from the bursa of Fabricius. B-lymphocytes mature into plasma cells, which synthesize humoral ANTIBODY. (See also IMMUNITY.)

T-l's, thymus-dependent lymphocytes, i.e., lymphocytes that pass through or are influenced by the thymus before migrating to the tissues; they are responsible for cell-mediated IMMUNITY and delayed hypersensitivity.

l. transforming factor (LTF), a lymphokine that causes transformation and clonal expansion of nonsensitized lymphocytes.

lymphocytoblast (lim″fo-si′to-blast) a lymphoblast.

lymphocytoma (lim″fo-si-to′mah) well-differentiated lymphocytic malignant LYMPHOMA.

lymphocytopenia (lim″fo-si″to-pe′ne-ah) reduction of the number of lymphocytes in the blood.

lymphocytopoiesis (lim″fo-si″to-poi-e′sis) the formation of lymphocytes. adj., **lymphocytopoiet′ic.**

lymphocytosis (lim″fo-si-to′sis) increase in the number of normal lymphocytes in the blood or in an effusion.

lymphoduct (lim′fo-dukt) a lymphatic vessel.

lymphogenous (lim-foj′ĕ-nus) 1. producing lymph. 2. produced from lymph or in the lymph vessels.

lymphoglandula (lim″fo-glan′du-lah), pl. *lymphoglan′dulae* [L.] a lymph node.

lymphogonia (lim″fo-go′ne-ah) large lymphocytes with a large nucleus, little chromatin, and nongranular cytoplasm.

lymphogram (lim′fo-gram) a roentgenogram of the lymphatic channels and lymph nodes.

lymphogranuloma (lim″fo-gran″u-lo′mah) Hodgkin's disease.

l. inguina′le, venereal l., l. vene′reum, a venereal disease caused by a strain of *Chlamydia trachomatis,* which affects the lymph organs in the genital area. The causative agent is usually transmitted by coitus, but may be spread by contaminated articles.

Seven to twelve days or longer after the body is infected, a small, hard sore appears in the genital area. The disease soon spreads from the local sore to the lymph nodes, particularly those in the groin. The lymph nodes may swell to the size of a walnut. As these swellings seldom break open and drain pus, they may remain for months. In women infected with the disease, the vulva may become greatly enlarged. The rectum may become narrowed, so that surgery is necessary for relief.

In the early stages of the disease, there may also be inflammation of the joints, skin rashes, and fever. Sometimes the brain and its covering membrane are affected. It is thought that after the initial sore heals, men may no longer transmit the disease. Women, however, may infect sexual partners for years.

Lymphogranuloma venereum may be successfully treated with antibiotics such as tetracycline.

lymphogranulomatosis (lim″fo-gran″u-lo″mah-to′sis) 1. infectious granuloma of the lymphatic system. 2. Hodgkin's disease.

lymphography (lim-fog′rah-fe) roentgenography of the lymphatic channels and lymph nodes, after injection of radiopaque material in a lymphatic vessel.

lymphoid (lim′foid) resembling or pertaining to lymph or to tissue of the lymphatic system.

l. cells, lymphocytes and plasma cells.

l. tissue, a lattice work of reticular tissue, the interspaces of which contain lymphocytes.

lymphoidectomy (lim″foi-dek′to-me) excision of lymphoid tissue, such as tonsils and adenoids.

lymphokine (lim′fo-kīn) a general term for soluble protein mediators released by sensitized lymphocytes on contact with antigen, and believed to play a role in macrophage activation, lymphocyte transformation, and cell-mediated IMMUNITY.

lymphokinesis (lim″fo-ki-ne′sis) 1. movement of endolymph in the semicircular canals. 2. the circulation of lymph in the body.

lymphology (lim-fol′o-je) the study of the lymphatic system.

lymphoma (lim-fo′mah) any neoplastic disorder of lymphoid tissue. Often used to denote malignant lymphoma, classifications of which are based on predominant cell type and degree of differentiation; various categories may be subdivided into nodular and diffuse types depending on the predominant pattern of cell arrangement.

African l., Burkitt's lymphoma.

Burkitt's l., a form of undifferentiated malignant lymphoma, usually manifested as a large osteolytic lesion in the jaw or as an abdominal mass (see also BURKITT'S LYMPHOMA).

clasmocytic l., histiocytic malignant lymphoma.

giant folliclar l., giant follicular lymphadenopathy.

granulomatous l., Hodgkin's disease.

lymphoblastic l., poorly-differentiated lymphocytic malignant lymphoma.

lymphocytic l., well-differentiated lymphocytic malignant lymphoma.

malignant l., histiocytic, a form in which the predominant cell is the primitive mesenchymal cell or one that has differentiated into the identifiable reticulum cell.

malignant l., mixed cell, a form containing proliferations of both histiocytes and lymphocytes.

malignant l., poorly-differentiated lymphocytic, a form in which the predominant cell is morphologically similar to the lymphoblast, containing a fine nuclear chromatin structure and one or more nucleoli. Called also lymphoblastoma.

malignant l., undifferentiated, a form in which relatively large stem cells with large nuclei, pale, scanty cytoplasm, and indistinct borders predominate.

malignant l., well-differentiated lymphocytic, a form in which the predominant cell is the mature lymphocyte. Called also lymphocytoma.

lymphomatosis (lim″fo-mah-to′sis) the formation of multiple lymphomas in the body.

lymphomatous (lim-fo′mah-tus) pertaining to, or of the nature of, lymphoma.

lymphopathia (lim″fo-path′e-ah) lymphopathy.
l. vene′reum, lymphogranuloma venereum.

lymphopathy (lim-fop′ah-the) any disease of the lymphatic system.

lymphopenia (lim″fo-pe′ne-ah) decrease in the number of lymphocytes of the blood.

lymphoplasmia (lim″fo-plaz′me-ah) absence of hemoglobin from the erythrocytes.

lymphopoiesis (lim″fo-poi-e′sis) the development of lymphocytes or of lymphoid tissue. adj., **lymphopoiet′ic.**

lymphoproliferative (lim″fo-pro-lif′er-ah″tiv) pertaining to or characterized by proliferation of lymphoid tissue.
l. syndrome, a general term applied to a group of diseases characterized by proliferation of lymphoid tissue, such as lymphocytic leukemia and malignant lymphoma.

lymphoreticular (lim″fo-rĕ-tik′u-lar) pertaining to the reticuloendothelial cells of lymph nodes.

lymphoreticulosis (lim″fo-rĕ-tik″u-lo′sis) proliferation of the reticuloendothelial cells of the lymph nodes.
benign l., cat-scratch disease.

lymphorrhagia, lymphorrhea (lim″fo-ra′je-ah; lim″fo-re′ah) flow of lymph from cut or ruptured lymphatic vessels.

lymphorrhoid (lim′fo-roid) a localized dilatation of a perianal lymph channel, resembling a hemorrhoid.

lymphosarcoma (lim″fo-sar-ko′mah) a general term applied to malignant neoplastic disorders of lymphoid tissue, but not including Hodgkin's disease.

lymphosarcomatosis (lim″fo-sar-ko″mah-to′sis) a condition characterized by the presence of multiple lesions of lymphosarcoma.

lymphostasis (lim-fos′tah-sis) stoppage of lymph flow.

lymphotaxis (lim″fo-tak′sis) the property of attracting or repulsing lymphocytes.

lymphotomy (lim-fot′o-me) the anatomy of the lymphatic system.

lymphotoxin (lim″fo-tok′sin) a substance liberated from specifically sensitized lymphocytes, as well as nonspecific stimulators, which has a cytotoxic effect on unrelated cells.

lymph-vascular (limf-vas′ku-lar) pertaining to lymphatic vessels.

lynestrenol (lin-es′trĕ-nōl) a progestin.

Lynoral (lin′or-al) trademark for a preparation of ethynylestradiol, an estrogenic compound.

Lyon hypothesis (li′on) the random and fixed inactivation (in the form of sex chromatin) of all X chromosomes in excess of one in mammalian cells at an early stage of embryogenesis, leading to mosaicism for X-linked genes in the female, since the paternal X chromosome is inactivated in some cells and the maternal one in the remainder.

lyophil (li′o-fil) a lyophilic substance.

lyophile (li′o-fil) 1. lyophil. 2. lyophilic.

lyophilic (li″o-fil′ik) having an affinity for, or stable in, solution.

lyophilization (li-of″ĭ-lĭ-za′shun) the creation of a stable preparation of a biologic substance by rapid freezing and dehydration of the frozen product under high vacuum.

lyophobe (li′o-fōb) a lyophobic substance.

lyophobic (li″o-fo′bik) not having an affinity for, or unstable in, solution.

lyotropic (li″o-trop′ik) readily soluble.

lypressin (li-pres′in) a synthetic preparation of lysine vasopressin used as an antidiuretic.

lyse (līz) 1. to cause or produce disintegration of a compound, substance, or cell. 2. to undergo lysis.

lysemia (li-se′me-ah) disintegration of the blood.

lysergic acid (li-ser′gik) a constituent of ergot alkaloids, obtained by hydrolysis, and from which LSD is derived.

lysergic acid diethylamide (li-ser′jik as′id di-eth′il-am″īd) a hallucinogenic drug better known as LSD.

lysergide (li′ser-jīd) LSD.

lysin (li′sin) an ANTIBODY capable of causing dissolution of cells, including hemolysin, bacteriolysin, etc.

lysine (li′sēn) a naturally occurring amino acid, essential for optimal growth in human infants and for maintenance of nitrogen equilibrium in adults.

lysinogen (li-sin′o-jen) lysogen.

lysis (li′sis) 1. destruction or decomposition, as of a cell or other substance, under the influence of a specific agent. 2. mobilization of an organ by division of restraining adhesions. 3. gradual abatement of the symptoms of a disease.

-lysis word element [Gr.], *dissolution.* adj., **-lyt′ic.**

lysocephalin (li″so-sef′ah-lin) a cephalin from which a fatty acid radical has been removed.

lysogen (li′so-jen) an antigen causing the formation of lysin; called also lysinogen.

lysogenesis (li″so-jen′ĕ-sis) 1. the production of lysis or lysins. 2. lysogenicity.

lysogenicity, lysogeny (li″so-jĕ-nis′ĭ-te; li-soj′ĭ-ne) 1. the ability to produce lysins or cause lysis. 2. the potentiality of a bacterium to produce bacteriophage. 3. the specific association of the phage genome (prophage) with the bacterial genome in such a way that only a few, if any, phage genes are transcribed.

lysokinase (li″so-ki′nās) a general term for substances of the fibrinolytic system that activate plasma proactivators.

Lysol (li′sol) trademark for a solution containing phenol derivatives; used as a disinfectant and antiseptic.

lysolecithin (li″so-les′ĭ-thin) a lecithin from which the terminal fatty acid radical has been removed.

lysosome (li′so-sōm) one of the minute bodies occurring in many types of cells, containing various hydrolytic enzymes and normally involved in the process of localized intracellular digestion. adj., **lysoso′mal.**

lysotype (li′so-tīp) phage type.

lysozyme (li′so-zīm) a crystalline, basic protein present in saliva, tears, egg white, and many animal fluids, which functions as an antibacterial enzyme.

lyssa (lis′ah) rabies. adj., **lys′sic.**

lyssoid (lis′oid) resembling rabies.

lyssophobia (lis″o-fo′be-ah) morbid fear of rabies.

lytic (lit′ik) pertaining to lysis or a lysin.

lyze (līz) lyse.

M

M symbol, *molar* (solution); the expressions M/10, M/100, etc., denote the strength of a solution in comparison with the molar, as tenth molar, hundredth molar, etc.

M. macerate, maximal, member, meter, minim, muscle, myopia; [L.] mil or mille (*thousand*), misce (*mix*), mistura (*mixture*).

m. meter.

m- symbol, *meta-*.

μ symbol, *micron.*

M.A. Master of Arts; meter angle; mental age.

ma. milliampere.

macerate (mas′er-āt) to soften by wetting or soaking.

maceration (mas″ĕ-ra′shun) the softening of a solid by soaking; wasting away, softening and fraying, as if by action of soaking; in obstetrics, the degenerative changes and eventual disintegration of a fetus retained in the uterus after its death.

macies (ma′shē-ēz) [L.] wasting.

macr(o)- word element [Gr.], *large; long.*

macrencephalia (mak″ren-sĕ-fa′le-ah) hypertrophy of the brain.

macroamylase (mak″ro-am′ĭ-lās) a complex in which normal serum amylase is bound to a variety of specific binding proteins, forming a complex too large for renal excretion.

macroamylasemia (mak″ro-am″ĭ-la-se′me-ah) the presence of macroamylase in the blood. adj., **macroamylase′mic.**

macrobiota (mak″ro-bi-o′tah) the macroscopic living organisms of a region. adj., **macrobiot′ic.**

macroblast (mak′ro-blast) an abnormally large, nucleated erythrocyte; a large young normoblast with megaloblastic features.

macroblepharia (mak″ro-blĕ-fa′re-ah) abnormal largeness of the eyelid.

macrocardius (mak″ro-kar′de-us) a fetus with an extremely large heart.

macrocephalous (mak″ro-sef′ah-lus) having an abnormally large head.

macrocephaly (mak″ro-sef′ah-le) abnormal enlargement of the cranium.

macrocheilia (mak″ro-ki′le-ah) excessive size of the lip.

macrocheiria (mak″ro-ki′re-ah) excessive size of the hands.

macrochemistry (mak″ro-kem′is-tre) chemistry in which the reactions may be seen with the naked eye.

macrocolon (mak″ro-ko′lon) megacolon.

macrocrania (mak″ro-kra′ne-ah) abnormal increase in size of the skull in relation to the face.

macrocyte (mak′ro-sīt) an abnormally large erythrocyte. adj., **macrocyt′ic.**

macrocythemia, macrocytosis (mak″ro-si-the′me-ah; mak″ro-si-to′sis) the presence of macrocytes in the blood.

macrodactyly (mak″ro-dak′tĭ-le) abnormal largeness of the fingers or toes.

macrodontia (mak″ro-don′she-ah) abnormal increase in size of one or more teeth. adj., **mac′rodont, macrodon′tic.**

macrofauna (mak″ro-faw′nah) the macroscopic animal organisms of a region.

macroflora (mak″ro-flo′rah) the macroscopic vegetable organisms of a region.

macrogamete (mak″ro-gam′ēt) the larger, female gamete of the malarial parasite.

macrogenitosomia (mak″ro-jen″ĭ-to-so′me-ah) excessive bodily development, with unusual enlargement of the genital organs.

m. prae′cox, macrogenitosomia occurring at an early age.

macroglia (mah-krog′le-ah) astroglia.

macroglobulin (mak″ro-glob′u-lin) a protein (globulin) of unusually high molecular weight, in the range of 1,000,000; observed in the blood in a number of diseases.

macroglobulinemia (mak″ro-glob″u-lin-e′me-ah) increased levels of macroglobulins in the blood.

Waldenström's m., a progressive syndrome of the endothelial system seen chiefly in males past age 50, associated with macroglobulinemia, adenopathy, hepatosplenomegaly, hemorrhagic phenomena, anemia, and lymphocytosis and plasmacytosis of bone marrow.

macroglossia (mak″ro-glos′e-ah) excessive size of the tongue.

macrognathia (mak″ro-nath′e-ah) abnormal overgrowth of the jaw. adj., **macrognath′ic.**

macrogyria (mak″ro-ji′re-ah) moderate reduction in the number of sulci of the cerebrum, sometimes with increase in the brain substance, resulting in excessive size of the gyri.

macrolide (mak′ro-līd) any antibiotic with molecules having many-membered lactone rings.

macromastia (mak″ro-mas′te-ah) excessive size of the breasts.

macromelia (mak″ro-me′le-ah) enlargement of one or more limbs.

macromelus (mah-krom′ĕ-lus) a fetus with abnormally large or long limbs.

macromere (mak′ro-mēr) one of the larger cells (blastomeres) formed in unequal cleavage of the fertilized ovum (at the vegetal pole).

macromethod (mak′ro-meth″od) a chemical test in which normal (not minute) quantities of the specimen substance are used.

macromolecule (mak″ro-mol′ĕ-kūl) a very large molecule having a polymeric chain structure, as in proteins, polysaccharides, etc. adj., **macromolec′ular.**

macromonocyte (mak″ro-mon′o-sīt) a giant monocyte.

macromyeloblast (mak″ro-mi′ĕ-lo-blast″) a large myeloblast.

macronormoblast (mak″ro-nor′mo-blast) a very large nucleated erythrocyte; macroblast.

macronychia (mak″ro-nik′e-ah) abnormally enlarged nails.

macrophage (mak′ro-fāj) any of the highly phagocytic cells in the wall of blood vessels and in loose connective tissue; they are usually immobile (histiocytes, or fixed macrophages), but when stimulated by inflammation become actively mobile (free macrophages). (See also IMMUNITY.)

m. activating factor (MAF), a lymphokine that induces in macrophages an increased content of lysosomal enzymes, more aggressive phagocytosis, and increased mitotic activity.

m. chemotactic factor (MCF), a lymphokine that attracts macrophages to the invasion site.

m. migration inhibiting factor (MIF), a lymphokine that inhibits migration of macrophages, causing them to accumulate at the site of antigen.

macrophthalmia (mak″rof-thal′me-ah) abnormal enlargement of the eyeball.

macropodia (mak″ro-po′de-ah) excessive size of the feet.

macropolycyte (mak″ro-pol′e-sīt) a hypersegmented polymorphonuclear leukocyte of greater than normal size.

macroprosopia (mak″ro-pro-so′pe-ah) excessive size of the face.

macropsia (mah-krop′se-ah) a disorder of visual perception in which objects appear larger than their actual size.

macrorrhinia (mak″ro-rin′e-ah) excessive size of the nose.

macroscopic (mak″ro-skop′ik) of large size; visible to the unaided eye.

macroscopy (mah-kros′ko-pe) examination with the unaided eye.

macrosigmoid (mak″ro-sig′moid) excessive size of the sigmoid colon.

macrosomatia, macrosomia (mak″ro-so-ma′sheah; mak″ro-so′me-ah) great bodily size.

macrostomia (mak″ro-sto′me-ah) excessive width of the mouth.

macrotia (mah-kro′she-ah) abnormal enlargement of the pinna of the ear.

macula (mak′u-lah), pl. *mac′ulae* [L.] 1. a stain, spot, or thickening; in anatomy, an area distinguishable by color or otherwise from its surroundings. 2. a macule: a discolored spot on the skin that is not raised above the surface. 3. a corneal scar, appreciated as a gray spot. 4. macula lutea. adj., **mac′ular, mac′ulate.**

mac′ulae acus′ticae, terminations of the vestibulocochlear nerve in the utricle and saccule.

m. atroph′ica, a white atrophic patch on the skin.

m. ceru′lea, a blue patch on the skin seen in pediculosis.

m. cor′neae, a circumscribed opacity of the cornea.

m. cribro′sa, a perforated spot or area; one of three perforated areas (inferior, medial, and superior) in the wall of the vestibule of the ear through which branches of the vestibulocochlear nerve pass to the saccule, utricle, and semicircular canals.

m. den′sa, a zone of heavily nucleated cells in the distal renal tubule.

m. fla′va, a yellow nodule at one end of a vocal cord.

m. follic′uli, the point on the surface of a vesicular ovarian follicle where rupture occurs.

m. germinati′va, germinal area; the part of the ovum where the embryo is formed.

m. lu′tea, m. ret′inae, an irregular yellowish depression on the retina, lateral to and slightly below the optic disk.

m. sac′culi, a thickening on the wall of the saccule where the epithelium contains hair cells that receive and transmit vestibular impulses.

m. sola′ris, a freckle.

m. utric′uli, a thickening in the wall of the utricle where the epithelium contains hair cells that receive and transmit vestibular impulses.

maculate (mak′u-lāt) spotted or blotched.

macule (mak′ūl) a macula.

maculocerebral (mak″u-lo-ser′ĕ-bral) pertaining to the macula lutea and the brain.

maculopapular (mak″u-lo-pap′u-lar) both macular and papular.

madarosis (mad″ah-ro′sis) loss of eyelashes or eyebrows.

Madelung's deformity (mah′dĕ-lo͞ongz) radical deviation of the hand secondary to overgrowth of the distal ulna or shortening of the radius.

Madelung's disease (mah′dĕ-lo͞ongz) 1. Madelung's deformity. 2. Madelungs's neck.

Madelung's neck (mah′dĕ-lo͞ongz) diffuse symmetrical lipomas of the neck.

Madura foot (mah-du′rah) maduromycosis of the foot.

maduromycosis (mah-du″ro-mi-ko′sis) a chronic disease due to various fungi or actinomycetes, affecting various body tissues, including the hands, legs and feet; called also mycetoma. The most common form affects the foot (Madura foot) and is characterized by sinus formation, necrosis, and swelling.

mafenide (maf′en-īd) a compound used in the topical treatment of superficial infections.

magaldrate (mag′al-drāt) a combination of aluminum hydroxide and magnesium hydroxide used as an antacid.

magenta (mah-jen′tah) fuchsin or other salt of rosaniline.

maggot (mag′ot) the soft-bodied larva of an insect, especially one living in decaying flesh.

magma (mag′mah) 1. a suspension of finely divided material in a small amount of water. 2. a thin, pastelike substance composed of organic material.

bentonite m., a preparation of bentonite and purified water, used as a suspending agent.

bismuth m., a water suspension of bismuth hydroxide and bismuth subcarbonate, used as an astringent and antacid.

magnesia m., magnesium hydroxide; used as a laxative and antacid.

Magnacort (mag′nah-kort) trademark for a preparation of hydrocortamate, used in treatment of dermatoses.

magnesia (mag-ne′zhah) magnesium oxide; aperient and antacid.

magnesium (mag-ne′ze-um) a chemical element, atomic number 12, atomic weight 24.312, symbol Mg. (See table of ELEMENTS.) Its salts are essential in nutrition, being required for the activity of many enzymes, especially those concerned with oxidative phosphorylation.

m. carbonate, an odorless, stable compound used as an antacid.

m. citrate, a mild cathartic.

m. hydroxide, a bulky white powder used as an antacid and cathartic.

m. oxide, a white powder used as an antacid.

m. phosphate, dibasic, a salt used as a mild saline laxative.

m. phosphate, tribasic, a white, odorless, tasteless powder used as an antacid.

m. stearate, a combination of magnesium with stearic and palmitic acids; used as a dusting powder and tablet lubricant.

m. sulfate, a cathartic; called also Epsom salt.

m. trisilicate, a combination of magnesium oxide and silicon dioxide with varying proportions of water; used as a gastric antacid.

magnet (mag′net) an object having polarity and capable of attracting iron.

magnetism (mag′nĕ-tizm) magnetic attraction or repulsion.

magnetotherapy (mag-ne″to-ther′ah-pe) treatment of disease by magnetic currents.

magnetropism (mag-net′ro-pizm) a growth response in a nonmotile organism under the influence of a magnet.

magnification (mag″nĭ-fĭ-ka′shun) 1. apparent increase in size, as under the microscope. 2. the process of making something appear larger, as by use of lenses. 3. the ratio of apparent (image) size to real size.

main (mān) [Fr.] hand.

m. en griffe (ma-non-grif′) clawhand.

Majocchi's disease (mah-yok′ēz) annular telangiectatic purpura.

Majocchi's granuloma (mah-yok′ēz) a form of tinea corporis, occurring chiefly on the lower legs due to *Trichophyton* infecting the hairs at the site of involvement, marked by raised, circumscribed, rather boggy granulomas, disseminated or arranged in chains; the lesions are slowly absorbed, or undergo necrosis, leaving depressed scars. Called also trichophytic granuloma.

mal (mal) [Fr.] illness; disease.

grand m., a generalized convulsive seizure attended by loss of consciousness (see also EPILEPSY).

m. de Meleda, symmetrical keratosis of the palms and soles associated with an ichthyotic thickening of the wrists and ankles.

m. de mer, seasickness.

petit m., momentary loss of consciousness without convulsive movements (see also EPILEPSY).

mala (ma′lah) the cheek or cheek bone. adj., **ma′lar.**

malabsorption (mal″ab-sorp′shun) impaired intestinal absorption of nutrients.

m. syndrome, a group of disorders marked by subnormal intestinal absorption of dietary constituents, and thus excessive loss of nutrients in the stool; it may be due to a digestive defect, a mucosal abnormality, or lymphatic obstruction.

malachite green (mal′ah-kīt) a dye used as a stain for bacteria and as an antiseptic for wounds.

malacia (mal-la′she-ah) 1. morbid softening or softness of a part or tissue; also used as a word termination, as in osteomalacia. 2. morbid craving for highly spiced foods.

malacoma (mal″ah-ko′mah) a morbidly soft part or spot.

malacoplakia (mal″ah-ko-pla′ke-ah) a circumscribed area of softening on the membrane lining a hollow organ, as the ureter, urethra, or renal pelvis.

m. vesi′cae, a flat yellow growth on the mucosa of the bladder.

malacosis (mal″ah-ko′sis) malacia.

malacosteon (mal″ah-kos′te-on) softening of the bones; osteomalacia.

malacotic (mal″ah-kot′ik) soft.

maladjustment (mal″ad-just′ment) in psychiatry, defective adaptation to the environment, marked by anxiety.

malady (mal′ah-de) a disease or illness.

malaise (mal-āz) [Fr.] a feeling of uneasiness or indisposition.

malalignment (mal″ah-līn′ment) displacement, especially of the teeth from their normal relation to the line of the dental arch.

malaria (mah-lār′e-ah) a serious infectious illness characterized by periodic chills and high fever. It responds well to modern drugs but can be chronic. adj., **malar′ial.**

It is endemic to parts of Africa, Asia, and Central and South America, and is estimated to occur at the rate of 100 million cases each year throughout the world. Epidemics usually occur in areas where mosquitoes persist in large numbers and the parasite is introduced into a region that is populated with persons who are not immune to malaria. Acute cases of malaria occur when nonimmune persons travel to regions where the disease is endemic.

A worldwide cooperative program begun about 20 years ago has met with limited success. Some difficulties encountered have been resistance of mosquitoes to insecticides, insufficient funding in some underdeveloped countries, resistance of plasmodia to antimalarial drugs, and the discovery that malaria in monkeys can be transmitted to man. In view of these difficulties recent efforts have been toward malaria control rather than eradication.

CAUSE. Malaria is caused by a protozoan parasite, *Plasmodium,* which is carried by the *Anopheles* mosquito. When the mosquito bites an infected person, it sucks in the parasites, which reside in the blood. In the mosquito the plasmodia multiply and travel to the salivary glands from which they are transmitted to the human bloodstream by the mosquito bite. Inside the human host they penetrate the erythrocytes, where they mature, reproduce and at complete maturity burst out of the blood cell. The life cycle varies according to the species of *Plasmodium.* For *P. vivax* it is 48 hours, *P. malariae* 72 hours, and *P. falciparum* 36 to 48 hours.

SYMPTOMS. There are usually no symptoms until several cycles have been completed. Then there is a simultaneous rupturing of erythrocytes by the entire brood, causing the characteristic chills followed in a few hours by fever. The temperature may rise to 104° or 105° F. (40° to 40.5° C.). As it subsides, there is profuse perspiring. Other symptoms are headache, nausea, body pains and, after the attack, exhaustion. The symptoms last from 4 to 6 hours and recur at regular intervals, depending upon the parasitic species and its cycle. If the attack occurs every other day, the disease is called tertian malaria; if it occurs at 3 day intervals, it is quartan malaria.

As the disease progresses, the attacks occur less frequently. Bouts of malaria last from 1 to 4 weeks but usually about 2 weeks. Relapses are common, with attacks ceasing and recurring at irregular intervals for several years, especially if untreated. Malaria is not usually fatal; when it is, it is almost always caused by the falciparum species.

TREATMENT. For many years, quinine was the standard treatment for malaria. The intensive research carried on since World War II has provided synthetic medicines such as chloroquine and amodiaquine that can either relieve the attack promptly or cure the infection. Quinine is still important in treatment of infection with drug-resistant plasmodia.

PREVENTION. There is no effective inoculation against malaria, but antimalarial drugs may be given prophylactically to persons traveling to areas where the disease is widespread. Preventive measures are concentrated on destroying the mosquito. This is done by filling in pools, swamps, and places containing stagnant water where mosquitoes breed, and by intensive use of DDT and other insecticides.

malariacidal (mah-lār″e-ah-si′dal) destructive to malarial plasmodia.

malariotherapy (mah-lār″e-o-ther′ah-pe) treatment of paresis by infecting the patient with the parasite of tertian malaria.

Malassezia (mal″ah-se′ze-ah) *Pityrosporon.*
M. fur′fur, *Pityrosporon orbiculare.*

malassimilation (mal″ah-sim″ĭ-la′shun) defective or faulty assimilation.

malate (ma′lāt) a salt of malic acid.

malaxate (mal′ak-sāt) to knead, as in making pills.

malaxation (mal″ak-sa′shun) an act of kneading.

male (māl) an individual of the sex that produces spermatozoa.

maleruption (mal″e-rup′shun) eruption of a tooth out of its normal position.

malformation (mal″for-ma′shun) defective formation; deformity.

malic acid (ma′lik) a crystalline acid from juices of many fruits and plants, and an intermediary product of carbohydrate metabolism in the body.

malignancy (mah-lig′nan-se) a tendency to progress in virulence. In popular usage, any condition that, if uncorrected, tends to worsen so as to cause serious illness or death. Cancer is the best known example.

malignant (mah-lig′nant) tending to become progressively worse and to result in death; having the properties of anaplasia, invasiveness, and metastasis; said of tumors.

malingerer (mah-ling′ger-er) one who is guilty of malingering.

malingering (mah-ling′ger-ing) willful, deliberate, and fraudulent feigning or exaggeration of the symptoms of illness or injury to attain a consciously desired end.

malleable (mal′e-ah-b′l) susceptible of being beaten out into a thin plate.

malleoincudal (mal″e-o-ing′ku-dal) pertaining to the malleus and incus.

malleolus (mah-le′o-lus), pl. *malle′oli* [L.] a rounded process, especially either of the two rounded prominences on either side of the ankle joint, at the lower end of the fibula (external, lateral, or outer malleolus) or of the tibia (inner, internal, or medial malleolus). adj. **malle′olar.**

malleotomy (mal″e-ot′o-me) 1. operative division of the malleus. 2. operative separation of the malleoli.

malleus (mal′e-us) the largest of the three ossicles of the ear; called also hammer. See Plate 15.

malnutrition (mal″nu-trish′un) poor nourishment resulting from improper diet or from some defect in metabolism that prevents the body from using its food properly. Extreme malnutrition may lead to starvation.

CAUSES. Although poverty is still the major cause of malnutrition, the condition is by no means confined to the underdeveloped parts of the world. Anyone can become undernourished if he seriously neglects his diet. A well balanced diet, the requirements of which vary slightly with a person's age, should include adequate amounts of protein, vitamins, minerals, and carbohydrates. For an explanation of the value of properly balanced diets, see NUTRITION.

Ignorance of the basic principles of nutrition is probably almost as great a cause of undernourishment as proverty. Misplaced faith in vitamin pills as a substitute for food, for example, can, if carried to extremes, cause undernourishment. So can over-reliance on excessively processed foods. Modern methods of processing and refining foods can sometimes cause a loss of valuable nutrients, as happens in the refining of certain grains, such as rice. However, this danger is recognized by both the government and the manufacturers who try to retain or restore the nutritional value of many foods. ALCOHOLISM, which frequently leads a person to rely on alcohol at the expense of food, is another cause of malnutrition.

People who want to gain or lose weight, or who, like vegetarians, avoid certain foods, may endanger their health by following an unbalanced diet that lacks essential nutrients. Anyone who plans to follow a special diet should talk the matter over with his physician.

Malnutrition can also stem from disease. If the organs of the digestive system that transform food into bone, tissue, blood, and energy fail to function properly, the body will not receive adequate nourishment. Such deficiencies can cause diabetes mellitus, certain liver diseases, and some anemias. The ENDOCRINE GLANDS and ENZYMES are also vital to the proper use of food by the body, and defects in their functioning may cause forms of malnutrition.

SYMPTOMS. In general, the symptoms of malnutrition are physical weakness, lassitude, and an increasing sense of detachment from the world. There are also specific symptoms that vary according to the essential substance lacking in the diet. For example, lack of vitamin A can result in NIGHT BLINDNESS, or poor vision in dim light. In the absence of adequate exposure to sunlight, a lack of vitamin D can cause RICKETS, which results in malformed limbs in infants and children because the bones fail to harden properly. A lack of vitamin C causes SCURVY, with symptoms of bleeding gums and easily bruised skin. Other vitamin deficiency diseases are BERIBERI, PELLAGRA, and SPRUE. If there is not enough iron in the diet, ANEMIA develops.

In starvation there are signs of multiple vitamin deficiency. There may be edema, abdominal distention, and excessive loss of weight. As starvation progresses, fat cells become small and accumulations of fat are depleted. The liver is reduced in size, the muscles shrivel, and the lymphoid tissue, gonads, and blood deteriorate.

Because the stomach and the intestinal tract may no longer be capable of digesting food of any bulk, treatment of starvation should begin by feeding the patient easily digested liquids, such as soups, in small quantities. If he is unable to eat or drink, the necessary nutrients can be supplied by intravenous infusion.

malocclusion (mal″ŏ-kloo′zhun) malposition of the teeth resulting in the faulty meeting of the teeth or jaws. The condition should be corrected because it predisposes to dental caries, may lead to digestive disorders and inadequate nutrition because of difficulty in chewing, and can cause serious psychologic effects if there is facial distortion. Corrective treatment is provided by an orthodontist, who may apply appropriate dental braces to improve the position of the teeth.

malpighian capsule (mal-pig′ĭ-an) a two-layered cellular envelope enclosing the tuft of capillaries constituting the glomerulus of the kidney; called also Bowman's capsule and glomerular capsule.

m. corpuscle, the funnel-like structure constituting the beginning of the structural unit of the kidney (nephron) and comprising the malpighian capsule and its partially enclosed glomerulus. Called also renal corpuscle.

m. layer, the basal layer and the prickle-cell layer of the skin considered together.

malposition (mal″po-zish′un) abnormal placement.

malpractice (mal″prak′tis) any professional misconduct, unreasonable lack of skill or fidelity in professional duties, or illegal or immoral conduct. Malpractice is one form of negligence, which in legal terms can be defined as the omission to do something that a reasonable man, guided by those ordinary considerations which ordinarily regulate human affairs, would do, or the doing of something that a reasonable and prudent man would not do. In medical and nursing practice, malpractice means bad, wrong, or injudicious treatment of a patient professionally; it results in injury, unnecessary suffering, or death to the patient. The court may hold that malpractice has occurred even though the physician or nurse acted in good faith. Also, malpractice and negligence may occur through omission to act as well as commission of an unwise or negligent act.

malpresentation (mal″prez-en-ta′shun) faulty fetal presentation.

malrotation (mal″ro-ta′shun) abnormal or pathologic rotation, as of the vertebral column.

malt (mawlt) a preparation of grain that contains dextrin, maltose, and diastase; it is nutritive and digestant, aiding in the digestion of starchy foods.

Malta fever (mawl′tah) brucellosis.

maltase (mawl′tās) α-glucosidase (see GLUCOSIDASE).

maltose (mawl′tōs) a sugar (disaccharide) formed when starch is hydrolyzed by amylase.

malum (ma′lum) [L.] a disease.

m. articulo′rum seni′lis, a painful degenerative state of a joint as a result of aging.

m. cox′ae seni′lis, osteoarthritis of the hip joint.

m. per′forans pe′dis, perforating ulcer of the foot.

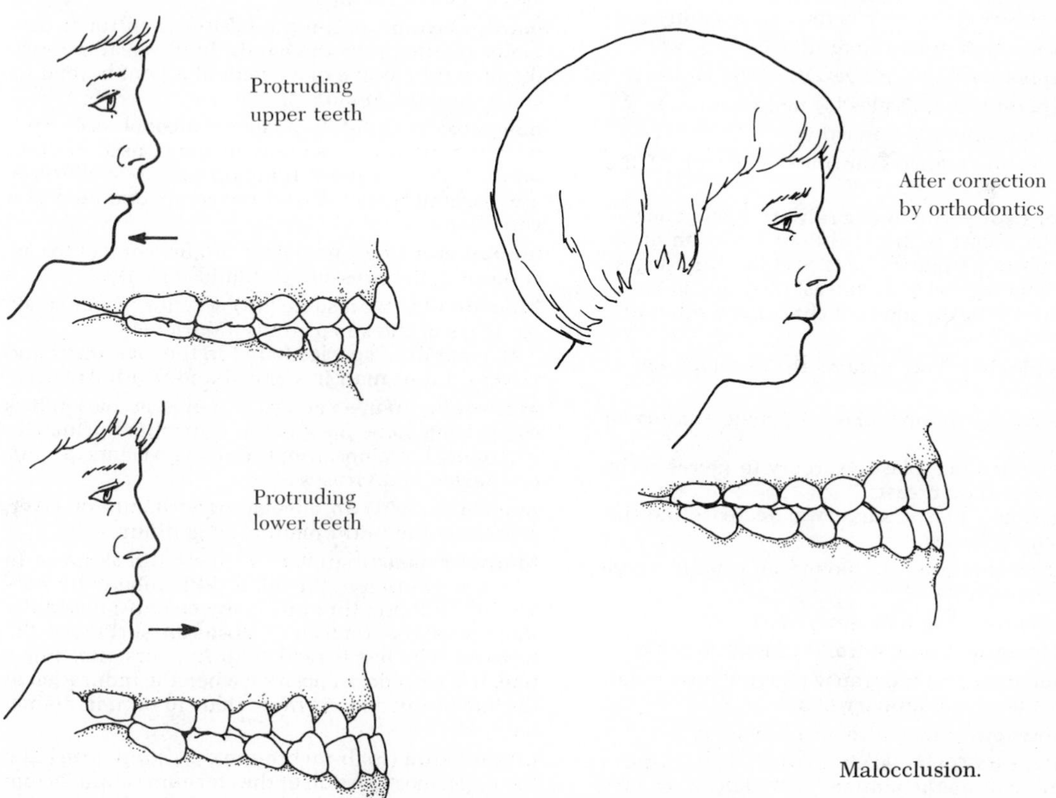

Malocclusion.

malunion (mal-ūn′yon) faulty union of the fragments of a fractured bone.

mamilla (mah-mil′ah), pl. *mamil′lae* [L.] 1. the nipple of the breast. 2. any nipple-like prominence. adj., **mam′illary.**

mamillated (mam′ĭ-lāt″ed) having nipple-like projections or prominences.

mamillation (mam″ĭ-la′shun) 1. the condition of being mamillated. 2. a nipple-like elevation or projection.

mamilliform (mah-mil′i-form) shaped like a nipple.

mamilliplasty (mah-mil′i-plas″te) theleplasty; plastic reconstruction of the nipples.

mamillitis (mam″i-li′tis) thelitis; inflammation of the nipple.

mamm(o)- word element [L], *breast; mammary gland.*

mamma (mam′ah), pl. *mam′mae* [L.] the milk-secreting gland of the female; mammary gland; the breast.

mammal (mam′al) an individual of the Mammalia, a division of vertebrates, including all that possess hair and suckle their young. adj., **mammal′ian.**

mammalgia (mah-mal′je-ah) pain in the mammary gland.

mammaplasty (mam′ah-plas″te) mammoplasty.

mammary (mam′ar-e) pertaining to the mammary gland or breast.

m. gland, the specialized gland of the skin of female mammals, which secretes milk for nourishment of the young, existing in a rudimentary state in the male (see also BREAST).

mammectomy (mah-mek′to-me) mastectomy.

mammilla (mah-mil′ah) mamilla.

mammiplasia (mam″ĭ-pla′ze-ah) mammoplasia.

mammiplasty (mam′ĭ-plas″te) mammoplasty.

mammitis (mah-mi′tis) mastitis.

mammogram (mam′o-gram) a radiograph of the breast.

mammography (mah-mog′rah-fe) roentgenography of the breast with or without injection of an opaque substance into its ducts. Simple mammography, without the use of a contrast medium, is sometimes used in the diagnosis of cancer and other disorders of the breast.

mammoplasia (mam″o-pla′ze-ah) development of breast tissue.

mammoplasty (mam′o-plas″te) plastic surgery of the breast.

augmentation m., plastic surgery to increase the size of the female breast.

reduction m., plastic surgery to decrease the size of the female breast.

mammose (mam′ōs) 1. having unusually large breasts. 2. mamillated.

mammotomy (mah-mot′o-me) mastotomy.

mammotrophic (mam″o-trof′ik) mammotropic.

mammotropic (mam″o-trop′ik) having a stimulating effect on the mammary gland.

mammotropin (mam″o-tro′pin) prolactin.

Mandelamine (man-del′ah-mēn) trademark for a preparation of methenamine mandelate, a urinary antiseptic.

mandelic acid (man-del′ik) a keto acid used as a urinary antiseptic in nephritis, pyelitis, and cystitis. It must be excreted in the urinary tract unchanged in order to have a bacteriostatic effect; therefore, a strongly acid urine should be maintained during its administration. To accomplish this, fluids may be limited and an acidifying agent given (see also ACID-ASH DIET). Citrus fruits and other foods producing an alkaline ash must be restricted. The average dose of mandelic acid or preparations containing this substance depends on the type of preparation used.

mandible (man′dĭ-b′l) the horseshoe-shaped bone forming the lower jaw. adj., **mandib′ular.** It consists of a central portion, which forms the chin and supports the lower teeth, and two perpendicular portions, or rami, which point upward from the back of the chin on either side and articulate with the temporal bones.

mandrin (man′drin) a metal guide for a flexible catheter.

manganese (mang′gah-nēs) a chemical element, atomic number 25, atomic weight 54.938, symbol Mn. (See table of ELEMENTS.) Its salts occur in the body tissue in very small amounts and serve as activators of liver arginase and other enzymes.

mange (mānj) a skin disease of domestic animals, due to mites.

mania (ma′ne-ah) a disordered mental state of extreme excitement; specifically, the manic type of manic-depressive psychosis. Also used as a word termination to denote obsessive preoccupation with something, as in tomomania. adj., **mani′acal, ma′nic.**

maniac (ma′ne-ak) one affected with mania.

manic-depressive (man″ik-de-pres′iv) marked by alternating periods of mania and depression (see also affective PSYCHOSIS).

manipulation (mah-nip″u-la′shun) skillful or dexterous treatment by the hands. In physical therapy, the forceful passive movement of a joint beyond its active limit of motion.

mannitol (man′ĭ-tol) a sugar alcohol occurring widely in nature, especially in fungi; used in diagnostic tests of kidney function and as a diuretic.

m. hexanitrate, a crystalline compound used as a vasodilator.

manometer (mah-nom′ĕ-ter) an instrument for ascertaining the pressure of liquids or gases.

Mansonella (man″so-nel′ah) a genus of nematode parasites of the superfamily Filarioidea.

M. ozzar′di, a species found in the mesentery and visceral fat of man in Central and South America.

Mansonia (man-so′ne-ah) a genus of mosquitoes comprising some 55 species, distributed primarily in tropical regions, important as vectors of microfilariae and viruses.

mantle (man′tl) an enveloping structure or layer, especially the brain mantle, or pallium.

Mantoux test (man-too′) a tuberculin skin test in which a solution of 0.1 ml. of PPD-tuberculin containing 5 tuberculin units is injected intradermally into either the anterior or posterior surface of the forearm. The test is read 48 to 72 hours after injection. It is considered positive when the induration at the site of injection is more than 10 mm. in diameter.

manubrium (mah-nu′bre-um), pl. *manu′bria* [L.] 1. the uppermost portion of the sternum (manu′brium ster′ni). 2. the largest process of the malleus, giving attachment to the tendon of the tensor muscle of the tympanum (manu′brium mal′lei).

manus (ma′nus), pl. *ma′nus* [L.] hand.

MAO monoamine oxidase.

maple bark disease a granulomatous interstitial pneumonitis due to inhalation of the spores from *Cryptostroma corticale,* a mold found beneath the bark of maple logs.

maple syrup urine disease a genetic disorder involving deficiency of an enzyme necessary in the metabolism of branched-chain amino acids, marked clinically by mental and physical retardation, feeding difficulties, and a characteristic odor of the urine.

marasmus (mah-raz′mus) a form of protein-calorie malnutrition occurring chiefly in the first year of life, with growth retardation and wasting of subcutaneous fat and muscle. adj., **maran′tic, maras′mic.**

marble bones osteopetrosis.

march foot painful swelling of the foot, usually with fracture of a metatarsal bone, after excessive foot strain.

Marchiafava-Micheli syndrome (mar″ke-ah-fah′va me-ka′le) the paroxysmal nocturnal form of intermittent HEMOGLOBINURIA.

Marezine (mar′ĕ-zēn) trademark for a preparation of cyclizine hydrochloride, an antihistamine.

Marfan's syndrome (mar-fahnz′) a hereditary disorder of connective tissue characterized by abnormal length of the extremities, especially of the fingers and toes, subluxation of the lens, congenital anomalies of the heart, and other deformities.

margination (mar″jĭ-na′shun) adhesion of leukocytes to blood vessel walls in the early stages of inflammation.

marginoplasty (mar′jin-o-plas″te) surgical restoration of a border, as of the eyelid.

margo (mar′go), pl. *mar′gines* [L.] border; margin.

Marie's disease (mah-rēz′) acromegaly.

Marie-Bamberger disease (mah-re′ bahm′berger) hypertrophic pulmonary osteoarthropathy.

Marie-Strümpell disease (mah-re′ strim′pel) rheumatoid spondylitis.

Marie-Tooth disease (mah-re′ tooth) progressive neuropathic (peroneal) muscular atrophy.

marijuana, marihuana (mar″i-wahn′ah) a preparation of the leaves and flowering tops of *Cannabis sativa,* the hemp plant, which contains a number of pharmacologically active principles (cannabinoids). *Hashish,* also derived from the hemp plant, is obtained from the clear resin secreted by the flowering tops of the plant. Hashish is thought to be four to eight times more potent than marijuana. Both drugs are used for their euphoric properties and are three to four times more potent when smoked and inhaled than when ingested.

Controversy over the legalization of marijuana in the United States continues at the time of this writing. It is known that the use of marijuana as a recreational drug in this country is exceeded only by the the use of alcohol and tobacco. Unfortunately, many years of widespread use are usually required for the full implications of the use of a drug to become apparent. Such has been the case with alcohol and tobacco, which many defenders of marijuana cite as examples of legal drugs that are "no better and no worse" than marijuana. Those opposed to marijuana agree that alcohol and tobacco are similar in some ways, but they too are detrimental to health. Their deleterious effects are well documented, but the search for evidence of the effects of marijuana must continue before it can be declared more or less harmful than the other two drugs.

Marplan (mar′plan) trademark for a preparation of isocarboxazid, an antidepressant.

marrow (mar′o) the soft, organic, spongelike material in the cavities of bones. Bone marrow is a network of blood vessels and special connective tissue fibers that hold together a composite of fat and blood-producing cells.

The chief function of marrow is to manufacture erythrocytes, leukocytes, and platelets. These blood cells normally do not enter the bloodstream until they are fully developed, so that the marrow contains cells in all stages of growth. If the body's demand for white cells is increased because of infection, the marrow responds immediately by stepping up production. The same is true if more red blood cells are needed, as in hemorrhage or anemia.

There are two types of marrow, red and yellow. The former produces the blood cells; the latter, which is mainly formed of fatty tissue, normally has no blood-producing function.

During infancy and early childhood all bone marrow is red. But gradually, as one gets older and less blood cell production is needed, the fat content of the marrow increases as some of the marrow turns from red to yellow. Red marrow continues to be present in adulthood only in the flat bones of the skull, the sternum, ribs, vertebral column, clavicle, humerus, and part of the femur. However, under certain conditions, as after hemorrhage, yellow marrow in other bones may again be converted to red and resume its cell-producing functions.

The marrow is occasionally subject to disease, as in aplastic anemia, which may be caused by destruction of the marrow by chemical agents or excessive x-ray exposure. Other diseases that affect the bone marrow are leukemia, pernicious anemia, myeloma, and metastatic tumors.

marsupialization (mar-su″pe-ah-lĭ-za′shun) conversion of a closed cavity, such as an abscess or cyst, into an open pouch, by incising it and suturing the edges of its wall to the edges of the wound.

marsupium (mar-su′pe-um), pl. *marsu′pia* [L.] pouch; the scrotum.

masculine (mas′ku-lin) pertaining to the male sex.

masculinity (mas″ku-lin′ĭ-te) the possession of masculine qualities.

masculinization (mas″ku-lin-ĭ-za′shun) the normal induction or development of male sex characters in the male; also, the induction or development of male secondary sex characters in the female.

masculinize (mas′ku-lĭ-nīz) to produce masculine qualities in women.

masculinovoblastoma (mas″ku-lin-o″vo-blas-to′mah) a rare, usually benign ovarian tumor composed of eosinophilic cells or cells with lipoid vacuoles, arising from ovarian cells or embryonic adrenal rest cells; it causes virilization. Called also adrenal rest tumor and lipoid cell tumor.

maser (ma′zer) a device that produces an extremely intense, small and nearly nondivergent beam of monochromatic radiation in the microwave region, with all the waves in phase.

mask (mask) 1. to cover or conceal, as the masking of the nature of a disorder by the presence of unassociated signs, organisms, etc.; in audiometry, to obscure or diminish a sound by the presence of another sound of different frequency. 2. an appliance for shading, protecting, or medicating the face.

leutic m., a brownish, blotchy pigmentation over the forehead, temples, and cheeks, sometimes occurring in tertiary syphilis.

m. of pregnancy, brown pigmentation of the forehead, cheeks and nose, sometimes seen in pregnancy; melasma gravidarum.

Venturi m., any of three types of masks used to administer controlled amounts of oxygen (see also OXYGEN therapy); each of these masks provides a constant concentration above that of the atmospheric concentration (21 per cent).

masochism (mas'o-kizm) a perversion in which infliction of physical or psychological pain gives sexual gratification to the recipient. adj., **masochis'tic.**

masochist (mas'o-kist) a person exhibiting or characterized by masochism.

mass (mas) 1. a lump or collection of cohering particles. 2. that characteristic of matter which gives it inertia.

body cell m., the total weight of the cells of the body, constituting the total mass of oxygen-utilizing, carbohydrate-burning, and energy-exchanging cells of the body; regarded as proportional to total exchangeable potassium in the body.

inner cell m., an internal cluster of cells at the animal pole of the blastocyst which develops into the body of the embryo.

intermediate cell m., nephrotome.

lean body m., that part of the body including all its components except neutral storage lipid; in essence, the fat-free mass of the body.

m. number, the number expressive of the mass of a nucleus, being the total number of nucleons—protons and neutrons—in the nucleus of an atom or nuclide; symbol A.

massa (mas'ah), pl. *mas'sae* [L.] mass (1).

massage (mah-sahzh') systematic therapeutic stroking or kneading of the body.

auditory m., massage of the tympanic membrane.

cardiac m., intermittent compression of the heart by pressure applied over the sternum (closed cardiac massage) or directly to the heart through an opening in the chest wall (open cardiac massage). (See also CARDIAC MASSAGE.)

vibratory m., massage by rapidly repeated light percussion with a vibrating hammer or sound.

masseter muscle (mah-se'ter) the muscle that closes the jaws; see table of MUSCLES.

masseur (mah-ser') [Fr.] a man who performs massage.

masseuse (mah"sōōs') [Fr.] a woman who performs massage.

massotherapy (mas"o-ther'ah-pe) treatment of disease by massage.

mast cell (mast) a connective tissue cell whose specific physiologic function is unknown. It elaborates granules that contain histamine, heparin, and, in the rat and mouse, serotonin.

m. c. disease, urticaria pigmentosa.

m. c. tumor, a benign, local aggregation of mast cells forming a nodulous tumor.

mastadenitis (mas"tad-ĕ-ni'tis) inflammation of a mammary gland; mastitis.

mastalgia (mas-tal'je-ah) pain in the breast.

mastatrophy (mas-tat'ro-fe) atrophy of the breast.

mastectomy (mas-tek'to-me) surgical removal of breast tissue. Mastectomy is usually performed to treat malignant breast tumors, although rarely it may be advisable to use the procedure for benign tumors and for other diseases of the breast, such as chronic cystic mastitis. (See also surgery of the BREAST.)

radical m., amputation of the breast with wide excision of the pectoral muscles and axillary lymph nodes.

Master "2-step" exercise test (mas'ter) a test of coronary circulation, electrocardiographic tracings being recorded while the subject repeatedly ascends and descends two steps, each 9 inches high, then immediately after and 2 and 6 minutes after cessation of the climbs. The amount of work (number of trips) is standardized for age, weight, and sex.

mastication (mas"tĭ-ka'shun) the act of chewing.

masticatory (mas'tĭ-kah-tor"e) 1. pertaining to mastication. 2. a substance to be chewed, but not swallowed.

Mastigophora (mas"tĭ-gof'o-rah) a subphylum of protozoa, including all those that have one or more flagella throughout most of their life cycle, and a simple, centrally located nucleus; many are parasitic in both invertebrates and vertebrates, including man.

mastigote (mas'tĭ-gōt) any member of the Mastigophora.

mastitis (mas"ti'tis) inflammation of the BREAST, occurring in a variety of forms and in varying degrees of severity.

Chronic cystic mastitis is the most common disorder of the breast resulting from hormonal imbalance. This condition generally occurs in women between the ages of 30 and 50. It is probably related to the activity of the ovaries and is rare after the menopause.

The disease is characterized by the formation of cysts which give a lumpy appearance to the breast. Symptoms may include pain and tenderness, which are usually aggravated before the menstrual period, at which time the cysts tend to enlarge. There may also be discharge from the nipple. Periodic change in the size of a lump or its rapid appearance and disappearance is common in cystic mastitis. Since there are times when it may be difficult to distinguish this condition from cancer of the breast, biopsy may be necessary. Treatment may involve removing fluid from the cysts.

To help relieve the pain associated with cystic mastitis a good supporting brassiere that fits well and is not constricting should be worn day and night. Care should be taken to avoid injury to the breasts.

Young girls whose breasts are maturing sometimes experience a painful swelling and hardness of the breast, known as puberty mastitis. Occasionally a cloudy liquid may be squeezed from the nipples. The condition, rarely serious, usually subsides within a few weeks. It is best to wear a brassiere that gives mild support but does not irritate.

Enlargement of one or both breasts, gynecomastia, is sometimes found in adolescent boys and old men. The condition is usually due to excessive estrogenic activity. Secretions may be extruded from the nipple.

A mild inflammation known as stagnation mastitis, or caked breast, may occur during the early lactation period. Glands of the breast can become congested with milk, with formation of painful lumps.

Acute mastitis may occur after childbirth, when it is known as puerperal mastitis. It is an infection resulting usually from the presence of staphylococci and, occasionally, streptococci, which enter through cracks in the skin of the breast, particularly of the nipples. In puerperal mastitis, the breasts are tender, red, and warm. They become swollen and painful, and the inflammation responds quickly to sulfonamide medicines or one of the antibiotics, but in some cases an abscess may develop which must be incised and drained.

A milk cyst, galactocele, sometimes develops during lactation. It is probably caused by obstruction of a duct. The cyst can be removed after the baby has been weaned.

There are other types of infectious mastitis not related to lactation. Inflammation of the breast sometimes accompanies mumps, particularly in adults.

Tuberculous mastitis usually occurs in young women and accompanies tuberculosis of the lungs or of the cervical lymph nodes. Treatment is with antibiotics, although surgery is sometimes necessary.

A condition that may occur at the time of the menopause or later in women who have had children is comedomastitis, which is distention of the milk-producing ducts caused by the caking of secretions. Some of the material may be discharged from the nipple. Eventually the condition may develop into plasma cell mastitis. The breast may be tender and painful, with lump formation, nipple retraction, change in the breast contour, and possibly a cloudy discharge from the nipple.

Persistent cases of mastitis may require mastectomy.

masto- (mas'to) word element [Gr.], *mammary gland; breast.*

mastocyte (mas'to-sīt) a mast cell.

mastocytoma (mas"to-si-to'mah) a benign, local aggregation of mast cells forming a nodulous tumor.

mastocytosis (mas'to-si-to'sis) an accumulation, local or systemic, of mast cells in the tissues; known as urticaria pigmentosa when widespread in the skin.

mastodynia (mas"to-din'e-ah) pain in the breast.

mastography (mas-tog'rah-fe) roentgenography of the breast; mammography.

mastoid (mas'toid) 1. breast or nipple-shaped. 2. the mastoid process. 3. pertaining to the mastoid process.

m. antrum, an air space in the mastoid portion of the temporal bone communicating with the middle ear and the mastoid cells.

m. bone, mastoid process.

m. cells, hollow spaces of various size and shape in the mastoid process of the temporal bone, communicating with the mastoid antrum and lined with a continuation of its mucous membrane.

m. process, the conical projection at the base of the mastoid portion of the temporal bone.

mastoidalgia (mas"toi-dal'je-ah) pain in the mastoid region.

mastoidectomy (mas"toi-dek'to-me) surgical removal of mastoid cells. The most frequent indication for mastoidectomy is chronic infection in the mastoid process occurring as a complication of chronic OTITIS MEDIA. The extent of surgery depends on extent of destruction. A radical mastoidectomy involves removal of diseased portions of the mastoid process as well as the incus and malleus of the middle ear and the tympanic membrane. The degree of hearing loss following mastoidectomy depends on the extent of surgery. In some cases tympanoplasty (plastic reconstruction of the middle ear) can preserve much of the hearing. (For nursing care after ear surgery, see EAR.)

mastoideocentesis (mas-toi"de-o-sen-te'sis) paracentesis of the mastoid cells.

mastoiditis (mas"toi-di'tis) inflammation of the mastoid antrum and cells. It is usually the result of an infection of the middle ear, with which the mastoid cells communicate. Mastoiditis most commonly follows sore throat and respiratory infection, but it can also be caused by such diseases as diphtheria, measles, and scarlet fever.

The symptoms include earache and a ringing in the ears. The mastoid process may become painful and swollen.

Treatment formerly was limited to mastoidectomy, in which infected cells are removed surgically. Today, however, the development of antibiotics has made it possible to check most cases of mastoiditis at an early stage, so that surgery usually is avoided.

mastoidotomy (mas"toi-dot'o-me) incision of the mastoid process of the temporal bone.

mastology (mas-tol'o-je) study of the mammary gland.

mastoncus (mas-tong'kus) a tumor or swelling of the breast.

masto-occipital (mas"to-ok-sip"ĭ-tal) pertaining to the mastoid process and occipital bone.

mastopathy (mas-top'ah-the) any disease of the mammary gland.

mastoparietal (mas"to-pah-ri'ĕ-tal) pertaining to the mastoid process and parietal bone.

mastopexy (mas'to-pek"se) surgical fixation of a pendulous breast.

mastoplasia (mas"to-pla'ze-ah) mammoplasia.

mastoplasty (mas'to-plas"te) mammoplasty.

mastoptosis (mas'to-to'sis) a pendulous condition of the breast.

mastorrhagia (mas"to-ra'je-ah) hemorrhage from the mammary gland.

mastoscirrhus (mas"to-skir'us) hardening of the mammary gland.

mastosquamous (mas"to-skwa'mus) pertaining to the mastoid and squama of the temporal bone.

mastotomy (mas-tot'o-me) incision of a mammary gland.

masturbation (mas"tur-ba'shun) sexual gratification by self-manipulation of the genitalia. Masturbation is too often thought of as shameful and unwholesome. Many harmful effects have mistakenly been attributed to it. We now know that the desire to masturbate is part of the normal process of sexual development. The real harm in masturbation is psychologic because it may evoke deep feelings of guilt, anxiety, and fear. A large number of boys and girls have experimented with masturbation during their growing years.

matching (mach′ing) comparison for the purpose of selecting objects having similar or identical characteristics.

m. of blood, comparing the blood of a contemplated donor with that of the recipient to ascertain whether their bloods belong to the same group.

cross m., determination of the compatibility of the blood of a donor and that of a recipient before transfusion by placing erythrocytes of the donor in the recipients's serum and erythrocytes of the recipient in the donor's serum. Absence of agglutination indicates that the two blood samples belong to the same group and are compatible.

materia medica (mah-tēr′e-ah med′ĭ-kah) pharmacology.

maternal (mah-ter′nal) pertaining to the female parent.

maternity (mah-ter′nĭ-te) motherhood.

matrix (ma′triks), pl. *mat′rices* [L.] 1. the groundwork on which anything is cast, or the basic material from which a thing develops.

bone m., the intercellular substance of bone, consisting of collagenous fibers, ground substance, and inorganic salts.

nail m., m. un′guis, the nail bed.

matter (mat′er) physical material having form and weight under ordinary conditions of gravity.

maturation (mat″u-ra′shun) 1. the stage or process of attaining maximal development; attainment of maximal intellectual and emotional development. In biology, a process of cell division during which the number of chromosomes in the germ cell is reduced to one-half the number characteristic of the species. 2. the formation of pus.

Maurer's dots (mow′rerz) irregular dots, staining red with Leishman's stain, seen in erythrocytes infected with *Plasmodium falciparum.*

maxilla (mak-sil′ah) pl. *maxil′lae* [*L.*], *maxil′las* one of two identical bones that form the upper jaw. The maxillae meet in the midline of the face and often are considered as one bone. They have been described as the architectural key of the face because all bones of the face except the mandible touch them. Together the maxillae form the floor of the orbit for each eye, the sides and lower walls of the nasal cavities, and the hard palate. The lower border of the maxilla supports the upper teeth. Each maxilla contains an air space called the maxillary sinus.

maxillofacial (mak-sil″o-fa′shal) pertaining to the maxilla and the face.

maxillomandibular (mak″sil″o-man-dib′u-lar) pertaining to the upper and lower jaws.

maxillotomy (mak″sĭ-lot′o-me) surgical sectioning of the maxilla which allows movement of all or part of the maxilla into the desired position.

maximum (mak′sĭ-mum) the greatest quantity, effect, or value possible or achieved under given circumstances. adj., **max′imal.**

tubular m., the highest rate in milligrams per minute at which the renal tubules can transfer artificially administered test substances; the maximal tubular excretory capacity. Abbreviated Tm.

Maxitate (mak′sĭ-tāt) trademark for preparations of mannitol hexanitrate, a vasodilator.

maze (māz) a complicated system of intersecting paths used in intelligence tests and in demonstrating learning in experimental animals.

M.B. Bachelor of Medicine.

M.C. [L.] *Ma′gister Chirur′giae* (Master of Surgery); Medical Corps.

Mc megacurie.

mc. millicurie.

μc. microcurie.

McArdle's disease (mak-ar′d′lz) glycogenosis (type V) in which a deficiency of muscle phosphorylase results in accumulation of glycogen in skeletal muscles, with muscle cramps and a depressed blood lactate level during exercise. Called also myophosphorylase deficiency glycogenosis.

McBurney's point (mak-ber′nēz) the point of special tenderness in acute appendicitis; situated about 2 inches from the right anterior superior spine of the ilium, on a line between this spine and the umbilicus. It corresponds with the normal position of the appendix.

McBurney's sign (mak-ber′nēz) special tenderness at McBurney's point; indicative of appendicitis.

mcg. microgram.

MCH mean corpuscular hemoglobin, an expression of the average hemoglobin content of a single cell in micromicrograms (picograms), obtained by multiplying the hemoglobin in grams by 10 and dividing by the number of erythrocytes (in millions).

MCHC mean corpuscular hemoglobin concentration, an expression of the average hemoglobin concentration in per cent, obtained by multiplying the hemoglobin in grams by 100 and dividing by the hematocrit determination.

mCi millicurie.

μCi microcurie.

McMurray's sign (mak-mur′ēz) occurrence of a cartilage click during manipulation of the knee; indicative of menisceal injury.

MCV 1. mean corpuscular volume, an expression of the average volume of individual red cells in cubic microns, obtained by multiplying the hematocrit determination by 10 and dividing by the number of erythrocytes (in millions). 2. mean clinical value, obtained by assigning a numerical value to the response noted in a number of patients receiving a specific treatment, adding these numbers and dividing by the number of patients treated.

M.D. Doctor of Medicine.

Md chemical symbol, *mendelevium.*

meal (mēl) a portion of food or foods taken at some particular and usually stated or fixed time. (See also TEST MEAL.)

mean (mēn) an average; a numerical value intermediate between two extremes.

measles (me′zelz) a highly contagious illness caused by a virus; called also rubeola. Measles is usually a childhood disease but it can be contracted at any age. Epidemics of measles usually recur every 2 or 3 years and are most common in the winter and spring. In spite of the availability of a vaccine and intensive effort on the part of public health personnel to eradicate the disease, the incidence of measles in the United States rose from approximately 23,000 cases in 1968 to more than 74,000 in 1971.

CAUSE. The virus that causes measles is spread by droplet infection. The virus can also be picked up by touching an article, such as a handkerchief, that an infected person has recently used.

The incubation period is usually 11 days, although it may be as few as 9 or as many as 14. The patient can transmit the disease from 3 or 4 days before the rash appears until the rash begins to fade, a total of about 7 or 8 days. One attack of measles usually gives a lifetime immunity to rubeola but not to German measles (RUBELLA), which is somewhat similar to ordinary measles.

SYMPTOMS. Measles symptoms generally appear in two stages. In the first stage the patient feels tired and uncomfortable, and may have a running nose, a cough, a slight fever, and pains in the head and back. The eyes may become reddened and sensitive to light. The fever rises a little each day.

The second stage begins at the end of the third or beginning of the fourth day. The patient's temperature is generally between 103° and 104° F. Koplik's spots, small white dots like grains of salt surrounded by inflamed areas, can often be seen on the gums and the inside of the cheeks. A rash appears, starting at the hairline and behind the ears and spreading downward, covering the body in about 36 hours. At first the rash consists of separate pink spots, about a quarter of an inch in diameter, but later some of the spots may run together, giving the patient a blotchy look. The fever usually subsides after the rash has spread. The rash turns brownish and fades after 3 or 4 days.

The most serious complication of rubeola is encephalitis, which occurs in about 0.1% of all cases and is responsible for an estimated 600 cases of mental retardation each year. Other complications include pneumonia, otitis media, and mastoiditis.

PATIENT CARE. The patient should be kept in bed as long as the rash and fever continue, and should get as much rest as possible. Aspirin, nose drops, and cough medicine may be prescribed during this stage. Water and fluids can be given for fever. The sickroom should be well ventilated and fairly warm. If the patient's eyes are sensitive to light, strong sunlight should be kept out of the room.

The rash may itch a great deal and prevent the patient from resting. If so, calamine lotion, cornstarch solution, or plain cool water will afford some relief. If the itching continues, antihistamine drugs may be necessary.

Measles can greatly lower the body's resistance to other infections such as bronchitis, pneumonia, and ear infection. If the patient's temperature remains high for more than 2 days after the rash fades, or if he complains of pain in the ear, throat, chest, or abdomen, medical attention should be obtained without delay.

PREVENTION. The first measles vaccine was developed and made available in the early 1960's. It consisted of killed viruses and is now known to have conferred little or no immunity and, in addition, made the person susceptible to the development of atypical measles when exposed to the disease. Children who received this type of vaccine should be given the newer live vaccine in order to be protected against the disease. The live measles virus vaccine confers lifelong immunity in 95% of those who receive potent vaccine. A 12 to 20% potency failure can occur when the vaccine is not stored and refrigerated properly.

The live vaccine usually is given when the child is one year of age. Until then the child is protected by the temporary immunity acquired from its mother. Children must be given the vaccine before exposure to measles, or within 48 hours after exposure, otherwise the vaccine is ineffective. If the vaccine cannot be given to a child exposed to measles, he is given measles immune globulin (MIG) or the standard immune serum globulin; a waiting period of three months is then necessary before he is given the measles vaccine. The vaccine is contraindicated during pregnancy.

A person with measles is placed under respiratory precautions from the time symptoms appear until seven days after the rash disappears.

A child with measles should be placed under respiratory ISOLATION as long as the disease lasts. Anyone with a cold or cough should be kept away from the patient because another infection can cause serious complications.

The best method is to isolate the child from 3 or 4 days before the rash appears until his temperature is normal and the rash has begun to fade. When the child is well again, the sickroom should be thoroughly cleaned and aired.

measure (mezh′er) see Tables of Weights and Measures in Appendix.

meatorrhaphy (me″ah-tor′ah-fe) suture of the cut end of the urethra to the glans penis after incision for enlarging the urinary meatus.

meatoscopy (me″ah-tos′ko-pe) visual examination of any meatus, especially the urinary meatus or the ureteral orifices.

meatotomy (me″ah-tot′o-me) incison of the urinary meatus in order to enlarge it.

meatus (me-a′tus), pl. *mea′tus* [L.] an opening or passage. adj., **mea′tal.**

acoustic m., m. acus′ticus, m. audito′rius, auditory m., a passage in the ear, one leading to the eardrum (external acoustic meatus) and one for passage of nerves and blood vessels (internal acoustic meatus).

m. na′si, m. of nose, one of the three portions of the nasal cavity on either side of the septum, inferior, middle, or superior (mea′tus na′si infe′rior, me′dius, supe′rior).

m. urina′rius, urinary m., the opening of the urethra on the body surface through which urine is discharged.

Mebaral (meb′ah-ral) trademark for a preparation of mephobarbital, an anticonvulsant with a slight hypnotic action.

mebendazole (mĕ-ben′dah-zōl) an anthelmintic, highly effective against *Trichuris trichura* (whipworm), *Enterobius vermicularis* (pinworm), and hookworm. Its action is achieved by blocking the glucose uptake of susceptible parasites.

mebeverine (mē-bev′er-ēn) a smooth muscle relaxant used as the hydrochloride salt.

mebutamate (meb′u-tam″āt) a compound used to reduce blood pressure.

mecamine (mek′ah-min) mecamylamine.

mecamylamine (mek″ah-mil′ah-min) a ganglionic blocking agent used in the form of the hydrochloride salt as an antihypertensive.

mechanics (mĕ-kan′iks) the science dealing with the motions of material bodies.

body m., the application of kinesiology to use of

the body in daily life activities and to the prevention and correction of problems related to posture.

mechanism (mek′ah-nizm) 1. a machine or machine-like structure. 2. the manner of combination of parts, processes, etc., which subserve a common function.

defense m., escape m., a mental mechanism by which psychic tension is diminished, e.g., repression, denial, overcompensation, rationalization, etc.

mental m., 1. the organization of mental operations. 2. an unconscious and indirect manner of gratifying a repressed desire.

mechanoreceptor (mek″ah-no-re-sep′tor) a nerve ending sensitive to mechanical pressures or distortions, as those responding to touch and muscle contractions.

mechanotherapy (mek″ah-no-ther′ah-pe) use of mechanical apparatus in treatment of disease or its results, especially in therapeutic exercises.

mechlorethamine (mĕ″klōr-eth′ah-mēn) a nitrogen mustard compound used as an antineoplastic agent.

Mecholyl (me′ko-lil) trademark for preparations of methacholine, a parasympathomimetic.

Meckel's diverticulum (mek′elz) a congenital sac or appendage occasionally found in the ileum; a relic of a fetal structure that connects the yolk sac with the intestinal cavity of the embryo.

meclizine (mek′lĭ-zēn) an antinauseant, used as the hydrochloride salt.

mecloqualon (mek″lo-kwal′ōn) a sedative and hypnotic.

meconium (mĕ-ko′ne-um) dark green mucilaginous material in the intestine of the full-term fetus; it constitutes the first stools passed by the newborn infant.

m. ileus, intestinal obstruction in the newborn due to the blocking of the bowels with thick meconium.

M.E.D. minimal effective dose; minimal erythema dose.

Medazepam (mĕ-daz′ĕ-pam) a minor tranquilizer.

Medex (med′eks) a physician assistant program for former military medical corpsmen; also, a graduate of such a program.

media (me′de-ah) [L.] 1. plural of *medium.* 2. middle, especially the middle coat of a blood vessel, or tunica media.

medial pertaining to or situated toward the midline.

medialis (me″de-a′lis) [L.] medial.

median (me′de-an) 1. situated in the median plane or in the midline of a body or structure. 2. the perpendicular line that divides the area of a frequency curve into two equal halves.

m. nerve, a nerve that originates in the brachial plexus and innervates muscles of the wrist and hand; see table of NERVES.

m. plane, an imaginary plane passing longitudinally through the body from front to back and dividing it into right and left halves.

mediastinal (me″de-as-ti′nal) of or pertaining to the mediastinum.

m. flutter, movement of the tissues and organs of the mediastinum back and forth with each movement of air in and out of an open sucking wound in the thoracic cavity. The condition can produce serious impairment of cardiopulmonary function and is fatal if not treated promptly. Symptoms are similar to those of mediastinal shift.

m. shift, a shifting or moving of the tissues and organs that comprise the mediastinum (heart, great vessels, trachea, and esophagus) to one side of the chest cavity. The condition occurs when a severe injury to the chest causes the entrapment of air in the pleural space (tension PNEUMOTHORAX). As the volume of air increases on the affected side, the lung collapses and the organs and tissues of the mediastinum are crowded to the opposite side of the chest. This can produce compression of the other lung and kinking or twisting of one or more of the great blood vessels, which in turn seriously impairs blood flow to and from the heart.

Symptoms of mediastinal shift include severe dyspnea, cyanosis, displacement of the trachea to one side, and distended neck veins. The immediate treatment is insertion of a hollow needle or trochar into the pleural space (THORACENTESIS) to provide an outlet for the escape of air and fluid. After the trapped air is released, closed chest drainage is initiated to allow for reexpansion of the lung.

mediastinitis (me″de-as″tĭ-ni′tis) inflammation of the mediastinum.

mediastinography (me″de-as″tĭ-nog′rah-fe) roentgenography of the structures of the mediastinum.

mediastinopericarditis (me″de-as″tĭ-no-per″ĭ-kar-di′tis) inflammation of the mediastinum and pericardium.

mediastinoscopy (me″de-as″tĭ-nos′ko-pe) endoscopic examination of the mediastinum.

mediastinotomy (me″de-as″tĭ-not′o-me) incision of the mediastinum.

mediastinum (me″de-ah-sti′num), pl. *mediasti′na* [L.] 1. a median septum or partition. 2. the mass of tissues and organs separating the sternum in front and the vertebral column behind, containing the heart and its large vessels, trachea, esophagus, thymus, lymph nodes, and other structures and tissues. It is divided into anterior, middle, posterior, and superior regions.

m. tes′tis, a partial septum of the testis formed near its posterior border by a continuation of the tunica albuginea.

medicable (med′ĭ-kah-b′l) subject to treatment with medicine with reasonable expectation of cure.

Medicaid (med′ĭ-kād) a state-operated program providing medical care to certain low-income persons; the state programs receive federal aid and are subject to federal guidelines.

medical laboratory technologist one who is skilled in the performance and interpretation of results of clinical laboratory procedures used in the diagnosis of disease and evaluation of patient progress. The medical laboratory technologist has completed four or more years of specialized education in medical technology. Graduates of programs approved by the American Medical Association are eligible to take certification examinations administered by the Board of Medical Technologists of the American Society of Clinical Pathology. Licensure is required by some states in the United States.

A second type of medical laboratory personnel is the *medical technician,* who has received formal training in a two-year associate degree program at a community college, a vocational technical school, or a private school.

In recent years there has been a trend toward academic programs to train *laboratory assistants.* Graduates of approved programs are eligible for state certification as Certified Laboratory Assistants (CLA).

Further information about medical laboratory personnel and their qualifications may be obtained by writing to the American Society of Medical Technologists, Suite 1600, Herman Professional Building, Houston, TX 77025; or to the American Medical Technologists, 710 Higgins Rd., Park Ridge, IL 60068.

medical record librarian one who supervises the indexing, recording, and storage of medical records and reports of patients admitted to hospitals and other health care agencies. She also prepares reports of births, deaths, transfers, and discharges of patients and the treatments received.

The registered record librarian (RRL) must have graduated from an approved school of medical record science and successfully completed the registration examination of the American Association of Medical Record Librarians, 211 East Chicago Ave., Chicago, IL 60611.

medicament (mĕ-dik′ah-ment, med′ĭ-kah-ment) a medicinal agent.

Medicare (med′ĭ-kār) a program of the Social Security Administration which provides medical care to the aged and to certain others.

medicated (med′ĭ-kāt″ed) imbued with a medicinal substance.

medication (med″ĭ-ka′shun) 1. administration of remedies. 2. a medicinal agent. 3. impregnation with a medicine.

medicinal (mĕ-dis′ĭ-nal) having healing qualities; pertaining to a medicine.

medicine (med′ĭ-sin) 1. any drug or remedy. 2. the art and science of the diagnosis and treatment of disease and the maintenance of health. 3. the nonsurgical treatment of disease.

aviation m., that branch of medicine which deals with the physiologic, medical, psychologic, and epidemiologic problems involved in flying.

clinical m., 1. the study of disease by direct examination of the living patient. 2. the last two years of the usual curriculum in a medical college.

experimental m., study of the science of healing diseases based on experimentation in animals.

family m., the medical specialty concerned with planning and provision of comprehensive primary health care for all family members, regardless of age or sex, on a continuing basis.

forensic m., the application of medical knowledge to questions of law; medical jurisprudence. Called also legal medicine.

group m., the practice of medicine by a group of physicians, usually representing various specialties, who are associated together for the cooperative diagnosis, treatment, and prevention of disease.

internal m., that dealing especially with diagnosis and medical treatment of diseases and disorders of internal structures of the body.

legal m., forensic medicine.

nuclear m., that branch of medicine concerned with the use of radionuclides in the diagnosis and treatment of disease.

patent m., a drug or remedy protected by a trademark, available without a prescription.

physical m., that branch of medicine using physical agents in the diagnosis and treatment of disease. It includes the use of heat, cold, light, water, electricity, manipulation, massage, exercise, and mechanical devices.

preclinical m., the subjects studied in medicine before the student observes actual diseases in patients.

preventive m., science aimed at preventing disease.

proprietary m., any chemical, drug, or similar preparation used in the treatment of diseases, if such article is protected against free competition as to name, product, composition, or process of manufacture by secrecy, patent, trademark, or copyright, or by other means.

psychosomatic m., the study of the interrelations between bodily processes and emotional life.

socialized m., a system of medical care regulated and controlled by the government. Called also state medicine.

space m., that branch of aviation medicine concerned with conditions to be encountered in space.

state m., socialized medicine.

tropical m., medical science as applied to diseases occurring primarily in the tropics and subtropics.

veterinary m., the diagnosis and treatment of the diseases of animals.

medicolegal (med″ĭ-ko-le′gal) pertaining to medicine and law, or to forensic medicine.

medionecrosis (me″de-o-nĕ-kro′sis) focal areas of destruction of the elastic tissue and smooth muscle of the tunica media of a blood vessel, especially of the aorta or its major branches.

mediotarsal (me″de-o-tar′sal) pertaining to the center of the tarsus.

Mediterranean anemia, disease (med″ĭ-tĕ-ra′ne-an) the homozygous form of β-THALASSEMIA.

Mediterranean fever, familial a hereditary disease usually occurring in Armenians and Sephardic Jews, and marked by short recurrent attacks of fever with pain in the abdomen, chest, or joints, and erythema resembling that seen in erysipelas; it is sometimes complicated by amyloidosis.

medium (me′de-um), pl. *me′dia, mediums* [L.] 1. an agent by which something is accomplished or an impulse is transmitted. 2. a substance providing the proper nutritional environment for the growth of microorganisms; called also culture medium.

contrast m., a radiopaque substance used in roentgenography to permit visualization of body structures.

culture m., a substance used to support the growth of microorganisms or other cells.

dioptric media, refracting media.

disperse m., dispersion m., the continuous phase of a colloid system; the medium in which a colloid is dispersed, corresponding to the solvent in a true solution.

refracting media, the transparent tissues and fluid in the eye through which light rays pass and by which they are refracted and brought to a focus on the retina.

medius (me′de-us) [L.] situated in the middle.

Medomin (med′o-min) trademark for a preparation of heptabarbital, a short- to intermediate-acting barbiturate.

medrogestone (med″ro-jes′tōn) a progestational agent.

Medrol (med′rol) trademark for a preparation of methylprednisolone, an anti-inflammatory steroid.

medroxyprogesterone (med-rok″sĭ-pro-jes′tĕ-rōn) a compound used as a progestational agent.

medulla (mĕ-dul′ah), pl. *medul′lae* [L.] the central or inner portion of an organ. adj., **med′ullary.**

adrenal m., the inner portion of the ADRENAL GLAND, where epinephrine is produced.

m. of bone, bone MARROW, contained in the medullary canal of bone.

m. oblonga′ta, that part of the hindbrain continuous with the pons above and the spinal cord below; it houses nerve centers for both motor and sensory nerves, where such functions as breathing and the beating of the heart are controlled (see also BRAIN).

m. os′sium, bone marrow.

renal m., the inner part of the substance of the kidney, composed chiefly of collecting tubules, and organized into a group of structures called the renal pyramids.

spinal m., m. spina′lis, spinal cord.

medullated (med′u-lāt″ed) myelinated; equipped with myelin sheaths.

medullization (med″u-lĭ-za′shun) the enlargement of the haversian canals in rarefying osteitis followed by their conversion into marrow channels; also the replacement of bone by marrow cells.

medulloadrenal (mĕ-dul″o-ah-dre′nal) pertaining to the adrenal medulla.

medulloblast (mĕ-dul′o-blast) an undifferentiated cell of the neural tube that may develop into either a neuroblast or spongioblast.

medulloblastoma (mĕ-dul″o-blas-to′mah) a brain tumor composed of medulloblasts.

medulloepithelioma (mĕ-dul″o-ep″ĭ-the″le-o′-mah) a brain tumor composed of primitive neuroepithelial cells lining the tubular spaces.

mega- (meg′ah) word element [Gr.], *large;* used in naming units of measurement to designate an amount 10^6 (one million) times the size of the unit to which it is joined, as megacuries (10^6 curies); abbreviation M.

megabladder (meg″ah-blad′er) permanent overdistention of the bladder.

megacaryocyte (meg″ah-kar′e-o-sīt″) megakaryocyte.

megacolon (meg″ah-ko′lon) dilatation and hypertrophy of the colon.

acquired m., colonic enlargement associated with chronic constipation, but with normal ganglion cell innervation.

aganglionic m., congenital m., that due to congenital absence of myenteric ganglion cells in a distal segment of the large bowel, with resultant loss of motor function in the aganglionic segment and massive hypertrophic dilatation of the normal proximal colon. Called also Hirschsprung's disease.

megacurie (meg″ah-ku′re) a unit of radioactivity, being one million (10^6) curies; abbreviated Mc.

megadyne (meg′ah-dīn) one million dynes.

megaesophagus (meg″ah-e-sof′ah-gus) dilatation and muscular hypertrophy of most of the esophagus, above a constricted, often atrophied, distal segment. See also ACHALASIA.

megahertz (meg′ah-hertz) one million (10^6) hertz; abbrevated MHz.

megakaryoblast (meg″ah-kar′e-o-blast) an immature megakaryocyte.

megakaryocyte (meg″ah-kar′e-o-sīt″) the giant cell of bone marrow; it is a large cell with a greatly lobulated nucleus, and is generally supposed to give rise to blood platelets.

megakaryocytosis (meg″ah-kar″e-o-si-to′sis) the presence of megakaryocytes in the blood or of excessive numbers in the bone marrow.

megakaryophthisis (meg″ah-kar″e-o-thi′sis) deficiency of megakaryocytes in bone marrow.

megal(o)- (meg′ah-lo) word element [Gr.], *large; abnormal enlargement.*

megalencephaly (meg″ah-len-sef′ah-le) macrencephalia; hypertrophy of the brain.

megalgia (meg-al′je-ah) a severe pain.

megaloblast (meg′ah-lo-blast″) a large, nucleated immature progenitor of an abnormal erythrocytic series; megaloblasts are present in the blood in certain anemias. adj., **megaloblas′tic.**

megalocardia (meg″ah-lo-kar′de-ah) cardiomegaly; enlargement of the heart.

megalocephaly (meg″ah-lo-sef′ah-le) abnormally increased size of the head.

megalocheiria (meg″ah-lo-ki′re-ah) abnormal largeness of the hands.

megalocornea (meg″ah-lo-kor′ne-ah) a developmental anomaly of the cornea, which is of abnormal size at birth and continues to grow, sometimes reaching a diameter of 14 or 15 mm. in the adult.

megalocystis (meg″ah-lo-sis′tis) an abnormally enlarged bladder.

megalocyte (meg′ah-lo-sīt″) an extremely large erythrocyte.

megalodactyly (meg″ah-lo-dak′tĭ-le) excessive size of the fingers or toes.

megaloenteron (meg″ah-lo-en′ter-on) enlargement of the intestine.

megaloesophagus (meg″ah-lo-e-sof′ah-gus) megaesophagus.

megalogastria (meg″ah-lo-gas′tre-ah) enlargement of the stomach.

megaloglossia (meg″ah-lo-glos′e-ah) macroglossia; hypertrophy of the tongue.

megalohepatia (meg″ah-lo-he-pat′e-ah) enlargement of the liver; hepatomegaly.

megalomania (meg″ah-lo-ma′ne-ah) a mental state characterized by delusions of exaggerated personal importance, wealth, power, etc.

megalomaniac (meg″ah-lo-ma′ne-ak) a person exhibiting megalomania.

megalomelia (meg″ah-lo-me′le-ah) abnormal largeness of the limbs.

megalonychosis (meg″ah-lo-nĭ-ko′sis) hypertrophy of the nails and their matrices.

megalopenis (meg″ah-lo-pe′nis) abnormal largeness of the penis.

megalophthalmos (meg″ah-lof-thal′mos) abnormally large size of the eyes; buphthalmos.

megalopodia (meg″ah-lo-po′de-ah) abnormal largeness of the feet.

megalopsia (meg″ah-lop′se-ah) macropsia.

megalosplenia (meg″ah-lo-sple′ne-ah) enlargement of the spleen; splenomegaly.

megalosyndactyly (meg″ah-lo-sin-dak′tĭ-le) a condition in which the digits are large and more or less webbed together.

megaloureter (meg″ah-lo-u-re′ter) enlargement of the ureter.

-megaly word element [Gr.], *enlargement.*

megarectum (meg″ah-rek′tum) a greatly dilated rectum.

megavitamin (meg″ah-vi′tah-min) a term denoting massive doses of vitamins.

megavolt (meg′ah-volt) one million volts.

megestrol (mĕ-jes′trōl) a synthetic progestational agent.

Megimide (meg′ĭ-mīd) trademark for a preparation of bemegride, an analeptic used in barbiturate poisoning.

meglumine (meg′loo-mēn) a crystalline base used in preparing salts of certain acids for use as diagnostic radiopaque media. Meglumine diatrizoate is used in angiocardiography and excretory urography; meglumine iodipamide is used in cholecystography; and meglumine iothalamate is used in cerebral angiography, excretory urography, and peripheral arteriography. Called also methylglucamine.

megohm (meg′ōm) one million ohms.

megophthalmos (meg″of-thal′mos) abnormally large eyes.

megrim (me′grim) migraine.

meibomian cyst (mi-bo′me-an) a small retention cyst of the meibomian gland, a sebaceous follicle of the eyelid; called also CHALAZION.

meiogenic (mi″o-jen′ik) promoting meiosis.

meiosis (mi-o′sis) a special method of cell division occurring in maturation of sex cells, wherein, over two successive cell divisions, each daughter nucleus receives half the number of chromosomes typical of the somatic cells of the species, so that the gametes are haploid. adj., **meiot′ic.**

melalgia (mel-al′je-ah) pain in the limbs.

melan(o)- word element [Gr.], *black; melanin.*

melancholia (mel″an-ko′le-ah) a mental state characterized by extreme sadness or depression, with inhibition of mental and physical activity. adj., **melanchol′ic.**

affective m., melancholia corresponding to the depressive phase of manic-depressive psychosis (see also affective PSYCHOSIS).

involutional m., an affective disorder occurring in late middle life, with agitation, worry, anxiety, somatic preoccupations, insomnia, and sometimes paranoid reactions.

mélangeur (ma-lan-zher′) [Fr.] an instrument for drawing and diluting specimens of blood for examination.

melaniferous (mel″ah-nif′er-us) containing melanin or other black pigment.

melanin (mel′ah-nin) a dark, sulfur-containing pigment normally found in the hair, skin, ciliary body, choroid of the eye, pigment layer of the retina, and certain nerve cells. It occurs abnormally in certain tumors, known as melanomas, and is sometimes excreted in the urine when such tumors are present (melanuria).

melanism (mel′ah-nizm) excessive deposit of melanin in the skin.

melanoameloblastoma (mel″ah-no-ah-mel″o-blas-to′mah) melanotic neuroectodermal tumor.

melanoblast (mel′ah-no-blast″) a cell that develops into a melanocyte.

melanoblastoma (mel″ah-no-blas-to′mah) melanotic neuroectodermal tumor.

melanocarcinoma (mel″ah-no-kar″sĭ-no′mah) malignant melanoma.

melanocyte (mel′ah-no-sīt″, mĕ-lan′o-sīt) the cell which produces the melanin-synthesizing organelle melanosome. adj., **melanocyt′ic.**

m.-stimulating hormone, MSH, a peptide from the anterior pituitary that influences the formation or deposition of melanin in the body.

melanoderma (mel″ah-no-der′mah) an abnormally increased amount of melanin in the skin.

melanodermatitis (mel″ah-no-der″mah-ti′tis) dermatitis with a deposit of melanin in the skin.

melanogen (mĕ-lan′o-jen) a colorless chromogen, convertible into melanin, which may occur in the urine in certain diseases.

melanogenesis (mel″ah-no-jen′ĕ-sis) the production of melanin.

melanoglossia (mel″ah-no-glos′e-ah) blackening and elongation of the papillae of the tongue; black tongue.

melanoid (mel′ah-noid) 1. resembling melanin. 2. a substance resembling melanin.

melanoleukoderma (mel″ah-no-lu″ko-der′mah) a mottled appearance of the skin.

m. col′li, a mottled appearance of the skin of the neck and adjacent regions, a rare manifestation of syphilis.

melanoma (mel″ah-no′mah) 1. any tumor composed of melanin-pigmented cells. 2. malignant melanoma.

juvenile m., a benign, pink to purplish red papule, usually on the face, especially the cheeks, most commonly originating before puberty; histologically, it suggests and has been mistaken for malignant melanoma.

malignant m., a malignant tumor, usually developing from a nevus and consisting of black masses of cells with a marked tendency to metastasis.

melanomatosis (mel″ah-no-mah-to′sis) the formation of melanomas throughout the body.

melanonychia (mel″ah-no-nik′e-ah) blackening of the nails by melanin pigmentation.

melanophage (mel′ah-no-fāj″) a histiocyte laden with phagocytosed melanin.

melanophore (mel′ah-no-fōr″) a pigment cell containing melanin, especially such a cell from fishes, amphibians, and reptiles.

melanoplakia (mel″ah-no-pla′ke-ah) pigmented patches on the mucous membrane of the mouth.

melanosarcoma (mel″ah-no-sar-ko′mah) malignant melanoma.

melanosis (mel″ah-no′sis) 1. a condition characterized by dark pigmentary deposits. 2. a disorder of pigment metabolism.

m. co′li, brown-black discoloration of the mucosa of the colon.

melanosome (mel′ah-no-sōm″) any of the granules within melanocytes that contain melanin.

melanotic (mel″ah-not′ik) characterized by the presence of melanin; pertaining to melanosis.

m. neuroectodermal tumor, a benign, rapidly

growing, dark tumor of the jaw and occasionally of other sites; almost always seen in infants. Called also melanoameloblastoma.

melanotrichia (mel″ah-no-trik′e-ah) abnormally increased pigmentation of the hair.

melanuria (mel″ah-nu′re-ah) the discharge of darkly stained urine.

melasma (mĕ-laz′mah) dark pigmentaion of the skin; called also chloasma.

m. addiso′nii, Addison's disease.

m. gravida′rum, that occurring on the face during pregnancy (mask of pregnancy).

melatonin (mel″ah-to′nin) a tryptamine derivative formed in the mammalian pineal body; it inhibits ovarian growth and estrus in certain mammals. It also causes concentration of melanophores in amphibians. Melatonin appears to be inactive in humans.

melena (mĕ-le′nah) darkening of the feces by blood pigments.

melengestrol (mel″en-jes′trōl) a progestin and antineoplastic.

melioidosis (mel″e-oi-do′sis) a glanders-like disease of rodents, transmissible to man, and caused by *Pseudomonas pseudomallei.*

melitagra (mel″ĭ-tag′rah) eczema with honeycomb crusts.

melitoptyalism (mel″ĭ-to-ti′ah-lizm) secretion of saliva containing glucose.

melituria (mel″ĭ-tu′re-ah) the presence of any sugar in the urine.

Mellaril (mel′ah-ril) trademark for preparations of thioridazine hydrochloride, a tranquilizer.

melomelus (mĕ-lom′ĕ-lus) a fetus with supernumerary limbs.

meloplasty (mel′o-plas″te) plastic surgery of the cheek.

melorheostosis (mel″o-re″os-to′sis) a form of osteosclerosis, with linear tracks extending through the long bones.

melotia (mĕ-lo′she-ah) congenital displacement of the auricle of the ear onto the cheek.

melphalan (mel′fah-lan) an alkylating antineoplastic agent.

member (mem′ber) a distinct part of the body, especially a limb.

membra (mem′bra) [L.] plural of *membrum.*

membrana (mem-bra′nah), pl. *membra′nae* [L.] membrane.

membrane (mem′brān) a thin layer of tissue that covers a surface, lines a cavity, or divides a space or organ. adj., **mem′branous.**

alveolodental m., periodontium.

arachnoid m., arachnoid; one of the layers of the meninges.

basement m., the delicate layer underlying the epithelium of mucous membranes and secreting glands.

basilar m., the lower boundary of the scala media of the ear.

Bowman's m., a thin layer of basement membrane between the outer layer of stratified epitheliium and the substantia propria of the cornea.

Bruch's m., the inner layer of the choroid, separating it from the pigmented layer of the retina.

cell m., the condensed protoplasm that forms the enveloping capsule of a cell. See also unit MEMBRANE.

decidual m's, deciduous m's, see DECIDUA.

Descemet's m., the posterior lining membrane of the cornea; it is a thin hyaline membrane between the substantia propria and the endothelial layer of the cornea.

diphtheritic m., the peculiar false membrane characteristic of diphtheria, formed by coagulation necrosis.

drum m., tympanic membrane.

false m., a membranous exudate, like the diphtheritic membrane.

fenestrated m., one of the perforated elastic sheets of the tunica intima and tunica media of arteries.

fetal m's, the membranes that protect the embryo and provide for its nutrition, respiration, and excretion: the yolk sac (umbilical vesicle), allantois, amnion, chorion, decidua, and placenta.

Henle's m., fenestrated membrane.

hyaline m., 1. a membrane between the outer root sheath and inner fibrous layer of a hair follicle. 2. basement membrane. 3. a homogeneous eosinophilic membrane lining alveolar ducts and alveoli, frequently found at necropsy in premature infants (see also HYALINE MEMBRANE DISEASE).

hyoglossal m., a fibrous lamina connecting the under surface of the tongue with the hyoid bone.

limiting m., one that constitutes the border of some tissue or structure.

mucous m., the membrane covered with epithelium that lines the tubular organs of the body.

nuclear m., the condensed double layer enclosing the nucleoplasm, separating it from the cytoplasm.

olfactory m., the olfactory portion of the mucous membrane lining the nasal fossa.

placental m., the semipermeable membrane that separates the fetal from the maternal blood in the placenta.

plasma m., cell membrane.

Reissner's m., the thin anterior wall of the cochlear duct, separating it from the scala vestibuli.

Scarpa's m., tympanic membrane, secondary.

semipermeable m., one permitting passage through it of some but not all substances.

serous m., the membrane lining the walls of the body cavities and enclosing the contained organs; it consists of mesothelium lying upon a connective tissue layer and it secretes a watery fluid.

synovial m., the inner of the two layers of the articular capsule of a synovial joint; composed of loose connective tissue and having a free smooth surface that lines the joint cavity.

tympanic m., the eardrum; the membrane marking the inner termination of the external acoustic meatus, separating it from the middle ear (see also TYMPANIC MEMBRANE).

tympanic m., secondary, the membrane enclosing the fenestra cochlearis; called also Scarpa's membrane.

unit m., a trilaminar structure common to all cell membranes, probably consisting of two layers of protein with a layer of lipid between them.

virginal m., hymen.

vitelline m., the external envelope of the ovum.

vitreous m., 1. Descemet's membrane. 2. hyaline membrane (1). 3. Bruch's membrane. 4. a delicate boundary layer investing the vitreous body.

membraniform (mem-bran′ĭ-form) resembling a membrane.

membranocartilaginous (mem″brah-no-kar″tĭ-laj′ĭ-nus) 1. developed in both membrane and cartilage. 2. partly cartilaginous and partly membranous.

membranoid (mem′brah-noid) resembling a membrane.

membrum (mem′brum), pl. *mem′bra* [L.] a limb or member of the body; an entire arm or leg.

m. mulie′bre, clitoris.

m. viri′le, penis.

memory (mem′o-re) the mental faculty that enables one to retain and recall previously experienced sensations, impressions, information, and ideas.

The ability of the brain to retain and to use knowledge gained from past experience is essential to the process of learning. Although the exact way in which the brain remembers is not completely understood, it is believed that a portion of the temporal lobe of the brain, lying in part under the temples, acts as a kind of memory center, drawing on memories stored in other parts of the brain.

There are many theories about the way memories are stored. Millions of nerve cells in special patterns are probably involved. One possible explanation for the vast number of memories and the ways the mind has access to them is the chemical one. Brain cells, like other cells in the body, are made up of giant protein molecules. Each living cell contains great numbers of these molecules. The brain alone contains a thousand billion billion (the figure 1 followed by 21 zeros) of them. The impulses that run along the nerves can change these molecules into new combinations, and each cell constantly reproduces these molecules exactly. This, then, could be a chemical way by which memories are stored: the nerve impulses of the experience leave traces in the minutely changed molecules within the cells. These molecules, as they disappear, are steadily reproduced, each according to its pattern. And so the memory trace would, theoretically, remain.

Memory Through Sense Impressions. Much of memory is based on the brain's ability to record impressions, images, and sensations received by the sense organs. A person remembers only a small portion of the sense impressions he receives; he is more apt to remember impressions that are pleasing to him, but this is only a general rule, and everyone remembers much that is unpleasant as well. But though the brain probably retains only about a tenth of the impressions it receives, even this amount adds up to an enormous store of memories. These memories of touch, taste, smell, sound, and sight become raw material that the brain can draw upon in many ways—to recall past experience, to apply it to present situations, to anticipate the nature of future events or to form new thoughts or concepts. As a person continues to have experiences and store up memories, the brain's association of memories becomes increasingly complex.

Sometimes a person may retain certain kinds of sense impressions more efficiently than others. Some persons, for example, have very accurate memories of things they hear, such as conversations or melodies. Others recall visual images more clearly. An extreme example of such aptitude is eidetic memory, in which a person is able to reproduce exact visual images of things he has seen.

Other Kinds of Remembering. The term memory is a general one, and it includes other kinds of remembering besides the collection of simple sense impressions. One of these is the ability to remember events that have just occurred and to add them to one's storehouse of memories. It is thought that this process begins when a new event stimulates a circular chain of electrical impulses in the brain. These impulses then stimulate each other, keeping the event part of one's conscious knowledge. Thinking about the event or mulling it over accentuates the impulses. Eventually the brain turns its attention to something new, but the impulses have left a record and made the event an enduring memory that can be clearly recalled. The ability to form memories of new events seems to be strongest in younger persons. Older persons may recall recent events poorly or with difficulty, while they are still able to remember the past clearly.

Memories of events, actions, or facts become stronger if the remembered thing is repeatedly experienced or used. This is why "cramming" may get students through an examination for a day but leave little residue of knowledge. Too much information at once cannot be effectively handled by memory. The repetition of actions contributes to the kind of memory that enables one to perform acts automatically. Many everyday actions and skills are performed in this way.

Distortion of Memory. Memories can easily be distorted. Experiments have shown that when a number of people observe an event and are later asked to describe it, no two persons describe it in exactly the same way. When a person has strong emotional feeling about an event, his memory of it is apt to be colored by his emotions. He may remember those aspects of the event that fit in with his own emotions and attitudes, and forget those that do not. Or he may unconsciously add to his recollection details that did not really happen. All of us have probably unconsciously altered the truth in this way at one time or another.

Another distortion of memory that may occur is the feeling that some situation is familiar and has previously been experienced, when in reality the situation is a completely new one. The person may feel he knows exactly what someone to whom he is talking will say next. It is not known exactly why one suddenly has the feeling, called *déja vu* (literally, "already seen"). Some psychologists suggest that this feeling may be because of some coincidental similarity between the new situation and a past experience.

Loss of Memory. Loss of memory, or AMNESIA, may be a symptom of damage to some area of the brain, or of a decrease in the brain's blood supply. It may also result from psychologic causes; certain experiences may be so distressing to recall that the brain relegates them to the subconscious mind.

Only rarely is all memory lost in amnesia. Sometimes an incident or a certain period in the patient's life is forgotten. Or he may recall events in the wrong order but remember each separate event accurately. Amnesia may take different forms, depending on what area of the brain has been injured; in amnesia of hearing, for example, the patient cannot remember spoken language, while in visual amnesia he has forgotten his written language.

menacme (mě-nak′me) the period of a woman's life which is marked by menstrual activity.

menadiol (men″ah-di′ol) a vitamin K analogue; its sodium diphosphate salt is used as a prothrombinogenic vitamin.

menadione (men″ah-di′ōn) a prothrombinogenic agent used as a vitamin K supplement.

menaphthone (men-af″thōn) menadione.

menarche (mě-nar′ke) establishment or beginning of the menstrual function. adj., **menar′cheal.**

Mendel's law (men′delz) in the inheritance of certain traits or characters, offspring are not intermediate in type between the parents, but inherit from one or the other parent in this respect. Thus, if a plant with the factor tallness (TT) is mated with one with the factor shortness (SS), then the offspring will inherit these factors in the ratio TT, 2Ts, SS. This law is usually expressed as the law of independent assortment and the law of segregation. Called also mendelian law.

Mendel-Bechterew reflex dorsal flexion of the second to fifth toes on percussion of the dorsum of the foot; in certain organic nervous disorders, planter flexion occurs.

mendelevium (men″dě-le′ve-um) a chemical element, atomic number 101, atomic weight 256, symbol Md. (See table of ELEMENTS.)

mendelian rate (men-de′le-an) an expression of the numerical relations of the occurrence of distinctly contrasted mendelian characteristics in succeeding generations of hybrid offspring.

Menetrier's disease (men″ě-tre-ārz′) excessive proliferation of the gastric mucosa, producing diffuse thickening of the wall; inflammatory changes may be associated. Called also giant hypertrophic gastritis.

Menformon (men′for-mon) trademark for a preparation of estrone, an estrogenic steroid.

Menière's disease (men″ě-ārz′) a disorder of the labyrinth of the inner ear; called also Menière's syndrome and sometimes spelled Meniere and Ménière. It is believed to result from dilation of the lymphatic channels in the cochlea. In about 90 per cent of cases only one ear is affected. The usual symptoms are tinnitus, heightened sensitivity to loud sounds, progressive loss of hearing, headache, and vertigo. In the acute stage there may be severe nausea with vomiting, profuse sweating, disabling dizziness, and nystagmus. Some attacks last only minutes, and others continue for hours; they may occur frequently or only several weeks apart.

The disease usually lasts a few years, with progressive loss of hearing in the affected ear; sometimes the symptoms stop before all hearing is lost. If loss of hearing in the affected ear does become complete, nausea symptoms are likely to disappear.

Menière's disease sometimes develops after an injury to the head or infection of the middle ear. Many cases, however, have no apparent cause. The disorder is most common among men between the ages of 40 and 60.

A low-salt diet, elimination or restriction of fluids, and vasodilating drugs are used in the treatment of this disorder. Sedatives are usually ordered to promote sleep and rest. If the ringing sensation becomes too disturbing to the patient, it may be masked (for example, by music piped in through earphones) to make sleeping easier.

Surgical treatment involves relief from accumulation of inner ear fluid in the endolymphatic sac. Procedures may be directed toward relief of pressure by the bony structures surrounding the sac, or toward opening the sac and diverting the flow of endolymph by means of a shunt to the mastoid bone or to the subarachnoid space.

mening(o)- word element [Gr.], *meninges; membrane.*

meningeal (mě-nin′je-al) pertaining to the meninges.

meningeorrhaphy (mě-nin″je-or′ah-fe) suture of membranes, especially the meninges.

meninges (mě-nin′jēz), plural of *meninx* [Gr.] the three membranes covering the brain and spinal cord: the dura mater, arachnoid, and pia mater. adj., **menin′geal.**

meningioma (mě-nin″je-o′mah) a hard, usually vascular tumor occurring mainly along the meningeal vessels and superior longitudinal sinus, invading the dura and skull and leading to erosion and thinning of the skull.

angioblastic m., angioblastoma.

meningism (men′in-jizm) 1. the symptoms and signs of meningitis associated with acute febrile illness or dehydration but without actual inflammation of the meninges. 2. a hysterical simulation of meningitis.

meningitis (men″in-ji′tis) inflammation of the meninges, the membranes that cover the brain and spinal cord.

There are several varieties of meningitis. The two most important are meningococcal meningitis (the commonest) and tuberculous meningitis. Others include aseptic meningitis and viral meningitis.

CAUSES. Meningococcal meningitis is caused by meningococci. It is generally the epidemic type and is very contagious because the bacteria are present in the throat as well as in the cerebrospinal fluid. It is transmitted by contact and by droplet infection. The incubation period for epidemic meningitis is 2 to 10 days.

In meningococcemia (Waterhouse-Friderichsen syndrome), the bacteria appear in the blood rather than the cerebrospinal fluid. The disease is associated with adrenal hemorrhage and may lead to destruction of the adrenal glands.

Tuberculous meningitis is produced by the same bacteria that cause tuberculosis of the lung. It results in a more chronic inflammation.

Aseptic meningitis occurs principally among young children during the warm months of the year. It is often referred to as "summer grippe." The infection is caused by enteroviruses (echoviruses) and is usually accompanied by a skin rash.

Viral meningitis in the United States and temperate climates generally is caused chiefly by mumps and poliomyelitis viruses, and less frequently by herpes simplex and other viruses.

SYMPTOMS AND TREATMENT. Whatever the type of infecting agent, the symptoms of meningitis are usually the same. The most characteristic are a violent persistent headache and vomiting, which are caused by increased intracranial pressure.

The patient may be delirious and suffer convulsions. He will hold his neck as rigidly as possible, because any movement of the neck muscles stretches the meninges and increases the pain of the headache.

In tuberculous meningitis, however, the symptoms develop gradually, taking a week or two to appear. Early symptoms are deceptive, particularly in children. They may include sore throat, a dull feeling, fever, general soreness, and a rash of red spots on the body.

Diagnosis is confirmed by LUMBAR PUNCTURE and identification of the causative organism in a sample of cerebrospinal fluid. Treatment is with antibiotics.

PATIENT CARE. The ISOLATION precautions and procedures necessary to prevent the spread of meningitis vary according to the type of meningitis. If the diagnosis is viral, serous, or nonbacterial meningitis (aseptic meningitis), *excretion precautions* are recommended during hospitalization. Meningococcal meningitis requires *respiratory isolation* until 24 hours after initiation of effective therapy, but other types of bacterial meningitis do not need to be handled with any special isolation techniques or precautions other than basic techniques of good personal hygiene and sanitation.

The environment should be quiet and nonstimulating so as to reduce irritability and promote relaxation. Noise is kept at a minimum and extremely bright lights in the patient's room should be avoided. Disorientation sometimes accompanies meningitis and demands constant attendance so that the patient does not injure himself.

Loss of sight or hearing, paralysis, and mental retardation are possible complications of meningitis. However, they are usually avoided by prompt treatment with antibiotics which destroy the organisms before permanent damage is done to the nervous system.

meningocele (mĕ-ning′go-sēl) hernial protrusion of meninges through a defect in the skull or vertebral column.

meningocerebritis (mĕ-ning″go-ser″ĕ-bri′tis) inflammation of the brain and meninges.

meningococcemia (mĕ-ning″go-kok-se′me-ah) the presence of meningococci in the blood, producing an acute fulminating disease or an insidious disorder persisting for months or years.

acute fulminating m., Waterhouse-Friderichsen syndrome.

meningococcidal (mĕ-ning″go-kok-si′dal) destroying meningococci.

meningococcus (mĕ-ning″go-kok′us), pl. *meningococ′ci* [Gr.] a microorganism of the species *Neisseria meningitidis,* the cause of some types of meningitis. adj., **meningococ′cal.**

meningocortical (mĕ-ning″go-kor′tĭ-kal) pertaining to the meninges and cortex of the brain.

meningocyte (mĕ-ning′go-sīt) a histiocyte of the meninges.

meningoencephalitis (mĕ-ning″go-en-sef″ah-li′tis) encephalomeningitis; inflammation of the brain and its meninges.

meningoencephalocele (mĕ-ning″go-en-sef′ah-lo-sēl″) hernial protrusion of the meninges and brain substance through a defect in the skull.

meningoencephalomyelitis (mĕ-ning″go-en-sef″-ah-lo-mi″ĕ-li′tis) inflammation of the meninges, brain, and spinal cord.

meningoencephalopathy (mĕ-ning″go-en-sef″-ah-lop′ah-the) noninflammatory disease of the cerebral meninges and brain.

meningomalacia (mĕ-ning″go-mah-la′she-ah) softening of a membrane.

meningomyelitis (mĕ-ning″go-mi″ĕ-li′tis) inflammation of the spinal cord and its meninges.

meningomyelocele (mĕ-ning-go-mi′e-lo-sēl″) hernial protrusion of the meninges and spinal cord through a defect in the vertebral column.

meningomyeloradiculitis (mĕ-ning″go-mi″ĕ-lo-rah-dik″u-li′tis) inflammation of the meninges, spinal cord, and spinal nerve roots.

meningopathy (men″in-gop′ah-the) any disease of the meninges.

meningoradicular (mĕ-ning″go-rah-dik′u-lar) pertaining to the meninges and the cranial or spinal nerve roots.

meningoradiculitis (mĕ-ning″go-rah-dik″u-li′tis) inflammation of the meninges and spinal nerve roots.

meningorhachidian (mĕ-ning″go-rah-kid′e-an) pertaining to the spinal cord and meninges.

meningorrhagia (mĕ-ning″go-ra′je-ah) hemorrhage from cerebral or spinal membranes.

meningorrhea (mĕ-ning″go-re′ah) effusion of blood between or upon the meninges.

meninx (me′ningks), pl. *menin′ges* [Gr.] a membrane, especially one of the membranes of the brain or spinal cord—the dura mater, arachnoid, and pia mater. adj., **menin′geal.**

meniscectomy (men″ĭ-sek′to-me) excision of a meniscus, as of the knee joint.

meniscitis (men″ĭ-si′tis) inflammation of a meniscus of the knee joint.

meniscocyte (mĕ-nis′ko-sīt) a sickle cell.

meniscocytosis (mĕ-nis″ko-si-to′sis) sickle cell anemia.

meniscus (mĕ-nis′kus), pl. *menis′ci* [L.] something of crescent shape, as the concave or convex surface of a column of liquid in a pipet or buret, or a crescent-shaped fibrocartilage (semilunar cartilage) in the knee joint. adj., **menis′ceal.**

meno- word element [Gr.], *menstruation.*

menoctone (mĕ-nok′tōn) an antimalarial agent.

menolipsis (men″o-lip′sis) temporary cessation of menstruation.

menometrorrhagia (men″o-met″ro-ra′je-ah) excessive uterine bleeding at and between menstrual periods.

menopause (men′o-pawz) the span of time during which the menstrual cycle wanes and gradually stops; called also change of life and climacteric. It is the period when ovaries stop functioning and therefore menstruation and childbearing cease. adj., **men′opausal.**

The menopause is a natural physiologic process that results from the normal aging of the ovaries. It occurs when the ovaries can no longer perform the function of ovulation and estrogen production. Because estrogen secretion stops, physiologic changes occur in the woman's body. The uterine tubes shrink in size and become less capable of movement. The uterus, the cavity of the uterus and the cervix also decrease in size. The vagina contracts and its folds become shallower. The clitoris and external sexual organs become smaller. There may be some thinning of the pubic and axillary hair. The breasts usually become less full and firm.

The average age of menopause for American women is between 47 and 49. Almost 75 per cent of women reach it while in their forties, but it may begin as early as 35 and can be delayed until as late as 55. If, for medical reasons, surgery of the reproductive organs becomes necessary, menopause may be brought on before the natural process has begun.

The length of time in which the menopause is completed varies among individual women, but its duration is usually from 6 months to 3 years.

SYMPTOMS AND TREATMENT. Most women pass through the menopause with little discomfort; only about 15 per cent of women experience distress. Occasionally during menopause some existing physical ailments may become exaggerated, and women of nervous temperament may show increased nervousness.

The first and most obvious sign of the menopause is change in the menstrual flow. In the majority of women, bleeding decreases with each period, and the periods are spaced farther apart. In some cases, there may be excessive bleeding during the regular period.

Bleeding may also occur between periods, either as a full flow, or in drops. Vaginal bleeding that occurs after menstruation has definitely stopped is not a normal part of the menopause.

A sensation of heat in the face and upper part of the body, called a "hot flash," is one of the commonest symptoms of menopause. Sometimes hot flashes are followed by sweating or chills. Some women feel just a few of these flashes for a short period of time. Others experience 10 or 20 a day.

Those few women who suffer psychologic reactions at this time may experience fatigue, crying spells, insomnia, inability to concentrate, or poor memory. More severe reactions may result in depression. At one time it was thought that the changes in the body's chemistry caused these reactions. Today, many physicians believe that the chemical changes only trigger reactions to other events that may occur at the same time of life. During her forties and fifties, a woman becomes aware of aging. She may be disturbed by the loss of relatives and friends or by her lessened family responsibilities as her children mature. Outside interests and community activities are recommended as a means of helping these women feel wanted and needed.

Hormone injections and mild sedatives or tranquilizers may be prescribed to relieve the more distressing symptoms of menopause. See also ESTROGEN for information on the risk of cancer in patients receiving hormone therapy.

menorrhagia (men″o-ra′je-ah) excessive menstruation. Its causes include uterine tumors, pelvic inflammatory disease, and abnormal conditions of pregnancy. Endocrine disturbances may produce functional menorrhagia. Excessive menstruation may cause anemia.

menorrhalgia (men″o-ral′je-ah) pain during menstruation (see also DYSMENORRHEA).

menoschesis (mĕ-nos′kĕ-sis, men″o-ske′sis) suppression of menstruation.

menostasis (mĕ-nos′tah-sis) amenorrhea.

menostaxis (men″o-stak′sis) a prolonged menstrual period.

menotropins (men″o-tro′pins) a purified extract of postmenopausal urine containing chiefly follicle-stimulating hormone with a trace of luteinizing hormone; used as a fertility drug.

menses (men′sēz) menstruation.

menstrual (men′stroo-al) pertaining to menstruation.

m. cycle, the period of the regularly recurring physiologic changes in the endometrium that culminate in its shedding (MENSTRUATION).

Menstrual cycles vary in length; the average is approximately 28 days. The menstrual flow generally lasts about 5 days, although this too varies from person to person. Women menstruate from puberty to menopause, except during pregnancy.

During the first 14 days of the menstrual cycle, a follicle containing an ovum develops in the ovaries. As the menstrual flow ceases, the lining of the uterus is stimulated by estrogen and begins to increase in thickness to prepare for reproduction.

On about the fourteenth day of the cycle, OVULATION takes place and the ovary discharges the ovum. At the time of ovulation, the ruptured follicle is transformed into a yellowish material called the corpus luteum, which in turn secretes progesterone. Progesterone acts on the endometrium, building up tissues with an enriched supply of blood to nourish the future embryo.

If conception does not take place, the estrogen level in the blood falls, the endometrium is no longer stimulated, and the uterus again becomes thinner. Blood circulation slows, blood vessels contract and the unused tissue breaks down into the bloody discharge known as menstruation. With its onset, the cycle starts again.

menstruation (men″stroo-a′shun) the periodic discharge from the vagina of blood and tissues from a nonpregnant uterus; the culmination of the MENSTRUAL CYCLE. Menstruation occurs every 28 days or so between puberty and menopause, except during pregnancy, and the flow lasts about 5 days, the times varying from woman to woman.

MENSTRUAL DIFFICULTIES. Some menstrual discomfort is common, but acute discomfort is usually indicative of some disorder. Among the disorders sometimes causing DYSMENORRHEA are myoma of the uterus, endometrial cysts, or displacement of the uterus. Menstrual pain may, in some cases, be related to tension or anxiety.

Excessive bleeding, or prolonged periods, called menorrhagia, is sometimes an indication of tumors, polyps, cancer, or inflammation.

Menstruation usually starts between the ages of 11 and 14 and continues into the forties. At first the periods may be irregular, but once they are established they usually occur in a fairly definite rhythm, at intervals of 21 to 35 days. In these regular cycles, there may be monthly variations of a few days, which are considered to be quite normal. These cycles may be influenced by changes in climate or living conditions, or by emotional factors. Slight irregularities, especially if they occur over a period of time, may be warnings of disturbance of either the thyroid or pituitary glands, or of tumors of the uterus or ovaries.

Occasionally menstruation does not occur at puberty. This condition is known as primary AMENORRHEA. It may be caused by underdevelopment or malformation of the reproductive organs, or by glandular disturbances, which generally can be corrected by the administration of hormones.

General ill health, a change in climate or living conditions, emotional shock or, frequently, either the hope or fear of becoming pregnant can sometimes stop menstruation after it has begun. This is called secondary amenorrhea. If this cessation is of short duration, it is not a cause for alarm. If it continues over a long period of time, and there is also the problem of infertility, hormone treatments may be necessary.

anovular m., anovulatory m., periodic uterine bleeding without preceding ovulation.

vicarious m., bleeding from extragenital mucous membrane at the time one would normally expect the menstrual period.

menstruum (men′stroo-um) a solvent medium.

mensuration (men″su-ra′shun) the process of measuring.

mental (men′tal) 1. pertaining to the mind. 2. pertaining to the chin.

m. hygiene, the science that deals with the development of healthy mental and emotional reactions.

m. mechanism, an unconscious and indirect manner of gratifying a repressed desire.

m. retardation, faulty or inadequate development of the brain which brings with it some degree of impaired adaptation in learning, social adjustment, or maturation, or in all three areas.

Mental retardation is not a disease; it is a general term for a wide range of conditions, resulting from many different causes. Many of these are directly related to various diseases, either in the mother during pregnancy, or in the infant; only some are hereditary. The general health of the mother and the economic situation of the family may also play a role in this condition.

Mental retardation is a relative term. Its meaning depends on what society demands of the individual in learning, skills, and social responsibility. Many people who are considered retarded in the complex modern world would get along normally in a simpler society.

DIAGNOSIS. There is no absolute measurement for retardation. At one time the different types were classified only according to the apparent severity of the retardation. Since the most practical standard was intelligence, the degree of retardation was based on the score of the patient on intelligence, or IQ, tests. The average person is considered to have an IQ of between 90 and 110. Those who score below 70 are considered mentally retarded.

In the past, the different groupings were classified in terms such as feebleminded, idiot, imbecile and moron. Today, most doctors use the following classifications: for IQ's from 50 to 70, mild; 35 to 50, moderate; 20 to 35, severe; under 20, profound. Whatever classifications are used, it is agreed that IQ measurements are only one of the factors to be considered in determining mental retardation. Others, such as the patient's adaptability to his surroundings, the services and training available to him, and the amount of control he has over his emotions, are also very important.

About 85 per cent of the patients who are considered mentally retarded are in the least severe, or mild group. Those in this group do not usually have any obvious physical defects and for this reason are not always easy to identify as mentally retarded while they are still infants. Sometimes such a child's mental defects do not show up until he enters school, where he has difficulty in learning and keeping up with others in his age group.

Many of those in the mild category, when they grow up, find employment or a place in society suitable to their abilities, and are no longer identified as mentally retarded. In general, most of those who are mildly retarded are much closer to being normal than abnormal.

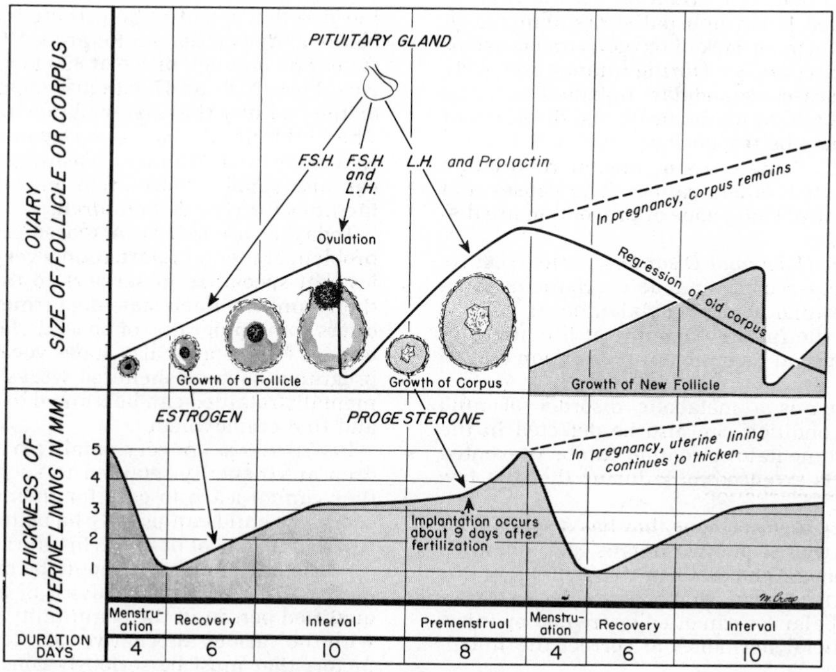

Average 28-day menstrual cycle. The cycle begins when hormones from the pituitary gland stimulate the development of an egg in a follicle inside one of the ovaries. About the fourteenth day, ovulation occurs: The follicle bursts, and the egg is discharged from the ovary. If the egg is not fertilized, the cycle ends in menstruation on the twenty-eighth day. If the egg is fertilized, pregnancy begins. (From Dorland's Illustrated Medical Dictionary. 25th ed. Philadelphia, W. B. Saunders Co., 1974.)

Many conditions that can cause severe retardation can be diagnosed during pregnancy, and in some cases proper treatment can lessen or even prevent retardation. Proper care for the mother during pregnancy and for the baby in his first months of life is also important.

CAUSES. There are many causes of mental retardation. Many are known, many are simply suspected. No apparent defect can be found in the vast majority of the mentally retarded. The specific cause of their retardation cannot be pinpointed. There are factors, however, that have been proved by research to contribute to retardation.

A child whose mother did not receive prenatal care is more likely to be retarded. Financial hardship, a broken home, a lack of intellectual stimulation in the family, or a deprived environment can play important roles. Unfavorable health factors, such as poor diet or insufficient medical care, can lead to poor physical condition, which may cause a lower level of performance.

Other physical factors may also be involved. A child born prematurely may occasionally not develop entirely normally. Heredity may play a part in some cases when certain combinations of parents' genes may result in faulty metabolism which affects the normal development of the brain.

The conditions that are known to cause mental retardation can occur at any time from conception through early childhood. At the time of conception, there may be genetic irregularities. During pregnancy, certain infections, such as rubella, syphilis, or meningitis, and other conditions such as glandular disorder, poor prenatal care, injury, or inadequate diet can lead to retardation. At the time of birth, prolonged labor, unusual stress, damage in the course of birth, or lack of oxygen can occasionally cause brain damage. During infancy and early childhood diseases, glandular imbalances, accidents, such as a blow on the head, and disorders of metabolism may be responsible.

PREVENTION. Some types of mental retardation can be prevented; others cannot. The causes and diseases that offer some hope of prevention are discussed below.

Metabolic or Hormonal Disorders. PHENYLKETONURIA, or PKU, is a congenital defect in the metabolism of the amino acid phenylalanine. If PKU is diagnosed in the first few months of life and controlled by a special diet, mental retardation can be prevented.

GALACTOSEMIA is a metabolic disorder of milk sugar. This condition can also be detected in the newborn, and mental retardation can be prevented if the infant is given no milk during the first few weeks of life.

A deficiency in a hormone that has a specific effect on the activities of other organs can have various consequences. The best known condition of this kind is HYPOTHYROIDISM, which results in CRETINISM. Hormone imbalances can often be treated by injections of artificial hormones to correct the imbalance.

Erythroblastosis Fetalis (Hemolytic Disease of the Newborn). Occasionally the blood of the mother and that of her unborn child may be incompatible because of a difference in the RH FACTOR. The infant suffering from erythroblastosis fetalis can be treated by exchange or intrauterine fetal TRANSFUSION.

Infections. If the mother contracts RUBELLA during pregnancy, especially during the first 3 months, it may result in defects of the baby's heart and eyes as well as damage to the brain.

SYPHILIS (but not gonorrhea) in the mother can cause mental retardation. This disease can be discovered by blood tests, and if it is treated soon enough, it may not damage the child.

MENINGITIS in childhood can result in severe damage to the brain. Fortunately, modern drugs can usually cure the disease and prevent mental retardation.

TREATMENT. Some types of mental retardation can be prevented or lessened by proper medical treatment; most, however, cannot. Almost all retarded children can benefit from special education and training which can lead to greater independence.

Parents who believe that their child is not developing at a proper rate or that he shows symptoms of retardation should consult their family physician or local child care clinic at once. It may be very difficult to face the fact that a child may be mentally retarded, but the sooner it is faced the better chance there is of developing a program to help the child make the best adjustment possible. A complete study of the child's condition can be arranged. From this, it will be possible to say how severe the retardation is and what improvement can be expected; a program of education and training for him will be planned. The doctor or agency will also be familiar with the kinds of help that are available in the community. Many public school systems now have special programs for retarded children, and help is available from other agencies, both public and private.

If there does not seem to be any organization in the area that can offer help, there is an office of the National Association for Retarded Children in every state. The national office at 420 Lexington Avenue, New York, N.Y. 10017, can also supply information on the facilities that are available in any local area. The Children's Bureau, U.S. Department of Health, Education and Welfare, Washington, D.C. 20201, can also supply information on schools and other facilities for retarded children.

Today, as a result of increased concern with the problem of mental retardation, every state has clinics that specialize in services to the retarded and their families. Each state department of education offers some programs of special classes for the retarded. Most states also have vocational training programs, such as sheltered workshops where the mentally retarded can be trained to do simple tasks and find employment.

INSTITUTIONS. A very small percentage of children are mentally retarded to such a degree that they cannot learn to care for themselves. In these cases, the child can usually be better cared for in a residential school or other institution.

A decision of this sort should be made by the parents with the help and advice of a professionally qualified person in the community who is familiar with the various alternatives available. Among the factors that must be seriously considered are how disruptive the child is to the home and other children, whether the family can give the child the care and attention he needs, whether an institution could better meet the child's needs, and whether the type and location of the institution are suitable.

It is always a difficult decision for parents to send a retarded child to an institution, but with professional guidance all factors can be taken into consideration, and the decision is likely to be one that brings the most benefit to everyone in the family.

menthol (men′thol) an alcohol from various mint oils or produced synthetically, used locally to relieve itching.

mentum (men′tum) [L.] chin.

mepacrine (mep′ah-krin) quinacrine hydrochloride, an antimalarial agent.

mepazine (mep′ah-zēn) a phenothiazine derivative used as a neuroleptic and antinauseant.

mepenzolate (me-pen′zo-lāt) an anticholinergic used in the form of the bromide to relieve abdominal pain, gaseous distention, and diarrhea associated with colonic disease.

meperidine hydrochloride (mĕ-per′ĭ-dēn) a fine, white crystalline powder used as a narcotic analgesic.

mephenoxalone (mef″en-ok′sah-lōn) a compound used as an antianxiety agent.

mephentermine (mĕ-fen′ter-mēn) a sympathomimetic and pressor agent.

mephenytoin (mef″en-ĭ′to-in) an anticonvulsant used in the treatment of epilepsy.

mephitic (mĕ-fit′ik) noxious; foul smelling.

mephobarbital (mef″o-bar′bĭ-tal) a white crystalline powder used as an anticonvulsant with a slight hypnotic action.

Mephyton (mef′ĭ-ton) trademark for preparations of vitamin K_1, used as a prothrombinogenic agent.

mepivacaine hydrochloride (mĕ-piv′ah-kān) a compound used as a local anesthetic.

Meprane (me′prān) trademark for preparations of promethestrol, a synthetic estrogen.

meprednisone (mĕ-pred′nĭ-sōn) an oral glucocorticoid used as an anti-inflammatory, antiallergic, and antineoplastic steroid.

meprobamate (mĕ-pro′bah-māt, mep″ro-bam′āt) a minor tranquilizer and skeletal muscle relaxant.

meprylcaine (mep′ril-kān) a compound used as a local anesthetic in dentistry.

mepyramine (me-pir′ah-mēn) pyrilamine, an antihistamine.

mEq. milliequivalent.

meralgia (mĕ-ral′je-ah) pain in the thigh.

m. paresthet′ica, a condition of numbness and tingling on the anterolateral aspect of the thigh, rarely accompanied by pain; it is due to entrapment of the lateral femoral cutaneous nerve at the inguinal ligaments.

meralluride (mer-al′u-rīd) a mercury compound used as a diuretic.

Meratran (mer′ah-tran) trademark for a preparation of pipradrol hydrochloride, a central nervous system stimulant.

merbromin (mer-bro′min) a topical antibacterial compound occurring as iridescent green scales or granules.

mercaptan (mer-kap′tan) an alcohol in which oxygen is replaced by sulfur.

mercaptomerin (mer-kap″to-mer′in) an organic mercurial diuretic.

sodium m., a compound used parenterally as a diuretic.

mercaptopurine (mer-kap″to-pu′rēn) a yellow crystalline compound used as an antineoplastic agent, primarily in acute leukemia.

mercocresol (mer″ko-kre′sol) a combination of cresol derivatives and an organic mercury, having germicidal, fungicidal, and bacteriostatic properties.

Mercodinone (mer″ko-di′nōn) trademark for a preparation of hydrocodone, an antitussive.

Mercuhydrin (mer″ku-hi′drin) trademark for preparations of meralluride, a mercurial diuretic.

mercurial (mer-ku′re-al) 1. pertaining to mercury. 2. a preparation containing mercury.

mercurialism (mer-ku′re-al-izm″) chronic mercury poisoning.

mercuric (mer-ku′rik) pertaining to mercury as a bivalent element; containing bivalent mercury.

m. chloride, mercury bichloride.

m. iodide, red, mercury biniodide, used as a topical antiseptic.

m. oxide, red, an orange-red crystalline powder used as an antiseptic.

m. oxide, yellow, a yellow to orange-yellow, heavy antiseptic powder used in ointment form for eye disorders.

Mercurochrome (mer-ku′ro-krōm) trademark for preparations of merbromin, a topical antibacterial compound.

mercurophylline (mer″ku-ro-fil′in) a white to slightly yellow, odorless powder used as a diuretic.

mercurous (mer′ku-rus) pertaining to mercury as a monovalent element; containing monovalent mercury.

m. chloride, a white, odorless, tasteless powder rarely used in pills or tablets as a cathartic, intestinal antiseptic, or to reduce edema, or, in an ointment, as a local antibacterial agent; called also calomel.

mercury (mer′ku-re) a chemical element, atomic number 80, atomic weight 200.59, symbol Hg. (See table of ELEMENTS.) Mercury forms two sets of classes of compounds: mercurous, in which a single atom of mercury combines with a monovalent radical, and mercuric, in which a single atom of mercury combines with a bivalent radical. Mercury and its salts have been employed therapeutically as purgatives; as alternatives in chronic inflammations; and as antisyphilitics, intestinal antiseptics, disinfectants, and astringents. They are absorbed by the skin and mucous membranes, causing chronic mercurial poisoning, or hydrargyria. The mercuric salts are more soluble and irritant than the mercurous. See also under mercurous and mercuric.

ammoniated m., a compound used as an antiseptic skin and ophthalmic ointment.

m. bichloride, a poisonous compound occurring as heavy, odorless crystals, crystalline masses or white powder; used in solution as a topical antiseptic and as a disinfectant.

m. chloride, mild, mercurous chloride.

m. oleate, a mixture of yellow mercuric oxide and oleic acid, used topically in various skin diseases.

m. poisoning, acute or chronic disease caused by mercury and its salts. The *acute* form, due to ingestion, is marked by severe abdominalgia, metallic taste in the mouth, vomiting, bloody diarrhea with watery stools, oliguria or anuria (usually at onset), and corrosion and ulceration of the entire digestive tract. The *chronic* form, due to absorption by the skin and mucous membranes, inhalation of vapors, or ingestion of mercury salts, is marked by stomatitis, metallic taste in the mouth, a blue line along the border of the gum, sore hypertrophied gums that bleed easy, loosening of the teeth, erethism, excessive secretion of saliva, tremors, and incoordination. Called also mercurialism and hydrargyrism.

merergastic (mer″er-gas′tik) pertaining to the simplest type of disorder of psychic function, marked by emotional instability and anxiety.

merethoxylline (mer″ĕ-thok′sĭ-lēn) a mercury compound used as a diuretic.

meridian (mĕ-rid′e-an) an imaginary line on the surface of a globe or sphere, connecting the opposite ends of its axis. adj., **merid′ional.**

mero- word element [Gr.] 1. *part.* 2. *thigh.*

meroblastic (mer-o-blas′tik) partially dividing; undergoing cleavage in which only part of the egg participates.

merocele (mer′o-sēl) femoral hernia.

merocrine (mer′o-krin) partly secreting: denoting that type of glandular secretion in which the secreting cell remains intact throughout the process of formation and discharge of the secretory products, as in the salivary and pancreatic glands; cf. apocrine and holocrine.

merogenesis (mer″o-jen′ĕ-sis) cleavage of an ovum.

merogony (mĕ-rog′o-ne) the development of only a portion of an ovum. adj., **merogon′ic.**

meromelia (mer″o-me′le-ah) congenital absence of a part, but not all, of a limb.

meromicrosomia (mer″o-mi″kro-so′me-ah) unusual smallness of some part of the body.

meromyosin (mer″o-mi′o-sin) a fragment of the myosin molecule isolated by treatment with proteolytic enzyme; there are two types, heavy (H-meromyosin) and light (L-meromyosin).

meropia (mĕ-ro′pe-ah) partial blindness.

merorachischisis (me″ro-rah-kis′kĭ-sis) fissure of part of the spinal cord.

merosmia (mĕ-roz′me-ah) inability to perceive certain odors.

merotomy (mĕ-rot′o-me) a cutting into segments.

merozoite (mer″o-zo′īt) one of the organisms formed by multiple fission (schizogony) of a sporozoite within the body of the host.

Merphene (mer′fēn) trademark for preparations of phenylmercuric nitrate, an antibacterial.

Merphenyl (mer′fen-il) trademark for preparations of phenylmercuric nitrate, an antibacterial.

mersalyl (mer′sah-lil) a white crystalline powder; a mercurial diuretic.

Merthiolate (mer-thi′o-lāt) trademark for preparations of thimerosal, an antibacterial.

mes(o)- (mez′o) word element [Gr.], *middle.*

mesangium (mes-an′je-um) the thin membrane supporting the capillary loops in renal glomeruli. adj., **mesan′gial.**

Mesantoin (mĕ-san′to-in) trademark for a preparation of mephenytoin, an anticonvulsant.

mesaortitis (mes″a-or-ti′tis) inflammation of the tunica media of the aorta.

mesarteritis (mes″ar-ter-i′tis) inflammation of the tunica media of an artery.

mesatipellic (mes-at″ĭ-pel′ik) having a round pelvis.

mescaline (mes′kah-lēn) a poisonous alkaloid derived from the flowering heads (mescal buttons) of a Mexican cactus, which produces hallucinations of sound and color (see also HALLUCINOGEN and DRUG ABUSE).

mescalism (mes′kah-lizm) intoxication due to mescal buttons or mescaline.

mesencephalitis (mes″en-sef″ah-li′tis) inflammation of the mesencephalon, or midbrain.

mesencephalon (mes″en-sef′ah-lon) 1. the midbrain. 2. the middle of the three primary brain vesicles of the embryo. adj., **mesencephal′ic.**

mesencephalotomy (mes″en-sef″ah-lot′o-me) surgical production of lesions in the midbrain for the relief of intractable pain.

mesenchyma (mĕ-seng′kĭ-mah) the meshwork of embryonic connective tissue in the mesoderm from which are formed the connective tissues of the body and also the blood vessels and lymph vessels. adj., **mesen′chymal.**

mesenchyme (mes′eng-kīm) mesenchyma.

mesenchymoma (mes″eng-ki-mo′mah) a mixed mesenchymal tumor composed of two or more cellular elements that are not commonly associated, exclusive of fibrous tissue.

mesenterectomy (mes″en-tĕ-rek′to-me) resection of the mesentery.

mesenteriopexy (mes″en-ter′e-o-pek″se) fixation or suspension of a torn mesentery.

mesenteriorrhaphy (mes″en-ter″e-or′ah-fe) suture of the mesentery.

mesenteriplication (mes″en-ter″ĭ-pli-ka′shun) the operation of taking a tuck in the mesentery to shorten it.

mesenteritis (mes″en-tĕ-ri′tis) inflammation of the mesentery.

mesenterium (mes″en-te′re-um) mesentery.

mesenteron (mes-en′ter-on) the midgut.

mesentery (mes′en-ter″e) a membranous fold attaching various organs to the body wall, especially the peritoneal fold attaching the small intestine to the dorsal body wall. adj., **mesenter′ic.**

mesiad (me′ze-ad) toward the middle or center.

mesial (me′ze-al) situated in the middle; median; nearer the middle line of the body or nearer the center of the dental arch.

mesially (me′ze-al″e) toward the median line.

mesiobuccal (me″ze-o-buk′kal) pertaining to or formed by the mesial and buccal surfaces of a tooth, or the mesial and buccal walls of a tooth cavity.

mesiocervical (me″ze-o-ser′vĭ-kal) pertaining to the mesial surface of the neck of a tooth.

mesioclusion (me″ze-o-kloo′zhun) anteroclusion; malrelation of the dental arches with the mandibular arch anterior to the maxillary arch (prognathism).

mesiodistal (me″ze-o-dis′tal) pertaining to the mesial and distal surfaces of a tooth.

mesiolabial (me″ze-o-la′be-al) pertaining to the mesial and labial surfaces of a tooth or a tooth cavity.

mesion (me′ze-on) the plane dividing the body into right and left symmetrical halves.

mesmerism (mez′mer-izm) hypnotism.

mesoappendix (mez″o-ah-pen′diks) the peritoneal fold connecting the appendix to the ileum.

mesoblast (mez′o-blast) the mesoderm, especially in the early stages.

mesobronchitis (mez″o-brong-ki′tis) inflammation of middle coat of the bronchi.

mesocardia (mez″o-kar′de-ah) location of the apex of the heart in the midline of the thorax.

mesocardium (mez″o-kar′de-um) 1. the part of the embryonic mesentery which connects the embryonic heart with the body wall in front and the foregut behind. 2. myocardium.

mesocecum (mez″o-se′kum) the occasionally occurring mesentery of the cecum.

mesocephalon (mez″o-sef′ah-lon) mesencephalon, or midbrain.

mesococcus (mez″o-kok′us), pl. *mesococ′ci* [L.] a spherical microorganism of medium size.

mesocolon (mez″o-ko′lon) the peritoneal process attaching the colon to the posterior abdominal wall, and called ascending, descending, or transverse, according to the portion of the colon to which it attaches.

pelvic m., sigmoid m., the peritoneum attaching the sigmoid colon to the posterior abdominal wall.

mesocolopexy (mez″o-ko′lo-pek″se) suspension or fixation of the colon.

mesocoloplication (mes″o-ko″lo-pli-ka′shun) plication of the mesocolon to limit its mobility.

mesocord (mez′o-kord) an umbilical cord adherent to the placenta.

mesoderm (mez′o-derm) the middle of the three primary germ layers of the embryo, lying between the ectoderm and entoderm; from it are derived the connective tissue, bone, cartilage, muscle, blood and blood vessels, lymphatics, lymphoid organs, notochord, pleura, pericardium, peritoneum, kidneys, and gonads. adj., **mesoder′mal, mesoder′mic.**

somatic m., the outer layer of the developing mesoderm.

splanchnic m., the inner layer of the developing mesoderm.

mesodiastolic (mez″o-di″ah-stol′ik) pertaining to the middle of the diastole.

mesoduodenum (mez″o-du″o-de′num) the mesenteric fold that in early fetal life encloses the duodenum.

mesoepididymis (mez″o-ep″ĭ-did′ĭ-mis) a fold of tunica vaginalis connecting the epididymis and testis.

mesogastrium (mez″o-gas′tre-um) the portion of the primitive mesentery that encloses the stomach and from which the greater omentum develops. adj., **mesogas′tric.**

mesoileum (mez″o-il′e-um) the mesentery of the ileum.

mesojejunum (mez″o-jĕ-ju′num) the mesentery of the jejunum.

mesolymphocyte (mez″o-lim′fo-sīt) a medium-sized lymphocyte.

mesomere (mez′o-mēr) 1. a blastomere of size intermediate between a macromere and a micromere. 2. a midzone of the mesoderm between the epimere and hypomere.

mesomerism (mĕ-zom′er-izm) the existence of organic chemical structures differing only in the position of electrons rather than atoms. adj., **mesomer′ic.**

mesometrium (mez″o-me′tre-um) the portion of the broad ligament below the mesovarium.

mesomorph (mez′o-morf, mes′o-morf) 1. an individual having the type of body build in which mesodermal tissues predominate: there is relative preponderance of muscle, bone, and connective tissue, usually with heavy, hard physique of rectangular outline. 2. a well-proportioned individual.

mesomorphy (mez″o-mor′fe) the condition of being a mesomorph. adj., **mesomor′phic.**

meson (me′zon, mes′on) 1. mesion. 2. any elementary particle having a mass intermediate between the mass of the electron and that of the proton.

mesonephroma (mez″o-nĕ-fro′mah) a malignant tumor of the female genital tract, usually the ovary, formerly thought to arise from mesonephric rests. Two types are recognized: one of müllerian duct derivation, the other an embryonal tumor occurring chiefly in children; the latter may also arise in the testis.

mesonephron (mez″o-nef′ron) mesonephros.

mesonephros (mez″o-nef′ros), pl. *mesoneph′roi* [Gr.] the excretory organ of the embryo, arising caudad to the pronephros and using its duct. adj., **mesoneph′ric.**

mesopexy (mez′o-pek″se) repair of the mesentery; mesenteriopexy.

mesophile (mez′o-fīl) a microorganism that grows best at 20° to 55° C.

mesophlebitis (mez″o-flĕ-bi′tis) inflammation of the tunica media of a vein.

Mesopin (mes′o-pin) trademark for a preparation of homatropine methylbromide, a parasympatholytic.

mesoporphyrin (mez″o-por′fĭ-rin) a crystalline iron-free porphyrin from heme obtained by a process of reduction.

mesorchium (mes-or′ke-um) the portion of the primitive mesentery enclosing the fetal testis, represented in the adult by a fold between the testis and epididymis. adj., **mesor′chial.**

mesorectum (mez″o-rek′tum) the fold of peritoneum connecting the upper portion of the rectum with the sacrum.

mesoridazine (mes″o-rid′ah-zēn) a member of the phenothiazine group used as a major tranquilizer.

mesoropter (mez″o-rop′ter) the normal position of the eyes with their muscles at rest.

mesorrhaphy (mez-or′ah-fe) suture of the mesentery.

mesosalpinx (mez″o-sal′pinks) the part of the broad ligament above the mesovarium, investing the uterine tube.

mesosigmoid (mez″o-sig′moid) the peritoneal fold by which the sigmoid flexure is attached to the abdominal wall.

mesosigmoidopexy (mez″o-sig-moi′do-pek″se) fixation of the mesosigmoid in prolapse of the rectum.

mesosome (mes′o-sōm) an invagination of the bacterial cell membrane, forming organelles thought to be the site of cytochrome enzymes and the enzymes of oxidative phosphorylation and the citric acid cycle.

mesosternum (mez″o-ster′num) the middle piece or body of the sternum.

mesotendineum, mesotendon (mez″o-ten-din′e-um; mez″o-ten′don) the connective tissue sheath attaching a tendon to its fibrous sheath.

mesothelial (mez″o-the′le-al) pertaining to the mesothelium.

mesothelioma (mez″o-the″le-o′mah) a tumor made up of cells derived from the mesothelium.

mesothelium (mez″o-the′le-um) the layer of flat cells, derived from the mesoderm, that lines the body cavity of the embryo. In the adult it forms the simple squamous-celled layer of the epithelium that covers the surface of all true serous membranes (peritoneum, pericardium, pleura).

mesovarium (mez″o-va′re-um) the portion of the broad ligament between the mesometrium and mesosalpinx, enclosing and holding the ovary in place.

mestranol (mes′trah-nōl) an estrogenic agent, used in combination with various progestogens as an oral contraceptive.

mesuprine (mes′u-prēn) a vasodilator and smooth muscle relaxant, used as the hydrochloride salt.

meta- word element [Gr.], (1) *change; transformation; exchange.* (2) *after; next.* (3) the 1,3-position in derivatives of benzene.

metabasis (mĕ-tab′ah-sis) change in the manifestations or course of a disease.

metabiosis (met″ah-bi-o′sis) the dependence of one organism upon another for its existence; commensalism.

metabolimeter (met″ah-bo-lim′ĕ-ter) an apparatus for measuring basal metabolism.

metabolism (mĕ-tab′o-lizm) the sum total of the physical and chemical processes and reactions taking place among the ions, atoms, and molecules of the body. adj., **metabol′ic.** Essentially these processes are concerned with the disposition of the nutrients absorbed into the blood following digestion.

There are two phases of metabolism: the anabolic and the catabolic phase. The anabolic, or constructive, phase is concerned with the conversion of simpler compounds derived from the nutrients into living, organized substances that the body cells can use. In the catabolic, or destructive, phase these organized substances are reconverted into simpler compounds, with the release of energy necessary for the proper functioning of the body cells.

The rate of metabolism can be increased by exercise; by elevated body temperature, as in a high fever, which can more than double the metabolic rate; by hormonal activity, such as that of thyroxine, insulin, and epinephrine; and by specific dynamic action that occurs following the ingestion of a meal.

The basal metabolic rate refers to the lowest rate obtained while an individual is at complete physical and mental rest. Metabolic rate usually is expressed in terms of the amount of heat liberated during the chemical reactions of metabolism. About 25 per cent of all energy from nutrients is utilized by the body to carry on its normal function; the remainder becomes heat. The unit for expressing the quantity of heat released is the Calorie (spelled with a capital C, which is equivalent to 1000 small calories). See also BASAL METABOLISM TEST.

Congenital defects of metabolic processes, known as inborn errors of metabolism, include TAY-SACHS DISEASE, GALACTOSEMIA, GLYCOGENOSIS, PHENYLKETONURIA and many others; all are rare.

basal m., the minimal energy expended for the maintenance of respiration, circulation, peristalsis, muscle tonus, body temperature, glandular activity, and the other vegetative functions of the body.

metabolite (mĕ-tab′o-līt) any substance produced during metabolism.

metabolize (mĕ-tab′o-līz) to subject to or be transformed by metabolism.

metabutethamine (met″ah-bu-teth′ah-min) a local anesthetic used in dentistry.

metabutoxycaine (met″ah-bu-tok′sĭ-kān) a compound used as a local anesthetic.

metacarpal (met″ah-kar′pal) 1. pertaining to the metacarpus. 2. a bone of the metacarpus.

metacarpectomy (met″ah-kar-pek′to-me) excision or resection of a metacarpal bone.

metacarpophalangeal (met″ah-kar″po-fah-lan′je-al) pertaining to the metacarpus and phalanges of the fingers.

metacarpus (met″ah-kar′pus) the part of the hand between the wrist and fingers, its skeleton being five bones (metacarpals) extending from the carpus to the phalanges. (See also table of BONES.)

metacentric (met″ah-sen′trik) having the centromere almost at the middle of the replicating chromosome.

metacercaria (met″ah-ser-ka′re-ah), pl. *metacerca′riae.* the encysted resting or maturing stage of a trematode parasite in the tissues of an intermediate host.

metachromasia (met″ah-kro-ma′ze-ah) 1. failure to stain true with a given stain. 2. the different coloration of different tissues produced by the same stain. 3. change of color produced by staining. adj., **metachromat′ic.**

metachromatism (met″ah-kro′mah-tizm) metachromasia.

metachromophil (met″ah-kro′mo-fil) not staining normally.

metacresol (met″ah-kre′sol) one of the three isomeric forms of cresol, the most strongly antiseptic of the group.

metagenesis (met″ah-jen′ĕ-sis) alteration of generations.

Metagonimus (met″ah-gon′ĭ-mus) a genus of trematodes, including *M. yokoga′wai,* which is parasitic in the small intestine of man and mammals in Japan, China, Indonesia, the Balkans, and Israel.

metal (met′al) any chemical element marked by luster, malleability, ductility, and conductivity of electricity and heat, and which will ionize positively in solution. adj., **metal′lic.**

alkali m., one of a group of monovalent elements including lithium, sodium, potassium, rubidium, and cesium.

m. fume fever, an occupational disorder with malaria-like symptoms occurring in those engaged in welding and other metallic operations and due to the volatilized metals. It includes brassfounder's fever (brass chill, brazier's chill) and spelter's fever (zinc chill, zinc fume fever).

metalbumin (met″al-bu′min) a substance found in ovarian cysts; pseudomucin.

metalloenzyme (mĕ-tal″o-en′zīm) any enzyme containing tightly bound metal atoms, e.g., the cytochromes.

metalloid (met′ah-loid) 1. any element with both metallic and nonmetallic properties. 2. any metallic element that has not all the characters of a typical metal.

metalloporphyrin (mĕ-tal″o-por′fĭ-rin) a combination of a metal with porphyrin, as in heme.

metalloprotein (mĕ-tal″o-pro′te-in) a protein molecule bound to a metal ion, e.g., hemoglobin.

metallurgy (met″al-ur′je) the science and art of using metals.

metalol (met′ah-lōl) an antiadrenergic agent (β-receptor antagonist).

metamer (met′ah-mer) a compound exhibiting, or capable of exhibiting, metamerism.

metamere (met′ah-mēr) one of a series of homologous segments of the body of an animal.

metamerism (mĕ-tam′er-izm) 1. a type of structural isomerism in which different radicals of the same chemical type are attached to the same polyvalent element and yet give rise to compounds having identical molecular formulae. 2. arrangement into metameres by the serial repetition of a structural pattern. adj., **metamer′ic.**

Metamine (met′ah-mēn) trademark for preparations of trolnitrate, a vasodilator.

metamorphopsia (met″ah-mor-fop′se-ah) defective vision, with distortion of the shape of objects looked at.

metamorphosis (met″ah-mor′fo-sis) change of structure or shape; particularly, transition from one developmental stage to another, as from larva to adult form. adj., **metamor′phic.**

fatty m., any normal or pathologic transformation of fat, including fatty infiltration and fatty degeneration.

platelet m., a series of progressive, irreversible structural alterations that platelets undergo during coagulation, dependent on the presence of divalent metallic ions.

retrograde m., conversion into a simpler or more primitive form.

structural m., viscous m., platelet metamorphosis.

metamyelocyte (met″ah-mi′ĕ-lo-sīt″) an immature polymorphonuclear leukocyte with a horseshoe- or sausage-shaped nucleus, developmentally preceded by the myelocyte and followed by the mature leukocyte.

Metandren (mĕ-tan′dren) trademark for preparations of methyltestosterone, an androgen.

metanephrine (met″ah-nef′rin) a urinary metabolite of epinephrine.

metanephros (met″ah-nef′ros), pl. *metaneph′roi* [Gr.] the permanent embryonic kidney, developing later than and caudad to the mesonephros. adj., **metaneph′ric.**

metaneutrophil (met″ah-nu′tro-fil) not staining normally with neutral stains.

metaphase (met′ah-fāz) the second stage of cell division (mitosis or meiosis), in which the chromosomes, each consisting of two chromatids, are arranged in the equatorial plane of the spindle prior to separation.

Metaphen (met′ah-fen) trademark for preparations of nitromersol, an antibacterial.

metaphysis (mĕ-taf′ĭ-sis), pl. *metaph′yses* [Gr.] the wider part at the end of the shaft of a long bone, adjacent to the epiphyseal disk. adj., **metaphys′eal.**

metaplasia (met″ah-pla′ze-ah) the change in the type of adult cells in a tissue to a form abnormal for that tissue, adj., **metaplas′tic.**

myeloid m., agnogenic, a condition characterized by foci of extramedullary hematopoiesis and by splenomegaly, immature red and white cells in the peripheral blood, and mild to moderate anemia.

metaplasm (met′ah-plazm) the inanimate particles of protoplasm; called also deutoplasm.

metapneumonic (met″ah-nu-mon′ik) succeeding or following pneumonia.

metaproterenol (met″ah-pro-ter′ĕ-nōl) a bronchodilator indicated in treatment of bronchial asthma, reversible bronchospasm of bronchitis, and emphysema. It is closely related to isoproterenol but is of longer duration and has fewer cardiovascular side effects.

metapsychology (met′ah-si-kol′o-je) the branch of speculative psychology that deals with the significance of mental processes that are beyond empirical verification.

metaraminol (met″ah-ram′ĭ-nol) an ephedrine compound used as a sympathomimetic and pressor agent.

metarhodopsin (met″ah-ro-dop′sin) an intermediate formed as rhodopsin absorbs light and eventually dissociates to opsin and *trans*-retinal.

metarubricyte (met″ah-roo″brĭ-sīt) an orthochromatic normoblast.

metastasis (mĕ-tas′tah-sis) 1. the transfer of disease from one organ or part to another not directly connected with it. It may be due either to the transfer of pathogenic microorganisms (e.g., tubercle bacilli) or to transfer of cells, as in malignant tumors. 2. pl. *metas′tases* [Gr.] a growth of pathogenic microorganisms or of abnormal cells distant from the site primarily involved by the morbid process. adj., **metastat′ic.** (See also CANCER.)

metastasize (mĕ-tas′tah-sīz) to form new foci of disease in a distant part by metastasis.

metasternum (met″ah-ster′num) the xiphoid process.

metatarsal (met″ah-tar′sal) 1. pertaining to the metatarsus. 2. a bone of the metatarsus.

metatarsalgia (met″ah-tar-sal′je-ah) pain in the metatarsus.

metatarsectomy (met″ah-tar-sek′to-me) excision or resection of a metatarsal bone.

metatarsophalangeal (met″ah-tar″so-fah-lan′je-al) pertaining to the metatarsus and the phalanges of the toes.

metatarsus (met″ah-tar′sus) the part of the foot between the ankle and the toes, its skeleton being the five bones (metatarsals) extending from the tarsus to the phalanges. (See also table of BONES.)

m. pri′mus va′rus, angulation of the first metatarsal bone toward the midline of the body, producing an angle sometimes of 20 degrees or more between its base and that of the second metatarsal bone.

metathalamus (met″ah-thal′ah-mus) the part of

the thalamencephalon composed of the medial and lateral geniculate bodies.

metathesis (mĕ-tath′ĕ-sis) 1. artificial transfer of a morbid process. 2. a chemical reaction in which an element or radical in one compound exchanges places with another element or radical in another compound.

metatrophic (met″ah-trof′ik) utilizing organic matter for food.

metaxalone (mĕ-taks′ah-lōn) a smooth muscle relaxant.

Metazoa (met″ah-zo′ah) the division of the animal kingdom that includes the multicellular animals, i.e., all animals except the Protozoa. adj., **metazo′al, metazo′an.**

metazoon (met″ah-zo′on), pl. *metazo′a* [Gr.] an individual organism of the Metazoa.

Metchnikoff theory (mech′nĭ-kof) the theory that bacteria and other harmful elements in the body are attacked and destroyed by cells called phagocytes, and that the contest between such harmful elements and the phagocytes produces inflammation. Name for Elie Metchnikoff (1845–1916), Russian zoologist in Paris and winner, with Ehrlich, of the Nobel prize for medicine and physiology in 1908.

metencephalon (met–en-sef′ah-lon), pl. *metenceph′ala* [Gr.] 1. the part of the central nervous system comprising the pons and cerebellum. 2. the anterior of two brain vesicles formed by specialization of the rhombencephalon in the developing embryo.

meteorism (me′te-o-rizm″) tympanites; drumlike distention of the abdomen caused by the presence of gas in the abdomen or intestines.

meteorotropism (me″te-o-rot′ro-pizm) the response to influence by meteorologic factors noted in certain biologic events, such as sudden death, attacks of angina, joint pain, insomnia, and traffic accidents. adj., **meteorotrop′ic.**

meter (me′ter) the basic unit of linear measure of the metric system, being the equivalent of 39.371 inches; abbreviated M.

-meter (me′ter) word element [Gr.], *instrument for measuring.*

metformin (met-for′min) an oral hypoglycemic.

methacholine chloride (meth″ah-ko′lēn) colorless or white crystals; a parasympathomimetic used in cardiovascular disease and as a diagnostic test for pheochromocytoma.

methacycline (meth″ah-si′klēn) a tetracycline analogue used as an oral broad-spectrum antibiotic.

methadone (meth′ah-dōn) a synthetic compound with pharmacologic properties qualitatively similar to those of morphine and heroin.

methallenestril (meth″al-ĕ-nes′tril) a nonsteroid estrogenic compound.

methalthiazide (meth″ah-thi′ah-zīd) a diuretic and antihypertensive.

methamphetamine (meth″am-fet′ah-mēn) a central nervous system stimulant and pressor drug; used as the hydrochloride salt. Abuse may lead to dependence. (See also AMPHETAMINE.)

methandriol (meth-an′dre-ol) a compound used as an anabolic stimulant.

methandrostenolone (meth-an″dro-sten′o-lōn) an anabolic steroid with androgenic effects.

methane (meth′ān) an inflammable, explosive gas from decomposition of organic matter.

methanol (meth′ah-nol) a mobile, colorless liquid widely used as a solvent; methyl alcohol.

methantheline bromide (mĕ-than′thĕ-lēn) an anticholinergic used to depress gastrointestinal activity.

methapyrilene (meth″ah-pir′ĭ-lēn) an antihistaminic with sedative action; the hydrochloride salt is used in the treatment of allergic disorders and insomnia, and as a local anesthetic.

methaqualone (meth″ah-qua′lōn) a nonbarbiturate hypnotic similar to barbituates in its effects.

metharbital (meth-ar′bĭ-tal) a long-acting barbiturate used as a central nervous system depressant with anticonvulsant action.

methazolamide (meth″ah-zo′lah-mīd) a carbonic anhydrase inhibitor given orally to reduce intraocular pressure.

methdilazine (meth-di′lah-zēn) a phenothiazine compound used as an antihistamine and antipruritic.

methemalbumin (met″hem-al-bu′min) a brownish pigment formed in the blood by the binding of albumin with heme; indicative of intravascular hemolysis.

methemoglobin (met-he″mo-glo′bin) a compound formed from hemoglobin by oxidation of the ferrous to the ferric state with essentially ionic bonds. A small amount of methemoglobin is present in the blood normally, but injury or toxic agents convert a larger proportion of hemoglobin into methemoglobin, which does not combine reversibly with oxygen.

methemoglobinemia (met-he″mo-glo″bĭ-ne′me-ah) methemoglobin in the blood, usually due to toxic action of drugs or other agents, or to hemolytic processes.

methemoglobinuria (met-he″mo-glo″bĭ-nu′re-ah) methemoglobin in the urine.

methenamine (mĕ-the′nah-min) a white crystalline powder used as a urinary antiseptic.

m. mandelate, a salt of methenamine and mandelic acid, used in infections of the urinary tract.

Methergine (meth′er-jin) trademark for preparations of methylergonovine, an oxytocic.

methicillin (meth″ĭ-sil′in) a semisynthetic penicillin which is highly resistant to inactivation by penicillinase; its sodium salt is used parenterally.

methimazole (meth-im′ah-zōl) a white to pale buff, crystalline powder, used as a thyroid inhibitor.

methiodal sodium (meth-i′o-dal) an odorless, white, crystalline, iodine-containing powder with a slightly saline taste, used as a radiopaque medium for roentgenography of the urinary tract.

methionine (mĕ-thi′o-nin) a sulfur-bearing amino acid essential for optimal growth in infants and for nitrogen equilibrium in adults; used therapeutically as a dietary supplement with lipotropic action.

methisazone (mĕ-this′ah-zōn) an antiviral agent used to prevent smallpox in those who come in contact with infected persons.

Methium (meth′e-um) trademark for preparations of hexamethonium, an antihypertensive.

methixene (mĕ-thiks′ēn) a smooth muscle relaxant used as an adjunct in gastrointestinal hypermotility and spasm.

methocarbamol (meth″o-kar′bah-mol) a compound used as a skeletal muscle relaxant.

methodology (meth″o-dol′o-je) the science dealing with principles of procedure in research and study.

methohexital (meth″o-hek′sĭ-tal) an ultra-short-acting barbiturate.

sodium m., a compound used intravenously to produce general anesthesia.

methopholine (meth″o-fo′lēn) an analgesic.

methopromazine (meth″o-pro′mah-zēn) methoxypromazine, a tranquilizer.

methotrexate (meth″o-trek′sāt) folic acid antagonist used as an antineoplastic agent; it is also used in the treatment of psoriasis.

methotrimeprazine (meth′o-tri-mep′rah-zēn) a non-narcotic analgesic and sedative given intramuscularly.

methoxamine (mĕ-thok′sah-mēn) a sympathomimetic amine used for its vasopressor effects.

methoxsalen (mĕ-thok′sah-len) an acrylic acid compound which induces melanin production on exposure of the skin to ultraviolet light; used in the treatment of idiopathic vitiligo and as a suntan accelerator and protectant.

methoxyflurane (mĕ-thok″se-floo′rān) a compound used as a general anesthetic administered by inhalation.

methoxyphenamine (mĕ-thok″se-fen′ah-mēn) a sympathomimetic drug used as a bronchodilator and nasal decongestant.

methoxypromazine (mĕ-thok″se-pro′mah-zēn) a phenothiazine derivative used as a tranquilizer.

methscopolamine (meth″sko-pol′ah-min) an anticholinergic.

methsuximide (meth-suk′sĭ-mīd) a white to grayish white crystalline powder used as an anticonvulsant to treat petit mal and psychomotor epilepsy.

methyclothiazide (meth″ĭ-klo-thi′ah-zīd) an orally effective diuretic and antihypertensive.

methyl (meth′il) the monovalent radical, $—CH_3$.

m. alcohol, a clear, colorless, inflammable liquid, CH_3OH, used as a solvent and fuel; it is poisonous if taken internally. Called also methanol and wood alcohol.

m. orange, an orange-yellow aniline dye, used as an indicator with a pH range of 3.2–4.4 and a color change from pink to yellow.

m. salicylate, a natural or synthetic wintergreen oil, used as a topical analgesic in rheumatic disorders, lumbago, and sciatica, and as a flavoring agent.

methylate (meth′ĭ-lāt) 1. a compound of methyl alcohol and a base. 2. to add a methyl group to a substance.

methylation (meth″ĭ-la′shun) the addition of methyl groups.

methylatropine (meth″il-at′ro-pēn) an atropine derivative; methylatropine nitrate, the quaternary ammonium derivative, has strong antimuscarinic effects and strong ganglionic blocking activity.

methylbenzethonium chloride (meth″il-ben″zĕ-tho′ne-um) an ammonium compound used as a local anti-infective; it is used mainly in prevention of dermatitis in infants. Soap inhibits its action.

methylcellulose (meth″il-sel′u-lōs) a methyl ester of cellulose; used as a bulk laxative and a suspending agent for drugs.

methylcytosine (meth″il-si′to-sin) a pyrimidine occurring in deoxyribonucleic acid.

methyldopa (meth″il-do′pah) an oral antihypertensive agent.

methyldopate hydrochloride (meth″il-do′pāt) an ethyl ester of methyldopa given by intravenous infusion for acute hypertensive crisis.

methylene blue (meth′ĭ-lēn) a synthetic organic compound, in dark green crystals or lustrous crystalline powder, used in treatment of methemoglobinemia, as an antidote in cyanide poisoning, as a stain in pathology and bacteriology, and as an antiseptic.

methylergonovine maleate (meth″il-er″go-no′vin) a compound used as an oxytocic.

methylglucamine (meth″il-gloo′kah-mīn) 1. a compound prepared from D-glucose and methylamine, used in the synthesis of pharmaceuticals. 2. meglumine.

methylhexaneamine (meth″il-hek-sān′ah-min) a compound used as an inhalant to relieve nasal congestion.

methylparaben (meth″il-par′ah-ben) a compound used as an antifungal preservative for drug solutions.

methylphenidate (meth″il-fen′i-dāt) a compound used as a mild central nervous system stimulant.

methylprednisolone (meth″il-pred-nis′o-lōn) a white, odorless, crystalline powder, a corticosteroid of the glucogenic type, having an anti-inflammatory action similar to that of prednisolone.

methylrosaniline chloride (meth″il-ro-zan′ĭ-lēn) gentian violet, a topical anti-infective, stain, and internal anthelmintic.

methyltestosterone (meth″il-tes-tos′tĕ-rōn) an orally effective, synthetic form of testosterone.

methylthiouracil (meth″il-thi″o-u′rah-sil) a white, odorless, crystalline powder, used as a thyroid inhibitor.

methyltransferase (meth″il-trans′fer-ās) any enzyme that catalyzes transmethylation.

methyprylon (meth″ĭ-pri′lon) a white, crystalline powder used as a sedative and hypnotic.

methysergide (meth″ĭ-ser′jīd) a potent serotonin antagonist used in the prophylaxis of migraine; also available as the maleate salt.

Meticortelone (met″ĭ-kor′tĕ-lōn) trademark for preparations of prednisolone, an anti-inflammatory agent.

Meticorten (met″ĭ-kor′ten) trademark for a preparation of prednisone, an anti-inflammatory agent.

metmyoglobin (met-mi″o-glo′bin) a compound formed from myoglobin by oxidation of the ferrous to the ferric state with essentially ionic bonds.

metopic (mĕ-top′ik) pertaining to the forehead.

metopon (met-o′pon) a morphine derivative, used as an analgesic.

metoxenous (mĕ-tok′sĕ-nus) requiring two hosts for the entire life cycle; said of parasites.

metra (me′trah) the uterus.

metra-, metro- word element [Gr.], *uterus.*

metralgia (me-tral′je-ah) pain in the uterus.

metratonia (me″trah-to′ne-ah) uterine atony.

metratrophia (me″trah-tro′fe-ah) atrophy of the uterus.

Metrazol (met′rah-zol) trademark for preparations of pentylenetetrazol, a central nervous system stimulant.

metrectasia (me″trek-ta′ze-ah) dilatation of the nonpregnant uterus.

metreurynter (me″troo-rin′ter) an inflatable bag for dilating the cervical canal of the uterus.

metreurysis (me-troo′rĭ-sis) dilation of the cervix uteri by means of the metreurynter.

metric (met′rik) 1. pertaining to measures or measurement. 2. having the meter as a basis.

m. system, a system of weights and measures based on the meter and having all units based on some power of 10. (See also Table of Weights and Measures in the Appendix.)

metritis (me-tri′tis) inflammation of the uterus.

m. dis′secans, metritis with necrosis of portions of the uterine wall.

puerperal m., infection of the uterus of the puerperal woman.

metrocele (me′tro-sēl) hernia of the uterus.

metrocolpocele (me″tro-kol′po-sēl) hernia of the uterus with vaginal prolapse.

metrocystosis (me″tro-sis-to′sis) formation of cysts in the uterus.

metrocyte (me′tro-sīt) a mother cell.

metrodynia (me″tro-din′e-ah) pain in the uterus.

metroleukorrhea (me″tro-lu″ko-re′ah) leukorrhea of uterine origin.

metrolymphangitis (me″tro-limf″an-ji′tis) inflammation of the uterine lymphatic vessels.

metromalacoma (me″tro-mal″ah-ko′mah) abnormal softening of the uterus.

metronidazole (mĕ″tro-nid′ah-zōl) a compound used as a trichomonacide.

metroparalysis (me″tro-pah-ral′ĭ-sis) paralysis of the uterus.

metropathia (me″tro-path′e-ah) any disorder of the uterus.

m. haemorrha′gica, essential uterine hemorrhage.

metropathy (me-trop′ah-the) any uterine disorder. adj., **metropath′ic.**

metroperitoneal (me″tro-per″ĭ-to-ne′al) pertaining to the uterus and peritoneum.

metroperitonitis (me″tro-per″ĭ-to-ni′tis) inflammation of the peritoneum about the uterus.

metrophlebitis (me″tro-flĕ-bi′tis) inflammation of the uterine veins.

Metropine (met′ro-pin) trademark for preparations of methylatropine, an anticholinergic.

metroplasty (me′tro-plas″te) reconstructive surgery on the uterus.

metroptosis (me″tro-to′sis) prolapse of the uterus.

metrorrhagia (me″tro-ra′je-ah) uterine bleeding, usually of normal amount, occurring at completely irregular intervals, the period of flow sometimes being prolonged.

metrorrhea (me″tro-re′ah) abnormal uterine discharge.

metrorrhexis (me″tro-rek′sis) rupture of the uterus.

metrosalpingitis (me″tro-sal″pin-ji′tis) inflammation of the uterus and uterine tubes.

metrosalpingography (me″tro-sal″ping-gog′rah-fe) hysterosalpingography; roentgenography of the uterus and uterine tubes.

metroscope (me′tro-skōp) an instrument for examining the uterus.

metrostaxis (me″tro-stak′sis) slight but persistent uterine bleeding.

metrostenosis (me″tro-stĕ-no′sis) stenosis of the uterus.

-metry word element [Gr.], *measurement.*

Metubine (mĕ-tu′bin) trademark for a preparation of dimethyl tubocurarine, a skeletal muscle relaxant.

Metycaine (met′ĭ-kān) trademark for preparations of piperocaine, a local anesthetic.

metyrapone (mĕ-ter′ah-pōn) a compound used as a

MULTIPLES AND SUBMULTIPLES OF THE METRIC SYSTEM

MULTIPLES AND SUBMULTIPLES	PREFIX	PRONUNCIATION	SYMBOL
$1,000,000,000,000 = 10^{12}$	tera	ter′a	T
$1,000,000,000 = 10^{9}$	giga	ji′ga	G
$1,000,000 = 10^{6}$	mega	meg′a	M
$1,000 = 10^{3}$	kilo	kil′o	k
$100 = 10^{2}$	hecto	hek′to	h
$10 = 10$	deka	dek′a	dk
[The unit = one]			
$0.1 = 10^{-1}$	deci	des′i	d
$0.01 = 10^{-2}$	centi	sen′ti	c
$0.001 = 10^{-3}$	milli	mil′i	m
$0.000\ 001 = 10^{-6}$	micro	mi′kro	μ
$0.000\ 000\ 001 = 10^{-9}$	nano	nan′o	n
$0.000\ 000\ 000\ 001 = 10^{-12}$	pico	pi′co	p
$0.000\ 000\ 000\ 000\ 001 = 10^{-15}$	femto	fem′to	f
$0.000\ 000\ 000\ 000\ 000\ 001 = 10^{-18}$	atto	at′to	a

International Committee on Weights and Measures, 1962. From Style Manual for Biological Journals.

diagnostic aid in determining anterior pituitary function (corticotropin secretion).

Mev million electron volts.

Meynet's nodes (ma-nāz′) nodules in the capsules of joints and in tendons in rheumatic conditions, especially in children.

M.F.D. minimum fatal dose.

Mg chemical symbol, *magnesium.*

mg. milligram.

μg. microgram.

mianserin (me-an′ser-in) a sertonin inhibitor and antihistaminic used as the hydrochloride salt.

mication (mi-ka′shun) a quick motion, such as winking.

micelle (mi-sel′) a supermolecular colloid particle, most often a packet of chain molecules in parallel arrangement.

miconazole nitrate (mi-kon′ah-zōl) a topical antifungal agent available in two formulations; one for dermatophytic infections such as athlete's foot, and the other for vulvovaginal candidiasis.

micr(o)- (mi′kro) word element [Gr.], *small;* used in naming units of measurement to designate an amount 10^{-6} (one-millionth) the size of the unit to which it is joined, e.g., microgram.

micrencephaly (mi″kren-sef′ah-le) abnormal smallness and underdevelopment of the brain.

microabscess (mi″kro-ab′ses) an abscess visible only under a microscope.

microaerophilic (mi″kro-a″er-o-fil′ik) growing best in the presence of very little free oxygen.

microaerotonometer (mi″kro-a″er-o-to-nom′ĕ-ter) an instrument for measuring the volume of gases in the blood.

microanalysis (mi″kro-ah-nal′ĭ-sis) the chemical analysis of minute quantities of material.

microanatomy (mi″kro-ah-nat′o-me) histology.

microaneurysm (mi″kro-an′u-rizm) a minute aneurysm occurring on a vessel of small size, as one in the retina of the eye or as occurs in thrombotic purpura.

microangiopathy (mi″kro-an″je-op′ah-the) a disorder involving the small blood vessels. adj., **microangiopath′ic.**

thrombotic m., formation of thrombi in the arterioles and capillaries.

microbe (mi′krōb) a microorganism, especially a pathogenic bacterium. adj., **micro′bial, micro′bic.**

microbicidal (mi-kro″bĭ-si′dal) destroying microbes.

microbicide (mi-kro′bĭ-sīd) an agent that destroys microbes.

microbiologist (mi″kro-bi-ol′o-jist) a specialist in microbiology.

microbiology (mi″kro-bi-ol′o-je) the study of microorganisms, including bacteria, fungi, viruses, and pathogenic protoza; bacteriology. adj., **microbiolog′ical.**

microbiota (mi″kro-bi-o′tah) the microscopic living organisms of a region. adj., **microbiot′ic.**

microblast (mi′kro-blast) an erythroblast of 5 microns or less in diameter.

microblepharia (mi″kro-blĕ-făr′e-ah) abnormal shortness of the vertical dimensions of the eyelids.

microbody (mi′kro-bod″e) any of the cytoplasmic particles found in kidney and liver cells and in certain other cells, surrounded by a limiting membrane, and containing dense crystalline-like inclusions and oxidases.

microbrachius (mi″kro-bra′ke-us) a fetus with abnormally small arms.

microcalorie (mi″kro-kal′o-re) small calorie; the heat required to raise 1 ml. of distilled water from 0 to 1° C.

microcardia (mi″kro-kar′de-ah) abnormal smallness of the heart.

microcentrum (mi″kro-sen′trum) centrosome.

microcephalus (mi″kro-sef′ah-lus) an individual with a very small head.

microcephaly (mi″kro-sef′ah-le) small size of the head in relation to the rest of the body. adj., **microcephal′ic.**

microcheilia (mi″kro-ki′le-ah) abnormal smallness of the lip.

microcheiria (mi″kro-ki′re-ah) abnormal smallness of the hands.

microchemistry (mi″kro-kem′is-tre) chemistry concerned with exceedingly small quantities of chemical substances.

microcinematography (mi″kro-sin″ĕ-mah-tog′rah-fe) moving picture photography of microscopic objects.

microcirculation (mi″kro-ser″ku-la′shun) the flow of blood through the fine vessels (arterioles, capillaries, and venules). adj., **microcirculato′ry.**

Micrococcaceae (mi″kro-kok-a′se-e) a family of bacteria containing six genera including *Staphylococcus* and *Micrococcus.*

Micrococcus (mi″kro-kok′us) a genus of gram-positive bacteria of the family Micrococcaceae found in soil, water etc.

micrococcus (mi″kro-kok′us), pl. *micrococ′ci* [Gr.] 1. any organism of the genus *Micrococcus.* 2. a very small, spherical microorganism.

microcolon (mi″kro-ko′lon) abnormal smallness of the colon.

microcoria (mi″kro-ko′re-ah) smallness of the pupil.

microcornea (mi″kro-kor′ne-ah) unusual smallness of the cornea, usually bilateral.

microcoulomb (mi″kro-koo′lomb) one-millionth of a coulomb.

microcrystalline (mi″kro-kris′tah-lin) made up of minute crystals.

microcurie (mi″kro-ku′re) one-millionth (10^{-6}) curie; abbreviated μCi or μc.

microcurie-hour (mi′kro-ku″re-owr″) a unit of dose equivalent to that obtained by exposure for one hour to radioactive material disintegrating at the rate of 3.7×10^4 atoms per second; abbreviated μc.-hr, or μC. hr.

microcyst (mi′kro-sist) a cyst visible only under a microscope.

microcyte (mi′kro-sīt) an erythrocyte 5 microns or less in diameter. adj., **microcyt′ic.**

microcythemia, microcytosis (mi″kro-si-the′me-ah; mi″kro-si-to′sis) a condition in which the erythrocytes are smaller than normal.

microdactyly (mi″kro-dak′tĭ-le) abnormal smallness of the fingers or toes.

microdetermination (mi″kro-de-ter″mĭ-na′shun) chemical examination of minute quantities of substance.

microdissection (mi″kro-dĭ-sek′shun) dissection of tissue or cells under the microscope.

microdontia (mi″kro-don′she-ah) abnormal smallness of the teeth.

microdrepanocytic (mi″kro-drep″ah-no-sit′ik) containing microcytic and drepanocytic elements, as in sickle cell-thalassemia disease.

microembolus (mi″kro-em′bo-lus), pl. *microem′boli* [L.] an embolus of microscopic size.

microerythrocyte (mi″kro-ĕ-rith′ro-sīt) microcyte.

microfarad (mi″kro-far′ad) one millionth (10^{-6}) farad; abbreviated μf.

microfauna (mi″kro-faw′nah) the microscopic animal organisms of a special region.

microfibril (mi″kro-fi′bril) an extremely small fibril.

microfilament (mi″kro-fil′ah-ment) any of the filaments about 60 angstroms in diameter, in the cytoplasmic ground substance.

microfilaremia (mi″kro-fil″ah-re′me-ah) the presence of microfilariae in the circulating blood.

microfilaria (mi″kro-fĭ-la″re-ah) the prelarval stage of Filariodea in the blood of man and in the tissues of the vector. This term is sometimes incorrectly used as a genus name, and is then spelled with a capital M.

m. bancrof′ti, the microfilaria of *Wuchereria bancrofti.*

m. streptocer′ca, the larval form of *Onchocerca volvulus,* found in cutaneous lesions of the natives of the Gold Coast.

microflora (mi″kro-flo′rah) the microscopic vegetable organisms of special region.

microgamete (mi″kro-gam′ēt) the smaller, male gamete of the malarial parasite.

microgastria (mi″kro-gas′tre-ah) congenital smallness of the stomach.

microgenia (mi″kro-je′ne-ah) abnormal smallness of the chin.

microgenitalism (mi″kro-jen′ĭ-tal″izm) smallness of the external genitalia.

microglia (mi-krog′le-ah) non-neural cells forming part of the adventitial structure of the central nervous system. They are migratory and act as phagocytes of waste products of the nervous system. adj., **microg′lial.**

microglioma (mi″kro-gli-o′mah) a tumor composed of microglial cells.

microglossia (mi″kro-glos′e-ah) abnormal smallness of the tongue.

micrognathia (mi″kro-nath′e-ah) abnormal smallness of the jaws, especially the lower jaw. adj., **micrognath′ic.**

microgram (mi′kro-gram) one-millionth (10^{-6}) gram, or one-thousandth (10^{-3}) milligram; abbreviated μg. or mcg.

micrograph (mi′kro-graf) 1. an instrument for recording very minute movements by making a greatly magnified photograph of the minute motions of a diaphragm. 2. a photograph of a minute object or specimen as seen through a microscope.

electron m., a graphic reproduction of an object as viewed with an electron microscope.

microgyria (mi″kro-ji′re-ah) abnormal smallness of convolutions of the brain.

microgyrus (mi″kro-ji′rus) an abnormally small, malformed convolution of the brain.

microhm (mi′krōm) one-millionth (10^{-6}) ohm.

microincineration (mi″kro-in-sin″er-a′shun) the oxidation of a small quantity of material, to eliminate organic matter and leave only the ash, for the purpose of analyzing the elements composing the material.

microinjector (mi″kro-in-jek′tor) an instrument for infusion of very small amounts of fluids or drugs.

microlesion (mi′kro-le″zhun) a minute lesion.

microliter (mi′kro-le″ter) one-millionth part of a liter, or one-thousandth of a milliliter; abbreviated μl.

microlith (mi″kro-lith) a minute concretion or calculus.

microlithiasis (mi″kro-lĭ-thi′ah-sis) the formation of minute concretions in an organ.

m. alveola′ris pulmo′num, pulmonary alveolar m., a condition simulating pulmonary tuberculosis, with deposition of minute calculi in the alveoli of the lungs.

micromanipulation (mi″kro-mah-nip″u-la′shun) the use of the micromanipulator.

micromanipulator (mi″kro-mah-nip′u-la″tor) an instrument for the moving, dissecting, etc., of minute specimens under the microscope.

micromastia (mi″kro-mas′te-ah) abnormal smallness of the breast.

micromelia (mi″kro-me′le-ah) abnormal smallness of one or more extremities.

micromelus (mi-krom′ĕ-lus) an individual with abnormally small limbs.

micromere (mi′kro-mēr) one of the small blastomeres formed by unequal cleavage of a fertilized ovum.

micrometer[1] (mi-krom′ĭ-ter) an instrument for making minute measurements.

micrometer[2] (mi′kro-me″ter) micron; one thousandth (10^{-3}) of a millimeter or one millionth (10^{-6}) of a meter. Abbreviated μm.

micromethod (mi′kro-meth″od) a technique dealing with exceedingly small quantities of material.

micrometry (mi-krom′ĕ-tre) measurement of microscopic objects.

micromicro- (mi″kro-mi′kro) word element designating 10^{-12} (one-trillionth), part of the unit to which it is joined; now supplanted by the prefix pico-.

micromicron (mi″kro-mi′kron) one-millionth (10^{-6}) micron, or 1 picometer; abbreviated $\mu\mu$.

micromillimeter (mi″kro-mil′ĭ-me″ter) one-millionth of a millimeter, or 1 nanometer; abbreviated μmm.

micromolecular (mi″kro-mo-lek′u-lar) composed of small molecules.

micromyelia (mi″kro-mi-e′le-ah) abnormal smallness of spinal cord.

micromyeloblast (mi″kro-mi′ĕ-lo-blast″) a small, immature myelocyte. adj., **micromyeloblas′tic.**

micron (mi′kron), pl. *mi′cra, mi′crons* [Gr.] micrometer; one thousandth (10^{-3}) millimeter or one millionth (10^{-6}) meter; abbreviated μ.

microneedle (mi″kro-ne′d′l) a fine glass needle used in micromanipulation.

micronodular (mi″kro-nod′u-lar) marked by the presence of small nodules.

micronucleus (mi″kro-nu′kle-us) 1. in ciliate protozoa, the smaller of two types of nucleus in each cell, which functions in sexual reproduction. (See also KINETOPLAST.) 2. a small nucleus. 3. nucleolus.

micronutrient (mi″kro-nu′tre-ent) a dietary element essential only in small quantities.

micronychia (mi″kro-nik′e-ah) abnormal smallness of the nails of the fingers or toes.

microorganism (mi″kro-or′gah-nizm) a microscopic organism; those of medical interest include bacteria, rickettsiae, viruses, fungi, and protozoa.

micropathology (mi″kro-pah-thol′o-je) 1. the sum of what is known about minute pathologic change. 2. pathology of diseases caused by microorganisms.

microphage (mi′kro-fāj) a small phagocyte; an actively motile neutrophilic leukocyte capable of phagocytosis.

microphakia (mi″kro-fa′ke-ah) abnormal smallness of the crystalline lens.

microphallus (mi″kro-fal′us) abnormal smallness of the penis.

microphone (mi′kro-fōn) a device to pick up sound for purposes of amplification or transmission.

microphonia (mi″kro-fo′ne-ah) marked weakness of voice.

microphotograph (mi″kro-fo′to-graf) a photograph of small size.

microphthalmia (mi″krof-thal′me-ah) abnormal smallness of the eyeball.

micropipet (mi″kro-pi″pet′) a pipet for handling small quantities of liquids (up to 1 ml.).

microplethysmography (mi″kro-pleth″is-mog′rah-fe) the recording of minute changes in the size of a part as produced by circulation of blood.

micropodia (mi″kro-po′de-ah) abnormal smallness of the feet.

microprobe (mi′kro-prōb″) a minute probe, as one used in microsurgery.

micropsia (mi-krop′se-ah) a disorder of visual perception in which objects appear smaller than their actual size.

micropyle (mi′kro-pīl) an opening through which a spermatozoon enters certain ova.

microradiography (mi″kro-ra″de-og′rah-fe) radiography under conditions that permit subsequent microscopic examination or enlargement of the radiograph up to several hundred linear magnifications.

microrespirometer (mi″kro-res″pĭ-rom′ĕ-ter) an apparatus for investigating oxygen utilization in isolated tissues.

microscope (mi′kro-skōp) an instrument used to obtain an enlarged image of small objects and reveal details of structure not otherwise distinguishable.

binocular m., one with two eyepieces, permitting use of both eyes simultaneously.

compound m., one consisting of two lens systems whereby the image formed by the system near the object is magnified by the one nearer the eye.

darkfield m., one so constructed that illumination is from the side of the field so that details appear light against a dark background.

electron m., one in which an electron beam, instead of light rays, is used to produce an image which may be viewed on a fluorescent screen or photographed. The electron microscope is able to produce much higher magnification than the light microscope.

light m., one in which the specimen is viewed under ordinary illumination.

operating m., one designed for use in performance of delicate surgical procedures, e.g., on the middle ear or small vessels of the heart.

phase m., phase-contrast m., a microscope that alters the phase relationships of the light passing through and that passing around the object, the contrast permitting visualization of the object without the necessity for staining or other special preparation.

simple m., one that consists of a single lens.

slit lamp m., a corneal microscope with a special attachment that permits examination of the endothelium on the posterior surface of the cornea.

stereoscopic m., a binocular microscope modified to give a three-dimensional view of the specimen.

x-ray m., one in which x-rays are used instead of light, the image usually being reproduced on film.

microscopic (mi″kro-skop′ik) of extremely small size; visible only by aid of a microscope.

microscopical (mi″kro-skop′ĭ-kal) pertaining to a microscope or to microscopy.

microscopist (mi-kros′ko-pist) a person skilled in using the microscope.

microscopy (mi-kros′ko-pe) examination with a microscope.

television m., a special technique in which a magnified image produced by a microscope is projected on a television screen.

microsecond (mi′kro-sek″und) one millionth (10^{-6}) of a second; abbreviated μs. or μsec.

microsome (mi′kro-sōm) any of the vesicular fragments of endoplasmic reticulum produced during homogenization of cells.

microsomia (mi″kro-so′me-ah) abnormally small size of the body.

microspectroscope (mi″kro-spek′tro-skōp) a spectroscope and microscope combined.

microspherocyte (mi″kro-sfe′ro-sīt) an erythrocyte whose diameter is less than normal, but whose thickness is increased.

microspherocytosis (mi″kro-sfe′ro-si-to′sis) the presence in the blood of an excessive number of microspherocytes.

microsphygmia (mi″kro-sfig′me-ah) that condition of the pulse in which it is perceived with difficulty by the finger.

microsplenia (mi″kro-sple′ne-ah) smallness of the spleen.

microsporid (mi-kros′po-rid) a secondary skin eruption which is an expression of hypersensitivity to *Microsporum* infection.

Microsporum (mi″kro-spo′rum) a genus of fungi that cause various diseases of the skin and hair, including the species *M. audoui′ni, M. ca′nis* (*lano′sum*), and *M. ful′vum* (*gyp′seum*).

microstomia (mi″kro-sto′me-ah) abnormally decreased size of the mouth.

microsurgery (mi″kro-ser′jer-e) dissection of minute structures under the microscope, with the use of extremely small instruments.

microsyringe (mi″kro-sĕr′inj) a syringe fitted with a screw-threaded micrometer for accurate measurement of minute quantities.

microtia (mi-kro′she-ah) abnormal smallness of the pinna of the ear.

microtome (mi′kro-tōm) an instrument for making thin sections for microscopic study.

freezing m., one for cutting frozen tissues.

rotary m., one in which wheel action is translated into a back-and-forth movement of the specimen being sectioned.

sliding m., one in which the specimen being sectioned is made to slide on a track.

microtomy (mi-krot′o-me) the cutting of thin sections.

microtonometer (mi″kro-to-nom′ĕ-ter) an instrument for measuring the oxygen and carbon dioxide tension of arterial blood.

microtrauma (mi″kro-traw′mah) a microscopic lesion or injury.

microtubule (mi″kro-tu′būl) a straight, hollow-appearing structure in the cytoplasm of a cell.

microvasculature (mi″kro-vas′ku-lah-chūr) the finer vessels of the body, as the arterioles, capillaries, and venules.

microvillus (mi″kro-vil′us), pl. *microvil′li.* a minute process of protrusion from the free surface of a cell, especially cells of the proximal convolution in renal tubules and of the intestinal epithelium.

microvolt (mi′kro-volt) one-millionth of a volt; abbreviated μv.

microwave (mi′kro-wāv) a wave typical of electromagnetic radiation between far infrared and radiowaves.

microzoon (mi″kro-zo′on), pl. *microzo′a* [Gr.] a microscopic animal organism.

micrurgy (mi′krur-je) manipulative technique in the field of a microscope. adj., **micrur′gic.**

micturate (mik′tu-rāt) urinate.

micturition (mik″tu-rish′un) urination.

midbrain (mid′brān) the short part of the brain stem just above the pons. It contains the nerve pathways between the cerebral hemispheres and the medulla oblongata, and also contains nuclei (relay stations or centers) of the third and fourth cranial nerves. The center for visual reflexes, such as moving the head and eyes, is located in the midbrain. Called also mesencephalon.

middle lobe syndrome atelectasis of the middle lobe of the right lung, with chronic pneumonitis, due to compression of the bronchus by tuberculous hilar lymph nodes.

midget (mij′et) a normal dwarf; an individual who is undersized but perfectly formed.

midgut (mid′gut) an intermediate region in the embryo between the foregut and hindgut, which is of only brief duration in man.

Midicel (mid′ĭ-sel) trademark for preparations of sulfamethoxypyridazine, a sulfonamide.

midline (mid′līn) the imaginary line that divides the body into right and left halves.

midwife (mid′wīf) a woman who assists at childbirth but who is not a physician.

nurse m., a professional nurse who specializes in the care of women throughout pregnancy, delivery, and the postpartum period.

midwifery (mid′wi-fer-e) the practice of a midwife.

migraine (mi′grān) a headache, usually severe, often limited to one side of the head, and sometimes accompanied by nausea and vomiting; called also a sick headache. adj., **mi′grainous.**

Although the cause is not completely understood, migraine is thought to be associated with constriction and then dilation of the cerebral arteries. It is also thought to have a psychologic aspect, since it occurs most often in persons with particular types of personalities and often follows emotional disturbances. Migraine tends to run in families. In women the headaches often occur during the menstrual periods.

The symptoms of migraine vary greatly not only from person to person but also from time to time in the same person. The headaches are usually intense and they frequently occur on one or the other side of the head. They are often accompanied by nausea and vomiting. A typical migraine attack begins with changes in vision, such as a flickering before the eyes, flashes of light, or a blacking out of part of the sight.

Aspirin is usually of little help in relieving migraine. Ergotamine tartrate is quite effective but has side effects, and weekly dosages must be limited. Psychotherapy may help to release the tensions that may be an underlying cause (see also BIOFEEDBACK).

abdominal m., migraine in which abdominal symptoms are prominent.

Mikedimide (mi-ked′ĭ-mīd) trademark for a preparation of bemegride, an analeptic used in barbiturate poisoning.

mikro- for words beginning thus, see those beginning *micro-*.

Mikulicz's disease (mik′u-lich″ez) a benign, chronic lymphocytic infiltration and enlargement of the lacrimal and salivary glands, of unknown origin.

Mikulicz's pad (mik′u-lich″ez) a pad made of folded gauze, for packing of viscera in surgical procedures.

mil (mil) contraction of milliliter.

miliaria (mil″e-a′re-ah) a cutaneous condition with retention of sweat, which is extravasated at different levels in the skin; called also prickly heat or heat rash. Treatment of miliaria is directed at reducing sweating generally by reducing the external heat load and avoiding irritating agents and tight clothing. Bland powders may be helpful.

miliary (mil′e-er″e) 1. like millet seeds. 2. characterized by the formation of lesions resembling millet seeds.

m. fever, an acute infectious disease characterized by fever, profuse sweating and the formation of a great many papules, succeeded by a crop of pustules; called also sweating sickness.

m. tuberculosis, an acute form of tuberculosis in which minute tubercles are formed in a number of organs of the body, owing to dissemination of the bacilli throughout the body by the bloodstream.

Milibis (mil′ĭ-bis) trademark for preparations of glycobiarsol, a compound used in amebiasis.

milieu (me-lyuh′) [Fr.] surroundings; environment.

m. extérieur (me-lyuh′ ek-sta′re-ur″) external environment.

m. intérieur (me-lyuh′ an-ta′re-ur″) internal environment; the blood and lymph in which the cells are bathed.

milium (mil′e-um), pl. *mil′ia* [L.] a whitish nodule in the skin, especially of the face, usually 1 to 4 mm. in diameter. Milia are spheroidal masses of lamellated keratin lying just under the epidermis, often associated with vellus hair follicles. Popularly called *whitehead.*

milk (milk) 1. a nutrient fluid produced by the mammary gland of many animals for nourishment of young mammals. 2. a liquid (emulsion or suspension) resembling the secretion of the mammary gland.

acidophilus m., milk fermented with cultures of *Lactobacillus acidophilus;* used in gastrointestinal disorders to modify the bacterial flora of the intestinal tract.

m.-alkali syndrome, ingestion of milk and absorbable alkali in excess amounts, resulting in kidney damage and elevated blood calcium levels.

m. of bismuth, a suspension of bismuth hydroxide and bismuth subcarbonate in water; used as an astringent and antacid.

casein m., a prepared milk containing very little salts and sugars and a large amount of fat and casein.

certified m., milk whose purity is certified by a committee of physicians or a medical milk commission.

condensed m., milk that has been partly evaporated and sweetened with sugar.

dialyzed m., milk from which the sugar has been removed by dialysis through a parchment membrane.

evaporated m., milk prepared by evaporation of half of its water content.

m. fever, 1. an endemic fever said to be due to the use of unwholesome cow's milk. 2. a form of paralysis due to a metabolic disorder affecting cows near delivery, and usually accompanied by hypocalcemia.

fortified m., milk made more nutritious by addition of cream, egg white, or vitamins.

homogenized m., milk treated so the fats form a permanent emulsion and the cream does not separate.

m. of magnesia, a suspension containing 7 to 8.5 per cent of magnesium hydroxide, used as an antacid and laxative.

modified m., cow's milk made to correspond to composition of human milk.

protein m., milk modified to have a relatively low content of carbohydrate and fat and a relatively high protein content.

witch's m., milk secreted in the breast of a newborn infant.

Milkman's syndrome (milk′manz) a generalized bone disease marked by multiple transparent stripes of absorption in the long and flat bones.

Miller-Abbott tube (mil′er ab′ot) a double-channel intestinal tube with an inflatable balloon at its distal end, used for diagnosing and treating obstructive lesions of the small intestine. The tube is inserted via a nostril and gently passed through the stomach and into the small intestine.

The Miller-Abbott tube is often used in the treatment of INTESTINAL OBSTRUCTION. Care must be used in irrigating the tube and in attaching it to a suction apparatus because of the possibility of confusing the two lumina. The lumen marked suction is used for irrigations and suction; the other lumen leads to the small rubber bag intended to hold the tube in place. The introduction of too large an amount of fluid into the bag would lead to rupture of the intestine.

milli- (mil′e) word element, *one-thousandth;* used in naming units of measurement to designate an amount 10^{-3} the size of the unit to which it is joined, e.g., milligram (0.001 gm).

milliampere (mil″e-am′pēr) one-thousandth of an ampere.

milliampere-minute (mil″e-am″pēr-min′ut) a unit of electricity equivalent to that delivered by a current of 1 milliampere strength acting for one minute.

millicoulomb (mil″i-koo′lom) one-thousandth (10^{-3}) coulomb; abbreviated mcoul.

millicurie (mil′ĭ-ku′re) one-thousandth (10^{-3}) curie; abbreviated mCi or mc.

millicurie-hour (mil′ĭ-ku′re-owr″) a unit of dose equivalent to that obtained by exposure for one hour to radioactive material disintegrating at the rate of 3.7×10^7 atoms per second; abbreviated mc.-hr.

milliequivalent (mil″e-e-kwiv′ah-lent) the number of grams of a solute contained in 1 milliliter of a normal solution; abbreviated mEq.

milligram (mil′ĭ-gram) one-thousandth of a gram; equivalent of 0.015432 grain avoirdupois or apothecaries' weight; abbreviated mg.

milliliter (mil′ĭ-le″ter) one-thousandth of a liter; equivalent of 16.23 minims; abbreviated ml.

millimeter (mil′ĭ-me″ter) one-thousandth of a meter; equivalent of 0.039 inch; abbreviated mm.

millimicro- (mil″ĭ-mi′kro) word element designating 10^{-3} (one-thousandth) of 10^{-6} (one-millionth), or 10^{-9} (one-billionth), part of the unit to which it is joined; now being supplanted by the prefix nano-.

millimicrocurie (mil″ĭ-mi″kro-ku′re) one-thousandth (10^{-3}) microcurie, or 10^{-9} curie; abbreviated mμc. Called also nanocurie.

millimicrogram (mil″ĭ-mi′kro-gram) a nanogram; one-thousandth (10^{-3}) microgram, or 10^{-9} gram; abbreviated mμg.

millimicron (mil″ĭ-mi′kron) nanometer; one-thousandth of a micron (10^{-6} mm., or 10 angstroms); abbreviated mμ.

millimole (mil′ĭ-mōl) one thousandth part of a mole; symbol mmol.

millinormal (mil″ĭ-nor′mal) having a concentration one-thousandth of normal; abbreviated mN.

milliosmole (mil″e-oz′mōl) one-thousandth of an osmole.

Millipore filter (mil′ĭ-por) trademark for a device used to filter nutrient solutions as they are administered intravenously.

millivolt (mil′ĭ-volt) one-thousandth of a volt; abbreviated mv.

Milontin (mi-lon′tin) trademark for preparations of phenuximide, an anticonvulsant.

Milpath (mil′path) trademark for a preparation of meprobamate and tridihexethyl chloride, a tranquilizer.

milphae, milphosis (mil'fe; mil-fo'sis) the falling out of the eyelashes.

Milroy's disease (mil'royz) hereditary permanent lymphedema of the legs due to lymphatic obstruction; called also congenital lymphedema.

Miltown (mil'town) trademark for a preparation of meprobamate, a tranquilizer.

min. minim; minimum; minute.

Minamata disease (min"ah-mah'tah) a severe neurologic disorder due to alkyl mercury poisoning, leading to severe permanent neurologic and mental disabilities or death; once prevalent among those who ate contaminated seafood from Minamata Bay, Japan.

mind (mīnd) the psyche; the faculty by which one is aware of surroundings and by which he is able to experience emotions, remember, reason, and make decisions.

mineral (min'er-al) any naturally occurring nonorganic homogeneous solid substance. There are 19 or more minerals forming the mineral composition of the body; at least 13 are essential to health. These minerals must be supplied in the diet and generally can be supplied by a varied or mixed diet of animal and vegetable products which meet the energy and protein needs. The Food and Nutrition Board of the National Research Council has established recommended daily intakes only for calcium and iron. These two minerals plus iodine are the three elements most frequently missing in the diet. Zinc, iron, copper, magnesium, and potassium are the five minerals that are most frequently involved in disturbances of metabolism.

Minerals are electropositive or electronegative. Combinations of electropositive and electronegative elements lead to the formation of salts such as sodium chloride and calcium phosphate.

m. oil, a mixture of liquid hydrocarbons from petroleum. Mineral oil is available in both light (light liquid petrolatum) and heavy (liquid, or heavy liquid, petrolatum) grades. Light mineral oil is used chiefly as a vehicle for drugs, but it may also be used as a cathartic and to cleanse the skin. Heavy mineral oil is used as a cathartic, solvent, and oleaginous vehicle. Prolonged use of mineral oil as a cathartic should be avoided because it prevents absorption of the fat-soluble vitamins. Lipid pneumonia caused by aspiration of the oil has been shown to occur in those who habitually take it, especially the elderly.

mineralization (min"er-al-ĭ-za'shun) the addition of mineral matter to the body.

mineralocorticoid (min"er-al-o-kor'tĭ-koid) any of the hormones of the adrenal cortex having effects on the electrolytes of the extracellular fluid, particularly sodium, potassium, and chloride. Aldosterone is the principal mineralocorticoid, and others are desoxycorticosterone and corticosterone, which is also a glucocorticoid. These hormones increase the renal tubular reabsorption of sodium and increase the renal tubular excretion of potassium. Thus, a deficiency of the mineralocorticoids results in excessive loss of sodium (and, consequently, water) in the urine and retention of potassium in the extracellular fluid.

The mineralocorticoids are essential to life because they indirectly affect the fluid and electrolyte balance of the body. Without them there is a decrease in blood volume which soon produces a diminished cardiac output followed by a shocklike state and eventually death.

The body increases the output of mineralocorticoids when the extracellular concentration of sodium falls below normal, or when increased blood pressure is needed to cope with physical stress (see also ALARM REACTION.)

minim (min'im) a unit of volume (liquid measure) in the apothecaries system, equivalent to 0.0616 ml.

Minin light (min'in) a lamp for therapeutic administration of violet and ultraviolet rays.

miocardia (mi"o-kar'de-ah) the contraction of the heart; systole.

miopus (mi'o-pus) a monster with two fused heads, one face being rudimentary.

miosis (mi-o'sis) excessive contraction of the pupil.

miotic (mi-ot'ik) 1. pertaining to, characterized by, or causing miosis. 2. an agent that causes contraction of the pupil.

miracidium (mi"rah-sid'e-um), pl. *miracid'ia* [Gr.] the free-swimming larva of a trematode parasite which emerges from an egg and penetrates the body of a snail host.

mire (mēr) [Fr.] a figure on the arm of an ophthalmometer the image of which is reflected on the cornea; used to measure corneal astigmatism.

miscarriage (mis-kar'ij) the lay term used to designate loss of the fetus before it is viable; spontaneous abortion. (See also ABORTION.)

miscible (mis'ĭ-bl) susceptible of being mixed.

misogamy (mĭ-sog'ah-me) morbid aversion to marriage.

misogyny (mĭ-soj'ĭ-ne) aversion to women.

misopedia (mis"o-pe'de-ah) morbid dislike of children.

Mitchell's disease (mich'elz) erythromelalgia.

mite (mīt) any arthropod of the order Acarina except the ticks; they are characterized by minute size, usually transparent or semitransparent body, and other features distinguishing them from the ticks. They may be free living or parasitic on animals or plants, and may produce various irritations of the skin.

harvest m., chigger.

itch m., mange m., *Sarcoptes scabiei.*

mithramycin (mith"rah-mi'sin) an antineoplastic antibiotic produced by *Streptomyces argillaceus* and *S. tanashiensis.*

mithridatism (mith'rĭ-da"tizm) acquisition of immunity to a poison by ingestion of gradually increasing amounts of it.

miticide (mi'tĭ-sīd) an agent destructive to mites.

mitochondria (mi"to-kon'dre-ah), sing., *mitochon'drion* [Gr.] small, spherical to rod-shaped components (organelles) of cytoplasm, the principal sites of oxidative reactions by which the energy in foodstuff is made available for endergonic processes in the cell. They contain enzymes of the Krebs cycle and fatty acid cycles and the respiratory pathway.

mitogen (mi'to-jen) an agent that induces mitosis. adj., **mitogen'ic.**

mitogenesis (mi"to-jen'ĕ-sis) the induction of mitosis in a cell.

mitome (mi'tōm) a thready network of protoplasm.

mitomycin (mi″to-mi′sin) a group of highly toxic antineoplastics (mitomycin A, B, and C) produced by *Streptomyces caespitosus,* indicated for palliative treatment of certain neoplasms that do not respond to surgery, radiation, and other drugs.

mitosis (mi-to′sis) the process by which a cell splits into two new cells, each daughter cell having the same number and kind of chromosomes as the parent cell. adj. **mitot′ic.**

The first step in mitosis is duplication of all genes and chromosomes. To accomplish this the cell must double its content of DEOXYRIBONUCLEIC ACID (DNA). Chromosomes are composed of the DNA molecule loosely bound with protein; genes are segments of the DNA molecule. Since the DNA molecule has the ability to duplicate itself (replication), it is possible for the cell to form two identical sets of chromosomes and genes. After they are duplicated they divide between the two separate nuclei that have formed. The final step in mitosis is the splitting of the parent cell into two identical daughter cells, each with a full complement of genes and chromosomes.

Most cells of the body are continually growing and reproducing, so that when the old cells die the new ones take their place; thus, mitosis is a continuous process. It is obvious that this reproduction must take place in an orderly manner, but the exact way in which cell growth and reproduction are regulated is not completely understood. Although certain cells such as the blood-forming cells of the bone marrow and the stratum germinativum of the skin grow and reproduce continually, other cells such as neurons (nerve cells) do not reproduce during a person's lifetime. Neoplastic disorders such as cancer are a result of the abnormal and unrestricted growth and reproduction of certain body cells.

Germ cells reproduce by the process of meiosis.

mitosome (mi′to-sōm) a body formed from the spindle fibers of the preceding mitosis; a spindle remnant.

mitral (mi′tral) shaped like a miter; pertaining to the mitral valve.

m. commissurotomy, surgical incision of thickened leaflets of a stenotic mitral valve (see also mitral COMMISSUROTOMY).

m. stenosis, a narrowing of the left atrioventricular orifice (mitral orifice). (See also mitral COMMISSUROTOMY.)

m. valve, the left atrioventricular valve, the valve between the left atrium and the left ventricle of the heart; it is composed of two cusps, anterior and posterior. Called also the bicuspid valve.

mitralization (mi″tral-i-za′shun) a straightening of the left border of the cardiac shadow, commonly seen radiographically in mitral stenosis.

mittelschmerz (mit′el-shmerts) [Ger.] pain midway between the menstrual periods.

Mittendorf's dot a congenital anomaly of the eye manifested as a small gray or white opacity just inferior and nasal to the posterior pole of the lens, representing the remains of the lenticular attachment of the hyaloid artery; it does not affect vision.

mixture (miks′tūr) a combination of different drugs or ingredients, as a fluid with other fluids or solids, or of a solid with a liquid.

Miyagawanella (mi″yah-gah″wah-nel′ah) a genus of organisms, the species of which are now assigned to the genus *Chlamydia* as follows: *M. lymphogranulomato′sis* and *M. bronchopneumo′niae* are assigned to *C. trachomatis,* and *M. bo′vis, M. fe′lis, M. illi′nii, M. louisia′nae, M. opos′sumi, M. ornitho′sis, M. o′vis, M. pe′coris, M. pneumo′niae,* and *M. psit′taci* are assigned to *C. psittaci.*

ml. milliliter.

M.L.A. Medical Library Association.

M.L.D. minimum lethal dose.

mm. millimeter; muscles.

mμ. millimicron

MMR measles, mumps, and rubella (vaccine).

Mn chemical symbol, *manganese.*

M'Naghten rule (mik-naw′ten) "to establish a defense on the ground of insanity, it must be clearly proved that at the time of committing the act the party accused was laboring under such a defect of reason from disease of the mind as not to know the nature or quality of the act he was doing, or, if he did know it, that he did not know he was doing what was wrong."

mnemonics (ne-mon′iks) improvement of memory by special methods or techniques. adj., **mnemon′ic.**

M.O. Medical Officer.

Mo chemical symbol, *molybdenum.*

mobilization (mo″bĭ-lĭ-za′shun) the rendering of a fixed part movable.

stapes m., surgical correction of immobility of the stapes in treatment of deafness.

Möbius' disease (me′be-oos) periodic migraine with paralysis of the oculomotor muscles.

modality (mo-dal′ĭ-te) 1. in homeopathy, a condition that modifies drug action; a condition under which symptoms develop, becoming better or worse. 2. a method of application of, or the employment of, any therapeutic agent; limited usually to physical agents. 3. a specific sensory entity, such as taste.

mode (mōd) in statistics, the value or item in a variations curve that shows the maximal frequency of occurrence.

Moderil (mod′er-il) trademark for a preparation of rescinnamine, a tranquilizer and antihypertensive.

modiolus (mo-di′o-lus) the central pillar or columella of the cochlea.

Modumate (mod′u-māt) trademark for a preparation of arginine and glutamic acid, a nutrient used for the treatment of ammonia intoxication due to liver failure.

M.O.H. Medical Officer of Health.

moiety (moi′ĕ-te) any equal part; a half; also any part or portion, as a portion of a molecule.

mol (mol) mole (2).

molal (mo′lal) containing one mole of solute per 1000 grams of solvent.

molality (mo-lal′ĭ-te) the number of moles of a solute per kilogram of pure solvent.

molar (mo′lar) 1. pertaining to a mass; not molecular. 2. adapted for grinding (see also TOOTH and see Plate 9). 3. containing 1 mole of solute per liter of solution.

molarity (mo-lar′ĭ-te) the number of moles of a solute per liter of solution.

mold (mōld) 1. any of a group of parasitic and saprophytic fungi causing a cottony growth on organic substances; also, the deposit of growth produced by such fungi.

molding (mōld′ing) the shaping of the fetal head to the size and shape of the birth canal.

mole (mōl) 1. a fleshy mass formed in the uterus by abortive development of an ovum. 2. that amount of a chemical compound whose mass in grams is equivalent to its formula mass. 3. a fleshy growth or blemish on the skin; a NEVUS.

hairy m., hairy nevus.

hydatid m., hydatidiform m., an abnormal pregnancy resulting from a pathologic ovum, with proliferation of the epithelial covering of the chorionic villi and dissolution and cystic cavitation of the avascular stroma of the villi. It results in a mass of cysts resembling a bunch of grapes.

pigmented m., nevus pigmentosus.

molecular (mo-lek′u-lar) of, pertaining to, or composed of molecules.

m. biology, study of the biochemical and biophysical aspects of structure and function of genes and other subcellular entities, and of such specific proteins as hemoglobins, enzymes, and hormones; it provides knowledge of cellular differentiation and metabolism and of comparative evolution.

m. weight, the weight of a molecule of a chemical compound as compared with the weight of an atom of carbon-12; it is equal to the sum of the weights of its constituent atoms.

molecule (mol′ĕ-kūl) a very small mass of matter; an aggregation of atoms composing the smallest unit of a compound possessing its characteristic properties.

molidone (mol′ĭ-dōn) a sedative and tranquilizer.

molimen (mo-li′men), pl. *molim′ina* [L.] a laborious effort made for the performance of any normal body function, especially that manifested by a variety of unpleasant symptoms preceding or accompanying menstruation.

Moll's glands (molz) sweat glands that have become arrested in their development, situated at the edges of the eyelids; called also ciliary glands.

mollities (mo-lish′e-ēz) abnormal softening.

m. os′sium, osteomalacia.

molluscum (mŏ-lus′kum) 1. any of various skin diseases marked by the formation of soft rounded cutaneous tumors. 2. molluscum contagiosum. adj., **mollus′cous.**

m. contagio′sum, a viral infection of the skin and occasionally of the conjunctiva. It is fairly common, usually affects children, and is mildly contagious. The source of infection and method of transmission often are unknown.

The disease is characterized by soft tumor-like lesions which first appear as papules with depressed centers containing a curdlike substance. If untreated the lesions may enlarge to the size of a bean. The lesions may occur over the entire body but affect chiefly the hands, face, and genitalia.

Treatment consists of curettage or light cauterization with an electric cautery.

mol. wt. molecular weight.

molybdenum (mo-lib′dĕ-num) a chemical element, atomic number 42, atomic weight 95.94, symbol Mo. (See table of ELEMENTS.)

momentum (mo-men′tum) the quantity of motion; the product of mass by velocity.

monad (mo′nad) 1. a single-celled protozoon or coccus. 2. a univalent radical or element. 3. in meiosis, one member of a tetrad.

monarthric (mon-ar′thrik) pertaining to a single joint.

monarthritis (mon″ar-thri′tis) inflammation of a single joint.

monarticular (mon″ar-tik′u-lar) pertaining to a single joint.

monathetosis (mon-ath″ĕ-to′sis) athetosis of one limb.

monatomic (mon″ah-tom′ik) 1. containing one atom. 2. univalent.

Mondor's disease (mon′dorz) phlebitis affecting the large subcutaneous veins normally crossing the lateral chest wall and breast from the epigastric or hypochondriac region to the axilla.

monecious (mon-e′shus) monoecious.

monesthetic (mon″es-thet′ik) affecting a single sense or sensation.

mongolian spot (mon-gōl′e-an) a smooth, brown to grayish blue nevus consisting of an excess of melanocytes, typically found at birth in the sacral region in Orientals, Negroes, American Indians, and many southern Europeans; it usually disappears during childhood.

mongolism (mon′go-lizm) a congenital condition involving some degree of mental retardation and various physical malformations. The name is based on characteristic facial traits resembling somewhat those of persons of the Mongolian race. The term mongolism is now considered to be inaccurate and undesirable and is being replaced by the term DOWN'S SYNDROME or trisomy 21. The latter name refers to the presence of three twenty-first chromosomes, found in those with Down's syndrome, instead of the usual pair.

mongoloid (mon′go-loid) 1. pertaining to or resembling the Mongols. 2. an individual with Down's syndrome (see MONGOLISM).

monilethrix (mo-nil′ĕ-thriks) a hereditary condition in which the hair is brittle and beaded.

Monilia (mo-nil′e-ah) former name of a genus of parasitic fungi, now called *Candida.*

monilial (mo-nil′e-al) pertaining to or caused by *Monilia* (*Candida*).

moniliasis (mo″nĭ-li′ah-sis) candidiasis.

moniliform (mo-nil′ĭ-form) beaded; having the appearance of a string of beads.

monitor (mon′ĭ-tor) 1. to check constantly on a given condition or phenomenon, e.g., blood pressure or heart or respiration rate. 2. an apparatus by which such conditions or phenomena can be constantly observed and recorded.

mono- (mon′o) word element [Gr.], *one; single; limited to one part; combined with one atom.*

monoamine (mon″o-am′ēn) an amine containing only one amino group.

m. oxidase, monoamine:oxygen oxidoreductase (deaminating). A cuproprotein enzyme that catalyzes the oxidation of amines into the corresponding aldehydes, ammonia, and hydrogen peroxide; called also amino oxidase.

m. oxidase inhibitors, MAO inhibitors, substances that inhibit the activity of monoamine oxidase, increasing catecholamine and 5-hydroxytryptophan levels in the brain; they are used as antidepressants and antihypertensives.

monobasic (mon″o-ba′sik) having but one atom of replaceable hydrogen.

monobenzone (mon″o-ben′zōn) a white, crystalline powder used as a depigmenting agent.

monoblast (mon′o-blast) the cell that is the precursor of the mature monocyte.

monoblastoma (mon″o-blas-to′mah) a tumor containing monoblasts and monocytes.

monoblepsia (mon″o-blep′se-ah) 1. a condition in which vision is better when only one eye is used. 2. blindness to all colors but one.

monobrachius (mon″o-bra′ke-us) a fetus with but one arm.

monocephalus (mon″o-sef′ah-lus) a monster with two bodies and one head.

monochorea (mon″o-ko-re′ah) chorea affecting but one part.

monochorial, monochorionic (mon″o-ko′re-al, mon″o-ko″re-on′ik) having a single chorion; said of identical twin fetuses.

monochromatic (mon″o-kro-mat′ik) pertaining to a single color.

monoclonal (mon″o-klo′nal) derived from a single cell; pertaining to a single clone.

monococcus (mon″o-kok′us) a form of coccus consisting of single cells.

monocontaminated (mon″o-kon-tam′ĭ-nāt″ed) infected by only one species of microorganisms or a single contaminating agent.

monocular (mon-ok′u-lar) 1. pertaining to one eye. 2. having but one eyepiece, as in a microscope.

monoculus (mon-ok′u-lus) 1. a bandage for one eye. 2. a cyclops.

monocyclic (mon″o-si′klik) in chemistry, having an atomic structure containing only one ring.

monocyte (mon′o-sīt) a mononuclear, phagocytic leukocyte, 13μ to 25μ in diameter, having an ovoid or kidney-shaped nucleus, containing chromatin, and an abundant cytoplasm filled with fine reddish and azurophilic granules. adj., **monocyt′ic.**

monocytopenia (mon″o-si-to-pe′ne-ah) deficiency of monocytes in the blood.

monocytosis (mon″o-si-to′sis) excess of monocytes in the blood.

monodactyly (mon″o-dak′tĭ-le) the presence of only one finger or toe on a hand or foot.

monodermoma (mon″o-der-mo′mah) a tumor developed from one germinal layer.

monodiplopia (mon″o-dĭ-plo′pe-ah) double vision in one eye.

Monodral (mon′o-dral) trademark for preparations of penthienate, used in parasympathetic blockade.

monoecious (mon-e′shus) having reproductive organs typical of both sexes in a single individual.

monoethanolamine (mon″o-eth″ah-nōl′ah-mēn) a moderately viscous liquid, used as a surfactant.

monogerminal (mon″o-jer′mĭ-nal) developed from one ovum; said of identical twins.

monoiodotyrosine (mon″o-i-o″do-ti′ro-sēn) an iodinated amino acid, an intermediate in the synthesis of thyroxine and triiodothyronine.

monolayer (mon″o-la′er) pertaining to or consisting of a single layer of molecules.

monolocular (mon″o-lok′u-lar) having but one cavity, as a cyst.

monomania (mon″o-ma′ne-ah) psychosis on a single subject or class of subjects.

monomelic (mon″o-mel′ik) affecting one limb.

monomer (mon′o-mer) a simple molecule of relatively low molecular weight, capable of reacting by repetition to form polymers.

fibrin m., the material resulting from the action of thrombin on fibrinogen, which then polymerizes to form fibrin.

monomeric (mon″o-mer′ik) 1. pertaining to a single segment. 2. in genetics, determined by a gene or genes at a single locus. 3. consisting of monomers.

monomolecular (mon″o-mo-lek′u-lar) pertaining to a single molecule or to a layer one molecule thick.

monomorphic (mon″o-mor′fik) existing in only one form.

monomphalus (mon-om′fah-lus) a double monster joined at the navel.

monomyoplegia (mon″o-mi″o-ple′je-ah) paralysis of a single muscle.

monomyositis (mon″o-mi″o-si′tis) inflammation of a single muscle.

mononeural (mon″o-nu′ral) supplied by a single nerve.

mononeuritis (mon″o-nu-ri′tis) inflammation of a single nerve.

m. mul′tiplex, simultaneous inflammation of several nerves remote from one another.

mononuclear (mon″o-nu′kle-ar) having only one nucleus.

mononucleosis (mon″o-nu″kle-o′sis) excess of mononuclear leukocytes (monocytes) in the blood.

infectious m., an acute infectious disease that causes changes in the leukocytes; called also glandular fever.

Mononucleosis is caused by the Epstein-Barr virus, and is usually transmitted by direct oral contact ("kissing disease"). It occurs more frequently in the spring and affects primarily children and young adults. Although epidemics have been reported, some authorities doubt that the disorder has been the same in all instances.

Symptoms. Generally, after an incubation period of uncertain duration (1 week to several weeks), headache, sore throat, mental and physical fatigue, severe weakness, and symptoms typical of influenza develop. Skin rashes may also occur.

Diagnosis can be confirmed by the finding of a marked increase in the number of mononuclear leukocytes present in the patient's blood. Another diagnostic test that indicates mononucleosis is the Paul-Bunnell heterophil agglutination test, which demonstrates the presence of certain antibodies capable of causing clumping of cells in a sample of sheep's blood.

Occasionally, in about 8 to 10 per cent of all cases of mononucleosis, the liver is involved and jaundice occurs, resulting in a condition that resembles infectious hepatitis. In rare cases, the heart, lungs and central nervous system may also be affected. The spleen may become enlarged; one of the complications, serious but rare, is rupture of the spleen. The lymph nodes and spleen may both remain enlarged for some time after other symptoms have disappeared.

TREATMENT. Treatment is chiefly symptomatic. Bed rest is especially important in the early stages of the disease, or later if the liver is involved. There is as yet no specific treatment for mononucleosis, and no immunization is available. Headache and sore throat may be relieved by aspirin and gargles.

Although the more obvious symptoms of mononucleosis may disappear after a period of rest, sufficient rest and curtailed activities must be maintained in order to improve the patient's severely weakened condition and to prevent recurrence of the disease. There is often mental as well as physical fatigue, especially among students, and in these cases some mental depression may accompany convalescence. A rest from schoolwork for a month or two is occasionally advisable in cases of this sort.

A vaccine is being developed that is expected to provide immunity to this disease.

mononucleotide (mon″o-nu′kle-o-tīd) a compound obtained by the digestion or hydrolytic decomposition of nucleic acid; it is composed of a base; (purine or pyrimidine), a sugar, and a phosphate group (see also NUCLEOTIDE).

flavin m. (FMN), a derivative of riboflavin that serves as a coenzyme for a number of oxidative enzymes.

monoparesis (mon″o-par′ĕ-sis) paresis of a single part.

monoparesthesia (mon″o-par″es-the′ze-ah) paresthesia of a single part.

monopathy (mo-nop′ah-the) a disease affecting a single part.

monophthalmus (mon″of-thal′mus) a fetus with one eye; cyclops.

monophyletic (mon″o-fi-let′ik) descended from a common ancestor or stem cell.

monoplegia (mon″o-ple′je-ah) paralysis of a single part. adj., **monople′gic.**

monopolar (mon″o-po′lar) having a single pole.

monops (mon′ops) a fetus with a single eye.

monopus (mon′o-pus) a fetus with only one foot.

monorchid (mon-or′kid) a person having only one testis in the scrotum.

monorchidism, monorchism (mon-or′kid-izm; mon′or-kizm) the condition of having only one testis or one descended testis.

monosaccharide (mon″o-sak′ah-rīd) a simple sugar; a carbohydrate that cannot be broken down to simpler substances by hydrolysis.

monosomy (mon″o-so′me) existence in a cell of only one instead of the normal diploid pair of a particular chromosome. adj., **monoso′mic.**

Monosporium (mon″o-spo′re-um) a genus of fungi.

M. apiosper′mum, a fungus that is one of the causative organisms of maduromycosis.

monostotic (mon″os-tot′ik) affecting a single bone.

monosymptomatic (mon″o-simp″to-mat′ik) manifested by only one symptom.

monosynaptic (mon″o-sĭ-nap′tik) pertaining to or passing through a single synapse.

Monotheamin (mon″o-the′ah-min) trademark for preparations of theophylline ethanolamine, a diuretic and bronchodilator.

monothermia (mon″o-ther′me-ah) a condition in which the body temperature remains the same throughout the day.

monotrichous (mon-ot′rĭ-kus) having a single flagellum; applied to a bacterial cell.

monovalent (mon″o-va′lent) 1. having a valence of one. 2. capable of binding with only one antigenic or antibody specificity.

monoxenous (mo-nok′sĕ-nus) requiring only one host to complete the life cycle.

monoxide (mon-ok′sīd) an oxide with one oxygen atom in the molecule.

monozygotic (mon″o-zi-got′ik) pertaining to or derived from a single zygote (fertilized ovum); said of TWINS.

mons (mons), pl. *mon′tes* [L.] a prominence.

m. pu′bis, the rounded fleshy prominence over the symphysis pubis in the female.

m. ven′eris, mons pubis.

monster (mon′ster) a fetus or infant with such pronounced developmental anomalies as to be grotesque and usually nonviable.

monstriparity (mon″strĭ-par′ĭ-te) the act of giving birth to a monster.

monstrosity (mon-stros′ĭ-te) 1. great congenital deformity. 2. a monster or teratism.

Monteggia's fracture (mon-tej′ahz) a fracture in the proximal half of the shaft of the ulna, with dislocation of the head of the radius (see also illustration accompanying FRACTURE).

Montgomery's glands (mont-gom′er-ēz) sebaceous glands in the mammary areola; called also areolar glands.

Montgomery straps (tapes) (mont-gom′er-e) straps made of lengths of adhesive tape, used to secure DRESSINGS that must be changed frequently.

monticulus (mon-tik′u-lus), pl. *montic′uli* [L.] a small eminence.

m. cerebel′li, the projecting part of the superior vermis cerebelli.

mood (mo͞od) a prevailing emotional tone or feeling.

morantel (mo-ran′tel) an anthelmintic used as the tartrate salt.

Moraxella (mo-rak-sel′ah) a genus of bacteria found as parasites and pathogens in warmblooded animals.

morbid (mor′bid) 1. pertaining to, affected with, or inducing disease; diseased. 2. unhealthy; unwholesome.

morbidity (mor-bid′ĭ-te) 1. the condition of being diseased. 2. the ratio of sick to well persons in a community.

morbific (mor-bif′ik) causing or inducing disease.

morbilli (mor-bil′i) [L.] measles.

morbilliform (mor-bil′ĭ-form) resembling measles.

morbus (mor′bus) [L.] disease.

morcellation (mor″sĕ-la′shun) division of a tumor or organ, followed by piecemeal removal.

mordant (mor′dant) 1. a substance capable of intensifying or deepening the reaction of a specimen to a stain. 2. to subject to the action of a mordant before staining.

Morgagni's hyperostosis (mor-gahn′yēz) frontal internal hyperostosis.

Morgagni's ventricle (mor-gahn′yēz) the space between the true and false vocal cords; called also ventricle of larynx.

morgue (morg) a place where dead bodies may be temporarily kept, for identification or until claimed for burial.

moria (mo′re-ah) a morbid tendency to joke.

moribund (mor′ĭbund) in a dying state.

Mornidine (mor′nĭ-dēn) trademark for preparations of pipamazine, an antiemetic.

morning sickness nausea and vomiting occurring during pregnancy, usually during the early months. Between 50 and 65 per cent of all women experience some degree of morning sickness at some time during pregnancy, and about one-third are affected to the point of vomiting. Morning sickness usually begins during the fifth or sixth week of pregnancy. Some cases may clear up in 1 to 3 weeks; others may persist until the fourteenth or sixteenth week.

In most cases, morning sickness begins with a feeling of nausea on arising. Despite its name, however, morning sickness is not always limited to the morning.

In rare cases—affecting about one woman in 200—HYPEREMESIS GRAVIDARUM, or pernicious vomiting of pregnancy, may develop. If unchecked, it may result in such symptoms as dehydration and weight loss, and may threaten the life of both mother and the unborn child.

CAUSES. The actual causes of morning sickness are not known. It is believed that hunger is a contributing factor. It is also thought that there may be a metabolic upset that occurs as a result of pregnancy and contributes to this condition. It is likely, however, that morning sickness is often psychologic in origin.

TREATMENT. Morning sickness is little more than a discomfort, and usually requires no treatment. If a woman can be diverted from thinking about it, the condition tends to lessen or to pass away entirely. If possible, a woman should have something light to eat before getting out of bed in the morning. This could be crackers or weak tea, possibly left on the bedside table at night, the tea in a thermos bottle; or better still, she should have breakfast in bed. After eating, she should rest for about 15 minutes before getting up.

Excessive fluid intake should be avoided. At meals, it is best to eat dry foods first. Liquids should be taken last and should be sipped in small quantities. Instead of three large meals, small meals should be eaten at more frequent intervals. It is also advisable to rest after each meal. Dry foods, such as crackers, or soft foods eaten every 2 hours until the nausea is over can also be helpful.

Sights, smells, and foods that may be disturbing should be avoided, as should greasy foods, fats, and butter. Also to be avoided are those vegetables which are hard to digest, such as cabbage, cauliflower, cucumbers, and onions. In certain cases, the physician may prescribe an antinauseant.

Moro reflex (mo′ro) flexion of an infant's thighs and knees, fanning and then clenching of fingers, with arms first thrown outward and then brought together as though embracing something; produced by a sudden stimulus, such as striking the table on either side of the child, and seen normally in the newborn. Called also embrace reflex.

moron (mo′ron) a mentally defective person whose mental age is between 8 and 12 years, usually requiring special training and supervision. The term is no longer acceptable as an expression of degree of MENTAL RETARDATION.

morphea (mor-fe′ah) [Gr.] a condition in which there is connective tissue replacement of the skin and sometimes of the subcutaneous tissues, marked by the formation of ivory white or pinkish patches, bands, or lines that are sometimes bordered by a purplish areola. The lesions are firm, but not hard, and are usually depressed; they may remain localized or may involute, leaving atrophy and scarring. Called also circumscribed or localized scleroderma.

morphine (mor′fēn) the principal and most active opium alkaloid, a narcotic analgesic and respiratory depressant, usually used as morphine sulfate. The use of morphine carries with it the dangers of addiction (see DRUG ADDICTION) and tolerance, so that increasingly larger doses are needed to achieve the desired effect. Since morphine is a powerful respiratory depressant, the drug should be withheld and the physician notified when the patient's respirations are less than 12 per minute.

morphinism (mor′fĭ-nizm) a morbid state due to habitual misuse of morphine.

morphium (mor′fe-um) morphine.

morphogenesis (mor″fo-jen′ĕ-sis) the developmental changes of growth and differentiation occurring in the organization of the body and its parts. adj., **morphogenet′ic.**

morphology (mor″fol′o-je) the science of the forms and structure of organized beings. adj., **morpholog′ic.**

morphometry (mor-fom′ĕ-tre) the measurement of forms.

-morphous word element [Gr.], *shape; form.*

Morquio's disease (syndrome) (mor-ke′ōz) a form of MUCOPOLYSACCHARIDOSIS becoming evident when the affected infant starts to walk, marked by severe dwarfism, prominent sternum, short neck, kyphosis, genu valgum, and waddling gait; mental retardation is absent or slight. Called also osteochondrodystrophy and familial osteochondrodystrophy.

Morquio-Ullrich disease (mor-ke′o-ool′rik) Morquio's disease.

mors (mors) [L.] death.

morsus (mor′sus) [L.] bite.

m. diab′oli, the fimbriated end of a uterine tube.

mortal (mor′tal) 1. destined to die. 2. causing or terminating in death; fatal.

mortality (mor-tal′ĭ-te) 1. the quality of being mortal. 2. the death rate; the ratio of total number of deaths to the total number of population. The mortality rate of a disease is the ratio of the number of deaths from a given disease to the total number of cases of that disease.

mortar (mor′tar) a vessel with a rounded internal surface, used with a pestle, for reducing a solid to a powder or producing a homogeneous mixture of solids.

mortification (mor″tĭ-fĭ-ka′shun) gangrene.

Morton's disease (mor′tunz) tenderness or pain in the metatarsophalangeal joint of the third or fourth toe.

Morton's neuralgia (mor′tunz) traumatic neuroma of the interdigital nerve of the foot.

morula (mor′u-lah) a solid mass of cells (blastomeres) resembling a mulberry, formed by cleavage of a fertilized ovum.

Morvan's disease (mor′vanz) a form of syringomyelia, with painless ulceration of the fingertips and analgesic paralysis and atrophy of the forearms and hands.

mosaic (mo-za′ik) a pattern made of numerous small pieces fitted together; in genetics, occurrence in an individual of two or more cell populations each having a different chromosome complement.

mosaicism (mo-za′ĭ-sizm) the presence in an individual of cells derived from the same zygote, but differing in chromosomal constitution.

mosquito (mos-ke′to) a blood-sucking winged insect, chiefly of the genus *Aedes, Anopheles,* or *Culex.* Certain species are responsible for the transmission of disease, including yellow fever and MALARIA.

motile (mo′til) having spontaneous but not conscious or volitional movement.

motility (mo-til′ĭ-te) the ability to move spontaneously.

motion sickness discomfort felt by some people on a moving boat, train, airplane, or automobile, or even on an elevator or a swing. The discomfort is caused by irregular and abnormal motion that disturbs the organs of balance located in the inner ear. There may be mild symptoms of nausea, dizziness, or headache, as well as pallor and cold perspiration. In more acute cases, there may be vomiting and sometimes prostration.

Though most people quickly adapt to travel by airplane, ship, and automobile, few are wholly immune to motion sickness. Even astronauts become ill if the inner ear organs of balance are continuously stimulated by unusual motion. Fortunately, most cases of motion sickness vanish quickly once the journey is over, leaving no ill effects.

CAUSES. The inner ear possesses three semicircular canals, located at right angles in three different planes. Man is accustomed to movement in the horizontal plane, which stimulates certain semicircular canals; but he is not accustomed to vertical movements, such as the motion of an elevator or a ship pitching at sea. These vertical movements stimulate the semicircular canals in an unusual way, producing the sensation of nausea, or motion sickness.

Anxiety, grief, or other emotions can also cause motion sickness. A person unaccustomed to traveling by boat or airplane may be apprehensive or nervous and therefore may develop symptoms of nausea. Some individuals with previous experience of motion sickness become ill on a boat at dock or on an airplane prior to take-off.

Airsickness usually occurs during a bumpy flight caused by stormy weather or turbulent air. However, it may also be triggered by poorly ventilated cabins, hunger, digestive upset, overindulgence in food and drink, and unpleasant odors, particularly tobacco smoke.

TREATMENT. Certain antihistamines have proved highly effective in treating symptoms of seasickness. Like nerve depressants, they may be used alone or in combination with mild sedatives. Those who suffer from motion sickness should ask their physician what he recommends before they embark on a trip. Symptoms may also be reduced if the seasick person rests lying down, with his head low, in a comfortable, well aired place.

PREVENTION. Being rested and in good health prior to a journey helps to prevent motion sickness. A cup of strong coffee taken just before departure may also be helpful. Alcoholic beverages in moderation make some people less nervous and thus help ward off motion sickness; however, in excess they can encourage the condition.

During a voyage by boat, it is advisable for the passenger to remain near the center of the ship, where there will be the least motion. Ample fresh air and exercise and avoidance of stuffy rooms and disagreeable smells are also good precautions. The traveler should keep comfortably warm and avoid overeating and rich foods.

For those traveling by air, a sedative or tranquilizer taken a half hour before departure, and small, easily digested meals taken during the flight help to prevent airsickness. The passenger who experiences motion sickness may benefit from reclining in his seat as far as possible and closing his eyes.

Carsickness is often relieved if the journey is interrupted for short walks in the fresh air and by keeping a window open. Children will frequently find it helpful to glance down, and to refrain from reading. Tobacco smoke can also be an aggravating factor.

motoceptor (mo′to-sep″tor) any muscle sense receptor.

motoneuron (mo″to-nu′ron) motor neuron; a neuron having a motor function; an efferent neuron conveying motor impulses.

lower m's, peripheral neurons whose cell bodies lie in the ventral gray columns of the spinal cord and whose terminations are in skeletal muscles.

peripheral m's, neurons in a peripheral reflex arc that receive impulses from interneurons and transmit them to voluntary muscles.

upper m's, neurons in the cerebral cortex that conduct impulses from the motor cortex to the motor nuclei of the cerebral nerves or to the ventral gray columns of the spinal cord.

motor (mo′tor) 1. pertaining to motion. 2. a muscle, nerve, or center that effects movements.

mottling (mot′ling) discoloration in irregular areas.

moulage (moo-lahzh′) [Fr.] a wax model of a structure or lesion.

mould (mōld) mold.

mounding (mownd′ing) the rising in a lump of a wasting muscle when struck.

mount (mownt) to prepare specimens and slides for study.

mountain fever 1. Colorado tick fever. 2. Rocky Mountain spotted fever. 3. brucellosis.

mountain sickness disturbances due to poor adjustment to high altitude. Symptoms include fatigability, shortness of breath, polycythemia, cyanosis and epistaxis.

mouse (mows) a small rodent, various species of which are used in laboratory experiments.

joint m., a movable fragment of synovial membrane, cartilage, or other body within a joint; usually associated with degenerative osteoarthritis and osteochondritis dissecans.

peritoneal m., a free body in the peritoneal cavity, probably a small detached mass or omentum, sometimes visible radiographically.

mouth (mowth) an opening, especially the oral cavity, forming the beginning of the DIGESTIVE SYSTEM.

In it the chewing of food takes place. The mouth is also the site of the organs of taste and the teeth, tongue, and lips. Not only is the mouth the entrance to the body for food and sometimes air, but it is a major organ of speech and emotional expression.

STRUCTURE. Except for the teeth, the interior of the mouth is covered with mucous membrane. This thin lining extends out from the front of the mouth to form the lips. Salivary glands lie above and below the mouth and produce saliva, a liquid that protects the delicate membranes and mixes with food in the first step of digestion of food.

The palate forms the roof of the mouth. The front two-thirds of the palate comprises the hard palate, and the back third, the soft palate. The soft palate is hinged to the hard palate and is flanked on both sides by the tonsils. In the middle of the soft palate is the uvula, a projection pointing down to the tongue. At the root of the tongue, below the uvula, lies the epiglottis.

DISORDERS. Because of its special functions the mouth is constantly exposed to infection and irritation. These can affect the whole mouth generally or only certain parts, such as the tongue.

Inflammation of the mouth, or STOMATITIS, can indicate the presence of either a mild or severe disease. Local conditions include THRUSH, TRENCH MOUTH, and herpes simplex. Generalized diseases can also give rise to inflammation of the mouth; these include diphtheria, tuberculosis, blood dyscrasias, vitamin deficiencies, and syphilis.

CANCER can afflict the sides of the mouth, the lips, the tongue and occasionally the salivary glands. Continued irritation, such as pipe smoking, is thought to be a cause of many mouth cancers. Any persistent sore or swelling should be promptly examined by a physician.

Birth defects affecting the mouth include CLEFT LIP AND CLEFT PALATE. Both have the same cause: failure of adjacent parts of the body to unite properly in fetal life. A cleft lip, or harelip, involves a split in the upper lip. Sometimes the cleft extends into the upper jaw, the floor of the nose and the palate. The resulting deformity of nose and mouth interferes with sucking and speech unless corrected by surgery. A cleft palate, which may cause difficulties in speaking and eating, signifies a cleavage in the uvula and the soft palate. Both conditions are successfully corrected by surgery.

trench m., inflammation of the gingivae and oral mucous membrane (see also TRENCH MOUTH).

mouth-to-mouth resuscitation a method of ARTIFICAL RESPIRATION in which the rescuer covers the patient's mouth with his own and breathes out vigorously.

mouthwash a solution for rinsing the mouth.

movement (mo͞ov′ment) 1. an act of moving; motion. 2. an act of defecation.

active m., movement produced by the person's own muscles.

ameboid m., movement like that of an ameba, accomplished by protrusion of cytoplasm of the cell.

associated m., movement of parts that act together, as the eyes.

brownian m., molecular m., the peculiar, rapid, oscillatory movement of fine particles suspended in a fluid medium.

passive m., a movement of the body or of the extremities of a patient performed by another person without voluntary motion on the part of the patient.

vermicular m's, the wormlike movements of the intestines in peristalsis.

moxa (mok′sah) a tuft of soft, combustible substance to be burned upon the skin as a cautery.

moxibustion (mok″sĭ-bus′chun) cauterization by the burning of a moxa.

M.P.D. maximum permissible dose.

M.P.H. Master of Public Health.

mr. milliroentgen.

M-R measles-rubella (vaccine).

M.R.L. Medical Record Librarian.

mRNA messenger RNA (ribonucleic acid).

MS multiple sclerosis.

M.S. Master of Science; Master of Surgery.

MSH melanocyte-stimulating hormone.

M.T. Medical Technologist.

μ (mu) micron.

Much's granules (mooks) granules and rods found in tuberculous sputum which do not stain by the usual processes for acid-fast bacilli, but do stain with Gram stain.

muciferous (mu-sif′er-us) secreting mucus.

muciform (mu′sĭ-form) resembling mucus.

mucigen (mu′sĭ-jen) a substance present in mucous cells, convertible into mucin and mucus.

mucilage (mu′sĭ-lij) an aqueous solution of a gummy substance, used as a vehicle or demulcent. adj., **mucilag′inous.**

mucilloid (mu′sil-oid) a preparation of a mucilaginous substance.

psyllium hydrophilic m., a powdered preparation of the mucilaginous portion of blond psyllium seeds, used in treatment of constipation.

mucin (mu′sin) mucopolysaccharide or glycoprotein that is the chief constituent of mucus.

mucinase (mu′sĭ-nās) an enzyme that acts upon mucin.

mucinogen (mu-sin′o-jen) a precursor of mucin.

mucinoid (mu′sĭ-noid) 1. resembling mucin. 2. mucoid (2).

mucinosis (mu″si-no′sis) a state with abnormal deposits of mucin in the skin, often associated with hypothyroidism (myxedema).

follicular m., a disease of unknown cause, characterized by plaques of folliculopapules and usually alopecia.

muciparous (mu-sip′ah-rus) secreting mucin.

mucocele (mu′ko-sēl) 1. dilation of a cavity with accumulated mucous secretion. 2. a mucous polyp.

mucocutaneous (mu″ko-ku-ta′ne-us) pertaining to mucous membrane and skin.

mucoenteritis (mu″ko-en″tĕ-ri′tis) mucous colitis.

mucoglobulin (mu″ko-glob′u-lin) one of the class of glycoproteins.

mucoid (mu′koid) 1. resembling mucus. 2. a mucus-like conjugated protein of animal origin, differing from mucin in solubility.

mucolytic (mu″ko-lit′ik) destroying or dissolving mucus.

mucomembranous (mu″ko-mem′brah-nus) pertaining to or composed of mucous membrane.

mucoperiosteum (mu″ko-per″e-os′te-um) periosteum having a mucous surface, as in parts of the auditory apparatus. adj., **mucoperios′teal.**

mucopolysaccharide (mu″ko-pol″ĭ-sak′ah-rīd) a group of polysaccharides that contain hexosamine, that may or may not be combined with protein and that, dispersed in water, form many of the mucins.

mucopolysaccharidosis (mu″ko-pol″ĭ-sak″ah-rĭ-do′sis) any of a group of genetically determined disorders due to a defect in mucopolysaccharide metabolism, marked by skeletal changes, mental retardation, visceral involvement, corneal clouding, with widespread tissue deposits and mucopolysacchariduria. HURLER'S SYNDROME is the prototype of this disorder.

mucopolysacchiduria (mu″ko-pol″ĭ-sak″ah-rĭ-du′re-ah) an excess of mucopolysaccharides in the urine.

mucoprotein (mu″ko-pro′te-in) a compound present in all connective and supporting tissues, containing, as prosthetic groups, mucopolysaccharides; soluble in water and relatively resistant to denaturation.

mucopurulent (mu″ko-pu′roo-lent) marked by an exudate containing both mucus and pus.

mucopus (mu′ko-pus) mucus blended with pus.

Mucor (mu′kor) a genus of saprophytic mold fungi; some species cause mucormycosis.

mucormycosis (mu″kor-mi-ko′sis) mycosis due to fungi of the order Mucorales, including species of *Absidia, Mucor,* and *Rhizopus,* usually occurring in debilitated patients, often beginning in the upper respiratory tract or lungs, from which mycelial growths metastasize to other organs.

mucosa (mu-ko′sah), pl. *muco′sae* [L.] mucous membrane. adj. **muco′sal.**

mucosanguineous (mu″ko-sang-gwin′e-us) composed of mucus and blood.

mucoserous (mu″ko-se′rus) composed of mucus and serum.

mucosin (mu-ko′sin) a form of mucin found in tenacious mucus.

mucosocutaneous (mu-ko″so-ku-ta′ne-us) pertaining to a mucous membrane and the skin.

mucous (mu′kus) pertaining to or resembling mucus; secreting mucus.

m. membrane, the membrane covered with epithelium that lines the tubular organs of the body.

mucoviscidosis (mu″ko-vis″ĭ-do′sis) a condition characterized by accumulation of extremely thick, tenacious mucus in the important mucus-secreting glands, involving especially the exocrine glands of the pancreas; called also CYSTIC FIBROSIS.

mucus (mu′kus) the free slime of the mucous membrane, composed of the secretion of its glands, various salts, desquamated cells, and leukocytes.

fertile m., see ovulation method of CONTRACEPTION.

müllerian duct (mil-e′re-an) either of the paired embryonic ducts developing into the vagina, uterus, and uterine tubes in the female, and becoming largely obliterated in the male. Called also paramesonephric duct.

multi- (mul′tĭ) word element [L.], *many.*

multiallelic (mul″te-ah-lel′ik) pertaining to or occupied by many different genes affecting the same or different hereditary characters.

multiarticular (mul″te-ar-tik′u-lar) pertaining to or affecting many joints.

multicapsular (mul″tĭ-kap′su-lar) having many capsules.

multicellular (mul″tĭ-sel′u-lar) composed of many cells.

multicuspidate (mul″tĭ-kus′pĭ-dāt) having numerous cusps.

multifactorial (mul″tĭ-fak-to′re-al) 1. of or pertaining to, or arising through the action of, many factors. 2. in genetics, arising as the result of the interaction of several genes.

multifocal (mul″tĭ-fo′kal) arising from or pertaining to many foci.

multiform (mul′tĭ-form) occurring in many forms; polymorphic.

multiglandular (mul″tĭ-glan′du-lar) affecting several glands.

multigravida (mul″tĭ-grav′ĭ-dah) a woman pregnant for the third (or more) time.

grand m., a woman who has had six or more previous pregnancies.

multilobar (mul″tĭ-lo′bar) having numerous lobes.

multilobular (mul″tĭ-lob′u-lar) having many lobules.

multilocular (mul″tĭ-lok′u-lar) having many compartments.

multinodular (mul″tĭ-nod′u-lar) having many nodules.

multinucleate (mul″tĭ-nu′kle-āt) having many nuclei.

multipara (mul-tip′ah-rah) a woman who has had two or more pregnancies resulting in viable offspring. adj., **multip′arous.**

grand m., a woman who has had six or more pregnancies that resulted in viable offspring.

multiparity (mul″tĭ-par′ĭ-te) the condition of being a multipara.

multiple (mul′tĭ-pl) manifold; occurring in various parts of the body at once.

m. myeloma, a primary malignant tumor of plasma cells usually arising in bone marrow, marked by circumscribed or diffuse tumor-like hyperplasia of the bone marrow, and usually associated with anemia and with Bence Jones protein in the urine. The patient complains of neuralgic pains; later painful swellings appear on the ribs and skull, and spontaneous fractures may occur. Called also Kahler's disease, myelopathic albumosuria, Bence Jones albumosuria, and lymphadenia ossea.

m. sclerosis, a disorder of the nervous system characterized by hardened patches scattered at random throughout the white matter of the brain and spinal cord. The various syndromes included under the term multiple sclerosis range from mild borderline cases to those that progress to severe disability.

The cause of multiple sclerosis has not been established, but it is believed to be viral in origin. It is hoped that in the near future serum will be developed that will provide immunity to the disease. It is the most common demyelinating disorder, affecting 10 persons per 100,000 in the southern United States and 60 per 100,000 in the North. The geographic distribution in European countries in similar. The disease occurs most often in adults between the ages of 20 and 40 years.

Multiple sclerosis is chronic; periods of improvement usually alternate with periods of worsening. The effects of multiple sclerosis vary with the portion of the nervous system affected. Since the location, extent, and duration of the injuries vary, it is difficult to describe a typical case of multiple sclerosis.

Often the first sign of the disease is a visual disturbance. The patient may "see double" or lose part of the visual field. Weakness and unusual fatigue are common. There may be a tremor or shaking of the limbs, interfering with fine movements such as writing or sewing. Speech may become slow or monotonous. Balance is sometimes impaired, and walking may be unsteady, or the knees may not bend, causing a stiff gait. There may be loss of bladder and bowel control. Finally, paralysis may occur in any part of the body.

Diagnosis in the early stages may be difficult.

TREATMENT. Multiple sclerosis seems to grow worse following any illness, and so good general care is necessary to keep up the body's health and resistance to disease. Physical therapy, including massage and exercise, may prevent the affected muscles from being unnecessarily weakened. Because this disease frequently grows worse when there are emotional disturbances, and because patients who are disabled by it may become depressed, psychotherapy may be helpful.

Patients with multiple sclerosis can often lead long, useful lives. The National Multiple Sclerosis Society, 257 Park Avenue South, New York, N.Y. 10010, provides information and assistance concerning all phases of this disease.

multipolar (mul″tĭ-po′lar) having more than two poles or processes.

multisynaptic (mul″tĭ-sĭ-nap′tik) pertaining to or relayed through two or more synapses.

multiterminal (mul″tĭ-ter′mĭ-nal) having several sets of terminals so that several electrodes may be used.

multivalent (mul″tĭ-va′lent) 1. combining with several univalent atoms. 2. active against several strains of an organism.

mummying (mum′e-ing) a form of physical restraint in which the entire body is enclosed in a sheet or blanket, leaving only the head exposed.

mumps (mumps) a communicable myxovirus disease that attacks one or both of the parotid glands, the largest of the three pairs of salivary glands; called also epidemic parotitis. Occasionally the submaxillary glands are also affected. Although older people may contract the disease, mumps usually strikes children between the ages of 5 and 15.

Mumps is spread by droplet infection. The disease is contagious in the infected person from 1 to 2 days before symptoms appear until 1 or 2 days after they disappear. The incubation period is usually 18 days, although it may vary from 12 to 26 days. One attack usually gives immunity.

SYMPTOMS. Often the first noticeable symptom of mumps is a swelling of one of the parotid glands. The swelling is frequently accompanied by pain and tenderness. Occasionally acid foods and beverages may cause an increase in the pain. In the first stage of mumps, the patient may have a fever of 100° to 104° F. Other common symptoms include loss of appetite, headache, and back pain.

The swelling increases for the first 2 or 3 days and then diminishes, disappearing by the sixth or seventh day. The swelling usually appears first on one side and then on the other, with as many as 12 days intervening. Sometimes both sides swell at once; occasionally the second side does not swell at all.

Sometimes the disease occurs virtually without symptoms. This mild form of mumps is responsible for the presence of antibodies and immunity in persons who cannot recall having had the disease and yet seem to be immune to it.

COMPLICATIONS. Mumps may affect other parts of the body as well as the salivary glands. In the male, when the testes are affected, the infection is known as orchitis. It strikes about one-third of those who contract mumps after the age of puberty. Orchitis may occur before the swelling of the parotid glands, but usually does not develop until about 7 to 10 days thereafter.

Involvement of the gonads in females is less common and more difficult to detect. Lower abdominal pain and enlargement of the ovaries are symptoms indicating involvement of the ovaries. The breasts may also be affected.

Mumps may affect the central nervous system. Acute meningoencephalitis is a complication in about 10 per cent of cases. It causes dizziness, vomiting, and headache. It may occur before the parotid glands swell or in the absence of other signs of mumps. No specific treatment is required, and the condition disappears without causing permanent damage.

Other less common complications are involvement of the auditory nerve (resulting in deafness), myelitis, and facial neuritis.

TREATMENT. Most children with mumps do not feel ill enough to be confined to bed, and it is sufficient if they remain quietly at home, unless there is a rise in temperature or a complication develops. When the swelling of the parotid glands disappears, the child may return to school. If both glands are involved, this time interval is approximately 7 days. A soft diet with plenty of fluids is recommended until fever and swelling vanish.

PREVENTION. Total isolation of the child is not essential. Males over the age of puberty should avoid contact with the patient. The mumps virus cannot survive for any length of time in open air, so it is unnecessary to take special precautions with the patient's clothing, bedding, dishes, or utensils.

The mumps vaccine induces antibodies in 95% of those inoculated and gives protection against the disease for about six years. It is not given to infants under one year of age, and is not recommended for persons allergic to eggs and neomycin. The vaccine does not afford protection if it is given during the incubation period following exposure and is contraindicated if another infection is present.

Mumps immune globulin may afford short-term immunity when there is an extraordinary need for protection. Its effectiveness is questionable.

iodine m., swelling of the salivary and lacrimal glands as a toxic reaction to iodine therapy.

Munchausen's syndrome (mun-chow′zenz) habitual seeking of hospital treatment for apparent acute illness, the patient giving a plausible and dramatic history, all of which is false.

mural (mu′ral) pertaining to or occurring in a wall of an organ or cavity.

muramidase (mu-ram′ĭ-dās) lysozyme.

Murchison-Pel-Ebstein fever (mur′chĭ-son-pel-eb′stīn) a type of fever typical of Hodgkin's disease, marked by irregular episodes of pyrexia of several days duration, with intervening periods in which the temperature is normal.

Murel (mu′rel) trademark for preparations of valethamate bromide, an antispasmodic and anticholinergic.

murine (mu'rēn) pertaining to or affecting mice or rats.

murmur (mer'mer) an auscultatory sound, particularly a periodic sound of short duration of cardiac or vascular origin.

aortic m., a sound indicative of disease of the aortic valve.

apex m., one heard over the apex of the heart.

arterial m., one in an artery, sometimes aneurysmal and sometimes constricted.

Austin Flint m., a loud presystolic murmur at the apex heard in aortic regurgitation.

blood m., one due to an abnormal, commonly anemic, condition of the blood.

cardiac m., any adventitious sound heard over the region of the heart.

cardiopulmonary m., one produced by the impact of the heart against the lung.

Carey-Coombs m., a rambling mid-diastolic murmur occurring in the early stages of rheumatic fever.

continuous m., a humming murmur heard throughout systole and diastole.

crescendo m., one marked by progressively increasing loudness.

Cruveilhier-Baumgarten m., one heard at the abdominal wall over veins connecting the portal and caval systems.

diastolic m., one at diastole, due to mitral obstruction or to aortic or pulmonic regurgitation.

Duroziez's m., a double murmur over the femoral or other large peripheral artery; due to aortic insufficiency.

ejection m., systolic murmurs heard predominantly in mid-systole, when ejection volume and velocity of blood flow are at their maximum.

Flint's m., Austin Flint murmur.

friction m., friction rub.

functional m., a cardiac murmur occurring in the absence of structural changes in the heart.

Gibson m., a long, rumbling sound occupying most of systole and diastole, usually localized in the second left interspace near the sternum, and usually indicative of patent ductus arteriosus.

Graham Steell m., one due to pulmonary regurgitation in patients with pulmonary hypertension and mitral stenosis.

heart m., any adventitious sound heard over the region of the heart.

hemic m., blood murmur.

machinery m., Gibson murmur.

mitral m., one due to disease of the mitral valve.

musical m., a cardiac murmur having a periodic harmonic pattern.

organic m., one due to structural change in the heart.

pansystolic m., one heard throughout systole.

prediastolic m., one occurring just before and with diastole, due to mitral obstruction or to aortic or pulmonary regurgitation.

presystolic m., one shortly before the onset of ventricular ejection, usually associated with a narrowed atrioventricular valve.

pulmonic m., one due to disease of the valves of the pulmonary artery.

regurgitant m., one due to a dilated valvular orifice with consequent regurgitation of blood through the valve.

seagull m., a raucous murmur resembling the call of a seagull, frequently heard in aortic insufficiency.

Still's m., a functional cardiac murmur of childhood, heard in midsystole.

systolic m., one occurring at systole, usually due to mitral or tricuspid regurgitation, or to aortic or pulmonary obstruction.

tricuspid m., one caused by disease of the tricuspid valve.

vascular m., one heard over a blood vessel.

vesicular m., the normal breath sounds heard over the lungs.

Murphy's sign (mur'fēz) a sign of gallbladder disease consisting of pain on taking a deep breath when the physician's fingers are on the approximate location of the gallbladder.

Musca (mus'kah) a genus of flies, including the common housefly, *M. domes'tica.*

musca (mus'kah), pl. *mus'cae* [L.] a fly.

mus'cae volitan'tes, specks seen as floating before the eyes.

muscarine (mus'kah-rin) a deadly alkaloid from various mushrooms, e.g., *Amanita muscaria* (the fly agaric), and also from rotten fish.

muscle (mus"l) a bundle of long slender cells, or fibers, that have the power to contract and hence to produce movement. Muscles are responsible for locomotion and play an important part in performing vital body functions. They also protect the contents of the abdomen against injury and help support the body (see also Plate 3).

Muscle fibers range in length from a few hundred

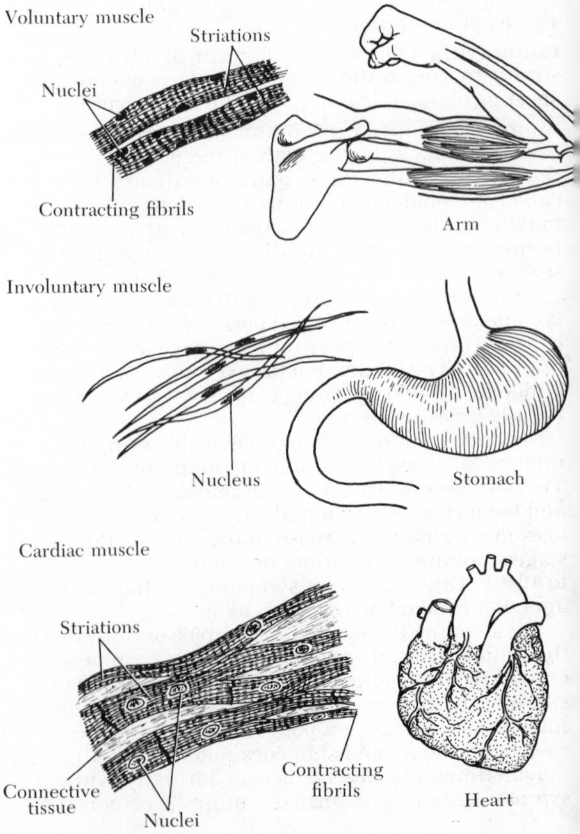

thousandths of an inch to several inches. They also vary in shape, and in color from white to deep red. Each muscle fiber receives its own nerve impulses, so that fine and varied motions are possible. Each has its small stored supply of glycogen, which it uses as fuel for energy. Muscles, especially the heart, also use free fatty acids as fuel. At the signal of an impulse traveling down the nerve, the muscle fiber changes chemical energy into mechanical energy, and the result is muscle contraction.

Some muscles are attached to bones by tendons. Others are attached to other muscles, and to skin—producing the smile, the wink and other facial expressions, for example. All or part of the walls of hollow internal organs, such as the heart, stomach, intestines, and blood vessels, are composed of muscles. The last stages of swallowing and of peristalsis are actually series of contractions by the muscles in the walls of the organs involved.

TYPES OF MUSCLE. There are three types of muscle—involuntary, voluntary, and cardiac. They are composed respectively of smooth, striated (or striped), and mixed smooth and striated tissue.

Muscles that are not under the control of the conscious part of the brain are called involuntary muscles. They respond to the nerve impulses of the autonomic nervous system. These involuntary muscles are the countless short-fibered, or smooth, muscles of the internal organs. They power the digestive tract, the pupils of the eyes, and all other involuntary mechanisms.

The muscles controlled by the conscious part of the brain are called voluntary muscles, and are striated. These are the skeletal muscles that enable the body to move, and there are more than 600 of them in the human body. The fibers of voluntary muscles are grouped together in a sheath of muscle cells. Groups of fibers are bundled together into fascicles and the bundles are surrounded by a tough sheet of connective tissue to form a muscle group like the biceps.

Unlike the involuntary muscles, which can remain in a state of contraction for long periods without tiring and are capable of sustained rhythmic contractions, the voluntary muscles are readily subject to fatigue. They also differ from the involuntary muscles in their need for regular and proper exercise.

The third kind of muscle, cardiac muscle, or the muscle of the heart, is involuntary and consists of striated fibers different from voluntary muscle fibers. The contraction and relaxation of cardiac muscle continue at a rhythmic pace until death unless the muscle is injured in some way. (See also HEART.)

PHYSIOLOGY OF MUSCLES. No muscle stays completely relaxed, and as long as a person is conscious, it remains slightly contracted. This condition is called tonus, or tone. It keeps the bones in place and enables a posture to be maintained. It allows a person to remain standing, sitting up straight, kneeling, or in any other natural position. Muscles also have elasticity. They are capable of being stretched and of performing reflex actions. This is made possible by the motor and sensory nerves which serve the muscles.

Muscles enable the body to perform different types of movement. Those that bend a limb at a joint, raising a thigh or bending an elbow, are called flexors. Those that straighten a limb are called extensors. There are others, the abductors, that make possible movement away from the midline of the body, whereas the adductors permit movement toward the midline. Muscles always act in opposing groups. In bending an elbow or flexing a muscle, for

(*Text continued on page 658.*)

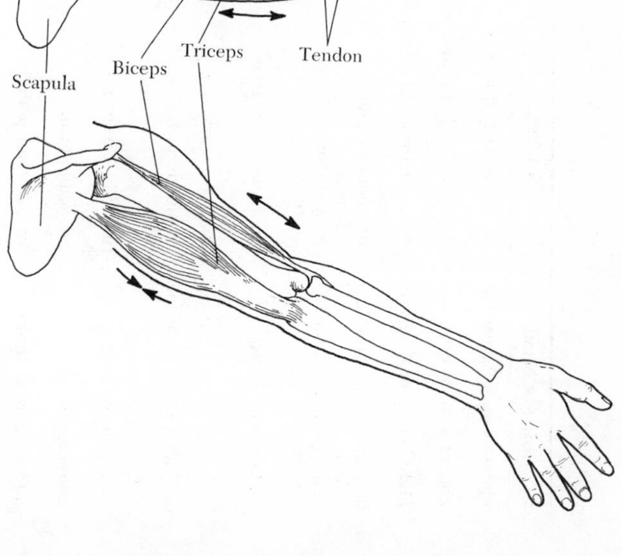

Voluntary muscles extend from one bone to another, effect movements by contraction and work on the principle of leverage. For every direct action made by a muscle, an antagonistic muscle effects an opposite movement. To flex the arm, the biceps contracts and the triceps relaxes; to extend the arm, the triceps contracts and the biceps relaxes.

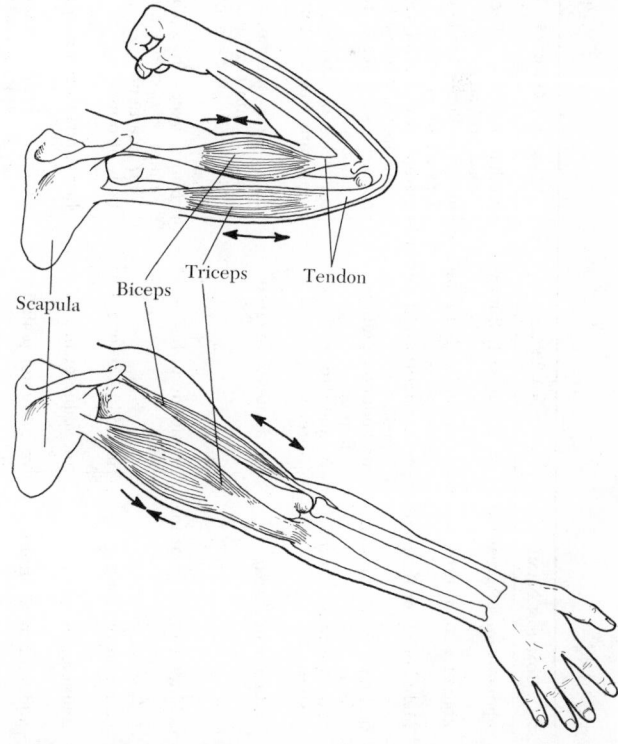

Table of Muscles

Common Name*	NA Term†	Origin*	Insertion*	Innervation	Action
abductor m. of great toe	m. abductor hallucis	medial tubercle of calcaneus, plantar fascia	medial side of base of proximal phalanx of great toe	medial plantar	abducts, flexes great toe
abductor m. of little finger	m. abductor digiti minimi manus	pisiform bone, tendon of ulnar flexor m. of wrist	medial side of base of proximal phalanx of little finger	ulnar	abducts little finger
abductor m. of little toe	m. abductor digiti minimi pedis	medial and lateral tubercle of calcaneus, plantar fascia	lateral side of base of proximal phalanx of little toe	lateral plantar	abducts little toe
abductor m. of thumb, long	m. abductor pollicis longus	posterior surfaces of radius and ulna	lateral side of base of first metacarpal bone and trapezium	posterior interosseous	abducts, extends thumb
abductor m. of thumb, short	m. abductor pollicis brevis	tubercles of scaphoid and trapezium, flexor retinaculum of hand	lateral side of base of proximal phalanx of thumb	median	abducts thumb
adductor m., great	m. adductor magnus	*deep part*–inferior ramus of pubis, ramus of ischium; *superficial part*–ischial tuberosity	*deep part*–linea aspera of femur; *superficial part*–adductor tubercle of femur	*deep part*–obturator; *superficial part*–sciatic	*deep part*–adducts thigh; *superficial part*–extends thigh
adductor m. of great toe	m. adductor hallucis	*oblique head*–long plantar ligament; *transverse head*–plantar ligaments	lateral side of base of proximal phalanx of great toe	lateral plantar	flexes, adducts great toe
adductor m., long	m. adductor longus	body of pubis	linea aspera of femur	obturator	adducts, rotates, flexes thigh
adductor m., short	m. adductor brevis	body and inferior ramus of pubis	upper part of linea aspera of femur	obturator	adducts, rotates, flexes thigh
adductor m. of thumb	m. adductor pollicis	*oblique head*–second metacarpal, capitate, and trapezoid; *transverse head*–front of third metacarpal	medial side of base of proximal phalanx of thumb	ulnar	adducts, opposes thumb
anconeus m.	m. anconeus	back of lateral epicondyle of humerus	olecranon and posterior surface of ulna	radial	extends forearm
antitragus m.	m. antitragicus	outer part of antitragus	caudate process of helix and anthelix	temporal, posterior auricular branches of facial	
arrector m's of hair	mm. arrectores pilorum	dermis	hair follicles	sympathetic	elevate hairs of skin
articular m. of elbow	m. articularis cubiti	a name applied to a few fibers of the deep surface of the triceps m. of arm that insert into the posterior ligament and synovial membrane of the elbow joint			
articular m. of knee	m. articularis genus	front of lower part of femur	upper part of capsule of knee joint	femoral	raises capsule of knee joint
aryepiglottic m.	m. aryepiglotticus	a name applied to inconstant fibers of oblique arytenoid m., from apex of arytenoid cartilage to lateral margin of epiglottis			
arytenoid m., oblique	m. arytenoideus obliquus	muscular process of arytenoid cartilage	apex of opposite arytenoid cartilage	recurrent laryngeal	closes inlet of larynx
arytenoid m., transverse	m. arytenoideus transversus	medial surface of arytenoid cartilage	medial surface of opposite arytenoid cartilage	recurrent laryngeal	approximates arytenoid cartilage
auricular m., anterior	m. auricularis anterior	superficial temporal fascia	cartilage of ear	facial	draws auricle forward
auricular m., posterior	m. auricularis posterior	mastoid process	cartilage of ear	facial	draws auricle backward
auricular m., superior	m. auricularis superior	galea aponeurotica	cartilage of ear	facial	raises auricle
biceps m. of arm	m. biceps brachii	*long head*–supraglenoid tubercle of scapula; *short head*–apex of coracoid process	tuberosity of radius, antebrachial fascia, ulna	musculocutaneous	flexes, supinates forearm

biceps m. of thigh	m. biceps femoris	*long head*–ischial tuberosity; *short head*–linea aspera of femur	head of fibula, lateral condyle of tibia	*long head*–tibial; *short head*–peroneal, popliteal	flexes, rotates leg laterally, extends thigh
brachial m.	m. brachialis	anterior aspect of humerus	coronoid process of ulna	musculocutaneous, radial	flexes forearm
brachioradial m.	m. brachioradialis	lateral supracondylar ridge of humerus	lateral surface of lower end of radius	radial	flexes forearm
bronchoesophageal m.	m. bronchoesophageus	a name applied to muscle fibers arising from wall of left bronchus, reinforcing musculature of esophagus			
buccinator m.	m. buccinator	buccinator ridge of mandible, alveolar processes of maxilla, pterygomandibular ligament	orbicular m. of mouth at angle of mouth	buccal branch of facial	compresses cheek and retracts angle of mouth
bulbocavernous m.	m. bulbocavernosus, m. bulbospongiosus	tendinous center of perineum, median raphe of bulb	fascia of penis or clitoris	pudendal	constricts urethra in male, vagina in female
canine m. *See* levator m. of angle of mouth					
ceratocricoid m.	m. ceratocricoideus	a name applied to muscle fibers from cricoid cartilage to inferior horn of thyroid cartilage			
chin m.	m. mentalis	incisive fossa of mandible	skin of chin	facial	wrinkles skin of chin
chondroglossus m.	m. chondroglossus	lesser horn and body of hyoid bone	substance of tongue	hypoglossal	depresses, retracts tongue
ciliary m.	m. ciliaris	*longitudinal division* (Brücke's m's)–junction of cornea and sclera; *circular division* (Müller's m.)–sphincter of ciliary body	outer layers of choroid and ciliary processes	short ciliary	makes lens more convex in visual accommodation
coccygeus m.	m. coccygeus	ischial spine	lateral border of lower part of sacrum, coccyx	third and fourth sacral	supports and raises coccyx
constrictor m. of pharynx, inferior	m. constrictor pharyngis inferior	undersurfaces of cricoid and thyroid cartilages	median raphe of posterior wall of pharynx	glossopharyngeal, pharyngeal plexus, external branch of superior laryngeal and recurrent laryngeal	constricts pharynx
constrictor m. of pharynx, middle	m. constrictor pharyngis medius	horns of hyoid bone, stylohyoid ligament	median raphe of posterior wall of pharynx	pharyngeal plexus of vagus, glossopharyngeal	constricts pharynx
constrictor m. of pharynx, superior	m. constrictor pharyngis superior	pterygoid plate, pterygomandibular raphe, mylohyoid ridge of mandible, mucous membrane of floor of mouth	median raphe of posterior wall of pharynx	pharyngeal plexus of vagus	constricts pharynx
coracobrachial m.	m. coracobrachialis	coracoid process of scapula	medial surface of shaft of humerus	musculocutaneous	flexes, adducts arm
corrugator m., superciliary	m. corrugator supercilii	medial end of superciliary arch	skin of eyebrow	facial	draws eyebrow downward and medially
cremaster m.	m. cremaster	inferior margin of internal oblique m. of abdomen	pubic tubercle	genital branch of genitofemoral	elevates testis
cricoarytenoid m., lateral	m. cricoarytenoideus lateralis	lateral surface of cricoid cartilage	muscular process of arytenoid cartilage	recurrent laryngeal	approximates vocal folds
cricoarytenoid m., posterior	m. cricoarytenoideus posterior	back of lamina of cricoid cartilage	muscular process of arytenoid cartilage	recurrent laryngeal	separates vocal folds
cricothyroid m.	m. cricothyroideus	front and side of cricoid cartilage	lamina and inferior horn of thyroid cartilage	external branch of superior laryngeal	tenses vocal folds

*m. = muscle; m's = (pl.) muscles
†m. = musculus; mm. = (L. pl.) musculi

Table of Muscles (*Continued*)

Common Name*	NA Term†	Origin*	Insertion*	Innervation	Action
deltoid m.	m. deltoideus	clavicle, acromion, spine of scapula	deltoid tuberosity of humerus	axillary	abducts, flexes, or extends arm
depressor m. of angle of mouth	m. depressor anguli oris	lateral border of mandible	angle of mouth	facial	pulls down angle of mouth
depressor m. of lower lip	m. depressor labii inferioris	anterior surface of lower border of mandible	orbicular m. of mouth and skin of lower lip	facial	depresses lower lip
depressor m. of septum of nose	m. depressor septi nasi	incisive fossa of maxilla	ala and septum of nose	facial	constricts nostril and depresses ala
depressor m., superciliary	m. depressor supercilii	a name applied to a few fibers of orbital part of orbicular m. of eye that are inserted into the eyebrow, which they depress			
detrusor urinae. *See* pubovesical m.					
diaphragm	diaphragma	back of xiphoid process, inner surfaces of lower 6 costal cartilages and lower 4 ribs, medial and lateral arcuate ligaments, bodies of upper lumbar vertebrae	central tendon of diaphragm	phrenic	increases volume of thorax in inspiration
digastric m.	m. digastricus	*anterior belly*–digastric fossa on lower border of mandible near symphysis; *posterior belly*–mastoid notch of temporal bone	intermediate tendon on hyoid bone	*anterior belly*–mylohyoid branch of inferior alveolar; *posterior belly*–digastric branch of facial	elevates hyoid bone, lowers jaw
dilator m. of pupil	m. dilator pupillae	a name applied to fibers extending radially from sphincter of pupil to ciliary margin		sympathetic	dilates iris
epicranial m.	m. epicranius	a name applied to muscular covering of scalp, including occipitofrontal and temporoparietal m's and galea aponeurotica			
erector m. of spine	m. erector spinae	a name applied to fibers of more superficial of deep muscles of back, originating from sacrum, spines of lumbar and eleventh and twelfth thoracic vertebrae, and iliac crest, which split and insert as iliocostal, longissimus, and spinal m's			
extensor m. of fingers	m. extensor digitorum	lateral epicondyle of humerus	extensor expansion of 4 medial fingers	deep branch of radial	extends wrist joint and phalanges
extensor m. of great toe, long	m. extensor hallucis longus	front of fibula, interosseous membrane	base of distal phalanx of great toe	deep peroneal	extends great toe, dorsiflexes ankle joint
extensor m. of great toe, short	m. extensor hallucis brevis	a name applied to portion of short extensor m. of toes that goes to great toe			
extensor m. of index finger	m. extensor indicis	posterior surface of ulna, interosseous membrane	extensor expansion of index finger	posterior interosseous	extends index finger
extensor m. of little finger	m. extensor digiti minimi	lateral epicondyle of humerus	extensor aponeurosis of little finger	deep branch of radial	extends little finger
extensor m. of thumb, long	m. extensor pollicis longus	posterior surface of ulna and interosseous membrane	back of distal phalanx of thumb	posterior interosseous	extends, adducts thumb
extensor m. of thumb, short	m. extensor pollicis brevis	posterior surface of radius	back of proximal phalanx of thumb	posterior interosseous	extends thumb
extensor m. of toes, long	m. extensor digitorum longus	anterior surface of fibula, lateral condyle of tibia, interosseous membrane	extensor expansion of 4 lateral toes	deep peroneal	extends toes

extensor m. of toes, short	m. extensor digitorum brevis	upper surface of calcaneus	extensor tendons of first, second, third, fourth toes	deep peroneal	extends toes
extensor m. of wrist, radial, long	m. extensor carpi radialis longus	lateral supracondylar ridge of humerus	back of base of second metacarpal bone	radial	extends, abducts wrist joint
extensor m. of wrist, radial, short	m. extensor carpi radialis brevis	lateral epicondyle of humerus	back of bases of second and third metacarpal bones	radial or its deep branch	extends, abducts wrist joint
extensor m. of wrist, ulnar	m. extensor carpi ulnaris	*humeral head* – lateral epicondyle of humerus; *ulnar head* – posterior border of ulna	base of fifth metacarpal bone	deep branch of radial	extends, abducts wrist joint
fibular m. *See* peroneal m.					
flexor m. of fingers, deep	m. flexor digitorum profundus	shaft of ulna, coronoid process, interosseous membrane	bases of distal phalanges of 4 medial fingers	anterior interosseous, ulnar	flexes distal phalanges
flexor m. of fingers, superficial	m. flexor digitorum superficialis	*humeroulnar head* – medial epicondyle of humerus, coronoid process of ulna; *radial head* – anterior border of radius	sides of middle phalanges of 4 medial fingers	median	flexes middle phalanges
flexor m. of great toe, long	m. flexor hallucis longus	posterior surface of fibula	base of distal phalanx of great toe	tibial	flexes great toe
flexor m. of great toe, short	m. flexor hallucis brevis	undersurface of cuboid, lateral cuneiform	both sides of base of proximal phalanx of great toe	medial plantar	flexes great toe
flexor m. of little finger, short	m. flexor digiti minimi brevis manus	hook of hamate bone, transverse carpal ligament	medial side of proximal phalanx of little finger	ulnar	flexes little finger
flexor m. of little toe, short	m. flexor digiti minimi brevis pedis	sheath of long peroneal	lateral surface of base of proximal phalanx of little toe	lateral plantar	flexes little toe
flexor m. of thumb, long	m. flexor pollicis longus	anterior surface of radius, medial epicondyle of humerus, coronoid process of ulna	base of distal phalanx of thumb	anterior interosseous	flexes thumb
flexor m. of thumb, short	m. flexor pollicis brevis	tubercle of trapezium, flexor retinaculum	lateral side of base of proximal phalanx of thumb	median, ulnar	flexes, adducts thumb
flexor m. of toes, long	m. flexor digitorum longus pedis	posterior surface of shaft of tibia	distal phalanges of 4 lateral toes	tibial	flexes toes, extends foot
flexor m. of toes, short	m. flexor digitorum brevis pedis	medial tuberosity of calcaneus, plantar fascia	middle phalanges of 4 lateral toes	medial plantar	flexes toes
flexor m. of wrist, radial	m. flexor carpi radialis	medial epicondyle of humerus	bases of second and third metacarpal bones	median	flexes, abducts wrist joint
flexor m. of wrist, ulnar	m. flexor carpi ulnaris	*humeral head* – medial epicondyle of humerus; *ulnar head* – olecranon and posterior border of ulna	pisiform bone, hook of hamate bone, base of fifth metacarpal bone	ulnar	flexes, adducts wrist joint
gastrocnemius m.	m. gastrocnemius	*medial head* – popliteal surface of femur, upper part of medial condyle, capsule of knee; *lateral head* – lateral condyle, capsule of knee	aponeurosis unites with tendon of soleus to form Achilles tendon	tibial	plantar flexes foot, flexes knee joint
gemellus m., inferior	m. gemellus inferior	tuberosity of ischium	internal obturator tendon	nerve to quadrate m. of thigh	rotates thigh laterally
gemellus m., superior	m. gemellus superior	spine of ischium	internal obturator tendon	nerve to internal obturator	rotates thigh laterally
genioglossus m.	m. genioglossus	superior genial tubercle	hyoid bone, undersurface of tongue	hypoglossal	protrudes, depresses tongue
geniohyoid m.	m. geniohyoideus	inferior genial tubercle	body of hyoid bone	a branch of first cervical nerve through hypoglossal	draws hyoid bone forward

TABLE OF MUSCLES (*Continued*)

COMMON NAME*	NA TERM†	ORIGIN*	INSERTION*	INNERVATION	ACTION
glossopalatine m. *See* palatoglossus m.					
gluteus maximus m., (gluteal m., greatest)	m. gluteus maximus	dorsal aspect of ilium, dorsal surfaces of sacrum, coccyx, sacrotuberous ligament	iliotibial tract of fascia lata, gluteal tuberosity of femur	inferior gluteal	extends, abducts, rotates thigh laterally
gluteus medius m., (gluteal m., middle)	m. gluteus medius	dorsal aspect of ilium between anterior and posterior gluteal lines	greater trochanter of femur	superior gluteal	abducts, rotates thigh medially
gluteus minimus m., (gluteal m., least)	m. gluteus minimus	dorsal aspect of ilium between anterior and posterior gluteal lines	greater trochanter of femur	superior gluteal	abducts, rotates thigh medially
gracilis m.	m. gracilis	body and inferior ramus of pubis	medial surface of shaft of tibia	obturator	adducts thigh, flexes knee joint
m. of helix, greater	m. helicis major	spine of helix	anterior border of helix	auriculotemporal, posterior auricular	tenses skin of acoustic meatus
m. of helix, smaller	m. helicis minor	anterior rim of helix	concha	temporal, posterior auricular	
hyoglossus m.	m. hyoglossus	body and greater horn of hyoid bone	side of tongue	hypoglossal	depresses, retracts tongue
iliac m.	m. iliacus	iliac fossa, ala of sacrum	greater psoas tendon, lesser trochanter of femur	femoral	flexes thigh. trunk on limb
iliococcygeus m.	m. iliococcygeus	a name applied to posterior portion of levator ani m., including fibers originating as far forward as obturator canal, and inserting on side of coccyx and in anococcygeal ligaments			
iliocostal m.	m. iliocostalis	a name applied to lateral division of erector m. of spine			
iliocostal m. of loins	m. iliocostalis lumborum	iliac crest	angles of lower 6 or 7 ribs	thoracic and lumbar	extends lumbar spine
iliocostal m. of neck	m. iliocostalis cervicis	angles of third, fourth, fifth, and sixth ribs	transverse processes of lower fourth, fifth, and sixth cervical vertebrae	cervical	extends cervical spine
iliocostal m. of thorax	m. iliocostalis thoracis	upper borders of angles of 6 lower ribs	angles of upper ribs and transverse process of seventh cervical vertebra	thoracic	keeps thoracic spine erect
iliopsoas m.	m. iliopsoas	a name applied collectively to iliac and greater psoas m's			
incisive m's of inferior lip	mm. incisivi labii inferioris	incisive fossae of mandible	angle of mouth	facial	make vestibule of mouth shallow
incisive m's of superior lip	m. incisivi labii superioris	incisive fossae of maxilla	angle of mouth	facial	make vestibule of mouth shallow
m. of incisure of helix	m. incisurae helicis	a name applied to inconstant slips of fibers continuing forward from m. of tragus to bridge notch of cartilaginous part of meatus			
infraspinous m.	m. infraspinatus	infraspinous fossa of scapula	greater tubercle of humerus	suprascapular	rotates arm laterally
intercostal m's	mm. intercostales	a name applied to the layer of muscle fibers separated from the internal intercostal m's by the intercostal nerves and vessels			
intercostal m's, external	mm. intercostales externi	inferior border of rib	superior border of rib below	intercostal	elevate ribs in inspiration
intercostal m's, internal	mm. intercostales interni	inferior border of rib and costal cartilage	superior border of rib and costal cartilage below	intercostal	act on ribs in expiration
interosseous m's of foot, dorsal	mm. interossei dorsales pedis	sides of adjacent metatarsal bones	base of proximal phalanges of second, third, and fourth toes	lateral plantar	flex, abduct toes

interosseous m's of hand, dorsal	mm. interossei dorsales manus	each by two heads from adjacent sides of metacarpal bones	extensor tendons of second, third, and fourth fingers	ulnar	abduct, flex proximal, extend middle and distal phalanges
interosseous m's, palmar	mm. interossei palmares	sides of first, second, fourth, and fifth metacarpal bones	extensor tendons of first, second, fourth, and fifth fingers	ulnar	adduct, flex proximal, extend middle and distal phalanges
interosseous m's, plantar	mm. interossei plantares	medial side of third, fourth, and fifth metatarsal bones	medial side of base of proximal phalanges of third, fourth, and fifth toes	lateral plantar	flex, abduct toes
interspinal m's	mm. interspinales	a name applied to short bands of muscle fibers extending on each side between spinous processes of contiguous vertebrae		spinal	extend vertebral column
intertransverse m's	mm. intertransversarii	a name applied to small muscles passing between transverse processes of adjacent vertebrae		spinal	bend vertebral column laterally
ischiocavernous m.	m. ischiocavernosus	ramus of ischium	crus of penis or clitoris	perineal branches of pudendal	maintains erection of penis or clitoris
latissimus dorsi m.	m. latissimus dorsi	spines of lower thoracic vertebrae, spines of lumbar and sacral vertebrae through attachment to thoracolumbar fascia, iliac crest, lower ribs, inferior angle of scapula	floor of intertubercular groove of humerus	thoracodorsal	adducts, extends, rotates humerus medially
levator m. of angle of mouth	m. levator anguli oris	canine fossa of maxilla	orbicular m. of mouth, skin at angle of mouth	facial	raises angle of mouth
levator ani m.	m. levator ani	a name applied collectively to important muscular components of pelvic diaphragm, arising mainly from back of body of pubis and running backward toward coccyx; includes pubococcygeus (levator m. of prostate in male and pubovaginal in female), puborectal, and iliococcygeus m's		third and fourth sacral	helps support pelvic viscera and resist increases in intra-abdominal pressure
levator m. of palatine velum	m. levator veli palatini	apex of pars petrosa of temporal bone and cartilage of auditory tube	aponeurosis of soft palate	pharyngeal plexus	raises and draws back soft palate
levator m. of prostate	m. levator prostatae	a name applied to part of anterior portion of pubococcygeus m., which in male is inserted into prostate and tendinous center of perineum		sacral, pudendal	supports, compresses prostate, helps control micturition
levator m's of ribs	mm. levatores costarum	transverse processes of seventh cervical and first 11 thoracic vertebrae	medial to angle of rib below	intercostal	aid elevation of ribs in respiration
levator m. of scapula	m. levator scapulae	transverse processes of 4 upper cervical vertebrae	vertebral border of scapula	third and fourth cervical	raises scapula
levator m. of thyroid gland	m. levator glandulae thyroideae	isthmus or pyramidal lobule of thyroid gland	body of hyoid bone	external branch of superior laryngeal	
levator m. of upper eyelid	m. levator palpebrae superioris	sphenoid bone above optic foramen	skin and tarsal plate of upper eyelid	oculomotor	raises upper eyelid
levator m. of upper lip	m. levator labii superioris	lower margin of orbit	musculature of upper lip	facial	raises upper lip
levator m. of upper lip and ala of nose	m. levator labii superioris alaeque nasi	frontal process of maxilla	skin and cartilage of ala of nose, upper lip	infraorbital branch of facial	raises upper lip, dilates nostril
long m. of head	m. longus capitis	transverse processes of third to sixth cervical vertebrae	basilar portion of occipital bone	cervical	flexes head

Table of Muscles (*Continued*)

Common Name*	NA Term†	Origin*	Insertion*	Innervation	Action
long m. of neck	m. longus colli	*superior oblique portion* – transverse processes of third to fifth cervical vertebrae; *inferior oblique portion* – bodies of first to third thoracic vertebrae; *vertical portion* – bodies of 3 upper thoracic and 3 lower cervical vertebrae	*superior oblique portion* – tubercle of anterior arch of atlas; *inferior oblique portion* – transverse processes of fifth and sixth cervical vertebrae; *vertical portion* – bodies of second to fourth cervical vertebrae	anterior cervical	flexes, supports cervical vertebrae
longissimus m. of head.	m. longissimus capitis	transverse processes of 4 or 5 upper thoracic vertebrae, articular processes of 3 or 4 lower cervical vertebrae	mastoid process of temporal bone	cervical	draws head backward, rotates head
longissimus m. of neck	m. longissimus cervicis	transverse processes of 4 or 5 upper thoracic vertebrae	transverse processes of second or third to sixth cervical vertebrae	lower cervical and upper thoracic	extends cervical vertebrae
longissimus m. of thorax	m. longissimus thoracis	transverse and articular proccesses of lumbar vertebrae and thoracolumbar fascia	transverse processes of all thoracic vertebrae, 9 or 10 lower ribs	lumbar and thoracic	extends thoracic vertebrae
longitudinal m. of tongue, inferior	m. longitudinalis inferior linguae	undersurface of tongue at base	tip of tongue	hypoglossal	changes shape of tongue in mastication and deglutition
longitudinal m. of tongue, superior	m. longitudinalis superior linguae	submucosa and septum of tongue	margins of tongue	hypoglossal	changes shape of tongue in mastication and deglutition
lumbrical m's of foot	mm. lumbricales pedis	tendons of long flexor m. of toes	medial side of base of proximal phalanges of 4 lateral toes	medial and lateral plantar	flex metatarsophalangeal joints, extend distal phalanges
lumbrical m's of hand	mm. lumbricales manus	tendons of deep flexor m. of fingers	extensor tendons of 4 lateral fingers	median, ulnar	flex metacarpophalangeal joints, extend middle and distal phalanges
masseter m.	m. masseter	*superficial part* – zygomatic process of maxilla, lower border of zygomatic arch; *deep part* – lower border and medial surface of zygomatic arch	*superficial part* – angle and ramus of mandible; *deep part* – upper half of ramus and lateral surface of coronoid process of mandible	masseteric, from mandibular division of trigeminal	raises mandible, closes jaws
multifidus m's	mm. multifidi	sacrum, sacroiliac ligament, mamillary processes of lumbar, transverse processes of thoracic, and articular processes of cervical vertebrae	spines of contiguous vertebrae above	spinal	extend, rotate vertebral column
mylohyoid m.	m. mylohyoideus	mylohyoid line of mandible	body of hyoid bone, median raphe	mylohyoid branch of inferior alveolar	elevates hyoid bone, supports floor of mouth
nasal m.	m. nasalis	maxilla	*alar part* – ala of nose; *transverse part* – by aponeurotic expansion with fellow of opposite side	facial	*alar part* – aids in widening nostril; *transverse part* – depresses cartilage of nose
oblique m. of abdomen, external	m. obliquus externus abdominus	lower 8 ribs at costal cartilages	crest of ilium, linea alba through rectus sheath	lower thoracic	flexes, rotates vertebral column, compresses abdominal viscera

oblique m. of abdomen, internal	m. obliquus internus abdominis	thoracolumbar fascia, iliac crest, iliac fascia, inguinal fascia	lower 3 or 4 costal cartilages, linea alba, conjoined tendon to pubis	lower thoracic	flexes, rotates vertebral column, compresses abdominal viscera
oblique m. of auricle	m. obliquus auriculae	cranial surface of concha	cranial surface of auricle above concha	posterior auricular, temporal	
oblique m. of eyeball, inferior	m. obliquus inferior bulbi	orbital surface of maxilla	sclera	oculomotor	abducts, rotates eyeball upward and outward
oblique m. of eyeball, superior	m. obliquus superior bulbi	lesser wing of sphenoid above optic foramen	sclera	trochlear	abducts, rotates eyeball downward and outward
oblique m. of head, inferior	m. obliquus capitis inferior	spinous process of axis	transverse process of atlas	spinal	rotates atlas and head
oblique m. of head, superior	m. obliquus capitis superior	transverse process of atlas	occipital bone	spinal	extends and moves head laterally
obturator m., external	m. obturatorius externus	pubis, ischium, external surface of obturator membrane	trochanteric fossa of femur	obturator	rotates thigh laterally
obturator m., internal	m. obturatorius internus	pelvic surface of hip bone and obturator membrane, margin of obturator foramen	greater trochanter of femur	fifth lumbar, first and second sacral	rotates thigh laterally
occipitofrontal m.	m. occipitofrontalis	*frontal belly*—galea aponeurotica; *occipital belly*—highest nuchal line of occipital bone	*frontal belly*—skin of eyebrow, root of nose; *occipital belly*—galea aponeurotica	*frontal belly*—temporal branch of facial; *occipital belly*—posterior auricular branch of facial	*frontal belly*—raises eyebrow; *occipital belly*—draws scalp backward
omohyoid m.	m. omohyoideus	superior border of scapula	body of hyoid bone	upper cervical through ansa cervicalis	depresses hyoid bone
opposing m. of little finger	m. opponens digiti minimi manus	hook of hamate bone	front of fifth metacarpal	eighth cervical through ulnar	abducts, flexes, rotates fifth metacarpal
opposing m. of thumb	m. opponens pollicis	tubercle of trapezium, flexor retinaculum	lateral side of first metacarpal	sixth and seventh metacarpal through median	flexes, opposes thumb
orbicular m. of eye	m. orbicularis oculi	*orbital part*—medial margin of orbit, including frontal process of maxilla; *palpebral part*—medial palpebral ligament; *lacrimal part*— posterior lacrimal crest	*orbital part*—near origin after encircling orbit; *palpebral part*—orbital tubercle of zygomatic bone; *lacrimal part*—lateral palpebral raphe	facial	closes eyelids, wrinkles forehead, compresses lacrimal sac
orbicular m. of mouth	m. orbicularis oris	a name applied to complicated sphincter muscle of mouth, comprising 2 parts: *labial part*—consisting of fibers restricted to lips; *marginal part*—consisting of fibers blending with those of adjacent muscles		facial	closes, protrudes lips
orbital m.	m. orbitalis	bridges inferior orbital fissure	fascia of inferior orbital fissure	sympathetic fibers	protrudes eye
palatoglossus m.	m. palatoglossus	undersurface of soft palate	side of tongue	pharyngeal plexus	elevates tongue, constricts fauces
palatopharyngeal m.	m. palatopharyngeus	posterior border of bony palate, palatine, aponeurosis	posterior border of thyroid cartilage, side of pharynx and esophagus	pharyngeal plexus	constricts pharynx, aids swallowing
palmar m., long	m. palmaris longus	medial epicondyle of humerus	flexor retinaculum, palmar aponeurosis	median	tenses palmar aponeurosis
palmar m., short	m. palmaris brevis	palmar aponeurosis	skin of medial border of hand	ulnar	assists in deepening hollow of palm
papillary m's	mm. papillares	a name applied to conical muscular projections from walls of cardiac ventricles, attached to cusps of atrioventricular valves by chordae tendineae			steady and strengthen atrioventricular valves and prevent eversion of their cusps

TABLE OF MUSCLES (*Continued*)

COMMON NAME*	NA TERM†	ORIGIN*	INSERTION*	INNERVATION	ACTION
pectinate m's	mm. pectinati	a name applied to small ridges of muscular fibers projecting from inner walls of auricles of heart, and extending in right atrium from auricle to crista terminalis			
pectineal m.	m. pectineus	pectineal line of pubis	pectineal line of femur	femoral, obturator	flexes, adducts thigh
pectoral m., greater	m. pectoralis major	clavicle, sternum, 6 upper costal cartilages, aponeurosis of external oblique m. of abdomen	crest of greater tubercle of humerus	lateral and medial pectoral	adducts, flexes, rotates arm medially
pector⁻ˡ m., smaller	m. pectoralis minor	second, third, fourth, and fifth ribs	coracoid process of scapula	medial and lateral pectoral	draws shoulder forward and downward, raises third, fourth, and fifth ribs in forced inspiration
peroneal m., long	m. peroneus longus	lateral condyle of tibia, head of fibula, lateral surface of fibula	medial cuneiform, first metatarsal	superficial peroneal	plantar flexes, everts, abducts foot
peroneal m., short	m. peroneus brevis	lateral surface of fibula	tuberosity of fifth metatarsal	superficial peroneal	everts, abducts, plantar flexes foot
peroneal m., third	m. peroneus tertius	anterior surface of fibula, interosseous membrane	fascia or base of fifth (or fourth) metatarsal	deep peroneal	everts, dorsiflexes foot
piriform m.	m. piriformis	ilium, second to fourth sacral vertebrae	greater trochanter of femur	first and second sacral	rotates thigh laterally
plantar m.	m. plantaris	popliteal surface of femur	Achilles tendon or back of calcaneus	tibial	plantar flexes foot, flexes leg
platysma	platysma	a name applied to a platelike muscle originating from the fascia of cervical region and inserting on mandible, and skin around mouth		cervical branch of facial	wrinkles skin of neck, depresses jaw
pleuroesophageal m.	m. pleuroesophageus	a name applied to a bundle of smooth muscle fibers, usually connecting esophagus with left mediastinal pleura			
popliteal m.	m. popliteus	lateral condyle of femur, lateral meniscus	posterior surface of tibia	tibial	flexes leg, rotates leg medially
procerus m.	m. procerus	fascia over nasal bones	skin of forehead	facial	draws medial angle of eyebrows down
pronator m., quadrate	m. pronator quadratus	anterior surface and border of distal third or fourth of shaft of ulna	anterior surface and border of distal fourth of shaft of radius	anterior interosseous	pronates forearm
pronator m., round	m. pronator teres	*humeral head* – medial epicondyle of humerus; *ulnar head* – coronoid process of ulna	lateral surface of radius	median	pronates and flexes forearm
psoas m., greater	m. psoas major	lumbar vertebrae	lesser trochanter of femur	second and third lumbar	flexes thigh or trunk
psoas m., smaller	m. psoas minor	last thoracic and first lumbar vertebrae	arcuate line of hip bone	first lumbar	assists greater psoas m.
pterygoid m., lateral (external)	m. pterygoideus lateralis	*upper head* – infratemporal surface of greater wing of sphenoid, infratemporal crest; *lower head* – lateral surface of lateral pterygoid plate	neck of mandible, capsule of temporomandibular joint	mandibular	protrudes mandible, opens jaws, moves mandible from side to side
pterygoid m., medial (internal)	m. pterygoideus medialis	medial surface of lateral pterygoid plate, tuber of maxilla	medial surface of ramus and angle of mandible	mandibular	closes jaws

pubococcygeus m.	m. pubococcygeus	a name applied to anterior portion of levator ani m., originating in front of obturator canal and inserting in anococcygeal ligament and side of coccyx		third and fourth sacral	helps support pelvic viscera and resist increases in intra-abdominal pressure
puboprostatic m.	m. puboprostaticus	a name applied to smooth muscle fibers contained within medial puboprostatic ligament, which pass from prostate anteriorly to pubis			
puborectal m.	m. puborectalis	a name applied to portion of levator ani m., with a more lateral origin from pubic bone, and continuous posteriorly with corresponding muscle of opposite side		third and fourth sacral	helps support pelvic viscera and resist increases in intra-abdominal pressure
pubovaginal m.	m. pubovaginalis	a name applied to part of anterior portion of pubococcygeus m., which is inserted into urethra and vagina		sacral and pudendal	helps control micturition
pubovesical m.	m. pubovesicalis	a name applied to smooth muscle fibers extending from neck of urinary bladder to pubis			
pyramidal m.	m. pyramidalis	body of pubis	linea alba	last thoracic	tenses abdominal wall
pyramidal m. of auricle	m. pyramidalis auriculae	a name applied to inconstant prolongation of fibers of m. of tragus to spine of helix			
quadrate m. of loins	m. quadratus lumborum	iliac crest, thoracolumbar fascia	twelfth rib, transverse processes of lumbar vertebrae	first and second lumbar, twelfth thoracic	flexes trunk laterally
quadrate m. of lower lip. *See* depressor m. of lower lip					
quadrate m. of sole	m. quadratus plantae	calcaneus, plantar fascia	tendons of long flexor m. of toes	lateral plantar	aids in flexing toes
quadrate m. of thigh	m. quadratus femoris	tuberosity of ischium	intertrochanteric crest and quadrate tubercle of femur	fourth and fifth lumbar, first sacral	adducts, rotates thigh laterally
quadrate m. of upper lip. *See* levator m. of upper lip					
quadriceps m. of thigh	m. quadriceps femoris	a name applied collectively to rectus m. of thigh and intermediate, lateral and medial vastus m's, inserting by a common tendon that surrounds patella and ends on tuberosity of tibia		femoral	extends leg upon thigh
rectococcygeus m.	m. rectococcygeus	a name applied to smooth muscle fibers originating on anterior surface of second and third coccygeal vertebrae and inserting on posterior surface of rectum		autonomic	retracts, elevates rectum
rectourethral m.	m. rectourethralis	a name applied to band of smooth muscle fibers in male, extending from perineal flexure of rectum to membranous part of urethra			
rectouterine m.	m. rectouterinus	a name applied to band of fibers in female, running between cervix uteri and rectum, in rectouterine fold			
rectovesical m.	m. rectovesicalis	a name applied to band of fibers in male, connecting longitudinal musculature of rectum with external muscular coat of bladder			
rectus m. of abdomen	m. rectus abdominis	pubic crest and symphysis	xiphoid process, fifth, sixth and seventh costal cartilages	lower thoracic	flexes lumbar vertebrae, supports abdomen
rectus m. of eyeball, inferior	m. rectus inferior bulbi	common tendinous ring	underside of sclera	oculomotor	adducts, rotates eyeball downard and medially
rectus m. of eyeball, lateral	m. rectus lateralis bulbi	common tendinous ring	lateral side of sclera	abducens	abducts eyeball
rectus m. of eyeball, medial	m. rectus medialis bulbi	common tendinous ring	medial side of sclera	oculomotor	adducts eyeball
rectus m. of eyeball, superior	m. rectus superior bulbi	common tendinous ring	upper side of sclera	oculomotor	adducts, rotates eyeball upward and medially
rectus m. of head, anterior	m. rectus capitis anterior	lateral mass of atlas	basilar part of occipital bone	first and second cervical	flexes, supports head
rectus m. of head, lateral	m. rectus capitis lateralis	transverse process of atlas	jugular process of occipital bone	first and second cervical	flexes, supports head

TABLE OF MUSCLES (*Continued*)

COMMON NAME*	NA TERM†	ORIGIN*	INSERTION*	INNERVATION	ACTION
rectus m. of head, posterior, greater	m. rectus capitis posterior major	spinous process of axis	occipital bone	suboccipital, greater occipital	extends head
rectus m. of head, posterior, smaller	m. rectus capitis posterior minor	posterior tubercle of atlas	occipital bone	suboccipital, greater occipital	extends head
rectus m. of thigh	m. rectus femoris	anterior inferior iliac spine, rim of acetabulum	base of patella, tuberosity of tibia	femoral	extends leg, flexes thigh
rhomboid m., greater	m. rhomboideus major	spinous processes of second, third, fourth and fifth thoracic vertebrae	vertebral margin of scapula	dorsal scapular	retracts and fixes scapula
rhomboid m., smaller	m. rhomboideus minor	spinous processes of seventh cervical and first thoracic vertebrae, lower part of nuchal ligament	vertebral margin of scapula at root of spine	dorsal scapular	retracts and fixes scapula
risorius m.	m. risorius	fascia over masseter	skin at angle of mouth	buccal branch of facial	draws angle of mouth laterally
rotator m's	mm. rotatores	a name applied to a series of small muscles deep in groove between spinous and transverse processes of vertebrae		spinal	extend and rotate vertebral column toward opposite side
sacrococcygeal m., dorsal (posterior)	m. sacrococcygeus dorsalis	a name applied to muscular slip passing from dorsal surface of sacrum to coccyx			
sacrococcygeal m., ventral (anterior)	m. sacrococcygeus ventralis	a name applied to musculotendinous slip passing from lower sacral vertebrae to coccyx			
sacrospinal m. *See* erector m. of spine.					
salpingopharyngeal m.	m. salpingopharyngeus	cartilage of auditory tube	posterior part of palatopharyngeus	pharyngeal plexus	raises pharynx
sartorius m.	m. sartorius	anterior superior iliac spine	upper part of medial surface of tibia	femoral	flexes thigh and leg
scalene m., anterior	m. scalenus anterior	transverse processes of third to sixth cervical vertebrae	scalene tubercle of first rib	second to seventh cervical	raises first rib, flexes cervical vertebrae laterally
scalene m., middle	m. scalenus medius	transverse processes of first to seventh cervical vertebrae	upper surface of first rib	second to seventh cervical	raises first rib, flexes cervical vertebrae laterally
scalene m. of pleura. *See* smallest scalene m.					
scalene m., posterior	m. scalenus posterior	transverse processes of fourth to sixth cervical vertebrae	second rib	second to seventh cervical	raises first and second ribs, flexes cervical vertebrae laterally
scalene m., smallest	m. scalenus minimus	a name applied to muscular band occasionally found between anterior and middle scalene m's			
semimembranous m.	m. semimembranosus	tuberosity of ischium	lateral condyle of femur, medial condyle and border of tibia	sciatic	flexes leg, extends thigh
semispinal m. of head	m. semispinalis capitis	transverse processes of upper thoracic and lower cervical vertebrae	occipital bone	suboccipital, greater occipital, branches of cervical	extends head
semispinal m. of neck	m. semispinalis cervicis	transverse processes of upper thoracic vertebrae	spinous processes of second to fifth (or fourth) cervical vertebrae	branches of cervical	extends, rotates vertebral column

semispinal m. of thorax	m. semispinalis thoracis	transverse processes of lower thoracic vertebrae	spinous processes of lower cervical and upper thoracic vertebrae	spinal	extends, rotates vertebral column
semitendinous m.	m. semitendinosus	tuberosity of ischium	upper part of medial surface of tibia	sciatic	flexes and rotates leg medially, extends thigh
serratus m., anterior	m. serratus anterior	8 upper ribs	vertebral border of scapula	long thoracic	draws scapula forward, rotates scapula to raise shoulder in abduction of arm
serratus m., posterior, inferior	m. serratus posterior inferior	spines of lower thoracic and upper lumbar vertebrae	4 lower ribs	ninth to twelfth (or eleventh) thoracic	lowers ribs in expiration
serratus m., posterior, superior	m. serratus posterior superior	nuchal ligament, spinous processes of upper thoracic vertebrae	second, third, fourth and fifth ribs	upper 4 thoracic	raises ribs in inspiration
soleus m.	m. soleus	fibula, tendinous arch, tibia	calcaneus by Achilles tendon	tibial	plantar flexes foot
sphincter m. of anus, external	m. sphincter ani externus	tip of coccyx, anococcygeal ligament	tendinous center of perineum	inferior rectal, perineal branch of fourth sacral	closes anus
sphincter m. of anus, internal	m. sphincter ani internus	a name applied to a thickening of circular layer of muscular tunic at caudal end of rectum			
sphincter m. of bile duct	m. sphincter ductus choledochi	a name applied to annular sheath of muscle fibers investing bile duct within wall of duodenum			
sphincter m. of hepatopancreatic ampulla	m. sphincter ampullae hepatopancreaticae	a name applied to annular band of muscle fibers investing hepatopancreatic ampulla			
sphincter m. of pupil	m. sphincter pupillae	a name applied to circular fibers of iris		parasympathetic through ciliary	constricts pupil
sphincter m. of pylorus	m. sphincter pylori	a name applied to a thickening of circular muscle of stomach around its opening into duodenum pylorus			
sphincter m. of urethra	m. sphincter urethrae	inferior ramus of pubis	median raphe behind and in front of urethra	perineal	compresses membranous urethra
sphincter m. of urinary bladder	m. sphincter vesicae urinariae	a name applied to circular layer of fibers surrounding internal urethral orifice		vesical	closes internal orifice of urethra
spinal m. of head	m. spinalis capitis	spinous processes of upper thoracic and lower cervical vertebrae	occipital bone	spinal	extends head
spinal m. of neck	m. spinalis cervicis	spinous process of seventh cervical vertebra, nuchal ligament	spinous processes of axis	branches of cervical	extends vertebral column
spinal m. of thorax	m. spinalis thoracis	spinous processes of upper lumbar and lower thoracic vertebrae	spinous processes of upper thoracic vertebrae	branches of spinal	extends vertebral column
splenius m. of head	m. splenius capitis	lower half of nuchal ligament, spinous processes of seventh cervical and upper thoracic vertebrae	mastoid part of temporal bone, occipital bone	cervical	extends, rotates head
splenius m. of neck	m. splenius cervicis	spinous process of upper thoracic vertebrae	transverse processes of upper cervical vertebrae	cervical	extends, rotates head and neck
stapedius m.	m. stapedius	interior of pyramidal eminence of tympanic cavity	neck of stapes	facial	dampens movement of stapes
sternal m.	m. sternalis	a name applied to muscular band occasionally found parallel to sternum on sternocostal head of greater pectoral m.			
sternocleidomastoid m.	m. sternocleidomastoideus	*sternal head*—manubrium; *clavicular head*—medial third of clavicle	mastoid process, superior nuchal line of occipital bone	accessory, cervical plexus	flexes vertebral column, rotates head to opposite side
sternocostal m. *See* transverse m. of thorax					

TABLE OF MUSCLES (*Concluded*)

COMMON NAME*	NA TERM†	ORIGIN*	INSERTION*	INNERVATION	ACTION
sternohyoid m.	m. sternohyoideus	manubrium sterni and/or clavicle	body of hyoid bone	ansa cervicalis	depresses hyoid bone and larynx
sternothyroid m.	m. sternothyroideus	manubrium sterni	lamina of thyroid cartilage	ansa cervicalis	depresses thyroid cartilage
styloglossus m.	m. styloglossus	styloid process	margin of tongue	hypoglossal	raises, retracts tongue
stylohyoid m.	m. stylohyoideus	styloid process	body of hyoid bone	facial	draws hyoid bone and tongue upward and backward
stylopharyngeus m.	m. stylopharyngeus	styloid process	thyroid cartilage, side of pharynx	glossopharyngeal, pharyngeal plexus	raises, dilates pharynx
subclavius m.	m. subclavius	first rib and its cartilage	lower surface of clavicle	nerve to subclavius	depresses lateral end of clavicle
subcostal m's	mm. subcostales	lower border of ribs	upper border of second or third rib below	intercostal	raise ribs in inspiration
subscapular m.	m. subscapularis	subscapular fossa of scapula	lesser tubercle of humerus	subscapular	rotates arm medially
supinator m.	m. supinator	lateral epicondyle of humerus, ligaments of elbow	radius	deep branch of radial	supinates forearm
supraspinous m.	m. supraspinatus	supraspinous fossa of scapula	greater tubercle of humerus	suprascapular	abducts arm
suspensory m.	m. suspensorius	a name applied to flat band of smooth muscle fibers originating from left crus of diaphragm and inserting continuous with muscular coat of duodenum at its junction with jejunum			
tarsal m., inferior	m. tarsalis inferior	inferior rectus m. of eyeball	tarsal plate of lower eyelid	sympathetic	widens palpebral fissure
tarsal m., superior	m. tarsalis superior	levator m. of upper eyelid	tarsal plate of upper eyelid	sympathetic	widens palpebral fissure
temporal m.	m. temporalis	temporal fossa and fascia	coronoid process of mandible	mandibular	closes jaws
temporoparietal m.	m. temporoparietalis	temporal fascia above ear	galea aponeurotica	temporal branches of facial	tightens scalp
tensor m. of fascia lata	m. tensor fasciae latae	iliac crest	iliotibial tract of fascia lata	superior gluteal	flexes, rotates thigh medially
tensor m. of palatine velum	m. tensor veli palatini	scaphoid fossa and spine of sphenoid	aponeurosis of soft palate, wall of auditory tube	mandibular	tenses soft palate, opens auditory tube
tensor m. of tympanum	m. tensor tympani	cartilaginous portion of auditory tube	handle of malleus	mandibular	tenses tympanic membrane
teres major m.	m. teres major	inferior angle of scapula	crest of lesser tubercle of humerus	lower subscapular	adducts, extends, and rotates arm medially
teres minor m.	m. teres minor	lateral margin of scapula	greater tubercle of humerus	axillary	rotates arm laterally
thyroarytenoid m.	m. thyroarytenoideus	medial surface of lamina of thyroid cartilage	muscular process of arytenoid cartilage	recurrent laryngeal	relaxes, shortens vocal folds
thyroepiglottic m.	m. thyroepiglotticus	lamina of thyroid cartilage	epiglottis	recurrent laryngeal	closes inlet to larynx
thyrohyoid m.	m. thyrohyoideus	lamina of thyroid cartilage	greater horn of hyoid bone	ansa cervicalis	raises and changes form of larynx
tibial m., anterior	m. tibialis anterior	lateral condyle and surface of tibia, interosseous membrane	medial cuneiform, base of first metatarsal	deep peroneal	dorsiflexes, inverts foot
tibial m., posterior	m. tibialis posterior	tibia, fibula, interosseous membrane	bases of second to fourth metatarsal bones and tarsal bones, except talus	tibial	plantar flexes, inverts foot
tracheal m.	m. trachealis	a name applied to transverse smooth muscle fibers filling gap at back of each cartilage of trachea		autonomic	lessens caliber of trachea
m. of tragus	m. tragicus	a name applied to short, flattened vertical band on lateral surface of tragus, innervated by auriculotemporal and posterior auricular nerves			

transverse m. of abdomen	m. transversus abdominis	lower 6 costal cartilages, thoracolumbar fascia, iliac crest	linea alba through rectus sheath, conjoined tendon to pubis	lower thoracic	compresses abdominal viscera
transverse m. of auricle	m. transversus auriculae	cranial surface of auricle	circumference of auricle	posterior auricular branch of facial	retracts helix
transverse m. of chin	m. transversus menti	a name applied to superficial fibers of depressor m. of angle of mouth which turn medially and cross to opposite side			
transverse m. of nape	m. transversus nuchae	a name applied to small muscle often present, passing from occipital protuberance to posterior auricular m.; it may be either superficial or deep to trapezius			
transverse m. of perineum, deep	m. transversus perinei profundus	ramus of ischium	tendinous center of perineum	perineal	fixes tendinous center of perineum
transverse m. of perineum, superficial	m. transversus perinei superficialis	ramus of ischium	tendinous center of perineum	perineal	fixes tendinous center of perineum
transverse m. of thorax	m. transversus thoracis	posterior surface of body of sternum and of xiphoid process	second to sixth costal cartilages	intercostal	perhaps narrows chest
transverse m. of tongue	m. transversus linguae	median septum of tongue	dorsum and margins of tongue	hypoglossal	changes shape of tongue in mastication and swallowing
transversospinal m.	m. transversospinalis	a name applied collectively to semispinal, multifidus, and rotator m's			
trapezius m.	m. trapezius	occipital bone, nuchal ligament, spinous processes of seventh cervical and all thoracic vertebrae	clavicle, acromion, spine of scapula	accessory, cervical plexus	elevates shoulder, rotates scapula to raise shoulder in abduction of arm, draws scapula backward
triangular m. *See* depressor m. of angle of mouth					
triceps m. of arm (triceps brachii m.)	m. triceps brachii	*long head*–infraglenoid tubercle of scapula; *lateral head*–posterior surface of humerus; *medial head*–posterior surface of humerus below groove for radial nerve	olecranon of ulna	radial	extends forearm; *long head* adducts, extends arm
triceps m. of calf (triceps surae m.)	m. triceps surae	a name applied collectively to gastrocnemius and soleus m's			
m. of uvula	m. uvulae	posterior nasal spine of palatine bone and aponeurosis of soft palate	uvula	pharyngeal plexus	raises uvula
vastus m., intermediate	m. vastus intermedius	anterior and lateral surfaces of femur	patella, common tendon of quadriceps m. of thigh	femoral	extends leg
vastus m., lateral	m. vastus lateralis	lateral aspect of femur	patella, common tendon of quadriceps m. of thigh	femoral	extends leg
vastus m., medial	m. vastus medialis	medial aspect of femur	patella, common tendon of quadriceps m. of thigh	femoral	extends leg
vertical m. of tongue	m. verticalis linguae	dorsal fascia of tongue	sides and base of tongue	hypoglossal	changes shape of tongue in mastication and deglutition
vocal m.	m. vocalis	angle between laminae of thyroid cartilage	vocal process of arytenoid cartilage	recurrent laryngeal	causes local variations in tension of vocal fold
zygomatic m., greater	m. zygomaticus major	zygomatic bone	angle of mouth	facial	draws angle of mouth upward and backward
zygomatic m., smaller	m. zygomaticus minor	zygomatic bone	orbicular m. of mouth, levator m. of upper lip	facial	draws upper lip upward and laterally

example, the biceps (flexor) contracts and the triceps (extensor) relaxes. The reverse happens in straightening the elbow.

A muscle that has contracted many times, and has exhausted its stores of glycogen and other substances, and accumulated too much lactic acid, becomes unable to contract further and suffers from what is called muscle fatigue. In prolonged exhausting work, fat in the muscles can also be used for energy, and as a consequence the muscles become leaner.

MUSCULAR DISORDERS AND DISEASES. Strenuous physical activity that strains and tears the fibers can cause such muscular disorders including strain, charley horse, and muscle cramps.

Muscles may become infected or inflamed by the invasion of organisms, such as the parasite *Trichinella spiralis,* which is taken into the body by eating uncooked or poorly cooked pork. It causes the disease called trichinosis. Another type of muscular inflammation is fibrositis.

In poliomyelitis and other diseases of the nervous system, the muscles are disabled because the nerves leading to them have been injured or destroyed. The muscles are not directly harmed, but because they can no longer be stimulated they eventually waste away from disuse. The group of diseases called the progressive muscular atrophies result from wasting.

MYASTHENIA GRAVIS involves primarily the muscles of the face, eyelids, larynx, and throat. The cause is an impairment of the conduction of nerve impulses to the muscles.

Some diseases directly disable the muscles. MUSCULAR DYSTROPHY weakens the muscles of the trunk and limbs. The muscles sometimes enlarge or they may weaken and atrophy.

Benign and malignant tumors may (rarely) develop in muscles, producing myomas.

agonistic m., one opposed in action by another muscle, called the antagonist.

antagonistic m., one that counteracts the action of another muscle (the agonist).

antigravity m's, those that by their tone resist the constant pull of gravity in the maintenance of normal posture.

appendicular m., one of the muscles of a limb.

articular m., one that has one end attached to the capsule of a joint.

cutaneous m., striated muscle that inserts into the skin.

extraocular m's, the six voluntary muscles that move the eyeball: superior, inferior, middle, and lateral recti, and superior and inferior oblique muscles.

extrinsic m., one that originates in another part than that of its insertion, as those originating outside the eye, which move the eyeball.

fixation m's, fixator m's, accessory muscles that serve to steady a part.

fusiform m., a spindle-shaped muscle.

hamstring m's, the muscles of the back of the thigh.

intraocular m's, the intrinsic muscles of the eyeball.

intrinsic m., one whose origin and insertion are both in the same part or organ, as those entirely within the eye.

orbicular m., one that encircles a body opening, e.g., the eye or mouth.

postaxial m., one on the dorsal side of a limb.

preaxial m., one on the ventral side of a limb.

red m., the darker-colored muscle tissue of some mammals, composed of fibers rich in sarcoplasm, but with only faint cross-striping.

m. relaxant, an agent that specifically aids in reducing muscle tension.

skeletal m's, striated muscles that are attached to bones and typically cross at least one joint.

sphincter m., a ringlike muscle that closes a natural orifice; called also sphincter.

synergic m's, synergistic m's, those that assist one another in action.

thenar m's, the abductor and flexor muscles of the thumb.

vestigial m., one that was once well developed but through evolution has become rudimentary.

visceral m., muscle fibers associated chiefly with the hollow viscera.

white m., the paler muscle tissue of some mammals, composed of fibers with little sarcoplasm and prominent cross-striping.

yoked m's, those that normally act simultaneously and equally, as in moving the eyes.

muscular (mus'ku-lar) 1. pertaining to a muscle. 2. having well developed muscles.

m. dystrophy, a group of genetically determined, painless, degenerative myopathies that are progressively crippling because muscles are gradually weakened and eventually atrophy. At present there is no specific cure. The disease can sometimes be arrested temporarily; not all forms of it are totally disabling.

The word dystrophy means faulty or imperfect nutrition. In muscular dystrophy the muscles suffer a vital loss of protein, and muscle fibers are replaced gradually by fat and connective tissue until, in the late stages of the disease, the voluntary muscle system becomes virtually useless. In muscular dystrophy all visible damage occurs in the muscles themselves, and thus the disease is markedly different from MULTIPLE SCLEROSIS, in which the muscles are rendered impotent by damage to the nerves that control them.

Muscular dystrophy, which is believed to affect almost a quarter of a million Americans, is hereditary, although the way it is inherited is not the same for all types of the disease. The disease (or a propensity for the disease) seems to be carried mainly by women who, while not suffering from it themselves, may pass it on to their offspring, usually their sons. A woman who has conceived a dystrophic child is likely to be a carrier, as may be a woman who has had a dystrophic relative such as an uncle.

CHILDHOOD MUSCULAR DYSTROPHY. Muscular dystrophy cannot be detected at birth. In most cases the symptoms begin to be noticeable about the second or third year. The child gradually finds it more difficult to play and get about. Then, as the weakening process of the disease continues, he relies on a wheel chair, and later must spend most of his time in bed. In many cases death comes before the age of 20 from respiratory ailments or heart failure.

This childhood type of disease—unfortunately the most common type—is known as the Duchenne type or progressive muscular dystrophy. It is also called pseudohypertrophic muscular dystrophy because at the beginning the muscles, especially those in the calves, appear healthy and bulging when actually they are already weakened and their size is due to an excess of fat.

OTHER TYPES. Another type of the disease sometimes begins in childhood but is much more likely to appear during the teens or twenties. When the first symptom is a failure of the musculature of the pelvic girdle, this type is referred to as limb-girdle muscular dystrophy. It usually proceeds more slowly than does the childhood form.

This same type may take the form of facioscapulohumeral muscular dystrophy (referring to the face, shoulder, and upper arm muscles), which is likely to manifest itself first in an almost imperceptible weakening of the facial muscles. It is also known as Landouzy-Déjerine muscular dystrophy. Muscle deterioration starts in childhood or early adulthood but it may proceed very gradually over a number of years, sometimes until late in life. Some patients may only be slightly handicapped.

Other, rarer types of muscular dystrophy have been identified, including a distal type that begins in the peripheral muscles of the extremities. Still another type affects only muscles of the eye. Sometimes two or more forms are present in the same patient.

MANAGEMENT OF MUSCULAR DYSTROPHY. There is almost never any pain in muscular dystrophy. The mind is not affected; patients have normal intelligence. As the small muscles often are the last to be damaged, patients may continue to use their fingers. Children with muscular dystrophy are able to enjoy many recreations, even when they must rely on crutches or wheelchairs. The disease is not contagious.

Recent experiments hold out some hope that the progress of the disease can be slowed down, at least temporarily, by the use of certain medications that contribute to a build-up of protein in the patient's body or strengthen his muscle-cell membranes to prevent excessive escape of protein. Physical therapy—exercises, including exercise of the lungs by deep breathing—can sometimes bolster the delaying action against muscular weakness. The aim of such exercise is not to restore muscle power (which cannot be done) but to ensure that the patient makes the best use of the good muscle tissue remaining.

The more active the patient is, the better he will be physically and mentally. Obesity should be avoided.

The Muscular Dystrophy Associations of America, 1790 Broadway, New York, N.Y. 10019, are concerned not only with research but with every aspect of the care and comfort of dystrophic patients and can offer many valuable suggestions.

muscularis (mus″ku-la′ris) [L.] relating to muscle, specifically a muscular layer or coat.

musculature (mus′ku-lah-tūr) the muscular system of the body, or the muscles of a particular region.

musculocutaneous (mus″ku-lo-ku-ta′ne-us) pertaining to muscle and skin.

musculomembranous (mus″ku-lo-mem′brah-nus) pertaining to muscle and membrane.

musculophrenic (mus″ku-lo-fren′ik) pertaining to (chest) muscles and the diaphragm.

musculoskeletal (mus″ku-lo-skel′ĕ-tal) pertaining to muscle and skeleton.

musculotendinous (mus″ku-lo-ten′dĭ-nus) pertaining to muscle and tendon.

musculotropic (mus″ku-lo-trop′ik) exerting its principal effect upon muscle.

musculus (mus′ku-lus), pl. *mus′culi* [L.] muscle.

musicotherapy (mu″zĭ-ko-ther′ah-pe) treatment of disease by music.

Musset's sign (mu-sāz) de Musset's sign.

mustard (mus′tard) an irritant compound derived from dried ripe seed of *Brassica nigra* or *B. juncea*.

nitrogen m's, highly toxic compounds, some of which are used in treatment of neoplastic disease (see also NITROGEN MUSTARD).

sulfur m., a synthetic compound with vesicant and other toxic properties.

Mustargen (mus′tar-jen) trademark for a preparation of mechlorethamine hydrochloride, an antineoplastic agent.

mutagen (mu′tah-jen) an agent that induces genetic mutation.

mutagenesis (mu″tah-jen′ĕ-sis) the induction of genetic mutation.

mutagenic (mu″tah-jen′ik) inducing genetic mutation.

mutagenicity (mu″tah-jĕ-nis′ĭ-te) the property of being able to induce genetic mutation.

mutant (mu′tant) 1. in genetics, a variation that breeds true, owing to genetic changes. 2. produced by mutation.

mutase (mu′tās) an enzyme that produces rearrangement of molecules.

mutation (mu-ta′shun) a permanent transmissible change in the genetic material. Also, an individual exhibiting such change; a sport.

induced m., a genetic mutation caused by external factors, experimentally or accidentally produced.

somatic m., a genetic mutation occurring in a somatic cell, providing the basis for a mosaic condition.

mute (mūt) 1. unable or unwilling to speak. 2. a person who cannot speak. In most cases, mutes are also deaf (deaf-mute).

mutism (mu′tizm) inability or refusal to speak. In almost all cases, mutes are unable to speak because their deafness has prevented them from hearing the spoken word. Speech is learned by imitating the speech of others. Even the child who is born with normal hearing and then loses it may lose part or all of his power of speech through loss of contact with the speech of others. In certain cases, mutism occurs because the voice organs themselves have been damaged or removed. This is particularly true in the case of cancer of the throat, in which LARYNGECTOMY is performed.

For information about training schools and educational institutions for the deaf-mute, both the National Association of Hearing and Speech Agencies, 919 18th Street, N.W., Washington, D.C. 20006, and the Volta Bureau, 1537 35th Street, N.W., Washington, D.C. 20007, may be consulted. The John Tracy Clinic, 806 West Adams Boulevard, Los Angeles, Calif. 90007, offers a free correspondence course that is designed to give assistance to the parents of deaf children below the age of 6.

akinetic m., a state in which the person makes no spontaneous movement or vocal sound, because of either neurologic or psychologic reasons.

hysterical m., hysterical inability to utter words.

muton (mu′ton) a gene when specified as the smallest hereditary element that can be altered by mutation.

mutualism (mu'tu-al-izm") the biologic association of two individuals or populations of different species, both of which are benefited by the relationship and sometimes unable to exist without it.

mutualist (mu'tu-al-ist) one of the organisms or species living in a state of mutualism.

M.V. [L.] *Medicus Veterinarius* (veterinary physician).

Mv chemical symbol, *mendelevium.*

mv. millivolt.

M.W.I.A. Medical Women's International Association.

Mx Medex.

my(o)- word element [Gr.], *muscle.*

myalgia (mi-al'je-ah) muscular pain.

epidemic m., epidemic pleurodynia.

Myanesin (mi-an'ě-sin) trademark for mephenesin, a muscle relaxant.

myasthenia (mi"as-the'ne-ah) muscular debility or weakness. adj., **myasthen'ic.**

angiosclerotic m., excessive muscular fatigue due to vascular changes; intermittent claudication.

m. gas'trica, weakness and loss of tone in the muscular coats of the stomach; atony of the stomach.

m. gra'vis, a chronic disease characterized by muscular weakness, caused by a chemical defect at the sites where the nerves and muscles interact (the myoneural junction). Normally, a chemical mediator called *acetylcholine* is released at the neural side of the myoneural junction; this chemical signals a muscular contraction and then is rapidly destroyed, allowing the muscle to relax in readiness for a subsequent contraction. The effectiveness of acetylcholine in patients with myasthenia gravis is greatly reduced, possibly because there is a decrease in the number of acetylcholine receptors on the motor end plate. An increase in the number of antibodies in the serum of myasthenia patients that react with muscle components suggest the disease might be an AUTOIMMUNE DISEASE.

People with myasthenia gravis find that certain muscles feel weak and tire quickly on exertion. Muscles frequently affected are those of the face, eyelids, larynx, and throat. The patient may first detect the onset of myasthenia gravis by the drooping of the eyelids or difficulty in such a relatively simple operation as chewing or even perhaps swallowing water.

There is no true paralysis of the muscles, and usually they do not atrophy. Severe forms of the disease, however, can be seriously disabling or even fatal because the vital muscles of swallowing or breathing may be affected.

Both medical and surgical treatments are helpful to many patients. The drugs neostigmine, physostigmine, and pyridostigmine have been used successfully to reverse the disordered chemical reaction at the myoneural junction. Removal of the thymus has also been found effective and in some instances it has even been curative.

PATIENT CARE. During acute episodes of myasthenia gravis the patient must be watched closely and his every need anticipated. He may not be able to call for help or do anything to help himself. Severe muscle weakness throws him completely at the mercy of those assigned to his care. An emergency tracheostomy set is kept at the bedside in case the trachea becomes obstructed with mucus that the patient is unable to remove by coughing. Frequent suctioning is often required, especially before meals.

myatonia (mi"ah-to'ne-ah) defective muscular tone.

m. congen'ita, amyotonia congenita.

myatrophy (mi-at'ro-fe) atrophy of a muscle.

myc(o)- word element [Gr.], *fungus.*

mycelium (mi-se'le-um,), pl. *myce'lia.* the mass of threadlike processes (hyphae) constituting the fungal thallas. adj., **myce'lial.**

mycetismus (mi"sě-tiz'mus) mushroom poisoning.

mycetogenic (mi-se"to-jen'ik) caused by fungi.

mycetoma (mi"sě-to'mah) a chronic disease caused by a variety of fungi, affecting the foot, hands, legs, and other parts; called also maduromycosis. The most common form is that of the foot (Madura foot), characterized by sinus formation, necrosis and swelling.

Mycobacterium (mi"ko-bak-te"re-um) a genus of gram-positive bacteria characterized by acid-fast staining.

M. bal'nei, the cause of swimming pool granuloma.

M. bo'vis, the bovine variety of tubercle bacillus, most commonly infecting cattle and acquired by man usually by ingestion of infected milk; uncommon in the United States because of strict testing of cattle.

M. kansas'ii, the etiologic agent of a tuberculosis-like disease in man.

M. lep'rae, the etiologic agent of leprosy.

M. tuberculo'sis, the causative agent of tuberculosis in man.

mycobacterium (mi"ko-bak-te"re-um,), pl. *mycobacte'ria* [L.] 1. an individual organism of the genus *Mycobacterium.* 2. a slender, acid-fast microorganism resembling the bacillus that causes tuberculosis.

anonymous mycobacteria, bacteria resembling the tubercle bacilli, found in pulmonary infections, usually of a chronic nature, in man, for which species names have not been established. Some are affected in color by exposure to light (chromogens), others are not (nonchromogens).

mycodermatitis (mi"ko-der"mah-ti'tis) fungal infection of the skin.

mycologist (mi-kol'o-jist) a specialist in mycology.

mycology (mi-kol'o-je) the study of fungi and fungus diseases.

mycomyringitis (mi"ko-mir"in-ji'tis) fungus inflammation of the eardrum.

Mycoplasma (mi"ko-plaz'mah) a genus of microorganisms including the pleuropneumonia-like organisms (PPLO) and separated into 15 species.

M. hom'inis, a species found associated with nongonococcal urethritis and reported to cause mild pharyngitis in humans.

M. mycoi'des, the type species, which causes pleuropneumonia in cattle (see also PLEUROPNEUMONIA-LIKE.)

M. pneumo'niae, a cause of primary atypical pneumonia; called also Eaton agent.

mycosis (mi-ko'sis) any disease caused by fungi.

m. fungoi'des, a chronic, malignant, lymphoreticular neoplasm of the skin and, in late stages, lymph nodes and viscera, with development of large, painful, ulcerating tumors.

mycostasis (mi-kos′tah-sis) prevention of growth and multiplication of fungi.

mycostat (mi′ko-stat) an agent that inhibits the growth of fungi.

Mycostatin (mi″ko-stat′in) trademark for a preparation of nystatin, an antifungal agent.

mycotic (mi-kot′ik) pertaining to a mycosis; caused by fungi.

mycotoxicosis (mi″ko-tok-sĭ-ko′sis) 1. poisoning due to a fungal or bacterial toxin. 2. poisoning due to ingestion of fungi.

mydriasis (mĭ-dri′ah-sis) great dilatation of the pupil.

mydriatic (mid″re-at′ik) 1. dilating the pupil. 2. a drug that dilates the pupil.

myectomy (mi-ek′to-me) excision of a muscle.

myectopia (mi″ek-to′pe-ah) displacement of a muscle.

myel(o)- word element [Gr.], *marrow* (often with specific reference to the spinal cord).

myelalgia (mi″ĕ-lal′je-ah) pain in the spinal cord.

myelapoplexy (mi″el-ap′o-plek″se) hemorrhage in the spinal cord.

myelatelia (mi″el-ah-te′le-ah) imperfect development of the spinal cord.

myelatrophy (mi″el-at′ro-fe) atrophy of the spinal cord.

myelemia (mi″el-e′me-ah) myelocytosis.

myelencephalon (mi″el-en-sef′ah-lon) 1. the part of the central nervous system comprising the medulla oblongata and lower part of the fourth ventricle. 2. the posterior of the two brain vesicles formed by specialization of the rhombencephalon in the developing embryo.

myelin (mi′ĕ-lin) 1. the lipid substance forming a sheath around the axons of certain nerve fibers; these nerve fibers are spoken of as myelinated or medullated fibers. 2. a lipoid substance found in the body, especially in certain degenerative diseases. adj., **myelin′ic.**

The myelin sheath is believed to influence the rate at which nerve impulses are conducted; transmission is always more rapid in myelinated fibers than in unmyelinated fibers.

Myelinated nerve fibers occur predominantly in the cranial and spinal nerves and compose the white matter of the brain and spinal cord. In fact, it is the myelin sheath that gives the whitish color to the areas of white matter. Unmyelinated fibers are abundant in the autonomic nervous system. The term gray matter refers to areas in the nervous system in which the nerve fibers are unmyelinated.

myelinated (mi′ĕ-lĭ-nāt′ed) having a myelin sheath.

myelination, myelinization (mi″ĕ-lĭ-na′shun; mi″ĕ-lin″ĭ-za′shun) production of myelin around an axon.

myelinolysis (mi″ĕ-lin-ol′ĭ-sis) destruction of myelin; demyelination.

myelinosis (mi″ĕ-lĭ-no′sis) fatty degeneration, with formation of myelin.

myelitis (mi″ĕ-li′tis) inflammation of the spinal cord (see also POLIOMYELITIS) or bone marrow (see also OSTEOMYELITIS). adj., **myelit′ic.**

ascending m., ascending myelopathy.

bulbar m., that involving the medulla oblongata.

central m., myelitis affecting chiefly the gray matter of the spinal cord.

disseminated m., that which has several distinct foci.

focal m., focal myelopathy.

sclerosing m., sclerosing myelopathy.

transverse m., transverse myelopathy.

traumatic m., traumatic myelopathy.

myeloblast (mi′ĕ-lo-blast″) an immature cell of bone marrow, not normally found in peripheral blood; it is the precursor of the promyelocyte, having evenly distributed chromatin, several nucleoli, and nongranular basophilic cytoplasm.

myeloblastemia (mi″ĕ-lo-blas-te′me-ah) myeloblasts in the peripheral blood.

myeloblastoma (mi″ĕ-lo-blas-to′mah) a focal malignant tumor composed of myeloblasts, observed in acute myelocytic leukemia.

myeloblastosis (mi″ĕ-lo-blas-to′sis) excess of myeloblasts in the blood.

myelocele (mi′ĕ-lo-sēl″) hernial protrusion of the spinal cord through a defect in the vertebral column.

myelocyst (mi′ĕ-lo-sist) a cyst developed from rudimentary medullary canals.

myelocystocele (mi″ĕ-lo-sis′to-sēl) hernial protrusion of spinal cord through a defect in the vertebral column.

myelocystomeningocele (mi″ĕ-lo-sis″to-mĕ-ning′-go-sēl) protrusion of cystic spinal cord and meninges through a defect in the vertebral column.

myelocyte (mi′ĕ-lo-sīt″) 1. an immature cell of the bone marrow, developed from the promyelocyte and developing into the metamyelocyte. In this stage, differentiation into specific cytoplasmic granules has begun. 2. any cell of the gray matter of the nervous system. adj., **myelocyt′ic.**

myelocythemia (mi″ĕ-lo-si-the′me-ah) an excess of myelocytes in the circulating blood.

myelocytoma (mi″ĕ-lo-si-to′mah) myeloma.

myelocytosis (mi″ĕ-lo-si-to′sis) increase of myelocytes in the blood.

myelodysplasia (mi″ĕ-lo-dis-pla′ze-ah) defective development of the spinal cord.

myeloencephalic (mi″ĕ-lo-en″se-fal′ik) pertaining to the spinal cord and brain.

myeloencephalitis (mi″ĕ-lo-en-sef″ah-li′tis) inflammation of the spinal cord and brain.

myelofibrosis (mi″ĕ-lo-fi-bro′sis) replacement of bone marrow by fibrous tissue.

myelogenesis (mi″ĕ-lo-jen′ĕ-sis) 1. development of the central nervous system. 2. the deposition of myelin around the axon.

myelogenic, myelogenous (mi″ĕ-lo-jen′ik; mi″ĕ-loj′ĕ-nus) produced in the bone marrow.

myelogeny (mi″ĕ-loj′ĕ-ne) development of the myelin sheaths of nerve fibers.

myelogone (mi′ĕ-lo-gōn″) a white blood cell of the myeloid series having a reticulate violaceous nucleus, well-stained nucleolus, and deep blue rim of cytoplasm. adj., **myelogon′ic.**

myelogram (mi′ĕ-lo-gram) 1. the film produced by myelography. 2. a graphic representation of the differential count of cells found in a stained representation of bone marrow.

myelography (mi″ĕ-log′rah-fe) roentgenography of the spinal cord after injection of a contrast medium into the subarachnoid space.

myeloid (mi′ĕ-loid) 1. pertaining to, derived from or resembling bone marrow. 2. pertaining to the spinal cord. 3. having the appearance of myelocytes, but not derived from bone marrow.

m. tissue, red bone marrow.

myeloidosis (mi″ĕ-loi-do′sis) formation of myeloid tissue, especially hyperplastic development of such tissue.

myelolipoma (mi″ĕ-lo-lip′o-mah) a rare benign tumor of the adrenal gland composed of adipose tissue, lymphocytes, and primitive myeloid cells.

myeloma (mi″ĕ-lo′mah) 1. a tumor composed of cells of the type normally found in the bone marrow. 2. multiple myeloma.

giant cell m., giant cell tumor (1).

multiple m., plasma cell m., a primary malignant tumor of plasma cells usually arising in bone marrow, marked by circumscribed or diffuse tumor-like hyperplasia of the bone marrow, and usually associated with anemia and with Bence Jones protein in the urine. The patient complains of neuralgic pains; later painful swellings appear on the ribs and skull, and spontaneous fractures may occur. Called also Kahler's disease, myelopathic albumosuria, Bence Jones albumosuria, and lymphadenia ossea.

myelomalacia (mi″ĕ-lo-mah-la′she-ah) morbid softening of spinal cord.

myelomatosis (mi″ĕ-lo-mah-to′sis) multiple myeloma.

myelomenia (mi″e-lo-me′ne-ah) vicarious menstruation into the spinal cord.

myelomeningitis (mi″ĕ-lo-men″in-ji′tis) inflammation of the spinal cord and meninges.

myelomeningocele (mi″ĕ-lo-mĕ-ning′go-sēl) hernial protrusion of the spinal cord and its meninges through a defect in the vertebral column.

myeloneuritis (mi″ĕ-lo-nu-ri′tis) inflammation of the spinal cord and peripheral nerves.

myelopathy (mi″ĕ-lop′ah-the) 1. any functional disturbance and/or pathological change in the spinal cord; often used to denote nonspecific lesions, as opposed to myelitis. 2. pathological bone marrow changes. adj., **myelopath′ic.**

ascending m., that progressing cephalad (upward) along the spinal cord.

descending m., a form progressing caudad (downward) along the spinal cord.

focal m., that affecting a small area only, or several small areas.

sclerosing m., a form marked by hardening of the spinal cord and overgrowth of the glia.

transverse m., a form affecting the entire cross-section of the spinal cord at one level.

traumatic m., that following injury to the spinal cord.

myelopetal (mi″ĕ-lop′ĕ-tal) moving toward the spinal cord.

myelophthisis (mi″ĕ-lo-thi′sis) 1. wasting of the spinal cord. 2. reduction of the cell-forming functions of bone marrow.

myeloplast (mi′ĕ-lo-plast″) any leukocyte of the bone marrow.

myelopoiesis (mi″ĕ-lo-poi-e′sis) the formation of marrow or the cells arising from it.

ectopic m., extramedullary m., formation of myeloid tissue outside bone marrow.

myeloproliferative (mi″ĕ-lo-pro-lif′er-ah″tiv) pertaining to or characterized by abnormal proliferation of bone marrow constituents.

m. syndrome, a group of diseases related histogenetically and marked, at varying times in varying degrees, by medullary and extramedullary proliferation of one or more lines of bone marrow constitutents, including myelocytic, erythroblastic, and megakaryocytic forms, in addition to various cells derived from the reticulum and mesenchymal elements.

myeloradiculitis (mi″ĕ-lo-rah-dik″u-li′tis) inflammation of the spinal cord and posterior nerve roots.

myeloradiculodysplasia (mi″ĕ-lo-rah-dik″u-lo-dis-pla′ze-ah) abnormal development of the spinal cord and spinal nerve roots.

myeloradiculopathy (mi″ĕ-lo-rah-dik″u-lop′ah-the) disease of the spinal cord and spinal nerve roots.

myelorrhagia (mi″ĕ-lo-ra′je-ah) spinal hemorrhage.

myelosarcoma (mi″ĕ-lo-sar-ko′mah) a sarcomatous growth made up of myeloid tissue or bone marrow cells.

myelosclerosis (mi″ĕ-lo-sklĕ-ro′sis) 1. sclerosis of the spinal cord. 2. obliteration of the marrow cavity by small spicules of bone. 3. myelofibrosis.

myelosis (mi″ĕ-lo′sis) 1. proliferation of bone marrow tissue, producing the blood changes of myelocytic leukemia. 2. formation of a tumor of the spinal cord.

erythremic m., a malignant blood dyscrasia, one of the myeloproliferative disorders, with progressive anemia, megaloblastic erythroid hyperplasia, myeloid dysplasia, hepatosplenomegaly, and hemorrhagic phenomena.

myelospongium (mi″ĕ-lo-spun′je-um) a network developing into the neuroglia.

myelosuppressive (mi″ĕ-lo-sŭ-pres′iv) 1. inhibitive to the function of bone marrow. 2. an agent that suppresses bone marrow function.

myelotomy (mi″ĕ-lot′o-me) severance of nerve fibers in the spinal cord.

myelotoxin (mi″ĕ-lo-tok′sin) a toxin that destroys bone marrow cells. adj., **myelotox′ic.**

myenteron (mi-en′ter-on) the muscular coat of the intestine. adj., **myenter′ic.**

Myerson's sign (mi′er-sunz) in Parkinson's disease, repeated blinking of the eyes on tapping the forehead.

myesthesia (mi″es-the′ze-ah) muscle sensibility.

myiasis (mi-i′ah-sis) invasion of the body by the larvae of flies, characterized as cutaneous (subdermal tissue), gastrointestinal, nasopharyngeal, ocular, or urinary, depending on the region invaded.

myko- for words beginning thus, see those beginning *myco-*.

Myleran (mil′er-an) trademark for a preparation of busulfan, an alkylating agent used in the treatment of myelocytic leukemia.

mylohyoid (mi″lo-hi′oid) pertaining to the hyoid bone and molar teeth.

myo- word element [Gr.], *muscle.*

myoalbumin (mi″o-al-bu′min) an albumin in muscle tissue.

myoarchitectonic (mi″o-ar″kĭ-tek-ton′ik) pertaining to the structural arrangement of muscle fibers.

myoatrophy (mi″o-at′ro-fe) muscular atrophy.

myoblast (mi′o-blast) an embryonic cell that becomes a cell of muscle fiber. adj., **myoblas′tic.**

myoblastoma (mi″o-blas-to′mah) a benign circumscribed tumor-like lesion of soft tissue (see granular cell TUMOR).

granular cell m., granular cell tumor.

myobradia (mi″o-bra′de-ah) slow reaction of muscle to stimulation.

myocardial (mi″o-kar′de-al) pertaining to the muscular tissue of the heart (the myocardium).

m. infarction, necrosis of the cells of an area of the heart muscle (myocardium) occurring as a result of oxygen deprivation, which in turn is caused by obstruction to the blood supply; commonly referred to as a "heart attack."

The myocardium receives its blood supply from the two large coronary arteries and their branches. Occlusion of one of these blood vessels (CORONARY OCCLUSION) is one of the major causes of myocardial infarction. The occlusion may result from the formation of a clot that develops suddenly when an atheromatous plaque ruptures through the sublayers of a blood vessel, or when the narrow, roughened inner lining of a sclerosed artery leads to thrombosis.

Other causes of myocardial infarction are related to a sudden increased need for blood supply to the heart, as in shock, hemorrhage, and severe physical exertion, and to restriction of blood flow through the aorta, as in aortic stenosis, which predisposes to the formation of emboli.

PATHOLOGY. The most common sites of myocardial infarction are in the left ventricle, that chamber of the heart which has the greatest work load. Tissue changes that occur in the myocardium are related to the extent to which the cells have been deprived of oxygen. Total deprivation results in an *area of infarction,* in which the cells die and the tissue becomes necrotic. Necrosis in this area is evident within 5 to 6 hours after the occlusion. In response to this necrosis the body increases its production of leukocytes, which aid in removal of the dead cells. As collateral circulation enlarges, it brings fibroblasts, which form connective tissues within the area of infarction. Usually, the formation of fibrous scar tissue is complete within two to three months.

Immediately surrounding the area of infarction is a less seriously damaged *area of injury.* It may deteriorate and thus extend the area of infarction or, with adequate collateral circulation, it may regain its function within 2 to 3 weeks.

The outermost area of damage is the *zone of ischemia,* which borders the area of injury. The cells in this area are weakened by decreased oxygen supply, but they can become functional again, usually within two to three weeks after the onset of occlusion.

All of the pathological changes described above can be identified by electrocardiography. The information thus obtained is used to prescribe the varying degrees of physical activity allowed the patient as he convalesces.

SYMPTOMS. The most outstanding symptom of myocardial infarction is a sudden painful sensation of pressure, often described as a "crushing pain" in the chest, occasionally radiating to the arms, throat, and back, and persisting for hours. Pallor, profuse perspiration, and other signs of shock are present. There may be nausea and vomiting, leading to the mistaken impression that the victim is suffering from acute indigestion. In almost all cases of severe myocardial infarction the patient is extremely apprehensive and has a sense of impending death.

Severity of symptoms depends on the size of the artery at the point of occlusion and the amount of myocardial tissue served by the artery. In some instances the artery may be small and the symptoms mild. In other cases the extent of damage is quite large and the attack is fatal.

Within 24 hours of the initial attack there is an elevated temperature and increased white cell count in response to the inflammatory process arising from necrosis of myocardial tissue. Death of the cells also brings about the release of certain enzymes which enter the general circulation. The levels of these enzymes in the blood can be determined by clinical laboratory tests. Within two to four hours after infarction the level of creatine phosphokinase (CPK) is increased. It reaches its peak in 24 to 36 hours and subsides to normal level in three days. The level of serum glutamic oxaloacetic transaminase (SGOT) increases rapidly in 4 to 6 hours, reaches its peak in 24 to 48 hours, and returns to normal in five days. In contrast to the rapid rise and decline of these two enzyme levels, lactic dehydrogenase (LDH) and serum hydroxybutyrate dehydrogenase (SHBD) levels begin to increase the first day after attack and persist at high levels for 10 to 20 days.

TREATMENT AND PATIENT CARE. Immediate care is concerned with combatting shock, relieving respiratory difficulty, and preventing further circulatory collapse. The victim should be kept lying down, and all tight clothing should be loosened to relieve dyspnea and promote comfort. Without delay, but in a calm, unharried manner, the patient is transported to a medical care facility. If the victim shows signs of CARDIAC ARREST, CARDIOPULMONARY RESUSCITATION efforts are begun immediately.

Medical treatment includes administration of an analgesic such as morphine sulfate and meperidine (Demerol); on occasion the physician may order atropine sulfate with morphine to prevent serious bradycardia. There is some controversy over the efficacy of oxygen therapy in the treatment of myocardial infarction; however, in almost all cases oxygen is administered for at least the first 24 hours.

Rest is essential to the repair of damaged myocardial cells, but this does not necessarily mean absolute bed rest. Whether the patient is placed on bed rest or allowed up in a chair depends on the preference of the physician. During the acute stage some physicians may prefer that the patient rest in a chair at the bedside. The patient is permitted to get out of bed with assistance and sit in the chair until he begins to feel fatigued. The amount of time he is allowed to sit up and become more physically active is gradually increased.

Adequate rest can only be achieved by the patient if he is free from mental anxiety and is attended by personnel who anticipate his needs and meet them cheerfully and willingly. The amount of rest needed and the degree of physical activity allowed depends on how extensive the area of infarction is thought to be, whether cardiac arrhythmias and other complications develop, and the response of the patient to increased physical activity. Careful monitoring of the pulse rate and blood pressure before and after each activity can provide information on which to evaluate the patient's tolerance for exercise and self-care activities.

Most patients with a myocardial infarction are cared for in a coronary care unit during the acute stage. It is important that the patient and his family be given a brief explanation of the various kinds of monitoring equipment in use and that they be reassured of each staff member's concern for the patient's welfare. There always is the danger that health care personnel become so engrossed in the operating of electronic gadgetry in the unit that they forget the patient's need to be recognized as a fellow human being.

As the patient's status improves he is gradually weaned away from intensive care and encouraged to do more for himself in preparation for the day when he will go home. For some patients this is a traumatic experience and they become very apprehensive about leaving the security of the monitors and the attention of the staff. It is possible that the stress of leaving the unit can cause development of complications. In some hospitals the transition from coronary care unit to home is made easier by transfer to a convalescent unit where the patient's response to activities is monitored and he is given instruction regarding his own care after discharge. Information about local coronary clubs, assistance in patient education, and availability of a Cardiac Work Evaluation Unit to determine the patient's readiness to return to work can be obtained by contacting the local unit of the American Heart Association.

myocardiograph (mi″o-kar′de-o-graf″) an instrument for making tracings of heart movements.

myocardiopathy (mi″o-kar″de-op′ah-the) any noninflammatory disease of the myocardium.

myocarditis (mi″o-kar-di′tis) inflammation of the muscular walls of the heart (the myocardium). The condition may result from bacterial or viral infections or it may be a toxic inflammation caused by drugs or toxins from infectious agents. Other systemic diseases that may be accompanied by myocarditis are TRICHINOSIS, SERUM SICKNESS, RHEUMATIC FEVER, and COLLAGEN DISEASES. In many cases the etiology is unknown.

SYMPTOMS. The most common symptoms of acute myocarditis are pain in the epigastric region or under the sternum, dyspnea, and cardiac arrhythmias. If the condition persists and becomes chronic, there is pain in the right upper quadrant of the abdomen, owing to hepatic congestion. The latter symptom is a sign of left ventricular failure and often is accompanied by edema and other signs of congestive heart failure.

TREATMENT. Acute myocarditis usually subsides when the primary illness improves. It is considered incidental to the systemic disease and, though it may be a serious manifestation of a systemic illness, acute myocarditis often does not require specific treatment. Steroids and pressor agents such as norepinephrine may be used to reduce the inflammatory process and maintain adequate arterial pressure.

If the heart involvement becomes chronic, treatment then must be aimed at management of the chronic heart failure. (See also congestive HEART FAILURE.)

myocardium (mi″o-kar′de-um) the middle and thickest layer of the heart wall, composed of cardiac muscle. adj., **myocar′dial.**

myocardosis (mi″o-kar-do′sis) any degenerative, noninflammatory disease of the myocardium.

myocele (mi′o-sēl) hernia of muscle through its sheath.

myocellulitis (mi″o-sel″u-li′tis) myositis with cellulitis.

myoceptor (mi′o-sep″tor) the end-plate.

myocerosis (mi″o-se-ro′sis) waxy degeneration of muscle.

Myochrysine (mi″o-kri′sin) trademark for a preparation of gold sodium thiomalate, an antiarthritic.

myoclonus (mi″o-klo′nus) shocklike contractions of part of a muscle, an entire muscle, or a group of muscles; usually a manifestation of a convulsive disorder. adj., **myoclon′ic.**

m. epilepsy, slowly progressive hereditary epilepsy beginning in childhood, with intermittent or continuous clonus of muscle groups, resulting in difficulties in voluntary movements; there is mental deterioration and the presence of Lafora bodies in various cells. Called also Lafora's disease and Unverricht's disease or syndrome.

palatal m., a condition characterized by a rapid rhythmic movement of one or both sides of the palate.

myocyte (mi′o-sīt) a cell of muscular tissue.

myocytoma (mi″o-si-to′mah) a tumor composed of myocytes.

myodemia (mi″o-de′me-ah) fatty degeneration of muscle.

myodystonia (mi″o-dis-to′ne-ah) disorder of muscular tone.

myoedema (mi″o-ĕ-de′mah) 1. mounding. 2. edema of a muscle.

myoelectric (mi″o-e-lek′trik) pertaining to the electric properties of muscle.

myoendocarditis (mi″o-en″do-kar-di′tis) combined myocarditis and endocarditis.

myoepithelioma (mi″o-ep″ĭ-the″le-o′mah) a tumor composed of outgrowths of myoepithelial cells from a sweat gland.

myoepithelium (mi″o-ep″ĭ-the′le-um) tissue made up of contractile epithelial cells. adj., **myoepithe′lial.**

myofascitis (mi″o-fah-si′tis) inflammation of a muscle and its fascia.

myofibril (mi″o-fi′bril) a muscle fibril, one of the slender threads of a muscle fiber, composed of numerous myofilaments. (See Plate 4.)

myofibroma (mi″o-fi-bro′mah) myoma combined with fibroma.

myofibrosis (mi″o-fi-bro′sis) replacement of muscle tissue by fibrous tissue.

myofibrositis (mi″o-fi″bro-si′tis) inflammation of the sheath of muscle fiber.

myofilament (mi″o-fil′ah-ment) any of the ultramicroscopic threadlike structures composing the myofibrils of striated muscle fibers; see Plate 4.

myogen (mi′o-jen) a water-soluble mixture of proteins from muscle.

myogenesis (mi″o-jen′ĕ-sis) the formation of muscle fibers and muscles in embryonic development. adj., **myogenet'ic.**

myogenic (mi″o-jen'ik) giving rise to or forming muscle tissue.

myogenous (mi-oj″ĕ-nus) originating in muscular tissue.

myoglia (mi-og'le-ah) a fibrillar substance formed by embryonic muscle cells.

myoglobin (mi″o-glo'bin) a ferrous protoporphyrin globin complex resembling hemoglobin that is present in muscle and that contributes to its color and acts as a storehouse of oxygen.

myoglobinuria (mi″o-glo″bin-u're-ah) the presence of myoglobin in the urine.

myoglobulin (mi″o-glob'u-lin) a globulin from muscle serum.

myogram (mi'o-gram) a record produced by myography.

myograph (mi'o-graf) an apparatus for recording the effects of muscular contraction.

myography (mi-og'rah-fe) 1. the use of myograph. 2. description of muscles. 3. radiography of muscle tissue after injection of a radiopaque medium. adj., **myograph'ic.**

myohematin (mi″o-hem'ah-tin) the cytochrome of muscle tissue.

myohemoglobin (mi″o-he″mo-glo'bin) myoglobin.

myoid (mi'oid) resembling muscle.

myoischemia (mi″o-is-ke'me-ah) local deficiency of blood supply in muscle.

myokinase (mi″o-ki'nās) adenylate kinase; an enzyme of muscle that catalyzes the phosphorylation of ADP to molecules of ATP and AMP.

myokinesimeter (mi″o-kin″ĕ-sim'ĕ-ter) an apparatus for measuring muscular contraction induced by electrical stimulation.

myokinetic (mi″o-ki-net'ik) pertaining to the motion or kinetic function of muscle, as contrasted with the myotonic or tonic function.

myokymia (mi″o-ki'me-ah) persistent quivering of the muscles.

myolipoma (mi″o-lĭ-po'mah) myoma with fatty elements.

myology (mi-ol'o-je) scientific study or description of the muscles and accessory structures (bursae and synovial sheath).

myolysis (mi-ol'ĭ-sis) degeneration of muscle tissue.

myoma (mi-o'mah) a tumor formed of muscle tissue. adj., **myom'atous.**

m. u'teri, m. of uterus, a benign tumor of the smooth muscle fibers of the uterus (see LEIOMYOMA UTERI).

myomalacia (mi″o-mah-la'she-ah) morbid softening of a muscle.

myomatosis (mi″o-mah-to'sis) the formation of multiple myomas.

myomectomy (mi″o-mek'to-me) 1. excision of a myoma. 2. myectomy.

myomelanosis (mi″o-mel″ah-no'sis) melanosis of muscle.

myomere (mi'o-mēr) myotome; the muscle plate or portion of a somite that develops into voluntary muscle.

myometer (mi-om'ĕ-ter) an apparatus for measuring muscle contraction.

myometritis (mi″o-me-tri'tis) inflammation of the myometrium.

myometrium (mi″o-me'tre-um) the smooth muscle coat of the uterus. adj., **myome'trial.**

myonecrosis (mi″o-nĕ-kro'sis) necrosis or death of individual muscle fibers.

myoneural (mi″o-nu'ral) pertaining to nerve terminations in muscles.

m. junction, the point of junction of a nerve fiber with the muscle that it innervates.

myoneuralgia (mi″o-nu-ral'je-ah) neuralgic pain in a muscle.

myopalmus (mi″o-pal'mus) muscle twitching.

myoparalysis (mi″o-pah-ral'ĭ-sis) paralysis of a muscle.

myoparesis (mi″o-pah-re'sis) slight muscle paralysis.

myopathy (mi-op'ah-the) any disease of a muscle. adj., **myopath'ic.**

centronuclear m., myotubular myopathy.

late distal m., hereditary muscular dystrophy starting in the hands and feet and spreading proximally.

myotubular m., a form marked by myofibers resembling those of early fetal muscle, i.e., myotubules.

nemaline m., a congenital abnormality of myofibrils in which small threadlike fibers are scattered through the muscle fibers; marked by hypotonia and proximal muscle weakness.

ocular m., a slowly progressive form affecting the extraocular muscles, with ptosis and progressive immobility of the eyes.

myope (mi'ōp) a person affected with myopia.

myopericarditis (mi″o-per″ĭ-kar-di'tis) inflammation of both the myocardium and pericardium.

myopia (mi-o'pe-ah) that error of refraction in which rays of light entering the eye parallel to the optic axis are brought to a focus in front of the retina, as a result of the eyeball being too long from front to back, so that vision for near objects is better than for far; called also nearsightedness and shortsightedness (see also VISION). adj., **myop'ic.**

Myopia generally appears before the age of 8, often becoming gradually worse until about the age of 20, when it ceases to change very much. In later years the nearsighted person may find he can read comfortably without his glasses.

In children, the most frequent symptoms of myopia are attempts to brush away blur, frequent rubbing of the eyes, and squinting at distant objects.

Myopia can almost always be corrected with eyeglasses. Eye exercises may be useful in helping the eyes adjust to glasses, but they cannot cure myopia.

There is no evidence that reading or watching television can cause or worsen nearsightedness if lighting conditions are satisfactory.

curvature m., myopia due to changes in curvature of the refracting surfaces of the eye.

index m., myopia due to abnormal refractivity of the media of the eye.

malignant m., pernicious m., progressive myopia with disease of the choroid, leading to retinal detachment and blindness.

progressive m., myopia that continues to increase in adult life.

myoplasm (mi'o-plazm) the contractile part of the muscle cell.

myoplasty (mi'o-plas"te) plastic surgery on muscle whereby portions of detached muscles are used, especially in the field of defects or deformities. adj., **myoplas'tic.**

myopsychopathy (mi"o-si-kop'ah-the) any neuromuscular affection associated with mental disorder.

myoreceptor (mi"o-re-sep'tor) a receptor situated in skeletal muscle that is stimulated by muscular contraction, providing information to higher centers regarding muscle position.

myorrhaphy (mi-or'ah-fe) suture of a muscle.

myorrhexis (mi"o-rek'sis) rupture of a muscle.

myosarcoma (mi"o-sar-ko'mah) a malignant tumor derived from myogenic cells.

myosclerosis (mi"o-sklĕ-ro'sis) hardening of muscle tissue.

myosin (mi'o-sin) one of the two main proteins of muscle. Myosin and actin are the proteins involved in contraction of muscle fibers.

myositis (mi"o-si'tis) inflammation of a voluntary muscle.

epidemic m., epidemic pleurodynia.

m. fibro'sa, a type in which there is a formation of connective tissue in the muscle.

multiple m., polymyositis.

m. ossif'icans, myositis marked by bony deposits in muscle.

trichinous m., that which is caused by the presence of *Trichinella spiralis.*

myospasm (mi'o-spazm) spasm of a muscle.

myotactic (mi"o-tak'tik) pertaining to the proprioceptive sense of muscles.

myotasis (mi-ot'ah-sis) stretching of muscle. adj., **myotat'ic.**

myotenositis (mi"o-tĕ"no-si'tis) inflammation of a muscle and tendon.

myotenotomy (mi"o-ten-ot'o-me) surgical division of the tendon of a muscle.

myotome (mi'o-tōm) 1. an instrument for dividing muscles. 2. the muscle plate or portion of a somite that develops into voluntary muscle. 3. a group of muscles innervated from a single spinal nerve.

myotomy (mi-ot'o-me) cutting or dissection of muscular tissue or of a muscle.

myotonia (mi"o-to'ne-ah) any disorder involving tonic spasm of muscle. adj., **myoton'ic.**

m. atroph'ica, myotonia dystrophica.

m. congen'ita, a hereditary disease marked by tonic spasm and rigidity of certain muscles when attempts are made to move them. The stiffness tends to disappear as the muscles are used.

m. dystroph'ica, a rare, slowly progressive, hereditary disease, marked by myotonia followed by muscular atrophy (especially of the face and neck), cataracts, hypogonadism, frontal balding, and cardiac disorders. Called also dystrophia myotonica.

myotonus (mi-ot'o-nus) tonic spasm of a muscle or a group of muscles.

myotrophic (mi'o-tro"fik) 1. increasing the weight of muscle. 2. pertaining to myotrophy.

myotrophy (mi-ot'ro-fe) nutrition of muscle.

myotropic (mi"o-trop'ik) having a special affinity for muscle.

myotube, myotubule (mi'o-tōōb; mi"o-too'būl) a developing skeletal muscle fiber with a centrally located nucleus. adj., **myotu'bular.**

myovascular (mi"o-vas'ku-lar) pertaining to muscle and blood vessels.

Myriapoda (mir"e-ap'o-dah) a class of arthropods, including the millipedes and centipedes.

myring(o)- (mĭ-ring'go) word element [L.], *tympanic membrane.*

myringa (mĭ-ring'gah) the tympanic membrane.

myringectomy (mir"in-jek'to-me) excision of the tympanic membrane; called also myringodectomy.

myringitis (mĭ-rin-ji'tis) inflammation of the tympanic membrane.

m. bullo'sa, bullous m., a form of viral otitis media in which serous or hemorrhagic blebs appear on the tympanic membrane and adjacent wall of the acoustic meatus.

myringodectomy (mĭ-ring"go-dek'to-me) myringectomy.

myringomycosis (mĭ-ring"go-mi-ko'sis) fungus disease of the tympanic membrane.

myringoplasty (mĭ-ring'go-plas"te) surgical reconstruction of the tympanic membrane.

myringostapediopexy (mĭ-ring"go-stah-pe'de-o-pek"se) fixation of the large lower portion of the tympanic membrane to the head of the stapes.

myringotomy (mir"ing-got'o-me) incision of the tympanic membrane.

myrrh (mer) the oleo-gum-resin from certain trees of Arabia and Africa, used as a protectant.

Mysoline (mi'so-lēn) trademark for preparations of primidone, an anticonvulsant.

mysophilia (mi"so-fil'e-ah) a form of paraphilia in which there is a lustful attitude toward excretions.

mysophobia (mis"o-fo'be-ah) morbid dread of contamination and filth.

Mytelase (mi'tĕ-lās) trademark for a preparation of ambenonium, a cholinesterase inhibitor.

mythomania (mith"o-ma'ne-ah) morbid tendency to lie or exaggerate.

mytilotoxin (mit"ĭ-lo-tok'sin) a neurotoxin from mussels, of the genus *Mytilus.*

myx(o)- word element [Gr.], *mucus; slime.*

myxadenitis (mik"sad-ĕ-ni'tis) inflammation of a mucus-secreting gland.

myxadenoma (mik"sad-ĕ-no'mah) an epithelial tumor with the structure of a mucous gland.

myxasthenia (mik"sas-the'ne-ah) deficient secretion of mucus.

myxedema (mik"sĕ-de'mah) a condition resulting from advanced hypothyroidism, or deficiency of thyroxine. It is the adult form of the disease known as CRETINISM in its congenital form. adj., **myxedem'atous.**

Caused by lack of iodine in the diet, by atrophy, surgical removal, or a disorder of the thyroid gland, or its destruction by radioactive iodine, or by deficient excretion of thyrotropin by the pituitary gland, myxedema is marked primarily by a growing puffiness and sogginess of the skin, involving a dry, waxy type of swelling (nonpitting edema) with abnormal deposits of mucin in the skin and distinctive facial changes (swollen lips and thickened nose).

Because thyroxine plays such an important role in the body's metabolism, lack of this hormone seriously upsets the balance of body processes. Among the symptoms associated with myxedema are excessive fatigue and drowsiness, headaches, weight gain, dryness of the skin, sensitivity to cold, and increasing thinness and brittleness of the nails. In women, menstrual bleeding may become irregular. Medical tests reveal slow tendon reflexes, low blood iodine, below-normal metabolism, and abnormal uptake of radioactive iodine by the thyroid.

In myxedema the body's defenses against infection are weakened. If the patient has heart disease, this is likely to worsen. Upset of the functions of the adrenal glands may become critical. In time, if myxedema is not brought under control, progressive mental deterioration may result in a psychosis marked by paranoid delusions.

Myxedema is treated by administration of thyroid extract or similar synthetic preparations. If treatment is begun soon after the symptoms appear, recovery may be complete. Delayed or interrupted treatment may mean permanent deterioration. In most instances, treatment with thyroid or synthetics must be continued throughout the patient's lifetime.

pretibial m., a localized myxedema associated with preceding hyperthyroidism occurring typically on the anterior surface of the legs.

myxedematoid (mik″sĕ-dem′ah-toid) resembling myxedema.

myxochondroma (mik″so-kon-dro′mah) chondroma with stroma resembling primitive mesenchymal tissue.

myxocyte (mik′so-sit) one of the cells of mucous tissue.

myxofibroma (mik″so-fi-bro′mah) a fibroma containing myxomatous tissue; called also fibroma myxomatodes and fibromyxoma.

myxofibrosarcoma (mik″so-fi″bro-sar-ko′mah) fibrosarcoma with myxomatous areas.

myxoid (mik′soid) resembling mucus.

myxolipoma (mik″so-lĭ-po′mah) lipoma with foci of myxomatous degeneration.

myxoma (mik-so′mah) a tumor composed of primitive connective tissue cells and stroma resembling mesencyhma. adj., **myxo′matous.**

odontogenic m., an uncommon tumor of the jaw, possibly produced by myxomatous degeneration of an odontogenic fibroma.

myxomatosis (mik″so-mah-to′sis) 1. the development of multiple myxomas. 2. myxomatous degeneration.

myxomyoma (mik″so-mi-o′mah) a myoma with myxomatous degeneration.

myxopoiesis (mik″so-poi-e′sis) the formation of mucus.

myxorrhea (mik″so-re′ah) a flow of mucus.

m. intestina′lis, excessive secretion of intestinal mucus.

myxosarcoma (mik″so-sar-ko′mah) a sarcoma containing myxomatous tissue.

myxovirus (mik″so-vi′rus) any of a group of RNA viruses, including the viruses of influenza, parainfluenza, mumps, and Newcastle disease, characteristically causing agglutination of chicken erythrocytes.

N

N 1. symbol, *refractive index.* 2. chemical symbol, *nitrogen.* 3. symbol, *normal* (solution); the expressions 2N (double normal), N/2 or 0.5N (half-normal), N/10 or 0.1N (tenth-normal), etc., denote the strength of a solution in comparison with the normal.

n 1. symbol, *refractive index.* 2. chemical symbol, *normal.*

NA Nomina Anatomica, the internationally approved official body of anatomical nomenclature.

Na chemical symbol, *sodium* (L. *natrium*).

Naboth's cysts (follicles) (na'bōths) cystlike formations due to occlusion of the lumina of glands in the mucosa of the uterine cervix, causing them to be distended with retained secretion. Called also nabothian cysts or follicles.

nabothian cysts (follicles) (nah-bo'the-an) Naboth's cysts.

nacreous (na'kre-us) having a pearl-like luster.

Nacton (nak'ton) trademark for a preparation of poldine, an anticholinergic.

NAD nicotinamide-adenine dinucleotide.

NADP nicotinamide-adenine dinucleotide phosphate.

naepaine (ne'pān) a local anesthetic; used as the hydrochloride salt.

nafcillin (naf-sil'in) a semisynthetic, acid- and penicillinase-resistant penicillin that is effective against staphylococcal infections.

Nägele's pelvis (na'gĕ-lēz) one contracted in an oblique diameter, with complete ankylosis of the sacroiliac synchondrosis of one side and imperfect development of the sacrum and coxa on the same side.

Nägele's rule (na'gĕ-lēz) a rule for calculating the estimated date of labor: Subtract 3 months from the first day of the last menstrual period and add 7 days.

nail (nāl) 1. a rod of metal, bone, or other material used for fixation of the ends of fractured bones. 2. a hardened or horny cutaneous plate overlying the dorsal surface of the distal end of a finger or toe. The nails are part of the outer layer of the skin. They are composed of hard tissue formed of keratin, the substance that gives skin its toughness.

CARE OF THE NAILS. The main care of the fingernails consists in keeping them trimmed and clean. Trimming may be done with nail scissors or clippers or by filing. With certain types of delicate nail, an emery board is preferable to a metal file. Hand lotion or cream applied to the cuticle helps to keep it soft and avoid hangnails. Wearing rubber gloves for housework and dishwashing helps to protect the nails from breaking.

Toenails seldom give trouble if they are cleaned and trimmed regularly and if shoes fit well. It is advisable to bathe the feet at least once a day and to clean dirt from under the toenails with a nailbrush. The toenails should be trimmed every 2 weeks or so by cutting them straight across rather than rounding them by cutting off their corners. This helps prevent ingrown toenails.

DISORDERS OF THE NAILS. Any change in the basic structure, shape, or appearance of the nails—such as softness, brittleness, furrowing, or speckling—may be a symptom of a disease affecting the whole body.

Certain disorders affect the nails themselves. They are readily exposed to outside sources of infection and are particularly vulnerable to injury in the course of daily life. Many of the diseases that afflict the skin may also affect the nail bed and be aggravated by the confining presence of the nail. Congenital defects and metabolic disturbances may affect the nails.

Infections. Most infections involving the nails originate in the folds of tissue around them. Inflammation of this area is called paronychia. It is a fairly common infection by staphylococci, streptococci, or other bacteria or by fungi, and causes painful swelling around the nail, with red, shiny skin. If untreated, paronychia may spread to the nail bed and cause inflammation there. This condition is known as onychia, and is more serious. The bacteria grow under the nail and can cause severe inflammation and pain. Onychia may also arise when the nail is injured and bacteria or fungi gain entrance to the tissue underneath. If the organisms that penetrate the nail produce pigments, the nail may change color as a result. In extreme cases onychia may also cause the nail to separate from its bed. Among the diseases from which paronychia and onychia may result are tuberculosis, diphtheria, and syphilis, and also skin diseases such as psoriasis, fungal diseases, and contact dermatitis.

Dermatitis is the most common disorder to involve the nails and often leads to the complete loss of the nail. After treatment the nail will generally grow back, but if the matrix is severely damaged a new nail may be deformed or may fail to grow.

Occasionally toenails become infected with the fungi that cause athlete's foot.

Injuries. A bruise on the nail can be extremely painful and may cause the nail to turn black and blue. Both effects are due to the accumulation of blood underneath. The nail may become detached from its bed or may fall off. Equally painful may be a splinter under the nail. A physician can relieve the pain of these injuries by releasing the accumulated blood with a small incision directly through the nail.

Burns and frostbite can injure the nails and in severe cases may destroy the matrix, so that regrowth is impossible. Too much exposure to radium or x-rays may injure the nail, making it brittle and easily breakable.

Nutritional and Metabolic Disturbances. The general condition of the body is readily reflected in the condition of the nails. Poor circulation may result in weak nails. Digestive disturbances may impair their growth, and vitamin deficiencies may cause them to become inflamed and sometimes to fall out.

Brittle nails may also be caused by metabolic disorders, for example, hypothyroidism.

Hereditary Defects. The shape and thickness of nails may be an inherited family trait. A child is sometimes born without nails or with one or more missing. In this case he will remain without them for life; however, hereditary deformities can be treated. For instance, the condition of excessively thick nails can be reduced if it is advisable.

Minor Disorders. Hangnails (shreds of skin at one side of a nail) are unsightly and can best be prevented from forming by gently pushing the cuticle instead of cutting it. A hangnail should be clipped off and treated with antiseptic to avoid the slight danger of infection.

n. extension, extension exerted on the distal fragment of a fractured bone by means of a nail or pin (Steinmann pin) driven into the fragment. Called also Steinmann extension.

ingrown n., aberrant growth of a toenail, with one or both lateral margins pushing deeply into adjacent soft tissue (see also INGROWN NAIL).

Smith-Petersen n., a flanged nail for fixing the head of the femur in fracture of the femoral neck.

spoon n., a nail with a concave surface.

Nalline (nal′ēn) trademark for a preparation of nalorphine.

nalorphine hydrochloride (nal′or-fēn) *N*-allylnormorphine; a narcotic antagonist used as an antidote in acute cases of narcotic overdose, but not in drug addiction. Nalorphine is a derivative of morphine and therefore its use is regulated by the Harrison antinarcotic act. It reverses respiratory depression, cardiac arrhythmias, and other symptoms of overdosage of morphine, meperidine, and methadone, but is ineffective against depression produced by barbiturates and general anesthetics.

The drug may be administered intravenously, intramuscularly, or subcutaneously. If the patient receiving the drug experiences serious withdrawal symptoms, he should be given the drug to which he is addicted because nalorphine does not eliminate withdrawal symptoms.

naloxone (nal-oks′ōn) a derivative of oxymorphone used in the form of the hydrochloride salt as a narcotic antagonist.

nandrolone (nan′dro-lōn) an androgenic, anabolic steroid; used as the decanoate and phenpropionate esters.

nanism (na′nizm) dwarfism.

nano- word element [Gr.], *dwarf; small size;* used in naming units of measurement to designate an amount 10^{-9} (one-billionth) the size of the unit to which it is joined, e.g., nanocurie.

nanocephaly (na″no-sef′ah-le) microcephaly. adj., **nanoceph′alous.**

nanocormia (na″no-kor′me-ah) abnormal smallness of the body or trunk.

nanocurie (na′no-ku″re) a unit of radioactivity, being 10^{-9} curie, or the quantity of radioactive material in which the number of nuclear disintegrations is 3.7×10, or 37, per second; abbreviated nc.

nanogram (na′no-gram) one-billionth (10^{-9}) gram.

nanoid (na′noid) dwarfish.

nanomelus (na-nom′ĕ-lus) micromelus.

nanosecond (na′no-sek″und) one billionth (10^{-9}) second abbreviated ns. or nsec.

nanosomia (na″no-so′me-ah) dwarfism.

nanous (na′nus) dwarfed; stunted.

nanus (na′nus) a dwarf.

nape (nāp) the back of the neck.

napelline (na-pel′in) an analgesic alkaloid from aconite.

naphazoline (naf-az′o-lēn) a sympathomimetic; used in the form of the hydrochloride salt as a vasoconstrictor to decongest nasal and ocular mucosae.

naphthalene (naf′thah-lēn) a hydrocarbon from coal tar oil; used as an antiseptic.

naphthol (naf′thol) a crystalline antiseptic substance from coal tar, occurring in two forms, alphanaphthol and betanaphthol. Excessive or continued use causes a toxic condition marked by anemia, jaundice, convulsions, and coma.

N.A.P.N.E.S. National Association for Practical Nurse Education and Services.

Naqua (nak′wah) trademark for a preparation of trichlormethiazide, a diuretic and antihypertensive.

narcissism (nar′sĭ-sizm) dominant interest in one's self; self-love. adj., **narcissis′tic.**

narco- word element [Gr.], *stupor; stuporous state.*

narcoanalysis (nar″ko-ah-nal′ĭ-sis) psychoanalysis with use of sedative drugs to help uncover unconscious material. Called also narcosynthesis.

narcohypnia (nar″ko-hip′ne-ah) numbness felt on waking from sleep.

narcohypnosis (nar″ko-hip-no′sis) hypnotic suggestions made while the patient is narcotized.

narcolepsy (nar′ko-lep″se) recurrent attacks of uncontrollable desire for sleep. adj., **narcolep′tic.**

narcosis (nar-ko′sis) a stuporous state induced by a drug.

basal n., basis n., narcosis with complete unconsciousness, amnesia, and analgesia.

narcosynthesis (nar″ko-sin′thĕ-sis) narcoanalysis.

narcotic (nar-kot′ic) 1. pertaining to or producing narcosis. 2. a drug that produces insensibility or narcosis.

Medically, the term narcotic includes any drug that has this effect. By legal definition, however, the term refers to habit-forming drugs—for example, opiates such as morphine and heroin and synthetic drugs such as meperidine (Demerol). Narcotics can be legally obtained only with a doctor's prescription. The sale or possession of narcotics for other than medical purposes is strictly prohibited by federal, state, and local laws, e.g. the Harrison antinarcotic act. (See also DRUG ABUSE.)

narcotine (nar′ko-tin) noscapine, a nonaddictive antitussive.

narcotize (nar′ko-tīz) to put under the influence of a narcotic.

Nardil (nar′dil) trademark for a preparation of phenelzine, an antidepressant.

nares (na′rēz), sing., *na′ris* [L.] the nostrils; the external openings of the nasal cavity.

Narone (nar′ōn) trademark for a preparation of dipyrone, an analgesic and antipyretic.

nasal (na′zal) pertaining to the nose.

n. concha, see nasal CONCHA.

n. septum, a plate of bone and cartilage covered with mucous membrane that divides the cavity of the nose (see also SEPTUM).

nascent (nas′ent, na′sent) 1. being born; just coming into existence. 2. just liberated from a chemical combination, and hence more reactive because uncombined.

nasion (na′ze-on) the middle point of the junction of the frontal and the two nasal bones (frontonasal suture).

naso- word element [L.], *nose.*

nasoantral (na″zo-an′tral) pertaining to the nose and maxillary antrum.

nasociliary (na″zo-sil″e-er″e) pertaining to the eyes, brow, and root of the nose.

nasofrontal (na″zo-frun′tal) pertaining to the nasal and frontal bones.

nasogastric tube (na″zo-gas′trik) a tube of soft rubber or plastic that is inserted through a nostril and into the stomach. The tube may be inserted for the purpose of instilling liquid foods or other substances, or as a means of withdrawing gastric contents. (See also TUBE FEEDING.)

nasolabial (na″zo-la′be-al) pertaining to the nose and lip.

nasolacrimal (na″zo-lak′rĭ-mal) pertaining to the nose and lacrimal apparatus.

naso-oral (na″zo-o′ral) pertaining to the nose and mouth.

nasopalatine (na″zo-pal′ah-tīn) pertaining to the nose and palate.

nasopharyngitis (na″zo-far″in-ji′tis) inflammation of the nasopharynx.

nasopharynx (na″zo-far′ingks) the part of the pharynx above the soft palate. adj., **nasopharyn′geal.**

nasosinusitis (na″zo-si″nŭ-si′tis) inflammation of the paranasal sinuses.

nasus (na′sus) [L.] nose.

natal (na′tal) 1. pertaining to birth. 2. pertaining to the nates (buttocks).

natality (na-tal′ĭ-te) the birth rate.

nates (na′tēz) [L., pl.] the buttocks.

natimortality (na″tĭ-mor-tal′ĭ-te) the proportion of stillbirths to the general birth rate.

National Association for Practical Nurse Education and Service the first national organization concerned solely with practical nurse education and the services rendered by the practical nurse, organized in 1941. Members of N.A.P.N.E.S. include professional and practical nurses, physicians, hospital administrators, other health and welfare workers, and interested lay citizens.

The organization maintains an accrediting program for state-approved schools of practical nursing, provides a consulting service for groups interested in starting a practical nurse program, prepares and publishes leaflets, booklets, and other educational materials for practical nurses, and sponsors regional workshops and summer school courses on practical nurse education and services.

The official publication of N.A.P.N.E.S. is the *Journal of Practical Nursing.* The headquarters is at 1465 Broadway, New York, NY 10036.

National Federation of Licensed Practical Nurses the only national organization with a membership consisting solely of licensed practical-vocational nurses. The organization was founded in 1949 and has its central office at 250 West 57th Street, New York, NY 10019. Membership is open to licensed practical-vocational nurses who are members of local, state, and territorial organizations through which the national organization functions.

N.F.L.P.N. lists its purposes as follows: to establish policy, to speak and act for licensed practical-vocational nurses, to conduct educational workshops and an annual convention, to represent licensed practical-vocational nurses in all affairs of practical nursing, and to promote their welfare and nursing skills through its official journal, *Nursing Care.*

National Formulary a book of standards for certain pharmaceuticals and preparations not included in the U.S.P.; revised every 5 years, and recognized as a book of official standards by the Pure Food and Drug Act of 1906. Abbreviated N.F.

National League for Nursing a national organization concerned with improving nursing education and nursing service at all levels. In 1952, after 10 years of study of existing nursing organizations, three national organizations and four committees agreed to combine and form the N.L.N. These organizations and committees were National League of Nursing Education, founded in 1893; National Organization for Public Health Nursing, founded in 1912; Association of Collegiate Schools of Nursing, founded in 1933; Joint Committee on Practical Nurses and Auxiliary Workers in Nursing, founded in 1945; Joint Committee on Careers in Nursing, founded in 1945; Joint Committee on Careers in Nursing, founded in 1948; National Committee for the Improvement of Nursing Services, founded in 1949; and the National Accrediting Service, founded in 1949.

There are two divisions of the N.L.N., one for individual members and one for agency members. Individual members may be professional and practical nurses, nurses' aides, and other professional and lay persons interested in fostering the development and improvement of nursing services or nursing education. An agency membership is available to any organization that provides a nursing service or conducts an educational program in nursing. An allied agency membership, without voting rights, is available as determined by the Board of Directors to interested organizations not engaged in providing nursing service or conducting an educational program in nursing.

The official magazine of the National League for Nursing is *Nursing Outlook.* Offices of the League are located at 10 Columbus Circle, New York, NY 10019.

natremia (na-tre′me-ah) hypernatremia.

natrium (na′tre-um) [L.] sodium (symbol Na).

natriuresis (na″tre-u-re′sis) the excretion of abnormal amounts of sodium in the urine.

natriuretic (na″tre-u-ret′ik) 1. pertaining to or promoting natriuresis. 2. an agent that promotes natriuresis.

natural childbirth a term used to describe an approach to LABOR and delivery in which the parents are prepared for the event so that the mother is awake and cooperative and the father is able to assume an active and supportive role during the birth of their child; also called prepared childbirth, educated childbirth, and cooperative childbirth.

The underlying concept for all methods of natural childbirth is education of the parents so that they can actively participate in and share the experience of childbirth. The methods of instruction may vary, but all proponents advocate a family-centered maternity care program. The benefits of this approach are believed to be a more comfortable pregnancy, a shorter period of labor, less trauma during birth, and a decrease in the morbidity and mortality rates among newborn infants.

Among the most widely used methods of childbirth is the LAMAZE METHOD, named after the French obstetrician Fernand Lamaze, who adapted the Russian psychoprophylactic method to his practice. The overall goal of psychoprophylaxis is use of the mind in the prevention of pain and, more specifically, the modification of the perception of pain. The Read method of preparation, based on the teaching and philosophy of Dr. Grantly Dick-Read, had its beginning earlier than the Lamaze method. The emphasis in the Read-based classes is on passivity of the mother and an interruption of the fear-tension-pain cycle. Other methods include the Erna Wright method, which originated in England, and the psychosexual method of Sheila Kitzinger, which includes marriage counseling and encompasses all family interrelationships and their effect on childbirth and feminine sexual response.

Although there are variations in the underlying philosophies and the specific techniques that are characteristic of each method, all are concerned with helping both parents understand the birth process and become familiar with their expected roles during labor and delivery, instruction in exercises that develop neuromuscular control, and physical conditioning exercises and specific breathing patterns that are employed during the three stages of labor. The father is given instruction in the ways in which he can support his wife and promote her comfort during labor. Many of the techniques learned in natural childbirth classes can be used to reduce the effects of stress and to relieve the discomfort associated with tension in many situations not related to childbirth. Most parents who have chosen natural childbirth describe it as an exhilarating and emotionally satisfying experience.

The two organizations concerned with preparation for natural childbirth are the International Childbirth Education Association (ICEA), Box 5852, Milwaukee, WI, and the American Society for Psycho-prophylaxis in Obstetrics (ASPO), Inc., 7 W. 96th St., New York, NY 10025. The ASPO has special membership categories for instructors and physicians. State and individual member groups of the ICEA have been organized in many communities. Additional help for parents seeking childbirth classes often can be obtained by contacting the local LA LECHE LEAGUE.

Naturetin (nat″u-re′tin) trademark for preparations of bendroflumethiazide, a diuretic and antihypertensive.

naturopath (na′tūr-o-path″) a practitioner of naturopathy.

naturopathy (na″tūr-op′ah-the) a drugless system of healing by the use of physical methods, such as light, air, water, etc.

nausea (naw′ze-ah) an unpleasant sensation vaguely referred to the epigastrium and abdomen, with a tendency to vomit. Nausea may be a symptom of a variety of disorders, some minor and some more serious.

Nausea is usually felt when nerve endings in the stomach and other parts of the body are irritated. The irritated nerves send messages to the center in the brain that controls the vomiting reflex. When the nerve irritation becomes intense, vomiting results.

Nausea and vomiting may be set off by nerve signals from many other parts of the body besides the stomach. For example, intense pain in almost any part of the body can produce nausea. The reason is that the nausea-vomiting mechanism is part of the involuntary autonomic nervous system. Nausea can also be precipitated by strong emotions.

nauseant (naw′ze-ant) 1. inducing nausea. 2. an agent causing nausea.

nauseate (naw′ze-āt) to affect with nausea.

nauseous (naw′shus, naw′ze-us) pertaining to or producing nausea or disgust.

navel (na′vel) the umbilicus, the scar marking the site of entry of the umbilical cord in the fetus.

navicular (nah-vik′u-lar) boat-shaped; applied to certain bones, as the navicular bone.

Nb chemical symbol, *niobium.*

nc. nanocurie.

N.C.I. National Cancer Institute.

Nd chemical symbol, *neodymium.*

N.D.A. National Dental Association.

Ne chemical symbol, *neon.*

nearsightedness (nēr-sīt′ed-nes) a condition in which vision for near objects is better than for distant ones; called also MYOPIA.

nearthrosis (ne″ar-thro′sis) a false or artificial joint.

nebramycin (neb″rah-mi′sin) an aminoglycoside antibiotic complex consisting of eight components, produced by *Streptomyces tenebrarius.*

nebula (neb′u-lah) 1. slight corneal opacity. 2. an oily preparation for use in an atomizer.

nebulization (neb″u-lĭ-za′shun) 1. conversion into a spray. 2. treatment by a spray.

nebulizer (neb′u-līz″er) an atomizer; a device for throwing a spray.

Necator (ne-ka′tor) a genus of HOOKWORMS.

N. america′nus, a species widely distributed in southern United States, Central and South America, and the Caribbean area; the New World, or American, HOOKWORM.

necatoriasis (ne-ka″to-ri′ah-sis) infection with organisms of the genus *Necator;* hookworm disease.

neck (nek) a constricted portion, such as the part connecting the head and trunk of the body, or the constricted part of an organ, as of the uterus (cervix uteri) or other structure.

anatomic n. of humerus, the constriction of the humerus just below its proximal articular surface.

n. of femur, the heavy column of bone connecting the head of the femur and the shaft.

surgical n. of humerus, the constricted part of the humerus just below the tuberosities.

n. of a tooth, the narrowed part of a tooth between the crown and the root.

uterine n., n. of uterus, cervix uteri.

webbed n., a thick skin fold on the side of the neck, from the mastoid region to the acromion. Called also pterygium colli.

wry n., torticollis.

necrectomy (nĕ-krek′to-me) excision of necrosed tissue.

necro- word element [Gr.], *death.*

necrobiosis (nek″ro-bi-o′sis) the physiologic death of cells; a normal mechanism in the constant turnover of many cell populations. adj., **necrobiot′ic.**

n. lipoi′dica diabetico′rum, a dermatosis characterized by patchy degeneration of the elastic and connective tissue of the skin with degenerated collagen occurring in irregular patches, especially in the dermis, most often on the mid or lower shins; usually associated with diabetes.

necrocytosis (nek″ro-si-to′sis) death and decay of cells.

necrogenic (nek″ro-jen′ik) productive of necrosis or death.

necrogenous (nĕ-kroj′ĕ-nus) originating or arising from dead matter.

necrology (nĕ-krol′o-je, ne-krol′o-je) statistics or records of death.

necrolysis (nĕ-krol′ĭ-sis) separation or exfoliation of necrotic tissue.

necromania (nek″ro-ma′ne-ah) necrophilia.

necroparasite (nek″ro-par′ah-sīt) an organism that lives in dead tissue.

necrophagous (ne-krof′ah-gus) feeding upon dead flesh.

necrophilia (nek″ro-fil′e-ah) morbid attraction to death or to dead bodies; coitus with a dead body; necromania.

necrophilic (nek″ro-fil′ik) 1. pertaining to necrophilia. 2. necrophilous.

necrophilous (nĕ-krof′ĭ-lus) showing a preference for dead tissue; said of microorganisms.

necrophobia (nek″ro-fo′be-ah) morbid dread of death or of dead bodies.

necropneumonia (nek″ro-nu-mo′ne-ah) gangrene of lung.

necropsy (nek′rop-se) examination of a body after death (see also AUTOPSY).

necrose (ne-krōs′) to become necrotic or to undergo necrosis.

necrosin (ne-kro′sin) a toxic substance occurring in inflammatory exudates.

necrosis (nĕ-kro′sis, ne-kro′sis) death of individual cells or groups of cells, or of localized areas of tissue. adj., **necrot′ic.**

aseptic n., necrosis without infection or inflammation.

Balser's fatty n., gangrenous pancreatitis with omental bursitis and disseminated patches of necrosis of fatty tissues.

caseous n., necrosis in which the tissue is soft, dry, and cheesy, occurring typically in tuberculosis.

central n., necrosis affecting the central portion of an affected bone, cell, or lobule of the liver.

cheesy n., that in which the tissue resembles cottage cheese; most often seen in tuberculosis and syphilis.

coagulation n., death of cells, the protoplasm of the cells becoming fixed and opaque by coagulation of the protein elements, the cellular outline persisting for a long time.

colliquative n., liquefactive necrosis.

fat n., necrosis of fatty tissue in small white areas.

liquefactive n., necrosis in which the necrotic material becomes softened and liquefied.

moist n., necrosis in which the dead tissue is wet and soft.

postpartum pituitary n., necrosis of the pituitary gland during the postpartum period, often associated with shock and excessive uterine bleeding during delivery, and leading to variable patterns of hypopituitarism.

subcutaneous fat n. of newborn, a benign condition seen in the first few weeks of life, in which there is induration of the subcutaneous fat.

Zenker's n., hyaline degeneration and necrosis of striated muscle; called also Zenker's degeneration.

necrospermia (nek″ro-sper′me-ah) a condition in which the spermatozoa of the semen are dead or motionless.

necrotizing (nek′ro-tīz″ing) causing necrosis.

necrotomy (nĕ-krot′o-me) 1. dissection of a dead body. 2. excision of a sequestrum.

necrotoxin (nek″ro-tok′sin) a factor or substance produced by certain staphylococci that kills tissue cells.

needle (ne′d′l) 1. a sharp instrument for suturing or puncturing. 2. to puncture or separate with a needle.

aneurysm n., one with a handle used in ligating blood vessels.

aspirating n., a long, hollow needle for removing fluid from a cavity.

cataract n., one used in removing a cataract.

discission n., a special form of cataract needle.

Hagedorn's n., a form of flat suture needle.

hypodermic n., a hollow, sharp-pointed needle to be attached to a hypodermic syringe for injection of solutions.

knife n., a slender knife with a needle-like point, used in ophthalmic operations.

ligature n., a long-handled, slender steel needle having an eye in its curved end, used for passing a ligature underneath an artery.

Reverdin's n., a surgical needle with an eye that can be opened and closed by means of a slide.

stop n., one with a shoulder that prevents too deep penetration.

negative (neg′ah-tiv) having a value of less than zero; indicating lack or absence, as chromatin-negative or Wassermann-negative; characterized by denial or opposition.

negativism (neg′ah-tĭ-vizm″) opposition to suggestion or advice; behavior opposite to that appropriate to a specific situation.

negatron (neg′ah-tron) a negatively charged electron.

Negri bodies (na′gre) oval or round bodies in the nerve cells of animals dead of rabies.

Neisseria (ni-se′re-ah) a genus of gram-negative bacteria (family Neisseriaceae).

N. gonorrhoe′ae, the etiologic agent of gonorrhea.

N. meningi′tidis, a prominent cause of meningitis and the specific etiologic agent of meningococcal meningitis.

Neisseriaceae (ni-se″re-a′se-e) a family of parasitic bacteria (order Eubacteriales).

nem (nem) a unit of nutrition equivalent to the nutritive value of 1 gm. of breast milk.

Nema (ne′mah) trademark for a preparation of tetrachloroethylene, an anthelmintic.

Nemathelminthes (nem″ah-thel-min′thēz) in some classifications, a phylum including the Acanthocephala and Nematoda.

nematocide (nem′ah-to-sīd″) 1. destroying nematodes. 2. an agent that destroys nematodes.

Nematoda (nem″ah-to′dah) a class of helminths (phylum Aschelminthes), the roundworms, many of which are parasites; in some classifications, considered to be a phylum, and sometimes known as Nemathelminthes, or a class of that phylum. (See also WORM.)

nematode (nem′ah-tōd) a roundworm; any individual organism of the class Nematoda.

Nembutal (nem′bu-tal) trademark for preparations of pentobarbital, a hypnotic and barbiturate.

neo- word element [Gr.], *new; recent.*

Neo-Antergan (ne″o-an′ter-gan) trademark for a preparation of pyrilamine, an antihistaminic.

neoantigen (ne″o-an′tĭ-jen) an intranuclear antigen, e.g., a T antigen, present in cells infected by oncogenic viruses.

neoarthrosis (ne″o-ar-thro′sis) nearthrosis.

neoblastic (ne″o-blas′tik) originating in or of the nature of new tissue.

neocerebellum (ne″o-ser″ĕ-bel′um) phylogenetically, the newer parts of the cerebellum, consisting of those parts predominately supplied by corticopontocerebellar fibers.

neocinetic (ne″o-si-net′ik) neokinetic.

neocortex (ne″o-kor′teks) neopallium.

neodymium (ne″o-dim′e-um) a chemical element, atomic number 60, atomic weight 144.24, symbol Nd. (See table of ELEMENTS.)

neogenesis (ne″o-jen′ĕ-sis) tissue regeneration. adj., **neogenet′ic.**

Neohetramine (ne″o-he′trah-min) trademark for a preparation of thonzylamine, an antihistaminic.

Neo-Hombreol (ne″o-hom′bre-ol) trademark for preparations of testosterone, an androgen.

Neohydrin (ne″o-hi′drin) trademark for a preparation of chlormerodrin, a mercurial diuretic.

neokinetic (ne″o-ki-net′ik) pertaining to the nervous motor mechanism regulating voluntary muscular control.

neologism (ne-ol′o-jizm) a newly coined word; in psychiatry, a word whose meaning may be known only to the patient using it.

neomembrane (ne″o-mem′brān) a false membrane.

neomycin (ne″o-mi′sin) an antibacterial substance produced by growth of *Streptomyces fradiae;* used as an intestinal antiseptic and in treatment of systemic infections due to gram-negative microorganisms.

neon (ne′on) a chemical element, atomic number 10, atomic weight 20.183, symbol Ne. (See table of ELEMENTS.)

neonatal (ne″o-na′tal) pertaining to the first 4 weeks after birth.

neonate (ne′o-nāt) a newborn infant up to 4 weeks old.

neonatologist (ne″o-na-tol′o-jist) a physician who specializes in neonatology.

neonatology (ne″o-na-tol′o-je) the branch of medicine dealing with disorders of the newborn infant.

neopallium (ne″o-pal′le-um) that part of the pallium (cerebral cortex) showing stratification and organization of the most highly evolved type; called also isocortex and neocortex.

neoplasia (ne″o-pla′ze-ah) the formation of a neoplasm.

neoplasm (ne′o-plazm) TUMOR; any new and abnormal growth, specifically one in which cell multiplication is uncontrolled and progressive. Neoplasms may be benign or malignant.

neoplastic (ne″o-plas′tik) pertaining to neoplasia or neoplasm.

Neorickettsia (ne″o-rĭ-ket′se-ah) a genus of rickettsiae (tribe Ehrlichieae).

N. helmin′thoeca, a species found in the salmon fluke (*Troglotrema salmincola*), a parasite of various fish, especially salmon and trout; it is the cause of hemorrhagic enteritis in those who ingest raw infected fish.

neostigmine (ne″o-stig′min) a cholinergic used orally as the bromide salt and parenterally as the methylsulfate salt in prevention and treatment of postoperative abdominal distention and urinary retention, in treatment of myasthenia gravis, glaucoma, and delayed menstruation, as a screening test for early pregnancy, and as an antidote for excessive curarization.

neostriatum (ne″o-stri-a′tum) the more recently developed part of the corpus striatum, comprising the caudate nucleus and the putamen.

Neo-Synephrine (ne″o-sĭ-nef′rin) trademark for a preparation of phenylephrine, an adrenergic.

neoteny (ne-ot′ĕ-ne) prolongation of the larval form in a sexually mature organism. adj., **neoten′ic.**

neothalamus (ne″o-thal′ah-mus) the part of the thalamus connected to the neopallium.

Neothylline (ne″o-thil′in) trademark for preparations of dyphylline, a diuretic, bronchodilator, and peripheral vasodilator.

nephelometer (nef″ĕ-lom′ĕ-ter) an instrument for measuring the concentration of substances in suspension.

nephelometry (nef″ĕ-lom′ĕ-tre) measurement of the concentration of a suspension by means of a nephelometer. adj., **nephelomet′ric.**

nephelopia (nef″ĕ-lo′pe-ah) a visual defect due to cloudiness of the cornea.

nephr(o)- word element [Gr.], *kidney.*

nephralgia (nĕ-fral′je-ah) pain in a kidney.

nephrectasia (nef″rek-ta′ze-ah) distention of the kidney.

nephrectomy (nĕ-frek′to-me) surgical removal of a kidney. The procedure is indicated when chronic disease or severe injury produces irreparable damage to the renal cells. Tumors, multiple cysts, and congenital anomalies may also necessitate removal of a kidney. A single kidney can carry on the functions formerly done by both kidneys, and thus a patient can survive nephrectomy in good health. (See also surgery of the KIDNEY.)

nephric (nef′rik) pertaining to the kidney.

nephridium (nĕ-frid′e-um), pl. *nephrid′ia* [L.] either of the paired excretory organs of certain invertebrates, having the inner end of the tubule opening into the coelomic cavity.

nephritic (nĕ-frit′ik) 1. pertaining to or affected with nephritis. 2. pertaining to the kidneys; renal. 3. an agent useful in kidney disease.

nephritis (nĕ-fri′tis) inflammation of the kidney; a focal or diffuse proliferative or destructive disease that may involve the glomerulus, tubule, or interstitial renal tissue. Called also Bright's disease. The most usual form is glomerulonephritis, that is, inflammation of the glomeruli, which are clusters of renal capillaries. Damage to the membranes of the glomeruli results in impairment of the filtering process, so that blood and proteins such as albumin pass out into the urine. Depending on the symptoms it produces, nephritis is classified as acute nephritis, chronic nephritis, or NEPHROSIS (called also the nephrotic syndrome).

ACUTE NEPHRITIS. Acute nephritis occurs most frequently in children and young people. The disease seems to strike those who have recently suffered from sore throat, scarlet fever, and other infections that are caused by streptococci, and it is believed to originate as an immune response on the part of the kidney.

An attack of acute nephritis may produce no symptoms. More often, however, there are headaches, a rundown feeling, back pain, and perhaps slight fever. The urine may look smoky, bloody, or wine-colored. Analysis of the urine shows the presence of erythrocytes, albumin, and casts. Another symptom is edema. If this occurs, the face or ankles are swollen, more so in the morning than in the evening. The blood pressure usually rises during acute nephritis, and in severe cases hypertension may be accompanied by convulsions.

Treatment consists chiefly of bed rest and a carefully controlled diet. Penicillin is often used if an earlier streptococcal infection is still lingering. Recovery is usually complete. In a small percentage of cases, however, acute nephritis resists complete cure. It may subside for a time and then become active again, or it may develop into chronic nephritis.

CHRONIC NEPHRITIS. Chronic nephritis may follow a case of acute nephritis immediately or it may develop after a long interval during which no symptoms have been present. Many cases of chronic nephritis occur in people who have never had the acute form of the disease.

The symptoms of chronic nephritis are often unpredictable, with great variations in different cases. But in almost every case of the disease there is steady, progressive, permanent damage to the kidneys.

Chronic nephritis generally moves through three stages. In the first stage, the latent stage, there are few outward symptoms, if any. There may be slight malaise, but often the only indication of the disease is the presence of albumin and other abnormal substances in the urine. If a blood count is made during this stage, anemia may be found. There is no special treatment during the latent stage of chronic nephritis. The patient can live a perfectly normal life. He should avoid extremes of fatigue and exposure, and should eat a well balanced diet.

There may be a second stage of chronic nephritis in which edema occurs. Excess body fluids collect in the face, legs, or arms. The main treatment in this stage consists of a high-protein, low-sodium diet. Steroid hormones may be helpful.

It is particularly important, at any stage of chronic nephritis, to avoid other infections, which will aggravate the condition.

At the final stage of chronic nephritis is UREMIA. At this point damage to the kidneys is so extensive that they begin to fail.

There is no known cure for chronic nephritis, although the progress of the disease can be delayed, so that the patient can live an almost normal life for years. Surgeons have had some success in transplanting a healthy kidney to replace a diseased one. So far, the difficulties in performing this operation are still great. Many patients are being helped by repeated purification of their uremic blood by treatment with an artificial KIDNEY.

glomerular n., glomerulonephritis.

interstitial n., nephritis with increase of interstitial tissue and thickening of vessel walls and malpighian corpuscles; sometimes due to alcohol or lead poisoning or gout.

parenchymatous n., nephritis affecting the parenchyma of the kidney.

salt-losing n., intrinsic renal disease causing abnormal urinary sodium loss in persons ingesting normal amounts of sodium chloride, with vomiting, dehydration, and vascular collapse.

scarlatinal n., an acute nephritis due to scarlet fever.

suppurative n., a form accompanied by abscess of kidney.

transfusion n., nephropathy following transfusion from an incompatible donor.

nephritogenic (nĕ-frit″o-jen′ik) causing nephritis.

nephroblastoma (nef″ro-blas-to′mah) a rapidly developing malignant mixed tumor of the kidneys, made up of embryonal elements, and occurring chiefly in children before the fifth year; called also Wilms' tumor.

nephrocalcinosis (nef″ro-kal″sĭ-no′sis) deposition of calcium phosphate in the renal tubules, resulting in renal insufficiency.

nephrocapsectomy (nef″ro-kap-sek′to-me) excision of the renal capsule.

nephrocardiac (nef″ro-kar′de-ak) pertaining to the kidney and the heart.

nephrocele (nef′ro-sēl) hernia of a kidney.

nephrocolic (nef″ro-kol′ik) 1. pertaining to the kidney and the colon. 2. renal colic.

nephrocoloptosis (nef″ro-ko″lop-to′sis) downward displacement of the kidney and colon.

nephrocystitis (nef″ro-sis-ti′tis) inflammation of the kidney and bladder.

nephrogenic (nef″ro-jen′ik) producing kidney tissue.

nephrogenous (nĕ-froj′ĕ-nus) arising in a kidney.

nephrogram (nef′ro-gram) a roentgenogram of the kidney.

nephrography (nĕ-frog′rah-fe) roentgenography of the kidney (see also PYELOGRAPHY).

nephroid (nef′roid) resembling a kidney.

nephrolith (nef′ro-lith) a calculus in a kidney.

nephrolithiasis (nef″ro-lĭ-thi′ah-sis) a condition marked by the presence of renal calculi.

nephrolithotomy (nef″ro-lĭ-thot′o-me) incision of kidney for removal of calculi.

nephrology (nĕ-frol′o-je) the branch of medicine dealing with the kidneys.

nephrolysin (nĕ-frol′ĭ-sin) nephrotoxin, a toxin destructive to kidney tissue.

nephrolysis (nĕ-frol′ĭ-sis) 1. freeing of a kidney from adhesions. 2. destruction of kidney substance. adj., **nephrolyt′ic.**

nephroma (nĕ-fro′mah) a tumor of kidney tissue.

nephromegaly (nef″ro-meg′ah-le) enlargement of the kidney.

nephron (nef'ron) the structural and functional unit of the KIDNEY, each nephron being capable of forming urine by itself. Each kidney is an aggregation of about a million nephrons. The specific function of the nephron is to remove from the blood plasma certain end products of metabolism, such as urea, uric acid, and creatinine, and also any excess sodium, chloride, and potassium ions. By allowing for reabsorption of water and some electrolytes back into the blood, the nephron also plays a vital role in the maintenance of normal fluid balance in the body.

The nephron is a complex system of arterioles, capillaries, and tubules. Blood is brought to the nephron via the afferent arteriole. As the blood flows through the glomerulus (a network of capillaries), about one-fifth of the plasma is filtered through the glomerular membrane and collects in the malpighian (Bowman's) capsule, which encases the glomerulus. The fluid then passes through the proximal tubule, from there into the loop of Henle, then into the distal tubule, and finally into the collecting tubule. As the fluid is making its tortuous journey through these various tubules, most of its water and some of the solutes are reabsorbed into the blood via the peritubular capillaries. The water and solutes remaining in the tubules become urine.

nephropathy (nĕ-frop'ah-the) any disease of the kidneys. adj., **nephropath'ic.**

nephropexy (nef'ro-pek"se) surgical fixation of a floating or hypermobile kidney (NEPHROPTOSIS). The care of a patient having this type of surgery is generally the same as that for any type of surgery of the kidney (see also KIDNEY). One important point is that after nephropexy the patient is positioned so that his chest is lower than his hips; this position relieves strain on the sutures and helps to maintain the kidney in a normal position.

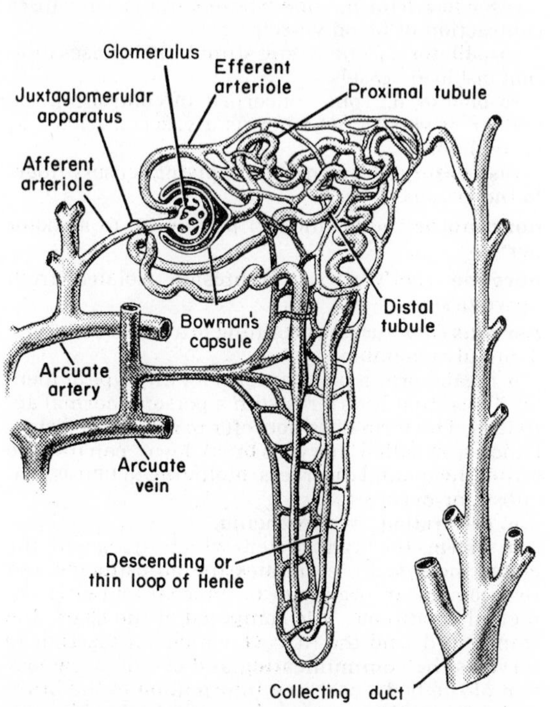

The nephron. (From Guyton, A. C.: Textbook of Medical Physiology. 5th ed. Philadelphia, W. B. Saunders Co., 1976.)

nephroptosis (nef"rop-to'sis) downward displacement of a kidney; called also floating, hypermobile, or wandering kidney. This is found most often in young adult women, especially those who are thin and long waisted. Displacement can occur when the kidney supports are weakened by a sudden strain or blow, or are congenitally defective.

Although the condition may not produce symptoms of a serious nature, it can lead to difficulties if there is kinking of the ureters, producing an obstruction to urinary flow from the kidneys to the bladder. In addition, the patient may have an increased susceptibility to infection.

Correction of nephroptosis is usually by NEPHROPEXY, surgical fixation of the floating kidney.

nephropyelitis (nef"ro-pi"ĕ-li'tis) inflammation of the kidney and its pelvis; pyelonephritis.

nephropyelography (nef"ro-pi"ĕ-log'rah-fe) roentgenography of the kidney (see also PYELOGRAPHY).

nephropyosis (nef"ro-pi-o'sis) suppuration of a kidney.

nephrorrhagia (nef"ro-ra'je-ah) hemorrhage from the kidney.

nephrorrhaphy (nef-ror'ah-fe) suture of the kidney.

nephrosclerosis (nef"ro-sklĕ-ro'sis) hardening of the kidney associated with hypertension and disease of the renal arterioles. It is characterized as benign or malignant depending on the severity and rapidity of the hypertension and arteriolar changes.

arteriolar n., that involving chiefly the arterioles, with degeneration of the renal tubules and fibrotic thickening of the glomeruli; the benign form is often associated with benign hypertension and hyaline arteriolosclerosis, the malignant with malignant hypertension and hyperplastic arteriolosclerosis.

nephrosis (nĕ-fro'sis) any kidney disease, especially disease marked by purely degenerative lesions of the renal tubules; called also nephrotic syndrome. adj., **nephrot'ic.**

Nephrosis probably represents one stage of NEPHRITIS. It is marked by excessive accumulation of fluid in the body, apparently due to the inability of the kidneys to regulate the body's water content properly. It is further characterized by a great loss of protein in the urine and decreased serum albumin. The disease may last for many years in children, without fatal result if serious infections and other disorders do not occur. In adults the disease is less common and more likely to become chronic.

The exact cause of nephrosis is not known. The disease may follow acute nephritis, either directly or after an interval as long as a number of years. It may follow or accompany some other disease of the kidneys. It may also occur in a person who has never had any kidney trouble at all. Some cases seem to be brought on by toxins, such as the venom of bees.

The chief symptom of nephrosis is edema, usually settling in the legs at first but then affecting the arms, face, and torso. The swelling may be enormous.

Despite his alarming appearance, however, the nephrosis patient usually recovers completely. Cortisone and related medicines are often very effective in reducing the edema, especially in children. There has also been success with certain immunosuppressive drugs.

amyloid n., chronic nephrosis with amyloid degeneration of the median coat of the arteries and glomerular capillaries.

lipid n., nephrosis marked by edema, albuminuria, and changes in the protein and lipids of the blood and accumulation of globules of cholesterol esters in the tubular epithelium of the kidney.

lower nephron n., renal insufficiency leading to uremia, due to necrosis of the lower nephron cells, blocking the tubular lumens of this region; seen after severe injuries, especially crushing injury to muscles (see also CRUSH SYNDROME).

nephrosonephritis (nĕ-fro″so-nĕ-fri′tis) renal disease with nephrotic and nephritic components.

nephrostoma (nĕ-fros′to-mah) one of the ciliated funnel-shaped orifices of the excretory tubules that open into the coelom in the embryo; best seen in lower vertebrates.

nephrostomy (nĕ-fros′to-me) creation of a permanent opening into the renal pelvis.

nephrotic syndrome (nĕ-frot′ik) a condition marked by massive edema, heavy proteinuria, hypoalbuminemia, and unusual susceptibility to intercurrent infections; called also NEPHROSIS.

nephrotome (nef′ro-tōm) one of the segmented divisions of the embryonic mesoderm connecting the somite with the lateral plates of unsegmented mesoderm; the source of much of the urogenital system.

nephrotomography (nef″ro-to-mog′rah-fe) body-section roentgenography for visualization of the kidney. adj., **nephrotomograph′ic.**

nephrotomy (nĕ-frot′o-me) incision of a kidney.

nephrotoxic (nef″ro-tok′sik) destructive to kidney cells.

nephrotoxin (nef″ro-tok′sin) a toxin having a specific destructive effect on kidney tissue.

nephrotropic (nef″ro-trop′ik) having a special affinity for kidney tissue.

nephrotuberculosis (nef″ro-tu-ber″ku-lo′sis) renal disease due to *Mycobacterium tuberculosis.*

neptunium (nep-tu′ne-um) a chemical element, atomic number 93, atomic weight 237, symbol Np. (See table of ELEMENTS.)

nerve (nerv) a macroscopic cordlike structure of the body, comprising a collection of nerve fibers that convey impulses between a part of the central nervous system and some other body region. For names of specific nerves of the body, see the table. (See also Plates 12, 13, and 14.)

Depending on their function, nerves are known as sensory, motor, or mixed. Sensory nerves, sometimes called afferent nerves, carry information from the outside world to the brain and spinal cord. Sensations of heat, cold, and pain are conveyed by the sensory nerves. Motor nerves, or efferent nerves, transmit impulses from the brain and spinal cord to the muscles. Mixed nerves are composed of both motor and sensory fibers, and transmit messages in both directions at once.

Together, the nerves make up the peripheral nervous system, as distinguished from the central nervous system, which consists of the brain and spinal cord. There are 12 pairs of CRANIAL NERVES, which carry messages to and from the brain. Spinal nerves arise from the spinal cord and pass out between the vertebrae; there are 31 pairs, 8 cervical, 12 thoracic, 5 lumbar, 5 sacral, and 1 coccygeal. The various nerve fibers and cells that make up the autonomic nervous system serve the glands, heart, blood vessels, and involuntary muscles of the internal organs.

accelerator n's, the cardiac sympathetic nerves, which, when stimulated, accelerate the action of the heart.

n. block, regional anesthesia secured by injection of an anesthetic in close proximity to the appropriate nerve.

depressor n., 1. an inhibitory nerve whose stimulation depresses a motor center. 2. a nerve that lessens activity of an organ.

excitor n., one that transmits impulses resulting in an increase in functional activity.

excitoreflex n., a visceral nerve that produces reflex action.

gangliated n., any nerve of the sympathetic nervous system.

inhibitory n., one that transmits impulses resulting in a decrease in functional activity.

pilomotor n's, those that supply the arrector muscles of hair.

pressor n., an afferent nerve whose irritation stimulates a vasomotor center and increases intravascular tension.

secretory n., an efferent nerve whose stimulation increases vascular activity.

somatic n's, the sensory and motor nerves supplying skeletal muscle and somatic tissues.

splanchnic n's, those of the blood vessels and viscera, especially the visceral branches of the thoracic, lumbar, and pelvic parts of the sympathetic trunks.

sudomotor n's, those that innervate the sweat glands.

sympathetic n's, 1. see sympathetic trunk. 2. any nerve of the sympathetic nervous system.

trophic n., one concerned with regulation of nutrition.

vasoconstrictor n., one whose stimulation causes contraction of blood vessels.

vasodilator n., one whose stimulation causes dilation of blood vessels.

vasomotor n., one concerned in controlling the caliber of vessels, whether as a vasoconstrictor or vasodilator.

vasosensory n., any nerve supplying sensory fibers to the vessels.

nervimotor (ner″vĭ-mo′tor) pertaining to a motor nerve.

nervone (ner′vōn) a cerebroside isolated from nerve tissue.

nervous (ner′vus) 1. pertaining to a nerve or nerves. 2. unduly excitable.

n. breakdown, a popular term for any type of mental illness that interferes with a person's normal activities. The term does not refer to a specific disturbance; a so-called "nervous breakdown" can include any of the mental disorders, including NEUROSIS, PSYCHOSIS, or DEPRESSION.

n. prostration, neurasthenia.

n. system, the organ system which, along with the endocrine system, correlates the adjustments and reactions of an organism to internal and environmental conditions. It is composed of the BRAIN, the spinal cord, and the NERVES, which act together to serve as the communicating and coordinating system of the body, carrying information to the brain and relaying instructions from the brain. The system has two main divisions: the central nervous system, composed of the brain and spinal cord; and the peripheral nervous system, which is subdivided into the voluntary and autonomic systems. (See also Plates 12, 13, and 14.)

THE NERVE CELL. The basic unit of the nervous system is the nerve cell, or NEURON. This highly specialized cell has many fibers extending from it which carry messages in the form of electrical charges and chemical changes. The fibers of some cells are only a fraction of an inch long, but those of others—for example, the sciatic nerve—extend for 2 or 3 feet. These fibers reach into muscles and organs throughout the body, to the ends of the fingers and toes, and cluster by the thousands in areas of the skin no larger than the head of a pin.

The nerve fibers come together from the extremities of the body and gather into cables running to and from the brain. Along the length of the spinal cord are a number of junctions where impulses or messages are sorted or relayed to higher centers.

The fibers of connecting nerve cells do not touch each other. Impulses are relayed from one to another by chemical means across the gap or synapse between them. In most cases an impulse must cross more than one synapse to cause the desired action.

In a REFLEX, the impulse is relayed from one nerve to another by a shortcut that produces a reaction without involving the brain. The knee jerk is an example of the simplest sort of reflex reaction. When the knee is tapped, the impulse travels through the sensory nerve that receives the tap, crosses a single synapse, and activates the motor nerve that controls the quadriceps muscle in the thigh, causing the leg to jerk up automatically.

A very different sort of reflex is the conditioned reflex. Conditioning is the process of building links or paths in the nervous system. When an action is done repeatedly the nervous system becomes familiar with the situation and learns to react automatically. A new reflex has been built into the system. Hundreds of daily actions are conditioned reflexes. Walking, running, going up and down stairs, and even buttoning a shirt all involve great numbers of complex muscle coordinations that have become automatic.

AUTONOMIC AND VOLUNTARY SYSTEMS. The peripheral nervous system in man evolved over many millennia, developing the ability to perform more and more complicated functions. It is divided into two specialized subsystems. The autonomic nervous system operates without conscious control as the caretaker of the body. The voluntary nervous system, which includes both motor and sensory nerves, controls the muscles and carries information to the brain.

The autonomic system is further specialized into two subsidiary systems: the sympathetic and the parasympathetic. The control centers of these systems lie in the hypothalamus. The sympathetic and parasympathetic nervous systems are continuously operative, functioning to adjust body processes to external and internal demands. (See also Plate 14.)

The sympathetic nervous system has in general an excitatory effect, and in response to danger or some other challenge, almost instantly puts body processes into high gear. This is done by the discharge of stimulating secretions at nerve junctions. These secretions, along with epinephrine discharged into the blood by the adrenal medulla, help start muscle action quickly. Glucose is released from the liver into the blood and thus is made available to all the body's muscles as a source of quick energy. The rates of heart and lung action increase, digestive activity slows down, blood vessels constrict, and sweating begins so that the body will be kept cool while under stress. Thus the body is prepared for an extraordinary effort.

The parasympathetic nervous system prevents body processes from accelerating to extremes. Acting more slowly than the sympathetic system, it causes the discharge of secretions that slow the heartbeat and lung action, restore digestive functioning, and limit the constriction of the blood vessels. Generally it acts as a damper, so that unless the challenge demands a prolonged effort, body processes will begin returning to normal.

The voluntary nervous system has nerves of two kinds, sensory and motor. The sensory nerves bring messages to the brain from all parts of the body. They are sorted in the spinal cord and sent on to the brain to be analyzed, acted upon, associated with other information and stored as memory.

Messages from the brain, often in response to information received by way of the sensory nerves, are delivered to the muscles by the motor nerves. One motor nerve with its branching fibers may control thousands of muscle fibers.

The different parts of the nervous system are constantly interacting, and are so well coordinated that man can think, feel, and act on many different levels and without serious confusion, all at the same time.

DISORDERS OF THE NERVOUS SYSTEM. The various organs of the nervous system may be affected by inflammatory processes, neoplastic disease, degenerative disease, and injury. These are referred to as neurologic disorders and may be manifested by paralysis, sensory malfunction, and convulsive seizures.

Inflammation of the meninges, the membranes covering the brain and spinal cord, is called MENINGITIS. The brain tissue itself may become inflamed (ENCEPHALITIS), may be deprived of adequate blood supply (cerebral thrombosis, cerebral hemorrhage, CEREBRAL VASCULAR ACCIDENT), or may be damaged by a violent blow to the head (HEAD INJURY, concussion, contusion). Malignant or benign tumors of the BRAIN can produce varying degrees of sensory and motor disorders.

The spinal cord may be affected by viral infections, as POLIOMYELITIS, or bacterial infections. In its late stage SYPHILIS may involve the brain and spinal cord. Accidental injury to the spinal cord can produce paralysis below the site of injury. A ruptured, or slipped, intervertebral DISK causes neurologic symptoms because it presses on the spinal cord.

Degenerative diseases affecting the nervous system include MYASTHENIA GRAVIS, MULTIPLE SCLEROSIS, and PARKINSON'S DISEASE.

EPILEPSY, which may or may not be traced to a brain lesion, is another disorder that affects the nervous system.

nervousness (ner′vus-nes) a state of excitability, with great mental and physical unrest.

nervus (ner′vus), pl. *ner′vi* [L.] nerve.

Nesacaine (nes′ah-kān) trademark for preparations of chloroprocaine, a local anesthetic.

nesidiectomy (nĕ-sid″e-ek′to-me) excision of the islet cells of the pancreas.

nesidioblast (nĕ-sid′e-o-blast″) any of the cells giving rise to islet cells of the pancreas.

(Text continued on page 694.)

Table of Nerves

COMMON NAME* [MODALITY]	NA TERM†	ORIGIN*	BRANCHES*	DISTRIBUTION*
abducent n. (6th cranial) [motor]	n. abducens	a nucleus in the pons, beneath floor of fourth ventricle		lateral rectus muscle of eyeball
accessory n. (11th cranial) [parasympathetic, motor]	n. accessorius	by cranial roots from side of medulla oblongata, and by spinal roots of spinal cord		internal branch to vagus, thereby to palate, pharynx, larynx, and thoracic viscera; external to sternocleidomastoid and trapezius muscles
acoustic n. *See* vestibulocochlear n.				
alveolar n., inferior [motor, general sensory]	n. alveolaris inferior	mandibular n.	inferior dental, mental, and inferior gingival nerves; mylohyoid n.	teeth and gums of lower jaw, skin of chin and lower lip, mylohyoid muscle and anterior belly of digastric muscle
alveolar n's, superior	nn. alveolares superiores	superior alveolar branches (anterior, middle, and posterior) that arise from infraorbital and maxillary n's, innervating teeth of upper jaw and maxillary sinus, and forming superior dental plexus		
ampullary n., anterior	n. ampullaris anterior	branch of vestibular part of eighth cranial (vestibulocochlear) n. that innervates ampulla of anterior semicircular duct, ending around hair cells of ampullary crest		
ampullary n., inferior. *See* ampullary n., posterior				
ampullary n., lateral	n. ampullaris lateralis	branch of vestibular part of eighth cranial (vestibulocochlear) n. that innervates ampulla of lateral semicircular duct, ending around hair cells of ampullary crest		
ampullary n., posterior	n. ampullaris posterior	branch of vestibular part of eighth cranial (vestibulocochlear) n. that innervates ampulla of posterior semicircular duct, ending around hair cells of ampullary crest		
ampullary n., superior. *See* ampullary n., anterior				
anococcygeal n's [general sensory]	nn. anococcygei	coccygeal plexus		sacrococcygeal joint, coccyx, skin over coccyx
auditory n. *See* vestibulocochlear n.				
auricular n's, anterior [general sensory]	nn. auriculares anteriores	auriculotemporal n.		skin of anterosuperior part of external ear
auricular n., great [general sensory]	n. auricularis magnus	cervical plexus – C2–C3	anterior and posterior branches	skin over parotid gland and mastoid process, and both surfaces of auricle
auricular n., posterior [motor, general sensory]	n. auricularis posterior	facial n.	occipital branch	posterior auricular and occipitofrontal muscles, skin of external acoustic meatus

auriculotemporal n. [general sensory]	n. auriculotemporalis	by two roots from mandibular n.	anterior auricular n., n. of external acoustic meatus, parotid branches, branch to tympanic membrane, branch communicating with facial n.; terminal branches superficial temporal to scalp	parotid gland, scalp in temporal region, tympanic membrane. *See also* auricular n., anterior, *and* n. of external acoustic meatus
axillary n. [motor, general sensory]	n. axillaris	posterior cord of brachial plexus–C5–C6	lateral superior brachial cutaneous n., muscular branches	deltoid and teres minor muscles, skin over back of arm
buccal n. [general sensory]	n. buccalis	mandibular n.		skin and mucous membrane of cheeks, gums, and perhaps first two molars and the premolars
cardiac n., cervical, inferior [sympathetic (accelerator), visceral afferent (chiefly pain)]	n. cardiacus cervicalis inferior	cervicothoracic ganglion		heart via cardiac plexus
cardiac n., cervical, middle [sympathetic (accelerator), visceral afferent (chiefly pain)]	n. cardiacus cervicalis medius	middle cervical ganglion		heart
cardiac n., cervical, superior [sympathetic (accelerator)]	n. cardiacus cervicalis superior	superior cervical ganglion		heart
cardiac n., inferior. *See* cardiac n., cervical, inferior				
cardiac n., middle. *See* cardiac n., cervical, middle				
cardiac n., superior. *See* cardiac n., cervical, superior				
cardiac n's, thoracic [sympathetic (accelerator), visceral afferent (chiefly pain)]	nn. cardiac thoracici	ganglia T2–T4 or T5 of sympathetic trunk	together with tympanic n. forms tympanic plexus	heart
caroticotympanic n's [sympathetic]	nn. caroticotympanici	internal carotid plexus	help form tympanic plexus	tympanic region, parotid gland
carotid n's, external [sympathetic]	nn. carotici externi	superior cervical ganglion		cranial blood vessels and glands via external carotid plexus
carotid n., internal [sympathetic]	n. caroticus internus	superior cervical ganglion		cranial blood vessels and glands via internal carotid plexus
cavernous n's of clitoris [parasympathetic, sympathetic, visceral afferent]	nn. cavernosi clitoridis	uterovaginal plexus		erectile tissue of clitoris

*n. = nerve; n's = (pl.) nerves.
†n. = [L.] nervus; nn. = [L. (pl.)] nervi.

TABLE OF NERVES—*Continued*

COMMON NAME* [MODALITY]	NA TERM†	ORIGIN*	BRANCHES*	DISTRIBUTION*
cavernous n's of penis [sympathetic, parasympathetic, visceral afferent]	nn. cavernosi penis	prostatic plexus		erectile tissue of penis
cerebral n's. *See* cranial n's				
cervical n's	nn. cervicales	the 8 pairs of n's that arise from cervical segments of spinal cord and, except last pair, leave vertebral column above correspondingly numbered vertebra; the ventral branches of upper 4, on either side, unite to form cervical plexus; those of lower 4, together with ventral branch of first thoracic n., form most of brachial plexus		
cervical n., transverse [general sensory]	n. transversus colli	cervical plexus—C2–C3	superior and inferior branches	skin on side and front of neck
ciliary n's, long [sympathetic, general sensory]	nn. ciliares longi	nasociliary n., from ophthalmic n.		dilator muscle of pupil, uvea, cornea
ciliary n's, short [parasympathetic, sympathetic, general sensory]	nn. ciliares breves	ciliary ganglion		smooth muscle and tunics of eye
clunial n's, inferior [general sensory]	nn. clunium inferiores	posterior femoral cutaneous n.		skin of lower part of buttock
clunial n's, middle [general sensory]	nn. clunium medii	plexus formed by lateral branches of dorsal branches of first 4 sacral nerves behind sacrum and coccyx		ligaments of sacrum and skin over posterior part of buttock
clunial n's, superior [general sensory]	nn. clunium superiores	lateral branches of dorsal branch of upper lumbar n's		skin of upper part of buttock
coccygeal n.	n. coccygeus	one of the pair of nerves arising from coccygeal segment of spinal cord		
cochlear n. *See* vestibulocochlear n.				
cranial n's	nn. craniales	the 12 pairs of n's connected with brain, including olfactory (I), optic (II), oculomotor (III), trochlear (IV), trigeminal (V), abducens (VI), facial (VII), vestibulocochlear (VIII), glossopharyngeal (IX), vagus (X), accessory (XI), and hypoglossal (XII) nerves		
cubital n. *See* ulnar n.				
cutaneous n. of arm, lateral, inferior [general sensory]	n. cutaneus brachii lateralis inferior	radial n.		skin of lateral surface of lower arm
cutaneous n. of arm, lateral, superior [general sensory]	n. cutaneus brachii lateralis superior	axillary n.		skin of back of arm

cutaneous n. of arm, medial [general sensory]	n. cutaneus brachii medialis	medial cord of brachial plexus (T1)		skin on medial and posterior aspects of arm
cutaneous n. of arm, posterior [general sensory]	n. cutaneus brachii posterior	radial n. in axilla		skin on back of arm
cutaneous n. of calf, lateral [general sensory]	n. cutaneus surae lateralis	common peroneal n.		skin of lateral side of back of leg, rarely may continue as sural n.
cutaneous n. of calf, medial [general sensory]	n. cutaneus surae medialis	tibial n.; usually joins peroneal communicating branch of common peroneal n. to form sural n.		may continue as sural n.
cutaneous n., dorsal, intermediate [general sensory]	n. cutaneus dorsalis intermedius	superficial peroneal n.	dorsal digital n's of foot	skin of front of lower third of leg and dorsum of foot; ankle; skin and joints of adjacent sides of third and fourth, and of fourth and fifth toes
cutaneous n., dorsal, lateral [general sensory]	n. cutaneus dorsalis lateralis	continuation of sural n.		skin and joints of lateral side of foot and fifth toe
cutaneous n., dorsal, medial [general sensory]	n. cutaneus dorsalis medialis	superficial peroneal n.		skin and joints of medial side of foot and big toe; adjacent sides of second and third toes
cutaneous n. of forearm, lateral [general sensory]	n. cutaneus antebrachii lateralis	continuation of musculocutaneous n.		skin over radial side of forearm; sometimes an area of skin of back of hand
cutaneous n. of forearm, medial [general sensory]	n. cutaneus antebrachii medialis	medial cord of brachial plexus (C8, T1)	anterior and ulnar	skin of front, medial, and posteromedial aspects of forearm
cutaneous n. of forearm, posterior [general sensory]	n. cutaneus antebrachii posterior	radial n.		skin of dorsal aspect of forearm
cutaneous n. of thigh, lateral [general sensory]	n. cutaneus femoris lateralis	lumbar plexus – L2–L3		skin of lateral aspect and front of thigh
cutaneous n. of thigh, posterior [general sensory]	n. cutaneus femoris posterior	sacral plexus – S1–S3	inferior clunial n's, perineal branches	skin of buttock, external genitalia, back of thigh and calf
digital n's, dorsal, radial. *See* digital n's of radial n., dorsal				
digital n's, dorsal, ulnar. *See* digital n's of ulnar n., dorsal				
digital n's of foot, dorsal [general sensory]	nn. digitales dorsales pedis	intermediate dorsal cutaneous n.		skin and joints of adjacent sides of third and fourth, and of fourth and fifth toes
digital n's of lateral plantar n., plantar, common [general sensory]	nn. digitales plantares communes nervi plantaris lateralis	superficial branch of lateral plantar n.	medial n. gives rise to 2 proper plantar digital n's	lateral one to short flexor muscle of little toe, skin and joints of lateral side of sole and little toe; medial one to adjacent sides of fourth and fifth toes

TABLE OF NERVES—*Continued*

COMMON NAME* [MODALITY]	NA TERM†	ORIGIN*	BRANCHES*	DISTRIBUTION*
digital n's of lateral plantar n., plantar, proper [motor, general sensory]	nn. digitales plantares proprii nervi plantaris lateralis	common plantar digital n's		short flexor muscle of little toe, skin and joints of lateral side of sole and little toe, and adjacent surfaces of fourth and fifth toes
digital n's of lateral surface of great toe and medial surface of second toe, dorsal [general sensory]	nn. digitales dorsales hallucis lateralis et digiti secundi medialis	medial terminal division of deep peroneal n.		skin and joints of adjacent sides of great and second toes
digital n's of medial plantar n., plantar, common [motor, general sensory]	nn. digitales plantares communes nervi plantaris medialis	medial plantar n.	muscular and proper plantar digital n's	flexor hallucis brevis muscle and first lumbrical muscles, skin and joints of medial side of foot and big toe, and adjacent sides of first and second, second and third, and third and fourth toes
digital n's of medial plantar n., plantar, proper [general sensory]	nn. digitales plantares proprii nervi plantaris medialis	common plantar digital n's		skin and joints of first toe, and adjacent sides of first and second, second and third, and third and fourth toes; the nerves extend to the dorsum to supply nail beds and tips of toes
digital n's of median n., palmar, common [motor, general sensory]	nn. digitales palmares communes nervi mediani	lateral and medial divisions of median n.	proper palmar digital n's	thumb, index, middle, and ring fingers, and first two lumbrical muscles
digital n's of median n., palmar, proper [motor, general sensory]	nn. digitales palmares proprii nervi mediani	common palmar digital n's		first two lumbrical muscles, skin and joints of both sides and palmar aspect of thumb, index, and middle fingers, radial side of ring finger, back of distal aspect of these digits
digital n's of radial n., dorsal [general sensory]	nn. digitales dorsales nervi radialis	superficial branch of radial n.		skin and joints of back of thumb, index finger, and part of middle finger, as far distally as digital phalanx
digital n's of ulnar n., dorsal [general sensory]	nn. digitales dorsales nervi ulnaris	dorsal branch of ulnar n.		skin and joints of medial side of little finger, dorsal aspects of adjacent sides of little and ring fingers and of ring and middle fingers
digital n's of ulnar n., palmar, common [general sensory]	nn. digitales palmares communes nervi ulnaris	superficial branch of ulnar n.	proper palmar digital n's	little and ring fingers
digital n's of ulnar n., palmar, proper [general sensory]	nn. digitales palmares proprii nervi ulnaris	the lateral of the two common palmar digital n's from superficial branch of ulnar n.		skin and joints of adjacent sides of fourth and fifth fingers

dorsal n. of clitoris [general sensory, motor]	n. dorsalis clitoridis	pudendal n.		deep transverse muscle of perineum, sphincter muscle of urethra, corpus cavernosum of clitoris, and skin, prepuce, and glans of clitoris
dorsal n. of penis [general sensory, motor]	n. dorsalis penis	pudendal n.		deep transverse muscle of perineum, sphincter muscle of urethra, corpus cavernosum of penis, and skin, prepuce, and glans of penis
dorsal scapular n. [motor]	n. dorsalis scapulae	brachial plexus – ventral branch of C5		rhomboid muscles and occasionally the levator muscle of scapula
ethmoidal n., anterior [general sensory]	n. ethmoidalis anterior	continuation of nasociliary n., from ophthalmic n.	internal, external, lateral, and medial nasal branches	mucosa of upper and anterior nasal septum, lateral wall of nasal cavity, skin of lower bridge and tip of nose
ethmoidal n., posterior [general sensory]	n. ethmoidalis posterior	nasociliary n., from ophthalmic n.		mucosa of posterior ethmoid cells and of sphenoidal sinus
n. of external acoustic meatus [general sensory]	n. meatus acustici externi	auriculotemporal n.		skin lining external acoustic meatus, and tympanic membrane
facial n. (7th cranial) [motor, parasympathetic, general sensory, special sensory]. *See* also intermediate n.	n. facialis	inferior border of pons, between olive and inferior cerebellar peduncle	stapedius n.; posterior auricular n.; parotid plexus; digastric, temporal, zygomatic, buccal, lingual, marginal mandibular, and cervical branches, and communicating branch with tympanic plexus	various structures of face, head, and neck (see also individual branches in this table)
femoral n. [general sensory, motor]	n. femoralis	lumbar plexus – L2–L4; descending behind inguinal ligament to femoral triangle	saphenous n., muscular and anterior cutaneous branches	skin of thigh and leg, muscles of front of thigh, and hip and knee joints (see also individual branches in this table)
fibular n. *See* entries under peroneal n.	n. fibularis (NA alternative for n. peroneus)			
frontal n. [general sensory]	n. frontalis	ophthalmic division of trigeminal n.; enters orbit through superior orbital fissure	supraorbital and supratrochlear n's	chiefly to forehead and scalp (see individual branches listed in this table)
genitofemoral n. [general sensory, motor]	n. genitofemoralis	lumbar plexus – L1–L2	genital and femoral branches	cremaster muscle, skin of scrotum or labium majus and of adjacent area of thigh and femoral triangle

TABLE OF NERVES—*Continued*

COMMON NAME* [MODALITY]	NA TERM†	ORIGIN*	BRANCHES*	DISTRIBUTION*
glossopharyngeal n. (9th cranial) [motor, parasympathetic, general sensory, special sensory, visceral sensory]	n. glossopharyngeus	several rootlets from lateral side of upper medulla oblongata, between olive and inferior cerebellar peduncle	tympanic n., pharyngeal, stylopharyngeal, tonsillar, and lingual branches, branch to carotid sinus, communicating branch with auricular branch of vagus n.	has two enlargements (superior and inferior ganglia) and supplies tongue, pharynx, and parotid nerve (see also individual branches in this table)
gluteal n., inferior [motor]	n. gluteus inferior	sacral plexus – L5–S2		gluteus maximus muscle
gluteal n., superior [motor, general sensory]	n. gluteus superior	sacral plexus – L4–S1		gluteus medius and minimus muscles, tensor fasciae latae, and hip joint
hemorrhoidal n's, inferior. *See* rectal n's, inferior				
hypogastric n.	n. hypogastricus (dexter et sinister)	a nerve trunk situated on either side (right and left), interconnecting superior and inferior hypogastric plexuses		
hypoglossal n. (12th cranial) [motor]	n. hypoglossus	several rootlets in anterolateral sulcus between olive and pyramid of medulla oblongata; passes through hypoglossal canal to tongue	lingual branches	styloglossus, hyoglossus, and genioglossus muscles, intrinsic muscles of tongue
iliohypogastric n. [motor, general sensory]	n. iliohypogastricus	lumbar plexus – L1 (sometimes T12)	lateral and anterior cutaneous branches	skin above pubis and over lateral side of buttock, and occasionally pyramidal muscle
ilioinguinal n. [general sensory]	n. ilioinguinalis	lumbar plexus – L1 (sometimes T12); accompanies spermatic cord through inguinal canal	anterior scrotal or labial branches	skin of scrotum or labia majora, and adjacent part of thigh
infraoccipital n. *See* suboccipital n.				
infraorbital n. [general sensory]	n. infraorbitalis	continuation of maxillary n., entering orbit through inferior orbital fissure, occupying in succession infraorbital groove, canal, and foramen	middle and anterior superior alveolar, inferior palpebral, internal and external nasal, and superior labial branches	incisor, cuspid, and premolar teeth of upper jaw, skin and conjunctiva of lower eyelid, mobile septum and skin of side of nose, mucous membrane of mouth, skin of upper lip
infratrochlear n. [general sensory]	n. infratrochlearis	nasociliary n., from ophthalmic n.	palpebral branches	skin of root and upper bridge of nose and lower eyelid, conjunctiva, lacrimal duct
intercostobrachial n's [general sensory]	nn. intercostobrachiales	second and third intercostal n's		skin on back and medial aspect of arm
intermediate n. [parasympathetic, special sensory]	n. intermedius	smaller root of facial n., between main root and vestibulocochlear n.	greater petrosal n., chorda tympani	lacrimal, nasal, palatine, submandibular, and sublingual glands, and anterior two thirds of tongue

interosseous n. of forearm, anterior [motor, general sensory]	n. interosseous [antebrachii] anterior	median n.		flexor pollicis longus, flexor digitorum profundus, and pronator quadratus muscles, wrist and intercarpal joints
interosseous n. of forearm, posterior [motor, general sensory]	n. interosseus [antebrachii] posterior	continuation of deep branch of radial n.		long abductor muscle of thumb, extensor muscles of thumb and index finger, and wrist and intercarpal joints
interosseous n. of leg [general sensory]	interosseus cruris	tibial n.		interosseous membrane and tibiofemoral syndesmosis
ischiadic n. *See* sciatic n.				
jugular n.	n. jugularis	a branch of the superior cervical which communicates with glossopharyngeal and vagus n's		
labial n's, anterior [general sensory]	nn. labiales anteriores	ilioinguinal n.		skin of anterior labial region of labia majora and adjacent part of thigh
labial n's, posterior [general sensory]	nn. labiales posteriores	pudendal n.		labium majus
lacrimal n. [general sensory]	n. lacrimalis	ophthalmic division of trigeminal n. entering orbit through superior orbital fissure		lacrimal gland, conjunctiva, lateral commissure of eye, skin of upper eyelid
laryngeal n., inferior [motor]	n. laryngeus inferior	recurrent laryngeal n., especially the terminal portion		intrinsic muscles of larynx, except cricothyroid communicates with internal laryngeal n.
laryngeal n., recurrent [parasympathetic, visceral afferent, motor]	n. laryngeus recurrens	vagus n. (chiefly the cranial part of the accessory n.)	inferior laryngeal n., tracheal, esophageal, and inferior cardiac branches	tracheal mucosa, esophagus, cardiac plexus (see also individual branches in this table)
laryngeal n., superior [motor, general sensory, visceral afferent, parasympathetic]	n. laryngeus superior	inferior ganglion of vagus n.	external, internal, and communicating branches	cricothyroid muscle and inferior constrictor muscle of pharynx, mucous membrane of back of tongue and larynx
lingual n. [general sensory]	n. lingualis	mandibular n., descending to tongue, first medial to mandible and then under cover of mucosa of mouth	sublingual n., lingual branch, branch to isthmus of fauces, branch communicating with hypoglossal n. and chorda tympani	anterior two thirds of tongue, adjacent areas of mouth, gums, isthmus of fauces
lumbar n's	nn. lumbales	the 5 pairs of n's that arise from lumbar segments of spinal cord, each pair leaving vertebral column below correspondingly numbered vertebrae; ventral branches of these nerves participate in formation of lumbosacral plexus		
mandibular n. (third division of trigeminal n.) [general sensory, motor]	n. mandibularis	trigeminal ganglion	meningeal branch, masseteric, deep temporal, lateral and medial pterygoid, buccal, auriculotemporal, lingual and inferior alveolar n's	extensive distribution to muscles of mastication, skin of face, mucous membrane of mouth, and teeth (see also individual branches in this table)

TABLE OF NERVES – *Continued*

COMMON NAME* [MODALITY]	NA TERM†	ORIGIN*	BRANCHES*	DISTRIBUTION*
masseteric n. [motor, general sensory]	n. massetericus	mandibular division of trigeminal n.		masseter muscle, temporomandibular joint
maxillary n. (second division of trigeminal n.) [general sensory]	n. maxillaris	trigeminal ganglion	meningeal branch, zygomatic n., posterior superior alveolar branches, infraorbital n., pterygopalatine n's, and indirectly branches of pterygopalatine ganglion	extensive distribution to skin of face and scalp, mucous membrane of maxillary sinus and nasal cavity, and teeth
median n. [general sensory]	n. medianus	lateral and medial cords of brachial plexus – C6–T1	anterior interosseous n. of forearm, common palmar digital n's, and muscular and palmar branches, and a communicating branch with ulnar n.	ultimately, skin on front of lateral part of hand, most of flexor muscles of front of forearm, most of short muscles of thumb, elbow joint, and many joints of hand
mental n. [general sensory]	n. mentalis	inferior alveolar n.	mental and inferior labial branches	skin of chin, lower lip
musculocutaneous n. [general sensory, motor]	n. musculocutaneus	lateral cord of brachial plexus – C5–C7	lateral cutaneous n. of forearm, muscular branches	coracobrachial, biceps, brachial muscles, elbow joint, skin of radial side of forearm
mylohyoid n. [motor]	n. mylohyoideus	inferior alveolar n.		mylohyoid muscle, anterior belly of digastric muscle
nasociliary n. [general sensory]	n. nasociliaris	ophthalmic division of trigeminal nerve	long ciliary, posterior ethmoidal, anterior ethmoidal, and infratrochlear n's and a communicating branch to ciliary ganglion	(see individual branches in this table)
nasopalatine n. [parasympathetic, general sensory]	n. nasopalatinus	pterygopalatine ganglion		mucosa and glands of most of nasal septum and anterior part of hard palate
obturator n. [general sensory, motor]	n. obturatorius	lumbar plexus – L3–L4	anterior, posterior, and muscular branches	gracilis and adductor muscles, skin of medial part of thigh, and hip joints
occipital n., greater [general sensory, motor]	n. occipitalis major	medial branch of dorsal branch of C2		semispinal muscle of head and skin of head as far forward as vertex
occipital n., lesser [general sensory]	n. occipitalis minor	superficial cervical plexus – C2–C3		ascends behind auricle and supplies some of the skin of side of head and on cranial surface of auricle

occipital n., third [general sensory]	n. occipitalis tertius	medial branch of dorsal branch of C3		skin of upper part of back of neck and head
oculomotor n. (3rd cranial) [motor, parasympathetic]	n. oculomotorius	brain stem, emerging medial to cerebral peduncles, running forward in the carvernous sinus	superior and inferior branches	entering orbit through superior orbital fissure, the branches supply levator muscle of upper lid, all extrinsic muscles except lateral rectus and superior oblique, and carry parasympathetic fibers from ciliary muscle to sphincter of pupil
olfactory n's (1st cranial) [special sensory]	nn. olfactorii	the n's of smell, consisting of about 20 bundles arising in the olfactory epithelium and passing through the cribriform plate of ethmoid bone to olfactory bulb		
ophthalmic n. (first division of trigeminal n.) [general sensory]	n. ophthalmicus	trigeminal ganglion	tentorial branches, frontal, lacrimal, nasociliary n's	eyeball and conjunctiva, lacrimal sac and gland, nasal mucosa and frontal sinus, external nose, eyelid, forehead, and scalp (see also individual branches in this table)
optic n. (2nd cranial) [special sensory]	n. opticus	the nerve of sight, consisting chiefly of axons and central processes of cells of the ganglionic layer of retina leaving the orbit through the optic canal, joining the optic chiasm (the medial ones crossing over to opposite side), and continuing as the optic tract		
palatine n., anterior. *See* palatine n., greater				
palatine n., greater [parasympathetic, sympathetic, general sensory]	n. palatinus major	pterygopalatine ganglion	posterior inferior [lateral] nasal branches	emerges through greater palatine foramen and supplies palate
palatine n's, lesser [parasympathetic, sympathetic, general sensory]	nn. palatini minores	pterygopalatine ganglion		emerge through lesser palatine foramen and supply soft palate and tonsil
perineal n's [general sensory, motor]	nn. perineales	pudendal n. in pudendal canal	muscular branches and posterior scrotal or labial nerves	muscular branches supply bulbospongiosus, ischiocavernosus, superficial transverse perinei muscles and bulb of penis and, in part, sphincter ani externi and levator ani; the scrotal (labial) n's supply the scrotum or labium majus
peroneal n., common [general sensory, motor]	n. peroneus communis	sciatic n. in lower thigh	supplies short head of biceps femoris muscle (while still incorporated in sciatic nerve), gives off lateral sural cutaneous n. and peroneal communicating branch descends in popliteal fossa, supplies knee and superior tibiofibular joints and anterior tibial muscle, and divides into superficial and deep peroneal n's	

TABLE OF NERVES—*Continued*

COMMON NAME* [MODALITY]	NA TERM†	ORIGIN*	BRANCHES*	DISTRIBUTION*
peroneal n., deep [general sensory, motor]	n. peroneus profundus	a terminal branch of common peroneal n.	winds around neck of fibula and descends on interosseous membrane to front of ankle; gives off muscular branches to tibialis anterior, extensor hallucis longus, extensor digitorum longus, and peroneus tertius muscles, and a twig to ankle joint; lateral terminal division supplies extensor digitorum brevis muscle and tarsal joints; medial terminal division (digital branch) divides into dorsal digital nerves for skin and joints of adjacent sides of big and second toes	
peroneal n., superficial [general sensory, motor]	n. peroneus superficialis	a terminal branch of common peroneal n.	descends in front of fibula, supplies long and short peroneal muscles and, in lower leg, divides into muscular branches, and medial and intermediate dorsal cutaneous n's (see also individual branches in this table)	
petrosal n., deep [sympathetic]	n. petrosus profundus	internal carotid plexus		joins greater petrosal n. to form n. of pterygoid canal, and supplies lacrimal, nasal, and palatine glands via pterygopalatine ganglion and its branches
petrosal n., greater [parasympathetic, general sensory]	n. petrosus major	intermediate n. via geniculate ganglion		running forward from geniculate ganglion, joins deep petrosal n. of pterygoid canal, and reaches lacrimal, nasal, and palatine glands and nasopharynx via pterygopalatine ganglion and its branches
petrosal n., lesser [parasympathetic]	n. petrosus minor	tympanic plexus		parotid gland via otic ganglion and auriculotemporal n.
phrenic n. [general sensory, motor]	n. phrenicus	cervical plexus—C4–C5	pericardial and phrenicoabdominal branches	pleura, pericardium, diaphragm, peritoneum, sympathetic plexuses
phrenic n's, accessory	nn. phrenici accessorii	inconstant contribution of fifth cervical n. to phrenic n.; when present, they run a separate course to root of neck or into thorax before joining phrenic n.		
plantar n., lateral [general sensory, motor]	n. plantaris lateralis	smaller of terminal branches of tibial n.	muscular, superficial, and deep branches	lying between first and second layers of muscles of sole, supplies quadratus plantae, abductor digiti minimi, flexor digiti minimi brevis, adductor hallucis, interossei, and second, third, and fourth lumbrical muscles, and gives off cutaneous and articular twigs to lateral side of sole and fourth and fifth toes (see also individual branches in this table)

plantar n., medial [general sensory, motor]	n. plantaris medialis	larger of terminal branches of tibial n.	common plantar digital n's and muscular branches	abductor hallucis, flexor digitorum brevis, flexor hallucis brevis, and first lumbrical muscles and cutaneous and articular twigs to medial side of sole and first to fourth toes (see also individual branches in this table)
pneumogastric n. *See* vagus n.				
pterygoid n., lateral [motor]	n. pterygoideus lateralis	mandibular n.		lateral pterygoid, tensor tympani, and tensor veli palatini muscles
pterygoid n., medial [motor]	n. pterygoideus medialis	mandibular n.		medial pterygoid muscle
n. of pterygoid canal [parasympathetic, sympathetic]	n. canalis pterygoidei	union of deep and greater petrosal n's		pterygopalatine ganglion and branches
pterygopalatine n's [general sensory]	nn. pterygopalatini	two nerves connecting maxillary n. to pterygopalatine ganglion; they are the sensory roots of the ganglion		
pudendal n. [general sensory, motor, parasympathetic]	n. pudendus	sacral plexus – S2–S4	enters pudendal canal, gives off inferior rectal n., then divides into perineal n. and dorsal n. of penis (clitoris)	muscles, skin, and erectile tissue of perineum (see also individual branches in this table)
radial n. [general sensory, motor]	n. radialis	posterior cord of brachial plexus – C6–C8, and sometimes C5 and T1	posterior cutaneous and inferior lateral cutaneous n's of arm, posterior cutaneous n. of forearm, muscular, deep, and superficial branches	descending in back of arm and forearm, ultimately distributed to skin on back of forearm, arm, and hand, extensor muscles on back of arm and forearm, and elbow joint and many joints of hand
rectal n's, inferior [general sensory, motor]	nn. rectales inferiores	pudendal n., or independently from sacral plexus		sphincter ani externus muscle, skin around anus, lining of anal canal up to pectinate line
recurrent n. *See* laryngeal n., recurrent				
saccular n.	n. saccularis	the branch of vestibular part of eighth cranial (vestibulocochlear) nerve that innervates macula of saccule		
sacral n's	nn. sacrales	the 5 pairs of n's that arise from sacral segments of spinal cord; the ventral branches of first 4 pairs participate in formation of sacral plexus		
saphenous n. [general sensory]	n. saphenus	termination of femoral n.	infrapatellar and medial crural cutaneous	knee joint, subsartorial and patellar plexuses, skin on medial side of leg and foot
sciatic n. [general sensory, motor]	n. ischiadicus	sacral plexus – L4–S3; leaves pelvis through greater sciatic foramen	divides into common peroneal and tibial n's, usually in lower third of thigh	(see individual branches in this table)
scrotal n's, anterior [general sensory]	nn. scrotales anteriores	ilioinguinal n.		skin of anterior scrotal region
scrotal n's, posterior [general sensory]	nn. scrotales posteriores	perineal n's		skin of scrotum

TABLE OF NERVES – *Continued*

COMMON NAME* [MODALITY]	NA TERM†	ORIGIN*	BRANCHES*	DISTRIBUTION*
spinal n's	nn. spinales	the 31 pairs of n's that arise from spinal cord, and pass between the vertebrae, including 8 cervical, 12 thoracic, 5 lumbar, 5 sacral, and 1 coccygeal		
splanchnic n., greater [preganglionic sympathetic, visceral afferent]	n. splanchnicus major	thoracic sympathetic trunk and thoracic ganglia T5–T10 of sympathetic trunk		descending through diaphragm or its aortic opening, ends in celiac ganglia and plexuses, with a splanchnic ganglion commonly near the diaphragm
splanchnic n., lesser [preganglionic sympathetic, visceral afferent]	n. splanchnicus minor	thoracic ganglia T9, T10 or sympathetic trunk	renal branch	pierces diaphragm, joins aorticorenal ganglion and celiac plexus, and communicates with renal and superior mesenteric plexuses
splanchnic n., lowest [sympathetic, visceral afferent]	n. splanchnicus imus	last ganglion of sympathetic trunk, or lesser splanchnic n.		aorticorenal ganglion and adjacent plexus
splanchnic n's, lumbar [preganglionic sympathetic, visceral afferent]	nn. splanchnici lumbales	lumbar ganglia or sympathetic trunk		upper nerves join celiac and adjacent plexuses, middle ones go to mesenteric and adjacent plexuses, lower ones descend to superior hypogastric plexus
splanchnic n's, pelvic [preganglionic parasympathetic, visceral afferent]	nn. splanchnici pelvini	sacral plexus – S3–S4		leaving sacral plexus, they enter inferior hypogastric plexus and supply pelvic organs
splanchnic n's, sacral [preganglionic sympathetic, visceral afferent]	nn. splanchnici sacrales	sacral part of sympathetic trunk		pelvic organs and blood vessels via inferior hypogastric plexus
stapedius n. [motor]	n. stapedius	facial n.		stapedius muscle
subclavian n. [motor, general sensory]	n. subclavius	upper trunk of brachial plexus – C5		subclavius muscle, sternoclavicular joint
subcostal n. [general sensory, motor]	n. subcostalis	ventral branch of T12		skin of lower abdomen and lateral side of gluteal region, parts of transverse, oblique, and rectus muscles, and usually pyramidal muscle, and adjacent peritoneum
sublingual n. [parasympathetic, general sensory]	n. sublingualis	lingual n.		sublingual gland and overlying mucous membrane

suboccipital n. [motor]	n. suboccipitalis	dorsal branch of C1		emerges above posterior arch of atlas, supplies muscles of suboccipital triangle and semispinal muscle of head
subscapular n. [motor]	n. subscapularis	posterior cord of brachial plexus – C5		usually two or more nerves, upper and lower, supplying subscapular and teres major muscles
supraclavicular n's, anterior. *See* supraclavicular n's, medial				
supraclavicular n's, intermediate [general sensory]	nn. supraclaviculares intermedii	cervical plexus – C3–C4		descends in posterior triangle, crosses clavicle, supplying skin over pectoral and deltoid regions
supraclavicular n's, lateral [general sensory]	nn. supraclaviculares laterales	cervical plexus – C3–C4		descends in posterior triangle, crosses clavicle, supplying skin of superior and posterior aspects of shoulder
supraclavicular n's, medial [general sensory]	nn. supraclaviculares mediales	cervical plexus – C3–C4		descends in posterior triangle, crosses clavicle, supplying skin of medial infraclavicular region
supraclavicular n's, middle. *See* supraclavicular n's, intermediate				
supraclavicular n's, posterior. *See* supraclavicular n's, lateral				
supraorbital n. [general sensory]	n. supraorbitalis	continuation of frontal n., from ophthalmic n.	lateral and medial branches	leaves orbit through supraorbital notch or foramen, supplying skin of upper eyelid, forehead, anterior part of scalp (to vertex), mucosa of frontal sinus
suprascapular n. [motor, general sensory]	n. suprascapularis	brachial plexus – C5–C6		descends through suprascapular and spinoglenoid notches, supplying acromioclavicular and shoulder joints, and supraspinous and infraspinous muscles
supratrochlear n. [general sensory]	n. supratrochlearis	frontal n., from ophthalmic n.		leaves orbit at end of supraorbital margin, supplying forehead and upper eyelid
sural n. [general sensory]	n. suralis	medial sural n. and communicating branch of common peroneal n.	lateral dorsal cutaneous n. and lateral calcaneal branches	skin on back of leg, and skin and joints on lateral side of foot and heel
temporal n's, deep [motor]	nn. temporales profundi	mandibular n.		temporal muscles
n. of tensor tympani [motor]	n. tensoris tympani	mandibular n. via n. to medial pterygoid muscle and otic ganglion		tensor muscle of tympanum

TABLE OF NERVES—*Concluded*

COMMON NAME* [MODALITY]	NA TERM†	ORIGIN*	BRANCHES*	DISTRIBUTION*
n. of tensor veli palatini [motor]	n. tensoris veli palatini	mandibular n. via n. to medial pterygoid muscle and otic ganglion		tensor muscle of palatine velum
thoracic n's	nn. thoracici	the 12 pairs of spinal n's that arise from thoracic segments of spinal cord, each pair leaving vertebral column below correspondingly numbered vertebra		body wall of thorax and upper part of abdomen
thoracic n., long [motor]	n. thoracicus longus	brachial plexus—ventral branches of C5–C7		descends behind brachial plexus to anterior serratus muscle
thoracodorsal n. [motor]	n. thoracodorsalis	posterior cord of brachial plexus—C7–C8		latissimus dorsi muscle
tibial n. [general sensory, motor]	n. tibialis	sciatic n. in lower thigh	interosseous n. of leg, medial cutaneous n. of calf, sural and medial and lateral plantar n's, and muscular and medial calcaneal branches	while still incorporated in sciatic n., supplies semimembranous and semitendinous muscles, long head of biceps, and adductor magnus muscle; supplies knee joint as it descends in popliteal fossa continuing into leg, supplies muscles and skin of calf, sole, and toes (see also individual branches in this table)
trigeminal n. (5th cranial) [general sensory, motor]	n. trigeminus	emerges from lateral surface of pons as a motor and a sensory root, the latter expanding into trigeminal ganglion, from which the 3 divisions of nerve arise (see mandibular n., maxillary n., and ophthalmic n.)		face, teeth, mouth, nasal cavity, muscles of mastication
trochlear n. (4th cranial) [motor]	n. trochlearis	fibers of each nerve (one on either side) decussate across median plane, and emerge from back of brain stem below corresponding inferior colliculus		runs forward in lateral wall of cavernous sinus, traverses superior orbital fissure, supplying superior oblique muscle of eyeball
tympanic n. [general sensory, parasympathetic]	n. tympanicus	inferior ganglion of glossopharyngeal n.	helps form tympanic plexus	mucous membrane of tympanic cavity, mastoid air cells, auditory tube, and, via lesser petrosal n. and otic ganglion, parotid gland
ulnar n. [general sensory, motor]	n. ulnaris	medial and lateral cords of brachial plexus—C7–T1	muscular, dorsal, palmar, superficial, and deep branches	ultimately to skin on front and medial part of hand, some flexor muscles on front of forearm, many short muscles of hand, elbow joint, many joints of hand
utricular n.	n. utricularis	the branch of vestibular part of eighth cranial (vestibulocochlear) n. that innervates macula of utricle		

utriculoampullary n.	n. utriculoampullaris	a n. that arises by peripheral division of vestibular part of eighth cranial (vestibulocochlear) n., and supplies utricle and ampullae of semicircular ducts		
vaginal n's [sympathetic, parasympathetic]	nn. vaginales	uterovaginal plexus		vagina
vagus n. (10th cranial) [parasympathetic, visceral afferent, motor, general sensory]	n. vagus	by numerous rootlets from lateral side of medulla oblongata in groove between olive and inferior cerebellar peduncle	superior and recurrent laryngeal n's, meningeal, auricular, pharyngeal, cardiac, bronchial, gastric, hepatic, celiac, and renal branches, pharyngeal, pulmonary, and esophageal plexuses, and anterior and posterior trunks	descending through jugular foramen, presents as a superior and an inferior ganglion, continues through neck and thorax into abdomen, supplying sensory fibers to ear, tongue, pharynx, and larynx, motor fibers to pharynx, larynx, esophagus, and parasympathetic and visceral fibers to thoracic and abdominal viscera (see also individual branches in this table)
vertebral n. [sympathetic]	n. vertebralis	cervicothoracic and vertebral		ascends with vertebral artery and gives fibers to spinal meninges, cervical n's, and posterior cranial fossa
vestibulocochlear n. (8th cranial)	n. vestibulocochlearis	emerges from brain between pons and medulla oblongata, at cerebellopontine angle and behind facial n.; it consists of 2 sets of fibers, the vestibular part from utricle, saccule, and semicircular ducts, and the cochlear part, from the cochlea, and is connected with the brain by corresponding superior and inferior roots		
vidian n. *See* n. of pterygoid canal				
vidian n., deep. *See* petrosal n., deep				
zygomatic n. [general sensory]	n. zygomaticus	maxillary n., entering orbit through inferior orbital fissure	zygomaticofacial and zygomaticotemporal branches	communicates with lacrimal nerve, supplying skin of temple and adjacent part of face

network (net'werk) a meshlike structure of interlocking fibers or strands.

neur(o)- word element [Gr.], *nerve.*

neurad (nu'rad) toward the neural axis or aspect.

neural (nu'ral) pertaining to a nerve or to the nerves.

neuralgia (nu-ral'je-ah) pain in a nerve or along the course of one or more nerves. adj., **neural'gic.** Neuralgia is usually a sharp, spasmlike pain that may recur at intervals. It is caused by inflammation of or injury to a nerve or group of nerves.

Inflammation of a nerve, or NEURITIS, may affect different parts of the body, depending upon the location of the nerve. TIC DOULOUREUX (called also trigeminal neuralgia) is due to involvement of the trigeminal nerve, with neuralgic pain over the jaw, cheek, and forehead.

Another form of neuralgia is SCIATICA, or pain occurring along the sciatic nerve. This pain is felt in the back and down the back of the thigh to the ankle. It may result from inflammation of or injury to the sciatic nerve, and is often associated with conditions such as arthritis of the spine, slipped intervertebral disk, diabetes mellitus, and gout.

n. facia'lis ve'ra, geniculate neuralgia.

Fothergill's n., tic douloureux (trigeminal neuralgia).

geniculate n., Hunt's n., neuralgia involving the geniculate ganglion, producing pain in the middle ear and external acoustic meatus.

idiopathic n., neuralgia of unknown etiology, not accompanied by any structural change.

intercostal n., neuralgia of the intercostal nerves, causing pain in the side.

mammary n., neuralgic pain in the breast.

Morton's n., pain in the metatarsus of the foot.

nasociliary n., pain in the eyes, brow, and root of the nose.

trifacial n., trigeminal n., tic douloureux.

neuraminidase (nūr″ah-min'ĭ-dās) an enzyme of the surface coat of myxoviruses that destroys the neuraminic acid of the cell surface during attachment, thereby preventing hemagglutination.

neuranagenesis (nu″ran-ah-jen'ĕ-sis) regeneration of nerve tissue.

neurapophysis (nu″rah-pof'ĭ-sis) a structure forming either side of the neural arch; also, the part supposedly homologous with this structure in a so-called cranial vertebra.

neurapraxia (nu″rah-prak'se-ah) a nerve lesion producing paralysis in the absence of peripheral degeneration.

neurarthropathy (nūr″ar-throp'ah-the) neuroarthropathy.

neurasthenia (nu″ras-the'ne-ah) a neurosis marked by chronic abnormal fatigability, lack of energy, feelings of inadequacy, moderate depression, inability to concentrate, loss of appetite, insomnia, etc. Popularly called nervous prostration. adj., **neurasthen'ic.**

neuratrophia (nu″rah-tro'fe-ah) impaired nutrition of the nervous system.

neuratrophic (nu″rah-trof'ik) characterized by atrophy of the nerves; also, a person so affected.

neuraxis (nu-rak'sis) 1. axon. 2. central nervous system. adj., **neurax'ial.**

neuraxon (nu-rak'son) axon.

neurectasia, neurectasis (nu″rek-ta'ze-ah; nu-rek'tah-sis) the surgical stretching of a nerve; neurotony.

neurectomy (nu-rek'to-me) excision of a part of a nerve.

neurectopia (nu″rek-to'pe-ah) displacement or abnormal situation of a nerve.

neurenteric (nu″ren-ter'ik) pertaining to the neural tube and archenteron of the embryo.

neurergic (nu-rer'jik) pertaining to or dependent on nerve action.

neurexeresis (nūr″ek-ser-e'sis) the operation of tearing out (avulsion) of a nerve.

neurilemma (nu″rĭ-lem'ah) the thin membrane spirally enwrapping the myelin layers of myelinated nerve fibers and the axons of unmyelinated nerve fibers. Called also sheath of Schwann.

neurilemmitis (nu″rĭ-lĕ-mi'tis) inflammation of the neurilemma.

neurilemoma (nu″rĭ-lĕ-mo'mah) a tumor of a peripheral nerve sheath (neurilemma); called also schwannoma.

neurinoma (nu″rĭ-no'mah) neurilemoma.

neuritis (nu-ri'tis), pl. *neurit'ides.* inflammation of a nerve; also used to denote noninflammatory lesions of the peripheral nervous system (see also NEUROPATHY). adj., **neurit'ic.** There are many forms with different effects. Some increase or decrease the sensitivity of the body part served by the nerve; others produce paralysis; some cause pain and inflammation. The cases in which pain is the chief symptom are generally called NEURALGIA.

Neuritis and neuralgia attack the peripheral nerves, the nerves that link the brain and spinal cord with the muscles, skin, organs, and all other parts of the body. These nerves usually carry both sensory and motor fibers; hence both pain and some paralysis may result. Treatment varies with the specific form of neuritis involved.

GENERALIZED NEURITIS. Certain toxic substances such as lead, arsenic, and mercury may produce a generalized poisoning of the peripheral nerves, with tenderness, pain, and paralysis of the limbs. Other causes of generalized neuritis include alcoholism, vitamin-deficiency diseases such as beriberi, and diabetes mellitus, thallium poisoning, some types of allergy, and some viral and bacterial infections, such as diphtheria, syphilis, and mumps.

Some attacks of generalized neuritis begin with fever and other symptoms of an acute illness. However, neuritis caused by lead or alcohol poisoning comes on very slowly over the course of weeks or months.

Usually an attack of generalized neuritis will subside by itself when the toxic substance is eliminated. Rest and a nutritious diet containing extra vitamins, especially of the B group, are helpful. Physical therapy may relieve the pain and paralysis. Generalized neuritis may be prevented through knowledge of the dangers of poor nutrition, industrial hazards, chronic alcoholism, and infections.

SPECIAL TYPES OF NEURITIS. Frequently, instead of a generalized irritation of the nerves, only one nerve is affected. BELL'S PALSY, or facial paralysis, results when the facial nerve is affected. It usually lasts only a few days or weeks. Sometimes, however, the cause is a tumor pressing on the nerve, or injury to the nerve by a blow, cut, or bullet. In that event, recovery depends on the success in treating the tumor or injury.

Sciatica. The sciatic nerve, which runs from the spinal cord down each leg, is the widest nerve in the body and one of the longest. It is exposed to many different kinds of injury in the back, in the pelvis, and along its course in the leg.

Inflammation of or injury to the sciatic nerve, with resultant SCIATICA, causes pain that travels down from the back or thigh into the feet and toes. Certain muscles of the leg may be partly or completely paralyzed, so that it is difficult to move the thigh or leg. A back injury, irritation from arthritis of the spine, or pressure on the nerve that occurs during certain types of work may be the cause. Certain diseases such as diabetes mellitus or gout may be the inciting factor. The most common cause is probably a herniated or slipped intervertebral disk.

Some cases of sciatica are idiopathic—that is, without known cause. However, because of the long, painful and disabling course of severe sciatica, it is worth considerable time and money to have every possible cause investigated and the underlying trouble corrected if possible. Sedatives and physical therapy may also be required to relieve the pain or disability.

Neuritis of the Spinal Nerves. Injury or disease may affect any of the many nerves traveling out from the spine. For example, inflammation of the nerves between the ribs causes pain in the chest that may resemble pleurisy or even coronary occlusion (heart attack). This is called intercostal neuritis or intercostal neuralgia. Similarly, the nerves traveling down the neck to the arm may be subject to various injuries or diseases. For example, too vigorous pulling on the nerves in the neck, as might occur in difficult obstetrical deliveries, causes the condition known as brachial paralysis.

Saturday Night Palsy. This is a pressure neuritis, so called because of its frequent occurrence in alcoholics. It is caused by prolonged compression of the radial nerve against a hard edge or surface, sometimes resulting in radial nerve paralysis with wristdrop.

Neuritis of the Cranial Nerves. Bell's palsy results from inflammation of the seventh cranial, or facial nerve. Another nerve, the fifth cranial, or trigeminal, nerve, also ends in the face and jaws, and may be the source of a neuralgia that causes spasms of pain on one side of the face. This is called TIC DOULOUREUX or trigeminal neuralgia. It may be set off by a draft of cold air, by chewing, or by other factors. Medicines and, if necessary, surgery can relieve this painful malady.

The nerves leading to the retina of the eye may be involved in various ailments. This condition, optic neuritis, is potentially dangerous to vision and requires immediate treatment. Any of the other cranial nerves may be affected by infections, tumors, and toxins. The antibiotic streptomycin occasionally causes damage to the eighth cranial nerve, which helps control the sense of balance in the inner ear. Any disturbance of vision, hearing, balance, swallowing, taste, or speech may be a sign of trouble in the cranial nerves, and should be brought to a physician's attention at once.

HERPES ZOSTER, or shingles, is also a nerve ailment caused by infection with the chickenpox virus, with symptoms of pain and small blisters following the path of the affected nerve.

endemic n., beriberi.

interstitial n., inflammation of the connective tissue of a nerve trunk.

multiple n., neuritis affecting several nerves at once; polyneuritis.

optic n., inflammation of the optic nerve, affecting the part of the nerve within the eyeball (neuropapillitis) or the part behind the eyeball (retrobulbar neuritis).

parenchymatous n., neuritis affecting primarily the axons and the myelin of the peripheral nerves.

retrobulbar n., optic neuritis affecting the part of the optic nerve behind the eyeball.

toxic n., neuritis due to some poison.

traumatic n., neuritis following and due to injury.

neuroanastomosis (nu″ro-ah-nas″to-mo′sis) surgical anastomosis of one nerve to another.

neuroanatomy (nu″ro-ah-nat′o-me) anatomy of the nervous system.

neuroarthropathy (nu″ro-ar-throp′ah-the) any disease of joint structures associated with disease of the central or peripheral nervous system.

neuroastrocytoma (nu″ro-as″tro-si-to′mah) a glioma composed mainly of astrocytes, found mostly in the floor of the third ventricle and the temporal lobes of the brain.

neurobiology (nu″ro-bi-ol′o-je) biology of the nervous system.

neurobiotaxis (nu″ro-bi′o-tak″sis) the theory that nerve cell bodies have a tendency during development to migrate toward the source of their stimulation. adj. **neurobiotac′tic.**

neuroblast (nu′ro-blast) an embryonic cell from which nervous tissue is formed.

neuroblastoma (nu″ro-blas-to′mah) sarcoma of nervous system origin, composed chiefly of neuroblasts, affecting mostly infants and children up to 10 years of age, usually arising in the autonomic nervous system (sympathicoblastoma) or in the adrenal medulla.

neurocanal (nu″ro-kah-nal′) vertebral canal.

neurocardiac (nu″ro-kar′de-ak) pertaining to the nervous system and the heart.

neurocentrum (nu″ro-sen′trum) one of the embryonic vertebral elements from which the spinous processes of the vertebrae develop. adj., **neurocen′tral.**

neurochemistry (nu″ro-kem′is-tre) that branch of neurology dealing with the chemistry of the nervous system.

neurochorioretinitis (nu″ro-ko″re-o-ret″ĭ-ni′tis) inflammation of the optic nerve, choroid, and retina.

neurochoroiditis (nu″ro-ko″roi-di′tis) inflammation of the optic nerve and choroid.

neurocirculatory (nu″ro-ser″ku-lah-to″re) pertaining to the nervous and circulatory systems.

neurocladism (nu-rok′lah-dizm) the formation of new branches by the process of a neuron; especially the force by which, in regeneration of divided nerves, the newly formed axons become attracted by the peripheral stump, so as to form a bridge between the two ends.

neuroclonic (nu″ro-klon′ik) marked by nervous spasm.

neurocranium (nu″ro-kra′ne-um) the part of the cranium enclosing the brain. adj., **neurocra′nial.**

neurocrine (nu′ro-krīn) 1. denoting an endocrine

influence on or by the nerves. 2. pertaining to neurosecretion.

neurocutaneous (nu″ro-ku-ta′ne-us) pertaining to nerves and skin, or the cutaneous nerves.

neurocyte (nu′ro-sīt) a nerve cell of any kind.

neurocytoma (nu″ro-si-to′mah) a brain tumor consisting of undifferentiated cells of nervous origin, i.e., cells resembling medullary neural epithelium. Called also neuroepithelioma.

neurodendrite, neurodendron (nu″ro-den′drīt; nu″ro-den′dron) dendrite.

neurodermatitis (nu″ro-der″mah-ti′tis) a general term for a dermatosis presumed to be caused by itching due to emotional causes. The term is also used to refer to LICHEN SIMPLEX CHRONICUS (circumscribed or localized neurodermatitis) and sometimes atopic DERMATITIS (disseminated neurodermatitis).

neurodynamic (nu″ro-di-nam′ik) pertaining to nervous energy.

neurodynia (nu″ro-din′e-ah) pain in a nerve.

neuroencephalomyelopathy (nu″ro-en-sef″ah-lo-mi″ĕ-lop′ah-the) disease involving the nerves, brain, and spinal cord.

neuroendocrine (nu″ro-en′do-krin) pertaining to neural and endocrine influence, and particularly to the interaction between the nervous and endocrine systems.

neuroendocrinology (nu″ro-en″do-krĭ-nol′o-je) the study of the interactions of the nervous and endocrine systems.

neuroepithelioma (nu″ro-ep″ĭ-the″le-o′mah) neurocytoma.

neuroepithelium (nu″ro-ep″ĭ-the′le-um) 1. epithelium made up of cells specialized to serve as sensory cells for reception of external stimuli. Called also sense, or sensory, epithelium. 2. the ectodermal epithelium, from which the cerebrospinal axis is derived.

neurofibril, neurofibrilla (nu″ro-fi′bril; nu″ro-fibril′ah) one of the delicate threads running in every direction through the cytoplasm of a nerve cell, extending into the axon and dendrites.

neurofibroma (nu″ro-fi-bro′mah) a tumor of peripheral nerves due to abnormal proliferation of Schwann cells. Called also fibroneuroma.

neurofibromatosis (nu″ro-fi″bro-mah-to′sis) a familial condition characterized by developmental changes in the nervous system, muscles, bones, and skin, and marked by the formation of neurofibromas over the entire body associated with patches of pigmentation; called also von Recklinghausen's disease.

neurogenesis (nu″ro-jen′ĕ-sis) the development of nervous tissue.

neurogenic (nu″ro-jen′ik) 1. forming nervous tissue, or stimulating nervous energy. 2. originating in the nervous system.

neurogenous (nu-roj′ĕ-nus) arising from the nervous system, or from some lesion of the nervous system.

neuroglia (nu-rog′le-ah) the supporting structure of nervous tissue, consisting, in the central nervous system, of astrocytes, oligodendrocytes, and microglia; called also glia. adj., **neurog′lial.**

neurogliocyte (nu-rog′le-o-sīt) one of the cells composing the neuroglia.

neuroglioma (nu″ro-gli-o′mah) a tumor composed of neuroglial tissue.

n. gangliona′re, ganglioneuroma.

neurogliosis (nu-rog″le-o′sis) a condition marked by numerous neurogliomas.

neurogram (nu′ro-gram) the imprint left on the brain by past mental experiences.

neurohistology (nu″ro-his-tol′o-je) histology of the nervous system.

neurohormone (nu′ro-hor″mōn) a hormone stimulating the neural mechanism.

neurohumor (nu″ro-hu′mor) a chemical substance formed in a neuron and able to activate or modify the function of a neighboring neuron, muscle, or gland. adj., **neurohu′moral.**

neurohypophysis (nu″ro-hi-pof′ĭ-sis) the posterior lobe of the PITUITARY GLAND. adj., **neurohypophys′eal.**

neuroid (nu′roid) resembling a nerve.

neuroinduction (nu″ro-in-duk′shun) mental suggestion.

neurokeratin (nu″ro-ker′ah-tin) a protein network seen in histological specimens of the myelin sheath.

neurolemma (nu″ro-lem′ah) neurilemma.

neurolemmitis (nu″ro-lĕ-mi′tis) neurilemmitis.

neurolemmoma (nu″ro-lĕ-mo′mah) neurilemoma.

neuroleptic (nu″ro-lep′tik) 1. denoting a neuropharmacologic agent having antipsychotic action affecting mainly psychomotor activity. 2. an agent producing such action.

neurologist (nu-rol′o-jist) a specialist in neurology.

neurology (nu-rol′o-je) that branch of medical science which deals with the nervous system, both normal and in disease. adj., **neurolog′ic.**

clinical n., that especially concerned with the diagnosis and treatment of disorders of the nervous system.

neurolysin (nu-rol′ĭ-sin) a cytolysin with a specific destructive action on neurons.

neurolysis (nu-rol′ĭ-sis) 1. release of a nerve sheath by cutting it longitudinally. 2. operative breaking up of perineural adhesions. 3. relief of tension upon a nerve obtained by stretching. 4. exhaustion of nervous energy. 5. destruction or dissolution of nerve tissue. adj., **neurolyt′ic.**

neuroma (nu-ro′mah) a tumor or new growth largely made up of nerve cells and nerve fibers. adj., **neurom′atous.**

acoustic n., a benign tumor within the auditory canal arising from the eighth cranial (acoustic) nerve.

amputation n., traumatic neuroma occurring after amputation of an extremity or part.

n. cu′tis, neuroma in the skin.

false n., one that does not contain nerve elements.

plexiform n., one made up of contorted nerve trunks.

n. telangiecto′des, one containing an excess of blood vessels.

traumatic n., an unorganized bulbous or nodular mass of nerve fibers and Schwann cells produced by hyperplasia of nerve fibers and their supporting tissues after accidental or purposeful sectioning of the nerve.

neuromalacia (nu″ro-mah-la′she-ah) morbid softening of the nerves.

neuromatosis (nu″ro-mah-to′sis) condition characterized by the presence of many neuromas.

neuromechanism (nu″ro-mek′ah-nizm) the structure and arrangement of the nervous system in regard to the regulation of the function of an organ.

neuromere (nu′ro-mēr) 1. any of a series of transitory segmental elevations in the wall of the neural tube in the developing embryo; also, such elevations in the wall of the mature rhombencephalon. 2. a part of the spinal cord to which a pair of dorsal roots and a pair of ventral roots are attached.

neuromuscular (nu″ro-mus′ku-lar) pertaining to the nerves and muscles.

neuromyelitis (nu″ro-mi″ĕ-li′tis) inflammation of nervous and medullary substance; myelitis attended with neuritis.

n. op′tica, combined demyelination of the optic nerve and spinal cord, with diminution of vision and possible blindness, flaccid paralysis of extremities, and sensory and genitourinary disturbances.

neuromyositis (nu″ro-mi″o-si′tis) neuritis blended with myositis.

neuron (nu′ron) nerve cell; any of the conducting cells of the nervous system, consisting of a cell body, containing the nucleus and its surrounding cytoplasm, and the axon and dendrites. (See Plate 12.) adj., **neuro′nal.** Neurons are highly specialized cells having two characteristic properties: irritability, which means they are capable of being stimulated; and conductivity, which means they are able to conduct impulses. They are composed of a cell body (neurosome or perikaryon), containing the nucleus and its surrounding cytoplasm and one or more processes (nerve fibers) extending from the body.

The processes or nerve fibers are actually extensions of the cytoplasm surrounding the nucleus of the neuron. A nerve cell may have only one such slender fiber extending from its body, in which case it is classified as unipolar. A neuron having two processes is bipolar, and one with three or more processes is multipolar. Most neurons are multipolar, this type of neuron being widely distributed throughout the central nervous system and autonomic ganglia. The multipolar neurons have a single process called an axon and several branched extensions called dendrites. The dendrites receive stimuli from other nerves or from a receptor organ, such as the skin or ear, and transmit them through the neuron to the axon. The axon conducts the impulses to the dendrite of another neuron or to an effector organ that is thereby stimulated to action.

Many processes are covered with a layer of lipid material called MYELIN. Peripheral nerve fibers have a thin outer covering called neurilemma.

TYPES OF NEURONS. Neurons that receive stimuli from the outside environment and transmit them toward the brain are called afferent or sensory neurons. Neurons that carry impulses in the opposite direction, away from the brain and other nerve centers to muscles, are called efferent or motor neurons, or motoneurons. Another type of nerve cell, the association or internuncial neuron, or interneuron, is found in the brain and spinal cord; these neurons conduct impulses from afferent to efferent neurons.

SYNAPSES. The point at which an impulse is transmitted from one neuron to another is called a synapse. The transmission is chemical in nature; that is, there is no direct contact between the axon of one neuron and the dendrites of another. The cholinergic nerves (parasympathetic nervous system) liberate at their axon endings a substance called acetylcholine, which acts as a stimulant to the dendrites of adjacent neurons. In a similar manner, the adrenergic nerves (sympathetic nervous system) liberate sympathin, a substance that closely resembles epinephrine and probably is identical to norepinephrine.

The synapse may involve one neuron in chemical contact with many adjacent neurons, or it may involve the axon terminals of one neuron and the dendrites of a succeeding neuron in a nerve pathway. There are many different patterns of synapses.

RECEPTOR END-ORGANS. The dendrites of the sensory neurons are designed to receive stimuli from various parts of the body. These dendrites are called receptor end-organs and are of three general types: exteroceptors, interoceptors, and proprioceptors. Their names give a clue to their specific function. The exteroceptors are located near the external surface of the body and receive impulses from the skin. They transmit information about the senses of touch, heat, cold, and other factors in the external environment. The interoceptors are located in the internal organs and receive information from the viscera, e.g., pressure, tension, and pain. The proprioceptors are found in muscles, tendons, and joints and transmit "muscle sense," by which one is aware of the position of his body in space.

NEURONS AND EFFECTORS. The axons of motor neurons form synapses with skeletal fibers to produce motion. These junctions are called motor end-plates or myoneural junctions. The axon of a motor neuron divides just before it enters the muscle fibers and forms synapses near the nuclei of muscle fibers. These motor neurons are called somatic efferent neurons. Visceral efferent neurons form synapses with smooth muscle, cardiac muscle, and glands.

Golgi n's, 1. (type I): pyramidal cells with long axons, which leave the gray matter of the central nervous system, traverse the white matter, and terminate in the periphery. 2. (type II): stellate neurons with short axons in the cerebral and cerebellar cortices and in the retina.

motor n., motoneuron.

postganglionic n's, neurons whose cell bodies lie in the autonomic ganglia and whose purpose is to relay impulses beyond the ganglia.

preganglionic n's, neurons whose cell bodies lie in the central nervous system and whose efferent fibers terminate in the autonomic ganglia.

neuronevus (nu″ro-ne′vus) a cellular or nevocytic nevus, especially a mature one with differentiation toward neural skin structures.

neuronophage (nu-ron′o-fāj) a phagocyte that destroys nerve cells.

neuronophagia (nu″ron-o-fa′je-ah) phagocytic destruction of nerve cells.

neuro-ophthalmology (nu″ro-of″thal-mol′o-je) that branch of ophthalmology dealing with portions of the nervous system related to the eye.

neuropapillitis (nu″ro-pap″ĭ-li′tis) optic NEURITIS affecting the part of the optic nerve within the eyeball.

neuroparalysis (nu″ro-pah-ral′ĭ-sis) paralysis due to disease of a nerve or nerves.

neuropathogenicity (nu″ro-path″o-jĕ-nis′ĭ-te) the quality of producing or the ability to produce pathologic changes in nerve tissue.

neuropathology (nu″ro-pah-thol′o-je) pathology of the nervous system.

neuropathy (nu-rop′ah-the) any functional disturbances and/or pathological changes in the peripheral nervous system; also used to denote nonspecific lesions, in contrast to inflammatory lesions (see also NEURITIS). adj., **neuropath′ic.**

ascending n., that progressing from the feet upwards to affect thigh, hip, trunk, etc.

descending n., that starting proximally (shoulder, hip) and spreading distally toward the limb extremities (hands, feet).

entrapment n., any of a group of neuropathies, e.g., carpal tunnel syndrome, due to mechanical pressure on a peripheral nerve.

progressive hypertrophic interstitial n., a slowly progressive familial disease beginning in early life, marked by hyperplasia of interstitial connective tissue, causing thickening of peripheral nerve trunks and posterior roots, and by sclerosis of the posterior columns of the spinal cord, with atrophy of distal parts of the legs and diminution of tendon reflexes and sensation. Called also Dejerine's disease and Dejerine-Sottas disease.

neuropharmacology (nu″ro-far″mah-kol′o-je) scientific study of the effects of drugs on the nervous system.

neurophthisis (nu-rof′thĭ-sis) wasting of nerve tissue.

neurophysiology (nu″ro-fiz″e-ol′o-je) physiology of the nervous system.

neuropil (nu′ro-pil) a dense feltwork of interwoven cytoplasmic processes of nerve cells (dendrites and axons) and of neuroglial cells in the central nervous system and some parts of the peripheral nervous system.

neuroplasm (nu′ro-plazm) the protoplasm of a nerve cell. adj., **neuroplas′mic.**

neuroplasty (nu′ro-plas″te) plastic repair of a nerve.

neuropodium (nu″ro-po′de-um) a bulbous termination of an axon in one type of synapse.

neuropore (nu′ro-pōr) an opening in the anterior or posterior end of the neural tube of the developing embryo that closes eventually.

neuropotential (nu″ro-po-ten′shal) nerve energy; nerve potential.

neuropsychiatrist (nu″ro-si-ki′ah-trist) a specialist in neuropsychiatry.

neuropsychiatry (nu″ro-si-ki′ah-tre) a branch of medicine combining neurology and psychiatry.

neuropsychopathy (nu″ro-si-kop′ah-the) a combined nervous and mental disease.

neuroradiology (nu″ro-ra″de-ol′o-je) radiology of the nervous system.

neurorecidive, neurorecurrence (nu″ro-res″ĭ-dēv′; nu″ro-re-ker′ens) neurorelapse.

neurorelapse (nu″ro-re-laps′) acute nervous symptoms precipitated by insufficient treatment of syphilis with arsphenamine.

neuroretinitis (nu″ro-ret″ĭ-ni′tis) inflammation of the optic nerve and retina.

neuroretinopathy (nu″ro-ret″ĭ-nop′ah-the) pathologic involvement of the optic disk and retina.

neuroroentgenography (nu″ro-rent″gen-og′rah-fe) neuroradiology.

neurorrhaphy (nu-ror′ah-fe) suture of a divided nerve.

neurosarcocleisis (nu″ro-sar″ko-kli′sis) an operation for neuralgia, done by relieving pressure on the affected nerve by partial resection of the bony canal through which it passes and transplanting the nerve among soft tissues.

neurosarcoma (nu″ro-sar-ko′mah) a sarcoma with neuromatous elements.

neurosclerosis (nu″ro-sklĕ-ro′sis) hardening of nerve tissue.

neurosecretion (nu″ro-se-kre′shun) secretory activities of nerve cells. adj., **neurosecre′tory.**

neurosis (nu-ro′sis), pl. *neuro′ses.* an emotional disorder that can interfere with a person's ability to lead a normal, useful life, or can impair his physical health; sometimes called psychoneurosis. adj., **neurot′ic.**

A neurosis is generally a milder form of mental illness than a PSYCHOSIS. Those persons with neurotic symptoms are usually in contact with reality; they are able to function in society even though they may feel uncomfortable or their efficiency may be impaired. By contrast, psychotic persons tend to withdraw from the real world into one of their own, or to act in strange, even bizarre, ways, and are often not aware of their illness.

CAUSES. Current theories agree that neuroses arise from mental conflicts rooted in a person's childhood. The budding personality handles these ever present conflicts by means of mental and defense mechanisms, including IDENTIFICATION, RATIONALIZATION, REPRESSION, PROJECTION, and others.

How each child uses these defense mechanisms in the process of maturing determines whether he will be healthy or neurotic. Symptoms such as obsessions, compulsions, phobias, and other behavior represent unsuccessful attempts to master these conflicts. These symptoms can be so mild as to be barely noticeable. They can sometimes even be useful: A compulsion for neatness makes a good craftsman. It is a rare person who does not at some time show some trace of neurotic symptoms or behavior. At the other extreme, neurotic patterns can be severe enough to warrant intensive treatment.

TYPES OF NEUROSES. Psychiatrists today prefer to call neuroses "reactions" because these conditions result from, or are reactions to, psychologic factors. At the time the word "neurosis" came into use, it was thought that disorders of the nervous system were responsible for neurotic symptoms, and the term is still very widely used to describe these conditions.

Types of neurosis include the neurotic character and the various specific neuroses. Specific neuroses may take a number of different forms, which are not necessarily clearly defined as separate. A person may have several different neurotic symptoms but usually one tends to dominate.

Neurotic Character. Practically everyone has unconscious conflicts to some extent. Most people take them in their stride. Some people, however, develop a neurotic character, and suffer from a general maladjustment to society. In most cases the neurotic cannot sustain satisfactory relationships in the world around him, though some of them are charming, attractive people. A neurotic character is more difficult to treat than a specific neurotic symptom. The patient with a specific neurosis usually senses that there is something wrong with him, but the patient with a neurotic character structure may not, since he has convinced himself his ways of behavior are reasonable.

Anxiety Neurosis. In this condition, the patient has periods of anxiety which can vary from mild uneasiness ("free-floating anxiety") to blind panic. The anxiety can produce a variety of physical symptoms such as sweating, dizziness, and shortness of breath.

Everyone occasionally experiences anxiety as a normal response to a dangerous or unusual situation. In anxiety neurosis the person feels the same emotion without any apparent reason. He cannot identify the source of the threat that produces his anxiety. The symptoms are the result of unconscious fears, which often are triggered by an apparently harmless stimulus that the patient unconsciously links with a deeply buried anxiety-producing experience.

Phobic Neurosis (Phobias). Phobic neurosis is an exaggerated fear. The feared objects, ideas, or situations are often symbolic of the unconscious conflict. They divert attention from the conflict, and thus help to keep it unconscious. The neurotic may make elaborate changes in his life to avoid the object of his fear, often with severe effects on his family and friends.

Before the roots of neurosis in psychologic conflicts were discovered, it was believed that the different phobias were separate conditions. Names were assigned to an almost endless list of fears. Some of these, such as claustrophobia, fear of enclosed spaces, have become fairly common words. Today, however, the treatment of phobic neurosis is concerned more with discovering and resolving the unconscious conflict that causes the fear than with the specific object that is feared.

Obsessive-Compulsive Neurosis. There are actually two different symptoms in this neurosis, although they are closely related and are often found in the same person. The obsessive symptom is an overwhelming intrusion of certain thoughts or desires into the mind. The patient does not know why these thoughts or desires keep intruding, but it is very difficult for him to eliminate them from his mind. The compulsive symptom is an uncontrollable urge to act in certain patterns. He does not know why he follows these patterns, but he is very uncomfortable if he does not.

The mild forms of these symptoms are familiar to most people. For example, most children play the game of avoiding the cracks on a sidewalk. As adults, they may find themselves doing this occasionally, perhaps when they are thinking over a problem. The neurotic who follows this pattern, however, will feel real anxiety if he steps on a crack in the sidewalk.

In phobias and obsessive-compulsive neurosis, the patient deflects, or displaces, the unresolved conflict onto an external object or action as a substitute. By doing this, the person tries to control the conflict magically and to eliminate his anxiety. The obsession or ritual probably represents a smokescreen which the mind throws up to keep the inner conflict from becoming conscious.

Depressive Neurosis. This is an excessively deep and long-lasting depression. It may be set off by an external event, such as the death of a loved one, or there may be no apparent cause.

Depression as such is not abnormal. The well-adjusted person, however, works out and absorbs his grief. He is soon able to resume his activities and reestablish social relationships. The neurotic is not able to escape his depression for any length of time.

The depressive neurotic suffers from a general slowing down of mental and physical activity. He may have symptoms such as insomnia, loss of appetite and lack of interest in outside activities. The condition can vary from very mild to extremely severe; in severe cases, the person may even attempt suicide.

Neurotic depression is closely associated with a lack of confidence and self-esteem and with an inability to express strong feelings. Repressed anger is thought to be a powerful contributor to depression. The person feels inadequate to cope with the situations that arise in everyday life and feels that he is insecure.

Dissociative Neurosis. In this condition, parts of the personality and memory become cut off from each other. At times, anxiety causes the person to forget who he is or what he is doing. When he regains his self-awareness, he does not recall what has taken place. An example of this is amnesia; a less severe form is sleepwalking.

A dissociative neurosis is very likely an attempt by the mind to shield itself from anxiety caused by an unresolved conflict. When the patient encounters a situation that may be symbolic of his inner conflict, he goes into a form of trance to avoid experiencing the conflict.

In a few extreme cases, dissociative neurosis may take the form of multiple personality. The change from one personality to another, with no conscious awareness of the other, takes place in situations of extreme emotional stress.

Conversion Neurosis. Conversion neurosis, or conversion reaction, is a severe form of hysteria, in which the person unconsciously converts his anxiety into a physical symptom. This symptom may be blindness, deafness, inability to speak, or paralysis of one or several limbs. The symptom is real, but there is no physical explanation for it. The symptom may disappear with as little apparent cause as it appeared.

The symptom in a conversion neurosis serves to spare the patient from dealing with an anxiety-producing situation that is too difficult to face. The best-known examples of this are shell shock and combat fatigue, in which the soldier becomes paralyzed and cannot participate in battle. The part of the body affected by conversion neurosis often has an important symbolic relationship to the patient's unconscious conflict. It may also be a part of the body which the patient considers weak.

Because the symptom is so obvious, a conversion neurosis is easily detected and diagnosed. It is a comparatively rare condition today.

PREVENTION. The formation of neurotic symptoms can be prevented to some extent. There is no doubt that a warm, secure home life, parental affection, and the proper balance between understanding and discipline promote a healthy soil for the sound development of the child. The overall solidity of the parents' relationship to their child is of enormous importance. However, other elements also play a role: Each child is born with different possibilities of reaction to the world around him. School and community influences are also meaningful. All these are also responsible to some degree for the mental health of everyone.

PSYCHOSOMATIC DISORDERS. Illnesses that result from the interaction of mind and body are known as psychosomatic disorders. They are an exaggerated physical reaction to emotional stress. Psychosomatic disorders usually affect only organs under the control of the autonomic nervous system, such as the digestive tract, the endocrine glands, the heart, the genitourinary, circulatory and respiratory systems, and the skin. Among illnesses known to be partly or completely psychosomatic illnesses are MIGRAINE, mucous COLITIS, ULCERATIVE COLITIS, peptic ULCER, SKIN allergies, and perhaps ASTHMA. Treatment must be directed at both the physical symptoms and the underlying psychologic cause. (See also PSYCHOSOMATIC DISEASE.)

TREATMENT. All neuroses are in part or entirely the result of unconscious conflicts and can be treated, even though the neurotic is entirely unaware of the conflicts. The form of treatment, PSYCHOTHERAPY, tries through many different methods to make the patient conscious of his unresolved conflict. Once he is aware of it, the therapist can help him resolve it.

neuroskeletal (nu″ro-skel′ĕ-tal) pertaining to nervous tissue and skeletal muscular tissue.

neuroskeleton (nu″ro-skel′ĕ-ton) endoskeleton.

neurosome (nu′ro-sōm) 1. the body of a nerve cell, or NEURON. 2. a small particle in the ground substance of the protoplasm of neurons.

neurospasm (nu′ro-spazm) nervous twitching of a muscle.

neurosplanchnic (nu″ro-splangk′nik) pertaining to the cerebrospinal and sympathetic nervous systems.

neurospongioma (nu″ro-spun″je-o′mah) neuroglioma.

neurospongium (nu″ro-spun′je-um) 1. the fibrillar component of neurons. 2. a meshwork of nerve fibrils, especially the inner reticular layer of the retina.

Neurospora (nu-ros′po-rah) a genus of fungi, comprising the bread molds, capable of converting tryptophan to niacin; used in genetic and enzyme research.

neurosurgeon (nu″ro-ser′jun) a physician who specializes in neurosurgery.

neurosurgery (nu″ro-ser′jer-e) surgery of the nervous system.

neurosuture (nu′ro-su″tūr) neurorrhaphy.

neurosyphilis (nu″ro-sif′ĭ-lis) syphilis of the nervous system.

paretic n., dementia paralytica.

tabetic n., tabes dorsalis.

neurotendinous (nu″ro-ten′dĭ-nus) pertaining to both nerve and tendon.

neurotherapy (nu″ro-ther′ah-pe) the treatment of nervous disorders.

neurotic (nu-rot′ik) 1. pertaining to or affected with a neurosis. 2. pertaining to the nerves. 3. a nervous person in whom emotions predominate over reason.

neuroticism (nu-rot′ĭ-sizm) a neurotic condition or trait.

neurotization (nu-rot″ĭ-za′shun) 1. regeneration of a nerve after its division. 2. the implantation of a nerve into a paralyzed muscle.

neurotmesis (nu″rot-me′sis) damage to a nerve, producing complete division of all the essential structures.

neurotome (nu′ro-tōm) 1. a needle-like knife for dissecting nerves. 2. neuromere.

neurotomy (nu-rot′o-me) dissection or cutting of nerves.

neurotony (nu-rot′o-ne) the surgical stretching of a nerve; neurectasia; neurectasis.

neurotoxicity (nu″ro-tok-sis′ĭ-te) the quality of exerting a destructive or poisonous effect upon nerve tissue. adj., **neurotox′ic.**

neurotoxin (nu″ro-tok′sin) a substance that is poisonous or destructive to nerve tissue.

neurotransmitter (nu″ro-trans′mit-er) a substance released at the synapse of a neuron that induces activity in susceptible cells.

neurotrauma (nu″ro-traw′mah) mechanical injury to nerve.

neurotrophy (nu-rot′ro-fe) nutrition and maintenance of tissues as regulated by nervous influence. adj., **neurotroph′ic.**

neurotropism (nu-rot′ro-pizm) 1. the quality of having a special affinity for nervous tissue. 2. the alleged tendency of regenerating nerve fibers to grow toward specific portions of the periphery. adj., **neurotrop′ic.**

neurotubule (nu″ro-too′būl) any of the long, straight, parallel tubules or canaliculi, 20 to 30 μm. in diameter, found in the axon, dendrites, and perikaryon of a neuron.

neurovaccine (nu″ro-vak′sēn) vaccine virus prepared by growing the virus in the brain of a rabbit.

neurovascular (nu″ro-vas′ku-ler) pertaining to both nervous and vascular elements, or to nerves controlling the caliber of blood vessels.

neurovisceral (nu″ro-vis′er-al) neurosplanchnic.

neurula (nu′roo-lah) the early embryonic stage following the gastrula, marked by the first appearance of the nervous system.

neurulation (nu″roo-la′shun) formation in the early embryo of the neural plate, followed by its closure with development of the neural tube.

Neusser's granules (noi′serz) basophil granules seen about the nuclei of leukocytes.

neutral (nu′tral) neither basic nor acid.

neutralize (nu′tral-īz) to render neutral.

Neutrapen (nu′trah-pen) trademark for a lyophilized preparation of penicillinase, an enzyme sometimes used to treat allergic reactions to penicillin.

neutrino (nu-tre′no) a subatomic particle with an extremely small mass and no electric charge.

neutrocyte (nu′tro-sīt) neutrophil (2).

neutron (nu′tron) an electrically neutral or uncharged particle of matter existing along with protons in the atoms of all elements except the mass 1 isotope of hydrogen.

neutropenia (nu″tro-pe′ne-ah) diminished number of neutrophils in the blood.

cyclic n., periodic neutropenia.

malignant n., agranulocytosis.

periodic n., a chronic form marked by regular, periodic episodic recurrences, associated with malaise, fever, stomatitis, and various infections.

neutrophil (nu′tro-fil) 1. a granular leukocyte having a nucleus with three to five lobes connected by threads of chromatin, and cytoplasm containing very fine granules; called also polymorphonuclear leukocyte. (See also HETEROPHIL.) 2. any cell, structure, or histologic element readily stainable with neutral dyes.

stab n., a neutrophilic leukocyte whose nucleus is not divided into segments.

neutrophilia (nu″tro-fil′e-ah) increase in the number of neutrophils in the blood.

neutrophilic (nu″tro-fil′ik) 1. pertaining to neutrophils. 2. stainable by neutral dyes.

nevocarcinoma (ne″vo-kar″sin-o′mah) malignant melanoma.

nevoid (ne′void) resembling a nevus.

nevoxanthoendothelioma (ne″vo-zan″tho-en″do-the″le-o′mah) a condition in which groups of yellow-brown papules or nodules occur on the extensor surfaces of the extremities of infants.

nevus (ne′vus), pl. *ne′vi* [L.] a circumscribed stable malformation of the skin and occasionally of the oral mucosa, which is not due to external causes; the excess (or deficiency) of tissue may involve epidermal, connective tissue, adnexal, nervous, or vascular elements; called also mole.

Most moles are either brown, black, or flesh-colored; they may appear on any part of the skin. They vary in size and thickness, and occur in groups or singly. Usually they are not disfiguring.

A nevus is usually not troublesome unless it is unsightly or unless it becomes inflamed or cancerous. Fortunately, nevi seldom become cancerous; when they do, the cause is often constant irritation. Any change in size, color, or texture of a mole, or any excessive itching or any bleeding, should be reported to a physician. Moles can be removed by surgery or by one of several other methods, such as the application of solid carbon dioxide, injections, and radium treatment.

n. arachnoi′deus, n. araneo′sus, n. ara′neus, one composed of dilated blood vessels radiating from a point in branches resembling the legs of a spider (see also vascular SPIDER).

blue n., a dark blue nodular lesion composed of closely grouped melanocytes and melanophages situated in the mid-dermis.

blue rubber bleb n., a hereditary condition marked by multiple bluish cutaneous hemangiomas with soft raised centers, frequently associated with hemangiomas of the gastrointestinal tract.

n. comedon′icus, a rare epidermal nevus marked by one or more patches 2 to 5 cm. or more in diameter, in which there are collections of large comedones or comedo-like lesions.

connective tissue n., any nevus occurring in the dermal connective tissue and characterized by nodules, papules, or plaques, or by combinations of such lesions. Histologically, there is inconstant focal or diffuse thickening and abnormal staining of collagen.

epidermal nevi, congenital skin tumors that do not contain melanocytes, which vary widely in appearance, size, and distribution, and which are commonly hyperkeratotic.

n. flam′meus, a diffuse, poorly defined area varying from pink to dark bluish red, involving otherwise normal skin; port-wine stain.

hairy n., a more or less pigmented nevus with hairs growing from its surface.

halo n., a pigmented nevus surrounded by a ring of depigmentation; called also leukoderma acquisitum centrifugum and Sutton's disease or nevus.

intradermal n., a nevocytic nevus in which the nevus cells occur in nests in the upper part of the dermis, with no evidence of the proliferative process by which they orginated.

n. of Ito, a mongolian spot in the distribution of the posterior supraclavicular and lateral cutaneous brachial nerves, over the shoulder.

junction n., a brownish, smooth, flat or slightly raised nevocytic nevus; histologically, there are nests of melanin-containing nevus cells at the dermoepidermal junction.

n. lipomato′sus, one that contains much fibrofatty tissue.

melanocytic n., any nevus, usually pigmented, composed of melanocytes.

nevocytic n., nevus-cell n., the common mole; a usually more or less hyperpigmented nevus, initially flat but soon becoming elevated, composed of nests of nevus cells.

n. of Ota, a mongolian spot, usually unilateral, involving the conjunctiva and eyelids, as well as adjacent facial skin, sclera, ocular muscles, and periosteum; rarely, malignant melanoma may develop, usually in the iris.

pigmented n., n. pigmento′sus, one containing melanin; the term is usually restricted to nevocytic nevi (moles), but may be applied to other pigmented nevi.

sebaceous n., sebaceous n. of Jadassohn, an epidermal nevus of the scalp or less often the face, frequently growing larger during puberty or early adult life, and rarely giving rise to a variety of new growths, including basal cell carcinoma.

spider n., nevus arachnoideus.

n. spi′lus, a smooth, tan to brown, macular nevus composed of melanocytes and speckled with smaller, darker macules.

n. spongio′sus al′bus, a white sponge nevus.

n. un′ius lat′eris, a verrucous epidermal nevus occurring as a linear band, patch, or streak, usually along the margin between two neuromeres on the side of the trunk.

n. vascular′is, n. vasculo′sus, a reddish swelling or patch on the skin due to hypertrophy of the skin capillaries: the term includes nevus flammeus, the elevated strawberry marks, blue rubber bleb nevus, vascular spider, and cavernous hemangioma.

white sponge n., a white spongy nevus of a mucous membrane, occurring as a hereditary condition.

newborn (nu′born) 1. recently born. 2. a human infant during the first 4 weeks after birth.

Newcastle disease (nu′kas-el) a viral disease of birds, including domestic fowl, characterized by respiratory and gastrointestinal or pneumonic and encephalitic symptoms; also transmissible to man.

newton (nu′ton) the SI unit of force; the force that, when acting continuously upon a mass of 1 kilogram, will impart to it an acceleration of 1 meter per second per second.

nexus (nek′sus) a bond, as between members of a series or group.

N.F. National Formulary, a publication of the American Pharmaceutical Association, revised at 5-year intervals, establishing official standards for therapeutically useful drugs.

N.F.L.P.N. National Federation of Licensed Practical Nurses.

ng. nanogram.

N.H.I. National Health Insurance; National Heart Institute.

N.H.L.I. National Heart and Lung Institute.

Ni chemical symbol, *nickel.*

niacin (ni′ah-sin) a water-soluble vitamin of the B complex found in various animal and plant tissues, especially liver, yeast, bran, peanuts, lean meats, fish, and poultry, and first prepared by the oxidation of nicotine. Called also nicotinic acid. It is important because of its biochemical role in the body, its pellagra-curative property, and its vasodilating action. A well balanced diet usually supplies more than the daily requirement. Niacinamide, a related compound, is usually used as the vitamin supplement, because niacin produces peripheral vasodilation with flushing of the skin. These effects are useful in some conditions, however, and niacin is used to improve peripheral circulation in MENIÈRE'S DISEASE, MIGRAIN, and peripheral vascular disease. It is also used to depress the blood cholesterol level.

niacinamide (ni″ah-sin-am′īd) the amide of niacin, differing from niacin in not having its vasodilating action, occurring naturally in the body and interconvertible with niacin; a preparation is used in treating pellagra.

NIAID National Institute of Allergy and Infectious Diseases.

nialamide (ni-al′ah-mīd) a monoamine oxidase inhibitor used as an antidepressant.

NIAMD National Institute of Arthritis and Metabolic Diseases.

Niamid (ni′ah-mid) trademark for a preparation of nialamide, an antidepressant.

niche (nich) a small recess, depression or indentation, especially a recess in the wall of a hollow organ that tends to retain contrast media, as revealed by roentgenography.

NICHHD National Institute of Child Health and Human Development.

nickel (nik′el) a chemical element, atomic number 28, atomic weight 58.71, symbol Ni. (See table of ELEMENTS.)

nicking (nik′ing) localized constriction of the retinal blood vessels.

niclosamide (nĭ-klo′sah-mīd) an anthelmintic.

Nicolas-Favre disease (ne-ko-lah′ fav′r) lymphogranuloma venereum.

Niconyl (ni′ko-nil) trademark for a preparation of isoniazid, used in the treatment of tuberculosis.

nicotinamide (nik″o-tin′ah-mīd) niacinamide.

n.-adenine dinucleotide (NAD), a coenzyme widely distributed in nature and involved in electron transfer in mitochondria; the products of its hydrolysis are 1 molecule each of adenine and nicotinamide and 2 each of *d*-ribose and phosphoric acid. Called also coenzyme I (CoI).

n.-adenine dinucleotide phosphate (NADP), a coenzyme required for a limited number of reactions, similar to nicotinamide-adenine dinucleotide, except for inclusion of 3 phosphate units. Called also coenzyme II (CoII).

nicotine (nik′o-tēn, nik′o-tin) a very poisonous alkaloid that in its pure state is a colorless, pungent, oily liquid, having an acrid burning taste. It is a constituent of tobacco, and is produced synthetically. In water solution, it is sometimes used as an insecticide and plant spray.

Although nicotine is highly toxic, the amount inhaled while smoking tobacco is too small to cause death. The nicotine in tobacco can, however, cause indigestion and increase in blood pressure, and dull the appetite. It also acts as a vasoconstrictor. Medical authorities link SMOKING with heart disease, lung cancer, and other diseases.

nicotinic acid (nik″o-tin′ik) NIACIN, the antipellagra factor of the vitamin B complex.

nicotinism (nik′o-tin-izm″) nicotine poisoning, marked by stimulation and subsequent depression of the central and autonomic nervous systems, with death due to respiratory paralysis.

nicoumalone (ni-koo′mah-lōn) acenocoumarol, an anticoagulant.

nictitation (nik″tĭ-ta′shun) the act of winking.

nidation (ni-da′shun) implantation of the fertilized ovum (zygote) in the endometrium of the uterus in pregnancy.

NIDR National Institute of Dental Research.

nidus (ni′dus), pl. *ni′di* [L.] 1. a nest; point of origin or focus of a morbid process. 2. nucleus (2). adj., **ni′dal.**

Niemann-Pick disease (ne′man pik) a rare hereditary disease with massive enlargement of the liver and spleen, brownish yellow discoloration of the skin, and nervous system dysfunction. Foamy reticular cells containing phospholipids infiltrate the liver, spleen, lungs, lymph nodes, and bone marrow. It occurs chiefly in Jewish chidren.

nifuroxime (ni″fūr-ok′sim) an antibacterial and antitrichomonal agent.

night blindness inability or a reduced ability to see in dim light. In night blindness, the eyes not only see more poorly in dim light, but are slower to adjust from brightness to dimness.

Depending on its brightness, light is perceived by either of two sets of visual cells located in the retina of the eye. One set, the cones, perceive bright light primarily; the other set, the rods, perceive dim light primarily. Dim light produces a change in a pigment called rhodopsin in the rods. This change causes nerve impulses to travel to the brain, where they register as visual impressions. Night blindness occurs when the rods lack rhodopsin.

One cause of night blindness is a deficiency of vitamin A—the primary source of rhodopsin. The defect in vision usually can be cured by proper diet plus therapeutic doses of the deficient vitamin.

In the elderly, there is sometimes a diminution of rhodopsin, with resulting night blindness. Other losses in vision may follow. Diminished blood supply to the eyes is thought to be a cause of this form of the condition. Treatment generally is only of limited effectiveness.

Night blindness sometimes accompanies glaucoma.

Nightingale (nīt′in-gāl″) Florence (1820–1910). Founder of modern nursing. Born in Florence, Italy, of wealthy English parents, Miss Nightingale in 1854 led a group of nurses to the Crimea to care for English troops, and proceeded to reorganize military nursing and sanitation in England and later in India. She contributed to the field of dietetics, and her skill as a statistician in gathering data won her election to the Royal Statistical Society and honorary membership in the American Statistical Association.

Nightingale Pledge an oath frequently taken by nurses at capping ceremonies or upon graduation from a school of nursing. It was written in 1893 by a committee of which Mrs. Lystra E. Gretter was chairman and was first administered to the 1893 graduating class of the Farrand Training School, Harper Hospital, Detroit, Michigan. It is as follows:

I solemnly pledge myself before God and in the presence of this assembly:

To pass my life in purity and to practice my profession faithfully.

I will abstain from whatever is deleterious and mischievous, and will not take or knowingly administer any harmful drug.

I will do all in my power to elevate the standard of my profession, and will hold in confidence all personal matters committed to my keeping and all family affairs coming to my knowledge in the practice of my profession.

With loyalty will I endeavor to aid the physician in his work, and devote myself to the welfare of those committed to my care.

nightmare (nīt′mār) a frightening dream, especially one that is so terrifying or disturbing that it causes the sleeper to wake up.

nightshade (nīt′shād) a plant of the genus *Solanum.*

deadly n., belladonna leaf.

NIGMS National Institute of General Medical Sciences.

nigra (ni′grah) [L. black] substantia nigra. adj., **ni′gral.**

nigrities (ni-grish′e-ēz) blackness.

n. lin′guae, black tongue.

nigrosin (ni′gro-sin) an aniline dye having a special affinity for ganglion cells.

N.I.H. National Institutes of Health.

nihilism (ni′ĕ-lizm) in psychiatry, the delusion of nonexistence of the self, part of the self, or of some object in external reality. adj., **nihilis′tic.**

nikethamide (nĭ-keth′ah-mīd) a central and respiratory stimulant.

Nikolsky's sign (nĭ-kol′skēz) in pemphigus vulgaris and some other bullous diseases, the outer epidermis separates easily from the basal layer on exertion of firm sliding manual pressure.

Nilevar (ni′le-var) trademark for preparations of norethandrolone, a synthetic androgen.

NIMH National Institute of Mental Health.

NINDB National Institute of Neurological Diseases and Blindness.

niobium (ni-o′be-um) a chemical element, atomic number 1, atomic weight 92.906, symbol Nb. (See table of ELEMENTS.)

Nionate (ni′o-nāt) trademark for a preparation of ferrous gluconate, a hematinic.

niphablepsia (nif″ah-blep′se-ah) snow blindness.

nipple (nip″l) the pigmented projection at the tip of each BREAST, which gives outlet to milk from the breast. Also, any similarly shaped structure. The nipples are located slightly to the side rather than in the middle of the breasts. Usually, the size of the nipple is in proportion to the size of the breast, but large nipples may be found on small breasts and vice versa. In men, the nipple is smaller than in women.

Surrounding the nipple is a pigmented area called the areola. The color of the areola varies with the complexion. In childless women, it is usually reddish. During pregnancy it increases in size and darkens in color, becoming almost black in brunettes. The color fades after the milk-producing period ends.

The tip of the female nipple contains tiny depressions that are openings of the lactiferous ducts. During pregnancy special care should be given the nipples. Any secretion that accumulates should be gently washed off. If the nipples are tender, the physician will advise the use of cold cream, cocoa butter, lanolin, or another emollient to increase their pliability.

If nipples are inverted, a woman may make them protrude by gently pressing with the fingers while applying cream or oil. It may be necessary to use a breast pump to evert the nipples.

PAGET'S DISEASE of the breast, a rare type of breast cancer, causes ulceration and itching of the nipple. A physician should be consulted immediately.

Nisentil (ni″sen-til) trademark for a preparation of alphaprodine, a narcotic analgesic.

Nissl bodies (granules) (nis″l) large granular bodies that stain with basic dyes, forming the substance of the reticulum of the cytoplasm of a nerve cell. Ribonucleoprotein is one of the main constituents.

nisobamate (ni″so-bam′āt) a minor tranquilizer, sedative, and hypnotic.

Nisulfazole (ni-sul′fah-zōl) trademark for a preparation of para-nitrosulfathiazole, an antibacterial.

nisus (ni′sus) [L.] an effort, strong tendency, or molimen.

nit (nit) the egg of a louse.

niter (ni′ter) potassium nitrate.

niton (ni′ton) radon.

Nitranitol (ni′trah-ni″tol) trademark for preparations of mannitol hexanitrate, a vasodilator.

nitrate (ni′trāt) any salt of nitric acid; organic nitrates are used in the treatment of angina pectoris.

nitre (ni′ter) potassium nitrate.

nitremia (ni-tre′me-ah) excess of nitrogen in the blood.

Nitretamin (ni-tre′tah-min) trademark for preparations of trolnitrate, a vasodilator.

nitric (ni′trik) pertaining to or containing nitrogen in one of its higher valences.

n. acid., a highly caustic, fuming acid that has a characteristic choking odor. It is sometimes used in the immediate treatment of animal bites to prevent rabies, and as a cauterizing agent in the eradication of various kinds of warts. It is also used in the form of its potassium and sodium salts. It can be fatal if swallowed, and large amounts of nitric acid applied to the skin can cause necrosis. The antidote for nitric acid poisoning is an alkali or sodium bicarbonate applied liberally.

nitride (ni′trīd) a binary compound of nitrogen with a metal.

nitrification (ni″trĭ-fĭ-ka′shun) the bacterial oxidation of ammonia and organic nitrogen to nitrites and nitrates in the soil.

nitrifying (ni′trĭ-fi″ing) oxidizing nitrites into nitrates; said of certain nitrogen bacteria.

nitrile (ni′tril) an organic compound containing trivalent nitrogen attached to one carbon atom, ·C⋮⋮N.

nitrite (ni′trīt) any salt of nitrous acid; organic nitrites are used in the treatment of angina pectoris.

Nitrobacter (ni″tro-bak′ter) a genus of bacteria (family Nitrobacteraceae) that oxidize nitrites to nitrates.

Nitrobacteraceae (ni″tro-bak″te-ra′se-e) a family of bacteria (order Pseudomonadales), deriving energy solely from oxidation of ammonia to nitrite, or of nitrite to nitrate; known informally as nitrifying bacteria.

nitrobenzene (ni″tro-ben′zēn) a poisonous benzol derivative.

nitrocellulose (ni″tro-sel′u-lōs) pyroxylin, a base that is dissolved in alcohol or ether to form collodion.

Nitrocystis (ni″tro-sis′tis) a genus of nitrifying bacteria (family Nitrobacteraceae), which are embedded in slime to form zooglea.

nitrodan (ni′tro-dan) an anthelmintic.

nitrofuran (ni″tro-fu′ran) any of a group of antibacterials, including nitrofurantoin, nitrofurazone, etc., that are effective against a wide range of bacteria.

nitrofurantoin (ni″tro-fu-ran′to-in) an antibacterial agent used in treatment of urinary tract infections.

nitrofurazone (ni″tro-fu′rah-zōn) a local anti-infective.

nitrogen (ni′tro-jen) a chemical element, atomic number 7, atomic weight 14.007, symbol N. (See table of ELEMENTS.) It is a gas constituting about four-fifths of common air; chemically it is almost inert.

n. balance, the state of the body in regard to ingestion and excretion of nitrogen. In negative nitrogen balance the amount of nitrogen excreted is greater than the quantity ingested; in positive nitrogen balance the amount excreted is smaller than the amount ingested.

n. cycle, the steps by which nitrogen is extracted from the nitrates of soil and water, incorporated as amino acids and proteins in the body of living organisms, and ultimately reconverted to nitrates (see also nitrogen CYCLE).

n. monoxide, nitrous oxide, a general anesthetic and analgesic.

n. mustards, a group of toxic, blistering alkylating agents, including nitrogen mustard itself (mechlorethamine hydrochloride) and related compounds; some have been used as antineoplastics in certain forms of cancer. Nitrogen mustards do not cure these conditions, but ease their effects by destroying mitotic cells—those newly formed by division—thereby affecting malignant tissue in its early stage of development, and leaving normal tissue unaffected. They are especially useful in the treatment of leukemia, in which they reduce the leukocyte count, and in cases in which the malignant disease is widespread throughout the body and therefore cannot be effectively treated locally by surgery or radiotherapy. In cases of lung cancer, mechlorethamine hydrochloride is usually injected directly into the lungs via the pulmonary circulation. Side effects, which tend to limit the usefulness of these drugs, include nausea, vomiting, and a decrease in bone marrow production.

nonprotein n., NPN, the nitrogenous constituents of the blood exclusive of the protein bodies, consisting of the nitrogen of urea, uric acid, creatine, creatinine, amino acids, polypeptides, and an undetermined part known as rest nitrogen.

Measurement of nonprotein nitrogen is used as a test of renal function. Normally nonprotein nitrogen substances are excreted by the kidneys as end products of protein metabolism; their accumulation in the blood may indicate kidney disease, urinary retention, decrease in urinary output, or circulatory disease that impairs the supply of blood to the kidneys. The normal range for nonprotein nitrogen is 15 to 35 mg. per 100 ml. of blood. No special preparation is necessary for this test.

nitrogenous (ni-troj′ĕ-nus) containing nitrogen.

nitroglycerin (ni″tro-glis′er-in) a chemical well known as an explosive but also possessing medical uses; called also glyceryl trinitrate.

Nitroglycerin is a vasodilator and is used medically to relieve certain types of pain, especially in the prophylaxis and treatment of ANGINA PECTORIS. Generally the nitroglycerin tablet is placed under the tongue when the attack occurs; it quickly dissolves and gives relief within 1 or 2 minutes. It is not effective when swallowed. It may cause transient palpitation, flushing, faintness, and perhaps headache.

The patient who is taking nitroglycerin should keep the medication with him at all times. It should be kept in a tightly closed, dark, glass container, free from heat and moisture. The drug is not addicting and there is no limit to the number that may be taken in a 24-hour period; however, no more than three tablets should be taken at 5 minute intervals during an attack. If no relief is obtained 15 minutes after the third tablet is taken, the physician should be notified immediately.

Nitroglyn (ni′tro-glin) trademark for a preparation of nitroglycerin, a vasodilator.

Nitrol (ni′trol) trademark for a preparation of nitroglycerin, a vasodilator.

nitromannite (ni″tro-man′īt) mannitol hexanitrate, a vasodilator.

nitromersol (ni″tro-mer′sol) a local anti-infective; used topically in tincture or solution.

nitrous (ni′trus) pertaining to or containing nitrogen in its lowest valence.

n. acid, an unstable compound with which free amino groups react to form hydroxyl groups and liberate gaseous nitrogen. It is used in the determination of urea, the N_2 being collected and measured. Also used in the form of its potassium and sodium salts.

n. oxide, a gas used by inhalation as a general anesthetic; called also laughing gas. (See also ANESTHETIC.)

Nitrovas (ni′tro-vas) trademark for a preparation of nitroglycerin, a vasodilator.

N.L.N. National League for Nursing.

N.M.S.S. National Multiple Sclerosis Society.

No chemical symbol, *nobelium.*

nobelium (no-be′le-um) a chemical element, atomic number 102, atomic weight 253, symbol No. (See table of ELEMENTS.)

Nocardia (no-kar′de-ah) a genus of bacteria (family Actinomycetaceae), including *N. asteroi′des,* which produces a tuberculosis-like infection in man, and *N. farci′na* (probably identical with *N. asteroides*), which produces a tuberculosis-like infection in cattle.

nocardial (no-kar′de-al) pertaining to or caused by *Nocardia.*

nocardiosis (no-kar″de-o′sis) infection with *Nocardia.*

noci- word element [L.], *harm; injury.*

nociassociation (no″se-ah-so″se-a′shun) unconscious discharge of nervous energy under the stimulus of trauma.

nociceptor (no″se-sep′tor) a receptor that is stimulated by injury; a receptor for pain. adj., **nocicep′tive.**

noci-influence (no″se-in′floo-ens) injurious or traumatic influence.

nociperception (no″se-per-sep′shun) the perception of traumatic stimuli.

noctalbuminuria (nok″tal-bu″mĭ-nu′re-ah) excess of albumin in the urine secreted at night.

Noctec (nok′tek) trademark for preparations of chloral hydrate, a hypnotic and sedative.

noctiphobia (nok″tĭ-fo′be-ah) morbid dread of night.

nocturia (nok-tu′re-ah) excessive urination at night.

node (nōd) a small mass of tissue in the form of a swelling, knot, or protuberance, either normal or pathological. adj., **no′dal.**

n. of Aschoff and Tawara, atrioventricular node.

atrioventricular (A-V) n., a collection of cardiac fibers at the base of the interatrial septum that transmits the cardiac impulse initiated by the sinoatrial node (see also ATRIOVENTRICULAR NODE).

Bouchard's n's, cartilaginous and bony enlargements of the proximal interphalangeal joints of the fingers in degenerative joint disease.

Delphian n., a lymph node encased in the fascia in the midline just above the thyroid isthmus, so called because it is exposed first at operation and, if diseased, is indicative of disease of the thyroid gland.

Flack's n., sinoatrial node.

Haygarth's n's, joint swellings in rheumatoid arthritis.

Heberden's n's, nodular protrusions on the phalanges at the distal interphalangeal joints of the fingers in osteoarthritis.

hemal n's, nodes with a rich content of erythrocytes within sinuses, found near large blood vessels along the ventral side of the vertebrae in various mammals, especially ruminants, having functions probably like those of the spleen; their presence in man is doubtful.

Keith's n., Keith-Flack n., sinoatrial node.

Legendre's n's, Bouchard's nodes.

lymph n., any of the accumulations of lymphoid tissue organized as definite lymphatic organs along the course of lymphatic vessels, consisting of an outer cortical and inner medullary part (see also LYMPH NODE).

Meynet's n's, nodules in the capsules of joints and in tendons in rheumatic conditions, especially in children.

Osler's n's, small, raised, swollen, tender areas, bluish or sometimes pink or red, occurring commonly in the pads of the fingers or toes, in the thenar or hypothenar eminences or the soles of the feet; they are practically pathognomonic of subacute bacterial endocarditis.

Parrot's n., bony nodes on the outer table of the skull of infants with congenital syphilis.

n's of Ranvier, constrictions of myelinated nerve fibers at regular intervals at which the myelin sheath is absent and the axon is enclosed only by Schwann cell processes (see Plate 12).

Schmorl's n., an irregular or hemispherical bone defect in the upper or lower margin of the body of a vertebra into which the nucleus pulposus of the intervertebral disk herniates.

sentinel n., signal n., an enlarged supraclavicular lymph node; often the first sign of a malignant abdominal tumor.

singer's n., a small, white nodule on the vocal cord; the condition occurs in persons who use their voices excessively.

sinoatrial (S-A) n., a collection of atypical muscle fibers in the wall of the right atrium where the rhythm of cardiac contraction is usually established; therefore also referred to as the pacemaker of the heart.

syphilitic n., a swelling on a bone due to syphilitic periostitis.

n. of Tawara, atrioventricular node.

teacher's n., singer's node.

Troisier's n., Virchow's n., sentinel node.

nodi (no′di) plural of *nodus.*

nodose (no′dōs) having nodes or projections.

nodosity (no-dos′ĭ-te) 1. a node. 2. the quality of being nodose.

nodular (nod′u-lar) marked with, or resembling, nodules.

nodulation (nod″u-la′shun) the formation of or presence of nodules.

nodule (nod′ūl) a small boss or node that is solid and can be detected by touch.

Albini's n's, gray nodules of the size of small grains, sometimes seen on the free edges of the atrioventricular valves of infants; they are remains of fetal structures.

apple jelly n's, minute, yellowish or reddish brown, translucent nodules, seen on diascopic examination of the lesions of lupus vulgaris.

Aschoff's n's, Aschoff's bodies.

Gamna n's, brown or yellow pigmented nodules seen in the spleen in certain cases of enlargement, such as Gamna's disease and siderotic splenomegaly.

Jeanselme's n's, juxta-articular n's, gummata of tertiary syphilis and of nonvenereal treponemal diseases, located on joint capsules, bursae, or tendon sheaths.

lymphatic n., 1. lymph node. 2. lymph follicle.

milker's n's, hard circumscribed nodules on the hands of those who milk cows affected with cowpox.

rheumatic n's, small, round or oval, mostly subcutaneous nodules made up chiefly of a mass of Aschoff bodies and seen in rheumatic fever.

Schmorl's n., Schmorl's node.

surfer's n's, hyperplastic, fibrosing granulomas occurring over bony prominences of the feet and legs as a result of repeated trauma from kneeling on surfboards.

typhus n's, minute skin nodules formed by perivascular infiltration of mononuclear cells in typhus.

n. of vermis, the part of the vermis of the cerebellum, on the ventral surface, where the inferior medullary velum attaches.

nodulus (nod′u-lus), pl. *nod′uli* [L.] nodule.

nodus (no′dus), pl. *no′di* [L.] node.

Noguchia (no-goo′che-ah) a genus of gram-negative bacteria (family Brucellaceae) found in the conjunctiva of man and animals having a follicular disease.

Noludar (nol'u-dar) trademark for preparations of methyprylon, a sedative.

noma (no'mah) gangrenous processes of the mouth or genitalia. In the mouth (cancrum oris, gangrenous stomatitis), it begins as a small gingival ulcer and results in gangrenous necrosis of surrounding facial tissues; on the genitalia (cancrum pudendi, noma pudendi, noma vulvae), it affects one labium majus and then the other.

nomenclature (no'men-kla"chur) terminology; a classified system of technical names, as of anatomical structures, organisms, etc.

binomial n., the system of designating plants and animals by two latinized words signifying the genus and species.

Nomina Anatomica (no'mi-nah an"ah-tom'ĭ-kah) the internationally approved official body of anatomic nomenclature; abbreviated NA.

nomogram (nom'o-gram) the graphic representation produced in nomography; a chart or diagram on which a number of variables are plotted, forming a computation chart for the solution of complex numerical formulae.

nomography (no-mog'rah-fe) a graphic method of representing the relation between any number of variables.

nomotopic (no"mo-top'ik) occurring at a normal place.

nonan (no'nan) recurring on the ninth day (every eight days).

non compos mentis (non kom'pos men'tis) [L.] not of sound mind.

nonconductor (non"kon-duk'tor) a substance that does not readily transmit electricity, light, or heat.

nondisjunction (non"dis-jungk'shun) failure (*a*) of two homologous chromosomes to pass to separate cells during the first division of meiosis, or (*b*) of the two chromatids of a chromosome to pass to separate cells during mitosis or during the second meiotic division. As a result, one daughter cell has two chromosomes or two chromatids, and the other has none.

nonelectrolyte (non"e-lek'tro-lit) a compound which, dissolved in water, does not separate into charged particles and is incapable of conducting an electric current.

nonigravida (no"ne-grav'ĭ-dah) a woman pregnant for the ninth time.

nonoxynol (no-noks'ĭ-nol) a group of compounds of the general composition, $C_{15}H_{24}O(C_2H_4O)_n$, which are assigned a number according to the value of *n*. Nonoxynol 4, 15, and 30 nonionic surfactants; nonoxynol 9 is a spermaticide.

nonprotein nitrogen (non-pro'te-in) NPN; the nitrogenous constituents of the blood exclusive of the protein bodies; measurement of NPN is used as a test of renal function. (See also nonprotein NITROGEN.)

nonsecretor (non"se-kre'tor) a person with A or B type blood whose body secretions do not contain the particular (A or B) substance.

nonunion (non-ūn'yun) failure of the ends of a fractured bone to unite.

nonviable (non-vi'ah-b'l) not capable of living.

Noonan's syndrome (noo'nanz) the male phenotype of Turner's syndrome, with short stature, webbed neck, low nuchal hairline, low-set ears, and cubitus valgus; valvular pulmonary stenosis, rather than coarctation of the aorta, is often present.

noopsyche (no'o-si"ke) the intellectual processes of the mind.

noracymethadol (nor"ah-sĭ-meth'ah-dōl) an analgesic, used as the hydrochloride salt.

noradrenalin (nor"ah-dren'ah-lin) · norepinephrine.

norbolethone (nor-bol'ĕ-thōn) an anabolic steroid.

nordefrin (nor'dĕ-frin) used as a vasoconstrictor in the form of the hydrochloride salt.

norepinephrine (nor"ep-ĭ-nef'rin) a hormone secreted by neurons which acts as a transmitter substance of the peripheral sympathetic nerve endings and probably of certain synapses in the central nervous system; also secreted by the adrenal medulla in response to splanchnic stimulation and released predominantly in response to hypotension. A synthetic compound (levarterenol) is used as a vasopressor.

norethandrolone (nor"eth-an'dro-lōn) a synthetic androgen equal to testosterone in anabolic activity, but having less androgenic activity.

norethindrone (nor-eth'in-drōn) a progestational agent similar in action to progesterone; also used in combination with mestranol as an oral contraceptive.

norethynodrel (nor"ĕ-thi'no-drel) a progestin, used alone as a gestational agent and, in combination with mestranol, as an oral contraceptive.

norflurane (nor-flo͞or'ān) an inhalation anesthetic.

norgestrel (nor-jes'trel) a potent progestin used as an antifertility agent.

Norisodrine (nor-i'so-drin) trademark for preparations of isoproterenol, a sympathomimetic, used chiefly as a bronchodilator.

Norlutin (nor-lu'tin) trademark for a preparation of norethindrone, a progestational agent.

norm (norm) a fixed or ideal standard.

norm(o)- word element [L.], *normal; usual; conforming to the rule.*

normal (nor'mal) 1. agreeing with the regular and established type. When said of a solution, it denotes one containing in each 1000 ml., 1 gram equivalent weight of the active substance (see also N [3]). 2. in bacteriology, not immunized or otherwise bacteriologically treated.

normetanephrine (nor"met-ah-nef'rin) metabolite of norepinephrine excreted in the urine and found in certain tissues.

normoblast (nor'mo-blast) a nucleated precursor cell in the erythrocytic series. adj., **normoblas'tic.** Four developmental stages are recognized: the PRONORMOBLAST; the basophilic normoblast (basophilic erythroblast), in which the cytoplasm is basophilic, the nucleus is large with clumped chromatin, and the nuclei have disappeared; the polychromatic normoblast (polychromatic erythroblast), in which the nuclear chromatin shows increased clumping and the cytoplasm begins to acquire hemoglobin and taken on an acidophilic tint; and the orthochromatic normoblast (acidophilic normoblast; orthochromatic erythroblast), the final stage before nuclear loss, in which the nucleus is small and ultimately becomes a blue-black homogeneous structureless mass.

normoblastosis (nor″mo-blas-to′sis) excessive production of normoblasts by the bone marrow.

normocalcemia (nor″mo-kal-se′me-ah) a normal level of calcium in the blood. adj., **normocalce′mic.**

normochromia (nor″mo-kro′me-ah) normal color of erythrocytes.

normocyte (nor′mo-sīt) an erythrocyte that is normal in size, shape, and color.

Normocytin (nor″mo-si′tin) trademark for preparations of concentrated crystalline vitamin B_{12} (cyanocobalamine).

normocytosis (nor″mo-si-to′sis) a normal state of the blood in respect to erythrocytes.

normoglycemia (nor″mo-gli-se′me-ah) normal glucose content of the blood. adj., **normoglyce′mic.**

normokalemia (nor″mo-kah-le′me-ah) a normal level of potassium in the blood. adj., **normokale′mic.**

normospermic (nor″mo-sper′mik) producing spermatozoa normal in number and motility.

normotensive (nor″mo-ten′siv) 1. characterized by normal tension, tone, or pressure, as by normal blood pressure. 2. a person with normal blood pressure.

normothermia (nor″mo-ther′me-ah) a normal state of temperature. adj., **normother′mic.**

normotonia (nor″mo-to′ne-ah) normal tone or tension. adj., **normoton′ic.**

normovolemia (nor″mo-vo-le′me-ah) normal blood volume.

Norodin (nor′o-din) trademark for a preparation of methamphetamine, a central nervous system stimulant.

Norrie's disease (nor′rēz) a hereditary disorder consisting of bilateral blindness from retinal malformation, mental retardation, and deafness.

nortriptyline (nor-trip′tĭ-lēn) an antidepressant, used as the hydrochloride salt.

nos(o)- word element [Gr.], *disease.*

noscapine (nos′kah-pēn) an alkaloid present in opium; used as a nonaddictive antitussive.

nose (nōz) the specialized structure of the face that serves both as the organ of smell and as a means of bringing air into the lungs. (See also Plate 16.) Air breathed in through the nose is warmed and filtered; that breathed through the mouth is not.

The nostrils, which form the external entrance of the nose, lead into the two nasal cavities, which are separated from each other by a partition (the nasal septum) formed of cartilage and bone. Three bony ridges project from the outer wall of each nasal cavity and partially divide the cavity into three air passages. At the back of the nose these passages lead into the pharynx. The passages also are connected by openings with the paranasal sinuses. One of the functions of the nose is to drain fluids discharged from the sinuses. The nasal cavities also have a connection with the ears by the eustachian tubes, and with the region of the eyes by the nasolacrimal ducts.

The interior of the nose is lined with mucous membrane. Most of this membrane is covered with minute hairlike projections called cilia. Moving in waves these cilia sweep out from the nasal passages the nasal mucus, which may contain pollen, dust, and bacteria from the air. The mucous membrane also acts to warm and moisten the inhaled air.

High in the interior of each nasal cavity is a small area of mucous membrane that is not covered with cilia. In this pea-sized area are located the endings of the nerves of smell, the olfactory receptors. These receptors sort out odors. Unlike the taste buds of the tongue, which distinguish between only four different tastes (salt, sweet, sour, and bitter), the olfactory receptors can detect innumerable different odors. This ability to smell contributes greatly to what we usually think of as taste, because much of what we consider flavor is really odor. (See also SMELL.)

DISORDERS OF THE NOSE. The mucous membrane

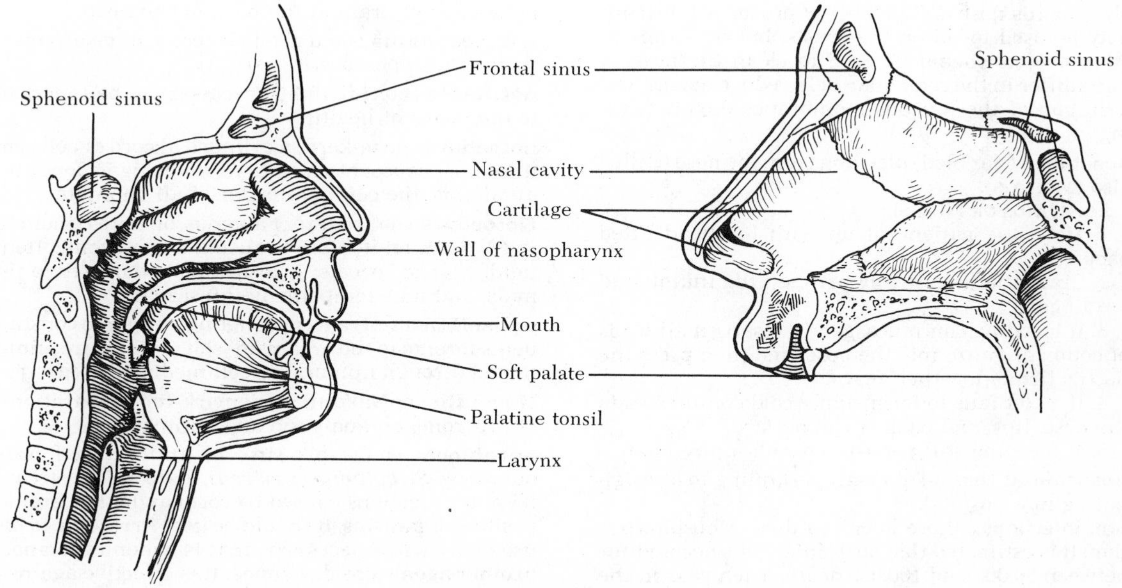

Nose and related structures.

of the nose is subject to inflammation; any such inflammation is called RHINITIS, a term derived from the Greek word *rhinos,* meaning nose. Rhinitis is often caused by an infection, as in the COMMON COLD, or by an allergy, particularly HAY FEVER. In both cases the symptoms are similar, including runny eyes, sneezing, a nasal discharge, and temporary stopping-up of the nasal passages. In such an infection, the nasal mucus is white or yellow in color.

Nasal polyps may obstruct the nasal passages and limit breathing through the nose. Enlarged adenoids also may interfere with nasal breathing.

Nosebleed may be caused by injury to the nose, or it may be a symptom of various diseases. (See also EPISTAXIS.)

Frequently the nasal septum may grow irregularly or be deflected to one side by an injury. This condition is known as deviated SEPTUM. The surgical procedure to correct deviations of the septum is called a submucous resection (SMR).

SURGERY OF THE NOSE. Nasal surgery is indicated in disorders of the nasal septum, polyps and other growths, and traumatic injury to the structures that interfere with normal nasal breathing. Cosmetic plastic surgery is also done to correct disfigurement that is disturbing to the patient.

Patient Care. Prior to surgery the patient is instructed in the kind of surgery anticipated and is informed of the immediate aftereffects of swelling and discoloration. He is told that the residual swelling may last for several weeks and success of the operation can not be assessed until after that time.

Immediately after surgery the greatest danger is hemorrhage. If the patient swallows repeatedly or spits up blood, excessive bleeding should be suspected. A Teflon splint or intranasal packing often is used to support the nasal structures and prevent the formation of hematoma, another complication that may develop.

Ice compresses are applied for 24 hours after surgery to reduce swelling and minimize bleeding. The patient is placed in semi-Fowler position during this time.

During convalescence the patient should avoid blowing his nose and picking at crusts. A lubricant may be used to soften the crusts, but no swabs or other objects should be used to clean the nose. A humidifier in the room may help reduce drying and irritation of the mucous membranes during healing.

nosebleed (nōz′blēd) bleeding from the nose (called also EPISTAXIS).

FIRST AID FOR NOSEBLEED

1. Have the patient sit up with his head tilted back.
2. Grasp the nose firmly between the thumb and forefinger.
3. If bleeding continues, gently insert small wads of cotton or gauze into the nose, and then press the nostils firmly together again.
4. If a clot fails to form, apply cold compresses to the nose, lips, and back of the neck.
5. If bleeding still persists, consult a physician.

nosocomial (nos″o-ko′me-al) pertaining to or originating in a hospital.

n. infections, those acquired during hospitalization. It is estimated that such infections account for between 50,000 and 100,000 deaths each year in the United States. The incidence of death and illness from nosocomial infections has become a major concern of the United States Public Health Service. According to recent studies by government and voluntary agencies, nosocomial infections occur most frequently in the genitourinary and respiratory tracts and in surgical wounds. The most common causative agents are *E. coli, Proteus, Pseudomonas,* and *Klebsiella,* among the gram-negative organisms, and *Staphylococcus* and *Enterococcus* among the gram-positive organisms.

nosogeny (no-soj′ĕ-ne) the development of a disease; pathogenesis.

nosoparasite (nos″o-par′ah-sīt) an organism found in a disease that it is able to modify, but not to produce.

nosophilia (nos″o-fil′e-ah) morbid desire to be sick.

nosophobia (nos″o-fo′be-ah) morbid dread of sickness or of a specific disease.

nosopoietic (nos″o-poi-et′ik) causing disease.

Nosopsyllus (nos″o-sil′us) a genus of fleas.

N. fascia′tus, the rat flea of North America and Europe, a carrier of murine typhus and probably of plague.

nosotaxy (nos′o-tak″se) the classification of disease.

nostril (nos′tril) either aperture (naris) of the nose.

nostrum (nos′trum) a quack, patent, or secret remedy.

Nostyn (nos′tin) trademark for a preparation of ectylurea, a sedative.

not(o)- word element [Gr.], *the back.*

notalgia (no-tal′je-ah) pain in the back.

notch (noch) an indentation, especially one on the edge of a bone or other organ.

aortic n., dicrotic n., a small downward deflection in the arterial pulse or pressure contour immediately following the closure of the semilunar valves, sometimes used as a marker for the end of systole or the ejection period.

parotid n., the notch between the ramus of the mandible and the mastoid process of the temporal bones.

tympanic n., Rivinus' incisure.

notencephalocele (no″ten-sef′ah-lo-sēl″) hernial protrusion of brain at the back of the head.

notencephalus (no″ten-sef′ah-lus) a fetus affected with notencephalocele.

notifiable (no″tĭ-fi′ah-b'l) necessary to be reported to the board of health.

notochord (no′to-kord) a cylindrical cord of cells on the dorsal aspect of an embryo, marking its longitudinal axis; the common factor of all chordates.

Notoedres (no″to-ed′rēz) a genus of mites, including *N. ca′ti,* an itch mite causing a persistent, often fatal, mange in cats; it also infests domestic animals, and may temporarily infest man.

not-self (not′self) a term denoting antigenic constituents foreign to the organism (self), which are eliminated through humoral or cell-mediated IMMUNITY.

Novaldin (no-val′din) trademark for preparations of dipyrone, an analgesic and antipyretic.

novobiocin (no″vo-bi′o-sin) an antibacterial produced by *Streptomyces niveus,* used in the treatment of infections caused by cocci and other gram-positive organisms. It should be kept in reserve to be used only when necessary, that is, when resistance to other agents has developed. It is effective against infections caused by penicillin-resistant microorganisms. However, organisms have been able to develop resistance to novobiocin rapidly. Leukopenia has been observed in some patients receiving the drug. Jaundice not uncommonly occurs in infants after novobiocin administration.

Novocain (no'vo-kān) trademark for preparations of procaine, a local anesthetic.

Novrad (nov'rad) trademark for preparations of levopropoxyphene, an antitussive.

noxious (nok'shus) hurtful; injurious.

Np chemical symbol, *neptunium.*

NPN nonprotein nitrogen.

ns. nanosecond.

N.S.A. Neurosurgical Society of America.

N.S.C.C. National Society for Crippled Children.

nsec. nanosecond.

N.S.N.A. National Student Nurse Association.

N.S.P.B. National Society for the Prevention of Blindness.

nucha (nu'kah) the nape, or back, of the neck. adj., **nu'chal.**

nuclear (nu'kle-ar) pertaining to a nucleus.

n. medicine, that branch of medicine concerned with the use of radionuclides in the diagnosis and treatment of disease.

nuclease (nu'kle-ās) any of a group of enzymes that split nucleic acids into nucleotides and other products.

nucleated (nu'kle-āt"ed) having a nucleus or nuclei.

nuclei (nu'kle-i) plural of *nucleus.*

nucleic acids (nu-kle'ik) substances found in the cells of all living tissue. They are extremely complex and of high molecular weight, containing phosphoric acid, sugars, and purine and pyrimidine bases. Two pentose sugars are involved as constituents of the nucleic acids: ribose and deoxyribose. Thus are derived the names of the nucleic acids RIBONUCLEIC ACID (RNA) and DEOXYRIBONUCLEIC ACID (DNA).

The nucleic acids and their derivatives are of great importance in metabolism, and though all of their functions are not yet completely understood, they appear to be concerned with controlling the general pattern of metabolism and acting as catalysts in many chemical reactions within the cell.

The nucleic acids, through the genetic code, are responsible for replication of cells and the control of cellular function. RNA, one form of which (mRNA), passes from the nucleus to the cytoplasm, plays a prominent role in the synthesis of proteins. The proteins formed under the direction of nucleic acids are structural proteins and enzymes, which promote various chemical reactions. These chemical activities supply energy to the cell and promote the synthesis of other substances important to cell growth and function.

The nucleic acids are also of great biologic significance. For example, DNA and RNA are the chemical repositories of genetic information and therefore affect the transmission of individual characteristics and functions from cell to cell and also from individual persons to their offspring.

nuclein (nu'kle-in) a decomposition product of nucleoprotein intermediate between native nucleoprotein and nucleic acid.

nucleocapsid (nu"kle-o-kap'sid) a unit of viral structure, consisting of a capsid with the enclosed nucleic acid.

nucleofugal (nu"kle-of'u-gal) moving away from a nucleus.

nucleohistone (nu"kle-o-his'tōn) a complex nucleoprotein made up of deoxyribonucleic acid and a histone, the principal constituents of chromatin.

nucleoid (nuk'kle-oid) 1. resembling a nucleus. 2. a nucleus-like body sometimes seen in the center of an erythrocyte. 3. the genetic material (nucleic acid) of a virus situated in the center of the virion.

nucleolonema (nu"kle-o"lo-ne'mah) a network of strands formed by organization of a finely granular substance, perhaps containing RNA, in the nucleolus of a cell.

nucleolus (nu-kle'o-lus), pl. *nucle'oli* [L.] a vacuole-like achromatic body, rich in RNA, within the nucleus of a cell; multiple nucleoli occur in some cells.

nucleon (nu'kle-on) a particle of an atomic nucleus; a proton or neutron, the total number of which constitutes the mass number of the isotope.

nucleonics (nu"kle-on'iks) the study of nucleons or of atomic nuclei and their reactions; nuclear physics.

nucleopetal (nu"kle-op'ĕ-tal) moving toward a nucleus.

nucleophilic (nu"kle-o-fil'ik) having an affinity for nuclei.

nucleoplasm (nu'kle-o-plazm") karyoplasm; the protoplasm of the nucleus of a cell.

nucleoprotein (nu"kle-o-pro'te-in) any of a class of conjugated proteins, consisting of nucleic acids and simple proteins (e.g., a histone).

nucleosidase (nu"kle-o-si'dās) an intracellular enzyme that is capable of causing the decomposition of nucleosides.

nucleoside (nu'kle-o-sīd) any of a class of compounds produced by hydrolysis of nucleotides, consisting of a sugar (a pentose or a hexose) and a purine or pyrimidine base.

nucleotidase (nu"kle-ot'ĭ-dās) an enzyme that splits nucleotides into nucleosides and phosphoric acid.

nucleotide (nu'kle-o-tīd) any of a group of compounds obtained by hydrolysis of nucleic acids, consisting of a purine or pyrimidine base linked to a sugar (ribose or deoxyribose), which in turn is esterified with phosphoric acid.

diphosphopyridine n., nicotinamide-adenine dinucleotide.

triphosphopyridine n., nicotinamide-adenine dinucleotide phosphate.

nucleotidyl (nu"kle-o-tīd'il) a nucleotide residue.

nucleotoxin (nu"kle-o-tok'sin) a toxin from cell nuclei, or one that affects cell nuclei.

nucleus (nu'kle-us), pl. *nu'clei* [L.] 1. a spheroid body within a cell, consisting of a thin nuclear membrane, organelles, one or more nucleoli, chromatin, linin, and nucleoplasm. The nucleus contains large quantities of DEOXYRIBONUCLEIC ACID (DNA), a nucleic acid that controls the synthesis of protein enzymes of the cytoplasm and also cellular reproduction. Because of its DNA content the nucleus is considered to be the control center of the cell. 2. a mass of gray matter in the central nervous system, especially such a mass marking the central termination of a cranial nerve. 3. in organic chemistry, the combination of atoms forming the central element or basic framework of the molecule of a specific compound or class of compounds. 4. the dense core of an atom; called also atomic nucleus. It has two major components: protons and neutrons. Traveling in orbit around the nucleus is a cloud of negatively charged particles called ELECTRONS. The number of protons in the atomic nucleus gives a substance its identity as a particular ELEMENT. adj., **nu'clear.**

n. ambig'uus, the nucleus of origin of motor fibers of the glossopharyngeal, vagus, and accessory nerves in the medulla oblongata.

arcuate nuclei, nu'clei, arcua'ti, small irregular areas of gray substance on the ventromedial aspect of the pyramid of the medulla oblongata.

atomic n., nucleus (3).

caudate n., n. cauda'tus, an elongated, arched gray mass closely related to the lateral ventricle throughout its entire extent, which, together with the putamen, forms the neostriatum.

cochlear nuclei, dorsal and ventral, the nuclei of termination of sensory fibers of the cochlear part of the vestibulocochlear (eighth cranial) nerve, which partly encircle the inferior cerebellar peduncle at the junction of the medulla oblongata and pons.

conjugation n., fertilization nucleus.

dentate n., n. denta'tus, the largest of the deep cerebellar nuclei lying in the white matter of the cerebellum.

diploid n., a cell nucleus containing the number of chromosomes typical of the somatic cells of the particular species.

fastigial n., n. fasti'gii, the most medial of the deep cerebellar nuclei, near the midline in the roof of the fourth ventricle.

fertilization n., one produced by fusion of the male and female pronuclei in the fertilized ovum.

free n., a cell nucleus from which the other elements of the cell have disappeared.

germ n., germinal n., pronucleus.

gonad n., micronucleus (1).

haploid n., a cell nucleus containing half of the number of chromosomes typical of the somatic cells of a particular species.

lenticular n., lentiform n., the part of the corpus striatum just lateral to the internal capsule, comprising the putamen and globus pallidus.

motor n., any collection of cells in the central nervous system giving origin to a motor nerve.

n. oliva'ris, olivary n., 1. a folded band of gray matter enclosing a white core and producing the elevation (olive) on the medulla oblongata. 2. olive (2).

n. of origin, any collection of nerve cells giving origin to the fibers, or a part of the fibers, of a peripheral nerve.

paraventricular n., n. paraventricula'ris, a band of cells in the wall of the third ventricle in the supraoptic part of the hypothalamus; many of its cells are neurosecretory in function and project to the neurohypophysis.

pontine nuclei, nu'clei pon'tis, groups of nerve cell bodies in the part of the pyramidal tract within the ventral part of the pons, upon which the fibers of the corticopontine tract synapse, and whose axons in turn cross to the opposite side and form the middle cerebellar peduncle.

n. pulpo'sus, pulpy n., a semifluid mass of fine white elastic fibers forming the center of an intervertebral disk.

red n., nucleus ruber.

reproductive n., micronucleus (1).

n. ru'ber, an oval mass of gray matter (pink in fresh specimens) in the anterior part of the tegmentum and extending into the posterior part of the hypothalamus; it receives fibers from the cerebellum. Called also red nucleus.

sensory n., the nucleus of termination of the afferent (sensory) fibers of a peripheral nerve.

sperm n., the male pronucleus.

supraoptic n., n. supraop'ticus, one just above the lateral part of the optic chiasm; many of its cells are neurosecretory in function and project to the neurohypophysis.

tegmental nuclei, several nuclear masses of the reticular formations of the pons and midbrain, especially of the latter, where they are in close approximation to the superior cerebellar peduncles.

thoracic n., n. thorac'icus, a column of cells in the posterior gray column of the spinal cord, extending from the 7th or 8th cervical segments to the 2nd or 3rd lumbar level.

vestibular nuclei, nu'clei vestibula'ris, the four cellular masses (superior, lateral, medial, and inferior) in the floor of the fourth ventricle, in which the branches of the eighth cranial (vestibulocochlear) nerve terminate.

nuclide (nu'klīd) a species of atom characterized by the charge, mass, number, and quantum state of its nucleus, and capable of existing for a measurable lifetime (usually more than 10^{-10} sec.).

nullipara (nu-lip'ah-rah) a woman who has not produced a viable offspring; PARA 0. adj., **nullip'arous.**

nulliparity (nul″ĭ-par'ĭ-te) the state of being a nullipara.

number (num'ber) a symbol, as a figure or word, expressive of a certain value or a specified quantity determined by count.

atomic n., a number expressive of the number of protons in an atomic nucleus, or the positive charge of the nucleus expressed in terms of the electronic charge; symbol A.

Avogadro's n., the number of particles of the type specified by the chemical formula of a certain substance in 1 gram-molecule of the substance; called also Avogadro's constant.

mass n., the number expressive of the mass of a nucleus, being the total number of nucleons—protons and neutrons—in the nucleus of an atom or nuclide.

numbness (num'nes) a lack or diminution of sensation in a part.

nummular (num'u-lar) 1. coin-sized and coin-shaped. 2. made up of round, flat disks. 3. arranged like a stack of coins.

Numorphan (nu-mor'fan) trademark for preparations of oxymorphone, a narcotic analgesic.

nunnation (nun-a'shun) the too frequent use of *n* sounds.

Nupercaine (nu'per-kān) trademark for preparations of dibucaine, a local anesthetic.

nurse (ners) 1. a person who makes a profession of caring for the sick, disabled or enfeebled, or of aiding in the maintenance of a state of health (see also NURSING PRACTICE). 2. to care for a sick or disabled person or to aid in the maintenance of health. 3. to nourish at the breast (see also BREAST FEEDING).

charge n., one who is in charge of a patient care unit of a hospital or similar health agency.

clinical n. specialist, primarily a clinician with a high degree of knowledge, skill, and competence in a specialized area of nursing. These skills are made directly available through the provision of nursing care to clients and indirectly available through guidance and planning of care with other nursing personnel. Clinical nurse specialists hold a master's degree in nursing, preferably with an emphasis in clinical nursing. Called also nurse specialist.

n. clinician, a professional nurse who has well-developed competencies in utilizing a broad range of cues. These cues are used for prescribing and implementing both direct and indirect nursing care and for articulating nursing therapies with other planned therapies. Nurse clinicians demonstrate expertise in nursing practice and insure ongoing development of expertise through clinical experience and continuing education. Generally minimal preparation for this role is the baccalaureate degree.

community n., in Great Britian, a public health nurse.

community health n., an especially prepared registered nurse whose work combines elements of both nursing and public health practice and takes place primarily outside the therapeutic institution (see also PUBLIC HEALTH NURSING).

general duty n., a registered nurse, usually one who has not undergone training beyond the basic nursing program, who sees to the general nursing care of patients in a hospital or other health agency.

graduate n., a graduate of a school of nursing; often used to designate one who has not been registered or licensed.

head n., charge nurse.

licensed practical n., licensed vocational n., a graduate of a school of practical nursing whose qualifications have been examined by a state board of nursing and who has been legally authorized to practice as a licensed practical or vocational nurse (L.P.N. or L.V.N.). According to the role definition proposed as a model by the American Nurses' Association, the definition of L.P.N. practice has been updated to include "the performance under the supervision of a registered nurse of those services required in observing and caring for the ill, injured, or infirm, in promoting preventive measures in community health, in acting to safeguard life and health, in administering treatment and medication prescribed by a physician or dentist or in performing other acts not requiring the skill, judgment, and knowledge of a registered nurse."

n.-midwife, a professional nurse who specializes in the care of women throughout pregnancy, delivery, and the postpartum period. The official organization, established in 1955, is the American College of Nurse-Midwives. The address is ACNM, 1000 Vermont Ave., N.W., Washington, DC 20005.

practical n., one who has had practical experience in nursing care but who is not a graduate of a nursing school; see also licensed practical NURSE.

private n., private duty n., one who attends an individual patient, usually on a fee-for-service basis, and who may specialize in a specific class of diseases.

probationer n., a person who has entered a school of nursing and is under observation to determine her fitness for the nursing profession; applied principally to nursing students enrolled in hospital schools of nursing.

public health n., a professional title being replaced in the United States by community health nurse (see also PUBLIC HEALTH NURSING).

Queen's Nurse, in Great Britain, a district nurse who has been trained at or in accordance with the regulations of the Queen Victoria Jubilee Institute for Nurses.

registered n., a graduate nurse registered and licensed to practice by a State Board of Nurse Examiners or other state authority. The Model Practice Act published by the American Nurses' Association defines the practice of nursing as performed by a registered nurse as "a process in which substantial specialized knowledge derived from the biological, physical, and behavioral sciences is applied to the care, treatment, counsel, and health teaching of persons who are experiencing changes in the normal health processes; or who require assistance in the maintenance of health or the management of illness, injury, or infirmity or in the achievement of a dignified death; and such additional acts as are recognized by the nursing profession as proper to be performed by a registered nurse."

scrub n., one who directly assists the surgeon in the operating room.

n. specialist, clinical nurse specialist.

visiting n., community health nurse.

wet n., a woman who breast-feeds the infant of another.

nursery (ner'sĕ-re) the department in a hospital where newborn infants are cared for.

day n., an institution devoted to the care of young children during the day.

nursing (ners'ing) the profession of performing the functions of a NURSE.

n. audit, a systematic procedure for assessing the quality of nursing care rendered to a specific patient population. The nursing audit developed partly in response to public demand for accountability for the kind of health care being provided, and partly as the result of a growing recognition among nurses of the need for professional self-regulation.

As in any type of audit, the nursing audit involves a thorough and systematic examination of patient records for the purpose of acquiring specific and relevant data. The observable data related to nursing activities are then applied to previously established criteria stated in terms of patient-centered outcomes. Deficiencies in patient care can thus be identified by comparing the actual nursing practice and the effects of the NURSING PROCESS to the established criteria. If deficiencies are identified, appropriate correction can then be taken. This may involve a change in staffing patterns, inservice education programs for members of the nursing staff, patient education programs, a change in available resources (both human and material), and a host of other actions designed to cope with the specific problems identified through the nursing audit.

The nursing audit provides a means of evaluating both the nursing process and the changes in the patient's health status that are a result of the nursing process. Because the implementation of an audit is greatly facilitated by the development of a data base, the identification of major problems the patient is experiencing, the recording of a plan of action, and the maintenance of progress notes to determine whether the plan of action is effectively achieving desired outcomes, it is clear that a PROBLEM-ORIENTED RECORD is essential to the assessment and improvement of patient care through nursing audits. (See also EVALUATION.)

n. diagnosis, see under DIAGNOSIS.

n. history, a written record providing data for assessing the nursing care needs of a patient.

n. practice, the performance for compensation of any act in the observation, care, and counsel of the ill, injured, or infirm, or in the maintenance of health or prevention of illness of others, or in the supervision and teaching of other personnel, or in the administration of medications and treatments as prescribed by a licensed physician or dentist, requiring substantial specialized judgment and skill and based on knowledge and application of the principles of biologic, physical, and social sciences.

According to the 1974 Congress for Nursing Practice, "practitioners of professional nursing are registered nurses who provide direct care to clients utilizing the NURSING PROCESS in arriving at decisions. They work in a collegial and collaborative relationship with other health professionals to determine health care needs and assume responsibility for nursing care. In the course of their practice they assess the effectiveness of actions taken, identify and carry out systematic investigations of clinical problems, and engage in periodic review of their own contributions to health care and those of their professional peers."

In addition: Nurse practitioners have advanced skills in the assessment of the physical and psychosocial health-illness status of individuals, families, or groups in a variety of settings through health and development history taking and physical examination. They are prepared for these special skills by formal continuing education which adheres to guidelines approved by the American Nurses' Association, or in a baccalaureate nursing program.

n. process, a systematic approach to the identification of a patient's nursing care problems and the utilization of nursing actions that effectively alleviate, minimize, or prevent the specific problems being presented or likely to develop. The nursing process begins with a search for data on which to base a nursing assessment or nursing diagnosis and is completed only after the process has been evaluated for effectiveness. It has been described as the essence of nursing.

There are certain assumptions that are basic to an understanding of the goals of the nursing process, and upon which the acceptance and successful employment of the process will depend. First, it is assumed that nurses recognize each patient as an individual with worth, dignity, and basic human needs. Each person has a right to service of high quality regardless of his socioeconomic status, cultural background, and religious beliefs.

The second assumption is that the patient or client and his family prefer a client-centered approach that actively seeks their input and respects their feelings and needs. Such an approach encourages them to enter into a partnership with members of the health care professions. It is also assumed that the focus of care will be on maintenance of health and prevention of disease.

Another assumption is that those nurses who engage in the nursing process will have current knowledge in their particular discipline and in such related fields as the physical and behavioral sciences. This implies, of course, continued informal study and formal education.

COMPONENTS OF THE PROCESS. Although the nursing process does follow a logical and systematic pattern, it also has a cyclical nature which sometimes demands that two or more components may be operating simultaneously. The components are not separate steps that must always follow a preordained sequence; there often is movement between and among the components.

The four major components of the nursing process are generally agreed to be: (1) assessment, (2) planning, (3) implementation, and (4) evaluation.

Assessment. The assessment phase of the process begins with data gathering and concludes with a nursing DIAGNOSIS stated in terms of client problems. Sources of data might be a nursing history, observation of and interviewing the patient and his family, reviewing the patient's medical records, and communication with other members of the health care team.

With the accumulated data at hand the nurse then organizes the information, analyzing it, finding relationships, and drawing inferences about the nature of the client's problems. While she is formulating inferences or conclusions about the client's problems and needs, she provides him with an opportunity to present his point of view in order to confirm the inferences drawn from the data. Throughout the nursing process it is essential that inferences be validated; otherwise much time and effort can be wasted in planning and implementing nursing activities which are of no use because they are not central to the client's real problems. If there is confirmation of the conclusions drawn from the data, a nursing diagnosis is made. The diagnosis provides the basis for formulation of a plan of care and should be shared with other nurses as well as with other members of the interdisciplinary health care team.

Planning. If no problems have been found during the assessment phase, the nurse and client sit down together to discuss plans for maintenance of wellness. It is the client's responsibility to implement the plan and to return for periodic assessments and identification of either new problems or the potential for them.

When problems are present and have been identified, priorities are set and specific actions are planned to meet the problems having the highest priorities. The nursing care plan should include all pertinent information about the client, the ordering of his problems, and expected outcomes of the prescribed nursing orders. The plan is shared with others who are appropriately concerned with the care of the client and the resolution of his problems.

The nursing care plan is not an inflexible and unchanging prescription for action. It is revised as often as necessary according to the reordering of priorities as indicated by the status of the patient.

Implementation. Nursing actions which implement the nursing care plan should include all aspects of patient care for which the nurse is prepared and willing to accept responsibility. In some instances implementation may include delegated medical therapy, and most certainly cannot ignore the nurse's attitude toward immediate intervention should the patient's condition warrant prompt and decisive action on the part of the nurse.

During implementation the nursing care plan is

tested for effectiveness and accuracy. Data gathering continues and plans may change on the basis of new information obtained.

The implementation phase concludes with the recording of the activities performed and the response of the patient.

Evaluation. The first three major components of the nursing process are all client-centered and so, too, must the phase of evaluation be concerned with the client's judgment about resolution of the identified problems. EVALUATION is conducted for the purpose of determining the effectiveness of the process and making decisions about whether the nursing actions taken should be employed in the same way in the future.

By accepting responsibility for evaluation of the process, the nurse demonstrates a professional attitude toward her clients and her own actions. She shows a willingness to be held accountable for what she does and to seek ways in which she can assure her clients of the optimum care that can be reasonably expected.

nutation (nu-ta'shun) the act of nodding, especially involuntary nodding.

nutgall (nut'gawl) an excrescence growing on certain oak trees, produced by insect eggs and larvae embedded in the plant tissues; a source of gallic and tannic acids.

nutrient (nu'tre-ent) 1. nourishing; aiding nutrition. 2. a nourishing substance, or food.

nutriment (nu'trĭ-ment) nourishment; nutritious material; food.

nutrition (nu-trish'un) 1. the sum of the processes involved in taking in nutriments and assimilating and utilizing them. 2. nutriment. adj., **nutri'tional.** It includes all the processes by which the body uses food for energy, maintenance, and growth. Nutrition is particularly concerned with those properties of food that build sound bodies and promote health. In this sense, good nutrition means a balanced diet containing adequate amounts of the essential nutritional elements that the body must have to function normally.

THE BALANCED DIET. To form the foundation for a good diet the Institute of Home Economics, United States Department of Agriculture, recommends the Basic Four Food Groups.

The essential ingredients of a balanced diet are proteins, vitamins, minerals, fats, and carbohydrates. The body can manufacture sugars from fats, and fats from sugars and proteins, depending on the need. But it cannot manufacture proteins from sugars and fats.

The most important constituents of proteins are the AMINO ACIDS. These complex organic compounds of nitrogen play a vital role in nutrition. The best sources of complete proteins—that is, proteins containing all the essential amino acids—are meat, fish, eggs, and dairy products. The amount of protein that a person actually needs, however, is much smaller than many people suppose.

Vitamins are special substances that are present, in varying amounts, in all food. Their absence from the diet can cause such diseases as beriberi (lack of vitamin B_1, or thiamine), pellagra (lack of the B vitamin niacin) and scurvy (lack of vitamin C, or ascorbic acid). (See also VITAMINS.)

The principal minerals needed by the body are calcium and phosphorus (to build bones and teeth) and iron (to assure a sufficient supply of erythrocytes). All three are plentiful in eggs, dairy products, lean meat, and enriched flour. Some sources of calcium are American cheese, Swiss cheese, molasses, turnip tops, and dandelion greens; of phosphorus, cereals, meat, and fish; of iron, kidney beans, navy beans, liver and other meats, beet greens, spinach, and whole-wheat bread.

The trace of iodine needed to prevent goiter is easily provided by iodized table salt. The minute amounts of magnesium, manganese, and copper that are necessary are found in any balanced diet.

For quick energy, the body should have sugars (carbohydrates) and starches (which the body converts into sugars). Fats and proteins can also provide energy and can be stored for future use, whereas sugars and starches cannot. Since the body can manufacture most of its own fat, fats are of secondary importance in a balanced diet.

AGE AND NUTRITION. Because the body's needs change as it grows and develops, good nutrition for a child or teenager is not the same as good nutrition for a mature or older person. Growing bodies need plentiful supplies of calcium, phosphorus, and other minerals to build strong bones and teeth, and abundant protein for firm muscles, energy, and stamina.

For children especially, breakfast is the key meal of the day. Expending as much energy as they do, children need a hearty morning meal, rich in vitamin C, calcium, iron, and thiamine, in order to offset the physical and mental fatigue that they usually feel before lunch time.

SPACING AND SERVING OF MEALS. Nutritionists generally consider breakfast the most important meal of the day because it ends the body's overnight fast and supplies the "fuel" for a person to get under way at top efficiency. If possible, meals should be spaced at regular intervals. They should never be rushed. This is especially true of the main daily meal.

nutritious (nu-trish'us) affording nourishment.

nutritive (nu'trĭ-tiv) pertaining to or promoting nutrition.

nutriture (nu'trĭ-tūr) the status of the body in relation to nutrition.

Nutting (nut'ing) M. Adelaide (1858–1948). A pioneer in establishing the foundations on which nursing as a modern profession rests. She was in the first graduating class at Johns Hopkins Hospital School of Nursing and eventually became Superintendent of Nurses and Principal of the School of Nursing. At Johns Hopkins, Miss Nutting instituted many reforms and advances in nursing education. She eliminated the 12-hour-duty day, abolished the monthly stipend for students, and instituted a 3-year course. Her purposes in instigating these changes were to release the student from financial obligation to the hospital so that exploitation of the student as a source of cheap labor could be abolished, and to provide the student with more time for study and learning.

nux (nuks) [L.] nut.

n. vom'ica, the dried ripe seed of *Strychnos nux-vomica,* containing several alkaloids, chiefly strychnine and brucine.

nyct(o)- word element [Gr.], *night; darkness.*

nyctalgia (nik-tal'je-ah) pain that occurs only in sleep.

nyctalope (nik'tal-lōp) a person affected with nyctalopia.

nyctalopia (nik"tah-lo'pe-ah) 1. night blindness. 2. in French (and incorrectly in English), day blindness.

nycterine (nik'ter-in) occurring at night.

nyctohemeral (nik"to-hem'er-al) pertaining to both day and night.

nyctophilia (nik"to-fil'e-ah) a preference for darkness or for night.

nyctophobia (nik"to-fo'be-ah) morbid dread of darkness.

nyctophonia (nik"to-fo'ne-ah) loss of voice during the day but not at night.

nyctotyphlosis (nik"to-tif-lo'sis) night blindness, or nyctalopia.

Nydrazid (ni'drah-zid) trademark for preparations of isoniazid, used in treatment of tuberculosis.

nylidrin (nil'ĭ-drin) a peripheral vasodilator; used as the hydrochloride salt.

nymph (nimf) a developmental stage in certain arthropods (e.g., ticks) between the larval form and the adult, and resembling the latter in appearance.

nymph(o)- word element [Gr.], *nymphae* (labia minora).

nympha (nim'fah,), p. *nym'phae* [L.] labium minus.

nymphectomy (nim-fek'to-me) excision of the nymphae (labia minora).

nymphitis (nim-fi'tis) inflammation of the nymphae (labia minora).

nymphomania (nim"fo-ma'ne-ah) excessive sexual desire in a woman, which may lead to promiscuous sexual behavior. This form of sexual deviation is usually the result of a psychologic inability to achieve sexual satisfaction. Since the condition originates in emotional rather than physical disturbance, it is the underlying emotional problem that should be treated.

nymphoncus (nim-fong'kus) swelling or enlargement of the nymphae (labia minora).

nymphotomy (nim-fot'o-me) surgical incision of the nymphae (labia minora) or clitoris.

nystagmiform (nis-tag'mĭ-form) resembling nystagmus.

nystagmograph (nis-tag'mo-graf) an instrument for recording the movements of the eyeball in nystagmus.

nystagmoid (nis-tag'moid) resembling nystagmus.

nystagmus (nis-tag'mus) involuntary, rapid, rhythmic movement (horizontal, vertical, rotatory, or mixed, i.e., of two types) of the eyeball. adj., **nystag'mic.**

aural n., labyrinthine nystagmus.

Cheyne's n., a peculiar rhythmical eye movement resembling Cheyne-Stokes respiration in rhythm.

dissociated n., that in which the movements in the two eyes are dissimilar.

end-position n., that occurring only at extremes of gaze.

fixation n., that occurring only on gazing fixedly at an object.

labyrinthine n., vestibular nystagmus due to labyrinthine disturbance.

latent m., that occurring only when one eye is covered.

lateral n., involuntary horizontal movement of the eyes.

optokinetic n., nystagmus induced by looking at a moving object.

pendular n., that which consists of to-and-fro movements of equal velocity.

retraction n., n. retracto'rius, a spasmodic backward movement of the eyeball occurring on attempts to move the eye; a sign of midbrain disease.

rotatory n., involuntary rotation of the eyes about the visual axis.

vertical n., involuntary up-and-down movement of the eyes.

vestibular n., nystagmus due to disturbance of the labyrinth or of the vestibular nuclei; the movements are usually jerky.

nystatin (nis'tah-tin) an antifungal agent produced by growth of *Streptomyces noursei;* used in treatment of infections due to *Candida albicans.*

nystaxis (nis-tak'sis) nystagmus.

nyxis (nik'sis) puncture, or paracentesis.

O

O chemical symbol, *oxygen.*

O. [L.] *oc'ulus* (eye); [L.] *octa'rius* (pint); opening.

o- symbol, *ortho-.*

O_2 1. chemical symbol, *molecular (diatomic) oxygen.* 2. symbol, *both eyes.*

O_3 chemical symbol, *ozone* (triatomic oxygen).

oasthouse urine disease (ōst'hows) Smith-Strang disease.

O.B. obstetrics.

ob- word element [L.], *against; in front of; toward.*

obcecation (ob″sĕ-ka'shun) incomplete blindness.

obesity (o-bēs'ĭ-te) excessive accumulation of fat in the body; increase in weight beyond that considered desirable with regard to age, height, and bone structure. adj., **obese'.**

EFFECTS OF OBESITY. Being overweight can affect physical and mental health. Too many extra pounds are a strain on the body, and can eventually shorten the span of life. Obesity is also unattractive, and this may create psychologic problems.

The overweight person is inviting a number of unnecessary complications. Some of these are an overworked heart; shortness of breath; a tendency to arteriosclerosis and high blood pressure or to diabetes mellitus; chronic back and joint pains from increased strain on joints and ligaments; a greater tendency to contract infectious diseases; and a reduced ability to exercise or enjoy sports. Carefully compiled statistics show that mortality from circulatory conditions is about 45 per cent higher in seriously overweight men than in those whose weight is reasonably close to normal, and death from such conditions is apt to occur sooner. Because of this increased risk, life insurance companies are reluctant to grant insurance to people greatly overweight.

Psychologically, too, the obese person is at a disadvantage. The show of good cheer sometimes associated with obese people usually masks unconscious—or even conscious—unhappiness and disappointment. Obesity can cause personality problems; in turn, emotional difficulties such as those caused by persistent loneliness, tension, or boredom sometimes find an outlet in compulsive overeating.

CAUSES. Most cases of obesity are due to an excessive intake of calories in proportion to expenditure of calories. Cultural factors, such as the abundance in the United States of purified high-caloric foods of low nutrient value, are among the most important contributing factors in the incidence of moderate overweight. Extreme obesity seems to be familial; in families in which both parents are obese, the children are very likely to be overweight also. Overweight children usually become overweight adults.

Endocrine and metabolic disturbances have been used by many persons as an excuse for their obesity, but these causes are relatively rare among the obese and most are probably secondary to the obesity.

Lack of exercise frequently is associated with obesity, particularly in women. Mental depression, which often occurs concomitantly with inactivity, may be exaggerated when there is loss of weight. Another behavioral aspect of obesity is the eating pattern. In many very obese persons the major caloric intake occurs during the evening meal or "bedtime snack." Early life patterns of eating and emotional responses to food are considered a major factor in obesity. Especially significant are the responses learned from the mother who rewarded good behavior with food, particularly food that is high in calories.

MANAGEMENT. Among the techniques currently in use in the management of overweight are: hospitalization with fasting, surgical intervention, self-help groups, behavioral techniques, and drugs to suppress the appetite or increase metabolism, or both.

Hospitalization with fasting usually is confined to select groups of patients with massive obesity that is resistant to other weight reducing measures and is not caused by endocrine dysfunction. It is essential that the clients be carefully supervised in a follow-up management program because many have a tendency to regain the lost pounds when they return home.

Surgical intervention, specifically INTESTINAL BYPASS (jejunoileal shunt), has proven to be hazardous for some patients and postoperative morbidity remains a serious limitation.

Self-help groups are considered by many health professionals to offer some of the best available techniques in weight reduction. The combination of low caloric diet and increased exercise, in conjunction with peer pressure and group interest, seems to be the most effective in bringing about gradual and permanent weight loss. Among the better known and more successful groups are TOPS (Take Off Pounds Sensibly) and Weight Watchers.

The emphasis in *behavior modification programs* is on understanding and changing behavior, stimuli, and REINFORCEMENT. The goal of the program is to alter gradually the maladaptive eating patterns and to increase the expenditures of calories through exercise. Results of studies have shown these techniques to be consistently better than other more conventional plans for medical management of obesity.

Drugs that inhibit appetite and increase metabolic rate have come under criticism in recent years. There is an increasing awareness of the dangers of drug dependency and abuse, and the deleterious side-effects of some of these drugs.

obex (o'beks) the ependyma-lined junction of the teniae of the fourth ventricle of the brain at the inferior angle.

objective (ob-jek'tiv) 1. perceptible by the external senses. 2. a result for whose achievement an effort has been made. 3. the lens or system of lenses of a microscope nearest the object that is being examined.

achromatic o., one in which the chromatic aberration is corrected for two colors and the spherical aberration for one color.

apochromatic o., one in which chromatic aberration is corrected for three colors and the spherical aberration for two colors.

immersion o., one designed to have its tip and the

coverglass over the specimen connected by a liquid instead of air.

obligate (ob'lĭ-gāt) not facultative; necessary; compulsory; pertaining to or characterized by the ability to survive only in a particular environment or to assume only a particular role, as an obligate anaerobe.

oblique (o-blēk') slanting; inclined.

obliquity (ŏ-blik'wĭ-te) the state of being oblique or slanting.

obliteration (ŏ-blit"ĕ-ra'shun) complete removal, by disease, degeneration, surgical procedure, irradiation, etc.

oblongata (ob"long-gah'tah) medulla oblongata (see also BRAIN). adj., **oblonga'tal.**

obsession (ob-sesh'un) any persistent unwanted idea or impulse that cannot be eliminated by reasoning. adj., **obses'sive.**

obsessive-compulsive (ob-ses'iv-kom-pul'siv) marked by a compulsion to repeatedly perform certain acts or carry out certain rituals. Obsessive-compulsive reaction is a type of NEUROSIS in which there is the intrusion of insistent, repetitious, and unwanted ideas or impulses to perform certain acts. The patient may feel compelled to wash his hands repeatedly, to utter certain words or phrases over and over again, or to carry out ritualistically other acts that interfere with his normal daily activities.

obstetrician (ob"stĕ-trish'an) a physician who specializes in obstetrics.

obstetrics (ob-stet'riks) the branch of medicine dealing with pregnancy, labor, and the puerperium. adj., **obstet'ric, obstet'rical.**

obstipation (ob"stĭ-pa'shun) intractable constipation.

obstruction (ob-struk'shun) the act of blocking or clogging; state of being clogged.

intestinal o., any hindrance to the passage of feces (see also INTESTINAL OBSTRUCTION).

obstruent (ob'stroo-ent) 1. causing obstruction. 2. any agent or agency that causes obstruction.

obtund (ob-tund') to render dull or blunt.

obtundent (ob-tun'dent) 1. having the power to dull sensibility or to soothe pain. 2. a soothing or partially anesthetic agent.

obturator (ob"tu-ra'tor) a disk or plate that closes an opening.

o. foramen, the large opening between the pubic bone and the ischium.

o. muscles, the muscles that rotate the thighs laterally (see also table of MUSCLES).

o. sign, pain on outward pressure on the obturator foramen as a sign of inflammation in the sheath of the obturator nerve, probably caused by appendicitis.

obtusion (ob-tu'zhun) a deadening or blunting of sensitivity.

occipital (ok-sip'ĭ-tal) pertaining to the occiput; located near the occipital bone, as the occipital lobe.

o. bone, the unpaired bone constituting the back and part of the base of the skull (see also table of BONES).

o. lobe, the most posterior portion of the cerebral hemisphere, forming a small part of its dorsolateral surface.

occipitalization (ok-sip"ĭ-tal-ĭ-za'shun) synostosis of the atlas with the occipital bone.

occipitocervical (ok-sip"ĭ-to-ser'vĭ-kal) pertaining to the occiput and neck.

occipitofrontal (ok-sip"ĭ-to-fron'tal) pertaining to the occiput and the face.

occiptomastoid (ok-sip"ĭ-to-mas'toid) pertaining to the occipital bone and mastoid process.

occipitomental (ok-sip"ĭ-to-men'tal) pertaining to the occiput and chin.

occipitoparietal (ok-sip"ĭ-to-pah-ri'ĕ-tal) pertaining to the occipital and parietal bones or lobes of the brain.

occipitotemporal (ok-sip"ĭ-to-tem'po-ral) pertaining to the occipital and temporal bones.

occipitothalamic (ok-sip"ĭ-to-thah-lam'ik) pertaining to the occipital lobe and thalamus.

occiput (ok'sĭ-put) the back part of the head.

occlude (o-klo͞od') to fit close together; to close tight; to obstruct or close off.

occlusal (ŏ-kloo'zal) pertaining to closure; applied to the masticating surfaces of the premolar and molar teeth, or to the contacting surfaces of opposing occlusion rims, or designating a position toward the hypothetical plane passing between the mandibular and maxillary teeth when the jaws are brought into approximation.

occlusion (ŏ-kloo'zhun) 1. the act of closure or state of being closed; an obstruction or a closing off. 2. the relation of the teeth of both jaws when in functional contact during activity of the mandible.

abnormal o., malocclusion.

central o., centric o., occlusion of the teeth when the mandible is in centric relation to the maxilla, with full occlusal surface contact of the upper and lower teeth in habitual occlusion.

coronary o., obstruction to the flow of blood through an artery of the heart (see also CORONARY OCCLUSION).

eccentric o., occlusion of the teeth when the lower jaw has moved from the centric position.

occlusive (ŏ-kloo'siv) pertaining to or effecting occlusion.

occult (ŏ-kult') obscure or hidden from view.

o. blood test, examination, microscopically or by a chemical test, of a specimen of feces, urine, gastric juice, etc., to determine the presence of blood not otherwise detectable. Feces are tested when intestinal bleeding is suspected but there is no visible evidence of blood in the stools.

occupational diseases (ok"u-pa'shun-al) diseases caused by various factors involved in one's occupation. The diseases vary with the type of work involved.

Dusts are a common cause of occupational diseases. Fine particles of silica can lead to SILICOSIS among miners, glassworkers, and persons involved in the manufacture of cement and similar materials. Another cause of occupational disease is poisonous gases and vapors, which can result in respiratory disorders and may also involve the blood and other body systems. Certain kinds of chemicals can affect the skin, causing some forms of DERMATITIS. Working conditions, such as high temperatures or humidity, excessive noise, changes in air pressure, or continuous exposure to sun and wind, can cause varied disorders such as HEAT EXHAUSTION, impaired hearing or vision, BENDS, or skin conditions.

Control and prevention of occupational diseases is

very much a major concern of the individual worker, management, the community health service, and the state and federal governments. It involves education of the worker on how to protect himself against occupational hazards; management's cooperation in supplying proper equipment and conditions; inspection and testing services performed by the government; the existence of adequate medical and first-aid services at the location of the work; adequate hospitalization facilities, insurance and compensation; and research into methods to provide safety and good health.

occupational therapy the use of any occupation for remedial purposes. It is defined by the American Occupational Therapy Association, Inc., as "the art and science of directing man's participation in selected tasks to restore, reinforce and enhance performance, facilitate learning of those skills and functions essential for adaptation and productivity, diminish or correct pathology and to promote and maintain health. Its fundamental concern is the development and maintenance of the capacity, throughout the life span, to perform with satisfaction to self and others those tasks and roles essential to productive living and to the mastery of self and environment."

The broad concerns of occupational therapy include all factors that facilitate the development of adaptive skills and increase performance capacity, and also those factors that may impede or restrict an individual's ability to function. In addition to those persons recovering from physical injury or illness, occupational therapy serves others who because of age, poverty, cultural differences, or psychologic and social disability, have difficulty coping with the tasks of living. The reference to occupation in the title is to be understood in the context of man's goal-directed use of time, energy, interest, and attention.

As is true of all types of therapeutic measures, the skills that are taught and the tasks prescribed for the client take into account his individual needs, abilities, and interests. This implies a thorough evaluation of his physical, mental, and emotional status and an acceptance of him as a person. In consultation with other members of the health care team, the occupational therapist designs a program of therapy that will lead to the goal of a productive life and satisfactory adjustment on the part of the patient.

ochrometer (o-krom′ĕ-ter) an instrument for measuring capillary blood pressure.

ochronosis (o″kro-no′sis) a peculiar discoloration of body tissues caused by deposit of alkapton bodies as the result of a metabolic disorder.

ocular o., brown or gray discoloration of the sclera, sometimes involving also the conjunctivae and eyelids.

octa- word element [Gr. L.], *eight.*

octabenzone (ok″tah-ben′zōn) a sun-screening agent.

octamethyl pyrophosphoramide (ok″tah-meth′il pir″o-fos-for′ah-mīd) a potent cholinesterase inhibitor and an insecticide.

octan (ok′tan) occurring on the eighth day (every seven days).

octapeptide (ok″tah-pep′tīd) a peptide which on hydrolysis yields eight amino acids.

octaploid (ok′tah-ploid) 1. pertaining to or characterized by octaploidy. 2. an individual or cell having eight sets of chromosomes.

octaploidy (ok′tah-ploi″de) the state of having eight sets of chromosomes (8n).

octavalent (ok″tah-va′lent) having a valency of eight.

octigravida (ok″tĭ-grav′ĭ-dah) a woman pregnant for the eighth time.

Octin (ok′tin) trademark for preparations of isometheptene, a sympathomimetic used as an antispasmodic and vasoconstrictor.

octipara (ok-tip′ah-rah) a woman who has had eight pregnancies that resulted in viable offspring; para VIII.

octodrine (ok′to-drēn) a vasoconstrictor and local anesthetic.

octoxynol (ok-toks′ĭ-nol) a viscous liquid used as a surfactant.

ocul(o)- word element [L.], *eye.*

ocular (ok′u-lar) 1. pertaining to the eye. 2. eyepiece (of a microscope).

oculist (ok′u-list) ophthalmologist.

oculocerebrorenal syndrome (ok″u-lo-sĕ-re″bro-re′nal) a hereditary syndrome of males, with vitamin D–refractory rickets, hydrophthalmia, congenital glaucoma and cataracts, mental retardation, and renal tubule dysfunction as evidenced by hypophosphatemia, acidosis, and aminoaciduria. Called also Lowe's disease.

oculocutaneous (ok″u-lo-ku-ta′ne-us) pertaining to or affecting both the eyes and the skin.

oculofacial (ok″u-lo-fa′shal) pertaining to the eyes and face.

oculogyration (ok″u-lo-ji-ra′shun) the movement of the eyeball about the anteroposterior axis.

oculomotor (ok″u-lo-mo′tor) pertaining to or affecting eye movements.

o. nerve, the third cranial nerve; it is mixed, that is, it contains both sensory and motor fibers. Various branches of the oculomotor nerve provide for muscle sense and movement in most of the muscles of the eye, for constriction of the pupil, and for accommodation of the eye (see also table of NERVES).

oculomotorius (ok″u-lo-mo-to′re-us) the oculomotor nerve.

oculomycosis (ok″u-lo-mi-ko′sis) any fungal disease of the eye.

oculonasal (ok″u-lo-na′zal) pertaining to the eye and the nose.

oculopupillary (ok″u-lo-pu′pĭ-ler″e) pertaining to the pupil of the eye.

oculozygomatic (ok″u-lo-zi″go-mat′ik) pertaining to the eye and the zygoma.

oculus (ok′u-lus), pl. *oc′uli* [L.] eye.

O.D. 1. Doctor of Optometry. 2. [L.] *oc′ulus dex′ter* (right eye).

odont(o)- word element [Gr.], *tooth.*

odontalgia (o″don-tal′je-ah) toothache.

odontectomy (o″don-tek′to-me) excision of a tooth.

odontic (o-don′tik) pertaining to the teeth.

odontoblast (o-don′to-blast) one of the connective tissue cells that deposit dentin and form the outer surface of the dental pulp adjacent to the dentin.

odontoblastoma (o-don″to-blas-to′mah) a tumor made up of odontoblasts.

odontoclast (o-don′to-klast) an osteoclast associated with absorption of the roots of deciduous teeth.

odontogenesis (o-don″to-jen′ĕ-sis) the origin and development of the teeth. adj., **odontogenet′ic.**

o. imperfec′ta, dentinogenesis imperfecta.

odontogenic (o-don″to-jen′ik) 1. forming teeth. 2. arising in tissues that give origin to the teeth.

odontogeny (o″don-toj′ĕ-ne) odontogenesis.

odontograph (o-don′to-graf) an instrument for recording the unevenness of the surface of tooth enamel.

odontography (o″don-tog′rah-fe) 1. a description of the teeth. 2. the use of the odontograph.

odontoid (o-don′toid) like a tooth.

odontology (o″don-tol′o-je) 1. scientific study of the teeth. 2. dentistry.

odontolysis (o″don-tol′ĭ-sis) the resorption of dental tissue.

odontoma (o″don-to′mah) any odontogenic tumor, especially a composite odontoma.

ameloblastic o., a rare neoplasm composed of enamel, dentin, and an odontogenic epithelium like that seen in ameloblastoma.

composite o., one consisting of both enamel and dentin in an abnormal pattern.

radicular o., one associated with a tooth root, or formed when the root was developing.

odontopathy (o″don-top′ah-the) any disease of the teeth.

odontosis (o″don-to′sis) formation or eruption of the teeth.

odontotomy (o″don-tot′o-me) incision of a tooth.

odynacusis (o-din″ah-ku′sis) painful hearing.

-odynia word element [Gr.], *pain.*

odynometer (o″din-om′ĕ-ter) an instrument for measuring pain.

odynophagia (o-din″o-fa′je-ah) painful swallowing of food.

oe- for words beginning thus, see also those beginning *e-*.

oedipal (ed′ĭ-pal) pertaining to the Oedipus complex.

Oedipus complex (ed′ĭ-pus) a term used originally in PSYCHOANALYSIS to signify the complicated conflicts and emotions felt by a child when, during a stage of his normal development as a member of the family circle, he becomes aware of a particularly strong, sexually tinged attachment to his mother; the term also applies to a similar attachment felt by a girl to her father (called also Electra complex). At the same time, the child tends to view the other parent as a rival and yearns to take that parent's place. This pattern, which was described by Sigmund Freud, is named from the legend of the mythical Greek hero, King Oedipus of Thebes, who unknowningly killed his father and married his mother.

According to psychoanalysts, a child enters the oedipal phase at about the third year and usually has solved his largely unconscious conflicts in a satisfactory way by the age of 5 or 6. He does this by turning his feelings of possessiveness toward one parent and competitiveness toward the other into a wish to be liked by both of them. Eventually, a child who has worked out his conflicts well can focus his affection on members of the opposite sex outside the family circle and can establish satisfactory marital relationships as an adult.

Freud's theory is generally accepted by psychiatrists, although many have developed supplementary theories for the behavior pattern he described.

oesophagostomiasis (e-sof″ah-go-sto-mi′ah-sis) infection with *Œsophagostomum.*

Œsophagostomum (e-sof″ah-gos′to-mum) a genus of nematode worms found in the intestines of various animals.

Oestrus (es′trus) a genus of botflies.

O. o′vis, a widespread species that deposits its larvae on the nostrils of sheep and goats, and which may cause ocular myiasis in man.

official (ŏ-fish′al) authorized by pharmacopeias and recognized formularies.

officinal (o-fis′ĭ-nal) regularly kept for sale in druggists' shops.

Oguchi's disease (o-goo′chēz) a form of hereditary night blindness occurring in Japan.

OH hydroxyl group; (with negative sign) hydroxyl ion; a hydroxide.

ohm (ōm) a unit of electric resistance, being that of a column of mercury 1 sq. mm. in cross section and 106.25 cm. long.

Ohm's law (ōmz) the strength of an electric current varies directly as the electromotive force and inversely as the resistance.

ohmmeter (ōm′me-ter) an instrument that measures electrical resistance in ohms.

oil (oil) 1. an unctuous, combustible substance that is liquid, or easily liquefiable, on warming, and is not miscible with water, but is soluble in ether. Such substances, depending on their origin, are classified as animal, mineral, or vegetable oils. Depending on their behavior on heating, they are classified as volatile or fixed. For specific oils, see the specific name, as CASTOR OIL. 2. a fat that is liquid at room temperature.

essential o., ethereal o., volatile oil.

fixed o., an oil that does not evaporate on warming and occurs as a solid, semisolid, or liquid.

volatile o., an oil that evaporates readily; such oils occur in aromatic plants, to which they give odor and other characteristics.

ointment (oint′ment) a semisolid preparation for external application to the body. Official ointments consist of medicinal substances incorporated in suitable vehicles (bases).

white o., mixture of white wax and white petrolatum; used as a vehicle for medications to be applied to the skin.

yellow o., a mixture of yellow wax and petrolatum; used as a vehicle for medications.

O.L. [L.] *oc′ulus lae′vus* (left eye).

-ol word termination indicating an alcohol or a phenol.

oleaginous (o″le-aj′ĭ-nus) oily; greasy.

oleandomycin (o″le-an″do-mi′sin) an antibiotic substance produced by growth of *Streptomyces antibioticus;* used chiefly in treatment of infections by gram-positive organisms.

oleate (o′le-āt) 1. a salt of oleic acid. 2. a solution of a substance in oleic acid.

olecranarthritis (o-lek″ran-ar-thri′tis) inflammation of the elbow joint.

olecranarthrocace (o-lek″ran-ar-throk′ah-se) tuberculosis of the elbow joint.

olecranarthropathy (o-lek″ran-ar-throp′ah-the) disease of the elbow joint.

olecranoid (o-lek′rah-noid) resembling the olecranon.

olecranon (o-lek′rah-non) the bony projection of the ulna at the elbow. adj., **olec′ranal.**

oleic acid (o-le′ik) a long-chain unsaturated fatty acid found in animal and vegetable fats.

oleo- word element [L.], *oil.*

oleoresin (o″le-o-rez′in) 1. a compound of a resin and a volatile oil, such as exudes from pines, etc. 2. a compound extracted from a drug by percolation with a volatile solvent, such as acetone, alcohol, or ether, and evaporation of the solvent.

oleotherapy (o″le-o-ther′ah-pe) treatment by injections of oil.

oleothorax (o″le-o-tho′raks) intrapleural injection of oil to compress the lung in pulmonary tuberculosis.

oleovitamin (o″le-o-vi′tah-min) a preparation of fat-soluble vitamins in fish liver or edible vegetable oil.

oleum (o′le-um), pl. *o′lea* [L.] oil.

olfact (ol′fakt) a unit of odor, the minimal perceptible odor, being the minimal concentration of a substance in solution that can be perceived by a large number of normal individuals, expressed in terms of grams per liter.

olfaction (ol-fak′shun) 1. the act of smelling. 2. the sense of smell.

olfactology (ol″fak-tol′o-je) the science of the sense of smell.

olfactometer (ol″fak-tom′ĕ-ter) an instrument for testing the sense of smell.

olfactory (ol-fak′to-re) pertaining to the sense of smell.

o. bulb, the bulblike extremity of the olfactory nerve on the undersurface of each anterior lobe of the cerebrum.

o. nerve, the first cranial nerve: it is purely sensory and is concerned with the sense of smell. The nerve cell bodies are situated in the olfactory area of the mucous membrane of the nose. The nerve fibers lead upward through openings in the ethmoid bone and connect with the cells of the olfactory bulb. From there the fibers pass inward to the cerebrum. (See also table of NERVES.)

olig(o)- word element [Gr.], *few; little; scanty.*

oligemia (ol″ĭ-ge′me-ah) deficiency in volume of the blood. adj., **olige′mic.**

oligochromemia (ol″ĭ-go-kro-me′me-ah) deficiency of hemoglobin in the blood.

oligochymia (ol″i-go-ki′me-ah) deficiency of chyme.

oligocythemia (ol″i-go-si-the′me-ah) deficiency of the cellular elements of the blood. adj., **oligocythe′mic.**

oligodactyly (ol″ĭ-go-dak′tĭ-le) congenital absence of one or more fingers or toes.

oligodendrocyte (ol″ĭ-go-den′dro-sīt) a cell of oligodendroglia.

oligodendroglia (ol″ĭ-go-den-drog′le-ah) 1. the non-neural cells of ectodermal origin forming part of the adventitial structure of the central nervous system. 2. the tissue composed of such cells.

oligodendroglioma (ol″ĭ-go-den″dro-gli-o′mah) a neoplasm derived from and composed of oligodendroglia.

oligodipsia (ol″ĭ-go-dip′se-ah) abnormally diminished thirst.

oligodontia (ol″ĭ-go-don′she-ah) congenital absence of some of the teeth.

oligodynamic (ol″ĭ-go-di-nam′ik) active in a small quantity.

oligogalactia (ol″ĭ-go-gah-lak′she-ah) deficient secretion of milk.

oligogenic (ol″ĭ-go-jen′ik) produced by a few genes at most; used in reference to certain hereditary characters.

oligohemia (ol″ĭ-go-he′me-ah) oligemia.

oligohydramnios (ol″ĭ-go-hi-dram′ne-os) deficiency in the amount of amniotic fluid.

oligohydruria (ol″ĭ-go-hi-droo′re-ah) abnormally high concentration of urine.

oligomenorrhea (ol″ĭ-go-men″o-re′ah) abnormally infrequent menstruation.

oligonucleotide (ol″ĭ-go-nu′kle-o-tīd) a polymer made up of a few (2–10) nucleotides.

oligophosphaturia (ol″ĭ-go-fos″fah-tu′re-ah) deficiency of phosphates in the urine.

oligophrenia (ol″ĭ-go-fre′ne-ah) mental deficiency. adj., **oligophren′ic.**

phenylpyruvic o., o. phenylpyru′vica, mental deficiency associated with PHENYLKETONURIA.

oligoplasmia (ol″ĭ-go-plaz′me-ah) deficiency of blood plasma.

oligopnea (ol″ĭ-gop′ne-ah) hypoventilation.

oligoptyalism (ol″ĭ-go-ti′ah-lizm) diminished secretion of saliva.

oligospermia (ol″ĭ-go-sper′me-ah) deficiency of spermatozoa in the semen.

oligotrophia, oligotrophy (ol″ĭ-go-tro′fe-ah; ol″ĭ-got′ro-fe) a state of poor (insufficient) nutrition.

oliguria (ol″ĭ-gu′re-ah) diminished urine secretion in relation to fluid intake.

olivary (ol′ĭ-ver″e) shaped like an olive.

o. body, o. nucleus, olive (2).

olive (ol′iv) 1. the tree *Olea europaea* and its fruit. 2. olivary body; a rounded elevation lateral to the upper part of each pyramid of the medulla oblongata.

olivifugal (ol″ĭ-vif′u-gal) moving or conducting away from the olive.

olivipetal (ol″ĭ-vip′ĕ-tal) moving or conducting toward the olive.

olivopontocerebellar (ol″ĭ-vo-pon″to-ser″ĕ-bel′ar) pertaining to the olive, the middle peduncles, and the cerebellar cortex.

Ollier's disease (ol″e-āz) enchondromatosis.

Ollier's layer (ol″e-āz′) the innermost layer of the periosteum; called also osteogenetic layer.

Ollier-Thiersch graft (ol″e-a-tērsh′) a very thin skin graft in which long, broad strips of skin, consisting of the epidermis, rete, and part of the corium, are used.

olophonia (ol″o-fo′ne-ah) defective speech due to malformed vocal organs.

-oma word element [Gr.], *tumor; neoplasm.*

omagra (o-mag′rah) gout in the shoulder.

omalgia (o-mal′je-ah) pain in the shoulder.

omarthritis (o″mar-thri′tis) inflammation of the shoulder joint.

omentectomy (o″men-tek′to-me) excision of all or part of the omentum.

omentitis (o″men-ti′tis) inflammation of the omentum.

omentofixation, omentopexy (o-men″to-fik-sa′-shun; o-men′to-pek″se) fixation of the omentum, especially to establish collateral circulation in portal obstruction.

omentorrhaphy (o″men-tor′ah-fe) suture or repair of the omentum.

omentum (o-men′tum), pl. *omen′ta* [L.] a fold of peritoneum extending from the stomach to adjacent abdominal organs. adj., **omen′tal.**

gastrocolic o., greater omentum.

gastrohepatic o., lesser omentum.

greater o., a peritoneal fold attached to the anterior surface of the transverse colon.

lesser o., a peritoneal fold joining the lesser curvature of the stomach and the first part of the duodenum to the porta hepatis.

o. ma′jus, greater omentum.

o. mi′nus, lesser omentum.

omitis (o-mi′tis) inflammation of the shoulder.

omnivorous (om-niv′o-rus) eating both plant and animal foods.

omoclavicular (o″mo-klah-vik′u-lar) pertaining to the shoulder and clavicle.

omodynia (o″mo-din′e-ah) pain in the shoulder.

omohyoid (o″mo-hi′oid) pertaining to the shoulder and the hyoid bone.

omphal(o)- word element [Gr.], *umbilicus.*

omphalectomy (om″fah-lek′to-me) excision of the umbilicus.

omphalelcosis (om″fal-el-ko′sis) ulceration of the umbilicus.

omphalic (om-fal′ik) pertaining to the umbilicus.

omphalitis (om″fah-li′tis) inflammation of the umbilicus.

omphaloangiopagus (om″fah-lo-an″je-op′ah-gus) twin fetuses, one of which derives its blood supply from the umbilicus or placenta of the other.

omphalocele (om′fal-o-sēl″) protrusion, at birth, of part of the intestine through a defect in the abdominal wall at the umbilicus.

omphalomesenteric (om″fah-lo-mes″en-ter′ik) pertaining to the umbilicus and mesentery.

omphalophlebitis (om″fah-lo-flĕ-bi′tis) inflammation of the umbilical veins.

omphalorrhagia (om″fah-lo-ra′je-ah) hemorrhage from the umbilicus.

omphalorrhea (om″fah-lo-re′ah) effusion of lymph at the umbilicus.

omphalorrhexis (om″fah-lo-rek′sis) rupture of the umbilicus.

omphalosite (om′fal-o-sīt″) the underdeveloped member of allantoidoangiopagous twins, joined to the more developed member (autosite) by the vessels of the umbilical cord.

omphalotomy (om″fah-lot′o-me) the cutting of the umbilical cord.

onanism (o′nah-nizm) incomplete sexual relations with withdrawal just before emission; sometimes used as a synonym for masturbation.

Onchocerca (ong″ko-ser′kah) a genus of nematode parasites (superfamily Filarioidea).

O. vol′vulus, a species causing human infection by invading the skin, subcutaneous tissues, and other tissues, producing fibrous nodules; blindness occurs after ocular invasion.

onchocerciasis (ong″ko-ser-ki′ah-sis) infection by nematodes of the genus *Onchocerca.*

onco- word element [Gr.], *tumor; swelling; mass.*

oncogenesis (ong″ko-jen″ĕ-sis) the production or causation of tumors. adj., **oncogenet′ic.**

oncogenic (ong″ko-jen′ik) giving rise to tumors or causing tumor formation; said especially of tumor-inducing viruses.

oncogenous (ong-koj′ĕ-nus) arising in or originating from a tumor.

oncology (ong-kol′o-je) the sum of knowledge regarding tumors; the study of tumors.

oncolysis (ong-kol′ĭ-sis) destruction or dissolution of a neoplasm. adj., **oncolyt′ic.**

oncoma (ong-ko′mah) a tumor.

oncosis (ong-ko′sis) a morbid condition marked by the development of tumors.

oncosphere (ong′ko-sfēr) the larva of the tapeworm contained within the external embryonic envelope and armed with six hooks.

oncotherapy (ong″ko-ther′ah-pe) the treatment of tumors.

oncotic (ong-kot′ik) pertaining to swelling.

oncotomy (ong-kot′o-me) incision of a tumor or swelling.

oncotropic (ong″ko-trop′ik) having special affinity for tumor cells.

oneir(o)- word element [Gr.], *dream.*

oneirodynia (o-ni″ro-din′e-ah) nightmare.

oneiric (o-ni′rik) pertaining to dreams.

oneirism (o-ni′rizm) a waking dream state.

oneirology (o″ni-rol′o-je) the science of dreams.

oneiroscopy (o″ni-ros′ko-pe) analysis of dreams for diagnosis of a patient's mental state.

onlay (on′la) a graft applied or laid on the surface of an organ or structure.

onomatology (on″o-mah-tol′o-je) the science of names and nomenclature.

onomatomania (on″o-mat″o-ma′ne-ah) mental derangement with regard to words or names.

onomatophobia (on″o-mat″o-fo′be-ah) morbid aversion to a certain word or name.

ontogeny (on″toj′ĕ-ne) the complete developmental history of an individual organism. adj., **ontogenet′ic, ontogen′ic.**

onyalai, onyalia (o″ne-al′a-e; o″ne-a′le-ah) a form of thrombopenic purpura due to a nutritional disorder occurring in Africa, marked by blebs on the buccal and palatal mucosa which contain semicoagulated blood.

onych(o)- word element [Gr.], *the nails.*

onychalgia (on″ĭ-kal′je-ah) pain in the nails.

onychatrophia (o-nik″ah-tro′fe-ah) atrophy of a nail or the nails.

onychauxis (on″ĭ-kawk′sis) hypertrophy of the nails.

onychectomy (on″ĭ-kek′to-me) excision of a nail or nail bed.

onychia (o-nik′e-ah) inflammation of the nail bed, resulting in loss of the nail.

onychitis (on″ĭ-ki′tis) inflammation of the matrix of a nail.

onychodystrophy (on″ĭ-ko-dis′tro-fe) malformation of a nail.

onychogenic (on″ĭ-ko-jen′ik) producing nail substance.

onychograph (o-nik′o-graf) an instrument for observing and recording the nail pulse and capillary circulation.

onychogryphosis, onychogryposis (on″ĭ-ko-grĭ-fo′sis; on″ĭ-ko-grĭ-po′sis) abnormal hypertrophy and curving of the nails, giving a clawlike appearance.

onychoheterotopia (on″ĭ-ko-het″er-o-to′pe-ah) abnormal location of the nails.

onychoid (on′ĭ-koid) resembling a fingernail.

onycholysis (on″ĭ-kol′ĭ-sis) loosening or separation of a nail from its bed; onychoschizia.

onychomadesis (on″ĭ-ko-mah-de′sis) complete loss of the nails.

onychomalacia (on″ĭ-ko-mah-la′she-ah) softening of the fingernail.

onychomycosis (on″ĭ-ko-mi-ko′sis) fungal disease of the nails; the nails become opaque, white, thickened, and friable.

onychopathy (on″ĭ-kop′ah-the) any disease of the nails.

onychophagia, onychophagy (on″ĭ-ko-fa′je-ah; on″ĭ-kof′ah-je) biting of the nails.

onychorrhexis (on″ĭ-ko-rek′sis) spontaneous splitting or breaking of the nails.

onychoschizia (on″ĭ-ko-skiz′e-ah) onycholysis.

onychosis (on″ĭ-ko′sis) disease or deformity of a nail or the nails.

onychotillomania (on″ĭ-ko-til″o-ma′ne-ah) neurotic picking or tearing at the nails.

onychotomy (on″ĭ-kot′o-me) incision into a fingernail or toenail.

onyx (on′iks) 1. a variety of hypopyon. 2. a fingernail or toenail.

oo- word element [Gr.], *egg; ovum.*

ooblast (o′o-blast) a primitive cell from which an ovum ultimately develops.

oocyst (o′o-sist) the encysted or encapsulated ookinete in the wall of a mosquito's stomach; also, the analagous stage in the development of any sporozoon.

oocyte (o′o-sīt) an immature ovum; it is derived from an oogonium, and is called a primary oocyte prior to completion of the first maturation division, and a secondary oocyte between the first and second maturation division.

oogenesis (o″o-jen′ĕ-sis) the development of mature ova from oogonia. adj., **oogenet′ic.**

oogonium (o″o-go′ne-um), pl. *oogo′nia* [Gr.] an ovarian egg during fetal development; near the time of birth it becomes a primary oocyte.

ookinesis (o″o-ki-ne′sis) the mitotic movements of an ovum during maturation and fertilization.

ookinete (o″o-kĭ-nēt′) the fertilized form of the malarial parasite in a mosquito's body, formed by fertilization of a macrogamete by a microgamete and developing into an oocyst.

oolemma (o″o-lem′ah) zona pellucida.

oophor(o)- word element [Gr.], *ovary.*

oophorectomy (o″of-o-rek′to-me) excision of one or both ovaries; called also ovariectomy. The procedure is done for tumors, severe infection, or other disorders of the ovary. Removal of the ovaries from a girl who has not yet reached puberty prevents the development of secondary sex characters. If the ovaries are removed from an adult woman, reproduction is not possible and the female sex hormones estrogen and progesterone are no longer produced.

oophoritis (o″of-o-ri′tis) inflammation of an ovary; ovaritis.

oophorocystectomy (o-of″o-ro-sis-tek′to-me) excision of an ovarian cyst.

oophorocystosis (o-of″o-ro-sis-to′sis) the formation of an ovarian cyst.

oophorohysterectomy (o-of″o-ro-his″ter-ek′to-me) excision of the ovaries and uterus.

oophoron (o-of′o-ron) an ovary.

oophoropexy (o-of′o-ro-pek″se) ovariopexy.

oophoroplasty (o-of′o-ro-plas″te) plastic repair of an ovary.

oophorostomy (o-of″o-ros′to-me) incision of an ovarian cyst for drainage purposes.

oophorotomy (o-of″o-rot′o-me) incision of an ovary.

ooplasm (o′o-plazm) cytoplasm of an ovum.

oosperm (o′o-sperm) a fertilized ovum.

ootid (o′o-tid) the cell produced by meiotic division of a secondary oocyte, which develops into the ovum. In mammals, this second maturation division is not completed unless fertilization occurs.

opacification (o-pah″sĭ-fĭ-ka′shun) the development of an opacity.

opacity (o-pas′ĭ-te) 1. the condition of being opaque. 2. an opaque area.

opalescent (o″pal-es′ent) showing a milky iridescence, like an opal.

opaque (o-pāk) impervious to light rays or, by extension, to roentgen rays or other electromagnetic radiation; neither translucent nor transparent.

opening (o′pen-ing) an aperture, orifice, or open space.

aortic o., 1. the aperture of the ventricle into the aorta. 2. the aperture in the diaphragm for passage of the descending aorta.

cardiac o., the opening from the esophagus into the stomach.

pyloric o., the opening between the stomach and duodenum.

operable (op′er-ah-b′l) subject to being operated upon with a reasonable degree of safety; appropriate for surgical removal.

operant (op′ĕ-rant) see instrumental (operant) CONDITIONING.

operate (op′er-āt) 1. to perform an operation. 2. the subject of an experiment who has undergone a specific surgical procedure.

operation (op″er-a′shun) any action performed with instruments or by the hands of a surgeon; a surgical procedure. 2. any effect produced by a therapeutic agent. For specific operations, see the specific name, as BLALOCK-TAUSSIG OPERATION.

cosmetic o., one intended to remove or correct a deformity in an esthetically acceptable manner.

exploratory o., incision into the body for determination of the cause of otherwise unexplainable symptoms.

flap o., any operation involving the raising of a flap of tissue.

radical o., one involving extensive resection of tissues for the complete extirpation of disease.

operative (op′er-a″tiv) 1. pertaining to an operation. 2. effective; not inert.

operculum (o-per′ku-lum), pl. *oper′cula* [L.] a lid or covering; the folds of pallium from the frontal, parietal, and temporal lobes of the cerebrum overlying the insula. adj., **oper′cular.**

dental o., the hood of gingival tissue overlying the crown of an erupting tooth.

trophoblastic o., the plug of trophoblast that helps close the gap in the endometrium made by the implanting blastocyst.

operon (op′er-on) a segment of a chromosome comprising an operator gene and closely linked structural genes having related functions, the activity of the latter being controlled by the operator gene through its interaction with a regulator gene.

ophiasis (o-fi′ah-sis) a form of alopecia areata involving the temporal and occipital margins of the scalp in a continuous band.

ophidism (o′fĭ-dizm) poisoning by snake venom.

ophryosis (of″re-o′sis) spasm of the eyebrow.

Ophthaine (of′thān) trademark for a preparation of proparacaine, a topical anesthetic.

ophthalm(o)- word element [Gr.], *eye.*

ophthalmagra (of″thal-mag′rah) sudden pain in the eye.

ophthalmalgia (of″thal-mal′je-ah) pain in the eye.

ophthalmectomy (of″thal-mek′to-me) excision of an eye; enucleation of the eyeball.

ophthalmencephalon (of″thal-men-sef′ah-lon) the retina, optic nerve, and visual apparatus of the brain.

ophthalmia (of-thal′me-ah) severe inflammation of the eye or of the conjunctiva or deeper structures of the eye.

Egyptian o., trachoma.

gonorrheal o., acute and severe purulent conjunctivitis due to gonorrheal infection.

o. neonato′rum, any hyperacute purulent conjunctivitis, e.g., gonorrheal ophthalmia, occurring during the first 10 days of life, usually contracted during birth from infected vaginal discharge of the mother. It is prevented by instilling silver nitrate or other chemicals in the eyes of the newborn.

phlyctenular o., phlyctenular keratoconjunctivitis.

sympathetic o., granulomatous inflammation of the uveal tract of the uninjured eye following a wound involving the uveal tract of the other eye, resulting in bilateral granulomatous inflammation of the entire uveal tract. Called also sympathetic uveitis.

ophthalmic (of-thal′mik) pertaining to the eye.

o. reaction, ophthalmoreaction.

ophthalmitis (of″thal-mi′tis) inflammation of the eyeball. adj., **opthalmit′ic.**

ophthalmoblennorrhea (of-thal″mo-blen″o-re′ah) gonorrheal ophthalmia.

ophthalmocele (of-thal′mo-sēl) exophthalmos.

ophthalmodonesis (of-thal″mo-do-ne′sis) trembling motion of the eyes.

ophthalmodynamometry (of-thal″mo-di″nah-mom′ĕ-tre) determination of the blood pressure in the retinal artery.

ophthalmodynia (of-thal″mo-din′e-ah) pain in the eye.

ophthalmoeikonometer (of-thal″mo-i″ko-nom′-ĕ-ter) an instrument used to determine both the refraction of the eye and the relative size and shape of the ocular images.

ophthalmography (of″thal-mog′rah-fe) description of the eye and its diseases.

ophthalmogyric (of-thal″mo-ji′rik) oculogyric.

ophthalmolith (of-thal′mo-lith) a lacrimal calculus.

ophthalmologist (of″thal-mol′o-jist) a physician who specializes in diagnosing and prescribing treatment for defects, injuries, and diseases of the EYE, and is skilled at delicate eye surgery, such as that required to remove cataracts; called also oculist or eye specialist.

ophthalmology (of″thal-mol′o-je) that branch of medicine dealing with the eye, its anatomy, physiology, pathology, etc. adj., **ophthalmolog′ic.**

ophthalmomalacia (of-thal″mo-mah-la′she-ah) abnormal softness of the eyeball.

ophthalmometer (of″thal-mom′ĕ-ter) an instrument used in ophthalmometry.

ophthalmometry (of″thal-mom′ĕ-tre) determination of the refractive powers and defects of the eye.

ophthalmomycosis (of-thal″mo-mi-ko′sis) any disease of the eye caused by a fungus.

ophthalmomyotomy (of-thal″mo-mi-ot′o-me) surgical division of the muscles of the eyes.

ophthalmoneuritis (of-thal″mo-nu-ri′tis) inflammation of the optic nerve.

ophthalmopathy (of″thal-mop′ah-the) any disease of the eye.

ophthalmoplasty (of-thal′mo-plas″te) plastic surgery of the eye or its appendages.

ophthalmoplegia (of-thal″mo-ple′je-ah) paralysis of the eye muscles. adj., **ophthalmople′gic.**

o. exter′na, paralysis of the extraocular muscles.

o. inter′na, paralysis of the iris and ciliary apparatus.

nuclear o., that due to a lesion of nuclei of motor nerves of eye.

Parinaud's o., paralysis of conjugate upward movement of the eyes without paralysis of convergence, associated with midbrain lesions.

partial o., that affecting some of the eye muscles.

progressive o., gradual paralysis of all the eye muscles.

total o., paralysis of all the eye muscles, both intraocular and extraocular.

ophthalmoptosis (of-thal″mop-to′sis) exophthalmos.

ophthalmoreaction (of-thal″mo-re-ak′shun) local reaction of the conjunctiva after instillation into the eye of toxins or organisms causing typhoid fever and tuberculosis, being more severe in those affected with these diseases. Called also ophthalmic reaction.

ophthalmorrhagia (of-thal″mo-ra′je-ah) hemorrhage from the eye.

ophthalmorrhea (of-thal″mo-re′ah) oozing of blood from the eye.

ophthalmorrhexis (of-thal″mo-rek′sis) rupture of an eyeball.

ophthalmoscope (of-thal′mo-skōp) an instrument for examining the interior of the eye. It sends a bright, narrow beam of light through the lens of the eye, and contains a perforated mirror and lenses through which the physician can examine interior parts of the eye. It is helpful in detecting possible disorders of the eyes, as well as disorders of other organs that are reflected in the condition of the eyes.

direct o., one that produces an upright, or unreversed, image of approximately 15 times magnification.

indirect o., one that produces an inverted, or reversed, direct image of two to five times magnification.

ophthalmoscopy (of″thal-mos′ko-pe) examination of the eye by means of the ophthalmoscope.

medical o., that performed for diagnostic purposes.

metric o., that performed for measurement of refraction.

ophthalmostasis (of″thal-mos′tah-sis) fixation of the eye with the ophthalmostat.

ophthalmostat (of-thal′mo-stat) an instrument for holding the eye steady during operation.

opthalmosteresis (of-thal″mo-stĕ-re′sis) loss of an eye.

ophthalmosynchysis (of-thal″mo-sin′kĭ-sis) effusion into the eye.

ophthalmotomy (of″thal-mot′o-me) incision of the eye.

ophthalmotrope (of-thal′mo-trōp) a mechanical eye that moves like a real eye.

ophthalmoxerosis (of-thal″mo-ze-ro′sis) xerophthalmia; abnormal dryness and thickening of the conjunctiva and cornea due to vitamin A deficiency or to local disease.

opianine (o-pi′ah-nin) noscapine, an antitussive.

opiate (o′pe-at) 1. any sedative narcotic containing opium or any of its derivatives. 2. any sedative or narcotic.

opiomania (o″pe-o-ma′ne-ah) intense craving for opium.

opipramol (o-pip′rah-mōl) an antidepressant and tranquilizer.

opisthorchiasis (o″pis-thor-ki′ah-sis) a diseased condition of the liver due to the presence of flukes of the genus *Opisthorchis.*

Opisthorchis (o″pis-thor′kis) a genus of flukes parasitic in the liver and biliary tract of various birds and mammals, including man.

O. sinen′sis, a species widely distributed in China, Japan, Korea, Taiwan, and Indochina; called also *Clonorchis sinensis.*

opisthotonos (o″pis-thot′o-nos) a form of spasm in which the head and heels are bent backward and the body bowed forward. adj. **opisthoton′ic.**

opium (o′pe-um) the air-dried milky exudation from unripe capsules of the opium poppy *Papaver somniferum* or its variety *album.* Opium contains some 25 alkaloids, the most important being morphine (from which heroin is derived), narcotine, codeine, papaverine, thebaine, and narceine; the alkaloids are used for their narcotic and analgesic effect. It is poisonous in large doses. Because it is highly addictive, opium production is restricted and its sale or possession for other than medical uses is strictly prohibited by federal, state, and local laws. (See also DRUG ABUSE.)

opocephalus (o″po-sef′ah-lus) a monster with ears fused to the head, one orbit, no mouth, and no nose.

opodidymus (o″po-did′ĭ-mus) a monster with two fused heads and sense organs partly fused.

Oppenheim's disease (op′en-hīmz) amyotonia congenita.

Oppenheim's gait (op′en-hīmz) a gait marked by irregular oscillation of the head, limbs, and body; seen in some cases of multiple sclerosis.

opportunistic (op″or-too-nis′tik) capable of adapting to a tissue or host other than the normal one; said of microorganisms.

opsin (op′sin) a protein of the retinal rods (scotopsin) and cones (photopsin) that combines with 11-*cis*-retinal to form visual pigments.

opsinogen (op-sin′o-jen) a substance (antigen) capable of producing the formation of opsonins. adj., **opsinog′enous.**

opsiuria (op″se-u′re-ah) excretion of urine more rapidly during fasting than after a meal.

opsoclonia, opsoclonus (op″so-clo′ne-ah; op″so-clo′nus) involuntary, nonrhythmic horizontal and vertical oscillations of the eyes.

opsogen (op′so-jen) opsinogen.

opsomania (op″so-ma′ne-ah) an abnormal craving for some special food.

opsonin (op-so′nin) an antibody that renders bacteria and other cells susceptible to phagocytosis. adj., **opson′ic.**

immune o., an antibody that sensitizes a particulate antigen to phagocytosis, after combination with the homologous antigen in vivo or in vitro.

opsonization (op″so-ni-za′shun) the rendering of bacteria and other cells subject to phagocytosis.

opsonize (op′so-nīz) to subject to opsonization.

opsonocytophagic (op″so-no-si″to-fa′jik) denoting the phagocytic activity of blood in the presence of serum opsonins and homologous leukocytes.

opsonometry (op″so-nom′ĕ-tre) measurement of the amount of opsonin present.

opsonotherapy (op″so-no-ther′ah-pe) treatment by use of bacterial vaccines to increase the opsonic index.

optesthesia (op″tes-the′ze-ah) visual sensibility; ability to perceive visual stimuli.

optic (op′tik) of or pertaining to the eye.

o. nerve, the second cranial nerve; it is purely sensory and is concerned with carrying impulses for the sense of sight. The rods and cones of the RETINA are connected with the optic nerve which leaves the eye slightly to the nasal side of the center of the retina. The point at which the optic nerve leaves the eye is called the blind spot because there are no rods and cones in this area. The optic nerve passes through the optic foramen of the skull and into the cranial cavity. It then passes backward and undergoes a division; those nerve fibers leading from the nasal side of the retina cross to the opposite side while those from the temporal side continue to the thalamus uncrossed. After synapsing in the thalamus the neurons convey visual impulses to the occipital lobe of the brain.

Degenerative and inflammatory lesions of the optic nerve occur as a result of infections, toxic damage to the nerve, metabolic or nutritional disorders, or trauma. Syphilis is the most frequent cause of infectious disorders of the optic nerve. Methanol (methyl alcohol) is highly toxic to the optic nerve and can cause total blindness. Diabetes mellitus and anemia are examples of metabolic and nutritional disorders that can lead to damage to the optic nerve and produce serious loss of vision.

Treatment of optic neuritis is aimed at control of the primary cause of the disorder. Cortisone and similar steroids are often used to relieve symptoms; however, nothing can be done to regain sight lost through damage to the nerve.

optical (op′tĭ-kal) pertaining to vision.

optician (op-tish′an) a specialist in opticianry. Although this is a very exact and intricate science, the optician does not need a state license to practice. He is not qualified to examine eyes or to prescribe the correct eyeglasses.

opticianry (op-tish′an-re) the translation, filling, and adapting of ophthalmic prescriptions, products, and accessories.

opticist (op′tĭ-sist) a specialist in the science of optics.

opticociliary (op″tĭ-ko-sil′e-er″e) pertaining to the optic and ciliary nerves.

opticokinetic (op″tĭ-ko-ki-net′ik) pertaining to movement of the eyes.

opticopupillary (op″tĭ-ko-pu′pĭ-ler″e) pertaining to the optic nerve and pupil.

optics (op′tiks) the science of light and vision.

opto- word element [Gr.], *visible; vision; sight.*

optogram (op′to-gram) the visual image formed on the retina by bleaching of visual purple under the influence of light.

optometer (op-tom′ĕ-ter) a device for measuring the power and range of vision.

optometrist (op-tom′ĕ-trist) a specialist in optometry; a professional person trained to examine the eyes and prescribe eyeglasses to correct irregularities in the vision. The optometrist uses various devices such as eye charts to determine the strength of the vision and to discover any irregularities such as ASTIGMATISM. He then prescribes the necessary correction. The optometrist is not a physician and is not qualified to diagnose or treat diseases or injuries of the eye, or to perform eye surgery.

optometry (op-tom′ĕ-tre) measurement of the powers of vision and the adaptation of lenses for the aid thereof, utilizing any means other than drugs.

optomyometer (op″to-mi-om′ĕ-ter) a device for measuring the power of ocular muscles.

O.R. operating room.

ora¹ (o′rah), pl. *o′rae* [L.] an edge or margin.

o. serra′ta ret′inae, the zigzag margin of the retina of the eye.

ora² (o′rah) [L.] plural of *os,* mouth.

orad (o′rad) toward the mouth.

oral (o′ral) pertaining to the mouth.

orange (or′anj) 1. the tree *Citrus aurantium* and its edible yellow fruit; the peel of two varieties is used in making various pharmaceuticals. 2. a color between yellow and red. 3. a dye or stain that produces an orange color.

methyl o., an orange-yellow aniline dye, used as an indicator with a pH range of 3.2–4.4 and a color change from pink to yellow.

orbicular (or-bik′u-lar) circular; rounded.

orbit (or′bit) 1. the bony cavity containing the eyeball and its associated muscles, vessels, and nerves; the ethmoid, frontal, lacrimal, nasal, palatine, sphenoid, and zygomatic bones and the maxilla contribute to its formation. 2. the path of an electron around the nucleus of an atom. adj., **or′bital.**

orbitonasal (or″bĭ-to-na′zal) pertaining to the orbit and nose.

orbitonometer (or″bĭ-to-nom′ĕ-ter) an instrument for measuring backward displacement of the eyeball produced by a given pressure on its anterior aspect.

orbitotomy (or″bĭ-tot′o-me) incision into the orbit.

orcein (or-se′in) a brownish-red coloring substance obtained from orcinol; used as a stain for elastic tissue.

orchi(o)- word element [Gr.], *testis.*

orchialgia (or″ke-al′je-ah) pain in a testis.

orchidectomy (or″kĭ-dek′to-me) orchiectomy.

orchidic (or-kid′ik) pertaining to a testis.

orchidorrhaphy (or″kĭ-dor′ah-fe) orchiopexy.

orchiectomy (or″ke-ek′to-me) excision of one or both testes. This procedure is sometimes necessary when a testis is seriously diseased or injured. It may be performed, also, in order to control cancer of the prostate.

If both testes are removed the ability to reproduce is ended. There is also a diminution in the production of the hormone testosterone. Orchiectomy does not interfere with the ability to have coitus but removal of the testes usually reduces sexual desire.

Removal of both testes before puberty prevents the development of secondary sex characters because of the deficiency of testosterone. If the procedure is performed after puberty, when the masculine characteristics are already developed, the changes that occur are much less extreme.

orchiepididymitis (or″ke-ep″ĭ-did″ĭ-mi′tis) inflammation of a testis and epididymis.

orchiocele (or′ke-o-sēl″) 1. hernial protrusion of a testis. 2. scrotal hernia. 3. tumor of a testis.

orchiomyeloma (or″ke-o-mi″ĕ-lo′mah) plasmacytoma of a testis.

orchiopathy (or″ke-op′ah-the) any disease of the testes.

orchiopexy (or′ke-o-pek″se) surgical fixation of an undescended testis in the scrotum. An incision is made over the inguinal canal and the testis is brought down into the scrotum. In most cases the surgeon applies traction by placing a suture in the lower scrotum and attaching the suture to the inner thigh by a piece of adhesive tape. This traction is continued for about 1 week.

PATIENT CARE. Preoperative care of the child is routine. During the postoperative period care must be taken to avoid disturbing the tension mechanism. Contamination of the suture line should be avoided, and if the child is not toilet trained, this usually requires leaving an indwelling catheter in place until the incision has healed.

orchioplasty (or′ke-o-plas″te) plastic surgery of a testis.

orchioscheocele (or″ke-os′ke-o-sēl) scrotal tumor with scrotal hernia.

orchiotomy (or″ke-ot′o-me) incision and drainage of a testis.

orchitis (or-ki′tis) inflammation of a testis. adj., **orchit′ic.** Orchitis is not a common disorder, but it can occur in a variety of infectious diseases, including syphilis, tuberculosis, glanders, leprosy, and certain of the parasitic diseases. It usually accompanies EPIDIDYMITIS. Acute orchitis may also occur in such diseases as typhoid fever, pneumonia, or mumps in adult males.

The symptoms of acute orchitis are swelling of one or both testes with pain and sensitivity to touch. In chronic orchitis there is no pain but the testes swell slowly and become hard.

orcinol (or′si-nol) an antiseptic principle derived mainly from lichens; used as a reagent.

order (or′der) a taxonomic category subordinate to a class and superior to a family (or suborder).

orderly (or′der-le) a male hospital attendant who does general work, attending especially to needs of male patients.

ordinate (or′dĭ-nāt) the vertical line in a graph along which is plotted one of the factors considered in the study, as temperature in a time-temperature study. The other line is called the abscissa.

Oretic (o-ret′ik) trademark for a preparation of hydrochlorothiazide, a diuretic.

Oreton (or′e-ton) trademark for preparations of testosterone, a male sex hormone.

orexigenic (o-rek″sĭ-jen′ik) increasing or stimulating the appetite.

orf (orf) a contagious pustular viral dermatitis of sheep, communicable to man.

organ (or′gan) a somewhat independent body part that performs a specific function or functions.

o. of Corti, the organ lying against the basilar membrane in the cochlear duct, containing special sensory receptors for hearing, and consisting of neuroepithelial hair cells and several types of supporting cells.

enamel o., a process of epithelium forming a cap over a dental papilla and developing into the enamel.

Golgi tendon o., any of the mechanoreceptors arranged in series with muscle in the tendons of mammalian muscles, being the receptor for stimuli responsible for the lengthening reaction.

lateral line o's, a system of sense organs arranged in longitudinal canals in the skin of fishes and amphibians, which are sensitive to changes in pressure and current and to vibrations of low frequency and thus aid in localizing objects.

reproductive o's, those concerned with reproduction (see also REPRODUCTIVE ORGANS).

sense o's, sensory o's, organs that receive stimuli that give rise to sensations, i.e., organs that translate certain forms of energy into nerve impulses which are perceived as special sensations.

spiral o., organ of Corti.

target o., the organ affected by a particular hormone.

vestigial o., an undeveloped organ that, in the embryo or in some remote ancestor, was well developed and functional.

o's of Zuckerlandl, para-aortic bodies.

organelle (or″gah-nel′) 1. a specific particle of membrane-bound organized living substance present in practically all cells, including mitochondria, the Golgi complex, etc. 2. one of the minute organs or protozoa concerned with such functions as locomotion, metabolism, or the like.

organic (or-gan′ik) 1. pertaining to an organ or organs. 2. having an organized structure. 3. arising from an organism. 4. pertaining to substances derived from living organisms. 5. denoting chemical substances containing carbon. 6. pertaining to or cultivated by use of animal or vegetable fertilizers, rather than synthetic chemicals.

o. acid, an acid containing the carboxyl group, COOH.

o. brain syndrome, any mental disorder, psychotic or nonpsychotic, caused by or associated with impairment of brain tissue function; it may be *acute* and reversible, arising in one previously psychologically normal and due to injury, infection, exogenous or endogenous intoxications, nutritional deficiency, etc., or *chronic,* resulting from or associated with relatively permanent and more or less irreversible diffuse organic impairment of brain tissue function.

o. chemistry, the scientific study of compounds containing carbon.

o. disease, a disease due to or accompanied by structural changes.

organism (or′gah-nizm) an individual animal or plant.

organization (or″gah-nĭ-za′shun) 1. the process of organizing or being organized. 2. the replacement of blood clots by fibrous tissue. 3. an organized body, group, or structure.

organizer (or′gah-nīz″er) a special region of the embryo that is capable of determining the differentiation of other regions.

primary o., the dorsal lip region of the blastopore.

organo- word element [Gr.], *organ.*

organogenesis, organogeny (or″gah-no-jen′ĕ-sis; or″gah-noj′ĕ-ne) the development or growth of organs.

organoid (or′gah-noid) 1. resembling an organ. 2. a structure that resembles an organ.

organology (or″gah-nol′o-je) the sum of what is known regarding the body organs.

organometallic (or″gah-no-mĕ-tal′ik) consisting of a metal combined with an organic radical.

organon (or′gah-non), pl. *or′gana* [Gr.] organ.

organotherapy (or″gah-no-ther′ah-pe) therapeutic administration of animal endocrine organs or their extracts.

organotropism (or-gah-not′ro-pizm) the special affinity of chemical compounds or pathogenic agents for particular tissues or organs of the body. adj., **organotrop′ic.**

organ-specific (or′gan-spĕ-sif′ik) restricted to, or having an effect only on, a particular organ, as an organ-specific antigen.

organum (or′gah-num), pl. *or′gana* [L.] an organ; a somewhat independent part of the body that performs a special function.

orgasm (or′gazm) the apex and culmination of sexual excitement.

orientation (o″re-en-ta′shun) the recognition of one's position in relation to time and space.

orifice (or′ĭ-fis) 1. the entrance or outlet of any body cavity. 2. any foramen, meatus, or opening. adj., **orific′ial.**

orificium (or″i-fish′e-um), pl. *orific′ia* [L.] orifice.

origin (or′ĭ-jin) the source or beginning of anything, especially the more fixed end or attachment of a muscle (as distinguished from its insertion), or the site of emergence of a peripheral nerve from the central nervous system.

Orinase (or′ĭ-nās) trademark for a preparation of tolbutamide, an oral hypoglycemic agent.

Ormond's disease (or′mondz) retroperitoneal fibrosis.

ornithine (or′nĭ-thēn) an amino acid obtained from arginine by splitting of urea; it is an intermediate in urea biosynthesis.

Ornithodoros (or″nĭ-thod′o-ros) a genus of soft-bodied ticks, many species of which are reservoirs and vectors of the spirochetes (*Borrelia*) of relapsing fevers.

ornithosis (or″nĭ-tho′sis) a disease of birds and domestic fowl, transmissible to man, caused by a strain of *Chlamydia psittaci;* the human disease is called PSITTACOSIS.

orofaciodigital syndrome (or″o-fa′she-o-dij′ĭ-tal) a syndrome occurring only in females, with mental retardation and anomalies of the mouth and tongue, the fingers, and frequently the face.

orolingual (o″ro-ling′gwal) pertaining to the mouth and tongue.

oronasal (o″ro-na′zal) pertaining to the mouth and nose.

oropharynx (o″ro-far′ingks) the part of the pharynx between the soft palate and the upper edge of the epiglottis.

orotic acid (o-rot′ik) an intermediate in the biosynthesis of pyrimidine nucleotides.

orotic aciduria (o-rot′ik) a hereditary defect of pyrimidine metabolism associated with excessive urinary excretion of orotic acid, and characterized by megaloblastic anemia, crystalluria, and frequently physical and mental retardation.

Oroya fever (o-ro′yah) the acute febrile anemic stage of Carrión's disease.

orphenadrine (or-fen′ah-drēn) a drug having antihistaminic, antitremor, and antispasmodic activities; its citrate and hydrochloride salts are used as skeletal muscle relaxants.

orth(o)- word element [Gr.], *straight; normal; correct.* In chemistry, *ortho-* indicates an isomer; also, a cyclic derivative having two substitutes in adjacent positions.

orthesis (or-the′sis), pl. *orthe′ses* [Gr.] orthosis.

orthetics (or-thet′iks) orthotics.

orthetist (or′thĕ-tist) orthotist.

orthocephalic (or″tho-sĕ-fal′ik) having a head with a vertical index of 70.1 to 75.

orthochorea (or″tho-ko-re′ah) choreic movements in the erect posture.

orthochromatic (or″tho-kro-mat′ik) staining normally.

orthodentin (or″tho-den′tin) straight-tubed dentin, as in mammalian teeth.

orthodontia, orthodontics (or″tho-don′she-ah; or″-tho-don′tiks) that branch of dentistry concerned with irregularities of teeth and malocclusion, and associated facial problems.

orthodontist (or″tho-don′tist) a dentist who specializes in orthodontics.

orthodromic (or″tho-drom′ik) conducting impulses in the normal direction; said of nerve fibers.

orthograde (or′tho-grād) carrying the body upright in walking.

orthometer (or-thom′ĕ-ter) an instrument for determining the relative protrusion of the eyeballs.

orthomyxovirus (or″tho-mik″so-vi′rus) a subgroup of myxoviruses that includes the viruses of human and animal influenza.

orthopedic (or″tho-pe′dik) pertaining to the correction of deformities of the musculoskeletal system; pertaining to orthopedics.

orthopedics (or″tho-pe′diks) that branch of surgery dealing with the preservation and restoration of the function of the skeletal system, its articulations, and associated structures.

orthopedist (or″tho-pe′dist) an orthopedic surgeon.

orthopercussion (or″tho-per-kush′un) percussion with the distal phalanx of the finger held perpendicularly to the body wall.

orthophenolase (or″tho-fe′no-lās) an enzyme in sweet potatoes that oxidizes catechol and orthocresol.

orthophoria (or″tho-fo′re-ah) normal equilibrium of the eye muscles, or muscular balance. adj., **orthophor′ic.**

orthopnea (or″thop-ne′ah) ability to breathe easily only in the upright position.

orthopneic position (or″thop-ne′ik) a position assumed to relieve orthopnea, in which the patient sits in an upright or semivertical position that is achieved by using two or more pillows to support his head and thorax, or he sits upright in a chair.

orthopraxis, orthopraxy (or″tho-prak′sis; or″tho-prak′se) mechanical correction of deformities.

orthopsychiatry (or″tho-si-ki′ah-tre) that branch of psychiatry that deals with mental and emotional development, embracing child psychiatry and mental hygiene.

orthoptic (or-thop′tik) correcting obliquity of one or both visual axes.

orthoptics (or-thop′tiks) treatment of STRABISMUS by exercise of the ocular muscles.

orthoscope (or′tho-skōp) an apparatus that neutralizes the corneal refraction by means of a layer of water; used in ocular examinations.

orthoscopic (or″tho-skop′ik) 1. affording a correct and undistorted view. 2. pertaining to orthoscopy.

orthoscopy (or-thos′ko-pe) examination by means of an orthoscope.

orthosis (or-tho′sis), pl. *ortho′ses* [Gr.] an orthopedic appliance or apparatus used to support, align, prevent, or correct deformities or to improve function of movable parts of the body.

orthostatic (or″tho-stat′ik) pertaining to or caused by standing erect.

orthostatism (or′tho-stat″izm) an erect standing position of the body.

orthotast (or'tho-tast) an apparatus for straightening curvatures of bone.

orthotic (or-thot'ik) serving to protect or to restore or improve function; pertaining to the use or application of an orthosis.

orthotics (or-thot'iks) the field of knowledge relating to orthoses and their use.

orthotist (or'tho-tist) a person skilled in orthotics and practicing its application in individual cases.

orthotonos, orthotonus (or-thot'o-nos) tetanic spasm that fixes the head, body, and limbs in a rigid straight line.

orthotopic (or"tho-top'ik) occurring at the normal place.

orthovoltage (or"tho-vol'tij) voltage in the range of 30 to 400 kv.

Orthoxine (or-thok'sēn) trademark for preparations of methoxyphenamine, a sympathomimetic drug.

O.S. [L.] *oc'ulus sinis'ter* (left eye).

Os chemical symbol, *osmium.*

os¹ (os), pl. *o'ra* [L.] 1. any body orifice. 2. the mouth.

os² (os), pl. *os'sa* [L.] a bone (see table of BONES).

osazone (o'sah-zōn) any one of a series of compounds obtained by heating sugars with phenylhydrazine and acetic acid.

osche(o)- word element [Gr.], *scrotum.*

oscheitis (os"ke-i'tis) inflammation of the scrotum.

oscheocele (os'ke-o-sēl") a swelling or tumor of the scrotum.

oscheoma (os"ke-o'mah) tumor of the scrotum.

oscheoplasty (os'ke-o-plas"te) plastic surgery of the scrotum.

oscillation (os"ĭ-la'shun) a backward and forward motion, like that of a pendulum; also vibration, fluctuation, or variation.

oscillo- word element [L.], *oscillation.*

oscillogram (ŏ-sil'o-gram) a graphic record made by an oscillograph.

oscillograph (ŏ-sil'o-graf) an instrument for recording electric oscillations.

oscillometer (os"ĭ-lom'ĕ-ter) an instrument for measuring oscillations.

oscillometry (os"ĭ-lom'ĕ-tre) the measurement of oscillations.

oscillopsia (os"ĭ-lop'se-ah) a visual sensation that stationary objects are swaying back and forth.

oscilloscope (ŏ-sil'o-skōp) an instrument that displays a visual representation of electrical variations on the fluorescent screen of a cathode-ray tube.

oscitation (os"ĭ-ta'shun) the act of yawning.

osculum (os'ku-lum) a small aperture or minute opening.

Osgood-Schlatter disease (oz'good shlat'er) osteochondrosis of the tuberosity of the tibia; called also Schlatter-Osgood disease.

OSHA an acronym for the Occupational Safety and Health Administration, which administers the Occupational Safety and Health Act of 1970. This Act of the United States Congress established minimum health and safety standards for workers and provides for the inspection of places of employment and the penalizing of employers who do not provide conditions that meet the established standards. Further information on OSHA can be obtained by writing to the: Office of Information Services, OSHA, U. S. Department of Labor, Washington, DC 20210.

-osis word element [Gr.], *disease, morbid state; abnormal increase.*

Osler's disease (ōs'lerz) 1. polycythemia vera. 2. hereditary hemorrhagic telangiectasia.

Osler's nodes (ōs'lerz) small, raised, swollen, tender areas, bluish or sometimes pink or red, occurring commonly in the pads of the fingers or toes, in the thenar or hypothenar eminences, or on the soles of the feet; they are practically pathognomonic of subacute bacterial endocarditis.

Osler-Vaquez disease (ōs'ler vah-ka') polycythemia vera.

osmatic (oz-mat'ik) pertaining to the sense of smell.

osmics (oz'miks) the science dealing with the sense of smell.

osmidrosis (oz"mĭ-dro'sis) the secretion of foul-smelling sweat; bromhidrosis.

osmium (oz'me-um) a chemical element, atomic number 76, atomic weight 190.2, symbol Os. (See table of ELEMENTS.)

osmolality (oz"mo-lal'ĭ-te) a property of a solution which depends on the concentration of the solute per unit of solvent.

serum o., a measure of the number of dissolved particles per unit of water in serum. In a solution, the fewer the particles of solute in proportion to the number of units of water (solvent), the less concentrated the solution. A low serum osmolality would be indicative of a higher than usual amount of water in relation to the amount of particles dissolved in it. It would be expected, then, that a low serum osmolality would accompany overhydration, or EDEMA, and an increased serum osmolality would be present in a state of DEHYDRATION.

Measurement of the serum osmolality gives information about the hydration status within the cells because of the osmotic equilibrium that is constantly being maintained on either side of the cell membrane (HOMEOSTASIS). Water moves freely back and forth across the membrane in response to the osmotic pressure being exerted by the molecules of solute in the intracellular and extracellular fluids. Serum osmolality reflects the status of hydration of the intracellular as well as the extracellular compartments and thus describes total body hydration. The normal value for serum osmolality is 270–300 mOsm./kg. water.

urine o., a measure of the number of dissolved particles per unit of water in the urine. A more accurate measure of urine concentration than specific gravity, urine osmolality is useful in diagnosing renal disorders of urinary concentration and dilution and in assessing status of hydration.

osmolar (oz-mo'lar) pertaining to the concentration of osmotically active particles in solution.

osmolarity (oz"mo-lar'ĭ-te) the concentration of osmotically active particles in solution.

osmole (oz'mōl) the standard unit of osmotic pressure, being the amount produced by one mole of solute in a liter of water.

osmometer (oz-mom'ĕ-ter) 1. a device for testing the sense of smell. 2. an instrument for measuring osmotic pressure.

osmophilic (oz"mo-fil'ik) having an affinity for solutions of high osmotic pressure.

osmophore (oz′mo-fōr) the group of atoms in a molecule of a compound that is responsible for its odor.

osmoreceptor (oz″mo-re-sep′tor) 1. a specialized sensory nerve ending sensitive to stimulation giving rise to the sensation of odors. 2. a specialized sensory nerve ending that is stimulated by changes in osmotic pressure of the surrounding medium.

osmoregulation (oz″mo-reg″u-la′shun) adjustment of internal osmotic pressure of a simple organism or body cell in relation to that of the surrounding medium. adj., **osmoreg′ulatory.**

osmose (oz′mōs) to diffuse by osmosis.

osmosis (oz-mo′sis, os-mo′sis) [Gr.] the passage of pure solvent from a solution of lesser to one of greater solute concentration when the two solutions are separated by a membrane which selectively prevents the passage of solute molecules, but is permeable to the solvent. adj., **osmot′ic.**

The process of osmosis and the factors that influence it are important clinically in the maintenance of adequate body fluids and in the proper balance between volumes of extracellular and intracellular fluids.

The term osmotic pressure refers to the amount of pressure necessary to stop the flow of water across the membrane. The hydrostatic pressure of the water exerts an opposite effect; that is, it exerts pressure in favor of the flow of water across the membrane. The osmotic pressure of the particles in a solute depends on the relative concentrations of the solutions on either side of the membrane, and on the area of the membrane. The osmotic pressure exerted by the nondiffusible particles in a solution is determined by the numbers of particles in a unit of fluid and not by the mass of the particles.

osphresiology (os-fre″ze-ol′o-je) the science of odors and sense of smell.

osphresiometer (os-fre″ze-om′ĕ-ter) an instrument for measuring acuteness of the sense of smell.

osphresis (os-fre′sis) the sense of smell. adj., **osphret′ic.**

ossein (os′e-in) the collagen of bone.

osseocartilaginous (os″e-o-kar″tĭ-laj′ĭ-nus) composed of bone and cartilage.

osseofibrous (os″e-o-fi′brus) made up of fibrous tissue and bone.

osseomucin (os″e-o-mu′sin) the ground substance that binds together the collagen and elastin fibrils of bone.

osseous (os′e-us) of the nature or quality of bone; bony.

ossicle (os′ĭ-kl) a small bone, especially one of those in the middle ear. adj., **ossic′ular.**

auditory o's, the small bones of the middle ear: incus, malleus, and stapes. (See Plate 15.)

ossiculectomy (os″ĭ-ku-lek′to-me) excision of one or more of the ossicles of the middle ear.

ossiculotomy (os″ĭ-ku-lot′o-me) incision of the auditory ossicles.

ossiculum (ŏ-sik′u-lum), pl. *ossic′ula* [L.] ossicle.

ossiferous (ŏ-sif′er-us) producing bone.

ossific (ŏ-sif′ik) forming or becoming bone.

ossification (os″ĭ-fĭ-ka′shun) formation of or conversion into BONE or a bony substance.

endochondral o., ossification that occurs in and replaces cartilage.

intramembranous o., ossification of bone that occurs in and replaces connective tissue.

ossify (os′ĭ-fi) to change or develop into bone.

oste(o)- word element [Gr.], *bone.*

ostealgia (os″te-al′je-ah) pain in the bones; osteodynia.

ostearthritis (os″te-ar-thri′tis) osteoarthritis.

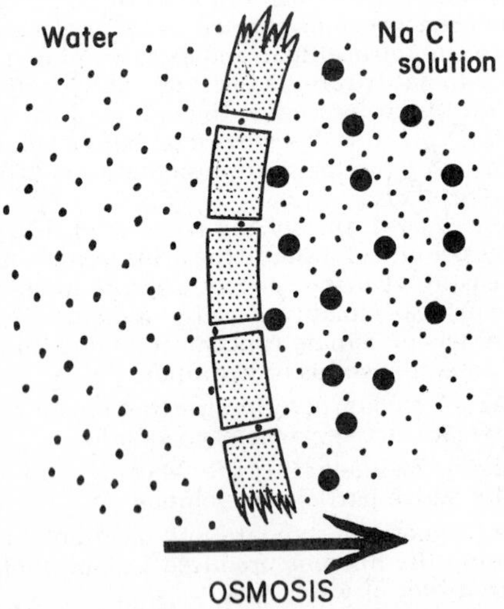

Osmosis at a cell membrane when a sodium chloride solution is placed on one side of the membrane and water on the other side. (From Guyton, A. C.: Textbook of Medical Physiology. 5th ed. Philadelphia, W. B. Saunders Co., 1976.)

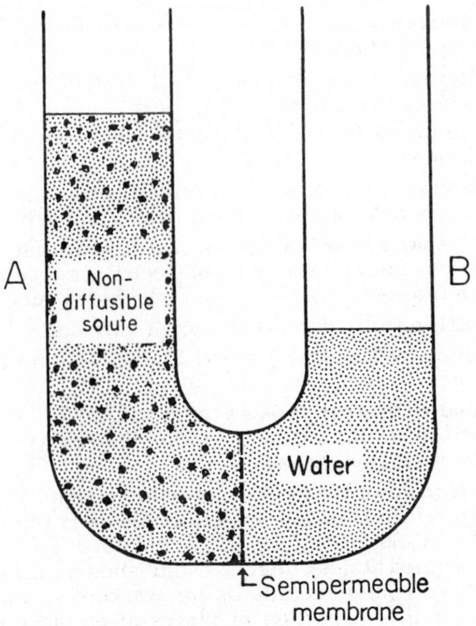

Demonstration of osmotic pressure on the two sides of a semipermeable membrane. (From Guyton, A. C.: Textbook of Medical Physiology. 5th ed. Philadelphia, W. B. Saunders Co., 1976.)

ostearthrotomy (os″te-ar-throt′o-me) excision of an articular end of a bone.

ostectomy (os-tek′to-me) excision of a bone or part of a bone.

osteectopia (os″te-ek-to′pe-ah) displacement of a bone.

ostein (os′te-in) ossein.

osteitis (os″te-i′tis) inflammation of bone. The term is used to describe a number of conditions; for instance, advanced cases of syphilis can lead to syphilitic osteitis.

condensing o., osteitis with hard deposits of earthy salts in affected bone.

o. defor′mans, rarefying osteitis of unknown cause leading to bowing of the long bones and deformation of the flat bones. The bones most commonly affected are the long bones of the legs, the lower spine, the pelvis, and the skull. Called also Paget's disease.

The disease is not common and usually does not occur in persons under the age of 30. Often symptoms are so mild they are unnoticed. When symptoms do occur, the earliest one is usually pain in the affected bone. The disease disturbs the growth of new bone tissue, with the result that bones often thicken, become soft, and coarsen in texture. In an advanced case, the weakened bone may be fractured by even a light blow. If the bones of the leg are affected, they become bowed under the body's weight. The person is stooped forward from spinal deformity. If the skull is affected, it may enlarge, causing headache. Nerves may be pinched by protruding bone, causing neuralgia or even deafness or blindness.

In most cases, no treatment is necessary. When there are complications, these can be treated, but almost all patients with this form of osteitis can expect to live out their normal life span.

o. fibro′sa cys′tica, rarefying osteitis with fibrous degeneration and the formation of cysts and the presence of fibrous nodules on the affected bones, due to osteoclastic activity secondary to HYPERPARATHYROIDISM. If a tumor of the parathyroid gland is the cause of the hyperparathyroidism, treatment includes removal of the tumor. When the disease is generalized, all the bones are affected (von Recklinghausen's disease). Orthopedic surgery may be necessary to correct severe bone deformities.

o. fragil′itans, osteogenesis imperfecta.

o. fungo′sa, chronic osteitis in which the haversian canals are dilated and filled with granulation tissue.

rarefying o., a bone disease in which the inorganic matter is diminished and the hard bone becomes cancellated.

sclerosing o., 1. sclerosing nonsuppurative osteomyelitis. 2. condensing osteitis.

ostempyesis (ost″em-pi-e′sis) suppuration within a bone.

osteoarthritis (os″te-o-ar-thri′tis) degenerative joint disease marked by degeneration of the articular cartilage, hypertrophy of bone at the margins, and changes in the synovial membrane; called also degenerative joint disease.

Osteoarthritis, as part of the normal aging process, is most likely to strike the joints that receive the most use or stress over the years. These include the knees, the joints of the big toes, and those of the lower part of the spine. Another common form of osteoarthritis affects the distal joints of the fingers; this form usually occurs in women.

Symptoms vary from mild to severe, depending on the amount of degeneration that has taken place. Osteoarthritis is caused by disintegration of the cartilage that covers the ends of the bones. As the cartilage wears away, the roughened surface of the bone is exposed, and pain and stiffness result. In severe cases the center of the bone wears away and a bony ridge is left around the edges. This ridge may restrict movement of the joint. Osteoarthritis is less crippling than rheumatoid arthritis, in which two bone surfaces may fuse, completely immobilizing the joint.

Treatment is aimed at preventing crippling deformities, relieving pain, and maintaining motion of the joint (see also treatment of ARTHRITIS).

osteoarthropathy (os″te-o-ar-throp′ah-the) any disease of the joints and bones.

hypertrophic pulmonary o., secondary hypertropic o., symmetrical osteitis of the four limbs, chiefly localized to the phalanges and terminal epiphyses of the long bones of the forearm and leg; it is often secondary to chronic lung and heart conditions.

osteoarthrosis (os″te-o-ar-thro′sis) chronic noninflammatory bone disease.

osteoarthrotomy (os″te-o-ar-throt′o-me) ostearthrotomy.

osteoblast (os′te-o-blast″) a cell arising from a fibroblast, which, as it matures, is associated with bone production.

osteoblastoma (os″te-o-blas-to′mah) a benign, rather vascular tumor of bone marked by formation of osteoid tissue and primitive bone.

osteocampsia (os″te-o-kamp′se-ah) curvature of a bone.

osteochondral (os″te-o-kon′dral) pertaining to bone and cartilage.

osteochondritis (os″te-o-kon-dri′tis) inflammation of bone and cartilage.

o. defor′mans juveni′lis, osteochondritis of the capitular head of the epiphysis of the femur.

o. defor′mans juvenil′lis dor′si, osteochondrosis of vertebrae.

o. dis′secans, osteochondritis resulting in the splitting of pieces of cartilage into the joint, particularly the knee joint or shoulder joint. The fragment of cartilage is called a joint mouse.

osteochondrodystrophy (os″te-o-kon″dro-dis′trofe) Morquio's disease.

familial o., a familial form of MUCOPOLYSACCHARIDOSIS becoming evident when the affected infant begins to walk (see also MORQUIO'S DISEASE).

osteochondrolysis (os″te-o-kon-drol′ĭ-sis) osteochondritis dissecans.

osteochondroma (os″te-o-kon-dro′mah) a benign bone tumor consisting of projecting adult bone capped by cartilage.

osteochondromatosis (os″te-o-kon″dro-mah-to′sis) the occurrence of multiple osteochondromas.

osteochondrosarcoma (os″te-o-kon″dro-sar-ko′mah) sarcoma blended with osteoma and chondroma.

osteochondrosis (os″te-o-kon-dro′sis) a disease of the growth ossification centers in children, beginning as a degeneration or necrosis followed by regeneration or recalcification; known by various names, depending on the bone involved.

o. defor′mans tib′iae, aseptic necrosis of the medial tibial condyle, producing lateral bowing of the leg.

osteoclasis (os″te-ok′lah-sis) surgical fracture or refracture of a bone.

osteoclast (os′te-o-klast″) 1. a large, multinuclear cell frequently associated with resorption of bone. 2. a surgical instrument used for osteoclasis. adj., **osteoclas′tic.**

osteoclastoma (os″te-o-klas-to′mah) giant cell tumor of bone.

osteocope (os′te-o-kōp″) severe pain in a bone. adj., **osteocop′ic.**

osteocranium (os″te-o-kra′ne-um) the fetal skull during the period of ossification, from early in the third month of gestation.

osteocystoma (os″te-o-sis-to′mah) a bone cyst.

osteocyte (os′te-o-sit″) an osteoblast that has become embedded within the bone matrix, occupying a flat oval cavity and sending, through openings in its walls, cytoplasmic processes that connect with other osteocytes in developing bone.

osteodentin (os″te-o-den′tin) dentin that resembles bone.

osteodermia (os″te-o-der′me-ah) osteoma cutis.

osteodiastasis (os″te-o-di-as′tah-sis) the separation of two adjacent bones.

osteodynia (os″te-o-din′e-ah) pain in a bone; ostealgia.

osteodystrophy (os″te-o-dis′tro-fe) abnormal development of bone.

renal o., a condition due to chronic kidney disease, marked by impaired kidney function, elevated serum phosphorus levels, and low or normal serum calcium levels, and by stimulation of parathyroid function, resulting in a variable admixture of bone disease, including osteitis fibrosa cystica, osteomalacia, osteoporosis, and sometimes osteosclerosis; if the onset is in childhood, renal dwarfism may result.

osteoepiphysis (os″te-o-ĕ-pif′ĭ-sis) any bony epiphysis.

osteofibroma (os″te-o-fi-bro′mah) osteoma blended with fibroma.

osteogen (os′te-o-jen″) the substance composing the inner layer of the periosteum, from which bone is formed.

osteogenesis (os″te-o-jen′ĕ-sis) the formation of bone; the development of the bones.

o. imperfec′ta, an inherited condition marked by abnormally brittle bones that are subject to fracture; osteogenesis imperfecta congenita occurs during intrauterine life and the child is born with deformities; in osteogenesis imperfecta tarda, the fractures occur when the child begins to walk. It is usually attended by blue coloration of the sclera (Lobstein's disease) and sometimes by otosclerotic deafness (van der Hoeve's syndrome).

osteogenic (os″te-o-jen′ik) derived from or composed of any tissue concerned in bone growth or repair.

osteogeny (os″te-oj′ĕ-ne) osteogenesis.

osteography (os″te-og′rah-fe) description of the bones.

osteohalisteresis (os″te-o-hah-lis″ter-e′sis) deficiency in mineral elements of bone.

osteoid (os′te-oid) 1. resembling bone. 2. the organic matrix of bone; young bone that has not undergone calcification.

osteolipochondroma (os″te-o-lip″o-kon-dro′mah) osteochondroma with fatty elements.

osteologist (os″te-ol′o-jist) a specialist in osteology.

osteology (os″te-ol′o-je) scientific study of the bones.

osteolysis (os″te-ol′ĭ-sis) dissoluton of bone; applied especially to the removal or loss of calcium from the bone. adj., **osteolyt′ic.**

osteoma (os″te-o′mah) a tumor, benign or malignant, composed of bony tissue; a hard tumor of bonelike structure developing on a bone (homoplastic osteoma) or other structures (heteroplastic osteoma).

BENIGN OSTEOMA. Benign tumors of bone are slow growing and often cause no symptoms. They frequently are first noticed as a swelling in the area; if they involve the joints symptoms result from decreased mobility. As the tumor develops, the patient experiences pain and tenderness, and pathologic fractures are not uncommon with large tumors. Treatment includes surgical removal of the tumor and repair of the affected bone. Some benign tumors require no treatment.

MALIGNANT OSTEOMA. Malignant bone tumors that arise from bone (sarcoma) are rare, only about 15 occurring per million persons. They are found most often in children and young adults.

Cancer that spreads to bone tissue from other parts of the body usually is carcinoma rather than sarcoma.

Cancer of the bone can spread to other organs of the body through the blood and lymph channels. It tends to metastasize to the lungs, and from the lungs to the brain or the organs of the abdomen.

Symptoms. Symptoms of bone cancer are pain, swelling, and disability in the area of the diseased bones. The pain at first is mild, stops and starts again, and then becomes increasingly severe. Swelling may appear soon after the first signs of pain, but often it cannot be seen until later. The disability may affect a nearby joint, such as the knee, shoulder, or hip. There may also be a hard, painful lump over which the skin moves freely. The skin temperature in the area may be slightly elevated.

Diagnosis and Treatment. Diagnosis of bone tumor is made after examination of x-ray film and a microscopic study of the suspected tissue. Malignant tumors can be treated by radiotherapy and surgery during the early stage of development. The prognosis for these tumors is grave, however. Hormone therapy and medication can also be helpful in certain types of the disease.

o. cu′tis, a condition in which bone-containing nodules form in the skin; called also osteodermia and osteosis cutis.

o. du′rum, o. ebur′neum, one containing hard bony tissue.

o. medulla′re, one containing marrow spaces.

osteoid o., a benign bone tumor of spongy bone occurring in the bones of the limbs and vertebrae in young persons.

o. spongio′sum, one containing cancellated bone.

osteomalacia (os″te-o-mah-la′she-ah) softening of the bones, resulting from impaired mineralization, with excess accumulation of osteoid, caused by a vitamin D deficiency in adults. adj., **osteomala′cic.** A similar condition in children is called RICKETS. The deficiency may be due to lack of exposure to ultraviolet rays, inadequate intake of vitamin D in the diet, or failure to absorb or utilize vitamin D.

The disease is characterized by decalcification of the bones, particularly those of the spine, pelvis, and lower extremities. X-ray examination reveals transverse, fracture-like lines in the affected bones and areas of demineralization in the matrix of the bone. As the bones soften they become bent, flattened, or otherwise deformed.

Treatment consists of administration of large daily doses of vitamin D and dietary measures to insure adequate calcium and phosphorus intake.

osteomatoid (os″te-o′mah-toid) resembling an osteoma.

osteomere (os′te-o-mēr″) one of a series of similar bony structures, such as the vertebrae.

osteometry (os″te-om′ĕ-tre) measurement of the bones.

osteomyelitis (os″te-o-mi″ĕ-li′tis) inflammation of bone, localized or generalized, due to a pyogenic infection. It may result in bone destruction, in stiffening of joints if the infection spreads to the joints, and, in extreme cases occurring before the end of the growth period, in the shortening of a limb if the growth center is destroyed.

Acute osteomyelitis is caused by bacteria that enter the body through a wound, spread from an infection near the bone, or come from a skin or throat infection. The infection usually affects the long bones of the arms and legs and causes acute pain and fever. It most often occurs in children and adolescents, particularly boys.

The onset may be quite sudden, with chills, high fever and severe pain. Signs and symptoms include a marked increase in leukocytes, tenderness, swelling, and redness of the skin over the bone involved, and bacteremia. About 10 to 14 days after the onset of symptoms, x-rays show signs of the bone infection.

Usually, antibiotic treatment will clear the infection. If not, the infection destroys areas of the bone involved and an abscess forms. Acute osteomyelitis may become chronic, especially if the patient has a low resistance to infection.

Tuberculous osteomyelitis is caused by tubercle bacilli that enter the bloodstream and settle in a bone. The disease progresses slowly and is chronic. Any bone may be infected but those most commonly involved are the vertebrae. Spinal tuberculosis, or POTT'S DISEASE, causes bone destruction and often spinal deformities. Other bones that may be affected are the long bones of the hands or feet.

TREATMENT. Treatment of acute osteomyelitis consists of administration of antibiotics and sometimes surgical drainage of the abscess. Fragments of dead bone (sequestra) that remain and prevent healing must be removed surgically. If the blood supply to the bone is not obstructed, the bone can grow back. Treatment of chronic osteomyelitis is similar to that for the acute type.

Tuberculous osteomyelitis is treated like other forms of TUBERCULOSIS and sometimes by surgical drainage and immobilization of the bones involved.

PATIENT CARE. Absolute rest of the affected part is essential to proper healing and prevention of deformity. Because of pain and local tenderness one must be very gentle in handling the patient. Proper positioning with pillows and sandbags helps relieve the discomfort and also keeps the affected limb in good alignment. When a cast has been applied to insure immobilization, the nursing care is the same as for any patient in a cast (see CAST). Drainage from the infected bone must be considered grossly contaminated and requires special precautions so that the infection is not spread to others.

Since most patients with osteomyelitis are children, some form of occupational therapy or diversionary activities must be devised to insure adequate rest for the affected bone. The parents must also be cautioned against letting the child indulge in strenuous exercise during the convalescent period at home. At all times during both the acute stage and the convalescent period the patient must be protected from other infections, which may result in a recurrence of symptoms. A well balanced diet, adequate periods of rest and other measures to promote the general well-being of the patient are important in overcoming the infection and preventing complications.

Garré's o., sclerosing nonsuppurative o., a chronic form involving the long bones, especially the tibia and femur, marked by a diffuse inflammatory reaction, increased density and spindle-shaped sclerotic thickening of the cortex, and an absence of suppuration.

osteomyelodysplasia (os″te-o-mi″ĕ-lo-dis-pla′ze-ah) a condition characterized by thinning of the osseous tissue of bones, increase in size of the marrow cavities, and associated leukopenia and fever.

osteon (os′te-on) the basic unit of structure of compact bone, comprising a haversian canal and its concentrically arranged lamellae.

osteonecrosis (os″te-o-nĕ-kro′sis) necrosis of a bone.

osteoneuralgia (os″te-o-nu-ral′je-ah) neuralgia of a bone.

osteopath (os′te-o-path″) a practitioner of OSTEOPATHY.

osteopathia (os″te-o-path′e-ah) osteopathy (1).

o. conden′sans dissemina′ta, osteopoikilosis.

o. stria′ta, an asymptomatic condition characterized radiographically by multiple condensations of cancellous bone tissue, giving a striated appearance.

osteopathology (os″te-o-pah-thol′o-je) any disease of bone.

osteopathy (os″te-op′ah-the) 1. any disease of a bone. 2. a system of therapy utilizing generally accepted physical, medicinal, and surgical methods of diagnosis and therapy, and emphasizing the importance of normal body mechanics and manipulative methods of detecting and correcting faulty structure. adj., **osteopath′ic.**

Osteopathy is founded on the theory that the body is capable of producing the remedies necessary to protect itself against disease and other toxic conditions when it is in normal structural relationship and has favorable environmental conditions and adequate nutrition.

During the past few decades, many changes have been made in the practice of osteopathy, bringing it closely into line with conventional medical practices. While still holding to the tenet that the body is a unit that possesses the inherent ability to overcome most curable diseases, osteopaths recognize that physical, chemical, and nutritional factors influence the state of health and that medicines and surgery are necessary in the treatment of disease.

Disorders that can be recognized are treated as distinct diseases, and manipulation may or may not be used as an adjunct to other treatment. Membership in the American Osteopathic Association requires a total of 150 continuing education hours every three years.

osteopenia (os″te-o-pe′ne-ah) any condition involving reduced bone mass.

osteoperiosteal (os″te-o-per″e-os′te-al) pertaining to bone and its periosteum.

osteoperiostitis (os″te-o-per″e-os-ti′tis) inflammation of a bone and its periosteum.

osteopetrosis (os″te-o-pĕ-tro′sis) a hereditary disease marked by abnormally dense bone, and by the common occurrence of fractures of affected bone. It may lead to obliteration of the marrow spaces, causing anemia. Called also Albers-Schönberg disease and marble bones.

osteophage (os′te-o-fāj) osteoclast.

osteophlebitis (os″te-o-flĕ-bi′tis) inflammation of the veins of a bone.

osteophony (os″te-of′o-ne) bone conduction.

osteophore (os′te-o-fōr″) a bone-crushing forceps.

osteophyma, **osteophyte** (os″te-o-fi′mah; os′te-o-fīt″) a bony excrescence or outgrowth.

osteoplasty (os′te-o-plas″te) plastic surgery of the bones.

osteopoikilosis (os″te-o-poi″kĭ-lo′sis) a mottled condition of bones, apparent radiographically, due to the presence of multiple sclerotic foci and scattered stippling. adj., **osteopoikilot′ic.**

osteoporosis (os″te-o-po-ro′sis) abnormal rarefaction of bone; it may be idiopathic or occur secondary to other diseases. adj., **osteoporot′ic.** The condition leads to thinning of the skeleton and decreased precipitation of lime salts. There also may be inadequate calcium absorption into the bone and excessive bone resorption.

The principal causes are lack of physical activity, lack of estrogens or androgens, and possibly a chronic low intake of calcium. There is almost always some degree of osteoporosis in senility. The condition may accompany endocrine disorders, bone marrow disorders, and nutritional disturbances.

Symptoms include pathologic fractures and collapse of the vertebrae without compression of the spinal cord. The latter is often discovered "accidentally" on x-ray examination made for some other reason.

Treatment varies with the cause but hormone therapy is helpful in most cases. Measures are taken to improve the nutritional status, and a diet high in protein and calcium is recommended. Patients should be kept active and those confined to bed must be given passive and active exercises. Prognosis usually is good when treatment is carried out diligently.

o. circumscrip′ta, demineralization occurring in localized areas of bone, especially in the skull.

o. of disuse, that occurring when the normal laying down of bone is slowed because of lack of the normal stimulus of functional stress on the bone.

post-traumatic o., loss of bone substance after an injury in which there is nerve damage, sometimes due to decreased blood supply caused by the neurogenic insult, or to disuse secondary to pain. Called also Sudeck's disease.

osteoradionecrosis (os″te-o-ra″de-o-nĕ-kro′sis) necrosis of bone as a result of excessive exposure to radiation.

osteorrhagia (os″te-o-ra′je-ah) hemorrhage from bone.

osteorrhaphy (os″te-or′ah-fe) fixation of fragments of bone with sutures or wires; called also osteosuture.

osteosarcoma (os″te-o-sar-ko′mah) osteogenic sarcoma. adj., **osteosarco′matous.**

osteosclerosis (os″te-o-sklĕ-ro′sis) the hardening, or abnormal density, of bone. adj., **osteosclerot′ic.**

o. congen′ita, achondroplasia.

o. frag′ilis, osteopetrosis; so called because of frequency of pathologic fracture of affected bones.

o. frag′ilis generalisa′ta, osteopoikilosis.

osteosis (os″te-o′sis) the formation of bony tissue.

o. cu′tis, osteoma cutis.

osteostixis (os″te-o-stik′sis) surgical puncture of a bone.

osteosuture (os″te-o-su′tūr) osteorrhaphy.

osteosynovitis (os″te-o-sin″o-vi′tis) synovitis with osteitis of neighboring bones.

osteosynthesis (os″te-o-sin′thĕ-sis) surgical fastening of the ends of a fractured bone.

osteotabes (os″te-o-ta′bēz) a disease, chiefly of infants, in which bone marrow cells are destroyed and the marrow disappears.

osteothrombosis (os″te-o-throm-bo′sis) thrombosis of the veins of a bone.

osteotome (os′te-o-tōm″) a chisel-like knife for cutting bone.

osteotomoclasis (os″te-o-to-mok′lah-sis) correction of bone curvature by partial division with the osteotome, followed by forcible fracture.

osteotomy (os″te-ot′o-me) incision or transection of a bone.

cuneiform o., removal of a wedge of bone.

linear o., the sawing or simple cutting of a bone.

ostitis (os-ti′tis) osteitis.

ostium (os′te-um), pl. *os′tia* [L.] a mouth or orifice; used in anatomic nomenclature as a general term to designate an opening into a tubular organ, or between two distinct body cavities. adj., **os′tial.**

o. abdomina′le, the fimbriated end of the uterine tube.

o. inter′num, ostium uterinum tubae.

o. pharyn′geum, the nasopharyngeal end of the eustachian tube.

o. pri′mum, an opening in the lower portion of the membrane dividing the embryonic heart into right and left sides. (See also CONGENITAL HEART DEFECT.)

o. secun′dum, an opening in the upper portion of the membrane dividing the embryonic heart into right and left sides, appearing later than the ostium primum. (See also CONGENITAL HEART DEFECT.)

tympanic o., o. tympan′icum, the opening of the eustachian tube on the carotid wall of the tympanic cavity.

o. u′teri, the external opening of the cervix of the uterus into the vagina.

o. uteri′num tu′bae, the point where the cavity of the uterine tube becomes continuous with that of the uterus.

o. vagi′nae, the external orifice of the vagina.

ostomate (os'to-māt) one who has undergone enterostomy or ureterostomy.

ostomy (os'to-me) general term for an operation in which an artificial opening is formed, as in colostomy, ureterostomy, etc. (See also STOMA.)

O.T. occupational therapy; Old tuberculin.

ot(o)- word element [Gr.], *ear.*

otalgia (o-tal'je-ah) pain in the ear; earache; otodynia.

OTC over the counter; applied to drugs not required by law to be sold on prescription only.

otectomy (o-tek'to-me) excision of tissues of the internal and middle ear.

othelcosis (ōt"hel-ko'sis) 1. ulceration of the auricle or external meatus of the ear. 2. suppuration of the middle ear.

othemorrhea (ōt"hem-o-re'ah) otorrhagia.

otic (o'tik) pertaining to the ear; aural.

otitis (o-ti'tis) inflammation of the ear. adj., **otit'ic.**

aviation o., a symptom complex due to difference between atmospheric pressure of the environment and air pressure in the middle ear; called also barotitis media.

o. exter'na, inflammation of the external ear.

furuncular o., the formation of furuncles in the external acoustic meatus.

o. inter'na, o. labyrin'thica, labyrinthitis.

o. mastoi'dea, inflammation of the mastoid spaces.

o. me'dia, inflammation of the middle ear. It occurs most commonly in infants and young children and frequently follows or accompanies an upper respiratory infection. The condition may be acute or chronic.

ACUTE OTITIS MEDIA. The principal symptoms are earache, loss of hearing, fever, and a feeling of fullness and pressure in the ear. As the infection progresses pressure builds up behind the tympanic membrane (eardrum) and may cause perforation or rupture of it. This is followed by drainage of exudate into the external acoustic meatus.

Treatment consists of bed rest, analgesics to relieve the pain, and systemic antibiotics. Surgical incision into the eardrum (myringotomy) may be necessary to relieve pressure and promote drainage. If acute otitis media is treated promptly it resolves with rare exception. If it is not treated successfully it will develop into chronic otitis media and the infection may spread to the mastoid cells, causing MASTOIDITIS.

CHRONIC OTITIS MEDIA. This condition is almost always associated with perforation of the eardrum. It may complicate an upper respiratory disease or be associated with MASTOIDITIS. Drainage from the ear, ringing in the ear, and loss of hearing are frequent symptoms.

Treatment is aimed at relief of the primary source of infection, which may be chronic sinusitis, enlarged tonsils and adenoids, nasal polyps, or nasal allergy. Antibiotic drugs and antiseptic or antibiotic ear drops are used to treat the infection. If suppuration continues and the mastoid process becomes involved, MASTOIDECTOMY is done.

o. sclerot'ica, otitis marked by hardening of the ear structures.

otoantritis (o"to-an-tri'tis) inflammation of the attic of the tympanum and the mastoid antrum.

Otobius (o-to'be-us) a genus of soft-bodied ticks parasitic in the ears of various animals and known also to infest man.

otoblennorrhea (o"to-blen"o-re'ah) mucous discharge from the ear.

otocephalus (o"to-sef'ah-lus) a monster lacking the lower jaw and having ears united below the face.

otocleisis (o"to-kli'sis) closure of the auditory passages.

otoconia (o"to-ko'ne-ah) statoconia.

otocranium (o"to-kra'ne-um) 1. the chamber in the petrous bone lodging the internal ear. 2. the auditory portion of the cranium adj., **otocra'nial.**

otocyst (o'to-sist) 1. the auditory vesicle of the embryo. 2. the organ of hearing in some lower animals.

otodynia (o"to-din'e-ah) pain in the ear; earache; otalgia.

otoencephalitis (o"to-en-sef"ah-li'tis) inflammation of brain extending from an inflamed middle ear.

otoganglion (o"to-gang'gle-on) the otic ganglion.

otogenic, otogenous (o"to-jen'ik; o-toj'ĕ-nus) originating within the ear.

otography (o-tog'rah-fe) description of the ear.

otolaryngology (o"to-lar"ing-gol'o-je) that branch of medicine dealing with disease of the ear, nose and throat; called also otorhinolaryngology.

otolith (o'to-lith) see STATOCONIA.

otologist (o-tol'o-jist) a specialist in otology.

otology (o-tol'o-je) the branch of medicine dealing with the ear and its anatomy, physiology, and pathology. adj., **otolog'ic.**

otomassage (o"to-mah-sahzh') massage of the middle ear and ossicles.

Oto-Microscope (o"to-mi'kro-skōp) trademark for an operating microscope devised to improve visualization of the surgical field in operations on the ear.

otomucormycosis (o"to-mu"kor-mi-ko'sis) mucormycosis of the ear.

otomycosis (o"to-mi-ko'sis) a fungal infection of the external auditory meatus and ear canal. The infection thrives in warm, moist climates and is encouraged by poor local hygiene and swimming. Symptoms include itching, which may be intense, pain, and a stinging sensation in the external acoustic meatus.

The condition is treated with antibiotics to prevent secondary infection and the administration of ear drops containing neomycin or polymyxin B sulfate. The area should be cleaned locally with dilute aluminum acetate solution combined with acetic acid before ear drops are applied.

otopathy (o-top'ah-the) any disease of the ear.

otopharyngeal (o"to-fah-rin'je-al) pertaining to the ear and pharynx.

otoplasty (o'to-plas"te) plastic sugery of the ear.

otopolypus (o"to-pol'ĭ-pus) a polyp in the ear.

otopyorrhea (o"to-pi"o-re'ah) a copious purulent discharge from the ear.

otorhinolaryngology (o"to-ri"no-lar"ing-gol'o-je) the branch of medicine dealing with disease of the ear, nose, and throat; called also otolaryngology.

otorhinology (o"to-ri-nol'o-je) the branch of medicine dealing with ear and nose.

otorrhagia (o"to-ra'je-ah) hemorrhage from the ear.

otorrhea (o″to-re′ah) a discharge from the ear.

otosclerosis (o″to-sklĕ-ro′sis) the formation of spongy bone in the capsule of the labyrinth of the ear, often causing the auditory ossicles to become fixed and less able to pass on vibrations when sound enters the ear. adj., **otosclerot′ic.** The ossicle chiefly involved in the condition is the stirrup or stapes, which becomes fixed to the oval window.

The cause of otosclerosis is still unknown. It may be hereditary, or perhaps related to vitamin deficiency or otitis media. An early symptom is ringing in the ears, but the most noticeable symptom is progressive loss of hearing.

This disease usually begins in the teens or early twenties. It strikes women about twice as often as men, and may be worsened by pregnancy. Approximately 10 million people in the United States are affected to a greater or lesser degree by otosclerosis.

Although no cure is known, recently developed surgical techniques can often restore hearing by freeing the stirrup or replacing it with other tissue. In this operation, STAPEDECTOMY, the stirrup is removed and replaced with grafted body tissue attached to a stainless steel wire or plastic tube.

In some cases of otosclerosis the hearing loss may be relieved by the use of a hearing aid.

otoscope (o′to-skōp) an instrument for inspecting or auscultating the ear.

otoscopy (o-tos′ko-pe) examination of the external acoustic meatus with an otoscope.

otosteal (o-tos′te-al) pertaining to the ossicles of the ear.

ototomy (o-tot′o-me) dissection of the ear.

ototoxic (o″to-tok′sik) having a deleterious effect upon the eighth cranial (vestibulocochlear) nerve or on the organs of hearing and balance.

ototoxicity (o″to-tok-sis′ĭ-te) the property of being ototoxic.

Otrivin (o′trĭ-vin) trademark for preparations of xylometazoline, a nasal decongestant.

Otto pelvis (ot′o) a pelvis in which the acetabulum is depressed, with protrusion of the femoral head into the pelvis.

O.U. [L.] *oc′uli uter′que* (each eye).

ouabain (wah-ba′in) a glycoside obtained chiefly from the plant *Strophanthus gratus,* used as a cardiotonic; its effect is similar to that of digitalis.

ounce (owns) a measure of weight in both the avoirdupois and the apothecaries' system; abbreviation oz. The ounce avoirdupois is 1/16 lb., or 437.5 gr., or 28.3495 gm. The apothecaries' ounce is 1/12 lb., or 480 gr., or 31.103 gm.; symbol ℥. (See also Table of Weights and Measures in the Appendix.)

fluid o., a unit of liquid measure of the apothecaries' system, being 8 fluid drams, or the equivalent of 29.57 ml.

outlet (owt′let) a means or route of exit or egress.

pelvic o., the inferior opening of the pelvis.

outpatient (owt-pa′shent) a patient who comes to the hospital, clinic, or dispensary for diagnosis and/or treatment but does not occupy a bed.

outpocketing (owt-pok′et-ing) evagination.

output (owt′poot) the yield or total of anything produced by any functional system of the body.

cardiac o., the effective volume of blood expelled by either ventricle of the heart per unit of time (usually volume per minute); it is equal to the stroke output multiplied by the number of beats per the time unit used in the computation.

energy o., the energy a body is able to manifest in work or activity.

stroke o., the amount of blood ejected by each ventricle at each beat of the heart.

urinary o., the amount of urine secreted by the kidneys (see also FLUID BALANCE).

ova (o′vah) plural of *ovum.*

ovalbumin (ov″al-bu′min) egg albumin.

ovalocyte (o′vah-lo-sīt″) elliptocyte, an elliptical erythrocyte.

ovalocytosis (o-val″o-si-to′sis) elliptocytosis.

ovari(o)- word element [L.], *ovary.* See also words beginning *oophor(o)-.*

ovarialgia (o-va″re-al′je-ah) pain in an ovary.

ovarian (o-va′re-an) pertaining to an ovary.

ovariectomy (o-va″re-ek′to-me) excision of an ovary (see also OOPHORECTOMY).

ovariocele (o-va′re-o-sēl″) hernia of an ovary.

ovariocentesis (o-va″re-o-sen-te′sis) surgical puncture of an ovary.

ovariocyesis (o-va″re-o-si-e′sis) ovarian pregnancy.

ovariopexy (o-va″re-o-pek′se) the operation of elevating and fixing an ovary to the abdominal wall.

ovariorrhexis (o-va″re-o-rek′sis) rupture of an ovary.

ovariosalpingectomy (o-va″re-o-sal″pin-jek′to-me) excision of an ovary and uterine tube.

ovariostomy (o-va″re-os′to-me) incision of an ovary, with drainage; oophorostomy.

ovariotomy (o-va″re-ot′o-me) surgical removal of an ovary, or removal of an ovarian tumor.

ovariotubal (o-va″re-o-tu′bal) pertaining to an ovary and uterine tube.

ovaritis (o″vah-ri′tis) inflammation of an ovary; oophoritis.

ovarium (o-va′re-um), pl. *ova′ria* [L.] ovary.

ovary (o′var-e) the female gonad; either of the sex glands in the female in which the ova are formed. adj., **ova′rian.** Almond-shaped and about the size of large walnuts, the two ovaries are located in the lower abdomen one on either side of the uterus.

FUNCTIONS OF THE OVARIES. The ovaries have two basic functions: ovulation and the production of hormones, chiefly estrogen and progesterone, which influence a woman's feminine physical characteristics and affect the reproductive process. (See also OVULATION and REPRODUCTION.)

DISORDERS OF THE OVARIES. One of the commonest disorders of the ovary is a cyst. Not all so-called ovarian cysts are true cysts; many are tumors. Ovarian cysts occur frequently and in a variety of sizes and types.

The commonest ovarian cysts are simple follicle retention cysts, small and frequently numerous cysts containing a clear fluid. Ordinarily follicle cysts disappear without treatment within 2 months. They do not change into malignant growths.

Another type of ovarian cyst, the mucinous cystadenoma, is in reality a tumor. These tumors may reach enormous size, creating pressure within the abdominopelvic cavity. Although these tumors are benign, they may become malignant.

DERMOID CYSTS of the ovary are usually benign although they may be subject to malignant change. They grow slowly and when opened after removal are found to be filled with a thick, yellow sebaceous fluid. Hair, teeth, bone, and other kinds of tissues are often found partially developed in the cyst.

Oophoritis (inflammation of an ovary) may be caused by infection reaching the ovary by way of the uterine tube. Tuberculous and streptococcal infections of the ovary are common, and the ovary may also become infected in GONORRHEA. Fever and pain, sometimes accompanied by swelling, are the usual symptoms. Sulfonamides and antibiotics usually can eliminate the infection, but if it fails to respond to treatment, surgery may become necessary. Surgical removal of an ovary is called OOPHORECTOMY, or ovariectomy.

Tumors of the ovary are generally classified as malignant or benign. They may arise from misplaced endometrial tissue or from the ovarian tissues. Malignant cells from other organs may travel to the ovary and set up a secondary malignant tumor in the ovary; an example is Krukenberg's tumor, which usually originates in the stomach.

Symptoms of an ovarian tumor usually do not present themselves until the tumor is fairly well advanced. Tumors in the early stage are usually found during a routine examination. Treatment of these tumors in all stages involves surgical removal or the use of radiotherapy or a combination of the two.

overbite (o′ver-bīt) extension of incisal ridges of the upper anterior teeth below the incisal ridges of the anterior teeth in the lower jaw when the jaws are closed normally.

overcompensation (o″ver-kom″pen-sa′shun) exaggerated correction of a real or imagined physical or psychologic defect.

overhydration (o″ver-hi-dra′shun) a state of excess fluids in the body.

overjet (o′ver-jet) extension of the incisal or buccal cusp ridges of the upper teeth labially or buccally to the ridges of the teeth in the lower jaw when the jaws are closed normally.

overlay (o′ver-la) a later component superimposed on a preexisting state or condition.

psychogenic o., an emotionally determined increment to a preexisting symptom or disability of organic or physically traumatic origin.

overventilation (o″ver-ven″tĭ-la′shun) hyperventilation.

ovi- word element [L.], *egg; ovum.*

ovicide (o′vĭ-sīd) an agent destructive to the ova of certain organisms.

oviduct (o′vĭ-dukt) a passage through which ova leave the maternal body or pass to an organ communicating with the exterior of the body (see also UTERINE TUBE). adj., **ovidu′cal, oviduct′al.**

oviferous (o-vif′er-us) producing ova.

oviform (o′vĭ-form) egg-shaped.

ovigenesis (o″vĭ-jen′ĕ-sis) oogenesis. adj., **ovigenet′ic.**

ovine (o′vīn) pertaining to, characteristic of, or derived from sheep.

oviparous (o-vip′ah-rus) producing eggs in which the embryo develops outside of the maternal body, as in birds.

oviposition (o″vĭ-po-zish′un) the act of laying or depositing eggs.

ovipositor (o″vĭ-pos′ĭ-tor) a specialized organ by which many female insects deposit their eggs.

ovisac (o′vĭ-sak) a graafian follicle.

ovo- word element [L.], *egg; ovum.*

Ovocylin (o″vo-sil′in) trademark for a preparation of estradiol, an estrogenic compound.

ovoflavin (o″vo-fla′vin) riboflavin derived from eggs.

ovoglobulin (o″vo-glob′u-lin) the globulin of white of egg.

ovomucoid (o″vo-mu′koid) a mucoid principle from egg albumin.

ovoplasm (o′vo-plazm) the cytoplasm of an unfertilized ovum.

ovotestis (o″vo-tes′tis) a gonad containing both testicular and ovarian tissue.

ovoviviparous (o″vo-vi-vip′ah-rus) bearing living young that hatch from eggs inside the maternal body, the embryo being nourished by food stored in the egg; said of lizards, etc.

ovular (o′vu-lar) pertaining to an ovule or an ovum.

ovulation (o″vu-la′shun) the discharge of the ovum from the GRAAFIAN FOLLICLE. adj., **ov′ulatory.** Normally, in an adult woman, ovulation occurs at intervals of about 28 days and alternates between the two ovaries. As a rule, only one ovum is produced, but occasionally ovulation produces two or more ova; if such ova subsequently become fertilized, the result may be multiple births, such as twins or triplets.

Ovulation takes place approximately at the midpoint of the menstrual cycle, 14 days after the onset of menstruation. During the preceding weeks, a graafian follicle, or cell cluster in the ovary containing the ovum, grows from the size of a pinhead to that of a pea. At the moment of ovulation, the follicle bursts open and the ovum is discharged.

The discharged ovum enters the UTERINE TUBE adjoining the ovary and moves toward the uterus; if it encounters a spermatozoon while it is still alive (about 48 hours), the two merge. Fertilization usually takes place in the uterine tube. The fertilized ovum then makes its way to the uterus, where it becomes embedded in the prepared wall as the first stage of growth of the new infant (see illustration, page 736, and see also REPRODUCTION). If fertilization does not take place the ovum loses its vitality and the blood and tissue lining the uterus are shed in the menstrual flow.

ovule (o′vūl) 1. the ovum within the graafian follicle. 2. any small, egglike structure.

ovum (o′vum), pl. *o′va* [L.] egg; the female reproductive or germ cell which, after fertilization, is capable of developing into a new member of the same species; sometimes applied to any stage of the fertilized germ cell during cleavage and even until hatching or birth of the new individual. The human ovum consists of protoplasm that contains some yolk, enclosed by a cell wall consisting of two layers, an outer one (zona pellucida, zona radiata) and an inner, thin one (vitelline membrane). There is a large nucleus (germinal vesicle) within which is a nucleolus (germinal spot). adj., **o′vular.**

centrolecithal o., one with the yolk concentrated at the center of the egg, surrounded by a peripheral shell of cytoplasm, and with an island of cystoplasm surrounding the nucleus.

holoblastic o., one that undergoes total cleavage.

isolecithal o., one with a small amount of yolk evenly distributed throughout the cytoplasm.

meroblastic o., one that undergoes partial cleavage.

primitive o., primordial o., any egg cell very early in its development.

telolecithal o., one with a comparatively large amount of yolk massed at one pole.

Owren's disease (ow'renz) parahemophilia.

oxacillin (ok"sah-sil'in) a semisynthetic penicillin used as the sodium salt in infections due to penicillin-resistant, gram-positive organisms.

Oxaine (ok'sān) trademark for a preparation of oxethazine, a gastric mucosal anesthetic.

oxalate (ok'sah-lāt) any salt of oxalic acid.

potassium o., colorless, odorless crystals used extensively as a reagent.

oxalemia (ok"sah-le'me-ah) excess of oxalates in the blood.

oxalic acid (ok-sal'ik) a poisonous, crystalline, dibasic acid found in various fruits and vegetables, and formed in the metabolism of ascorbic acid in the body; used as a chemical reagent in pharmacy, industry, and the arts. It is highly toxic and if ingested should be neutralized by the administration of lime water (calcium hydroxide solution) or other convenient source of calcium, which reacts with the acid to form insoluble calcium oxalate.

oxalism (ok'sah-lizm) poisoning by oxalic acid or by an oxalate.

oxalosis (ok"sah-lo'sis) primary hyperoxaluria.

oxaluria (ok"sah-lu're-ah) hyperoxaluria.

oxanamide (ok-san'ah-mīd) a tranquilizer.

oxandrolone (ok-san'dro-lōn) an androgenic steroidal lactone used to accelerate anabolism and/or to arrest excessive catabolism.

oxazepam (oks-az'ĕ-pam) a minor tranquilizer.

oxethazaine (ok-seth'ah-zān) a gastric mucosal anesthetic.

oxidant (ok'sĭ-dant) the electron acceptor in an oxidation-reduction (redox) reaction.

oxidase (ok'sĭ-dās) any of a class of enzymes that catalyze the reduction of molecular oxygen independently of hydrogen peroxide.

oxidation (ok"sĭ-da'shun) the act of oxidizing or state of being oxidized. adj., **oxida'tive.** Chemically it consists in the increase of positive charges on an atom or the loss of negative charges. Univalent oxidation indicates loss of one electron; divalent oxidation, the loss of two electrons. The opposite reaction to oxidation is reduction.

oxidation-reduction (ok"sĭ-da'shun-re-duk'shun) the chemical reaction whereby electrons are removed (oxidation) from atoms of the substance being oxidized and transferred to those being reduced (reduction).

oxide (ok'sīd) a compound of oxygen with an element or radical.

oxidize (ok'sĭ-dīz) to cause to combine with oxygen or to remove hydrogen.

oxidoreductase (ok"sĭ-do-re-duk'tās) a class of enzymes that catalyze the reversible transfer of electrons from one substance to another (oxidation-reduction, or redox reaction).

oxim, oxime (ok'sim) any of a series of compounds formed by action of hydroxylamine on an aldehyde or ketone.

oximeter (ok-sim'ĕ-ter) a photoelectric device for determining the oxygen saturation of the blood.

oxolinic acid (ok"so-lin'ik) a long-acting antibacterial agent, derived from quinolone, used orally in

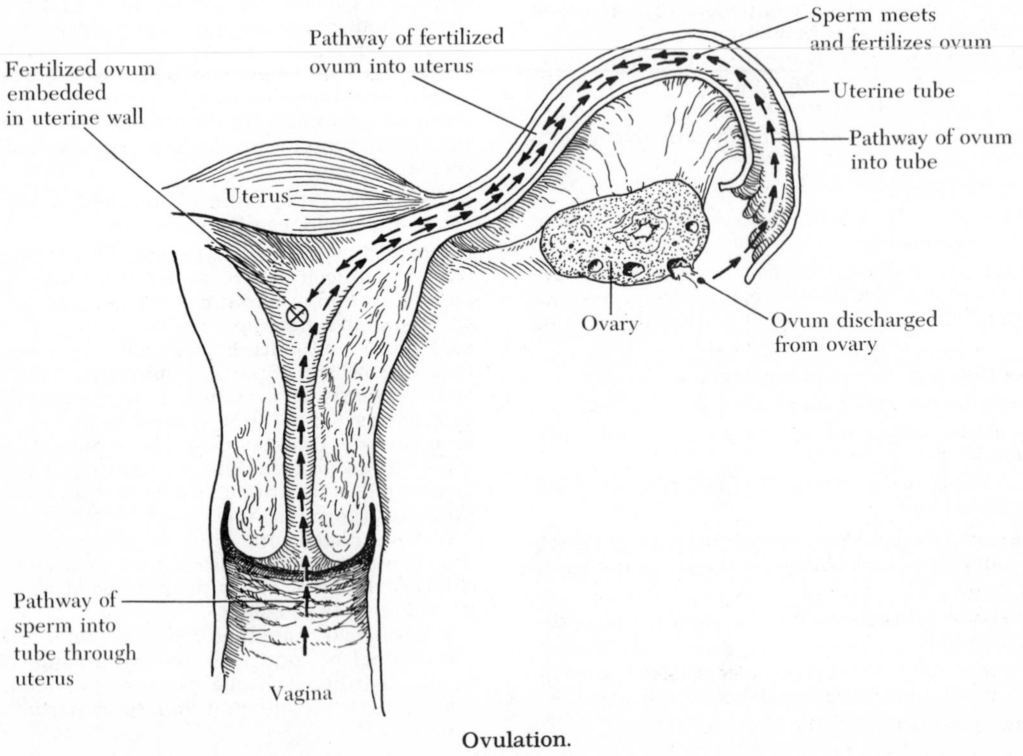

Ovulation.

the treatment of urinary tract infections caused by susceptible gram-negative organisms.

oxophenarsine (ok″so-fen-ar′sin) an antitrypanosomal agent.

oxprenolol (oks-pren′o-lōl) a coronary vasodilator.

Oxsoralen (ok-sor′ah-len) trademark for preparations of methoxsalen, a pigment stimulant.

oxtriphylline (oks-trif′ĭ-lēn) a theophylline derivative used as a bronchodilator.

oxy- word element [Gr.], *sharp; quick; sour; presence of oxygen in a compound.*

oxyblepsia (ok″sĭ-blep′se-ah) unusual acuity of vision.

Oxycel (ok′sĭ-sel) trademark for preparations of oxidized cellulose.

oxycephaly (ok-sĭ-sef′ah-le) a high, pointed condition of the skull, with a vertical index of 77 or more. adj., **oxycephal′ic.**

oxychloride (ok″sĭ-klo′rīd) an element or radical combined with oxygen and chlorine.

oxychromatic (ok″sĭ-kro-mat′ik) staining with acid dyes; acidophilic.

oxychromatin (ok″sĭ-kro′mah-tin) that part of chromatin that stains with acid aniline dyes.

oxycinesia (ok″sĭ-si-ne′ze-ah) pain on motion.

oxyesthesia (ok″se-es-the′ze-ah) abnormal acuteness of the senses.

oxygen (ok′sĭ-jen) a chemical element, atomic number 8, atomic weight 15.999, symbol O. (See table of ELEMENTS.) It is a colorless and odorless gas that makes up about 20 per cent of the atmosphere. In combination with hydrogen, it forms water; by weight, 90 per cent of water is oxygen. It is the most abundant of all the elements of nature. Large quantities of it are distributed throughout the solid matter of the earth, because the gas combines readily with many other elements. With carbon and hydrogen, oxygen forms the chemical basis of much organic material.

Oxygen is essential in sustaining all kinds of life. Among the higher animals, it is obtained from the air and drawn into the lungs by the process of RESPIRATION. (See also BLOOD GAS ANALYSIS.)

OXYGEN BALANCE AND "OXYGEN DEBT." The need of every cell for oxygen requires a balance in supply and demand. But this balance need not be exact at all times. In fact, in strenuous exercise the oxygen needs of muscle cells are greater than the amount the body can absorb even by the most intense breathing. Thus, during athletic competition, the participants make use of the capacity of muscles to function even though their needs for oxygen are not fully met. When the competition is over, however, the athletes will continue to breathe heavily until the muscles have been supplied with sufficient oxygen. This temporary deficiency is called oxygen debt.

EFFECTS AND TREATMENT OF OXYGEN LACK. Total deprivation of the supply of oxygen to the body causes death within minutes. Severe curtailment of oxygen, as during ascent to high altitudes or in certain illnesses, may bring on a variety of symptoms of HYPOXIA, or oxygen lack. A number of poisons, among them cyanide and carbon monoxide, and also large overdoses of sedatives disrupt the oxygen distribution system of the body. Such disruption occurs also in various illness, such as anemia and diseases of lungs, heart, kidneys, and liver.

o. therapy, supplemental oxygen administered for the purpose of relieving hypoxemia and preventing damage to the tissue cells as a result of oxygen lack (HYPOXIA). Oxygen can be toxic and therefore, as with a drug, its dosage and mode of administration are based on an assessment of the needs of the individual patient. Although many types of hypoxia can be treated successfully by the administration of oxygen, not all cases respond to this therapy. There also is the possibility that the injudicious use of oxygen can produce serious and permanent damage to the body tissues. The administration of oxygen should never be considered a "routine" or harmless procedure.

ADVERSE EFFECTS OF OXYGEN. Although it is true that all living organisms require oxygen to maintain life, excessive amounts can be detrimental. For example, an environment of 100 per cent oxygen inhibits the growth of living tissue cultures, and laboratory experiments have shown that hyperoxygenation of the body tissues can cause irreversible damage. It is now known that high concentrations of inhaled oxygen can result in collapse of alveoli because of the displacement of nitrogen by the oxygen. RETROLENTAL FIBROPLASIA in premature infants was found to be caused by excessively high levels of oxygen in the blood.

Another serious complication of high-oxygen concentration therapy is the development of a hyaline membrane, a condition that results from a deficiency of pulmonary surfactant, a substance that is vitally important to normal expansion and deflation of the alveoli. Prolonged exposure to inspired oxygen concentrations in excess of 50 per cent can impair the production of this surfactant in a patient of any age. The result is a loss of lung compliance and reduction of the transport of oxygen across the alveolar membrane.

The danger of oxygen toxicity can be minimized by a careful assessment of each patient's need for oxygen therapy and the systematic monitoring of blood gases to determine patient response and effectiveness of treatment. (See also BLOOD GAS ANALYSIS.)

Symptoms of oxygen toxicity are substernal distress, nausea and vomiting, malaise, fatigue, and numbness and tingling of the extremities.

INDICATIONS FOR OXYGEN THERAPY. In general, the clinical situations in which the administration of supplemental oxygen is indicated are: (1) Profound but potentially reversible hypoxia that appears amenable to the short-term administration of high concentrations of oxygen. Examples would include the patient who is apneic, suffering from cardiovascular collapse, or is a victim of carbon monoxide poisoning. (2) Conditions in which there is a need to reduce the work load of the cardiovascular and pulmonary systems and at the same time assure an adequate supply of oxygen to the tissues. Congestive heart failure, myocardial infarction, and such acute pulmonary diseases as pulmonary embolism and pneumonia are examples of the type of clinical situations that are best treated by the administration of moderate levels of oxygen concentration. (3) Evidence of hypoventilation, whether from anesthesia and sedation, CHRONIC OBSTRUCTIVE PULMONARY DISEASE (COPD), or other conditions. The patient who is hypoventilating is in danger of suffering from an adverse effect of oxygen therapy because increased oxygenation can lead to decreased respiratory effort. In other words, the oxygen acts as a respiratory depressant and therefore has the potential of contributing to rather than overcoming the problem of hypoxia. If there is evidence that the patient is hypoventilating, it may be necessary to administer the oxygen by assisted or controlled ventilation.

DOSAGE AND METHOD OF ADMINISTRATION. If one bears in mind that oxygen can act like a drug and should be prescribed and administered as such, it is apparent that vague orders about its administration are never acceptable. There must be specific written orders for flow rate and mode of administration. Decisions about the initial dosage, as well as any changes in mode of administration and dosage, including the discontinuance of oxygen therapy, should be based on evaluation of the P_{O_2}, the P_{CO_2}, and the blood pH (BLOOD GAS ANALYSIS).

The clinical signs and symptoms of hypoxemia may vary from patient to patient, and they should not be depended upon as valid indications of oxygen insufficiency. This is especially true of cyanosis, a symptom that depends on local circulation to the area, the red cell count, and hemoglobin level.

In addition to the data obtained from blood gas analyses, an oxygen analyzer should be used occasionally to check inspired oxygen concentration.

In general, the dosage and mode of administration fall into the following categories. *High concentrations* above 50 per cent usually are prescribed when there is a need for the delivery of high levels of oxygen for a short period of time to overcome acute hypoxia, as in cardiovascular failure and pulmonary edema. The flow rate may be as high as 12 liters per minute, administered through a close-fitting face mask with or without a rebreathing bag, or via an endotracheal tube.

Moderate concentrations of oxygen are indicated when the patient is suffering from impaired circulation of oxygen, as in congestive heart failure and pulmonary embolism, or from increased need for oxygen, as in thyrotoxicosis, in which the increased metabolic rate creates a need for more oxygen. The rate of flow should be 4 to 8 liters per minute, administered through a Venturi mask that delivers concentrations above 23 per cent, or in a dosage of 3 to 5 liters per minute through a nasal cannula.

Low concentrations of oxygen are indicated when the patient is receiving oxygen therapy over an extended period of time, as in CHRONIC OBSTRUCTIVE PULMONARY DISEASE, and there is the possibility of hypoventilation and the danger of increased CO_2 retention. The rate of flow should be 1–4 liters per minute, administered through a nasal cannula, or via a Venturi mask that delivers either 24, 28, or 35 per cent concentration of oxygen.

Other methods of oxygen administration include the nasal catheter and the oxygen tent. The nasal catheter can cause some discomfort to the patient, and since it is no more and no less effective than the cannula, most therapists prefer to use the catheter only for restless and uncooperative patients. The oxygen tent is considered by many to be obsolete, its use being limited to the administration of oxygen to children who cannot or will not tolerate other modes of delivery, and to cases in which the objective is to provide oxygen and humidity or humidity alone.

PATIENT CARE. No matter what mode of administration is used, it is essential that the inspired air be moisturized. This is necessary to prevent drying of the respiratory mucosa and thickening of secretions that can further inhibit the flow of air through the air passages. Humidity may be provided by humidifying the oxygen with water, or by aerosoling the water into fine particles and adding it to the oxygen. Most patients need 60 to 65 per cent relative humidity at room temperature. Patients with endotracheal tubes require as close to 100 per cent humidity as possible.

Oxygen is not an explosive gas, but it does support combustion and presents a serious fire hazard. All electrical equipment should be checked for defects that could produce sparks. All appliances that transmit house current must be kept outside an oxygen tent, and all equipment with exposed switches and meters must be considered potential sources of fire. Static electricity is a minimal risk which can be further reduced by maintaining a relatively high humidity in the oxygen tent. Smoking in the immediate area of oxygen administration is prohibited and there should be signs informing visitors and others of this restriction.

When the patient is wearing a mask for an extended period of time, his discomfort can be minimized by removing the mask and washing and drying his face at least every eight hours. To be effective the mask must fit snugly and follow the contour of the face. This means that reddened areas will appear where the mask has pressed against the skin. These areas should be gently massaged and the skin lightly powdered to reduce friction.

Nasal catheters have a tendency to produce irritation of the nasal mucosa and therefore require frequent changing, using alternate nostrils. The patient may be more comfortable if some type of nonoily lubricant is applied to the nasal mucosa. Patients who have suffered stroke, are very elderly, or are deeply comatose may have diminished or absent epiglottal reflexes. In these cases the flow of oxygen may be directed into the stomach via the esophagus. This presents the very real danger of gastric rupture at worst, and severe distention which may further aggravate breathing difficulties at best. For such patients it is suggested that a mode of oxygen administration other than nasal catheter be chosen.

A program of infection control is especially important in the prevention of cross-infection from the equipment that is used to administer oxygen. Some humidifiers and nebulizers heat the water to 122° F. (53° C.) so as to increase water vapor and facilitate humidification. These may serve as sources of infection because they provide an excellent medium for the growth of bacteria and molds. There is less danger of this happening when disposable equipment is used, but this does not preclude the need for a systematic development of policies and procedures to prevent and control the spread of infection. Each and every person involved in the care of the patient must be aware of this program and cooperate in its implementation.

The termination of oxygen therapy is never done abruptly. The patient is gradually weaned from the oxygen administration by alternating periods of oxygen supplemented inspiration with periods of breathing without the additional oxygen.

oxygenase (ok′sĭ-jen-ās″) any enzyme of the oxidoreductase class that catalyzes the incorporation of both atoms of molecular oxygen into the substrate.

oxygenation (ok″sĭ-jĕ-na′shun) saturation with oxygen.

hyperbaric o., exposure to oxygen under conditions of greatly increased pressure (see also HYPERBARIC OXYGENATION).

oxygenator (ok″sĭ-jĕ-na″tor) an apparatus by which oxygen is introduced into the blood during circulation outside the body, as during open-heart surgery. (See also HEART-LUNG MACHINE.)

bubble o., a device in which pure oxygen is bubbled through an extracorporeal reservoir of blood, either directly or through a filter.

film o., a device, encased in a container of oxygen, that makes possible reduction of a thin film of blood to facilitate the exchange of gases.

rotating disk o., a type of film oxygenator in which a series of parallel disks rotate through an extracorporeal pool of venous blood in a container of oxygen; gaseous exchange occurs between the thin film of blood on the exposed surface of the disks and the oxygen in the container.

screen o., a type of film oxygenator in which the venous blood is passed over a series of screens in a container of oxygen, gaseous exchange taking place in the thin film of blood produced on the screens.

oxygeusia (ok″sĭ-gu′ze-ah) extreme acuteness of the sense of taste.

oxyhematoporphyrin (ok″sĭ-hem″ah-to-por′fĭ-rin) a pigment sometimes found in the urine, closely allied to hematoporphyrin.

oxyhemoglobin (ok″sĭ-he″mo-glo′bin) hemoglobin charged with oxygen.

oxyhemoglobinometer (ok″sĭ-he″mo-glo″bĭ-nom′ĭ-ter) an instrument for measuring the oxygen content of the blood.

oxyiodide (ok″se-i′o-dīd) an element or radical combined with oxygen and iodine.

oxylalia (ok″sĭ-la′le-ah) rapidity of speech.

Oxylone (ok′sĭ-lōn) trademark for a preparation of fluorometholone, an anti-inflammatory glucocorticoid.

oxymetazoline (ok″sĭ-met-az′o-lēn) a vasoconstrictor used topically as the hydrochloride salt in nasal congestion.

oxymetholone (ok″sĭ-meth′o-lōn) a steroid compound used to treat patients with wasting effects after a long illness.

oxymorphone (ok″sĭ-mor′fōn) a narcotic analgesic, used as the hydrochloride salt.

oxymyoglobin (ok″sĭ-mi″o-glo′bin) myoglobin charged with oxygen.

oxyopia (ok″se-o′pe-ah) abnormal acuteness of sight.

oxypertine (ok″sĭ-per′tēn) an antidepressant.

oxyphenbutazone (ok″sĭ-fen-bu′tah-zōn) a nonsteroid anti-inflammatory agent.

oxyphencyclimine (ok″sĭ-fen-si′klĭ-mēn) an anticholinergic with antisecretory, antimotility, and antispasmodic actions; the hydrochloride salt is used in the treatment of peptic ulcer and other gastrointestinal disorders.

oxyphenonium (ok″sĭ-fĕ-no′ne-um) an anticholinergic used as the bromide ester in the treatment of peptic ulcer and gastrointestinal hypermotility or spasm.

oxyphil (ok′sĭ-fil) 1. Hürthle cell. 2. oxyphilic.

oxyphilic, oxyphilous (ok″sĭ-fil′ik; ok-sif′ĭ-lus) stainable with an acid dye.

oxyphonia (ok″sĭ-fo′ne-ah) an abnormally sharp quality or pitch of the voice.

oxypurine (ok″sĭ-pu′rēn) a purine containing oxygen.

oxypurinol (ok″sĭ-pūr′ĭ-nol) a xanthine oxidase inhibitor.

oxytetracycline (ok″sĭ-tet-rah-si′klēn) a broad-spectrum antibiotic substance isolated from the elaboration products of *Streptomyces rimosus*.

oxytalan (oks-it′ah-lan) a connective tissue fiber found in the periodontal membrane.

oxytocia (ok″sĭ-to′se-ah) rapid labor.

oxytocic (ok″sĭ-to′sik) 1. pertaining to, marked by, or promoting oxytocia. 2. an agent that promotes rapid labor by stimulating contractions of the myometrium.

oxytocin (ok″sĭ-to′sin) a hypothalamic hormone stored in and released from the posterior pituitary, or prepared synthetically. It acts as a powerful stimulant to the pregnant uterus, especially toward the end of gestation. The hormone also causes milk to be expressed from the alveoli into the lactiferous ducts during suckling.

Injection of oxytocin may be used to induce labor or strengthen the uterine contractions during labor. It is administered with care so as to avoid trauma to the mother or infant by hyperactivity of the uterine muscles during labor. Oxytocin also may be administered intravenously by slow drip and it is sometimes applied to the mucous membranes of the nasal cavity and absorbed into the bloodstream.

oxyuriasis (ok″se-u-ri′ah-sis) infection with *Enterobius vermicularis* (in humans) or with other oxyurids; enterobiosis.

oxyuricide (ok″se-u′rĭ-sīd) an agent that kills oxyurids.

oxyurid (ok″se-u′rid) a pinworm, seatworm, or threadworm; an individual organism of the superfamily Oxyuroidea.

Oxyuris (ok″se-u′ris) a genus of nematode intestinal parasites (superfamily Oxyuroidea).

O. vermicula′ris, *Enterobius vermicularis*.

Oxyuroidea (ok″sĭ-u″roi-de′ah) a superfamily of small nematodes–the pinworms, seatworms, or threadworms–usually parasitic in the cecum and colon of vertebrates, but may infect invertebrates.

oz. ounce.

ozena (o-ze′nah) a condition of the nose associated with a foul-smelling discharge.

ozone (o′zōn) a bluish explosive gas or blue liquid, being an allotropic form of oxygen, O_3; it is antiseptic and disinfectant, and irritating and toxic to the pulmonary system.

ozonometer (o″zo-nom′ĕ-ter) an apparatus for measuring the ozone in the atmosphere.

ozostomia (o″zo-sto′me-ah) foulness of the breath.

P

P chemical symbol, *phosphorus.*

P. position; presbyopia; [L.] *prox'imum* (near); pulse; [L.] *punc'tum* (point); pupil.

P_1 parental generation.

P_2 pulmonic second sound (see HEART SOUNDS).

p- symbol, *para-*.

Pa chemical symbol, *protactinium.*

PAB, PABA para-aminobenzoic acid, used as a sunscreen and in bacterial culture media.

pabulum (pab'u-lum) food or aliment.

Pacatal (pak'ah-tal) trademark for a preparation of mepazine, a neuroleptic and antinauseant.

pacemaker (pās'māk-er) that which sets the pace at which a phenomenon occurs; the term usually refers to the cardiac pacemaker.

The cardiac or so-called "normal" pacemaker of the HEART is the sinoatrial node, a small mass of specialized muscle tissue in the heart near the junction with the superior vena cava. It sets a rhythm of contraction and relaxation that is followed by the other portions of the heart. Thus the heartbeat is established.

The normal rhythm, 60 to 100 contractions per minute, is increased by physical or emotional stress, and decreases during rest. The pace varies from person to person and is affected by abnormal conditions such as heart injuries and generalized infections. If the normal pacemaker fails to function, its regulating task may be taken over by another small mass of special muscular tissue, the atrioventricular node.

In women, the uterus contains two pacemakers that control uterine contractions. These regulating centers are located near the openings of the uterine tubes. When the child is ready to be born, the pacemakers set off a series of rhythmic contractions in the uterus that gradually force the baby out into the birth canal.

ELECTRONIC PACEMAKERS. In some types of heart disease in which the heart's pacemaker is malfunctioning, an electronic device known as an *artificial cardiac pacemaker* may be employed to regulate the heart beat. The electronic pacemaker contains batteries, transistors, and other components designed to send a very brief stimulus to the heart via a soft plastic cable attached to the heart muscle. The pacemaker regulates the beat of the heart causing the myocardium to contract at a rate of 60 to 70 beats per minute.

Indications. Any person who has had one or more attacks of Adams-Stokes syndrome caused by heart block or tachycardia and does not respond to drug therapy is a candidate for a pacemaker. Other indications include extremely slow heart rates due to sinus bradycardia, or the carotid sinus syndrome.

Types. The *temporary* or *external* pacemaker is very similar to a small transistor radio. Its components are a pulse generator and an electrode catheter. The pulse generator remains outside the body and the leads from it are directed to the heart through the catheter, usually inserted through a large systemic vein (transvenously). Other less frequently used methods are insertion of the electrodes through the chest wall into the myocardium and the direct application of the electrodes to the external chest wall. The latter technique is painful to the patient and can cause burns of the chest. The use of a temporary external pacemaker often is an emergency or semiemergency procedure.

Temporary pacemakers are also routinely used after cardiac surgery. In this instance two tiny wires are loosely sewn to the epicardium and a third is sewn into subcutaneous tissue. The wires exit through an incision in the chest wall and are attached to the pulse generator. They are easily removed when they are no longer needed.

The *permanent* or *implantable* pacemaker is very small, about half the size of a pack of cigarettes. The pulse generator is sewn into a subcutaneous pocket located beneath the clavicle or under the axilla. The wires that connect the pulse generator to the heart muscle are inserted transvenously. Permanent cardiac pacemakers may be used for months to years.

Pacemakers may be designed to send impulses at a fixed rate or only on demand. The simplest pacemaker is the *fixed rate* or asynchronous type. It sends electrical stimuli to the heart at a predetermined rate regardless of the needs of the heart. Because it may compete with the patient's own natural pacemaker and initiate ventricular tachycardia or ventricular fibrillation, this type of device is less acceptable than the *demand* pacemaker. The demand pacemaker avoids competition by stimulating the heart at a pre-fixed rate only if the patient's rate falls below a predetermined level.

Work is constantly being done on improving the design and method of applying cardiac pacemakers. It is expected that with continued research the pacemakers will become smaller and longer lasting and the insertion of leads will be less traumatic.

wandering p., a condition in which the site of origin of the impulses controlling the heart rate shifts from the head of the sinoatrial node to a lower part of the node or to another part of the atrium.

pachy- word element [Gr.], *thick.*

pachyacria (pak"e-a'kre-ah) enlargement of the soft parts of the extremities.

pachyblepharon (pak"ĭ-blef'ah-ron) thickening of the eyelids.

pachycephaly (pak"ĭ-sef'ah-le) abnormal thickness of the bones of the skull. adj., **pachycephal'ic.**

pachycheilia (pak"ĭ-ki'le-ah) thickening of the lips.

pachychromatic (pak"ĭ-kro-mat'ik) having the chromatin in thick strands.

pachydactyly (pak"ĭ-dak'tĭ-le) enlargement of the fingers and toes.

pachyderma (pak"ĭ-der'mah) abnormal thickening of the skin. adj., **pachyder'matous.**

p. circumscrip'ta, p. laryn'gis, localized warty epithelial thickenings on the vocal cords.

p. ves'icae, thickening of the mucous membrane of the bladder.

pachydermatocele (pak"ĭ-der-mat'o-sēl) plexiform

neuroma attaining large size, producing an elephantiasis-like condition.

pachydermoperiostosis (pak″ĭ-der″mo-per″e-os-to′sis) pachyderma affecting the face and scalp, thickening of the bones of the distal extremities, and clubbing of the fingers and toes.

pachyglossia (pak″ĭ-glos′e-ah) abnormal thickness of the tongue.

pachygyria (pak″ĭ-ji′re-ah) macrogyria.

pachyhematous (pak″ĭ-hem′ah-tus) pertaining to or having thickened blood.

pachyleptomeningitis (pak″ĭ-lep″to-men″in-ji′tis) inflammation of the dura mater and pia mater.

pachymeningitis (pak″ĭ-men″in-ji′tis) inflammation of the dura mater; perimeningitis.

pachymeningopathy (pak″ĭ-men″in-gop′ah-the) noninflammatory disease of the dura mater.

pachymeninx (pak″ĭ-me′ninks) the dura mater.

pachynsis (pah-kin′sis) an abnormal thickening. adj., **pachyn′tic.**

pachyonychia (pak″e-o-nik′e-ah) abnormal thickening of the nails.

p. congen′ita, a hereditary congenital anomaly marked by great thickening of the nails, hyperkeratosis of palms and soles, and leukoplakia.

pachyperiostitis (pak″ĭ-per″e-os-ti′tis) periostitis of long bones resulting in abnormal thickness of affected bones.

pachyperitonitis (pak″ĭ-per″ĭ-to-ni′tis) inflammation and thickening of the peritoneum.

pachypleuritis (pak″ĭ-ploo-ri′tis) fibrothorax.

pachysalpingitis (pak″ĭ-sal″pin-ji′tis) chronic interstitial inflammation of the muscular coat of the oviduct producing thickening; called also mural salpingitis and parenchymatous salpingitis.

pachysalpingo-ovaritis (pak″ĭ-sal-ping″go-o″var-i′tis) chronic inflammation of the ovary and oviduct, with thickening.

pachysomia (pak″ĭ-so′me-ah) thickening of parts of the body.

pachytene (pak′ĭ-tēn) in meiosis, the stage following synapsis, in which the homologous chromosome threads shorten, thicken, and intertwine.

pachyvaginalitis (pak″ĭ-vaj″ĭ-nal-i′tis) inflammation and thickening of the tunica vaginalis of the testis.

pachyvaginitis (pak″ĭ-vaj″ĭ-ni′tis) chronic vaginitis with thickening of the vaginal walls.

pack (pak) 1. treatment by wrapping a patient in blankets or sheets, or a limb in towels, wet or dry and either hot or cold; referred to as wet, dry, hot, or cold pack, respectively. Also, the blankets, sheets, or towels used for this purpose. 2. a tampon.

packer (pak′er) an instrument for introducing a dressing into a cavity or a wound.

packing (pak′ing) 1. the filling of a wound or cavity with gauze, sponge, or other material. 2. the material used for this purpose.

Pa_{CO_2} symbol for partial pressure of carbon dioxide in the arterial blood (see also BLOOD GAS ANALYSIS).

pad (pad) a cushion-like mass of soft material.

abdominal p., a pad for the absorption of discharges from abdominal wounds, or for packing off abdominal viscera to improve exposure during surgery.

dinner p., a pad placed over the stomach before a plaster jacket is applied; the pad is then removed to leave space under the jacket to take care of expansion of the stomach after eating.

fat p., a large pad of fat lying behind and below the patella.

knuckle p′s, nodular thickenings of the skin on the dorsal surface of the interphalangeal joints.

Mikulicz′s p., a pad made of folded gauze, for packing off viscera in surgical procedures.

sucking p., suctorial p., a lobulated mass of fat that occupies the space between the masseter muscle and the external surface of the buccinator muscle. It is well developed in infants.

pae- for words beginning thus, see those beginning *pe-*.

Paget′s disease (paj′ets) any of the three diseases named after Sir James Paget (1814–1899). One is a bone disease that is called also OSTEITIS DEFORMANS. The second is a rare, inflammatory cancerous affection of the areola and nipple. The third is an extramammary counterpart of the latter disease, which usually involves the vulva, and sometimes other sites, such as the perianal and axillary regions.

pagetoid (paj′ĕ-toid) resembling Paget′s disease.

Pagitane (paj′ĭ-tān) trademark for a preparation of cycrimine, an anticholinergic used in the treatment of Parkinson′s disease.

-pagus word element [Gr.], *conjoined twins.*

PAH, PAHA para-aminohippuric acid, used in testing renal function. Normal values for males are 561 to 833 ml./min., and for females 492 to 696 ml./min.

pain (pān) a feeling of distress, suffering, or agony, caused by stimulation of specialized nerve endings. Its purpose is chiefly protective; it acts as a warning that early tissue damage is taking place somewhere in the body.

The receptors for the stimulus of pain are specific groups of myelinated and unmyelinated nerve fibers abundantly distributed near the surface of the body, and to a lesser degree in the internal organs. Some of the internal organs such as the lungs and uterus have comparatively few receptors, and therefore are relatively insensitive to painful stimuli. The distribution of pain receptors in the mucosa of the intestinal tract apparently is similar to that in the skin, and the mucosa is quite sensitive to irritation or other painful stimuli.

Superficial pain is felt when a stimulus reaches the cutaneous receptors near the surface of the body. It is felt as a sudden, sharp pain at the site of the stimulation. Deep pain arises from stimulation of receptors in the internal structures such as the muscles and viscera, and tends to be duller, of longer duration, and less localized.

When the receptors are stimulated, the impulses are transmitted along nerve fibers that feed into the spinal ganglia. They then travel upward along nerve fibers to the thalamus. Here the pain impulses are integrated and the individual becomes aware of the painful stimulus. The impulses are finally transmitted to the sensory portion of the cerebral cortex where the pain is analyzed and its location and intensity are determined.

REACTIONS TO PAIN. There are two types of reaction to pain: physical and psychologic. The physical reaction is usually an automatic response to superficial pain resulting from stimulation of the sympathetic nervous system and producing an outpouring of epinephrine. There is a shift of blood from the skin, brain, and intestinal tract toward the muscles; the blood pressure increases and the pulse rate rises. This reaction soon subsides if the pain persists and remains intense. The individual then becomes weak, shows signs of shock, and may become nauseated and vomit. He most often seeks rest and quiet and becomes withdrawn.

The psychologic aspects of pain are more complex and difficult to determine. An individual's reaction to pain depends on many factors, such as his previous experience with pain, his training in regard to proper and acceptable responses to pain and discomfort, his state of health, and the presence or absence of fatigue. Anxiety and tension generally increase sensitivity to pain. A person's attention to, or degree of distraction from, the presence of painful stimuli can also affect his reaction to the pain.

PATIENT CARE. Pain is a subjective symptom, that is, the patient is relied on to determine and describe the intensity, location, and characteristics of the pain he is feeling. By observation of the patient's general posture, facial expressions, and outward symptoms of physical reaction to pain it is sometimes possible to determine whether or not discomfort or distress is present. By being aware of the psychologic aspects of pain such as anxiety and tension, one can do much to relieve or lessen to some degree the distress suffered by a patient. Denying or expressing doubt that the pain actually exists, or implying that a patient is not acting in an acceptable manner when something is causing him suffering, only serves to increase his discomfort. His anxiety and tension can be greatly reduced if one shows appreciation of the fact that pain is present and indicates a willingness to try to help him gain relief. Simple measures such as smoothing the bed linen, rearranging the pillows, or changing the patient's position can show such a willingness. It also may help the patient if he is allowed to talk about his feelings toward the pain or the cause of it.

When analgesic drugs have been ordered "as needed" the patient should know that they are available to him and that they will be given promptly if he requests them. If he is forced to wait until someone else decides when he needs them, he may become resentful, angry, and tense, and the effect of the medication when it is finally given will be diminished. Of course, one must guard against addiction or habituation in patients with chronic disorders necessitating frequent administration of narcotics and analgesics.

Since pain is a symptom and therefore of value in diagnosis, it is important to keep accurate records of the observations of the patient having pain. These observations should include the following: the nature of the pain, that is, whether it is described by the patient as being sharp, dull, burning, aching, etc.; the location of the pain, if the patient is able to determine this; the time of onset and the duration, and whether or not certain nursing measures and drugs are successful in obtaining relief; and the relation to other circumstances, such as the position of the patient, occurrence before or after eating, and stimuli in the environment such as heat or cold that may trigger the onset of pain.

abdominal p., pain occurring in the area between the chest and pelvis; it is usually a signal that something is wrong with one of the organs within the abdominal cavity.

One of the most frequent causes of abdominal pain is stomach or intestinal distress caused by some indiscretion such as overeating, eating too much rich food, or eating when one is tired or emotionally upset. Pain from such a cause is usually transient and will clear up as soon as the digestive disorder resolves. Whenever abdominal pain is severe or persistent, or whenever it is accompanied by fever, vomiting, rectal bleeding, or diarrhea, there are urgent reasons for seeking medical attention.

There are certain questions a doctor will usually ask about abdominal pain in order to find its cause:

1. Is the pain a new one or has it occurred before, and if so, how often?
2. Is there any specific area of the abdomen where the pain began, and has it remained there or moved elsewhere?
3. Does the pain ease or disappear after eating?
4. Is it accompanied by nausea or diarrhea?
5. Is it a dull pain, a sharp pain, or a crampy pain?
6. Is the pain eased by walking about or by lying down?

bearing-down p., pain accompanying uterine contractions during the second stage of LABOR.

boring p., a sensation as of being pierced with a long, slender twisting object.

false p's, ineffective pains during pregnancy that resemble labor pains, not accompanied by cervical dilatation; called also false labor. (See also BRAXTON-HICKS CONTRACTIONS.)

fulgurant p's, lightning pains.

gas p's, pains caused by distention of the stomach or intestine by accumulations of air or other gases (see also GAS PAINS).

growing p., pains peculiar to youth (see also GROWING PAINS).

hunger p., pain coming on at the time for feeling hunger for a meal; a symptom of gastric disorder.

intermenstrual p., pain accompanying ovulation, occurring during the period between the menses, usually about midway.

labor p's, the rhythmic pains of increasing severity and frequency due to contraction of the uterus at childbirth. (See also LABOR.)

lancinating p., sharp darting pain.

lightning p's, the cutting pains of tabes dorsalis; called also fulgurant pains.

phantom p., pain felt as if it were arising in an absent (amputated) limb. (See also AMPUTATION.)

referred p., pain in a part other than that in which the cause that produced it is situated.

root p., pain caused by disease of the sensory nerve roots and occurring in the cutaneous areas supplied by the affected roots.

terebrant p., terebrating p., boring pain.

painful bruising syndrome autoerythrocyte sensitization syndrome.

palat(o)- word eleement [L.], *palate.*

palate (pal'at) the roof of the mouth. adj., **pal'atal.** The front portion braced by the upper jaw bones (maxillae) is known as the hard palate and forms the partition between the mouth and the nose. The fleshy part arching downward from the hard palate to the throat is called the soft palate and separates the mouth and the upper throat cavity, or pharynx. When one swallows, the rear of the soft palate swings up against the back of the pharynx and blocks the passage of food and air to the nose. A fleshy lobe called the uvula hangs from the middle of the soft palate.

cleft p., congenital fissure of median line of palate (see also CLEFT LIP).

palatitis (pal″ah-ti′tis) inflammation of the palate.

palatoglossal (pal″ah-to-glos′al) pertaining to the palate and tongue.

palatognathous (pal″ah-tog′nah-thus) having a congenitally cleft palate.

palatomaxillary (pal″ah-to-mak′sĭ-ler-e) pertaining to the palate and maxilla.

palatopharyngeal (pal″ah-to-fah-rin′je-al) pertaining to the palate and pharynx.

palatoplasty (pal′ah-to-plas″te) plastic reconstruction of the palate.

palatoplegia (pal″ah-to-ple′je-ah) paralysis of the palate.

palatorrhaphy (pal″ah-tor′ah-fe) surgical correction of a cleft palate.

palatoschisis (pal″ah-tos′kĭ-sis) cleft palate.

palatum (pal-ah′tum) [L.] palate.

pale(o)- word element [Gr.], *old.*

paleencephalon (pa″le-en-sef′ah-lon) the (phylogenetically) old brain; all of the brain except the cerebral cortex and its dependences.

paleocerebellum (pa″le-o-ser″ĕ-bel′um) originally, the phylogenetically older parts of the cerebellum; the term is now applied specifically to those parts whose afferent inflow is predominantly supplied by spinocerebellar fibers. adj., **paleocerebel′lar.**

paleocortex (pa″le-o-kor′teks) paleopallium.

paleogenetic (pa″le-o-jĕ-net′ik) originated in the past; not newly acquired; said of traits, structures, etc., of species.

paleokinetic (pa″le-o-ki-net′ik) old kinetic; a term applied to the nervous motor mechanism concerned in automatic associated movements.

paleopallium (pa″le-o-pal′e-um) that part of the pallium (cerebral cortex) developing with the archipallium in association with the olfactory system; it is phylogenetically older and less stratified than the neopallium, and composed chiefly of the piriform cortex and parahippocampal gyrus. Called also paleocortex.

paleopathology (pa″le-o-pah-thol′o-je) study of disease in bodies that have been preserved from ancient times.

paleostriatum (pa″le-o-stri-a′tum) the phylogenetically older portion of the corpus striatum, represented by the globus pallidus. adj., **paleostria′tal.**

paleothalamus (pa″le-o-thal′ah-mus) the phylogenetically older part of the thalamus, i.e., the medial portion which lacks reciprocal connections with the neopallium.

pali(n)- word element [Gr.], *again; pathologic repetition.*

palikinesia (pal″ĭ-ki-ne′ze-ah) pathologic repetition of movements.

palilalia (pal″ĭ-la′le-ah) a condition in which a phrase or word is repeated with increasing rapidity.

palindromia (pal″in-dro′me-ah) a recurrence or relapse. adj., **palindrom′ic.**

palinesthesia (pal″in-es-the′ze-ah) the return of sensation after anesthesia or coma.

palingraphia (pal″in-graf′e-ah) pathologic repetition of words or phrases in writing.

palinphrasia (pal″in-fra′ze-ah) pathologic repetition of words or phrases in speaking.

palladium (pah-la′de-um) a chemical element, atomic number 46, atomic weight 106.4, symbol Pd. (See table of ELEMENTS.)

pallanesthesia (pal″an-es-the′ze-ah) loss or absence of pallesthesia.

pallesthesia (pal″es-the′ze-ah) sensibility to vibrations; the peculiar vibrating sensation felt when a vibrating tuning-fork is placed against a subcutaneous bony prominence of the body. adj., **pallinesthet′ic.**

palliate (pal′e-āt) to relieve symptoms.

palliative (pal′e-a″tiv) affording relief; also, a drug that so acts.

pallidectomy (pal″ĭ-dek′to-me) extirpation of the globus pallidus.

pallidotomy (pal″ĭ-dot′o-me) creation of lesions in the globus pallidus for treatment of extrapyramidal disorders.

pallidum (pal′ĭ-dum) the globus pallidus of the brain. adj., **pal′lidal.**

pallium (pal′e-um) the cerebral cortex viewed in its entirety, i.e., the mantle of gray matter covering both cerebral hemispheres. Also, the cerebral cortex during its development.

pallor (pal′or) paleness, as of the skin.

palm (pahm) the hollow or flexor surface of the hand. adj., **pal′mar.**

palma (pahl′mah), pl. *pal′mae* [L.] palm.

palmaris (pahl-ma′ris) palmar.

palmitic acid (pal-mit′ik) a saturated fatty acid from animal and vegetable fats. (See also STEARIC ACID.)

palmus (pahl′mus) 1. palpitation. 2. clonic spasm of leg muscles, producing a jumping motion.

palpable (pal′pah-b'l) perceptible by touch.

palpate (pal′pāt) to perform palpation.

palpation (pal-pa′shun) the act of feeling with the hand; the application of the fingers with light pressure to the surface of the body for the purpose of determining the condition of the parts beneath in physical diagnosis.

palpebra (pal′pĕ-brah), pl. *pal′pebrae* [L.] eyelid. adj., **pal′pebral.**

palpebritis (pal″pĕ-bri′tis) blepharitis.

palpitation (pal″pĭ-ta′shun) a heartbeat that is unusually rapid, strong or irregular enough to make a person aware of it—usually over 120 per minute, as opposed to the normal 60 to 100 per minute. In most cases, palpitation is the result of excitement or nervousness, of strong exertion or of taking certain medications. There are also palpitations that result from various types of heart disorders such as paroxysmal tachycardia and flutter, abnormal rhythms in which the heart executes runs of rapid beats. Another is atrial fibrillation, in which the beats are rapid but irregular, seeming to occur at random.

These palpitations may be caused by organic heart disease, but they also can result from other factors. Similarly, emotional pressures rather than organic changes may cause the so-called "nervous heart," or functional heart disease.

palsy (pawl′ze) paralysis.

Bell's p., facial paralysis due to lesion of the facial nerve, resulting in characteristic facial distortion (see also BELL'S PALSY).

birth p., birth paralysis.

cerebral p., a persisting qualitative motor disorder appearing before age 3, due to nonprogressive damage of the brain (see also CEREBRAL PALSY).

Erb's p., Erb-Duchenne paralysis.

facial p., Bell's palsy.

Saturday night p., paralysis of the extensor muscles of the wrist and fingers, so called because of its frequent occurrence in alcoholics. It is most often due to prolonged compression of the radial (musculospiral) nerve, and, depending upon the site of nerve injury, sometimes accompanied by weakness and extension of the elbow. Called also musculospiral or radial paralysis.

shaking p., paralysis agitans.

paludism (pal'u-dizm) malaria.

Paludrine (pal'u-drin) trademark for a preparation of proguanil, an antimalarial drug.

Pamine (pam'ēn) trademark for preparations of methscopolamine bromide, an anticholinergic.

Pamisyl (pam'ĭ-sil) trademark for preparations of aminosalicylic acid, used in treatment of tuberculosis.

pampiniform (pam-pin'ĭ-form) shaped like a tendril.

pan- word element [Gr.], *all.*

panacea (pan"ah-se'ah) a remedy for all diseases.

panagglutinin (pan"ah-gloo'tĭ-nin) an agglutinin that agglutinates the erythrocytes of all human blood groups.

panangiitis (pan"an-je-i'tis) inflammation involving all the coats of a vessel.

panarthritis (pan"ar-thri'tis) inflammation of all the joints.

panatrophy (pan-at'ro-fe) atrophy of several parts; diffuse atrophy.

pancarditis (pan"kar-di'tis) diffuse inflammation of the heart.

Pancoast's syndrome (pan'kōsts) 1. roentgenographic shadow at the apex of the lung, neuritic pain in the arm, atrophy of the muscles of the arm and hand, and Horner's syndrome, observed in tumor near the apex of the lung, due to involvement of the brachial plexus. 2. osteolysis in the posterior part of one or more ribs and sometimes involving also the corresponding vertebra.

pancolectomy (pan"ko-lek'to-me) excision of the entire colon, with creation of an outlet from the ileum on the body surface.

pancreas (pan'kre-as) a large, elongated, racemose gland located transversely behind the stomach, between the spleen and duodenum. (See also Plate 9.) It is composed of both endocrine and exocrine tissue. The islands of Langerhans, being endocrine in nature, secrete two hormones: insulin, which plays a major role in carbohydrate metabolism, and glucagon, which has an effect opposite to that of insulin. The exocrine cells of the pancreas secrete pancreatic juice, which contains enzymes essential to the digestive processes. A system of ducts within the organ collects these secretions and empties them into the duodenum.

DISORDERS OF THE PANCREAS. Failure of the islands of Langerhans to produce sufficient amounts of insulin results in DIABETES MELLITUS. Disturbances in the exocrine functions of the pancreas produce serious digestive disorders. The pancreas can also be the seat of cancerous growth, and occasionally the pancreatic ducts are blocked by stones; either condition may require surgery. Various factors, not yet fully understood, may result in acute pancreatitis, a condition in which the fluids digest the tissue of the organ itself. This self-digesting may also be set off if the flow in the ducts is reversed and bile enters the pancreas, activating the enzymes in its secretions. Excessive alcohol intake also may be implicated in pancreatitis. Sudden severe abdominal pain, vomiting, and fever can accompany pancreatitis. Treatment may involve surgery, though bed rest and antibiotics are frequently prescribed. Chronic pancreatitis, a less serious disorder, sometimes occurs after gallbladder diseases.

CYSTIC FIBROSIS, a serious congenital disease, is characterized by a deficiency in the secretion of pancreatic juice, and an increase in its viscosity.

annular p., a developmental anomaly in which the pancreas forms a ring entirely surrounding the duodenum.

pancreatalgia (pan"kre-ah-tal'je-ah) pain in the pancreas.

pancreatectomy (pan"kre-ah-tek'to-me) excision of the pancreas.

pancreatic (pan"kre-at'ik) pertaining to the pancreas.

p. duct, the main excretory duct of the pancreas, which usually unites with the common bile duct before entering the duodenum at the major duodenal papilla (see also BILE DUCTS).

pancreatico- word element [Gr.], *pancreatic duct.*

pancreaticoduodenal (pan"kre-at"ĭ-ko-du"o-de'nal) pertaining to the pancreas and duodenum.

pancreaticoduodenostomy (pan"kre-at"ĭ-ko-du"o-dĕ-nos'to-me) anastomosis of the pancreatic duct to a different site on the duodenum.

pancreaticoenterostomy (pan"kre-at"ĭ-ko-en"ter-os'to-me) anastomosis of the pancreatic duct to the intestine.

pancreaticogastrostomy (pan"kre-at"ĭ-ko-gas-tros'to-me) anastomosis of the pancreatic duct to the stomach.

pancreaticojejunostomy (pan"kre-at"ĭ-ko-jĕ-joo-nos'to-me) anastomosis of the pancreatic duct to the jejunum.

pancreatin (pan'kre-ah-tin) a substance from the pancreas of the hog or ox containing enzymes, principally amylase, protease, and lipase; used as a digestive aid.

pancreatitis (pan"kre-ah-ti'tis) inflammation of the PANCREAS.

acute hemorrhagic p., a condition due to autolysis of pancreatic tissue caused by escape of enzymes into the substance, resulting in hemorrhage into the parenchyma and surrounding tissues.

pancreato- word element [Gr.], *pancreas.*

pancreatoduodenectomy (pan"kre-ah-to-du"o-dĕ-nek'to-me) excision of the head of the pancreas along with the encircling loop of the duodenum.

pancreatogenous (pan"kre-ah-toj'ĕ-nus) arising in the pancreas.

pancreatography (pan"kre-ah-tog'rah-fe) roentgenography of the pancreas, performed during surgery by injecting contrast medium into the pancreatic duct.

pancreatolithectomy (pan-kre″ah-to-lĭ-thek′to-me) excision of a calculus from the pancreas.

pancreatolithiasis (pan-kre″ah-to-lĭ-thi′ah-sis) the presence of calculi in the ductal system or parenchyma of the pancreas.

pancreatolithotomy (pan-kre″ah-to-lĭ-thot′o-me) incision of the pancreas for the removal of calculi.

pancreatolysis (pan″kre-ah-tol′ĭ-sis) destruction of pancreatic tissue. adj., **pancreatolyt′ic.**

pancreatotomy (pan″kre-ah-tot′o-me) incision of the pancreas.

pancreatotropic (pan-kre″ah-to-trop′ik) having a special affinity for the pancreas.

pancreolithotomy (pan″kre-o-lĭ-thot′o-me) pancreatolithotomy.

pancreolysis (pan″kre-ol′ĭ-sis) pancreatolysis.

pancreozymin (pan′kre-o-zi″min) a hormone of the duodenal mucosa that stimulates the external secretory activity of the pancreas, especially its production of amylase; identical with cholecytokinin.

pancuronium (pan″ku-ro′ne-um) a skeletal muscle relaxant used as the bromide salt.

pancytopenia (pan″si-to-pe′ne-ah) abnormal depression of all the cellular elements of the blood.

pandemic (pan-dem′ik) a widespread epidemic disease; widely epidemic.

panencephalitis (pan″en-sef″ah-li′tis) encephalitis, probably of viral origin, which produces intranuclear or intracytoplasmic inclusion bodies that result in parenchymatous lesions of both the gray and white matter of the brain.

panendoscope (pan-en′do-skōp) a cystoscope that gives a wide view of the bladder.

panesthesia (pan″es-the′ze-ah) the sum of the sensations experienced. adj., **panesthet′ic.**

panhypopituitarism (pan-hi″po-pĭ-tu′ĭ-tar-izm″) generalized hypopituitarism due to absence or damage to the pituitary gland, which in its complete form, leads to absence of gonadal function and insufficiency of thyroid and adrenal function. When cachexia is a prominent feature, it is called SIMMONDS' DISEASE or pituitary cachexia.

panhysterectomy (pan″his-tĕr-ek′to-me) total hysterectomy.

panhysterosalpingectomy (pan″his-ter-o-sal″-pin-jek′to-me) excision of the uterus, cervix, and oviducts.

panhysterosalpingo-oophorectomy (pan″his-ter-o-sal-ping″go-o″of-o-rek′to-me) excision of the uterus, cervix, oviducts, and ovaries.

panic (pan′ik) extreme and unreasoning fear and anxiety.

panimmunity (pan″ĭ-mu′nĭ-te) immunity to several bacterial and viral infections.

Panmycin (pan-mi′sin) trademark for preparations of tetracycline, an antibiotic.

panmyeloid (pan-mi′ĕ-loid) pertaining to all elements of the bone marrow.

panmyelophthisis (pan-mi″ĕ-lof′thĭ-sis) aplastic anemia.

panmyelosis (pan-mi″ĕ-lo′sis) proliferation of all the elements of the bone marrow.

panniculitis (pah-nik″u-li′tis) inflammation of the panniculus adiposus, especially of the abdomen.

nodular nonsuppurative p., relapsing febrile nonsuppurative p., a disease marked by fever and the formation of crops of tender nodules in the subcutaneous fatty tissues. Called also Weber-Christian or Christian-Weber disease.

panniculus (pah-nik′u-lus), pl. *pannic′uli* [L.] a layer of membrane.

p. adipo′sus, the subcutaneous fat; a layer of fat underlying the corium.

p. carno′sus, a muscular layer in the superficial fascia of certain lower animals; represented in man mainly by the platysma.

pannus (pan′us) 1. superficial vascularization of the cornea with infiltration of granulation tissue. 2. an inflammatory exudate overlying synovial cells on the inside of a joint capsule, usually occurring in rheumatoid arthritis or related articular rheumatism.

panophobia (pan″o-fo′be-ah) fear of everything; vague and persistent dread of an unknown evil.

panophthalmitis (pan″of-thal-mi′tis) inflammation of all the eye structures or tissues.

panosteitis (pan″os-te-i′tis) inflammation of every part of a bone.

panotitis (pan″o-ti′tis) inflammation of all the parts or structures of the ear.

Panparnit (pan-par′nit) trademark for a preparation of caramiphen, an anticholinergic used in parkinsonism.

panphobia (pan-fo′be-ah) panophobia.

pansinusitis (pan″si-nŭ-si′tis) inflammation involving all the paranasal sinuses.

Panstrongylus (pan-stron′jĭ-lus) a genus of hemipterous insects, species of which are vectors of trypanosomes.

pant(o)- word element [Gr.], *all; the whole.*

pantalgia (pan-tal′je-ah) pain over the whole body.

pantetheine (pan″tĕ-the′in) an amide of pantothenic acid, an intermediate in the biosynthesis of CoA, a growth factor for *Lactobacillus bulgaricus,* and a cofactor in certain enzyme complexes.

pantothenate (pan-to′then-āt) any salt of pantothenic acid.

pantothenic acid (pan″to-then′ik) a vitamin of the B complex present in all living tissues, almost entirely in the form of a coenzyme A (CoA). This coenzyme has many metabolic roles in the cell, and a lack of pantothenic acid can lead to depressed metabolism of both carbohydrates and fats. The daily requirement for this vitamin is not known and no definite deficiency syndrome has been recognized in man, perhaps because of its wide occurrence in almost all foods. However, some symptoms attributed to deficiency of other B-complex vitamins may be due to a lack of pantothenic acid.

pantotropic, pantropic (pan″to-trop′ik; pan-trop′-ik) having affinity for tissues derived from all three of the germ layers (ectoderm, entoderm, and mesoderm).

panzootic (pan″zo-ot′ik) occurring pandemically among animals.

Pa_{O_2} symbol for partial pressure of oxygen in arterial blood (see also BLOOD GAS ANALYSIS).

Pap test (smear) (pap) Papanicolaou test.

papain (pah-pa′in, pah-pi′in) a proteolytic enzyme from the latex of papaw, *Carica papaya.*

Papanicolaou test (smear) (pap″ah-nik″o-la′oo) a

simple, painless test used most commonly to detect cancer of the uterus and cervix; often called Pap test or smear. The test is based on the discovery by Dr. George N. Papanicolaou (1883–1962) that malignant uterine tumors slough off cancerous cells into surrounding vaginal fluid.

The Papanicolaou technique, an exfoliative cytological staining procedure, is used also in diagnosis of lung, stomach, and bladder cancers and in evaluating endocrine function. The test can be performed on any body excretion (urine, feces), secretion (sputum, prostatic fluid, vaginal fluid), or tissue scraping (as from the uterus or the stomach). The sample is removed from the area being examined, placed on a glass slide, stained, and then studied under a microscope for evidence of abnormal, or cancerous, cells.

In 5 minutes, the Pap test can reveal uterine or cervical cancer at a stage in which it produces no visible symptoms, has done no damage and usually can be completely cured. The American Cancer Society recommends that all women over 30 have a routine Papanicolaou test once a year.

Papaver (pah-pav′er) a genus of herbs, the poppies. *P. somnif′erum* and its variety *al′bum* are the source of opium.

papaverine (pah-pav′er-in) an alkaloid obtained from opium and prepared synthetically; the hydrochloride salt is used as a smooth muscle relaxant.

papilla (pah-pil′ah), pl. *papil′lae* [L.] a small, nipple-shaped projection or elevation. adj., **pap′illary.**

circumvallate p., vallate papilla.

conical p., one of the sparsely scattered elevations on the tongue, often considered to be modified filiform papillae.

papillae of corium, conical extensions of the fibers, capillary blood vessels, and sometimes nerves of the corium into corresponding spaces among downward- or inward-projecting rete ridges on the undersurface of the epidermis.

dental p., dentinal p., the small mass of condensed mesenchyme capped by each of the enamel organs.

duodenal p., either of the small elevations (major and minor) on the mucosa of the duodenum, the major at the entrance of the conjoined pancreatic and common bile ducts, the minor at the entrance of the accessory pancreatic duct.

filiform p., one of the threadlike elevations covering most of the tongue surface.

foliate p., one of the parallel mucosal folds on the tongue margin at the junction of its body and root.

fungiform p., one of the knoblike projections of the tongue scattered among the filiform papillae.

gingival p., the triangular pad of the gingiva filling the space between the proximal surfaces of two adjacent teeth.

hair p., the fibrovascular mesodermal papilla enclosed within the hair bulb.

incisive p., an elevation at the anterior end of the raphe of the palate.

lacrimal p., an elevation on the margin of either eyelid, near the medial angle of the eye.

lingual papillae, elevations on the surface of the tongue, containing the taste buds; the conical, filiform, foliate, fungiform, and vallate papillae.

mammary p., the nipple of the breast.

optic p., optic disk.

palatine p., incisive papilla.

p. pi′li, hair papilla.

renal p., the blunted apex of a renal pyramid.

tactile papillae, tactile corpuscles.

urethral p., a slight elevation in the vestibule of the vagina at the external orifice of the uretha.

vallate p., one of the 8 to 12 large papillae arranged in a V near the base of the tongue.

p. of Vater, Vater's p., major duodenal papilla.

papillectomy (pap″ĭ-lek′to-me) excision of a papilla.

papilledema (pap″il-ĕ-de′mah) edema and hyperemia of the optic disk, usually associated with increased intracranial pressure; called also choked disk.

papillitis (pap″ĭ-li′tis) inflammation of a papilla, especially of the optic disk.

papilloadenocystoma (pap″ĭ-lo-ad″ĕ-no-sis-to′-mah) papillary cystadenoma.

papillocarcinoma (pap″ĭ-lo-kar″sĭ-no′mah) papillary carcinoma.

papilloma (pap″ĭ-lo′mah) a benign tumor derived from epithelium. Papillomas may arise from skin, mucous membranes, or glandular ducts. adj., **papillo′matous.**

papillomatosis (pap″ĭ-lo″mah-to′sis) development of multiple papillomas.

papilloretinitis (pap″ĭ-lo-ret″ĭ-ni′tis) inflammation of the optic nerve and disk.

papovavirus (pap″o-vah-vi′rus) a group of relatively small, ether-resistant DNA viruses, many of which are oncogenic or potentially oncogenic.

papulation (pap″u-la′shun) the formation of papules.

papule (pap′ūl) a small circumscribed, solid, elevated lesion of the skin. adj., **pap′ular.**

papulopustular (pap″u-lo-pus′tu-lar) marked by papules and pustules.

papulosis (pap″u-lo′sis) the presence of multiple papules.

papulosquamous (pap″u-lo-skwa′mus) both papular and scaly.

papulovesicular (pap″u-lo-vĕ-sik′u-lar) marked by papules and vesicles.

papyraceous (pap″ĭ-ra′shus) like paper.

par (par) [L.] pair.

para (par′ah) [L.] a woman who has produced one or more viable offspring. Used with numerals to designate the number of pregnancies that have resulted in the birth of viable offspring, as para 0 (none —nullipara), para I (one—unipara), para II (two —bipara), para III (three—tripara), para IV (four— quadripara). The number is not indicative of the number of offspring produced in the event of a multiple birth.

para- word element [Gr.], *beside; beyond; accessory to; apart from; against.* In chemistry, a prefix indicating the substitution in a derivative of the benzene ring of two atoms linked to opposite carbon atoms in the ring; abbreviated *p-*.

para-aminobenzoic acid (par″ah-am″ĭ-no-ben-zo′ik) PAB or PABA; a derivative of benzoic acid, classified as a vitamin of the B complex group but not yet proved essential in the diet of human beings. PABA antagonizes the action of sulfonamides and should not be used in combination with them. Derivatives of para-aminobenzoic acid include local anesthetics such as procaine (Novocain).

para-aminohippuric acid (par″ah-am″ĭ-no-hĭ-pu′-

rik) PAH or PAHA; a derivative of para-aminobenzoic acid used to measure the effective renal plasma flow and to determine the functional capacity of the renal tubular excretory mechanism. Called also aminohippuric acid. (See also PAH, PAHA.)

para-aminosalicylic acid (par″ah-am″ĭ-no-sal″ĭ-sil′ik) PAS or PASA; a derivative of benzoic acid used in treatment of tuberculosis. Called also aminosalicylic acid. It enhances the potency of streptomycin and delays development of bacilli resistant to streptomycin. Gastrointestinal irritation accompanied by anorexia, nausea, and vomiting may be reduced by administering the drug together with food at mealtime.

para-anesthesia (par″ah-an″es-the′ze-ah) anesthesia of the lower part of the body.

para-aortic bodies (par″ah-a-or′tik) enclaves of chromaffin cells near the sympathetic ganglia along the abdominal aorta, serving as chemoreceptors responsive to oxygen, carbon dioxide, and hydrogen in concentration, and which help control respiration. Tumors of these structures produce symptoms similar to those of PHEOCHROMOCYTOMA. Called also organs of Zuckerkandl.

parabiosis (par″ah-bi-o′sis) 1. the union of two individuals, as conjoined twins, or of experimental animals by surgical operation. 2. temporary suppression of conductivity and excitability. adj., **parabiot′ic.**

parablepsia (par″ah-blep′se-ah) false or perverted vision.

parabulia (par″ah-bu′le-ah) perversion of will.

paracasein (par″ah-ka′se-in) the chemical product of the action of rennin on casein.

paracenesthesia (par″ah-sen″es-the′ze-ah) any disturbance of the general sense of well-being.

paracentesis (par″ah-sen-te′sis) surgical puncture of a cavity for the aspiration of fluid. adj., **paracentet′ic.**

abdominal p., insertion of a trocar through a small incision and into the abdominal cavity, to remove fluids or inject a therapeutic agent. The procedure is most often done to remove excess fluid in the peritoneal cavity of a patient with CIRRHOSIS of the liver.

Before the procedure the patient is instructed to empty his bladder, to reduce the danger of accidental puncture of the bladder. The skin below the umbilicus and overlying the rectus muscle is cleansed with an antiseptic. A local anesthetic is used to anesthetize the skin and underlying tissues at the site of insertion of the trocar. During the procedure the patient may be placed in a sitting position with his feet resting on a foot stool or on the floor. His back and arms should be well supported. The container for collecting the drainage is placed at the patient's feet. As the fluid is being withdrawn the patient is observed for symptoms of fainting or shock.

The amount and character of the fluid obtained is recorded and a specimen is saved if the physician requests laboratory examination of the fluid. After the trocar is removed a sterile dressing is applied to the site.

thoracic p., surgical puncture and drainage of the thoracic cavity (see also THORACENTESIS).

paracephalus (par″ah-sef′ah-lus) a fetus with a defective head and imperfect sense organs.

parachlorophenol (par″ah-klo″ro-fe′nol) a local anti-infective used in dentistry.

paracholera (par″ah-kol′er-ah) a disease resembling Asiatic cholera but not caused by *Vibrio cholerae.*

parachordal (par″ah-kor′dal) beside the notochord.

parachromatopsia (par″ah-kro″mah-top′se-ah) color blindness.

Paracoccidioides (par″ah-kok-sid″ĭ-oi′dēz) a genus of fungi that proliferate by multiple budding yeast cells in the tissues.

P. brasilien′sis, the etiologic agent of paracoccidioidomycosis. Called also *Blastomyces brasiliensis.*

paracoccidioidomycosis (par″ah-kok-sid″e-oi″do-mi-ko′sis) an often fatal, chronic granulomatous disease caused by *Paracoccidioides brasiliensis.* The disease is endemic in Brazil and occurs in other parts of South America, in Central America, and in the arid southwestern regions of the United States. Infection primarily involves the lungs, but spreads to the skin, mucous membranes, lymph nodes, and internal organs. Amphotericin B is the specific drug used for treatment. Called also South American blastomycosis.

paracolitis (par″ah-ko-li′tis) inflammation of the outer coat of the colon.

Paracort (par′ah-kort) trademark for a preparation of prednisone, a glucocorticoid.

Paracortol (par″ah-kor′tol) trademark for a preparation of prednisolone, a glucocorticoid.

paracusis (par″ah-ku′sis) any perversion of hearing.

paracystic (par″ah-sis′tik) situated near the bladder.

paracystitis (par″ah-sis-ti′tis) inflammation of tissues around the bladder.

paradental (par″ah-den′tal) 1. having some association with dentistry. 2. periodontal.

paradidymis (par″ah-did′ĭ-mis) a small, vestigial structure found occasionally in the adult in the anterior part of the spermatic cord.

Paradione (par″ah-di′ōn) trademark for preparations of paramethadione, an anticonvulsant.

paradipsia (par″ah-dip′se-ah) a perverted appetite for fluids.

paradoxical respiration (par″ah-dok′se-kal) a type of breathing in which all or part of a lung inflates during inspiration and balloons out during expiration; the opposite of normal chest motion. Called also paradoxical motion. The condition seriously inhibits the movement of gases during respiration and can produce severe and even fatal cardiovascular disturbances and respiratory insufficiency if not quickly relieved by emergency treatment.

Paradoxical respiration or paradoxical motion of the lung usually results from traumatic injury to the thorax (FLAIL CHEST) in which several ribs are fractured in two or more places and are no longer attached by bony cartilage to the rest of the rib cage. The condition can also be seen following surgical removal of several ribs and in paralysis of the diaphragm.

paraffin (par′ah-fin) a purified mixture of solid hydrocarbons obtained from petroleum.

liquid p., liquid petrolatum (mineral oil).

paraffinoma (par″ah-fĭ-no′mah) a chronic granuloma produced by prolonged exposure to paraffin.

Paraflex (par′ah-fleks) trademark for a preparation of chlorzoxazone, a skeletal muscle relaxant.

paragammacism (par″ah-gam′ah-sizm) faulty enunciation of *g, k,* and *ch* sounds.

paraganglioma (par″ah-gang″gle-o′mah) a tumor of the tissue composing the paraganglia.

paraganglion (par″ah-gang′gle-on), pl. *paragan′glia* [Gr.] a collection of chromaffin cells derived from neural ectoderm, occurring outside the adrenal medulla, usually near the sympathetic ganglia and in relation to the aorta and its branches. Most secrete epinephrine or norepinephrine.

parageusia (par″ah-gu′ze-ah) perversion of the sense of taste. adj., **parageu′sic.**

paraglobulin (par″ah-glob′u-lin) a globulin from blood serum, blood cells, lymph, and various connective tissues.

paraglossia (par″ah-glos′e-ah) inflammation of the oral tissues under the tongue.

paragonimiasis (par″ah-gon″ĭ-mi′ah-sis) infection with flukes of the genus *Paragonimus.*

Paragonimus (par″ah-gon′ĭ-mus) a genus of trematode parasites, having two invertebrate hosts, the first a snail, the second a crab or crayfish.

P. westerman′i, the lung fluke, occurring especially in Asia; it is found in cysts in the lungs, and sometimes the pleura, abdominal cavity, liver, and elsewhere in man and lower animals who ingest infected freshwater crayfish and crabs.

paragrammatism (par″ah-gram′ah-tizm) a disorder of speech, with confusion in the use and order of words and grammatical forms.

paragranuloma (par″ah-gran″u-lo′mah) the most benign form of Hodgkin's disease, largely confined to the lymph nodes.

paragraphia (par″ah-graf′e-ah) impairment of ability to express thoughts in writing.

parahemophilia (par″ah-he″mo-fil′e-ah) a hereditary hemorrhagic tendency due to deficiency of CLOTTING factor V.

parahormone (par″ah-hōr′mōn) a substance, not a true hormone, that has a hormone-like action in controlling the functioning of some distant organ.

parainfluenza virus (par″ah-in″floo-en′zah) one of a group of viruses isolated from patients with upper respiratory tract disease of varying severity.

parakeratosis (par″ah-ker″ah-to′sis) persistence of the nuclei of keratinocytes as they rise into the horny layer of the skin, marked by scaling.

parakinesia (par″ah-ki-ne′se-ah) perversion of motor powers; in ophthalmology, irregular action of an individual ocular muscle.

paralalia (par″ah-la′le-ah) a disorder of speech, especially the production of a vocal sound different from the one desired, or the substitution in speech of one letter for another.

paralambdacism (par″ah-lam′dah-sizm) faulty enunciation of the *l* sound.

paralbumin (par″al-bu′min) an albumin or protein substance found in ovarian cysts.

paraldehyde (pah-ral′dĕ-hīd) a polymerization product of acetaldehyde, used as a hypnotic, especially in the treatment of alcoholism.

paralexia (par″ah-lek′se-ah) impairment of reading ability, with transposition of words and syllables into meaningless combinations.

paralgesia (par″al-je′ze-ah) an abnormal and painful sensation.

parallagma (par″ah-lag′mah) displacement of a bone or of the fragments of broken bone.

parallax (par′ah-laks) an apparent displacement of an object due to change in the observer's position.

parallergy (par-al′er-je) a condition in which an allergic state, produced by specific sensitization, predisposes the body to react to other allergens with clinical manifestations that differ from the original reaction. adj., **paraller′gic.**

paralogia (par″ah-lo′je-ah) derangement of the reasoning faculty, marked by illogical or delusional speech.

paralysis (pah-ral′ĭ-sis) loss or impairment of motor function in a part due to a lesion of the neural or muscular mechanism; also, by analogy, impairment of sensory function (sensory paralysis). Called also palsy. Paralysis is a symptom of a wide variety of physical and emotional disorders rather than a disease in itself.

TYPES OF PARALYSIS. Paralysis results from damage to parts of the nervous system. The kind of paralysis resulting, and the degree, depend on whether the damage is to the central nervous system or the peripheral nervous system.

If the central nervous system is damaged, paralysis frequently affects the movement of a limb as a whole, not the individual muscles. The more common forms of central paralysis are HEMIPLEGIA, in which the whole of one side of the body, including the face, arm, and leg, is affected, and PARAPLEGIA in which both legs and possibly the trunk are affected. In central paralysis the tone of the muscles is increased (spasticity).

If the peripheral nervous system is damaged, individual muscles or groups of muscles in a particular part of the body, rather than a whole limb, are more likely to be affected. The muscles are flaccid, and there is often impairment of sensation.

CAUSES OF CENTRAL PARALYSIS. A CEREBROVASCULAR ACCIDENT, or stroke, is one of the commonest causes of central paralysis. Although there is usually some permanent disability, much can be done to rehabilitate the patient.

Paralysis produced by damage to the spinal cord can be the result of direct injuries, tumors, and infectious diseases.

Paralysis in children may be a result of failure of the brain to develop properly in intrauterine life or of injuries to the brain, as in the case of CEREBRAL PALSY. Congenital SYPHILIS may also leave a child partially paralyzed.

There is no organic basis for the paralysis resulting from hysteria. This type of paralysis is a result of emotional disturbance or mental illness.

CAUSES OF PERIPHERAL PARALYSIS. Until the recent development of immunizing vaccines, the most frequent cause of peripheral paralysis in children was POLIOMYELITIS. NEURITIS, inflammation of a nerve, can produce paralysis. Causes can be physical, as with cold or injury; chemical, as in lead poisoning; or disease states, such as diabetes mellitus or infection. Paralysis caused by neuritis frequently disappears when the disorder causing it is corrected.

p. of accommodation, paralysis of the ciliary muscles of the eye so as to prevent accommodation.

p. ag'itans, a form of parkinsonism of unknown etiology; it is a slowly progressive disease usually occurring in late life, marked by masklike facies, tremor, slowing of voluntary movements, festinating gait, peculiar posture, and muscle weakness (see also PARKINSON'S DISEASE).

ascending p., spinal paralysis that progresses upward.

birth p., that due to injury received at birth.

brachial p., paralysis of an arm from damage to the brachial plexus.

bulbar p., that due to changes in motor centers of the medulla oblongata; the chronic form is marked by progressive paralysis and atrophy of the lips, tongue, pharynx, and larynx, and is due to degeneration of the nerve nuclei of the floor of the fourth ventricle.

central p., any paralysis due to a lesion of the brain or spinal cord.

cerebral p., paralysis caused by some intracranial lesion (see also CEREBRAL PALSY).

compression p., that caused by pressure on a nerve.

conjugate p., loss of ability to perform some parallel ocular movements.

crossed p., paralysis affecting one side of the face and the other side of the body.

decubitus p., paralysis due to pressure on a nerve from lying for a long time in one position.

diver's p., decompression sickness (BENDS).

Duchenne's p., 1. Erb-Duchenne paralysis. 2. progressive bulbar paralysis.

Erb-Duchenne p., paralysis of the upper roots of the brachial plexus due to destruction of the fifth and sixth cervical roots, without involvement of the small muscles of the hand. Called also Erb's palsy.

facial p., weakening or paralysis of the facial nerve, as in BELL'S PALSY.

familial periodic p., a hereditary disease with recurring attacks of rapidly progressive flaccid paralysis, associated with a fall in (hypokalemic type), a rise in (hyperkalemic type), or normal (normokalemic type) serum potassium levels.

flaccid p., paralysis with loss of muscle tone of the paralyzed part and absence of tendon reflexes.

immunological p., the absence of immune response to a specific antigen.

infantile p., the major form of poliomyelitis.

infantile cerebral ataxic p., a congenital condition due to defective development of the frontal regions of the brain, affecting all extremities.

ischemic p., local paralysis due to stoppage of circulation.

Klumpke's p., Klumpke-Dejerine p., atrophic paralysis of the lower arm and hand, due to lesion of the eighth cervical and first dorsal nerves.

Landry's p., Guillain-Barré syndrome.

lead p., wristdrop due to lead poisoning.

mixed p., combined motor and sensory paralysis.

motor p., paralysis of the voluntary muscles.

musculospiral p., Saturday night palsy.

obstetric p., birth paralysis.

progressive bulbar p., the chronic form of bulbar paralysis; called also Duchenne's disease or paralysis.

pseudobulbar muscular p., pseudohypertrophic muscular dystrophy.

pseudohypertrophic muscular p., pseudohypertrophic muscular dystrophy.

radial p., Saturday night palsy.

sensory p., loss of sensation resulting from a morbid process.

spastic p., paralysis with rigidity of the muscles and heightened deep muscle reflexes.

spastic spinal p., lateral sclerosis.

tick p., progressive ascending flaccid motor paralysis following the bite of certain ticks, usually *Dermacentor andersoni,* in children and domestic animals in Oregon, British Columbia, and other parts of the world.

Volkmann's p., ischemic paralysis.

paralytic (par″ah-lit′ik) 1. pertaining to paralysis. 2. a person affected with paralysis.

p. ileus, adynamic ileus.

paralyzant (par′ah-līz″ant) 1. causing paralysis. 2. a drug that causes paralysis.

paramania (par″ah-ma′ne-ah) parathymia in which the patient manifests joy by complaining.

paramastigote (par′ah-mas′tĭ-gōt) having an accessory flagellum by the side of a larger one.

paramastitis (par″ah-mas-ti′tis) inflammation of tissues around the mammary gland.

Paramecium (par″ah-me′she-um) a genus of ciliate protozoa.

paramecium (par″ah-me′she-um), pl. *parame′cia.* any organism of the genus *Paramecium.*

paramedical (par″ah-med′ĭ-kal) having some connection with or relation to the science or practice of medicine; adjunctive to the practice of medicine in the maintenance or restoration of health and normal functioning. The paramedical services include physical, occupational, and speech therapy, etc., and the activity of social workers.

paramenia (par″ah-me′ne-ah) disordered or difficult menstruation.

parameter (pah-ram′ĕ-ter) 1. an arbitrary constant whose values characterize the mathematical expressions into which it enters. 2. a variable whose measure is indicative of a quantity or function that cannot itself be precisely determined by direct methods.

paramethadione (par″ah-meth″ah-di′ōn) an anticonvulsant used in petit mal epilepsy.

paramethasone (par″ah-meth′ah-sōn) a glucocorticoid used as the 21-acetate ester for its anti-inflammatory and antiallergic effects.

parametric (par″ah-met′rik) near the uterus.

parametritis (par″ah-me-tri′tis) inflammation of the parametrium.

parametrium (par″ah-me′tre-um) loose connective tissue between the two layers of the broad ligament of the uterus, adj., **parame′trial.**

paramimia (par″ah-mim′e-ah) the use of improper or inappropriate gestures when speaking.

paramnesia (par″am-ne′ze-ah) 1. perversion of memory in which the person believes he remembers events or circumstances that never happened; called also retrospective falsification. 2. a state in which words are remembered, but are used without a comprehension of their meaning.

paramucin (par″ah-mu′sin) a colloid substance from ovarian cysts, differing from mucin and pseudomucin in that it reduces Fehling's solution before boiling with acid.

paramutation (par″ah-mu-ta′shun) a permanent transmissible change in an allele after passage through a heterozygote.

paramyloidosis (par-am″ĭ-loi-do′sis) accumulation of an atypical form of amyloid in tissues.

paramyoclonus (par″ah-mi-ok′lo-nus) a condition characterized by myoclonic contractions of various muscles.

p. mul′tiplex, a condition characterized by sudden shocklike contractions.

paramyotonia (par″ah-mi″o-to′ne-ah) a disease marked by tonic spasms due to disorder of muscular tonicity, especially a hereditary and congenital affectation.

p. congen′ita, myotonia congenita.

paramyxovirus (par″ah-mik″so-vi′rus) any of a subgroup of myxoviruses, including the viruses of human and animal parainfluenza, mumps, and Newcastle disease.

paranasal sinuses (par″ah-na′zal) mucosa-lined air cavities in bones of the skull, communicating with the nasal cavity (see also SINUS and Plate 16).

paranephric (par″ah-nef′rik) 1. near the kidney. 2. pertaining to the adrenal gland.

paranephritis (par″ah-nĕ-fri′tis) 1. inflammation of the adrenal gland. 2. inflammation of the connective tissue around the kidney.

paranephros (par″ah-nef′ros), pl. *paraneph′roi* [Gr.] an adrenal gland.

paranesthesia (par″an-es-the′ze-ah) para-anesthesia.

paraneural (par″ah-nu′ral) alongside a nerve.

para-nitrosulfathiazole (par″ah-ni″tro-sul″fah-thi′ah-zōl) a sulfonamide used by rectal instillation as an adjunct in the treatment of ulcerative colitis and proctitis.

paranoia (par″ah-noi′ah) a mental disorder characterized by well systematized delusions of persecution, illusions of grandeur, or a combination of both. adj., **parano′ic.** It is a chronic disease that develops over months and years and for which there is usually no cure.

In the acute stage of the disease, the paranoiac regards himself as being very important and distinguished, or he believes he is being plotted against by others, and in his imagination he builds up an elaborate system of "evidence" to support this belief. This imaginary system is kept separate from the paranoiac's everyday attitudes and activities; hence his outward behavior may appear normal. The extent of his illness remains mostly hidden, though it may erupt occasionally into crimes of violence.

Symptoms of paranoia sometimes appear in lesser degrees in SCHIZOPHRENIA. In slight to moderate form, paranoid personality traits are found in many neurotic persons who are excessively suspicious of other people's motives and are quick to take offense at imagined wrongs. (See also PSYCHOSIS.)

paranoiac (par″ah-noi′ak) a person affected with paranoia.

paranoid (par′ah-noid) 1. resembling paranoia. 2. paranoiac.

paranomia (par″ah-no′me-ah) aphasia marked by inability to name objects felt (myotactic paranomia) or seen (visual paranomia).

paranosis (par″ah-no′sis) the primary advantage that is to be gained by illness.

paranucleus (par″ah-nu′kle-us) a body sometimes seen in cell protoplasm near the nucleus. adj., **paranu′clear.**

paraparesis (par″ah-pah-re′sis) a partial paralysis of the lower extremities.

paraphasia (par″ah-fa′ze-ah) partial aphasia in which the patient employs wrong words, or uses words in wrong and senseless combinations (*choreic paraphasia*).

paraphemia (par″ah-fe′me-ah) aphasia marked by the employment of the wrong words.

paraphia (par-a′fe-ah) perversion of the sense of touch; parapsis.

paraphilia (par″ah-fil′e-ah) expression of the sexual instinct in practices that are socially prohibited or unacceptable, or biologically undesirable (see also SEXUAL DEVIATION).

paraphimosis (par″ah-fi-mo′sis) retraction of a phimotic foreskin, causing swelling of the glans.

paraphrasia (par″ah-fra′ze-ah) disorderly arrangement of spoken words.

paraplasm (par′ah-plazm) 1. any abnormal growth. 2. hyaloplasm (1).

paraplastic (par″ah-plas′tik) exhibiting a perverted formative power; of the nature of a paraplasm (1).

paraplectic (par″ah-plek′tik) paraplegic.

paraplegia (par″ah-ple′je-ah) paralysis of the legs and, in some cases, the lower part of the body. adj., **paraple′gic.** Paraplegia is a form of central nervous system paralysis, in which the paralysis affects all the muscles of the parts involved.

In the majority of cases, paraplegia results from disease or injury of the spinal cord that causes interference with nerve paths connecting the brain and the muscles. Conditions that may result in such interference include physical injuries, hemorrhage, tuberculosis, tumor, and syphilis.

In paraplegia, the loss of ability to use the legs may be accompanied by a loss of sensation in them and, in some cases, by loss of control over the bowels and bladder. Fortunately, much has been learned about the techniques of restoring paraplegics to normal activity, and today many are able to resume useful and productive lives.

PATIENT CARE. Because rehabilitation is the ultimate goal for a paraplegic patient, the patient care during the early stages of the disorder must be particularly concerned with preventing complications that may stand in the way of successful rehabilitation. These complications include DECUBITUS ULCERS, respiratory disorders, orthopedic deformities, urinary infections or calculi, and gastrointestinal disorders.

The psychologic and emotional aspects of paraplegia also must be considered. Many times the paraplegic patient is suddenly thrust into the role of dependence because of accidental injury to the spinal cord. This means that he must make a tremendous adjustment to his condition in a short time. His mental attitude and emotional response to paralysis will greatly affect the success of attempts at rehabilitation.

During the early stages of his illness the patient may not be able to assist in his daily personal care, but as his condition improves and the physician allows more physical activity he must be encouraged to do as much as possible for himself. As he learns to become less dependent on others, his attitude toward his future will improve.

If it is anticipated that the patient will be confined

to a wheelchair or will use crutches, he is taught transfer techniques so that he can move himself from bed to chair and from chair to other surfaces. Wheelchairs and crutches are prescribed according to the individual patient's body build and weight, and the purpose for which they are to be used. The patient is instructed in correct CRUTCH walking if he will be using them; if he is to be using a wheelchair, he is taught how to operate the chair to receive maximum benefit from it. Mastering these techniques can enhance his mobility, increase his independence, and give him a certain degree of confidence that can greatly improve his outlook.

Care of the Skin. The type of bed used and the positioning of the patient with paraplegia will depend on the cause and extent of the paralysis and the preference of the physician. Patients with spinal cord injuries may be placed in traction or the spinal cord may be hyperextended by placing the patient's head at the foot of the bed and adjusting the bed. In some cases the physician may request a special orthopedic frame such as the STRYKER FRAME or CircOlectric bed. These devices facilitate daily care but the patient still must be turned frequently (as allowed by the physician) and receive special skin care to avoid the development of decubitus ulcers (pressure sores).

Since the patient has no feeling below the point of damage to the spinal cord, he will not be aware of discomfort or other signs of pressure. Injections should not be given in the area of paralysis because of limited absorption of the drug and decreased circulation to the part.

Respiratory Disorders. Hypostatic pneumonia and other respiratory problems are guarded against by deep breathing exercises. Coughing and frequent changing of position may be contraindicated and the physician must be consulted before these measures are taken. The patient should be protected from respiratory infections, such as the COMMON COLD, which can have serious complications in a paraplegic who is confined to bed.

Orthopedic Deformities. Until the patient is allowed out of bed and can engage in some form of physical activity his joints should be put through their full RANGE OF MOTION at least once a day. Proper positioning of the feet and legs will help prevent contractures, footdrop, and ankylosis.

A therapeutic EXERCISE program, including passive and active exercises, is initiated to maintain any remaining muscle function and to restore as much muscle activity in the affected parts as possible. If the patient is to use crutches or wheelchair he must strengthen his arm and shoulder muscles in preparation for transfer techniques. HYDROTHERAPY and DIATHERMY may be utilized to promote relaxation of muscle spasms and tension and to facilitate implementation of the exercise program.

Urinary Problems. Urinary infections and the formation of calculi, particularly in the bladder, present very real problems for the patient with paralysis in the lumbosacral area. If he has no control over urination, an indwelling catheter may seem to be the technique of choice for keeping him dry, but it also predisposes him to infection. A thorough assessment of the patient's status and his potential for achieving bladder control should be made before a final choice is made.

Ideally, the patient learns to achieve bladder control through an intensive BLADDER TRAINING program designed to fit his individual needs. Whether this can be accomplished depends on the extent of nerve damage suffered and the degree of success in avoiding such complications as infection and calculi. The achievement of bladder control is more difficult than bowel control, but every effort must be made to help the patient accomplish as much as possible and to avoid whenever feasible the use of artificial collecting and drainage devices.

Patients with neurogenic or cord bladder are unaware of the need to void and therefore require training to initiate voiding. In some patients the bladder empties by reflex, and training involves techniques to make reflex emptying more effective. If the lesion causing paralysis is at the 2nd, 3rd, or 4th sacral segment, the bladder is flaccid and training must be aimed at avoiding overdistention and dribbling. Some patients may never be able to achieve bladder control to any appreciable degree, requiring the use of catheters, penile clamps, or other collecting devices. URETEROSTOMY and ureteroileostomy may be required in some cases.

The formation of bladder stones results from incomplete emptying of the bladder, with pooling of urine and inadequate elimination of wastes. To minimize the formation of stones it is recommended that the patient receive between 2500 and 3000 ml. of fluid every 24 hours. Since an alkaline urine supports the growth of bacteria and the formation of stones, an excess of citrus fruit juices should be avoided. Cranberry juice provides an acid urine and may be used to counteract the effect of citrus juices. The high calcium content of milk also may foster stone formation and carbonated drinks irritate the bladder. A wide variety of liquids can be most effective in avoiding the formation of stones.

Gastrointestinal Complications. A flaccid bowel produces abdominal distention and predisposes the patient to fecal impaction. If the bowel paralysis is temporary, the distention may be relieved by a rectal tube and injections of neostigmine or other drugs to stimulate peristalsis. If the lumbar region is permanently paralyzed, the patient will have fecal incontinence as well as frequent accumulations of flatus and fecal material in the lower intestine. Rehabilitation of the patient then requires working out some method of bowel control so that regularity of defecation can be accomplished.

As in bladder training, the program for BOWEL TRAINING is designed according to the individual needs of the patient and his ability to work with those who are trying to help him. It is essential that an assessment be made of the patient's status in regard to nerve damage and potential for rehabilitation. In addition, it is important to know about the patient's previous bowel habits in regard to frequency and time of day for a movement.

The training program also should include attention to fluid and food intake. The patient learns to avoid foods that produce diarrhea and flatus, and to rely upon a daily intake of fluids sufficient to insure soft, formed stools. Adequate physical exercise also is helpful in establishing regularity of defecation. Rectal suppositories and digital stimulation at regular intervals may be necessary to stimulate evacuation at a time convenient for the patient.

paraplegiform (par″ah-plej′ĭ-form) resembling paraplegia.

parapoplexy (par-ap′o-plek″se) a condition resembling apoplexy.

parapraxia (par″ah-prak′se-ah) 1. irrational behavior. 2. inability to perform purposive movements properly.

paraprotein (par″ah-pro′te-in) immunoglobulin produced by a clone of neoplastic plasma cells proliferating abnormally, e.g., myeloma proteins and cryoglobulins.

paraproteinemia (par″ah-pro″te-ĭ-ne′me-ah) the presence in the blood of paraproteins.

parapsis (par-ap′sis) perversion of the sense of touch; paraphia.

parapsoriasis (par″ah-so-ri′ah-sis) a group of slowly developing, persistent, maculopapular scaly erythrodermas, devoid of subjective symptoms and resistant to treatment.

parapsychology (par″ah-si-kol′o-je) the branch of psychology dealing with psychical effects and experiences that appear to fall outside the scope of physical law, e.g., telepathy and clairvoyance.

parareflexia (par″ah-re-flek′se-ah) any disorder of the reflexes.

pararhotacism (par″ah-ro′tah-sizm) faulty enunciation of *r* sound.

pararosaniline (par″ah-ro-zan′ĭ-lin) a basic dye; a triphenylmethane derivative, one of the components of basic fuchsin.

pararrhythmia (par″ah-rith′me-ah) parasystole.

pararthria (par-ar′thre-ah) imperfect utterance of words.

parasacral (par″ah-sa′kral) situated near the sacrum.

Parasal (par′ah-sal) trademark for preparations of para-aminosalicylic acid, used in treatment of tuberculosis.

parasigmatism (par″ah-sig′mah-tizm) faulty enunciation of *s* and *z* sounds.

parasinoidal (par″ah-si-noi′dal) situated along the course of a sinus.

parasite (par′ah-sīt) 1. a plant or animal that lives upon or within another living organism at whose expense it obtains some advantage (see also SYMBIOSIS). adj., **parasit′ic.** Among the many parasites in nature, a few feed upon human hosts, causing diseases ranging from the mildly annoying to the severe and even fatal. Parasites include multicelled and single-celled animals, fungi, and bacteria. Viruses are sometimes considered to be parasites.

accidental p., one that parasitizes an organism other than the usual host.

facultative p., one that may be parasitic upon another organism but can exist independently.

incidental p., accidental parasite.

malarial p., *Plasmodium.*

obligate p., obligatory p., one that is entirely dependent upon a host for its survival.

periodic p., one that parasitizes a host for short periods.

temporary p., one that lives free of its host during part of its life cycle.

parasitemia (par″ah-si-te′me-ah) the presence of parasites, especially malarial forms, in the blood.

parasiticide (par″ah-sit′ĭ-sīd) destructive to parasites; also, an agent that is destructive to parasites.

parasitism (par′ah-si″tizm) 1. symbiosis in which one population (or individual) adversely affects another, but cannot live without it. 2. infection or infestation with parasites.

parasitize (par′ah-sĭ-tīz″) to live on or within a host as a parasite.

parasitogenic (par″ah-si″to-jen′ik) due to parasites.

parasitologist (par″ah-si-tol′o-jist) a person skilled in parasitology.

parasitology (par″ah-si-tol′o-je) the scientific study of parasites and parasitism.

parasitotropic (par″ah-si″to-trop′ik) having affinity for parasites.

paraspadias (par″ah-spa′de-as) a congenital condition in which the urethra opens on one side of the penis.

parasternal (par″ah-ster′nal) beside the sternum.

parasympathetic nervous system (par″ah-sim″pah-thet′ik) part of the autonomic NERVOUS SYSTEM, the preganglionic fibers of which leave the central nervous system with cranial nerves III, VII, IX, and X and the first three sacral nerves; postganglionic fibers are distributed to the heart, smooth muscles, and glands of the head and neck, and thoracic, abdominal, and pelvic viscera. (See also Plate 14.)

parasympatholytic (par″ah-sim″pah-tho-lit′ik) anticholinergic: producing effects resembling those of interruption of the parasympathetic nerve supply of a part; having a destructive effect on the parasympathetic nerve fibers or blocking the transmission of impulses by them. Also, an agent that produces such effects.

parasympathomimetic (par″ah-sim″pah-tho-mi-met′ik) cholinergic: producing effects resembling those of stimulation of the parasympathetic nerve supply of a part. Also, an agent that produces such effects.

parasynapsis (par″ah-sĭ-nap′sis) the union of chromosomes side by side during meiosis.

parasynovitis (par″ah-sin″o-vi′tis) inflammation of the tissues about a synovial sac.

parasystole (par″ah-sis′to-le) a cardiac irregularity attributed to the interaction of two foci independently initiating cardiac impulses at different rates. Called also pararrhythmia.

paratenon (par″ah-ten′on) the fatty areolar tissue filling the interstices of the fascial compartment in which a tendon is situated.

parathion (par″ah-thi′on) an agricultural insecticide highly toxic to humans and animals.

parathormone (par″ah-thōr′mōn) parathyroid hormone.

parathymia (par″ah-thi′me-ah) perverted, contrary, or inappropriate emotions.

parathyroid (par″ah-thi′roid) 1. situated beside the thyroid gland. 2. one of the thyroid glands.

p. glands, small bodies in the region of the thyroid gland, occurring in a variable number of pairs, commonly two. They are part of the endocrine system. Their secretion, parathyroid hormone, controls the metabolism of CALCIUM and PHOSPHORUS in the body.

The parathyroid glands are subject to two major disorders: HYPERPARATHYROIDISM and HYPOPARATHYROIDISM.

parathyroidectomy (par″ah-thi″roi-dek′to-me) excision of a parathyroid gland.

parathyrotropic (par″ah-thi″ro-trop′ik) having an affinity for the parathyroid glands.

paratope (par′ah-tōp) the site on the antibody molecule that attaches to an antigen.

Some Animal Parasites Harmful to Man

Parasite *(Approximate Length)* Areas of Occurrence	Condition Caused	Usual Source of Infection	Prevention
INTERNAL PARASITES			
AMEBA *(1/25,000 in.–microscopic)* Tropics; occasionally U.S.	Amebic dysentery	Contaminated food and drink	Avoiding unsanitary food and drink
MALARIA PARASITE *(1/3,000 in.–microscopic)* Tropics; southern U.S.	Malaria	Mosquito bites	Mosquito control; protection against bites
BLOOD FLUKE *(1/4–1/2 in.)* Tropics; rare in U.S.	Schistosomiasis (disease of liver, intestine, bladder)	Water (organism can penetrate skin)	Avoiding contaminated water
TAPEWORM *(6–60 ft.)* Most countries; beef tapeworm common in U.S.	Tapeworm (in intestine)	Raw or poorly cooked beef, pork or fish	Cooking meat and fish
HOOKWORM *(1/4–1/2 in.)* Warm regions; common in southern U.S.	Hookworm disease (ancylostomiasis)	Contaminated soil	Wearing shoes; avoiding direct contact with infected soil
ASCARIS ROUNDWORM *(6–12 in.)* Parts of southern U.S.; wherever sanitation is poor	Intestinal disorder (ascariasis)	Raw vegetables and fruits	Cooking fruits and vegetables
PINWORM *(1/12–1/2 in.)* Throughout world	Pinworm infection (enterobiasis)	Contaminated food; contact with infected person	Personal cleanliness
TRICHINA WORM *(1/16–1/6 in.)* Throughout world; common in U.S.	Trichinosis	Poorly cooked pork	Thorough cooking of pork products
FILARIA WORM *(1 1/2–4 in.)* Tropics	Filariasis	Mosquito bites	Avoiding mosquito bites
SKIN PARASITES			
ITCH MITE *(1/100 in.)* Most countries, including U.S.	Scabies	Contact with infected person	Cleanliness of body and clothing; avoiding contact with infected person
LICE *(1/25–1/8 in.)* Most countries, including U.S.	Itching of skin (pediculosis); also may carry disease germ	Contact with human carrier, clothing, bedding	Cleanliness of body and clothing; avoiding contact with infected person
TICKS *(1/10–1/2 in.)* Most countries, including U.S.	Skin infestation; also may carry rabbit fever, other diseases	Tick-infested areas	Avoiding tick-infested areas or wearing heavy tight-fitting clothing
FLEAS *(1/12–1/8 in.)* Most countries, including U.S.	Skin irritation; also may carry disease germs	Animal and human carriers	Cleanliness; avoiding close contact with carriers

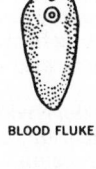

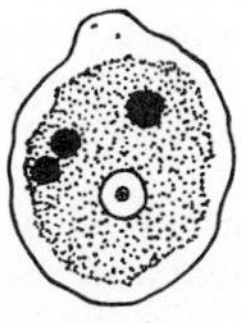
AMEBA

BLOOD FLUKE

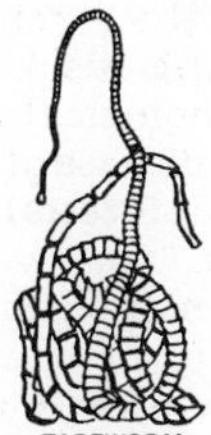
TAPEWORM

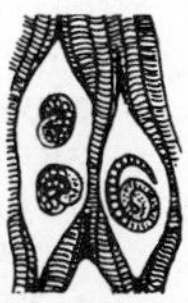
TRICHINA WORMS

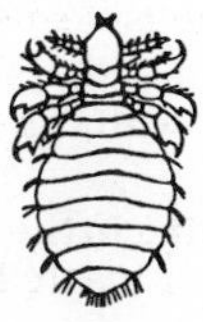
LOUSE

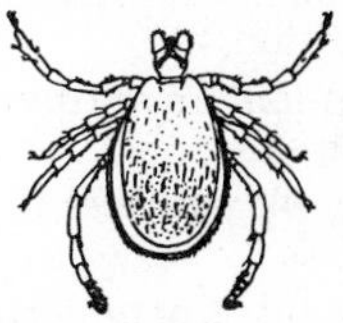
TICK

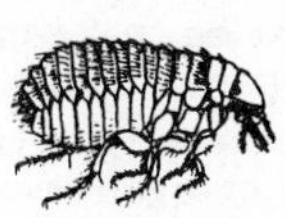
FLEA

paratrophy (par-at′ro-fe) dystrophy.

paratuberculosis (par″ah-too-ber″ku-lo′sis) a tuberculosis-like disease not due to *Mycobacterium tuberculosis.*

paratyphoid (par″ah-ti′foid) infection caused by *Salmonella* of all groups except *S. typhosa.* The disease is usually milder and has a shorter incubation period, more abrupt onset, and a lower mortality rate than does typhoid. Clinically and pathologically, the two diseases cannot be distinguished. (See also TYPHOID FEVER.)

paraurethral (par″ah-u-re′thral) near the urethra.

paravaginitis (par″ah-vaj″ĭ-ni′tis) inflammation of the tissues alongside the vagina.

paravertebral (par″ah-ver′tĕ-bral) near the vertebrae.

paravitaminosis (par″ah-vi″tah-mĭ-no′sis) vitamin deficiency without the usual symptoms.

Paré (par-a′) Ambroise (1510–1590). French surgeon. As an army surgeon treating gunshot wounds, Paré discontinued the application of boiling oils as was customary at that time. He invented many new surgical instruments and reintroduced the use of ligatures to tie off the blood vessels for amputation. He described carbon monoxide poisoning and has been cited as probably the first to think of flies as transmitters of infectious disease. In obstetrics he did podalic versions and induced labor for uterine hemorrhage. He introduced reimplantation of the teeth in dentistry, and wrote a small book on medical jurisprudence.

Paredrine (par′ah-drēn) trademark for preparations of hydroxyamphetamine, a sympathomimetic nasal decongestant, pressor, and mydriatic.

paregoric (par″ĕ-gor′ik) a mixture of powdered opium, anise oil, benzoic acid, camphor, and glycerin, in diluted alcohol, used as an antiperistaltic, especially in the treatment of diarrhea.

parenchyma (pah-reng′kĭ-mah) the essential or functional elements of an organ, as distinguished from its stroma or framework. adj., **paren′chymal, parenchym′atous.**

parenchymatitis (par″eng-kim″ah-ti′tis) inflammation of a parenchyma.

Parenogen (par-en′o-gen) trademark for a preparation of fibrinogen, CLOTTING factor I, essential for blood clotting.

parenteral (pah-ren′ter-al) not through the alimentary canal, e.g., by subcutaneous, intramuscular, intrasternal, or intravenous injection.

parepididymis (par″ep-ĭ-did′ĭ-mis) paradidymis.

paresis (pah-re′sis, par′ĕ-sis) 1. slight or incomplete paralysis. 2. dementia paralytica. adj., **paret′ic.**

general p., a chronic syphilitic meningoencephalitis (see also DEMENTIA PARALYTICA).

paresthesia (par″es-the′ze-ah) morbid or perverted sensation; an abnormal sensation, as burning, prickling, formication, etc.

pargyline (par′gĭ-lēn) an antihypertensive, used as the hydrochloride salt.

paries (pa′re-ez), pl. *pari′etes* [L.] a wall, as of an organ or cavity.

parietal (pah-ri′ĕ-tal) 1. of or pertaining to the walls of an organ or cavity. 2. pertaining to or located near the parietal bone.

p. bone, one of two quadrilateral bones forming the sides and roof of the cranium (see also table of BONES).

p. lobe, the upper central portion of the cerebral hemisphere, between the frontal and occipital lobes, and above the temporal lobe. It is the receptive area for fine sensory stimuli, and the highest integration and coordination of sensory information is carried on in this area. Damage to the parietal lobe can produce defects in vision and aphasia.

parietofrontal (pah-ri″ĕ-to-fron′tal) pertaining to the parietal and frontal bones, gyri, or fissures.

parietography (pah-ri″ĕ-tog′rah-fe) roentgenographic visualization of the walls of an organ.

Parinaud's oculoglandular syndrome (pah-rĭ-nōz′) a general term applied to conjunctivitis, usually unilateral and of the follicular type, followed by tenderness and enlargement of the preauricular lymph nodes; often due to leptotrichosis but may be associated with other infections. Called also leptothricosis conjunctivae.

Parinaud's ophthalmoplegia (pah-rĭ-nōz′) paralysis of conjugate upward movement of the eyes without paralysis of convergence, associated with midbrain lesions.

parity (par′ĭ-te) 1. para; the condition of a woman with respect to her having borne viable offspring. 2. equality; close correspondence or similarity.

Parkinson's disease (par′kin-sunz) a slowly progressive disease usually occurring in later life, characterized pathologically by degeneration within the nuclear masses of the extrapyramidal system, and clinically by masklike facies (PARKINSON'S FACIES), a characteristic tremor of resting muscles, a slowing of voluntary movements, a festinating gait, peculiar posture, and muscular weakness. When this symptom complex occurs secondarily to another disorder, the condition is called PARKINSONISM.

SYMPTOMS. Parkinson's disease usually appears gradually and progresses slowly. At first the victim may be troubled by mild tremors of the hands and nodding of the head. He may notice that his movements are somewhat slower and more difficult than usual. Then loss of mobility in the face produces the characteristic masklike facies. As the disease advances, the tremors increase and may involve the whole body, although generally they are not apparent with intentional movements. The muscles become stiffer, making movement increasingly difficult. The gait becomes shuffling and festinating. The back tends to become bent forward in a stooped position. Parkinson's disease does not affect the mental capacity.

TREATMENT. In general, treatment is symptomatic, supportive, and palliative. Most patients require lifelong management consisting of drug therapy, supportive psychotherapy, physical therapy, and rarely, surgical intervention. Newer forms of treatment now give hope for freedom from the progressive disability that once was the expected outcome.

Since the patient's mental outlook and motivation can affect the extent to which he can successfully cope with his disability, it is important that he receive psychological support. He should know the nature of the disease affecting him and be given realistic hopes for forestalling or preventing its more serious effects.

Some benefits can be derived from physical therapy in the form of applications of heat and massage to alleviate muscle cramps and relieve the tension headaches that often accompany rigidity of the cervical muscles. The patient also is instructed in simple EXERCISES that he can perform at home.

The use of levodopa in the treatment of Parkinson's disease is determined by the severity of the disease and the patient's ability to tolerate the drug. It is contraindicated when there is evidence of prior mental illness and in patients suffering from angina pectoris or transient ischemic cerebral attacks. It is given with caution to patients having a history of arrhythmias associated with myocardial disease. Patients receiving levodopa require nutritional counseling because dietary habits can greatly affect the drug's action. Protein intake requires special attention because levodopa, an amino acid, must compete with the dietary amino acids for absorption through the intestinal epithelium and across the blood-brain barrier. Alcohol intake also must be limited because in large amounts it can antagonize the effects of levodopa.

Synthetic anticholinergic drugs also may be given in the treatment of Parkinson's disease. Antidepressants, when used in combination with anticholinergic drugs or levodopa, may be beneficial.

The best candidates for surgical treatment are those who exhibit unilateral involvement. The procedure involves either electrocoagulation or freezing of tissues to interrupt the neural pathways in the ventrolateral nucleus of the thalamus which appear essential for the production of symptoms, and at a site where normal sensory and motor function will not be affected. The advent of newer pharmacological modes of therapy that have produced satisfying results has decreased the number of cases requiring surgery.

Parkinson's facies (par′kin-sunz) a stolid mask-like expression of the face, with infrequent blinking; it is pathognomonic of PARKINSON'S DISEASE.

parkinsonian (par″kin-sun′e-an) pertaining to parkinsonism.

p. syndrome, any disorder manifesting the symptoms of PARKINSON'S DISEASE.

parkinsonism (par′kin-sun-izm″) any disorder manifesting the symptoms of PARKINSON'S DISEASE. Any such symptom complex occurring secondarily to another disorder, such as encephalitis, cerebral arteriosclerosis, poisoning with certain toxins, and neurosyphilis.

Parnate (par′nāt) trademark for a preparation of tranylcypromine, an antidepressant.

paroccipital (par″ok-sip′ĭ-tal) beside the occipital bone.

paromomycin (par′o-mo-mi″sin) a broad-spectrum antibiotic derived from *Streptomyces rimosus* var. *paromomycinus;* the sulfate salt is used as an antiamebic.

paromphalocele (par″om-fal′o-sēl) hernia near the navel.

paronychia (par″o-nik′e-ah) inflammation involving the folds of tissue surrounding the fingernail. The causative organisms may be bacteria or fungi, which usually gain entrance through a hangnail or break in the skin due to improper manicuring. Acute infections are treated with hot compresses and the application of an antibiotic or fungicidal ointment. A pocket of purulent material may require incision with a scalpel to promote drainage and healing. Chronic infections are more difficult to cure and may require the application of a corticosteroid ointment. If the infection is widespread and difficult to treat topically, removal of the nail may be necessary. (See also NAIL.)

paroophoron (par″o-of′o-ron) an inconstantly present, small group of coiled tubules between the layers of the mesosalpinx, being a remnant of the excretory part of the mesonephros.

parophthalmia (par″of-thal′me-ah) inflammation of the connective tissue around the eye.

paropsis (par-op′sis) a disorder of vision.

parorchidium (par″or-kid′e-um) displacement of a testis or testes.

parorexia (par″o-rek′se-ah) nervous perversion of the appetite, with craving for special articles of food or for articles not suitable for food.

parosmia (par-oz′me-ah) perversion of the sense of smell.

parostosis (par″os-to′sis) ossification of tissues outside of the periosteum.

parotid (pah-rot′id) near the ear.

p. glands, the largest of the three main pairs of salivary glands, located on either side of the face, just below and in front of the ears. From each gland a duct, the parotid duct (sometimes called Stensen's duct), runs forward across the cheek and opens on the inside surface of the cheek opposite the second molar of the upper jaw.

The parotid glands are made up of groups of cells clustered around a globular cavity, resembling a bunch of grapes. Small ducts draining each cavity join the ducts of neighboring cavities to form large ducts, which in turn join the parotid duct.

From the system of ducts flows the thin, watery secretion of the parotid glands called saliva, which plays an important role in the process of digestion. As food is chewed the saliva with which it is mixed and moistened makes it possible for the food to be reduced to a substance that can be swallowed.

Controlled by the autonomic nervous system, the secretion of the salivary glands begins whenever the sensory nerves of the mouth, or in some cases nerves located elsewhere in the body, are stimulated.

Salivation may be an involuntary reflex, as when food or even inedible material placed in the mouth starts the flow of the secretion from the glands, or it may be a conditioned reflex, as when the flow is started by the sight, smell, or thought of food.

DISORDERS OF THE PAROTID GLANDS. The most common disease affecting the parotid glands is MUMPS, or epidemic parotitis.

Swelling and tenderness may also result from infections caused by other viruses or bacteria in the glands. Less often, these symptoms indicate a blockage of a duct by either infection or a calculus, in which case the swelling is likely to fluctuate, especially at mealtimes. Though stubborn or recurring cases sometimes require surgery, stones often can be removed by massage. For infections, antibiotics and warm compresses are the usual treatment.

Occasionally additional glandular masses grow in or near a parotid gland. The majority of such growths are mixed tumors, so called because they contain cartilage or other material as well as the usual glandular material. Usually they are benign; occasionally they may be malignant and require surgery.

parotidectomy (pah-rot″ĭ-dek′to-me) excision of a parotid gland.

parotiditis, parotitis (pah-rot″ĭ-di′tis, par″o-ti′tis) inflammation of the parotid gland.

contagious p., epidemic p., MUMPS; an acute, communicable viral disease involving chiefly the parotid gland, but frequently affecting other oral glands or the pancreas or gonads.

parovarian (par″o-va′re-an) 1. beside the ovary. 2. pertaining to the parovarium (epoophoron).

parovarium (par″o-va′re-um) epoophoron; a vestigial structure associated with the ovary.

paroxysm (par′ok-sizm) 1. a sudden recurrence or intensification of symptoms. 2. a spasm or seizure. adj., **paroxys′mal.**

Parrot's node (par-ōz′) bony nodes on the outer table of the skull of infants with congenital syphilis.

Parrot's pseudoparalysis (par-ōz′) pseudoparalysis of one or more extremities in infants, due to syphilitic osteochondritis of an epiphysis.

parrot fever an infection transmitted to man by birds; called also PSITTACOSIS.

Parry's disease (par′ēz) Graves' disease.

pars (pars), pl. *par′tes* [L.] a division or part.

p. mastoi′dea, the mastoid portion of the temporal bone, being the irregular, posterior part.

p. petro′sa, the petrous portion of the temporal bone, containing the inner ear and located at the base of the cranium.

p. pla′na, the thin part of the ciliary body; the ciliary disk.

p. squamo′sa, the flat, scalelike, anterior and superior portion of the temporal bone.

p. tympan′ica, the tympanic portion of the temporal bone, forming the anterior and inferior walls and part of the posterior wall of the external acoustic meatus.

Parsidol (par′sĭ-dol) trademark for a preparation of ethopropazine, used in treatment of Parkinson's disease.

parthenogenesis (par″thĕ-no-jen′ĕ-sis) asexual reproduction in which an egg develops without being fertilized by a spermatozoon, as in certain lower animals, especially arthropods; it may occur as a natural phenomenon or be induced by chemical or mechanical stimulation (artificial parthenogenesis). adj., **parthenogenet′ic.**

particle (par′tĭ-k′l) an extremely small mass of material. (See also ALPHA PARTICLES and BETA PARTICLES.)

Dane p., a particle 42 nm. in diameter, containing hepatitis B (HB) antigen on its surface (HB S) and in its core (HB C).

particulate (par-tik′u-lāt) composed of separate particles.

parturient (par-tu′re-ent) giving birth or pertaining to birth; by extension, a woman in LABOR.

parturiometer (par-tu″rĭ-om′ĕ-ter) a device used in measuring the expulsive power of the uterus.

parturition (par″tu-rish′un) the act or process of giving birth to a child. (See also LABOR.)

parulis (pah-roo′lis) a subperiosteal abscess of the gum.

parumbilical (par″um-bil′ĭ-kal) alongside the navel.

parvicellular (par″vĭ-sel′u-lar) composed of small cells.

parvovirus (par″vo-vi′rus) a group of extremely small, morphologically similar, ether-resistant DNA viruses, including the adeno-associated viruses.

PAS, PASA para-aminosalicylic acid, used in treatment of tuberculosis.

Pasteur (pas-ter′) Louis (1822–1895). French chemist and bacteriologist, founder of microbiology and developer of the method of vaccination by attenuated virus. He was born at Dôle, Jura.

By optical investigation of racemic acid, he discovered a new class of isomeric substances which led to work by others on stereochemistry and for which he received the ribbon of the Legion of Honor. Pasteur came to the rescue of the wine industry by his interest in fermentation, and showed that spoiling of wine caused by microorganisms could be prevented by partial heat sterilization (pasteurization), a process now applied to many perishable foods. Experimental foundation was given to his ideas of fermentation and the long-accepted theory of spontaneous generation was disposed of once and for all. Later he came to the rescue of the silkworm industry and found methods for detecting and preventing pébrine and flâcherie, the two diseases that were destroying it. He turned his attention then to anthrax, chicken cholera, and hydrophobia (rabies), and developed preventive inoculations against them. The Pasteur Institute was opened shortly thereafter and institutions were founded all over the world for inoculation against rabies.

Pasteur effect (pas-ter′) the decrease in the rate of glucose utilization and the suppression of lactate accumulation by tissues or microorganisms in the presence of oxygen.

Pasteur-Chamberland filter (pas-ter′-shahm-ber-lah′) a hollow column of unglazed porcelain through which liquids are forced by pressure or by vacuum exhaustion.

Pasteurella (pas″tĕ-rel′ah) a genus of gram-negative bacteria (family Brucellaceae).

P. multoci′da, the etiologic agent of the hemorrhagic septicemias.

P. pes′tis, the etiologic agent of plague.

P. tularen′sis, *Francisella tularensis.*

pasteurellosis (pas″ter-ĕ-lo′sis) infection with organisms of the genus *Pasteurella.*

pasteurization (pas″tūr-ĭ-za′shun) heating of milk or other liquids to a temperature of 60° C. (140° F.) for 30 minutes, killing pathogenic bacteria and considerably delaying other bacterial development.

patch (pach) a small area differing from the rest of a surface.

Peyer's p's, whitish, oval, elevated patches closely packed lymph follicles in mucous and submucous layers of the small intestine.

p. test, a test for hypersensitivity in which filter paper or gauze saturated with the substance in question is applied to the skin, usually on the forearm. A positive reaction is reddening or swelling at the site. (See also SKIN TEST.)

patella (pah-tel′ah), pl. *patel′lae* [L.] a triangular bone at the knee; the kneecap (see also table of BONES).

patellar (pah-tel′ar) of or pertaining to the patella.

p. ligament, the continuation of the central portion of the tendon of the quadriceps femoris muscle distal to the patella, extending from the patella to the tuberosity of the tibia; called also patellar tendon.

p. reflex, involuntary contraction of the quadriceps muscle and jerky extension of the leg when the patellar ligament is sharply tapped. It is often used as a test of nervous system function. Called also KNEE JERK and quadriceps reflex.

patellectomy (pat″ĕ-lek′to-me) excision of the patella.

patelliform (pah-tel′ĭ-form) shaped like the patella.

patellofemoral (pah-tel″o-fem′o-ral) pertaining to the patella and femur.

patency (pa′ten-se) the condition of being wide open.

patent (pa′tent) 1. open, unobstructed, or not closed. 2. apparent, evident.

p. ductus arteriosus, abnormal persistence of an open lumen in the ductus arteriosus, between the aorta and the pulmonary artery, after birth. The ductus arteriosus is open during prenatal life, allowing most of the blood of the fetus to bypass the lungs, but normally this channel closes shortly before birth. When the ductus arteriosus remains open, it places special burdens on the left ventricle and causes a diminished blood flow in the aorta.

The symptoms of patent ductus arteriosus are usually so slight they are not noticed until the child is older and more active. He then begins to experience dyspnea on exertion. If the ductus is large there may be retardation of growth.

Treatment is surgical, preferably when the child is from 4 to 10 years of age. The open ductus arteriosus is ligated. Prognosis for this condition, when not accompanied by other congenital heart defects, is excellent.

p. medicine (pat′ent), a drug or remedy protected by a trademark, available without a prescription.

path(o)- word element [Gr.], *disease.*

pathergasia (path″er-ga′ze-ah) mental malfunction, implying functional or structural damage, marked by abnormal behavior.

pathergy (path′er-je) 1. a condition in which the application of a stimulus leaves the organism unduly susceptible to subsequent stimuli of a different kind. 2. a condition of being allergic to several antigens. adj., **pather′gic.**

pathfinder (path′find-er) 1. an instrument for locating urethral strictures. 2. a dental instrument for tracing the course of root canals.

pathobiology (path″o-bi-ol′o-je) pathology.

pathoclisis (path″o-klis′is) a specific sensitivity to specific toxins, or a specific affinity of certain toxins for certain systems or organs.

pathogen (path′o-jen) any disease-producing agent or microorganism. adj., **pathogen′ic.**

pathogenesis (path″o-jen′ĕ-sis) the development of morbid conditions or of disease; more specifically the cellular events and reactions and other pathologic mechanisms occurring in the development of disease. adj., **pathogenet′ic.**

pathogenicity (path″o-jĕ-nis′ĭ-te) the quality of producing or the ability to produce pathologic changes or disease.

pathogeny (pah-thoj′ĕ-ne) pathogenesis.

pathognomonic (path″og-no-mon′ik) specifically distinctive or characteristic of a disease or pathologic condition; denoting a sign or symptom on which a diagnosis can be made.

pathologic (path′o-loj′ik) indicative of or caused by some morbid condition.

pathological (path″o-loj′ĭ-k′l) pertaining to pathology; pathologic.

pathologist (pah-thol′o-jist) a specialist in pathology.

pathology (pah-thol′o-je) that branch of medicine treating of the essential nature of disease, especially of the changes in body tissues and organs which cause or are caused by disease.

clinical p., pathology applied to the solution of clinical problems, especially the use of laboratory methods in clinical diagnosis.

comparative p., that which considers human disease processes in comparison with those of the lower animals.

experimental p., the study of artificially induced pathologic processes.

oral p., that which treats of conditions causing or resulting from morbid anatomic or functional changes in the structures of the mouth.

surgical p., the pathology of disease processes that are surgically accessible for diagnosis or treatment.

pathomimesis (path″o-mi-me′sis) malingering.

pathomorphism (path″o-mor′fizm) perverted or abnormal morphology.

pathonomia (path″o-no′me-ah) the science of the laws of disease.

pathophysiology (path″o-fiz″e-ol′o-je) the physiology of disordered function.

pathopsychology (path″o-si-kol′o-je) the psychology of mental disease.

pathosis (pah-tho′sis) a diseased condition.

pathway (path′wa) a course usually followed. In neurology, the nerve structures through which a sensory impression is conducted to the cerebral cortex (afferent pathway), or through which an impulse passes from the brain to the skeletal musculature (efferent pathway). Also used alone to indicate a sequence of reactions that convert one biological material to another (metabolic pathway).

biosynthetic p., the sequence of enzymatic steps in the synthesis of a specific end-product in a living organism.

Embden-Meyerhof p. (of glucose metabolism), the series of enzymatic reactions in the anaerobic conversion of glucose to lactic acid, resulting in energy in the form of adenosine triphosphate (ATP).

pentose phosphate p., a pathway of hexose oxidation in which glucose-6-phosphate undergoes two successive oxidations by NADP, the final forming a pentose phosphate.

-pathy word element [Gr.], *morbid condition* or *disease;* generally used to designate a noninflammatory condition.

patient (pa′shent) a person who is ill or is undergoing treatment for disease.

Patrick's test (pat′riks) the thigh and knee of the supine patient are flexed, the external malleolus rests on the patella on the opposite leg, and the knee is depressed; production of pain indicates arthritis of the hip. Also known as *fabere sign,* from the initial letters of movements necessary to elicit it, i.e., *f*lexion, *ab*duction, *e*xternal *r*otation, and *e*xtension.

patrilineal (pat″rĭ-lin′e-al) descended through the male line.

patulin (pat′u-lin) a toxic antibiotic from various fungi, especially *Aspergillus* and *Penicillium;* used as an antimicrobial.

patulous (pat′u-lus) spread widely apart; open; distended.

Paul-Bunnell test (pawl bun-el′) a method of testing for the presence of heterophil antibodies in the blood for the diagnosis of infectious mononucleosis, based on the agglutination of sheep erythrocytes by the inactivated serum of patients with the disease.

pause (pawz) an interruption, or rest.

compensatory p., the pause after a premature ventricular systole, related to blockage of one beat of the basic pacemaker of the heart.

Paveril (pav′er-il) trademark for preparations of dioxyline, a vasodilator.

pavor (pa′vor) terror.

p. diur′nus, attacks of fear in children during a daytime nap.

p. noctur′nus, a nightmare of children causing them to cry out in fright and awake in panic.

P.B. *Pharmacopoeia Britannica* (British Pharmacopoeia).

Pb chemical symbol, lead (L. *plumbum*).

PBI protein-bound iodine (see PROTEIN-BOUND IODINE TEST).

p.c. [L.] *post ci′bum* (after meals).

PCG phonocardiogram.

Pco_2 carbon dioxide partial pressure or tension; also written P_{CO_2}, pCO_2, or pCO_2 (see RESPIRATION and BLOOD GAS ANALYSIS).

P.C.V. packed-cell volume, the volume of packed red cells in milliliters per 100 ml. of blood.

Pd chemical symbol, *palladium*.

p.d. potential difference; prism diopter.

peanut oil (pe′nut) a refined fixed oil from seed kernels of cultivated varieties of *Arachis hypogaea;* used as a solvent for drugs.

pearl (perl) 1. a small medicated granule, or a glass globule with a single dose of volatile medicine, as amyl nitrite. 2. a rounded mass of tough sputum, as seen in the early stages of an attack of bronchial asthma.

epidermic p's, epithelial p's, rounded concentric masses of epithelial cells found in certain papillomas and epitheliomas.

Laënnec's p's, soft casts of the smaller bronchial tubes expectorated in bronchial asthma.

pecazine (pe′kah-zēn) mepazine, a tranquilizer.

pectase (pek′tās) pectinesterase.

pecten (pek′ten), pl. *pec′tines* [L.] 1. a comb; in anatomy, applied to certain comblike structures. 2. a narrow zone in the anal canal, bounded above by the pectinate line. adj., **pectin′eal.**

p. os′sis pu′bis, pectineal line.

pectenitis (pek″tĕ-ni′tis) inflammation of the pecten of the anus.

pectenosis (pek″tĕ-no′sis) stenosis of the anal canal due to an inelastic ring of tissue between the anal groove and anal crypts.

pectin (pek′tin) a homosaccharidic polymer of sugar acids of fruit that forms gels with sugar at the proper pH; a purified form obtained from the acid extract of the rind of citrus fruits or from apple pomace is used as a protectant and in cooking. adj., **pec′tic.**

pectinase (pek′tĭ-nās) polygalacturonase.

pectinate (pek′tĭ-nāt) comb-shaped.

p. line, the line marking the junction of the zone of the anal canal lined with stratified squamous epithelium and the zone lined with columnar epithelium.

pectineal (pek-tin′e-al) pertaining to the os pubis.

pectinesterase (pek″tin-es′ter-ās) an enzyme that catalyzes the hydrolysis of methyl ester groups of pectic substances, releasing the free acid.

pectiniform (pek-tin′ĭ-form) comb-shaped.

pectoral (pek′tor-al) 1. of or pertaining to the chest or breast. 2. relieving disorders of the respiratory tract, as an expectorant.

p. muscles, four muscles of the chest (see table of MUSCLES).

pectoralis (pek″to-ra′lis) [L.] pertaining to the chest or breast; pectoral.

pectoriloquy (pek″to-ril′o-kwe) transmission of the sound of spoken words through the chest wall, indicating the presence of a cavity or solidification of pulmonary structures.

pectose (pek′tōs) a principle in unripe fruits and plants from which pectin is derived.

pectus (pek′tus) the breast, chest, or thorax.

p. carina′tum, a malformation of the chest wall in which the sternum is abnormally prominent; called also pigeon chest or chicken breast.

Moderate cases cause no difficulties and require no treatment. In severe cases, the deformity of the chest may interfer with lung and heart action, causing dyspnea on exercise and increased susceptibility to respiratory infections. Serious malformations can usually be corrected by surgery.

p. excava′tum, a congenital malformation of the chest wall characterized by a pronounced funnel-shaped depression with its apex over the lower end of the sternum; called also funnel chest.

The condition is caused by a shortening of the central portion of the diaphragm, which pulls the sternum backward during inhalation, and by the growth of ribs. Except in mild cases, it decreases the ability of the child to engage in sustained exercise. It delays recovery from coughs and colds, reduces the ability to eat a full meal, so that most patients are underweight, and often produces a functional heart murmur. Noisy breathing may occur during sleep. A child may also develop an emotional problem because of embarrassment over the deformity.

The deformity can be satisfactorily corrected by surgery.

ped(o)- word element, (1) [Gr.], *child;* (2) [L.], *foot.*

pedal (ped′al) pertaining to the foot or feet.

pederast (ped′er-ast) one who practices pederasty.

pederasty (ped″er-as′te) homosexual anal intercourse between men and boys as the passive partners.

pedia- word element [Gr.], *child.*

pediatrician (pe″de-ah-trish′an) a specialist in pediatrics.

pediatrics (pe″de-at′riks) that branch of medicine dealing with the child and its development and care and with the diseases of children and their treatment. adj., **pediat′ric.**

pedicellation (ped″ĭ-sĕ-la′shun) the development of a pedicle.

pedicle (ped'ĭ-k'l) a footlike, stemlike, or narrow basal part or structure, such as a narrow strip by which a graft of tissue remains attached to the donor site.

vertebral p., one of the paired parts of the vertebral arch that connect a lamina to the vertebral body.

pediculation (pĕ-dik"u-la'shun) 1. the process of forming a pedicle. 2. infestation with lice.

pediculicide (pĕ-dik'u-lĭ-sīd) 1. destroying lice. 2. an agent that destroys lice.

pediculosis (pĕ-dik"u-lo'sis) infestation with lice. (See also LOUSE.)

pediculous (pĕ-dik'u-lus) infested with lice.

Pediculus (pĕ-dik'u-lus) a genus of lice.

P. huma'nus, a species that feeds on human blood and is an important vector of relapsing fever, typhus, and trench fever; two subspecies are recognized: *P. humanus* var. *capitis* (head louse) found on the scalp hair, and *P. humanus* var. *corporis* (body, or clothes, louse) found elsewhere on the body.

pedodontia, pedodontics (pe"do-don'she-ah; pe"do-don'tiks) that branch of dentistry dealing with the teeth and mouth conditions of children.

pedodontist (pe"do-don'tist) a dentist who specializes in pedodontics.

pedodynamometer (pe"do-di"nah-mom'ĕ-ter) an instrument for measuring leg strength.

pedophilia (pe"do-fil'e-ah) abnormal fondness for children; sexual activity of adults with children. adj., **pedophil'ic.**

peduncle (pe-dung'k'l) a stemlike connecting part, especially, (*a*) a collection of nerve fibers coursing between different regions in the central nervous system, or (*b*) the stalk by which a nonsessile tumor is attached to normal tissue. adj., **pedun'cular.**

cerebellar p's, three sets of paired bundles (superior, middle, and inferior) connecting the cerebellum to the midbrain, pons, and medulla oblongata, respectively.

cerebral p., the ventral half of the midbrain, divisible into a dorsal part (*tegmentum*) and a ventral part (*crus cerebri*), which are separated by the substantia nigra.

pineal p., habenula (2).

pedunculated (pe-dung'ku-lāt"ed) having a peduncle.

pedunculotomy (pe-dung"ku-lot'o-me) incision of a cerebral peduncle.

pedunculus (pe-dung'ku-lus) peduncle.

peg (peg) a projecting structure.

rete p's, inward projections of the epidermis into the dermis, as seen histologically in verticle sections.

Peganone (peg'ah-nōn) trademark for a preparation of ethotoin, an anticonvulsant.

Pel-Ebstein disease (pel eb'stīn) Hodgkin's disease.

pelage (pel'ij, pĕ-lahzh') [Fr.] the hairy coat of mammals; the hairs of the body, limbs, and head, collectively.

peliosis (pe"le-o'sis) purpura.

pellagra (pĕ-la'grah, pĕ-lag'rah) a syndrome caused by a diet seriously deficient in niacin (or by failure to convert tryptophan to niacin). Most persons with pellagra also suffer from defiencies of vitamin B_2 (riboflavin) and other essential vitamins and minerals. adj., **pellag'rous.**

Pellagra occurs in many areas of the world. Until recent years, it was the major form of acute vitamin deficiency in the southeastern United States. It is now sharply on the decline in the United States, largely as a result of the efforts of the Public Health Service. The disease also occurs in persons suffering from alcoholism and drug addiction.

SYMPTOMS. Chief symptoms of pellagra are various skin, digestive, and mental disturbances. The mouth becomes inflamed and the tongue red and sore; cracks and sores appear in the skin around the mouth. The skin on the back of the hands may become red, thick, and scaly, as may that of the neck and chest—areas exposed to sunlight and the chafing of clothes.

Vomiting and loss of appetite occur. Diarrhea often appears early and becomes worse as the disease progresses, thus hampering treatment by preventing effective absorption of essential vitamins.

Mental symptoms are variable. In some cases, there may be only insomnia and minor depression. In other cases, the sufferer may become stuporous, or on the contrary become violent and irrational. Headache, irritability, and general anxiety may also be present.

TREATMENT. Treatment of pellagra consists of an improved diet, often combined with large doses of niacinamide. In acute cases, niacinamide must be administered by injection and must be accompanied by large doses of other vitamins.

The patient's diet should include meat (particularly liver), whole-grain cereals, and peanuts, all of which are especially good sources of niacin. In severe cases of pellagra, bed rest is required. Skin lesions are treated with antibiotics.

pellagroid (pĕ-lag'roid) resembling pellagra.

Pellegrini's disease, Pellegrini-Stieda disease (pel"a-gre'nēz; pel"a-gre'ne-ste'dah) calcification of the medial collateral ligament of the knee due to trauma.

pellet (pel'et) a small pill or granule.

pellicle (pel'ĭ-k'l) a thin scum forming on the surface of liquids.

pellucid (pĕ-lu'sid) translucent.

pelvic (pel'vik) pertaining to the pelvis.

p. bone, hip bone, comprising the ilium, ischium and pubis (see also table of BONES).

p. diameter, any diameter of the pelvis, such as the diagonal conjugate, joining the posterior surface of the pubis to the tip of the sacral promontory; the external conjugate, joining the depression under the last lumbar spine to the upper margin of the pubis; the true (internal) conjugate, the anteroposterior diameter of the pelvic inlet, measured from the upper margin of the pubic symphysis to the sacrovertebral angle; the oblique, joining the one sacroiliac articulation to the iliopubic eminence of the other side; the transverse (of inlet), joining the two most widely separated points of the pelvic inlet; the transverse (of outlet), joining the medial surfaces of the ischial tuberosities.

p. inlet, the superior opening of the pelvis.

p. outlet, the inferior opening of the pelvis.

pelvicephalometry (pel"vĭ-sef"ah-lom"ĕ-tre) measurement of the fetal head in relation to the maternal pelvis.

pelvifixation (pel″vĭ-fik-sa′shun) surgical fixation of a displaced pelvic organ.

pelvimeter (pel-vim′ĕ-ter) an instrument for measuring the pelvis.

pelvimetry (pel-vim′ĕ-tre) measurement of the capacity and diameter of the pelvis, either internally or externally or both, with the hands or with a pelvimeter.

pelviotomy (pel″ve-ot′o-me) 1. incision or transection of a pelvic (hip) bone. 2. pyelotomy; incision of the renal pelvis.

pelviperitonitis (pel″vĭ-per″ĭ-to-ni′tis) inflammation of the pelvic peritoneum.

pelvirectal (pel″vĭ-rek′tal) pertaining to the pelvis and rectum.

pelvis (pel′vis), pl. *pel′ves.* the lower (caudal) portion of the trunk of the body, forming a basin bounded anteriorly and laterally by the hip bones and posteriorly by the sacrum and coccyx. Also applied to any basin-like structure, e.g., the renal pelvis.

The bony pelvis is formed by the sacrum, the coccyx, and the ilium, pubis, and ischium, bones that form the hip and pubic arch. These bones are separate in the child, but become fused by adulthood.

The pelvis is subjected to more stress than any other body structure. The upper part of the pelvic girdle, which is somewhat flared, supports the weight of internal organs in the upper part of the body.

Pelvic structures in men and women differ both in shape and in relative size. The male pelvis is heart-shaped and narrow and proportionately heavier and stronger than the female, so that it is better suited for lifting and running. The female pelvis is constructed to accommodate the fetus during pregnancy and to facilitate its downward passage through the pelvic cavity in childbirth. The most obvious difference between the male and female pelvis is in the shape. A woman's hips are wider and her pelvic cavity is round and relatively large. Even among women, moreover, there are differences in the shape of the pelvis, and these differences must be taken into account in childbirth. During pregnancy the capacity of the pelvis and the PELVIC DIAMETERS are measured, so that possible complications during labor can be avoided.

android p., one with a wedge-shaped inlet and narrow anterior segment typically found in the male.

anthropoid p., one whose anteroposterior diameter equals or exceeds the transverse diameter.

assimilation p., one in which the ilia articulates with the vertebral column higher (high assimilation pelvis) or lower (low assimilation pelvis) than normal, the number of lumbar vertebrae being correspondingly decreased or increased.

beaked p., one with the pelvic bones laterally compressed and their anterior junction pushed forward.

brachypellic p., a short oval type of pelvis, in which the transverse diameter exceeds the anteroposterior diameter by 1 to 3 cm.

contracted p., one showing a decrease of 1.5 to 2 cm. in an important diameter; when all dimensions are proportionately diminished, it is a generally contracted pelvis.

cordate p., a heart-shaped pelvis.

dolichopellic p., a long, oval pelvis with the anteroposterior diameter greater than the transverse diameter.

extrarenal p., see renal PELVIS.

false p., the part of the pelvis superior to a plane passing through the ileopectineal lines.

flat p., one in which the anteroposterior dimension is abnormally reduced.

frozen p., a condition, due to infection or carcinoma, in which the adnexa and uterus are fixed in the pelvis.

funnel p., one with a normal inlet but a greatly narrowed outlet.

gynecoid p., the normal female pelvis: a rounded oval pelvis with well rounded anterior and posterior segments.

infantile p., a generally contracted pelvis with an oval shape, a high sacrum, and inclination of the walls; called also juvenile pelvis.

p. jus′to ma′jor, an unusually large gynecoid pelvis, with all dimensions increased.

p. jus′to mi′nor, a small gynecoid pelvis, with all dimensions symmetrically reduced.

juvenile p., infantile pelvis.

kyphotic p., a deformed pelvis marked by increase of the conjugate diameter at the brim with decrease of the transverse diameter at the outlet.

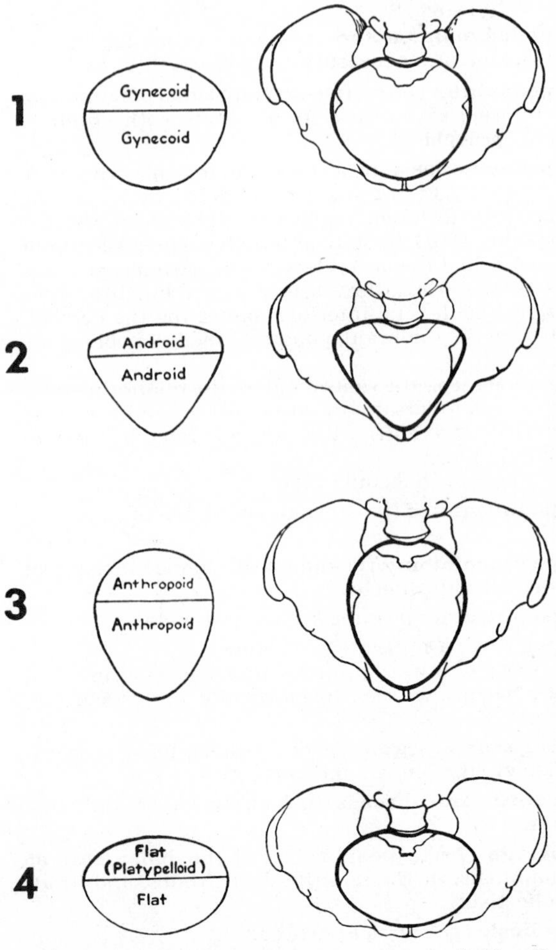

Pure types of pelvic inlets according to Caldwell, Moloy, and D'Esopo. (From Davis, M. E., and Rubin, R.: De Lee's Obstetrics for Nurses. 18th ed. Philadelphia, W. B. Saunders Co., 1966.)

p. ma'jor, false pelvis.

mesatipellic p., a round type of pelvis, in which the transverse diameter is equal to the anteroposterior diameter or exceeds it by no more than 1 cm.

p. mi'nor, true pelvis.

Nägele's p., one contracted in an oblique diameter, with complete ankylosis of the sacroiliac synchondrosis on one side and imperfect development of the sacrum and coxa on the same side.

Otto p., one in which the acetabulum is depressed, with protrusion of the femoral head into the pelvis.

platypellic p., platypelloid p., one shortened in the anteroposterior aspect, with a flattened transverse, oval shape.

rachitic p., one distorted as a result of rickets.

renal p., the funnel-shaped expansion of the upper end of the ureter into which the renal calices open; it is usually within the renal sinus, but under certain conditions, a large part of it may be outside the kidney (*extrarenal pelvis*).

Robert's p., a transversely contracted pelvis caused by osteoarthritis affecting both sacroiliac joints, the inlet becoming a narrow wedge.

scoliotic p., one deformed as a result of scoliosis.

split p., one with a congenital separation at the symphysis pubis.

spondylolisthetic p., one deformed by sliding of the lower lumbar vertebrae over the sacrum and into the pelvis.

true p., the part of the pelvis inferior to a plane passing through the ileopectineal lines.

pelvospondylitis (pel″vo-spon″dĭ-li′tis) inflammation of the pelvic portion of the spine.

p. ossif'icans, rheumatoid spondylitis.

pemoline (pem′o-lēn) a central nervous system stimulant.

pemphigoid (pem′fĭ-goid) 1. resembling pemphigus. 2. a group of skin disorders similar to but clearly distinguishable from pemphigus.

bullous p., a chronic, generalized, usually nonfatal, bullous skin eruption usually seen in elderly persons.

pemphigus (pem′fĭ-gus) a distinctive group of diseases characterized by successive crops of large bullae ("water blisters"); the name is derived from the Greek word for blister: *pemphix*. A rare disease, it is also a serious one that requires prompt treatment. It can occur in acute or chronic form. The term pemphigus generally refers to pemphigus vulgaris.

Clusters of blisters usually appear first near the nose and mouth—sometimes inside them—and then gradually spread over the skin of the rest of the body. When the blisters burst, they leave round patches of raw and tender skin. The skin itches, burns and gives off an offensive odor. The patient loses appetite and weight. If the disease is allowed to progress, it may cause extreme weakness, prostration and shock, accompanied by chills, sweating, fever, and often pneumonia.

The cause of pemphigus is unknown. It seems to occur only in adults.

The patient must be hospitalized from the beginning and given antibiotics and sometimes blood transfusions. He suffers intense discomfort and may need to suck anesthetic tablets to allay pain around the mouth while eating.

Progress has been made in the treatment of this disease through the persistent use of cortisone, administered orally, and of the pituitary extract ACTH, administered intramuscularly. Fatalities, once fairly common, now can usually be averted. The disease is difficult to control, however, and therapy sometimes must be maintained for years to prevent continuing attacks.

benign familial p., a hereditary, recurrent vesiculobullous dermatitis, usually involving the axillae, groin, and neck, with crops of lesions that regress over several weeks or months. Called also Hailey-Hailey disease.

p. erythemato'sus, a chronic form in which the lesions, limited to the face and chest, resemble those of disseminated lupus erythematosus.

p. folia'ceus, a chronic, generalized, vesicular and scaling eruption somewhat resembling dermatitis herpetiformis or, later in its course, exfoliative dermatitis.

p. veg'etans, a variant of pemphigus vulgaris in which the bullae are replaced by verrucoid hypertrophic vegetative masses.

p. vulga'ris, a rare relapsing disease with suprabasal, intraepidermal bullae of the skin and mucous membranes; invariably fatal if untreated (see PEMPHIGUS).

pempidine (pem′pĭ-dēn) a ganglionic blocking agent used in hypertension.

pendulous (pen′du-lus) hanging loosely; dependent.

penetrance (pen′ĕ-trans) the frequency with which a heritable trait is manifested by individuals carrying the principal gene or genes conditioning it.

penetrometer (pen″ĕ-trom′ĕ-ter) an instrument for measuring the penetrating power of x-rays; qualimeter.

-penia word element [Gr.], *deficiency*.

penicillamine (pen″ĭ-sil-am′in) a product of penicillin which chelates copper and other metals; used mainly to remove excess copper from the body in hepatolenticular degeneration.

penicillic acid (pen″ĭ-sil′ik) an antibiotic substance isolated from cultures of various species of *Penicillium* and *Aspergillus*.

penicillin (pen″ĭ-sil′in) an antibiotic substance extracted from cultures of certain molds of the genera *Penicillium* and *Aspergillus* that have been grown on special media. It is also prepared synthetically.

Penicillin was discovered by Sir Alexander Fleming in 1929 at St. Mary's Hospital in London. During World War II it came into general use and was hailed as a "wonder drug" because of its ability to control certain types of bacterial infections. Since the discovery of penicillin many other antibiotics have been developed, some of them more effective than penicillin against certain types of organisms. Penicillin is known as a narrow-spectrum antibiotic, which means that it is effective against relatively few organisms. (See also ANTIBIOTIC.)

Many different preparations of penicillin are available today; the choice of preparation depends on the specific needs in a particular case. Penicillin is prepared in a number of salts, but aluminum, calcium, potassium, and sodium are the most common. It exists in several types: F, G, K, O, V, and X. Type G is most commonly used. Type V is a synthetic penicillin. Procaine penicillin G is a preparation modified to prolong its effectiveness. Benzathine penicillin G has a long-sustained action and is used orally or parenterally. Dimethoxyphenyl penicillin (methicillin) and oxacillin are semisynthetic penicillins that are highly resistant to inactivation by penicillinase. Phenoxymethyl penicillin (phenethicillin) is a preparation for oral administration.

Penicillin is administered intramuscularly, orally, in liquid or tablet form, and topically in ointments. Oral administration requires larger doses of the drug because absorption is incomplete.

Allergic reaction to penicillin occurs in some persons. The reaction may be slight—a stinging or burning sensation at the site of injection—or it can be more serious—severe dermatitis or even anaphylactic shock, which may be fatal.

penicillinase (pen″ĭ-sil′ĭ-nās) an enzyme produced by bacteria that inactivates penicillin, thus increasing resistance to the antibiotic; a purified form from *Bacillus cereus* is used in the treatment of reactions to penicillin.

Penicillium (pen″ĭ-sil′e-um) a genus of fungi.

penicilloyl-polylysine (pen″ĭ-sil′oil-pol″ĕ-li′sēn) an agent prepared from polylysine and a penicillic acid; intradermal reaction elicits a wheal and erythema response in those sensitive to penicillin.

penicillus (pen″ĭ-sil′us), pl. *penicil′li* [L.] any of the brushlike groups of arterial branches in the lobules of the spleen.

penile (pe′nīl) of or pertaining to the penis.

penis (pe′nis) the external male organ of urination and copulation.

The body of the penis consists of three cylindrical-shaped masses of erectile tissue which run the length of the penis. Two of the masses lie alongside each other and end behind the head of the penis. The third mass lies underneath them. This latter mass contains the urethra. The penis terminates in an oval or cone-shaped body, the glans penis, which contains the exterior opening of the urethra.

The glans penis is covered by a loose skin, the foreskin or prepuce, which enables it to expand freely during erection. The skin ends just behind the glans penis and folds forward to cover it. The inner surface of the foreskin contains glands that secrete a lubricating fluid called smegma which makes it easy for the penis to expand and retract past the foreskin.

Disorders of the Penis. Disorders of the penis are rare. One of the most common complaints is phimosis, due to tight foreskin, which may make erection painful. This condition can be easily remedied by circumcision.

Among the most common diseases of the penis are those caused by venereal infections, such as syphilis and gonorrhea. Cancer of the penis is rare and rarely occurs in a man who has been circumcised.

penitis (pe-ni′tis) inflammation of the penis.

penniform (pen′ĭ-form) shaped like a feather.

Penrose drain (pen′rōz) a drain made by drawing a strip of gauze or surgical sponge into a tube of gutta-percha; called also cigarette drain.

pent(a)- word element [Gr.], *five.*

pentaerythritol (pen″tah-e-rith′rĭ-tol) a vasodilator, used in the form of the tetranitrate salt in the treatment of angina pectoris.

pentagastrin (pen″tah-gas′trin) a synthetic pentapeptide consisting of β-alanine and C-terminal tetrapeptide of gastrin; used as a test of gastric secretory function.

pentamidine (pen-tam′ĭ-dēn) a trypanosomicide, used as the isethionate salt in the prophylaxis and treatment of African trypanosomiasis and in the treatment of leishmaniasis.

pentapeptide (pen″tah-pep′tīd) a polypeptide containing five amino acids.

pentaploid (pen′tah-ploid) 1. pertaining to or characterized by pentaploidy. 2. an individual or cell having five sets of chromosomes.

pentaploidy (pen′tah-ploi″de) the state of having five sets of chromosomes (5n).

pentavalent (pen″tah-va′lent, pen-tav′ah-lent) having a valence of five.

pentazocine (pen-taz′o-sēn) a synthetic narcotic used as an analgesic.

penthienate (pen-thi′ĕ-nāt) an anticholinergic; the bromide is used as an antispasmodic in peptic ulcer.

Penthrane (pen′thrān) trademark for a preparation of methoxyflurane, an inhalation anesthetic.

Pentids (pen′tidz) trademark for preparations of potassium penicillin G.

pentobarbital (pen″to-bar′bĭ-tal) a short- to intermediate-acting barbiturate; used as a hypnotic and sedative in the form of the sodium salt.

pentolinium (pen″to-lin′e-um) a ganglionic blocking agent used primarily as an antihypertensive in the form of the tartrate salt. Dosage is adjusted according to observations of blood pressure as well as toxic effects. These side effects include cardiovascular collapse and must be treated immediately with epinephrine or levarterenol.

pentose (pen′tōs) a monosaccharide containing five carbon atoms in a molecule.

pentoside (pen′to-sīd) a compound (glycoside) of pentose with another substance.

pentosuria (pen″to-su′re-ah) a benign inborn error of metabolism due to a defect in the activity of the enzyme L-xylulose dehydrogenase, resulting in high levels of L-xylulose in the urine.

Pentothal (pen′to-thal) trademark for a preparation of thiopental, used as an anesthetic.

pentylenetetrazol (pen″tĭ-lēn-te′trah-zol) a convulsant analeptic.

Pen-Vee (pen′ve) trademark for a preparation of phenoxymethyl penicillin.

peotillomania (pe″o-til″o-ma′ne-ah) constant but nonmasturbatory, pulling at the penis.

peplomer (pep′lo-mer) a subunit of a peplos.

peplos (pep′lohs) the lipoprotein envelope of some types of virions, assembled in some cases from subunits (peplomers).

peppermint (pep′er-mint) the dried leaves and flowering tops of *Mentha piperita,* used as a flavoring vehicle for drugs.

pepsin (pep′sin) a proteolytic enzyme that is the principal digestive component of gastric juice. It acts as a catalyst in the chemical breakdown of protein to form a mixture of polypeptides; it is formed from pepsinogen in the presence of acid or, autocatalytically, in the presence of pepsin itself. Pepsin also has milk-clotting action similar to that of rennin and thereby facilitates the digestion of milk protein.

pepsinogen (pep-sin′o-jen) a zymogen secreted by the chief cells of the gastric glands and converted into pepsin in the presence of gastric acid or of pepsin itself.

peptic (pep'tik) pertaining to pepsin or to digestion or to the action of gastric juices.

p. ulcer, an ulceration of the mucous membrane of the esophagus, stomach, or duodenum, caused by the action of the acid gastric juice. There are two kinds of peptic ulcers: *Gastric* ulcers occur in the stomach; *duodenal* ulcers occur in the duodenum, the part of the small intestine nearest the stomach.

It is estimated that 3 out of every 1000 people have peptic ulcers. Ulcers develop at any age, though rarely in children under ten. They occur in people of all races and occupations; in men more than in women; and most frequently in tense, hard-driving, or anxious persons. (See also ULCER.)

peptidase (pep'tĭ-dās) any of a subclass of proteolytic enzymes that catalyze the hydrolysis of peptide linkages.

peptide (pep'tīd, pep'tid) any of a class of compounds of low molecular weight which yield two or more amino acids on hydrolysis; known as di-, tri-, tetra-, (etc.) peptides, depending on the number of amino acids in the molecule. Peptides form the constituent parts of proteins.

peptidolytic (pep"tĭ-do-lit'ik) capable of splitting up peptide bonds.

peptogenic (pep"to-jen'ik) 1. producing pepsin or peptones. 2. promoting digestion.

peptolysis (pep-tol'ĭ-sis) the splitting up of peptone. adj., **peptolyt'ic.**

peptone (pep'tōn) a derived protein, or a mixture of cleavage products produced by partial hydrolysis of native protein. adj., **pepton'ic.**

peptonize (pep'to-nīz) to convert a native protein into peptone.

peptotoxin (pep"to-tok'sin) any toxin or poisonous base developed from a peptone; also, a poisonous alkaloid or ptomaine occurring in certain peptones and putrefying proteins.

per- word element [L.], (1) *throughout; completely; extremely;* (2) in chemistry, a *large amount; combination of an element in its highest valence.*

peracid (per-as'id) an acid containing more than the usual quantity of oxygen.

peracute (per"ah-kūt) very acute.

Perandren (per-an'dren) trademark for a preparation of testosterone, a male sex hormone.

per anum (per a'num) [L.] through the anus.

Perazil (per'ah-zil) trademark for preparations of chlorcyclizine, an antihistaminic.

percept (per'sept) the object perceived; the mental image of an object in space perceived by the senses.

perception (per-sep'shun) the conscious mental registration of a sensory stimulus. adj., **percep'tive.**

depth p., the ability to recognize depth or the relative distances to different objects in space.

extrasensory p., knowledge of, or response to, an external thought or objective event not achieved as the result of stimulation of the sense organs; abbreviated E.S.P.

perceptive (per-sep'tiv) related to or important in the function of perception.

perceptivity (per"sep-tiv'ĭ-te) ability to receive sense impressions.

percolate (per'ko-lāt) 1. to strain; to submit to percolation. 2. a liquid that has been submitted to percolation. 3. to trickle slowly through a substance.

percolation (per"ko-la'shun) the extraction of soluble parts of a drug by passing a solvent liquid through it.

percolator (per"ko-la'tor) a vessel used in percolation.

Percorten (per-kor'ten) trademark for preparations of desoxycorticosterone, a corticosteroid.

percuss (per-kus') to perform percussion.

percussible (per-kus'ĭ-b'l) detectable on percussion.

percussion (per-kush'un) in medical diagnosis, striking a part of the body with short, sharp blows of the fingers in order to determine the size, position, and density of the underlying parts by the sound obtained. Percussion is most commonly used on the chest and back for examination of the heart and lungs. For example, since the heart is not resonant and the adjacent lungs are, when the examiner's fingers strike the chest over the heart the sound waves will change in pitch. This serves as a guide to the precise location and size of the heart.

auscultatory p., auscultation of the sound produced by percussion.

immediate p., that in which the blow is struck directly against the body surface.

mediate p., that in which a pleximeter is used.

palpatory p., a combination of palpation and percussion, affording tactile rather than auditory impressions.

percussor (per-kus'or) an instrument for performing percussion.

percutaneous (per"ku-ta'ne-us) performed through the skin.

perencephaly (per"en-sef'ah-le) porencephaly.

perfectionism (per-fek'shun-izm) the setting of impossible high standards for oneself.

perforans (per'fo-rans) [L.] penetrating; a term applied to various muscles and nerves.

perforation (per"fo-ra'shun) a hole or break in the containing walls or membranes of an organ or structure of the body. Perforation occurs when erosion, infection, or other factors create a weak spot in the organ and internal pressure causes a rupture. It also may result from a deep penetrating wound caused by trauma.

A perforated ULCER is a complication of duodenal and gastric ulcers. It requires immediate surgical correction to prevent hemorrhage, shock, and peritonitis.

Perforation of the eardrum occurs when an infectious process of the middle ear creates an increase in pressure behind the tympanic membrane. Although perforation may occur spontaneously in OTITIS MEDIA, and is advantageous because it allows for adequate drainage of exudate and relieves pain, it is not desirable because the ragged edges of the perforation may not heal as they should for the eardrum to remain intact. Surgical incision of the eardrum (myringotomy) is preferred to spontaneous perforation.

The eardrum also may be perforated when a sharp object is inserted into the external acoustic meatus or when extreme pressure from the outside, such as occurs when swimming or diving in deep water, causes the tympanic membrane to rupture.

Gallbladder perforation sometimes occurs as a complication of CHOLECYSTITIS and GALLSTONES. When the gallbladder is infected, necrosis may progress to the point of destroying the wall of the gallbladder, so that the bile spills out into the abdominal cavity. Gallstones may cause complete obstruction of the cystic duct so that the flow of bile is dammed up and the gallbladder becomes inflamed and eventually ruptures. Treatment of gallbladder perforation usually involves cholecystectomy.

Intestinal perforation is a complication of typhoid fever, ULCERATIVE COLITIS, INTESTINAL OBSTRUCTION, and other disorders in which there is inflammation of the intestinal wall or obstruction of the intestinal lumen. The condition is treated surgically with resection of the affected portion of intestine.

perfusate (per-fu′zāt) a liquid that has been subjected to perfusion.

perfusion (per-fu′zhun) 1. the act of pouring through or over; especially the passage of a fluid through the vessels of a specific organ. 2. a liquid poured through or over an organ or tissue.

peri- word element [Gr.], *around; near.* See also words beginning *para-*.

periacinal, periacinous (per″e-as′ĭ-nal; per″e-as′ĭ-nus) around an acinus.

Periactin (per″e-ak′tin) trademark for preparations of cyproheptadine, an antihistamine and antiserotonin.

periadenitis (per″e-ad″ĕ-ni′tis) inflammation of tissues around a gland.

p. muco′sa necrot′ica recur′rens, the more severe form of aphthous stomatitis, marked by recurrent attacks of aphtha-like lesions that begin as small, firm nodules, which enlarge, ulcerate, and heal by scar formation, leaving numerous atrophied scars on the oral mucosa. Called also Sutton's disease.

perianal (per″e-a′nal) around the anus.

periangiitis (per″e-an″je-i′tis) inflammation of the tissue around a blood or lymph vessel.

periangiocholitis (per″e-an″je-o-ko-li′tis) inflammation of tissues around the bile ducts; pericholangitis.

periaortitis (per″e-a″or-ti′tis) inflammation of tissues around the aorta.

periapical (per″e-a′pĭ-kal) surrounding the apex of the root of a tooth.

periappendicitis (per″e-ah-pen″dĭ-si′tis) inflammation of the vermiform appendix and surrounding tissues.

periarterial (per″e-ar-te′re-al) around an artery.

periarteritis (per″e-ar″ter-i′tis) inflammation of the outer coat of an artery and of the tissues surrounding it.

p. gummo′sa, accumulation of gummas in the blood vessels in syphilis.

p. nodo′sa, an inflammatory disease of the coats of small and medium-sized arteries, marked by a variety of systemic symptoms (see also COLLAGEN DISEASES). Called also Kussmaul's disease.

periarthritis (per″e-ar-thri′tis) inflammation of the tissues around a joint.

periarticular (per″e-ar-tik′u-lar) situated around a joint.

periaxial (per″e-ak′se-al) around an axis.

periaxillary (per″e-ak′sĭ-ler″e) around the axilla.

periblast (per′ĭ-blast) the portion of the blastoderm of telolecithal eggs, the cells of which lack complete cell membranes.

peribronchial (per″ĭ-brong′ke-al) around a bronchus or bronchi.

peribronchiolar (per″ĭ-brong″ke-o′lar) around the bronchioles.

peribronchiolitis (per″ĭ-brong″ke-o-li′tis) inflammation of the tissues around the bronchioles.

peribronchitis (per″ĭ-brong-ki′tis) a form of bronchitis consisting of inflammation and thickening of the tissues around the bronchi.

pericardiac (per″ĭ-kar′de-ak) pertaining to the pericardium; around the heart.

pericardial (per″ĭ-kar′de-al) pertaining to the pericardium.

p. rub, a scraping or grating noise heard with the heart beat, usually a to-and-fro sound, associated with an inflamed pericardium.

pericardicentesis (per″ĭ-kar″dĭ-sen-te′sis) surgical puncture of the pericardial cavity with aspiration of fluid.

pericardiectomy (per″ĭ-kar″de-ek′to-me) excision of a portion of the pericardium.

pericardiocentesis (per″ĭ-kar″de-o-sen-te′sis) pericardicentesis.

pericardiolysis (per″ĭ-kar″de-ol′ĭ-sis) the operative freeing of adhesions between the visceral and parietal pericardium.

pericardiophrenic (per″ĭ-kar″de-o-fren′ik) pertaining to the pericardium and diaphragm.

pericardiopleural (per″ĭ-kar″de-o-ploo′ral) pertaining to the pericardium and pleura.

pericardiorrhaphy (per″ĭ-kar″de-or′ah-fe) suture of the pericardium.

pericardiostomy (per″ĭ-kar″de-os′to-me) creation of an opening into the pericardium, usually for drainage of effusions.

pericardiotomy (per″ĭ-kar″de-ot′o-me) incision of pericardium.

pericarditis (per″ĭ-kar-di′tis) inflammation of the pericardium. adj., **pericardit′ic.**

TYPES OF PERICARDITIS. There are many forms of pericarditis. Acute pericarditis is usually secondary to some other bacterial infection, for example, osteomyelitis, lung abscess, or pneumonia. It may also occur without bacterial infection, resulting from a tumor, rheumatic heart disease, uremia, or coronary thrombosis, or it may be the aftermath of a chest wound in which the pericardium is pierced. Acute pericarditis may be dry, or fibrinous, in which a fibrinous exudate forms on the serous membrane, or it may occur with effusion, that is, with accumulation of fluid in the pericardial cavity.

Occasionally the pericardium is affected directly by what appears to be a virus; this condition is called acute nonspecific pericarditis. Another form, chronic pericarditis, is usually adhesive—that is, the heart is anchored to surrounding tissues by adhesions. It sometimes follows acute pericarditis, but often the cause is unknown. In the constrictive form of chronic pericarditis, which may be tuberculous in origin, calcium and fibrous deposits may form around the heart and interfere with its movements. This form may be extremely serious and difficult to cure.

SYMPTOMS AND TREATMENT. The symptoms of acute pericarditis vary with the cause but usually include chest pain and dyspnea, an increase in the pulse rate, and a rise in temperature. In dry pericarditis distinct sounds of friction caused by deposits of fibrin may be heard through a stethoscope. In the effusive form, the excess accumulation of pericardial fluid can be detected by x-rays or electrocardiography. The excess fluid is sometimes drained by pericardicentesis.

Treatment of acute pericarditis is directed mainly at curing its original cause. Antibiotics have proved successful in treating bacterial pericarditis. Many patients with nonspecific pericarditis with effusion are helped dramatically by cortisone medications.

In the constrictive form of chronic pericarditis there may be dyspnea and pain in the heart region, plus symptoms elsewhere in the body, such as edema, enlargement of the liver, or distention of the neck veins. The best means of treatment is surgery to remove the constrictions and permit free heart action.

pericardium (per″ĭ-kar′de-um) the fibroserous sac enclosing the heart and the roots of the great vessels, composed of external (fibrous) and internal (serous) layers.

adherent p., one abnormally connected with the heart by dense fibrous tissue.

fibrous p., the external layer of the pericardium, consisting of dense fibrous tissue.

parietal p., the parietal layer of the serous pericardium, which is in contact with the fibrous pericardium.

serous p., the inner, serous portion of pericardium, consisting of two layers, visceral and parietal; the space between the layers is the pericardial cavity.

visceral p., the inner layer of the serous pericardium, which is in contact with the heart and roots of the great vessels. Called also epicardium.

pericecal (per″ĭ-se′kal) around the cecum.

pericecitis (per″ĭ-se-si′tis) inflammation of the tissues around the cecum.

pericellular (per″ĭ-sel′u-lar) surrounding a cell.

pericementitis (per″ĭ-se″men-ti′tis) periodontitis.

pericholangitis (per″ĭ-ko″lan-ji′tis) inflammation of tissues surrounding the bile ducts; periangiocholitis.

pericholecystitis (per″ĭ-ko″le-sis″ti′tis) inflammation of tissues around the gallbladder.

perichondritis (per″ĭ-kon-dri′tis) inflammation of the perichondrium.

perichondrium (per″ĭ-kon′dre-um) the layer of fibrous connective tissue investing all cartilage except the articular cartilage of synovial joints. adj., **perichon′dral.**

perichordal (per″ĭ-kor′dal) surrounding the notochord.

perichoroidal (per″ĭ-ko-roi′dal) surrounding the choroid coat of the eye.

Periclor (per′ĭ-klōr) trademark for a preparation of petrichloral, a hypnotic and sedative.

pericolic (per″ĭ-kol′ik) around the colon.

pericolitis, pericolonitis (per″ĭ-ko-li′tis; per″ĭ-ko″lon-i′tis) inflammation around the colon, especially of its peritoneal coat.

pericolpitis (per″ĭ-kol-pi′tis) inflammation of the tissues around the vagina; perivaginitis.

periconchal (per″ĭ-kong′kal) around the concha.

pericorneal (per″ĭ-kor′ne-al) around the cornea.

pericoronal (per″ĭ-kŏ-ro′nal) around the crown of a tooth.

pericranitis (per″ĭ-kra-ni′tis) inflammation of the pericranium.

pericranium (per″ĭ-kra′ne-um) the periosteum of the skull. adj., **pericra′nial.**

pericystitis (per″ĭ-sis-ti′tis) inflammation of tissues about the bladder.

pericyte (per′ĭ-sīt) one of the peculiar elongated, contractile cells found wrapped about precapillary arterioles outside the basement membrane.

pericytial (per″ĭ-si′shal) around a cell.

periderm (per′ĭ-derm) the outer layer of the bilaminar fetal epidermis, generally disappearing before birth.

peridesmitis (per″ĭ-dez-mi′tis) inflammation of the peridesmium.

peridesmium (per″ĭ-dez′me-um) the areolar membrane that covers the ligaments.

perididymis (per″ĭ-did′ĭ-mis) the tunica vaginalis testis, the membrane covering the front and sides of the testis and epididymis.

perididymitis (per″ĭ-did″ĭ-mi′tis) inflammation of the tunica vaginalis testis.

peridiverticulitis (per″ĭ-di″ver-tik″u-li′tis) inflammation around an intestinal diverticulum.

periductal (per″ĭ-duk′tal) around a duct.

periduodenitis (per″ĭ-du″o-dĕ-ni′tis) inflammation around the duodenum.

periencephalitis (per″e-en-sef″ah-li′tis) inflammation of the surface of the brain.

periencephalomeningitis (per″e-en-sef″ah-lo-men″in-ji′tis) inflammation of the cerebral cortex and meninges.

perienteritis (per″e-en″tĕ-ri′tis) inflammation of the peritoneal coat of the intestines.

periesophagitis (per″e-e-sof″ah-ji′tis) inflammation of the tissues around the esophagus.

perifistular (per″ĭ-fis′tu-lar) around a fistula.

perifollicular (per″ĭ-fŏ-lik′u-lar) surrounding a follicle.

perifolliculitis (per″ĭ-fŏ-lik″u-li′tis) inflammation around the hair follicles.

perigangliitis (per″ĭ-gang″gle-i′tis) inflammation around a ganglion.

perigastric (per″ĭ-gas′trik) around the stomach; pertaining to the peritoneal coat of the stomach.

perigastritis (per″ĭ-gas-tri′tis) inflammation of the peritoneal coat of the stomach.

perihepatic (per″ĭ-hĕ-pat′ik) around the liver.

perihepatitis (per″ĭ-hep″ah-ti′tis) inflammation of the peritoneal coat of the liver and the surrounding tissue.

perijejunitis (per″ĭ-je″joo-ni′tis) inflammation around the jejunum.

perikaryon (per″ĭ-kar′e-on) the cell body of a neuron.

perilabyrinthitis (per″ĭ-lab″ĭ-rin-thi′tis) inflammation of the tissues around the labyrinth.

perilaryngitis (per″ĭ-lar″in-ji′tis) inflammation of the tissues around the larynx.

perilymph, perilympha (per′ĭ-limf; per″ĭ-lim′fah) the fluid contained in the space separating the membranous and osseous labyrinths of the ear.

perilymphangitis (per″ĭ-lim″fan-ji′tis) inflammation around a lymphatic vessel.

perimeningitis (per″ĭ-men″in-ji′tis) pachymeningitis; inflammation of the dura mater.

perimeter (pĕ-rim′ĕ-ter) 1. the boundary of a two-dimensional figure. 2. an apparatus for determining the extent of the peripheral visual field.

perimetrium (per″ĭ-me′tre-um) the serous membrane enveloping the uterus.

perimetry (pĕ-rim′ĕ-tre) determination of the extent of the peripheral visual field. adj., **perimet′ric.**

perimyelitis (per″ĭ-mi″ĕ-li′tis) inflammation of (*a*) the pia of the spinal cord, or (*b*) the endosteum.

perimyositis (per″ĭ-mi″o-si′tis) inflammation of connective tissue around a muscle.

perimysiitis (per″ĭ-mis″e-i′tis) inflammation of the perimysium.

perimysium (per″ĭ-mis′e-um) connective tissue demarcating a fascicle of skeletal muscle fibers. (See also Plate 4.) adj., **perimys′ial.**

perinatal (per″ĭ-na′tal) relating to the period shortly before and after birth; from the twenty-ninth week of gestation to 1 to 4 weeks after birth.

perineal (per″ĭ-ne′al) pertaining to the perineum.

perineocele (per″ĭ-ne′o-sēl) a hernia between the rectum and the prostate or between the rectum and the vagina.

perineoplasty (per″ĭ-ne′o-plas″te) plastic repair of the perineum.

perineorrhaphy (per″ĭ-ne-or′ah-fe) suture of the perineum.

perineotomy (per″ĭ-ne-ot′o-me) incision of the perineum.

perineovaginal (per″ĭ-ne″o-vaj′ĭ-nal) pertaining to or communicating with the perineum and vagina.

perinephric (per″ĭ-nef′rik) around the kidney.

perinephritis (per″ĭ-nĕ-fri′tis) inflammation of the perinephrium.

perinephrium (per″ĭ-nef′re-um) the peritoneal envelope and other tissues around the kidney. adj., **perineph′rial.**

perineum (per″ĭ-ne′um) the pelvic floor and associated structures occupying the pelvic outlet, bounded anteriorly by the pubic symphysis, laterally by the ischial tuberosities, and posteriorly by the coccyx. During childbirth the perineum may be torn, resulting in possible damage to the urinary meatus and anal sphincter. To avoid a perineal tear, the obstetrician often cuts the perineum just before delivery and sutures the incision after delivery of the infant and the placenta. This procedure is called an episiotomy. Surgical repair of a torn or lacerated perineum is called perineorrhaphy.

perineuritis (per″ĭ-nu-ri′tis) inflammation of the perineurium.

perineurium (per″ĭ-nu′re-um) the connective tissue sheath surrounding each bundle of nerve fibers (fascicle) in a peripheral nerve. (See also Plate 12.) adj., **perineu′rial.**

periocular (per″e-ok′u-lar) around the eye.

periodic (pe″re-od′ik) repeated or recurring at intervals.

periodicity (pe″re-o-dis′ĭ-te) recurrence at regular intervals of time.

periodontal (per″e-o-don′tal) around a tooth; pertaining to the periodontium.

p. disease, any disease or disorder of the periodontium (see also PERIODONTITIS and PERIODONTOSIS).

periodontics (per″e-o-don′tiks) the branch of dentistry dealing with the study and treatment of diseases of the periodontium.

periodontist (per″e-o-don′tist) a dentist who specializes in periodontics.

periodontitis (per″e-o-don-ti′tis) inflammation of the periodontium. The condition is caused by residual food, bacteria, and calcium deposits (tartar) that collect in the spaces between the gum and lower part of the tooth crown. If it continues unchecked the infection will spread to the bone in which the teeth are rooted. The bone then resorbs and the teeth are slowly detached from their supporting tissues. Peridontitis is the major cause of tooth loss after the age of 35. It almost always has it inception in early childhood and already is present in over half the population of high school students in the United States.

Periodontitis is treated with local cleansing and scraping of the area, establishment of drainage for exudate, and oxygenating mouthwashes. Antibiotic drugs are indicated if the symptoms are severe. Extraction of the affected teeth may be necessary if the lesion is advanced.

periodontium (per″e-o-don′she-um) the tissues investing and supporting the teeth, including the cementum, periodontal ligament, alveolar bone, and gingiva. In NA, restricted to the periodontal ligament.

periodontoclasia (per″e-o-don″to-kla′ze-ah) any degenerative or destructive disease of the periodontium.

periodontosis (per″e-o-don-to′sis) a degenerative, noninflammatory condition of the periodontium, characterized by destruction of the tissues.

periomphalic (per″e-om-fal′ik) situated around the umbilicus.

perionychium (per″e-o-nik′e-um) the epidermis bordering a nail.

perioophoritis (per″e-o″of-o-ri′tis) inflammation of the tissues around the ovary.

perioophorosalpingitis (per″e-o-of″o-ro-sal″pin-ji′tis) inflammation of the tissues around ovary and oviduct.

periophthalmic (per″e-of-thal′mik) around the eye.

perioptometry (per″e-op-tom′ĕ-tre) measurement of acuity of peripheral vision or of the limits of the visual field.

perioral (per″e-o′ral) around the mouth.

periorbita (per″e-or′bĭ-tah) the periosteum of the bones forming the orbit, or eye socket. adj., **perior′bital.**

periorbitis (per″e-or-bi′tis) inflammation of the periorbita.

periorchitis (per″e-or-ki′tis) inflammation of the tunica vaginalis testis; vaginalitis.

periosteitis (per″e-os″te-i′tis) periostitis.

periosteoma (per″e-os-te-o′mah) a morbid bony growth surrounding a bone.

periosteomyelitis (per″e-os″te-o-mi″ĕ-li′tis) inflammation of the entire bone, including periosteum and marrow.

periosteophyte (per″e-os′te-o-fīt″) a bony growth on the periosteum.

periosteotomy (per″e-os″te-ot′o-me) incision of the periosteum.

periosteum (per″e-os′te-um) a specialized connective tissue covering all bones of the body, and possessing bone-forming potentialities. Periosteum also serves as a point of attachment for certain muscles. The connective tissues of the muscle fuse with the fibrous layers of periosteum. adj., **perios′teal.**

periostitis (per″e-os-ti′tis) inflammation of the periosteum.

dental p., periodontitis.

diffuse p., widespread periostitis of the long bones.

periostosis (per″e-os-to′sis) abnormal deposition of periosteal bone.

periotic (per″e-o′tik) 1. situated about the ear, especially the internal ear. 2. the petrous and mastoid portions of the temporal bone, at one stage a distinct bone.

peripachymeningitis (per″ĭ-pak″ĭ-men″in-ji′tis) inflammation of the substance between the dura mater and the bony covering of the central nervous system.

peripancreatitis (per″ĭ-pan″kre-ah-ti′tis) inflammation of tissues around the pancreas.

peripapillary (per″ĭ-pap′ĭ-ler″e) around the optic papilla.

periphacitis (per″ĭ-fah-si′tis) inflammation of the capsule of the eye lens.

peripherad (pĕ-rif′er-ad) toward the periphery.

peripheral (pĕ-rif′er-al) pertaining to or situated at or near the periphery.

p. nervous system, the portion of the NERVOUS SYSTEM consisting of the nerves and ganglia outside the brain and spinal cord.

p. vision, vision produced by stimulation of receptors in the retina outside the macula lutea; called also indirect vision.

periphery (pĕ-rif′er-e) an outward structure or surface; the portion of a system outside the central region.

periphlebitis (per″ĭ-flĕ-bi′tis) inflammation of the tissues around a vein, or the external coat of a vein.

periplocin (per″ĭ-plo′sin) a cardiotonic glycoside from the woody vine *Periploca graeca.*

periplocymarin (per″ĭ-plo-si′mah-rin) a cardiac glycoside from the woody vine *Periploca graeca.*

periportal (per″ĭ-por′tal) situated around the portal vein.

periproctitis (per″ĭ-prok-ti′tis) inflammation of tissues around the rectum and anus.

periprostatic (per″ĭ-pros-tat′ik) around the prostate.

periprostatitis (per″ĭ-pros″tah-ti′tis) inflammation of the tissues around the prostate.

peripylephlebitis (per″ĭ-pi″le-flĕ-bi′tis) inflammation of tissues around the portal vein.

peripyloric (per″ĭ-pi-lo′rik) around the pylorus.

perirectal (per″ĭ-rek′tal) around the rectum.

perirectitis (per″ĭ-rek-ti′tis) periproctitis.

perirenal (per″ĭ-re′nal) around the kidney.

perirhinal (per″ĭ-ri′nal) around the nose.

perisalpingitis (per″ĭ-sal″pin-ji′tis) inflammation of tissues around the uterine tube.

periscopic (per″ĭ-skop′ik) affording a wide range of vision.

perisigmoiditis (per″ĭ-sig″moi-di′tis) inflammation of the peritoneum of the sigmoid flexure.

perisinusitis (per″ĭ-si″nŭ-si′tis) inflammation of the tissues around a sinus.

perispermatitis (per″ĭ-sper″mah-ti′tis) inflammation of tissues around the spermatic cord.

perisplanchnic (per″ĭ-splangk′nik) around a viscus or the viscera.

perisplanchnitis (per″ĭ-splangk-ni′tis) inflammation of tissues around the viscera.

perisplenic (per″ĭ-splen′ik) around the spleen.

perisplenitis (per″ĭ-sple-ni′tis) inflammation of the peritoneal surface of the spleen.

perispondylitis (per″ĭ-spon″dĭ-li′tis) inflammation of tissues around a vertebra.

peristalsis (per″ĭ-stal′sis) the wormlike movement by which the alimentary canal or other tubular organs having both longitudinal and circular muscle fibers propel their contents, consisting of a wave of contraction passing along the tube for variable distances. adj., **peristal′tic.**

When food is swallowed, it passes into the esophagus. Muscular contractions in the wall of the esophagus work the food downward, pushing it into the stomach. Here peristaltic contractions not only move the food in small amounts into the intestine but also aid in the disintegration of the food and help mix it with gastric juice. Peristalsis forces the food through the intestine for further digestion until the food waste finally reaches the rectum, from which it is periodically discharged from the body. The waves of peristalsis are irregular; they are stronger at some times than others. They are also weaker in some people, notably the elderly.

Although the normal peristaltic wave is downward, it is sometimes reversed. Reverse peristaltic action may be triggered by mild digestive upsets or more serious disorders, such as an obstruction in the stomach or intestines.

peristaphyline (per″ĭ-staf′ĭ-līn) around the uvula.

perisynovial (per″ĭ-sĭ-no′ve-al) around a synovial structure.

peritectomy (per″ĭ-tek′to-me) excision of a ring of conjunctiva around the cornea in treatment of pannus.

peritendineum (per″ĭ-ten-din′e-um) connective tissue investing larger tendons and extending between the fibers composing them.

peritendinitis, peritenonitis (per″ĭ-ten″dĭ-ni′tis; per″ĭ-ten″o-ni′tis) inflammation of the sheath of a tendon; TENOSYNOVITIS.

perithelioma (per″ĭ-the″le-o′mah) hemangiopericytoma.

perithelium (per″ĭ-the′le-um) the connective tissue layer surrounding the capillaries and smaller vessels.

perithyroiditis (per″ĭ-thi″roi-di′tis) inflammation of the capsule of the thyroid.

peritomy (pĕ-rit′o-me) 1. surgical incision of the conjunctiva and subconjunctival tissue about the whole circumference of the cornea. 2. circumcision.

peritoneal (per″ĭ-to-ne′al) pertaining to the peritoneum.

p. cavity, the space between the parietal and visceral layers of the peritoneum.

p. dialysis, the employment of the peritoneum surrounding the abdominal cavity as a dialyzing membrane for the purpose of removing waste products or toxins accumulated as a result of renal failure. Certain crystalloids such as urea; creatinine; electrolytes; and some drugs, such as the salicylates, bromides, and barbiturates, can be removed. Peritoneal dialysis is used as an alternative to the artificial KIDNEY in the treatment of renal failure.

Fluid equal in osmolarity and chemical content with normal blood and tissue fluid is introduced into the peritoneal cavity via a catheter. The dialyzing fluid is left in the peritoneal cavity for 20 minutes to 1 hour. This period is referred to as the equalization period or dialysis phase and is followed by drainage of the fluid from the peritoneum. Then a new exchange is begun. The exchange is continued for a variable period of time, depending on the diagnosis and the patient's symptoms. Dialysis is usually discontinued after the patient's blood chemistry approaches a normal level.

INDICATIONS. Renal failure, whether acute or chronic, is the most frequent indication for peritoneal dialysis. Since certain drugs can be removed by dialysis, some types of acute drug poisoning are treated by this method.

Peritoneal dialysis cannot be employed when there is severe abdominal trauma, adhesions, or severe coagulation defects. Such complications as peritonitis, bleeding, intestinal perforation, and excessive loss of plasma protein may occur. Peritoneal dialysis is more expensive and time-consuming and less efficient than the artificial kidney.

PATIENT CARE. To avoid complications strict adherence to aseptic technique is essential. If there is any break in the tubing connections during the procedure the peritoneal cavity must be considered contaminated. If the tubing becomes blocked the physician should be notified immediately.

An *exchange record* is kept of the fluid that is introduced into and withdrawn from the peritoneal cavity. The amount withdrawn is expected to closely approximate or be slightly more than the amount introduced. The exchange record contains information about the starting time of infusion, amount infused, concentration of fluid and drugs added, finishing time of infusion, starting time of drainage, volume of drainage, and total patient fluid loss (−) or retention (+) up to the time of recording. Since this last item is frequently a source of error, it is essential that all personnel involved in the dialysis procedure know how the recording is done. Daily weight on a stretcher scale facilitates calculation of fluid loss or gain.

The peritoneal drainage fluid is observed for cloudiness and the presence of blood or other abnormal constituents. The vital signs are recorded at frequent intervals so that early signs of shock or the development of an infection can be discovered. Respiratory difficulty may develop as a result of pressure of the fluid against the diaphragm. Mild dyspnea may be relieved by elevating the head of the bed. Severe dyspnea may necessitate immediate drainage of the fluid from the peritoneal cavity and notification of the physician.

peritonealgia (per″ĭ-to″ne-al′je-ah) pain in the peritoneum.

peritoneocentesis (per″ĭ-to″ne-o-sen-te′sis) paracentesis of the abdominal (peritoneal) cavity.

peritoneoclysis (per″ĭ-to″ne-ok′lĭ-sis) injection of fluid into the peritoneal cavity.

peritoneopathy (per″ĭ-to″ne-op′ah-the) any disease of the peritoneum.

peritoneopericardial (per″ĭ-to-ne″o-per″ĭ-kar′de-al) pertaining to the peritoneum and pericardium.

peritoneoscope (per″ĭ-to′ne-o-skōp″) an endoscope for use in peritoneoscopy.

peritoneoscopy (per″ĭ-to″ne-os′ko-pe) visual examination of the organs of the abdominal (peritoneal) cavity with a peritoneoscope.

peritoneotomy (per″ĭ-to″ne-ot′o-me) incision into the peritoneum.

peritoneum (per″ĭ-to-ne′um) the serous membrane lining the walls of the abdominal and pelvic cavities (parietal peritoneum) and investing contained viscera (visceral peritoneum), the two layers enclosing a potential space, the peritoneal cavity.

peritonitis (per″i-to-ni′tis) inflammation of the peritoneum.

ACUTE PERITONITIS. Acute peritonitis may be produced by inflammation of abdominal organs, by irritating substances from a perforated gallbladder or gastric ulcer, by rupture of a cyst, or by irritation from blood, as in cases of internal bleeding.

Symptoms and Diagnosis. Immediate and intense pain is felt at the site of infection, followed usually by fever, vomiting, and extreme weakness. The abdomen becomes rigid and sensitive to the touch. The patient may suffer mental confusion, fever, prostration, or shock. Although antibiotics have greatly reduced the mortality rate of acute peritonitis, the infection should be treated and controlled immediately; it can be fatal if neglected.

Diagnosis is based on manual examination, x-ray films, and blood tests.

Treatment. The basic treatment for acute peritonitis is a combination of surgery, antibiotics, and other measures. The peritoneal cavity often must be opened and the toxic material removed. The original source of infection, such as an inflamed appendix, may have to be removed, or an abscess caused by the peritonitis may have to be drained. Antibiotics such as penicillin, streptomycin, or tetracycline are used to fight the infection itself.

The patient usually takes nothing by mouth. Fluids are given intravenously. Narcotics and sedatives are often used to relieve pain and insure rest. Treatment may also include blood transfusions and suction through a nasogastric tube to relieve abdominal pressure and to prevent accumulation of gas in the intestines.

CHRONIC PERITONITIS. The chronic form of this disease is comparatively rare, and is often associated with tuberculosis. Less frequently it may result from longstanding irritation caused by the presence in the abdomen of a foreign body such as gunshot.

In general, symptoms of chronic peritonitis are milder than those of acute peritonitis. Symptoms of tuberculous peritonitis are abdominal pain, low-grade fever, constipation, and general ill health, including loss of weight and appetite. Treatment depends on the underlying cause and the severity of the condition.

adhesive p., peritonitis characterized by adhesions between adjacent serous structures.

bile p., biliary p., that due to the presence of bile in the peritoneum; choleperitoneum.

silent p., asymptomatic peritonitis.

peritonsillar (per″ĭ-ton′sĭ-lar) around a tonsil.

peritonsillitis (per″ĭ-ton″sĭ-li′tis) inflammation of peritonsillar tissues.

peritracheal (per″ĭ-tra′ke-al) around the trachea.

Peritrate (per′ĭ-trāt) trademark for a preparation of pentaerythritol, a vasodilator used in treatment of angina pectoris.

peritrichous (pĕ-rit′rĭ-kus) 1. having flagella around the entire surface; said of bacteria. 2. having flagella around the cytostome only; said of Ciliophora.

periumbilical (per″e-um-bil′ĭ-kal) around the umbilicus.

periureteral (per″ĭ-u-re′ter-al) around the ureter.

periureteritis (per″ĭ-u-re″tĕ-ri′tis) inflammation of tissues around the ureter.

periurethral (per″ĭ-u-re′thral) around the urethra.

periuterine (per″ĭ-u′ter-in) around the uterus.

perivaginal (per″ĭ-vaj″ĭ-nal) around the vagina.

perivaginitis (per″ĭ-vaj″ĭ-ni′tis) inflammation of tissues around the vagina; pericolpitis.

perivascular (per″ĭ-vas′ku-lar) around a vessel.

perivasculitis (per″ĭ-vas″ku-li′tis) inflammation of a perivascular sheath and surrounding tissue.

perivesical (per″ĭ-ves′ĭ-kal) around the bladder.

perivesiculitis (per″ĭ-vĕ-sik″u-li′tis) inflammation of tissues around the seminal vesicles.

perlèche (per-lesh′) inflammation with exudation, maceration, and fissuring at the labial commissures.

permeability (per″me-ah-bil′ĭ-te) the property or state of being permeable.

permeable (per′me-ah-b′l) not impassable; pervious; allowing passage.

permease (per′me-ās) the genetically controlled mechanism responsible for active transport of nutrient substances across the bacterial membrane.

pernicious (per-nish′us) tending to a fatal issue.

p. anemia, a form of anemia caused by lack of the intrinsic factor, which normally is produced by the stomach mucosa. The deficiency results in inadequate and abnormal formation of erythrocytes, and failure to absorb vitamin B_{12}. Some persons with pernicious anemia show only mild symptoms and are not particularly aware of the illness; in others the condition becomes very serious and, if it remains untreated, it can be fatal.

SYMPTOMS. A pale, colorless complexion is typical of all anemias, including pernicious anemia. Jaundice also occurs in pernicious anemia, with soreness and reddening of the tongue, difficulty in swallowing, and digestive disturbances, including diarrhea. Other symptoms may include fatigability, heart palpitation, and dyspnea. Changes in the nerves and spinal cord may produce numbness and tingling in the fingers and toes, and the gait may become unsteady. The involvement of the nerves can be completely cured if it has existed for less than 6 months, but may be incurable if it is of long standing. In advanced cases, mental disturbances may also occur. Laboratory tests reveal abnormalities in the erythrocytes in the blood and in the bone marrow. Gastric analysis shows an absence of hydrochloric acid and perhaps even an absence of gastric juice.

TREATMENT. Pernicious anemia is successfully treated by regular injections of vitamin B_{12}, given several times a week at first and monthly after the condition has been brought under control. This treatment must be lifelong to prevent relapse. The injections do not cure the disease but arrest it by providing the body directly with the necessary vitamin that it fails to absorb from the digestive tract. Special diets, liver extract, and other medications taken by mouth usually are not required since the basic defect is not dietary deficiency but improper use of food ingested.

Pernicious anemia is believed to be inherited. The disease occurs usually after the age of 35, and it is more common in persons of Scandinavian, Irish, and English descent. Although no cure is known, most patients who continue with treatments can look forward to a normal life span with good health and normal activities.

See also ANEMIA for patient care.

pernio (per′ne-o) chilblain.

pero- word element [Gr.], *deformity; maimed.*

perobrachius (pe″ro-bra′ke-us) a fetus with deformed arms.

perocephalus (pe″ro-sef′ah-lus) a fetus with a deformed head.

perochirus (pe″ro-ki′rus) a fetus with deformed hands.

peromelia (pe″ro-me′le-ah) congenital deformity of the limbs.

peromelus (pe″rom′ĕ-lus) a fetus with deformed limbs.

peroneal (per″o-ne′al) pertaining to the fibula or to the outer side of the leg; fibular.

p. nerve, common, a nerve originating in the sciatic nerve and innervating the calf and foot. (See also table of NERVES.)

peropus (pe′ro-pus) a fetus with malformed legs and feet.

peroral (per-o′ral) performed or administered through the mouth.

per os (per os) [L.] by mouth.

peroxidase (pĕrok′sĭdās) any of a group of iron-porphyrin enzymes that catalyze the oxidation of some organic substrates in the presence of hydrogen peroxide.

peroxide (pĕ-rok′sīd) that oxide of any element containing more oxygen than any other; more correctly applied to compounds having such linkage as —O—O—.

hydrogen p., H_2O_2, an antiseptic with a mildly antibacterial action. A 3 per cent solution foams on touching skin or mucous membrane and appears to have a mechanical cleansing action.

peroxisome (pĕ-roks′ĭ-sōm) a cellular microbody isolated from mitochondrial and lysosomal fractions that contains urate oxidase, amino acid oxidase, catalase, and other enzymes.

perphenazine (per-fen′ah-zēn) a phenothiazine compound used as a tranquilizer and antiemetic.

per primam (intentionem) (per pri′mam in-ten″she-o′nem) [L.] by first intention (see HEALING).

per rectum (per rek′tum) by way of the rectum.

Persantine (per-san′tēn) trademark for preparations of dipyridamole, a coronary vasodilator.

per secundam (intentionem) (per se-kun′dam in-ten″she-o′nem) [L.] by second intention (see HEALING).

perseveration (per-sev″er-a′shun) persistent repetition of the same verbal or motor response to varied stimuli; continuance of activity after cessation of the causative stimulus.

persona (per-so′nah) Jung's term for the personality "mask" or facade presented by a person to the outside world, as opposed to the anima, the unconscious, or inner being, of a person.

personality (per″sŏ-nal′ĭ-te) that which constitutes, distinguishes, and characterizes a person as an entity over a period of time; the total reaction of a person to his environment. Many factors that determine personality are inherited; they are shaped and modified by the individual's environment. Students of human behavior have long debated whether inherited traits or life experiences play the greater role in molding personality. They all agree, however, on the influence of the early years on personality development.

EARLY LIFE AND PERSONALITY. The infant comes into the world completely dependent on others for his basic needs. His feelings of security in a relationship with his mother, or an adequate substitute, is the cornerstone of his mental health in later years.

As a child develops, he needs to learn and to meet the day-to-day problems of life, and to master them. In resolving these challenges, he chooses his solutions from many possibilities. He must substitute other ways of behavior for his many natural antisocial impulses. Psychologists have studied how these choices are made and use technical terms to describe them, such as repression and sublimation. The behavior patterns chosen result in certain character traits which will influence a child's way of meeting the world—whether he will lead or follow, be conscientious or reckless, imitate his parents or prefer to be as different from them as possible, or take a realistic, flexible path between these extremes. The sum total of these traits represents the personality.

THE WELL ADJUSTED PERSONALITY. A well adjusted individual is one who adjusts himself to his surroundings, the world he lives in, and the people in it. If he cannot, he makes realistic efforts to change the situation. He also uses his abilities constructively and successfully.

The well adjusted person is realistic. He faces facts whether they are pleasant or unpleasant and deals with them instead of merely worrying about them or denying them.

The mature person is independent. He forms reasoned opinions and then acts on them. He seeks a reasonable amount of information and advice before making a decision. Once the decision is made, he is willing to face the consequences of it. He does not attempt to force others to make decisions for him.

An ability to love others is typical of the well adjusted individual. On the other hand, the mature person is also able to enjoy receiving love and affection. He can accept a reasonable dependence on others.

The well adjusted individual has the ability to make long-range choices and to forego immediate pleasures for the sake of these long-range goals. He is also able to reevaluate these goals and change them if necessary.

The mature person can get angry, but his anger is directed at rational targets. When the occasion demands, he can be stirred to fierce anger, but he never loses sight of the reason for his anger or of what he hopes to accomplish with it. He is not a chronic worrier. He usually likes his work and does it well, but it is not his entire life.

Finally, the mature person has the capacity for continued emotional growth. He continues to deepen his understanding of others throughout his life.

Naturally, few people meet all these qualifications of the ideally developed prsonality, just as few people are in perfect physical health.

DISORDERS OF PERSONALITY. In addition to specific types of mental illness, such as NEUROSIS and PSYCHOSIS, there are a number of what are known as personality or character disorders. In general these are difficult both to diagnose and to treat.

Terms that are often used to describe persons with disturbed personalities are neurotic or neurotic character. Such persons are able to function in their daily life, but are emotionally and psychologically "crippled" by inadequate or unstable personalities, and their chances of forming good relationships and fulfilling their potentialities are poor. Among the patterns often encountered in such persons are either passive or aggressive reactions to life, in which the person is excessively dependent on other people or hostile to them. Sometimes his behavior represents a combination of both attitudes. Other personality types have traits that show some similarity to the symptoms of the three major types of psychosis—schizophrenia, paranoia, and affective psychosis—although these people are not psychotic. They are referred to as schizoid, paranoid, or cyclothymic personalities.

A special form of personality disorder is the PSYCHOPATHIC PERSONALITY, or sociopathic personality. A person with this disorder shows abnormal behavior patterns, although they differ from the patterns observed in neurosis and psychosis. He may have a greatly exaggerated sense of self-importance, and his emotions are often very shallow. Some of the problems of the psychopathic personality can include sexual deviation, alcoholism, and drug addiction. Certain kinds of criminals belong in this group.

Although personality disorders are more difficult to treat than other forms of mental illness, a great deal can be done in many cases. Since these disorders are the result of unresolved emotional conflicts, often dating back to childhood, the treatment attempts to uncover the roots of these conflicts and to help the patient resolve them. The various techniques for doing this are included under the term PSYCHOTHERAPY.

alternating p., see multiple PERSONALITY.

antisocial p., a personality disorder in which repetitive antisocial behavior is associated with ego eccentricity, lack of guilt or anxiety, and imperviousness to punishment. Called also psychopathic personality.

cyclothymic p., a personality marked by alternate moods of elation and dejection.

double p., dual p., see multiple PERSONALITY.

multiple p., a dissociative reaction in which an individual adopts two or more personalities alternatively, in none of which is he aware of the experiences of the other(s).

psychopathic p., antisocial personality.

schizoid p., a personality disorder marked by timidness, self-consciousness, introversion, feelings of isolation and loneliness, and failure to form close interpersonal relationships; the individual is frequently ambitious, meticulous, and a perfectionist.

perspiration (per″spĭ-ra′shun) 1. sweating; the excretion of moisture through the pores of the skin. 2. sweat; the salty fluid, consisting largely of water, excreted by the sweat glands in the skin.

The body has approximately 2 million sweat glands. The secretory portion is located in the corium and is connected to the epidermis by a long straight duct. The largest of these glands are in the armpits and groin, but the greatest number per square inch is found on the soles of the feet and the palms of the hands.

In midsummer temperatures—or during strenuous exertion or unusual emotional stress—the body's perspiration output may exceed several quarts per day. On a cool day without exertion or emotional stress, the body loses well over a pint of perspiration. This kind of sweating is known medically as "insensible" perspiration because it is virtually unnoticeable; as the sweat reaches the surface of the skin, it evaporates immediately. When sweating becomes noticeable, it is known as "sensible" perspiration.

FUNCTIONS. The chief role of sweat glands and perspiration is to maintain the body temperature at a constant level. Thus the skin is cooled as perspiration evaporates. The blood in the capillaries of the skin likewise is cooled before it courses back into the body.

The sweat glands have a minor excretory function. Perspiration contains water, sodium chloride, and small amounts of urea, lactic acid, and potassium ions. It also contains antibacterial substances that defend the body against infection.

ABNORMAL PERSPIRATION. Malfunctioning of the sweat glands is somewhat unusual and seldom is cause for alarm unless accompanied by another disease. For example, profuse sweating (diaphoresis) may accompany such diseases as tuberculosis, rickets, and malaria. Night sweats may be a sign of serious disease. Excessive perspiration may also be generated temporarily by shock or by motion sickness or hormonal changes during menopause.

The commonest serious problem from excessive sweating is probably the temporary loss of salt, resulting in a sodium deficiency.

Excessive sweating, or hyperhidrosis, that is not accompanied by disease is sometimes hereditary and is difficult to treat. Diminished or total absence of sweating, or anhidrosis, may occur in the elderly and in those with pronounced thyroid deficiency or severe skin disease. In treating anhidrosis the primary step is to try to cure the condition causing it.

In CYSTIC FIBROSIS the sweat contains an abnormally high content of sodium chloride, and excessive sweating in these patients must be guarded against. In the rare malady called chromhidrosis, the perspiration turns black, blue, green, red, yellow, or a combination of colors. The cause is unknown although certain bacteria may be responsible.

persulfate (per-sul′fāt) a salt of persulfuric acid.

persulfuric acid (per″sul-fu′rik) an oxidized form of sulfuric acid.

per tertiam (intentionem) (per ter′she-am in-ten″she-o′nem) [L.] by third intention (see HEALING).

Perthes' disease (per′tēz) osteochondrosis of the epiphysis of the head of the femur.

Pertophrane (per′to-frān) trademark for a preparation of desipramine, an antidepressent.

per tubam (per tu′bam) [L.] through a tube.

pertussis (per-tus′is) an infectious disease due to *Bordetella pertussis,* and characterized by coryza, bronchitis, and a typical explosive cough ending in crowing or whooping inspiration (see also WHOOPING COUGH).

pertussoid (per-tus′oid) 1. resembling whooping cough. 2. an influenzal cough resembling that of whooping cough.

per vaginam (per vah-ji′nam) [L.] through the vagina.

perversion (per-ver′zhun) deviation from the normal course.

sexual p., sexual deviation, or paraphilia.

pervert (per′vert) a deviant person, especially a paraphiliac.

pes (pes), pl. *pe′des* [L.] foot; the terminal organ of the leg, or lower limb; any footlike part.

p. abduc′tus, a deformity in which the anterior part of the foot is displaced and lies laterally to the vertical axis of the leg.

p. adduc′tus, a deformity in which the anterior part of the foot is displaced and lies medially to the vertical axis of the leg.

p. ca′vus, a foot with an abnormally high longitudinal arch, either congenital or caused by contractures or disturbed muscle balance.

p. hippocam′pi, a formation of two or three elevations on the ventricular surface of the hippocampus.

p. pla′nus, flatfoot.

p. val′gus, flatfoot.

p. va′rus, a permanent toeing-in position of the foot; pigeon toe; talipes varus.

pessary (pes′ah-re) 1. an instrument placed in the vagina to support the uterus or rectum or as a contraceptive device. 2. a medicated vaginal suppository.

pesticide (pes′tĭ-sīd) a poison used to destroy pests of any sort.

pestilence (pes′tĭ-lens) a virulent contagious epidemic or infectious epidemic disease. adj., **pestilen′tial.**

pestle (pes′t′l) an instrument with a rounded end, used in a mortar to reduce a solid to a powder or produce a homogeneous mixture of solids.

-petal word element [L.], *directed* or *moving toward.*

petechia (pe-te′ke-ah), pl. *pete′chiae* [L.] a minute, pinpoint, nonraised, perfectly round, purplish red spot caused by intradermal or submucous hemorrhage, which later turns blue or yellow. adj., **pete′chial.**

pethidine (peth′ĭ-dēn) meperidine, a narcotic analgesic drug.

petiole (pet′e-ōl) a stem, stalk, or pedicle.

epiglottic p., the pointed lower end of the epiglottic cartilage, attached to the thyroid cartilage.

petiolus (pĕ-ti′o-lus) petiole.

Petit's ligament (ptēz) uterosacral ligament.

petit mal (pĕ-te′ mahl) a relatively mild epileptic attack occurring in children, contrasting with grand mal, a major attack. In petit mal, the affected person loses consciousness only momentarily. Often the only outward signs of the attack are twitching of the eyes and mouth and a brief lapse of attention. The facial expression is blank and empty. (See also EPILEPSY.)

petrichloral (pet″rĭ-klo′ral) a hypnotic and sedative.

pétrissage (pa-trĭ-sahzh′) [Fr.] foulage.

petrolatum (pet″ro-la′tum) a purified mixture of hydrocarbons obtained from petroleum; used as a base for ointments, protective dressings, and soothing applications to the skin. Called also petroleum jelly. Two types of liquid petrolatum are recognized, light and heavy (see MINERAL OIL).

petroleum (pĕ-tro′le-um) a thick natural oil obtained from beneath the earth. It consists of a mixture of various hydrocarbons of the paraffin and olefin series.

p. jelly, petrolatum.

petromastoid (pet″ro-mas′toid) 1. pertaining to the petrous portion of the temporal bone and its mastoid process. 2. otocranium (2).

petrosal (pĕ-tro′sal) pertaining to the pars petrosa, or petrous portion of the temporal bone.

petrositis (pet″ro-si′tis) inflammation of the pars petrosa or petrous portion of the temporal bone.

petrosphenoid (pet″ro-sfe′noid) pertaining to the petrous portion of the temporal bone and to the sphenoid bone.

petrosquamous (pet″ro-skwa′mus) pertaining to the petrous and squamous portions of the temporal bone.

petrous (pet′rus) resembling rock or stone; stony.

p. bone, the pars petrosa, or petrous portion of the temporal bone (see also table of BONES).

Peutz-Jeghers syndrome familial gastrointestinal polyposis, especially in the small bowel, associated with mucocutaneous pigmentation.

pexis (pek′sis) 1. the fixation of matter by a tissue. 2. surgical fixation, usually by suturing. adj., **pex′ic.**

-pexy word element [Gr.], *surgical fixation.* adj., **-pec′tic.**

Peyer's patches (pi′erz) whitish, oval, elevated patches of closely packed lymph follicles in mucous and submucous layers of the small intestine.

peyote (pa-o′te) a stimulant drug from mescal buttons, the flowering heads of the cactus *Lophophora williamsii,* whose active principle is mescaline; used by North American Indians in certain ceremonies to produce an intoxication marked by feelings of ecstasy (see also HALLUCINOGEN).

Peyronie's disease (pa-ron-ēz′) induration of the corpora cavernosa of the penis, producing a fibrous chordee.

Pezzer's catheter a self-retaining catheter with a bulbous extremity.

Pfeiffer's disease (pfi′ferz) infectious mononucleosis.

pg. picogram.

PGA pteroylglutamic (folic) acid.

pH symbol, *hydrogen ion concentration;* expresses degree to which a solution is acidic or alkaline. An acid is a substance that can give up a hydrogen ion (H^+); a base is a substance that can accept H^+. The symbol pH connotes the negative logarithm, or p, of the H ion. Because it is a negative logarithm, a higher pH indicates a lower hydrogen ion concentration. The cation H^+ is the basic constituent of all acids; thus, a high hydrogen ion concentration, and inversely a low pH, indicates acidity. A lower H^+ concentration, and a higher pH, indicates alkalinity.

The pH range extends from 0 ("pure" acid) to 14 ("pure" base): pH 7.0 indicates neutrality; a pH of less than 7 indicates acidity, and a pH of more than 7 indicates alkalinity. The pH is used as a measure of whether the body is maintaining a normal ACID-BASE BALANCE. A favorable pH is essential to the functioning of enzymes and other biochemical systems. The body's fluids are normally somewhat alkaline, the pH being between 7.35 and 7.45. A pH above 7.8 or below 6.8 is generally fatal.

phac(o)- word element [Gr.], *lens.* See also words beginning *phako-.*

phacitis (fah-si′tis) phakitis.

phacoanaphylaxis (fak″o-an″ah-fi-lak′sis) hypersensitivity to the protein of the crystalline lens of the eye, induced by escape of material from the lens capsule.

phacocele (fak′o-sēl) hernia of the eye lens.

phacocystectomy (fak″o-sis-tek′to-me) excision of part of the lens capsule for cataract.

phacocystitis (fak″o-sis-ti′tis) inflammation of the capsule of the eye lens.

phacoemulsification (fak″o-e-mul″sĭ-fĭ-ka′shun) a technique of CATARACT extraction, utilizing high-frequency ultrasonic vibrations combined with controlled irrigation to maintain normal pressure in the anterior chamber, and suction to remove lens fragments and irrigating fluid.

phacoerysis (fak″o-er′ĭ-sis) removal of the eye lens in cataract by suction.

phacoid (fak′oid) shaped like a lens.

phacoiditis (fak″oi-di′tis) phakitis.

phacolysis (fah-kol′ĭ-sis) dissolution or discission of the crystalline lens. adj., **phacolyt′ic.**

phacomalacia (fak″o-mah-la′she-ah) softening of the eye lens; a soft cataract, that is, one without a hard nucleus.

phacometachoresis (fak″o-met″ah-ko-re′sis) displacement of the eye lens.

phacosclerosis (fak″o-sklĕ-ro′sis) hardening of the eye lens; a hard cataract, that is, one with a hard nucleus.

phacoscope (fak′o-skōp) an instrument for viewing accommodative changes of the eye lens.

phacotoxic (fak″o-tok′sik) exerting a deleterious effect upon the crystalline lens.

phag(o)- word element [Gr.], *eating; ingestion.*

phage (fāj) bacteriophage.

p. type, an intraspecies type of bacterium demonstrated by phage typing; called also lysotype and phagotype.

p. typing, characterization of bacteria, extending to strain differences, by demonstration of susceptibility to one or more (a spectrum) races of bacteriophage; widely applied to staphylococci, typhoid bacilli, etc., for epidemiological purposes.

phagedena (faj″ĕ-de′nah) rapidly spreading and sloughing ulceration.

-phagia, -phagy word element [Gr.], *eating; swallowing.*

phagocyte (fag′o-sīt) any cell that ingests microorganisms or other cells and foreign particles. adj., **phagocyt′ic.**

phagocytin (fag″o-si′tin) a bactericidal substance from neutrophilic leukocytes.

phagocytize (fag′o-sĭ-tīz) phagocytose.

phagocytoblast (fag″o-si′to-blast) a cell giving rise to phagocytes.

phagocytolysis (fag″o-si-tol′ĭ-sis) destruction of phagocytes. adj., **phagocytolyt′ic.**

phagocytose (fag″o-si′tōs) to envelop and destroy bacteria and other foreign material; phagocytize.

phagocytosis (fag″o-si-to′sis) the engulfing of microorganisms or other cells and foreign particles by phagocytes.

phagodynamometer (fag″o-di″nah-mom′ĕ-ter) an apparatus for measuring the force exerted in chewing food.

phagokaryosis (fag″o-kar″e-o′sis) phagocytosis allegedly effected by the cell nucleus.

phagomania (fag″o-ma′ne-ah) an insatiable craving for food or an obsessive preoccupation with the subject of eating.

phagosome (fag′o-sōm) a membrane-bound vesicle in a phagocyte containing the phagocytized material.

phagotype (fag′o-tīp) phage type.

phak(o)- see *phac(o)-*.

phakitis (fa-ki′tis) inflammation of the crystalline lens of the eye.

phakoma (fah-ko′mah) 1. an occasional small, grayish white tumor seen microscopically in the retina in tuberous sclerosis. 2. a patch of myelinated nerve fibers seen very infrequently in the retina in neurofibromatosis.

phakomatosis (fak″o-mah-to′sis) any of four hereditary syndromes (neurofibromatosis, tuberous sclerosis, Sturge-Weber syndrome, and von Hippel-Lindau disease) marked by disseminated hamartomas of the eye, skin, and brain.

phalangeal (fah-lan′je-al) pertaining to a phalanx.

phalangectomy (fal″an-jek′to-me) excision of a phalanx.

phalangitis (fal″an-ji′tis) inflammation of one or more phalanges.

phalanx (fa′langks), pl. *phalan′ges* [Gr.] any bone of a finger or toe. adj., **phalan′geal.** (See also table of BONES.)

phallectomy (fal-ek′to-me) amputation of the penis.

phallic (fal′ik) pertaining to the penis.

phallitis (fal-i′tis) penitis.

phallocampsis (fal″o-kamp′sis) curvature of the penis during erection.

phalloidin, phalloidine (fah-loid′in) a hexapeptide poison from the mushroom *Amanita phalloides,* which causes asthenia, vomiting, diarrhea, convulsions, and death.

phallus (fal′us) the penis. adj., **phal′lic.**

phanerosis (fan″er-o′sis) the process of becoming visible.

Phanodorn (fan′o-dorn) trademark for a preparation of cyclobarbital, a barbiturate.

phantasm (fan′tazm) phantom (1).

phantom (fan′tom) 1. an image or impression not evoked by actual stimuli. 2. a model of the body or of a specific part thereof. 3. a device for simulating the *in vivo* effect of radiation on tissues.

p. pain, pain felt as if it were arising in an absent (amputated) limb. (See also AMPUTATION.)

phar., pharm. pharmacy; pharmaceutical; pharmacopeia.

pharmac(o)- word element [Gr.], *drug; medicine.*

pharmaceutical (far″mah-su′tĭ-kal) 1. pertaining to pharmacy or drugs. 2. a medicinal drug.

pharmaceutics (far″mah-su′tiks) 1. pharmacy (1). 2. pharmaceutical preparations.

pharmacist (far′mah-sist) one who is licensed to prepare and sell or dispense drugs and compounds, and to make up prescriptions. Called also druggist.

pharmacodiagnosis (far″mah-ko-di″ag-no′sis) use of drugs in diagnosis.

pharmacodynamics (far″mah-ko-di-nam′iks) the study of the action of drugs on living systems. adj., **pharmacodynam′ic.**

pharmacogenetics (fahr″mah-ko-jĕ-net′iks) the study of the relationship between genetic factors and the nature of responses to drugs.

pharmacognosy (fahr″mah-kog′no-se) the branch of pharmacology dealing with natural drugs and their constituents.

pharmacologist (fahr″mah-kol′o-jist) a specialist in pharmacology.

pharmacology (fahr″mah-kol′o-je) the scientific study of the action of drugs on living systems. adj., **pharmacolog′ic.**

pharmacomania (far″mah-ko-ma′ne-ah) uncontrollable desire to take or to administer drugs.

pharmacopeia (far″mah-ko-pe′ah) an authoritative treatise on drugs and their preparations. (See also U.S.P.) adj., **pharmacopei′al.**

pharmacophobia (far″mah-ko-fo′be-ah) morbid dread of medicines or drugs.

pharmacophore (far′mah-ko-for″) the group of atoms in the molecule of a drug responsible for the drug's action.

pharmacopoeia (far″mah-ko-pe′ah) pharmacopeia.

pharmacopsychosis (far″mah-ko-si-ko′sis) a group of mental diseases due to alcohol, drugs, or poisons.

pharmacotherapy (far″mah-ko-ther′ah-pe) treatment of disease with medicines.

pharmacy (far′mah-se) 1. the art of preparing, compounding, and dispensing medicines. 2. a place for the preparation, compounding, and dispensing of drugs and medicinal supplies.

pharyng(o)- word element [Gr.], *pharynx.*

pharyngalgia (far″ing-gal′je-ah) pain in the pharynx.

pharyngeal (far-rin′je-al) pertaining to the pharynx.

p. reflex, gag reflex.

pharyngectomy (far″in-jek′to-me) excision of part of the pharynx.

pharyngemphraxis (far″in-jem-frak′sis) obstruction of the pharynx.

pharyngismus (far″in-jiz′mus) muscular spasm of the pharynx.

pharyngitis (far″in-ji′tis) inflammation of the pharynx. adj., **pharyngit′ic.**

Acute pharyngitis usually appears suddenly and runs its course in a few days or a week. Symptoms, more severe in children, are dry, sore throat, fatigue, and mild fever. Often, swallowing is painful, the head aches, and there is a harsh cough and a persistent desire to clear the throat. The throat frequently becomes swollen and covered with a thick mucous material. Sometimes there is pain in the ears, or hoarseness. In most cases, treatment is similar to that for a cold: rest, liquids, aspirin, and, when prescribed, antibiotics.

Chronic pharyngitis is the result of continuous reinfection or chronic irritation of exposed parts of the throat. It is similar to acute pharyngitis, but less severe. The simple catarrhal form can be caused by smoking, dust, smog, or constant breathing through the mouth.

Symptomatic treatment includes hot saline gargles, liquid diet, and an increase in fluid intake. Sulfonamides or antibiotics may be prescribed when a bacterial infection is present.

The symptoms of pharyngitis can occur during the early stages of such diseases as scarlet fever, measles, and whooping cough.

pharyngocele (fah-ring'go-sēl) a herniation or cystic deformity of the pharynx.

pharyngoconjunctival fever (fah-ring"go-kon"-jung-ti'val) an epidemic disease due to an adenovirus, occurring chiefly in school children, with fever, pharyngitis, conjunctivitis, rhinitis, and enlarged cervical lymph nodes.

pharyngodynia (fah-ring"go-din'e-ah) pain in the pharynx.

pharyngoesophageal (fah-ring"go-e-sof"ah-je'al) pertaining to the pharynx and esophagus.

pharyngoglossal (fah-ring"go-glos'al) pertaining to the pharynx and tongue.

pharyngokeratosis (fah-ring"go-ker"ah-to'sis) keratosis of the pharynx.

pharyngolaryngitis (fah-ring"go-lar"in-ji'tis) inflammation of the pharynx and larynx.

pharyngomycosis (fah-ring"go-mi-ko'sis) any fungal infection of the pharynx.

pharyngonasal (fah-ring"go-na'zal) pertaining to the pharynx and nose.

pharyngoparalysis (fah-ring"go-pah-ral'ĭ-sis) paralysis of the pharyngeal muscles; pharyngoplegia.

pharyngoperistole (fah-ring"go-pĕ-ris'to-le) pharyngostenosis.

pharyngoplasty (fah-ring'go-plas"te) plastic repair of the pharynx.

pharyngoplegia (fah-ring"go-ple'je-ah) pharyngoparalysis.

pharyngorhinitis (fah-ring"go-ri-ni'tis) inflammation of the nasopharynx.

pharyngorrhea (far"ing-go-re'ah) mucous discharge from the pharynx.

pharyngoscleroma (fah-ring"go-skle-ro'mah) scleroma of the pharynx.

pharyngoscope (fah-ring'go-skōp) an instrument for inspecting the pharynx.

pharyngoscopy (far"ing-gos'ko-pe) direct visual examination of the pharynx.

pharyngospasm (fah-ring'go-spazm) spasm of the pharyngeal muscles.

pharyngostenosis (fah-ring"go-stĕ-no'sis) narrowing of the pharynx; pharyngoperistole.

pharyngotomy (far"ing-got'o-me) incision of the pharynx.

pharynx (far'ingks) the throat; the musculomembranous cavity, about 5 inches long, behind the nasal cavities, mouth, and larynx, communicating with them and with the esophagus.

The pharynx includes many individual structures and may be divided into three areas: the nasopharynx (top), oropharynx (center, behind the mouth), and laryngopharynx (bottom). The nasopharynx, connected with the nasal cavities, provides a passage for air during breathing; it also contains the openings of the eustachian tubes through which air enters the middle ear. The oropharynx and laryngopharynx provide passageways for both air and food. The pharynx also functions as a resonating organ in speech.

The pharynx is separated from the mouth by the soft palate and its fleshy V-shaped extension or flap, the uvula, which hangs from the top of the back of the mouth, above the root of the tongue. In swallowing, the uvula lifts up, closing off the nasopharynx as food passes from the mouth through the lower parts of the pharynx to the esophagus. On each side of the entrance to the pharynx from the mouth, and behind the nasal passage, are the TONSILS and ADENOIDS, masses of lymphoid tissue.

The most common disorders of the pharynx are PHARYNGITIS and the inflammation and discomfort resulting from TONSILLITIS.

phase (fāz) 1. one of the aspects or stages through which a varying entity may pass. 2. In physical chemistry, a component that is homogeneous of itself, bounded by an interface, and mechanically separable from other phases of the system.

continuous p., in a heterogeneous system, the component in which the disperse phase is distributed, corresponding to the solvent in a true solution.

disperse p., the discontinuous portion of a heterogeneous system, corresponding to the solute in a true solution.

phasmid (faz'mid) 1. either of the two caudal chemoreceptors occurring in certain nematodes (Phasmidia). 2. any nematode containing phasmids.

Phe-Mer-Nite (fe'mer-nīt) trademark for preparations of phenylmercuric nitrate, used as a bacteriostatic.

Phemerol (fe'mer-ol) trademark for preparations of benzethonium, a local antiseptic.

phenacaine (fen'ah-kān) a topical anesthetic.

phenacemide (fĕ-nas'ĕ-mīd) an anticonvulsant used in psychomotor and grand mal epilepsy.

phenacetin (fĕ-nas'ĕ-tin) a white crystalline powder with antipyretic properties but used primarily as an analgesic in the relief of common aches and pains such as headache, neuralgia, and dysmenorrhea. Called also acetophenetidin. The drug must be used with caution because its continued overdose can lead to serious renal and hematologic complications. Preparations of phenacetin must be labeled with the following warning: Do not take regularly for more than 10 days unless directed to do so by a physician.

phenaglycodol (fen"ah-gli'ko-dol) a sedative.

phenanthrene (fe-nan'thrēn) a colorless, crystalline hydrocarbon.

phenazocine (fĕ-naz'o-sēn) a narcotic analgesic, used as the hydrobromide salt.

phenazopyridine (fen"ah-zo-pēr'ĭ-dēn) a urinary analgesic, used as the hydrochloride salt.

phencarbamide (fen-kar′bah-mīd) an anticholinergic.

phencyclidine (fen-si′klĭ-dēn) an anesthetic.

phenelzine (fen′el-zēn) an antidepressant, used as the sulfate salt.

Phenergan (fen′er-gan) trademark for preparations of promethazine, an antihistaminic.

phenethicillin (fĕ-neth″ĭ-sil′in) phenoxymethyl penicillin.

phenformin (fen-for′min) a synthetic hypoglycemic drug whose action is not yet completely understood; it is not related to other hypoglycemic agents such as tolbutamide or chlorpropamide in activity and chemical structure. Phenformin is no longer approved for use in the United States.

phenindamine (fĕ-nin′dah-min) an antihistaminic, used as the tartrate salt.

phenindione (fen-in′di-ōn) an anticoagulant.

pheniramine (fĕ-nir′ah-min) an antihistaminic, used as the maleate salt.

Phenistix (fen′ĭ-stiks) trademark for a reagent strip impregnated with ferric chloride and glacial acetic acid; used in screening tests for phenylketonuria and in detection of salicylates and chlorpromazine in the urine.

phenmetrazine (fen-met′rah-zēn) a central nervous stimulant, used as an anorexic in the form of the hydrochloride salt.

phenobarbital (fe″no-bar′bĭ-tal) a hypnotic, anticonvulsant, and sedative.

phenocopy (fe′no-kop″e) 1. an environmentally induced phenotype mimicking one usually produced by a specific genotype. 2. an individual exhibiting such a phenotype; the simulated trait in a phenocopy.

phenol (fe′nol) 1. an extremely poisonous compound obtained by distillation of coal tar or produced synthetically; used as an antimicrobial. Called also carbolic acid. Ingestion or absorption of phenol through the skin causes colic, weakness, collapse, and local irritation and corrosion. Phenol should be properly labeled and stored to avoid accidental poisoning. 2. any organic compound containing one or more hydroxyl groups attached to an aromatic or carbon ring.

p. coefficient, a measure of the bactericidal activity of a chemical compound in relation to phenol. The activity of the compound is expressed as the ratio of dilution in which it kills in 10 minutes but not in 5 minutes under the specified conditions. It can be determined in the absence of organic matter, or in the presence of a standard amount of added organic matter.

liquefid p., phenol maintained in liquid state by the presence of 10 per cent of water; used in diluted form in preparations for use on the skin.

p. red, phenolsulfonphthalein.

phenolphthalein (fe″nol-thal′ēn) a cathartic.

phenolsulfonphthalein (fe″nol-sul″fōn-thal′ēn) PSP, a dye used in testing kidney function, particularly renal blood flow and tubular function. The PSP test is less accurate than some other renal function tests because damage to the kidney cells must be rather extensive before positive results are obtained. The dye is given intravenously or intramuscularly; in both instances the patient may have a light breakfast and one glass of water, but no coffee or tea. In the intravenous test, the patient first drinks a glass of water and a urine specimen is collected 15 minutes later. At this time he drinks another glass of water, and then urine specimens are collected 1 hour and 2 hours after the dye has been administered. The intramuscular test is similar except that the last two urine specimens are collected 1 hour and 10 minutes, and 2 hours and 10 minutes, after injection of the dye.

phenomenon (fĕ-nom′ĕ-non), pl. *phenom′ena.* any sign or objective symptom; any observable occurrence or fact. For specific phenomena, see specific names, as RAYNAUD'S PHENOMENON.

phenopropazine (fe″no-pro′pah-zēn) ethopropazine, used to produce parasympathetic blockade and to reduce tremors in Parkinson's disease.

phenothiazine (fe″no-thi′ah-zēn) a veterinary anthelmintic; also used to denote a group of major tranquilizers resembling phenothiazine in molecular structure.

phenotype (fe′no-tīp) 1. the outward, visible expression of the hereditary constitution of an organism. 2. an individual exhibiting a certain phenotype; a trait expressed in a phenotype. adj., **phenotyp′ic.**

Phenoxene (fĕ-nok′sēn) trademark for a preparation of chlorphenoxamine, used to reduce muscular rigidity in parkinsonism.

phenoxybenzamine (fĕ-nok″se-ben′zah-mēn) an adrenergic blocking agent; the hydrochloride salt is used as a vasodilator and sometimes as an antihypertensive.

phenozygous (fe″no-zi′gus) having the calvaria narrower than the face, so that the zygomatic arches are visible when the head is viewed from above.

phenprocoumon (fen-pro′koo-mon) an anticoagulant of the coumarin type.

phensuximide (fen-suk′sĭ-mīd) an anticonvulsant.

phentermine (fen′ter-mēn) an anorexic.

phentetiothalein (fen″tĕ-ti′o-thal′e-in) a compound whose sodium salt is used as a radiopaque medium and as a test of liver function.

phentolamine (fen-tol′ah-mēn) a potent alpha-adrenergic blocking agent; it blocks the hypertensive action of epinephrine and norepinephrine and most responses of smooth muscles that involve alpha-adrenergic cell receptors. Its hydrochloride and mesylate salts are used in the diagnosis of hypertension due to pheochromocytoma.

Phenurone (fen′u-rōn) trademark for a preparation of phenacemide, an anticonvulsant.

phenyl (fen′il, fe′nil) the monovalent radical, C_6H_5. adj., **phenyl′ic.**

phenylalanine (fen″il-al′ah-nīn) a naturally occurring amino acid essential for optimal growth in infants and for nitrogen equilibrium in human adults.

phenylbutazone (fen″il-bu′tah-zōn) a drug with analgesic, antipyretic, and anti-inflammatory properties, used as an antirheumatic.

phenylephrine (fen″il-ef′rin) an adrenergic used as the hydrochloride salt for its potent vasoconstrictor properties.

phenylhydrazine (fen″il-hi′drah-zēn) a reagent for sugars, ketones, and aldehydes; the hydrochloride salt is used in the treatment of polycythemia vera.

phenylketonuria (fen″il-ke″to-nu′re-ah) PKU, a

Exchange Lists for Low Phenylalanine Diet

Food	Amount
List I – Lofenalac	
30 Mg. Phenylalanine – 2 Equivalents†	
Lofenalac‡ (dry)	4 tbsp.
Lofenalac (reconstituted)	1 c.
List II – Vegetables	
15 Mg. Phenylalanine – 1 Equivalent	
Beans, green	
Strained and chopped	1 1/2 tbsp.
Regular	3 tbsp.
Beets	
Strained	2 tbsp.
Regular	3 tbsp.
Cabbage, raw, shredded	4 tbsp.
Carrots	
Strained and chopped	3 tbsp.
Raw	1/4 large
Canned	4 tbsp.
Celery, raw	1 1/2 small stalks
Cucumber, raw	1/3 medium
Lettuce, head	2 leaves
Spinach, creamed – strained and chopped	1 1/2 tbsp.
Squash	
Winter	
Strained	3 tbsp.
Chopped	6 tbsp.
Cooked	2 tbsp.
Summer, cooked	4 tbsp.
Tomato	
Raw	1/4 small
Canned	2 tbsp.
Juice	2 1/2 tbsp.
List III – Fruits	
15 Mg. Phenylalanine – 1 Equivalent	
Apple	2 medium-large
Apricots, dried	4 large halves
Banana	1/2 med.
Cantaloupe	1/2 c. diced
Dates, dried	2
Fruit cocktail, canned	2 1/2 tbsp.
Grapefruit	
Sections	1/3 c.
Juice	1/3 c.
Orange	1 medium
Sections	2/3 c.
Juice	3 tbsp.
Grape juice	1/3 c.
Lemon juice	3 tbsp.
Nectarine	1 medium
Peaches	
Raw	1 medium
Canned in syrup	1 1/2 halves
Strained	5 tbsp.
Chopped	7 tbsp.
Pears	
Raw	1 1/3 medium
Canned in syrup	3 halves
Strained and chopped	10 tbsp.
Pears and pineapple, strained and chopped	7 tbsp.
Pineapple	
Raw	1/3 c.
Canned in syrup	1 1/2 small slices
Juice	1/2 c.
Plums, canned in syrup	1 1/2 medium
Plums with tapioca	
Strained	5 tbsp.
Chopped	7 tbsp.
Prunes	
Cooked	2 large
Juice	1/3 c.
Strained	3 tbsp.
Raisins	2 tbsp.
Strawberries	3 large
Tangerine	2/3 small
Watermelon	2/3 c.
List IV – Breads	
30 Mg. Phenylalanine – 2 Equivalents	
Barley cereal, Gerber's, dry	2 1/3 tbsp.
Biscuits[a]	1 small
Cereal food, Gerber's, dry	2 tbsp.
Cookies, arrowroot	1 1/2
Corn	2 tbsp.
Cornflakes	1/3 c.
Crackers	
Barnum animal	6
Saltines	3
Cream of Wheat, cooked	2 tbsp.
Farina, cooked	2 1/2 tbsp.
Mixed cereal, pablum, dry	1 2/3 tbsp.
Oatmeal	
Gerber's strained	1 2/3 tbsp.
Pablum, dry	1 2/3 tbsp.
Potatoes, Irish	2 1/2 tbsp.
Rice Flakes, Quaker	1/3 c.
Rice Krispies, Kellogg's	1/3 c.
Rice, Puffed, Quaker	1/2 c.
Sugar Crisps	1/4 c.
Sweet potatoes or yams	
Cooked	3 tbsp.
Strained	4 tbsp.
Wafers, sugar, Nabisco	6
Wheat, Puffed, Quaker	1/3 c.
List V – Fats	
5 Mg. Phenylalanine – 1/3 Equivalent	
Butter	1 tsp.
Cream, heavy	1 tsp.
Margarine	1 tbsp.
Mayonnaise	1 1/2 tbsp.
Olives, ripe	1 large
List VI – Desserts	
30 Mg. Phenylalanine – 2 Equivalents	
Cookies	
Rice flour	2
Corn starch	2
Ice cream[a]	
Chocolate	1/3 c.
Pineapple	1/3 c.
Strawberry	1/3 c.
Vanilla	1/3 c.
Puddings[a]	1/3 c.
Sauce, Hershey syrup	2 tbsp.
List VII – Free Foods; Little or No Phenylalanine; May Be Used as Desired	
Candy	
Butterscotch	–
Cream mints	–
Fondant	–
Gum drops	–
Hard	–
Jelly beans	–
Lollipops	–
Cornstarch	–
Guava butter	–
Honey	–
Jams, jellies, and marmalades	–
Molasses	–
Oil	–

EXCHANGE LISTS FOR LOW PHENYLALANINE DIET *(Concluded)*

FOOD	AMOUNT	FOOD	AMOUNT
Sauces		*List VIII – Foods to Avoid; High Phenylalanine Content; May Be Used Only Occasionally in Very Small Portions*	
Lemon[a]	–	Breads, most	–
White[a]	–	Cheeses of all kinds	–
Syrups		Eggs	–
Corn	–	Legumes, dried	–
Maple	–	Meat, poultry, fish	–
Sugar		Milk#	–
Brown	–	Nuts	–
White	–	Nut butters	–
Tapioca	–		

From Krause, M. V.: Food, Nutrition and Diet Therapy. 4th ed. Philadelphia, W. B. Saunders Co., 1966; adapted from Phenylketonuria. Children's Bureau Pub. No. 388, U. S. Department of Health, Education, and Welfare, Social Security Adm., Washington, D.C., 1961, and Miller, G. T., et al.: Phenylalanine content of fruit. J. Amer. Diet. Ass., 46:43, 1965.

†One equivalent may be defined as providing 15 mg. phenylalanine.

‡Mead Johnson & Company.

[a]Special recipe must be used.

#Milk is high in phenylalanine (1 oz. contains 50 mg.), but it may be ordered in infants to keep phenylalanine blood levels up to normal.

congenital disease due to a defect in the metabolism of the amino acid phenylalanine. adj., **phenylketonu'ric.** The condition is hereditary and is transmitted recessively through apparently healthy parents who, if tested, will show signs of the disease. It results from lack of an enzyme, phenylalanine hydroxylase, necessary for the conversion of the amino acid phenylalanine into tyrosine. Thus there is accumulation of phenylalanine in the blood with eventual excretion of phenylpyruvic acid in the urine. If untreated, the condition results in mental retardation and other abnormalities.

Persons with phenylketonuria are usually blue-eyed and blond, with defective pigmentation, the skin being excessively sensitive to light and tending to eczema. Other manifestations besides mental retardation are tremors, poor muscular coordination, excessive perspiration, a mousy odor, and perhaps convulsions.

DIAGNOSIS. Screening of newborns for PKU entails a simple test using a urine-wet diaper and Phenistix. The screening is required by law in most states in the United States and in all provinces in Canada. It should be pointed out that not all infants exhibiting excess metabolities in the urine have "classic" PKU. The simple screening test must be followed by more extensive clinical laboratory evaluations to distinguish between the variants of PKU. These variants have been named *hyperphenylalanemia without phenylketonuria* and *atypical PKU.*

The current criteria for establishment of a diagnosis of classic PKU are: (1) a rise in plasma phenylalanine during the first few weeks of life from a level of 1 to 4 mg. per cent at birth to 20 mg. per cent or higher; (2) a normal serum tyrosine level; and (3) urine that contains ortho-hydroxyphenylactic acid during the newborn period, and later contains phenylketones. Diagnosis of variants of the disease depends in part on values of plasma phenylalanine, family history, clinical course, and the infant's response to ingestion of natural protein.

TREATMENT. Restriction of the infant's diet to control the effects of PKU is prescribed on the basis of the individual child's requirements for phenylalanine, protein, and calories. Effectiveness of the special diet must be evaluated by frequent determinations for phenylalanine blood levels; otherwise the child may suffer from serious dietary deficiencies.

The development of a palatable hydrolysate preparation (Lofenalac) has facilitated implementation of the prescribed treatment. About 90 per cent of the protein requirement is derived from this dietary protein substitute.

Although PKU cannot be cured, its effects can be counteracted or prevented altogether by proper management. Research has shown that the mean intelligence quotient of children treated within the first month of life is about 28 points higher than that of either siblings or matched pairs who were treated after the first month or who were never treated.

phenylmercuric (fen″il-mer-ku′rik) denoting a compound containing the radical C_6H_5Hg—, forming various antiseptic, antibacterial, and fungicidal salts; compounds of the acetate and nitrate salts are used as bacteriostatics, and the former is also used as a herbicide.

phenylpropanolamine (fen″il-pro″pah-nol′ah-min) an adrenergic used chiefly as a nasal and sinus decongestant in the form of the hydrochloride salt.

phenylpropylmethylamine (fen″il-pro″pil-meth″il-am′ēn) a vasoconstrictor; its hydrochloride salt is used as a nasal decongestant.

phenylpyruvic acid (fen″il-pi-roo′vik) an intermediate product of the metabolism of phenylalanine in the body.

phenylthiocarbamide (fen″il-thi″o-kar-bam′īd) phenylthiourea.

phenylthiourea (fen″il-thi″o-u-re′ah) a compound used in genetics research, the ability to taste it being determined by a single dominant gene. The compound is intensely bitter to approximately 70 per cent of the population, and nearly tasteless to the rest.

phenyltoloxamine (fen″il-to-lok′sah-mēn) an antihistaminic.

phenyramidol (fen″ĭ-ram′ĭ-dol) an analgesic and

skeletal muscle relaxant; used as the hydrochloride salt.

phenytoin (fen′ĭ-to-in) an anticonvulsant used in the treatment of all forms of epilepsy except petit mal; called also diphenylhydantoin.

pheochrome (fe′o-krōm) chromaffin.

pheochromoblast (fe″o-kro′mo-blast) any of the embryonic structures that develop into chromaffin (pheochrome) cells.

pheochromocyte (fe″o-kro′mo-sīt) a chromaffin cell.

pheochromocytoma (fe″o-kro″mo-si″to′mah) a small chromaffin cell tumor, usually located in the adrenal medulla but occasionally occurring in chromaffin tissue of the sympathetic paraganglia. It is relatively rare and has a tendency to occur in families. The tumor is potentially fatal, but the condition can be cured if diagnosed early, before there has been irreparable damage to the cardiovascular system.

SYMPTOMS. Because the tumor is composed of cells similar to the secreting cells of the adrenal medulla, it is capable of secreting epinephrine and norepinephrine. The symptoms of the tumor are therefore directly related to excessive amounts of these two hormones in the tissues and blood.

The cardinal symptom is hypertension. In some cases the blood pressure is consistently high with slight fluctuations, and in others the hypertension is intermittent with periods of normal blood pressure. Other symptoms include severe headache, sweating, visual blurring, apprehension, tachycardia, and postural hypotension.

DIAGNOSIS. Pheochromocytoma must be differentiated from several other disorders such as essential hypertension and thyrotoxicosis, which it closely resembles. Diagnosis is based on the patient's symptoms and the findings of specific chemical and pharmacologic tests. The test considered most reliable is direct assay of epinephrine and norepinephrine in the plasma and urine following an attack. Another test involving measurement of vanillylmandelic acid (VMA) and of metanephrine and normetanephrine in urine is considered satisfactory. The level of these substances in the urine in patients with pheochromocytoma is almost twice the upper limits of normal.

Two types of pharmacologic tests may be used; one provokes an increase in blood pressure, the other causes a fall in blood pressure. The provocative test uses histamine or methacholine to stimulate action of the tumor and thereby provoke an attack. This test must be given with extreme caution and only when the patient is between attacks and his blood pressure is near normal (less than 170/110 mm. of mercury).

For the patient with sustained hypertension the test of choice involves the administration of an adrenolytic agent such as phentolamine, which will produce hypotension. If, after administration of the drug, the blood pressure decreases to near normal within 3 to 4 minutes and remains depressed for several minutes more, the diagnosis of pheochromocytoma is confirmed.

The pharmacologic tests have largely been replaced by the more reliable and less hazardous hormonal assays. The presence of pheochromocytoma often can be confirmed by radiologic studies.

TREATMENT. Surgical removal of the tumor, or tumors if there are more than one, is necessary for complete remission of symptoms. There are two possible complications of surgery: a sudden rise in blood pressure and development of tachycardia due to discharge of pressor agents as the tumor is being manipulated, and severe hypotension and shock following removal of the tumor. These hazards have been substantially reduced in recent years by the preoperative administration of sedatives and antihypertensive drugs, and the use of blood or plasma to maintain adequate blood volume.

If surgery has involved resection of a portion of the adrenal cortex, it may be necessary for the patient to receive adrenocortical hormones by injection.

PATIENT CARE. Once the diagnosis of pheochromocytoma has been established, the patient is prepared for surgery. The preoperative period may extend for several weeks while attempts are made to stabilize the blood pressure and hormonal imbalances. The patient should be kept in a quiet atmosphere and usually is given sedatives, such as phenobarbital, to promote rest. His blood pressure is taken at frequent intervals and recorded. These readings are used later as a basis for comparison during the postoperative period. They also alert the physician to extremes in blood pressure that are characteristic in this disorder.

A day or two before surgery the patient may be given repeated doses of phentolamine (Regitine) to block the vasoconstricting effects of epinephrine and norepinephrine. The blood pressure may be drastically affected and therefore must be monitored frequently for signs of instability and dangerous extremes.

Postoperatively the patient must again be watched for the development of severe hypertension, which can lead to cerebral vascular accident, and for extreme hypotension with circulatory collapse and profound shock.

If the adrenal cortex has been resected during surgery, hormonal imbalances are likely to occur. These include HYPOGLYCEMIA, addisonian crisis and extreme diuresis, and electrolyte and fluid imbalance. The hypoglycemia is most likely to occur in patients who have had symptoms of diabetes mellitus prior to surgery, and is treated with infusions of glucose solution. Adrenocortical hormones may be administered by slow intravenous drip, the rate of flow being adjusted according to blood pressure readings and other reactions of the patient. The patient's status is closely monitored so that disturbances in ELECTROLYTE and FLUID BALANCE, extremes in blood pressure, and disorders of metabolism can be recognized early and treated promptly.

Ph.G. Graduate in Pharmacy.

pheromone (fer′o-mōn) a substance secreted to the outside of the body and perceived (as by smell) by other individuals of the same species, releasing specific behavior in the percipient.

-philia word element [Gr.], *affinity for; morbid fondness of.* adj., **-phil′ic.**

Philadelphia (Ph^1) chromosome see Philadelphia CHROMOSOME.

philtrum (fil′trum) the vertical groove in the median portion of the upper lip.

phimosis (fi-mo′sis) constriction of the orifice of the prepuce so that it cannot be drawn back over the glans. adj., **phimot′ic.**

pHisoHex (fi′so-heks) trademark for an emulsion

containing hexachlorophene; used as a skin cleanser.

phleb(o)- word element [Gr.], *vein.*

phlebangioma (fleb″an-je-o′mah) a venous aneurysm.

phlebarteriectasia (fleb″ar-te″re-ek-ta′ze-ah) general dilatation of veins and arteries.

phlebectasia (fleb″ek-ta′ze-ah) dilation of a vein or veins; a varicosity.

phlebectomy (flĕ-bek′to-me) excision of a vein, or a segment of a vein.

phlebemphraxis (fleb″em-frak′sis) stoppage of a vein by a plug or clot.

phlebismus (flĕ-biz′mus) obstruction and consequent turgescence of veins.

phlebitis (flĕ-bi′tis) inflammation of a vein. adj., **phlebit′ic.** It is relatively common, especially in the veins of the lower limbs.

Phlebitis is not serious when the inflammation is located in a superficial vein since these veins are numerous enough to permit the flow of blood to be rechanneled, so that the inflamed vein is bypassed. When a deep vein is involved, however, phlebitis is potentially more dangerous. It can also have serious consequences if it occurs in certain areas such as the veins of the cranium, where it may lead to cerebral abscesses.

CAUSES. The causes of phlebitis are uncertain. The disease sometimes occurs for no apparent reason; at other times, it seems to follow a variety of other disorders—for example, circulatory difficulties, blood disorders, and obesity. Phlebitis may be a complication of pneumonia, typhoid fever, or other general infections. It may also be a result of injury to a vein, either after an accident or occasionally as an aftermath of surgery.

Once in about a hundred births phlebitis develops in a newly delivered mother; in such cases it usually appears about 10 days after delivery. This form of phlebitis is commonly called "milk leg," because it is associated with the onset of milk production by the mother.

Phlebitis may also develop when circulation is sluggish after long periods of staying in bed without proper exercising of the limbs and frequent changing of position.

SYMPTOMS AND TREATMENT. When phlebitis occurs in a superficial vein, there is usually pain and tenderness. This may be so slight at first that the tenderness is felt only when pressure is applied to the painful area. As the inflammation increases, the pain becomes more acute, especially during walking or other exercise.

The inflamed area swells and becomes red and warm. A tender cordlike mass may form under the skin; it may grow smaller as the condition subsides, but occasionally lasts for some time.

When the inflammation occurs in a deep vein and affects the vein's inner lining, there may be formation of a thrombus on the vein wall. This condition is known as thrombophlebitis. When clots in the veins interfere with the normal flow of blood, fluid accumulates and causes edema.

If phlebitis is superficial, the patient usually does not have to be confined to bed. Frequently, a supportive elastic dressing is used until the vein is healed.

When deeper veins are affected, however, or if the inflammation is severe, bed rest is required to prevent the clot from being dislodged. Antibiotics are sometimes prescribed to combat infection. Anticoagulants are used and the extremity is elevated to prevent further clots or propagation of the existing clot. In some extreme cases, or when an embolism is likely to occur, surgery may be necessary as a preventive measure.

In persons prone to thrombophlebitis, anticoagulation is used as a preventive measure, particularly when long periods of bed rest are required, such as after surgery.

phleboclysis (flĕ-bok′lĭ-sis) injection of fluid into a vein; venoclysis (see also INTRAVENOUS INFUSION).

phlebogram (fleb′o-gram) 1. a radiogram of a vein filled with contrast medium. 2. a phlebographic or sphygmographic tracing of the venous pulse.

phlebograph (fleb′o-graf) an instrument for recording the venous pulse.

phlebography (flĕ-bog′rah-fe) 1. radiography of a vein filled with contrast medium. 2. the graphic recording of the venous pulse. 3. a description of the veins.

phlebolith (fleb′o-lith) a venous calculus or concretion.

phlebolithiasis (fleb″o-lĭ-thi′ah-sis) the development of phleboliths.

phlebomanometer (fleb″o-mah-nom′ĕ-ter) an instrument for the direct measurement of venous blood pressure.

phlebophlebostomy (fleb″o-flĕ-bost′to-me) operative anastomosis of one vein to another, as of the portal vein and inferior vena cava.

phleboplasty (fleb′o-plas″te) plastic repair of a vein.

phleborrhaphy (flĕ-bor′ah-fe) suture of a vein.

phleborrhexis (fleb″o-rek′sis) rupture of a vein.

phlebosclerosis (fleb″o-sklĕ-ro′sis) fibrous thickening of the walls of veins.

phlebostasis (flĕ-bos′tah-sis) 1. retardation of blood flow in veins. 2. temporary sequestration of a portion of blood from the general circulation by compressing the veins of an extremity.

phlebothrombosis (fleb″o-throm-bo′sis) the development of venous thrombi in the absence of associated inflammation of the vessel wall, as opposed to thrombophlebitis, in which there are inflammatory changes in the vessel wall.

Phlebotomus (flĕ-bot′o-mus) a genus of biting flies, called sandflies, the females of which are blood sucking. They are vectors of various diseases, including kala-azar (*P. argen′tipes, P. chinen′sis, P. marti′ni, P. pernicio′sus*), Carrión's disease (*P. nogu′chi, P. verruca′rum*), cutaneous leishmaniasis (*P. sergen′ti*), and phlebotomus fever (*P. papatas′ii*).

phlebotomus fever (flĕ-bot′o-mus) a febrile viral disease of short duration, transmitted by the sandfly *Phlebotomus papatasii,* with dengue-like symptoms, occurring in Mediterranean and Middle East countries. Called also sandfly fever.

phlebotomy (flĕ-bot′o-me) incision of a vein.

phlegm (flem) viscid mucus excreted in abnormally large quantities from the respiratory tract.

phlegmasia (fleg-ma′ze-ah) inflammation.

p. al′ba do′lens, phlebitis of the femoral vein, with swelling of the leg, usually without redness (milk leg), occasionally following parturition or an acute febrile illness.

p. al'ba do'lens puerpera'rum, phlebitis of the femoral vein in puerperal women.

p. ceru'lea do'lens, an acute fulminating form of deep venous thrombosis, with pronounced edema and severe cyanosis of the extremity.

phlegmatic (fleg-mat'ik) of dull and sluggish temperament.

phlegmon (fleg'mon) cellulitis. adj., **phleg'monous.**

phlog(o)- word element [Gr.], *inflammation.*

phlogogenic (flo"go-jen'ik) producing inflammation.

phlorhizin (flo-ri'zin) a bitter glycoside from the root bark of apple, cherry, plum, and pear trees, which causes glycosuria by blocking the renal tubular reabsorption of glucose.

phloroglucin (flo"ro-gloo'sin) the aglycone of many glycosides, obtained from the bark of apple and other trees; used as a reagent for hydrochloric acid in gastric juice and as a decalcifier of bone specimens.

phlyctena (flik-te'nah) 1. a small blister made by a burn. 2. a small vesicle containing lymph seen on the conjunctiva in certain conditions. adj., **phlyc'tenar.**

phlyctenoid (flik'tĕ-noid) resembling a phlyctena.

phlyctenular (flik-ten'u-lar) associated with the formation of phlyctenules, or of vesicle-like prominences.

phlyctenule (flik'ten-ūl) a minute vesicle; an ulcerated nodule of the cornea or conjunctiva.

phlyctenulosis (flik-ten"u-lo'sis) a condition marked by formation of phlyctenules.

phobia (fo'be-ah) any persistent abnormal dread or fear that appears to result from repressed inner conflicts of which the affected person is not aware. Used as a word ending designating abnormal or morbid fear of or aversion to the subject indicated by the stem to which it is affixed. adj., **pho'bic.**

A person with a phobia reacts uncontrollably and unreasonably to the situation of which he is afraid. A wide variety of exaggerated fears can exist in neurotic persons (see also NEUROSIS).

Some typical phobias are: acrophobia—fear of heights; agoraphobia—fear of open or public places; astraphobia—fear of lightning; cenotophobia—morbid fear of new things or new ideas; claustrophobia—morbid fear of closed places; hemophobia—fear of blood; xenophobia—morbid dread of strangers.

phobophobia (fo"bo-fo'be-ah) morbid fear of being afraid.

phocomelia (fo"ko-me'le-ah) congenital absence of the proximal portion of a limb or limbs, the hands or feet being attached to the trunk by a small, irregularly shaped bone. adj., **phocome'lic.**

phocomelus (fo-kom'ĕ-lus) an individual exhibiting phocomelia.

phon(o)- word element [Gr.], *sound; voice; speech.*

phonal (fo'nal) pertaining to the voice.

phonasthenia (fo"nas-the'ne-ah) weakness of the voice; difficult phonation from fatigue.

phonation (fo-na'shun) the utterance of vocal sounds.

phonatory (fo"nah-to're) subserving or pertaining to phonation.

phoneme (fo'nēm) the smallest distinct unit of sound in speech; the basic unit of spoken language.

phonendoscope (fo-nen'do-skōp) a stethoscopic device that intensifies auscultatory sounds.

phonetic (fo-net'ik) pertaining to the voice or to articulate sounds.

phonetics (fo-net'iks) the science of vocal sounds.

phoniatrics (fo"ne-at'riks) the treatment of speech defects.

phonic (fon'ik, fo'nik) pertaining to the voice.

phonism (fo'nizm) a sensation of hearing produced by the effect of something seen, felt, tasted, smelled, or thought of.

phonocardiogram (fo"no-kar'de-o-gram") the record produced by phonocardiography.

phonocardiograph (fo"no-kar'de-o-graf") the instrument used in phonocardiography.

phonocardiography (fo"no-kar"de-og'rah-fe) the graphic recording of the sounds produced by action of the heart. adj., **phonocardiograph'ic.**

Phonocardiography involves picking up, through a highly sensitive microphone, sonic vibrations from the heart which are then converted into electrical energy and fed into a galvanometer, where they are recorded on paper. The procedure is most useful when there is evidence of heart murmurs or unusual heart sounds, such as gallops, that are difficult to discern by the human ear.

phonocatheter (fo"no-kath'ĕ-ter) a catheter with a device in its tip for picking up and transmitting sound.

phonogram (fo'no-gram) a graphic record of a sound.

phonomassage (fo"no-mah-sahzh') the treatment of ear disease by an apparatus which carries a more or less musical vibration into the auditory canal, stimulating the ossicles.

phonometer (fo-nom'ĕ-ter) a device for measuring the intensity of sounds.

phonomyoclonus (fo"no-mi-ok'lŏ-nus) myoclonus in which a sound is heard on auscultation of an affected muscle, indicating fibrillar contractions.

phonomyogram (fo"no-mi'o-gram) a record produced by phonomyography.

phonomyography (fo"no-mi-og'rah-fe) the recording of sounds produced by muscle contraction.

phonopathy (fo-nop'ah-the) any disease of the organs of speech.

phonophobia (fo"no-fo'be-ah) morbid dread of sounds or of speaking aloud.

phonophotography (fo"no-fo-tog'rah-fe) photographic recording of the movements of a diaphragm set up by sound waves.

phonopneumomassage (fo"no-nu"mo-mah-sahzh') air massage of the middle ear.

phonopsia (fo-nop'se-ah) a visual sensation caused by the hearing of sounds.

phonoreceptor (fo"no-re-sep'tor) a receptor for sound stimuli.

phonorenogram (fo"no-re'no-gram) a record of the sounds produced by pulsation of the renal artery obtained by a phonocatheter passed through a ureter into the renal pelvis.

phonostethograph (fo"no-steth'o-graf) an instrument by which chest sounds are amplified, filtered, and recorded.

-phore word element [Gr.], *a carrier.*

-phoresis word element [Gr.], *transmission.*

phoria (fo′re-ah) any tendency to deviation of the eyes from the normal when fusional stimuli are absent or fusion is otherwise prevented; a latent or usually unmanifested tropia. (See also HETEROPHORIA.)

phorometer (fo-rom′ĕ-ter) an instrument for measuring heterophoria, and more generally the relative strength of the ocular muscles.

Phoroptor (fo-rop′ter) trademark for a phorometer fitted with a battery of cylindrical lenses.

phose (fōz) a subjective visual sensation, as of light or color.

phosgene (fos′jēn) a suffocating and highly poisonous war gas, carbonyl chloride, $COCl_2$.

phosphagen (fos′fah-jen) a group of compounds, including phosphocreatine and phosphoarginine, that are present in tissue and that yield high-energy phosphate on cleavage.

Phosphaljel (fos′fal-jel) trademark for a preparation of aluminum phosphate gel, an antacid, astringent, and demulcent.

phosphatase (fos′fah-tās) any of a group of enzymes capable of catalyzing the hydrolysis of esterified phosphoric acid, with liberation of inorganic phosphate, found in practically all tissues, body fluids, and cells, including erythrocytes and leukocytes.

acid p., a type showing optimal activity at a pH between 3 and 6; found in erythrocytes, prostatic tissue, spleen, kidney, and other tissues.

alkaline p., a type showing optimal activity at a pH of about 9.3; found in bone, liver, kidney, leukocytes, adrenal cortex, and other tissues.

phosphate (fos′fāt) any salt or ester of phosphoric acid. adj., **phosphat′ic.**

Phosphates are widely distributed in the body, the largest amounts being in the bones and teeth. They are continually excreted in the urine and feces, and must be replaced in the diet. Inorganic phosphates function as buffer salts to maintain the ACID-BASE BALANCE in blood, saliva, urine, and other body fluids. The principal phosphates in this buffer system are monosodium and disodium phosphate. Organic phosphates, in particular adenosine triphosphate (ATP), take part in a series of reversible reactions involving phosphoric acid, lactic acid, glycogen, and other substances, which furnish the energy expended in muscle contraction. This is thought to occur through the hydrolysis of the so-called high-energy phosphate bond present in ATP, phosphocreatine, and certain other body compounds.

acid p., any in which only one or two of the hydrogen atoms have been replaced.

calcium p., a compound containing calcium and the phosphate radical (PO_4).

creatine p., phosphocreatine.

normal p., one in which all the hydrogen atoms of the acid have been replaced.

triple p., a calcium, ammonium, and magnesium phosphate, sometimes found in urine.

phosphatemia (fos″fah-te′me-ah) an excess of phosphates in the blood.

phosphaturia (fos″fah-tu′re-ah) an excess of phosphates in the urine.

phosphene (fos′fēn) an objective visual sensation that occurs with the eyes closed, and in the absence of retinal stimulation by visible light.

phosphide (fos′fīd) a binary compound of phosphorus and another element or radical.

phosphite (fos′fīt) any salt of phosphorous acid.

phosphoamidase (fos″fo-am′ĭ-dās) an enzyme that catalyzes the conversion of phosphocreatine to creatine and orthophosphate.

phosphoarginine (fos″fo-ar′jĭ-nin) an arginine–phosphoric acid compound homologous with phosphocreatine, but found in invertebrate muscles.

phosphocreatine (fos″fo-kre′ah-tin) a creatine–phosphoric acid compound occurring in muscle, being the most important storage form of high-energy phosphate, the energy source in muscle contraction.

phosphofructokinase (fos″fo-fruk″to-ki′nās) an enzyme of spermatozoa, which enables them to utilize fructose as an energy source.

phospholipase (fos″fo-lip′ās) any of four enzymes (phospholipase A to D) which catalyze the hydrolysis of a phospholipid.

phospholipid, phospholipin (fos″fo-lip′id; fos″fo-lip′in) a lipid containing phosphorus, which on hydrolysis yields fatty acids, glycerin, and a nitrogenous compound. Lecithin, cephalin, and sphingomyelin are examples.

phosphonecrosis (fos″fo-nĕ-kro′sis) necrosis of the jaw bone due to exposure to phosphorus; called also phossy jaw.

phosphoprotein (fos″fo-pro′te-in) a conjugated protein in which phosphoric acid is esterified with a hydroxy amino acid.

phosphorated (fos′fo-rāt″ed) charged or combined with phosphorus.

phosphorescence (fos″fo-res′ens) the emission of light without appreciable heat; the property of continuing to be luminous in the dark after exposure to light or other radiation. adj., **phosphores′cent.**

phosphoribokinase (fos″fo-ri″bo-ki′nās) an enzyme that catalyzes the conversion of ATP and ribose 5-phosphate to ADP and ribose 1,5-diphosphate.

phosphoribulokinase (fos″fo-ri″bu-lo-ki′nās) an enzyme that catalyzes the conversion of ATP and D-ribulose 5-phosphate to ADP and D-ribulose 1,5-diphosphate.

phosphoric acid (fos-for′ik) a crystalline acid formed by oxidation of phosphorus; its salts are called phosphates.

phosphorism (fos′fo-rizm) chronic PHOSPHORUS poisoning.

phosphorolysis (fos″fo-rol′ĭ-sis) cleavage of a chemical bond with simultaneous addition of the elements of phosphoric acid to the residues.

phosphorous acid (fos′for-us) a dibasic reducing acid; its salts are called phosphites.

phosphoruria (fos″for-u′re-ah) free phosphorus in the urine.

phosphorus (fos′for-us) a chemical element, atomic number 15, atomic weight 30.974, symbol P. (See table of ELEMENTS.) Phosphorus, in combination with calcium, oxygen, and hydrogen, forms the substance of bones. It also plays an important role in cell metabolism. It is obtained by the body from milk products, cereals, meat, and fish, and its use by the body is controlled by vitamin D and calcium.

Phosphorus is very inflammable and exceedingly poisonous. Inhalation of its vapor by workers in chemical industries may cause necrosis of the mandible (phosphonecrosis or phossy jaw). Free phosphorus causes fatty degeneration of the liver and other viscera.

^{32}P, radioactive p., radiophosphorus.

phosphoryl (fos′fōr-il) the trivalent chemical radical ≡P:O.

phosphorylase (fos-for′ĭ-lās) an enzyme that, in the presence of inorganic phosphate, catalyzes the conversion of glycogen into glucose-1-phosphate.

phosphorylation (fos″for-ĭ-la′shun) the process of introducing the trivalent PO (phosphoryl) group into an organic molecule.

phosphotransacetylase (fos″fo-trans″ah-set′ĭ-lās) an enzyme which catalyzes the transfer of an acetyl group between acetylphosphate and acetylcoenzyme A.

phosphotransferase (fos″fo-trans′fer-ās) any of a class of enzymes that catalyze the transfer of a phosphate group.

phot(o)- word element [Gr.], *light*.

photalgia (fo-tal′je-ah) pain, as in the eye, caused by light.

photic (fo′tik) pertaining to light.

photism (fo′tizm) a visual sensation produced by the effect of something heard, felt, tasted, smelled, or thought of.

photobiology (fo″to-bi-ol′o-je) the branch of biology dealing with the effect of light on organisms.

photobiotic (fo″to-bi-ot′ik) living only in the light.

photocatalysis (fo″to-kah-tal′ĭ-sis) promotion or stimulation of a chemical reaction by light. adj., **photocatalyt′ic.**

photocatalyst (fo″to-kat′ah-list) a substance, e.g., chlorophyll, that brings about a chemical reaction on exposure to light.

photochemistry (fo″to-kem′is-tre) the branch of chemistry that deals with the chemical properties or effects of light rays or other radiation. adj., **photochem′ical.**

photochromogen (fo″to-kro′mo-jen) a microorganism whose pigmentation develops as a result of exposure to light. adj., **photochromogen′ic.**

photocoagulation (fo″to-ko-ag″u-la′shun) condensation of protein material by controlled use of light rays, as in treatment of pathologic conditions of the eye, such as retinal detachment.

photodermatitis, photodermatosis (fo″to-der″mah-ti′tis; fo″to-der″mah-to′sis) an abnormal state of the skin in which light is an important causative factor.

photodynamics (fo″to-di-nam′iks) the science of the activating effects of light. adj., **photodynam′ic.**

photodynia (fo″to-din′e-ah) photalgia.

photofluorography (fo″to-floo″or-og′rah-fe) the photographic recording of fluoroscopic images on small films, using a fast lens, a procedure used in mass roentgenography of the chest. Called also fluorography and fluororoentgenography.

photogenic (fo″to-jen′ik) 1. produced by light. 2. emitting or producing light.

photokinetic (fo″to-ki-net′ik) moving in response to the stimulus of light.

photolysis (fo-tol′ĭ-sis) chemical decomposition by light. adj., **photolyt′ic.**

photolyte (fo′to-līt) a substance decomposed by light.

photometer (fo-tom′ĕ-ter) a device for measuring the intensity of light.

photometry (fo-tom′ĕ-tre) measurement of the intensity of light.

photomicrograph (fo″to-mi′kro-graf) a photograph of an object as seen through an ordinary light microscope.

photon (fo′ton) a particle (quantum) of radiant energy.

photo-opthalmia (fo″to-of-thal′me-ah) ophthalmia caused by exposure to intense light, as in snow blindness.

photoperceptive (fo″to-per-sep′tiv) able to perceive light.

photoperiod (fo″to-pēr′e-od) the period of time per day that an organism is exposed to daylight (or to artificial light). adj., **photoperiod′ic.**

photoperiodism (fo-to-pēr″e-o-dizm) the physiologic and behavioral reactions brought about in organisms by changes in the duration of daylight and darkness.

photophilic (fo″to-fil′ik) thriving in light.

photophobia (fo″to-fo′be-ah) abnormal visual intolerance to light. adj., **photopho′bic.**

photophthalmia (fo″tof-thal′me-ah) photo-ophthalmia.

photopia (fo-to′pe-ah) day vision. adj., **photop′ic.**

photopsia (fo-top′se-ah) an appearance as of sparks or flashes, in retinal irritation.

photopsin (fo-top′sin) the protein moiety of the cones of the retina that combines with retinal to form photochemical pigments.

photopsy (fo-top′se) photopsia.

photoptarmosis (fo″to-tar-mo′sis) sneezing caused by the influence of light.

photoptometer (fo″top-tom′ĕ-ter) an instrument for measuring visual acuity by determining the smallest amount of light that will render an object just visible.

photoreactivation (fo″to-re-ak″tĭ-va′shun) reversal of the biological effects of ultraviolet radiation on cells by subsequent exposure to visible light.

photoreception (fo″to-re-sep′shun) the process of detecting radiant energy, usually of wavelengths between 0.39 and 0.77 μm., being the range of visible light.

photoreceptive (fo″to-re-sep′tiv) sensitive to stimulation by light.

photoreceptor (fo″to-re-sep′tor) a nerve end-organ or receptor sensitive to light.

photoretinitis (fo″to-ret″ĭ-ni′tis) retinitis due to exposure to intense light.

photoscan (fo′to-skan) a two-dimensional representation (map) of the gamma rays emitted by a radioisotope, revealing its varying concentration in a body tissue, differing from a scintiscan only in that the printout mechanism is a light source exposing a photographic film.

photosensitive (fo″to-sen′sĭ-tiv) exhibiting abnormally heightened sensitivity to sunlight.

photosensitization (fo″to-sen″sĭ-ti-za′shun) the development of abnormally heightened reactivity of the skin to sunlight.

photostable (fo′to-sta″b′l) unchanged by the influence of light.

photosynthesis (fo″to-sin′thĕ-sis) a chemical combination caused by the action of light; specifically the formation of carbohydrates from carbon dioxide and water in the chlorophyll tissue of plants under the influence of light. adj., **photosynthet′ic.**

phototaxis (fo″to-tak′sis) the movement of cells and microorganisms under the influence of light. adj., **phototac′tic.**

phototherapy (fo″to-ther′ah-pe) treatment of disease by exposure to light as, for example, bilirubinemia in the newborn.

phototoxic (fo″to-tok′sik) having a toxic effect triggered by exposure to light.

phototrophic (fo″to-trof′ik) utilizing light in metabolism, as in certain plants and bacteria.

phototropism (fo-tot′ro-pizm) 1. the tendency of an organism to turn or move toward (positive phototropism) or away from (negative phototropism) light. 2. change of color produced in a substance by the action of light. adj., **phototrop′ic.**

photuria (fo-tu′re-ah) excretion of urine having a luminous appearance.

phren(o)- word element [Gr.], (1) *diaphragm;* (2) *mind.*

phrenalgia (frĕ-nal′je-ah) 1. pain in the diaphragm. 2. melancholia.

phrenemphraxis (fren″em-frak′sis) surgical crushing of the phrenic nerve, phrenicotripsy.

phrenetic (frĕ-net′ik) maniacal.

phrenic (fren′ik) pertaining to the diaphragm or to the mind.

p. nerve, a major branch of the cervical plexus. It extends through the thorax to provide innervation of the diaphragm. Nerve impulses from the inspiratory center in the brain travel down the phrenic nerve, causing contraction of the diaphragm, and inspiration occurs.

phrenicectomy (fren″ĭ-sek′to-me) resection of the phrenic nerve.

phrenicoexeresis (fren″ĭ-ko-ek-ser′ĕ-sis) avulsion of the phrenic nerve.

phrenicotomy (fren″ĭ-kot′o-me) surgical division of the phrenic nerve, causing a one-sided paralysis of the diaphragm with immobilization and compression of a diseased lung.

phrenicotripsy (fren″ĭ-ko-trip′se) phrenemphraxis.

phrenitis (frĕ-ni′tis) 1. delirium or frenzy. 2. diaphragmitis.

phrenocolic (fren″o-kol′ik) pertaining to the diaphragm and colon.

phrenogastric (fren″o-gas′trik) pertaining to the diaphragm and stomach.

phrenohepatic (fren″o-hĕ-pat′ik) pertaining to the diaphragm and liver.

phrenology (frĕ-nol′o-je) the study of the faculties and qualities of mind from the shape of the skull.

phrenoplegia (fren″o-ple′je-ah) 1. a sudden attack of mental disorder. 2. loss or paralysis of the mental faculties. 3. paralysis of the diaphragm.

phrenosin (fren′o-sin) a cerebroside containing cerebronic acid attached to the sphingosine.

phrenotropic (fren″o-trop′ik) exerting its principal effect upon the mind.

phrynoderma (frin″o-der′mah) a follicular hyperkeratosis probably due to deficiency of vitamin A or of essential fatty acids.

phthalylsulfacetamide (thal″il-sul″fah-set′ah-mīd) an intestinal antibacterial.

phthalylsulfathiazole (thal″il-sul″fah-thi′ah-zōl) an intestinal antibacterial.

phthalylsulfonazole (thal″il-sul-fon′ah-zōl) phthalylsulfacetamide.

phthiriasis (thĭ-ri′ah-sis) infestation with lice of the species *Phthirus pubis.*

Phthirus (thir′us) a genus of lice.

P. pu′bis, the pubic, or crab, louse, a species of louse that infests the pubic hair and sometimes the eyebrows and eyelashes.

phthisis (thi′sis) 1. a wasting of the body. 2. tuberculosis.

p. bul′bi, shrinkage of the eyeball.

grinder's p., a combination of tuberculosis and pneumoconiosis occurring in grinders in the cutlery trade.

miner's p., pneumoconiosis of coal workers.

phyco- word element [Gr.], *seaweed; algae.*

phycobilin (fi″ko-bil′in) a group of protein-linked pigments found in the red and the blue-green algae.

phycochrome (fi′ko-krōm) a blue-green pigment from algae.

phycocyanin (fi″ko-si′ah-nin) a blue chromoprotein found in blue-green algae.

phycoerythrin (fi″ko-er′ĭ-thrin) a red chromoprotein found in red algae.

phycology (fi-kol′o-je) the scientific study of algae.

Phycomycetes (fi″ko-mi-se′tēz) a group of fungi comprising the common water, leaf, and bread molds.

phycomycosis (fi″ko-mi-ko′sis) any of a group of acute fungal diseases caused by members of the Phycomycetes.

phylloquinone (fil″o-kwin′ōn) phytonadione, a vitamin K preparation.

phylogeny (fi-loj′ĕ-ne) the complete developmental history of a race or group of organisms. adj., **phylogenet′ic, phylogen′ic.**

phylum (fi′lum), pl. *phy′la* [L., Gr.] a primary division of the plant or animal kingdom, including organisms that are assumed to have a common ancestry.

phyma (fi′mah), pl. *phy′mata* [Gr.] a skin tumor or tubercle.

physiatrics (fiz″e-ah′triks) that branch of medicine using PHYSICAL THERAPY, physical agents, such as light, heat, water, and electricity, and mechanical apparatus, in the diagnosis, prevention, and treatment of bodily disorders.

physiatrist (fiz″e-ah′trist) a physician who specializes in physiatrics.

physic (fiz′ik) 1. the art of medicine and therapeutics. 2. a medicine, especially a cathartic.

physical (fiz′ĭ-kal) pertaining to the body, to material things, or to physics.

p. examination, examination of the bodily state of

a patient by ordinary physical means, as inspection, palpation, percussion, and auscultation.

p. therapist, one who is skilled in the physical therapeutic arts in the treatment of such disorders as fractures, sprains, muscle tension, and paralysis. Among the procedures used are exercise, hydrotherapy, massage, and other body manipulations.

Persons seeking certification as physical therapists must have completed a course of study in an approved school of physical therapy and should successfully pass the state examination required in many states of the United States. Applicants for membership in the American Physical Therapy Association and registration with the American Registry of Physical Therapists must meet the above criteria. An exception to these requirements may be made in the case of a person who becomes a physical therapist with one of the branches of the Armed Forces. The address of the American Physical Therapy Association is 1740 Broadway, New York, NY 10019.

p. therapy, the treatment of bodily ailments by various physical or nonmedicinal means. This usually includes the use of heat, water, exercise, massage, and electric current.

Physical therapy attempts to relieve pain and to improve or restore muscular function. Its ultimate goal is to train the disabled individual in the safest and most effective means of performing essential activities.

EXERCISE is the most widely used means of treatment in physical therapy. Methods may vary widely because exercises are designed to fit the patient's individual needs and abilities. Exercise makes it possible to increase the mobility of a joint, to strengthen a muscle, and to train a voluntary muscle to contract and relax in coordination with other muscles. Exercise may be either active or passive.

In some instances, exercises are carried out under water (HYDROTHERAPY). This is particularly true in cases of poliomyelitis. Special pools are often used to train muscles because the buoyancy of the water requires less effort from weakened muscles and allows a greater range of movement. (See also HUBBARD TANK.)

HEAT is a very important agent in many types of physical therapy. It stimulates circulation and relieves pain in the area being treated. Heat may be applied by means of infrared rays, high-frequency electric currents (DIATHERMY), hot moist compresses, immersion in hot water, or through the use of melted paraffin. Heat is of particular value in the treatment of arthritis.

Massage is frequently used as an adjunct of exercise. It helps improve circulation and relieves local pain or muscle spasms. Electrotherapy, or the use of electrical currents of low intensity, is sometimes employed to make muscles contract spontaneously. This is important in training weakened muscles.

physician (fĭ-zish′un) an authorized practitioner of medicine, as one graduated from a college of medicine or osteopathy and licensed by the appropriate board (see also DOCTOR).

attending p., one who attends a hospital at stated times to visit the patients and give directions as to their treatment.

family p., a medical specialist who plans and provides the comprehensive primary health care of all members of a family, regardless of age or sex, on a continuous basis.

resident p., a graduate and licensed physician learning a specialty through in-hospital training.

physicochemical (fiz″ĭ-ko-kem′ĭ-kal) pertaining to both physics and chemistry.

physics (fiz′iks) the study of the laws and phenomena of nature, especially of forces and general properties of matter and energy.

physio- word element [Gr.], *nature; physiology; physical.*

physiochemical (fiz″e-o-kem′ĭ-kal) pertaining to both physiology and chemistry.

physiognomy (fiz″e-og′no-me) 1. the determination of mental or moral character and qualities by the face. 2. the countenance, or face. 3. the facial expression and appearance as a means of diagnosis.

physiologic, physiological (fiz″e-o-loj′ik; fiz″e-o-loj′ĭ-kal) pertaining to physiology; normal; not pathologic.

physiologist (fiz″e-ol′o-jist) a specialist in physiology.

physiology (fiz″e-ol′o-je) 1. the science which treats of the functions of the living organism and its parts, and of the physical and chemical factors and processes involved. 2. the basic processes underlying the functioning of a species or class of organism, or any of its parts or processes.

cell p., scientific study of phenomena involved in cell growth and maintenance, self-regulation and division of cells, interactions between nucleus and cytoplasm, and general behavior of protoplasm.

comparative p., the study of organ functions in various animals to find fundamental relations in the physiology of all animals.

general p., that concerned with establishment of the general principles of functional mechanisms underlying life processes of all organisms.

morbid p., pathologic p., the study of disordered functions or of function in diseased tissues.

special p., the physiology of particular organs.

physiopathologic (fiz″e-o-path″o-loj′ik) pertaining to pathologic physiology.

physiotherapist (fiz″e-o-ther′ah-pist) physical therapist.

physiotherapy (fiz″e-o-ther′ah-pe) physical therapy.

physique (fĭ-zēk′) the body organization, development, and structure.

physo- word element [Gr.], *air; gas.*

physohematometra (fi″so-hem″ah-to-me′trah) gas and blood in the uterine cavity.

physohydrometra (fi″so-hi″dro-me′trah) gas and serum in the uterine cavity.

physometra (fi″so-me′trah) gas in the uterine cavity.

physopyosalpinx (fi″so-pi″o-sal′pinks) gas and pus in the oviduct.

physostigmine (fi″so-stig′min) an alkaloid usually obtained from the dried ripe seed of *Physostigma venenosum;* used as a topical miotic in the form of the base and of the salicylate and sulfate salts.

phyt(o)- word element [Gr.], *plant; an organism of the vegetable kingdom.*

phytase (fi′tās) an enzyme of plants that catalyzes the hydrolysis of phytic acid to inositol and phosphoric acid.

phytoagglutinin (fi″to-ah-gloo′tĭ-nin) an agglutinin of plant origin.

phytobezoar (fi″to-be′zōr) a bezoar composed of vegetable fibers.

phytochemistry (fi″to-kem′is-tre) study of chemical processes occurring in plants, the nature of plant chemicals, and various applications of such chemicals to science and industry.

phytogenous (fi-toj′ĕ-nus) derived from plants, or caused by a vegetable growth.

phytohemagglutinin (fi″to-hem″ah-gloo′tĭ-nin) a hemagglutinin of plant origin.

phytohormone (fi″to-hōr′mōn) plant hormone; any of the hormones produced in plants which are active in controlling growth and other functions at a site remote from their place of production.

phytoid (fi′toid) resembling a plant.

phytol (fi′tol) an unsaturated aliphatic alcohol present in chlorophyll as an ester; used in the preparation of vitamins E and K.

phytomenadione (fi″to-men″ah-di′ōn) phytonadione.

phytonadione (fi″to-nah-di′ōn) a vitamin K preparation used as a prothrombinogenic agent.

phytoparasite (fi″to-par″ah-sīt) any parasitic vegetable organism.

phytopathogenic (fi″to-path″o-jen′ik) producing disease in plants.

phytopathology (fi″to-pah-thol′o-je) 1. the pathology of plants. 2. pathology of diseases caused by bacteria.

phytophotodermatitis (fi″to-fo″to-der″mah-ti′tis) phototoxic dermatitis due to contact with certain plants and subsequent exposure to sunlight.

phytoplankton (fi″to-plank′ton) the minute plant (vegetable) organisms which, with those of the animal kingdom, make up the plankton of natural waters.

phytoplasm (fi′to-plazm) protoplasm of plants.

phytoprecipitin (fi″to-pre-sip′ĭ-tin) a precipitin formed in response to vegetable antigen.

phytosis (fi-to′sis) any disease caused by a phytoparasite.

phytosterol (fi″to-ste′rol) a sterol of vegetable origin.

phytotoxic (fi″to-tok′sik) 1. pertaining to phytotoxin. 2. poisonous to plants.

phytotoxin (fi″to-tok′sin) an exotoxin produced by certain species of higher plants; any toxin of plant origin.

pia-arachnitis (pi″ah-ar″ak-ni′tis) leptomeningitis; inflammation of the leptomeninges, or pia mater and arachnoid.

pia-arachnoid (pi″ah-ah-rak′noid) the pia mater and arachnoid considered together as one organ.

pial (pi′al) pertaining to the pia mater.

pia mater (pi′ah ma′ter) [L.] the innermost of the three meninges covering the brain and spinal cord.

piarachnitis (pi″ar-ak-ni′tis) leptomeningitis; pia-arachnitis.

piarachnoid (pi″ar-ak′noid) pia-arachnoid.

pica (pi′kah) craving for unnatural articles of food; a depraved appetite.

Pick's cells (piks) round, oval, or polyhedral cells with foamy, lipid-containing cytoplasm, found in the bone marrow and spleen in Niemann-Pick disease.

Pick's disease (piks) 1. lobar atrophy. 2. ascites and fibrotic liver disease associated with constrictive pericarditis.

pickwickian syndrome (pik-wik′e-an) obesity, somnolence, hypoventilation, and erythrocytosis.

pico- designating 10^{-12} (one trillionth) part of the unit to which it is joined.

picogram (pi′ko-gram) one trillionth (10^{-12}) gram. Abbreviated pg.

picometer (pi″ko-me′ter) a unit of length, 10^{-12} meter. Abbreviated pm.

picornavirus (pi-kor″nah-vi′rus) an extremely small, ether-resistant RNA virus, one of the group comprising the enteroviruses and the rhinoviruses.

picrate (pik′rāt) any salt of picric acid.

picric acid (pik′rik) a substance used as dye, tissue fixative, antiseptic, astringent, and stimulant of epithelialization; it can be detonated on percussion or by heating above 300° C. Called also trinitrophenol.

picrocarmine (pik″ro-kar′min) a histological stain consisting of a mixture of carmine, ammonia, distilled water, and aqueous solution of picric acid.

picrotoxin (pik″ro-tok′sin) an active principle from the seed of *Anamirta cocculus,* used as a central and respiratory stimulant in barbiturate poisoning.

piebaldism (pi-bawld′izm) a condition in which the skin is partly brown and partly white, as in partial albuminism and vitiligo.

piedra (pe-a′drah) a fungal disease of the hair in which white or black nodules of fungi form on the shafts.

Pierre Robin syndrome (pe-yair′ ro-bah′) micrognathia occurring in association with cleft palate, glossoptosis, and absent gag reflex.

piesesthesia (pi-e″zes-the′ze-ah) the sense by which pressure stimuli are felt.

piesimeter (pi″e-sim′ĕ-ter) an instrument for testing the sensitiveness of the skin to pressure.

-piesis word element [Gr.], *pressure.* adj., **-pies′ic.**

pigeon chest prominence of the sternum and rib cartilage; called also PECTUS CARINATUM and pigeon breast.

pigeon toe a foot condition in which the toes turn inward; called also pes varus. Severe cases are considered a form of CLUBFOOT.

pigment (pig′ment) 1. any coloring matter of the body. 2. a stain or dyestuff. 3. a paintlike medicinal preparation to be applied to the skin. adj., **pig′mentary.**

bile p., any one of the coloring matters of the bile, including bilirubin, biliverdin, etc.

blood p., any one of the pigments derived from hemoglobin, including heme, hematoidin, etc.

respiratory p's, substances, e.g., hemoglobin, myoglobin, or cytochromes, which take part in the oxidative processes of the animal body.

pigmentation (pig″men-ta′shun) the deposition of coloring matter; the coloration or discoloration of a part by a pigment.

hematogenous p., pigmentation produced by accumulation of hemoglobin derivatives, such as hematoidin or hemosiderin.

pigmented (pig′ment-ed) colored by deposit of pigment.

pigmentolysin (pig″men-tol′ĭ-sin) a lysin that destroys pigment.

pigmentophage (pig-men′to-fāj) any pigment-destroying cell, especially such a cell of the hair.

piitis (pi-i′tis) inflammation of the pia mater.

pilar, pilary (pi′lar; pil′ah-re) pertaining to the hair.

pile (pīl) 1. a hemorrhoid. 2. in nucleonics, a chain-reacting fission device for producing slow neutrons and radioisotopes.

sentinel p., a hemorrhoid-like thickening of the mucous membrane at the lower end of an anal fissure.

piles (pīlz) hemorrhoids.

pileus (pil′e-us) caul.

pili (pi′li) plural of *pilus.*

pill (pil) a small globular or oval medicated mass to be swallowed; a tablet.

enteric-coated p., one enclosed in a substance that dissolves only when it has reached the intestines.

hexylresorcinol p., one containing hexylresorcinol, with a rupture-resistant coating which disintegrates in the digestive tract.

pillar (pil′ar) a supporting column, usually occurring in pairs.

p's of the fauces, folds of mucous membrane at the sides of the fauces.

pillion (pil′yon) a temporary artificial leg.

pilo- word element [L.], *hair; composed of hair.*

pilocarpine (pi″lo-kar′pin) a cholinergic alkaloid from leaves of *Pilocarpus jaborandi* and *P. microphyllus;* used as an ophthalmic miotic in the form of its hydrochloride and nitrate salts.

pilocystic (pi″lo-sis′tik) hollow or cystlike, and containing hair; said of dermoid tumors.

piloerection (pi″lo-e-rek′shun) erection of the hair.

pilojection (pi″lo-jek′shun) introduction of one or more hairs into an aneurysmal sac, to promote formation of a blood clot.

pilomatrixoma (pi″lo-ma-trik′so-mah) a benign, circumscribed, calcifying epithelial neoplasm derived from hair matrix cells, manifested as a small firm intracutaneous spheroid mass, usually on the face, neck, or arms.

pilomotor (pi″lo-mo′tor) causing movement of the hairs; pertaining to the arrector muscles, the contraction of which produces cutis anserina (goose flesh) and piloerection.

p. nerves, the nerves supplying the arrector muscles of the hair.

pilonidal (pi″lo-ni′dal) having a nidus of hairs.

p. cyst, a hair-containing sacrococcygeal dermoid cyst or sinus, often opening at a postnatal dimple. The cyst is believed to result from an infolding of skin in which hair continues to grow. These cysts cause no symptoms unless they become infected, which is quite likely because of their location. Pain and swelling, with the formation of an abscess, are the symptoms of an infected pilonidal cyst. Treatment consists of surgical removal.

pilose (pi′lōs) hairy; covered with hair.

pilosebaceous (pi″lo-se-ba′shus) pertaining to the hair follicles and sebaceous glands.

pilus (pi′lus), pl. *pi′li* [L.] 1. a hair. 2. fimbria (2).

p. cunicula′tus (pl. *pi′li cunicula′ti*), burrowing hair.

p. incarna′tus (pl. *pi′li incarna′ti*), ingrown hair.

p. tor′tus (pl. *pi′li tor′ti*), twisted hair.

pimelitis (pim″ĕ-li′tis) inflammation of the adipose tissue.

pimelopterygium (pim″ĕ-lo-ter-ij′e-um) a fatty outgrowth on the conjunctiva.

pimelosis (pim″ĕ-lo′sis) 1. conversion into fat. 2. obesity.

piminodine (pi-min′o-dēn) a narcotic analgesic, used as the esylate ester.

pimple (pim′p′l) a papule or pustule.

pin (pin) a slender, elongated piece of metal used for securing fixation of parts.

Steinmann p., a metal rod for the internal fixation of fractures. (See also STEINMANN EXTENSION.)

pincement (pans-maw′) [Fr.] pinching of the flesh in massage.

pindolol (pin′do-lōl) a vasodilator.

pineal (pin′e-al) 1. shaped like a pine cone. 2. pertaining to the pineal body.

p. body, p. gland, a small, conical structure attached by a stalk to the posterior wall of the third ventricle of the cerebrum, believed by many to be an endocrine gland. In certain amphibians and reptiles the gland is thought to function as a light receptor. In most mammals, including man, it appears to be the major or unique site of melatonin biosynthesis. The effect of melatonin on the body and the exact function of the pineal body remain obscure.

pinealectomy (pin″e-ah-lek′to-me) excision of the pineal body.

pinealism (pin′e-al-izm) the condition due to deranged secretion of the pineal body.

pinealoblastoma (pin″e-ah-lo-blas-to′mah) pinealoma in which the pineal cells are not well differentiated.

pinealocyte (pin′e-ah-lo-sīt) an epithelioid cell of the pineal body.

pinealoma (pin″e-ah-lo′mah) a tumor of the pineal body composed of neoplastic nests of large epithelial cells; it may cause hydrocephalus, precocious puberty, and gait disturbances.

Pinel (pe-nel′) Philippe (1745–1826). French physician, born at Saint-André, Tarn. In his *Traité médico-philosophique sur l'aliénation mentale* he advocated more humane treatment of the insane. As head physician first of the Bicêtre and then of Salpêtrière, he abandoned the use of restraining chains and was able to put into practice a number of other reforms.

pinguecula (ping-gwek′u-lah), pl. *pinguec′ulae* [L.] a small, benign, yellowish spot on the bulbar conjunctiva, seen usually in the elderly.

piniform (pin′ĭ-form) conical or cone-shaped.

pink disease acrodynia.

pinkeye (pink′i) a contagious inflammation of the conjunctiva caused by *Hemophilus aegypticus;* called also acute contagious CONJUNCTIVITIS.

pinna (pin′ah) the projecting part of the ear lying outside the head; auricle. adj., **pin′nal.**

pinocyte (pin′o-sīt) a cell that exhibits pinocytosis.

pinocytosis (pin″o-si-to′sis) a mechanism by which cells ingest extracellular fluid and its contents; it involves the formation of invaginations by the cell membrane, which close and break off to form fluid-filled vacuoles in the cytoplasm. adj., **pinocytot'ic.**

pinosome (pin'o-sōm) the intracellular vacuole formed by pinocytosis.

pint (pīnt) a unit of liquid measure in the apothecaries' system, 16 fluid ounces or equivalent to 473.17 milliliters.

pinta (pin'tah) a treponemal infection characterized by bizarre pigmentary changes in the skin occurring in tropical America; it is effectively treated by penicillin.

p. fever, a disease observed in northern Mexico, identical with Rocky Mountain spotted fever.

pinworm (pin'werm) any oxyurid, especially *Enterobius vermicularis* (see also WORM).

pipamazine (pi-pam'ah-zēn) a phenothiazine derivative used as an antiemetic.

Pipanol (pip'ah-nol) trademark for a preparation of trihexyphenidyl, used as an anticholinergic and in treatment of Parkinson's disease.

pipazethate (pi-paz'ĕ-thāt) an antitussive.

pipenzolate (pi-pen'zo-lāt) an anticholinergic used as the bromide salt in peptic ulcer and gastritis.

piperacetazine (pi″per-ah-set'ah-zēn) a tranquilizer.

piperazine (pi-per'ah-zēn) a compound, various salts of which are used as anthelmintics.

piperidine (pi-per'ĭ-dēn) a colorless liquid used as a pharmaceutical intermediate.

piperidolate (pi″per-id'o-lāt) an anticholinergic used as a gastrointestinal antispasmodic in the form of the hydrochloride salt.

piperocaine (pi'per-o-kān) a local anesthetic, used as the hydrochloride salt.

piperoxan (pi″per-oks'an) an α-adrenergic blocking agent used in the diagnosis and surgical removal of pheochromocytoma.

pipet, pipette (pi-pet') [Fr.] 1. a glass or transparent plastic tube used in measuring or transferring small quantities of liquid or gas. 2. to dispense by means of a pipette.

Pipizan (pi'pĭ-zan) trademark for a preparation of piperazine, an anthelmintic.

pipradrol (pi'prah-drol) a central stimulant; used as the hydrochloride salt.

Piptal (pip'tal) trademark for preparations of pipenzolate, an anticholinergic.

piriform (pir'ĭ-form) pear-shaped.

Pirquet's reaction (per-kāz') appearance of a papule with a red areola 24–48 hours after introduction of two small drops of Old tuberculin by slight scarification of the skin; a positive test indicates previous infection with tubercle bacilli.

pisiform (pi'sĭ-form) resembling a pea in size and shape.

pit (pit) 1. a hollow fovea or indentation. 2. a pockmark. 3. to indent, or to become and remain for a few minutes indented, by pressure.

anal p., proctodeum.

auditory p., a distinct depression in each auditory placode, marking the beginning of the embryonic development of the internal ear.

lens p., a pitlike depression in the fetal head where the lens develops.

nasal p., olfactory p., a depression appearing in the olfactory placodes in the early stages of development of the nose.

p. of stomach, the epigastric fossa or epigastric region.

pitch (pich) 1. a dark, more or less viscous residue from distillation of tar and other substances. 2. natural asphalt of various kinds. 3. the quality of sound dependent on the frequency of vibration of the waves producing it.

pitchblend (pich'blend) a black mineral containing uranium oxide; from it are obtained radium, polonium, and uranium.

pithecoid (pith'ĕ-koid) apelike.

pithing (pith'ing) destruction of the brain and spinal cord by thrusting a blunt needle into the vertebral canal and cranium, done on animals to destroy sensibility preparatory to experimenting on their living tissue.

Pitocin (pĭ-to'sin) trademark for a solution of oxytocin for injection; used to stimulate uterine contraction.

Pitressin (pĭ-tres'in) trademark for a solution of vasopressin for injection. It has the pressor actions of posterior pituitary extract.

pitting (pit'ing) 1. the formation, usually by scarring, of a small depression. 2. the removal from erythrocytes, by the spleen, of such structures as iron granules, without destruction of the cells. 3. remaining indented for a few minutes after removal of firm-finger-pressure, distinguishing fluid edema from myxedema.

pituicyte (pĭ-tu'ĭ-sīt) any of the distinctive fusiform cells composing most of the neurohypophysis.

pituitarism (pĭ-tu'ĭ-tar-izm″) disorder of pituitary function (see also HYPERPITUITARISM and HYPOPITUITARISM).

pituitary (pĭ-tu'ĭ-tār″e) 1. pertaining to the pituitary gland. 2. pituitary gland. 3. a preparation of the pituitary glands of animals, used therapeutically.

p. gland, the master gland of the endocrine system, so called because it controls hormone production of other endocrine glands; called also hypophysis, or hypophysis cerebri.

This pea-sized gland lies in a small recess (the sella turcica) at the base of the brain and is connected to the HYPOTHALAMUS by the hypophyseal (pituitary) stalk. The hypothalamus controls many of the secretory functions of the pituitary gland by secreting hormonal substances which in turn stimulate production of pituitary hormones. Information concerned with the well-being of an individual and gathered by the nervous system is transmitted by the hypothalamus, which then regulates secretion of pituitary hormones. The activities of the nervous system and the endocrine system are thereby correlated.

The pituitary gland is divided physiologically into two portions, each portion producing a number of different hormones. The adenohypophysis, called also the anterior lobe, produces at least seven hormones, six of which have their primary action on other endocrine glands. The neurohypophysis, called also the posterior lobe, is not as well understood, but is known to release two important hormones that are secreted by the hypothalamus. All the endocrine glands interact with one another to some extent, but only the pituitary has the special function of stimulating other members of the system to produce their particular hormones.

Hormones of the Adenohypophysis (Anterior Lobe). *Growth Control.* The hormones from the adenohypophysis exert their influence indirectly, except for growth hormone (somatotropin), which acts directly on the tissues of the body. This hormone insures proper growth and development of the skeleton.

Overproduction of growth hormone, which is usually due to a tumor of the pituitary gland, leads to GIGANTISM, a disorder that produces overly tall but well proportioned persons who are usually of normal strength and mental ability. If the overproduction of growth hormone occurs after a person has reached adulthood, he will grow no taller, but certain parts of his bony structure will grow abnormally, especially the cheek bones, jaw bone, hands, and feet. This condition is called ACROMEGALY. Treatment for it, and for gigantism, is by IRRADIATION or surgical removal (hypophysectomy) of the pituitary gland.

At the other end of the scale is DWARFISM. Although dwarfism may be the result of other disorders, underproduction of growth hormone of the pituitary gland is one of the more common causes.

Weight Control. Failure of the pituitary to produce sufficient hormones can lead to a rare condition of malnourishment and premature senility known as SIMMONDS' DISEASE. A slightly different kind of pituitary deficiency can cause a rare condition called Fröhlich's syndrome in children; the symptoms are obesity, mental dullness, and underdevelopment of the reproductive organs. If the condition occurs after puberty, fat may accumulate around certain portions of the body, particularly the hips.

Treatment of pituitary underproduction is by the administration of pituitary extract.

Control of Other Glands. In addition to growth hormone, six other hormones have been isolated from the adenohypophysis.

Thyrotropin (called also thyroid-stimulating hormone, or TSH) controls secretion of the hormone thyroxine from the thyroid gland. Corticotropin (adrenocorticotropic hormone, or ACTH) controls secretion of cortisol (hydrocortisone) from the cortex of the ADRENAL GLAND. By way of a feedback device, the secretion of cortisol from the adrenal cortices regulates the release of ACTH from the adenohypophysis. Thus a high level of cortisol in the blood inhibits the secretion of ACTH.

Follicle-stimulating hormone (FSH) affects the reproductive organs of both the female and the male. It stimulates the growth of the ovarian follicle and secretion of estrogen in the female and maintains the formation of spermatozoa in the male. FSH is called a gonadotropic hormone because it controls the GONADS. Another gonadotropic hormone is luteinizing hormone (LH). In the female, LH acts with FSH to bring about maturation of the ovarian follicle; it also initiates rupture of the mature follicle so that the ovum is released, acts upon the cells of the capsule surrounding the follicle to cause formation of the corpus luteum, and stimulates these cells to produce progesterone. In the male, LH is called interstitial cell-stimulating hormone (ICSH); it stimulates the development and functioning of the Leydig or interstitial cells of the testes and thereby controls testicular production of testosterone.

Lactogenic or luteotropic hormone (LTH) is also known by such names as luteotropin, prolactin, and mammotropin. It has two known functions in the female. It stimulates the corpus luteum to produce progesterone and stimulates the production of milk in the mammary glands. (The ejection of milk from the mammary glands is controlled by oxytocin, a secretion of the hypothalamus which is stored in and released from the neurohypophysis.)

Melanocyte-stimulating hormone (MSH) is believed to influence the formation or deposition of melanin in the body.

Pituitary Hormones

Name and Source	Synonyms	Function
Adenohypophysis (anterior lobe)		
TSH	Thyroid-stimulating hormone; thyrotropin	Stimulates thyroid growth and secretion
ACTH	Adrenocorticotropic hormone; corticotropin	Stimulates adrenocortical growth and secretion
STH	Growth hormone; somatotropin	Accelerates body growth
FSH	Follicle-stimulating hormone	Stimulates growth of ovarian follicle and estrogen secretion in the female and spermatogenesis in the male
LH	Luteinizing hormone (in the female); interstitial cell-stimulating hormone, ICSH (in the male)	Stimulates ovulation and luteinization of ovarian follicles in the female and production of testosterone in the male
LTH	Luteotropic hormone; luteotropin, prolactin; mammotropin; lactogenic hormone	Maintains the corpus luteum and stimulates secretion of milk
MSH	Melanocyte-stimulating hormone	Stimulates melanocytes causing pigmentation
Neurohypophysis (posterior lobe)		
Antidiuretic hormone (ADH)	Vasopressin	Promotes water retention by way of the renal tubules and stimulates smooth muscle of blood vessels and digestive tract
Oxytocin		Stimulates contraction of smooth muscle in the uterus

From Jacob, S. W., and Francone, C. A.: Structure and Function in Man. 2nd ed. Philadelphia, W. B. Saunders Co., 1970.

HORMONES OF THE NEUROHYPOPHYSIS (POSTERIOR LOBE). The neurohypophysis stores and releases two hypothalamic hormones. Vasopressin, or antidiuretic hormone (ADH), decreases the rate of urine formation by stimulating reabsorption of water by the renal tubules, and therefore is important in the maintenance of fluid balance; it also increases blood pressure (pressor effect), stimulates contraction of the intestinal musculature and increases peristalsis, and exerts some influence on the uterus. Underproduction of this hormone results in excessive urination and a rare disorder called diabetes insipidus (not to be confused with diabetes mellitus).

The other hormone released by the neurohypophysis is oxytocin. It is necessary for contraction of the uterus during labor and delivery; the exact mechanism responsible for its release at the time it is needed is not known. Oxytocin also is secreted during suckling and causes ejection of milk from the mammary glands.

Both vasopressin and oxytocin are available for therapeutic use. Vasopressin is used as a test substance in diagnosing and treating diabetes insipidus. Oxytocin is given to induce labor, and also to cause contraction of the uterus after delivery of the placenta. A powdered preparation of posterior pituitary is occasionally used as a nasal snuff to treat diabetes insipidus, and posterior pituitary injection is available for subcutaneous injection.

Pituitrin (pĭ-tu′ĭ-trin) trademark for a preparation of posterior pituitary injection.

pityriasis (pit″ĭ-ri′ah-sis) originally, a group of skin diseases marked by the formation of fine, branny scales, but now used only with a modifier.

p. al′ba, a chronic condition with patchy scaling and hypopigmentation of the skin of the face.

p. ro′sea, a dermatosis marked by scaling pink oval macules arranged with the long axes parallel to the cleavage lines of the skin.

p. ru′bra pila′ris, a chronic inflammatory skin disease marked by pink scaling macules and fine acuminate, horny, follicular papules, beginning usually with severe seborrhea of the scalp and seborrheic dermatitis of the face, and associated with keratoderma of the palms and soles.

p. versic′olor, tinea versicolor.

pityroid (pit′ĭ-roid) furfuraceous; branny.

Pityrosporon (pit″ĭ-ros′po-ron) a genus of yeastlike fungi, including *P. orbic′ulare,* a species customarily found on normal skin but capable of causing tinea versicolor in susceptible hosts.

PKU phenylketonuria.

placebo (plah-se′bo) [L.] an inactive substance or preparation given to satisfy the patient's symbolic need for drug therapy, and used in controlled studies to determine the efficacy of medicinal substances. Also, a procedure with no intrinsic therapeutic value, performed for such purposes.

placenta (plah-sen′tah), pl. *placentas* or *placen′tae* [L.] an organ characteristic of true mammals during pregnancy, joining mother and offspring, providing endocrine secretion and selective exchange of soluble bloodborne substances through apposition of uterine and trophoblastic vascularized parts. Called also afterbirth. adj., **placen′tal.**

In anatomic nomenclature the placenta consists of a uterine and a fetal portion. The chorion, the superficial or fetal portion, is surfaced by a smooth, shining membrane continuous with the sheath of the umbilical cord (amnion). The deep, or uterine, portion is divided by deep sulci into lobes of irregular outline and extent (the cotyledons). Over the maternal surface of the placenta is stretched a delicate, transparent membrane of fetal origin. Around the periphery of the placenta is a large vein (the marginal sinus), which returns a part of the maternal blood from the organ.

The major function of the placenta is to allow diffusion of nutrients from the mother's blood into the fetus's blood and diffusion of waste products from the fetus back to the mother. This two-way exchange takes place across the placental membrane, which is semipermeable; that is, it acts as a selective filter, allowing some materials to pass through and holding back others.

In the early months of pregnancy the placenta acts as a nutrient storehouse and helps to process some of the food substances that nourish the fetus. Later, as the fetus grows and develops, these metabolic functions of the placenta are gradually taken on by the fetal liver.

The placenta secretes both estrogens and progesterone. After birth of the infant the placenta is cast off from the uterus and expelled via the birth canal.

abrup′tio placen′tae, premature separation of a normally situated placenta. Mild abruptio placentae usually occurs during labor when the cervix uteri is partially dilated. Symptoms include change in the character of the patient's labor, external bleeding, and fetal distress.

Serious abruptio placentae occurs most often before the onset of labor. Symptoms include sudden, severe pain in the region of the uterus, some external bleeding, and indications of fetal distress. Treatment is symptomatic unless there is an indication of severe hemorrhage or fetal death, in which case a cesarean section is indicated.

p. accre′ta, one abnormally adherent to the uterine wall, with partial or complete absence of the decidua basalis.

battledore p., one with the umbilical cord inserted at the edge.

p. circumvalla′ta, one encircled with a dense, raised, white nodular ring, the attached membranes being doubled back over the edge of the placenta.

p. fenestra′ta, one that has spots where placental tissue is lacking.

p. incre′ta, placenta accreta with penetration of the uterine wall.

p. membrana′cea, one that is abnormally thin and spread over an unusually large area of the uterine wall.

p. percre′ta, placenta accreta with invasion of the uterine wall to the serosal layer, sometimes causing rupture of the uterus.

p. prae′via, one located in th lower uterine segment, so that it partially or entirely covers the internal os, instead of in the proper position higher on the uterine wall. Any expansion of the cervix may cause tearing of placental tissue and bleeding. This condition is life threatening to both mother and fetus, and may require delivery by cesarean section.

p. reflex′a, one in which the margin is thickened, appearing to turn back on itself.

p. spu′ria, an accessory portion without blood vessels connecting it with the main placenta.

p. succenturia′ta, an accessory portion with an artery and a vein connecting it with the main placenta.

placentation (plas″en-ta′shun) the series of events following implantation of the embryo and leading to development of the placenta.

placentitis (plas″en-ti′tis) inflammation of the placenta.

placentography (plas″en-tog′rah-fe) radiological visualization of the placenta after injection of a contrast medium.

indirect p., that done to measure the space between the placenta and the presenting fetal head to determine the presence of placenta previa.

placentoid (plah-sen′toid) resembling the placenta.

placentolysin (plas″en-tol′ĭsin) an antibody (cytolysin) formed in reaction to injection of placenta cells.

Placidyl (plas′ĭ-dil) trademark for a preparation of ethchlorvynol, a sedative.

placode (plak′ōd) a platelike structure, especially a thickening of the ectoderm marking the site of future development in the early embryo of an organ of special sense, e.g., the *auditory placode* (ear), *lens placode* (eye), and *olfactory placode* (nose).

placoid (plak′oid) platelike or plaquelike.

plagiocephaly (pla″je-o-sef′ah-le) bizarre distortion of the shape of the skull resulting from irregular closure of the cranial sutures. adj., **plagiocephal′ic.**

plague (plāg) an acute febrile, infectious, highly fatal disease caused by the bacillus *Pasteurella pestis.* It is primarily a disease of rats, and is usually spread to human beings by fleas. The more common form of plague is the bubonic. There is also a pneumonic type, which can be spread directly from man to man by droplet infection.

Plague is a devastating disease. Three outbreaks of plague in history have wiped out whole populations. The first of these spread over Europe in the sixth century A.D. in a tremendous cycle of pestilence that lasted for more than 50 years. The second, called the Black Death, was perhaps the most deadly outbreak the world has known. It swept over Europe in the 14th century, and more than one-quarter of the European population—25 million people—perished. The Great Plague of London in 1665 was a relatively minor outbreak. A third great epidemic raged in the Orient at the turn of the 20th century. The greatest toll was in India, where there were more than 12 million deaths from 1896 to 1933.

Some cases have spread to the United States. Extensive epidemics have been prevented in this country by strict quarantines and by sanitation measures that have been enforced since the disease was traced to rat and wild rodent fleas.

BUBONIC PLAGUE. Bubonic plague is characterized by acutely inflamed and painful swellings of the lymph nodes, or buboes, usually in the groin.

The disease strikes suddenly with chills and fever. Children may have convulsions. There is vomiting and thirst, generalized pain, headache, and mental dullness. Delirium may also be present.

After the third day, black spots, which give the disease the name "black death," may appear. Tender, enlarged lymph nodes are usually seen between the second and fifth days. Some cases of bubonic plague are mild. The more virulent cases last 5 or 6 days, and are usually fatal. If the patient survives past the tenth or twelfth day, there is a good chance of recovery.

The mortality rate for untreated cases runs between 25 and 50 per cent, but has reached as high as 90 per cent. Until recently, little could be done for the disease. Today, however, streptomycin, when used early enough, has cut the mortality rate to 5 per cent. Sulfadiazine is less effective.

PNEUMONIC PLAGUE. Pneumonic plague usually occurs during outbreaks of bubonic plague and may be a direct complication of it. There is extensive involvement of the lungs and the sputum contains many organisms. At one time, pneumonic plague was always fatal. Now, with streptomycin, the chances of recovery are good if treatment is begun within 24 hours.

PREVENTION. The most important measure in controlling plague is the extermination of rats. This is especially necessary around shipping areas, in warehouses, and on docks. Rat control for ships arriving from plague areas is vital.

Where there is an outbreak of plague, strict quarantine measures are called for, as well as the use of insecticides to protect inhabitants of the stricken area against fleas. Immunization with plague vaccine is desirable. Persons who have been in contact with active cases of plague are given preventive medicines.

hemorrhagic p., severe bubonic plague with petechial hemorrhages.

sylvatic p., plague in wild rodents, such as the ground squirrel, which serve as a reservoir from which man may be infected.

plane (plān) 1. a flat surface determined by the position of three points in space. 2. a specified level, as the plane of anesthesia. 3. to rub away or abrade (see also PLANING and PLASTIC SURGERY). 4. a superficial incision in the wall of a cavity or between tissue layers, especially in plastic surgery, made so that the precise point of entry into the cavity or between the layers can be determined.

coronal p., frontal plane.

datum p., a given horizontal plane from which craniometric measurements are made.

frontal p., any plane passing longitudinally through the body from side to side, at right angles to the median plane and dividing the body into front and back parts. Called also coronal plane.

horizontal p., one passing through the body at right angles to the median and frontal planes, and dividing the body into upper and lower parts.

median p., one passing longitudinally through the body from front to back and dividing it into right and left halves.

sagittal p., a vertical plane through the body parallel to the median plane (or to the sagittal suture) and dividing the body into left and right portions.

transverse p., one passing horizontally through the body, at right angles to the sagittal and frontal planes, and dividing the body into upper and lower portions.

vertical p., one perpendicular to a horizontal plane, dividing the body into left and right, or front and back portions.

planigraphy (plah-nig′rah-fe) a method of body-section roentgenography that shows in detail structures lying in a predetermined plane of the body while blurring structures in other planes, produced by movement of the film and x-ray tube in certain specified directions. adj., **planigraph′ic.**

planing (pla′ning) abrasion of disfigured skin to promote reepithelization with minimal scarring; done by mechanical means (dermabrasion) or by application of a caustic (chemabrasion). (See also PLASTIC SURGERY.)

plankton (plangk'ton) the minute, free-floating organisms living in practically all natural waters.

planned parenthood birth control.

planoconcave (pla"no-kon'kāv) flat on one side and concave on the other.

planoconvex (pla"no-kon'veks) flat on one side and convex on the other.

planography (plah-nog'rah-fe) planigraphy.

planta pedis (plan'tah pe'dis) the sole of the foot.

Plantago (plan-ta'go) a genus of herbs, including *P. in'dica, P. psyl'lium* (Spanish psyllium), and *P. ova'ta* (blond psyllium); (see also psyllium hydrophilic MUCILLOID and plantago SEED).

plantalgia (plan-tal'je-ah) pain in the sole of the foot.

plantar (plan'tar) pertaining to the sole of the foot.

p. wart, a common WART located on the sole of the foot. Plantar warts are epidermal tumors caused by a virus which may be picked up by going barefoot. Unlike other warts, this type is usually sensitive to pressure; it may feel tender when touched and may be painful during walking. Called also verruca plantaris.

plantaris (plan-ta'ris) [L.] plantar.

plantigrade (plan'tĭ-grād) walking or running flat on the full sole of the foot; characteristic of man and of such quadrupeds as the bear.

planula (plan'u-lah) a larval coelenterate.

planum (pla'num), pl. *pla'na* [L.] plane.

plaque (plak) any patch or flat area.

atheromatous p., a deposit of predominantly fatty material in the lining of blood vessels occurring in atherosclerosis.

bacterial p., dental p., a deposit of material on a tooth surface, which may serve as a medium for bacterial growth or as a nucleus for formation of a dental calculus.

Hollenhorst p's, atheromatous emboli containing cholesterol crystals in the retinal arterioles, a sign of impending serious cardiovascular disease.

Plaquenil (pla'kwĕ-nil) trademark for a preparation of hydroxychloroquine, used especially as a lupus erythematosus suppressant.

plasm (plazm) 1. plasma. 2. formative substance (cytoplasm, hyaloplasm, etc.).

germ p., the line of cells which by successive division gives rise to the gametes.

plasma (plaz'mah) the fluid portion of the blood in which corpuscles are suspended. Plasma is to be distinguished from serum, which is plasma from which the fibrinogen has been separated in the process of clotting. adj., **plasmat'ic.**

Of the total volume of blood, 55 per cent is made up of plasma. It is a clear, straw-colored liquid, 92 per cent water, in which are contained plasma proteins, inorganic salts, foods, gases, waste materials from the cells, and various hormones, secretions, and enzymes. These substances are transported to or from the tissues of the body by the plasma.

Plasma obtained from blood donors is given to those suffering from loss of blood or from shock to help maintain adequate blood pressure. Since plasma can be dried and stored in bottles, it can be transported almost anywhere, ready for immediate use after addition of the appropriate fluid. Plasma can be given to anyone, regardless of blood type. (See also BLOOD, SERUM, and TRANSFUSION.)

antihemophilic human p., normal human plasma that has been processed promptly to preserve the antihemophilic properties of the original blood; used for temporary correction of bleeding tendency in hemophilia.

normal human p., sterile plasma obtained by pooling approximately equal amounts of the liquid portion of citrated whole blood from eight or more adult humans; used as a blood volume replenisher.

p. volume expander, a solution transfused instead of blood to increase the volume of fluid circulating in the blood vessels. Called also artificial plasma extender.

plasmablast (plaz'mah-blast) the immature precursor of a plasmacyte, or plasma cell.

plasmacyte (plaz'mah-sīt) a spherical or ellipsoidal cell with a single nucleus containing chromatin, an area of perinuclear clearing, and generally abundant, sometimes vacuolated cytoplasm. Plasmocytes are involved in the synthesis, storage, and release of antibody. Called also plasmocyte and plasma cell.

plasmacytoma (plaz"mah-si-to'mah) any focal neoplasm of plasmacytes, including those of multiple myeloma. Isolated plasmacytomas may occur outside the bone marrow (extramedullary plasmacytomas), affecting such tissues as the nasal, oral, and pharnygeal mucosa and the viscera.

plasmacytosis (plaz"mah-si-to'sis) an excess of plasmacytes in the blood.

plasmagene (plaz'mah-jēn) a self-reproducing copy of a nuclear gene persisting in the cytoplasm of a cell.

plasmalemma (plaz"mah-lem'ah) cell membrane.

plasmapheresis (plaz"mah-fĕ-re'sis) removal of blood, separation of the blood cells by centrifugation, and reinjection of the packed cells suspended in citrate-saline or other suitable medium; used as a means of obtaining plasma and in the treatment of certain pathologic conditions.

plasmatorrhexis (plaz"mah-to-rek'sis) bursting of a cell from internal pressure.

plasmic (plaz'mik) plasmatic; pertaining to or of the nature of plasma.

plasmin (plaz'min) the active principle of the fibrinolytic or clot-lysing system, a proteolytic enzyme with a high specificity for fibrin and the particular ability to dissolve formed fibrin clots.

plasminogen (plaz-min'o-jen) the inactive precursor of plasmin, occurring in plasma and converted to plasmin by the action of urokinase; called also profibrinolysin.

plasmocyte (plaz'mo-sīt) plasmacyte.

plasmocytoma (plaz"mo-sĭ-to'mah) plasmacytoma.

plasmodesma (plaz"mo-dez'mah), pl. *plasmodes'mata.* a bridge of cytoplasm connecting adjacent cells.

plasmodicidal (plaz-mo"dĭ-si'dal) destructive to plasmodia; malariacidal.

Plasmodium (plaz-mo'de-um) a multispecies genus of sporozoa parasitic in the erythrocytes of various animals; four species, *P. falcip'arum, P. mala'riae, P. ova'le,* and *P. vi'vax,* cause the four specific types of malaria in man.

plasmodium (plaz-mo'de-um), pl. *plasmo'dia* [Gr.] 1. a parasite of the genus *Plasmodium.* 2. a multinucleate continuous mass of protoplasm. adj., **plasmo'dial.**

plasmogen (plaz'mo-jen) bioplasm (2); the more vital or essential part of the cytoplasm.

plasmolysis (plaz-mol'ĭ-sis) contraction of cell protoplasm due to loss of water by osmosis. adj., **plasmolyt'ic.**

plasmoma (plaz-mo'mah) plasmacytoma.

plasmon (plaz'mon) the hereditary factors of the egg cytoplasm.

plasmorrhexis (plaz″mo-rek'sis) a morphologic change in erythrocytes, consisting in the escape from the cells of round, shiny granules and splitting off of particles; called also erythrocytorrhexis.

plasmoschisis (plaz-mos'kĭ-sis) the splitting up of cell protoplasm.

plasmotropism (plaz-mot'ro-pizm) destruction of erythrocytes in the liver, spleen, or marrow, as contrasted with their destruction in the circulation. adj., **plasmotrop'ic.**

plaster (plas'ter) 1. a mixture of materials that hardens; used for immobilizing or making impressions of body parts. 2. an adhesive substance spread on fabric or other suitable backing material, for application to the skin, often containing some medication, such as an anodyne or rubefacient.

adhesive p., adhesive tape.

p. of Paris, calcium sulfate dihydrate, reduced to a fine powder; the addition of water produces a porous mass used in making casts and bandages to support or immobilize body parts, and in dentistry for taking dental impressions.

salicylic acid p., a mixture of 10 to 40 per cent salicylic acid in a suitable base; used as a keratolytic.

Plastibell (plas'tĭ-bel) trademark for a bell-shaped device used as a guide in the removal of the foreskin in CIRCUMCISION. The Plastibell is slipped over the glans, and the foreskin is then pulled over and secured tightly around the bell. After the tissue is trimmed from the glans, the handle of the Plastibell is snapped off, leaving the bell in place; within 5 to 10 days the bell and the remnant of the foreskin become detached, leaving a healed edge.

plastic (plas'tik) 1. tending to build up tissues to restore a lost part. 2. capable of being molded. 3. a substance produced by chemical condensation or by polymerization. 4. material that can be molded.

p. surgery, surgery concerned with the restoration, reconstruction, correction, or improvement in the shape and appearance of body structures that are defective, damaged, or misshapened by injury, disease, or anomalous growth and development. This kind of surgery has been practiced for thousands of years. Artificial noses and ears have been found on Egyptian mummies. Medical records show that the ancient Hindus reconstructed noses by using skin flaps lifted from the cheek or forehead—a technique that was often practiced, since it was a custom to mutilate the noses of persons who broke the laws.

SKIN GRAFTING. The most common procedure of plastic surgery is skin GRAFTING. This is the replacement of severely damaged skin in one area with healthy skin obtained from another area of the patient's body or from the body of a skin donor. Some grafting is done to prevent the formation of disfiguring scars, such as those that may form on the face from severe burns. If burns or other injuries are extensive, grafting can prevent extensive scarring with tissue that is unsightly and cannot perform all the necessary functions of normal skin. Skin contractures can thus be avoided.

A skin graft can sometimes be made by the simple procedure of cutting a piece of healthy skin from one part of the body, such as the back or the thigh, and stitching it to the injured area. Small arteries from the tissues surrounding the injured area then grow into the graft, nourish it with blood and promote normal growth. If the area to be covered is large, a number of separate patches may be stitched to it, forming islands of skin that will enlarge with healing until the entire area is covered. This is called "postage stamp" or pinch grafting.

In some cases, in order to ensure a good blood supply to the patch, or for other reasons, the surgeon may employ a modern version of the technique used by the ancient Hindus—the pedicle graft. He cuts a flap of skin only partly free from the healthy area in the patient's body, then attaches the loose end to the damaged area. Still fed by its natural blood supply, the flap remains healthy while its cut edge grows into and begins to cover the area of damaged skin. Meanwhile, the area from which the flap was cut and folded away is healing and growing new skin. Soon the surgeon can cut the flap free, and both the graft and the area from which the flap was taken can heal completely.

When the damaged area and the flap are awkwardly located, this technique can involve inconvenience to the patient. His arm, for example, may have to be strapped against his head to provide a skin flap for his face. This sometimes can be avoided by a delayed graft, a plate of skin moved from the healthy area to the damaged one by stages, without at any stage being entirely cut loose from the blood supply.

REPAIRING MOUTH AND OTHER DEFECTS. Among common defects that can be corrected by plastic surgery are CLEFT LIP and CLEFT PALATE. Others are webbed fingers and toes, protruding or missing ears, receding chins, and injured noses. In addition, the shape of various types of noses can be altered for the sake of appearance.

FACIAL RECONSTRUCTION. In facial reconstruction, missing bone and muscle, and sometimes skin, are replaced by substitutes. Sometimes the reconstruction is made with bone or cartilage taken from another part of the body, or sometimes it is made by artificial means.

Use of Prostheses. Often the substitute for missing tissue is a prosthesis, a replacement not made from living tissue. A prosthesis may be inserted beneath the skin (to build out a receding chin, for instance) or attached to the skin surface (for example, to replace an ear).

Prostheses attached to, not inserted beneath, the skin frequently are employed to fill out depressed or missing facial areas, the after effects of accidents, cancer, or war injuries. In building such a replacement, the surgeon first makes an impression of the face and a plaster cast of the impression. The substitute part is molded in wax or clay in the plaster cast, and from this model the actual replacement part is made. Such parts, molded and painted to match the texture and color of the skin, have been used to replace many structures, including missing ears and noses.

Use of Cartilage, Skin, and Bone. Noses and ears also have been reconstructed with rib cartilage and skin grafts. Eyebrows have been made by the use of skin grafts from the scalp, and chest deformities repaired by the use of bone chips from other parts of the body.

Sometimes a nose is remodeled to correct a hump or hook, or a saddle nose (a depression on the ridge), or a twisted nose. Incisions are made inside to avoid causing outside scars, and the surgeon either removes excess cartilage or bone, or inserts it, according to the improvement wanted. Cartilage and bone may be obtained from other parts of the body, usually the ribs or hip. After the operation, the skin over the nose adapts to the new structure.

Dermabrasion. Skin blemishes such as acne scars and pits can be "sandpapered" or planed. This technique, called dermabrasion, seeks to correct superficial blemishes and to remove superficial accumulations of pigment. However, as dermabrasion can occasionally cause increased scarring or introduce variation in skin color and texture, such treatment is infrequently performed today.

FACE LIFTING. This operation is performed to make an aging face look younger. The technical term for this is rhytidoplasty, or plastic surgery for the removal of wrinkles. If such as operation is performed by a reputable surgeon it can be moderately successful, but only temporarily. Reoperation is often necessary. The operation is usually done by opening skin flaps in the region around the ears and undermining the skin of the cheeks and jaws. The eyelids and the area of the eyebrows may be operated on in association with the primary operation.

plasticity (plas-tis′ĭ-te) the quality of being plastic, or capable of being molded.

plastid (plas′tid) 1. any elementary constructive unit, as a cell. 2. any specialized organ of the cell other than the nucleus and centrosome, such as chloroplast or amyloplast.

-plasty (plas′te) word element [Gr.], *formation* or *plastic repair of.*

plate (plāt) 1. a flat structure or layer, as a flat layer of bone. 2. dental plate.

axial p., the primitive streak of the embryo.

bite p., biteplate.

deck p., roof plate.

dental p., a plate of acrylic resin, metal, or other material that is fitted to the shape of the mouth, and serves for the support of artificial teeth.

dorsal p., roof plate.

epiphyseal p., the thin plate of cartilage between the epiphysis and the shaft of a long bone; it is the site of growth in length and is obliterated by epiphyseal closure.

equatorial p., the collection of chromosomes at the equator of the spindle in mitosis.

floor p., the unpaired ventral longitudinal zone of the neural tube; called also ventral plate.

foot p., the flat portion of the stapes.

medullary p., neural plate.

muscle p., myotome (2).

neural p., a thickened band of ectoderm in the midbody region of the developing embryo, which develops into the neural tube; called also medullary plate.

polar p's, platelike bodies at the end of the spindle in certain forms of mitosis.

roof p., the unpaired dorsal longitudinal zone of the neural tube; called also dorsal plate and deck plate.

sole p., a mass of protoplasm in which a motor nerve ending is embedded.

tarsal p., one of the plates of connective tissue forming the framework of either (upper or lower) eyelid.

ventral p., floor plate.

platelet (plāt′let) a small disk or platelike structure, especially the smallest of the formed elements in blood. Blood platelets (called also thrombocytes) are disk-shaped, non-nucleated blood elements with a very fragile membrane; they tend to adhere to uneven or damaged surfaces. They average about 250,000 per cubic millimeter of blood and are principally concerned with coagulation of blood and the contraction of a blood clot. They are formed in red bone marrow and the rate of their formation seems to be governed by the amount of oxygen in the blood and the presence of nucleic acid derivatives from injured tissue.

direct p. count, estimation of the number of platelets per cubic millimeter of blood directly from whole blood.

p. factors, factors important in hemostasis which are contained in or attached to the platelets: platelet factor 1 is adsorbed CLOTTING factor V from the plasma; platelet factor 2 is an accelerator of the thrombin-fibrinogen reaction; platelet factor 3 plays a role in the generation of intrinsic prothrombin converting principle; platelet factor 4 is capable of inhibiting the activity of heparin.

indirect p. count, the count of the total number of platelets per cubic millimeter of blood by counting the platelets on a stained blood film.

platinum (plat′ĭ-num) a chemical element, atomic number 78, atomic weight 195.09, symbol Pt. (See table of ELEMENTS.)

platy- word element [Gr.], *broad; flat.*

platybasia (plat″ĭ-ba′ze-ah) malformation of the base of the skull, with upward displacement of the upper cervical vertebrae and bony impingement on the brain stem. It is accompanied by neurologic signs referable to the medulla oblongata, cervical spinal cord, and cranial nerves. Called also basilar impression.

platycelous (plat″ĭ-se′lus) having one surface flat and the other concave, referring to vertebrae.

platycephalic, platycephalous (plat″ĭ-sĕ-fal′ik; plat″ĭ-sef′ah-lus) having a wide, flat head.

platycoria (plat″ĭ-ko′re-ah) a dilated condition of the pupil of the eye.

platyhelminth (plat″ĭ-hel′minth) one of the Platyhelminthes; a flatworm.

Platyhelminthes (plat″ĭ-hel-min′thēz) a phylum of acoelomate, dorsoventrally flattened, bilaterally symmetrical animals, commonly known as flatworms; it includes the classes Cestoidea (tapeworms) and Trematoda (flukes). (See also WORM.)

platyhieric (plat″ĭ-hi-er′ik) having a wide sacrum, with a sacral index above 100.

platypellic, platypelloid (plat″ĭ-pel′ik; plat″ĭ-pel′oid) having a broad pelvis.

platypodia (plat″ĭ-po′de-ah) flatfoot.

platyrrhine (plat′ĭ-rīn) having a broad nose, with a nasal index above 53.

platysma (plah-tiz′mah) a subcutaneous neck muscle extending from the neck to the clavicle; it acts to wrinkle the skin of the neck and to depress the jaw. (See also table of MUSCLES.)

pledget (plej'et) a small compress or tuft.

-plegia word element [Gr.], *paralysis; a stroke.*

pleiotropism, pleiotropy (pli-ot'ro-pizm; pli-ot'ro-pe) the production by a single gene of multiple phenotypic effects.

pleochromatism (ple"o-kro'mah-tizm) the property of some crystals of transmitting one color in one position and the complementary color in a position at right angles to the first. adj., **pleochromat'ic.**

pleocytosis (ple"o-si-to'sis) the presence of a greater than normal number of cells, as of more than the normal number of lymphocytes in cerebrospinal fluid.

pleomastia (ple"o-mas'te-ah) the presence of supernumerary mammary glands or nipples; polymastia.

pleomorphism (ple"o-mor'fizm) the assumption of various distinct forms by a single organism or within a species. adj., **pleomor'phic, pleomor'phous.**

pleonasm (ple'o-nazm) an excess of parts.

pleonectic (ple"o-nek'tik) characterized by having a higher than normal O_2 content at a given Po_2; said of blood.

pleonexia (ple"o-nek'se-ah) 1. morbid desire for acquisition; morbid greediness. 2. the condition of being pleonectic.

pleonosteosis (ple"on-os"te-o'sis) abnormally increased ossification.

Léri's p., a hereditary syndrome of premature and excessive ossification, with short stature, limitation of movement, broadening and deformity of digits, and mongolian facies.

plessesthesia (ples"es-the'ze-ah) palpatory percussion.

plessimeter (plĕ-sim'ĕ-ter) pleximeter.

plessor (ples'or) plexor.

plethora (pleth'o-rah) a general term denoting a red florid complexion, or specifically, an excessive amount of blood. adj., **plethor'ic.**

plethysmograph (plĕ-thiz'mo-graf) an instrument for recording variations in the volume of an organ, part, or limb, and in the amount of blood present or passing through it for recording variations in the size of parts and in the blood supply.

plethysmography (pleth"iz-mog'rah-fe) the determination of changes in volume by means of a plethysmograph.

pleur(o)- word element [Gr.], *pleura; rib; side.*

pleura (ploo'rah), pl. *pleu'rae* [Gr.] the serous membrane investing the lungs (pulmonary pleura) and lining the walls of the thoracic cavity (parietal pleura), the two layers enclosing a potential space, the pleural cavity. adj., **pleu'ral.**

pleuracotomy (ploo"rah-kot'o-me) incision into the pleural cavity.

pleuralgia (ploo-ral'je-ah) pain in the pleura or in the side. adj., **pleural'gic.**

pleurapophysis (ploo"rah-pof'ĭ-sis) a rib, or a vertebral process corresponding to a rib.

pleurectomy (ploo-rek'to-me) excision of a portion of the pleura.

Pleur-evac trademark for a disposable underwater-seal unit designed for drainage of the pleural cavity; it has a graduated collection chamber, permitting immediate and accurate measurement of the amount of drainage from the pleural cavity via the CHEST TUBE.

pleurisy, pleuritis (ploo'rĭ-se; ploo-ri'tis) inflammation of the pleura; it may be caused by infection, injury, or tumor. It may be a complication of lung diseases, particularly of pneumonia, or sometimes of tuberculosis, lung abscess, or influenza. The symptoms are cough, fever, chills, sharp, sticking pain that is worse on inspiration, and rapid shallow breathing. adj., **pleurit'ic.**

TYPES OF PLEURISY. The membranous pleura that encases each lung is composed of two close-fitting layers; between them is a lubricating fluid. If the fluid content remains unchanged by the disease, the pleurisy is said to be dry. If the fluid increases abnormally, it is a wet pleurisy, or pleurisy with effusion. (See also pleural EFFUSION.)

In dry pleurisy the two layers of membrane may become congested and swollen and rub against each other with a grating effect as the lungs inflate and deflate with breathing. This can be painful. Although only the outer layer causes pain (the inner layer has no pain nerves), the pain may be severe enough to necessitate the use of a strong analgesic.

Wet pleurisy is less likely to cause pain, because there usually is no chafing. But the fluid may interfere with breathing by compressing the lung. In some cases the lung is permanently displaced, failing to return to full capacity because of thickening of the pleura.

If the excess fluid of wet pleurisy becomes infected, with formation of pus, the condition is known as purulent pleurisy or EMPYEMA.

Inflammation of the part of the pleura that covers the diaphragm is called diaphragmatic pleurisy.

TREATMENT. The most effective measures against pleurisy are antibiotics, heat applications, and bed rest. When there is intense pain on breathing, the physician may strap the chest to limit its movement.

pleurocele (ploo'ro-sēl) hernia of lung tissue or of pleura.

pleurocentesis (ploo"ro-sen-te'sis) paracentesis of the pleural cavity.

pleurocentrum (ploo"ro-sen'trum) the lateral element of the vertebral column.

pleuroclysis (ploo-rok'lĭ-sis) injection of fluids into the pleural cavity.

pleurodynia (ploo"ro-din'e-ah) paroxysmal pain in the intercostal muscles.

epidemic p., an epidemic disease due to coxsackievirus B, marked by a sudden attack of violent pain in the chest, fever, and a tendency to recrudescence on the third day; called also devil's grip and Bornholm disease.

pleurogenic, pleurogenous (ploo"ro-jen'ik; ploor-oj'ĕ-nus) originating in the pleura.

pleurography (ploo-rog'rah-fe) roentgenography of the pleural cavity.

pleurohepatitis (ploo"ro-hep"ah-ti'tis) hepatitis with inflammation of a portion of the pleura near the liver.

pleurolith (ploo'ro-lith) a concretion in the pleura.

pleurolysis (ploo-rol'ĭ-sis) surgical separation of the pleura from its attachments.

pleuroparietopexy (ploo"ro-pah-ri'ĕ-to-pek"se) the operation of fixing the visceral pleura to the parietal pleura, thus binding the lung to the chest wall.

pleuropericardial (ploor″o-per″ĭ-kar′de-al) pertaining to the pleura and pericardium.

pleuropericarditis (ploo″ro-per″ĭ-kar-di′tis) inflammation involving the pleura and the pericardium.

pleuroperitoneal (plo͞or″o-per″ĭ-to-ne′al) pertaining to the pleura and peritoneum.

pleuropneumonia (ploo″ro-nu-mo′ne-ah) 1. pneumonia accompanied by pleurisy. 2. an infectious disease of cattle, combining pneumonia and pleurisy, due to *Mycoplasma mycoides* (see also PLEUROPNEUMONIA-LIKE).

pleuropneumonia-like organisms PPLO, a term applied to a group of filtrable microorganisms similar to *Mycoplasma mycoides,* the cause of pleuropneumonia in cattle. (See also MYCOPLASMA.)

pleurothotonos (ploo″ro-thot′o-nus) tetanic bending of the body to one side.

pleurotomy (ploo-rot′o-me) incision of the pleura.

pleurovisceral (ploo″ro-vis′er-al) pertaining to the pleura and viscera.

plexiform (plek′sĭ-form) resembling a plexus or network.

pleximeter (plek-sim′ĕ-ter) 1. a plate to be struck in mediate percussion. 2. diascope.

plexitis (plek-si′tis) inflammation of a nerve plexus.

plexor (plek′sor) a hammer used in diagnostic percussion; plessor.

plexus (plek′sus), pl. *plex′us, plex′uses* [L.] a network or tangle, chiefly of veins or nerves. adj., **plex′al.**

brachial p., a nerve plexus originating from the ventral branches of the last four cervical and the first thoracic spinal nerves. It gives off many of the principal nerves of the shoulder, chest, and arms.

cardiac p., the plexus around the base of the heart, chiefly in the epicardium, formed by cardiac branches from the vagus nerves and the sympathetic trunks and ganglia, and made up of sympathetic, parasympathetic, and visceral afferent fibers that innervate the heart.

carotid p's, nerve plexuses surrounding the common, external, and internal carotid arteries.

celiac p., solar plexus.

cervical p., a nerve plexus formed by the ventral branches of the first four cervical spinal nerves and supplying the structures in the region of the neck. One important branch is the phrenic nerve, which supplies the diaphragm.

choroid p., the ependyma lining the ventricles of the brain with the vascular fringes of the pia mater invaginating them; it is concerned with formation of the cerebrospinal fluid.

coccygeal p., a nerve plexus formed by the ventral branches of the coccygeal and fifth sacral nerve and by a communication from the fourth sacral nerve, giving off the anococcygeal nerves.

cystic p., a nerve plexus near the gallbladder.

dental p., either of two plexuses (inferior and superior) of nerve fibers, one from the inferior alveolar nerve, situated around the roots of the lower teeth, and the other from the superior alveolar nerve, situated around the roots of the upper teeth.

lumbar p., one formed by the ventral branches of the second to fifth lumbar nerves in the psoas major muscle (the branches of the first lumbar nerve often are included).

lumbosacral p., the lumbar and sacral plexuses considered together, because of their continuous nature.

myenteric p., a nerve plexus situated in the muscular layers of the intestines.

nerve p., a plexus composed of intermingled nerve fibers.

pampiniform p., 1. a plexus of veins from the testis and the epididymis, constituting part of the spermatic cord. 2. a plexus of ovarian veins in the broad ligament of the uterus.

sacral p., a plexus arising from the ventral branches of the last two lumbar and first four sacral spinal nerves.

solar p., a network of ganglia and nerves supplying the abdominal viscera (see also SOLAR PLEXUS); called also celiac plexus.

tympanic p., a network of nerve fibers supplying the mucous lining of the tympanum, mastoid air cells, and pharyngotympanic tube.

plica (pli′kah), pl. *pli′cae* [L.] a ridge or fold.

plicate (pli′kāt) plaited or folded.

plication (pli-ka′shun) the operation of taking tucks in a structure to shorten it.

plicotomy (pli-kot′o-me) surgical division of the posterior fold of the tympanic membrane.

plombage (plom-bahzh′) [Fr.] the filling of a space or cavity in the body with inert material.

PLT *p*sittacosis-*l*ymphogranuloma venereum-*t*rachoma (group) (see CHLAMYDIA).

plug (plug) an obstructing mass.

epithelial p., mass of ectodermal cells that temporarily closes the external naris of the fetus.

mucous p., a plug formed by secretions of mucous glands, of the cervix uteri and closing the cervical canal during pregnancy.

plumbic (plum′bik) pertaining to lead.

plumbism (plum′bizm) a chronic form of poisoning caused by absorption of lead or lead salts (see also LEAD POISONING).

plumbum (plum′bum) [L.] lead (symbol Pb).

Plummer-Vinson syndrome (plum′er vin′son) dysphagia with glossitis, hypochromic anemia, splenomegaly, and atrophy of the mouth, pharynx, and upper end of the esophagus.

pluri- word element [L.], *many.*

pluriglandular (ploor″ĭ-glan′du-lar) pertaining to several glands or their secretions.

plurigravida (ploor″ĭ-grav′ĭ-dah) multigravida; a woman pregnant for the third (or more) time.

plurilocular (ploor″ĭ-lok′u-lar) multilocular; having many cells or compartments.

pluripara (ploo-rip′ah-rah) multipara; a woman who has had two or more pregnancies that resulted in viable offspring.

pluriparity (ploor″ĭ-par′ĭ-te) multiparity; the condition of being a pluripara (multipara).

pluripotentiality (ploor″ĭ-po-ten″she-al′ĭ-te) ability to develop in any one of several different ways, or to affect more than one organ or tissue. adj., **pluripo′tent, pluripoten′tial.**

plutonium (ploo-to′ne-um) a chemical element, atomic number 94, atomic weight 242, symbol Pu. (See table of ELEMENTS.)

Pm chemical symbol, *promethium.*

-pnea word element [Gr.], *respiration; breathing.* adj., **-pne'ic.**

pneo- word element [Gr.], *breath; breathing.*

pneogram (ne'o-gram) the tracing obtained by the pneograph; called also spirogram.

pneograph (ne'o-graf) a device for registering chest movements in respiration; called also spirograph.

pneometer (ne-om'ĕ-ter) a device for measuring the air inspired and expired; called also pneumometer and spirometer.

pneoscope (ne'o-skōp) pneograph.

pneum(o)- word element [Gr.], *air* or *gas; lung.*

pneumarthrogram (nu-mar'thro-gram) a film obtained by pneumarthrography.

pneumarthrography (nu"mar-throg'rah-fe) roentgenography of a joint after it has been injected with air as a contrast medium; pneumoarthrography.

pneumarthrosis (nu"mar-thro'sis) gas or air in a joint.

pneumat(o)- word element [Gr.], *air* or *gas; lung.*

pneumatic (nu-mat'ik) pertaining to air or respiration.

pneumatization (nu"mah-tĭ-za'shun) the formation of air cavities in tissue, especially such formation in the temporal bone.

pneumatocele (nu-mat'o-sēl) 1. hernia of lung tissue. 2. a usually benign, thin-walled, air-containing cyst of the lung. 3. a tumor or sac containing gas, especially a gaseous swelling of the scrotum.

pneumatogram (nu-mat'o-gram) pneogram.

pneumatograph (nu-mat'o-graf) pneograph.

pneumatometer (nu"mah-tom'ĕ-ter) pneometer.

pneumatometry (nu"mah-tom'ĕ-tre) measurement of the air inspired and expired.

pneumatorrhachis (nu"mah-tor'ah-kis) the presence of gas in the vertebral canal.

pneumatosis (nu"mah-to'sis) air or gas in an abnormal location in the body.

p. cystoi'des intestina'lis, a condition characterized by the presence of thin-walled, gas-containing cysts in the wall of the intestines.

pneumatotherapy (nu"mah-to-ther'ah-pe) treatment by rarefied or compressed air.

pneumaturia (nu"mah-tu're-ah) gas or air in the urine.

pneumectomy (nu-mek'to-me) pneumonectomy.

pneumoangiogram (nu"mo-an'je-o-gram") a composite of radiographs obtained by pneumoencephalography and cerebral angiography.

pneumoangiography (nu"mo-an"je-og'rah-fe) roentgenography of the blood vessels of the lungs.

pneumoarthrography (nu"mo-ar-throg'rah-fe) roentgenography of a joint after injection of air or gas as a contrast medium; pneumarthrography.

pneumocephalus (nu"mo-sef'ah-lus) air in the intracranial cavity.

pneumococcemia (nu"mo-kok-se'me-ah) pneumococci in the blood.

pneumococcidal (nu"mo-kok-si'dal) destroying pneumococci.

pneumococcosis (nu"mo-kok-o'sis) infection with pneumococci.

pneumococcosuria (nu"mo-kok"o-su're-ah) pneumococci in the urine.

pneumococcus (nu"mo-kok'us), pl. *pneumococ'ci.* an individual organism of the species *Diplococcus pneumoniae,* which is the commonest cause of lobar pneumonia; it is a small, slightly elongated, encapsulated coccus, one end of which is pointed or lance-shaped, and commonly occurs in pairs; 80 serologic strains or types have been differentiated. adj., **pneumococ'cal.**

pneumoconiosis (nu"mo-ko"ne-o'sis) any of a group of lung diseases resulting from inhalation of particles of industrial substances, such as the dust of iron ore or coal, and permanent deposition of substantial amounts of such particles in the lungs. The diseases vary in severity but all are occupational diseases, acquired by workers in the course of their jobs.

Symptoms of the pneumoconioses include shortness of breath, chronic cough, and expectoration of mucus containing the offending particles.

SILICOSIS is probably the best known and most severe of these diseases. Asbestosis, caused by inhalation of asbestos fibers, is probably second only to silicosis in severity. Prevention and early diagnosis are important, for no effective treatment is available. Anthracosilicosis is caused by the inhalation of coal dust and silica and is similar in its development and its effects to silicosis. Beryllium lung disease or berylliosis is found in workers exposed to beryllium in the manufacture of fluorescent lamps, and in members of their families who are contaminated by the chemicals in the worker's clothing. Other types of pneumoconiosis include aluminum pneumoconiosis, cadmium worker's disease, and siderosis.

Pneumocystis (nu"mo-sis'tis) a genus of organisms of uncertain status, but considered to be protozoa. *P. cari'nii* is the causative agent of interstitial plasma cell pneumonia.

pneumocystography (nu"mo-sis-tog'rah-fe) roentgenography of the urinary bladder after injection of air or gas.

pneumoderma (nu"mo-der'mah) subcutaneous emphysema; air or gas in subcutaneous tissues.

pneumodynamics (nu"mo-di-nam'iks) the dynamics of the respiratory process.

pneumoencephalogram (nu"mo-en-sef'ah-lo-gram") the film produced by pneumoencephalography.

pneumoencephalography (nu"mo-en-sef"ah-log'-rah-fe) radiographic visualization of the fluid-containing structures of the brain after cerebrospinal fluid is intermittently withdrawn by lumbar puncture and replaced by air, oxygen, or helium.

pneumoenteritis (nu"mo-en"ter-i'tis) inflammation of the lungs and intestine.

pneumography (nu-mog'rah-fe) 1. an anatomical description of the lungs. 2. graphic recording of the respiratory movements. 3. radiography of a part after injection of a gas.

pneumohemopericardium (nu"mo-he"mo-per"ĭ-kar'de-um) air or gas and blood in the pericardium.

pneumohemothorax (nu"mo-he"mo-tho'raks) gas or air and blood in the pleural cavity.

pneumohydrometra (nu"mo-hi"dro-me'trah) gas and fluid in the uterus.

pneumohydropericardium (nu"mo-hi"dro-per"ĭ-kar'de-um) air or gas with fluid in the pericardium.

pneumohydrothorax (nu″mo-hi″dro-tho′raks) air or gas with fluid in the thoracic cavity.

pneumolith (nu′mo-lith) a pulmonary concretion.

pneumolithiasis (nu″mo-lĭ-thi′ah-sis) the presence of concretions in the lungs.

pneumomediastinum (nu″mo-me″de-ah-sti′num) the presence of air or gas in tissues of the mediastinum, occurring pathologically or introduced intentionally.

pneumometer (nu-mom′ĕ-ter) spirometer.

pneumomycosis (nu″mo-mi-ko′sis) any fungal disease of the lungs.

pneumomyelography (nu″mo-mi″ĕ-log′rah-fe) radiography of the spinal canal after withdrawal of cerebrospinal fluid and injection of air or gas.

pneumonectomy (nu″mo-nek′to-me) excision of lung tissue, of an entire lung (total pneumonectomy) or less (partial pneumonectomy), or of a single lobe (lobectomy). (See also surgery of the LUNG.)

pneumonia (nu-mo′ne-ah) inflammation of the lung with consolidation and exudation. Pneumonia once was a common cause of death and killed one out of four victims. It is still a serious disease, especially in infants and the elderly, who are most vulnerable. The general mortality rate has been drastically reduced, however, because of new medicines and modern methods of treatment.

TYPES AND SYMPTOMS. Infectious pneumonia may be caused by either bacteria or viruses. It may be primary or secondary (a complication of another disease) and may involve one or both lungs. It is most frequently caused by the pneumococcus (*Diplococcus pneumoniae*). The microorganisms that give rise to pneumonia are always present in the upper respiratory tract. They cause no harm unless resistance is severely lowered by some other factor, such as a severe cold, disease, alcoholism, or general poor health. Age is also a factor. When resistance is lowered or the conditions are favorable, the pneumococci invade the lungs.

Lobar Pneumonia. Pneumonia that affects a segment or an entire lobe of the lung is called lobar pneumonia. When both lungs are affected, the disease is called bilateral, or double, pneumonia. Whole sections of the lung tissue become solidified by inflammatory material, so that air cannot enter the alveoli. A chest x-ray is usually made to confirm the diagnosis and determine the extent of the disease.

Lobar pneumonia strikes suddenly. The symptoms are a cough, sharp chest pains (due to accompanying PLEURISY), blood-streaked or brownish sputum, and a high fever that generally starts with a chill. Pulse and respiration increase to almost twice their normal rates.

Bronchial Pneumonia (Bronchopneumonia). Bronchopneumonia is a less dramatic form of pneumonia that is more prevalent than lobar pneumonia. The area affected is usually smaller than in the lobar type. The inflammation is localized in or around the bronchi, and causes the lung to be spotted with clusters of infected tissue. The symptoms appear gradually and are usually milder than in lobar pneumonia. The temperature rises more slowly and does not go as high, and there is no crisis as in lobar pneumonia.

Bronchopneumonia is rarely fatal except in patients with heart disease or other complications. It is often more difficult to treat, however; relapses are common and can be serious. Diagnosis is also more difficult because the causes are varied.

Staphylococcic pneumonia is a very serious form of the disease and is occasionally fatal.

Primary Atypical Pneumonia. This type of pneumonia occurs chiefly in young adults who are otherwise healthy. It is often found in military camps and is due to various viruses or to *Mycoplasma pneumoniae.*

In the past this type of pneumonia often went undetected. The symptoms are similar to those of a cold. There may be headache, fever, a dry cough, generalized aches, and a feeling of extreme fatigue. X-ray examination of the lungs will reveal evidence of infection.

Other Types. Other kinds of pneumonia are caused by inhalation of poisonous gases (chemical pneumonia), accidental inhalation of food or liquids while unconscious (aspiration pneumonia), a blow or injury to the chest that interferes with normal respiration (traumatic pneumonia), or inhalation of oily substances (lipid or lipoid pneumonia). Hypostatic pneumonia, which is due to lying on the back, frequently occurs in elderly bedridden patients. Interstitial pneumonia is a chronic form in which there is an increase of the interstitial tissue and a decrease of the proper lung tissue, with induration.

PREVENTION. Many debilitated and elderly patients are prime candidates for the development of pneumonia, as are those who are physically inactive and immobile and those who suffer from acute and chronic pulmonary disease. It is possible to prevent pneumonia in many susceptible persons by being aware of factors that predispose one to the disease and by taking precautionary measures.

In the postoperative period it is important to position the patient properly and watch him closely while he is recovering from anesthesia so that he does not aspirate vomitus or other material into his lungs. The same precautions are essential for all patients in varying stages of unconsciousness and coma and in those who have poorly functioning gag reflexes. Early ambulation is another preventive measure to be used in postoperative and postpartal patients unless contraindicated. All patients who are immobilized for any reason should be turned regularly to avoid hypostatic pneumonia. Oversedation and overenthusiastic use of cough depressants can make a person more susceptible to pneumonia. The infectious agents that can cause pneumonia must be considered a constant hazard; vigorous adherence to the principles of cleanliness and personal hygiene are necessary to avoid the introduction of these agents into the respiratory tract of the susceptible person.

PATIENT CARE. Bed rest is of primary importance in assisting the body to combat the infection and in preventing unnecessary strain on the lungs and respiratory system. The fever presents problems of dehydration. Fluids are given frequently by mouth, or intravenously if necessary. An accurate record must be kept of the patient's intake and output. Bowel elimination must be checked regularly since the peristaltic action of the intestines may be affected in severe pneumonia. Delirium is not uncommon because of the high fever and requires careful observation of the patient and measures to prevent self-injury (see also DELIRIUM).

Mouth care is given regularly to combat dryness

and cracking of the lips, which occur as a result of fever and dehydration.

To relieve the chest pain caused by PLEURISY in pneumonia, it may help to have the patient lie on the affected side so that the side is splinted during coughing episodes. It is also helpful to place the hands on the patient's chest and apply pressure as a means of splinting the chest as the patient coughs.

The temperature, pulse, and respiration are checked and recorded at least every 4 hours. When the temperature falls the patient usually perspires profusely, requiring frequent changing of his gown and the bed linens. He must be protected from drafts and kept warm during this time.

p. al'ba, a fatal desquamative pneumonia of the newborn due to congenital syphilis, with fatty degeneration of the lungs, which appear pale and virtually airless.

desquamative p., chronic pneumonia with hardening of the fibrous exudate and proliferation of the interstitial tissue and epithelium.

desquamative interstitial p., chronic pneumonia with desquamation of large alveolar cells and thickening of the walls of distal air passages; marked by dyspnea and nonproductive cough.

Friedländer's p., Friedländer's bacillus p., a form characterized by massive mucoid inflammatory exudates in a lobe of the lung, due to *Klebsiella pneumoniae.*

influenzal p., influenza virus p., an acute, severe, usually fatal disease due to influenza virus, with high fever, prostration, sore throat, aching pains, profound dyspnea and anxiety, and massive edema and consolidation. The term is also applied to influenza complicated by bacterial pneumonia.

interstitial plasma cell p., a form affecting infants and debilitated persons, including those receiving certain drugs, in which cellular detritus containing plasma cells appears in lung tissue; it is caused by *Pneumocystis carinii.*

varicella p., that developing after the skin eruption in varicella (chickenpox) and apparently due to the same virus; symptoms may be severe, with violent cough, hemoptysis, and severe chest pain.

pneumonic (nu-mon'ik) pertaining to the lung or to pneumonia.

p. plague, a form of PLAGUE with extensive involvement of the lungs.

pneumonitis (nu"mo-ni'tis) inflammation of lung tissue.

pneumono- word element [Gr.], *lung.*

pneumonocentesis (nu-mo"no-sen-te'sis) surgical puncture of a lung for aspiration.

pneumonocyte (nu-mon'o-sīt) collective term for the alveolar epithelial cells (great alveolar cells and squamous alveolar cells) and alveolar phagocytes of the lungs.

pneumonolysis (nu"mo-nol'ĭ-sis) division of tissues attaching the lung to the wall of the chest cavity, to permit collapse of the lung.

pneumonopathy (nu"mo-nop'ah-the) any lung disease.

pneumonopexy (nu-mo'no-pek"se) fixation of the lung to the thoracic wall.

pneumonorrhaphy (nu"mon-or'ah-fe) suture of the lung.

pneumonosis (nu"mo-no'sis) any lung disease.

pneumonotomy (nu"mo-not'o-me) incision of the lung.

pneumopericardium (nu"mo-per"ĭ-kar'de-um) the presence of air or gas in the pericardial cavity.

pneumoperitoneum (nu"mo-per"ĭ-to-ne'um) the presence of air or gas in the peritoneal cavity, occurring pathologically or introduced intentionally.

pneumoperitonitis (nu"mo-per"ĭ-to-ni'tis) peritonitis with accumulation of air or gas in the peritoneal cavity.

pneumopleuritis (nu"mo-ploo-ri'tis) inflammation of the lungs and pleura.

pneumopyelography (nu"mo-pi"ĕ-log'rah-fe) roentgenography after injection of oxygen or air into the renal pelvis.

pneumopyopericardium (nu"mo-pi"o-per"ĭ-kar'de-um) air or gas and pus in the pericardium.

pneumopyothorax (nu"mo-pi"o-tho'raks) air or gas and pus in the pleural cavity.

pneumoradiogrphy (nu"mo-ra"de-og'rah-fe) radiography of a part after injection of oxygen or other gas as contrast material.

pneumoretroperitoneum (nu"mo-ret"ro-per"ĭ-to-ne'um) the presence of air or gas in the retroperitoneal space.

pneumorrhagia (nu"mo-ra'je-ah) hemorrhage from the lungs; severe hemoptysis.

pneumotachograph (nu"mo-tak'o-graf) an instrument for recording the velocity of respired air.

pneumotachometer (nu"mo-tah-kom'ĕ-ter) a transducer for measuring expired air flow.

pneumotaxic (nu"mo-tak'sik) regulating the respiratory rate.

pneumotherapy (nu"mo-ther'ah-pe) 1. treatment of disease of the lungs. 2. pneumatotherapy.

pneumothorax (nu"mo-tho'raks) accumulation of air or gas in the pleural cavity, resulting in collapse of the lung on the affected side. The condition may occur spontaneously, as in the course of a pulmonary disease, or it may follow trauma to, and perforation of, the chest wall. *Artificial pneumothorax* is a surgical procedure sometimes used in the treatment of tuberculosis or following pneumonectomy; it involves the injection of measured amounts of air into the pleural cavity to collapse the lung and immobilize it while healing takes place (see also surgery of the LUNG).

SPONTANEOUS PNEUMOTHORAX. This condition sometimes occurs when there is an opening on the surface of the lung allowing leakage of air from the bronchi into the pleural cavity. Most often it occurs when an emphysematous bulla or other weakened area on the lung ruptures. Normally the pleural cavity is an airtight compartment with a negative pressure. When air enters the pleural cavity the lung collapses, producing shortness of breath, mediastinal shift toward the unaffected side (see also MEDIASTINAL SHIFT).

Other symptoms of spontaneous pneumothorax are a sudden sharp chest pain, fall in blood pressure, weak and rapid pulse, and cessation of normal respiratory movements on the affected side of the chest.

Spontaneous pneumothorax may require no specific treatment beyond bed rest and the administration of oxygen to relieve dyspnea. The patient usually is more comfortable if he is allowed to sit up. In some cases THORACENTESIS and aspiration of air from the pleural cavity may be necessary. This allows for reexpansion of the lung. If air continues to leak from the defect in the lung surface a continuous closed-drainage apparatus is set up (see also CHEST TUBES). As soon as the lung lesion heals and the lung is reexpanded, the patient is allowed to resume his usual activities.

Tension pneumothorax is a particularly dangerous form of pneumothorax that occurs when air escapes into the pleural cavity from a bronchus but cannot regain entry into the bronchus. As a result, continuously increasing air pressure in the pleural cavity causes progressive collapse of the lung tissue. Emergency treatment—aspiration of air from the pleural cavity—is necessary in this disorder. If untreated, increased pressure within the pleural cavity will cause lung collapse and MEDIASTINAL SHIFT.

pneumotomy (nu-mot′o-me) pneumonotomy.

pneumoventriculography (nu″mo-ven-trik″u-log′rah-fe) pneumoencephalography.

P.O. [L.] *per os* (by mouth; orally).

Po chemical symbol, *polonium.*

Po_2 oxygen partial pressure (tension); also written P_{O_2}, pO_2, and pO_2 (see also BLOOD GAS ANALYSIS).

pock (pok) a pustule, especially of smallpox.

pockmark (pok′mark) a depressed scar left by a pustule.

pod(o)- word element [Gr.], *foot.*

podagra (po-dag′rah) gouty pain in the great toe.

podalgia (po-dal′je-ah) pain in the feet.

podalic (po-dal′ik) accomplished by means of the feet, as podalic version.

podarthritis (pod″ar-thri′tis) inflammation of the joints of the feet.

podencephalus (pod″en-sef′ah-lus) a monster without a cranium, the brain hanging by a pedicle.

podiatrist (po-di′ah-trist) chiropodist; a specialist in podiatry.

podiatry (po-di′ah-tre) chiropody; the specialized field dealing with the study and care of the foot, including its anatomy, pathology, medical and surgical treatment, etc.

podium (po′de-um), pl. *po′dia* [L.] a footlike process, such as an extension of the protoplasm of a cell.

podocyte (pod′o-sīt) an epithelial cell of the visceral layer of a renal glomerulus, having a number of footlike radiating processes (pedicles).

pododynamometer (pod″o-di″nah-mom′ĕ-ter) a device for determining the strength of the leg muscles.

pododynia (pod″o-din′e-ah) neuralgic pain of the heel and sole; burning pain without redness in the sole of the foot.

podology (po-dol′o-je) podiatry.

podophyllin (pod″o-fil′in) podophyllum resin.

podophyllum (pod″o-fil′um) the dried rhizome and roots of *Podophyllum peltatum.*

p. resin, a mixture of resins from podophyllum, used as a topical caustic in the treatment of certain papillomas.

pogoniasis (po″go-ni′ah-sis) excessive growth of the beard, or growth of a beard on a woman.

pogonion (po-go′ne-on) the anterior midpoint of the chin.

-poiesis word element [Gr.], *formation.* adj., **-poiet′ic.**

poikilo- word element [Gr.], *varied; irregular.*

poikiloblast (poi′kĭ-lo-blast″) an abnormally shaped erythroblast.

poikilocyte (poi′kĭ-lo-sīt″) an abnormally shaped erythrocyte.

poikilocytosis (poi″kĭ-lo-si-to′sis) the presence of poikilocytes in the blood.

poikiloderma (poi″kĭ-lo-der′mah) a condition characterized by pigmentary and atrophic changes in the skin, giving it a mottled appearance.

poikilotherm (poi′kĭ-lo-therm″) an animal that exhibits poikilothermy; a cold-blooded animal.

poikilothermy (poi″kĭ-lo-ther′me) the state of having body temperature that varies with that of the environment. adj., **poikilother′mal, poikilother′mic.**

point (point) 1. a small area or spot; the sharp end of an object. 2. to approach the surface, like the pus of an abscess, at a definite spot or place.

p. A, a roentgenographic, cephalometric landmark, determined on the lateral head film; it is the most retruded part of the curved bony outline from the anterior nasal spine to the crest of the maxillary alveolar process.

auricular p., the center of the opening of the external acoustic meatus.

p. B, a roentgenographic, cephalometric landmark, determined on the lateral head film; it is the most posterior midline point in the concavity between the infradentale and pogonium.

boiling p., the temperature at which a liquid will boil: at sea level, 100° C., or 212° F.

boiling p., normal, the temperature at which a liquid boils at one atmosphere pressure.

cardinal p's, 1. the points on the different refracting media of the eye that determine the direction of the entering or emerging light rays. 2. four points within the pelvic inlet—the two sacroiliac articulations and the two iliopectineal eminences.

corresponding p's, points upon the two retinas whose impressions unite to produce a single perception; cf. disparate points.

craniometric p's, the established points of reference for measurement of the skull.

dew p., the temperature at which moisture in the atmosphere is deposited as dew.

disparate p's, points on the two retinas on which incident light rays do not produce the same impression; cf. corresponding points.

far p., the remotest point at which an object is clearly seen when the eye is at rest.

fixation p., the point on which the vision is fixed.

freezing p., the temperature at which a liquid begins to freeze; for water, 0° C., or 32° F.

ice p., the temperature of equilibrium between ice and air-saturated water under one atmosphere pressure.

isoelectric p., the pH of a solution at which a dipolar ion does not migrate in an electric field.

isoionic p., the pH of a solution at which the number of cations equals the number of anions.

jugal p., the point at the angle formed by the masseteric and maxillary edges of the zygomatic bone; called also jugale.

lacrimal p., a small aperture situated on a slight elevation at the medial end of the eyelid margin, through which tears from the lacrimal lake enter the lacrimal canaliculi. (See also LACRIMAL APPARATUS.)

p. of maximal impulse, the point on the chest where the impulse of the left ventricle is felt most strongly, normally in the fifth costal interspace inside the mamillary line.

McBurney's p., a point of special tenderness in appendicitis, about $\frac{1}{2}-2$ inches from the right anterior iliac spine on a line between the spine and the navel.

melting p., the minimum temperature at which a solid begins to liquefy.

near p., the nearest point of clear vision, the absolute near point being that for either eye alone with accommodation relaxed, and the relative near point that for the two eyes together with employment of accommodation.

nodal p's, two points on the axis of an optical system situated so that a ray falling on one will produce a parallel ray emerging through the other.

pressure p's, various locations on the body at which digital pressure may be applied to control hemorrhage.

trigger p., a spot on the body at which pressure or other stimulus gives rise to specific sensations or symptoms.

Valleix's p's, tender points along the course of certain nerves in neuralgia; called also puncta dolorosa.

pointillage (pwahn-te-yahzh′) [Fr.] massage with the points of the fingers.

poison (poi′zun) a substance that, on ingestion, inhalation, absorption, application, injection, or development within the body, in relatively small amounts, may cause structural damage or functional disturbance.

Corrosives are poisons that destroy tissues directly. They include the mineral acids, such as nitric acid, sulfuric acid, and hydrochloric acid; the caustic alkalis, such as ammonia, sodium hydroxide (lye), sodium carbonate, and sodium hypochlorite; and carbolic acid (phenol).

Irritants are poisons that inflame the mucous membranes by direct action. These include arsenic, copper sulfate, salts of lead, zinc, and phosphorus, and many others.

Nerve toxins act on the nerves or affect some of the basic cell processes. This large group includes the narcotics, such as opium, heroin, and cocaine, and the barbiturates, anesthetics, and alcohols.

Blood toxins act on the blood and deprive it of oxygen. They include carbon monoxide, carbon dioxide, hydrocyanic acid, and the gases used in chemical warfare. Some blood toxins destroy the blood cells or the platelets.

See also POISONING and names of individual poisons.

p. ivy, oak, and sumac, common plants of the genus *Rhus* (or *Toxicodendron*) that cause allergic skin reactions. The poison contained in their leaves, roots, and berries is an oily substance called urushiol. It has no effect on some people; in others, momentary or even indirect contact may cause painful rashes and blisters.

POISON IVY. Poison ivy (*Rhus radicans*) grows in the form of climbing vines, shrubs that trail on the ground, and shrubbery that grows upright without any support. The vine clings to stone and brick houses and climbs trees and poles. It flourishes abundantly along fences, paths, and roadways, and is often partly hidden by other foliage.

Recognition. The poison ivy plant is attractive and is often picked as a decoration by unsuspecting flower gatherers. Although poison ivy comes in many forms and displays seasonal changes, it has one constant characteristic: The leaves always grow in clusters of three, one at the end of the stalk, the other two opposite one another.

Transmission. The plant is particularly potent in the spring and early summer when it is full of oily resinous sap. This forms an invisible film upon the human skin on contact. Direct contact is not always necessary. Some cases of poison ivy dermatitis are caused by the handling of clothing or garden implements that have been contaminated by the sap, sometimes months earlier; dogs and cats may carry it on their fur. Many people are so sensitive that smoke from a brush fire containing poison ivy brings on a rash.

Symptoms. After exposure, the symptoms of poison ivy dermatitis may develop in a matter of hours, though sometimes they do not appear for several days. There is reddening on the hands, neck, face, legs, or whatever parts of the body have been exposed, with considerable itching. Small blisters form which later become larger and eventually exude a watery fluid. The skin then becomes crusty and dry. After a few weeks all symptoms spontaneously disappear.

Treatment. An attack of poison ivy dermatitis can sometimes be avoided if the skin is scrubbed immediately after contact with ordinary yellow laundry soap, which has a high alkaline content. The skin should be lathered several times and rinsed each time in running water. This may remove all or at least part of the poison ivy film before it is able to penetrate the skin.

If, despite precautions, dermatitis does develop, various treatments may relieve the itching. One is to apply a compress soaked in Burow's solution (obtainable at any drugstore), diluted in the proportion of one part solution to 15 parts cool water. Another standard remedy is calamine lotion.

If the inflammation becomes unusually severe or is accompanied by fever, a physician should be consulted. He may prescribe one of the cortisone preparations, which may be taken orally, injected, or applied locally as a cream.

Immunization. In general, programs of desensitizing and immunization must be started well in advance of potential contact with poison ivy, and must be repeated at regular intervals, often weekly for 4 or 5 weeks. There is some doubt as to their effectiveness.

POISON OAK. Poison oak (*Rhus diversiloba* or *R. toxicodendron*), sometimes known as oakleaf ivy, is not related to the oak tree but does bear a close kinship to poison ivy. The eastern and western varieties resemble each other quite closely.

Poison oak is usually a low-growing shrub and seldom a climbing vine. It has three leaves, like poison ivy, but they are lobed and bear a slight resemblance to small oak leaves. The berries are white and small, resembling those of poison ivy.

Poison oak causes the same symptoms as poison ivy, except that they are usually milder. There is redness of the skin, but blisters are less frequent.

Prevention, treatment, and immunization are the same as for poison ivy dermatitis.

POISON SUMAC. Although poison sumac (*Rhus vernix*) goes by other names, such as swamp sumac, poison elder, poison ash, poison dogwood, and thunderwood, there is only one variety of it.

Sometimes, however, poison sumac is confused with the several harmless kinds of sumac.

Poison sumac is a coarse woody shrub or small tree, and it has white berries, which distinguish it from the several harmless varieties of sumac, which have red berries.

Symptoms and treatment are similar to those of poison ivy dermatitis.

poisoning (poi′zun-ing) the morbid condition produced by a poison. The poison may be swallowed, inhaled (as in CARBON DIOXIDE POISONING), injected by a stinging insect as in a BEE STING, or spilled or otherwise brought into contact with the skin.

SYMPTOMS. The symptoms of poisoning vary greatly according to the poison taken and the time that has elapsed. Some poisons cause no immediate symptoms. In general, poisoning should be suspected in the following instances: (1) a revealing odor such as alcohol on the breath; (2) discoloration of the mouth or lips; (3) evidence of eating leaves or wild berries; (4) severe pain or a burning sensation in the mouth and throat; (5) nausea or vomiting; (6) convulsions; (7) confusion or disturbance of sight; (8) unconsciousness or deep sleep; (9) sudden illness, when an open bottle or container of medicine or poisonous chemicals is found nearby.

FIRST AID. In all cases of poisoning, speed in treatment is an essential, but deliberate speed and calm thinking will avoid hasty decisions that may result in ineffective if not harmful treatment.

It is not advisable to force the victim to drink a large amount of water or other liquid in an effort to neutralize an ingested poison. This may only serve to increase absorption. The victim of an inhaled poison does require immediate removal to fresh air and artificial respiration to restore breathing. When the skin has been contaminated by a poison, immediate and repeated drenching of the area with cool water is necessary to remove the poison.

Supportive measures that can be beneficial to any poison victim include maintenance of an open AIRWAY, keeping the victim quiet (especially if he is likely to have convulsions, as in strychnine poisoning), and maintaining body heat to avoid SHOCK.

Swallowed Poisons. In general, the rule of thumb is to induce vomiting except under the following conditions: (1) if the victim has swallowed a corrosive poison, such as a strong acid or alkali, in which case there is severe pain, a burning sensation in the mouth and throat, and vomiting, (2) if the victim has swallowed a petroleum product, such as gasoline, kerosene, or cigarette lighter fluid, (3) if the victim has swallowed iodine or strychnine, and (4) if the victim has convulsions, is in a coma, or is unconscious.

The administration of an emetic, usually syrup of ipecac followed by a glass of warm water, is the best way to induce vomiting. Attempts through radio, television, newspapers, and an annual "poison prevention week," to urge mothers of small children to keep this medication on hand have not been completely successful; however, it should be available at home or a nearby drugstore or a neighbor's house. If no ipecac can be obtained, the victim should be taken immediately to a hospital or physician's office. Efforts to induce vomiting by putting a finger or a spoon at the back of the throat are usually not successful, but may be tried if no emetic drug is available. When induced vomiting is unsuccessful or undesirable, LAVAGE may be employed to remove the stomach contents and wash out the remaining poison.

Many poisons have a specific antidote that can effectively counteract the action of the poison or neutralize it. The "universal antidote" may be of doubtful value because the tannic acid and magnesium may dilute the third ingredient, activated charcoal, and reduce its effectiveness as an absorbent. Activated charcoal is another product that should be kept in the households where small children live. This substance is given in doses of 10 times the estimated ingested dose as a 25 per cent solution in 8 ounces of water. It is given after the syrup of ipecac dosage, but is not useful in alcohol and insecticide poisoning.

Inhaled Poisons. General first-aid treatment for poisoning by such gases as carbon monoxide, hydrocyanic acid, and methane consists of dragging or carrying the victim to fresh air and administering artificial respiration, if breathing is irregular or has stopped. The rescuer should be careful not to risk being overcome himself. In telephoning the hospital, police, or fire department for help, one should specify the nature of the accident so that the proper emergency equipment may be brought. The victim should be wrapped in blankets to maintain body temperature, and be kept quiet. If he has convulsions, he should be kept in a semidark room and care should be taken to avoid jarring him.

External Poisons. If the skin has been contaminated by a chemical, the poison should be washed off immediately with water from a faucet, shower, or hose, and any contaminated clothing should be removed at the same time.

If the poison is in the eye, the eyelids should be held open while a gentle, continuous stream of water is poured into the eye.

PREVENTION OF POISONING. *In poisoning, prevention is far better than any treatment.* To prevent poisoning, the American Medical Association recommends the following precautions:

1. Keep all medicines, household chemicals, and other poisonous substances locked up. There is no place "out of reach of children."
2. Never transfer poisonous substances to unlabeled containers, or food containers such as milk or soda bottles, or cereal boxes.
3. Never reuse containers of chemical products.
4. Never store poisonous substances on the same shelves used for storing food. Confusion might be fatal.
5. Never leave discarded medicines within the reach of children or pets. Pour contents down the drain or toilet or incinerator. Rinse the container.
6. Always read the label before using any chemical product.
7. Do not give or take medicines in the dark.
8. Never tell children the medicine you are giving them is candy.
9. When preparing the baby's formula, taste the ingredients. Never store boric acid, salt, or talcum near the formula ingredients.

There are more than 500 Poison Control Centers throughout the United States. In case of poisoning, information concerning antidotes can be obtained by telephone from the nearest center.

blood p., septicemia.

food p., a group of acute illnesses due to ingestion of contaminated food (see also FOOD POISONING).

Polaramine (po-lar′ah-mēn) trademark for preparations of dexchlorpheniramine, an antihistaminic.

polarimeter (po″lah-rim′ĕ-ter) a device for measuring the rotation of plane polarized light.

polarimetry (po″lah-rim′ĕ-tre) measurement of the rotation of plane polarized light.

polariscope (po-lar′ĭ-skōp) an instrument for the study of polarization.

polarity (po-lar′ĭte) the condition of having poles or of exhibiting opposite effects at the two extremities.

polarization (po″lar-ĭ-za′shun) the production of that condition in light in which its vibrations are parallel to each other in one plane, or in circles and ellipses.

polarizer (po′lah-rīz″er) an appliance for polarizing light.

poldine (pol′dēn) an anticholinergic used as the methylsulfate salt to reduce gastric secretion of hydrochloric acid.

pole (pōl) 1. either extremity of any axis, as of the fetal ellipse or a body organ. 2. either one of two points that have opposite physical qualities (electric or other). adj., **po′lar.**

animal p., that pole of an ovum to which the nucleus is approximated, and from which the polar bodies pinch off.

cephalic p., the end of the fetal ellipse at which the head of the fetus is situated.

frontal p., the most prominent part of the anterior end of each hemisphere of the brain.

germinal p., animal pole.

negative p., the terminal of an electric cell that has the lower potential, and toward which the current flows; cathode.

occipital p., the posterior end of the occipital lobe of the brain.

pelvic p., the end of the fetal ellipse at which the breech of the fetus is situated.

positive p., the terminal of an electic cell that has the higher potential, and from which the current flows; anode.

temporal p., the prominent anterior end of the temporal lobe of the brain.

vegetal p., vegetative p., vitelline p., that pole of an ovum at which the greater amount of food yolk is deposited.

poli(o)- word element [Gr.], *gray matter.*

polio (po′le-o) poliomyelitis.

polioclastic (po″le-o-klas′tik) destroying the gray matter of the nervous system.

poliodystrophia (po″le-o-dis-tro′fe-ah) poliodystrophy.

p. cer′ebri, a rare disease of young children, marked by neuron degeneration of the cerebral cortex and elsewhere, with progressive mental deterioration, motor disturbances, sometimes cortical deafness and blindness, and early death. Called also Alper's disease.

poliodystrophy (po″le-o-dis′tro-fe) atrophy of the cerebral gray matter.

polioencephalitis (po″le-o-en-sef″ah-li′tis) inflammatory disease of the gray matter of the brain.

inferior p., bulbar paralysis.

polioencephalomeningomyelitis (po″le-o-en-sef″ah-lo-mĕ-ning″go-mi″ĕ-li′tis) inflammation of the gray matter of the brain and spinal cord and of the meninges.

polioencephalomyelitis (po″le-o-en-sef″ah-lo-mi″ĕ-li′tis) inflammation of the gray matter of the brain and spinal cord.

polioencephalopathy (po″le-o-en-sef″ah-lop′ah-the) any disease of the gray matter of the brain.

poliomyelitis (po″le-o-mi″ĕ-li′tis) an acute, contagious viral disease that attacks the central nervous system, injuring or destroying the nerve cells that control the muscles and sometimes causing paralysis; called also polio and infantile paralysis. Paralysis most often affects the legs but can involve any muscles, including those that control breathing and swallowing. Since the development and the use of vaccines against poliomyelitis, the disease has become far less common. However, the number of cases among very young infants who have not been immunized is on the rise.

Poliomyelitis is a very serious disease, but it is not often fatal. Paralysis develops in about half of all patients with polio, and of these about half recover completely. Only a small percentage of patients have serious symptoms; many cases are so mild that they are undiagnosed and never reported.

There are three known types of poliovirus, each causing a different type of the disease. Most paralytic cases are caused by type 1. Poliovirus is found in the throat of a patient for the first few days of the disease, and in his intestines for a longer period, sometimes as long as 17 weeks. The disease spreads by means of droplets of moisture from an infected person's throat or by waste products from his intestines. The contagious period is 7 or more days from the time of onset of the disease.

The poliovirus is short-lived, and cannot survive long in the air. The incubation period of polio is from 1 to 2 weeks, and occasionally as long as 3 weeks. Members of the family or other contacts may be carriers, but only for a short period of time.

SYMPTOMS. The early symptoms of polio include fever, headache, vomiting, sore throat, pain and stiffness in the back and neck, and drowsiness. In the nonparalytic type, the fever usually lasts about 7 days, and the stiffness fades away in 3 to 5 days. In paralytic polio, some weakness or paralysis of the arms or legs begins 1 to 7 days after the first symptoms. The first sign of bulbar polio, which affects the muscles of swallowing and breathing, is difficulty in swallowing, speaking, and breathing. This usually occurs in the first 3 days of the disease.

TREATMENT. There is at present no cure for polio; once the disease begins it must be allowed to run its course. Supportive care is important, however, and proper symptomatic treatment can reduce discomfort and prevent some crippling aftereffects. Applications of HEAT in the form of hot wet packs, DIATHERMY, warm baths in the form of HYDROTHERAPY, and gentle exercising can reduce pain caused by muscle spasms and prevent deformities. During the acute stage of the disease bed rest is essential and the patient is kept warm and quiet.

PREVENTION. The first safe, effective vaccine against polio was developed under the direction of Dr. Jonas E. Salk, and is referred to as the Salk vaccine. This early vaccine, which used killed polio viruses to stimulate production and release of antibodies has been replaced in the United States by the Sabin vaccine. This is a live vaccine, an oral preparation of attenuated viruses available in trivalent and monovalent forms. The preferred trivalent form of polio vaccine (TOPV) contains organisms of types 1, 2, and 3 polio in one solution. The monovalent vaccine is recommended for use only in epidemics when the type of polio is known.

The American Academy of Pediatrics recommends that infants be given TOPV drops at 2, 4, and 6 months, at 18 months, and at age 4 to 6, immediately before entrance to school. Older children and teenagers who have not been immunized should receive the first two immunizations 6 to 8 weeks apart and the final one 3 to 12 months later. A single booster dose is recommended for adults before traveling to areas where polio is endemic or if they live in a community that experiences an outbreak.

Unfortunately, in spite of the availability of the vaccine many persons have not been adequately immunized against polio. Nationwide surveys have shown a decline in the percentage of children under the age of five who have been fully or even partially immunized.

REHABILITATION. A person who has been paralyzed by an acute case of polio can often be restored to activity through proper treatment. New techniques of physical therapy have been remarkably successful in educating patients to use individual muscles again. (See also EXERCISE.) In some cases, reconstructive surgery on the affected limb is valuable. Orthopedic devices, such as braces, supports, and special shoes, may also be helpful.

The National Foundation (formerly the National Foundation for Infantile Paralysis) can give advice on all aspects of treatment and rehabilitation for polio victims. The Foundation also gives financial aid to polio patients who are unable to afford proper treatment. The headquarters of the National Foundation are at 800 Second Avenue, New York, N.Y. 10017; there are local offices in many communities across the country.

PATIENT CARE. The patient with poliomyelitis is cared for under "excretion precautions" until the acute phase is over. Further ISOLATION is not considered necessary. While on complete bed rest the patient should lie on a firm mattress and be positioned properly to avoid orthopedic deformities. When his position is changed he must be turned gently, with his joints supported, and care must be taken not to grasp the muscles, which are extremely tender and painful and have a tendency toward spasms when stimulated. The paralysis of the affected limbs is a result of involvement of the motor nerves; the sensory nerves are not involved and thus the patient has no loss of sensory perception and can experience pain.

Warm, moist packs are applied to the affected limbs to reduce muscle spasm and relieve pain. Later, as the acute symptoms subside, the physician may order physical therapy measures such as massage and passive exercises to avoid contractures and maintain muscle tone.

If the poliomyelitis is of the bulbar type, affecting the muscles of respiration, a VENTILATOR will be used to maintain adequate ventilation of the lungs. A TRACHEOSTOMY is sometimes necessary to facilitate breathing and maintain a patent airway. Swallowing difficulties may require TUBE FEEDING or intravenous infusion to provide adequate nutrition. The patient with bulbar poliomyelitis must have someone in constant attendance during the acute stage of his illness.

Fears and anxieties about the outcome of his illness are quite common in a patient with poliomyelitis. Most persons, even children, are usually aware of the crippling effects of this disease. The health care team must help the patient and his family in their adjustment to the changes poliomyelitis may bring about in their lives.

poliomyelopathy (po″le-o-mi″ĕ-lop′ah-the) any disease of the gray matter of the spinal cord.

poliosis (po″le-o′sis) permature grayness of the hair.

poliovirus (po″le-o-vi′rus) the causative agent of poliomyelitis, separable, on the basis of specificity of neutralizing antibody, into three serotypes designated types 1, 2, and 3.

pollen (pol′en) the male fertilizing element of flowering plants.

pollenosis (pol″ĕ-no′sis) pollinosis.

pollex (pol′eks) [L.] thumb.

pollinosis (pol″ĭ-no′sis) an allergic reaction to pollen; hay fever.

pollution (pŏ-lu′shun) defiling or making impure, especially contamination by noxious substances.

polonium (po-lo′ne-um) a chemical element, atomic number 84, atomic weight 210, symbol Po. (See table of ELEMENTS.)

poloxalkol (pol-ok′sal-kol) a pharmacologically inert oxyalkylene polymer used as a fecal softener.

polus (po′lus), pl. *po′li* [L.] pole.

poly- word element [Gr.], *many; much.*

polyadenitis (pol″e-ad″ĕ-ni′tis) inflammation of several glands.

polyadenosis (pol″e-ad″ĕ-no′sis) disorder of several glands, particularly endocrine glands.

polyangiitis (pol″e-an″je-i′tis) inflammation involving multiple blood or lymph vessels.

polyarteritis (pol″e-ar″tĕ-ri′tis) a condition marked by multiple sites of inflammatory and destructive lesions in the arterial system (see also PERIADENITIS NODOSA).

polyarthric (pol″e-ar′thrik) polyarticular.

polyarthritis (pol″e-ar-thri′tis) inflammation of several joints.

chronic villous p., chronic inflammation of the synovial membrane of several joints.

p. rheumat′ica, rheumatic fever.

polyarticular (pol″e-ar-tik′u-lar) affecting many joints; polyarthric.

polyatomic (pol″e-ah-tom′ik) made up of several atoms.

polybasic (pol″e-ba′sik) having several replaceable hydrogen atoms.

polycarbophil (pol″e-kar′bo-fil) polyacrylic acid cross-linked with divinyl glycol; used as a gastrointestinal absorbent.

polychemotherapy (pol″e-ke″mo-ther′ah-pe) simultaneous administration of several chemotherapeutic agents.

polycholia (pol″e-ko′le-ah) excessive flow or secretion of bile.

polychondritis (pol″e-kon-dri′tis) inflammation of many cartilages of the body.

chronic atrophic p., p. chron′ica atro′phicans, relapsing p., an acquired disease of unknown origin, chiefly involving various cartilages and showing both chronicity and a tendency to recurrence; it is marked by inflammatory and degenerative lesions of various cartilaginous structures.

polychromasia (pol″e-kro-ma′ze-ah) 1. variation in the hemoglobin content of erythrocytes. 2. polychromatophilia.

polychromatic (pol″e-kro-mat′ik) many-colored.

polychromatocyte (pol″e-kro-mat′o-sīt) a cell stainable with various kinds of stains.

polychromatophil (pol″e-kro-mat′o-fil) a structure stainable with many kinds of stains.

polychromatophilia (pol″e-kro-mat″o-fil′e-ah) 1. the property of being stainable with various stains; affinity for all sorts of stains. 2. a condition in which the erythrocytes, on staining, show various shades of blue combined with tinges of pink. adj., **polychromatophil′ic.**

polychromemia (pol″e-kro-me′me-ah) increase in the coloring matter of the blood.

polyclinic (pol″e-klin′ik) a hospital and school where diseases and injuries of all kinds are studied and treated.

polyclonal (pol″e-klōn′al) derived from different cells; pertaining to several clones.

polyclonia (pol″e-klo′ne-ah) a disease marked by many clonic spasms; called also polymyoclonus.

polycoria (pol″e-ko′re-ah) more than one pupil in an eye.

polycrotism (po-lik′ro-tizm) the quality of having several secondary waves to each beat of the pulse. adj., **polycrot′ic.**

Polycycline (pol″e-si′klēn) trademark for preparations of tetracycline, an antibiotic.

polycyesis (pol″e-si-e′sis) multiple pregnancy.

polycystic (pol″e-sis′tik) containing many cysts.

polycythemia (pol″e-si-the′me-ah) an increase in the total cell mass of the blood.

There are two distinct forms of the disease. In primary polycythemia (called also polycythemia vera), the cause for the red cell increase is not understood. There is hyperplasia of the cell-forming tissues of the bone marrow, with resultant elevation of the erythrocyte count and hemoglobin level, and an increase in the number of leukocytes and platelets. The condition has been compared to leukemia and regarded as a malignant neoplastic disease.

Secondary polycythemia is a physiologic condition resulting from a decreased oxygen supply to the tissues. The body attempts to compensate for the oxygen deficiency by manufacturing more hemoglobin and red blood cells. Living at high altitudes can produce polycythemia, as can severe chronic lung and heart disorders, especially congenital heart defects.

SYMPTOMS. The symptoms of both primary and secondary polycythemia are much the same. The increased erythrocyte production results in thickening of the blood and an increased tendency toward clotting. The viscosity of the blood limits its ability to flow properly, diminishing the supply of blood to the brain and to other vital tissues. This may cause mental sluggishness, irritability, headache, dizziness, fainting, disturbances of sensation in the hands and feet, and a feeling of fullness in the head. There may be episodes of acute pain as spontaneous clots occur in the blood vessels.

The spleen becomes enlarged. The smaller veins become more prominent, so that the skin has a bluish hue. The secondary form is often accompanied by enlargement of the tips of the fingers (clubbing).

In another form, polycythemia hypertonica, called also Gaisböck's disease, there is no spleen enlargement, but hypertrophy of the heart and increased blood pressure.

TREATMENT. Treatment is aimed at reducing the red cell count and decreasing the blood volume. It includes both the modern techniques of radiation therapy and the ancient practice of bloodletting. In mild cases periodic bloodletting may be the only treatment necessary. More recent methods use radioactive phosphorus or nitrogen mustard and other alkylating agents.

In secondary polycythemia, successful treatment of the causative illness will relieve the polycythemia.

polydactylism, polydactyly (pol″e-dak′til-izm; pol″e-dak′tĭ-le) the presence of supernumerary fingers or toes.

polydipsia (pol″e-dip′se-ah) excessive thirst.

polydysplasia (pol″e-dis-pla′ze-ah) faulty development of several tissues, organs, or systems.

polyemia (pol″e-e′me-ah) excessive blood in the body.

polyendocrine (pol″e-en′do-krīn) pertaining to several endocrine glands.

polyesthesia (pol″e-es-the′ze-ah) a sensation as if several points were touched on application of a stimulus to a single point.

polyethylene (pol″e-eth′ĭ-lēn) polymerized ethylene, $(CH—CH_2)_n$, a synthetic plastic material, forms of which have been used in reparative surgery.

p. glycol, a polymer of ethylene oxide and water, available in liquid form (polyethylene glycol 300 or 400) or as waxy solids (polyethylene glycol 1540 or 4000), used in various pharmaceutical preparations as a water-soluble ointment base.

polygalactia (pol″e-gah-lak′she-ah) excessive secretion of milk.

polygalacturonase (pol″e-gah-lak-tu′ro-nās) an enzyme that catylyzes the hydrolysis of pectin to sugars and galacturonic acid.

polygene (pol′ĕ-jēn) a group of nonallelic genes that interact to influence the same character with additive effect.

polygenic (pol″e-jen′ik) pertaining to or determined by several different genes.

polyglandular (pol″e-glan′du-lar) pertaining to or affecting several glands.

polyglycolic acid (pol″e-gli-ko′lik) a polymer of glycolic acid used as an absorbable suture material.

polygnathus (po-lig′nah-thus) a double monster in which a parasitic twin is attached to the autosite's jaw.

polygram (pol′e-gram) a tracing made by a polygraph.

polygraph (pol′e-graf) an apparatus for simultaneously recording several mechanical or electrical impulses, such as blood pressure, pulse, and respiration, and variations in electrical resistance of the skin; popularly known as a lie-detector.

polygyria (pol″e-ji′re-ah) a condition in which there is more than the normal number of convolutions in the brain.

polyhedral (pol″e-he′dral) having many sides or surfaces.

polyhidrosis (pol″e-hĭ-dro′sis) hyperhidrosis.

polyhydramnios (pol″e-hi-dram′ne-os) hydramnios.

polyhydric (pol″e-hi′drik) containing more than two hydroxyl groups.

polyinfection (pol″e-in-fek′shun) infection with more than one organism.

Polykol (pol′e-kol) trademark for preparations of poloxalkol, a fecal softener.

polyleptic (pol″e-lep′tik) having many remissions and excerbations.

polylysine (pol″e-li′sen) a polypeptide composed of lysine molecules in peptide linkage (see PENICILLOYL-POLYLYSINE).

polymastia (pol″e-mas′te-ah) the presence of supernumerary mammary glands or nipples; pleomastia.

polymelus (po-lim′ĕ-lus) an individual with supernumerary limbs.

polymenorrhea (pol″e-men″o-re′ah) abnormally frequent menstruation.

polymer (pol′ĭ-mer) a compound, usually of high molecular weight, formed by combination of simpler molecules (monomers).

addition p., one formed by repeated combination of the smaller molecules without formation of any other product.

condensation p., one formed by repeated combination of the smaller molecules, with simultaneous elimination of water or other simple compound, e.g., nylon.

polymerase (pol-im′er-ās) an enzyme that catalyzes polymerization.

polymeric (pol″ĭ-mer′ik) exhibiting the character of a polymer.

polymerization (po-lim″er-ĭ-za′shun, pol″ĭ-mer″ĭ-za′shun) the combining of several simpler compounds to form a polymer.

polymicrobial, polymicrobic (pol″e-mi-kro′be-al; pol″e-mi-kro′bik) marked by the presence of several species of microorganisms.

polymicrogyria (pol″e-mi″kro-ji′re-ah) a brain malformation marked by development of numerous microgyri.

polymorph (pol′e-morf) a colloquial term for a polymorphonuclear leukocyte.

polymorphic (pol″e-mor′fik) occurring in several or many forms; appearing in different forms in different developmental stages.

polymorphism (pol″e-mor′fizm) the quality of existing in several different forms.

polymorphocellular (pol″e-mor″fo-sel′u-lar) having cells of many forms.

polymorphonuclear (pol″e-mor″fo-nu′kle-ar) 1. having a nucleus so deeply lobed or so divided as to appear to be multiple. 2. a polymorphonuclear leukocyte (see also NEUTROPHIL [1]).

polymorphous (pol″e-mor′fus) polymorphic.

polymyalgia (pol″e-mi-al′je-ah) pain involving many muscles.

polymyoclonus (pol″e-mi-ok′lo-nus) 1. a fine or minute muscular tremor. 2. polyclonia.

polymyopathy (pol″e-mi-op′ah-the) any disease affecting several muscles simultaneously.

polymyositis (pol″e-mi″o-si′tis) inflammation of several or many muscles at once, attended by weakness, pain, tension, edema, deformity, insomnia, and sweats.

polymyxin (pol″e-mik′sin) a generic term for antibiotics derived from various strains of *Bacillus polymyxa*, several closely related compounds being designated by letters.

p. B, a bacteriostatic and bactericidal, effective mainly against gram-negative organisms. It is used as the sulfate salt, and is especially effective against *Pseudomonas aeruginosa*, which may cause septicemia, meningitis, urinary tract infections, and middle ear infections. Toxicity is low but there may be some damage to kidney and nerve cells.

Polymyxin is administered parenterally or orally. Oral preparations are not used for systemic infections because the drug is poorly absorbed from the intestinal tract. It may be administered topically in the ear; before application the external acoustic meatus should be cleaned and dried thoroughly.

polynesic (pol″ĭ-ne′sik) occurring in many foci.

polyneural (pol″e-nu′ral) pertaining to or supplied by many nerves.

polyneuralgia (pol″e-nu-ral′je-ah) neuralgia of several nerves.

polyneuritis (pol″e-nu-ri′tis) inflammation of many nerves simultaneously.

acute febrile p., acute idiopathic p., acute infectious p., acute postinfectious p., an acute, rapidly progressive, ascending paralysis, beginning in the feet and ascending to the other muscles, often occurring after an enteric or respiratory infection (see also GUILLAIN-BARRÉ SYNDROME).

polyneuromyositis (pol″e-nu″ro-mi-o-si′tis) inflammation involving the muscles and peripheral nerves, with loss of reflexes, sensory loss, and paresthesias.

polyneuropathy (pol″e-nu-rop′ah-the) a disease involving several nerves.

erythredema p., a condition occurring in infants, marked by swollen bluish red hands and feet and disordered digestion, followed by multiple arthritis and muscular weakness; called also acrodynia.

polyneuroradiculitis (pol″e-nu″ro-rah-dik″u-li′-tis) inflammation of spinal ganglia, nerve roots, and peripheral nerves.

polynuclear (pol″e-nu′kle-ar) 1. polynucleate. 2. polymorphonuclear.

polynucleate (pol″e-nu′kle-āt) having many nuclei.

polynucleotidase (pol″e-nu″kle-o-ti′dās) an enzyme that catalyzes the depolymerization of nucleic acids.

polynucleotide (pol″e-nu′kle-o-tīd) any polymer of mononucleotides.

polyodontia (pol″e-o-don′she-ah) the presence of supernumerary teeth.

polyonychia (pol″e-o-nik′e-ah) the presence of supernumerary nails.

polyopia (pol″e-o′pe-ah) visual perception of several images of a single object.

polyorchidism (pol″e-or′kĭ-dizm) the presence of more than two testes.

polyorchis (pol″e-or′kis) a person exhibiting polyorchidism.

polyorchism (pol″e-or′kizm) polyorchidism.

polyostotic (pol″e-os-tot′ik) affecting several bones.

polyotia (pol″e-o′she-ah) the presence of more than two ears.

polyovulatory (pol″e-ov′u-lah-tor″e) discharging several ova in one ovarian cycle.

polyoxyl stearate (pol″e-oks′il) a group of surfactants consisting of a mixture of mono- and diesters of stearate and polyoxyethylene diols; they are numbered according to the average polymer length of oxyethylene units, e.g., polyoxyl 40 stearate.

polyp (pol′ip) any growth or mass protruding from a mucous membrane. Polyps may be attached to a membrane by a thin stalk, in which case they are known as pedunculated polyps, or may have a broad base (sessile polyps). They are usually an overgrowth of normal tissue, but sometimes polyps are true tumors—that is, masses of new tissue separate from the supporting membrane. Usually benign, they may lead to complications or eventually become malignant.

Polyps may occur wherever there is mucous membrane: in the nose, ears, mouth, lungs, heart, stomach, intestines, urinary bladder, uterus, and cervix.

Polyps are most commonly found in the uterus, where they may cause excessive menstrual flow and sometimes sterility. They are often removed by surgery.

Cervical polyps are more dangerous than uterine polyps since they are more likely to become malignant.

Nasal polyps grow in the nasal cavity or in the sinuses. They are produced by local irritation, sometimes as a result of an allergy. They are not dangerous, but if they grow large enough to extend into the nose, they sometimes cause stuffiness and headaches. It is necessary to treat the allergy or any other source of irritation responsible for the growth of polyps. If the polyps continue to be troublesome, surgery may be necessary.

Polyps occasionally occur on the gingiva between the teeth. Here again, the only problem is discomfort; they may easily be removed. Much the same is true of the raspberry-shaped polyp occasionally found in the ear.

Polyps in the stomach are rarer but more serious. A polyp can cause pain if the stalk is sufficiently long for the polyp to be drawn into the duodenum. Usually, however, no pain is felt. When stomach polyps are discovered, they should be removed by surgery. Although usually benign, they may become malignant in time.

Polyps also form in the intestines. Usually they appear there in middle age, but some infants are born with polyps in the large intestine. Multiple intestinal polyps may be a hereditary disorder. In most cases they cause no symptoms unless they become large enough to obstruct the intestine or become ulcerated so that they bleed. When they do, symptoms may include cramping pains in the lower abdomen, diarrhea, and the passage of blood and mucus.

Whether or not they cause symptoms, intestinal polyps should be removed by surgery, since any one of them may become malignant. Although all causes of intestinal cancer have not yet been discovered, it is believed that polyps are often a contributing factor.

In males, polyps sometimes occur in the urethra, usually as the result of some disorder of the prostate. They are not likely to develop into cancer, but they may cause a discharge from the urethra and make urination difficult or frequent. They do not affect sexual potency or vigor. Although these polyps can be removed by surgery, they are more often removed by fulguration.

In women, a urethral polyp, or caruncle, is a small growth on the mucous membrane of the urethra. It may cause pain on urination, vaginal discharge, or bleeding Caruncles are easily removed by fulguration.

polyparesis (pol″e-pah-re′sis) dementia paralytica.

polypathia (pol″e-path′e-ah) the presence of several diseases at one time.

polypectomy (pol″e-pek′to-me) excision of a polyp.

polypeptidase (pol″e-pep′tĭ-dās) an enzyme that catalyzes the hydrolysis of polypeptides.

polypeptide (pol″e-pep′tīd) a compound containing two or more amino acids linked by a peptide bond; called dipeptide, tripeptide, etc., depending on the number of amino acids present.

polypeptidemia (pol″e-pep″tĭ-de′me-ah) the presence of polypeptides in the blood.

polyphagia (pol″e-fa′je-ah) excessive ingestion of food.

polyphalangia, polyphalangism (pol″e-fah-lan′je-ah; pol″e-fah-lan′jizm) excess of phalanges in a finger or toe.

polypharmacy (pol″e-far′mah-se) 1. the administration of many drugs together. 2. administration of excessive medication.

polyphenoloxidase (pol″e-fe″nol-ok′sĭ-dās) a copper-containing enzyme that oxidizes phenols and their amino compounds to quinones.

polyphobia (pol″e-fo′be-ah) abnormal fear of many things.

polyphrasia (pol″e-fra′ze-ah) morbid volubility.

polyplastic (pol″e-plas′tik) 1. containing many structural or constituent elements. 2. undergoing many changes of form.

polyplegia (pol″e-ple′je-ah) paralysis of several muscles.

polyploid (pol′e-ploid) 1. characterized by polyploidy. 2. an individual or cell characterized by polyploidy.

polyploidy (pol′e-ploi″de) the state of having more than two sets of homologous chromosomes.

polypnea (pol″ip-ne′ah) hypernea.

polypodia (pol″e-po′de-ah) the presence of supernumerary feet.

polypoid (pol′y-poid) resembling a polyp.

polyporous (pol-ip′o-rus) having many pores.

polyposia (pol″ĭ-po′ze-ah) ingestion of abnormally increased amounts of fluids for long periods of time.

polyposis (pol″ĭ-po′sis) the formation of numerous polyps.

familial p., a hereditary condition marked by multiple adenomatous polyps with high malignant potential, lining the intestinal mucosa, especially that of the colon, beginning at about puberty. Multiple intestinal polyps occur in Gardner's, Peutz-Jeghers, Canada-Cronkhite, and Turcot's syndromes.

polypous (pol′ĭ-pus) polyp-like.

polyptychial (pol″e-ti′ke-al) arranged in several layers.

polypus (pol′ĭ-pus), pl. *pol′ypi* [L.] polyp.

polyradiculitis (pol″e-rah-dik″u-li′tis) inflammation of the nerve roots.

polyradiculoneuritis (pol″e-rah-dik″u-lo-nu-ri′tis) acute infectious polyneuritis that involves the peripheral nerves, the spinal nerve roots, and the spinal cord.

polyribosome (pol″e-ri′bo-sōm) a cluster of ribosomes connected with messenger RNA; they play a role in peptide synthesis.

polysaccharide (pol″e-sak′ah-rīd) a carbohydrate which, on acid hydrolysis, yields 10 or more monosaccharides.

immune p's, polysaccharides that can function as specific antigens.

polyscelia (pol″e-se′le-ah) the presence of more than two legs.

polyserositis (pol″e-se″ro-si′tis) general inflammation of serous membranes, with effusion.

polysinusitis (pol″e-si″nŭ-si′tis) inflammation of several sinuses.

polysomaty (pol″e-so′mah-te) having reduplicated chromatin in the nucleus.

polysome (pol′e-sōm) polyribosome.

polysomia (pol″e-so′me-ah) doubling or tripling of the fetal body.

polysomus (pol″e-so′mus) a monster exhibiting polysomia. adj., **polyso′mic.**

polysomy (pol″e-so′me) an excess of a particular chromosome.

polysorbate 80 (pol″e-sor′bāt) an oleate ester of sorbitol and its anhydride (sorbitan) condensed with polymers of ethylene oxide, consisting of approximately 20 oxyethylene units; it is a surfactant used as an emulsifying, dispersing, and solubilizing agent.

polyspermia (pol″e-sper′me-ah) 1. excessive secretion of semen. 2. polyspermy.

polyspermy (pol″e-sper′me) fertilization of an ovum by more than one spermatozoon; occurring normally in certain species (physiologic polyspermy) and sometimes abnormally in others (pathologic polyspermy).

polystichia (pol″e-stik′e-ah) two or more rows of eyelashes on an eyelid.

polystyrene (pol″e-sti′rēn) the resin produced by polymerization of styrol, a clear resin of the thermoplastic type, used in the construction of denture bases.

polysynaptic (pol″e-sĭ-nap′tik) pertaining to or relayed through two or more synapses.

polysyndactyly (pol″e-sin-dak′tĭ-le) hereditary association of polydactyly and syndactyly.

polytene (pol′e-tēn) composed of or containing many strands of chromatin (chromonemata).

polyteny (pol″e-te′ne) reduplication of chromonemata in the chromosome without separation into distinct daughter chromosomes.

polythelia (pol″e-the′le-ah) the presence of supernumerary nipples.

polythiazide (pol″e-thi′ah-zīd) a diuretic and antihypertensive.

polytocous (po-lit′ŏ-kus) giving birth to several offspring at one time.

polytrichia (pol″e-trik′e-ah) hypertrichosis; excessive hairiness.

polyuria (pol″e-u′re-ah) excessive excretion of urine.

polyvalent (pol″e-va′lent) multivalent; having more than one valence.

p. vaccine, one prepared from more than one strain or species of microorganisms.

polyvinylpyrrolidone (pol″e-vi″nil-pi-rol′ĭ-dōn) PVP, povidone.

Pompe's disease (pomps) glycogenosis (type II) in which the deficiency of the enzyme α-1,4-glucosidase results in generalized glycogen accumulation, with cardiomegaly, cardiorespiratory failure, and death. Children affected with this disease appear imbecilic and hypotonic. Called also generalized glycogenosis.

pompholyx (pom′fo-liks) an intensely pruritic skin eruption on the sides of the digits or on the palms and soles, consisting of small, discrete, round vesicles, typically occurring in repeated self-limited attacks. Called also dyshidrosis and cheiropompholyx.

POMR Problem-Oriented Medical Record (see PROBLEM-ORIENTED RECORD).

pomum (po′mum), pl. *po′ma* [L.] apple.

p. ada′mi, the prominence on the throat caused by thyroid cartilage; Adam's apple.

pons (ponz) 1. that part of the metencephalon lying between the medulla oblongata and the midbrain, ventral to the cerebellum (see also brain stem, under BRAIN). 2. any slip of tissue connecting two parts of an organ.

p. varo′lii, pons (1).

ponticulus (pon-tik′u-lus), pl. *pontic′uli* [L.] delicate plates of white matter passing across the anterior end of the pyramid, just below the pons. adj., **pontic′ular.**

pontine (pon′tīn) pertaining to the pons.

pontobulbar (pon″to-bul′bar) pertaining to the pons and the region of the medulla oblongata dorsad to it.

Pontocaine (pon′to-kān) trademark for preparations of tetracaine, a local and spinal anesthetic.

pontocerebellar (pon″to-ser″ĕ-bel′ar) pertaining to the pons and cerebellum.

popliteal (pop″lĭ-te′al) pertaining to the area behind the knee.

POR Problem-Oriented Record.

poradenitis (pōr″ad-ĕ-ni′tis) inflammation of lymph nodes with formation of small abscesses.

porcine (pōr′sīn) pertaining to swine.

pore (pōr) a small opening or empty space.

porencephalia (po″ren-sĕ-fa′le-ah) porencephaly.

porencephalitis (po″ren-sef″ah-li′tis) porencephaly with inflammation of the brain.

porencephalous (po″ren-sef′ah-lus) characterized by porencephaly.

porencephaly (po″ren-sef′ah-le) development or presence of abnormal cysts or cavities in the brain tissue, usually communicating with a lateral ventricle. adj., **porencephal′ic, porenceph′alous.**

porocele (po′ro-sēl) scrotal hernia with thickening of the coverings of the testes.

porokeratosis (po″ro-ker″ah-to′sis) a hereditary dermatosis marked by a centrifugally spreading hypertrophy of the stratum corneum around the sweat pores, followed by atrophy. Also known as porokeratosis of Mibelli. adj., **porokeratot′ic.**

poroma (po-ro′mah) a tumor arising in a pore.

eccrine p., a benign tumor arising from the intradermal portion of an eccrine sweat duct, usually on the sole.

porosis (po-ro'sis) 1. formation of the callus in repair of a fractured bone. 2. cavity formation.

porosity (po-ros'ĭ-te) the condition of being porous; a pore.

porotomy (po-rot'o-me) meatotomy.

porous (po'rus) penetrated by pores and open spaces.

porphin (por'fin) the fundamental ring structure of four linked pyrrole nuclei around which porphyrins, hemin, cytochromes, and chlorophyll are built.

porphobilinogen (por"fo-bi-lin'o-jen) an intermediary product in the biosynthesis of heme.

porphyria (por-fēr'e-ah; por-fi're-ah) a genetic disorder characterized by a disturbance in porphyrin metabolism with resultant increase in the formation and excretion of porphyrins (uroporphyrin and coproporphyrin) or their precursors; called also hematoporphyria. Porphyrins, in combination with iron, form hemes, which in turn combine with specific proteins to form hemoproteins. Hemoglobin is a hemoprotein, as are many other substances that are essential to normal functioning of the cells and tissues of the body.

Two general types of porphyria are known: erythropoietic porphyrias, which are concerned with the formation of erythrocytes in the bone marrow; and hepatic porphyrias, which are responsible for liver dysfunction.

The manifestations of porphyria include gastrointestinal, neurologic and psychologic symptoms, cutaneous photosensitivity, pigmentation of the face (and later of the bones), and anemia with enlargement of the spleen. Large amounts of porphyrins are excreted in the urine and feces.

Treatment of this condition has been primarily symptomatic and varies in its effectiveness. Photosensitivity may be controlled by avoiding exposure to light. Removal of the spleen is useful in some cases of the erythropoietic type of porphyria. Drug therapy includes the use of phenothiazines, chlorpromazine and promazine in particular. These drugs allay pain and nervousness and apparently allow a period of remission from symptoms. Corticotropin has been successful in some cases.

Patients with porphyria must not be given barbiturates, sulfonamides, alcohol, or chloroquine as these chemicals may precipitate or intensify attacks. It is recommended that patients with this disease carry with them at all times some means of identifying themselves as having porphyria so that in an emergency they will not be given a drug that may precipitate an attack, and possibly cause death.

porphyrin (por'fĭ-rin) any of a group of iron- or magnesium-free cyclic tetrapyrrole derivatives, occurring universally in protoplasm, and forming the basis of the respiratory pigments of animals and plants. Porphyrins, in combination with iron, form hemes.

porphyrinuria (por"fĭ-rĭ-nu're-ah) an excess of porphyrin in the urine.

porta (por'tah), pl. *por'tae* [L.] an entrance or gateway, especially the site where blood vessels and other supplying or draining structures enter an organ.

p. hep'atis, the transverse fissure on the visceral surface of the liver, where the portal vein and hepatic artery enter and the hepatic ducts leave. Called also portal fissure and transverse fissure.

portacaval (por"tah-ka'val) pertaining to or connecting the portal vein and inferior vena cava.

portal (por'tal) 1. an avenue of entrance; porta. 2. pertaining to an entrance, especially the porta hepatis.

p. circulation, a general term denoting the circulation of blood through larger vessels from the capillaries of one organ to those of another; applied especially to the passage of blood from the gastrointestinal tract and spleen through the portal vein to the liver. (See also CIRCULATORY SYSTEM.)

p. of entry, the pathway by which bacteria or other pathogenic agents gain entry to the body.

p. vein, a short, thick trunk formed by the union of the superior mesenteric and splenic veins behind the neck of the pancreas; it ascends to the right end of the porta hepatis, where it divides into successively smaller branches, following branches of the hepatic artery, until it forms a capillary system of sinusoids that permeates the entire substance of the liver.

portio (por'she-o), pl. *portio'nes* [L.] a part or division.

p. du'ra, the facial nerve.

p. interme'dia, intermediate.

p. mol'lis, vestibulocochlear nerve.

p. vagina'lis, the portion of the uterus that projects into the vagina.

portogram (por'to-gram) the film obtained by portography.

portography (por-tog'rah-fe) roentgenography of the portal vein after injection of opaque material.

portal p., portography after injection of opaque material into the superior mesenteric vein or one of its branches, the abdomen being opened.

splenic p., portography after percutaneous injection of opaque material into the substance of the spleen.

port-wine stain nevus flammeus.

porus (po'rus), pl. *po'ri* [L.] an opening or pore.

p. acus'ticus exter'nus, the outer end of the external acoustic meatus.

p. acus'ticus inter'nus, the opening of the internal acoustic meatus in the cranial cavity.

p. op'ticus, the opening in the sclera for passage of the optic nerve.

-posia word element [Gr.], *intake of fluids.*

position (po-zish'un) 1. a bodily posture or attitude. 2. the relationship of a given point on the presenting part of the fetus to a designated point of the maternal pelvis; see accompanying table. (See also PRESENTATION.)

anatomic p., that of the human body, standing erect, with palms facing forward, used as the position of reference in designating the site or direction of structures of the body.

Bonner's p., flexion, abduction, and outward rotation of the thigh in coxitis.

Bozeman's p., the knee-elbow position with straps used for support.

Brickner p., the wrist is tied to the head of the bed to obtain abduction and external rotation for shoulder disability.

decubitus p., that of the body lying on a horizontal surface, designated according to the aspect of the body touching the surface as dorsal decubitus (on the back), left or right lateral decubitus (on the left or right side), and ventral decubitus position (on the anterior surface).

Fowler's p., the head of the patient's bed is raised 18 to 20 inches above the level, with the knees also elevated.

genucubital p., knee-elbow position.

genupectoral p., knee-chest p., the patient rests on his knees and chest. The head is turned to one side, and the arms are extended on the bed, the elbows flexed and resting so that they partially bear the weight of the patient. The abdomen remains unsupported, though a small pillow may be placed under the chest.

knee-elbow p., the patient resting on his knees and elbows with his chest elevated.

lithotomy p., the patient lies on his back with the legs well separated, the thighs acutely flexed on the abdomen and the legs on the thighs. Stirrups may be used to support the feet and legs.

orthopneic p., the patient assumes an upright or semivertical position by using two or more pillows to support his head and chest from the recumbent position, or he sits upright in a chair. Used when the patient has difficulty in breathing except in the upright position (orthopnea).

POSITIONS OF THE FETUS IN VARIOUS PRESENTATIONS

CEPHALIC PRESENTATION

Vertex—occiput the point of direction
- Left occipitoanterior (L.O.A.)
- Left occipitotransverse (L.O.T.)
- Right occipitoposterior (R.O.P.)
- Right occipitotransverse (R.O.T.)
- Right occipitoanterior (R.O.A.)
- Left occipitoposterior (L.O.P.)

Face—chin the point of direction
- Right mentoposterior (R.M.P.)
- Left mentoanterior (L.M.A.)
- Right mentotransverse (R.M.T.)
- Right mentoanterior (R.M.A.)
- Left mentotransverse (L.M.T.)
- Left mentoposterior (L.M.P.)

Brow—the point of direction
- Right frontoposterior (R.F.P.)
- Left frontoanterior (L.F.A.)
- Right frontotransverse (R.F.T.)
- Right frontoanterior (R.F.A.)
- Left frontotransverse (L.F.T.)
- Left frontoposterior (L.F.P.)

BREECH OR PELVIC PRESENTATION

Complete breech—sacrum, the point of direction (feet crossed and thighs flexed on abdomen)
- Left sacroanterior (L.S.A.)
- Left sacrotransverse (L.S.T.)
- Right sacroposterior (R.S.P.)
- Right sacroanterior (R.S.A.)
- Right sacrotransverse (R.S.T.)
- Left sacroposterior (L.S.P.)

Incomplete breech—sacrum the point of direction. Same designations as above, adding the qualifications footling, knee, etc.

TRANSVERSE LIE OR SHOULDER PRESENTATION

Shoulder—scapula the point of direction

Left scapuloanterior (L. Sc. A.) Right scapuloanterior (R. Sc. A.)	Back anterior positions
Right scapuloposterior (R. Sc. P.) Left scapuloposterior (L. Sc. P.)	Back posterior positions

Rose's p., a supine position with the head over the table edge in full extension.

Sims' p., the patient lies on his left side with the left thigh slightly flexed, and the right thigh acutely flexed on the abdomen. The left arm is drawn behind the body with the body inclined forward. The right arm may be positioned according to the patient's comfort.

Trendelenburg's p., the patient lies on his back, on a plane inclined 45 degrees with the head lower than the rest of the body. The legs and knees flexed over the adjustable lower section of the table or bed, which is lowered. The patient is well supported to prevent slipping.

positive (poz'ĭ-tiv) having a value greater than zero; indicating existence or presence, as chromatin-positive or Wassermann-positive; characterized by affirmation or cooperation.

positron (poz'ĭ-tron) a positively charged electron.

posology (po-sol'o-je) the science of dosage or a system of dosage. adj., **posolog'ic.**

post- word element [L.] *after; behind.*

postaxial (pōst-ak'se-al) behind an axis; in anatomy, referring to the medial (ulnar) aspect of the upper arm, and the lateral (fibular) aspect of the lower leg.

postbrachial (pōst-bra'ke-al) on the posterior part of the upper arm.

postcardiotomy (pōst-kar"de-ot'o-me) occurring after open-heart surgery.

postcava (pōst-ka'vah) the inferior vena cava. adj., **postca'val.**

postcibal (pōst-si'bal) after eating.

postclavicular (pōst-klah-vik'u-lar) behind the clavicle.

postcoital (pōst-ko'ĭ-tal) after coitus.

postcommissurotomy syndrome (pōst-kom"ĭ-shūr-ot'o-me) fever, chest pain, pleuritis, pericarditis, and pneumonia, occurring frequently in patients who have undergone mitral commissurotomy, and sometimes related to cytomegalic inclusion disease.

postcordial (pōst-kor'de-al) behind the heart.

postcornu (pōst-kor'nu) the posterior horn of the lateral ventricle.

postdiastolic (pōst-di"as-tol'ik) after diastole.

postdicrotic (pōst"di-krot'ic) after the dicrotic elevation of the sphygmogram.

postencephalitic (pōst"en-sef"ah-lit'ik) occurring after or as a consequence of encephalitis.

postepileptic (pōst"ep-ĭ-lep'tik) following an epileptic attack.

posterior (pos-tēr'e-or) directed toward or situated at the back; opposite of anterior.

postero- word element [L.], *the back; posterior to.*

posteroanterior (pos"ter-o-an-tēr'e-or) directed from the back toward the front.

posteroexternal (pos"ter-o-ek-ster'nal) situated on the outside of a posterior aspect.

posteroinferior (pōst"er-o-in-fe're-or) behind and below.

posterolateral (pos"ter-o-lat'er-al) situated on the side and toward the posterior aspect.

posteromedian (pos"ter-o-me'de-an) situated on the middle of a posterior aspect.

posterosuperior (pos"ter-o-su-pēr'e-or) situated behind and above.

postesophageal (pōst″e-sof″ah-ge′al) behind the esophagus; retroesophageal.

postganglionic (pōst″gang-gle-on′ik) distal to a ganglion.

posthepatitic (post″hep-ah-tit′ik) occurring after or as a consequence of hepatitis.

posthioplasty (pos′the-o-plas″te) plastic repair of the prepuce.

posthitis (pos-thi′tis) inflammation of the prepuce.

posthypnotic (pōst″hip-not′ik) following the hypnotic state.

postictal (pōst-ik′tal) following a seizure.

postmaturity (pōst″mah-chu′rĭ-te) the condition of an infant after a prolonged gestation period. adj., **postmature′**.

postmenopausal (pōst″men-o-paw′zal) after the menopause.

postmitotic (pōst″mi-tot′ik) occurring after or pertaining to the time following mitosis.

post mortem (pōst mor′tem) [L.] after death.

postmortem (pōst-mor′tem) performed or occurring after death.

postnatal (pōst-na′tal) occurring after birth, with reference to the newborn.

postoperative (pōst-op′er-ah-tiv, pōst-op′er-a″tiv) after a surgical operation.

p. care, care of the patient following a surgical procedure. Immediately after surgery the patient usually is transferred to a recovery room. This is a special unit within the operating room suite, designed to facilitate management of the patient recovering from anesthesia, and staffed with personnel experienced in this type of patient care.

Immediately after surgery, the patient requires constant attendance. A patient AIRWAY must be maintained so that respiration is adequate and of normal character. An endotracheal tube and VENTILATOR may be used to assist the patient with respiratory difficulties. The skin is observed for color, turgor, and dryness. A flaccid, parchment-like skin indicates dehydration; cold clammy skin may be symptomatic of shock, and cyanosis and local discoloration are indicative of oxygen deficiency as a result of an obstructed airway or impaired circulation. The pulse, respirations, and blood pressure are checked every 15 minutes or oftener; notes are made as to their quality, rate, and rhythm.

The position of the patient may be governed by the type of surgery done, but ideally the patient should be placed on his side with a pillow to his back for support. The uppermost leg is slightly flexed to relieve tension on the abdominal muscles and may be supported with a small pillow. The side position allows for drainage of mucus or other material in the mouth and lessens the danger of aspirations of vomitus. During vomiting the head is kept turned to the side and suctioning is used as necessary to clear the air passages. The patient's position should be changed at least every 2 hours unless there is a contraindication, and pressure areas are gently massaged. When repositioning the patient, all movements should be gentle and slow, as sudden overstimulation can cause a drop in blood pressure.

While the patient is awakening from anesthesia the hospital personnel must use caution in their conversations and statements made about the patients in the unit. With his senses dulled and his reasoning hampered by drugs and anesthesia, the patient may misinterpret the sounds and statements he hears. Noise must be kept at a minimum, voices should be kept low, and whispering (which is rude at any time) is especially disturbing to the patient recovering from anesthesia.

In many cases a catheter, nasogastric tube, or drainage tube is inserted during surgery. The purposes of these should be understood by the nurse and it is usually the nurse's responsibility to connect them to the proper drainage and suction apparatus. Dressings around drainage tubes should be observed for excess drainage or bleeding and reinforced as necessary.

Other physical aspects of postoperative care are outlined in the table. See also specific operative procedures (e.g., COLOSTOMY) and specific organs (e.g., surgery of the KIDNEY or LUNG). For complications that may arise during the postoperative period, see also SHOCK, HEMORRHAGE, THROMBOSIS, EMBOLISM, and CARDIAC ARREST.

postoral (pōst-o′ral) in the back part of the mouth.

postparalytic (pōst″par-ah-lit′ik) following an attack of paralysis.

post partum (pōst par′tum) [L.] after parturition.

postpartum (pōst-par′tum) occurring after childbirth, with reference to the mother.

p. pituitary necrosis, necrosis of the pituitary during the postpartum period, often associated with shock and excessive uterine bleeding during delivery, and leading to variable patterns of hypopituitarism. Called also Sheehan's syndrome.

postpericardiectomy syndrome (post-per″e-kar″de-ek′to-me) delayed pericardial or pleural reaction, with fever, chest pains, and signs of pleural and/or pericardial inflammation, following opening of the pericardium.

postprandial (pōst-pran′de-al) after a meal.

postpuberal, postpubertal (pōst-pu′ber-al; pōst-pu′ber-tal) after puberty.

postpubescent (pōst″pu-bes′ent) after puberty.

postradiation (pōst″ra-de-a′shun) following exposure to radiation.

postsphygmic (pōst-sfig′mik) after the pulse wave.

p. interval, p. period, the short period (0.08 second) of ventricular diastole, after the sphygmic period, and lasting until the atrioventricular valves open.

poststenotic (post″stĕ-not′ik) located or occurring distal to or beyond a stenosed segment.

postsynaptic (post″sĭ-nap′tik) distal to or occurring beyond a synapse.

posttraumatic (post″traw-mat′ik) following injury.

postulate (pos′tu-lāt) anything assumed or taken for granted.

Koch's p's, a statement of the kind of experimental evidence required to establish the causative relation of a given microorganism to a given disease. The conditions are: 1, the microorganism is present in every case of the disease; 2, it is to be cultivated in pure culture; 3, inoculation of such culture must produce the disease in susceptible animals; 4, it must be obtained from such animals, and again grown in a pure culture.

postural (pos′tu-ral) pertaining to posture or position.

p. drainage, a technique in which the patient assumes one or more positions that will facilitate the drainage of secretions from the bronchial airways. The procedure utilizes the force of gravity to move secretions toward the trachea, where they can be coughed up more easily.

The choice of position is based on radiologic studies and auscultatory evidence of pooled secretions. Variations of the most effective position are adapted to the patient's general physical condition, his tolerance, and pulmonary status.

Before postural drainage is attempted the patient should have been instructed in and able to perform diaphragmatic breathing and effective coughing. (See also CHRONIC OBSTRUCTIVE PULMONARY DISEASE.) If he has difficulty in removing secretions, a suction machine should be on hand to remove secretions the patient cannot expectorate. When severe dyspnea or exhaustion occur during the postural drainage the treatment should not be continued. Other contraindications are a full stomach (the procedure is never done immediately after a meal) and unstable vital signs. Mouth care is given after each treatment to remove the foul taste frequently accompanying removal of the stagnant mucus from the bronchial tree.

Percussion or "clapping," and vibration are often done in conjunction with postural drainage. *Percussion* involves a rhythmic striking of the chest wall over the area being drained. It is done with the hands cupped; the fingers are flexed and the thumbs are held tightly against the index fingers. If done properly, a hollow sound is heard and there is no discomfort to the patient.

Vibration is done immediately after percussion and is directed to the same area. While the patient performs a prolonged exhalation through pursed lips, the therapist presses the flat of her hands against the thorax in a downward movement toward the midline of the body. This is repeated four or five times. While neither percussion nor vibration are difficult techniques to master, anyone attempting to assist the patient in this manner should have instruction and practice before attempting them. The purpose of both activities is to dislodge plugs of mucus, allowing air to penetrate behind them and thus aid in their removal.

posture (pos'tūr) an attitude of the body. Good posture cannot be defined by any rigid formula. It is usually considered to be the natural and comfortable bearing of the body in normal, healthy persons. This generally means that in a standing position the body is naturally, but not rigidly, straight, and that in a sitting position the back is comfortably straight.

Good standing and sitting posture helps promote normal functioning of the body's organs and increases the efficiency of the muscles, thereby mini-

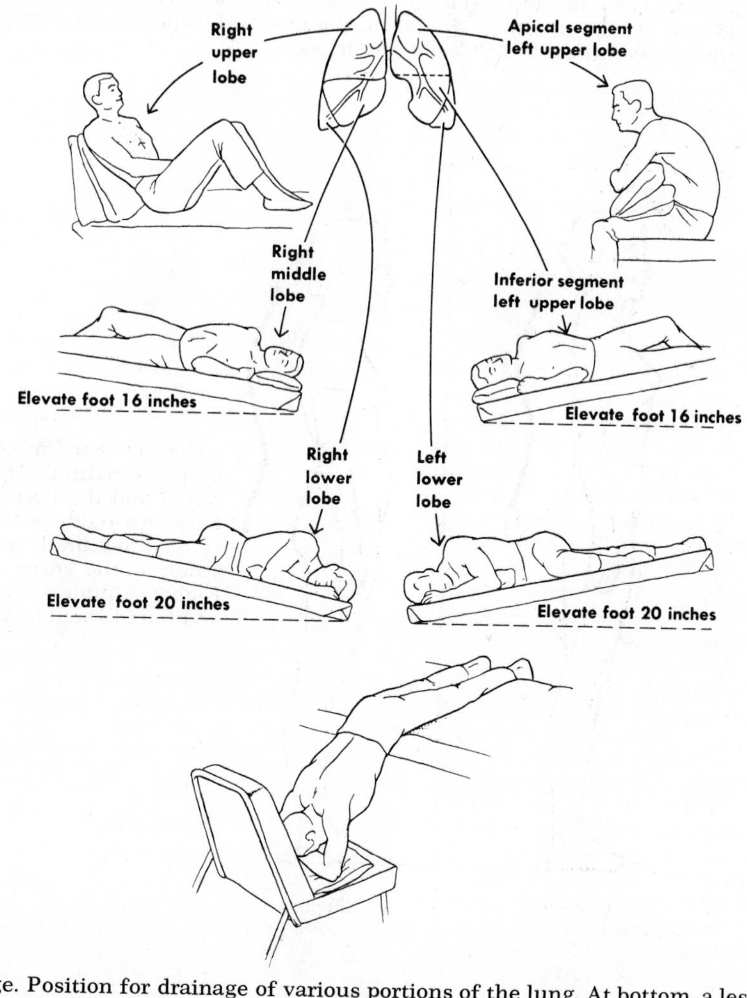

Postural drainage. Position for drainage of various portions of the lung. At bottom, a less specific position that is frequently used. (From Shafer, K. N., et al.: Medical-Surgical Nursing. 6th ed. St. Louis, C. V. Mosby Co., 1975.)

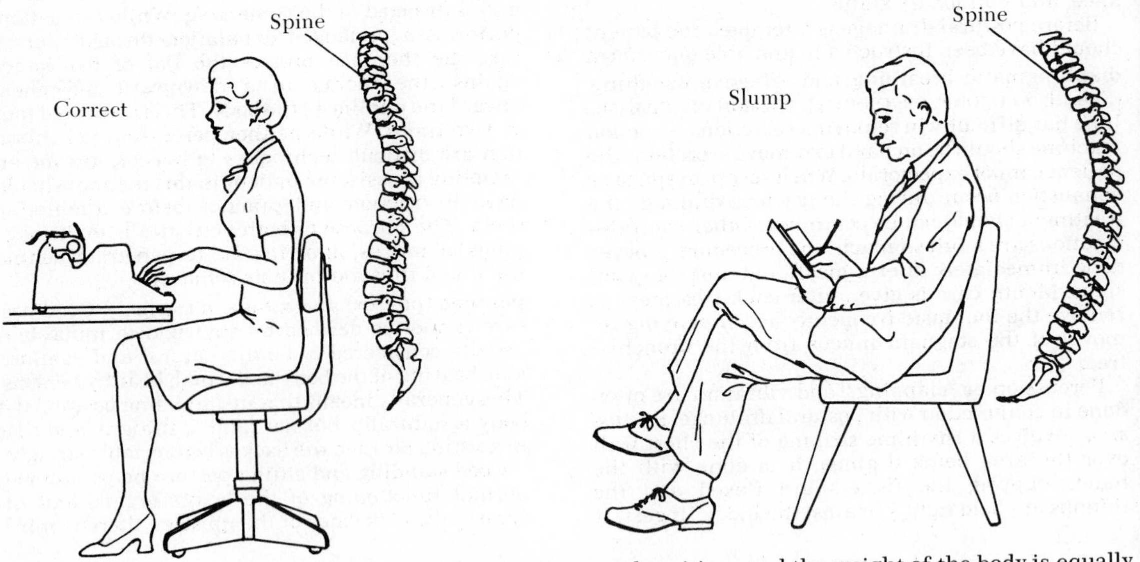

Left, good sitting posture: the spine and feet are in normal positions and the weight of the body is equally distributed. Right, slouching puts too much weight on the end of the spine, compresses internal organs, strains muscles, and interferes with the circulation in the legs.

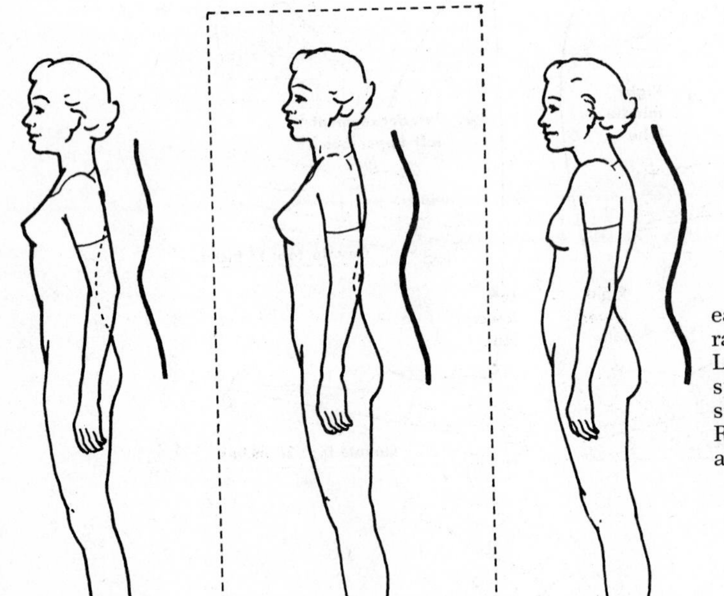

Correct standing posture, center, is easy and natural. The chest is slightly raised and the buttocks are tucked in. Left, too-rigid posture. Keeping the spine unnaturally straight can cause strain on the knees and back muscles. Right, slumping can lead to backache and round shoulders.

mizing fatigue. Good posture is also important to good appearance. Clothes fit better, movements become more graceful, and an impression of poise is achieved.

Maintenance of good posture for a patient confined to bed or wheelchair is essential to the patient's general well-being and also is important in the prevention of deformities of the muscles and bones. The patient should be observed for evidence of "slumping," in which the normal curves of the spine are exaggerated. The rib cage should be supported so that the ribs are elevated and there is no constriction of the chest wall. Pillows are arranged under the shoulders and head so that the chin is not forced downward on the chest. Excessive extension of the ankles should be avoided by adequate support against the soles of the feet. The legs should be supported so that the weight of one does not fall on the other. The arms are supported so that they do not lie across the chest or pull the shoulders into a "rounded" position. Frequent changing of position and adequate exercise of the limbs are also essential to the maintenance of good posture and the prevention of deformities.

postuterine (pōst-u′ter-in) behind the uterus.

postvaccinal (pōst-vak′sĭ-nal) occurring after inoculation for smallpox.

potable (po′tah-b'l) fit to drink.

potash (pot′ash) impure potassium carbonate.

caustic p., potassium hydroxide.

sulfurated p., a mixture of potassium polysulfides and potassium thiosulfate; a source of sulfide in pharmaceuticals.

potassemia (pot″ah-se′me-ah) hyperkalemia.

potassium (po-tas′e-um) a chemical element, atomic number 19, atomic weight 39.102, symbol K. (See table of ELEMENTS.) In combination with other minerals in the body, potassium forms alkaline salts that are important in body processes and play an essential role in maintenance of the acid-base and water balance in the body. All body cells, especially muscle tissue, require a high content of potassium. A proper balance between sodium, calcium, and potassium in the blood plasma is necessary for proper cardiac function.

Since most foods contain a good supply of potassium, potassium deficiency (hypokalemia) is unlikely to be caused by an unbalanced diet. Possible causes include Cushing's syndrome (due to an adrenal gland disorder) and Fanconi's syndrome (the result of a congenital kidney defect). The cause could also be an excessive dose of cortisone or prolonged vomiting or diarrhea. Signs of potassium deficiency can include weakness and lethargy, rapid pulse, nausea, diarrhea, and tingling sensations.

If the body absorbs enough potassium but the element is not distributed properly, various disorders may develop. Thus an abnormally low content of potassium in the blood may result in an intermittent temporary paralysis of the muscles, known as familial periodic paralysis.

Potassium deficiency can be treated by means of medication containing potassium salts. If the difficulty lies in the body's use of potassium, treatment is concerned with the primary cause of the deficiency.

p. acetate, a systemic and urinary alkalizer.

p. aminosalicylate, an antibacterial used against tubercle bacilli.

p. bicarbonate, an electrolyte replenisher.

p. bitartrate, a cathartic.

p. carbonate, a salt used chiefly in pharmaceutical and chemical manufacturing procedures.

p. chloride, a compound used orally or intravenously as an electrolyte replenisher.

p. citrate, a diuretic, expectorant, and systemic alkalizer.

p. gluconate, an electrolyte replenisher used in the prophylaxis and treatment of hypokalemia.

p. guaiacolsulfonate, an expectorant.

p. hydroxide, a powerful alkaline and caustic compound, used as an alkalinizing agent and occasionally as an escharotic in bites of rabid animals.

p. iodide, an expectorant and antithyroid agent.

p. nitrate, a diuretic used in the prophylaxis and treatment of potassium deficiency and digitalis intoxication; called also niter and saltpeter.

p. nitrite, a compound sometimes used in place of potassium nitrate.

p. oxalate, a salt used extensively as a reagent.

p. permanganate, a topical anti-infective, oxidizing agent, and antidote for many poisons.

p. phenethicillin, an oral penicillin.

p. phosphate, a cathartic.

p. sodium tartrate, a compound used as a saline cathartic and also in combination with sodium bicarbonate and tartaric acid (Seidlitz powders, a cathartic).

p. tartrate, a mild cathartic.

potency (po′ten-se) power; especially (1) the ability of the male to perform coitus; (2) the power of a medicinal agent to produce the desired effects; (3) the ability of an embryonic part to develop and complete its destiny. adj., **po′tent.**

potential (po-ten′shal) 1. existing and ready for action, but not active. 2. electric tension or pressure.

action p., the electrical activity developed in a muscle or nerve cell during activity.

after-p., the period following termination of the spike potential.

membrane p., the electric potential that exists on the two sides of a membrane or across the wall of a cell.

resting p., the potential difference across the membrane of a normal cell at rest.

spike p., the initial, very large change in potential of an excitable cell membrane during excitation.

potentiation (po-ten″she-a′shun) enhancement of one agent by another so that the combined effect is greater than the sum of the effects of each one alone.

potion (po′shun) a large dose of liquid medicine.

Pott's curvature (pots) abnormal posterior curvature of the spine occurring as a result of Pott's disease.

Pott's disease (pots) tuberculosis of the spine, usually beginning as a tuberculous osteomyelitis of the vertebrae and progressing to damage of the intervertebral disks. If erosion continues unchecked, there is complete destruction of the affected vertebrae.

Symptoms include stiffness of the back, pain on motion, prominence of the spinous process of certain vertebrae, and occasionally abscess formation, paralysis, and abdominal pain. Diagnosis is confirmed by demonstration of *Mycobacterium tuberculosis* (the tubercle bacillus) in the affected bone.

Treatment includes administration of antibacterial drugs such as isoniazid and streptomycin. Para-aminosalicylic acid (PAS) may be used instead of streptomycin if streptomycin is contraindicated. Surgical fixation of the affected vertebrae (spinal fusion) may be required for correction of orthopedic deformities such as KYPHOSIS (hunchback) which may occur as a result of Pott's disease.

Pott's fracture (pots) fracture of the lower part of the fibula with serious injury of the lower tibial articulation.

pouch (powch) a pocket-like space, cavity, or sac, e.g., one formed by bending back of the peritoneum on the surfaces of adjoining organs.

abdominovesical p., the pouchlike reflection of the peritoneum from the abdominal wall to the anterior surface of the bladder.

Douglas' p., Douglas' cul-de-sac.

Prussak's p., a recess in the tympanic membrane between the flaccid part of the membrane and the neck of the malleus.

Rathke's p., a diverticulum from the embryonic buccal cavity from which the anterior lobe of the pituitary gland is developed.

rectouterine p., Douglas' cul-de-sac.

Seesel's p., an outpouching of the embryonic pharynx rostrad to the pharyngeal membrane and caudal to Rathke's pouch.

poudrage (poo-drahzh') [Fr.] application of a powder to a surface, as done to promote fusion of serous membranes (e.g., two layers of pericardium or pleura).

poultice (pōl'tis) a soft, moist, mass about the consistency of cooked cereal, spread between layers of muslin, linen, gauze, or towels and applied hot to a given area in order to create moist local heat or counterirritation.

pound (pownd) a unit of weight in the avoirdupois (453.6 gm., or 16 ounces) or apothecaries' (373.2 gm., or 12 ounces) system.

Poupart's ligament (poo-parts') inguinal ligament.

povidone (po'vĭ-don) polyvinylpyrrolidine, a synthetic polymer used as a dispersing and suspending agent; it has also been used as a plasma volume expander.

povidone-iodine (po'vĭ-dōn-i'o-dīn) a complex produced by reacting iodine with the polymer povidone; used as a topical anti-infective.

powder (pow'der) an aggregation of particles obtained by grinding or triturating a solid.

aromatic p., powder of cinnamon, ginger, cardamon seed, and myristica.

dusting p., a fine powder used as a talc substitute.

effervescent p's, compound, Seidlitz powders.

Goa p., a brownish yellow to umber brown powder deposited in the wood of the Brazilian tree *Andira araroba;* the source of chrysarobin.

Seidlitz p's, a mixture of sodium bicarbonate, potassium sodium tartrate, and tartaric acid; used as a cathartic.

senna p., compound, a powder prepared from fennel oil, sucrose, powdered senna, powdered glycyrrhiza, and washed sulfur; used as a laxative.

pox (poks) any eruptive or pustular disease, especially one caused by a virus, e.g., chickenpox, cowpox, etc.

poxvirus (poks-vi'rus) any of a group of morphologically similar and immunologically related DNA viruses, including the virus of vaccinia (cowpox), smallpox, and those producing pox diseases in lower animals.

P.P.D. purified protein derivative (tuberculin).

PPLO pleuropneumonia-like organisms.

p.p.m. parts per million.

Pr chemical symbol, *praseodymium.*

prae- for words beginning thus, see those beginning *pre-.*

pragmatagnosia (prag"mat-ag-no'ze-ah) inability to recognize formerly known objects.

pragmatamnesia (prag"mat-am-ne'ze-ah) loss of power of remembering the appearance of objects.

pralidoxime (pral"ĭ-doks'ēm) a cholinesterase reactivator, whose salts are used in treatment of organophosphate poisoning; it also has limited value in counteracting carbamate-type cholinesterase inhibitors.

pramoxine (pram-ok'sēn) a topical anesthetic.

prandial (pran'de-al) pertaining to a meal.

Pranone (pra'nōn) trademark for a preparation of ethisterone, a progestational steroid.

Prantal (pran'tal) trademark for preparations of diphemanil, an anticholinergic.

praseodymium (pra"ze-o-dim'e-um) a chemical element, atomic number 59, atomic weight 140.907, symbol Pr. (See table of ELEMENTS.)

Prausnitz-Küstner reaction (prows'nits kist'ner) a local hypersensitivity reaction induced by intradermal injection into a normal person of serum from a hypersensitive individual; injection 24 hours later of the antigen to which the donor is allergic results in a wheal-and-flare response.

praxiology (prak"se-ol'o-je) the science or study of conduct.

prazepam (praz'ĕ-pam) a muscle relaxant.

pre- word element [L.], *before* (in time or space).

preagonal (pre-ag'o-nal) immediately before the death agony.

preanesthesia (pre"an-es-the'ze-ah) preliminary anesthesia; light anesthesia or narcosis induced by medication as a preliminary to administration of a general anesthetic.

preanesthetic (pre"an-es-thet'ik) 1. pertaining to preanesthesia. 2. an agent that produces preanesthesia.

preantiseptic (pre"an-tĭ-sep'tik) pertaining to the time before the discovery of antisepsis.

preauricular (pre"aw-rik'u-lar) in front of the auricle of the ear.

preaxial (pre-ak'se-al) situated before an axis; in anatomy, referring to the lateral (radial) aspect of the upper arm, and the medial (tibial) aspect of the lower leg.

precancer (pre'kan-ser) a condition that tends to become malignant (see CANCER). adj., **precan'cerous.**

precapillary (pre-kap'ĭ-ler"e) a vessel lacking complete coats, intermediate between an arteriole and a capillary.

precava (pre-ka'vah) the superior vena cava. adj., **preca'val.**

prechordal (pre-kor'dal) in front of the notochord.

precipitant (pre-sip'ĭ-tant) a substance that causes precipitation.

precipitate (pre-sip'ĭ-tāt) 1. to cause settling in solid particles of a substance in solution. 2. a deposit of solid particles settled out of a solution. 3. occurring with undue rapidity, as precipitate labor.

precipitation (pre-sip″ĭ-ta′shun) the act or process of precipitating.

precipitin (pre-sip′ĭ-tin) an antibody to soluble antigen that specifically aggregates the macromolecular antigen *in vivo* or *in vitro* to give a visible precipitate.

p. reaction, a reaction involving the specific serologic precipitation of an antigen in solution with its specific antiserum in the presence of electrolytes. The reaction is used in the typing of pneumococcus strains, in testing whether blood is human or animal, and for diagnostic purposes.

precipitinogen (pre-sip″ĭ-tin′o-jen) a soluble antigen that stimulates the formation of and reacts with a precipitin.

preclinical (pre-klin′ĭ-kal) before a disease becomes clinically recognizable.

precocity (pre-kos′ĭ-te) unusually early development of mental or physical traits. adj., **preco′cious.**

precognition (pre″kog-nish′un) the extrasensory perception of a future event.

precoma (pre-ko′mah) the neuropsychiatric state preceding coma, as in hepatic encephalopathy. adj., **precom′atose.**

preconscious (pre-kon′shus) not present in consciousness, but readily recalled into it; foreconscious.

preconvulsive (pre″kon-vul′siv) preceding convulsions.

precordia, precordium (pre-kor′de-ah; pre-kor′de-um) the region over the heart and lower thorax; adj., **precor′dial.**

precostal (pre-kos′tal) in front of the ribs.

precuneus (pre-ku′ne-us), pl. *precu′nei* [L.] a small convolution on the medial surface of the parietal lobe of the cerebrum.

precursor (pre-ker′sor) something that precedes. In biological processes, a substance from which another, usually more active or mature substance is formed. In clinical medicine, a sign or symptom that heralds another.

prediabetes (pre-di″ah-be′tēz) a state of latent impairment of carbohydrate metabolism in which the criteria for diabetes mellitus are not all satisfied.

prediastole (pre″di-as′to-le) the interval immediately preceding diastole. adj., **prediastol′ic.**

predicrotic (pre″di-krot′ik) occurring before the dicrotic wave of the sphygmogram.

predigestion (pre″di-jes′chun) partial artificial digestion of food before its ingestion into the body.

predisposition (pre-dis″po-zish′un) a latent susceptibility to disease which may be activated under certain conditions.

prednisolone (pred-nis′o-lōn) a glucocorticoid used as an anti-inflammatory and antiallergic agent.

prednisone (pred′nĭ-sōn) a glucocorticoid used like prednisolone.

preeclampsia (pre″e-klamp′se-ah) a toxemia of late pregnancy, characterized by hypertension, albuminuria, and edema, but without convulsions (see also ECLAMPSIA).

prefrontal (pre-frun′tal) 1. situated in the anterior part of the frontal region or lobe. 2. the central part of the ethmoid bone.

preganglionic (pre″gang-gle-on′ik) proximal to a ganglion.

pregenital (pre-jen′ĭ-tal) antedating the emergence of genital interests.

pregnancy (preg′nan-se) the condition of having a developing embryo or fetus in the body, after union of an ovum and spermatozoon. Human pregnancy lasts about 9 months, although it may vary considerably from that average.

CONCEPTION. Once a month an ovum matures in one of the ovaries and travels down the nearby uterine tube to the uterus. This process is called ovulation. If coitus takes place within a day or two of ovulation, one of the spermatozoa may unite with the ovum and fertilize it. The fertilized ovum then implants itself in the wall of the uterus, which is richly supplied with blood, and begins to grow. (See also OVULATION, REPRODUCTION, and UTERINE TUBE.)

SIGNS OF PREGNANCY. Usually the first indication of pregnancy is a missed menstrual period. Unless the period is more than 10 days late, however, this is not a definite indication, since many factors, including a strong fear of pregnancy, can delay menstruation. Nausea, or "morning sickness," usually begins in the fifth or sixth week of pregnancy. About 4 weeks after conception, changes in the breasts become noticeable: there may be a tingling sensation in the breasts, the nipples enlarge, and the areolae (the darkened areas around the nipples) may become darker. Frequent urination, another early sign, is the result of expansion of the uterus, which presses on the bladder.

Other signs of pregnancy include softening of the cervix and filling of the cervical canal with a plug of mucus. Early in labor this plug is expelled and there is slight bleeding; expulsion of the mucous plug is known as "show" and indicates the beginning of cervical dilatation. Chadwick's sign of pregnancy refers to a bluish color of the vagina which is a result of increased blood supply to the area.

When the abdominal wall becomes stretched there may be a breaking down of elastic tissues resulting in depressed areas in the skin which are smooth and reddened. These markings are called striae gravidarum. In subsequent pregnancies the old striae appear as whitish streaks and frequently do not disappear completely.

There are several fairly accurate laboratory tests for pregnancy. The so-called "rabbit" and "frog" tests are based on the fact that a pregnant woman's urine contains a hormone that causes certain changes in the test animal (see also PREGNANCY TESTS). Recently developed blood tests utilize the technique of radioassay to verify pregnancy and are said to have almost 100 per cent accuracy within a few days after the first missed menstrual period.

GROWTH OF THE FETUS. The average pregnancy lasts about 280 days, or 40 weeks, from the date of conception to childbirth. Since the exact date of conception usually is not known, the physician determines an approximate date of birth by taking the date of the beginning of the last menstrual period, adding 7 days, counting back 3 months, and advancing the date arrived at to the following year. This is approximate, since pregnancy may be shorter than the average or can last as long as 300 days.

The stages of growth of the fetus are fairly well defined. At the end of the first month, the fetus has grown beyond microscopic size. After 2 months, it is a little over an inch long, its face is formed, and its limbs are partly formed. By the end of the third month, the fetus is 3 inches long and weighs about an ounce. The limbs, fingers, toes, and ears are fully formed, and the sex can be distinguished.

After 4 months, the fetus is about 8 inches long and weighs nearly half a pound. The mother can feel its movements, and usually the physician can hear its heartbeat. The eyebrows and eyelashes are formed, and the skin is pink and covered with fine hair. By the end of the fifth month, the fetus is 12 inches long and weighs 1 lb. It now has hair on its head. At the end of the sixth month, the fetus is 14 inches long and weighs nearly 2 lb. Its skin is very wrinkled.

After 7 months, the fetus is 16 inches long and weighs about 3 lb., with more fat under its skin. In the male, the testes have descended into the scrotum. By the end of the eighth month, the fetus is 18 inches long, weighs about 5 lb., and has a good chance of survival if it is born at that time. At the end of 9 months, the average length of the fetus is 20 inches, and the average weight is 7 lb.

CARE OF THE UNBORN INFANT. A host of influences can adversely affect the growth and development of the unborn and his chances for survival and good health after birth. The diet of the mother should be nutritious and well-balanced so that the infant receives the necessary food elements for development and maturity of the body structures. It is especially important that the mother receive adequate protein in her diet, a deficiency of which can hamper the infant's intellectual development. Supplemental iron and vitamins usually are recommended during pregnancy.

There is now less emphasis on severe restriction of the mother's dietary intake to maintain a limited weight gain. It is generally agreed that the average gain should be about 24 pounds during pregnancy and that either starvation diets or forced feedings can be unhealthy for the mother and hazardous for the unborn infant. Ideally, the mother should achieve normal weight before she becomes pregnant because obesity increases by at least 60 per cent the possibility of ECLAMPSIA and other serious complications of pregnancy. Mothers who are underweight are more likely to deliver immature babies who, by virtue of their physiologic immaturity, are more likely to suffer from birth defects, HYALINE MEMBRANE DISEASE, and other developmental disorders of the newborn.

Other factors affecting the unborn child include certain drugs taken by the mother during pregnancy. A well known example is thalidomide, which inhibits the growth of the extremities of the fetus and results in gross deformities. Many drugs, including prescription as well as nonprescription medications, are now believed to be capable of causing fetal abnormalities. In addition, consumption of alcohol during pregnancy may result in FETAL ALCOHOL SYNDROME. Most obstetricians recommend that all drugs be avoided during pregnancy excepting those essential to the control of disease in the mother.

Diseases that increase the risk of obstetrical complications include diabetes, heart disease, hypertension, kidney disease, and anemia. Rubella (German measles) can be responsible for many types of birth defects, particularly if the mother contracts it in the first 3 months of pregnancy. Venereal diseases can have tragic effects on the baby, even though the symptoms in the mother are minor at the time of pregnancy. SYPHILIS is particularly dangerous because it is one of the few diseases that can be transmitted to the fetus in the uterus. The child is either stillborn or born infected, and rarely escapes physical or mental defects or both. Successful treatment of the mother before the fifth month of pregnancy will prevent infection in the infant.

During the birth process the infant may be infected with GONORRHEA as it passes through the birth canal. Gonorrheal infection of the eyes can cause blindness. HERPES SIMPLEX Type II involving the genitals of the mother can also be transmitted to the infant at birth. The mortality and morbidity rate for such infected infants is extremely high; in fact, such infection is almost always fatal.

The age of the mother is also an important factor in the well-being of the unborn infant. The mortality and morbidity rate for infants born of mothers below the age of 15 and above 40 are much higher than for those of mothers between these age limits.

Recently developed tests to monitor fetal health have taken much of the guesswork out of predicting the chances of survival and health status of the fetus after birth. Such tests and evaluation techniques include AMNIOCENTESIS, chemical and hormonal assays, ultrasound examinations, electronic surveillance of fetal vital signs and reaction to uterine contractions, and analyses of the infant's blood during labor.

PRENATAL CARE. The care of the mother during her entire pregnancy is important to her well-being and that of her unborn infant. It will help provide ease and safety during pregnancy and childbirth. The physician learns about the patient's physical condition and medical history, and can detect possible complications before they become serious.

On the first prenatal visit the patient's medical history is taken in considerable detail, including any diseases or operations she has had, the course of previous pregnancies, if any, and whether there is a family history of multiple births or of diabetes mellitus or other chronic diseases. The first visit also includes a thorough physical examination and measurement of the pelvis. Blood samples are taken for a serologic test for syphilis and for laboratory tests such as an erythrocyte count, hemoglobin determination, and blood typing. Urine is tested for albumin and sugar and examined microscopically. On subsequent visits the patient brings a urine specimen, collected upon arising that morning, to be tested for albumin. At each prenatal visit her blood pressure is taken and recorded and she is weighed.

Patients who are considered "high-risk" mothers usually are sent to a specialist and the infant is delivered at a regional hospital where sophisticated monitoring equipment and laboratory tests are available, and specially trained personnel can attend to the needs of the mother and her infant.

Discomforts and Complications. MORNING SICKNESS usually appears in the early months of pregnancy and rarely lasts beyond the third month. Often it requires no treatment, or can be relieved by such simple measures as eating dry crackers and tea before rising. Indigestion and heartburn are best prevented by avoiding foods that are difficult to digest, such as cucumbers, cabbage, cauliflower, spinach, and onions, and rich foods. Milk of magnesia may provide relief. Constipation usually can be corrected by diet or a mild laxative like milk of magnesia. Stronger laxatives should not be used unless prescribed by the physician.

A visit to a dentist early in pregnancy is a good idea to forestall any possibility of infection arising from tooth decay. Pregnancy does not encourage tooth decay.

HEMORRHOIDS sometimes occur in pregnancy because of pressure from the enlarged uterus on the veins in the rectum. The physician should be consulted for treatment.

VARICOSE VEINS also result from pressure of the uterus, which restricts the flow of blood from the legs and feet. Lying flat with the feet raised on a pillow several times a day will help relieve swelling and pain in the legs. In more difficult cases the physician may prescribe an elastic bandage or support stockings.

Backache during pregnancy is caused by the heavy abdomen pulling on muscles that are not normally used, and can be relieved by rest, a maternity corset, and sensible shoes.

Swelling of the feet and ankles usually is relieved by rest and by remaining off the feet for a day or two. If the swelling does not disappear, the physician should be informed since it may be an indication of a more serious complication.

Shortness of breath is common in the later stages of pregnancy. If at any time it becomes so extreme that the woman cannot climb a short flight of stairs without discomfort, the physician should be consulted. If a mild shortness of breath interferes with sleep, lying in a half-sitting position, supported by several pillows, may help.

The more serious complications of pregnancy include PYELITIS, HYPEREMESIS GRAVIDARUM, TOXEMIA and ECLAMPSIA, and PLACENTA PRAEVIA and ABRUPTIO PLACENTAE.

abdominal p., ectopic pregnancy within the peritoneal cavity.

ampullar p., ectopic pregnancy in the ampulla of the uterine tube.

cervical p., ectopic pregnancy within the cervical canal.

combined p., simultaneous intrauterine and extrauterine pregnancies.

cornual p., pregnancy in a horn of the uterus.

ectopic p., **extrauterine p.**, development of the fertilized ovum outside the cavity of the uterus. The site of implantation usually is one of the uterine tubes. As the fetus grows the tube ruptures, presenting the danger of hemorrhage. Symptoms include vaginal bleeding and severe pain on one side of the abdomen. Prompt surgery is necessary to remove the tube and control bleeding.

false p., development of all the signs of pregnancy without the presence of an embryo.

interstitial p., pregnancy in that part of the uterine tube within the wall of the uterus.

intraligamentary p., ectopic pregnancy within the broad ligament.

multiple p., the presence of more than one fetus in the uterus at the same time.

mural p., interstitial pregnancy.

ovarian p., pregnancy occurring in an ovary.

phantom p., false pregnancy due to psychogenic factors.

p. tests, laboratory procedures for early determination of pregnancy. Within one week after the first missed menstrual period human CHORIONIC GONADOTROPIN (HCG), a hormone secreted by the placenta, is present in the blood and urine of a pregnant woman. It can be detected by biologic tests, in which urine (or serum) is injected into laboratory animals, by immunologic tests, and by radioreceptor assay.

In the Aschheim-Zondek (AZ) test, immature female mice are used, and changes in their ovaries are observed within 100 hours if HCG is present in the urine injected.

The Friedman test makes use of a female rabbit, and ovarian changes are observed within 48 hours after injection of urine from a pregnant woman.

Male frogs are used in the Galli Mainini test; sperm are found in their urine 1 to 4 hours after injection of urine containing HCG.

In the immunologic tests, urine is mixed with antihuman chorionic gonadotropin serum; if the urine does *not* contain HCG (absence of pregnancy), an antigen-antibody reaction (agglutination) will occur. These tests take only a few minutes or a few hours.

A relatively new technique for detection of HCG and luteinizing hormone (LH) is that of radioreceptor-assay, developed by Dr. Brij Saxena. This test is reported to be almost 100 per cent reliable in diagnosing pregnancy one week after conception. The test requires only a few drops of finger blood and, through the use of a gamma counter to indicate radioactivity, can yield results in one hour.

tubal p., ectopic pregnancy within a uterine tube.

tuboabdominal p., ectopic pregnancy occurring partly in the fimbriated end of the uterine tube and partly in the abdominal cavity.

tubo-ovarian p., pregnancy at the fimbria of the uterine tube.

pregnane (preg′nān) a crystalline saturated steroid hydrocarbon; *β-pregnane* is the form from which several hormones, including progesterone, are derived; *α-pregnane* is the form excreted in the urine.

pregnanediol (preg″nān-di-ol) a crystalline, biologically inactive dihydroxy derivative of pregnane, formed by reduction of progesterone and found especially in urine of pregnant women.

pregnanetriol (preg″nān-tri′ol) a metabolite of 17-hydroxyprogesterone; its excretion in the urine is greatly increased in certain disorders of the adrenal cortex.

pregnant (preg′nant) with child; gravid; having a developing embryo or fetus within the uterus.

pregnene (preg′nēn) a compound that forms the chemical nucleus of progesterone.

pregneninolone (preg″nēn-in′o-lōn) ethisterone, a progestational steroid.

prehallux (pre-hal′uks) a supernumerary bone of the foot growing from the medial border of the scaphoid.

prehemiplegic (pre″hem-ĭ-ple′jik) preceding hemiplegia.

prehensile (pre-hen′sil) adapted for grasping or seizing.

prehension (pre-hen′shun) the act of grasping.

prehypophysis (pre″hi-pof′ĭ-sis) the anterior lobe of the hypophysis, or pituitary gland.

preictal (pre-ik′tal) occurring before a stroke, seizure, or attack.

preicteric (pre″ik-ter′ik) preceding the appearance of jaundice (icterus).

preinvasive (pre″in-va′siv) not yet invading tissues outside the site of origin.

preleukemia (pre″loo-ke′me-ah) a stage of bone marrow dysfunction preceding the development of acute myelogenous leukemia. adj., **preleuke′mic.**

prelimbic (pre-lim′bik) in front of a limbus.

premalignant (pre″mah-lig′nant) precancerous.

premature (pre″mah-tūr′) born or interrupted before the state of maturity; occurring before the proper time.

p. infant, one with a gestational age of less than 37 weeks. The premature infant may be classifid as *large premature* if he weights more than 1500 gm. and his gestational age is between 32 and 37 weeks or *small premature* if he weighs less than 1500 gm. and his gestation age is less than 32 weeks. The prematurity of an infant is determined by the criterion of *stage of maturity* rather than weight, because his physiological development bears a direct relationship to the kinds of difficulties he will experience outside the uterus and the kind of care he must receive if he is to survive. Causes of premature birth include diseased condition in the mother, multiple births, and induced labor.

Some infants of normal gestational age weigh much less at birth than expected because of failure to thrive and to gain weight within the uterus. They appear undernourished and many have suffered neurologic damage from hypoxia during the prenatal period or at the time of birth. These infants do not present the same problems as do premature infants. To avoid confusion between premature infants and those who weigh less than expected at birth, the term "small-for-dates" infant is used. This simply implies that according to the period of gestation as calculated according to the mother's last menstrual period, the infant weighs less than expected. The main difficulties these infants encounter are (1) poor temperature control because of a deficit of insulating body fat, (2) hypoglycemia due to low glycogen reserves, and (3) susceptibility to infection because of a deficit of immune bodies.

In addition to the criterion of gestational age, some signs of prematurity in a newborn include smooth soles of the feet, with only one or two creases across the ball of the foot and a smooth heel. The full-term infant has deep creases across the sole of his feet. "Cotton-wool hair," in which it is difficult to distinguish one strand of hair from another, is common until the 38th week of gestation. Since cartilage in the ear develops in the ninth month, a soft, somewhat shapeless ear may indicate prematurity.

Care of the premature infant is concerned with helping him cope with life outside the uterus until he has matured sufficiently and is able to function on his own. He has very weak or absent sucking and swallowing reflexes and thus must be fed by gavage, or intravenously, if he is unable to tolerate oral feedings. A deficiency of body fat and immature body temperature controls require an environment designed to maintain his body temperature at normal levels. To accomplish this he is placed in an incubator and his body temperature is monitored.

A common difficulty in premature infants is RESPIRATORY DISTRESS SYNDROME (RDS) occurring as a result of HYALINE MEMBRANE DISEASE. Oxygen is administered very carefully to avoid the hazards of RETROLENTAL FIBROPLASIA and oxygen toxicity. (See also OXYGEN THERAPY.) A suction machine and artificial VENTILATOR usually are needed to maintain adequate exchange of respiratory gases and prevent an acid-base imbalance. An elevated level of bilirubin in the blood and resultant jaundice may occur in the premature infant. In some institutions all premature infants are routinely placed under phototherapy units. Because of the premature infant's lowered resistance to infection and his lack of sufficient immunity to infectious diseases, it is imperative that precautions be taken to avoid introducing pathogenic bacteria into his environment. These precautions include isolation of the infant and minimal handling. Those who care for the infant must wear masks, caps, and gowns, and must adhere to the strict policies of handwashing and other infection control measures.

The care of the premature infant requires specialized training in the specific needs of these infants and the therapeutic procedures and techniques that their care demands. The mortality rate of premature infants has decreased in the past two decades, but it still remains disturbingly high.

prematurity (pre″mah-tūr′ĭ-te) underdevelopment; the condition of a premature infant.

premaxilla (pre-mak′sĭ-lah) a separate element derived from the median nasal processes in the embryo, which later fuses with the maxilla (see also INCISIVE BONE).

premaxillary (pre-mak′sĭ-ler″e) 1. situated in front of the maxilla proper. 2. incisive bone.

p. bone, premaxilla.

premedication (pre″med-ĭ-ka′shun) preliminary medication, particularly internal medication to produce narcosis prior to general anesthesia.

premenarchal (pre″mĕ-nar′kal) occurring before establishment of menstruation.

premenstrual (pre-men′stroo-al) preceding menstruation.

p. tension, a complex of symptoms sometimes occurring in the 10 days before menstruation, including emotional instability and irritability, pain in the breasts, headache, nausea, anorexia, constipation, pelvic discomfort, edema, and abdominal distention.

The causes of these symptoms are not fully understood but are believed to be associated with a disturbed salt balance, resulting in the accumulation of water in the tissues just before menstruation. Psychogenic factors may contribute. Emotional and physical symptoms usually disappear with the onset of menstruation. If symptoms are habitually troublesome, restriction of fluid and salt intake and a diuretic may be prescribed. Tranquilizers and reassurance that the condition is not serious are also helpful.

premenstruum (pre-men′stroo-um) the period immediately before menstruation.

premolar (pre-mo′lar) in front of the molar teeth (see also TOOTH).

premorbid (pre-mor′bid) occurring before the development of disease.

premunition (pre″mu-nish′un) resistance to infection by the same or closely related pathogen established after an acute infection has become chronic, and lasting as long as the infecting organisms are in the body. adj., **premu′nitive.**

premyeloblast (pre-mi′ĕ-lo-blast″) a precursor of a myeloblast.

premyelocyte (pre-mi′ĕ-lo-sīt) promyelocyte.

prenatal (pre-na′tal) preceding birth.

p. care, care of the pregnant woman before delivery of the infant (see also PREGNANCY).

preneoplastic (pre″ne-o-plas′tik) before the formation of a tumor.

prenylamine (prĕ-nil′ah-mēn) a coronary vasodilator.

preoperative (pre-op′er-ah-tiv, pre-op′er-a″tiv) preceding an operation.

p. care, the psychologic and physiologic preparation of a patient before operation. The preoperative period may be extremely short, as with an emergency operation, or it may encompass several weeks during which diagnostic tests, specific medications and treatments, and measures to improve the patient's general well-being are employed in preparation for surgery.

PSYCHOLOGIC ASPECTS. Although each patient reacts in his own unique way to the news that he is going to have surgery, all patients experience some degree of anxiety and fear—fear of the unknown, worry over disability or death, and apprehension about the insecurity of his and his family's future.

Much of this anxiety can be relieved if the various aspects of his preoperative and postoperative care and the type of surgery planned are explained to the patient. The surgeon usually explains the surgical procedure and assists the patient in planning rehabilitation. The anesthesiologist usually reviews the type of anesthesia to be used and the general effects it will have on the patient. The nursing staff explains the hospital routine, specific nursing procedures necessary, the purpose of diagnostic tests required, and the types of equipment that will be used during the preoperative and postoperative periods. The nurse can demonstrate interest in the patient and his family by answering questions (or referring them to the surgeon), and giving them a general idea of how long the patient will be away from his room during surgery and recovery from anesthesia. It is reassuring for them to know, for example, that oxygen administration, blood transfusions, and the use of a nasogastric tube or catheter do not necessarily indicate a critical situation. The use of various pieces of equipment that seem "routine" to the hospital staff may be extremely upsetting to the patient and his family if they do not understand why the equipment is necessary.

Spiritual reinforcement during this period may be very important to some patients, and though the nurse must be careful not to give the impression of prying into the patient's private affairs, she must also show a willingness to assist him and his family in obtaining a spiritual advisor if they indicate a desire for her to do so. The nurse must always respect the individual patient's beliefs and convictions even though she may not share them, and must support the patient in his search for spiritual reassurance and guidance.

LEGAL ASPECTS. Any patient undergoing surgery, whether it is expected to be major or minor surgery, must sign an operative permit. He has the right to know the type of surgery intended and its expected outcome, aftereffects, and possible complications. If he is underage, mentally incompetent, or unconscious, the permit is signed by a relative or guardian. The permit protects the patient against unwanted surgery and operative procedures he does not understand. It protects the hospital staff and surgeon from legal claims that the surgery was done without the patient's permission or knowledge of what was to be done. The signed operative permit is placed in the patient's chart and is sent to the operating room with him.

PREVENTIVE ASPECTS. During the preoperative period the patient should be instructed in coughing, turning, deep breathing, and exercises of the extremities. These techniques can be most effective in preventing many of the complications of surgery. Exercises to strengthen specific muscles in preparation for rehabilitation, as following AMPUTATION, for example, are begun well in advance so that the patient is in optimal condition to begin a program of rehabilitation as soon after surgery as possible. Other topics of instruction will depend on the anticipated needs of the patient during his recovery from surgery.

PHYSIOLOGIC ASPECTS. Except in emergency situations every effort is made to have the patient in a state of optimal health before surgery is performed. Specific diets, protein and vitamin supplements, and other measures to improve the nutritional status may be employed. Intravenous infusions and transfusions of whole blood or plasma may be necessary to improve the fluid and electrolyte status and blood volume. Infections should be brought under control before surgery if they cannot be eliminated completely. Accurate records of the patient's vital signs, blood pressure, and urinary output will assist the surgeon in diagnosing and correcting conditions that may adversely affect the patient's physiologic response to an operative procedure.

PHYSICAL PREPARATION. The skin and hair are harborers of infection and require special attention before surgery. The particular area to be shaved and cleansed will depend on the wishes of the surgeon and the accepted hospital procedure. Generally, it is desirable to shave and cleanse with an antiseptic an area larger than the proposed incision. An exception may be the head or face, especially the eyebrows, which are never shaved. If large amounts of hair must be removed from the head, the hair should be saved so that it can be used for a hairpice later if the patient so desires.

A depilatory cream may be substituted for shaving, depending on hospital policy. Some surgeons do not require removal of the hair at all, especially in some types of gynecologic surgery.

In some types of orthopedic surgery preparation of the skin may start as much as 24 hours before the operation. The operative site is wrapped in sterile towels or dressings; in some cases the dressings are removed at regular intervals and an antiseptic is applied. This type of skin preparation must be done according to specific directions from the surgeon.

Restriction of food and fluids varies. Usually the patient is allowed a light evening meal and then given nothing by mouth after midnight the night before surgery. Other procedures for preparation of the gastrointestinal tract may include enemas and insertion of a nasogastric tube.

PREOPERATIVE MEDICATIONS. Generally there are three types of drugs used prior to surgery: sedatives, such as one of the barbiturates, to promote relaxation and rest and to stabilize the blood pressure and pulse; drying agents, such as atropine and scopolamine, which decrease secretion of mucus in the mouth and throat; and narcotics, such as morphine and meperidine hydrochloride (Demerol), which promote relaxation and enhance the effects of the anesthetic.

Preoperative medications must be given at the exact time ordered because their strength, action, and duration are planned according to the type of anesthesia used.

IMMEDIATE PREOPERATIVE CARE. Most institutions use a check list or clearance record for surgical procedures. This eliminates the danger of overlooking some aspect of the immediate preoperative preparation. Such an omission might delay surgery or result in legal problems. The operative permit must be signed by the patient or his guardian or legal representative. This permit is necessary to protect the surgeon against claims of unauthorized surgery, and to protect the patient against surgery he would not willingly endorse.

The preoperative check list includes such items as laboratory tests and their findings, history and physical examination records, disposal of valuables, removal of dentures and their disposition, vital signs and blood pressure of the patient immediately before he goes to the operating room and, other specific information such as consultation for sterilization and operative permit.

Unless a urinary catheter has been inserted, the patient is offered the bedpan just before he is taken to the operating room. Hairpins, bobbie pins, and combs are removed from the hair and the head is covered with a cap or scarf. As the patient leaves the unit he is reassured that everything is in order and that everyone concerned with his care is interested in him and the outcome of his operation.

preoral (pre-o'ral) in front of the mouth.

preparalytic (pre"par-ah-lit'ik) preceding paralysis.

prepatellar (pre"pah-tel'ar) in front of the patella.

preprandial (pre-pran'de-al) before meals.

prepuberal, prepubertal (pre-pu'ber-al; pre-pu'ber-tal) before puberty; pertaining to the period of accelerated growth preceding gonadal maturity.

prepubescent (pre"pu-bes'ent) prepubertal.

prepuce (pre'pūs) foreskin; a cutaneous fold over the glans penis. adj., **prepu'tial.**

p. of clitoris, a fold capping the clitoris formed by union of the labia minora and the clitoris.

preputiotomy (pre-pu"she-ot'o-me) incision of the prepuce of the penis to relive phimosis.

preputium (pre-pu'she-um) prepuce.

prepyloric (pre"pi-lor'ik) just proximal to the pylorus.

presacral (pre'sa-kral) anterior to the sacrum.

presby- word element [Gr.], *old age.*

presbyatrics (pres"be-at'riks) geriatrics.

presbycardia (pres"bĭ-kar'de-ah) impairment of cardiac function attributed to aging, with senescent changes in the body and no evidence of other cause of heart disease.

presbycusis (pres"bĭ-ku'sis) progressive, bilaterally symmetrical perceptive hearing loss occurring with age.

presbyope (pres'be-ōp) one who is affected with presbyopia.

presbyophrenia (pres"be-o-fre'ne-ah) loss of memory, disorientation, and confabulation, occurring in old age; called also Wernicke's syndrome.

presbyopia (pres"be-o'pe-ah) diminution of accommodation of the lens of the eye occurring normally with aging, and usually resulting in hyperopia, or farsightedness. adj., **presbyop'ic.** Presbyopia is caused by a loss of elasticity in the crystalline lens of the eye. The lens focuses images on the retina with the aid of muscles that stretch it to make it less convex or relax it to make it more spherical and thus more convex. As it ages, the lens may lose its ability to become convex enough to accommodate to nearby objects. This condition usually begins around the age of 40. Presbyopia can most often be comfortably corrected through the use of eyeglasses.

prescription (pre-skrip'shun) a written directive, as for the compounding or dispensing and administration of drugs, or for other service to a particular patient.

Federal law divides medicines into two main classes: prescription medicines and over-the-counter medicines. Dangerous, powerful, or habit-forming medicines to be used under a physician's supervision can be sold only by prescription. The prescription must be written by a physician; otherwise the pharmacist is forbidden to prepare and fill it.

There are four parts to a drug prescription. The first is the symbol ℞ from the Latin *recipe,* meaning "take." This is the superscription. The second part is the inscription, specifying the ingredients and their quantities. The third part is the subscription, which tells the pharmacist how to compound the medicine. The signature is the last part, and it is usually preceded by an S to represent the Latin *signa,* meaning "mark." The signature is where the physician indicates what instructions are to be put on the outside of the package to tell the patient when and how to take the medicine and in what quantities.

The pharmacist keeps a file of all the prescriptions he fills.

presenile (pre-se'nīl) pertaining to a condition resembling senility, but occurring in early or middle life.

presentation (prez"en-ta'shun) lie; the relationship of the long axis of the fetus to that of the mother. (See also POSITION.)

breech p., presentation of the fetal buttocks or feet in labor; the feet may be alongside the buttocks (complete breech presentation); the legs may be extended against the trunk and the feet lying against the face (frank breech presentation); or one or both feet or knees may be prolapsed into the maternal vagina (incomplete breech presentation).

cephalic p., presentation of any part of the fetal head in labor, whether the vertex, face, or brow.

compound p., prolapse of an extremity of the fetus alongside the head in cephalic presentation or of one or both arms alongside a presenting breech at the beginning of labor.

footling p., presentation of the fetus with one foot (single footling) or two feet (double footling) prolapsed into the maternal vagina.

funic p., presentation of the umbilical cord in labor.

longitudinal p., that in which the long axis of the fetus lies parallel to that of the mother, with either the head or breech the presenting part.

oblique p., that in which the long axis of the fetal body lies obliquely to that of the mother; the shoulder presents first.

placental p., placenta praevia.

shoulder p., oblique presentation or transverse lie.

transverse p., transverse lie.

preservative (pre-zer'vah-tiv) a substance added to

a product to destroy or inhibit multiplication of microorganisms.

presomite (pre-so′mīt) referring to embryos before the appearance of somites.

presphenoid (pre-sfe′noid) the anterior portion of the body of the sphenoid bone.

presphygmic (pre-sfig′mik) preceding the pulse wave.

p. interval, p. period, the first phase of ventricular systole, being the period (0.04–0.06 sec.) immediately after closure of the atrioventricular valves and lasting until the semilunar valves open.

prespinal (pre-spi′nal) in front of the spine.

pressor (pres′or) tending to increase blood pressure.

pressoreceptive (pres″o-re-sep′tiv) sensitive to stimuli due to vasomotor activity; pressosensitive.

pressoreceptor (pres″o-re-sep′tor) a receptor or nerve ending sensitive to stimuli of vasomotor activity.

pressosensitive (pres″o-sen′sĭ-tiv) pressoreceptive.

pressure (presh′ur) stress or strain, by compression, expansion, pull, thrust, or shear.

arterial p., the blood pressure in the arteries.

atmospheric p., the pressure exerted by the atmosphere, about 15 lb. to the square inch at sea level.

blood p., the pressure of the blood on the walls of the arteries, dependent on the energy of the heart action, elasticity of the arterial walls, and volume and viscosity of the blood; the maximum or systolic pressure occurs near the end of the stroke output of the left ventricle, and the minimum or diastolic late in ventricular diastole (see also BLOOD PRESSURE).

capillary p., the blood pressure in the capillaries.

central venous p., the pressure of blood in the right atrium (see also CENTRAL VENOUS PRESSURE).

cerebrospinal p., the pressure of the cerebrospinal fluid, normally 100 to 150 mm. as measured by the manometer.

intracranial p., the pressure of the subarachnoidal fluid.

intraocular p., the pressure exerted against the outer coats by the contents of the eyeball.

negative p., pressure less than that of the atmosphere.

oncotic p., the osmotic pressure of a colloid in solution.

osmotic p., the potential pressure of a solution directly related to its solute osmolar concentration; it is the maximum pressure developed by osmosis in a solution separated from another by a semipermeable membrane, i.e., the pressure that will just prevent OSMOSIS between two such solutions.

partial p., pressure exerted by each of the constituents of a mixture of gases.

p. points, various locations on the body at which digital pressure may be applied for the control of hemorrhage.

positive p., pressure greater than that of the atmosphere.

pulse p., the difference between the systolic and diastolic pressures.

p. sore, decubitus ulcer.

venous p., the blood pressure in the veins.

presternum (pre-ster′num) the manubrium; the upper part of the sternum.

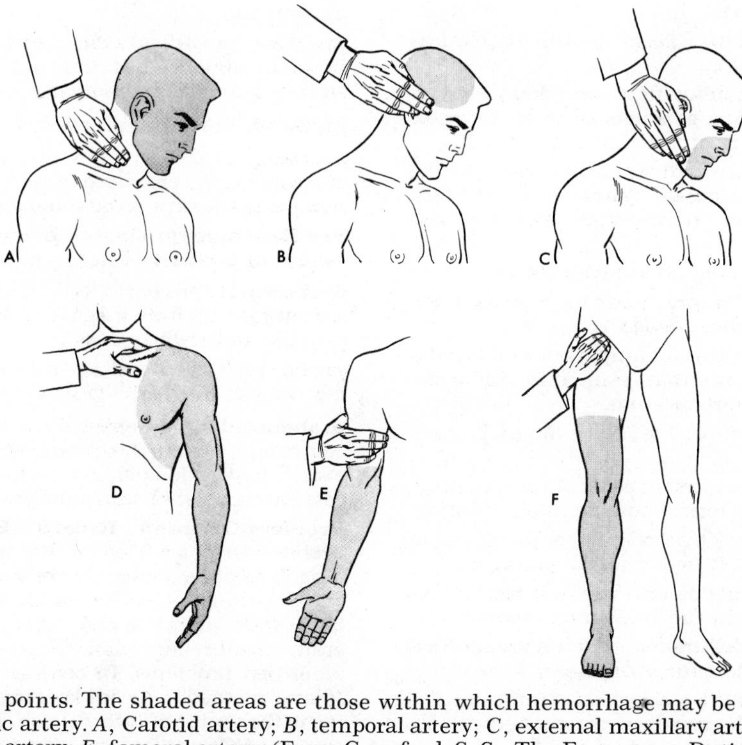

Digital pressure points. The shaded areas are those within which hemorrhage may be controlled by pressure on the specific artery. *A*, Carotid artery; *B*, temporal artery; *C*, external maxillary artery; *D*, subclavian artery; *E*, brachial artery; *F*, femoral artery. (From Crawford, S. S.: The Emergency Duties of the Industrial Nurse. Nursing Clin. N. Amer., 2:271, 1967.)

presuppurative (prē-sup′u-ra″tiv) preceding suppuration.

presymptomatic (pre″simp-to-mat′ik) existing before the appearance of symptoms.

presynaptic (pre″sĭ-nap′tik) situated or occurring proximal to a synapse.

presystole (pre-sis′to-le) the interval just before systole.

presystolic (pre″sis-tol′ik) preceding systole.

pretarsal (pre-tar′sal) in front of the tarsus.

pretibial (pre-tib′e-al) in front of the tibia.

p. fever, leptospirosis due to *Leptospira autumnalis,* marked by a rash on the pretibial region, with lumbar and postorbital pain, malaise, coryza, and fever. Called also Fort Bragg fever.

prevalence (prev′ah-lens) the total number of cases of a specific disease in existence in a given population at a certain time.

preventive (pre-ven′tiv) serving to avert the occurrence of; prophylactic.

p. medicine, science aimed at preventing disease.

prevertebral (pre-ver′tĕ-bral) in front of a vertebra.

prevesical (pre-ves′ĭ-kal) anterior to the bladder.

prezygotic (pre″zi-got′ik) occurring before completion of fertilization.

priapism (pri′ah-pizm) persistent abnormal erection of the penis, accompanied by pain and tenderness. It is seen in diseases and injuries of the spinal cord, and may be caused by vesical calculus and certain injuries to the penis.

prickle cell (prik″l) a cell with delicate radiating processes connecting with similar cells, being a dividing keratinocyte of the prickle-cell layer of the epidermis.

prickly heat miliaria.

prilocaine (pril′o-kān) a local anesthetic, used as the hydrochloride salt.

primaquine (pri′mah-kwin) a compound used as an antimalarial, being gametocidal to all forms of malarial parasites; used as the phosphate salt.

primate (pri′māt) an individual belonging to the highest order of mammals, Primates (pri-ma′tēz), which includes man and the apes, monkeys, and lemurs.

primidone (pri′mĭ-dōn) an anticonvulsant.

primigravida (pri″mĭ-grav′ĭ-dah) a woman pregnant for the first time; gravida I.

primipara (pri-mip′ah-rah) unipara; a woman who has had one pregnancy that resulted in viable offspring, para I. adj., **primip′arous.**

primiparity (pri″mĭ-par′ĭ-te) the state of being a primipara.

primitive (prim′ĭ-tiv) first in point of time; existing in a simple or early form; showing little evolution.

primordial (pri-mor′de-al) original or primitive; of the simplest and most undeveloped character.

primordium (pri-mor′de-um) the first beginnings of an organ or part in the developing embryo.

Prinadol (prin′ah-dol) trademark for a preparation of phenazocine, a narcotic analgesic.

principle (prin′sĭ-p′l) 1. a chemical component. 2. a substance on which certain of the properties of a drug depend. 3. a law of conduct.

active p., any constituent of a drug that helps to confer upon it a medicinal property.

antianemia p., the constituent in liver and certain other tissues (vitamin B_{12}) that produces the hematopoietic effect in pernicious anemia.

immediate p., any of the more or less complex substances of definite chemical constitution into which a heterogenous substance can be readily resolved.

pleasure p., the automatic instinct or tendency to avoid pain and secure pleasure.

proximate p., immediate principle.

reality p., in freudian terminology, the mental activity that develops to control the pleasure principle under the pressure of necessity or the demands of reality.

Prinzmetal's angina (prinz-met′alz) a variant of angina pectoris in which the attacks occur during rest, exercise capacity is well preserved, and attacks are associated electrocardiographically with elevation of the ST-segment.

Priodax (pri′o-daks) trademark for a preparation of iodoalphionic acid, used as a contrast medium in cholecystography.

Priscoline (pris′ko-lēn) trademark for preparations of tolazoline, a peripheral vasodilator and smooth muscle relaxant.

Privine (pri′vēn) trademark for preparations of naphazoline, a vasoconstrictor.

p.r.n. [L.] *pro re na′ta* (according to circumstances).

pro- word element [L., Gr.], *before; in front of; favoring.*

proaccelerin (pro″ak-sel′er-in) clotting factor V.

proactinomycin (pro-ak″tin-o-mi′sin) a group of antibiotics, designated A, B, and C, from cultures of *Nocardia gardneri,* active against gram-positive bacteria.

proactivator (pro-ak′tĭ-va″tor) a precursor of an activator; a factor that reacts with an enzyme to form an activator.

proatlas (pro-at′las) a rudimentary vertebra which in some animals lies in front of the atlas; sometimes seen in many as an anomaly.

proband (pro′band) propositus.

probang (pro′bang) a flexible rod with a ball, tuft, or sponge at the end; used to apply medications to or remove matter from the esophagus or larynx.

Pro-Banthine (pro-ban-thīn) trademark for preparations of propantheline, an anticholinergic.

probarbital (pro-bar′bĭ-tal) an intermediate-acting barbiturate used as a sedative in the form of the calcium and sodium salts.

probe (prōb) a long, slender instrument for exploring wounds or body cavities or passages.

probenecid (pro-ben′ĕ-sid) a white, crystalline compound, used in the treatment of GOUT to promote excretion of uric acid; also used to increase serum concentration of certain antibiotics and other drugs.

Problem-Oriented Record (POR) called also Problem-Oriented Medical Record (POMR), an approach to patient care record keeping that focuses on the patient's specific health problems requiring immediate attention, and the structuring of a cooperative health care plan designed to cope with the identified problems. In contrast to the traditional "diary" method of record keeping organized according to the source of information (physicians, nurses, etc.), the POR utilizes progress sheets that integrate all written notes under labeled problems.

The POR system of record keeping was first introduced in the late 1960's by Dr. Lawrence L. Weed. The purpose of the system is to improve patient care by employing the systematic analysis and logical documentation of the care rendered by various members of the health care team. When properly implemented, the problem-oriented approach is expected to provide a more effective means of communication among the members of the health care team (including the patient), and to facilitate the coordination of preventive care, health maintenance, and continuity of care. Other areas affected by the POR include cost of health care delivery, evaluation and control of the quality of care rendered, and medical-legal aspects related to informed consent by the patient.

By eliminating much of the duplication of time and effort spent by health care professionals in acquiring and recording patient care data, the POR system can reduce significantly the overall cost of health care. Other costs related to the preparation of insurance forms, record reviews for quality control, and duplication of patient records, can be reduced substantially by the more efficient and less cumbersome problem-oriented system. The accumulation of specific and objective data relative to patient care is a major step toward the establishment of explicit criteria against which the preformance of health care providers can be measured. The objective evaluation of performance is especially important in the certification and recertification of health care personnel.

Although the details of implementing a POR system may vary according to the setting in which it is to be used and the type of clientele being served, there are four components that are basic to the problem-oriented record. These are the *database, problem list, plan,* and *notes.*

THE DATABASE. In the traditional system of recording, pertinent information about the patient's history and present status is scattered throughout the patient's chart. The POR system contains only one database section in which input from a variety of sources is recorded. The information recorded in the database section pertains to the particular patient in the particular setting, that is, hospital, outpatient clinic, other health care setting, and includes his general history, physical examination findings, physiologic and laboratory data, nursing history, and observations about lifestyle and current status. Data is acquired for the purpose of identifying current (active) major problems, which are *flagged* in the database and then described under a titled *notes* section. Minor and inactive problems are described within the database.

As time goes on, the acquisition of new information about the patient requires additional notes on the database forms. In the event such additions become extensive, the original database form may be "retired" to an inactive record and a new database generated for the active record. The active database serves as a concise and relevant record of the patient's current status, and thus facilitates continuity of care and coordination of plans for his care as he moves through various inpatient and outpatient agencies and institutions.

The patient's contribution to the database usually involves the completion of any of a number of forms designed to elicit information about his personal and family medical history. The patient accepts responsibility for answering the questions presented as accurately as possible; however, he may need assistance in completing the forms so as to avoid trivial and "false-positive" clues to the exact nature of his problems.

The database and the more extensive data about his major problems constitute the "complete data set," that is, a complete work-up.

THE PROBLEM LIST. The active problem list contains those major problems currently needing attention for further observation, diagnosis, management, or patient education. It serves as the basis for a plan of care. The problems may fall into the area of psychologic, social, and economic factors, as well as the more familiar physical diagnosis. For example, the problem identified could be congestive heart failure, if this has been established previously as a documented diagnosis, or it may be only a symptom, an abnormal laboratory finding, a risk factor, or some other problem that must be dealt with. As problems are resolved or new problems added, the problem list may be retired to an inactive record and a new list prepared.

The problem list is the first document encountered in the patient's chart. It serves as a guide to the current and important health problems of the patient. Its purpose is to draw attention to the problem areas so that they will not be overlooked. In order for the problem list to serve the purpose for which it is intended, it is necessary to use language that is concise and explicit. If a diagnosis has been made, that should be written, but if there are several manifestations of an illness, they should be incorporated into a single definition that is as brief and accurate as possible. The manifestations themselves may be listed separately on a flow sheet or narrative notes elsewhere in the chart. It is important to remember that the problem list is just that, a list, and not a detailed explanation of the difficulties the patient is experiencing.

THE PLAN. This is a plan of action that is derived from the problems which have been identified and that serves as a focus for patient care. The written plan is entered on the progress notes under each labeled problem. Specific physicians' plans and nursing plans should be integrated to avoid duplication and to provide a means of coordinating and communicating the care plan. The physician-generated plans are those related to diagnostic studies and therapy, the traditional physician's "orders." The nurse-generated plans are concerned with observations, activity, diet, and patient education.

The plan as recorded in the problem-oriented record is intended to eliminate the unnecessary writing of trivia and is focused on the reporting of exceptional and relevant infomation only. Routine procedures and data such as the daily bath, respiratory rate, and bowel movements can be deleted from the permanent record if they are not related to the patient's problems. They may be entered on work sheets that are discarded at the time of discharge. Should an abnormality or difficulty in carrying out routine care be detected, it is entered as a problem on the problem list.

NOTES. In the problem-oriented approach there is only one section for progress notes. Physicians, nurses, and all other health care personnel directly participating in the care of the patient use the progress notes to document their observations, assessments, nursing care plans, physician's orders, etc.

As a device for conceptualizing the process of recording progress notes, Weed and others suggest the SOAP structuring of notes. The *S* indicates subjective data obtained from the patient and his significant others. The *O* designates objective data obtained by observation, physical examination, diagnostic studies, etc. The *A* refers to assessment of the patient's status through analysis of the problem, possible interaction of problems, and changes in the status of problems. The *P* designates plan.

Progress notes need not be daily records of each problem. It usually is not necessary to record every problem every day, and all of the complements of SOAP need not be written daily. The goal of problem-oriented recording is to keep writing at a minimum and to record only that which is relevant to the patient's problems and important to communication and continuity of care.

probucol (pro'bu-kol) a bis-phenol compound taken orally to lower elevated serum cholesterol levels.

procainamide (pro-kān'ah-mīd) a cardiac depressant used as the hydrochloride salt in the treatment of cardiac arrhythmias.

procaine (pro'kān) a local anesthetic; the hydrochloride salt is used in solution for infiltration, nerve block, and spinal anesthesia.

procarboxypeptidase (pro"kar-bok"se-pep'tĭ-dās) the inactive precursor of carboxypeptidase, which is converted to the active enzyme by the action of trypsin.

procelous (pro-se'lus) having the anterior surface concave; said of vertebrae.

procentriole (pro-sen'tre-ōl) the immediate precursor of centrioles and ciliary basal bodies.

procephalic (pro"sĕ-fal'ik) pertaining to the anterior part of the head.

procercoid (pro-ser'koid) a larval stage of fish tapeworms.

process (pros'es) 1. a prominence or projection, as from a bone. 2. a series of operations or events leading to achievement of a specific result; also, to subject to such a series to produce desired changes.

acromial p., acromion.

alveolar p., the part of the bone in either the maxilla or mandible that surrounds and supports the teeth.

basilar p., a quadrilateral plate of the occipital bone projecting superiorly and anteriorly from the foramen magnum.

caudate p., the right of the two processes on the caudate lobe of the liver.

ciliary p's, meridionally arranged ridges or folds projecting from the crown of the ciliary body.

clinoid p., any of the three (anterior, medial, and posterior) processes of the sphenoid bone.

coracoid p., a curved process arising from the upper neck of the scapula and overhanging the shoulder joint; called also coracoid.

coronoid p., 1. the anterior part of the upper end of the ramus of the mandible. 2. a projection at the proximal end of the ulna.

ensiform p., xiphoid process.

ethmoid p., a bony projection above and behind the maxillary process of the inferior nasal concha.

frontonasal p., an expansive facial process in the embryo that develops into the forehead and bridge of the nose.

malar p., zygomatic process of the maxilla.

mamillary p., a tubercle on each superior articular process of a lumbar vertebra.

mastoid p., a conical projection at the base of mastoid portion of temporal bone.

nursing p., a systematic approach to the identification of a patient's nursing care problems (see also NURSING PROCESS).

odontoid p., a toothlike projection of the axis that articulates with the atlas.

pterygoid p., one of the wing-shaped processes of the sphenoid bone.

spinous p. of vertebrae, a part of the vertebrae projecting backward from the arch, giving attachment to muscles of the back.

styloid p., a long, pointed projection, particularly a long spine projecting downward from the inferior surface of the temporal bone.

uncinate p., any hooklike process, as of vertebrae, the lacrimal bone, or the pancreas.

xiphoid p., the pointed process of cartilage, supported by a core of bone, connected with the lower end of the sternum; called also xiphoid.

zygomatic p., a projection from the frontal or temporal bone, or from the maxilla, by which they articulate with the zygoma.

processus (pro-ses'us), pl. *proces'sus* [L.] process.

prochlorpemazine (pro"klor-pem'ah-zēn) prochlorperazine.

prochlorperazine (pro"klōr-per'ah-zēn) a phenothiazine derivative used as a major tranquilizer and antiemetic.

prochondral (pro-kon'dral) occurring before the formation of cartilage.

procidentia (pro"sĭ-den'she-ah) a state of prolapse, especially prolapse of the uterus.

procoagulant (pro"co-ag'u-lant) 1. tending to promote coagulation. 2. a precursor of a natural substance necessary to coagulation of the blood.

proconvertin (pro"kon-ver'tin) clotting factor VII.

procreation (pro"kre-a'shun) the act of begetting or generating.

proct(o)- word element [Gr.], *rectum;* see also words beginning *rect(o)-*.

proctalgia (prok-tal'je-ah) pain in the rectum; proctodynia.

proctatresia (prok"tah-tre'ze-ah) imperforate anus.

proctectasia (prok"tek-ta'ze-ah) dilatation of the rectum or anus.

proctectomy (prok-tek'to-me) excision of the rectum.

procteurynter (prok"tu-rin'ter) a baglike device used to dilate the rectum.

proctitis (prok-ti'tis) inflammation of the rectum.

proctocele (prok'to-sēl) hernial protrusion of part of the rectum into the vagina; rectocele.

proctoclysis (prok-tok'lĭ-sis) slow introduction of large quantities of liquid into the rectum.

proctocolonoscopy (prok"to-ko"lon-os'ko-pe) inspection of the interior of the rectum and lower colon.

proctocolpoplasty (prok"to-kol'po-plas"te) repair of a rectovaginal fistula.

proctocystotomy (prok"to-sis-tot'o-me) removal of a bladder calculus through the rectum.

proctodeum (prok"to-de'um) the ectodermal depression of the caudal end of the embryo, which becomes the anal canal; called also anal pit.

proctodynia (prok″to-din′e-ah) pain in the rectum; proctalgia.

proctology (prok-tol′o-je) the branch of medicine concerned with disorders of the rectum and anus. adj., **proctolog′ic.**

proctoparalysis (prok″to-pah-ral′ĭ-sis) paralysis of the anal and rectal muscles; proctoplegia.

proctoplasty (prok′to-plas″te) plastic repair of the rectum and anus.

proctoplegia (prok″to-ple′je-ah) proctoparalysis.

proctoptosis (prok″top-to′sis) prolapse of the rectum.

proctorrhaphy (prok-tor′ah-fe) suture of the rectum.

proctorrhea (prok″to-re′ah) a mucous discharge from the anus.

proctoscope (prok′to-skōp) a speculum or tubular instrument with illumination for inspecting the rectum.

proctoscopy (prok-tos′ko-pe) inspection of the lower part of the intestine with a proctoscope. The examination is usually done prior to rectal surgery, and it may be a part of the physical examination of a patient with hemorrhoids, rectal bleeding, or other symptoms of a rectal disorder.

PATIENT CARE. Before the examination, the lower bowel is cleansed so that visualization of the rectal mucosa will be possible. Cleansing is done by enema or insertion of a rectal suppository or both. If the patient has an extremely irritated bowel, this preparation may be omitted. Cathartics are not given as they tend to cause collection of liquid stool in the area being examined. The patient is instructed to eat a light meal the evening before proctoscopy is scheduled, and breakfast is omitted or limited to liquids.

For the examination the patient is placed in knee-chest position and draped so that the rectal orifice is exposed. If the patient cannot maintain this position, the physician may allow him to lie on his side in Sims' position. The proctoscope is lubricated before insertion. Although the procedure may be uncomfortable and tiring for the patient there should be no pain beyond mild abdominal cramps, associated with proctoscopy.

After the examination is completed the patient should be allowed to rest before returning to his home or hospital room.

proctosigmoidectomy (prok″to-sig″moi-dek′to-me) excision of the rectum and sigmoid colon; rectosigmoidectomy.

proctosigmoiditis (prok″to-sig″moi-di′tis) inflammation of the rectum and sigmoid colon.

proctosigmoidoscopy (prok″to-sig″moi-dos′ko-pe) examination of the rectum and sigmoid colon with the sigmoidoscope.

proctospasm (prok′to-spazm) spasm of the rectum.

proctostenosis (prok″to-stĕ-no′sis) stricture of the rectum.

proctostomy (prok-tos′to-me) surgical creation of a permanent artificial opening from the body surface into the rectum.

proctotomy (prok-tot′o-me) incision of the rectum, usually for anal or rectal stricture.

proctovalvotomy (prok″to-val-vot′o-me) incision of the rectal valves.

procumbent (pro-kum′bent) prone; lying on the face.

procursive (pro-ker′siv) tending to run forward.

procyclidine (pro-si′klĭ-dēn) a skeletal muscle relaxant used as the hydrochloride salt in the treatment of parkinsonism.

prodrome (pro′drōm) a premonitory symptom; a symptom indicating the onset of a disease. adj., **prodro′mal, prodro′mic.**

productive (pro-duk′tiv) producing or forming; said especially of an inflammation that produces new tissue or of a cough that brings forth sputum or mucus.

proencephalus (pro″en-sef″ah-lus) a fetus with a protrusion of the brain through a frontal fissure.

proenzyme (pro-en′zīm) zymogen; an inactive precursor of an enzyme.

proerythroblast (pro″ĕ-rith′ro-blast) pronormoblast.

proestrus (pro-es′trus) the period of heightened follicular activity preceding estrus.

profadol (pro′fah-dōl) a non-narcotic analgesic.

profenamine (pro-fen′ah-mēn) ethopropazine, an antiparkinsonian agent.

Professional Standards Review Organization (PSRO) an organization established to monitor health care services paid for through Medicare, Medicaid, and Maternal and Child Health programs to assure that services provided are medically necessary, meet professional standards, and are provided in the most economic medically appropriate health care agency or institution.

The PSRO's are an outcome of the Social Security Amendment of 1972 (Public Law 92-603) which requires the setting up of PSRO's to monitor health care services paid for, wholly or in part, under provisions of the Social Security Act.

The procedures for establishing and maintaining a PSRO are described in the *PSRO Program Manual*, issued by the Department of Health, Education and Welfare. The three major mechanisms as cited in the manual are: "(a) concurrent admission certification and continued care review, (b) medical care evaluation studies, and (c) analysis of hospital, practitioner, and patient profiles." Final decisions regarding the professional conduct of physicians must, by law, be made only by licensed physicians.

The PSRO's serve specific geographic areas and each PSRO develops or selects its own norms of care, diagnosis, and treatment. The norms are based on typical patterns of practice in the area being served, including typical lengths of stay for institutional care by age and diagnosis.

profibrinolysin (pro-fi″brĭ-nol′ĭ-sin) plasminogen, the precursor of fibrinolysin.

profile (pro′fīl) a simple outline, as of the side view of the head or face; by extension, a graph representing quantitatively a set of characteristics determined by tests.

proflavine (pro-fla′vin) a constituent of acriflavine, $C_{13}H_{11}N_3$, used as a topical and urinary antiseptic in the form of the hemisulfate salt.

profundus (pro-fun′dus) [L.] deep.

progastrin (pro-gas′trin) an inactive precursor of gastrin.

progeria (pro-je′re-ah) premature old age, a condition occurring in childhood marked by small stature, absence of facial and pubic hair, wrinkled skin, gray hair, and eventual development of atherosclerosis.

progestational (pro″jes-ta′shun-al) preceding gestation; referring to changes in the endometrium preparatory to implantation of the developing ovum should fertilization occur.

p. agent, a group of hormones secreted by the corpus luteum and placenta and, in small amounts, by the adrenal cortex, including progesterone, Δ^4-3-ketopregnen-20(α)-ol, and Δ^4-3-ketopregnene-20(β)-ol; agents having progestational activity are also produced synthetically.

p. hormones, substances, including PROGESTERONE, that are concerned mainly with preparing the endometrium for nidation of the fertilized ovum if conception has occurred.

progesterone (pro-jes′tĕ-rōn) a steroid with progestational activity, isolated from human ovaries, adrenal cortex, and placenta. A synthetic preparation is used in the treatment of functional uterine bleeding, menstrual cycle abnormalities, and threatened abortion.

Progesterone plays a major part in the menstrual cycle. During the maturation of the ovum, estrogen, the principal female sex hormone, is produced at a high rate. At ovulation estrogen production is sharply reduced, and the ovary then creates within itself a special endocrine structure called the corpus luteum whose sole function is to produce progesterone. Unless fertilization takes place, the corpus luteum disappears when it has performed its function.

The progesterone produced by the corpus luteum is promptly carried by the blood to the uterus, as was the estrogen that preceded it. Both hormones now work to prepare the uterus for possible conception.

In pregnancy, progesterone acts in a way that protects the embryo and fosters growth of the placenta. By decreasing the frequency of uterine contractions it helps to prevent expulsion of the implanted ovum. It also promotes secretory changes in the mucosa of the uterine tubes, thereby helping to provide nutrition for the fertilized ovum as it travels through the tube on its way to the uterus.

Another function of progesterone is promotion of the development of the mammary glands in preparation for lactation. Lactogenic hormone, from the anterior lobe of the PITUITARY GLAND, stimulates production of the milk, and progesterone prepares the glands for secretion.

Progesterone also has an indirect effect on the fluid and electrolyte balance of the body by blocking the effect of aldosterone.

Diminished secretion of progesterone can lead to menstrual difficulties in nonpregnant women and spontaneous abortion in pregnant women.

progestin (pro-jes′tin) originally, the crude hormone of the corpus luteum; it has since been isolated in pure form and is now known as PROGESTERONE. Certain synthetic and natural progestational agents are called progestins.

progestogen (pro-jes′to-jen) any substance having progestational activity.

proglossis (pro-glos′is) the tip of the tongue.

proglottid, proglottis (pro-glot′id; pro-glot′is) one of the segments making up the body of a tapeworm (see also STROBILA).

prognathism (prog′nah-thizm) abnormal protrusion of one or both jaws, especially the lower jaw, the gnathic index being above 103. adj., **prognath′ic, prog′nathous.**

prognathous (prog′nah-thus, prog-na′thus) having projecting jaws.

prognose (prog-nōs) to give a prognosis.

prognosis (prog-no′sis) a forecast of the probable course and outcome of a disorder. adj., **prognos′tic.**

progranulocyte (pro-gran′u-lo-sīt″) promyelocyte.

progravid (pro-grav′id) denoting the phase of the endometrium in which it is prepared for pregnancy.

progressive (pro-gres′iv) advancing; increasing in scope or severity.

proguanil (pro-gwan′il) an antimalarial effective against *Plasmodium falciparum;* used as the hydrochloride salt.

Progynon (pro-jin′on) trademark for preparations of estradiol, an estrogen.

proinsulin (pro-in′su-lin) a precursor of insulin, having low biologic activity.

projection (pro-jek′shun) 1. a throwing forward, especially the reference of impressions made on the sense organs to their proper source, so as to locate correctly the objects producing them. 2. a connection between the cerebral cortex and other parts of the nervous system or organs of special sense. 3. the act of extending or jutting out, or a part that juts out. 4. a mental mechanism whereby emotionally unacceptable traits are denied by a person as his own and regarded (projected) as belonging to the external world or to someone else. It is often called the "blaming" mechanism because in using it one seeks to place the blame for his inadequacies upon someone else. In its extreme form projection can lead to hostility and physical attack upon others when the person mistakenly perceives these persons as responsible for his mental anguish.

prokaryon (pro-kar′e-on) 1. nuclear material scattered in the cytoplasm of the cell, rather than bounded by a nuclear membrane; found in some unicellular organisms, such as bacteria. 2. prokaryote.

prokaryote (pro-kar′e-ōt) an organism without a true nucleus, the nuclear material being scattered in the cytoplasm of the cell, and which reproduces by cell division.

prolabium (pro-la′be-um) the prominent central part of the upper lip.

prolactin (pro-lak′tin) a hormone secreted by the anterior pituitary that promotes the growth of breast tissue and stimulates and sustains milk production in postpartum mammals, and shows luteotropic activity in certain mammals; called also lactogenic hormone, luteotropic hormone, LTH, and mammotropin. It is identical with luteotropin.

prolamine (pro-lam′in) any of a class of simple proteins insoluble in water and absolute alcohol, but soluble in 70 to 80 per cent ethyl alcohol; obtained principally from cereal seeds.

prolapse (pro′laps) 1. the falling down, or downward displacement, of a part or viscus. 2. to undergo such displacement.

p. of cord, protrusion of the umbilical cord ahead of the presenting part of the fetus in labor.

p. of the iris, protrusion of the iris through a wound in the cornea.

rectal p., p. of rectum, protrusion of the rectal mucous membrane through the anus.

p. of uterus, downward displacement of the uterus

so that the cervix is within the vaginal orifice (first-degree prolapse), the cervix is outside the orifice (second-degree prolapse), or the entire uterus is outside the orifice (third-degree prolapse).

prolapsus (pro-lap′sus) [L.] prolapse.

prolepsis (pro-lep′sis) recurrence of a paroxysm before the expected time. adj., **prolep′tic.**

prolidase (pro′lĭ-dās) an enzyme that catalyzes the hydrolysis of the imide bond between an α-carboxyl group and proline or hydroxyproline.

proliferation (pro-lif″ĕ-ra′shun) the reproduction or multiplication of similar forms, especially of cells. adj., **prolif′erative, prolif′erous.**

proligerous (pro-lij′er-us) producing offspring.

prolinase (pro′lĭ-nās) an enzyme that catalyzes the hydrolysis of dipeptides containing proline or hydroxyproline as N-terminal groups.

proline (pro′lēn) a naturally occurring amino acid.

Prolixin (pro-lik′sin) trademark for preparations of fluphenazine, a major tranquilizer.

Proluton (pro-lu′ton) trademark for preparations of progesterone.

prolymphocyte (pro-lim′fo-sīt) a cell of the lymphocytic series intermediate between the lymphoblast and lymphocyte.

promastigote (pro-mas′tĭ-gōt) the morphologic stage in the development of certain protozoa, characterized by a free anterior flagellum and resembling the typical adult form of *Leptomonas.*

promazine (pro′mah-zēn) a phenothiazine derivative used as a major tranquilizer in the form of the hydrochloride salt.

promegakaryocyte (pro″meg-ah-kar′e-o-sīt″) a developmental form of the platelet-producing megakaryocyte series, intermediate between the megakaryoblast and the megakaryocyte.

promegaloblast (pro-meg′ah-lo-blast″) the earliest form in the abnormal erythrocyte maturation sequence occurring in vitamin B_{12} and folic acid deficiencies; it corresponds to the pronormoblast, and develops into a megaloblast.

promethazine (pro-meth′ah-zēn) a phenothiazine derivative used as an antihistaminic, antiemetic, and tranquilizer in the form of the hydrochloride salt.

promethestrol (pro-meth′es-trol) a synthetic estrogenic agent; used as the dipropionate ester.

promethium (pro-me′the-um) a chemical element, atomic number 61, atomic weight 147, symbol Pm. (See table of ELEMENTS.)

Promin (pro′min) trademark for a preparation of glucosulfone, a leprostatic and tuberculostatic.

promine (pro′mēn) a substance widely distributed in animal cells, characterized by its ability to promote cell division and growth.

prominence (prom′ĭ-nens) a protrusion or projection.

promonocyte (pro-mon′o-sīt) a cell of the monocytic series intermediate between the monoblast and monocyte, with coarse chromatin structure and one or two nucleoli.

promontory (prom′on-tor″e) a projecting process or eminence.

promoxolane (pro-mok′so-lān) a skeletal muscle relaxant and tranquilizer.

promyelocyte (pro-mi′ĕ-lo-sīt″) a precursor of the granular leukocytes, intermediate between myeloblast and myelocyte, containing a few, as yet undifferentiated, cytoplasmic granules.

pronate (pro′nāt) to subject to pronation.

pronation (pro-na′shun) the act of assuming the prone position, or the state of being prone. Applied to the hand, turning the palm backward (posteriorly) or downward, performed by medial rotation of the forearm. Applied to the foot, a combination of eversion and abduction movements taking place in the tarsal and metatarsal joints and resulting in lowering of the medial margin of the foot, hence of the longitudinal arch.

pronator (pro-na′tor) a muscle that pronates.

prone (prōn) lying face downward, or on the ventral surface.

pronephros (pro-nef′ros), pl. *proneph′roi* [Gr.] the primordial kidney; an excretory structure or its rudiments developing in the embryo before the mesonephros; its duct is later used by the mesonephros, which arises caudal to it.

Pronestyl (pro-nes′til) trademark for preparations of procainamide, a cardiac depressant.

pronormoblast (pro-nor′mo-blast) the earliest erythrocyte precursor, having a relatively large nucleus containing several nucleoli, surrounded by a small amount of cytoplasm (see also NORMOBLAST). Called also proerythroblast and rubriblast.

pronucleus (pro-nu′kle-us) the haploid nucleus of a sex cell.

female p., the haploid nucleus of the fully mature ovum which loses its nuclear envelope and liberates its chromosomes to meet the synapsis with those from the male pronucleus.

male p., the nuclear material of the head of a spermatozoon, after it has penetrated the ovum and acquired a pronuclear membrane.

prootic (pro-ot′ik) in front of the ear.

Propadrine (pro′pah-drēn) trademark for a preparation of phenylpropanolamine, a nasal and sinus decongestant.

propagation (prop″ah-ga′shun) reproduction. adj., **prop′agative.**

propane (pro′pān) a gaseous hydrocarbon from petroleum and natural gas.

propantheline (pro-pan′thĕ-lēn) an anticholinergic used as the bromide salt, especially in the treatment of peptic ulcer.

proparacaine (pro-par′ah-kān) a topical anesthetic used as the hydrochloride salt.

propepsin (pro-pep′sin) pepsinogen; the inactive precursor of pepsin.

properdin (pro′per-din) a relatively heat-labile, normal serum protein (a euglobulin) that, in the presence of COMPLEMENT component C3 and magnesium ions, acts nonspecifically against gram-negative bacteria and viruses and plays a role in lysis of erythrocytes. It migrates as a beta-globulin, and although not an antibody, may act in conjunction with complement-fixing ANTIBODY.

prophage (pro′fāj) the latent stage of a BACTERIOPHAGE in a LYSOGENIC BACTERIUM, in which the viral GENOME becomes inserted into a specific portion of the host chromosome and is duplicated into each cell generation.

prophase (pro′fāz) the first stage of cell replication in either meiosis or mitosis.

prophenpyridamine (pro″fen-pi-rid′ah-mēn) pheniramine, an antihistaminic.

prophylactic (pro″fĭ-lak′tik) 1. tending to ward off disease; pertaining to prophylaxis. 2. an agent that tends to ward off disease.

prophylaxis (pro″fĭ-lak′sis) prevention of disease; preventive treatment.

propiolactone (pro″pe-o-lak′tōn) a disinfectant.

propiomazine (pro″pe-o-ma′zēn) a phenothiazine derivative used as a tranquilizer in the form of the hydrochloride salt.

propionic acid (pro″pe-on′ik) $CH_3CH_2 \cdot COOH$, found in chyme and sweat, and one of the products of bacterial fermentation of wood pulp waste; its salts (calcium and sodium propionate) are used as local antifungals, and to inhibit mold growth in bakery and dairy products.

proplasmacyte (pro-plaz′mah-sīt) a cell intermediate between the plasmablast and the plasmacyte (plasma cell).

proplastid (pro-plas′tid) an organelle that develops into a plastid as the cell matures.

proplexus (pro-plek′sus) the choroid plexus of the lateral ventricle of the brain.

propositus (pro-poz′ĭ-tus), pl. *propos′iti* [L.] the original person presenting a mental or physical disorder who serves as the basis for a hereditary or genetic study; called also proband.

propoxycaine (pro-pok′se-kān) a local anesthetic, used as the hydrochloride salt.

propoxyphene (pro-pok′se-fēn) an analgesic used as the hydrochloride and napsylate salts. Called also dextropropoxyphene.

propranolol (pro-pran′o-lōl) a β-adrenergic blocking agent used in the treatment of cardiac arrhythmias and hypertrophic subaortic stenosis.

proprietary medicine (pro-pri′ĕ-ter″e) any chemical, drug, or similar preparation used in the treatment of diseases, if such article is protected against free competition as to name, product, composition, or process of manufacture by secrecy, patent, trademark, or copyright, or by other means.

proprioceptor (pro″pre-o-sep′tor) any of the sensory nerve endings that give information concerning movements and position of the body; they occur chiefly in muscles, tendons, and the labyrinth. adj., **propriocep′tive.**

proptometer (pro-tom′ĕ-ter) an instrument for measuring the degree of exophthalmos.

proptosis (prop-to′sis) forward displacement or bulging, especially of the eye.

propulsion (pro-pul′shun) 1. a tendency to fall forward in walking. 2. festination.

propyl (pro′pil) the univalent radical CH_3CH_2-CH_2— from propane.

propylene (pro′pĭ-lēn) a gaseous hydrocarbon having anesthetic properties.

p. glycol, a colorless, viscous liquid, used as a substitute for glycerin.

propylhexedrine (pro″pil-hek′sĕ-drēn) an adrenergic given by inhalation to decongest nasal mucosa.

propyliodone (pro″pil-i′o-dōn) a radiopaque medium used in bronchography.

propylparaben (pro″pil-par′ah-ben) used as an antifungal preservative.

propylthiouracil (pro″pil-thi″o-u′rah-sil) a thyroid inhibitor.

pro re nata (pro ra nah′tah) [L.] according to circumstances; abbreviated p.r.n.

prorennin (pro-ren′in) the zymogen (proenzyme) in the gastric glands that is converted to rennin.

prorubricyte (pro-roo′brĭ-sīt) basophilic normoblast.

pros(o)- word element [Gr.], *forward; anterior.*

proscillaridin A (pro″sil-ar′ĭ-din) a cardiac glycoside used as a cardiotonic.

prosecretin (pro″se-kre′tin) the precursor of secretin.

prosection (pro-sek′shun) carefully programmed dissection for demonstration of anatomic structure.

prosector (pro-sek′tor) one who performs prosection.

prosencephalon (pros″en-sef′ah-lon) the forebrain.

prosodemic (pros″o-dem′ik) passing directly from one person to another instead of reaching a large number at once, through such means as water supply: said of a disease progressing in that way.

prosop(o)- word element [Gr.], *face.*

prosopagnosia (pros″o-pag-no′se-ah) inability to recognize the faces of other people or one's own features in a mirror.

prosopalgia (pros″o-pal′je-ah) trigeminal neuralgia (TIC DOULOUREUX). adj., **prosopal′gic.**

prosopectasia (pros″o-pek-ta′ze-ah) oversize of the face.

prosoplasia (pros″o-pla′ze-ah) 1. abnormal differentiation of tissue. 2. development into a higher state of organization or function.

prosopodiplegia (pros″o-po-di-ple′je-ah) paralysis of the face and one lower extremity.

prosoponeuralgia (pros″o-po-nu-ral′je-ah) facial neuralgia.

prosopoplegia (pros″o-po-ple′je-ah) facial paralysis. adj., **prosopople′gic.**

prosoposchisis (pros″o-pos′kĭ-sis) congenital fissure of the face.

prosopospasm (pros′o-po-spazm″) spasm of the facial muscles.

prosoposternodymia (pros″o-po-ster″no-dim′e-ah) a double monster joined face to face and sternum to sternum.

prosopothoracopagus (pros″o-po-tho″rah-kop′ah-gus) twin fetuses fused from the face to the thorax.

prostaglandin (pros″tah-glan′din) a group of naturally occurring, chemically related, long-chain hydroxy fatty acids that stimulate contractility of the uterine and other smooth muscle tissues and have the ability to lower blood pressure and to affect the action of certain hormones. First found in semen, they have since been found in cells throughout the body and in menstrual fluid. There are four types, F, E, A, and B, the degree of saturation of the side chain of each being designated by subscripts 1, 2, and 3.

Prostaglandin injections into the amniotic sac, an in-hospital procedure, have been used as an ABORTION technique in pregnancies after the 16th week. About 30 minutes after an injection of prostaglandin F_2, contractions begin, and abortion takes place within 19–20 hours.

prostatalgia (pros″tah-tal′je-ah) pain in the prostate.

prostate (pros′tāt) an accessory reproductive organ in the male, located next to and under the bladder and completely surrounding the urethra. It is about the size of a walnut and consists of a median and two lateral lobes. adj., **prostat′ic.**

The prostate secretes a thin, slightly alkaline fluid that flows through ducts into the urethra. This fluid is secreted continuously, and the excess passes from the body in the urine. The rate of secretion increases greatly during sexual stimulation and the fluid contributes to the bulk of the semen.

DISORDERS OF THE PROSTATE. Enlargement of the prostate (benign prostatic hypertrophy) is a common complaint in men over 50 years of age. Because of its position around the urethra, enlargement of the prostate quickly interferes with the normal passage of urine from the bladder. Urination becomes increasingly difficult, and the bladder never feels completely emptied. If left untreated, continued enlargement of the prostate eventually obstructs the bladder completely, and emergency measures become necessary to empty the bladder. If the prostate is markedly enlarged, chronic constipation may result. The usual remedy is PROSTATECTOMY.

In men over 60 years of age, cancer of the prostate may occur. The symptoms are similar to those of prostatic enlargement. If the malignancy is discovered in time, the gland can be removed before the cancer has a chance to spread. Symptoms of cancer of the prostate usually respond to estrogens or to orchiectomy.

Inflammation of the prostate (prostatitis) usually responds to antimicrobial therapy; if it does not, a prostatic abscess may form, which can be incised and drained surgically.

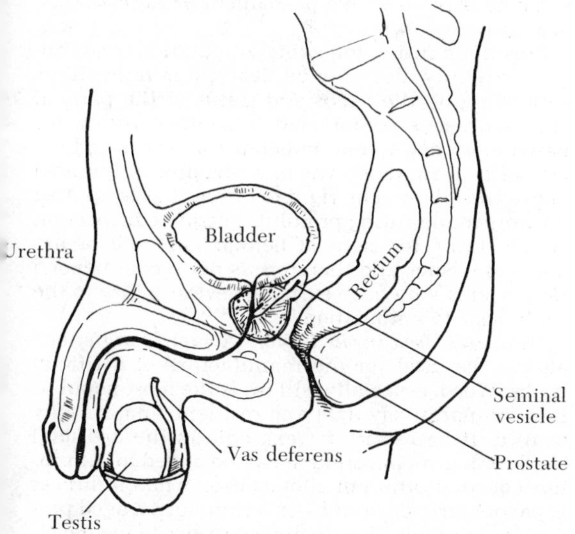

Prostate.

prostatectomy (pros″tah-tek′to-me) excision of all or part of the prostate. There are several alternate methods of performing this surgical procedure. In suprapubic prostatectomy the gland is removed through an abdominal incision. The bladder is also incised and the gland is removed from above. This procedure is preferred when the prostate is greatly enlarged. In perineal prostatectomy an incision is made into the perineum and the gland is removed from below. Disadvantages of this method include frequent contamination of the wound and the likelihood of incontinence and rectal injury as complications. The most popular and least traumatic method of removal of an enlarged prostate is transurethral resection. A surgical incision is not involved since the surgeon approaches the prostate via the urethra, using a cystoscope and removing small pieces of obstructing gland tissue with an electric wire.

PATIENT CARE. Preoperatively the patient must be watched for signs of urinary retention and bladder distention. An indwelling catheter is often inserted to prevent this difficulty; if so, its purpose should be explained to the patient. Care must be used in the administration of sedatives and hypnotics since many of these patients are elderly and are likely to suffer from mental confusion and other adverse effects from drugs of this type. It may be necessary to use side rails on the bed, especially at night, to prevent accidents and injury to the patient.

Immediately after surgery the patient is observed for signs of hemorrhage, a primary danger of prostatectomy. Though the urinary drainage can be expected to be bright red for the first 24 hours after surgery, excessive bleeding must be reported immediately. An increasingly darker color may indicate an increase in blood content in the drainage.

In addition, special attention is given the catheter leading from the bladder to insure adequate drainage at all times. Severe pain in the bladder region may indicate obstruction of the catheter by blood clots or bits of tissue. Irrigations, when done to remove the obstruction, demand strict aseptic technique to avoid the introduction of infectious microorganisms into the urinary tract and the surgical wound. Severe abdominal pain and rigidity may indicate perforation of the bladder.

The surgical wound of a suprapubic prostatectomy demands frequent attention since the bladder has been incised and there is almost constant drainage of urine onto the surgical dressings. Frequent changing of these dressings is necessary to prevent irritation of the surrounding skin and the development of unpleasant odors. Infection is a particular hazard in both suprapubic and perineal prostatectomy patients.

prostatism (pros′tah-tizm) the signs and symptoms associated with prostatic lesions that produce malfunction of the urinary tract.

prostatitis (pros″tah-ti′tis) inflammation of the prostate. adj., **prostatit′ic.**

prostatocystitis (pros″tah-to-sis-ti′tis) inflammation of the neck of the bladder (prostatic urethra) and the bladder cavity.

prostatocystotomy (pros″tah-to-sis″tot′o-me) incision of the bladder and prostate.

prostatodynia (pros″tah-to-din′e-ah) pain in the prostate.

prostatolith (pros-tat′o-lith) a calculus in the prostate.

prostatolithotomy (pros″tah-to-lĭ-thot′o-me) incision of the prostate for removal of a calculus.

prostatomegaly (pros″tah-to-meg′ah-le) hypertrophy of the prostate.

prostatorrhea (pros″tah-to-re′ah) catarrhal discharge from the prostate.

prostatotomy (pros″tah-tot′o-me) surgical incision of the prostate.

prostatovesiculectomy (pros″tah-to-vĕ-sik″u-lek′to-me) excision of the prostate and seminal vesicles.

prostatovesiculitis (pros″tah-to-vĕ-sik″u-li′tis) inflammation of the prostate and seminal vesicles.

prosthesis (pros′thĕ-sis, pros-the′sis), pl. *prosthe′ses* [Gr.] 1. the replacement of an absent part by an artifical substitute. 2. an artificial substitute for a missing part, such as an eye, leg, or tooth, used for functional or cosmetic reasons, or both.

ARTIFICIAL LIMB. Recent advances in the field of surgical amputation and the art of designing artificial limbs have made it possible for a person who has lost a limb to be equipped with a prosthesis that functions so efficiently, and so closely resembles the original in appearance, that he is able to resume normal activities with his handicap passing virtually unnoticed.

Fitting an Artificial Limb. Since the early 1960's, when immediate fitting of a lower limb was first introduced in France, surgeons throughout the world have had two alternatives for the fitting of a prosthesis: *immediate* fitting and *delayed* fitting. Prior to this time there was extensive preparation of the stump, sometimes lasting from three months to a year, involving stump wrapping and conditioning. During this process severe orthopedic complications frequently developed and the mental attitude of the patient often was so negatively affected as to make rehabilitation difficult if not impossible.

Today the patient may be fitted with a prosthesis immediately after the limb is removed and before he leaves the operating room. He awakens from anesthesia to find the stump encased in a rigid dressing similar to a cast and designed to accommodate a temporary prosthesis. With this device he can begin ambulation the first postoperative day and avoid many of the complications connected with inactivity. Not all patients can begin ambulation this early, however, and not all amputees are good candidates for immediate fitting of a prosthesis. Another disadvantage to immediate fitting is the hazard of wound disruption and skin breakdown, and slippage of the rigid dressing from the stump. This latter situation can cause rapid development of edema of the stump, with resultant stress on the suture line and disruption of the wound.

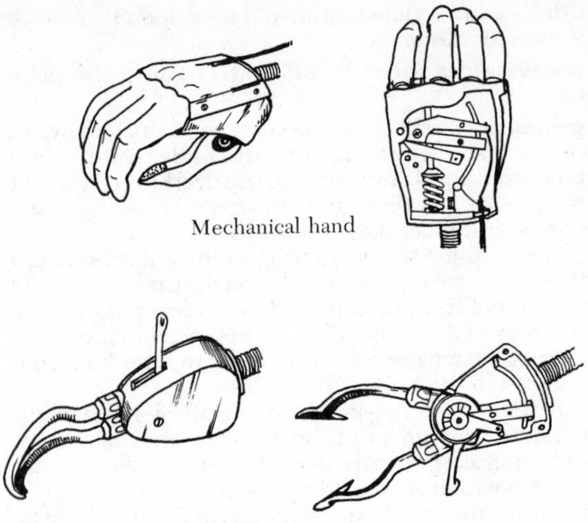

Artificial hands. The hook is the more efficient, but the mechanical hand, sometimes covered by a glove, provides both cosmetic value and utility.

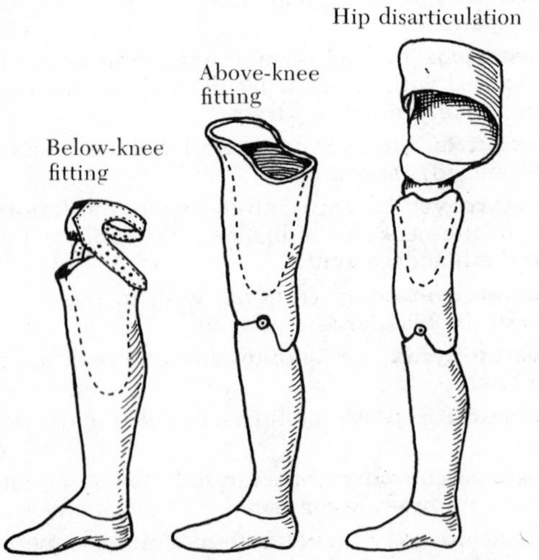

Artificial legs.

Delayed fitting involves conventional wrapping of the stump and delay in using a temporary prosthesis until the 2nd or 3rd week after surgery, when the stump has healed sufficiently to allow partial weight-bearing. By the 6th week, if all goes well, the patient begins full weight-bearing and by the 10th week he is fitted with a permanent prosthesis. (See also AMPUTATION.)

Prosthetic fitting following amputation of an upper extremity also may be delayed or immediate, depending on the needs and status of the patient. Some surgeons recommend immediate fitting for patients with amputation below the elbow and delayed fitting for those who have the limb amputated above the elbow. The rigid dressing that is applied for immediate fitting prohibits adequate inspection of the stump for signs of hemorrhage and breakdown of tissues and therefore is not recommended for patients who have suffered severe injury to the limb prior to amputation.

Materials Used in the Limb. A variety of materials can be used for the manufacture of artificial limbs. Wood, especially willow, is the most popular. It is comparatively light and resilient, and is easily shaped. If necessary, for example in the artificial limb for a growing child, it can be added to. Aluminum or an aluminum alloy is used when lightness is particularly desirable—in a limb for an aged person, for example. Plastic limbs are also being developed. Leather and various metals are used for reinforcement and control.

Powering the Limb. Most artificial limbs are powered by the muscles, either those remaining in the stump or other available muscles. The muscles of the stump often can be considerably strengthened by physical therapy. Muscle power can be reinforced by means of springs, straps, gears, locks, levers, or, in some cases, hydraulic mechanisms.

The Artificial Leg. The most commonly fitted artificial limb is the knee-jointed leg, used by persons whose legs have been amputated above the knee. This prosthesis is powered by the hip and remaining thigh muscles, which kick the leg forward. The key points in such a limb are the socket, where it fits onto the stump, the knee, and the ankle. The possibility of walking with a normal gait depends primarily on the successful alignment of the socket joint; the knee usually consists of a joint centered slightly behind that of the natural leg, as this has been found to afford greater stability; sometimes the ankle joint is omitted and flexibility of the ankle achieved by the use of a rubber foot.

The Artificial Arm. The choice of a particular artificial arm depends largely on the person's occupation. There is a wide variety of types, ranging from the purely functional, which will enable a person to perform heavy work, to the purely cosmetic, which aims only at looking as natural as possible. Those persons whose work requires them to do heavy lifting are often fitted with a "pegarm," a short arm without an elbow joint, which is easily controlled and has great leverage.

The Artificial Hand. There are a great many different types of artificial hands. Many artificial arms are so constructed that they can be fitted with a selection of different hands, depending on the type of work to be done. It is generally agreed by experts that the various types of hooks offer the greatest functional efficiency. These reproduce the most powerful function of natural hands—the pressure between thumb and forefinger. But there are hands that combine a certain amount of utility with cosmetic value, often by means of a cosmetic glove covering a mechanical hand; and there are also hands designed simply for appearance, though these usually offer some support as well.

Most hooks and hands are mechanically connected to the opposite shoulder and operated by a shrugging motion. However, a procedure known as kineplasty employs the person's own arm and chest muscles to work the device. In this method, selected muscles are tunneled under by surgery and lined by skin. Pegs adapted to the tunnels can then be made to move an artificial hand mechanism. Kineplasty is employed when skill rather than strength is desired.

PROTECTING THE STUMP. In a person with an artificial limb, there is always a danger that the stump will become irritated or infected. He will probably wear a sock to cover the stump, and this should be washed daily; the stump itself should also be washed regularly and carefully, particularly between skin folds. And when the artificial limb is not being used the stump should, if possible, be exposed to the fresh air.

prosthetic (pros-thet′ik) serving as a substitute; pertaining to prostheses or to prosthetics.

prosthetics (pros-thet′iks) the field of knowledge relating to prostheses, their design, use, etc.

prosthetist (pros′thĕ-tist) a person skilled in prosthetics and practicing its application.

prosthodontics (pros″tho-don′tiks) that branch of dentistry concerned with the construction of artificial appliances designed to restore and maintain oral function by replacing missing teeth and sometimes other oral structures or parts of the face.

prosthodontist (pros″tho-don′tist) a specialist in prosthodontics.

prostholith (pros′tho-lith) a preputial concretion or calculus.

Prostigmin (pro-stig′min) trademark for preparations of neostigmine, a cholinergic.

Prostin F2 Alpha (pros′tin) trademark for a preparation of dinoprost tromethamine, a prostaglandin used as an abortifacient.

prostration (pros-tra′shun) extreme exhaustion or lack of energy or power.

heat p., a condition caused by exposure to excessive heat (see also HEAT EXHAUSTION).

nervous p., neurasthenia.

protactinium (pro″tak-tin′e-um) a chemical element, atomic number 91, atomic weight 231, symbol Pa. (See table of ELEMENTS.)

protamine (pro′tah-min) any of a class of simple proteins, soluble in water, not coagulated by heat, and precipitated from aqueous solution by addition

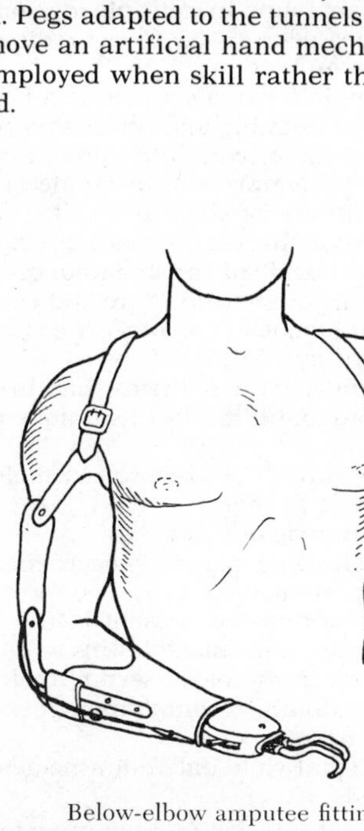

Below-elbow amputee fitting

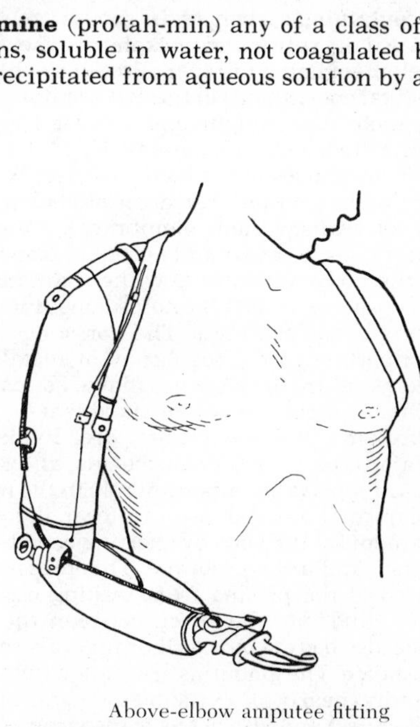

Above-elbow amputee fitting

Artificial arms. Most are mechanically controlled and are connected by straps to the opposite shoulder.

of alcohol, found combined with nucleic acids in the sperm of certain fish, and having the property of neutralizing heparin. Protamine sulfate is used as an antidote to heparin overdosage.

protanope (pro′tah-nōp) a person exhibiting protanopia.

protanopia (pro″tah-no′pe-ah) red blindness; imperfect perception of red, with confusion of reds and greens. adj., **protanop′ic.**

protean (pro′te-an) changing form or assuming different shapes.

protease (pro′te-ās) any proteolytic enzyme.

protectant, protective (pro-tek′tant; pro-tek′tiv) 1. affording defense or immunity. 2. an agent affording defense against harmful influence.

protective isolation a type of ISOLATION designed to prevent contact between potentially pathogenic microorganisms and uninfected persons who have seriously impaired resistance. Called also reverse isolation. The National Communicable Disease Center recommends protective isolation precautions for patients suffering from agranulocytosis, severe and extensive dermatitis, certain types of lymphomas and leukemias, and those who are receiving immunosuppressive therapy.

Those entering the room should wear gowns, masks, and under some circumstances, booties and caps. The hands must be washed with an antimicrobial soap or detergent and water on entering and leaving the room. Gloves are worn by all persons having direct contact with the patient. In some cases the linen is sterilized prior to use in the patient's immediate environment.

It is essential that all health care personnel, visitors, and the patient himself understand the purpose of protective isolation and the need for conscientious adherence to the precautionary rules in order to protect the patient from an infection.

protein (pro′te-in) any of a group of organic compounds containing carbon, hydrogen, oxygen, nitrogen, and usually sulfur and phosphorus, the characteristic element being nitrogen. Proteins, which are the principal constituents of the cell protoplasm, are of high molecular weight and consist largely of chains of AMINO ACIDS. adj., **protein′ic.**

Protein substances in the body are essential to its structure and function. For example, such structures as cell walls, various membranes, connective tissue, and muscles are mainly protein. None of the cells of the body can survive without an adequate supply of protein; in fact, proteins constitute about 20 per cent of the cell mass. The hormones, which are so important in the regulation of metabolism, are proteins, as are the enzymes that act as catalysts in the chemical reactions of metabolism.

The proteins in blood plasma are divided into three major types: ALBUMIN, GLOBULINS, and FIBRINOGEN. Albumin plays an important role in the maintenance of normal distribution of water in the various compartments of the body by exerting osmotic pressure at the capillary membrane. This pressure prevents fluid of the plasma from leaking out of the capillaries and into the space between the tissue cells. (See also body FLUIDS.) Albumin is also a transport substance. The globulins are vital to the process of immunity (nearly all ANTIBODIES are gamma globulin molecules) and also act as transporters of various substances from one part of the body to another. Fibrinogen is essential to the blood clotting mechanism.

Food proteins are of great nutritional importance since they are necessary for the building and repair of all kinds of body tissues, especially of muscles and organs such as the heart, liver, and kidneys. Major sources of protein are animal products such as meat, eggs, fish, and milk.

The digestion of protein foods begins in the stomach, is continued in the duodenum, and is completed in the small intestine. The end products of protein digestion, amino acids, pass into the blood, some to be used as structural proteins for the building of body tissues, others to be used as enzymes, and the rest to be carried to various parts of the body as a reserve. If a ready supply of carbohydrates is not available, some proteins may be converted into needed energy.

SYMPTOMS OF PROTEIN DEFICIENCY. Severe protein deficiency undermines general health, and is usually manifest in weakness, poor resistance, and swelling of body tissues (nutritional edema) due to accumulation of fluid in the tissue spaces. Protein starvation can result from lack of protein in the diet—in persons who, from lack of available supplies of protein foods or through ignorance, satisfy their hunger with large amounts of carbohydrates and little else. Kwashiorkor is a disorder of infants and young children whose diet is deficient in protein. The illness develops soon after weaning when the child no longer receives a protein supply from his mother's milk.

Sometimes deficiency develops when digestive disorders or infections interfere with proper digestion. A congenital defect in metabolism such as PHENYLKETONURIA may lead to inability to make proper use of the protein that is available in the diet.

The first step in treatment of protein deficiency is correction of the deficiency in the diet. If the protein deficiency is secondary to another disorder, treatment is aimed at relief of the primary cause of the deficiency.

Bence Jones p., a low-molecular weight, heat-sensitive urinary protein found in multiple myeloma; it coagulates when heated to 45°–55° C. and redissolves partially or wholly on boiling.

carrier p., one which, when coupled to a hapten, renders it capable of eliciting an immune response.

conjugated p's, those in which the protein molecule is united with nonprotein molecule(s) (the prosthetic group) otherwise than as a salt.

C-reactive p., a globulin that forms a precipitate with the C-polysaccharide of the pneumonococcus; its demonstration in the serum is an indicator of inflammation of infectious or noninfectious origin (see also C-REACTIVE PROTEIN).

denatured p., one whose structure has been so changed, as by heat, that it has lost its unique properties.

derived p's, derivatives of the protein molecule formed by hydrolytic changes.

immune p's, immunoglobulins.

native p., an unchanged, naturally occurring animal or vegetable protein.

plasma p's, all the proteins present in the blood plasma, including the immunoglobulins.

serum p., proteins in the blood serum, including immunoglobulins, albumin, complement, coagulation factors, and enzymes.

simple p's, those that yield only α-amino acids on complete hydrolysis.

proteinaceous (pro″te-in-a′shus) pertaining to or of the nature of protein.

proteinase (pro'te-in-ās") any enzyme that catalyzes the splitting of interior peptide bonds in a protein; an endopeptidase.

protein-bound iodine test PBI; a laboratory test done to determine thyroid function by measuring the amount of iodine precipitated with plasma proteins. The hormone thyroxine contains iodine which is bound to blood proteins (protein-bound). Thus measurement of the amount of protein-bound iodine in the blood aids in determining the thyroid's production of thyroxine. Most normal values fall in the range of 4 to 6 mcg. per 100 ml. of blood; however, the spectrum of normality is wide (3.5 to 8 mcg. per 100 ml.) so that the PBI test is limited in borderline cases. A decreased PBI indicates HYPOTHYROIDISM, an increased PBI indicates HYPERTHYROIDISM.

Many factors can alter the outcome of this test, and it is most reliable in patients with normal thyroid function. In spite of its drawbacks, the PBI is still considered useful in the total picture of diagnostic tests for thyroid dysfunction.

Preparation for the test is minimal; neither restriction of intake of foods or fluids nor limitation of physical activity is required. Because seafoods contain iodine, it is recommended that these not be eaten by the patient several weeks prior to the test. It is also important that the patient not receive iodine in any artificial form, as in dyes used for x-ray studies, prescribed medications, cough syrups, gargles, or other patent medicines. Estrogens and contraceptive pills and mercurials also must be withheld because they cause an abnormally high reading.

proteinemia (pro"te-ĭ-ne'me-ah) excess of protein in the blood.

proteinosis (pro"te-ĭ-no'sis) the accumulation of excess protein in the tissues.

lipid p., a hereditary defect of lipid metabolism marked by yellowish deposits of hyaline lipid carbohydrate mixture on the inner surface of the lips, under the tongue, on the oropharynx and larynx, and skin lesions.

pulmonary alveolar p., a chronic lung disease in which the distal alveoli become filled with a bland, eosinophilic, probably endogenous proteinaceous material that prevents ventilation of affected areas.

proteinuria (pro"te-ĭ-nu're-ah) an excess of serum proteins ih the urine.

proteolipid (pro"te-o-lip'id) a combination of a peptide or protein with a lipid, having the solubility characteristics of lipids.

proteolysis (pro"te-ol'ĭ-sis) the splitting of proteins by hydrolysis of the peptide bonds, with formation of smaller polypeptides.

proteolytic (pro"te-o-lit'ik) 1. pertaining to, characterized by, or promoting proteolysis. 2. a proteolytic enzyme.

proteometabolism (pro"te-o-mĕ-tab'o-lizm) the metabolism of protein.

proteopeptic (pro"te-o-pep'tik) digesting protein.

proteose (pro'te-ōs) any of a group of derived proteins intermediate between native proteins and peptones.

proteosuria (pro"te-o-su're-ah) the presence of proteose in the urine.

Proteus (pro'te-us) a genus of gram-negative, motile bacteria usually found in fecal and other putrefying matter, including *P. morga'ni,* found in the intestines and associated with summer diarrhea of infants, and *P. vulga'ris,* often found as a secondary invader in various localized suppurative pathologic processes; it is a cause of cystitis.

prothipendyl (pro-thi'pen-dil) a tranquilizer and sedative.

prothrombin (pro-throm'bin) a glycoprotein present in the plasma that is converted into thrombin by extrinsic thromboplastin during the second stage of blood CLOTTING; called also clotting factor II.

p. consumption, a clinical laboratory test done to determine thromboplastin generating capacity, which provides information about the first stage of coagulation. When clotting of a normal blood sample occurs, prothrombin is converted to thrombin, thus there should be little or no prothrombin in the serum after the clot is formed. If, however, there is deficiency of blood coagulation, some of the prothrombin will not be utilized (consumed). Abnormal results of the test are found in deficiencies of the first-stage factors of coagulation (factors VIII and IX), and in the presence of circulating anticoagulants, thrombocytopenia, and any other condition leading to inadequate generation of thromboplastin.

p. time, a test to measure the activity of clotting factors V, VII, and X, prothrombin, and fibrinogen; abbreviation Pro time or PT. Deficiency of any of these factors leads to a prolongation of the one-stage prothrombin times, as will circulating anticoagulants that are active against factors V, VII, or against thromboplastin.

The test is considered basic to any study of the coagulation process and is also widely used for guidance in establishing and maintaining anticoagulant therapy. Test results are best understood when both the patient's and the control times are reported. The therapeutic range for coagulation therapy is usually 2 to 3 times that of the normal (12 to 15 sec.) control.

prothrombinase (pro-throm'bin-ās) thromboplastin.

prothrombinogenic (pro-throm"bĭ-no-jen'ik) promoting the production of prothrombin.

protist (pro'tist) any member of the Protista.

Protista (pro-tis'tah) a kingdom comprising bacteria, algae, slime molds, fungi, and protozoa; it includes all single-celled organisms.

protistology (pro"tis-tol'o-je) microbiology.

protium (pro'te-um) the mass 1 isotope of hydrogen, symbol ^{1}H; ordinary, or light, hydrogen.

proto- word element [Gr.], *first.*

protoblast (pro'to-blast) 1. a cell with no cell wall; an embryonic cell. 2. the nucleus of an ovum. 3. a blastomere from which a particular organ or part develops. adj., **protoblas'tic.**

protocol (pro'to-kol) the original notes made on a necropsy, an experiment, or on a case of disease.

protodiastolic (pro"to-di"ah-stol'ik) pertaining to early diastole, i.e., immediately following the second heart sound.

protoduodenum (pro"to-du"o-de'num) the first or proximal portion of the duodenum, extending from the pylorus to the duodenal papilla.

protofibril (pro"to-fi'bril) the first elongated unit appearing in formation of any type of fiber.

protogaster (pro"to-gas'ter) archenteron.

protokylol (pro"to-ki'lol) a sympathomimetic used as a bronchodilator in the form of the hydrochloride salt.

proton (pro′ton) an elementary particle of mass number 1, with a positive charge equal to the negative charge of the electron; a constituent particle of every nucleus, the number of protons in the nucleus of each ATOM of a chemical element being indicated by its atomic number.

protoneuron (pro″to-nu′ron) the first neuron in a peripheral reflex arc.

protoplasm (pro′to-plazm) the viscid, translucent colloid material, the essential constituent of the living cell, including cytoplasm and nucleoplasm. adj., **protoplas′mic.**

protoplast (pro′to-plast) a bacterial or plant cell deprived of its rigid wall but with its plasma membrane intact; the cell is dependent for its integrity on an isotonic or hypertonic medium.

protoporphyria (pro″to-por-fēr′e-ah) porphyria marked by excessive protoporphyrin in erythrocytes, plasma, and feces, and by intense itching, erythema, and edema on short exposure to sunlight; skin lesions usually fade without scarring or pigmentation but a chronic weatherbeaten appearance is characteristic. Called also erythropoietic protoporphyria.

protoporphyrin (pro″to-por′fĭ-rin) a porphyrin whose iron complex united with protein occurs in hemoglobin, myoglobin, and certain respiratory pigments.

protoporphyrinuria (pro″to-por″fĭ-rĭ-nu′re-ah) protoporphyrin in the urine.

prototroph (pro′to-trōf) an organism with the same growth factor requirements as the ancestral strain; said of microbial mutants. adj., **prototroph′ic.**

prototype (pro′to-tīp) the original type or form that is typical of later individuals or species.

protoveratrine (pro″to-ver′ah-trēn) an antihypertensive alkaloid isolated from *Veratrum album* and *V. viride,* occurring in two forms, A and B.

protovertebra (pro″to-ver′tĕ-brah) 1. somite. 2. the caudal half of a somite forming most of the vertebra.

protoxide (pro-tok′sīd) that one of a series of oxides of the same element which contains the least amount of oxygen.

Protozoa (pro″to-zo′ah) a phylum comprising the simplest forms of the animal kingdom, consisting of unicellular organisms ranging in size from microscopic to macroscopic. It includes the Sarcodina, Mastigophora, Ciliophora, and Sporozoa. Pathogenic protozoa include the *Plasmodium* of human malaria, *Trypanosoma gambiense* of African trypanosomiasis (African sleeping sickness), *Entamoeba histolytica* of amebic dysentery, and *Balantidium coli* and *Isospora belli,* both of which cause diarrhea in man.

protozoacide (pro″to-zo′ah-sīd) destructive to protozoa; an agent destructive to protozoa.

protozoal (pro″to-zo′al) pertaining to or caused by protozoa.

protozoan (pro″to-zo′an) 1. of or pertaining to protozoa. 2. an organism belonging to the Protozoa.

protozoiasis (pro″to-zo-i′ah-sis) any disease caused by protozoa.

protozoology (pro″to-zo-ol′o-je) the scientific study of protozoa.

protozoon (pro″to-zo′on), pl. *protozo′a* [Gr.] any member of the protozoa.

protozoophage (pro″to-zo′o-fāj) a cell having phagocytic action on protozoa.

protraction (pro-trak′shun) a forward projection of a facial structure; in mandibular protraction the gnathion is anterior to the orbital plane; in maxillary protraction the subnasion is anterior to the orbital plane.

protractor (pro-trak′tor) an instrument for extracting foreign bodies from wounds.

protrusion (pro-troo′zhun) extension beyond the usual limits, or above a plane surface.

protuberance (pro-tu′ber-ans) a projecting part, or prominence.

protuberantia (pro-tu′ber-an′she-ah), pl. *protuberan′tiae* [L.] protuberance.

proud flesh exuberant amounts of soft, edematous, granulation tissue developing during healing of large surface wounds.

Provera (pro-ver′ah) trademark for preparations of medroxyprogesterone, a progestational agent.

provertebra (pro-ver′tĕ-brah) somite.

provirus (pro-vi′rus) the genome of an animal virus integrated (by crossing over) into the chromosome of the host cell, and thus replicated in all of its daughter cells.

provitamin (pro-vi′tah-min) a substance, e.g., ergosterol, from which the animal organism can form a vitamin.

proximad (prok′sĭ-mad) in a proximal direction.

proximal (prok′sĭ-mal) nearest to a point of reference, as to a center or median line or to the point of attachment or origin.

proximalis (prok″sĭ-ma′lis) [L.] proximal.

proximate (prok′sĭ-mit) immediate; nearest.

proximoataxia (prok″sĭ-mo-ah-tak′se-ah) ataxia of the proximal part of an extremity.

proximobuccal (prok″sĭ-mo-buk′al) pertaining to the proximal and buccal surfaces of a posterior tooth.

prozone (pro′zōn) the phenomenon exhibited by some sera, in which agglutination or precipitation occurs at higher dilution ranges, but is not visible at lower dilutions or when undiluted.

pruriginous (proo-rij′ĭ-nus) of the nature of prurigo or tending to cause prurigo.

prurigo (proo-ri′go) [L.] any of several itchy skin eruptions in which the characteristic lesion is dome-shaped with a small transient vesicle on top, followed by crusting or lichenification.

p. mi′tis, prurigo of a mild type.

p. nodula′ris, a form of neurodermatitis, usually occurring on the extremities in middle-aged women, marked by discrete, firm, rough-surfaced, dark brownish-gray, intensely itchy nodules.

p. sim′plex, papular urticaria.

pruritogenic (proo″rĭ-to-jen′ik) causing pruritus, or itching.

pruritus (proo-ri′tus) itching. adj., **prurit′ic.** It is common in many types of skin disorders, especially allergic inflammation and parasitic infestations. Systemic diseases that may cause pruritus include DIABETES MELLITUS (pruritus vulvae) and liver disorders with jaundice. Hemorrhoids are often accompanied by rectal pruritus. Emotional distress plays an important role in the development and control of this disturbing symptom. Unless pruritus is relieved the patient may become exhausted from lack of sleep.

Cleanliness, soothing ointments or lotions, sodium bicarbonate baths, and sometimes tranquilizing drugs are used in the relief of pruritus. Since it is a symptom of some other disorder, complete cure of pruritus depends on cure of the primary illness.

p. a'ni, intense chronic itching in the anal region.

essential p., that occurring without known cause.

p. seni'lis, itching in the aged, due to degeneration of the skin.

symptomatic p., that which occurs secondarily to another condition.

p. vul'vae, intense itching of the external genitalia in the female.

Prussak's pouch (proo'sahks) a recess in the tympanic membrane between the flaccid part of the membrane and the neck of the malleus.

psammoma (sah-mo'mah) a tumor, especially a meningioma, which contains psammoma BODIES.

psammosarcoma (sam"o-sar-ko'mah) a sarcoma containing granular material.

pseud(o)- word element [Gr.], *false.*

pseudarthritis (soo"dar-thri'tis) a hysterical joint affection.

pseudarthrosis (soo"dar-thro'sis) a pathologic entity characterized by deossification of a weight-bearing long bone, followed by bending and pathologic fracture, with inability to form normal callus leading to existence of the "false joint" that gives the condition its name.

pseudencephalus (soo"den-sef'ah-lus) a fetus with a tumor in place of the brain.

pseudesthesia (soo"des-the'ze-ah) a subjective sensation occurring in the absence of the appropriate stimuli; an imaginary sensation.

pseudoacanthosis nigricans (soo"do-ak"an-tho'sis ni'grĭ-kans) a benign form of acanthosis nigricans associated with obesity; the obesity is sometimes due to endocrine disturbance.

pseudoagraphia (soo"do-ah-graf'e-ah) a condition in which the patient can copy writing, but cannot write except in a meaningless and illegible manner.

pseudoallele (soo"do-ah-lēl') one of two or more genes that are seemingly allelic, but which can be shown to have distinctive but closely linked loci. adj., **pseudoallel'ic.**

pseudoanemia (soo"do-ah-ne'me-ah) marked pallor with no evidence of anemia.

pseudoaneurysm (soo"do-an'u-rizm) an appearance resembling an aneurysm, but due to enlargement and tortuosity of a vessel.

pseudoangina (soo"do-an'jĭ-nah) a nervous disorder resembling angina.

pseudoankylosis (soo"do-ang"kĭ-lo'sis) a false ankylosis.

pseudoapoplexy (soo"do-ap'o-plek"se) a condition resembling apoplexy, but without cerebral hemorrhage.

pseudobulbar (soo"do-bul'bar) apparently, but not really, due to a bulbar lesion.

pseudocartilaginous (soo"do-kar"tĭ-laj'ĭ-nus) resembling cartilage.

pseudocast (soo'do-kast) an accidental formation of urinary sediment resembling a true cast.

pseudocele (soo'do-sēl) pseudocoele.

pseudochancre (soo"do-shang'ker) an indurated lesion resembling chancre.

pseudocholesteatoma (soo"do-ko"les-te"ah-to'mah) a horny mass of epithelial cells resembling cholesteatoma in the tympanic cavity in chronic middle ear inflammation.

pseudochorea (soo"do-ko-re'ah) a state of general incoordination resembling chorea.

pseudochromesthesia (soo"do-kro"mes-the'ze-ah) a false sensation of color.

pseudochromhidrosis (soo"do-krōm"hĭ-dro'sis) discoloration of sweat by surface contaminants, such as pigment-producing bacteria or chemical substances on the skin.

pseudocirrhosis (soo"do-sĭ-ro'sis) a condition suggestive of, but not due to cirrhosis; often due to pericarditis (pericardial pseudocirrhosis). (See also PICK'S DISEASE [2].)

pseudocoarctation (soo"do-ko"ark-ta'shun) a condition radiographically resembling coarctation but without compromise of the lumen, as occurs in a congenital anomaly of the aortic arch.

pseudocoele (soo"do-sēl) the fifth ventricle of the brain.

pseudocolloid (soo"do-kol'oid) a mucoid substance sometimes found in ovarian cysts.

p. of lips, Fordyce's disease.

pseudocoloboma (soo"do-kol"o-bo'mah) a line or scar on the iris resembling a coloboma.

pseudocoxalgia (soo"do-kok-sal'je-ah) osteochondrosis of the capitular epiphysis of the femur.

pseudocrisis (soo"do-kri'sis) sudden but temporary abatement of febrile symptoms.

pseudocroup (soo"do-kro͞op) laryngismus stridulus; sudden laryngeal spasm with crowing inspiration.

pseudocyesis (soo"do-si-e'sis) false pregnancy; development of all the signs of pregnancy without the presence of an embryo.

pseudocylindroid (soo"do-sĭ-lin'droid) a shred of mucin in the urine resembling a cylindroid.

pseudocyst (soo"do-sist) an abnormal dilated space resembling a cyst but not lined with epithelium.

pseudodementia (soo"do-de-men'she-ah) a state of general apathy resembling dementia, but with no actual defect of intelligence.

pseudodiphtheria (soo"do-dif-the're-ah) the presence of a false membrane not due to *Corynebacterium diphtheriae.*

pseudoedema (soo"do-ĕ-de'mah) a puffy state resembling edema.

pseudoemphysema (soo"do-em"fĭ-se'mah) a condition resembling emphysema, but due to temporary obstruction of the bronchi.

pseudoephedrine (soo"do-ĕ-fed'rin) one of the optical isomers of ephedrine; the hydrochloride salt is used as a nasal decongestant.

pseudofracture (soo"do-frak'chur) roentgenographic appearance of a thickened periosteum and new bone formation over what looks like an incomplete fracture.

pseudoganglion (soo"do-gang'gle-on) an enlargement on a nerve resembling a ganglion.

pseudogeusesthesia (soo"do-gūs"es-the'ze-ah) a

false sensation of taste associated with a sensation of another modality.

pseudogeusia (soo″do-gu′ze-ah) a sensation of taste occurring in the absence of a stimulus or inappropriate to the exciting stimulus.

pseudoglioma (soo″do-gli-o′mah) any condition mimicking retinoblastoma, e.g., retrolental fibroplasia or exudative retinopathy.

pseudoglobulin (soo″do-glob′u-lin) any of a class of globulins characterized by being soluble in water in the absence of neutral salts and thus not a euglobulin.

pseudogout (soo″do-gowt) a condition resembling gout, but with calcium salt rather than urate crystals in the synovial fluid.

pseudohemophilia (soo″do-he″mo-fil′e-ah) angiohemophilia.

pseudohermaphrodite (soo″do-her-maf′ro-dīt) an individual exhibiting pseudohermaphroditism.

pseudohermaphroditism (soo″do-her-maf′ro-di-tizm″) a state in which the gonads are of one sex but one or more contradictions exist in the morphologic criteria of sex. In female pseudohermaphroditism, the individual is a genetic and gonadal female with partial masculinization; in male pseudohermaphroditism, the individual is a genetic and gonadal male with incomplete masculinization. Pseudohermaphroditism is not to be confused with hermaphroditism, in which the individual possesses both ovarian and testicular tissue.

pseudohernia (soo″do-her′ne-ah) an inflamed sac or gland simulating strangulated hernia.

pseudohypertrophy (soo″do-hi-per′tro-fe) increase in size without true hypertrophy. adj., **pseudohypertroph′ic.**

pseudohypoparathyroidism (soo″do-hi″po-par″-ah-thi′roi-dizm) a hereditary condition clinically resembling hypoparathyroidism, but caused by failure of response to, rather than deficiency of, parathyroid hormone; it is marked by hypocalcemia and hyperphosphatemia and commonly by short stature, obesity, short metacarpals, and ectopic calcification.

pseudoisochromatic (soo″do-i″so-kro-mat′ik) seemingly of the same color throughout: applied to solutions for testing color blindness, containing two pigments or colors which will be distinguished by the normal eye, but not by the color blind.

pseudojaundice (soo″do-jawn′dis) yellowness of the skin due to blood changes and not to liver disease.

pseudologia (soo″do-lo′je-ah) the writing of anonymous letters to people of prominence, to one's self, etc.

p. fantas′tica, a tendency to tell extravagant and fantastic falsehoods centered about one's self.

pseudomania (soo″do-ma′ne-ah) 1. false or pretended mental disorder. 2. pathologic lying.

pseudomelanosis (soo″do-mel″ah-no′sis) pigmentation of tissues after death by blood pigments.

pseudomembrane (soo″do-mem′brān) false membrane.

Pseudomonas (soo″do-mo′nas) a genus of bacteria, some species of which are pathogenic for plants and vertebrates.

P. aerugino′sa, the only species that is pathogenic for man; it produces the blue-green pigment, pyocyanin, which gives the color to "blue pus," and causes various human diseases.

P. mal′lei, the causative agent of glanders, a disease of horses that is communicable to man.

P. pseudomal′lei, the causative agent of melioidosis, a disease of rodents occasionally transmitted to man.

pseudomucin (soo″do-mu′sin) a mucin-like substance found in ovarian cysts.

pseudomyxoma (soo″do-mik-so′mah) a mass of epithelial mucus resembling a myxoma.

p. peritone′i, the presence in the peritoneal cavity of mucoid material from a ruptured ovarian cyst or a ruptured mucocele of the appendix.

pseudoneuritis (soo″do-nu-ri′tis) a congenital hyperemic condition of the optic papilla.

pseudopapilledema (soo″do-pap″il-ĕ-de′mah) anomalous elevation of the optic disk.

pseudoparalysis (soo″do-pah-ral′ĭ-sis) apparent loss of muscular power without real paralysis.

arthritic general p., a condition resembling dementia paralytica, dependent on intracranial atheroma in arthritic patients. Called also Klippel's disease.

Parrot's p., syphilitic p., pseudoparalysis of one or more extremities in infants, due to syphilitic osteochondritis of an epiphysis.

pseudoparaplegia (soo″do-par″ah-ple′je-ah) spurious paralysis of the lower limbs, as in hysteria or malingering.

pseudoparesis (soo″do-pah-re′sis) a hysterical or nonorganic condition simulating paresis.

pseudopelade (soo″do-pe′lād) patchy alopecia roughly simulating alopecia areata; it may be due to various diseases of the hair follicles, some of which are associated with scarring.

pseudoplegia (soo″do-ple′je-ah) hysterical paralysis.

pseudopodium (soo″do-po′de-um) a temporary protrusion of the cytoplasm of an ameba, serving for purposes of locomotion or to engulf food.

pseudopolyp (soo″do-pol′ip) a hypertrophied tab of mucous membrane resembling a polyp, but caused by ulceration surrounding intact mucosa.

pseudopolyposis (soo″do-pol″ĭ-po′sis) numerous pseudopolyps in the colon and rectum, due to longstanding inflammation.

pseudopregnancy (soo″do-preg′nan-se) false pregnancy; development of all the signs of pregnancy without the presence of an embryo.

pseudo-pseudohypoparathyroidism (soo″do-soo″do-hi″po-par″ah-thi′roi-dizm) an incomplete form of pseudohypoparathyroidism, marked by the same constitutional features but by normal levels of calcium and phosphorus in the blood serum.

pseudopterygium (soo″do-tĕ-rij′e-um) an adhesion of the conjunctiva to the cornea following a burn or other injury.

pseudoptosis (soo″do-to′sis) decrease in the size of the palpebral aperture.

pseudoreaction (soo″do-re-ak′shun) a false or deceptive reaction; in intradermal skin tests, a reaction not due to the specific test substance but to protein in the medium employed in producing the toxin.

pseudorickets (soo″do-rik′ets) renal osteodystrophy.

pseudoscarlatina (soo″do-skar″lah-te′nah) a septic condition with fever and eruption resembling scarlet fever.

pseudosclerosis (soo″do-sklĕ-ro′sis) a condition with the symptoms but without the lesions of multiple sclerosis.

Westphal-Strümpell p., hepatolenticular degeneration.

pseudosmia (soo″doz′me-ah) a sensation of odor without the appropriate stimulus.

pseudotetanus (soo″do-tet′ah-nus) persistent muscular contractions resembling tetanus but not associated with *Closdridium tetani.*

pseudotruncus arteriosus (soo″do-trunk′us ar-te″re-o′sus) the most severe form of tetralogy of Fallot.

pseudotumor (soo″do-tu′mor) phantom tumor.

p. cer′ebri, cerebral edema and raised intracranial pressure without neurological signs except occasional sixth-nerve palsy.

pseudoxanthoma elasticum (soo″do-zan-tho′mah e-las′tĭ-kum) a dermatosis marked clinically by small yellowish macules and papules, individual or confluent, or massed into plaques, and histologically by masses of swollen, calcified elastic fibers with degeneration of the collagen fibers in the lower and middle dermis and in the gastrointestinal tract and heart.

p.s.i. pounds per square inch.

psilocin (si′lo-sin) a hallucinogenic substance closely related to psilocybin.

psilocybin (si″lo-si′bin) a HALLUCINOGEN having indole characteristics, isolated from the mushroom *Psilocybe mexicana.*

psittacosis (sit″ah-ko′sis) a disease due to a strain of *Chlamydia psittaci,* first seen in parrots and later found in other birds and domestic fowl. It is transmissible to man. (See also ORNITHOSIS.)

The etiologic organism is inhaled into the body and attacks the respiratory tract. The first symptoms appear after an incubation period of 6 to 15 days and include fever, sore throat, headache, loss of appetite, chills, and profuse sweating. Later there may be coughing, difficulty in breathing, abdominal distress, and often splenomegaly. Prostration may occur. Infiltrates may appear in the chest x-ray. Special laboratory tests are necessary for accurate diagnosis.

Psittacosis usually runs its course in 2 or 3 weeks. Complications may be avoided by the administration of such antibiotics as tetracycline and penicillin. Fatalities are uncommon.

psoitis (so-i′tis) inflammation of a psoas muscle or its sheath.

psoralen (sor′ah-len) any of the constituents of certain plants (e.g., *Psoralea corylifolia*) that have the ability to produce photoxic dermatitis when an individual is first exposed to it and then to sunlight; certain perfumes and drugs (e.g., methoxsalen) contain psoralens.

psoriasis (so-ri′ah-sis) a usually chronic, hereditary, recurrent skin disease marked by discrete bright red macules, papules, or patches covered with lamellated silvery scales. adj., **psoriat′ic.** The lesions appear most often on the knees, elbows, and scalp, and sometimes in the form of dot-shaped marks on the fingernails. The chest, abdomen, backs of arms and legs, palms of hands, and soles of feet are other locations frequently affected.

It may occur in association with rheumatoid arthritis, although the connection is not clear.

Some cases of psoriasis are acute; most cases are chronic and recurrent. Early attacks may respond well to treatment, only to reappear.

TREATMENT. There is at present no cure available and all treatments must be used with caution to avoid permanent damage to the skin. A folic acid antagonist, methotrexate, is the most widely used systemic agent in the treatment of psoriasis and is successful in the control of severe psoriasis. Topically, corticosteroids, tar preparations, and psoralens are also used.

PSP phenolsulfonphthalein, a dye used in testing kidney function.

PSRO Professional Standards Review Organization.

psych(o)- word element [Gr.], *mind.*

psychalgia (si-kal′je-ah) pain of mental or hysterical origin; pain attending or due to mental effort. adj., **psychal′gic.**

psychanopsia (si″kah-nop′se-ah) psychic blindness.

psychataxia (si″kah-tak′se-ah) a disordered mental state with confusion, agitation, and inability to fix the attention.

psyche (si′ke) the mind; the human faculty for thought, judgment, and emotion; the mental life, including both conscious and unconscious processes. adj., **psy′chic.**

psychedelic (si″kĕ-del′ik) pertaining to or causing hallucinations, distortions of perception, and, sometimes, psychotic-like behavior; also, a drug producing such effects. Psychedelic drugs such as LSD and mescaline cause hallucinations and altered mental function. They are highly controversial and potentially dangerous and should be used for experimental purposes only, and under the direct supervision of a competent authorized investigator. (See also HALLUCINOGEN.)

psychiatrist (si-ki′ah-trist) a physician who specializes in psychiatry.

psychiatry (si-ki′ah-tre) the branch of medicine that deals with the study, treatment, and prevention of mental illness. adj., **psychiat′ric.**

descriptive p., that based on observation and study of external factors that can be seen, heard, or felt.

dynamic p., the study of emotional processes, their origins and the mental mechanisms underlying them.

forensic p., that dealing with the legal aspects of mental disorders.

orthomolecular p., the study of mental disease on the basis of the molecular environment of the brain.

psychic (si′kik) pertaining to the mind or psyche.

psychoanaleptic (si″ko-an″ah-lep′tik) exerting a stimulating effect on the mind.

psychoanalysis (si″ko-ah-nal′ĭ-sis) a technique for diagnosing and treating mental illness originally developed by Dr. Sigmund Freud. adj., **psychoanalyt′ic.** Psychoanalysis is a well known form of PSYCHOTHERAPY, a term that covers all psychologic techniques used in the treatment of mental illness.

Psychoanalysis is based on Freud's theories of the

TABLE OF SCHOOLS OF PSYCHIATRY

- I. Reconstructive
  - A. Psychoanalysis – Sigmund Freud
  - B. Neo-Freudian, modifications of psychoanalysis.
    1. Active analytic techniques – Sandor Ferenczi, Wilhelm Stekel, the Chicago school (especially Franz Alexander and Thomas French)
    2. Analytic play therapy – Anna Freud, Melanie Klein
    3. Analytical psychology – Carl Jung
    4. Character analysis, orgone therapy – Wilhelm Reich
    5. Cognitive – Jean Piaget
    6. Developmental – Erik Erikson
    7. Ego psychology – Paul Federn, Edoardo Weiss, Heinz Hartmann, Ernst Kris, Rudolph Loewenstein
    8. Existential analysis – Ludwig Binswanger
    9. Holistic analysis – Karen Horney
    10. Individual psychology – Alfred Adler
    11. Transactional analysis – Eric Berne
    12. Washington cultural school – Harry Stack Sullivan, Erich Fromm, Clara Thompson
    13. Will therapy – Otto Rank
  - C. Group Approaches
    1. Orthodox psychoanalytic – S. R. Slavson
    2. Psychodrama – Jacob L. Moreno
    3. Psychoanalysis in groups – Alexander Wolf
    4. Valence systems – Walter Bion
- II. Reeducative and Supportive, Individual and Group
  1. Client-centered (non-directive) – Carl Rogers
  2. Conditioning, behavior therapy, behavior modification
     - a. aversion therapy – N. V. Kantorovich
     - b. behaviorism – John B. Watson
     - c. classical conditioning – Ivan Pavlov
     - d. operant conditioning – Burrhus F. Skinner
     - e. sexual counseling – William Masters, Virginia Johnson
     - f. systematic desensitization – Joseph Wolpe
  3. Family therapy – Nathan Ackerman
  4. Gestalt – Wolfgang Kohler, Kurt Lewin, Fritz Perls
  5. Logotherapy – Victor Frankl
  6. Psychobiology (distributive analysis and synthesis) – Adolf Meyer
  7. Zen (satori) – Alan Watts

From *A Psychiatric Glossary*. 4th ed. American Psychiatric Association, 1975.

way the mind develops and functions. Briefly, these theories state that during early childhood the child has a number of instinctual impulses and desires that are in conflict with what is expected of him by his family and the society in which he lives. In the process of resolving these conflicts he represses the feelings he must curb, or blocks them out of his conscious mind. Some of these repressed desires continue to exist in his unconscious mind, however. When they continue to exist as conflicts, they may erupt into NEUROSIS.

A neurotic adult will tend to respond to people in terms of his childhood feelings toward members of his family, even though these responses are not appropriate to the situation. Without realizing it, he is going through adult life still fighting the battles of childhood. His unresolved conflicts prevent him from seeing others as they are and reacting to them in an appropriate way.

Psychoanalysis attempts, in Freud's words, "to make the unconscious conscious." Its goal is to help the patient become aware of and resolve his childhood conflicts, so that he can react to his life situation as it is and not in terms of these conflicts. The psychoanalyst does not instruct or advise the patient; he helps him to instruct himself.

TECHNIQUES. One of the techniques that Freud developed to aid this process is free association. When a person is trying to focus on an emotional disturbance, he often has stray thoughts that seem to be meaningless but offer clues to the real nature of this difficulty. These thoughts can be organized by the analyst and interpreted to indicate the unconscious process involved. In psychoanalysis, the patient is asked to say whatever comes to his mind, however trivial or "unspeakable" it may seem. In order to make free association easier, the patient lies in a relaxed position on a couch facing away from the analyst.

Another important technique of psychoanalysis is interpretation of dreams. A person's dreams are an expression of his unconcious wishes and drives, which are disguised, appear as symbols, and give valuable indications of unconscious fears and conflicts. With the help of the analyst, the patient free-associates about his dreams, and tries to understand their real content and to learn what is behind the disguise.

Hypnosis is sometimes used to elicit experiences that have been repressed.

During the course of analysis, the patient tends to react to the analyst in terms of his childhood conflicts. This is called transference. Since the analyst is a neutral figure, when the patient reacts to his analyst in unreasonable ways, accusing him, for example of being cruel, the analyst can point out to the patient that this is how he must have felt about his father. Again, the patient might be able to find excuses for his fear of his neighbors in various ways, but be unable to find an excuse for his similar fear of the analyst. He may then realize that others of his fears are also groundless and based on unconscious conflicts.

Psychoanalysis is ordinarily a very prolonged, intensive form of treatment. It usually involves several sessions a week for a year or more.

psychoanalyst (si″ko-an′ah-list) a practitioner of psychoanalysis.

psychobiology (si″ko-bi-ol′o-je) study of the interrelations of body and mind in the formation and functioning of personality. adj., **psychobiolog′ical.**

psychocortical (si″ko-kor′tĭ-kal) pertaining to the mind and the cerebral cortex.

psychodelic (si″ko-del′ik) psychedelic.

psychodiagnosis (si″ko-di″ag-no′sis) the diagnostic use of psychologic testing.

psychodrama (si″ko-drah′mah) group PSYCHOTHERAPY in which patients dramatize their individual conflicting situations of daily life.

psychodynamics (si″ko-di-nam′iks) the science of human behavior and motivation.

psychogalvanic reflex (si″ko-gal-van′ik) a decrease in electrical resistance of the body due to emotional or mental agitation.

psychogalvanometer (si″ko-gal″vah-nom′ĕ-ter) a galvanometer for recording the electrical agitation produced by emotional stresses.

psychogenesis (si″ko-jen′ĕ-sis) 1. mental development. 2. the production of a symptom or illness by psychic, as opposed to organic, factors.

psychogenic (si″ko-jen′ik) having an emotional or psychologic origin.

psychogram, psychograph (si′ko-gram; si′ko-graf) 1. a chart for recording graphically the personality traits of an individual. 2. a written description of the mental functioning of an individual.

psychokinesis (si″ko-ki-ne′sis) the production or alteration of motion by directed thought processes.

psycholepsy (si″ko-lep′se) a condition characterized by sudden changes of mood.

psycholeptic (si″ko-lep′tik) a drug that affects the mental state.

psychology (si-kol′o-je) the science dealing with the mind and mental processes, especially in relation to human and animal behavior. adj., **psycholog′ic, psycholog′ical.**

analytic p., psychology by introspective methods, as opposed to experimental psychology.

clinical p., the use of psychologic knowledge and techniques in the treatment of persons with emotional difficulties.

criminal p., the study of the mentality, the motivation, and the social behavior of criminals.

depth p., psychoanalysis.

dynamic p., psychology stressing the element of energy in mental processes.

experimental p., the study of the mind and mental operations by the use of experimental methods.

genetic p., psychology dealing with the development of the mind in the individual and with its evolution in the race.

gestalt p., gestaltism; the theory that the objects of mind, as immediately presented to direct experience, come as complete unanalyzable wholes or forms that cannot be split into parts.

physiologic p., psychology applying the facts taught in neurology to show the relation between the mental and neural.

social p., psychology treating of the social aspects of mental life.

psychometrician (si″ko-mĕ-trish′an) a person skilled in psychometry.

psychometrics, psychometry (si″ko-met′riks; si-kom′ĕ-tre) the testing and measuring of mental and psychologic ability, efficiency, potentials, and functioning. adj., **psychomet′ric.**

psychomotor (si″ko-mo′tor) pertaining to motor effects of cerebral or psychic activity.

p. epilepsy, EPILEPSY manifested by impaired consciousness of variable degree, the patient carrying out a series of coordinated acts that are out of place, bizarre, and serve no useful purpose and for which he is amnesic.

psychoneurosis (si″ko-nu-ro′sis) neurosis. adj., **psychoneurot′ic.**

psychonomy (si-kon′o-me) the science of the laws of mental activity.

psychopath (si′ko-path) a person who has a psycopathic personality.

psychopathic (si″ko-path′ik) antisocial; pertaining to a psychopath.

p. personality, a type of personality disorder, characterized by a conspicuous disregard for the rights or needs of others; called also sociopathic personaltiy. The behavior patterns of the psychopath are not typical of either NEUROSIS or PSYCHOSIS, and differ somewhat from those of other types of personality disorders.

There is no sharp dividing line between the normal and the psychopathic personality. The psychopath shows a lack of emotional maturity, an unwillingness to take responsibility and emotional instability. Unlike the neurotic person, he expresses his conflict in antisocial acts so that society suffers, rather than the psychopath himself.

CHARACTERISTICS. The chief characteristic of a psychopath is an apparent lack of conscience. He expresses his conflicts in various ways, including compulsive lying, stealing, and certain other types of antisocial or criminal activity. He may suffer from alcoholism or drug addiction; sexual deviation may also be an expression of psychopathic personality.

Like other types of mental illness, a psychopathic personality probably has many roots in the emotions and experiences of early childhood, but their form of expression is different. A psychopathic personality affects the entire structure of the character, so that the person feels that everyone else is out of step. If the patient is a criminal, he may honestly believe that anyone who is not a criminal is merely stupid. Those with psychopathic personalities often seem to be unable to learn from experience.

TREATMENT. Unfortunately, it is extremely difficult to treat a patient with a psychopathic personality. The techniques of PSYCHOTHERAPY depend on the cooperation of the patient, and this in turn depends on his willingness to admit that something is wrong with him. This is an admission that those with psychopathic personalities are rarely willing or able to make. They seldom accept psychiatric help, and since they are legally sane, they cannot be compelled to undergo treatment.

psychopathology (si″ko-pah-thol′o-je) the branch of medicine dealing with the causes and processes of mental disorders.

psychopathy (si-kop′ah-the) any disease of the mind.

psychopharmacology (si″ko-far″mah-kol′o-je) the study of the action of drugs on the mind. adj., **psychopharmacolog′ic.**

psychophysical (si″ko-fiz′ĭ-kal) pertaining to the mind and its relation to physical manifestations.

psychophysics (si″ko-fiz′iks) scientific study of the quantitative relations between characteristics or patterns of physical stimuli and the sensations induced by them.

psychophysiology (si″ko-fiz″e-ol′o-je) scientific study of the interaction and interrelations of psychic and physiologic factors. adj., **psychophysiolog′ic.**

psychoplegic (si″ko-ple′jik) an agent lessening cerebral activity or excitability.

psychoprophylaxis (si″ko-pro″fĭ-lak′sis) psychophysical training aimed at preventing pain and modifying the perception of painful sensations associated with normal uncomplicated childbirth. (See also NATURAL CHILDBIRTH.)

psychosensory (si″ko-sen′so-re) perceiving and interpreting sensory stimuli.

psychosexual (si″ko-seks′u-al) pertaining to the psychic or emotional aspects of sex.

psychosis (si-ko′sis), pl. *psycho′ses.* any major mental disorder of organic or emotional origin, marked by derangement of the personality and loss of contact with reality, often with delusions, hallucinations, or illusions. adj., **psychot′ic.**

A psychotic person may live in his own private world, completely out of touch with reality. He cannot cope with the demands of the real world, and he withdraws from it. In general, this loss of contact with reality is one of the more obvious differences between psychosis and NEUROSIS.

About half the hospital beds in the United States today are occupied by patients with mental illness, almost all of them sufferers from psychosis. Psychosis disables as many Americans per year as heart disease and cancer combined.

TYPES OF PSYCHOSIS. Psychoses are usually classified as functional psychoses, those for which no physical cause has been discovered, and organic psychoses, which are the result of organic damage to the brain.

The main types of functional psychosis are schizophrenia, paranoia, affective psychosis, and involutional reaction.

Schizophrenia. This is the most widespread form of psychosis. About half of all patients hospitalized for mental illness are schizophrenics. This condition was formerly called dementia praecox, or "early insanity," because it usually appears between the ages of 15 and 30.

The schizophrenic is apt to be shy, dreamy, bored, and lacking in physical and mental energy. When he becomes unable to find a solution for a painful situation, he retreats into a world he imagines as he would like it to be. The schizophrenic becomes unable to distinguish fact from imagination and uninterested in doing so. As a result, his actions may seem very strange unless they are understood as the product of a dream world. For example, one symptom of schizophrenia is the use of neologisms, or made-up words that are meaningless to the listener. Hallucinations and delusions may occur, as may CATALEPSY.

Certain types of schizophrenia respond more readily to treatment than do others. In all types, early treatment is extremely important, as the prospects for recovery seem to be closely connected with the duration of the condition.

Paranoia. This psychosis, which is much less common than schizophrenia, is characterized by delusions of persecution or grandiose delusions. A person suffering from it becomes more and more deluded, seeing hidden meanings to support his conviction that others are plotting against him, or to substantiate his belief that he is a person of great importance. He often uses an intricate form of logic to try to explain his delusions.

There are many degrees of paranoid reaction. Paranoid attitudes also appear in one type of schizophrenia.

In paranoia, unlike other psychoses, the entire personality is not affected; the patient does not lose contact with reality, but tends rather to misinterpret reality in terms of his delusion.

Affective Psychosis. This psychosis is characterized by greatly exaggerated emotional reactions. It is called a manic-depressive reaction because of the conspicuous mood swings that are characteristic of the condition. Although there are two possible phases, manic and depressive, the disorder takes many forms, sometimes entirely manic, or entirely depressive, with many variations. In an extremely mild form the affective reaction is not a true psychosis.

During the manic phase, the patient's energy and optimism seem boundless, mental activity and talking are accelerated, physical activity becomes greatly increased; lack of judgment, combined with overenthusiasm, may make the patient dangerous to himself and to others. During the depressive phase, the patient's mental activity is greatly retarded, he may sit or lie inert, scarcely able to move or speak (see also CATALEPSY). The danger of suicide may be present. In some cases the patient appears greatly agitated even though he is extremely depressed.

Affective psychosis tends to recur. Many patients seem to recover spontaneously and then exhibit symptoms again after a period of more or less normal behavior.

Involutional Reaction. This is a psychotic reaction that occurs in late middle age. It was formerly thought to be related to the menopause in women and its emotional counterpart, the climacteric, in men. Characteristics of this type of psychosis include agitation, depression, feelings of guilt, paranoia, preoccupation with minor symptoms of physical disorders, severe insomnia, and suicidal tendencies. The course of the illness tends to be prolonged.

CAUSES. There is still much to be learned about the causes of functional psychoses. The roots of these conditions may be in the patient's early emotional experiences, or in his physical make-up, or in his environment. The high incidence of psychosis in certain families with a history of mental illness suggests that heredity may also play some role. However, it should be remembered that children whose parents are mentally disturbed and untreated may absorb psychotic ways of responding emotionally and viewing reality, in the same way that young children learn healthy ways of dealing with the real world from their environment.

The causes of organic psychoses are much better understood. Among the physical causes that can lead to psychosis are infectious diseases which involve the brain, certain deficiency diseases, lead poisoning, tumors, interference with the brain's blood supply, and wounds and blows that injure the brain. In a very few cases, epilepsy may lead to some mental deterioration. These organic psychoses are more resistant to treatment than are those with a functional basis.

TREATMENT. In most cases, patients with psychosis must be treated in a mental hospital. The major form of treatment is PSYCHOTHERAPY, in which the patient is helped to understand and deal with his condition. However, this method will not work when the patient is out of contact with reality, and completely absorbed in his own fantasies and hallucinations.

In such cases, chemotherapy, the use of drugs to control the patient's emotions and behavior, may be very helpful. Important among these drugs are chlorpromazine hydrochloride (Thorazine) and certain other phenothiazine derivatives. They act to calm the patient and often to help him become more rational.

The treatment of psychosis has been revolutionized by the development of two other types of drugs, the tranquilizers and the antidepressants or "psychic elevators." These medicines do not cure the conditions; they merely control the symptoms. In many cases, they make it possible to treat the patients while they continue to live at home.

Another type of treatment that is sometimes used is SHOCK THERAPY. The patient is rendered unconscious briefly by electric shock or drugs. This treatment often helps bring patients with melancholia or schizophrenia back to reality, thus making it possible to use the techniques of psychotherapy.

In a very few cases that are not helped by any other form of treatment, psychosurgery may be used. In this treatment, the connection between different parts of the brain is surgically severed. The result is a lessening of emotional reactions and tensions. Many doctors object to psychosurgery because of the negative aspects of its results, and the operation is used as a last resort.

alcoholic p., mental disorder caused by excessive use of alcohol.

depressive p., one characterized by mental depression, melancholy, despondency, inadequacy, and feelings of guilt.

exhaustion p., a psychosis due to some exhausting or depressing occurrence, as a surgical operation.

gestational p., a psychosis developing during pregnancy.

Korsakoff's p., a syndrome marked by amnesia, confabulation, and peripheral neuritis, usually associated with alcoholism and believed to be a chronic form of Wernicke's syndrome (see also KORSAKOFF'S SYNDROME).

polyneuritic p., Korsakoff's psychosis.

senile p., mental deterioration in old age, with organic brain changes, the symptoms including impaired memory for recent events, confabulation, irritability, etc. Called also senile dementia.

situational p., one caused by an unbearable situation over which the patient has no control.

toxic p., psychosis due to the ingestion of toxic agents or to the presence of toxins within the body.

psychosolytic (si″ko-so-lit′ik) relieving or abolishing psychotic symptoms.

psychosomatic (si″ko-so-mat′ik) pertaining to the interrelations of mind and body; having bodily symptoms of psychic, emotional, or mental origin.

p. illness, traditionally, an illness that can be traced to an emotional cause. It is becoming increasingly more recognized, however, that emotional factors play a role in the development of nearly all organic illnesses and that the physical symptoms experienced by the patient are related to many interdependent factors, including the psychological and cultural. The physical manifestations of an illness, unless caused by mechanical trauma, cannot be divorced from a person's emotional life. He responds in his own unique way to stress; his emotions affect his sensitivity to trauma and to irritating elements in his environment, his susceptibility to infection, and his ability to recover from the effects of his illness. It is believed by some behavioral scientists that regardless of their origin, many psychosomatic symptoms are useful in some way to the patient, perhaps as a means of getting attention from others or as a way of finding relief from the pressures of a stressful situation.

Among the illnesses recognized to be pecipitated or exacerbated by emotional stimuli are ASTHMA, MIGRAINE HEADACHE, ANOREXIA NERVOSA, INSOMNIA, neurodermatitis, HYPERTENSION, and some urinary and intestinal disorders, such as ENURESIS and regional ILEITIS. In recent years attempts to utilize the techniques of behavior therapy to treat these and other illnesses whose symptoms are related to the autonomic system have met with some degree of success. Clients are taught new ways of coping with stress and new patterns of behavior. Among the techniques used by behavior therapists are BIOFEEDBACK, relaxation training, classical CONDITIONING, and operant conditioning using social and material reinforcements.

psychosurgery (si″ko-ser′jer-e) brain surgery done to relieve mental and psychic symptoms.

psychotherapy (si″ko-ther′ah-pe) any of a number of related techniques for treating mental illness by psychologic methods. These techniques are similar in that they all rely mainly on establishing communication between the therapist and the patient as a means of understanding and modifying the patient's behavior. On occasion, drugs may be used, but only in order to make this communication easier.

FORMS OF PSYCHOTHERAPY. Perhaps the best known form of psychotherapy is PSYCHOANALYSIS, the technique developed by Dr. Sigmund Freud. Psychoanalysis attempts, through free association and dream interpretation, to reveal and resolve the unconscious conflicts that are at the root of mental illness.

Closely related to psychoanalysis is analytically oriented therapy, or "brief therapy." This uses some of the techniques of psychoanalysis, but tends to concentrate on the patient's present-life difficulties rather than on the unconscious roots of these difficulties.

One widely used technique is group therapy. Six to ten patients meet regularly to discuss their problems under the guidance of a group therapist. Group therapy is based on the principle of transference—that is, a patient tends to react to others in terms of his childhood attitudes toward family members. During group therapy, he may react to one member of the group as a hated rival brother, and to another as a dominating mother. In the give-and-take of discussion, he will begin to recognize the distortions in these reactions, and to see similar distortions in his day-to-day relationships with other people. Group therapy is generally combined with individual therapy and can help reduce the cost to each patient. It is also widely used in mental hospitals, where it has helped relieve the great shortage of trained therapists.

Adjunctive therapy, such as occupational therapy and music therapy, is helpful in relieving tensions and emotional problems that are associated with a feeling of uselessness. Psychodrama, in which patients act out fantasies or real-life situations, may provide a means of communication for patients who are not capable of expressing their problem by speech.

Play therapy is a form of psychotherapy adapted to children. It is very difficult to induce an emotionally disturbed or even a normal child to talk about his problems. Play therapy provides an alternative. The child reveals himself when he plays with toys provided by the therapist and acts out his fantasies. The therapist helps him "get things out of his system," accepting him warmly as he is, and guiding him toward a solution to his problems. Since these are closely related to the way he is treated at home, play therapy is usually combined with some form of therapy for the parents. Recently experiments have been made with family group therapy, in which the entire family meets regularly with the therapist. This new technique sometimes appears to have remarkable results.

psychotic (si-kot′ik) 1. pertaining to, characterized by, or caused by psychosis. 2. a person exhibiting psychosis.

psychotogenic (si-kot″o-jen′ik) producing a psychosis.

psychotomimetic (si-kot″o-mi-met′ik) characterized by or producing symptoms similar to those of a psychosis.

psychotropic (si″ko-trop′ik) exerting an effect upon the mind; said especially of drugs.

psychr(o)- word element [Gr.], *cold.*

psychralgia (si″kral′je-ah) a painful sensation of cold.

psychrometer (si-krom′ĕ-ter) an instrument for measuring the moisture of the atmosphere.

psychrophile (si′kro-fīl) a psychrophilic organism.

psychrophilic (si″kro-fil′ik) fond of cold; said of bacteria that grow best in the cold (15°–20° C.).

psychrophore (si′kro-fōr) a double catheter for applying cold.

psychrotherapy (si″kro-ther′ah-pe) treatment of disease by applying cold.

psyllium (sil′e-um) a plant of the genus *Plantago* (see also psyllium hydrophilic MUCILLOID and plantago [psyllium] SEED).

Pt chemical symbol, *platinum.*

pt. pint.

PTA plasma thromboplastin antecedent, clotting factor XI.

ptarmic (tar′mic) causing sneezing.

ptarmus (tar′mus) spasmodic sneezing.

PTC plasma thromboplastin component, clotting factor IX.

pterin (ter′in) any of a class of nitrogenous compounds, including aminopterin and xanthopterin, first observed in butterfly wings.

pteroylglutamic acid (ter″o-il-gloo-tam′ik) folic acid.

pterygium (tĕ-rij′e-um) a winglike structure, especially an abnormal triangular fold of membrane in the interpalpebral fissure, extending from the conjunctiva to the cornea.

p. col′li, webbed neck; a thick skin fold on the side of the neck, from the mastoid region to the acromion.

pterygoid (ter′ĭ-goid) shaped like a wing.

p. bone, pterygoid process.

p. process, either of the two processes of the sphenoid bone descending from the points of junction of the great wings and body of the bone, and each consisting of a lateral and medial plate.

pterygomandibular (ter″ĭ-go-man-dib′u-lar) pertaining to the pterygoid process and the mandible.

pterygomaxillary (ter″ĭ-go-mak′sĭ-ler″e) pertaining to a pterygoid process and the maxilla.

pterygopalatine (ter″ĭ-go-pal′ah-tīn) pertaining to a pterygoid process and the palatine bone.

ptilosis (ti-lo′sis) falling out of the eyelashes.

ptomaine (to′mān, to-mān′) any of an indefinite class of toxic bases, usually considered to be formed by the action of bacterial metabolism on proteins.

p. poisoning, a term commonly misapplied to FOOD POISONING. Contrary to popular belief, ptomaines are not injurious to the human digestive system, which is quite capable of reducing them to harmless substances. Decomposed foods are often responsible for food poisoning, however, because they may harbor certain forms of poison-producing bacteria.

ptosed (tōst) affected with ptosis.

ptosis (to′sis) 1. prolapse of an organ or part. 2. paralytic drooping of the upper eyelid. adj., **ptot′ic.**

-ptosis word element [Gr.], *downward displacement.* adj., **-ptot′ic.**

ptyal(o)- word element [Gr.], *saliva.*

ptyalagogue (ti-al′ah-gog) sialagogue.

ptyalectasis (ti″ah-lek′tah-sis) 1. a state of dilatation of a salivary duct. 2. surgical dilation of a salivary duct.

ptyalin (ti′ah-lin) α-amylase occurring in saliva.

ptyalism (ti′ah-lizm) excessive secretion of saliva.

ptyalocele (ti-al′o-sēl) a cystic tumor containing saliva.

ptyalogenic (ti″ah-lo-jen′ik) formed from or by the action of saliva.

ptyaloreaction (ti″ah-lo-re-ak′shun) a reaction occurring in or performed on the saliva.

ptyalorrhea (ti″ah-lo-re′ah) ptyalism.

Pu chemical symbol, *plutonium.*

pubarche (pu-bar′ke) the first appearance of pubic hair.

puberty (pu′ber-te) the period during which the secondary sex characteristics begin to develop and the capability of sexual reproduction is attained. Puberty in a girl is marked by broadening of the hips, development of the breasts, the appearance of pubic hair, and the onset of menstruation. At puberty a boy's shoulders broaden, his voice deepens, and pubic and facial hair appears. Girls usually reach puberty between the ages of 11 and 13, and boys between 13 and 15; the timing varies widely among individuals, however.

precocious p., unusually early sexual maturation, either idiopathic or pathologic.

pubes (pu′bēz), sing. *pu′bis* [L.] 1. the hairs growing over the pubic region. 2. the pubic region.

pubescence (pu-bes′ens) 1. puberty. 2. lanugo.

pubescent (pu-bes′ent) 1. arriving at the age of puberty. 2. covered with down or lanugo.

pubic (pu′bik) pertaining to or lying near the pubes.

pubiotomy (pu″be-ot′o-me) surgical separation of the pubis (pubic bone) lateral to the symphysis.

pubis (pu′bis), pl. *pu′bes* [L.] the anterior portion of the hip bone, a distinct bone in early life; called also pubic bone.

public health (pub′lik) the field of medicine that is concerned with safeguarding and improving the physical, mental, and social well-being of the community as a whole.

The United States Public Health Service (U.S.P.H.S.) is a tax-supported federal health agency that is a unit of the Department of Health, Education and Welfare. State and county public health agencies function under the supervision of and with financial support from the national Public Health Service.

Programs carried out by the U.S.P.H.S. include research programs, quarantine regulations, medical and psychiatric examinations of immigrants, Civil Defense programs, and financial and technical aid to local health departments to support training programs for personnel and improve the health of citizens of the community.

p. h. nursing, the branch of nursing concerned with providing nursing care and health guidance to individuals and families in the home and school, at work, and at medical and health centers. The public health nurse is employed by a local agency or the United States Public Health Service. She works to implement such programs as school and preschool health programs, immunization and treatment of communicable diseases, maternal and child health clinics, and home visits for the purpose of providing health education and nursing care. She frequently participates in educational programs for nurses, allied professional workers, and civic organizations, and is involved in studying and planning and putting into action local and national health programs.

pubofemoral (pu″bo-fem′o-ral) pertaining to the pubis and femur.

puboprostatic (pu″bo-pros-tat′ik) pertaining to the pubis and prostate.

pubovesical (pu″bo-ves′ĭ-kal) pertaining to the pubis and bladder.

pudendum (pu-den′dum), pl. *puden′da* [L.] the external genitalia of humans, especially of the female, including the mons pubis, labia majora and minora, vestibule, and clitoris. Called also pudendum femininum, pudendum muliebre, and VULVA. adj., **puden′dal, pu′dic.**

puerile (pu′er-il) pertaining to a child or to childhood; childish.

puerpera (pu-er′per-ah) a woman who has just given birth to a child.

puerperal (pu-er′per-al) pertaining to a puerpera or to the puerperium.

p. fever, an infectious disease of childbirth; called also puerperal sepsis and childbed fever.

Until the mid-19th century, this dreaded, then mysterious illness sometimes swept through a hospital maternity ward, killing most of the new mothers. Today strict aseptic hospital techniques have made the disease uncommon in most parts of the world, except in unusual circumstances such as illegally induced abortion.

Puerperal fever results from an infection, usually streptococcal, originating in the birth canal and affecting the endometrium. This infection can spread throughout the body, causing septicemia. The preliminary symptoms are fever, chills, excessive bleeding, foul lochia, and abdominal and pelvic pain. In acute stages, the pain spreads to the legs and chest; complications may be serious or even fatal.

Treatment consists mainly of administration of antibiotics, and in most instances they promptly clear up the infection. If the disease has progressed to an acute stage before treatment begins, blood transfusions may be necessary.

p. metritis, infection of the uterus in a puerperal woman.

puerperalism (pu-er′per-al-izm″) a morbid condition incident to childbirth.

puerperium (pu″er-pe′re-um) the period or state of confinement after childbirth.

Pulex (pu′leks) a genus of fleas, several species of which transmit the microorganism causing plague.

P. ir′ritans, a widely distributed species, known as the human flea, which infests domestic animals as well as man, and may act as an intermediate host of certain helminths.

pulicicide (pu-lis′ĭ-sīd) an agent destructive to fleas.

pullulation (pul″u-la′shun) development by sprouting, or budding.

pulmo (pul′mo), pl. *pulmo′nes* [L.] lung.

pulmo- word element [L.], *lung.*

pulmoaortic (pul″mo-a-or′tik) pertaining to the lungs and aorta.

pulmonary (pul′mo-ner″e) pertaining to the lungs, or to the pulmonary artery.

p. artery, the large artery originating from the superior surface of the right ventricle of the heart and passing diagonally upward to the left across the route of the aorta. The pulmonary trunk divides between the fifth and sixth thoracic vertebrae, forming the right pulmonary artery, which enters the right lung, and the left pulmonary artery, which enters the left lung.

p. circulation, the circulation of blood to and from the lungs. Unoxygenated blood from the right ventricle flows through the right and left pulmonary arteries to the right and left lung. After entering the lungs, the branches subdivide, finally emerging as capillaries which surround the alveoli and release the carbon dioxide in exchange for a fresh supply of oxygen. The capillaries unite gradually and assume the characteristics of veins. These veins join to form the pulmonary veins, which return the oxygenated blood to the left atrium. (See also CIRCULATORY SYSTEM.)

p. edema, an effusion of serous fluid into the pulmonary interstitial tissues and air sacs (see also pulmonary EDEMA).

p. embolism, obstruction of the pulmonary artery or one of its branches by an embolus (see also EMBOLISM).

p. function tests, specific evaluation techniques and procedures done for the purpose of assessing ventilatory status. The data obtained from these tests may be used in conjunction with BLOOD GAS ANALYSIS and other clinical findings to follow the course of a pulmonary disease, to aid in the management of a patient having thoracic surgery, and as a screening technique to detect pulmonary dysfunction. The tests cannot be used to establish the cause of a pulmonary disease and, because of a wide range in normal variability, they are not reliable for locating minor localized changes in the respiratory tract and lungs.

The patient must be willing and able to cooperate fully during the testing procedures; otherwise the results will be meaningless. He should be well instructed in the part he is to play in the testing and he must be mentally competent to follow the instructions given. If the patient is too weak, disoriented, or otherwise unable or unwilling to cooperate, the information obtained will not be a reliable index of his true pulmonary status. The tests should not be done while the patient has a respiratory infection or is recovering from one. Depressant or stimulating drugs can affect the outcome of the tests and should be withheld or the testing deferred until the patient is no longer under their influence.

Most pulmonary function testing procedures involve a battery of tests so as to obtain as accurate an evaluation as possible. Some of the tests are relatively simple while others require sophisticated machinery and highly trained specialists. Gas volume measurements include VITAL CAPACITY, which measures total lung volume; MAXIMAL BREATHING CAPACITY, which measures the maximal amount of air a subject can breathe in 60 seconds; INSPIRATORY RESERVE VOLUME and EXPIRATORY RESERVE VOLUME, which measure the maximal volume of air that can be inspired and expired after a quiet inhalation and exhalation. These and other gas volume tests utilize the SPIROMETER to measure the volume of gas.

Pulmonary capacities are determined by combining two or more of the pulmonary volumes. For example, the vital capacity of the lung is determined by adding the inspiratory reserve volume to the tidal volume and the expiratory reserve volume. The total of these three volumes comprises the vital capacity of the lungs, which is about 4600 ml.

The *body plethysmograph* is a sophisticated technique requiring an airtight chamber large enough to accommodate the subject. The volume of air within the chamber is known and, as the subject breathes, the changes in gas volume are measured. The changes provide information about the inspiratory and expiratory volume of the lungs; changes in alveolar pressure that occur as the subject breathes can be calculated.

Other pulmonary function tests measure oxygen consumption and carbon dioxide elimination and the *respiratory quotient,* which is determined by dividing the value of carbon dioxide eliminated by that of oxygen consumption. In EXERCISE TESTING the subject performs certain exercises while ventilation tests are done. *Bronchospirometry* utilizes a double-lumen catheter that is passed into the trachea and permits the separate measurement and analysis of the tidal volume, minute volume, vital capacity, and oxygen consumption of each lung.

p. valve, the pocket-like structure that guards the orifice between the right ventricle and the pulmonary artery.

p. vein, the large vein (right and left branches) that carries oxygenated blood from the lungs to the left atrium of the heart.

pulmonic (pul-mon′ik) pulmonary.

pulmonitis (pul″mo-ni′tis) inflammation of the lung; pneumonitis; pneumonia.

pulmotor (pul′mo-tor) an apparatus for forcing oxygen into the lungs, and inducing artificial respiration.

pulp (pulp) any soft, juicy animal or vegetable tissue. adj., **pul′pal.**

p. canal, root canal.

dental p., the richly vascularized and innervated connective tissue inside the pulp cavity of a tooth.

digital p., a cushion of soft tissue on the palmar or plantar surface of the distal phalanx of a finger or toe.

red p., splenic p., the dark reddish brown substance filling the interspaces of the splenic sinuses.

tooth p., dental pulp.

white p., sheaths of lymphatic tissue surrounding the arteries of the spleen.

pulpa (pul′pah), pl. *pul′pae* [L.] pulp.

pulpectomy (pul-pek′to-me) removal of dental pulp.

pulpefaction (pul″pĕ-fak′shun) conversion into pulp.

pulpitis (pul-pi′tis), pl. *pulpit′ides* [L.] inflammation of dental pulp; endodontitis.

pulpy (pul′pe) soft; of the consistency of pulp.

pulsatile (pul′sah-tīl) characterized by a rhythmic pulsation.

pulsation (pul-sa′shun) a throb, or rhythmic beat, as of the heart.

pulse (puls) the beat of the heart as felt through the walls of the arteries. What is usually meant by pulse is the pulsation felt in the radial artery at the wrist. Other sites of pulsation include the side of the neck (carotid artery), the elbow (brachial artery), the temple (temporal artery), the anterior side of the hip bone (femoral artery), the back of the knee (popliteal artery), and the instep (dorsalis pedis artery).

What is felt is not the blood pulsing through the arteries (as is commonly supposed) but a shock wave that travels along the fibers of the arteries as the heart contracts. This shock wave is generated by the pounding of the blood as it is ejected from the heart under pressure. It is analogous to the hammering sound heard in steampipes as the steam is admitted into the pipes under pressure. A pulse in the veins is too weak to be felt, although sometimes it is measured by sphygmograph; the tracing obtained is called a phlebogram.

The pulse is usually felt just inside the wrist below the thumb by placing two or three fingers lightly upon the radial artery. The thumb is never used to take a pulse because its own pulse is likely to be confused with the one being taken. Pressure should be light; if the artery is pressed too hard, the pulse will disappear entirely. The number of beats felt in exactly 1 minute is the pulse rate.

In taking a pulse, the rate, rhythm, and force of the pulse are noted. The average rate in an adult is between 60 and 80 beats per minute. The rhythm is checked for possible irregularities, which may be an indication of the general condition of the heart and the circulatory system.

An instrument for registering the movements, form, and force of the arterial pulse is called a sphygmograph. The sphygmographic tracing (or pulse tracing) consists of a curve having a sudden rise (primary elevation) followed by a sudden fall, after which there is a gradual descent marked by a number of secondary elevations.

abdominal p., that over the abdominal aorta.

alternating p., one with regular alteration of weak and strong beats without changes in cycle length.

anacrotic p., one in which the ascending limb of the tracing shows a transient drop in amplitude.

anadicrotic p., one in which the ascending limb of the tracing shows two small additional waves or notches.

bigeminal p., one in which two beats occur in rapid succession, the groups of two being separated by a longer interval.

brachial p., that which is felt over the brachial artery at the inner aspect of the elbow; palpated before taking blood pressure to determine location of the stethoscope.

carotid p., the pulse felt over the carotid artery, which lies between the larynx and the sternocleidomastoid muscle in the neck; frequently used to assess effectiveness of cardiac massage during cardiopulmonary respiration (CPR). It can be felt by pushing the muscle to the side and pressing against the larynx, or, if the patient is dyspneic, by palpating the pulse at the groove in the muscle.

catadicrotic p., one in which the descending limb of the tracing shows two small notches.

Corrigan's p., a jerky pulse with full expansion and sudden collapse.

p. deficit, the difference between the apical pulse and the radial pulse. Obtained by having one person count the apical pulse as heard through a stethoscope over the heart and a second person counting the radial pulse at the same time.

dicrotic p., one in which the tracing shows two marked expansions in one beat of the artery.

dorsalis pedis p., the pulse felt on the top of the foot, between the first and second metatarsal bones. In 8 to 10 per cent of the population this pulse cannot be detected.

entoptic p., a phose occurring with each heart beat.

femoral p., that which is located at the site where the femoral artery passes through the groin in the femoral triangle.

hard p., one characterized by high tension.

jerky p., one in which the artery is suddenly and markedly distended.

paradoxical p., one that markedly decreases in size during inspiration, as often occurs in constrictive pericarditis.

pistol-shot p., one in which the arteries are subject to sudden distention and collapse.

plateau p., one that is slowly rising and sustained.

popliteal p., the pulse palpated at the indentation in the back of the knee. Most easily detected when the patient is lying in the prone position with the knee flexed about 45 degrees.

posterior tibialis p., the pulse that is felt just posterior to the ankle bone on the inner aspect of the ankle.

p. pressure, the difference between the systolic and diastolic pressures.

Quincke's p., alternate blanching and flushing of the nail bed due to pulsation of subpapillary arteriolar and venous plexuses, as seen in aortic insufficiency.

radial p., that felt over the radial artery at the wrist.

Riegel's p., one which is smaller during respiration.

thready p., one that is very fine and scarcely perceptible.

tricrotic p., one in which the tracing shows three marked expansions in one beat of the artery.

trigeminal p., one with a pause after every third beat.

undulating p., one giving the sensation of successive waves.

vagus p., a slow pulse.

venous p., the pulsation over a vein, especially over the right jugular vein.

wiry p., a small, tense pulse.

pulse generator the power source for a cardiac pacemaker system, usually fueled by lithium or plutonium-238. It supplies electrical impulses to the implanted electrodes, either at a fixed rate or in some programmed pattern. (See also PACEMAKER.)

pulseless disease (puls'les) progressive obliteration of the brachiocephalic trunk and left subclavian and left common carotid arteries above their origin in the aortic arch, leading to loss of the pulse in both arms and carotids and to symptoms associated with ischemia of the brain, eyes, face, and arms. Called also Takayasu's arteritis or disease.

pulsion (pul'shun) a pushing outward.

pulsus (pul'sus) [L.] pulse.

p. alter'nans, alternating pulse.

p. bigem'inus, bigeminal pulse.

p. ce'ler, a swift, abrupt pulse.

p. dif'ferens, inequality of the pulse observable at corresponding sites on either side of the body.

p. paradox'us, paradoxical pulse.

p. par'vus et tar'dus, a small hard pulse that rises and falls slowly.

p. tar'dus, an abnormally slow pulse.

pultaceous (pul-ta'shus) like a poultice; pulpy.

pulverulent (pul-ver'u-lent) powdery; dusty.

pulvinar (pul-vi'nar) the posterior medial part of the posterior end of the thalamus.

pumice (pum'is) a substance consisting of silicates of aluminum, potassium, and sodium; used in dentistry as an abrasive.

pump (pump) 1. an apparatus for drawing or forcing liquid or gas. 2. to draw or force liquids or gases.

air p., one for exhausting or forcing in air.

blood p., a machine used to propel blood through the tubing of extracorporeal circulation devices.

breast p., a pump for taking milk from the breast.

p. oxygenator, heart-lung machine.

sodium p., the mechanism of active transport by which sodium is extruded from a cell to maintain electrolyte balance across the cell membrane.

stomach p., a pump for removing the contents from the stomach.

punchdrunk (punch'drunk) a traumatic encephalopathy of prizefighters resulting from cumulative cerebral concussions, with general slowing of mental functions, bouts of confusion, and scattered memory loss.

punctate (pungk'tāt) spotted; marked with points or punctures.

punctiform (pungk'tĭ-form) like a point.

punctograph (punk'to-graf) an instrument for radiographic localization of foreign bodies.

punctum (pungk'tum), pl. *punc'ta* [L.] a point or small spot.

p. cae'cum, blind spot.

punc'ta doloro'sa, Valleix's points.

p. lacrima'le (pl. *punc'ta lacrima'lia*), an opening of a lacrimal duct on the edge of the eyelid.

p. prox'imum, near point.

p. remo'tum, far point.

punc'ta vasculo'sa, minute red spots that mark the cut surface of white matter of the brain.

puncture (pungk'tur) the act of piercing or penetrating with a pointed object or instrument; a wound so made.

cisternal p., puncture of the cisterna cerebellomedullaris just below the occipital bone to obtain a specimen of cerebrospinal fluid (see also CISTERNAL PUNCTURE).

lumbar p., puncture of the subarachnoid space in the region of the lumbar vertebrae (see also LUMBAR PUNCTURE).

spinal p., puncture of the spinal canal (see also SPINAL PUNCTURE).

sternal p., removal of bone marrow from the manubrium of the sternum through a spinal puncture needle (see also STERNAL PUNCTURE).

P.U.O. pyrexia of unknown origin.

pupa (pu′pah), pl. *pu′pae* [L.] the second stage in the development of an insect, between the larva and the imago. adj., **pu′pal.**

pupil (pu′pil) the opening in the center of the iris (see Plate 15).

Adie's p., one that responds to accommodation and convergence in a slow, delayed fashion, as in ADIE'S SYNDROME.

Argyll Robertson p., one that is miotic and responds to accommodation effort, but not to light.

fixed p., a pupil that does not react either to light or on convergence, or in accommodation.

Hutchinson's p., one that is dilated while the other not.

tonic p., Adie's pupil.

pupilla (pu-pil′ah) [L.] pupil.

pupillometer (pu″pĭ-lom′ĕ-ter) an instrument for measuring the width or diameter of the pupil.

pupillometry (pu″pĭ-lom′ĕ-tre) measurement of the diameter or width of the pupil of the eye.

pupilloplegia (pu″pĭ-lo-ple′je-ah) Adie's pupil.

pupilloscopy (pu″pĭ-los′ko-pe) skiametry; retinoscopy.

pupillostatometer (pu″pĭ-lo-stah-tom′ĕ-ter) an instrument for measuring the distance between the pupils.

purgation (per-ga′shun) catharsis; purging effected by a cathartic medicine.

purgative (per′gah-tiv) 1. cathartic (1); causing bowel evacuation. 2. a cathartic, particularly one stimulating peristaltic action.

purge (perj) 1. a purgative medicine or dose. 2. to cause free evacuation of feces.

purinase (pu′rĭ-nās) an enzyme that catalyzes purine conversions.

purine (pu′rēn) a compound, not found in nature, but variously substituted to produce a group of compounds, purines or purine bases, of which uric acid is a metabolic end product.

p.-free diet, a diet sometimes used in the treatment of GOUT, omitting meat, fowl, and fish, but using eggs, cheese, and vegetables. The following foods are especially high in purines: kidney, liver, sweetbreads, sardines, anchovies, and meat extracts.

Purinethol (pu′rēn-thol) trademark for a preparation of mercaptopurine, an antineoplastic agent.

Purkinje's cells (pur-kin′jēz) large, branched cells of the middle layer of the brain.

Purkinje's fibers (pur-kin′jēz) modified cardiac muscle fibers in the subendothelial tissue, concerned with conducting impulses to the heart.

Purodigin (pu″ro-dij′in) trademark for a preparation of crystalline digitoxin, a heart stimulant.

puromycin (pu″ro-mi′sin) an antineoplastic and antitrypanosomal antibiotic produced by *Streptomyces alboniger.*

purple (pur′p′l) 1. a color between blue and red. 2. a substance of this color used as a dye or indicator.

visual p., rhodopsin.

purpura (per′pu-rah) a hemorrhagic disease characterized by extravasation of blood into the tissues, under the skin and through the mucous membranes, and producing spontaneous ecchymoses (bruises) and petechiae (small red patches) on the skin. When the disorder is accompanied by a decrease in the circulating platelets, it is called thrombocytopenic purpura; when there is no decrease in the platelet count, it is called nonthrombocytopenic purpura. adj., **purpu′ric.**

There are two general types of purpura: primary or idiopathic thrombocytopenic purpura, in which the cause is unknown, and secondary or symptomatic thrombocytopenic purpura, which may be associated with exposure to drugs or other chemical agents, systemic diseases such as anemia and leukemia, diseases affecting the bone marrow or spleen, and infectious diseases such as rubella (German measles).

SYMPTOMS. The outward manifestations and laboratory findings of purpura are similar. There is evidence of bleeding under the skin, with easy bruising and the development of petechiae. In the acute form there may be bleeding from any of the body orifices, such as hematuria, nosebleed, vaginal bleeding, and bleeding gums. In the thrombocytopenic form, PLATELET count is below 100,000 per cubic millimeter of blood and may go as low as 10,000 per cubic millimeter (normal count is about 250,000 per cubic millimeter). The bleeding time is prolonged and clot retraction is poor. Coagulation time is normal.

TREATMENT. Differential diagnosis is necessary to determine the type of purpura present and to eliminate the cause if it can be determined. General measures include protection of the patient from trauma, elective surgery, and tooth extractions, any one of which may lead to severe or even fatal hemorrhage. In the thrombocytopenic form, corticosteroids may be administered when the purpura is moderately severe and of short duration. Splenectomy is indicated when other, more conservative measures fail and is successful in a majority of cases. In some instances, especially in children, there may be spontaneous and permanent recovery from idiopathic purpura.

allergic p., anaphylactic p., Schönlein-Henoch purpura.

annular telangiectatic p., a rare form in which punctate erythematous lesions coalesce to form an annular or serpiginous pattern. Called also Majocchi's disease.

fibrinolytic p., purpura associated with increased fibrinolytic activity of the blood.

p. ful′minans, a form of nonthrombocytopenic purpura seen mainly in children, usually after an infectious disease, marked by fever, shock, anemia, and sudden, rapidly spreading symmetrical skin hemorrhages of the lower limbs, often associated with extensive intravascular thromboses and gangrene.

p. hemorrha′gica, idiopathic thrombocytopenic purpura.

Henoch's p., Schönlein-Henoch purpura in which abdominal symptoms predominate.

nonthrombocytopenic p., purpura without any decrease in the platelet count of the blood. In such cases the cause of purpura is either abnormal capillary fragility or a clotting factor deficiency.

Schönlein's p., Schönlein-Henoch purpura in which articular systems predominate; called also Schönlein's disease.

Schönlein-Henoch p., nonthrombocytopenic purpura of unknown cause, most often seen in children, associated with various clinical symptoms, such as urticaria and erythema, arthropathy and arthritis, gastrointestinal symptoms, and renal involvement. Called also Schönlein-Henoch disease.

p. seni'lis, dark purplish red ecchymoses occurring on the forearms and backs of the hands in the elderly.

thrombocytopenic p., purpura associated with a decrease in the number of platelets in the blood.

thrombotic thrombocytopenic p., a disease marked by thrombocytopenia, hemolytic anemia, neurological manifestations, azotemia, fever, and thromboses in terminal arterioles and capillaries.

purpureaglycoside (per-pu″re-ah-gli′ko-sīd) a cardiac glycoside from the leaves of *Digitalis purpurea.*

p. C, deslanoside.

purpurin (per′pu-rin) 1. a red coloring matter of the urine; called also uroerythrin. 2. a dye from madder root.

purulence (pu′roo-lens) the formation or presence of pus.

purulent (pu′roo-lent) containing or forming pus.

puruloid (pu′roo-loid) resembling pus.

pus (pus) a protein-rich liquid inflammation product made up of cells (leukocytes), a thin fluid (liquor puris), and cellular debris.

blue p., pus with a bluish tint, produced by *Pseudomonas aeruginosa.*

pustula (pus′tu-lah), pl. *pus′tulae* [L.] pustule.

pustulation (pus″tu-la′shun) the formation of pustules.

pustular (pus′tu-lar) pertaining to or of the nature of a pustule; consisting of pustules.

pustule (pus′tūl) a small, elevated, circumscribed, pus-containing lesion of the skin.

pustulosis (pus″tu-lo′sis) a condition marked by an eruption of pustules.

putamen (pu-ta′men) the larger and more lateral part of the lenticular nucleus.

Putnam-Dana syndrome (put′nam-da′nah) see subacute combined DEGENERATION of spinal cord.

putrefaction (pu″trĕ-fak′shun) enzymatic decomposition, especially of proteins, with the production of foul-smelling compounds, such as hydrogen sulfide, ammonia, and mercaptans. adj., **putrefac′tive.**

putrefy (pu′trĕ-fi) to undergo putrefaction.

putrescence (pu-tres′ens) the condition of undergoing putrefaction. adj., **putres′cent.**

putrescine (pu-tres′in) a poisonous bacterial decomposition product found in decaying meat, formed by decarboxylation or ornithine.

putrid (pu′trid) rotten; putrified.

PVP polyvinylpyrrolidone (see POVIDONE).

PVP-I povidone-iodine.

pyarthrosis (pi″ar-thro′sis) suppuration within a joint cavity; acute suppurative arthritis.

pyel(o)- word element [Gr.], *renal pelvis.*

pyelectasis (pi″ĕ-lek′tah-sis) dilatation of the renal pelvis.

pyelitis (pi″ĕ-li′tis) inflammation of the renal pelvis, the outer basin-like portion of the kidney at the attachment of the ureter. adj., **pyelit′ic.**

Pyelitis is a fairly common disease, and usually can be diagnosed and cured without great difficulty. Prompt and effective treatment is necessary to prevent the spread of infection and the development of pyelonephritis, a severely disabling disease in the chronic form, in which damage to the kidney cells may lead to high blood pressure and uremia.

CAUSE. Pyelitis is usually caused by a microorganism such as *Escherichia coli* or (less often) streptococcus or staphylococcus, which may invade the kidneys by way of the blood. Pyelitis may also arise from an infection of the bladder (CYSTITIS).

The disease is most common among young children, affecting females far more often than males because the urethra is considerably shorter in the female than in the male. This favors ascending infections from the outside to enter the bladder. Female children not properly trained in their toilet habits will, after bowel movements, rub the toilet tissue from the anus forward toward the vagina rather than vice versa. In this way the bacteria so commonly found in fecal matter find their way into the urinary bladder and from there to the pelvis of the kidney.

Any urinary obstruction can sharply increase the chances of the development of pyelitis, since obstruction interferes with the normal ability of the kidney to rid the body of harmful bacteria.

SYMPTOMS. Probably the most common symptoms of pyelitis are frequency and urgency of urination and dysuria. Other possible symptoms include fever, chills, headache, and pain in one or both sides of the lower back. Pyelitis may also be present without any outward symptoms, but urinalysis will reveal many pus cells and occasionally erythrocytes.

TREATMENT. Pyelitis and pyelonephritis can usually be treated quite successfully with sulfonamides. Certain antibiotics are also helpful, and so are the urinary antiseptics. If the disease is treated promptly, the patient can look forward to early and complete recovery.

cystic p., pyelitis with formation of multiple submucosal cysts.

pyelocaliectases (pi″ĕ-lo-kal″e-ek′tah-sis) dilation of the renal pelvis and calices.

pyelocystis (pi″ĕ-lo-sis-ti′tis) inflammation of the renal pelvis and bladder.

pyelogram (pi′ĕ-lo-gram″) the film produced by pyelography.

pyelography (pi″ĕ-log′rah-fe) roentgenography of the kidney and ureter after injection of a contrast medium, introduced by the intravenous or retrograde method. Preparation of the patient for pyelography includes clearing the intestinal tract of as much fecal material and gas as possible so that there can be adequate visualization of the urinary tract structures. Usually this is accomplished by administration of castor oil and enemas. The evening before the examination the patient is given a light meal and then all foods and fluids are restricted after 9:00 P.M.

In the intravenous method the contrast medium is injected intravenously at designated intervals and x-ray films are taken to observe the rate of excretion, the concentration of the contrast medium in the pelvis and calices of the kidney, and the outline of the ureters and urinary bladder. The possibility of an allergic reaction to the contrast medium must always be considered. Drugs such as epinephrine and hydrocortisone should be on hand for use in the event of a serious allergic reaction. The patient may experience a mild transitory sensation of warmth, flushing of the face, or a salty taste in the mouth, but these should last only a few moments. Symptoms of ANAPHYLACTIC SHOCK demand immediate treatment.

Retrograde pyelography involves introduction of the contrast medium by way of ureteral catheters. This procedure may be done when special studies of certain parts of the urinary tract are indicated, or when adequate concentration of the contrast medium cannot be achieved by the intravenous method.

pyelolithotomy (pi″ĕ-lo-lĭ-thot′o-me) incision of the renal pelvis for removal of calculi.

pyelonephritis (pi″ĕ-lo-nĕ-fri′tis) inflammation of the kidney and renal pelvis (see also PYELITIS and NEPHRITIS). Called also nephropyelitis.

pyelonephrosis (pi″ĕ-lo-nĕ-fro′sis) any disease of the kidney and its pelvis.

pyelopathy (pi″ĕ-lop′ah-the) any disease of the renal pelvis.

pyeloplasty (pi′ĕ-lo-plas″te) plastic repair of the renal pelvis.

pyeloplication (pi″ĕ-lo-pli-ka′shun) reduction in size of a dilated renal pelvis by surgical infolding of its walls.

pyelostomy (pi″ĕ-los′to-me) the operation of forming an opening in the renal pelvis for the purpose of temporarily diverting the urine from the ureter.

pyelotomy (pi″ĕ-lot′o-me) incision of the renal pelvis.

pyelovenous (pi″ĕ-lo-ve′nus) pertaining to the renal pelvis and renal veins.

pyemesis (pi-em′ĕ-sis) the vomiting of pus.

pyemia (pi-e′me-ah) septicemia in which secondary foci of suppuration occur and multiple abscesses are formed. adj., **pye′mic.**

arterial p., a form due to the dissemination of septic emboli from the heart.

cryptogenic p., that in which the source of infection is in an unidentified tissue.

Pyemotes (pi″ĕ-mo′tēz) a genus of parasitic mites.

P. ventrico′sus, a species that attacks certain insect larvae found on straw, grain, and other plants, and causes a dermatitis in man (grain itch).

pyencephalus (pi″en-sef′ah-lus) abscess of the brain.

pygal (pi′gal) pertaining to the buttocks.

pygalgia (pi-gal′je-ah) pain in the buttocks.

pygoamorphus (pi″go-ah-mor′fus) asymmetrical conjoined twins, in which the parasite is an amorphous mass attached to the sacral region of the autosite.

pygodidymus (pi″go-did′ĭ-mus) a fetus with double hips and pelvis.

pygomelus (pi-gom′ĕ-lus) a fetus with a supernumerary limb or limbs attached to or near the buttocks.

pygopagus (pi-gop′ah-gus) conjoined twins fused in the sacral region.

pykn(o)- word element [Gr.], *thick; compact; frequent.*

pyknic (pik′nik) having a short, thick, stocky build.

pyknocyte (pik′no-sīt) a distorted and contracted, occasionally spiculed erythrocyte.

pyknocytosis (pik″no-si-to′sis) conspicuous increase in the number of pyknocytes.

pyknodysostosis (pik″no-dis″os-to′sis) a hereditary syndrome of dwarfism, osteopetrosis, and skeletal anomalies of the cranium, digits, and mandible.

pyknometer (pik-nom′ĕ-ter) an instrument for determining the specific gravity of fluids.

pyknomorphous (pik″no-mor′fus) having the stained portions of the cell body compactly arranged.

pyknophrasia (pik″no-fra′ze-ah) thickness of speech.

pyknosis (pik-no′sis) a thickening, especially degeneration of a cell in which the nucleus shrinks in size and the chromatin condenses to a solid, structureless mass or masses. adj., **pyknot′ic.**

pyle- word element [Gr.], *portal vein.*

pylephlebectasis (pi″le-flĕ-bek′tah-sis) dilatation of the portal vein.

pylephlebitis (pi″le-flĕ-bi′tis) inflammation of the portal vein.

pylethrombophlebitis (pi″le-throm″bo-flĕ-bi′tis) thrombosis and inflammation of the portal vein.

pylethrombosis (pi″le-throm-bo′sis) thrombosis of the portal vein.

pylor(o)- word element [Gr.], *pylorus.*

pyloralgia (pi″lo-ral′je-ah) pain in the region of the pylorus.

pylorectomy (pi″lo-rek′to-me) excision of the pylorus.

pyloric (pi-lor′ik) pertaining to the pylorus or to the pyloric part of the stomach.

p. stenosis, obstruction of the pyloric orifice of the stomach; it may be congenital as in hypertrophic pyloric stenosis, or acquired, due to peptic ulceration or prepyloric carcinoma.

The initial symptom is vomiting, mild at first but becoming increasingly more forceful. It can occur both during and after feedings. Diagnosis may be confirmed by x-ray examination using a barium meal.

Treatment is usually surgical, involving longitudinal splitting of the muscle (pyloromyotomy).

pylorodiosis (pi-lor″o-di-o′sis) dilatation of a pyloric stricture with the fingers during a surgical operation.

pyloroduodenitis (pi-lor″o-du″o-dĕ-ni′tis) inflammation of the pyloric and duodenal mucosa.

pylorogastrectomy (pi-lor″o-gas-trek′to-me) excision of the pylorus and adjacent portion of the stomach.

pyloromyotomy (pi-lor″o-mi-ot′o-me) incision of the longitudinal and circular muscles of the pylorus.

pyloroplasty (pi-lor′o-plas″te) plastic surgery of the pylorus, especially for pyloric stricture, to provide a larger communication between the stomach and duodenum.

Finney p., enlargement of the pyloric canal by establishment of an inverted U-shaped anastomosis between the stomach and duodenum after longitudinal incision.

Heineke-Mikulicz p., enlargement of a pyloric stricture by incising the pylorus longitudinally and suturing the incision transversely.

pyloroscopy (pi-lor-os′ko-pe) endoscopic inspection of the pylorus.

pylorospasm (pi-lor′o-spazm) spasm of the pylorus or of the pyloric portion of the stomach.

pylorostenosis (pi-lor″o-stĕ-no-sis) pyloric stenosis.

pylorostomy (pi″lor-os′to-me) surgical formation of an opening through the abdominal wall into the stomach near the pylorus.

pylorotomy (pi″lor-ot′o-me) incision of the pylorus.

pylorus (pi-lor′us) the distal aperture of the stomach, opening into the duodenum. The term pylorus is variously used to mean the pyloric part of the stomach, and the pyloric antrum, canal, opening, or sphincter. A ring of muscles, the pyloric sphincter, serves as a "gate," closing the opening from the stomach to the intestine. It opens periodically, allowing the contents of the stomach to move into the duodenum. The pylorus contains many glands that help produce hydrochloric acid.

Occasionally, in infants, the pyloric muscle is greatly enlarged and thickened, so that emptying of the stomach is prevented. This condition, hypertrophic pyloric obstruction or PYLORIC STENOSIS, can be corrected by surgery.

pyo- word element [Gr.], *pus.*

pyocele (pi′o-sēl) a collection of pus, as in the scrotum.

pyocephalus (pi″o-sef′ah-lus) the presence of purulent fluid in the cerebral ventricles.

pyochezia (pi″o-ke′ze-ah) the presence of pus in the feces.

pyococcus (pi″o-kok′us) a pus-forming coccus.

pyocolpocele (pi″o-kol′po-sēl) a vaginal tumor containing pus.

pyocolpos (pi″o-kol′pos) pus in the vagina.

pyocyanase (pi″o-si′ah-nās) an antibacterial substance from cultures of *Pseudomonas aeruginosa* (*pyocyanea*); bactericidal for many bacteria and lytic for some (*Vibrio cholerae*).

pyocyanic (pi″o-si-an′ik) pertaining to blue pus, or to *Pseudomonas aeruginosa.*

pyocyanin (pi″o-si′ah-nin) a blue-green antibiotic pigment produced by *Pseudomonas aeruginosa;* it gives the color to "blue pus."

pyocyst (pi′o-sist) a cyst containing pus.

pyoderma (pi″o-der′mah) any purulent skin disease.

p. gangreno′sum, a rapidly evolving cutaneous ulcer or ulcers, with undermining of the border. Once regarded as a complication peculiar to ulcerative colitis, it is now known to occur in other wasting diseases.

pyodermia (pi″o-der′me-ah) pyoderma.

pyogenesis (pi″o-jen′ĕ-sis) the formation of pus.

pyogenic (pi″o-jen′ik) producing pus.

pyohemia (pi″o-he′me-ah) pyemia.

pyohemothorax (pi″o-he″mo-tho′raks) pus and blood in the pleural cavity.

pyoid (pi′oid) resembling or like pus.

pyolabyrinthitis (pi″o-lab″ĭ-rin-thi′tis) inflammation of the labyrinth of the ear, with suppuration.

pyometra (pi″o-me′trah) an accumulation of pus within the uterus.

pyometritis (pi″o-me-tri′tis) purulent inflammation of the uterus.

pyonephritis (pi″o-nĕ-fri′tis) purulent inflammation of the kidney.

pyonephrolithiasis (pi″o-nef″ro-lĭ-thi′ah-sis) pus and calculi in the kidney.

pyonephrosis (pi″o-nĕf-ro′sis) suppurative destruction of the renal parenchyma, with total or almost complete loss of kidney function.

pyo-ovarium (pi″o-o-va′re-um) an abscess of the ovary.

pyopericarditis (pi″o-per″ĭ-kar-di′tis) purulent pericarditis.

pyopericardium (pi″o-per″ĭ-kar′de-um) pus in the pericardium.

pyoperitoneum (pi″o-per″ĭ-to-ne′um) pus in the peritoneal cavity.

pyoperitonitis (pi″o-per″ĭ-to-ni′tis) purulent inflammation of the peritoneum.

pyophthalmitis (pi″of-thal-mi′tis) purulent inflammation of the eye.

pyophysometra (pi″o-fi″so-me′trah) pus and gas in the uterus.

pyopneumocholecystitis (pi″o-nu″mo-ko″le-sis-ti′tis) distention of the gallbladder, with the presence of pus and gas.

pyopneumohepatitis (pi″o-nu″mo-hep″ah-ti′tis) abscess of the liver with pus and gas in the abscess cavity.

pyopneumopericardium (pi″o-nu″mo-per″ĭ-kar′de-um) pus and gas in the pericardium.

pyopneumoperitonitis (pi″o-nu″mo-per″ĭ-to-ni′tis) peritonitis with the presence of pus and gas.

pyopneumothorax (pi″o-nu″mo-tho′raks) pus and air or gas within the pleural cavity.

pyoptysis (pi-op′tĭ-sis) expectoration of purulent matter.

pyopyelectasis (pi″o-pi″ĕ-lek′tah-sis) dilatation of the renal pelvis with pus.

pyorrhea (pi″o-re′ah) a copious discharge of pus.

p. alveola′ris, a purulent inflammation of the dental periosteum, with progressive necrosis of the alveoli and looseness of the teeth (see also PERIODONTITUS).

pyosalpingitis (pi″o-sal″pin-ji′tis) purulent salpingitis.

pyosalpingo-oophoritis (pi″o-sal-ping″go-o″of-o-ri′tis) purulent inflammation of the uterine tube and ovary.

pyosalpinx (pi″o-sal′pinks) an accumulation of pus in a uterine tube.

pyostatic (pi″o-stat′ik) arresting suppuration; an agent that arrests suppuration.

pyothorax (pi″o-tho′raks) an accumulation of pus in the thorax (see also EMPYEMA).

pyoureter (pi″o-u-re′ter) pus in the ureter.

pyoxanthine (pi″o-zan′thēn) a brownish pigment from oxidation of pyocyanine.

pyoxanthose (pi″o-zan′thōs) a yellow pigment produced by the oxidation of pyocyanin.

pyramid (pir′ah-mid) a pointed or cone-shaped structure or part.

p. of cerebellum, pyramid of vermis.

p. of light, a triangular reflection seen upon the tympanic membrane.

malpighian p's, renal pyramids.
p's of the medulla oblongata, either of two rounded masses, one on either side of the median fissure of the medulla oblongata.
renal p's, the conical masses constituting the medulla of the kidney, the base toward the cortex and culminating at the summit in the renal papilla.
p. of thyroid, an occasional third lobe of the thyroid gland, extending upward from the isthmus.
p. of tympanum, the hollow elevation in the inner wall of the middle ear that contains the stapedius muscle.
p. of vermis, the part of the vermis cerebelli between the tuber vermis and the uvula.

pyramidal (pi-ram′ĭ-dal) shaped like a pyramid.
p. tracts, collections of motor nerve fibers arising in the brain and passing down through the spinal cord to motor cells in the anterior horns.

pyramis (pir′ah-mis), pl. *pyram′ides* [Gr.] pyramid.

pyran (pi′ran) a cyclic compound in which the ring consists of 5 carbon atoms and 1 oxygen atom.

pyranose (pi′rah-nōs) a hexose having a ring structure analogous to pyran.

pyrantel (pĭ-ran′tel) an anthelminthic, used as the pamoate and tartrate salts.

pyrathiazine (pi″rah-thi′ah-zēn) a phenothiazine derivative; the hydrochloride salt is used as an antihistaminic.

pyrazinamide (pi″rah-zin′ah-mīd) a tuberculostatic antibacterial.

pyrectic (pi-rek′tik) 1. pertaining to fever; feverish. 2. a fever-inducing agent.

pyretic (pi-ret′ik) pertaining to fever.

pyretogenesis (pi-re″to-jen′ĕ-sis) the origin and causation of fever.

pyretogenous (pi″rĕ-toj′ĕ-nus) 1. caused by high fever. 2. pyrogenic.

pyretotherapy (pi-re″to-ther′ah-pe) 1. treatment by artificially increasing the patient's body temperature. 2. the treatment of fever.

pyrexia (pi-rek′se-ah) a fever, or febrile condition. adj., **pyrex′ial.**

Pyribenzamine (pir″ĭ-ben′zah-mēn) trademark for preparations of tripelennamine, an antihistaminic.

pyridine (pir′ĭ-dēn, pir′ĭ-din) 1. a substance derived from coal tar and also from tobacco and various organic matter. 2. any of a group of substances homologous with normal pyridine.

pyridostigmine (pir″ĭ-do-stig′mēn) a cholinesterase inhibitor; the bromide salt is used in the treatment of myasthenia gravis.

pyridoxal (pir″ĭ-dok′sal) a form of vitamin B_6.

pyridoxamine (pir″ĭ-doks′ah-mēn) one of the three active forms of vitamin B_6.

pyridoxine (pir″ĭ-dok′sēn) one of the forms of vitamin B_6, chiefly used, as the hydrochloride salt, in the prophylaxis and treatment of vitamin B_6 deficiency. It is also used in counteracting the neurotoxic effects of isoniazid, and sometimes in the treatment of myasthenia gravis.

pyrilamine (pi-ril′ah-mēn) an antihistaminic, used as the hydrochloride salt.

pyrimethamine (pi″rĭ-meth′ah-mēn) an antimalarial used especially for suppressive prophylaxis.

pyrimidine (pi-rim′ĭ-dēn) an organic compound that is the fundamental form of the pyrimidine bases, including uracil, cytosine, and thymine.

pyrithiamine (pir″ĭ-thi′ah-min) an analogue of thiamine which by metabolic competition can cause symptoms of thiamine deficiency.

pyro- word element [Gr.], *fire; heat;* (in chemistry) *produced by heating.*

pyrogallol (pi″ro-gal′ol) pyrogallic acid, derived from gallic acid and used externally as an antimicrobial and irritant.

pyrogen (pi′ro-jen) an agent that causes fever. adj., **pyrogen′ic.**

pyroglobulinemia (pi″ro-glob″u-lin-e′me-ah) the presence in the blood of an abnormal globulin constituent that is precipitated by heat.

pyromania (pi″ro-ma′ne-ah) obsessive preoccupation with fire; a morbid compulsion to set fires.

pyrometer (pi-rom′ĕ-ter) a device for measuring high degrees of heat.

Pyronil (pi′ro-nil) trademark for a preparation of pyrrobutamine, an antihistaminic.

pyronine (pi′ro-nin) a red aniline histologic stain.

pyrophobia (pi″ro-fo′be-ah) morbid dread of fire.

pyrophosphatase (pi″ro-fos′fah-tās) any enzyme that catalyzes the hydrolysis of central pyrophosphate linkages.

pyrophosphate (pi″ro-fos′fāt) any salt of pyrophosphoric acid.

pyrosis (pi-ro′sis) HEARTBURN; a burning sensation in the esophagus and stomach, with sour eructation.

pyrotic (pi-rot′ik) caustic; burning.

pyroxylin (pi-rok′sĭ-lin) a product of the action of a mixture of nitric and sulfuric acids on cotton, consisting chiefly of cellulose tetranitrate; a necessary ingredient of collodion.

pyrrobutamine (pir″o-bu′tah-min) an antihistaminic.

pyrrocaine (pir′o-kān) a local anesthetic used in dentistry as the hydrochloride salt.

pyrrole (pir′ōl) a basic, cyclic substance, obtained by destructive distillation of various animal substances.

pyrrolidine (pĭ-rol′ĭ-din) a simple base obtained from tobacco or prepared from pyrrole.

pyruvate (pi′roo-vāt) a salt or ester of pyruvic acid; in biochemistry, the term is used interchangeably with pyruvic acid.

pyruvic acid (pi-roo′vik) a compound formed in the body in aerobic metabolism of carbohydrate; also formed by dry distillation of tartaric acid.

pyrvinium (pir-vin′e-um) an anthelmintic used for intestinal pinworms in the form of the pamoate salt.

pyuria (pi-u′re-ah) pus in the urine.

PZI protamine zinc insulin.

Q

Q. quadrant.

q.d. [L.] *qua'que di'e* (every day).

Q fever a febrile rickettsial infection caused by *Coxiella burnetii.* The causative microorganisms are found on the hides of sheep and cattle, and it is thought that human beings contract the disease by breathing in the dried microorganisms carried in dust particles in the air. In Australia, where the disease was first described, it is transmitted by ticks. Symptoms include sudden high fever, chills, headache, muscle pains, and coughing. The disease usually is quickly brought under control by antibiotics. The Q stands for query.

q.h. [L.] *qua'que ho'ra* (every hour).

q.i.d. [L.] *qua'ter in di'e* (four times a day).

q.q.h. [L.] *qua'que quar'ta ho'ra* (every 4 hours).

QRS complex a group of waves depicted on an electrocardiogram; called also the QRS wave. It actually consists of three distinct waves created by the passage of the cardiac electrical impulse through the ventricles and occurs at the beginning of each contraction of the ventricles. In a normal ELECTROCARDIOGRAM the R wave is the most prominent of the three; the Q and S waves may be extremely weak and sometimes are absent.

One abnormality of the QRS complex is increased voltage resulting from enlargement of heart muscle, which produces increased quantities of electric current. This enlargement is caused by an excessive work load for some part of the heart and usually is due to a defect in the heart valves or great vessels near the heart.

A low-voltage QRS complex may result from local intraventricular block, toxic conditions of the heart, and fluid in the pericardium. Pleural effusion and emphysema also can cause a decrease in the voltage of the QRS complex.

q.s. [L.] *quan'tum sa'tis* (a sufficient amount).

qt. quart.

quack (kwak) one who misrepresents his ability and experience in diagnosis and treatment of disease or the effects to be achieved by his treatment.

quackery (kwak'er-e) the practice or methods of a quack.

quadr(i)- word element [L.], *four.*

quadrangular (kwod-rang'gu-lar) having four angles.

quadrant (kwod'rant) 1. one-fourth of the circumference of a circle. 2. one of four corresponding parts, or quarters, as of the surface of the abdomen or of the field of vision.

quadrantanopia (kwod″ran-tah-no'pe-ah) defective vision or blindness in one fourth of the visual field.

quadrantanopsia (kwod″ran-tah-nop'se-ah) quandrantanopia.

quadrate (kwod'rāt) square or squared.

quadriceps (kwod'rĭ-seps) having four heads. **q. muscle,** a name applied collectively to four muscles, the rectus of the thigh and intermediate lateral and medial great muscles, inserting by a common tendon that surrounds the patella and ends on the tuberosity of the tibia, and acting to extend the leg upon the thigh. (See Plate 3.)

quadrigemina (kwod″rĭ-jem'ĭ-nah) the corpora quadrigemina.

quadrigeminal (kwod″rĭ-jem'ĭ-nal) fourfold; in four parts; forming a group of four.

quadrilateral (kwod″rĭ-lat'er-al) having four sides.

quadrilocular (kwod″rĭ-lok'u-lar) having four cavities.

quadripara (kwod-rip'ah-rah) a woman who has had four pregnancies that resulted in viable offspring; para IV.

quadripartite (kwod″rĭ-par'tīt) divided into four.

quadriplegia (kwod″rĭ-ple'je-ah) paralysis of all four limbs; tetraplegia. adj., **quadriple'gic.**

PATIENT CARE. The quadriplegic patient is paralyzed from the neck down and is, therefore, subject to the many problems associated with immobility and loss of sensation. The immediate goal of care is the prevention of infection and the maintenance of the integrity of the body systems so that optimum rehabilitation can be achieved. The extent to which the patient may eventually achieve mobility in a wheelchair and some degree of independence is greatly affected by the caliber of care received and the motivation and drive of the individual patient.

Mechanical devices such as braces and crutches are helpful in compensating for the loss of muscular function. PHYSICAL THERAPY procedures and techniques and OCCUPATIONAL THERAPY are essential aspects of patient care and are vital to the attainment of the goals of REHABILITATION. (See also PARAPLEGIA.)

Patient education is especially important to the long-range goal of prevention of serious complications. The patient and his family should be aware of the early signs and symptoms of breakdown of the skin (DECUBITUS ULCER), FECAL IMPACTION, a developing infection, and urinary difficulties. As with any type of long-term care, the patient should be medically evaluated periodically and his care should be under the supervision of a visiting nurse. In spite of the many difficulties that may be encountered by the paralyzed patient, it is possible for these patients to lead useful and personally rewarding lives.

quadrisect (kwod'rĭ-sekt) to cut into four parts.

quadritubercular (kwod″rĭ-tu-ber'ku-lar) having four tubercles or cusps.

quadrivalent (kwod″rĭ-va'lent, kwod-riv'ah-lent) having a valence of four.

quadruped (kwod'roo-ped) 1. four-footed. 2. an animal having four feet.

quadruplet (kwah-drup'let, kwah-droo'plet, kwod'roo-plet) one of four offspring produced at one birth.

qualimeter (kwah-lim'ĭ-ter) an instrument for measuring the penetrating power of x-rays; penetrometer.

quality assurance in the health care field, a pledge to the public by those within the various health disciplines that they will work toward the goal of an optimal achievable degree of excellence in the services rendered to every patient. Since the 1960's there has been an increasing emphasis on the individual citizen's right to health and the obligation of individual members of the health care team to hold themselves accountable to the public for the caliber of care they provide.

A quality assurance program takes into account the need to define that which is to be measured. Quality assurance implies a clear understanding of what is meant by "quality" and a valid and reliable method for evaluating the care that is provided. (See also EVALUATION.) In the health care field, evaluation of practice operates within the parameters of *outcome, cost-benefit,* and *access* to the health care delivery system. Outcome represents a measurable change in the health/illness status of the patient that is the end result of the care the patient received. Cost-benefit refers to the expenditure of money, time, and effort in providing health care and the relationship this cost bears to the actual benefits to the recipient. Access to health care refers to its availability, the ease with which one can obtain the kind of health care he needs.

Implementation of a quality assurance program involves the development of criteria based on acceptable standards of care and norms of professional behavior. The norms are established by members of the profession who are expert in the care of specific patient populations. The health/illness criteria should be patient-centered: they must express in positive terms what it is a patient should be able to do as a direct result of the care he has received. For example, in the area of nursing care, an elderly patient with "night incontinence" should remain dry throughout the night as a result of an individualized BLADDER TRAINING program, or a patient who is bedridden should be able to maintain joint motion as a result of a daily range-of-motion exercise program.

The development of outcome criteria is an essential first step in a quality assurance program. The criteria are then used as the "yardstick" against which actual practice and its results can be evaluated. Evaluation is conducted by a review committee, preferably one composed of practitioners in the area of health care being evaluated. A *retrospective review* measures actual documented outcomes against desirable and valued outcomes. Data for documentation of actual outcomes are obtained from the medical records of a specific patient population after the patients have been discharged. A *concurrent review* evaluates patient care while it is in progress. Documentation of the caliber of care being delivered is obtained through review of the patient's chart, interview, observation, and examination of the patient. The advantage of concurrent review is that it can provide opportunities for improvement of patient care while it is in progress.

The ultimate goal of both retrospective and concurrent review is improvement of patient care. If, at the time of review, a deficiency is detected in either the health care process or the health/illness status of the patient, an effort is made to correct the difference between "what should be" and "what actually is." It is this promise to evaluate thoroughly and to employ the results of the evaluation for continuous improvement of patient care that is the essence of quality assurance.

quantimeter (kwon-tim'ĕ-ter) an instrument for measuring the quantity of roentgen rays generated by a Coolidge tube.

quantivalence (kwon-tiv'ah-lens) valence (1).

quantum (kwon'tum), pl. *quan'ta* [L.] an elemental unit of energy; the amount emitted or absorbed at each step when energy is emitted or absorbed by atoms or molecules.

q. theory, radiation and absorption of energy occur in quantities (quanta) which vary in size with the frequency of the radiation.

quarantine (kwor'an-tēn) 1. a place or period of detention of ships coming from infected or suspected ports. 2. restrictions placed on entering or leaving premises where a case of communicable disease exists.

quart (kwort) one-fourth of a gallon (946 ml.); abbreviated qt.

quartan (kwor'tan) 1. recurring in 4-day cycles (every third day). 2. a variety of intermittent fever of which the paroxysms recur on every third day (see MALARIA).

double q., a quartan fever of which the recurrences are alternately severe and relatively mild.

triple q., a fever in which the paroxysms occur every day because of infection with three different groups of quartan parasites.

quartile (kwor'tīl, kwor'til) one of the values establishing the division of a series of variables into fourths, or the range of items included in such a segment.

quartipara (kwor-tip'ah-rah) quadripara; a woman who has had four pregnancies that resulted in viable offspring; para IV.

quater in die (kwah'ter in de'a) [L.] four times a day.

quaternary (kwah'ter-ner"e, kwah-ter'ner-e) 1. fourth in a series. 2. made up of four elements or groups.

Queckenstedt's test (kwek'en-stets") when the veins in the neck are compressed on one or both sides there is a rapid rise in the pressure of the cerebrospinal fluid of healthy persons, and this rise quickly disappears when pressure is taken off the neck. But when there is a block in the spinal canal the pressure of the cerebrospinal fluid is affected little or not at all by the maneuver.

Quelicin (kwel'ĭ-sin) trademark for a preparation of succinylcholine, a muscle relaxant.

quercetin (kwer'sĕ-tin) a form of rutin and other glycosides, used to reduce abnormal capillary fragility.

Quervain's disease (kār'vanz) inflammation of the long abductor and short extensor tendons of the thumb, with swelling and tenderness. Called also de Quervain's disease.

Quiactin (kwi-ak'tin) trademark for a preparation of oxanamide, a tranquilizer.

Quick hippuric acid excretion test (kwik) measurement of hippuric acid in the urine after ingestion of a standard dose of benzoic acid.

Quick one-stage prothrombin time test (kwik) a method of determining the integrity of the prothrombin complex in the blood; used in controlling anticoagulant therapy.

Quick tourniquet test (kwik) estimation of capillary fragility by counting the number of petechiae appearing in a limited area on the flexor surface of the forearm after obstruction to the circulation by a blood pressure cuff applied to the upper arm.

quickening (kwik′en-ing) the first perceptible movement of the fetus in the uterus, appearing usually in the sixteenth to eighteenth week of pregnancy.

quinacrine (kwin′ah-krin) an anthelmintic for tapeworms, used as the hydrochloride salt.

quinalbarbitone (kwin″al-bar′bĭ-tōn) secobarbital, a short- to intermediate-acting barbiturate.

Quincke's disease (kwink′ez) angioneurotic edema.

Quincke's pulse (kwink′ez) alternate blanching and flushing of the nail bed due to pulsation of subpapillary arteriolar and venous plexuses, as seen in aortic insufficiency.

quinestrol (kwin-es′trōl) a long-acting estrogen.

quinethazone (kwin-eth′ah-zōn) a diuretic.

quingestanol (kwin-jes′tah-nōl) a long-acting progestin.

quinic acid (kwin′ik) a crystalline compound from cinchona, coffee, and cranberries; it is converted by the body to benzoic acid and excreted as hippuric acid.

quinidine (kwin′ĭ-din) the dextrorotatory isomer of quinine, used in treatment of cardiac arrhythmias.

quinine (kwi′nīn) an alkaloid from cinchona used as an antimalarial, especially against *Plasmodium falciparum;* also used for its analgesic, oxytocic, antipyretic, and sclerosing properties, and for alleviating muscle contractures and cramps.

q. and urea hydrochloride, a double salt of quinine and urea hydrochlorides; used in treatment of malaria and as a sclerosing agent for internal hemorrhoids.

q. and urethan injection, a sterile solution containing quinine hydrochloride and urethan; a sclerosing agent for varicose veins.

q. salicylate, a salt used as an antipyretic and antirheumatic.

q. sulfate, a white crystalline salt, more largely used as a remedy than any other of the cinchona alkaloid salts.

quininism (kwin′ĭ-nizm) cinchonism; poisoning from cinchona bark or its alkaloids.

quinone (kwi-nōn′, kwin′ōn) a principle obtained by oxidizing quinic acid.

quinquevalent (kwing″kwĕ-va′lent, kwing-kwev′-ah-lent) pentavalent; having a valence of five.

quinsy (kwin′ze) peritonsillar abscess.

quint- word element [L.], *five.*

quintan (kwin′tan) recurring every 5 days (every fourth day).

q. fever, trench fever.

quintipara (kwin-tip′ah-rah) a woman who has had five pregnancies that resulted in viable offspring; para V.

quintuplet (kwin′too-plet) one of five offspring produced at one birth.

Quotane (kwo′tān) trademark for a preparation of dimethisoquin, a local anesthetic.

quotid. [L.] *quotid′ie* (every day).

quotidian (kwo-tid′e-an) 1. recurring every day. 2. a form of intermittent malarial fever with daily recurrent paroxysms.

double q., a fever having two daily paroxysms.

quotient (kwo′shent) a number obtained by division.

achievement q., the achievement age divided by the mental age, indicating progress in learning.

caloric q., the heat evolved (in calories) divided by the oxygen consumed (in milligrams) in a metabolic process.

intelligence q., I.Q., a numerical expression of intellectual capacity obtained by multiplying the mental age of the subject, ascertained by testing, by 100 and dividing by his chronologic age.

respiratory q., an expression of the ratio of the volume of expired carbon dioxide to the volume of oxygen absorbed by the lungs per unit of time.

R

R 1. symbol, *roentgen*. 2. a symbol used in general chemical formulae to represent an organic radical.

R. Rankine (scale), Réaumur (scale); [L.] *remo'tum* (far); respiration; *Rickettsia;* right.

℞ symbol [L.], *rec'ipe* (take); prescription; treatment.

Ra chemical symbol, *radium.*

rabbit fever tularemia.

rabiate, rabid (ra'be-āt, rab'id) affected with rabies; pertaining to rabies.

rabies (ra'bēz, ra'be-ēz) an acute infectious viral disease communicated to man by the bite of an infected animal and affecting the brain and the nervous system; called also hydrophobia.

Rabies is transmitted by warm-blooded animals, especially dogs, foxes, and bats. The virus is often present in the saliva of affected animals and is transmitted chiefly through bite wounds and occasionally through open wounds or sores.

After the virus enters the body it travels along the nerve trunk to the brain; the farther the bite is from the head, the longer it takes the virus to reach the brain. The incubation period varies from 2 weeks to as long as 6 months. The bitten person must start treatment with antirabies vaccine and serum before the virus reaches the brain. The disease must be prevented because it is almost invariably fatal.

PREVENTION. All warm-blooded family pets—including dogs, cats, and monkeys—should be vaccinated against rabies periodically.

It is also essential to learn to recognize a rabid animal. In the early "anxiety" stages, a rabid animal may have a change of temperament. Many, including wild animals, may become unusually friendly. The rabid animal may next enter a "furious" stage, in which it wanders about biting everything that moves, and even some things that do not move, such as sticks and stones. It then develops paralysis of the throat, which makes swallowing difficult. The name hydrophobia, "fear of water," was given to the disease because it was observed that stricken animals avoid water. Actually, they do not do so because of fear, but because they cannot swallow. Saliva often drips from the animal's mouth and may be whipped into a foam.

Some animals pass directly from the anxiety stage to paralysis without becoming violent. This is called the "dumb" form of rabies. The animal may appear to have something caught in his throat. Usually, a dog with something in his throat tries to remove it himself, but a rabid dog will not. Eventually all of the rabid animal's muscles become paralyzed and it dies.

TREATMENT. When a person is bitten by an animal the wound should be washed thoroughly with soap and water, and then treated like any other wound. It is extremely important to go to a physician immediately. If at all possible, steps should be taken to find out if the biting animal has rabies. The animal should be confined for observation. When the biting animal must be killed in order to capture it, care must be taken to see that the head is not damaged, so that the brain can be examined to establish a diagnosis. There are times when the biting animal cannot be caught for observation. If so, the bitten person must be given antirabies treatment immediately.

Preventive treatment of suspected rabies is based on immunization by a series of vaccine injections. When bites are in areas close to the head or in areas with many nerve endings, such as the hands, the virus may reach the brain very quickly. In such cases treatment should start immediately, even though the suspected animal is still being observed. Along with the vaccine, such patients are often given immune serum to establish passive immunity.

In man, rabies causes pain, fever, mental derangement, vomiting, profuse secretion of sticky saliva, convulsions, and difficulty in breathing and swallowing. Treatment is palliative and includes sedation of the patient and provision of a quiet environment to reduce anxiety and relieve pain, administration of a powerful muscle relaxant (curare-like drugs) to reduce muscular contractions, and supportive measures to maintain urinary and respiratory function. Death occurs in 2 to 5 days.

race (rās) a class or breed of animals; a group of individuals having certain characteristics in common, owing to a common inheritance.

racemase (ra'sĕ-mās) an enzyme that catalyzes the racemization of an optically active substance.

racemate (ra'sĕ-māt) a racemic compound.

racemic (ra-se'mik) optically inactive, being composed of equal amounts of dextrorotatory and levorotatory isomers.

racemization (ras"ĕ-mĭ-za'shun) the transformation of one-half of the molecules of an optically active compound into molecules that possess exactly the opposite (mirror-image) configuration, with complete loss of rotatory power because of the statistical balance between equal numbers of dextrorotatory and levorotatory molecules.

racemose (ras'ĕ-mōs) shaped like a bunch of grapes.

racephedrine (ra-sef'ĕ-drin) the racemic form of ephedrine; the hydrochloride salt is used as a sympathomimetic.

rachi(o)- word element [Gr.], *spine.*

rachialgia (ra"ke-al'je-ah) pain in the spine.

rachianesthesia (ra"ke-an"es-the'ze-ah) loss of sensation produced by injection of an anesthetic into the spinal canal.

rachicentesis (ra"kĭ-sen-te'sis) puncture into the lumbar spinal canal (see also SPINAL PUNCTURE).

rachidial, rachidian (rah-kid'e-al; rah-kid'e-an) pertaining to the spine.

rachigraph (ra'kĭ-graf) an instrument for recording the outlines of the spine and back.

rachilysis (rah-kil'ĭ-sis) correction of lateral curvature of the spine by combined traction and pressure.

rachiocampsis (ra"ke-o-kamp'sis) spinal curvature.

rachiometer (ra"ke-om'ĕ-ter) an apparatus for measuring spinal curvature.

rachiomyelitis (ra″ke-o-mi″ĕ-li′tis) inflammation of the spinal cord.

rachiotomy (ra″ke-ot′o-me) incision of a vertebra or the vertebral column.

rachipagus (ra-kip′ah-gus) twin fetuses joined at the vertebral column.

rachis (ra′kis) the vertebral column.

rachischisis (rah-kis′kĭ-sis) congenital fissure of the vertebral column.
r. poste′rior, spina bifida.

rachitic (rah-kit′ik) pertaining to rickets.

rachitis (rah-ki′tis) rickets.

rachitogenic (rah-kit″o-jen′ik) causing rickets.

rachitomy (rah-kit′o-me) the surgical or anatomic opening of the spinal canal.

rad (rad) acronym for *radiation absorbed dose;* a unit of measurement of the absorbed dose of ionizing radiation. It corresponds to an energy transfer of 100 ergs per gram of any absorbing material (including tissue).

rad. [L.] *ra′dix* (root).

radectomy (rah-dek′to-me) excision of a portion of the root of a tooth.

radiability (ra″de-ah-bil′ĭ-te) the property of being readily penetrated by roentgen or other rays.

radiad (ra′de-ad) toward the radius or radial side.

radial (ra′de-al) 1. pertaining to the radius. 2. radiating; spreading outward from a common center.
r. artery, an artery in the forearm, wrist, and hand; the one usually used for taking the PULSE.

radialis (ra″de-a′lis) [L.] radial.

radiant (ra′de-ant) 1. diverging from a center. 2. emitting rays, as of light or heat.

radiate (ra′de-āt) 1. to diverge or spread from a common point. 2. arranged in a radiating manner.

radiatio (ra″de-a′she-o), pl. *radiatio′nes* [L.] a radiating structure. In anatomy, a collection of nerve fibers connecting different portions of the brain.

radiation (ra″de-a′shun) 1. divergence from a common center. 2. a structure made up of diverging elements, especially a tract of the central nervous system made up of diverging fibers. 3. electromagnetic waves, such as those of visible light, infrared rays, ultraviolet rays, x-rays, and gamma rays, or streams of atomic particles such as alpha and beta particles.

Sources of radiation include natural or "background" radiation, such as cosmic rays from outer space, and the naturally occurring radioactive substances found in the earth. Man-made radiations result from artificially produced nuclear reactions in stable elements which are then changed to radioactive substances. (See also RADIOACTIVITY.)

KINDS OF RADIATION. Radiations are particulate and nonparticulate; that is, they may be made up of particles such as neutrons and protons, which are fragments of the nuclei of disintegrating atoms, or they may consist of electromagnetic waves, which have no mass. Particulate radiations may consist of ALPHA PARTICLES or BETA PARTICLES. Most radioactive isotopes (RADIOISOTOPES) emit particulate radiations and at the same time also release electromagnetic rays (GAMMA RAYS).

Both particulate and nonparticulate radiations are capable of penetrating and being absorbed into matter. Alpha particles are the least penetrating; beta particles slightly more penetrating; and the gamma rays, like x-rays, are capable of completely penetrating the body. This ability to penetrate matter and change the basic structure of cells of the body is used beneficially in the treatment of tumors and other medical conditions.

X-rays, called also roentgen rays, are a form of radiation consisting of energy waves of very short wavelength, which gives them their special penetrating power. They are produced by bombarding a tungsten target with highspeed electrons in a Coolidge tube. They are not visible to the human eye, but, like ordinary light, they may be captured as a visible image on film or on the specially coated screen of a FLUOROSCOPE. The degree of penetration of x-rays depends partly on the density of the matter at which they are aimed and partly on the voltage used. Equipment used for x-ray diagnosis is usually lower in voltage than that used for x-ray therapy.

The application of radiation, whether by x-ray or radioactive substances, for treatment of various illnesses is called RADIOTHERAPY or therapeutic radiation.

RADIATION HAZARDS. Harmful effects of uncontrolled radiation include serious disturbances of bone marrow and other blood-forming organs, burns, and sterility. There may be permanent damage to the germ plasm or GENES, which results in genetic mutations. The mutations can be transmitted to future generations. Radiation also may produce harmful effects on the embryo or fetus, bringing about fetal death or malformations. Studies of groups of persons exposed to long-term radiation have shown that radiation acts as a carcinogen; that is, it can produce cancer, especially leukemia. Radiation also apparently shortens the life span of those exposed to it over a period of time, and predisposes persons to the development of cataracts.

Exposure to large doses of radiation over a short period of time produces a group of symptoms known as the acute radiation syndrome. These symptoms include general malaise, nausea, and vomiting, followed by a period of remission of symptoms. Later, the patient develops more severe symptoms such as fever, hemorrhage, fluid loss, anemia, and central nervous system involvement. The symptoms then gradually subside or become more severe, and may lead to death.

RADIATION PROTECTION. In order to avoid the radiation hazards mentioned above, one must be aware of three basic principles of time, distance, and shielding involved in protection from radiation. Obviously, the longer one stays near a source of radiation the greater will be his exposure. The same is true of proximity to the source; the closer one gets to a source of radiation the greater the exposure.

Shielding is of special importance when, as in the case of physicians and hospital personnel involved in radiotherapy, time and distance cannot be completely utilized as safety factors. In such instances lead, which is an extremely dense material, is utilized as a protective device. The walls of diagnostic x-ray rooms are lined with lead, and lead containers are used for radium, cobalt-60, and other radioactive materials used in radiotherapy. X-ray therapists, radiologists and other personnel concerned with use of x-rays can obtain additional protection by wearing lead aprons and gloves.

Monitoring devices such as the film badge or pocket monitor are worn by persons working near sources of radiation. These devices contain special photographic film that is sensitive to radiation and thus serve as a guide to the amount of radiation to which a person has been exposed. For monitoring large areas in which radiation hazards may pose a problem, survey meters such as the Geiger counter may be used. The survey meter also is useful in finding sources of radiation such as a radium implant, which might be lost.

Sensible use of these protective and monitoring devices can greatly reduce unnecessary exposure to radiation and allow for full realization of the many benefits of radiation.

corpuscular r., particles emitted in nuclear disintegration, including alpha and beta particles, protons, neutrons, positrons, and deuterons.

electromagnetic r., energy, unassociated with matter, that is transmitted through space by means of waves (electromagnetic waves) traveling in all instances at 3×10^{10} cm., or 186,284 miles per second, but ranging in length from 10^{11} cm. (electrical waves) to 10^{-12} cm. (cosmic rays) and including radio waves, infrared, visible light and ultraviolet, x-rays, and gamma rays.

infrared r., the portion of the spectrum of electromagnetic radiation of wavelengths ranging between 0.75 and 1000 μm. (see also INFRARED RAYS).

interstitial r., energy emitted by radium or radon inserted directly into the tissue.

ionizing r., corpuscular or electromagnetic radiation that is capable of producing ions, directly or indirectly, in its passage through matter.

pyramidal r., fibers extending from the pyramidal tract to the cortex.

r. sickness, a condition sometimes occurring in patients who have received therapeutic doses of radiation. Its severity varies with the individual and his physical condition, the body areas exposed, and the amount, kind, and intensity of the exposure. The disease may be so slight that the exposed person scarcely notices it, or it may cause severe symptoms. With modern techniques and increased knowledge about radiation, there is a lower incidence of severe radiation sickness than formerly.

The systemic reactions to radiation include a general feeling of malaise, loss of appetite or nausea and vomiting, and headache. These symptoms tend to subside when the therapy is discontinued, leaving no permanent effect on the patient.

r. striothalam'ica, a fiber system joining the thalamus and the hypothalamic region.

tegmental r., fibers radiating laterally from the nucleus ruber.

thalamic r., fibers streaming out through the lateral surface of the thalamus, through the internal capsule to the cerebral cortex.

ultraviolet r., the portion of the spectrum of electromagnetic radiation of wavelengths ranging between 0.39 and 0.18 μm. (see also ULTRAVIOLET RAYS).

radical (rad'ĭ-kal) 1. directed to the cause; going to the root or source of a morbid process. 2. a group of atoms that enters into and goes out of chemical combination without change and that forms one of the fundamental constituents of a molecule.

acid r., the electronegative element that combines with hydrogen to form an acid.

alcohol r., all of the alcohol molecule except the hydroxyl group (—OH).

color r., chromophore.

radicle (rad'ĭ-k'l) one of the smallest branches of a vessel or nerve.

radicotomy (rad"ĭ-kot'o-me) rhizotomy; division or transection of a nerve root.

radiculalgia (rah-dik"u-lal'je-ah) pain due to disorder of the spinal nerve roots.

radicular (rah-dik'u-lar) pertaining to a root or radicle.

radiculitis (rah-dik"u-li'tis) inflammation of a spinal nerve root, especially of the portion of the root that lies between the spinal cord and the spinal canal.

radiculoganglionitis (rah-dik"u-lo-gang"gle-o-ni'tis) inflammation of the posterior spinal nerve roots and their ganglia.

radiculomedullary (rah-dik"u-lo-med'u-ler"e) affecting the nerve roots and spinal cord.

radiculomeningomyelitis (rah-dik"u-lo-mĕ-ning"go-mi"ĕ-li'tis) inflammation of the nerve roots, meninges, and spinal cord.

radiculomyelopathy (rah-dik"u-lo-mi"ĕ-lop'ah-the) disease of the nerve roots and spinal cord.

radiculoneuritis (rah-dik"u-lo-nu-ri'tis) acute febrile polyneuritis.

radiculoneuropathy (rah-dik"u-lo-nu-rop'ah-the) disease of the nerve roots and spinal nerves.

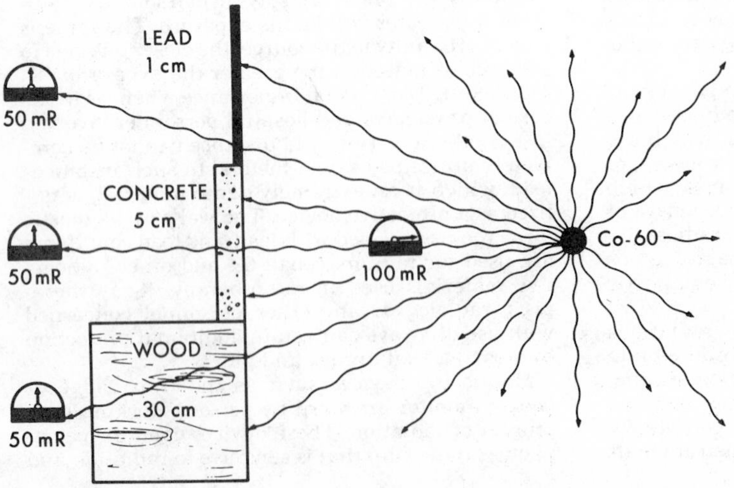

Comparison of efficacy of various materials for radiation shielding. (From Boeker, E. H.: The nurse in radiation protection. Nursing Clin. N. Amer., 2:23, 1967.)

radiculopathy (rah-dik″u-lop′ah-the) disease of the nerve roots.

radiectomy (ra″de-ek′to-me) excision of the root of a tooth.

radio- word element [L.], *ray; radiation; emission of radiant energy; radium; radius* (bone of the forearm); affixed to the name of a chemical element to designate a radioactive isotope of that element.

radioactinium (ra″de-o-ak-tin′e-um) a substance formed by the disintegration of actinium.

radioactive (ra″de-o-ak′tiv) characterized by radioactivity.

radioactivity (ra″de-o-ak-tiv′ĭ-te) the emission of particulate or electromagnetic radiations consequent to the disintegration of the nuclei of unstable or radioactive elements. These emissions or radiations include ALPHA PARTICLES, BETA PARTICLES, and GAMMA RAYS.

The property of radioactivity occurs naturally in a number of elements. In general, the chemical elements of atomic number above 83 are radioactive. Stable elements that are not naturally radioactive can be made so by bombarding isotopes of the element with high-velocity particles. When an element is unstable, whether naturally or artificially, the ratio of protons to neutrons in its atoms is uneven. Each atom attempts to achieve stability by giving off particles from its nucleus and thus it begins to disintegrate, releasing both nuclear particles and electromagnetic radiations. Since these radiations interact with matter, including the cells of the body, they can be used in medical therapy. (See also RADIATION and RADIOTHERAPY.)

The amount of radioactivity of a given substance can be measured by determining the rate at which a given number of atoms disintegrate in a given period of time. The basic unit of measurement used for radioactivity is the curie (Ci). One-thousandth of a curie is a millicurie; one-millionth of a curie is a microcurie; and one-trillionth of a curie is a picocurie. These units of measure are used to calculate the dosage of radioactivity needed for various therapeutic procedures in much the same way that units of measure such as the gram or milligram are used to measure dosage of medications. (See also RADIOISOTOPE.)

radioautogram (ra″de-o-aw′to-gram) autoradiogram.

radioautography (ra″de-o-aw-tog′rah-fe) autoradiography.

radiobicipital (ra″de-o-bi-sip′ĭ-tal) pertaining to the radius and biceps muscle of the arm.

radiobiologist (ra″de-o-bī-ol′o-jist) an expert in radiobiology.

radiobiology (ra″de-o-bi-ol′o-je) the branch of science concerned with effects of light and of ultraviolet and ionizing radiations on living tissue or organisms.

radiocalcium (ra″de-o-kal′se-um) a radioactive isotope of calcium, ^{45}Ca, with a half-life of 180 days; used as a tracer in the study of calcium metabolism.

radiocarbon (ra″de-o-kar′bon) a radioactive isotope of carbon; the isotope of mass 14 (^{14}C) is used in many diagnostic procedures and physiologic investigations; with a half-life of 5568 years, it has provided a means of determining the age of many ancient substances and articles.

radiocardiogram (ra″de-o-kar′de-o-gram″) the graphic record produced by radiocardiography.

radiocardiography (ra″de-o-kar″de-og′rah-fe) graphic recording of variation with time of the concentration, in a selected chamber of the heart, of a radioactive isotope, usually injected intravenously.

radiocarpal (ra″de-o-kar′pal) pertaining to the radius and carpus.

radiochemistry (ra″de-o-kem′is-tre) the branch of chemistry dealing with radioactive materials.

radiocinematograph (ra″de-o-sin″ĕ-mat′o-graf) an apparatus combining the moving picture camera and the x-ray machine, making possible moving pictures of the internal organs.

radiocurable (ra″de-o-kūr′ah-b'l) curable by radiation.

radiocystitis (ra″de-o-sis-ti′tis) inflammatory tissue changes in the urinary bladder caused by irradiation.

radiode (ra′de-ōd) an apparatus for therapeutic application of radioactive substances.

radiodermatitis (ra″de-o-der″mah-ti′tis) a cutaneous inflammatory reaction to exposure to biologically effective levels of ionizing radiation; x-ray dermatitis.

radiodiagnosis (ra″de-o-di″ag-no′sis) diagnosis by means of x-rays or gamma rays.

radioecology (ra″de-o-e-kol′o-je) the science dealing with the effects of radiation on species of plants and animals in natural communities or ecosystems.

radioelectrocardiogram (ra″de-o-e-lek″tro-kar′de-o-gram″) the tracing obtained by radioelectrocardiography.

radioelectrocardiograph (ra″de-o-e-lek″tro-kar′de-o-graf″) the apparatus used in radioelectrocardiography.

radioelectrocardiography (ra″de-o-e-lek″tro-kar″de-og′rah-fe) the recording of alterations in the electric potential of the heart, with impulses beamed by radio waves from the subject to the recording device by means of a small transmitter attached to the patient.

radioelement (ra″de-o-el′ĕ-ment) any chemical element having radioactive properties.

radioencephalogram (ra″de-o-en-sef′ah-lo-gram″) a curve showing the passage of an injected tracer through the cerebral blood vessels as revealed by an external scintillation counter.

radioencephalography (ra″de-o-en-sef″ah-log′rah-fe) the recording of changes in the electric potential of the brain without direct attachment between the recording apparatus and the subject, the impulses being beamed by radio waves from the subject to the receiver.

radiogold (ra′de-o-gold″) a RADIOISOTOPE of gold, especially ^{198}Au, which has a half-life of 2.7 days and emits gamma and beta radiation.

radiogram (ra′de-o-gram″) radiograph.

radiograph (ra′de-o-graf″) the film produced by radiography.

radiography (ra″de-og′rah-fe) the making of film records (radiographs) of internal structures of the body by exposure of film specially sensitized to x-rays or gamma rays. adj., **radiograph′ic.**

radiohumeral (ra″de-o-hu′mer-al) pertaining to the radius and humerus.

radioimmunity (ra″de-o-ĭ-mu′nĭ-te) diminished sensitivity to radiation.

radioimmunoassay (ra″de-o-im″u-no-as′a) immunoassay using a radioactive-labeled substance that reacts with the substance under test.

radioimmunodiffusion (ra″de-o-im″u-no-dif-fu′zhun) immunodiffusion conducted with radioisotope-labeled antibodies or antigens.

radioiodine (ra″de-o-i′o-dīn) a RADIOISOTOPE of iodine; ^{131}I and ^{125}I are used in diagnosis and treatment of disease of the thyroid gland and in scintiscanning of the lungs, liver, etc. Called also radioactive iodine.

radioiron (ra″de-o-i′ern) a radioisotope of iron; a mixture of ^{55}Fe and ^{59}Fe has been used in blood studies.

radioisotope (ra″de-o-i′so-tōp) a radioactive form of an element. A radioisotope consists of unstable atoms that emit rays of energy or streams of atomic particles. Radioisotopes occur naturally, as in the cases of radium and uranium, or may be created artificially.

Scientists create artificial radioisotopes by bombarding stable atoms of an element with subatomic particles in a nuclear reactor or in an atom smasher, or cyclotron. When the nucleus of a stable atom is charged by bombarding particles, the atom usually becomes unstable, or radioactive, and is said to be "labeled" or "tagged."

Radioisotopes are used in medicine for both diagnosis and treatment. In general, the therapeutic use of radioisotopes is reserved for older persons, aged 40 and over, because of the possible danger of radiation-induced chromosomal change. (See also RADIOTHERAPY.)

The most widely used radioisotopes in medicine are forms of iodine, phosphorus, gold, iron, and cobalt.

RADIOACTIVE IODINE. When taken into the body, iodine salts concentrate in the thyroid gland. The amount of ^{131}I (radioactive iodine) absorbed by the gland, as measured by a Geiger counter or similar instrument, can reveal whether the gland is functioning normally or is underactive or overactive. In exophthalmic GOITER and HYPERTHYROIDISM, radiation from ^{131}I is used to destroy excessive thyroid tissue. Similarly, ^{131}I is used to destroy malignant cells in some kinds of cancer of the thyroid.

RADIOACTIVE PHOSPHORUS. Radioactive phosphorus (^{32}P) gravitates to actively growing tissues, particularly those involved in manufacturing blood cells; its radiation is therefore used to destroy erythrocytes in polycythemia vera. Phosphorus-32 is also useful in the treatment of chronic leukemia and some other forms of cancer.

RADIOACTIVE GOLD. A radioisotope of gold (^{198}Au) is used to relieve some types of cancer that are not subject to surgery, such as inoperable cancer of the prostate. A further use is the treatment of certain malignant conditions in body cavities of the chest and abdominal regions. Gold-198 may also be used to reduce or destroy a tumor of the pituitary gland.

RADIOACTIVE IRON. Since iron forms part of hemoglobin, radioactive iron (^{59}Fe) is useful in studying the dynamics of hemoglobin formation and breakdown, as in anemia.

RADIOACTIVE COBALT. Radioactive cobalt (^{60}Co) is used in radiotherapy for localized cancer. It can be produced relatively cheaply and in compact equipment, and provides radiation of high intensity. Cobalt-60 is also used in measuring vitamin B_{12} absorption in pernicious anemia.

radiologic technologist one who specializes in the use of x-rays and radioactive isotopes in the diagnosis and treatment of disease, and who works under the supervision of a radiologist.

The registered technologist must pass the examination administered by the American Registry for Radiologic Technologists. Programs of study may vary from one year to eighteen months and may be located in vocational-technical schools or in hospitals. Such schools are approved by the American Medical Association in cooperation with the American College of Radiology.

The address of the American Society of Radiologic Technologists is 645 N. Michigan Ave., Chicago, Illinois 60611.

radiologist (ra″de-ol′o-jist) a physician specializing in radiology.

radiology (ra″de-ol′o-je) the branch of medical science dealing with use of x-rays, radioactive substances, and other forms of radiant energy in diagnosis and treatment of disease. adj., **radiolog′ic, radiolog′ical.**

radiolucent (ra″de-o-lu′sent) permitting the passage of radiant energy, such as x-rays, yet offering some resistance to it, the representative areas appearing dark on the exposed film.

radiometer (ra″de-om′ĕ-ter) 1. an instrument for estimating roentgen-ray quantity. 2. an instrument in which radiant heat and light may be directly converted into mechanical energy. 3. an instrument for measuring the penetrating power of radiant energy.

radiomimetic (ra″de-o-mi-met′ik) producing effects similar to those of ionizing radiations.

radion (ra′de-on) a particle given off by radioactive matter.

radionecrosis (ra″de-o-nĕ-kro′sis) tissue destruction due to radiant energy.

radioneuritis (ra″de-o-nu-ri′tis) neuritis from exposure to radiant energy.

radionuclide (ra″de-o-nu′klid) a radioactive nuclide; one that disintegrates with the emission of corpuscular or electromagnetic radiations.

radiopacity (ra″de-o-pas′ĭ-te) the quality or property of obstructing the passage of radiant energy, such as x-rays, the representative areas appearing light or white on the exposed film. adj., **radiopaque′.**

radiopathology (ra″de-o-pah-thol′o-je) the pathology of radiation effects on tissues.

radiopelvimetry (ra″de-o-pel-vim′ĕ-tre) measurement of the pelvis by radiography.

radiophosphorus (ra″de-o-fos′fo-rus) either of two radioactive isotopes of phosphorus, ^{32}P and ^{33}P; the former, a pure beta emitter, has a half-life of 14.3 days and is used in solution or colloidal form in erythrocyte studies and in the treatment of polycythemia vera and chronic leukemia.

radiopotentiation (ra″de-o-po-ten″she-a′shun) the action of a drug in enhancing the effects of irradiation.

radioreceptor (ra″de-o-re-sep′tor) a receptor for the stimuli that are excited by radiant energy, such as light and heat.

radioresistance (ra″de-o-re″zis′tans) resisting the

effects of radiation, especially in reference to the treatment of malignancy. adj., **radioresist′ant.**

radioresponsive (ra″de-o-re-spon′siv) reacting favorably to irradiation.

radioscopy (ra″de-os′ko-pe) fluoroscopy.

radiosensitivity (ra″de-o-sen″sĭ-tiv′ĭ-te) sensitivity, as of the skin, tumor tissue, etc., to radiant energy, such as x-ray or other radiations. adj., **radiosen′sitive.**

radiosodium (ra″de-o-so′de-um) a radioactive isotope of sodium; ^{24}Na and ^{22}Na are used in the study of blood flow, water balance, and peripheral vascular diseases.

radiosurgery (ra″de-o-ser′jer-e) surgical treatment in which radium is used.

radiotelemetry (ra″de-o-tĕ-lem′ĕ-tre) measurement based on data transmitted by radio waves from the subject to the recording apparatus.

radiotherapist (ra″de-o-ther′ah-pist) a specialist in radiotherapy.

radiotherapy (ra″de-o-ther′ah-pe) the use of x-rays, radiation from radioactive substances, and other similar forms of radiant energy in the treatment of cancer and other diseases.

X-RAYS, or roentgen rays, are energy waves of very short wavelength that have many properties, including the power to injure or destroy tissue, such as the growths produced by cancer. Therapeutic radiation ordinarily does not destroy cancer cells directly; only the very highest dose will kill the cells outright. Radiation somehow alters the cell so that it cannot reproduce. The irradiated cell eventually ages and dies, leaving no new cells behind. Radium, the first radioactive substance to be used in medical treatment, spontaneously gives off rays that affect the growth of tissue. Other substances not normally radioactive, such as cobalt, can be made radioactive (see RADIOISOTOPE) and are widely used in medicine.

The purpose of radiotherapy is to deliver a definite amount of radiation to a specific location. The prescribed dosage should be sufficient to treat the lesion, but not great enough to damage permanently the normal tissue surrounding the lesion. Radiotherapy is often used in conjunction with surgical treatment or with drugs, or with a combination of the two, especially in the treatment of cancer.

Certain sources of radioactivity lend themselves to specific locations or types of malignant disease or other medical disorders. Radium, for example, can be utilized as an implant directly into a malignant tumor located in the mouth or uterine cavity. Cobalt-60 and cesium-137 emit high-energy gamma rays and are often housed in shielded units that are located a distance from the patient. The unit, called a teletherapy unit, is designed so that a beam of gamma radiation can be aimed at a designated part of the patient's body. This type of radiotherapy is particularly useful in the treatment of deep-seated malignancies that are not readily accessible for implantation. Liquid radioisotopes, such as colloid suspensions of radioactive gold (radiogold) or phosphorus, can be instilled into the pleural or peritoneal cavity for local irradiation. Other radioisotopes in liquid form, such as radioactive iodine, are administered on the basis of the affinity of a body organ for a particular element.

X-rays are employed for a variety of disorders. High-voltage x-rays can be used for deep-seated malignancies; low-voltage x-rays are useful in the treatment of skin lesions that require only surface penetration over a relatively large area.

PATIENT CARE. Hospital personnel concerned with the care of patients receiving radiotherapy must be aware of the hazards of radiation and the protective policies and procedures established to reduce these hazards. Most institutions and clinics provide a safety program under the leadership of a radiation physicist or radiation safety officer. Since radiation cannot be seen or felt, it is extremely important to observe all rules outlined in the program.

Sources of radiation that may be of particular concern to health care personnel include: radioactive substances such as radium and cobalt-60 that are used as implants and serve as internal sources of radiation; external sources of radiation such as x-ray machines and cobalt-60 therapy units; and liquid radioisotopes such as iodine-131 and suspensions of radioactive gold or phosphorus.

Generally speaking, the degree of exposure to radiation depends on three factors: (1) the distance between the source of radiation and the individual, (2) the amount of time an individual is exposed to radiation, and (3) the type of shielding provided. (See also RADIATION.)

When a therapist must remain with a patient while he receives diagnostic or therapeutic x-rays, the therapist should wear a lead apron and lead gloves. The therapist must be aware of, and observe carefully, the policies and procedures established for personnel in and around x-ray rooms and the rooms that house teletherapy units. After the treatment is finished the patient will not serve as a source of radiation.

Internal implants can present certain hazards to those involved in bedside care of patients receiving this type of radiotherapy. The hospital staff should be instructed in the amount of time it is safe to remain close to the patient.

Another factor to be considered is accidental removal or dislodgment of a radioactive implant. Most patients are confined to bed and refused bathroom privileges, but it is still possible for a radium needle or radon seeds, for example, to be accidentally removed from the body. Should an implant become dislodged the physician or radiation safety officer must be notified immediately. Under no circumstances should a radioactive substance be handled with the bare hands. A lead container and long-handled forceps should be kept at the patient's bedside in the event an implant should become dislodged. It can then be picked up immediately and placed in the container. Dressings, bed linen, bedpans, and emesis basins should be checked with a radiation detection instrument after each use or before disposal.

Liquid radioactive substances require additional precautions since these substances can enter the body of a worker through the skin, or by ingestion or inhalation. Not all types of radioactive materials require the same precautions. For example, radioactive iodine is excreted in the urine for several days after it has been administered to the patient. In addition it appears in the patient's sweat, tears and saliva; thus all articles such as bed linens and toothbrush used by the patient must be considered a possible radiation hazard. Radiophosphorus acts in the same way. Colloidal gold usually is instilled into a body cavity and is not absorbed as are iodine and phosphorus. However, the radioactive gold emits gamma rays that penetrate beyond the patient's body and present a radiation hazard.

Care of the skin is of particular importance when a patient is receiving radiation from x-ray or teletherapy unit. Before the series of treatments is begun, the skin is washed with soap and water to remove all traces of ointments or lotions from the skin. Powders, ointments, and other applications containing metals such as zinc absorb x-rays and increase damage to the skin.

Once the treatments are begun, the areas marked as "ports" or areas of entry for radiation are not washed or rubbed with alcohol or lotion. These ports of entry are extremely sensitive and subject to breakdown as would be a minor burn. It is important to avoid any friction or pressure on the area. No medications, lotions, or powders may be applied to the area without written orders from the physician.

Local reactions to radiation from internal sources include irritation of mucous membranes lining the mouth, pharynx, vagina, or bladder. The affected area becomes inflamed and tender. If the irritation continues, a grayish white membrane may form over the area. Bleeding also may occur as the underlying tissues become irritated.

In most cases the oral and pharyngeal mucosa heals rapidly once the radiation is discontinued. During radiotherapy frequent mouth washes, good oral hygiene, and soothing gargles may help eliminate the distressing symptoms.

If the vaginal mucosa is irritated, the physician may order douches to cleanse the area and promote healing. Because the area is greatly irritated, douching must be done with extreme gentleness. The occurrance of bleeding is usually a contraindication to douching and should be reported to the physician.

Irritation of the bladder mucosa may result in difficulty in voiding and painful urination. This should be reported so that urinary antiseptics may be ordered to relieve the symptoms and reduce the danger of infection.

Diarrhea, constipation, or blood in the stool indicates irritation of the bowel mucosa in patients receiving radiotherapy for conditions of the lower abdomen or pelvis. An oil retention enema or analgesic suppository may be ordered to relieve the irritation.

Since nausea frequently occurs in patients receiving radiotherapy a high-calorie liquid diet given in small frequent feedings is usually best. Patients unable to swallow because of involvement of the mouth or throat are fed by nasogastric tube.

The distressing side effects of radiotherapy are often aggravated by the patient's mental attitude toward this type of treatment. It is often helpful to have the patient and his family discuss their feelings and express their anxieties about radiation. They should be given a simple explanation of the purpose of the treatment and helped to understand that the discomforts associated with radiotherapy are not indicative of a lack of success or an unusual reaction to radiotherapy. This type of treatment may be more acceptable to the patient if it is pointed out to him that surgery and other types of therapy are also accompanied by discomforts and inconveniences and that these side effects are only temporary.

radiothermy (ra″de-o-ther′me) short-wave diathermy.

radiotoxemia (ra″de-o-tok-se′me-ah) toxemia produced by a radioactive substance, or resulting from radiotherapy.

radiotransparent (ra″de-o-trans-pār′ent) permitting the passage of x-rays or other forms of radiation.

radiotropic (ra″de-o-trop′ik) influenced by radiation.

radioulnar (ra″de-o-ul′nar) pertaining to the radius and ulna.

radium (ra′de-um) a chemical element, atomic number 88, atomic weight, 226, symbol Ra. (See table of ELEMENTS.) Radium is highly radioactive and is found in uranium minerals. Radium salts emit, besides heat and light, three distinct kinds of radiation (alpha, beta, and gamma rays) and also a radioactive gas called radon.

Radium is used in the treatment of malignant diseases, particularly those that are readily accessible, for example, tumors of the cervix uteri, mouth, or tongue. In the form of needles or pellets, it can be inserted in the tumorous tissue (interstitial implantation) and left in place until its rays penetrate and alter the structure of the malignant cells. It can also be used in the form of plaques applied to the diseased tissue. Large amounts of radium are used as a source of GAMMA RAYS, which are capable of deep penetration of matter. Radium rays have been used in the treatment of lupus, eczema, psoriasis, xanthoma, mycosis fungoides, and other skin diseases; for the removal of papillomas, granulomas, and nevi; for palliative treatment in carcinoma and sarcoma; and in myelogenous and lymphatic leukemia. (See also RADIOTHERAPY.)

radius (ra′de-us), pl. *ra′dii* [L.] 1. a line radiating from a center, or a circular limit defined by a fixed distance from an established point or center. 2. in anatomy, the bone on the outer or thumb side of the forearm.

radix (ra′diks), pl. *rad′ices* [L.] root.

radon (ra′don) a chemical element, atomic number 86, atomic weight 222, symbol Rn. (See table of ELEMENTS.) Radon is a colorless, gaseous, radioactive element produced by the disintegration of radium.

rage (rāj) a state of violent anger.

sham r., an outburst of motor activity resembling the outward manifestations of fear and anger, occurring in decorticated animals and in certain pathologic conditions in man.

rale (rahl) an abnormal respiratory sound heard in auscultation and indicating some pathologic condition.

amphoric r., a coarse, musical, and tinkling rale due to the splashing of fluid in a cavity connected with a bronchus.

clicking r., a small sticky sound heard on inspiration, due to the passage of air through secretions in the smaller bronchi.

crackling r., subcrepitant rale.

crepitant r., a fine dry, crackling sound like that made by rubbing hairs between the fingers; heard at the end of inspiration in the early stages of pneumonia.

dry r., a whistling, musical, or squeaky sound, heard in asthma and bronchitis.

moist r., a sound produced by fluid in the bronchial tubes.

sibilant r., a high-pitched hissing sound due to viscid secretions in the bronchial tubes or to thickening of the tube walls; heard in asthma and bronchitis.

subcrepitant r., a fine, moist rale associated with fluid in the bronchioles.

ramal (ra'mal) pertaining to a ramus.

rami (ra'mi) [L.] plural of *ramus.*

Ramibacterium (ra″me-bak-te′re-um) a genus of bacteria found in the intestinal tract and occasionally associated with purulent infections.

ramification (ram″ĭ-fĭ-ka′shun) 1. distribution in branches. 2. a branch or set of branches.

ramify (ram′ĭ-fi) 1. to branch; to diverge in different directions. 2. to traverse in branches.

ramisection (ram″ĭ-sek′shun) section of the appropriate rami communicantes of the sympathetic nervous system.

ramose (ra′mōs) branching; having many branches.

ramulus (ram′u-lus), pl. *ram′uli* [L.] a small branch or terminal division.

ramus (ra′mus), pl. *ra′mi* [L.] a branch, as of a nerve, vein, or artery.

r. commu′nicans (pl. *ra′mi communican′tes*), a branch connecting two nerves or two arteries.

rancid (ran′sid) having a musty, rank taste or smell; applied to fats that have undergone decomposition, with the liberation of fatty acids.

range (rānj) the difference between the upper and lower limits of a variable or of a series of values.

r. of accommodation, the alteration in the refractive state of the eye produced by accommodation. It is the difference in diopters between the refraction by the eye adjusted for its far point and that when adjusted for its near point. Called also amplitude of accommodation.

r. of audibility, the range between the extremes of vibration beyond which the human ear perceives no sound: lower limit, 16 to 20 cycles per second; upper limit, 18,000 to 20,000 cycles per second.

r. of motion, the range, measured in degrees of a circle, through which a joint can be extended and flexed. (See also RANGE OF MOTION EXERCISES.)

ranine (ra′nīn) pertaining to (a) a frog; (b) a ranula, or to the lower surface of the tongue; (c) the sublingual vein.

Rankine scale (ran′kin) an absolute scale on which the unit of measurement corresponds with that of the FAHRENHEIT SCALE, but the ice point is at 459.67 degrees (459.67° R.).

Rankine thermometer (ran′kin) a thermometer employing the RANKINE SCALE.

ranula (ran′u-lah) a cystic tumor beneath the tongue due to obstruction and dilatation of the sublingual or submaxillary gland or of a mucous gland. adj., **ran′ular.**

pancreatic r., a retention cyst of the pancreatic duct.

raphe (ra′fe) a seam; used in anatomic nomenclature as a general term to designate the line of union of the halves of various symmetrical parts.

abdominal r., linea alba.

rapport (rah-por′) a relation of harmony and accord, as between patient and physician.

rarefaction (rar″ĕ-fak′shun) the condition of being or becoming less dense.

rash (rash) a temporary eruption on the skin.

butterfly r., a skin eruption across the nose and adjacent areas of the cheeks in the pattern of a butterfly, as in lupus erythematosus and seborrheic dermatitis.

diaper r., dermatitis occurring in infants on the areas covered by the diaper.

drug r., dermatitis medicamentosa.

heat r., miliaria.

raspberry mark congenital hemangioma.

ratbite fever either of two distinct diseases that may be transmitted to man by the bite of an infected rat and less commonly by the bite of an infected squirrel, weasel, dog, cat, or pig. The more common of the two fevers in the United States is Haverhill fever, so named because the first epidemic to be studied occurred in Haverhill, Mass. The other form, sodoku, rarely occurs in the United States but is observed frequently in Japan and other Eastern countries. Although when both diseases were originally identified they followed the bite of a rat or similar animal, there are also other modes of transmission.

Haverhill fever is caused by *Streptobacillus moniliformis.* If the disease follows a rat bite, a fluid-filled sore appears at the site of the bite within 10 days. High fever alternates with periods of normal temperature at intervals of 24 to 48 hours, and there is swelling of regional lymph nodes. The joints—usually the large joints—become reddened, swollen, and painful. There may be back pain, and a spotty, measles-like skin rash.

Sodoku, or spirillar ratbite fever, is caused by *Spirillum minus.* The original bite heals promptly, but within 5 to 28 days the site becomes swollen and takes on a dusky, purplish hue. In sodoku, there is usually no joint inflammation and the rash is patchy rather than spotty. Otherwise the symptoms are similar to those characteristic of Haverhill fever.

Treatment for both forms of ratbite fever is with penicillin, streptomycin, or other antibiotics.

rate (rāt) the speed or frequency with which an event or circumstance occurs per unit of time, population, or other standard of comparison.

attack r., the rate at which new cases of a specific disease occur.

basal metabolism r., an expression of the rate at which oxygen is utilized in a fasting subject at complete rest as a percentage of a value established as normal for such a subject. Abbreviated BMR. (See also BASAL METABOLISM TEST.)

birth r., the number of births during one year for the total population (crude birth rate), for the female population (refined birth rate), or for the female population of childbearing age (true birth rate).

case r., morbidity rate.

case fatality r., the number of deaths due to a specific disease as compared to the total number of cases of the disease.

death r., the number of deaths per stated number of persons (1000 or 10,000 or 100,000) in a certain region in a certain time period.

dose r., the amount of any therapeutic agent administered per unit of time.

erythrocyte sedimentation r., an expression of the extent of settling of erythrocytes in a vertical column of blood per unit of time (see also SEDIMENTATION RATE).

fatality r., the number of deaths caused by a specific circumstance or disease, expressed as the absolute or relative number among individuals encountering the circumstance or having the disease.

glomerular filtration r., an expression of the quantity of glomerular filtrate formed each minute in the nephrons of both kidneys, calculated by measuring the clearance of specific substances, e.g., inulin or creatinine.

growth r., an expression of the increase in size of an organic object per unit of time.

heart r., the number of contractions of the cardiac ventricles per unit of time.

metabolic r., an expression of the amount of oxygen consumed by the body cells.

morbidity r., the number of cases of a given disease occurring in a specified period per unit of population.

mortality r., death rate; the mortality rate of a disease is the ratio of the number of deaths from a given disease to the total number of cases of that disease.

pulse r., the number of pulsations noted in a peripheral artery per unit of time; normally between 60 and 80 per minute in an adult.

respiration r., the number of movements of the chest wall per unit of time, indicative of inspiration and expiration; normally 16 to 20 per minute in an adult.

sedimentation r., the rate at which a sediment is deposited in a given volume of solution, especially when subjected to the action of a centrifuge. (See also SEDIMENTATION RATE.)

Rathke's pouch (rahth'kez) a diverticulum from the embryonic buccal cavity from which the anterior pituitary is developed.

ratio (ra'she-o) [L.] an expression of the quantity of one substance or entity in relation to that of another; the relationship between two quantities expressed as the quotient of one divided by the other.

A-G r., albumin-globulin r., the ratio of albumin to globulin in blood serum, plasma, cerebrospinal fluid, or urine.

arm r., a figure expressing the relation of the length of the longer arm of a mitotic chromosome to that of the shorter arm.

cardiothoracic r., the ratio of the transverse diameter of the heart to the internal diameter of the chest at its widest point just above the dome of the diaphragm.

lecithin-sphingomyelin r., the ratio of lecithin to sphingomyelin in amniotic fluid (see also LECITHIN-SPHINGOMYELIN RATIO).

sex r., the number of males in a population per number of females, usually stated as the number of males per 100 females.

rational (rash'un-al) based upon reason; characterized by possession of one's reason.

rationalization (rash"un-al-ĭ-za'shun) a defense mechanism in which a person finds logical reasons (justification) for his behavior while ignoring the real reasons. It is a form of self-deception unconsciously employed to make tolerable certain feelings, behavior, and motives that would otherwise be intolerable. Everyone employs rationalization at some time or other and in most instances it is a relatively harmless behavior pattern; the danger lies in deceiving oneself habitually so that eventually harmful or destructive behavior can be justified in one's mind.

Rau-Sed (row'sed) trademark for a preparation of reserpine, an antihypertensive.

Rauwiloid (row'wi-loid) trademark for preparations of alseroxylon, an antihypertensive.

Rauwolfia (raw-wol'fe-ah) a genus of tropical trees and shrubs, including over 100 species and providing numerous alkaloids, notable reserpine, of medical interest.

rauwolfia (raw-wol'fe-ah) any member of the genus *Rauwolfia;* the dried root, or extract of the dried root, of *Rauwolfia*.

r. serpenti'na, the dried root of *Rauwolfia serpentina,* sometimes with fragments of rhizome and other parts, used as an antihypertensive and sedative.

ray (ra) a line emanating from a center, as a more or less distinct portion of radiant energy (light or heat), proceeding in a specific direction.

actinic r., a light ray that produces chemical changes.

alpha r's, α-r's, high-speed helium nuclei ejected from radioactive substances; they have less penetrating power than beta rays. (See also ALPHA PARTICLES.)

beta r's, β-r's, electrons ejected from radioactive substances with velocities as high as 0.98 of the velocity of light; they have more penetrating power than alpha rays, but less than gamma rays. (See also BETA PARTICLES.)

border r's, grenz rays.

caloric r., radiant energy that is converted into heat when applied to the body.

cathode r., negative particles of electricity streaming out in a vacuum tube at right angles to the surface of the cathode and away from it irrespective of the anode's position, moving in a straight line unless deflected by a magnet; by striking on solids they generate roentgen rays.

cosmic r's, very penetrating radiations that apparently move through interplanetary space in every direction.

digital r., a digit of the hand or foot and corresponding metacarpal or metatarsal bone, regarded as a continuous unit.

gamma r's, γ-r's, electromagnetic radiation of short wavelengths emitted by an atomic nucleus during a nuclear reaction, consisting of high energy photons, having no mass and no electric charge, and traveling with the speed of light and with great penetrating power. (See also GAMMA RAYS.)

grenz r's, very soft electromagnetic radiation of wavelengths of about 2 angstroms.

hertzian r's, electromagnetic waves with a greater wavelength than a light wave, used in wireless transmission of signals, speech, etc.

infrared r's, radiations just beyond the red end of the spectrum, having wavelengths of 0.75–1000 μm. (see also INFRARED).

medullary r., a cortical extension of a bundle of tubules from a renal pyramid.

Millikan r's, cosmic rays.

roentgen r's, x-rays.

ultraviolet r's, radiant energy beyond the violet end of the visible spectrum, of 0.39 to 0.18 μm. wavelength (see also ULTRAVIOLET RAYS).

x-r's, electromagnetic radiation of wavelengths ranging between 5.0×10^{-6} and 5.0×10^{-4} μm. (including grenz rays). (See also X-RAYS.)

x-r's, diagnostic, x-rays of wavelengths of 1.2×10^{-5} to 3.0×10^{-5} μm.

x-r's, therapeutic, x-rays of wavelength of 5.0 × 10^{-6} to 1.2 × 10^{-5} μm.

Raynaud's disease (ra-nōz′) a primary or idiopathic vasospastic disorder characterized by bilateral and symmetrical pallor and cyanosis of the fingers, with or without local gangrene. In some cases both the hands and feet may be affected, and rarely the disease may involve the nose, chin, or cheeks. The cause of Raynaud's disease is unknown. Attacks are precipitated by cold or emotional upset and relieved by warmth. The condition occurs almost exclusively in young women, especially those who are experiencing tension and emotional pressure.

Attacks often end spontaneously or upon application of warmth. As the disease progresses, however, small gangrenous ulcers may develop on the fingertips and, eventually, permanent disability of the hands can result from contractures, severe pain, and changes in the skin. The latter condition (sclerodactylia) is characterized by a tightening of the skin so that it appears stretched over the fingers, a decrease of mobility, and a smoothness and abnormal shine to the skin.

Mild cases of Raynaud's disease can be controlled by avoidance of cold and injury to the fingers, high-calorie diet, relief of mental stress and, if necessary, elimination of the habit of smoking. More severe cases may require sympathectomy to prevent conduction of sympathetic nerve impulses which stimulate constriction of the local blood vessels. Vasodilating drugs are sometimes useful in preventing attacks if they are taken before exposure to cold, but they are not successful in all cases and act primarily to provide only a temporary relief of symptoms. Some cases have responded favorably to the employment of BIOFEEDBACK to increase circulation to the affected parts.

Raynaud's phenomenon (ra-nōz′) episodic, symmetrical constriction of small arteries of the extremities, resulting in cyanosis or pallor of the part, followed by hyperemia, producing a red color.

Rb chemical symbol, *rubidium.*

RBC red blood cells; red blood (cell) count (see BLOOD COUNT).

R.B.E. relative biological effectiveness; effectiveness of other types of radiation compared with that of one roentgen of gamma rays or x-rays.

R.D.H. Registered Dental Hygienist.

RDS respiratory distress syndrome.

Re chemical symbol, *rhenium.*

reabsorb (re″ab-sorb′) to absorb again; to undergo or to subject to reabsorption; to resorb.

reabsorption (re″ab-sorp′shun) 1. the act or process of absorbing again, as the absorption by the kidneys of substances (glucose, proteins, sodium, etc.) already secreted into the renal tubules. 2. resorption.

react (re-akt′) 1. to respond to a stimulus. 2. to enter into chemical action.

reaction (re-ak′shun) 1. opposite action or counteraction; the response of a part to stimulation. 2. the phenomena caused by the action of chemical agents; a chemical process in which one substance is transformed into another substance or substances. 3. in psychology, the mental or emotional state that develops in any particular situation. For specific reactions, see under the specific name, as PIRQUET'S REACTION.

adjustment r., one elicited by a change in situation or environment, sometimes evidenced as a transient personality disorder.

alarm r., all of the nonspecific phenomena elicited by exposure to stimuli affecting large portions of the body and to which the organism is not adapted; rapid involution of lymphoid tissues due to hormonal action is a striking manifestation (see also ALARM REACTION).

allergic r., a local or general reaction characterized by altered reactivity of the animal body to an antigenic substance (see also ALLERGY).

antigen-antibody r., the specific combination of antigen with homologous antibody resulting in the reversible formation of antigen-antibody complexes that differ in solubility according to the antigen-antibody ratio (see also ANTIGEN).

anxiety r., a neurotic reaction characterized by abnormal apprehension or uneasiness.

Arias-Stella r., nuclear and cellular hypertrophy of the endometrial epithelium associated with ectopic pregnancy.

biuret r., see BIURET.

chain r., one that is self-propagating; a chemical process in which each time a free radical is destroyed a new one is formed.

conversion r., a condition in which motor or sensory symptoms are used to symbolize intrapsychic conflict (see also CONVERSION REACTION).

cross r., interaction between an antibody and an antigen that is closely related to the one which specifically stimulated synthesis of the antibody.

defense r., a mental reaction that shuts out from consciousness ideas not acceptable to the ego.

r. of degeneration, the reaction to electrical stimulation of muscles whose nerves have degenerated, consisting of loss of response to a faradic stimulation in a muscle, and to galvanic and faradic stimulation in the nerve.

delayed r., a reaction, such as an allergic reaction, occurring hours to days after exposure to an inducer.

dissociative r., a neurotic reaction in which such dissociated behavior as amnesia, fugues, somnambulism, and dream states occur.

false negative r., an erroneously negative reaction to a test.

false positive r., an erroneously positive reaction to a test, especially a positive response to a test for syphilis due to some disease other than syphilis.

gross stress r., an acute emotional reaction to severe environmental stress.

hemianopic pupillary r., in certain cases of hemianopia, light thrown upon one side of the retina causes the iris to contract, while light thrown upon the other side arouses no response.

immune r., 1. immune response. (See IMMUNITY and IMMUNE RESPONSE.) 2. formation of a papule and areola without development of a vesicle following smallpox vaccination.

lengthening r., reflex elongation of extensor muscles that permits flexion of a limb.

leukemic r., leukemoid r., a peripheral blood picture resembling leukemia or indistinguishable from it on the basis of morphologic appearance alone, characterized by immature leukocytes in the blood.

ophthalmic r., ophthalmoreaction.

Prausnitz-Küstner r., a local hypersensitivity reaction induced by intradermal injection into a normal person of serum from a hypersensitive individual; injection 24 hours later of the antigen to which the donor is allergic results in a wheal-and-flare response.

precipitin r., a reaction involving the specific serologic precipation of an antigen in solution with its specific antiserum in the presence of electrolytes. The reaction is used in the typing of pneumococcus strains, in testing whether blood is human or animal, and for diagnostic purposes.

stress r., 1. alarm reaction. 2. gross stress reaction.

r. time, the time elapsing between the application of a stimulus and the resulting reaction.

transfusion r., a group of symptoms due to agglutination of the recipient's blood cells when blood for transfusion is incorrectly matched, or when the recipient has a hypersensitivity to some element of the donor blood (see also TRANSFUSION).

Wassermann r., a test for syphilis based upon fixation of complement.

wheal-flare r., a cutaneous sensitivity rection to skin injury or administration of antigen, due to histamine production and marked by edematous elevation and erythematous flare.

reaction-formation (re-ak'shun-for-ma'shun) a psychic mechanism by which a person unconsciously assumes an attitude which is the reverse of, and a substitute for, a repressed antisocial impulse.

reactivity (re″ak-tiv'ĭ-te) the process or property of reacting.

Reactrol (re-ak'trol) trademark for a preparation of clemizole, an antihistaminic.

reading (rēd'ing) understanding of written or printed symbols representing words.

lip r., speech r., understanding of speech through observation of the speaker's lip movements.

reagent (re-a'jent) a substance used to produce a chemical reaction so as to detect, measure, produce, etc., other substances.

reagin (re'ah-jin) 1. antibody of a specialized immunoglobulin class (IgE) which attaches to tissue cells of the same species from which it is derived, and which interacts with its antigen to induce the release of histamine and other vasoactive amines. A form of cytotropic antibody, it is present in the serum of naturally hypersensitive individuals and can confer specific immediate hypersensitivity in nonreactive individuals. 2. a complement-fixing antibody interacting with cardiolipin in the Wassermann reaction. adj., **re'aginic.**

atopic r., the antibody responsible for hypersensitivity reactions to specific substances with manifestations such as asthma and eczema.

reality orientation a technique employed to rehabilitate those suffering from a moderate to severe degree of disorientation. More information can be obtained by writing to the Publication Services Division of the American Psychiatric Association, 1700 Eighteenth St. N.W., Washington, DC 20009.

Réaumur scale (ra″o-mer') a temperature scale with the ice point at 0 and the normal boiling point of water at 80 degrees (80° R.).

Réaumur thermometer (ra″o-mer') a thermometer employing the Réaumur scale.

recapitulation theory ontogeny recapitulates phylogeny, i.e., an organism, in the course of its development goes through the same successive stages (in abbreviated form) as did the species in its evolutionary development.

receptaculum (re″sep-tak'u-lum), pl. *receptac'ula* [L.] a vessel or receptable.

r. chy'li, cisterna chyli.

receptor (re-sep'tor) 1. a chemical grouping on the surface of an immunologically competent cell with the capability of combining specifically with antigen. 2. a sensory nerve ending that responds to various stimuli.

adrenergic r's, postulated sites on effector organs innervated by postganglionic adrenergic fibers of the sympathetic nervous system, classified as α-adrenergic and β-adrenergic receptors according to their reaction to norepinephrine and epinephrine respectively, and to certain blocking and stimulating agents.

cholinergic r's, receptor sites on effector organs innervated by cholinergic nerve fibers and which respond to the acetylcholine secreted by these fibers.

recess (re-ses') a small, empty space or cavity.

recessive (re-ses'iv) tending to recede; in genetics, incapable of expression unless the responsible allele is carried by both members of a set of homologous chromosomes. 2. a recessive allele or trait.

r. gene, one that produces an effect in the organism only when it is transmitted by both parents. (See also HEREDITY.)

recessus (re-ses'us), pl. *reces'sus* [L.] a recess.

recidivation (re-sid″ĭ-va'shun) 1. the relapse or recurrence of a disease. 2. the repetition of an offense or crime.

recidivism (re-sid'ĭ-vizm) a tendency to relapse, especially the tendency to return to a life of crime.

recidivist (re-sid'ĭ-vist) a person who tends to relapse, especially one who tends to return to criminal habits after treatment or punishment.

recipe (res'ĭ-pe) 1. [L.] take: used at the head of a prescription, indicated by the symbol ℞. 2. a formula for the preparation of a combination of ingredients.

recipient (re-sip'e-ent) one who receives, as a blood transfusion, or a tissue or organ graft.

universal r., a person thought to be able to receive blood of any "type" without agglutination of the donor cells.

Recklinghausen's disease (rek'ling-how″zenz) 1. neurofibromatosis. 2. see OSTEITIS FIBROSA CYSTICA.

recombination (re″kom-bĭ-na'shun) the reunion, in the same or different arrangement, of formerly united elements that have been separated; in genetics, the formation of new gene combinations due to crossing over by homologous chromosomes.

recompression (re″kom-presh'un) return to normal environmental pressure after exposure to greatly diminished pressure.

recon (re'kon) the smallest unit of genetic material capable of recombination.

recrement (rek'rĕ-ment) saliva, or other secretion, that is reabsorbed into the blood. adj., **recrementi'tous.**

recrudescence (re″kroo-des'ens) recurrence of symptoms after temporary abatement; a recrudescence occurs after some days or weeks, a relapse after weeks or months. adj., **recrudes'cent.**

recruitment (re-kro͞ot'ment) 1. the gradual increase to a maximum in a reflex when a stimulus of unaltered intensity is prolonged. 2. in audiology, an abnormal increase in loudness caused by a very slight increase in sound intensity, as in Menière's disease.

rect(o)- word element [L.], *rectum.* See also words beginning *proct(o)-*.

rectal (rek′tal) pertaining to the rectum.

rectalgia (rek-tal′je-ah) proctalgia; pain in the rectum.

rectectomy (rek-tek′to-me) excision of the rectum.

rectification (rek″tĭ-fĭ-ka′shun) 1. the act of making straight, pure, or correct. 2. redistillation of a liquid to purify it.

rectified (rek′tĭ-fīd) refined; made straight.

rectitis (rek-ti′tis) proctitis; inflammation of the rectum.

rectoabdominal (rek″to-ab-dom′ĭ-nal) pertaining to the rectum and abdomen.

rectocele (rek′to-sēl) hernial protrusion of part of the rectum into the vagina.

rectocolitis (rek″to-co-li′tis) coloproctitis; inflammation of the rectum and colon.

rectolabial (rek″to-la′be-al) relating to the rectum and a labium majus.

rectopexy (rek′to-pek″se) proctopexy.

rectoplasty (rek′to-plas″te) proctoplasty.

rectoscope (rek′to-skōp) proctoscope.

rectosigmoid (rek″to-sig′moid) the lower portion of the sigmoid colon and the upper portion of the rectum.

rectosigmoidectomy (rek″to-sig″moi-dek′to-me) excision of the rectosigmoid colon; proctosigmoidectomy.

rectostomy (rek-tos′to-me) the operation of forming a permanent opening into the rectum for the relief of stricture of the rectum.

rectourethral (rek″to-u-re′thral) pertaining to or communicating with the rectum and urethra.

rectouterine (rek″to-u′ter-in) pertaining to the rectum and uterus.

rectovaginal (rek″to-vaj′ĭ-nal) pertaining to the rectum and vagina.

rectovesical (rek″to-ves′ĭ-kal) pertaining to or communicating with the rectum and bladder.

rectovestibular (rek″to-ves-tib′u-lar) pertaining to or communicating with the rectum and the vestibule of the vagina.

rectovulvar (rek″to-vul′var) pertaining to or communicating with the rectum and vulva.

rectum (rek′tum) the distal portion of the large intestine, beginning anterior to the third sacral vertebra as a continuation of the sigmoid and ending at the anal canal. The feces, the solid waste products of digestion, are formed in the large intestine and are gradually pushed down into the rectum by the muscular action of the intestine. Distention of the rectum by the accumulating feces sets up nerve impulses that indicate to the brain the need to empty the bowels.

The rectum is between 6 and 8 inches long, with the anal canal making up the last inch. The anus is kept closed—except during the evacuation process—by muscular rings, the anal sphincters.

In a rectal examination, the examiner palpates the rectum by inserting a gloved and lubricated finger into the rectum. The examination helps in determining whether there are masses in the rectum or pelvic region, and in determining the size and texture of the prostate in men. More extensive examination of the interior surface of the rectum may be done by PROCTOSCOPY.

rectus (rek′tus) [L.] straight.

recumbent (re-kum′bent) lying down.

recuperation (re-koo″per-a′shun) recovery of health and strength.

recurrence (re-ker′ens) the return of symptoms after a remission.

recurrent (re-ker′ent) returning after a remission; reappearing.

r. fever, relapsing fever.

recurvation (re″kur-va′shun) a backward bending or curvature.

red (red) 1. one of the primary colors, produced by the longest waves of the visible spectrum. 2. a red dye or stain.

r. blood cell, erythrocyte.

Congo r., a dark red or brownish powder used as a diagnostic aid in amyloidosis.

cresol r., an indicator, being yellow at pH 7.2 and red at pH 8.8.

methyl r., an indicator, being red at pH 4.4 and yellow at pH 6.0.

neutral r., an indicator, being red at pH 6.8 and yellow at pH 8.0.

phenol r., phenolsulfonphthalein.

scarlet r., an azo dye having some power to stimulate cell proliferation; it has been used to enhance wound healing.

vital r., a dye injected into the circulation to estimate blood volume by determining the concentration of the dye in the plasma.

redia (re′de-ah), pl. *re′diae* [L.] a larval stage of certain trematode parasites, which develops in the body of a snail host and gives rise to daughter rediae, or to the cercariae.

redintegration (red″in-tĕ-gra′shun) 1. the restoration or repair of a lost or damaged part. 2. a psychic process in which part of a complex stimulus provokes the complete reaction that was previously made only to the complex stimulus as a whole.

Redisol (red′ĭ-sol) trademark for a preparation of crystalline cyanocobalamin (vitamin B_{12}).

redox (red′oks) oxidation-reduction.

reduce (re-dūs′) 1. to restore to the normal place or relation of parts, as to reduce a fracture. 2. to undergo reduction. 3. to decrease in weight or size.

reducible (re-du′sĭ-b′l) permitting of reduction.

reductant (re-duk′tant) the electron donor in an oxidation-reduction (redox) reaction.

reductase (re-duk′tās) an enzyme that has a reducing action on chemicals.

reduction (re-duk′shun) 1. the correction of a fracture, luxation, or hernia. 2. the addition of hydrogen to a substance, or more generally, the gain of electrons; the opposition of oxidation.

r. of chromosomes, the passing of the members of a chromosome pair to the daughter cells during meiosis, each daughter cell receiving half the diploid number.

closed r., the manipulative reduction of a fracture without incision.

open r., reduction of a fracture after incision into the fracture site.

reduplication (re-du″plĭ-ka′shun) 1. a doubling back. 2. the recurrence of paroxysms of a double type. 3. a developmental anomaly resulting in the doubling of an organ or part, with a connection between them at some point and the excess part usually a mirror image of the other.

Reed (rēd) Walter (1851–1902). American bacteriologist, born in Gloucester County, Virginia. As a military physician, Reed was appointed during the Spanish-American War chief of a committee to investigate typhoid fever epidemic in the army camps. In 1899, when yellow fever was particularly severe in Cuba, he again was appointed chairman of a committee to study its method of transmission, and he proved by thorough experimentation that yellow fever was carried only by a certain species of mosquito, *Aedes aegypti.*

reef (rēf) an infolding or tuck of tissue, as a tuck made in plication.

reentry (re-en'tre) in cardiology, a postulated mechanism by which a premature beat can be coupled to the normal beat.

refection (re-fek'shun) recovery; repair.

refine (re-fīn) to purify or free from foreign matter.

reflection (re-flek'shun) a turning or bending back, as the folds produced when a membrane passes over the surface of an organ and then passes back to the body wall that it lines.

reflector (re-flek'tor) a device for reflecting light or sound waves.

reflex (re'fleks) a reflected action or movement; the sum total of any particular automatic response mediated by the nervous system.

A reflex is built into the nervous system and does not need the intervention of conscious thought to take effect.

The knee jerk is an example of the simplest type of reflex. When the knee is tapped, the nerve that receives this stimulus sends an impulse to the spinal cord, where it is relayed to a motor nerve. This causes the quadriceps muscle at the front of the thigh to contract and jerk the leg up. This reflex, or simple reflex arc, involves only two nerves and one synapse. The leg begins to jerk up while the brain is just becoming aware of the tap.

Other simple reflexes, the stretch reflexes, help the body maintain its balance. Every time a muscle is stretched, it reacts with a reflex impulse to contract. As a person reaches or leans, the skeletal muscles tense and tighten, tending to hold him and keep him from falling. Even in standing still, the stretch reflexes in the skeletal muscles make many tiny adjustments to keep the body erect.

The "hot-stove" reflex is more complex, calling into play many different muscles. Before the hand is pulled away, an impulse must go from the sensory nerve endings in the skin to a center in the spinal cord, from there to a motor center, and then out along the motor nerves to shoulder, arm, and hand muscles. Trunk and leg muscles respond to support the body in its sudden change of position, and the head and eyes turn to look at the cause of the injury. All this happens while the person is becoming aware of the burning sensation. A reflex that protects the body from injury, as this one does, is called a nociceptive reflex. Sneezing, coughing, and gagging are similar reflexes in response to foreign bodies in the nose and throat, and the wink reflex helps protect the eyes from injury.

A conditioned reflex is one acquired as the result of experience. When an action is done repeatedly the nervous system becomes familiar with the situation and learns to react automatically, and a new reflex is built into the system. Walking, running, and typewriting are examples of activities that require large numbers of complex muscle coordinations that have become automatic.

abdominal r's, contractions of the abdominal muscles about the navel on stimulating the abdominal skin. It indicates that the spinal cord from the eighth to the twelfth dorsal nerve is intact.

accommodation r., the coordinated changes that occur when the eye adapts itself for near vision; they are constriction of the pupil, convergence of the eyes, and increased convexity of the lens.

Achilles r., plantar extension of the foot elicited by a tap on the Achilles tendon, preferably while the

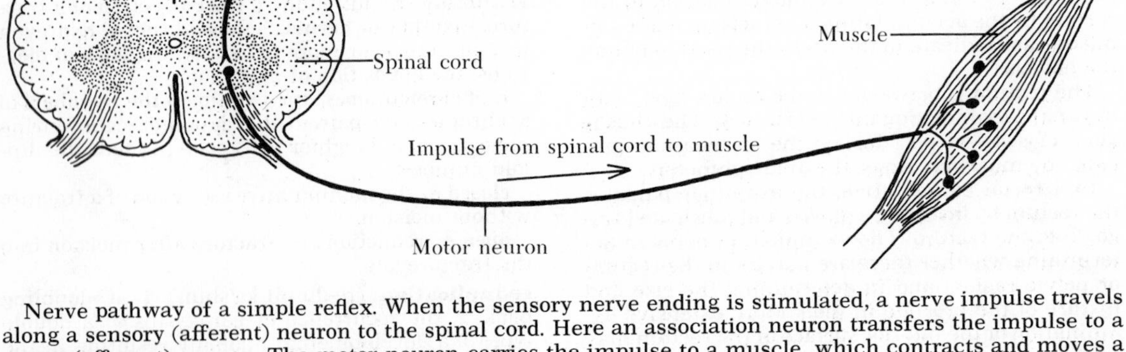

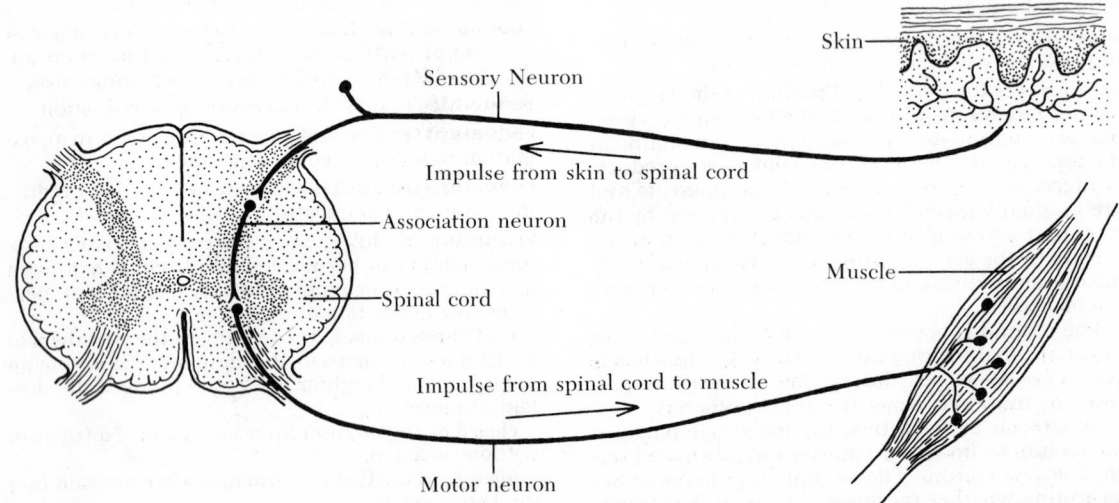

Nerve pathway of a simple reflex. When the sensory nerve ending is stimulated, a nerve impulse travels along a sensory (afferent) neuron to the spinal cord. Here an association neuron transfers the impulse to a motor (efferent) neuron. The motor neuron carries the impulse to a muscle, which contracts and moves a body part.

patient kneels on a bed or chair, the feet hanging free over the edge; called also ankle jerk and triceps surae reflex.

anal r., contraction of the anal sphincter on irritation of the anal skin.

ankle r., Achilles reflex.

auditory r., any reflex caused by stimulation of the auditory nerve; especially momentary closure of both eyes produced by a sudden sound.

Babinski's r., dorsiflexion of the big toe and fanning of the other toes when the sole of the foot is scraped (see also BABINSKI REFLEX).

biceps r., contraction of the biceps muscle when its tendon is tapped.

Brain's r., quadrupedal extensor reflex.

carotid sinus r., slowing of the heart beat on pressure on the carotid artery at the level of the cricoid cartilage (see also CAROTID SINUS SYNDROME).

Chaddock's r., in lesions of the pyramidal tract, stimulation below the external malleolus causes extension of the great toe (see also CHADDOCK'S REFLEX).

chain r., a series of reflexes, each serving as a stimulus to the next one, representing a complete activity.

ciliary r., the movement of the pupil in accommodation.

ciliospinal r., dilation of the ipsilateral pupil on painful stimulation of the skin at the side of the neck.

clasp-knife r., lengthening reaction; reflex elongation of extensor muscles which permits flexion of a limb.

conditioned r., conditioned response. (See also CONDITIONING.)

conjunctival r., closure of the eyelid when the conjunctiva is touched.

corneal r., reflex closure of the eyelids on irritation of the cornea (see also CORNEAL REFLEX).

cough r., the sequence of events initiated by the sensitivity of the lining of the passageways of the lung and mediated by the medulla as a consequence of impulses transmitted by the vagus nerve, resulting in coughing, i.e., the clearing of the passageways of foreign matter.

cremasteric r., contraction of the ipsilateral cremaster muscle, drawing the testis upward, when the upper inner aspect of the thigh is stroked longitudinally.

deep r., one elicited by a sharp tap on the appropriate tendon or muscle to induce brief stretch of the muscle.

digital r., Hoffmann's sign (2).

embrace r., Moro reflex.

gag r., elevation of the soft palate and retching elicited by touching the back of the tongue or the wall of the pharynx; called also pharyngeal reflex.

gastrocolic r., increase in intestinal peristalsis after food enters the empty stomach.

gastroileal r., increase in ileal motility and opening of the ileocecal valve when food enters the empty stomach.

grasp r., flexion or clenching of the fingers or toes on stimulation of the palm of the hand or sole of the foot.

Hering-Breuer r's, inflation and deflation reflexes that help regulate the rhythmic ventilation of the lungs, thereby preventing overdistention and extreme deflation (see also HERING-BREUER REFLEXES).

Hoffmann's r., Hoffmann's sign (2).

jaw r., jaw-jerk r., closure of the mouth caused by a downward blow on the passively hanging chin; rarely seen in health but very noticeable in corticospinal tract lesions.

knee r., knee jerk.

light r., 1. constriction of the pupil when a light is shown into the same (direct light reflex) or the opposite eye (indirect or consensual light reflex). 2. a luminous image reflected when light strikes the normal tympanic membrane.

lung r's, Hering-Breuer reflexes.

Magnus and de Kleijn neck r's, extension of both ipsilateral limbs, or one, or part of a limb, and increase of tonus on the side to which the chin is turned when the head is rotated to the side, and flexion with loss of tonus on the side to which occiput points. Essentially a sign of decerebrate rigidity.

Mayer's r., opposition and adduction of the thumb combined with flexion at the metacarpophalangeal joint and extension at the interphalangeal joint, on downward pressure of the index finger.

Mendel-Bechterew r., dorsal flexion of the second to fifth toes on percussion of the dorsum of the foot; in certain organic nervous disorders, plantar flexion occurs.

Moro r., flexion of an infant's thighs and knees, fanning and then clenching of fingers, with arms first thrown outward and then brought together as though embracing something; produced by a sudden stimulus and seen normally in the newborn (see also MORO REFLEX).

myotatic r., stretch reflex.

nociceptive r's, reflexes initiated by painful stimuli.

palatal r., swallowing caused by stimulation of the palate.

patellar r., knee jerk.

pharyngeal r., gag reflex.

pilomotor r., the production of goose flesh on stroking the skin.

plantar r., plantar flexion of the foot when the ankle is grasped firmly and the lateral border of the sole is stroked or scratched from the heel toward the toes.

proprioceptive r., a reflex that is initiated by stimuli arising from some function of the reflex mechanism itself.

psychogalvanic r., decreased electrical resistance of the body due to emotional or mental agitation.

pupillary r., a change in size of the pupil in response to various stimuli (change in illumination or point of fixation, or emotional stimulation).

quadriceps r., contraction of the quadriceps muscle and extension of the leg elicited by tapping the patellar ligament when the leg hangs loosely flexed at a right angle (see also KNEE JERK).

quadrupedal extensor r., extension of a hemiplegic flexed arm on assumption of the quadrupedal position.

red r., a luminous red appearance seen upon the retina in retinoscopy.

righting r., the ability to assume an optimal position when there has been a departure from it.

Rossolimo's r., in pyramidal tract lesions, plantar flexion of the toes on tapping their plantar surface.

spinal r., any reflex action mediated through a center of the spinal cord.

startle r., Moro reflex.

stretch r., reflex contraction of a muscle in response to passive longitudinal stretching.

sucking r., sucking movements of the lips of an

infant elicited by touching the lips or the skin near the mouth.

superficial r., one elicited by stimulation of superficial nerve endings, as in the skin.

swallowing r., swallowing caused by stimulation of the palate; called also palatal reflex.

tendon r., contraction of a muscle caused by percussion of its tendon.

tonic neck r., extension of the arm and sometimes of the leg on the side to which the head is forcibly turned, with flexion of the contralateral limbs; seen normally in the newborn.

triceps r., contraction of the belly of the triceps muscle and slight extension of the arm when the tendon of the muscle is tapped directly, with the arm flexed and fully supported and relaxed.

triceps surae r., Achilles reflex.

reflexogenic (re-flek″so-jen′ik) producing or increasing reflex action.

reflexograph (re-flek′so-graf) an instrument for recording a reflex.

reflexometer (re″flek-som′ĕ-ter) an instrument for measuring the force required to produce myotactic contraction.

reflux (re′fluks) a backward or return flow.

hepatojugular r., distention of the jugular vein induced by applying manual pressure over the liver; it suggests insufficiency of the right heart.

vesicoureteral r., backward flow of urine from the bladder into a ureter.

refract (re-frakt′) 1. to cause to deviate. 2. to ascertain errors of ocular refraction.

refraction (re-frak′shun) 1. the act or process of refracting; specifically, the determination of the refractive errors of the eye and their correction with glasses. 2. the deviation of light in passing obliquely from one medium to another of different density.

double r., refraction in which incident rays are divided into two refracted rays.

dynamic r., refraction of the eye during accommodation.

ocular r., the refraction of light produced by the media of the normal eye and resulting in the focusing of images upon the retina.

static r., refraction of the eye when its accommodation is paralyzed.

refractionist (re-frak′shun-ist) one skilled in determining the refracting power of the eyes and correcting refracting defects.

refractive (re-frak′tiv) pertaining to or subserving a process of refraction; having the power to refract.

refractometer (re″frak-tom′ĕ-ter) 1. an instrument for measuring the refractive power of the eye. 2. an instrument for determining the indexes of refraction of various substances, particularly for determining the strength of lenses for spectacles.

refractory (re-frak′to-re) not readily yielding to treatment.

r. period, the period of depolarization and repolarization of the cell membrane after excitation; during the first portion (absolute refractory period), the nerve or muscle fiber cannot respond to a second stimulus, whereas during the relative refractory period, it can respond only to a strong stimulus.

refrangible (re-fran′jĭ-b′l) susceptible of being refracted.

refresh (re-fresh′) to freshen or make raw again; to denude a wound of epithelium to enhance tissue repair.

refrigerant (re-frij′er-ant) 1. relieving fever and thirst. 2. a cooling remedy.

refrigeration (re-frij″ĕ-ra′shun) therapeutic application of low temperature (see also HYPOTHERMIA).

refusion (re-fu′zhun) the temporary removal and subsequent return of blood to the circulation (see also HEART-LUNG MACHINE).

regeneration (re-jen″ĕ-ra′shun) the natural renewal of a structure, as of a lost tissue or part.

regimen (rej′ĭ-men) a strictly regulated scheme of diet, exercise, or other activity designed to achieve certain ends.

regio (re′je-o), pl. *regio′nes* [L.] region; a plane area with more or less definite boundaries; used in anatomic nomenclature as a general term to designate certain areas on the surface of the body within certain defined boundaries.

region (re′jun) a plane with more or less definite boundaries; called also regio.

abdominal r′s, the areas into which the anterior surface of the abdomen is divided, including the epigastric, hypochondriac (right and left), inguinal (right and left), lateral (right and left), pubic, and umbilical.

facial r′s, the areas into which the face is divided, including the buccal (side of oral cavity), infraorbital (below the eye), mental (chin), nasal (nose), oral (lips), orbital (eye), parotideomasseter (angle of the jaw), and zygomatic (cheek bone).

lumbar r., the region of the back lying lateral to the lumbar vertebrae.

pectoral r., the areas into which the anterior surface of the chest is divided, including the axillary, infraclavicular, and mammary.

perineal r., the region underlying the pelvic outlet, including the anal and urogenital.

precordial r., the part of the anterior surface of the body covering the heart and the pit of the stomach.

pubic r., the middle portion of the most inferior region of the abdomen, located below the umbilical region and between the inguinal regions.

regional (re′jun-al) pertaining to a certain region or regions.

r. anesthesia, insensibility caused by interrupting the sensory nerve conductivity of any region of the body (see also ANESTHETIC).

r. enteritis, inflammation of the terminal portion of the ileum; called also regional ileitis and Crohn's disease.

registrant (rej′is-trant) a nurse listed on the books of a registry as available for duty.

registrar (rej′is-trar) 1. an official keeper of records. 2. in British hospitals, a resident specialist who acts as assistant to the chief or attending specialist.

registration (rej″is-tra′shun) the act of recording; in dentistry, the making of a record of the jaw relations present or desired, in order to transfer them to an articulator to facilitate proper construction of a dental prosthesis.

registry (rej′is-tre) 1. an office where a nurse's name may be listed as being available for duty. 2. a central agency for collection of pathologic material and related data in a specified field of pathology, so organized that the data can be properly processed and made available for study.

Regitine (rej′ĭ-tēn) trademark for a preparation of

phentolamine, an adrenolytic used to test for the presence of PHEOCHROMOCYTOMA.

regression (re-gresh′un) 1. return to a former or earlier state. 2. subsidence of symptoms or of a disease process. 3. in biology, the tendency in successive generations toward the mean. 4. a mental mechanism utilized to resolve conflict or frustration by returning to a behavior that was successful in earlier years. adj., **regres′sive.** Everyone uses this mechanism at some time, usually when under stress, resorting to tears, tantrums, or other childish behavior to obtain certain goals or relieve frustrations. Some degree of regression frequently accompanies physical illness and can be expected in patients who are hospitalized for a physical disorder. Patients who are mentally ill may exhibit regression to an extreme degree, reverting all the way back to infantile behavior (atavistic regression).

regurgitant (re-ger′jĭ-tant) flowing back.

regurgitation (re-ger″jĭ-ta′shun) a backward flowing, as the casting up of undigested food, or the backflow of blood through a defective heart valve.

valvular r., backflow of blood through the orifices of the heart valves owing to imperfect closing of the valves (valvular insufficiency); named, according to the valve affected, aortic, mitral, pulmonic, or tricuspid regurgitation.

rehabilitation (re″hah-bil″ĭ-ta′shun) the process of restoring a person's ability to live and work as normally as possible after a disabling injury or illness. It aims to help the patient achieve maximum possible physical and psychologic fitness and regain the ability to care for himself. It offers assistance with the learning or relearning of skills needed in everyday activities, with occupational training and guidance and with psychologic readjustment.

Rehabilitation is an integral part of convalescence. Proper food, medication, and hygiene and suitable exercise provide the physical basis for recovery. The patient is encouraged to be active physically and mentally to the extent recommended by the physician. PHYSICAL THERAPY, OCCUPATIONAL THERAPY, and vocational training are used extensively in the rehabilitation of severely handicapped individuals.

rehabilitee (re″hah-bil′ĭ-te) the subject of rehabilitation.

rehalation (re″hah-la′shun) rebreathing.

rehydration (re″hi-dra′shun) the restoration of water or fluid content to a body or to a substance that has become dehydrated.

reimplantation (re″im-plan-ta′shun) replacement of tissue or a structure in the site from which it was previously lost or removed.

reinfection (re″in-fek′shun) a second infection by the same agent.

reinforcement (re″in-fors′ment) the increasing of force or strength. In behavioral science, the process of presenting a reinforcing stimulus so as to strengthen a response. Reinforcement is central in operant CONDITIONING.

A positive reinforcer is a stimulus that is added to the environment immediately after the desired response has been exhibited. It serves to strengthen the response, that is, to increase the likelihood of its occurring again. Examples of a positive reinforcer are food, money, a special privilege, or some other reward that is satisfying to the subject.

A negative reinforcer is a stimulus that is withdrawn (subtracted) from the environment immediately after the response, and the withdrawal serves to strengthen the response.

r. of reflex, strengthening of a reflex response by the patient's performance of some unrelated action during elicitation of the reflex.

reinnervation (re″in-er-va′shun) the operation of grafting a live nerve to restore the nerve supply of an organ or paralyzed muscle.

reintegration (re″in-tĕ-gra′shun) 1. biological integration. 2. the resumption of normal mental and physical activity after disappearance of the catatonic state or other psychic disturbance.

Reiter's disease (ri′terz) a disease of males marked by initial diarrhea followed by urethritis, conjunctivitis, and migratory polyarthritis and frequently accompanied by keratotic lesions of the skin.

rejection (re-jek′shun) the immune reaction of the recipient to foreign tissue cells (antigens) after homograft TRANSPLANTATION, with the production of antibodies and ultimate destruction of the transplanted organ.

relapse (re-laps′) the return of a disease weeks or months after its apparent cessation.

relapsing fever (re-laps′ing) any one of a group of similar infectious diseases transmitted to man by the bites of lice and ticks, and marked by alternating periods of normal temperature and periods of fever relapse. The diseases in the group are caused by several different species of spirochetes belonging to the genus *Borrelia.* Called also recurrent fever.

SYMPTOMS AND DIAGNOSIS. Generally, relapsing fever starts with a sudden high fever of 104° to 105° F., accompanied by chills, headache, muscle aches, nausea, and vomiting. There may also be jaundice and a rash. The attack lasts 2 or 3 days, after which the symptoms disappear by crisis, with profuse sweating accompanying the rapid drop in temperature. In elderly people this may be accompanied by collapse, in which the heart and respiratory system function poorly. After 3 or 4 days there is a relapse and the symptoms return in their former severity. The cycle continues through four or more attacks before the disease has run its course. Relapsing fevers are rarely fatal, but they can be serious.

TREATMENT AND PREVENTION. Treatment is with antibiotics. Sponge baths and aspirin help to control the fever and comfort the patient.

Although tick-borne relapsing fever still occurs in the western United States as well as in other parts of the world, the louse-borne fever is now largely confined to underdeveloped parts of Asia, Africa, and Latin America. Improved public sanitation and louse and tick control account for the decline in the incidence of the disease.

relaxant (re-lak′sant) 1. causing relaxation. 2. an agent that causes relaxation.

muscle r., an agent that specifically aids in reducing muscle tension.

relaxation (re″lak-sa′shun) a lessening of tension.

relaxin (re-lak′sin) a factor that produces relaxation of the symphysis pubis and dilation of the cervix uteri in certain animal species. A pharmaceutical preparation, extracted from the ovaries of pregnant sows, has been used in treatment of dysmenorrhea and premature labor, and to facilitate labor at term.

Releasin (re-le′sin) trademark for a preparation of relaxin.

REM rapid eye movement, a phase of SLEEP associated with dreaming and characterized by rapid movements of the eyes.

rem (rem) *r*oentgen-*e*quivalent-*m*an: the amount of any ionizing radiation which has the same biological effectiveness of 1 rad of x-rays; 1 rem = 1 rad × RBE (relative biological effectiveness).

remedy (rem′ĕ-de) anything that cures or palliates disease. adj., **reme′dial.**

specific r., one that is invariably effective in treatment of a certain condition.

remineralization (re-min″er-al-i-za′shun) restoration of mineral elements, as of calcium salts to bone.

remission (re-mish′un) diminution or abatement of the symptoms of a disease; the period during which such diminution occurs.

remittence (re-mit′ens) temporary abatement, without actual cessation, of symptoms.

remittent (re-mit′ent) having periods of abatement and of exacerbation.

ren (ren), pl. *re′nes* [L.] kidney.

r. mo′bilis, hypermobile kidney; nephroptosis.

renal (re′nal) pertaining to the kidney.

r. clearance tests, laboratory tests that determine the ability of the kidney to remove certain substances from the blood.

r. pelvis, the funnel-shaped expansion of the upper end of the ureter into which the renal calices open; it is usually the renal sinus, but under certain conditions, a large part of it may be outside the kidney (*extrarenal pelvis*).

Rendu-Weber-Osler disease (ron-du′ web′er ōs′ler) hereditary hemorrhagic telangiectasia.

reniform (ren′ĭ-form) kidney-shaped.

renin (re′nin) a proteolytic enzyme liberated by renal ischemia or by diminished pulse pressure; it converts angiotensinogen into angiotensin.

renipelvic (ren″ĭ-pel′vik) pertaining to the pelvis of the kidney.

reniportal (ren″ĭ-por′tal) pertaining to the portal system of the kidney.

renipuncture (ren″ĭ-pungk′tūr) surgical incision of the capsule of the kidney; done for relief of albuminuric pain.

rennet (ren′et) an extract of calf's stomach that contains rennin and is used for curdling the milk in cheese-making.

rennin (ren′in) the milk-curdling enzyme found in the gastric juice of human infants (before pepsin formation) and abundantly in that of the calf and other ruminants; a preparation from the stomach of the calf is used to coagulate milk protein to facilitate its digestion. Rennin catalyzes the conversion of casein from a soluble to an insoluble form (paracasein or curd).

renninogen (rĕ-nin′o-jen) prorennin; the proenzyme in the gastric glands that is converted into rennin.

renogastric (re″no-gas′trik) pertaining to the kidney and stomach.

renography (re-nog′rah-fe) radiography of the kidney.

renointestinal (re″no-in-tes′tĭ-nal) pertaining to the kidney and intestine.

renopathy (re-nop′ah-the) any disease of the kidneys; nephropathy.

renoprival (re″no-pri′val) pertaining to or caused by lack of kidney function.

renotropic (re″no-trop′ik) having a special affinity for kidney tissue.

reovirus (re″o-vi′rus) any of a group of ether-resistant RNA viruses isolated from healthy children, children with febrile and afebrile upper respiratory disease, children with diarrhea, and many animals.

rep (rep) *r*oentgen-*e*quivalent-*p*hysical, a unit of radiation equivalent to the absorption of 93 ergs per gram of water or soft tissue.

repair (re-pār) the physical or mechanical restoration of damaged tissues, especially the replacement of dead or damaged cells in a body tissue or organ by healthy new cells.

plastic r., restoration of anatomic structure by means of tissue transferred from other sites or derived from other individuals, or by other substance.

repellent (re-pel′ent) able to repel or drive off; also, an agent that repels.

repercussion (re″per-kush′un) 1. the driving in of an eruption or the scattering of a swelling. 2. ballottement.

replantation (re″plan-ta′shun) restoration of an organ or other body structure to its original site.

replication (rĕ″plĭ-ka′shun) 1. a turning back of a part so as to form a duplication. 2. repetition of an experiment to ensure accuracy. 3. the process of duplicating or reproducing, as replication of an exact copy of a polynucleotide strand of DNA or RNA.

repolarization (re″po-lar-ĭ-za′shun) the reestablishment of polarity, especially the return of cell membrane potential to resting potential after depolarization.

repositor (re-poz′ĭ-tor) an instrument used in returning displaced organs to the normal position.

repression (re-presh′un) the act of restraining, inhibiting, or suppressing; in psychiatry, a defense mechanism whereby a person unconsciously banishes unacceptable ideas, feelings or impulses from consciousness. A person using repression to obtain relief from mental conflict is unaware that he is "forgetting" unpleasant situations as a way of avoiding them. If employed to extreme, repression may lead to increased tension and irresponsible behavior that the person himself cannot understand or explain. Psychoanalysis frequently is employed to explore the causes and relieve tension resulting from repressed feelings of guilt, hostility, or rejection.

coordinate r., parallel diminution of the concentrations of the several enzymes of a metabolic pathway, resulting from increases in the level of repressor.

enzyme r., interference, usually by the end product of a pathway, with synthesis of the enzymes of that pathway.

repressor (re-pres′or) that which restrains or inhibits; a specific protein molecule coded for by a regulatory gene, which acts through the cytoplasm to repress the synthesis of a specific protein.

reproduction (re″pro-duk′shun) 1. the process by which a living entity or organism produces a new individual of the same kind. 2. the creation of a similar object or situation; duplication; replication.

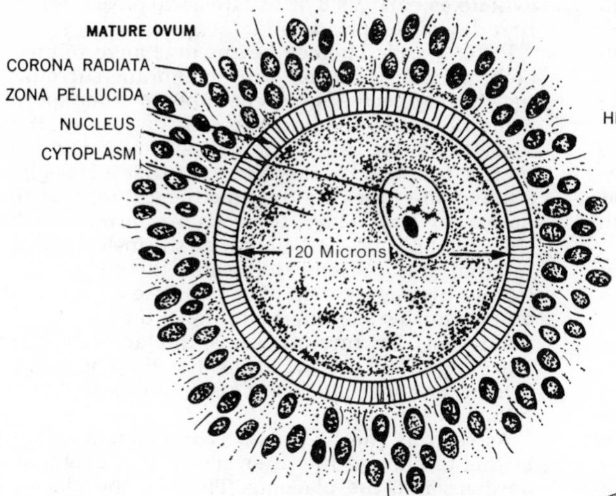

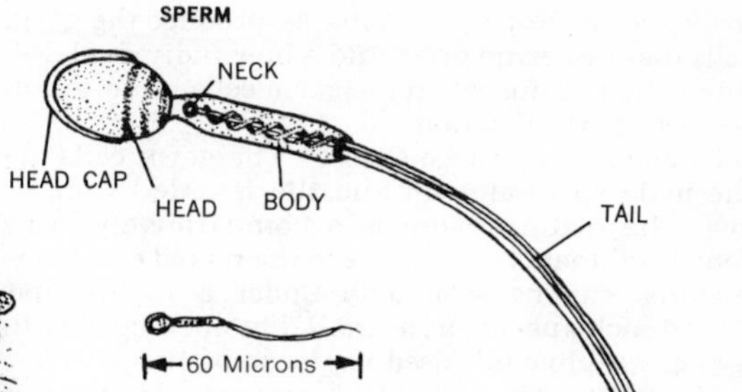

Note the relative sizes of the sperm and ovum.

Only one of millions of sperm cells that the male introduces into the female actually fertilizes an ovum, shown here in diagrammatic cross section. The sperm propel themselves with their tails. The fertilized ovum rapidly divides and redivides; the resulting cell mass is called the morula.

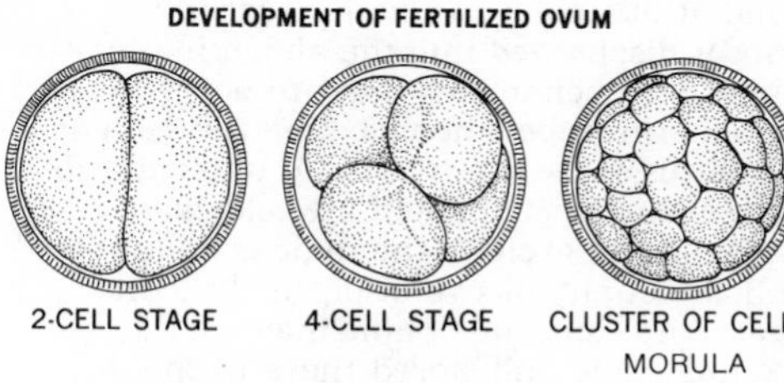

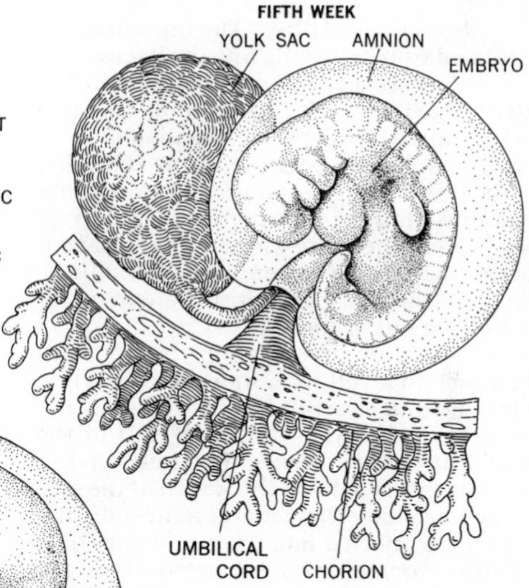

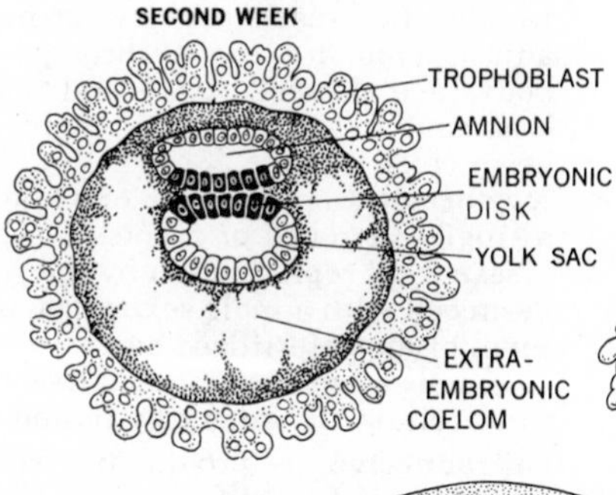

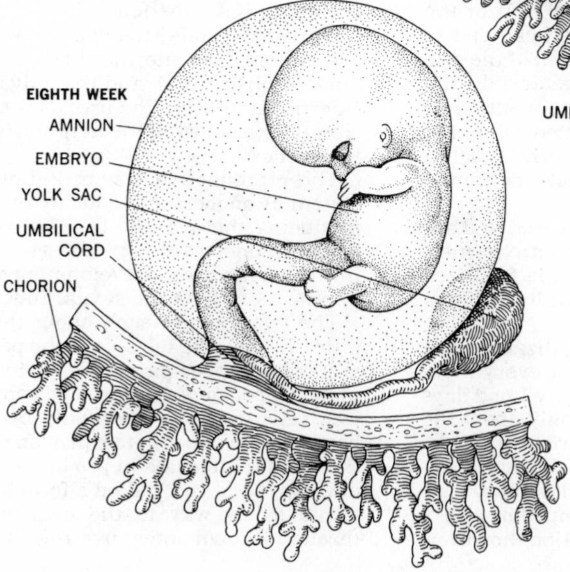

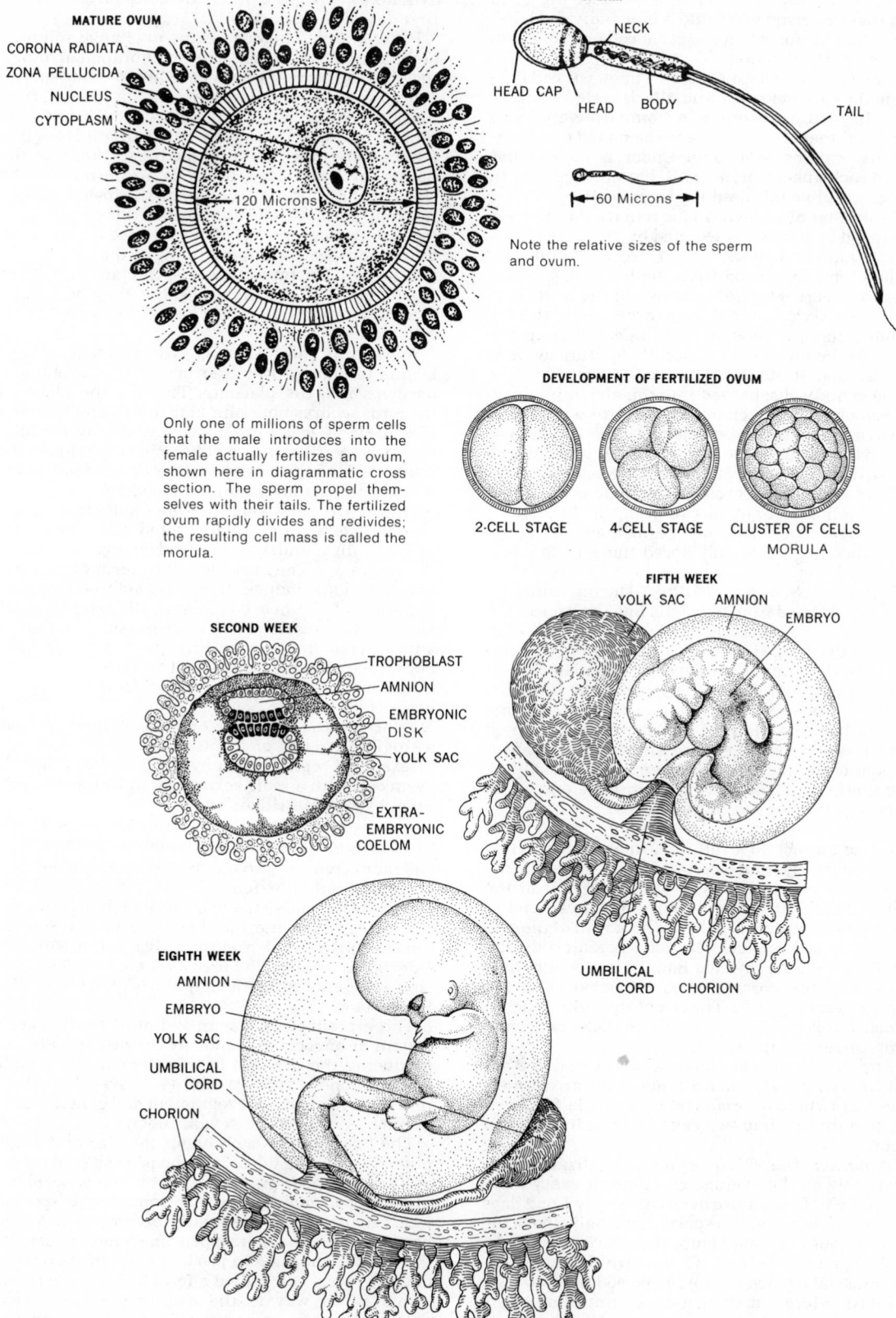

The gonads, or sex glands—the ovaries in the female and the testes in the male—produce the germ cells that unite and grow into a new individual. Reproduction begins when the germ cells unite, a process called fertilization.

PRODUCTION OF GERM CELLS. The germ cells are the male spermatozoon and the female ovum, or egg. The mature ovum is a comparatively large round cell that is just visible to the naked eye. Spermatozoa can be seen only under a microscope, where each appears as a small, flattened head with a long whiplike tail used for locomotion.

Maturation of an ovum is a remarkable process controlled by hormones secreted by the female's endocrine glands. The MENSTRUAL CYCLE is ordinarily 28 days long, measured from the beginning of one menstrual period to the beginning of the next. During the first 2 weeks of the usual cycle, one of the ova becomes mature enough to be released from the ovary. At the time of OVULATION the mature ovum is released and at this point can be fertilized.

The ovum is discharged into the abdominal cavity. Somehow, by mechanisms that are not clear, it moves into a uterine tube. Then it begins the descent toward the uterus. If the ovum remains unfertilized, menstrual bleeding occurs about 2 weeks later.

There is no sexual cycle in the male comparable to the cyclical activity of ovulation in the female. Mature sperm are constantly being made in the testes of the adult male and stored there in the duct system.

FERTILIZATION, OR CONCEPTION. During coitus, semen is ejaculated from the penis into the back of the vagina near the cervix uteri. About a teaspoonful of semen is discharged with each ejaculation, containing several hundred millions of spermatozoa. Of this enormous number of sperm, only one is needed to fertilize the egg. Yet the obstacles to be overcome are considerable. Many of the sperm are deformed and cannot move. Others are killed by the acid secretions of the vagina (the semen itself is alkaline). The sperm must then swim against the current of secretions flowing out of the uterus.

The sperm swim on the average between an eighth of an inch to a full inch in a minute. When one or more vigorous sperm are able to reach the ovum, which is normally in the outer half of the uterine tube, fertilization occurs. The head end of the sperm plunges through the thick wall of the egg, leaving its tail outside. The genetic materials, the chromosomes, are injected into the egg, where they unite with the chromosomes inherited from the mother (see HEREDITY). The sex of the child is determined at this instant; it depends on the sex chromosome carried by the sperm.

If by chance two eggs have been released and are fertilized by two sperm, fraternal TWINS are formed. Identical twins are produced by a single fertilized egg that divides into two eggs early in its development.

Ovulation and Fertilization. Fertilization can occur only on the average of 4 days of every menstrual cycle. The mature ovum lives only 1 or 2 days after ovulation, and the sperm have only about the same amount of time before they perish in the female reproductive tract. To fertilize the ovum, coitus must take place within the period that begins 1 or 2 days before ovulation and lasts until 1 or 2 days after ovulation. There is much variation, however, in the time when ovulation occurs. Most women ovulate between the twelfth and the sixteenth days after the beginning of the last period, but others ovulate as early as 8 or as late as 20 days after the first day of the period.

PREGNANCY. The egg begins to change immediately after fertilization. The membrane surrounding the egg becomes impenetrable to other sperm. Soon the egg is dividing into a cluster of two, then four, then more cells, as it makes its way down the uterine tube toward the uterus. At first it looks like a bunch of grapes. By the time the egg reaches the uterus, in 3 to 5 days, the cells are formed in the shape of a minute ball, hollow on the inside with an internal bump at one side where the embryo will form. This aggregation of cells, called a blastocyst, quickly buries itself in the lining of the uterus (implantation). On rare occasions, implantation takes place not in the uterine lining, but elsewhere in an ectopic, or abnormal, site. This produces an ECTOPIC PREGNANCY.

As soon as the blastocyst is implanted, its wall begins to change into a structure that eventually develops into the placenta. Through the placenta the fetus secures nourishment from the mother and rids itself of waste products. Essentially the placenta is a filtering mechanism by which the mother's blood is brought close to the fetal blood without the actual mixing of blood cells.

During the early stages of pregnancy, the future child grows at an extremely rapid rate. The mother's body must undergo profound changes to support this organism. The muscles of the uterus grow, vaginal secretions change, the blood volume expands, the work of the heart increases, the mother gains weight, the breasts prepare for nursing, and other adjustments are made throughout the mother's body. (See also PREGNANCY and LABOR.)

asexual r., reproduction without the fusion of germ cells.

cytogenic r., production of a new individual from a single germ cell or zygote.

sexual r., reproduction by the fusion of a female germ cell with a male sexual cell or by the development of an unfertilized egg.

somatic r., production of a new individual from a multicellular fragment by fission or budding.

reproductive (re″pro-duk′tiv) subserving or pertaining to reproduction.

r. organs, female, the ovaries, which produce the ova, or eggs; the uterine tubes; the uterus; the vagina, or birth canal; and the vulva, comprising the external genitalia. The breasts are a secondary sex character, enclosing the mammary glands (see also Plate 11).

The reproductive system is linked to the body's system of endocrine glands by the ovaries. Besides producing the ova, the ovaries secrete the female sex hormones ESTROGEN and PROGESTERONE, which influence the body's development and general functioning as well as the sexual function.

The two ovaries, each about the size of a small plum, lie one on each side of the pear-shaped uterus at its wide upper part. When a female is born, her undeveloped ovaries already contain the specialized cells that can eventually become ova. At puberty these ova begin to ripen, one a month; usually the ovaries alternate in producing them. As the undeveloped egg cell, called a follicle, begins to ripen, it makes its way to the ovary's surface, breaks through its own outer covering, and is released. Release of an egg cell, called OVULATION occurs about once in 28 days.

After its separation from the ovary the ovum is drawn into the nearby uterine tube through its fringed, flared opening, and is moved along by rhythmic contractions of the tube's walls and by the cilia of its mucous membrane lining. In the course of its passage the ovum ripens fully, and if fertilization occurs it usually takes place while the ovum is moving through the uterine tube.

The other end of the tube opens directly into the uterus. This muscular organ is capable of stretching to contain a fertilized ovum as it grows through the 9 months of pregnancy. Its mucous membrane lining is also specially adapted to hold the unborn infant securely and to nourish it. When the ovum arrives, the hormones estrogen and progesterone produced in the ovary have previously stimulated the uterus to prepare its lining with extra blood vessels. If the egg has not been fertilized, it loses its vitality, the hormone supply ceases, and the extra blood and tissues are discharged from the body through the vagina, in the menstrual flow. If fertilization, or conception, has taken place, the growth of a new life has begun; menstruation does not occur, and in fact ceases entirely during the 9 months (approximately 280 days) of pregnancy.

The lower end of the uterus forms an opening called the cervix, or neck, which protrudes into the birth canal, or vagina. Enclosed by muscles and lined with mucous membrane, the vagina measures on the average about 3 inches in length. In coitus it receives the male copulatory organ, the penis, and the discharge of sperm during ejaculation. Like the uterus, the vagina undergoes changes during pregnancy that enable it to stretch to many times its usual size, allowing the infant to pass through it in childbirth.

The exterior opening of the vagina and the surrounding organs make up the vulva. The vulva consists of the labia majora (the major lips), the labia minora (the minor lips), the vestibule, and the clitoris. Somewhat anterior to the vulva lies a triangular fatty pad covered with pubic hair, the mons veneris. Between the clitoris and the entry to the vagina is the opening of the urethra, from which urine is excreted. The anus lies to the rear of the vaginal opening. In a virgin, a membrane called the hymen usually closes off a part of the opening to the vagina.

The labia majora envelop the labia minora, and these join together at the clitoris, a rudimentary, dimunutive, penis-like organ that has a purely erotic function. Like the penis, the clitoris has a foreskin and many nerve endings. The area that surrounds the entry to the vagina and lies within the labia minora is the vestibule. At each side of the vaginal opening and elsewhere in the vestibule, glands secrete lubricating fluids to facilitate coitus.

A woman's breasts serve to provide milk for the newborn infant. At puberty the breasts increase in size; during pregnancy they become much larger and start to secrete milk shortly after childbirth.

DISORDERS OF THE FEMALE REPRODUCTIVE ORGANS. Bacterial and other infections, tumors, and birth injuries can affect the female reproductive organs. Growths, or tumors, can develop in all parts of the female reproductive tract. These are most often benign and may not require treatment, but they should be examined periodically in case they grow large and affect the organs, or become malignant.

In the OVARY, cysts or tumors can develop without symptoms. When diagnosed, an ovarian tumor is usually removed surgically; cysts, however, often remain without excessive harm or pain. The neighboring uterine tubes may also be the site of growths, though such tumors usually result from the involvement of some other organ. The UTERUS, particularly the cervix, is one of the most frequent locations of tumors. In the uterus they are usually leiomyomas, which may attain considerable size. These are, however, quite readily diagnosed and, when found early enough, are treated successfully by surgery.

In the reproductive system, the BREASTS are the most common site of growths of all kinds, both cysts and tumors, the latter both benign and malignant. A variety of sores and abscesses may afflict the breasts, especially in their milk-producing periods. Any lump or other irregularity within or on a breast should receive prompt medical attention.

The most prevalent bacterial diseases of a woman's reproductive organs are the venereal infections. Of these the most serious are SYPHILIS and GONORRHEA. Venereal diseases are almost always contracted through coitus.

A number of bacterial, protozoa, and fungal infections can occur within the vagina or in the area of the vulva. These cause discharges and irritation and can usually be readily treated following a correct diagnosis.

Difficult childbirth can produce deformations of the reproductive organs, particularly of the uterus.

r. organs, male, the external genitalia, accessory glands that secrete special fluids and the ducts through which these organs and glands are connected to each other and through which the spermatozoa are ejaculated during coitus.

EXTERNAL GENITALIA. The penis, testes, and scrotum (the sac that contains the testes) are together known as the external genitalia. The penis is the organ through which semen is transferred into the female during coitus. Semen is a carrier for the spermatozoa, which are produced in the testes. The testes also produce the male hormone testosterone, which gives a sexually mature male his distinctively masculine characteristics and his sexual energy and drive.

The testes are suspended from the spermatic cord, which also connects the testes with the other parts of the reproductive system. This cord consists of blood vessels, nerves and ducts, all enclosed in connective tissue (see also Plate 11).

ACCESSORY GLANDS. The accessory reproductive glands include the prostate, two seminal vesicles, and two bulbourethral glands, known also as Cowper's glands.

The PROSTATE is located below and against the urinary bladder. It completely surrounds the urethra. It produces a thin, clear, slightly alkaline fluid that neutralizes the normal acidity of the urethra caused by the continual passage of urine. This fluid enables the spermatozoa to pass through the urethra unharmed.

The seminal vesicles are two glands located just above and to the rear of the prostate. These glands consist of many small sacs, or pockets, in which is produced and stored the thick, milky fluid that is ejaculated during the male orgasm. The fluid serves as the carrier for the sperm and is the major constituent of the semen.

The two bulbourethral glands, which are about the size of peas, secrete a clear, sticky fluid that lubricates the urethra, thus making it easier for the semen to pass through it during ejaculation.

DUCTS. The spermatozoa are led from the testes to the urethra through a system of ducts. First, there are two convoluted tubes, one lying on top of each testis and connected directly to it. Each tube is called an epididymis. Mature spermatozoa produced in the testes are stored in each epididymis.

Each epididymis is connected to a vas deferens, a part of the spermatic cord that conducts the spermatozoa to the duct lying close to the bladder.

The vasa deferentia join with ducts leading from the seminal vesicles just before the urethra. The combined duct is called the ejaculatory duct. This duct passes through the prostate and joins with the urethra. The urethra then conducts the semen through the penis.

DISCHARGE OF SEMEN. The tissues that form the mass of the penis are called erectile tissue. This tissue is spongy in nature and filled with innumerable hollow spaces. There is also a network of veins and arteries within the penis. Sexual excitement causes the muscles surrounding the veins to contract, thereby restricting the flow of blood from the penis. At the same time, the muscles surrounding the arteries relax, permitting the free flow of blood into the penis at the full pressure of the circulatory system. The result is that the spongy tissue fills with blood and the penis swells in size and becomes stiff and erect.

Sexual excitement also stimulates the accessory glands to secrete larger amounts of their fluids. When the sexual tension becomes acute enough, as a result of coitus, masturbation, or purely mental stimulation (as in "wet dreams"), there is a series of reflex contractions of the reproductive organs. The muscles surrounding the seminal ducts, the prostate, and the seminal vesicles contract convulsively; this causes the semen to be ejaculated forcibly from the penis. There is first an ejaculation of the fluid from the prostate, followed immediately by the semen. About 2 or 3 ml. of semen is ejaculated. This volume of semen is believed to contain between 200 and 500 million sperm, only one of which is necessary to fertilize the ovum.

DISORDERS OF THE MALE REPRODUCTIVE ORGANS. For disorders that affect particular organs, see PENIS, PROSTATE, and CRYPTORCHIDISM. Since the male reproductive organs are connected so closely with each other, an infection in one is likely to spread throughout the entire reproductive system. This is particularly true of venereal diseases, such as SYPHILIS and GONORRHEA, which are contracted almost always through coitus.

repulsion (re-pul′shun) 1. the act of driving apart or away; a force that tends to drive two bodies apart. 2. in genetics, the occurrence on opposite chromosomes in a double heterozygote of the two mutant alleles of interest.

RES reticuloendothelial system.

rescinnamine (re-sin′ah-min) an alkaloid from various species of *Rauwolfia;* used as an antihypertensive and tranquilizer.

resect (re-sekt′) to excise part of an organ or other structure.

resection (re-sek′shun) excison of a portion of an organ or other structure.

gastric r., partial gastrectomy.

transurethral r., resection of the prostate by means of an instrument passed through the urethra.

wedge r., removal of a triangular mass of tissue, as from the ovary.

resectoscope (re-sek′to-skōp) an instrument for transurethral prostatic resection.

resectoscopy (re″sek-tos′ko-pe) transurethral resection of the prostate.

reserpine (res′er-pēn) an active alkaloid from various species of *Rauwolfia,* used as an antihypertensive, tranquilizer, and sedative.

reserve (re-zerv′) 1. to hold back for future use. 2. a supply, beyond that ordinarily used, that may be utilized in emergency.

alkali r., alkaline r., the amount of buffer compounds in the blood that are capable of neutralizing acids, such as sodium bicarbonate and proteins. Since the bicarbonates are the most important of these buffers, the term blood bicarbonate is often preferred to alkali reserve. (See also ALKALI RESERVE.)

cardiac r., the potential ability of the heart to perform work beyond that necessary under basal conditions.

reservoir (rez′er-vwar) 1. a storage place or cavity. 2. an alternate host or passive carrier of a pathogenic organism.

resident (rez′ĭ-dent) a graduate and licensed physician receiving training in a specialty in a hospital.

residual (re-zid′u-al) remaining or left behind.

r. urine, urine remaining in the bladder after voiding; seen with bladder outlet obstruction and disorders affecting nerves controlling bladder function.

residue (rez′ĭ-doo) a remainder; that which remains after the removal of other substances.

residuum (re-zid′u-um), pl. *resid′ua* [L.] a residue or remainder.

resin (rez′in) 1. a solid or semisolid, amorphous organic substance of vegetable origin or produced synthetically. True resins are insoluble in water, but are readily dissolved in alcohol, ether, and volatile oils. 2. rosin. adj., **res′inous.**

acrylic r's, products of the polymerization of acrylic or methacrylic acid or their derivatives, used in fabrication of medical prostheses and dental restorations and appliances.

activated r., self-curing resin.

anion-exchange r., see ion-exchange resin.

autopolymer r., self-curing resin.

cation-exchange r., see ion-exchange resin.

cholestyramine r., a synthetic, strongly basic anion-exchange resin in the chloride form which chelates bile salts in the intestine, thus preventing their reabsorption; used in the symptomatic relief of pruritus associated with bile stasis.

ion-exchange r., a high-molecular-weight insoluble polymer of simple organic compounds capable of exchanging its attached ions for other ions in the surrounding medium; classified as (*a*) cation- or anion-exchange resins, depending on which ions the resin exchanges (the former are used to restrict intestinal sodium absorption in edematous states, and the latter as antacids in ulcer treatment); and (*b*) carboxylic, sulfonic, etc., depending on the nature of the active groups.

podophyllum r., a mixture of resins from podophyllum, used as a topical caustic in the treatment of certain papillomas.

quick-cure r., self-curing r., any resin that can be

polymerized by addition of an activator and a catalyst without the use of external heat.

synthetic r., an amorphous, organic solid or semisolid material produced by polymerization or condensation of simpler compounds.

resistance (re-zis′tans) 1. opposition, or counteracting force, as opposition of a conductor to passage of electricity or other energy or substance. 2. the natural ability of a normal organism to remain unaffected by noxious agents in its environment (see also IMMUNITY). 3. in studies of respiration, an expression of the opposition to flow of air produced by the tissues of the air passages, in terms of pressure per amount of air per unit of time. 4. in psychoanalysis, opposition to the coming into consciousness of repressed material.

peripheral r., resistance to the passage of blood through the small blood vessels, especially the arterioles.

resolution (rez″o-lu′shun) 1. subsidence of a pathologic state, as the subsidence of an inflammation, or the softening and disappearance of a swelling. 2. perception as separate of two adjacent points; in microscopy, the smallest distance at which two adjacent objects can be distinguished as separate.

resolvent (re-zol′vent) promoting resolution or the dissipation of a pathologic growth. 2. an agent that promotes resolution.

resolving power (re-zol′ving) the ability of the eye or of a lens to make small objects that are close together separately visible, thus revealing the structure of an object.

resonance (rez′o-nans) 1. the prolongation and intensification of sound produced by transmission of its vibrations to a cavity, especially such a sound elicited by percussion. Decrease of resonance is called *dullness;* its increase, *flatness.* 2. a vocal sound heard on auscultation. 3. mesomerism.

amphoric r., a sound resembling that produced by blowing over the mouth of an empty bottle.

skodaic r., increased percussion resonance at the upper part of the chest, with flatness below it.

tympanic r., drumlike reverberation of a cavity filled with air.

tympanitic r., the peculiar sound elicited by percussing a tympanitic abdomen.

vesicular r., normal pulmonary resonance.

vocal r., the sound of ordinary speech as heard through the chest wall.

resonant (rez′o-nant) giving an intense, rich sound on percussion; exhibiting resonance.

resonator (rez′o-na″tor) 1. an instrument used to intensify sounds. 2. an electric circuit in which oscillations of a certain frequency are set up by oscillations of the same frequency in another circuit.

resorb (re-sorb′) to dissolve and assimilate; to reabsorb.

resorcin (rĕ-zor′sin) resorcinol.

resorcinism (rĕ-zor′sĭ-nizm) chronic poisoning by resorcinol, resulting in methemoglobinemia, paralysis, and damage to the capillaries, kidneys, heart, and nervous system.

resorcinol (rĕ-zor′sĭ-nol) a keratolytic applied topically to the skin; the monoacetate salt is used as a keratolytic and antiseborrheic applied topically to the scalp.

resorcinolphthalein (rĕ-zor″sĭ-nol-thal′ēn) fluorescein, a dye used in certain diagnostic procedures, as for example the detection of corneal abrasions.

resorption (re-sorp′shun) 1. the lysis and assimilation of a substance, as of bone. 2. reabsorption.

respirable (rĕ-spīr′ah-b′l) suitable for respiration.

respiration (res″pĭ-ra′shun) the exchange of oxygen and carbon dioxide between the atmosphere and the body cells, including inspiration and expiration, diffusion of oxygen from the pulmonary alveoli to the blood and of carbon dioxide from the blood to the alveoli, and the transport of oxygen to and carbon dioxide from the body cells. (See also Plates 5 and 6.)

THE RESPIRATORY SEQUENCE. The sequence of the respiration process begins as air enters the corridors of the nose or mouth, where it is warmed and moistened. The air then passes through the pharynx, larynx, and trachea and into the bronchi.

The bronchi branch in the lungs into smaller and smaller bronchioles, ending in clusters of tiny air sacs. There are 750 million of these alveoli, as these sacs are called, in the lungs. The blood flows through the lungs in the pulmonary circulation. Through the thin membrane of the network of capillaries around the alveoli, the air and the blood exchange oxygen and carbon dioxide. The carbon dioxide molecules migrate from the erythrocytes in the capillaries through the porous membrane into the air in the alveoli, while the oxygen molecules cross from the air into the red blood cells.

The erythrocytes proceed through the circulatory system, carrying the oxygen in loose combination with HEMOGLOBIN and giving it up to the body cells that need it. In cellular respiration the blood cells release oxygen and pick up carbon dioxide. The lungs dispose of the carbon dioxide, left there by the red blood cells, in the process of breathing. With each breath, about one-sixth of the air in the lungs is exchanged for new air.

BREATHING. The lungs inflate and deflate some 16 to 20 times a minute. Their elastic tissue allows them to expand and contract like a bellows worked by the diaphragm and the intercostal muscles. The diaphragm contracts, flattening itself downward, and thus enlarges the thoracic cavity. At the same time the ribs are pulled up and outward by the action of the narrow but powerful intercostal muscles that expand and contract the rib cage. As the chest expands, the air rushes in.

Exhalation occurs when the respiratory muscles relax and the chest returns automatically to its minimum size, expelling the air (see also LUNG).

Automatic Breathing Controls. The automatic control of breathing stems from poorly defined areas known as the respiratory centers, located in the medulla oblongata and pons. From there, impulses are sent down the spinal cord to the nerves that control the diaphragm, and to the intercostal muscles. Chemical and reflex signals control these nerve centers. (See HERING-BREUER REFLEXES.)

The chemical controls of breathing are mainly dependent on the level of carbon dioxide in the blood. The response is so sensitive that if the carbon dioxide in the blood increases two-tenths of 1 per cent, the respiratory rate increases automatically to double the amount of air taken in, until the excess of carbon dioxide is eliminated. It is not lack of oxygen but excess of carbon dioxide that causes this instant and powerful reaction.

The P_{CO_2}, or carbon dioxide tension, of arterial blood normally is 38 to 40 mm. of mercury. When the P_{CO_2} increases, the respiratory centers are stimulated and breathing becomes more rapid; conversely, decrease of the P_{CO_2} slows the rate of respiration. The P_{CO_2} acts both directly on the respiratory centers of the brain and on the carotid and aortic bodies, chemoreceptors that are responsive to changes in blood P_{CO_2}, P_{O_2}, and pH (see also BLOOD GAS ANALYSIS).

PROTECTIVE RESPIRATORY MECHANISMS. The lungs are constantly exposed to the surrounding atmosphere. Twenty times a minute, more or less, they take in a gaseous mixture, along with whatever foreign particles happen to be floating in it and at whatever temperature it may be. To compensate, the lungs have some remarkable protective devices.

On its way through the nasal passage, the cold air from outside is preheated by a large supply of blood, which gives off warmth through the thin mucous membrane that lines the respiratory tract. This same mucous lining is always moist, and dry air picks up moisture as it passes.

Dust, soot, and bacteria are filtered out by a barrier of cilia, tiny threadlike growths that line the passageways of the respiratory tract. The cilia catch not only foreign particles but also mucus produced by the respiratory passages themselves. Since the movement of the cilia is always toward the outside, they push the interfering matter upward, away from the delicate lung tissues, so that it can be expectorated or swallowed. Particles that are too large for the cilia to dispose of usually stimulate a sneeze or a cough, which forcibly expels them.

Sneezing and coughing are reflex acts in response to stimulation of nerve endings in the respiratory passages. The stimulus for a cough comes from the air passages in the throat; for a sneeze, from those in the nose.

abdominal r., inspiration and expiration accomplished mainly by the abdominal muscles and diaphragm.

aerobic r., oxidative transformation of certain substrates into secretory products, the released energy being used in the process of assimilation.

anaerobic r., respiration in which energy is released by chemical reactions in which free oxygen takes no part.

artificial r., that maintained by force applied to the body (see also ARTIFICIAL RESPIRATION).

Biot's r., rapid, short breathing, with pauses of several seconds.

cell r., the processes in the living cell by which organic substances are oxidized and chemical energy is released.

Cheyne-Stokes r., breathing characterized by rhythmic waxing and waning of respiration depth, with regularly recurring apneic periods (see also CHEYNE-STOKES RESPIRATION).

cogwheel r., breathing with jerky inspiration.

diaphragmatic r., that performed mainly by the diaphragm.

electrophrenic r., induction of respiration by electric stimulation of the phrenic nerve.

external r., the exchange of gases between the lungs and the blood.

internal r., the exchange of gases between the body cells and the blood.

Kussmaul's r., air hunger.

paradoxical r., that in which a lung, or a portion of a lung, is deflated during inspiration and inflated during expiration (see also PARADOXICAL RESPIRATION).

tissue r., internal respiration.

respirator (res′pĭ-ra″tor) an apparatus to qualify the air breathed through it, or a device for giving artificial respiration or to assist in pulmonary ventilation (see also VENTILATOR).

r. shock, circulatory SHOCK due to interference with the flow of blood through the great vessels and chambers of the heart, causing pooling of blood in the veins and the abdominal organs and a resultant vascular collapse. The condition sometimes occurs as a result of increased intrathoracic pressure in patients who are being maintained on a mechanical VENTILATOR.

respiratory (re-spi′rah-to″re, res′per-ah-to″re) pertaining to respiration.

r. distress syndrome (of newborn) (RDS), a condition most often seen in premature infants, infants of diabetic mothers and of those who experienced bleeding during pregnancy, infants delivered by cesarean section, and infants who experienced asphyxia during birth; it is marked by dyspnea and cyanosis, and includes two patterns: In HYALINE MEMBRANE DISEASE, affected infants often die of respiratory distress in the first few days of life and at autopsy have a hyaline-like membrane lining the terminal respiratory passages. In idiopathic respiratory distress of the newborn, affected infants may live, but in those who die, only resorption atelectasis is seen.

r. failure, a life-threatening condition in which respiratory function is inadequate to maintain the body's need for oxygen supply and carbon dioxide removal while at rest; called also acute ventilatory failure. The condition usually occurs when a patient with CHRONIC OBSTRUCTIVE PULMONARY DISEASE develops an infection or otherwise suffers an additional strain on his already seriously impaired respiratory functions. Inadequate or unsuccessful treatment of RESPIRATORY INSUFFICIENCY from a variety of causes can lead to respiratory failure.

Early symptoms include dyspnea, wheezing, and apprehension; cyanosis is rarely present. As the condition worsens the patient becomes drowsy and mentally confused and may slip into coma. BLOOD GAS ANALYSIS is an important tool is diagnosing respiratory failure and assessing effectiveness of treatment. The condition is a medical emergency that can rapidly progress to irreversible cardiopulmonary failure and death. Treatment is concerned with improving ventilation and oxygenation of tissues, restoring and maintaining fluid and electrolyte balance (see also FLUID BALANCE) and ACID-BASE BALANCE, and stabilizing cardiac function.

r. insufficiency, a condition in which respiratory function is inadequate to meet the body's needs when increased physical activity places extra demands on it. Insufficiency occurs as a result of progressive degenerative changes in the alveolar structure and the capillary tissues in the pulmonary bed, as, for example, in CHRONIC OBSTRUCTIVE PULMONARY DISEASE and pulmonary fibrosis. Treatment is essentially supportive and symptomatic. If the condition is not successfully managed it may progress to RESPIRATORY FAILURE.

r. quotient, the ratio of the volume of expired carbon dioxide to the volume of oxygen absorbed by the lungs per unit of time.

r. syncytial virus, a virus isolated from children with bronchopneumonia and bronchitis, characteristically causing syncytium formation in tissue culture.

r. system, the group of specialized organs whose specific function is to provide for the transfer of oxygen from the air to the blood and of waste carbon dioxide from the blood to the air. The organs of the system include the NOSE, the PHARYNX, the LARYNX, the TRACHEA, the bronchi, and the LUNGS. (See also RESPIRATION and Plates 5 and 6.)

RESPIRATORY DISORDERS. Of the numerous disorders that affect the respiratory system, the most frequent is the COMMON COLD, a viral infection of the upper respiratory tract. Common upper respiratory disorders also include HAY FEVER and other allergic reactions.

Other diseases that affect the respiratory tract include INFLUENZA, WHOOPING COUGH, and DIPHTHERIA. Some more generalized diseases, such as MEASLES, are also accompanied by respiratory symptoms. A respiratory inflammation or infection, such as a cold, may spread to other parts of the respiratory system and may be a cause of a number of related symptoms and disorders. For example, one condition that may stem from a cold or from other causes is SINUSITIS, inflammation of the paranasal sinuses.

In children in particular, enlarged ADENOIDS may block the rear of the nasal passages and make breathing through the nose difficult. The tonsils at the sides of the throat are also very susceptible to infection and enlargement (see also TONSILLITIS). When inflammation affects the larynx, or voice box, the condition is known as LARYNGITIS, and if it attacks the bronchial tubes, it is called BRONCHITIS. Another disorder that affects the bronchial tubes is ASTHMA, which causes contraction and mucous plugging of the tubes and hinders breathing. Asthma is frequently an allergic reaction (see also CHRONIC OBSTRUCTIVE PULMONARY DISEASE).

Some of the most serious respiratory disorders arise as complications in a number of types of heart disease. Pulmonary embolism also causes serious respiratory distress.

Inflammation of the lungs is known as PNEUMONIA. PLEURISY occurs when the coverings of the lungs, the pleurae, become inflamed. A serious infectious disease that may attack the lungs is TUBERCULOSIS. A LUNG ABSCESS, an inflammation in which there is localized accumulation of pus and destruction of tissue, may sometimes be a complication of tuberculosis or pneumonia.

A very serious disease that has become increasingly prevalent in the 20th century is LUNG CANCER. Other parts of the respiratory system may also be affected by cancer. For information on other respiratory disorders, see the separate articles on the various respiratory organs.

r. therapist, registered, see respiratory THERAPIST, registered.

r. therapy, the technical speciality concerned with the treatment of cardiopulmonary disorders; formerly called inhalation therapy.

There are two basic types of respiratory therapy personnel: (1) the registered respiratory therapist (ARRT), who is a graduate of a college/hospital affiliation program, holds at least an associate degree, and has passed the national examinations of the National Board of Respiratory Therapy (see also under THERAPIST); and (2) the certified respiratory therapy technician (CRTT) who has completed a one-year program in respiratory therapy, has had one year of on-the-job training, and has passed the Technician Certification Board examination (see also under TECHNICIAN).

The bulk of direct patient care is usually provided by the CRTT, while the ARRT has administrative, supervisory, or teaching responsibilities. All respiratory therapy personnel work under the direction and supervision of a physician.

r. therapy technician, certified, see respiratory therapy TECHNICIAN, certified.

respirometer (res″pĭ-rom′ĕ-ter) an instrument for determining the nature of the respiration.

response (re-spons′) any action or change of condition evoked by a stimulus.

anamnestic r., the rapid reappearance of antibody in the blood following introduction of an antigen to which the subject had previously developed a primary immune response.

autoimmune r., the immune response in which antibodies or immune lymphoid cells are produced against the body's own tissues.

conditioned r., an acquired response developed by regular association of some physiological function with an unrelated outside event (see also CONDITIONED REPONSE and CONDITIONING).

galvanic skin r., the alteration in the electrical resistance of the skin associated with sympathetic nerve discharge.

immune r., specifically altered reactivity of the animal body after exposure to antigen, manifested as antibody-production, cell-mediated immunity, or as immunologic tolerance. Called also immune reaction. (See also IMMUNE RESPONSE.)

reticulocyte r., increase in the formation of reticulocytes in reponse to a bone marrow stimulus.

triple r. (of Lewis), a physiologic reaction of the skin to stroking with a blunt instrument: first a red line develops at the site of stroking, owing to the release of histamine or a histamine-like substance, then a flare develops around the red line, and lastly a wheal is formed as a result of local edema.

unconditioned r., an unlearned response, i.e., one that occurs naturally (see also CONDITIONING).

rest (rest) 1. repose after exertion. 2. a fragment of embryonic tissue retained within the adult organism.

restenosis (re″stĕ-no′sis) recurrent stenosis, especially of a cardiac valve after surgical correction of the primary condition.

false r., stenosis recurring after failure to divide either commissure of a cardiac valve beyond the area of incision of the papillary muscles.

restibrachium (res″tĭ-bra′ke-um) the inferior peduncle of the cerebellum.

restiform (res′tĭ-form) shaped like a rope.

restis (res′tis) the inferior peduncle of the cerebellum.

restitution (res″tĭ-too′shun) the spontaneous realignment of the fetal head with the fetal body, after delivery of the head.

restoration (res″to-ra′shun) 1. induction of a return to a previous state, as a return to health or replacement of a part to normal position. 2. partial or complete reconstruction of a body part, or the device used in its place.

restorative (rĕ-stōr′ah-tiv) 1. promoting a return to health or to consciousness. 2. a remedy that aids in restoring health, vigor, or consciousness.

restraint (re-strānt′) forcible control, as by means of a straitjacket.

resuscitation (rĕ-sus″ĭ-ta′shun) restoration to life or consciousness of one apparently dead, or whose respirations have ceased (see also ARTIFICIAL RESPIRATION).

cardiopulmonary r., an emergency technique used in cardiac arrest to reestablish heart and lung function until more advanced life support is available (see also CARDIOPULMONARY RESUSCITATION).

resuscitator (rĕ-sus′ĭ-ta″tor) an apparatus for initiating respiration in persons whose breathing has stopped.

retainer (re-tān′er) an appliance or device that keeps a tooth or partial denture in proper position.

retardate (rĕ-tar′dāt) a mentally retarded person.

retardation (re″tar-da′shun) delay; hindrance; delayed development.

mental r., subnormal general intellectual development, associated with impairment either of learning and social adjustment or of maturation, or of both (see also MENTAL RETARDATION).

retardin (rĕ-tar′din) a hormone from the pancreas that regulates fat metabolism and neutralizes the toxic action of thyroxine.

retching (rech′ing) a strong involuntary effort to vomit.

rete (re′te), pl. *re′tia* [L.] a network or meshwork, especially of blood vessels.

arterial r., r. arterio′sum, an anastomotic network of minute arteries, just before they become capillaries.

articular r., a network of anastomosing blood vessels in or around a joint.

r. malpig′hii, the innermost stratum of epidermis.

r. mirab′ile, a vascular network formed by division of an artery or vein into many smaller vessels that reunite into a single vessel.

r. tes′tis, the network of channels formed in the mediastinum of the testis by the seminiferous tubules.

r. veno′sum, an anastomotic network of small veins.

retention (rĕ-ten′shun) the process of holding back or keeping in a position, as persistence in the body of material normally excreted.

r. of urine, accumulation of urine within the bladder because of inability to urinate.

reticular (rĕ-tik′u-lar) resembling a net.

r. activating system, the system of cells of the reticular formation of the medulla oblongata that receive collaterals from the ascending sensory pathways and project to higher centers; they control the overall degree of central nervous system activity, including wakefulness, attentiveness, and sleep; abbreviated RAS.

reticulated (rĕ-tik′u-lāt″ed) reticular.

reticulation (rĕ-tik″u-la′shun) the formation or presence of a network.

reticulemia (rĕ-tik″u-le′me-ah) the presence in the blood of increased numbers of immature erythrocytes.

reticulin (rĕ-tik′u-lin) a scleroprotein present in the connective fibers of reticular tissue, closely related to collagen in composition.

reticulocyte (rĕ-tik′u-lo-sit″) a young erythrocyte showing a basophilic reticulum under vital staining.

reticulocytopenia (rĕ-tik″u-lo-si″to-pe′ne-ah) a deficiency of reticulocytes in the peripheral blood.

reticulocytosis (rĕ-tik″u-lo-si-to′sis) an excess of reticulocytes in the peripheral blood.

reticuloendothelial (rĕ-tik″u-lo-en″do-the′le-al) pertaining to the reticuloendothelium or to the reticuloendothelial system.

r. system, a network of cells and tissues found throughout the body, especially in the blood, general connective tissue, spleen, liver, lungs, bone marrow, and lymph nodes. They have both endothelial and reticular attributes and the ability to take up colloidal dye particles. Some of the reticuloendothelial cells found in the blood and in the general connective tissue are unusually large in size. These cells are concerned in blood cell formation and destruction, storage of fatty materials, and metabolism of iron and pigment, and they play a role in inflammation and immunity. Some of the cells are motile —that is, capable of spontaneous motion—and phagocytic—they can ingest and destroy unwanted foreign material.

The reticuloendothelial cells of the SPLEEN possess the ability to dispose of disintegrated erythrocytes. They do not, however, destroy hemoglobin, which is liberated in the process.

The reticuloendothelial cells located in the blood cavities of the LIVER are called Kupffer cells. These cells, together with the cells of the general connective tissue and bone marrow, are capable of transforming into bile pigment the hemoglobin released by disintegrated erythrocytes.

DISORDERS OF THE RETICULOENDOTHELIAL SYSTEM. The reticuloendothelial system can be the site of a variety of diseases, all of which are rare. They are generally treated by x-ray therapy and steroids, among other methods. The prospects for recovery cannot always be predicted.

The disorders include Gaucher's disease, Letterer-Siwe disease, eosinophilic granuloma, and HAND-SCHÜLLER-CHRISTIAN DISEASE. A rare illness called Niemann-Pick disease strikes mainly children of Jewish origin.

reticuloendothelioma (rĕ-tik″u-lo-en″do-the″le-o′mah) malignant lymphoma.

reticuloendotheliosis (rĕ-tik″u-lo-en″do-the″le-o′sis) hyperplasia of reticuloendothelial tissue.

reticuloendothelium (rĕ-tik″u-lo-en″do-the′le-um) the tissue of the reticuloendothelial system.

reticulohistiocytoma (rĕ-tik′u-lo-his″te-o-si-to′mah) a granulomatous aggregation of lipid-laden histiocytes and multinucleated giant cells.

reticuloma (rĕ-tik″u-lo′mah) histiocytic malignant lymphoma.

reticulopenia (rĕ-tik″u-lo-pe′ne-ah) reticulocytopenia.

reticulopodium (rĕ-tik″u-lo-po′de-um) a thread-like, branching pseudopodium.

reticulosarcoma (rĕ-tik″u-lo-sar-ko′mah) malignant lymphoma, histiocytic or undifferentiated.

reticulosis (rĕ-tik″u-lo′sis) an abnormal increase in cells derived from or related to the reticuloendothelial cells.

familial histiocytic r., histiocytic medullary r., a fatal hereditary disorder marked by anemia, granulocytopenia, thrombocytopenia, phagocytosis of blood cells, diffuse proliferation of histiocytes, and enlargement of the liver, spleen, and lymph nodes.

reticulum (rĕ-tik′u-lum), pl. *retic′ula* [L.] 1. a small network, especially a protoplasmic network in cells. 2. reticular tissue.

endoplasmic r., an ultramicroscopic organelle of nearly all higher plant and animal cells, consisting of a system of membrane-bound cavities in the cytoplasm, occurring in two types: granular or rough-surfaced, bearing large numbers of ribosomes on its outer surface, and agranular or smooth-surfaced.

sarcoplasmic r., a form of agranular reticulum in the sarcoplasm of striated muscle, comprising a system of smooth-surfaced tubules surrounding each myofibril.

retiform (rĕ'tĭ-form, ret'ĭ-form) reticular.

retina (ret'ĭ-nah) the innermost of the three tunics of the eyeball, surrounding the vitreous body and continuous posteriorly with the optic nerve. The retina is composed of light-sensitive neurons arranged in three layers; the first layer is made up of rods and cones and the other two transmit impulses from the rods and cones to the OPTIC NERVE. The rods are sensitive in dim light, and the cones are sensitive in bright light and are responsible for color vision. (See also EYE.)

Retinopathies are pathologic conditions of the retina; they occur in conjunction with certain systemic disorders, such as hypertension, nephritis, toxemia of pregnancy, and diabetes mellitus.

DETACHMENT OF THE RETINA is complete or partial separation of the retina from the choroid, the middle coat of the eyeball. It occurs most often in persons with MYOPIA (nearsightedness), but it also can result from trauma to the head.

retinaculum (ret"ĭ-nak'u-lum), pl. *retinac'ula* [L.] 1. a structure that retains an organ or tissue in place. 2. an instrument for retracting tissues during surgery.

flexor r. of hand, a fibrous band forming the carpal tunnel, through which pass the tendons of the flexor muscles of the hand and fingers.

r. morgag'ni, a ridge formed by the coming together of segments of the ileocecal valve.

r. ten'dinum, a tendinous restraining structure, such as an annular ligament.

retinal (ret'ĭ-nal) 1. pertaining to the retina. 2. the aldehyde of retinol, having vitamin A activity. One isomer (11-*cis* retinal) combines with opsin in the retinal rods (scotopsin) to form rhodopsin (visual purple); another, all-*trans* retinal, or visual yellow, results from the bleaching of rhodopsin by light, in which the 11-*cis* form is converted to the all-*trans* form. Retinal also combines with opsins in the retinal cones to form the three pigments responsible for color vision.

retine (ret'ēn) a substance stated to be widely distributed in animal cells, capable of inhibiting cell division and growth.

retinene (ret'ĭ-nēn) an ocular pigment derived from vitamin A and formed by the bleaching action of light on rhodopsin. It occurs in two forms: $retinene_1$ is retinal (2), and $retinene_2$ is dehydroretinal.

retinitis (ret"ĭ-ni'tis) inflammation of the retina.

r. circina'ta, circinate r., circinate retinopathy.

r. discifor'mis, a bilateral, degenerative retinal disease, with an elevated grayish white mass in the macular area.

exudative r., Coats' disease.

r. haemorrha'gica, retinitis with profuse retinal hemorrhage.

r. pigmento'sa, a group of diseases, often hereditary, marked by progressive loss of retinal response, retinal atrophy, attenuation of retinal vessels, star-shaped deposits of pigment, and progressive contraction of the visual field.

r. prolif'erans, a condition that may result from intraocular hemorrhage, with the formation of fibrous bands extending into the vitreous from the retina; retinal detachment may result.

suppurative r., retinitis due to pyemic infection.

retinoblastoma (ret"ĭ-no-blas-to'mah) a tumor arising from retinal cells.

retinochoroiditis (ret"ĭ-no-ko"roi-di'tis) inflammation of the retina and choroid.

r. juxtapapilla'ris, a small area of inflammation on the fundus of the eye near the papilla; seen in young healthy individuals.

retinoid (ret'ĭ-noid) resembling the retina.

retinol (ret'ĭ-nol) vitamin A_1; the form of vitamin A found in mammals, which is reversibly dehydrogenated by enzymatic action into its aldehyde, retinal.

retinomalacia (ret"ĭ-no-mah-la'she-ah) softening of the retina.

retinopapillitis (ret"ĭ-no-pap"ĭ-li'tis) inflammation of retina and optic disk (papilla).

retinopathy (ret"ĭ-nop'ah-the) any noninflammatory disease of the retina.

circinate r., a condition in which a circle of white spots encloses the macula, leading to complete foveal blindness.

diabetic r., retinal manifestations of diabetes mellitus, including microaneurysms and punctate exudates.

exudative r., Coats' disease.

hypertensive r., exudates, hemorrhages, and vascular sclerosis in the retina due to hypertension.

r. of prematurity, retrolental fibroplasia.

retinoschisis (ret"ĭ-nos'kĭ-sis) splitting of the retina, occurring in the nerve fiber layer (in juvenile form), or in the external plexiform layer (in adult form).

retinoscope (ret'ĭ-no-skōp") skiascope; an instrument used in retinoscopy.

retinoscopy (ret"ĭ-nos'ko-pe) skiametry; observation of the pupil and retina under a beam of light projected into the eye, as a means of determining refractive errors of the eye.

retinosis (ret"ĭ-no'sis) any degenerative, noninflammatory condition of the retina.

retort (rĕ-tort') a globular, long-necked vessel used in distillation.

retothelium (re"to-the'le-um) reticuloendothelium.

retractile (rĕ-trak'til) susceptible of being drawn back.

retraction (rĕ-trak'shun) the act of drawing back, or condition of being drawn back.

clot r., the drawing away of a blood clot from a vessel wall, a function of blood platelets.

retractor (rĕ-trak'tor) 1. an instrument for holding open the edges of a wound. 2. a muscle that retracts.

retro- word element [L.], *behind; backward.*

retroaction (ret"ro-ak'shun) action in a reversed direction; reaction.

retroauricular (ret"ro-aw-rik'u-lar) behind the auricle of the ear.

retrobulbar (ret"ro-bul'bar) behind the eyeball.

retrocecal (ret″ro-se′kal) behind the cecum.

retrocervical (ret″ro-ser′vĭ-kal) behind the cervix uteri.

retrocession (ret″ro-sesh′un) a going backward; backward displacement.

retrocolic (ret″ro-kol′ik) behind the colon.

retrocollic (ret″ro-kol′ik) pertaining to the back of the neck; nuchal.

retrocollis (ret″ro-kol′is) spasmodic torticollis in which the head is drawn back.

retrocursive (ret″ro-ker′siv) marked by stepping backward.

retrodeviation (ret″ro-de″ve-a′shun) a general term including retroversion, retroflexion, retroposition, etc.

retrodisplacement (ret″ro-dis-plās′ment) backward or posterior displacement.

retroesophageal (ret″ro-ĕ-sof″ah-je′al) behind the esophagus.

retroflexion (ret″ro-flek′shun) the bending of an organ so that its top is thrust backward: specifically, the bending backward of the body of the uterus upon the cervix.

retrogasserian (ret″ro-gas-se′re-an) pertaining to the sensory (posterior) root of the trigeminal (gasserian) ganglion.

retrognathia (ret″ro-nath′e-ah) underdevelopment of the maxilla and/or mandible. adj., **retrognath′ic.**

retrograde (ret′ro-grād) going backward; retracting a former course; catabolic.

r. pyelography, radiography of the kidney after introduction of contrast medium through the ureter.

retrogression (ret″ro-gresh′un) degeneration; deterioration; regression; return to an earlier, less complex condition.

retroinsular (ret″ro-in′su-lar) behind the island of Reil of the cerebral cortex.

retrolental (ret″ro-len′tal) behind the lens of the eye.

r. fibroplasia, a condition peculiar to premature infants and characterized by the presence of opaque tissue behind the lens, leading to detachment of the retina and arrest of growth of the eye. It is the chief cause of blindness in the newborn. The cause of the condition is OXYGEN poisoning; a high concentration of oxygen causes spasm of the retinal vessels, which eventually leads to exudation of blood and serum through the vessel walls. To prevent this occurrence it is recommended that the concentration of oxygen in the incubator not exceed 40 per cent, and that administration of oxygen be discontinued as soon as possible.

retrolingual (ret″ro-ling′gwal) behind the tongue.

retromammary (ret″ro-mam′ar-e) behind the mammary gland.

retromandibular (ret″ro-man-dib′u-lar) behind the lower jaw.

retromastoid (ret″ro-mas′toid) behind the mastoid process.

retromorphosis (ret″ro-mor-fo′sis) retrograde metamorphosis.

retronasal (ret″ro-na′zal) pertaining to the back part of the nose.

retro-ocular (ret″ro-ok′u-lar) behind the eye.

retroparotid (ret″ro-pah-rot′id) behind the parotid gland.

retroperitoneal (ret″ro-per′ĭ-to-ne′al) behind the peritoneum.

r. fibrosis, deposition of fibrous tissue in the retroperitoneal space, producing vague abdominal discomfort, and often causing blockage of the ureters, with resultant hydronephrosis and impaired renal function, which may result in renal failure. Called also Ormond's disease.

retroperitoneum (ret″ro-per″ĭ-to-ne′um) the retroperitoneal space; the space between the peritoneum and the posterior abdominal wall.

retroperitonitis (ret″ro-per″ĭ-to-ni′tis) inflammation in the retroperitoneal space.

retropharyngeal (ret″ro-fah-rin′je-al) behind the pharynx.

retropharyngitis (ret″ro-far″in-ji′tis) inflammation of posterior part of the pharynx.

retroplasia (ret″ro-pla′ze-ah) retrograde metaplasia; degeneration of a tissue or cell into a more primitive type.

retroposed (ret″ro-pōsd′) displaced backward.

retroposition (ret″ro-po-zish′un) backward displacement.

retropulsion (ret″ro-pul′shun) 1. a driving back, as of the fetal head in labor. 2. tendency to walk backward, as in some cases of tabes dorsalis. 3. an abnormal gait in which the body is bent backward.

retrotarsal (ret″ro-tar′sal) behind the tarsus of the eye.

retrouterine (ret″ro-u′ter-in) behind the uterus.

retroversion (ret″ro-ver′zhun) the tipping backward of an entire organ, as of the uterus.

Reuss's color charts (rois′ez) charts with colored letters printed on colored backgrounds; used for testing color vision.

Reverdin's needle (ra-ver-danz′) a surgical needle with an eye that can be opened by means of a slide.

reversal (rĕ-ver′sal) a turning or change in the opposite direction.

sex r., a change in characteristics from those typical of one sex to those typical of the other.

reverse isolation see PROTECTIVE ISOLATION.

reverse transcriptase an enzyme of RNA viruses that catalyzes the transcription of RNA to DNA, which is then incorporated into the genome of the host cell. (See also CANCER.)

reversion (rĕ-ver′zhun) 1. a returning to a previous condition; regression. 2. in genetics, inheritance from some remote ancestor of a character that has not been manifest for several generations.

revulsant (rĕ-vul′sant) revulsive.

revulsion (rĕ-vul′shun) the drawing of blood from one part to another, as in counterirritation; the diminution of morbid action in any part of the body by irritation in another.

revulsive (rĕ-vul′siv) 1. causing revulsion. 2. an agent causing revulsion.

Reye's syndrome an acute and often fatal disease of childhood characterized by acute edema of the brain, hypoglycemia, and fatty infiltration and dysfunction of the liver. The disease may follow a variety of common viral infections, but the relationship between the viral infection and pathologic changes in the brain and liver is not known.

Within several hours to several days after a mild

gastrointestinal disturbance or upper respiratory infection, the patient presents with symptoms of persistent vomiting followed by delirium, convulsions, and coma. There are no meningeal or focal neurologic signs present, and the cerebrospinal fluid protein is normal.

Treatment is aimed at the correction of HYPOGLYCEMIA, ACIDOSIS, and electrolyte imbalance. Measures are employed to reduce intracranial pressure and to correct metabolic abnormalities. There is no specific medication or treatment that will cure the disease. Survivors may suffer from the effects of brain damage.

Reduction in the mortality rate, which has been reported as low as 25 per cent and as high as 80 per cent, is believed to be the result of improved management and the correct diagnosis of milder cases that were formerly misdiagnosed.

Rezipas (rez'ĭ-pas) trademark for a preparation of para-aminosalicylic acid, used in treatment of tuberculosis.

Rf chemical symbol, *rutherfordium.*

R.F.A. right frontoanterior (position of the fetus).

R.F.P. right frontoposterior (position of the fetus).

R.F.T. right frontotransverse (position of the fetus).

Rh 1. chemical symbol, *rhodium.* 2. symbol for Rhesus factor (see RH FACTOR).

Rh factor genetically determined antigens (agglutinogens) present on the surface of erythrocytes. There are at least eight different variations of these agglutinogens, and each of the agglutinogens is called an Rh factor (named for the rhesus monkey used in early experiments). If any one of these factors is present in an individual's red blood cells, he is said to be Rh positive (D positive, Rh_0); if the factor is absent he is said to be Rh negative (D negative, dd, or Hr_0). Approximately 85 per cent of all Caucasoids are Rh positive, and 15 per cent are Rh negative. Other races, such as Indians of North America, Negroes, Japanese, and Chinese, are 99 to 100 per cent Rh positive.

The presence or absence of an Rh factor is especially important in blood transfusions and in pregnancy because mixing of two types of blood may result in the agglutination (clumping together) of red blood cells, with plugging of the capillaries and destruction of the red blood cells. This agglutination is an immune reaction and depends on the formation of antibodies against the specific agglutinogen (Rh factor) present in the erythrocytes. It should be pointed out that this immune reaction does not occur immediately, but depends on the gradual formation of antibodies; the response also is more severe in some persons than in others. Thus there may be no difficulty in the first transfusion of Rh-incompatible blood, but on repeated exposure to the Rh factor, the Rh-negative individual becomes "sensitized" to the agglutinogens in Rh-positive blood and builds up a greater quantity of antibodies.

In pregnancy difficulty may arise when the mother is Rh negative and the fetus is Rh positive. The Rh antigens (agglutinogens) in the fetal tissues diffuse through the placental membrane and enter the mother's blood. Her body reacts by forming anti-Rh agglutinins, which diffuse back through the placental membrane into the fetal circulation and cause clumping of the fetal erythrocytes. This condition is called ERYTHROBLASTOSIS FETALIS, or hemolytic disease of the newborn. When the erythrocytes are destroyed, hemoglobin leaks into the plasma, producing jaundice and anemia. *In utero,* the hemo-

globin is metabolized by the mother mainly; however, post partum, the neonate cannot detoxify the excess hemoglobin pigments (bilirubin) and they may destroy nerve tissue and produce brain damage—a condition called kernicterus. The antibodies also may damage many other cells of the body.

The fetal-maternal reaction is similar to an Rh-produced transfusion reaction in that the agglutination varies in severity and usually occurs gradually. An Rh-negative mother having her first Rh-positive child usually does not build up sufficient antibodies (agglutinins) to cause harm to the fetus, but in subsequent pregnancies with Rh-positive infants she may. The incidence of erythroblastosis fetalis in infants of Rh-negative mothers depends on the number of Rh-positive children she has. If the father of the children is Rh positive and heterozygous (about 55 per cent are) about one-fourth of the offspring will be Rh negative and will not stimulate the production of antibodies in the mother.

Scientific advances have helped reduce the risk to the Rh-positive infants of Rh-negative mothers. (See also AMNIOCENTESIS, and exchange and intrauterine TRANSFUSION.) Recently it has become possible to immunize Rh-negative mothers after their first pregnancy against future Rh-incompatibility reactions. Immediately after parturition, anti-Rh antibody (RhoGAM) is injected into the mother; it combines with Rh-positive erythrocytes or substances from the fetus that have entered the maternal circulation, and renders them inert—that is, no longer capable of eliciting maternal antibody formation. Immunization must be repeated after each birth.

rhabd(o)- word element [Gr.], *rod; rod-shaped.*

Rhabditis (rab-di'tis) a genus of minute nematodes found mostly in damp earth, and as an accidental parasite in man.

rhabdocyte (rab'do-sīt) metamyelocyte.

rhabdoid (rab'doid) resembling a rod; rod-shaped.

rhabdomyoblastoma (rab"do-mi"o-blas-to'mah) rhabdomyosarcoma.

rhabdomyolysis (rab"do-mi-ol'ĭ-sis) disintegration of striated muscle fibers with excretion of myoglobin in the urine.

rhabdomyoma (rab"do-mi-o'mah) a tumor containing striated muscle fibers.

rhabdomyosarcoma (rab"do-mi"o-sar-ko'mah) a highly malignant tumor of striated muscle derived from primitive mesenchymal cells and characterized by anaplastic striated cells.

Rhabdonema (rab"do-ne'mah) Rhabditis.

rhabdosarcoma (rab"do-sar-ko'mah) rhabdomyosarcoma.

rhabdovirus (rab"do-vi'rus) any of a group of morphologically similar bullet-shaped or bacilliform RNA viruses.

rhachi- for words beginning thus, see those beginning *rachi-.*

rhagades (rag'ah-dēz) fissures, cracks, or fine scars in the skin, especially such lesions around the mouth or other regions subjected to frequent movement.

rhaphe (ra'fe) raphe.

rhenium (re'ne-um) a chemical element, atomic

number 75, atomic weight 186.2, symbol Re. (See table of ELEMENTS.)

rheo- word element [Gr.], *electric current; flow* (as of fluids).

rheobase (re'o-bās) the minimum potential of electric current necessary to produce stimulation. adj., **rheoba'sic.**

rheology (re-ol'o-je) the science of the deformation and flow of matter, such as the flow of blood through the heart and blood vessels.

rheonome (re'o-nōm) an apparatus for determining the effect of irritation on a nerve.

rheostat (re'o-stat) an apparatus for regulating resistance in an electric circuit.

rheostosis (re″os-to'sis) a condition of hyperostosis marked by the presence of streaks in the bones; melorheostosis.

rheotaxis (re″o-tak'sis) orientation of an organism in a stream of liquid, with its long axis parallel with the direction of flow, designated negative (moving in the same direction) or positive (moving in the opposite direction).

rhestocythemia (res″to-si-the'me-ah) the occurrence of broken-down erythrocytes in the blood.

rheum (rōōm) any watery or catarrhal discharge.

rheumarthritis (roo″mar-thri'tis) rheumatoid arthritis.

rheumatalgia (roo″mah-tal'je-ah) chronic rheumatic pain.

rheumatic (roo-mat'ik) pertaining to or affected with rheumatism.

r. fever, a disease associated with the presence of hemolytic streptococci in the body. It is called rheumatic fever because two of the commonest symptoms are fever and pain in the joints similar to that of rheumatism. Rheumatic fever is relatively common and occurs particularly among children between 5 and 15 years of age. Young adults in the early twenties are also susceptible, although less so.

CAUSES. Rheumatic fever is a delayed sequela of an upper respiratory infection caused by the Group A hemolytic streptococcus that causes such common childhood illnesses as scarlet fever, tonsillitis, "strep throat," and ear infections. Rheumatic fever is only one of several complications that can result from a streptococcal infection.

The connection between rheumatic fever and a previous streptococcal infection has been proved only indirectly. That is, in almost all cases of rheumatic fever there is evidence of a previous streptococcal infection; and when these infections have been treated promptly, the occurrence of rheumatic fever has declined sharply. There is evidence that the symptoms of rheumatic fever may result from an antigen-antibody reaction to one or more of the products of the hemolytic streptococcus, but the exact way in which this occurs is not known. Rheumatic fever has been classified as an AUTOIMMUNE DISEASE.

Rheumatic fever tends to run in families, and there may be a hereditary predisposition to the disease. Economic and environmental conditions such as damp, cold climate and poor health habits may be contributing factors.

SYMPTOMS. The initial symptoms usually appear 1 to 4 weeks after the streptococcal infection has occurred. The actual onset of the disease may be either gradual or sudden. The symptoms vary widely and may be of any degree of severity.

The commonest initial complaints are a slight fever, a feeling of tiredness, a vague feeling of pain in the limbs, and nosebleeds. If the disease takes an acute form, the fever may reach 104° F. (40° C.) by the second day and continue for several weeks, although the usual course of the fever is about 2 weeks. On the other hand, the fever may be quite mild.

Joint pain develops at any stage of the disease and lasts from a few hours to several weeks. The joints swell and are tender to the touch. The pain and swelling often subside in one group of joints and arise in another. As the pain subsides, the joints return to normal.

Other symptoms may include spasmodic twitching movements known as Sydenham's chorea, often called St. Vitus's dance; it is most common in girls between the ages of 6 and 11. A rash caused by the fever may appear upon the body. Nodules may be seen or felt under the skin at the elbow, knee, and wrist joints, and along the spine. Among the most serious signs is the development of a heart murmur and cardiac decompensation.

HEART DAMAGE. The seriousness of rheumatic fever lies primarily in the permanent damage it can do to the heart. The disease tends to recur; and these recurrent attacks may further weaken the heart.

The usual cardiac complication of rheumatic fever is endocarditis—inflammation of the inner lining of the heart, including the membrane over the valves. As a valve heals, its edges may become so scarred and stiff that they fail to close properly. As a result, blood leaks through the valve when it is closed, producing the sound characteristic of a heart murmur. The valves may become thickened with scar tissue, so that the amount of blood that can flow through the heart is restricted. If there is severe stenosis of the mitral valve and the patient develops symptoms of congestive heart failure, surgery to enlarge the valve (COMMISSUROTOMY) may be indicated.

TREATMENT. The main purposes of treatment are reduction of fever and pain and promotion of the natural healing processes; no means have yet been discovered for fighting the disease directly. Until the introduction of antibiotics and hormone extracts, the chief medications were aspirin and other salicylates. Penicillin is prescribed if there is evidence of a ongoing streptococcal infection or the chance of exposure to streptococcal infection. Prednisone may be prescribed to reduce the pain and swelling in the joints, but its effect on the ultimate course of the disease is controversial. If pain is severe, analgesic drugs may be given.

Bed rest is an important part of the treatment, particularly if the disease has caused heart damage. Depending upon the severity of the disease, the patient may be kept in bed for months, and prolonged convalescence may be needed.

PATIENT CARE. In the acute phase of rheumatic fever rest is most important to reduce the work load of the heart. The patient should be made as comfortable as possible and disturbed only when necessary. The care should be planned so that long periods of complete rest are possible. Proper positioning with adequate support of the limbs and maintenance of good body alignment is essential to rest and the prevention of complications.

The temperature, pulse, and respirations are checked and recorded at least every 4 hours during the day. The volume and rhythm as well as the rate of the pulse should be noted. The blood pressure is taken once a day. Fluid intake may be restricted if there is edema, and sodium intake may also be limited; in either case the reason for the restriction should be explained to the patient. A record is kept of the intake and output.

Frequent back care and good oral hygiene are needed to promote comfort and relaxation. When turning the patient, one should be gentle and slow, avoiding unnecessary handling of the joints, which may be tender and swollen.

During the convalescence period the patient is allowed a gradual return to physical activities. The amount of activity depends on the physician's orders and is based on the patient's pulse rate, erythrocyte sedimentation rate, and C-reaction protein test. Measures must be taken to avoid respiratory infections, which will retard the progress of the patient. Small, frequent feedings that provide a well-balanced diet are usually preferred to three meals a day, which may be only partially eaten by a patient who is not engaging in a normal amount of physical activity.

As the need for rest is decreased, some provision must be made for diversional activities that will help eliminate boredom and keep the child content. The psychologic effects of a prolonged period of enforced dependence on others must also be considered. The parents and the child will need encouragement and help in the transition from total dependence to relative independence.

PREVENTION. Preventive care is extremely important, especially when rheumatic fever has once occurred, since it tends to return unless precautionary steps are taken. The patient is given penicillin, orally every day or by intramuscular injection once a month, for many years in order to prevent streptococcal infection. A good nutritious diet and sufficient sleep are important. Administration of antibiotics to all patients with history of rheumatic fever undergoing even minor surgery, including tooth extraction, is important in preventing bacterial endocarditis.

It is believed that prompt and effective treatment of "strep throat" among the general population will prevent many cases of rheumatic fever.

r. heart disease, the most important and constant manifestation of rheumatic fever, consisting of inflammatory changes with valvular deformities.

rheumatid (roo′mah-tid) any skin lesion etiologically associated with rheumatism.

rheumatism (roo′mah-tizm) any of a variety of disorders marked by inflammation, degeneration, or metabolic derangement of the connective tissue structures, especially the joints and related structures, and attended by pain, stiffness, or limitation of motion; a term applied by laymen to such disorders as ARTHRITIS, OSTEOARTHRITIS, BURSITIS, and SCIATICA. See also Table accompanying ARTHRITIS.

acute articular r., rheumatic fever.

muscular r., fibrositis.

palindromic r., repeated attacks of arthritis and periarthritis without fever and without causing irreversible joint changes.

rheumatoid (roo′mah-toid) resembling rheumatism.

r. arthritis, a form of arthritis, the cause of which is unknown, although infection, hypersensitivity, hormone imbalance, and psychologic stress have been suggested as possible causes. The disease is most common in persons 20 to 40 years old (it is relatively uncommon in children), and more than two-thirds of the patients are women.

SYMPTOMS. Rheumatoid arthritis is marked by stiff, sore jonts, usually in the fingers, wrists, knees, ankles, or toes. Swelling, redness, and tenderness occur in the soft tissue surrounding the affected joints. In acute stages, the patient may feel severe pain, fatigue, and general weakness caused by rheumatoid changes in the muscles, and there may be fever. The affected joints become painful, swollen, and stiff, and the pain tends to migrate to other joints. Later, nodules may develop under the skin at sites of bony prominences.

The course of rheumatoid arthritis is unpredictable. Symptoms may stop abruptly for reasons as little understood as the causes of the disease; they usually recur just as unexpectedly. In general, joint and muscle symptoms are particularly troublesome after the patient has been inactive physically, and lessen when he resumes normal activity. Chronic rheumatoid arthritis may result in permanent deformity and immobility of joints.

TREATMENT. Proper care and early treatment are essential to recovery and to the prevention of permanent damage to the joints. Though no specific cure has been found for rheumatoid arthritis, most patients respond well to treatment involving salicylates, cortisone, and gold salts and carefully regulated programs of alternating rest and therapeutic exercise (see ARTHRITIS). The disease is progressive and likely to recur, sometimes with increasing intensity. In about 15 per cent of the cases, some degree of permanent stiffness eventually develops.

RHEUMATOID ARTHRITIS IN CHILDREN. About 5 per cent of all patients with rheumatoid arthritis are children, with the onset of the illness occurring between the ages of 2 and 4 years. The disease is self-limited, usually lasting about 3 years. It begins quite abruptly with a spiking fever to as high as 106° F. (41.1° C.), pain and swelling of joints, and a rash. During the clinical course there often are periods of remission followed by sudden exacerbations of symptoms. Treatment is the same as for adults.

Because of the nature of the disease and the age of the patient, a long-term plan of home care is necessary. The parents, local physician, and community agencies concerned with chronic illness should participate in the planning and care of the child so that a coordinated and disciplined program can be carried out.

r. factor, a protein of high molecular weight in the serum of most patients with rheumatoid arthritis, detectable by serologic tests.

r. spondylitis, rheumatoid arthritis of the spine, affecting young males predominantly and producing pain and stiffness as a result of inflammation of the sacroiliac, intervertebral, and costovertebral joints; it may progress to cause complete spinal and thoracic rigidity. Called also Bechterew's disease and Marie-Strümpell disease.

rheumatologist (roo″mah-tol′o-jist) a specialist in rheumatology.

rheumatology (roo″mah-tol′o-je) the study of rheumatism.

rhexis (rek′sis) the rupture of a blood vessel or of an organ.

rhigosis (rĭ-go′sis) the perception of cold.

rhin(o)- word element [Gr.], *nose; noselike structure.*

rhinal (ri'nal) pertaining to the nose.

rhinalgia (ri-nal'je-ah) pain in the nose.

rhinencephalon (ri"nen-sef'ah-lon) 1. the part of the brain once thought to be concerned entirely with olfactory mechanisms, including olfactory nerves, bulbs, tracts, and subsequent connections (all olfactory in function) and the limbic system (not primarily olfactory in function); homologous with olfactory portions of the brain in lower animals. 2. one of the parts of the embryonic telencephalon.

rhinesthesia (ri"nes-the'ze-ah) the sense of smell.

rhineurynter (ri"nu-rin'ter) a dilatable rubber bag for distending a nostril.

rhinion (rin'e-on) the lower end of the suture between the nasal bones.

rhinitis (ri-ni'tis) inflammation of the mucous membrane of the nose. It may be mild and chronic, or acute.

Viruses, bacteria, and allergens are responsible for the varied manifestations of rhinitis. Often a viral rhinitis is complicated by a bacterial infection caused by streptococci, staphylococci, and pneumococci or other bacteria. Hay fever, an acute type of allergic rhinitis, is also subject to bacterial complications. Many factors assist the invasion of the mucous membranes by bacteria, including allergens, excessive dryness, exposure to dampness and cold, excessive inhalation of dust, and injury to the nasal cilia due to viral infection.

In general, rhinitis is not serious, but some forms may be contagious. The mucous membrane of the nose becomes swollen and there is a nasal discharge. Some types are accompanied by fever, muscle aches, and general discomfort with sneezing and running eyes. Breathing through the nose may become difficult or impossible. Often rhinitis is accompanied by inflammation of the throat and sinuses. If bacterial infection develops, the nasal discharge is thick and contains pus.

In acute rhinitis, the medical term for the COMMON COLD, the best treatment consists of rest, preferably in bed, a well-balanced diet, and sufficient fluids. Aspirin will relieve headache and fever.

Chronic rhinitis may result in a permanent thickening of the nasal mucosa. Treatment is aimed at eliminating the primary cause of rhinitis and administration of decongestants to relieve nasal congestion.

allergic r., anaphylactic r., any allergic reaction of the nasal mucosa, occurring perennially (nonseasonal allergic RHINITIS) or seasonally (HAY FEVER).

atrophic r., chronic rhinitis with wasting of the mucous membrane and glands.

r. caseo'sa, that with a caseous, gelatinous, and fetid discharge.

fibrinous r., rhinitis with development of a false membrane.

hypertrophic r., that with thickening and swelling of the mucous membrane.

membranous r., chronic rhinitis with a membranous exudate.

nonseasonal allergic r., allergic rhinitis occurring continuously or intermittently all year round, due to exposure to a more or less ever-present allergen, marked by sudden attacks of sneezing, swelling of the nasal mucosa with profuse watery discharge, itching of the eyes, and lacrimation. Called also nonseasonal, or perennial, hay fever.

purulent r., chronic rhinitis with formation of pus.

vasomotor r., 1. nonallergic rhinitis in which transient changes in vascular tone and permeability (with the same symptoms of allergic rhinitis) are brought on by such stimuli as mild chilling, fatigue, anger, and anxiety. 2. any condition of allergic or nonallergic rhinitis, as opposed to infectious rhinitis.

rhinoantritis (ri"no-an-tri'tis) inflammation of the nasal cavity and maxillary sinus.

rhinocanthectomy (ri"no-kan-thek'to-me) rhinommectomy.

rhinocephalus (ri"no-sef'ah-lus) a fetus exhibiting rhinocephaly.

rhinocephaly (ri"no-sef'ah-le) a developmental anomaly characterized by the presence of a proboscis-like nose above eyes partially or completely fused into one.

rhinocheiloplasty (ri"no-ki'lo-plas"te) plastic surgery of the nose and lip.

rhinocleisis (ri"no-kli'sis) obstruction of the nasal passage.

rhinodacryolith (ri"no-dak're-o-lith") a lacrimal concretion in the nasal duct.

rhinodynia (ri"no-din'e-ah) pain in the nose.

rhinogenous (ri-noj'ĕ-nus) arising in the nose.

rhinokyphosis (ri"no-ki-fo'sis) an abnormal hump on the ridge of the nose.

rhinolalia (ri"no-la'le-ah) a nasal quality of speech from some disease or defect of the nasal passages.

r. aper'ta, that due to too great opening of the nasal passages.

r. clau'sa, that due to undue closure of the nasal passages.

rhinolaryngitis (ri"no-lar"in-ji'tis) inflammation of the mucosa of the nose and larynx.

rhinolith (ri'no-lith) a nasal calculus.

rhinolithiasis (ri"no-lĭ-thi'ah-sis) a condition associated with formation of rhinoliths.

rhinologist (ri-nol'o-jist) a specialist in rhinology.

rhinology (ri-nol'o-je) the sum of knowledge about the nose and its diseases.

rhinometer (ri-nom'ĕ-ter) an instrument for measuring the nose or its cavities.

rhinommectomy (ri"nom-mek'to-me) excision of the inner canthus of the eye.

rhinomycosis (ri"no-mi-ko'sis) fungal infection of the nasal mucosa.

rhinonecrosis (ri"no-nĕ-kro'sis) necrosis of the nasal bones.

rhinopathy (ri-nop'ah-the) any disease of the nose.

rhinopharyngitis (ri"no-far"in-ji'tis) inflammation of the nasopharynx.

rhinophonia (ri"no-fo'ne-ah) a nasal twang or quality of voice.

rhinophore (ri'no-fōr) a nasal cannula to facilitate breathing.

rhinophycomycosis (ri"no-fi"ko-mi-ko'sis) a fungal disease caused by *Entomophora coronata*, marked by formation of large polyps in the subcutaneous tissues of the nose and paranasal sinuses; orbital involvement and unilateral blindness may follow. Cerebral involvement is common.

rhinophyma (ri"no-fi'mah) a form of rosacea marked by redness, sebaceous hyperplasia, and nodular swelling and congestion of the skin of the nose.

rhinoplasty (ri′no-plas″te) plastic surgery of the nose.

rhinopolypus (ri″no-pol′ĭ-pus) a nasal polyp.

rhinorrhagia (ri″no-ra′je-ah) nosebleed; epistaxis.

rhinorrhea (ri″no-re′ah) the free discharge of a thin nasal mucus.

cerebrospinal r., discharge of cerebrospinal fluid through the nose, usually due to skull fracture.

rhinosalpingitis (ri″no-sal″pin-ji′tis) inflammation of the mucosa of the nose and eustachian tube.

rhinoscleroma (ri″no-sklĕ-ro′mah) a granulomatous disease involving the nose and nasopharynx. The growth forms hard patches or nodules, which tend to enlarge and are painful to the touch. The disease occurs in Egypt, eastern Europe, and Central and South America. It is ascribed to the presence of *Klebsiella rhinoscleromatis.*

rhinoscope (ri′no-skōp) a speculum for use in nasal examination.

rhinoscopy (ri-nos′ko-pe) examination of the nose with a speculum, through either the anterior nares or the nasopharynx.

rhinosporidiosis (ri″no-spo-rid″e-o′sis) a fungal disease caused by *Rhinosporidium seeberi,* marked by large polyps on the mucosa of the nose, eyes, ears, and sometimes the penis and vagina.

rhinotomy (ri-not′o-me) incision into the nose.

rhinovirus (ri″no-vi′rus) a subgroup of the picornaviruses, considered to be etiologically associated with the common cold and certain other upper respiratory ailments. Called also coryzavirus.

rhizo- (ri′zo) word element [Gr.], *root.*

rhizoid (ri′zoid) resembling a root.

rhizome (ri′zōm) the subterranean root stem of a plant.

rhizomelic (ri″zo-mel′ik) pertaining to the hips and shoulders (the roots of the limbs).

rhizomeningomyelitis (ri″zo-mĕ-ning″go-mi″ĕ-li′tis) radiculomeningomyelitis; inflammation of the nerve roots, meninges, and spinal cord.

rhizoneure (ri′zo-nūr) a nerve cell forming a nerve root.

Rhizopoda (ri-zop′o-dah) a class of protozoa of the subphylum Sarcodina, having pseudopodia, and including the amebae.

rhizopodium (ri″zo-po′de-um), pl. *rhizopo′dia* [Gr.] a filamentous pseudopodium, characterized by branching and anastomosis of the branches.

rhizotomy (ri-zot′o-me) division or transection of a nerve root, either within the spinal canal or outside it.

rhod(o)- (ro′do) word element [Gr.], *red.*

rhodium (ro′de-um) a chemical element, atomic number 45, atomic weight 102.905, symbol Rh. (See table of ELEMENTS.)

rhodogenesis (ro″do-jen′ĕ-sis) regeneration of rhodopsin after its bleaching by light.

rhodophylaxis (ro″do-fi-lak′sis) the property of the retinal epithelium of facilitating rhodogenesis. adj., **rhodophylac′tic.**

rhodoporphyrin (ro″do-por′fĭ-rin) a porphyrin derived from chlorophyll.

rhodopsin (ro-dop′sin) visual purple: a photosensitive purple-red chromoprotein in the retinal rods that is bleached to visual yellow (all-*trans* retinal) by light, thereby stimulating retinal sensory endings. Lack of rhodopsin results in NIGHT BLINDNESS. Vitamin A is the primary source of rhodopsin.

RhoGAM (ro′gam) trademark for a preparation of Rh_0 (D antigen) immune globulin. The gamma globulin is derived from the plasma of women previously immunized to the Rh_0 (D) antigen and is administered after each Rh-incompatible pregnancy. The gamma globulin prevents the formation of antibodies after delivery or abortion (see also RH FACTOR).

rhombencephalon (romb″en-sef′ah-lon) 1. the hindbrain, including the medulla oblongata, pons, and cerebellum. 2. the most caudal of the three primary vesicles formed in embryonic development of the brain, which later divides into the metencephalon and the myelencephalon.

rhombocoele (rom′bo-sēl) the terminal expansion of the canal of the spinal cord.

rhomboid (rom′boid) shaped like a rectangle that has been skewed to one side so that the angles are oblique.

rhonchus (rong′kus) a rattling in the throat; also, a dry, coarse rale in the bronchial tubes, due to a partial obstruction. adj., **rhon′chal, rhon′chial.**

rhubarb (roo′barb) the dried rhizome and root of *Rheum officinale;* used in fluidextract or aromatic tincture as a cathartic.

Rhus (rus) a genus of trees and shrubs, many of them poisonous. Contact with certain species produces a severe dermatitis. The most important poisonous species are *R. diversilo′ba* and *R. toxicoden′dron,* or poison oak, *R. ra′dicans,* or poison ivy, and *R. ver′nix,* or poison sumac. Most species of *Rhus* are sometimes classified in the genus *Toxicodendron.* (See also POISON IVY, OAK, AND SUMAC.)

rhythm (rith′m) a measured movement; the recurrence of an action or function at regular intervals. adj., **rhyth′mic, rhyth′mical.**

alpha r., a uniform rhythm of waves in the normal electroencephalogram, showing an average frequency of 10 per second, typical of a normal person awake in a quiet resting state. Called also Berger's rhythm. (See also ELECTROENCEPHALOGRAPHY.)

beta r., a rhythm in the electroencephalogram consisting of waves smaller than those of the alpha rhythm, having an average frequency of 25 per second, typical during periods of intense activity of the nervous system. (See also ELECTROENCEPHALOGRAPHY.)

biological r's, the cyclic changes that occur in physiological processes of living organisms; called also biorhythms. These rhythms are so persistent throughout the living kingdom that they probably should be considered a fundamental characteristic of life, as are growth, reproduction, metabolism, and irritability. Many of the physiological rhythms occurring in humans about every 24 hours (circadian rhythm) have been known for centuries. Examples include the peaks and troughs that are manifested in body temperature, vital signs, brain function, and muscular activity. Biochemical analyses of urine, blood enzymes, and plasma serum also have demonstrated rhythmic fluctuations in a 24-hour period.

It has long been believed that the cyclic changes observed in plants and animals were totally in response to environmental changes and, as such, were exogenous or of external origin. This hypothesis is now being rejected by some chronobiologists who hold that the biological rhythms are intrinsic to the organisms, and that the organisms possess their own physiological mechanism for keeping time. This mechanism has been called the "biological clock." An example of adjustment of the biological clock in humans is recovery from "jet lag." This phenomenon, also known as jet syndrome, occurs when humans are transported by jet plane across time zones. It is characterized by fatigue and lowered efficiency, which persist until the "biological clock" adjusts to the new environmental cycle.

Biological rhythms are responsive to, or synchronous with, environmental cycles, but it is generally agreed among chronobiologists that the rhythmic changes in environmental factors do not create biological rhythms, even though they are capable of influencing them. Even in the absence of such environmental stimuli as light, darkness, temperature, gravity, and electromagnetic field, biological rhythms continue to maintain their cyclic nature for a period of time. Seasonal changes in morbidity and mortality in humans were formerly considered to be exclusively related to environmental changes; however, this hypothesis is now being challenged by chronobiologists, who contend that circannual (yearly) biological rhythms can and do have an effect on the incidence of heart attacks, insulin needs in diabetics, and other endocrine and related disorders.

It is expected that with continued research in the fields of the physical and behavioral sciences and pharmacology, additional information on the biological rhythms in humans and the enzymatic activity in drug metabolism will greatly influence future modes of treatment and the scheduling of all forms of therapy, including elective surgery and psychotherapy.

circadian r., the regular recurrence in cycles of about 24 hours from one stated point to another, as certain biological activities which occur at that interval, regardless of constant darkness or other environmental conditions.

circannual r., the recurrence of a phenomenon in cycles of about one year.

circamensual r., that which occurs in cycles of about one month (30 days).

circaseptan r., that which occurs in cycles of about seven days (one week).

coupled r., heart beats occurring in pairs, the second beat of the pair usually being a ventricular premature beat.

delta r., 1. electroencephalographic waves having a frequency below $3\frac{1}{2}$ per second, typical in deep sleep, in infancy, and in serious brain disorders (see also ELECTROENCEPHALOGRAPHY). 2. delta waves.

escape r., a heart rhythm initiated by lower centers when the sinoatrial node fails to initiate impulses, its rhythmicity is depressed, or its impulses are completely blocked.

gallop r., an auscultatory finding of three or four heart sounds, the extra sounds by convention being in diastole and related to atrial contraction (fourth sound, presystolic gallop), to early rapid filling of a ventricle with an altered ventricular compliance (protodiastolic gallop), or to concurrence of atrial contraction and ventricular early rapid filling (summation gallop).

gamma r., a rhythm in the waves in the electroencephalogram having a frequency of 50 per second. (See also ELECTROENCEPHALOGRAPHY.)

nodal r., heart rhythm initiated in the specialized junctional tissue, i.e., the atrioventricular node and the main (His) bundle.

nyctohemeral r., a day and night rhythm.

pendulum r., alternation in the rhythm of the heart sounds in which the diastolic sound is equal in time, character, and loudness to the systolic sound, the beat of the heart resembling the tick of a watch.

sinus r., normal heart rhythm originating in the sinoatrial node.

theta r., electroencephalographic waves having a frequency of 4 to 7 per second, occurring mainly in children but also in adults under emotional stress. (See also ELECTROENCEPHALOGRAPHY.)

ventricular r., the ventricular contractions which occur in cases of complete heart block.

rhythmicity (rith-mis′ĭ-te) in cardiology, the ability to beat, or the state of beating, rhythmically without external stimuli.

rhytidectomy (rit″ĭ-dek′to-me) excision of skin for elimination of wrinkles.

rhytidoplasty (rit′ĭ-do-plas″te) plastic surgery for the elimination of wrinkles.

rhytidosis (rit′ĭ-do′sis) a wrinkling, as of the cornea.

rib (rib) any one of the paired bones, 12 on either side, extending from the thoracic vertebrae toward the median line on the ventral aspect of the trunk, forming the major part of the thoracic skeleton. Called also costa. (See table of BONES.)

abdominal r's, asternal r's, false ribs.

cervical r., a supernumerary rib arising from a cervical vertebra.

false r's, the five lower ribs on either side, not attached directly to the sternum.

floating r's, the two lower false ribs on either side, usually without ventral attachment.

slipping r., one whose attaching cartilage is repeatedly dislocated.

true r's, the seven upper ribs on either side, attached to both vertebrae and sternum.

vertebral r's, floating ribs.

vertebrocostal r's, the three upper false ribs on either side, attached to vertebrae and costal cartilages.

vertebrosternal r's, true ribs.

riboflavin (ri″bo-fla′vin) vitamin B_2, a yellow crystalline powder, apparently concerned in the metabolism of all living cells.

Symptoms of riboflavin deficiency (ariboflavinosis) include general weakness, weight loss, lesions at the corners of the mouth, on the lips and around the nose, reddening and soreness of the tip and edges of the tongue, corneal and other eye changes, and seborrheic dermatitis.

Foods with the highest content of riboflavin are liver, kidney, heart, brewer's yeast, milk, eggs, greens, and enriched cereals. Riboflavin deficiency is most common among people of the southeastern United States and other regions, such as Asia and the West Indies, where the diet is likely to contain relatively large quantities of corn, potatoes, and rice, which lack riboflavin. A well-balanced diet will prevent riboflavin deficiency; it will also correct the disorder, with the help of supplementary doses of riboflavin and other vitamins.

ribonuclease (ri″bo-nu′kle-ās) an enzyme that catalyzes the depolymerization of ribonucleic acid.

ribonucleic acid (ri″bo-nu-kle′ik) RNA, a NUCLEIC ACID present in all living cells which controls cellular protein synthesis and replaces DNA as a carrier of genetic codes in some viruses. RNA is similar in composition to DNA with two exceptions. The sugar in RNA is ribose; in DNA it is deoxyribose. In RNA the pyrimidine uracil replaces the thymine in DNA.

The structure of RNA varies from helical to uncoiled strands of varying lengths, depending on the number of nucleotide units forming the strand. This variance in structure is evident in the different types of RNA. For example, transfer RNA (tRNA) contains only about 75 nucleotide units, while other types may contain thousands of units.

Messenger RNA (mRNA) receives its name from its function of carrying the genetic code from the nucleus of the cell to the cytoplasm, where most cellular functions take place. The transfer of the genetic code from DNA to mRNA is called transcription. Molecules of mRNA migrate to the ribosomes, where the manufacture of proteins occurs. The strands of RNA contain codons, some of which signal when formation of a particular protein should stop and the formation of another start.

Transfer RNA (tRNA), also called soluble RNA, brings about the transfer of specific amino acid molecules to protein molecules during the synthesis of proteins. Each of the 20 common amino acids found in protein molecules has a corresponding type of transfer RNA. Thus, a specific tRNA carries the appropriate amino acid to its appropriate place in the chain of the protein molecule being synthesized.

Ribosomal RNA is so called because it is found in the ribosomes and in some way affects the linking of amino acids into protein molecules.

ribonucleoprotein (ri″bo-nu″kle-o-pro′te-in) a substance composed of both protein and ribonucleic acid.

ribonucleoside (ri″bo-nu′kle-o-sīd) a nucleoside in which the purine or pyrimidine base is combined with ribose.

ribonucleotide (ri″bo-nu′kle-o-tīd) a nucleotide in which the purine or pyrimidine base is combined with ribose.

ribose (ri′bōs) an aldopentose present in ribonucleic acid (RNA).

r. nucleic acid, ribonucleic acid.

ribosome (ri′bo-sōm) any of the intracellular ribonucleoprotein particles concerned with protein synthesis; they consist of reversibly dissociable units and are found either bound to cell membranes or free in the cytoplasm. They may occur singly or occur in clusters (polyribosomes).

ribosyl (ri′bo-sil) a glycosyl radical formed from ribose.

ribulose (ri′bu-lōs) the 2-ketose isomer of ribose.

Richards (rich′ardz) Melinda Ann (1841–1930). "America's first trained nurse," the first graduate of the Training School of the New England Hospital in Boston, in 1873. She devoted her life to active nursing and to the training of other nurses.

ricin (ri′sin) a phytotoxin in the seeds of the castor oil plant (*Ricinus communis*), inhalation or ingestion of which causes intoxication, producing superficial inflammation of the respiratory mucosa with hemorrhages into the lungs, or edema of the gastrointestinal tract with hemorrhages.

Ricinus communis (ris′ĭ-nus kom-u′nis) the plant whose seeds afford castor oil.

rickets (rik′ets) a condition of infancy and childhood caused by deficiency of vitamin D, which leads to altered calcium and phosphorus metabolism and consequent disturbance of ossification of bone. Because of the widespread use of vitamin D-fortified milk, together with the additional vitamins that most infants are given, the disease is now uncommon in the United States.

Since the action of sunlight on the skin produces vitamin D in the human body, rickets often occurs in parts of the world where the winter is especially long, and where smoke and fog constantly intercept the sun. Negroes and other dark-skinned people are somewhat more susceptible to the disease if they live in areas with little sunlight, since the pigment in the skin blocks absorption of the sun's rays.

When a vitamin D deficiency occurs in adults, it produces a condition known as OSTEOMALACIA, softening of the bone.

SYMPTOMS. A major symptom of rickets is softening (decalcification) of the bones. In children, this can produce various degrees of deformity, including nodules on the ribs and flexibility and bending of bones. Bowleg and knock-knee and an improperly developed or misshapen skull of a squared or boxed appearance are typical. The ability of the bones to support the body is seriously impaired.

PREVENTION. A proper diet that includes vitamin D-fortified milk is usually sufficient to prevent rickets. Ordinary milk contains adequate amounts of calcium but is a poor source of vitamin D. Small amounts of the vitamin are present in eggs, and in such fish as cod, herring, tuna, sardines, and salmon. Sunlight and other sources of ultraviolet light are beneficial.

TREATMENT. Treatment of an active case of rickets involves the administration of vitamin D concentrate. The response to treatment usually is rapid.

There is a type of vitamin D–resistant rickets in which excessive loss of calcium and phosphorus does not respond to the usual doses of vitamin D. This condition is often familial. Treatment involves massive doses of vitamin D and calcium supplements in the diet.

adult r., a rickets-like disease affecting adults.

fetal r., achondroplasia.

late r., that occurring in older children.

renal r., renal osteodystrophy.

tardy r., late rickets.

vitamin D–resistant r., a condition almost indistinguishable from ordinary rickets clinically but resistant to unusually large doses of vitamin D; it is often familial but may occur sporadically. In hypophosphatemic vitamin D–resistant rickets, hypophosphatemia is the main characteristic, while in hypocalcemic vitamin D–resistant rickets, the serum concentration of phosphate is within normal limits or nearly so, and the concentration of calcium is abnormally low.

Rickettsia (rĭ-ket′se-ah) a genus of small, rod-shaped to round microorganisms found in the cytoplasm of tissue cells of lice, fleas, ticks, and mites, and transmitted to man by their bites.

The diseases caused by rickettsiae can be classified in groups: the spotted fever group (ROCKY MOUNTAIN SPOTTED FEVER, boutonneuse fever, and rickettsialpox); the TYPHUS group (epidemic typhus and endemic typhus); a tsutsugamushi group (scrub

TYPHUS); and a miscellaneous group, including Q FEVER and trench fever.

Rickettsial diseases are not common in communities with high sanitary standards, since prevention depends on controlling the rodent and insect populations. Major epidemics have occurred, especially in times of war when standards of sanitation drop.

rickettsia (rĭ-ket′se-ah), pl. *rickett′siae.* an individual organism of the family Rickettsiaceae.

Rickettsiaceae (ri-ket″se-a′se-e) a family of the order Rickettsiales.

rickettsial (rĭ-ket′se-al) pertaining to or caused by rickettsiae.

Rickettsiales (rĭ-ket″se-a′lēz) an order of microorganisms occurring as elementary bodies, usually found intercellularly. Parasitic for vertebrates and invertebrates, which serve as vectors, they may be pathogenic for man and other animals.

rickettsialpox (rik-et′se-al-poks″) a febrile disease marked by a vesiculopapular eruption, resembling chickenpox clinically, caused by *Rickettsia akari* and transmitted by mites. Called also Kew Gardens spotted fever.

rickettsicidal (rĭ-ket″sĭ-si′dal) destructive to rickettsiae.

ridge (rij) a linear projection or projecting structure; a crest.

dental r., any linear elevation on the crown of a tooth.

dermal r's, cristae cutis, ridges of the skin produced by the projecting papillae of the corium on the palm of the hand and sole of the foot, producing a fingerprint and footprint characteristic of the individual; called also dermal ridges.

genital r., the more medial part of the urogenital ridge, giving rise to the gonad.

interureteric r., a fold on mucous membrane extending across the bladder between the ureteric orifices.

mammary r., an ectodermal thickening in early embryos, along which the mammary glands subsequently develop.

mesonephric r., the more lateral portion of the urogenital ridge, giving rise to the mesonephros.

oblique r., a variable linear elevation obliquely crossing the occlusive surface of a maxillary molar.

urogenital r., a longitudinal ridge in the embryo, lateral to the mesentery.

Riedel's lobe (re′delz) an anomalous tongue-shaped mass of tissue projecting from the right lobe of the liver.

Rieder cell leukemia (re′der) myeloblastic leukemia in which the blood contains asynchronously developed cells with immature cytoplasm and a lobulated, relatively more mature nucleus.

Riegel's pulse (re′gelz) a pulse that is smaller during respiration.

rifamide (rif′ah-mīd) a semisynthetic antibacterial derived from rifamycin B, used in treatment of pulmonary tuberculosis.

rifampicin (rif-am″pĭ-sin) rifampin.

rifampin (rif′am-pin) a semisynthetic antibacterial derived from rifamycin SV, used in treatment of pulmonary tuberculosis and carriers of *Neisseria meningitidis.* The use of rifampin in the treatment of leprosy is being investigated.

rifamycin (rif″ah-mi′sin) any of a family of antibiotics isolated from broths of *Streptomyces mediterranei,* effective against tubercle bacilli and certain other bacteria; the various forms are designated rifamycin B, C, D, E, O, S, SV, and X.

Rift Valley fever a febrile disease with dengue-like symptoms, due to an arbovirus transmitted by mosquitoes or by contact with diseased animals; first observed in the Rift Valley, Kenya.

rigidity (rĭ-jid′ĭ-te) inflexibility or stiffness.

clasp-knife r., increased tension in the extensor of a joint when it is passively flexed, giving way suddenly on exertion of further pressure; seen especially in upper motor neuron disease.

cogwheel r., tension in a muscle that gives way in little jerks when the muscle is passively stretched; seen in paralysis agitans.

decerebrate r., rigid extension of the limbs as a result of decerebration; in man it also occurs as a result of lesions in the upper brain stem.

rigor (rig′or, ri′gor) a chill; rigidity.

r. mor′tis, the stiffening of a dead body accompanying depletion of adenosine triphosphate in the muscle fibers.

rima (ri′mah), pl. *ri′mae* [L.] a cleft or crack.

r. glot′tidis, the elongated opening between the true vocal cords and between the arytenoid cartilages.

r. o′ris, the opening of the mouth.

r. palpebra′rum, palpebral fissure.

r. puden′di, the space between the labia majora; called also pudendal fissure.

Rimifon (rim′ĭ-fon) trademark for a preparation of isoniazid, used in treatment of tuberculosis.

rimula (rim′u-lah), pl. *rim′ulae* [L.] a minute fissure, as of the spinal cord or brain.

ring (ring) 1. any annular or circular organ, structure, or area. 2. in chemistry, a collection of atoms united in a continuous or closed chain.

abdominal r., external, an opening in the aponeurosis of the external oblique muscle for the spermatic cord or round ligament.

abdominal r., internal, an aperture in the transverse fascia for the spermatic cord or round ligament.

Albl's r., a ring-shaped shadow in radiographs of the skull, caused by aneurysm of a cerebral artery.

Bandl's r., pathologic retraction ring.

benzene r., the hexagon representing the arrangement of carbon atoms in a molecule of benzene, different compounds being derived by replacement of the hydrogen atoms by different elements or compounds.

Cannon's r., a focal contraction seen radiographically at the mid-third of the transverse colon, marking an area of overlap between the superior and inferior nerve plexuses.

conjunctival r., a ring at the junction of the conjunctiva and cornea.

constriction r., a contracted area of the uterus, where the resistance of the uterine contents is slight, as over a depression in the contour of the fetus, or below the presenting part.

deep inguinal r., an aperture in the transverse fascia for the spermatic cord or the round ligament.

Kayser-Fleischer r., a gray-green to red-gold pigmented ring at the outer margin of the cornea, seen in progressive lenticular degeneration and pseudosclerosis.

retraction r., pathologic, a complication of prolonged labor marked by failure of relaxation of the circular fibers at the internal opening of the cervix, obstructing delivery of the infant.

retraction r., physiologic, the demarcation between the upper, contracting portion of the uterus in labor and the lower, dilating part.

Schwalbe's r., a circular ridge composed of collagenous fibers surrounding the outer margin of Descemet's membrane.

superficial inguinal r., an opening in the aponeurosis of the external oblique muscle for the spermatic cord or the round ligament.

tympanic r., the bony ring forming part of the temporal bone at birth and developing into the tympanic plate.

umbilical r., the orifice in the abdominal wall of the fetus for transmission of the umbilical vein and arteries.

vascular r., a congenital anomaly of the aortic arch and its tributaries, the vessels forming a ring about the trachea and esophagus and causing varying degrees of compression.

Ringer's solution (ring′erz) a sterile solution of sodium chloride, potassium chloride, and calcium chloride in purified water, a physiologic salt solution for topical use.

ringworm (ring′werm) the popular name for a fungal infection of the skin, even though it is not caused by a worm and is not always ring-shaped in appearance. Called also TINEA.

Ringworm is caused by a group of related fungi of different types. These parasites feed on the body's waste products of dead skin and perspiration. They attack the skin in various areas, especially in body folds, such as the armpit and crotch. One type found between the toes is called ATHLETE'S FOOT; another affects the soles and toenails.

Some forms of ringworm, usually found in children and frequently traced to exposure to infected pets, attack the scalp and exposed areas of the body, particularly the arms and legs. These infections appear as reddish patches, often scaly or blistered, and may cause destruction of the hair shaft. They sometimes become ring-shaped as the infection spreads out while its center heals or seems to heal. There is itching and soreness.

The fungi are highly contagious and are spread by humans, animals, and even objects, such as combs or towels handled by infected persons. Scratching is almost certain to pass the infection from one part of the body to another.

Ringworm is treated with antifungal drugs. Prevention is largely a matter of cleanliness. All parts of the body should be washed with soap and water, expecially hairy areas and body folds where perspiration is likely to collect. Thorough drying is as important as bathing, for the fungi thrive in warm dampness.

Rinne test (rin′nĕ) a test of hearing made with tuning forks, comparing the duration of perception by bone conduction and by air conduction. In the normal ear, the fork is heard twice as long by air conduction as by bone conduction.

Risa-131 (ri′sah) trademark for a preparation of iodinated I-131 serum albumin, used for measuring blood volume and cardiac output.

ristocetin (ris″to-se′tin) an antibiotic derived from culture of *Nocardia lurida;* used in treatment of infections by gram-positive cocci.

risus (ri′sus) [L.] laughter.

r. sardon′icus, a grinning expression produced by spasm of the facial muscles.

Ritalin (rit′ah-lin) trademark for preparations of methylphenidate, a mild central nervous system stimulant and antidepressant.

Ritter's disease (rit′erz) dermatitis exfoliativa neonatorum.

Rivinus' incisure (re-ve′nus) a defect in the upper tympanic part of the temporal bone, filled by the upper portion of the tympanic membrane.

riziform (riz′ĭ-form) resembling grains of rice.

R.L.L. right lower lobe (of lung).

R.L.Q. right lower quadrant (of abdomen).

R.M.A. right mentoanterior (position of the fetus).

R.M.P. right mentoposterior (position of the fetus).

R.M.T. right mentotransverse (position of the fetus).

R.N. Registered Nurse.

Rn chemical symbol, *radon.*

RNA ribonucleic acid.

RNase ribonuclease.

R.O.A. right occipitoanterior (position of the fetus).

Robalate (ro′bah-lāt) trademark for preparations of dihydroxyaluminum aminoacetate, an antacid.

Robaxin (ro-bak′sin) trademark for preparations of methocarbamol, a skeletal muscle relaxant.

Robb (rob) Isabel Hampton (1860–1910). An early leader in nursing education, the first "principal" of Johns Hopkins School of Nursing in Baltimore and a founder of the forerunner of the American Nurses' Association.

Robert's pelvis (ro′bārts) a transversely contracted pelvis caused by osteoarthritis affecting both sacroiliac joints, the inlet becoming a narrow wedge.

Roccal (ro′kal) trademark for a preparation of benzalkonium, a disinfectant and germicide.

Rocky Mountain spotted fever an infectious disease marked by fever, headache, muscle pain, rash, and mental symptoms. It occurs in Rocky Mountain regions, southeastern coastal states, and Long Island and Cape Cod. Called also tick fever, and it is also known by various names according to the geographic area.

Rocky Mountain spotted fever belongs to a group of insect-borne fevers caused by microscopic parasites known as rickettsiae, which attack the cells lining small blood vessels. The species, *Rickettsia rickettsii,* responsible for Rocky Mountain spotted fever is transmitted from rodent to man by various ticks.

SYMPTOMS. After the bite of the infected tick, there is an incubation period of 3 to 10 days before the major symptoms set in. Within a day or two after the bite, the victim may feel somewhat ill and lose his appetite. The actual onset is marked by chills or chilly sensations, fever, headache, pain behind the eyes, joint and muscle pain, and photophobia. Other symptoms are nausea, vomiting, sore throat, and abdominal pain. Some patients become highly irritable and delirious, or so lethargic that they may lapse into a stupor or coma. Usually 3 to 5 days after the onslet a rash appears on the wrists and ankles, then spreads to the trunk and limbs and occasionally to the face.

The appearance and progress of small red spots that eventually become larger sores distinguish Rocky Mountain spotted fever from the several diseases it resembles in its other symptoms (measles, typhoid fever, typhus).

TREATMENT AND PREVENTION. Like other rickettsial diseases, Rocky Mountain spotted fever responds readily to treatment with tetracyclines and chloramphenicol. If untreated, it can be extremely serious and often fatal. Preventive measures are directed mainly against the disease-carrying ticks and rodents.

rod (rod) a straight, slim mass of substance; specifically, one of the retinal rods.

Corti's r's, rodlike bodies in a double row in the inner ear, having their heads joined and their bases on the basilar membrane widely separated so as to form a spiral tunnel.

retinal r's, highly specialized cylindrical segments of the visual cells containing rhodopsin; together with the retinal cones, they form the light-sensitive elements of the retina.

rodenticide (ro-den′tĭ-sīd) 1. destructive to rodents. 2. an agent destructive to rodents.

Roentgen (rent′gen) Wilhelm Conrad (1845–1923). German physicist, born at Lennep (Rhineland). For his accidental discovery of x-rays in 1895, while experimenting with a cathode-ray tube, he received the first Nobel prize for physics in 1901.

roentgen (rent′gen) the international unit of x- or γ-radiation; it is the quantity of x- or γ-radiation such that the associated corpuscular emission per 0.001293 gm. of air produces, in air, ions carrying 1 electrostatic unit of electrical charge of either sign. Abbreviated R.

r. ray, x-ray.

roentgenkymogram (rent″gen-ki′mo-gram) the film obtained by roentgenkymography.

roentgenkymograph (rent″gen-ki′mo-graf) the apparatus used in roentgenkymography.

roentgenkymography (rent″gen-ki-mog′rah-fe) a technique of graphically recording the movements of an organ on a single x-ray film.

roentgenogram (rent′gen-o-gram″) a film produced by roentgenography.

roentgenography (rent″gĕ-nog′rah-fe) the taking of pictures (roentgenograms) of internal structures of the body by passage of x-rays through the body to act on specially sensitized film. adj., **roentgenograph′ic.**

body-section r., a special technique to show in detail images and structures lying in a predetermined plane of tissue, while blurring or eliminating detail in images in other planes; various mechanisms and methods for such roentgenography have been given various names, e.g., laminagraphy, tomography, etc.

mucosal relief r., a technique for revealing any abnormality of the intestinal mucosa, involving injection and evacuation of a barium enema, followed by inflation of the intestine with air under light pressure. The light coating of barium on the inflated intestine in the roentgenogram reveals clearly even small abnormalities.

serial r., the making of several exposures of a particular area at arbitrary intervals.

spot-film r., the making of localized instantaneous roentgenographic exposures during fluoroscopy.

roentgenologist (rent″gĕ-nol′o-jist) a specialist in roentgenology; radiologist.

roentgenology (rent″gĕ-nol′o-je) that branch of radiology dealing with the diagnostic and therapeutic use of roentgen rays (x-rays).

roentgenometry (rent″gĕ-nom′ĕ-tre) 1. measurement of the intensity of x-rays. 2. the direct measurement of structures shown in the roentgenogram with or without the necessity of correcting for magnification.

roentgenoscope (rent′gen-o-skōp″) a fluoroscope; an apparatus for examining the body by means of the fluorescent screen excited by x-rays.

roentgenoscopy (rent″gĕ-nos′ko-pe) examination by means of roentgen rays (x-rays); fluoroscopy.

roentgenotherapy (rent″gen-o-ther′ah-pe) treatment by roentgen rays (x-rays).

roflurane (ro-floo̅r′ăn) an inhalation anesthetic.

Roger's disease (ro-zhāz′) a ventricular septal defect; the term is usually restricted to small, asymptomatic defects.

Rokitansky's disease acute yellow atrophy of the liver.

Rolando's fissure (ro-lan′dōz) fissure of Rolando.

Rolicton (ro-lik′ton) trademark for a preparation of amisometradine, a diuretic.

rolitetracycline (ro″le-tet″rah-si′klēn) an antibiotic compound used for intravenous or intramuscular injection.

ROM range of motion (see under EXERCISE).

rombergism (rom′berg-izm) the tendency of a patient to sway when he stands still with feet close together and eyes closed; associated with loss of position sense.

Romilar (ro′mil-ar) trademark for preparations of dextromethorphan, an antitussant.

rongeur (ron-zher′) [Fr.] an instrument for cutting tissue, particularly bone.

room (ro̅o̅m) a place in a building enclosed and set apart for occupancy or for the performance of certain procedures.

delivery r., one in which infants are delivered.

intensive therapy r., intensive care unit, a hospital unit in which are concentrated special equipment and skilled personnel for seriously ill patients requiring immediate and continuous care and observation.

labor r., predelivery room.

operating r., one especially equipped for the performance of surgical operations.

postdelivery r., a recovery room for the care of obstetric patients immediately after delivery.

predelivery r., a hospital room where an obstetric patient remains during the first stage of labor, i.e., from the time contractions begin until she is ready for delivery.

recovery r., a hospital unit adjoining operating or delivery rooms, with special equipment and personnel for the care of patients immediately after operation or childbirth.

root (ro̅o̅t) 1. the descending and subterranean part of a plant. 2. that portion of an organ, such as a tooth, hair, or nail, that is buried in the tissues, or by which it arises from another structure.

anterior r., ventral root.

r. canal, that part of the pulp cavity extending from the pulp chamber to the apical foramen. Called also pulp canal.

dorsal r., the posterior, or sensory, division of each spinal nerve, attached centrally to the spinal cord and joining peripherally with the ventral root to form the nerve before it emerges from the intervertebral foramen.

motor r., ventral root.

posterior r., dorsal root.

sensory r., dorsal root.

ventral r., the anterior, or motor, division of each spinal nerve, attached centrally to the spinal cord and joining peripherally with the dorsal root to form the nerve before it emerges from the intervertebral foramen.

R.O.P. right occipitoposterior (position of the fetus).

Rorschach test (ror'shahk) one for disclosing personality traits and conflicts by the patient's interpretation of 10 cards bearing symmetrical ink blots in various colors and shading.

rosacea (ro-za'she-ah) a chronic disease affecting the skin of the nose, forehead, and cheeks, marked by flushing, followed by red coloration due to capillary dilatation, with the appearance of papules and acne-like pustules; called also acne rosacea and brandy face.

rosaniline (ro-zan'ĭ-lin) a substance from coal tar, the basis of various dyes and stains.

rosary (ro'zah-re) a structure resembling a string of beads.

rachitic r., a succession of beadlike prominences along the costal cartilages, in rickets.

Rose's position (ro'zez) a supine position with the head over the table edge in full extension.

Rosenbach test (ro'zen-bahk) detection of cold hemolysins by hemoglobinuric response to immersion of the hands or feet in ice water.

roseola (ro-ze'o-lah, ro″ze-o'lah) [L.] 1. any rose-colored rash. 2. roseola infantum.

r. infan'tum, a fairly common acute viral disease that usually occurs in children less than 24 months old; called also exanthem subitum, it attacks suddenly but disappears in a few days, leaving no permanent marks.

Diagnosis is difficult because the sole symptom at first, beyond irritability and drowsiness, is fever. There may be convulsions, and generally the fever is very high; 104° F. (40° C.) is not unusual. Despite the high fever, the disease is quite mild. Treatment consists only of such standard measures as aspirin and tepid sponge baths to allay the fever.

As the fever subsides, in 3 or 4 days, and the disease is apparently at an end, a pink-reddish rash breaks out, usually on the body. This is completely unlike the course of other childhood diseases, such as measles, scarlet fever, and chickenpox, in which the rash is present during the most intense phase of the illness.

The rash of roseola infantum does not persist for more than a few days, and, in fact, may disappear in a few hours. Very often it is so transitory that it is entirely missed. Once the disease is over, the child is believed to be immune for life against further attacks.

syphilitic r., an eruption of rose-colored spots in early secondary syphilis.

r. typho'sa, rose spots.

rosette (ro-zet') any structure or formation resembling a rose, such as (1) the clusters of polymorphonuclear leukocytes around a globule of lipid nuclear material, as observed in the test for disseminated lupus erythematosus, or (2) a figure formed by the chromosomes in an early stage of mitosis.

rosin (roz'in) the solid resin obtained from species of *Pinus,* a genus of trees; used in preparation of ointments and plasters.

Rossolimo's reflex (ros″o-le'mōz) in pyramidal tract lesions, plantar flexion of the toes on tapping their plantar surface.

rostellum (ros-tel'um) a small protuberance or beak, especially the fleshy protuberance of the scolex of a tapeworm, which may or may not bear hooks.

rostrad (ros'trad) 1. toward a rostrum; nearer the rostrum in relation to a specific point of reference. 2. cephalad.

rostral (ros'tral) 1. pertaining to or resembling a rostrum; having a rostrum or beak. 2. rostrad.

rostrate (ros'trāt) beaked.

rostrum (ros'trum,), pl. *ros'tra* [L.] a beak-shaped process.

R.O.T. right occipitotransverse (position of the fetus).

rot (rot) decay.

rotation (ro-ta'shun) the process of turning around an axis. In obstetrics, the turning of the fetal head (or presenting part) for proper orientation to the pelvic axis. It should occur naturally, but if it does not it must be accomplished manually or instrumentally by the obstetrician.

rotenone (ro'tĕ-nōn) a poisonous compound from derris root and other roots; used as an insecticide and as a scabicide.

Roth's spot (rōts) round or oval white spots sometimes seen in the retina early in the course of subacute bacterial endocarditis.

rotoxamine (ro-toks'ah-mēn) an antihistaminic.

rotula (rot'u-lah) 1. the patella. 2. any disklike bony process. 3. a lozenge or troche.

rotular (rot'u-lar) patellar.

roughage (ruf'ij) coarse, largely indigestible material, such as bran, cereals, fruit, and vegetable fibers, that acts as an irritant to stimulate intestinal evacuation.

rouleau (roo-lo'), pl. *rouleaux'* [Fr.] a roll of red blood cells resembling a pile of coins.

roundworm (round'werm) any of various types of parasitic nematode worms, somewhat resembling the common earthworm, which sometimes invade the human intestinal tract and multiply there. Very common among them is the pinworm, or seatworm, which infects 10 per cent of the population of North America. Others include the ascarids, the hookworm, and trichina, which causes TRICHINOSIS. These worms can all impair health to varying degrees, but proper treatment will generally eliminate them. (See also WORMS.)

Roux-en-Y (roo-ahn-wi) denoting any Y-shaped anastomosis in which the small intestine is included.

R.P.F. renal plasma flow.

rpm revolutions per minute.

R.Q. respiratory quotient.

-rrhage, -rrhagia (rāj, ra'je-ah) word element [Gr.], *excessive flow.* adj., **-rrhag'ic.**

-rrhea (re'ah) word element [Gr.], *profuse flow;* adj., **-rrhe'ic.**

rRNA ribosomal RNA (ribonucleic acid).

R.S.A. right sacroanterior (position of the fetus).

R.Sc.A. right scapuloanterior (positon of the fetus).

R.Sc.P. right scapuloposterior (position of the fetus.)

R.S.N.A. Radiological Society of North America.

R.S.P. right sacroposterior (position of the fetus).

R.S.T. right sacrotransverse (position of the fetus).

Ru chemical symbol, *ruthenium.*

rub (rub) friction rub, an auscultatory sound caused by the rubbing together of two serous surfaces.

pericardial r., a scraping or grating noise heard with the heart beat, usually a to-and-fro sound, associated with an inflamed pericardium.

rubber-dam (rub′er-dam) a sheet of thin latex rubber used by dentists to isolate a tooth from the fluids of the mouth during dental treatment, and occasionally in surgical procedures to isolate certain tissues or structures. Called also dam.

rubefacient (roo″bĕ-fa′shent) 1. reddening the skin. 2. an agent that reddens the skin.

rubella (roo-bel′ah) a mild systemic disease caused by a virus and characterized by a fever and a transient rash; called also German measles and 3-day measles.

If a pregnant women contracts rubella, especially during the first trimester, the virus can damage the developing offspring. The location and extent of the congenital anomaly that can result are determined in large measure by the developmental stage of the embryo at the time the virus attacks. Congenital heart defects, cataract, mental retardation, and deafness are some of the more common defects resulting from maternal rubella.

Rubella is not as contagious as chickenpox or measles, but there are frequent epidemics among school children, usually during the spring and early summer. The virus is spread by direct contact and by droplet infection. The patient can transmit the disease from the first appearance of symptoms until the rash disappears, usually a total of 3 or 4 days. The incubation period of rubella is usually 16 to 18 days.

Rubella begins with a slight cold, some fever, and a sore throat. The lymph nodes just behind the ears and at the back of the neck may swell, causing some soreness or pain when the head is moved. The rash appears first on the face and scalp, and spreads to the body and arms the same day. Rubella rash is similar to that of MEASLES, although the spots usually do not run together. The rubella rash fades after 2 or 3 days, although in a few cases the disease may last as long as a week.

TREATMENT AND PREVENTION. Except for complications that may result if the disease is contracted during pregnancy, other complications are quite rare. The patient may be kept in bed for the duration of the illness, but no special treatment, medicine, or diet is necessary unless the patient has a high fever. One attack of German measles usually gives lifetime immunity to the disease, although a second attack does occasionally occur.

A vaccine against rubella is available. It is given in a single subcutaneous injection to children more than a year old. It is never given to a pregnant woman, or to any woman who might become pregnant in the succeeding 2 months.

r. syndrome, congenital anomalies in an infant due to rubella infection in the mother during early pregnancy.

rubeola (roo-be′o-lah, ru″be-o′lah) a synonym of measles in English and of German measles in French and Spanish.

rubeosis (roo″be-o′sis) redness.

r. i′ridis, a condition characterized by a new formation of vessels and connective tissue on the surface of the iris, frequently seen in diabetics.

ruber (roo′ber) [L.] red.

rubescent (roo-bes′ent) growing red; reddish.

rubidium (roo-bid′e-um) a chemical element, atomic number 37, atomic weight 85.47, symbol Rb. (See table of ELEMENTS.)

Rubin test (roo′bin) a test for patency of the uterine tubes, made by transuterine inflation with carbon dioxide gas. Called also tubal insufflation.

Rubner's test (ro͞ob′nerz) 1. one for carbon monoxide in the blood. 2. one for lactose, dextrose, maltose, and levulose in the urine.

rubor (roo′bor) [L.] redness, one of the cardinal signs of inflammation.

Rubramin (roo′brah-min) trademark for preparations of cyanocobalamin (vitamin B_{12}) activity concentrate.

rubriblast (roo′brĭ-blast) pronormoblast.

rubric (roo′brik) red; specifically, pertaining to the red nucleus.

rubricyte (roo′brĭ-sīt) polychromatic normoblast.

rubrospinal (roo″bro-spi′nal) pertaining to the red nucleus and the spinal cord.

rubrothalamic (roo″bro-thah-lam′ik) pertaining to the red nucleus and the thalamus.

rubrum (roo′brum) [L.] red.

r. scarlati′num, scarlet red.

rudiment (roo′dĭ-ment) 1. an organ or part having little or no function but which has functioned at an earlier stage of the same individual or in his ancestors. 2. primordium.

rudimentary (roo″dĭ-men′ter-e) 1. imperfectly developed. 2. vestigial.

rudimentum (roo″dĭ-men′tum) rudiment; in NA, the first indication of a structure in the course of its embryonic development.

ruga (roo′gah), pl. *ru′gae* [L.] a ridge or fold.

rugose (roo′gōs) marked by ridges; wrinkled.

rugosity (roo-gos′ĭ-te) 1. the condition of being rugose. 2. a fold, wrinkle, or ruga.

R.U.L. right upper lobe (of lung).

rule (ro͞ol) a statement of conditions commonly observed in a given situation, or of a prescribed procedure to obtain a given result. For specific rules, see specific name, as M'NAGHTEN RULE.

rumbatron (rum′bah-tron) a high efficiency radio oscillator in which atoms are shattered and which employs electrons as the bombarding particles.

ruminant (roo′mĭ-nant) 1. chewing the cud. 2. an animal that has a stomach with four complete cavities, and that characteristically regurgitates undigested food from the rumen, the first stomach, and masticates it when at rest.

rumination (roo″mĭ-na′shun) 1. in man, the regurgitation of food after almost every meal, part of it being vomited and the rest swallowed; a condition seen in infants. 2. persistent meditation on a certain subject.

rump (rump) the buttock or gluteal region.

runt disease (runt) a syndrome produced by immunologically competent cells in a foreign host that is unable to reject them, resulting in gross retardation of host development and in death.

rupia (roo'pe-ah) thick, dark, raised, lamellated, adherent crusts on the skin, somewhat resembling oyster shells, as in late recurrent secondary syphilis. adj., **ru'pial.**

rupture (rup'tūr) 1. tearing or disruption of tissue. 2. hernia.

R.U.Q. right upper quadrant (of abdomen).

Rush (rush) Benjamin (1745–1813). American physician, born in Philadelphia, and educated at Princeton and the University of Edinburgh. He helped found the Philadelphia Dispensary in 1786, and was physician to Pennsylvania Hospital, where he introduced clinical instruction. Rush protested against improper treatment of the insane until the legislature made provision for construction of a ward for them at Pennsylvania Hospital. He served as a surgeon in the Continental army, and founded with James Pemberton the first anti-slave society in America. As a member of the Continental Congress, Rush was a signer of the Declaration of Independence, and in 1787 he was a member of the Pennsylvania convention that adopted the Federal Constitution. He was appointed Treasurer of the United States Mint in Philadelphia in 1799.

rush (rush) peristaltic rush; a powerful wave of contractile activity that travels very long distances down the small intestine, caused by intense irritation or unusual distention.

Russell's viper venom (rus'elz) the venom of Russell's viper (*Vipera russelli*), which acts *in vitro* as an instrinsic thromboplastin and is useful in defining deficiencies of blood clotting factor X.

ruthenium (roo-the'ne-um) a chemical element, atomic number 44, atomic weight 101.07, symbol Ru. (See table of ELEMENTS.)

rutherford (ruth'er-ford) a unit of radioactive disintegration, representing one million disintegrations per second.

rutherfordium (ruth"er-for'de-um) a chemical element, atomic number 104, atomic weight 261, symbol Rf. (See table of ELEMENTS.)

R.V. residual volume.

℞, Rx [L.] symbol *rec'ipe* (take); prescription; treatment.

rye (ri) the cereal plant *Secale cereale,* and its nutritious seed.

ergotized r., spurred r., see ERGOT.

S

S chemical symbol, *sulfur.*

S. [L.] *se'mis* (half); sight; [L.] *sig'na* (mark); [L.] *sin'ister* (left).

S.A.B. Society of American Bacteriologists.

Sabin (sa'bin) Albert Bruce (born 1906). American virologist, born in Bialystok, Russia; he came to the United States in 1921, and is known for his discovery of an oral vaccine against poliomyelitis.

S. vaccine, an oral vaccine against POLIOMYELITIS consisting of three types of live, attenuated polioviruses. It is given in a capsule, in candy, on a lump of sugar, in milk, or by medicine dropper, and is especially convenient for administration to children and large groups of people.

A unique advantage of the Sabin vaccine is its potential effectiveness in checking the transmission of paralytic viruses from one person to another. Polioviruses reside first in the intestinal tract, from which they spread to other areas, eventually reaching the nervous system and causing paralysis. In a person who has been vaccinated by injection (with Salk vaccine), the viruses are destroyed by antibodies before they reach the nervous system but after they have moved out of the intestine; viruses in the intestine are not destroyed and, still infectious, pass out of the body.

Sabin vaccine, taken orally, stimulates the production of antibodies in the digestive system as well as in other systems of the body; viruses in the intestine are destroyed, not passed on. Thus persons who have received the Sabin vaccine become neither infected nor carriers, whereas those who have received the Salk vaccine can be carriers of the viruses even though they are not themselves infected.

sabulous (sab'u-lus) gritty or sandy.

saburra (sah-bur'ah) sordes; foulness of the mouth or stomach.

saburral (sah-bur'al) 1. pertaining to saburra. 2. gritty, gravelly.

sac (sak) a pouch; a baglike organ or structure.

air s., alveolar sac.

alveolar s's, the spaces into which the alveolar ducts open distally, and with which the alveoli communicate. See Plate 6.

amniotic s., the sac enclosing the fetus suspended in the amniotic fluid; the amnion.

conjunctival s., the potential space, lined by conjunctiva, between the eyelids and the eyeball.

endolymphatic s., the blind, flattened cerebral end of the endolymphatic duct.

heart s., the pericardium.

hernial s., the peritoneal pouch that encloses protruding intestine.

lacrimal s., the dilated upper end of the nasolacrimal duct. See also LACRIMAL APPARATUS.

yolk s., the extraembryonic membrane connected with the midgut; in vertebrates below true mammals, it contains a yolk mass.

saccade (sah-kād') the series of involuntary, abrupt, rapid, small movements or jerks of both eyes simultaneously in changing the point of fixation. adj., **saccad'ic.**

saccate (sak'āt) 1. shaped like a sac. 2. contained in a sac.

saccharase (sak'ah-rās) β-fructofurinosidase.

saccharate (sak'ah-rāt) a salt of saccharic acid.

saccharated (sak'ah-rāt″ed) sugary; charged with sugar.

saccharic acid (sah-kar'ik) a dibasic acid formed by the action of nitric acid on dextrose or carbohydrates containing dextrose.

saccharide (sak'ah-rīd) one of a series of carbohydrates, including the sugars; they are divided into monosaccharides, disaccharides, trisaccharides, and polysaccharides according to the number of saccharide groups composing them.

sacchariferous (sak″ah-rif'er-us) containing sugar.

saccharimeter (sak″ah-rim'ĕ-ter) a device for estimating the proportion of sugar in a solution.

saccharin (sak'ah-rin) a white, crystalline compound several hundred times sweeter than sucrose; used as a noncaloric sweetening agent, but now proved to be carcinogenic in test animals.

calcium s., an artificial sweetening agent.

saccharogalactorrhea (sak″ah-ro-gah-lak″to-re'ah) secretion of milk containing an excess of sugar.

saccharolytic (sak″ah-ro-lit'ik) capable of splitting up sugar.

saccharometabolic (sak″ah-ro-met″ah-bol'ik) pertaining to the metabolism of sugar.

saccharometabolism (sak″ah-ro-mĕ-tab'o-lizm) the metabolism of sugar.

saccharometer (sak″ah-rom'ĕ-ter) saccharimeter.

Saccharomyces (sak″ah-ro-mi'sēz) a genus of protophytes, the yeast fungi. They are oval, unicellular organisms characterized by budding. Only two species are pathogenic for man: *S. al'bicans* (*Candida albicans*) and *S. neofor'mans* (*Cryptococcus neoformans*).

saccharose (sak'ah-rōs) ordinary cane sugar, or sucrose.

saccharum (sak'ah-rum) [L.] sugar, especially sucrose.

s. lac'tis, lactose.

sacciform (sak'sĭ-form) shaped like a bag or sac.

saccular (sak'u-lar) pertaining to or resembling a sac.

sacculated (sak'u-lāt″ed) containing saccules.

sacculation (sak″u-la'shun) 1. a saccule, or pouch. 2. the quality of being sacculated. 3. the formation of pouches.

saccule (sak'ūl) a little bag or sac; a small, pouch-like cavity, especially the smaller of the two divisions of the membranous labyrinth of the inner ear.

laryngeal s., sacculus laryngis.

sacculus (sak'u-lus), pl. *sac'uli* [L.] a saccule.

s. laryn'gis, a diverticulum extending upward from the front of the ventricle of the larynx.

saccus (sak'us), pl. *sac'ci* [L.] a sac.

sacr(o)- word element [L.], *sacrum.*

sacrad (sa′krad) toward the sacrum.

sacral (sa′kral) pertaining to the sacrum.

sacralgia (sa-kral′je-ah) pain in the sacrum.

sacralization (sa″kral-ĭ-za′shun) anomalous fusion of the fifth lumbar vertebra with the first segment of the sacrum.

sacrectomy (sa-krek′to-me) excision or resection of the sacrum.

sacrococcygeal (sa″kro-kok-sij′e-al) pertaining to the sacrum and coccyx.

sacrocoxalgia (sa″kro-kok-sal′je-ah) a painful condition of the sacrum and coccyx.

sacrocoxitis (sa″kro-kok-si′tis) inflammation of the sacroiliac joint.

sacrodynia (sa″kro-din′e-ah) pain in the sacral region.

sacroiliac (sa″kro-il′e-ak) pertaining to the sacrum and the ilium, or the joint formed by these two bones, or to the lower part of the back where these bones meet on both sides of the back. The ilium is the upper part of the hip bone. The sacrum, near the end of the spine, forms a wedge-shaped joint within the open portion of the ilium.

The tight joint allows little motion and is subject to great stress, as the body's weight pushes downward and the legs and pelvis push upward against the joint. The sacroiliac joint must also bear the leverage demands made by the trunk of the body as it turns, twists, pulls, and pushes. When these motions, especially during weight lifting, place an excess of stress on the ligaments that bind the joint and on the connecting muscles, strain may result.

s. **disease,** chronic tuberculous inflammation of the sacroiliac joint.

sacroiliitis (sa″kro-il″e-i′tis) inflammation of the sacroiliac joint.

sacrolumbar (sa″kro-lum′bar) pertaining to the sacrum and loins.

sacrosciatic (sa″kro-si-at′ik) pertaining to the sacrum and ischium.

sacrospinal (sa″kro-spi′nal) pertaining to the sacrum and vertebral column.

sacrouterine (sa″kro-u′ter-in) pertaining to the sacrum and uterus.

sacrovertebral (sa″kro-ver′tĕ-bral) pertaining to the sacrum and vertebrae.

sacrum (sa′krum) the triangular-shaped bone at the base of the spine formed usually by five fused vertebrae that are wedged dorsally between the two hip bones. See also table of BONES.

sadism (sad′izm) a form of sexual perversion in which sexual satisfaction is gained by inflicting pain on others. adj., **sadis′tic.** It can manifest itself in many ways other than during the sexual act. Sadism is a mental disturbance and should be treated by psychotherapy.

sadist (sad′ist) a person who practices sadism.

sadomasochism (sad″o-mas′o-kizm) a state characterized by both sadistic and masochistic tendencies. adj., **sadomasochis′tic.**

sadomasochist (sad″o-mas′o-kist) a person exhibiting sadomasochism.

sagittal (saj′ĭ-tal) 1. shaped like an arrow. 2. situated in the direction of the sagittal suture; said of an anteroposterior plane or section parallel to the median plane of the body.

sagittalis (saj″ĭ-ta′lis) [L.] sagittal.

sago (sa′go) starch from the pith of various palm trees.

Saint Anthony's fire 1. ergotism. 2. an infection of the skin and subcutaneous tissues; called also ERYSIPELAS.

Saint Vitus's dance Sydenham's chorea.

Saint's triad (sāntz) hiatus hernia, colonic diverticula, and cholelithiasis.

sal (sal) [L.] salt.

s. **ammo′niac,** ammonium chloride.

s. **so′da,** sodium carbonate.

s. **volat′ile,** ammonium carbonate.

Sala's cells (sal′ahz) star-shaped cells of connective tissue in the fibers that form the sensory nerve endings situated in the pericardium.

salicylamide (sal″ĭ-sil-am′īd) a white, crystalline powder used as an analgesic.

salicylanilide (sal″ĭ-sil-an′ĭ-līd) a white or slightly pink crystalline compound used as an antifungal agent.

salicylate (sal′ĭ-sil″āt, sah-lis′ĭ-lāt) a salt of salicylic acid.

salicylated (sal′ĭ-sil-āt″ed) impregnated or charged with salicylic acid.

salicylazosulfapyridine (sal″ĭ-sil″ah-zo-sul″fah-pir′ĭ-din) a sulfonamide-related salicylic acid compound used in treatment of chronic ulcerative colitis.

salicylic acid (sal″ĭ-sil′ik) a hydroxyl derivative of benzoic acid. In its pure form it is used as a keratolytic agent to induce peeling of skin or skin lesions. It is prepared in ointments, creams, and collodions containing from 3 to 20 per cent salicylic acid, depending on the effect desired.

The sodium salt of salicylic acid, sodium salicylate, is used mainly as an antirheumatic and antipyretic. Acetylsalicylic acid (ASPIRIN) is a widely used analgesic, antipyretic, and antirheumatic.

Since salicylic acid is an irritant to skin and mucous membranes, preparations taken internally may produce gastrointestinal upsets with prolonged use or overdosage.

salicylism (sal′ĭ-sil″izm) toxic symptoms caused by salicylic acid.

salifiable (sal″ĭ-fi′ah-b′l) capable of combining with an acid to form a salt.

salimeter (sah-lim′ĕ-ter) a hydrometer for determining the strength of saline solutions.

saline (sa′līn) salty; of the nature of a salt.

s. **solution,** a solution of salt (sodium chloride) in purified water. Physiologic saline solution is a 0.9 per cent solution of sodium chloride and water and is isotonic, i.e., of the same osmotic pressure as blood serum. It is sometimes given intravenously to replace lost sodium and chloride. Excessive quantities may cause edema, elevated blood sodium levels, and loss of potassium from the tissue fluid.

saliva (sah-li′vah) the enzyme-containing secretion of the salivary glands.

salivant (sal′ĭ-vant) causing flow of saliva.

salivary (sal′ĭ-ver-e) pertaining to the saliva.

s. **gland,** any of the glands in the mouth that secrete saliva. The major ones are the three pairs of glands known as the parotid, submaxillary, and sublingual glands (see Plate 9). There are other smaller salivary glands within the cheeks and tongue.

The largest of the salivary glands are the parotids, located below and in front of each ear. Saliva secreted by these is discharged into the mouth through openings in the cheeks on each side opposite the upper teeth. The submaxillary glands, located inside the lower jaw, discharge saliva upward through openings into the floor of the mouth. The sublingual glands, beneath the tongue, also discharge saliva into the floor of the mouth.

The saliva is needed to moisten the mouth, to lubricate food for easier swallowing, and to provide the enzyme (ptyalin) necessary to begin food breakdown in the preliminary stage of digestion. The salivary glands produce about 3 pints of saliva daily.

The salivary glands are controlled by the nervous system. Normally they respond by producing saliva within 2 or 3 seconds after being stimulated by the sight, smell, or taste of food. This quick response is a reflex action.

In mumps (parotitis), the parotids become inflamed and swollen. Occasionally, salivary glands produce too much saliva; this condition is called ptyalism, and is the result of local irritation from dental appliances or of disturbances of digestion or of the nervous system or other causes. Certain diseases, drugs such as morphine or atropine, and nutritional deficiency of vitamin B can result in decreased secretion of saliva.

s. gland inclusion disease, cytomegalic inclusion disease.

salivation (sal″ĭ-va′shun) 1. the secretion of saliva. 2. ptyalism.

Salk (sawlk) Jonas Edward (born 1914). American physician, born in New York City. He developed a vaccine for the prevention of poliomyelitis, and is director of the Salk Institute for Biological Studies.

S. vaccine, a preparation of killed polioviruses of three types given in a series of intramuscular injections to immunize against POLIOMYELITIS.

Salmonella (sal″mo-nel′ah) a genus of gram-negative bacteria including the typhoid-paratyphoid bacilli and bacteria usually pathogenic for lower animals which are often transmitted to man.

S. enterit′idis, a common cause of gastroenteritis in man.

S. paraty′phi, the usual etiologic agent of paratyphoid.

S. ty′phi, S. typho′sa, the causative organism of typhoid fever, occurring only in man.

S. typhimu′rium, the causative agent of mouse typhoid and of food poisoning in man.

salmonella (sal″mo-nel′ah), pl. *salmonel′lae.* any organism of the genus *Salmonella.* adj., **salmonel′lal.**

salmonellosis (sal″mo-nel-o′sis) infection with *Salmonella,* especially (1) paratyphoid and (2) a form of FOOD POISONING due to certain species of *Salmonella.*

salping(o)- word element [Gr.], *tube (eustachian tube* or *uterine tube).*

salpingectomy (sal″pin-jek′to-me) excision of a uterine tube.

salpingemphraxis (sal″pin-jem-frak′sis) obstruction of a eustachian tube.

salpingian (sal-pin′je-an) pertaining to the eustachian or the uterine tube.

salpingion (sal-pin′je-on) a point at the apex of the petrous bone on the lower surface.

salpingitis (sal″pin-ji′tis) 1. inflammation of a uterine tube. 2. inflammation of the eustachian tube.

mural s., pachysalpingitis.

parenchymatous s., pachysalpingitis.

salpingocele (sal-ping′go-sēl) hernial protrusion of a uterine tube.

salpingocyesis (sal-ping″go-si-e′sis) development of the embryo within a uterine tube; tubal pregnancy.

salpingography (sal″ping-gog′rah-fe) radiography of the uterine tubes after intrauterine injection of a radiopaque medium.

salpingolithiasis (sal-ping″go-lĭ-thi′ah-sis) the presence of calcareous deposits in the wall of the uterine tubes.

salpingolysis (sal″ping-gol′ĭ-sis) surgical separation of adhesions involving the uterine tubes.

salpingo-oophorectomy (sal-ping″go-o″of-o-rek′to-me) excision of a uterine tube and ovary.

salpingo-oophoritis (sal-ping″go-o″of-o-ri′tis) inflammation of a uterine tube and ovary.

salpingo-oophorocele (sal-ping″go-o-of′o-ro-sēl″) hernia of a uterine tube and ovary.

salpingopexy (sal-ping′go-pek″se) fixation of a uterine tube.

salpingopharyngeal (sal″ping-go-fah-rin′je-al) pertaining to the auditory tube and the pharynx.

salpingoplasty (sal-ping′go-plas″te) plastic repair of a uterine tube.

salpingostomy (sal″ping-gos′to-me) 1. formation of an opening or fistula into a uterine tube for the purpose of drainage. 2. surgical restoration of the patency of a uterine tube.

salpingotomy (sal″ping-got′o-me) surgical incision of a uterine tube.

salpinx (sal′pinks) 1. a uterine tube. 2. a eustachian tube.

salt (sawlt) 1. sodium chloride, or common salt. 2. any compound of a base and an acid. 3. (plural, *salts*) a saline purgative.

acid s., a salt in which some of the replaceable hydrogen atoms remain in the molecule, giving it the properties of an acid.

basic s., a salt with hydroxyl groups in the molecule, giving it the properties of a base.

bile s′s, salts of the bile acids that aid in digestion and absorption of fats and absorption of fat-soluble vitamins.

buffer s., a salt in the blood that is able to absorb slight excesses of acid or alkali with little or no change in the hydrogen ion concentration.

double s., a salt in which the hydrogen atoms of the acid have been replaced by two metals or basic radicals.

Epson s., magnesium sulfate, a cathartic.

Glauber′s s., sodium sulfate.

haloid s., a binary compound of a halogen—i.e., of chlorine, iodine, bromine, fluorine.

neutral s., normal s., a salt in which all the hydrogen of the acid has been replaced; it is neither acid nor basic.

Rochelle s., potassium sodium tartrate, a cathartic.

smelling s′s, aromatic ammonium carbonate, a stimulant and restorative.

saltation (sal-ta′shun) the action of leaping, especially (1) chorea, or the dancing which sometimes accompanies it; (2) conduction along myelinated nerves; (3) in genetics, an abrupt variation in species; a mutation. adj., **sal′tatory.**

salting out (sawl′ting-owt) the separation of protein fractions in the serum or plasma by precipitation in increasing concentrations of neutral salts.

salt-losing crisis (syndrome) vomiting, dehydration, hypotension, and sudden death due to very large sodium losses from the body. It may be seen in abnormal losses of sodium into the urine (as in congenital adrenal hyperplasia, adrenocortical insufficiency, or one of the forms of salt-losing NEPHRITIS) or in large extrarenal sodium losses, usually from the gastrointestinal tract.

salubrious (sah-lu′bre-us) conducive to health; wholesome.

saluresis (sal″u-re′sis) excretion of sodium and chloride in the urine.

saluretic (sal″u-ret′ik) 1. pertainig to saluresis. 2. an agent that promotes saluresis.

salutary (sal′u-tār″e) healthful.

salve (sav) ointment.

Salyrgan (sal′er-gan) trademark for a preparation of mersalyl, a mercurial diuretic.

S.A.M.A. Student American Medical Association.

samarium (sah-ma′re-um) a chemical element, atomic number 62, atomic weight 150.35, symbol Sm. (See table of ELEMENTS.)

sanative (san′ah-tiv) curative; healing.

sanatorium (san″ah-to′re-um) an institution for treatment of sick persons, especially a private hospital for convalescents or patients who are not extremely ill; often applied to an institution for the treatment of tuberculosis.

sanatory (san′ah-tor″e) conducive to health.

sand (sand) material occurring in fine gritty particles.

brain s., acervulus cerebri; sandy matter about the pineal gland and other parts of the brain.

sandfly (sand′fli) various two-winged flies, especially those of the genus *Phlebotomus,* which are important vectors in the transmission of leishmaniasis and phlebotomus fever, known also as sandfly fever.

Sandhoff's disease (sand′hofz) a variant of Tay-Sachs disease marked by a progressively more rapid course, due to a defect in the enzymes hexosaminidase A and B.

Sandril (san′dril) trademark for preparations of reserpine, an antihypertensive and tranquilizer.

sane (sān) sound in mind.

sangui- word element [L.], *blood.*

sanguifacient (sang″gwĭ-fa′shent) forming blood.

sanguine (sang′gwin) 1. abounding in blood. 2. ardent; hopeful.

sanguineous (sang-gwin′e-us) bloody; abounding in blood.

sanguinolent (sang-gwin′o-lent) of a bloody tinge.

sanguis (sang′gwis) [L.] blood.

sanguivorous (sang-gwiv′o-rus) blood-eating; said of female mosquitoes that prefer blood to other nutrients.

sanies (sa′ne-ēz) a fetid ichorous discharge containing serum, pus, and blood. adj., **sa′nious.**

saniopurulent (sa″ne-o-pu′roo-lent) partly sanious and partly purulent.

sanioserous (sa″ne-o-se′rus) partly sanious and partly serous.

sanitarian (san″ĭ-ta′re-an) one skilled in sanitation and public health science.

sanitarium (san″ĭ-ta′re-um) an institution for the promotion of health. The word was originally coined to designate the institution established by the Seventh Day Adventists at Battle Creek, Michigan, to distinguish it from institutions providing care for mental or tuberculous patients.

sanitary (san′ĭ-tār″e) promoting or pertaining to health.

sanitation (san″ĭ-ta′shun) the establishment of conditions favorable to health.

sanitization (san″ĭ-tĭ-za′shun) the process of making or the quality of being made sanitary.

sanitize (san′ĭ-tīz) to clean and sterilize.

sanity (san″ĭ-te) soundness, especially soundness of mind.

San Joaquin Valley fever the primary form of COCCIDIOIDOMYCOSIS.

santonin (san′to-nin) a lactone from the unexpanded flower heads of *Artemisia cina;* used as an anthelmintic.

Sa_{O_2} symbol for percentage of available hemoglobin that is saturated with oxygen (see BLOOD GAS ANALYSIS).

sap (sap) the natural fluid substance of animal or vegetable tissue.

cell s., hyaloplasm (1).

nuclear s., karyolymph.

saphena (sah-fe′nah) the small saphenous or the great saphenous vein.

saphenous (sah-fe′nus) pertaining to or associated with a saphena; applied to certain arteries, nerves, veins, etc.

great s. vein, the longest vein in the body, extending from the dorsum of the foot to just below the inguinal ligament, where it opens into the femoral vein.

small s. vein, a vein in the back of the ankle passing up the back of the leg to the knee joint.

sapo (sa′po) [L.] soap; a compound of fatty acids with an alkali.

saponaceous (sa″po-na′shus) soapy; of soaplike feel or quality.

saponification (sah-pon″ĭ-fĭ-ka′shun) conversion of an oil or fat into a soap by combination with an alkali. In chemistry, the term now denotes the hydrolysis of an ester by an alkali, resulting in the production of a free alcohol and an alkali salt of the ester acid.

saponin (sap′o-nin) a group of glycosides widely distributed in the plant world and characterized by (1) their property of forming durable foam when their watery solutions are shaken, (2) their ability to dissolve erythrocytes even in high dilutions and (3) their having the compound sapogenin as their aglycones.

sapophore (sap′o-fōr) the group of atoms in the molecule of a compound that gives the substance its characteristic taste.

sapphism (saf′izm) homosexual behavior in the female; lesbianism.

sapr(o)- word element [Gr.], *rotten; putrid; decay; decayed material.*

saprophyte (sap′ro-fīt) any organism, such as a bacterium, living upon dead or decaying organic matter. adj., **saprophyt′ic.**

saprozoic (sap″ro-zo′ik) living on decayed organic matter; said of animals, especially protozoa.

sarc(o)- word element [Gr.], *flesh.*

sarcoblast (sar′ko-blast) a primitive cell that develops into a muscle cell.

sarcocele (sar′ko-sēl) any fleshy swelling or tumor of the testis.

sarcocyst (sar′ko-sist) any member of, or any cyst formed by, *Sarcocystis.*

Sarcocystis (sar″ko-sis′tis) a genus of parasitic sporozoa (order Sarcosporidia), found in cysts (sarcosporidian cysts, or sarcocysts) in the muscle tissue of mammals, birds, and reptiles. *S. lindeman′ni* is the species that infects man.

Sarcodina (sar″ko-di′nah) a subphylum of Protozoa, including all the amebae, both free-living and parasitic, characterized by the ability to produce pseudopodia during most of the life cycle; flagella, when present, develop only during the early stages.

sarcoid (sar′koid) 1. tuberculoid; characterized by noncaseating epithelioid cell tubercles. 2. pertaining to or resembling sarcoidosis. 3. sarcoidosis.

Boeck's s., a type of multiple benign sarcoid characterized by its superficial nature and showing a predilection for the face, arms and shoulders.

sarcoidosis (sar″koi-do′sis) a chronic, progressive, generalized granulomatous reticulosis that may affect any part of the body but most frequently involving the lymph nodes, liver, spleen, lungs, skin, eyes, and small bones of the hands and feet, characterized by the presence in all affected organs or tissues of epithelioid cell tubercles, which become converted, in the older lesions, into a rather hyaline featureless fibrous tissue.

s. cor′dis, involvement of the heart in sarcoidosis, with lesions ranging from a few asymptomatic granulomas to widespread infiltration of the myocardium by large masses of sarcoid tissue.

muscular s., sarcoidosis involving the skeletal muscles, with sarcoid tubercles, interstitial inflammation with fibrosis, and disruption and atrophy of the muscle fibers.

sarcolemma (sar″ko-lem′ah) the delicate elastic sheath covering every striated muscle fiber. adj., **sarcolem′mic, sarcolem′mous.**

sarcoma (sar-ko′mah) a tumor, often highly malignant, composed of cells derived from connective tissue such as bone and cartilage, muscle, blood vessel, or lymphoid tissue. These tumors usually develop rapidly and metastasize through the lymph channels. adj., **sarco′matous.**

The different types of sarcomas are named for the specific tissue they affect: fibrosarcoma—in fibrous connective tissue; lymphosarcoma—in lymphoid tissues; osteosarcoma—in bone; chondrosarcoma—in cartilage; rhabdosarcoma—in muscle; liposarcoma—in fat cells.

Abernethy's s., a malignant fatty tumor occurring mainly on the trunk.

alveolar soft part s., one with a reticulated fibrous stroma enclosing groups of sarcoma cells enclosed in alveoli walled with connective tissue.

botryoid s., s. botryoi′des, an embryonal rhabdomyosarcoma arising in submucosal tissue, usually in the upper vagina, cervix uteri, or neck of urinary bladder in young children and infants, presenting grossly as a polypoid grapelike structure.

endometrial stromal s., a pale, polypoid, fleshy, malignant tumor of the endometrial stroma.

Ewing's s., Ewing's tumor.

giant cell s., a malignant form of giant cell tumor of bone.

Kaposi's s., a multifocal, metastasizing, malignant reticulosis with features resembling those of angiosarcoma, principally involving the skin, although visceral lesions may be present; it usually begins on the distal parts of the extremities, most often on the toes or feet, as reddish blue or brownish soft nodules and tumors.

osteogenic s., a malignant primary tumor of bone composed of a malignant connective tissue stroma with evidence of osteoid, bone, and/or cartilage formation; depending upon the dominant component, classified as osteoblastic, fibroblastic, or chondroblastic.

reticulum cell s., a form of malignant lymphoma in which the dominant cell type is derived from the reticuloendothelium.

sarcomatoid (sar-ko′mah-toid) resembling a sarcoma.

sarcomatosis (sar-ko″mah-to′sis) a condition characterized by development of many sarcomas.

sarcomatous (sar-ko′mah-tus) pertaining to or of the nature of a sarcoma.

sarcomere (sar′ko-mēr) the unit of length of a myofibril.

sarcomphalocele (sar″kom-fal′o-sēl) a fleshy tumor of the umbilicus.

sarcoplasm (sar′ko-plazm) the interfibrillary matter of striated muscle. adj., **sarcoplas′mic.**

sarcoplast (sar′ko-plast) an interstitial cell of a muscle, itself capable of being transformed into a muscle.

sarcopoietic (sar″ko-poi-et′ik) forming muscle.

Sarcoptes (sar-kop′tēz) a widely distributed genus of mites, including the species *S. scabie′i,* the itch mite, the cause of scabies in man; different varieties of the organism cause mange in different animals.

sarcosis (sar-ko′sis) abnormal increase of flesh.

Sarcosporidia (sar″ko-spo-rid′e-ah) an order of sporozoa parasitic in the cardiac and striated muscles of vertebrates. It includes the genus *Sarcocystis,* a source of human infection.

sarcosporidiosis (sar-ko′spo-rid″e-o′sis) infection with sporozoa of the genus *Sarcocystis.*

sarcostosis (sar″kos-to′sis) ossification of fleshy tissue.

sarcotubules (sar″ko-too′būlz) the membrane-limited structures of the sarcoplasm, forming a canalicular network around each myofibril.

sarcous (sar′kus) pertaining to flesh or muscle tissue.

sardonic (sar-don′ik) noting a kind of spasmodic or satanic grin or involuntary smile, the risus sardonicus.

sat. saturated.

satellite (sat′ĕ-līt) 1. in genetics, a knob of chromatin connected by a stalk to the short arm of certain chromosomes. 2. a minor, or attendant, lesion situated near a large one. 3. a vein that closely accompanies an artery.

satellitosis (sat″ĕ-li-to′sis) accumulation of neuroglial cells about neurons; seen whenever neurons are damaged.

saturated (sat′u-rāt-ed) 1. having all affinities of its elements satisfied (saturated compound). 2. holding all of a solute that can be held in a solution by the solvent (saturated solution).

saturation (sat″u-ra′shun) the state of being saturated, or the act of saturating.

saturnine (sat′ur-nīn) pertaining to lead.

saturnism (sat′urn-izm) lead poisoning; plumbism.

satyriasis (sat″ĭ-ri′ah-sis) pathologic or exaggerated sexual desire in the male.

saucerization (saw″ser-ĭ-za′shun) 1. the excavation of tissue to form a shallow shelving depression, usually performed to facilitate drainage from infected areas of bone. 2. the shallow saucer-like depression on the upper surface of a vertebra which has suffered a compression fracture.

saxitoxin (sak″sĭ-tok′sin) a neurotoxin from poisonous mussels, clams, and plankton.

Sayre's jacket (sa′erz) a plaster-of-Paris jacket used as a support for the vertebral column.

Sb chemical symbol, *antimony* (L. *stibium*).

Sc chemical symbol, *scandium.*

s.c. subcutaneously.

scab (skab) 1. the crust of a superficial sore. 2. to become covered with a crust or scab.

scabicide (ska′bĭ-sīd) 1. lethal to *Sarcoptes scabiei,* the cause of scabies. 2. an agent lethal to *Sarcoptes scabiei.*

scabies (ska′bēz, ska′be-ēz) a contagious skin disease caused by the itch mite, *Sarcoptes scabiei.* Scabies, sometimes called "the itch," is most likely to erupt in folds of the skin, as in the groin, beneath the breasts, or between the toes or fingers.

The adult itch mite has a rounded body about one-fiftieth of an inch long. Scabies is caused by the female, which burrows beneath the skin and digs a short tunnel parallel to the surface, in which it lays its eggs. The eggs hatch in a few days, after which the baby mites find their way to the skin surface, where they live their brief lives until they too are ready to burrow and lay their eggs.

SYMPTOMS. During the initial tunnel-digging and egg-laying, the human host may be oblivious to what is happening. There is little itching. The very slight skin discoloration may be mistaken for any one of numerous other skin disorders.

In about a week, the itching becomes intense because of hypersensitivity to the mite. The itch is much worse at night. The tunnels in the skin can now be discerned as slightly elevated grayish white lines. The mite itself can often be seen—with the aid of a magnifying glass—as an infinitesimal white speck at the end of the tunnel. Blisters and pustules also may develop on the skin near the tunnel.

TRANSMISSION. Scabies is easily transmitted from person to person by direct skin contact or to a limited extent by contact with clothing of infected persons. Epidemics are fairly common in such places as camps, barracks, and institutions. It is unusual for one member of a family not to communicate it to the others.

The period of communicability lasts until the itch mites and eggs are totally destroyed, a period of 1 to 2 weeks, depending on the effectiveness of the treatment used.

TREATMENT AND PREVENTION. The usual therapy begins with a hot bath and thorough scrubbing to open and expose the burrows. This is followed by the application of some type of DDT preparation.

The patient's underwear and bedclothing must be changed and laundered daily until all the itch mite eggs are hatched out and the mites eliminated.

Good personal hygiene and wearing fresh and clean clothing are the two most effective ways to prevent scabies.

Norwegian s., a variety characterized by immense numbers of mites and marked scaling of the skin.

scabietic (ska″be-et′ik) pertaining to scabies.

scabieticide (ska″be-et′ĭ-sīd) scabicide.

scala (ska′lah), pl. *sca′lae* [L.] a ladder-like structure, applied especially to various passages of the cochlea.

s. me′dia, the cochlear duct: a space in the ear between Reissner's membrane and the basilar membrane.

s. tym′pani, the part of the cochlea below the spiral lamina.

s. vestib′uli, the part of the cochlea above the spiral lamina.

scald (skawld) a burn caused by a hot liquid or a hot, moist vapor; to burn in such fashion.

scale (skāl) 1. a thin flake or compacted platelike body, as of cornified epithelial cells. 2. a scheme or device by which some property may be measured (as hardness, weight, linear dimension). 3. to remove incrustations or other material from a surface, as from the enamel of teeth.

absolute s., a temperature scale with zero at the absolute zero of temperature.

Baumé s., a graduated scale for indicating the specific gravity of a liquid.

Celsius s., a temperature scale with zero at the freezing point of water and the normal boiling point of water at 100 degrees. (For equivalents of Celsius and Fahrenheit temperatures, see Appendix.)

centigrade s., one with 100 gradations or steps between two fixed points, as the Celsius scale.

Fahrenheit s., a temperature scale with the freezing point of water at 32 and the normal boiling point of water at 212 degrees. (For equivalents of Fahrenheit and Celsius temperatures, see Appendix.)

French s., one used for denoting the size of catheters, sounds, and other tubular instruments, each unit being approximately 0.33 mm. in diameter.

Kelvin s., an absolute scale on which the unit of measurement corresponds to that of the Celsius (centigrade) scale, but the ice point is at 273.15 degrees (273.15° K.).

Rankine s., an absolute scale on which the unit of measurement corresponds with that of the Fahrenheit scale, but the ice point is at 459.67 degrees (459.67° R.).

Réaumur s., a temperature scale on which zero represents the freezing point and 80 degrees the boiling point of water.

scalene muscles (ska′lēn) four muscles (anterior, middle, posterior, smallest) of the upper thorax that raise the first and second ribs and thus aid in respiration.

scalenectomy (ska″le-nek′to-me) resection of a scalene muscle.

scalenotomy (ska″le-not′o-me) division of the scalene muscles for the purpose of restricting respiratory activity of the upper part of the thorax; used in treatment of pulmonary tuberculosis.

scalenus syndrome, scalenus anticus syndrome see CERVICAL RIB SYNDROME.

scaler (skāl′er) a dental instrument for removal of calculus from teeth.

scalp (skalp) that part of the skin of the head (exclusive of the face) which is usually covered by a growth of hair.

scalpel (skal′pel) small surgical knife usually having a convex edge.

scaly (skāl′e) characterized by scales; scalelike.

scan (skan) scintiscan.

scandium (skan′de-um) a chemical element, atomic number 21, atomic weight 44.956, symbol Sc. (See table of ELEMENTS.)

scanner (skan′er) scintiscanner.

scanning (skan′ing) 1. close visual examination of a small area or of different isolated areas. 2. a manner of utterance characterized by somewhat regularly recurring pauses.

radioisotope s., production of a two-dimensional record of the emissions of a radioactive isotope concentrated in a specific organ or tissue of the body, as brain, kidney, or thyroid gland.

total body s., utilization of an x-ray unit and COMPUTERIZED AXIAL TOMOGRAPHY (CAT) to examine a cross section of the entire body. As the unit revolves in a half circle around the part of the body being examined, the images produced by varying densities of tissues, fluids, and bone are passed to a computer. The computer then assigns a digit to each density gradient and translates the digits into a televised picture on the screen. The "picture" is a complete cross section of the part of the body being scanned.

Total body scanning does not require the injection of a radiopaque substance, nor is there a need for use of a radioactive material to produce a record of the findings.

The total body scanner is particularly useful in visualizing organs in the retroperitoneal space, for example, the pancreas, liver, spleen, and ovaries, and the abdominal section of the aorta. At the present time, total body scanners are found only in large medical centers.

scanography (skan-og′rah-fe) a method of making radiographs by the use of a narrow slit beneath the tube, so that, as the x-ray tube moves over the target, all the rays of the central beam pass through the part being radiographed at the same angle.

scapha (ska′fah), pl. *sca′phae* [L.] the curved depression separating the helix and antihelix.

scaphocephaly (skaf″o-sef′ah-le) abnormal length and narrowness of the skull as a result of premature closure of the sagittal suture; usually accompanied by mental retardation. adj., **scaphocephal′ic, scaphoceph′alous.**

scaphoid (skaf′oid) shaped like a boat; see table of BONES.

scaphoiditis (skaf″oi-di′tis) inflammation of the scaphoid bone.

scapula (skap′u-lah), pl. *scap′ulae* [L.] the flat triangular bone in the back of the shoulder; the shoulder blade. See table of BONES.

winged s., one having a prominent vertebral border usually owing to weakness of one of the muscles holding the scapula in place.

scapulalgia (skap″u-lal′je-ah) pain in the scapular region.

scapular (skap′u-lar) pertaining to the scapula.

scapulectomy (skap″u-lek′to-me) excision or resection of the scapula.

scapuloclavicular (skap″u-lo-klah-vik′u-lar) pertaining to the scapula and clavicle.

scapulohumeral (skap″u-lo-hu′mer-al) pertaining to the scapula and humerus.

scapulopexy (skap′u-lo-pek″se) surgical fixation of the scapula.

scapulothoracic (skap″u-lo-tho-ras′ik) pertaining to the scapula and thorax.

scar (skar) cicatrix; a mark remaining after the healing of a wound, such as one caused by injury, illness, smallpox vaccination, or surgery.

Beneath the skin is a fibrous connective tissue known as subcutaneous tissue and composed of cells called fibroblasts, which after injury are stimulated to grow into granulation tissue, which knits the wound together. Dense masses of granulation tissue form scar tissue. (See also HEALING and KELOID.)

scarification (skar″ĭ-fĭ-ka′shun) production in the skin of many small superficial scratches or punctures, as for introduction of vaccine.

scarificator (skar′ĭ-fĭ-ka″tor) scarifier.

scarifier (skar′ĭ-fi″er) an instrument with many sharp points, used in scarification.

scarlatina (skar″lah-te′nah) scarlet fever. adj., **scarlat′inal.**

s. angino′sa, scarlet fever with severe throat symptoms.

s. haemorrha′gica, a form in which there is extravasation of blood into the skin and mucous membranes.

s. malig′na, a variety with severe symptoms and great prostration.

scarlatinella (skar-lat″ĭ-nel′ah) Duke's disease.

scarlatiniform (skar″lah-tin′ĭ-form) resembling scarlet fever.

scarlet fever (skar′let) an acute contagious childhood disease caused by a hemolytic streptococcus; called also scarlatina. Scarlet fever follows a streptococcal infection of the throat, skin, middle ear, or some other part of the body. The disease is most common in late winter and spring.

Scarlet fever is usually spread by droplet infection. Objects the infected person has used, such as clothes, dishes, or toys, may carry the streptococcus but this mode of transmission is rare. Occasionally a widespread outbreak may be caused by milk or food that has been infected by a person carrying the streptococcus.

Scarlet fever was formerly a very common and serious disease. In recent years, the number and severity of cases have greatly decreased. Complications are much less common, largely as a result of the development and use of antibiotics.

SYMPTOMS. The incubation period is usually 2 to 5 days, although it may be as few as 1 or as many as 7 days. Symptoms vary a great deal. In some patients there is only sore throat and swelling of the lymph nodes of the neck. The tonsils may be covered by a patchy purulent discharge. The bright red rash from which the disease takes its name appears on the second day; it may be mild or widely spread, depending on the strain of the causative streptococcus. There may be nausea and vomiting. The skin usually feels hot and dry, and there also may be headache and chills. In mild cases the temperature may rise to about 101° F. (38° C.) and in severe cases to 103° (39.4° C.) or even 105° F. (40.5° C.).

If there are no complications, the temperature will slowly return to normal. The rash fades in about a week, and the skin peels; this peeling is usually most pronounced on the palms and soles. In all, the active stage of the disease lasts about 7 days.

TREATMENT. Because of the contagious nature of the disease, the patient should be isolated. Antibiotics, usually penicillin, are administered. This treatment is continued for about 10 days to avoid relapse. Aspirin may be used to relieve headache, fever, and sore throat.

COMPLICATIONS. Among the possible complications of scarlet fever are swelling of the lymph nodes of the neck, infection of the ears and sinuses, kidney disease, pneumonia, and rheumatic fever. Any of these complications may be serious. However, since the development of antibiotics, they have become increasingly rare. Prompt and adequate treatment greatly reduces the danger of complications.

PREVENTION. If a child who has not had scarlet fever is exposed to it, prompt treatment with antibiotics may prevent the disease altogether. The short incubation period of scarlet fever makes immediate treatment necessary.

A person who has been exposed to scarlet fever and has not developed symptoms by the end of 7 days can assume that he was not infected. If symptoms do develop, he should be treated immediately. Cases of scarlet fever must be reported to local health authorities.

A vaccine that gives some immunity to scarlet fever has been developed but it confers immunity for only about 6 months. Since scarlet fever has become a much milder disease than it was in the past, this vaccine is not often necessary.

Contact with a patient with scarlet fever or with any objects he uses should be avoided. The patient's clothes and bedding should be washed separately immediately after use, or soaked in a disinfectant for 2 hours if they are to be washed with those of other members of the family. Any toys, books, or other objects that the patient uses should be thoroughly aired or washed with soap and hot water.

The active stage of scarlet fever is over as soon as the fever is gone. The patient's skin may peel during the convalescent period but he can no longer pass the disease on to others. If the case was mild, the patient can usually return to his normal activities in 7 to 10 days.

If there is any persistent discharge from a body opening, such as a running ear, contagion may still be possible, although if the patient has been treated properly with antibiotics, the streptococci will usually have been destroyed.

After the patient has recovered, his room should be thoroughly cleaned and aired. Dust-catching surfaces, such as floors, tables, and window sills, should be washed with soap and hot water. If the patient has been using a private bathroom, it should be washed and disinfected as well. (See also ISOLATION TECHNIQUE.)

Scarpa's fascia (skar′pahz) the deep, membranous layer of the subcutaneous abdominal fascia.

Scarpa's foramen (skar′pahz) an opening behind the upper medial incisor, for the nasopalatine nerve.

Scarpa's ganglion (skar′pahz) vestibular ganglion.

Scarpa's membrane (skar′pahz) secondary tympanic membrane.

Scarpa's triangle (skar′pahz) femoral triangle.

SCAT SHEEP CELL AGGLUTINATION TEST, a test for infectious mononucleosis.

scatology (skah-tol′o-je) study and analysis of feces, as for diagnostic purposes. adj., **scatolog′ic.**

scatophagy (skah-tof′ah-je) the eating of dung.

scatoscopy (skah-tos′ko-pe) examination of the feces.

scatter (skat′er) the diffusion or deviation of x-rays produced by a medium through which the rays pass.
  back s., backward diffusion of x-rays.

scattergram (skat′er-gram) a graph in which the values found in a statistical study are represented by disconnected, individual symbols.

Sc.D. Doctor of Science.

Scheie's syndrome (shāz) a type of MUCOPOLYSACCHARIDOSIS considered to be an atypical form of Hurler's syndrome, in which the principal sign is marked progressive corneal clouding; hirsutism, joint stiffness, mild deformities of the bones that may only affect the hands, disease of the aorta, and wide-mouthed facies occur, but there is no mental retardation.

schema (ske′mah) a plan, outline, or arrangement.

Scheuermann's disease (shoi′er-manz) osteochondrosis of the vertebral epiphyses in juveniles.

Schick test (shik) intracutaneous injection of diluted diphtheria toxin equal to one-fiftieth of the minimum lethal dose. Lack of immunity to diphtheria is indicated by redness and edema at the injection site on the fifth to seventh day.

Schilder's disease (shil′derz) a subacute or chronic leukoencephalopathy of children and adolescents, with massive destruction of the white substance of the cerebral hemispheres; clinical symptoms include blindness, deafness, bilateral spasticity, and mental deterioration. Called also encephalitis periaxialis diffusa and progressive subcortical encephalopathy.

Schilling test (shil′ing) a test for gastrointestinal absorption of vitamin B_{12}; a measured amount of radioactive vitamin B_{12} is given orally, followed by a parenteral flushing dose of the nonradioactive vitamin, and the percentage of radioactivity is determined in the urine excreted over a 24-hour period. A low urinary excretion that becomes normal after the test is repeated with intrinsic factor is diagnostic of primary pernicious anemia.

Schimmelbusch's disease (shim′el-boosh″ez) cystic disease of the breast.

schindylesis (shin″dĭ-le′sis) an articulation in which a thin plate of one bone is received into a cleft in another, as in the articulation of the perpendicular plate of the ethmoid bone with the vomer.

Schirmer's test (sher′merz) a test for keratoconjunctivitis sicca; a piece of filter paper is inserted into the conjunctival sac over the lower eyelid with the end of the paper hanging down on the outside. If the projecting paper remains dry after 15 minutes, deficient tear formation is indicated.

schist(o)- word element [Gr.], *cleft; split.*

schistocelia (shis″to-se′le-ah) congenital fissure of the abdomen.

schistocephalus (shis″to-sef′ah-lus) a fetus with a cleft head.

schistocormus (shis″to-kor′mus) a fetus with a cleft trunk.

schistocyte (shis″to-sīt) a fragment of an erythrocyte, commonly observed in the blood in hemolytic anemia.

schistocytosis (shis″to-si-to′sis) an accumulation of schistocytes in the blood.

schistoglossia (shis″to-glos′e-ah) cleft tongue.

schistomelus (shis-tom′ĕ-lus) a fetus with a cleft limb.

schistoprosopus (shis″to-pros′o-pus) a fetus with a cleft face.

Schistosoma (shis″to-so′mah) a genus of trematodes, including several species parasitic in the blood of man and domestic animals. The organisms are called schistosomes or blood flukes. Larvae (cercariae) enter the body of the host by way of the digestive tract, or through the skin from contact with contaminated water, and migrate in the blood to small blood vessels of organs of the intestinal or urinary tract; they attach themselves to the blood vessel walls and mature and reproduce. The intermediate host is snails of various species.

S. haemato′bium, a species endemic in north, central and west Africa and the Near East; the organisms are found in the venules of the urinary bladder wall, and eggs may be isolated from the urine.

S. japon′icum, a species geographically confined to the Far East, and found chiefly in the venules of the intestine.

S. manso′ni, a species widely distributed in Africa and parts of South America; the organisms are found in the host's mesenteric veins, and eggs may be found in the feces.

schistosome dermatitis (shis′to-sōm) dermatitis caused by penetration of the skin by larvae (cercariae) of organisms of the genus *Schistosoma.*

schistosomiasis (shis″to-so-mi′ah-sis) infection with flukes of the genus *Schistosoma;* called also bilharziasis. The disease is rare in North America, but is a significant health problem in many parts of the world, including the Near East, Africa, the Far East, South America and the West Indies, and Puerto Rico. The various species cause different forms of the disease; *S. mansoni* and *S. japonicum* produce intestinal symptoms, and *S. haematobium* produces hematuria and other urinary symptoms.

Treatment includes correction of anemia and other nutritional disorders caused by the parasites, and destruction of adult worms by administration of antimony and stibophen. Improvement in sanitation and snail control are the chief preventive measures.

schistosomicide (shis″to-so′mĭ-sīd) an agent that destroys schistosomes.

schistosomus (shis″to-so′mus) a fetus with a cleft abdomen.

schistothorax (shis″to-tho′raks) congenital fissure of the chest or sternum.

schiz(o)- word element [Gr.], *divided; division.*

schizaxon (skiz-ak′son) an axon that divides into two nearly equal branches.

schizogenesis (skiz″o-jen′ĕ-sis) reproduction by fission.

schizogony (skĭ-zog′o-ne) the asexual reproduction of a sporozoan parasite (sporozoite) by multiple fission within the body of the host, giving rise to merozoites, as in malaria. adj., **schizogon′ic.**

schizogyria (skiz″o-ji′re-ah) a condition in which the cerebral convolutions have wedge-shaped cracks.

schizoid (skiz′oid) 1. resembling schizophrenia: a term applied to a shut-in, unsocial, introspective personality. 2. a person of schizoid personality.

schizomycete (skiz″o-mi-sēt′) an organism of the class Schizomycetes.

Schizomycetes (skiz″o-mi-se′tēz) a taxonomic class comprising the bacteria; they are typically unicellular organisms, considered plants which commonly multiply by cell division, and which may be free living, saprophytic, parasitic, or even pathogenic, the last causing disease in plants or animals.

schizont (skiz′ont) the stage in the development of the malarial parasite following the trophozoite whose nucleus divides into many smaller nuclei.

schizonychia (skiz″o-nik′e-ah) splitting of the nails.

schizophasia (skiz″o-fa′ze-ah) incomprehensible, disordered speech.

schizophrenia (skiz″o-fre′ne-ah) a broad term encompassing a large group of mental disorders, usually of psychotic proportions, that have in common disturbances in feeling, thought, and behavior. adj., **schizophren′ic.** The symptoms presented by the schizophrenic patient may vary from mild episodes of aberrant behavior brought on by a stressful, anxiety-producing situation, to profound mental disturbances requiring intensive and prolonged therapy and hospitalization.

The disorder of thought that is common to all types of schizophrenia is characterized by an impairment in the formation of abstract concepts that may lead to misinterpretation of reality and withdrawal into a concrete frame of reference. There may or may not be *delusions* and *hallucinations.*

Schizophrenia (literally "splitting of the mind") was formerly called *dementia praecox,* which means early insanity, implying that the condition has its onset early in life. Early onset is usually characteristic of schizophrenia, but not always. Neither term adequately covers the many different patterns of mental and emotional disturbances usually included in the group.

TYPES. Schizophrenia is sometimes classified according to probable cause and expected prognosis. *Process* or *nuclear* schizophrenia is thought to be due to an organic or chemical predisposition, characterized by a prolonged deterioration of behavior, and having a poor prognosis. *Reactive schizophrenia* is thought to be of environmental origin, having occurred as a reaction to some events in the patient's life, and presenting less severe thought disorders. The prognosis for recovery from reactive schizophrenia is much better than that of process schizophrenia.

Another classification for schizophrenia, one that is more commonly used by North American psychiatrists, is based on the symptoms presented by the patient and the age at which these symptoms occur. For example, *childhood schizophrenia* appears before puberty, is concerned with self (*autism*), and is marked by a withdrawal from social interaction with others. *Hebephrenic schizophrenia* derives its name from the inappropriate laughter, giggling, and regressive behavior that is characteristic of this type. (See below for these and other types.) The various types of schizophrenia recognized by most psychiatrists are not to be thought of as precisely categorized disease entities. There may be much overlapping of symptoms, and frequently the symptomatic behavior of the schizophrenic patient may be present in other types of mental illness, particularly in the manic-depressive group.

ETIOLOGY. Within recent years there has been intensive research into the possible origins of schizophrenia, especially in regard to environomental or social causes as opposed to biochemical and genetic causes. Among the many studies that have been done to determine biochemical changes associated with schizophrenia, some of the most promising are those concerned with the fact that schizophrenia is manifested by decreased levels of *serotonin* in the brain. Experimental studies of the effects of LSD show a profound antagonism between this compound and sertonin, and it is suggested that LSD and similar hallucinogenic compounds produce psychotic behavior because they interfere with the binding of serotonin to either RNA or DNA sites in the brain.

Currently there is no conclusive eveidence to substantiate a claim for any specific, identifiable cause of schizophrenia. The general view is that there are many possible and varied causes, most likely involving both physical and psychological factors.

TREATMENT. A variety of therapeutic measures may be used to help the schizophrenic patient cope with reality and the demands of everyday living. The combination of therapies will depend on the needs of the individual patient, his age and family background, the environment in which he must live, and the preferences of the attending psychiatrist and psychologist. Among the kinds of therapy utilized are psychoanalysis, medications to alter and control extremes of mood, behavior therapy employing CONDITIONING and REINFORCEMENT, family counseling and support, and some form of shock therapy.

catatonic s., a psychotic reaction characterized by uncooperative or impulsive behavior and motor disturbances, especially excitement, stupor, or CATALEPSY. Called also catatonia.

hebephrenic s., a psychotic state characterized by shallow and inappropriate affect, unpredictive giggling, silly behavior and mannerisms, and profound regression. Called also hebephrenia.

paranoid s., a psychotic state marked by delusions of grandeur or persecution; often accompanied by hallucinations.

process s., severe progressive schizophrenia with a poor prognosis, attributed by many to organic brain changes.

simple s., schizophrenia marked by apathy, lack of initiative, and withdrawal.

schizotrichia (skiz″o-trik′e-ah) splitting of the hairs at the ends.

Schlatter-Osgood disease (shlat′er oz′good) osteochondrosis of the tuberosity of the tibia. Called also Osgood-Schlatter disease.

Schlemm's canal (schlemz) a circular canal at the junction of the sclera and cornea (see also venous SINUS of sclera).

Schmorl's disease (shmorlz) herniation of the nucleus pulposus.

Schmorl's node (nodule) (shmorlz) an irregular or hemispherical bone defect in the upper or lower margin of the body of a vertebra into which the nucleus pulposus of the intervertebral disk herniates.

Schönlein's purpura (disease) (shān′līnz) Schönlein-Henoch purpura in which articular symptoms predominate.

Schönlein-Henoch purpura (disease) (shān′līn-hen′ōk) nonthrombocytopenic purpura of unknown cause, most often seen in children, associated with various clinical symptoms, such as urticaria and erythema, arthropathy and arthritis, gastrointestinal symptoms, and renal involvement.

Schüffner's dots (granules) (shif′nerz) small granules seen in erythrocytes infected with *Plasmodium vivax* when stained by certain methods.

Schüller's disease (shil′erz) Hand-Schüller-Christian disease.

Schüller-Christian disease (shil′er-kris′chan) Hand-Schüller-Christian disease.

Schwabach test (shvah′bak) a test of hearing made with tuning forks of 256, 512, 1024, and 2048 cycle frequency, the duration of perception of the patient by bone conduction being compared with that of the examiner.

Schwalbe's ring (shvahl′bez) a circular ridge composed of collagenous fibers surrounding the outer margin of Descemet's membrane.

schwannoma (shwah-no′mah) neurilemoma.

sciage (se-ahzh′) [Fr.] a sawing movement in massage.

sciatic (si-at′ik) pertaining to the ischium.

s. nerve, a nerve extending from the base of the spine down the thigh, with branches throughout the lower leg and foot. It is the widest nerve of the body and one of the longest. Inflammation of the sciatic nerve causes pain along its course, or SCIATICA.

sciatica (si-at′ĭ-kah) neuralgia along the course of the sciatic nerve. The term is popularly used to describe a number of disorders directly or indirectly affecting the sciatic nerve. Because of its length, the nerve is exposed to many different kinds of injury, and inflammation of the nerve or injury to it causes pain that travels down from the back or thigh along its course in the leg and into the foot and toes. Certain muscles of the legs may be partly or completely paralyzed by such a disorder.

True sciatic neuritis is comparatively rare. It can be caused by certain toxic substances, such as lead and alcohol, and occasionally by various other factors. Sciatic pain can be produced by a number of conditions other than inflammation of the nerve. Probably the most common cause is a slipped, or herniated, DISK. A back injury, irritation from arthritis of the spine, or pressure on the nerve from certain types of exertion may also be the cause. Occasionally certain diseases such as diabetes mellitus, gout, and vitamin deficiencies may be the inciting factor. In rare cases, pain may be referred over connected nerve pathways to the sciatic nerve from a disorder in another part of the body. Some cases are idiopathic. Because of the long, painful, and disabling course of severe sciatica, the underlying cause should be investigated and corrected when possible.

sciеropia (si″er-o′pe-ah) a defect of vision in which objects appear in a shadow.

scintigram (sin′tĭ-gram) scintiscan.

scintillation (sin″tĭ-la′shun) 1. the emission of sparks. 2. the sensation of sparks before the eyes. 3. a particle emitted in disintegration of a radioactive element.

scintiscan (sin′tĭ-skan) a two-dimensional representation (map) of the gamma rays emitted by a radioisotope, revealing its concentration in a specific organ or tissue.

scintiscanner (sin″tĭ-skan′er) the system of equipment used to make a scintiscan.

scirrho- word element [Gr.], *hard.*

scirrhoid (skir′oid) resembling scirrhous carcinoma.

scirrhous (skir′us) hard or indurated.

s. carcinoma, carcinoma with a hard structure owing to the formation of dense connective tissue in the stroma.

scirrhus (skir′us) scirrhous carcinoma.

scissura (sĭ-su′rah), pl. *scissu′rae* [L.] an incisure; a splitting.

scler(o)- word element [Gr.], *hard; sclera.*

sclera (skle′rah) the tough, white outer coat of the eyeball, covering approximately the posterior five-sixths of its surface, continuous anteriorly with the cornea and posteriorly with the external sheath of the optic nerve. adj., **scle′ral.**

blue s., abnormal blueness of the sclera, a prominent feature of osteogenesis imperfecta; also seen in certain other conditions.

scleradenitis (sklēr″ad-ĕ-ni′tis) inflammation and hardening of a gland.

sclerectasia (sklēr″ek-ta′ze-ah) a bulging state of the sclera.

sclerectoiridectomy (skle-rek″to-ir″ĭ-dek′to-me) excision of part of the sclera and of the iris.

sclerectoiridodialysis (skle-rek″to-ir″ĭ-do-di-al′ĭ-sis) sclerectomy and iridodialysis.

sclerectomy (sklĕ-rek′to-me) 1. excision of part of the sclera. 2. removal of sclerosed parts of the middle ear after otitis media.

scleredema (sklēr″ĕ-de′mah) edematous hardening of the skin; see also AUTOIMMUNE DISEASE and COLLAGEN DISEASE.

s. adulto′rum, Buschke's s., hardening of the skin and subcutaneous tissues, affecting chiefly the head, neck, and trunk, rarely the extremities.

s. neonato′rum, sclerema neonatorum.

sclerema (sklĕ-re′mah) induration of the subcutaneous fat.

s. adipo′sum, s, neonato′rum, an often fatal condition characterized by diffuse, rapidly spreading, nonedematous, tallow-like hardening of the subcutaneous tissues in the first few weeks of life.

scleriritomy (skle″rĭ-rit′o-me) incision of the sclera and iris in anterior staphyloma.

scleritis (sklĕ-ri′tis) inflammation of the sclera. It may be superficial (episcleritis) or deep.

anterior s., inflammation of the sclera adjoining the limbus of the cornea.

posterior s., scleritis involving the retina and choroid.

scleroblastema (skle″ro-blas-te′mah) the embryonic tissue from which bone is formed.

sclerochoroiditis (skle″ro-ko″roi-di′tis) inflammation of the sclera and choroid.

sclerocornea (skle″ro-kor′ne-ah) the sclera and cornea regarded as one.

sclerodactyly (skle″ro-dak′tĭ-le) scleroderma of the fingers and toes.

scleroderma (skle″ro-der′mah) an insidious chronic disorder characterized by progressive collagenous fibrosis of many organs and systems, usually beginning with the skin (see also COLLAGEN DISEASES).

circumscribed s., morphea.

sclerogenous (sklĕ-roj′ĕ-nus) producing sclerosis or a hard tissue or material.

scleroiritis (skle″ro-i-ri′tis) inflammation of the sclera and iris.

sclerokeratitis (skle″ro-ker″ah-ti′tis) inflammation of the sclera and cornea.

scleroma (sklĕ-ro′mah) a hardened patch or induration of skin or mucous membrane.

respiratory s., rhinoscleroma.

scleromalacia (skle″ro-mah-la′she-ah) degeneration (softening) of the sclera, occurring in patients with rheumatoid arthritis.

scleromyxedema (skle″ro-mik″sĕ-de′mah) a variant of lichen myxedematosus characterized by a generalized eruption of the nodules and diffuse thickening of the skin.

scleronyxis (skle″ro-nik′sis) surgical puncture of the sclera.

sclero-oophoritis (skle″ro-o″of-o-ri′tis) sclerosing inflammation of the ovary.

sclerophthalmia (skle″rof-thal′me-ah) encroachment of the sclera upon the cornea so that only a portion of the central part remains clear.

scleroplasty (skle′ro-plas″te) plastic repair of the sclera.

scleroprotein (skle″ro-pro′te-in) a simple protein characterized by its insolubility and its fibrous structure; it usually serves a supportive or protective function in the body.

sclerosant (skle-ro′sant) a chemical irritant producing inflammation and eventual fibrosis.

sclerose (skle′rōs) to become, or cause to become, hardened.

sclerosis (sklĕ-ro′sis) an induration or hardening, especially hardening of a part from inflammation and in disease of the interstitial substance. The term is used chiefly for such a hardening of the nervous system. adj., **sclerot′ic.**

amyotrophic lateral s., degeneration of the anterior horn cells and pyramidal tract, with muscular atrophy (see also AMYOTROPHIC LATERAL SCLEROSIS).

arteriolar s., arteriolosclerosis.

disseminated s., multiple sclerosis.

familial centrolobar s., a progressive familial form of leukoencephalopathy, marked by nystagmus, ataxia, tremor, parkinsonian facies, dysarthria, and mental deterioration.

lateral s., a form seated in the lateral columns of the spinal cord. It may be primary, with spastic paraplegia, rigidity of the limbs, and increase of the tendon reflexes but no sensory disturbances, or secondary to myelitis, with paraplegia and sensory disturbance.

multiple s., demyelination of the white matter of the brain and spinal cord occurring in scattered patches, and resulting in a chronic disabling condition characterized by visual disturbances, weakness, tremors, and finally paralysis (see also MULTIPLE SCLEROSIS).

tuberous s., a congenital hereditary disease with tumors on the surfaces of the lateral ventricles of the brain and sclerotic patches on its surface, and marked by mental deterioration and epileptic attacks.

scleroskeleton (skle″ro-skel′ĕ-ton) the part of the bony skeleton formed by ossification in ligaments, fasciae and tendons.

sclerostenosis (skle″ro-stĕ-no′sis) induration or hardening combined with contraction.

sclerostomy (sklĕ-ros′to-me) surgical creation of an opening through the sclera for the relief of glaucoma.

sclerotherapy (skle″ro-ther′ah-pe) injection of sclerosing solutions in the treatment of hemorrhoids or other varicose veins.

sclerothrix (skle′ro-thriks) abnormal hardness and dryness of the hair.

sclerotica (sklĕ-rot′ĭ-kah) [L.] sclera.

sclerotitis (skle″ro-ti′tis) scleritis.

sclerotium (sklĕ-ro′she-um) a hard blackish mass formed by certain fungi, as ergot.

sclerotome (skle′ro-tōm) 1. an instrument used in incision of the sclera. 2. the area of a bone innervated from a single spinal segment. 3. one of the paired masses of mesenchymal tissue, separated from the ventromedial part of a somite, which develop into vertebrae and ribs.

sclerotomy (sklĕ-rot′o-me) incision of the sclera.

anterior s., the opening of the anterior chamber of the eye, chiefly done for the relief of glaucoma.

posterior s., an opening made into the vitreous through the sclera, as for detachment of the retina or the removal of a foreign body.

sclerous (skle′rus) hard; indurated.

S.C.M. State Certified Midwife.

scolex (sko′leks), pl. *sco′lices* [Gr.] the attachment organ of a tapeworm, generally considered the anterior, or cephalic, end.

scoli(o)- word element [Gr.], *crooked; twisted.*

scoliokyphosis (sko″le-o-ki-fo′sis) combined lateral (scoliosis) and posterior (kyphosis) curvature of the spine.

scoliorachitic (sko″le-o-rah-kit′ik) affected with scoliosis and rickets.

scoliosiometry (sko″le-o-se-om′ĕ-tre) measurement of spinal curvature.

scoliosis (sko″le-o′sis) lateral curvature of the vertebral column. adj., **scoliot′ic.**

Scoliosis may begin during infancy, and the curvature usually occurs in the upper part of the infant's spine and grows progressively more marked. More often the condition develops about the age of 12; this form is ten times more common in girls than in boys. The first visible sign is likely to be unevenness of the hips or shoulders. In general, the earlier the condition begins, the more severe the curvature finally becomes. The malformation tends to progress no further once the spine has reached full growth, i.e., about the age of 15 for girls and 17 for boys.

CAUSES. Habitually poor posture over a long period of time is a common cause of scoliosis; the faulty posture may be accompanied by lack of muscle tone and general physical inactivity. Unevenness in the length of the legs may lead to lateral curvature of the spine. This can usually be corrected by adding a lift to the shoe worn on the foot of the shorter leg. Diseases that affect the spine, such as RICKETS, or that weaken the muscles supporting the vertebral column can bring about scoliosis. In the majority of cases, particularly in adolescents, the original cause is unknown.

TREATMENT. The type of treatment depends on the cause and degree of the malformation. Corrective exercises may eliminate the condition in some cases; in others, braces, casts, or surgery may be necessary.

scopolamine (skl-pol′ah-mēn) an anticholinergic alkaloid derived from various plants, used in parasympathetic blockade and as a central nervous system depressant. It has been used during labor because of its tendency to cause amnesia.

scopometer (sko-pom′ĕ-ter) an instrument for measuring the turbidity of solutions, i.e., the density of a precipitate.

scopophilia (sko″po-fil′e-ah) 1. the derivation of sexual pleasure from looking at genitalia; voyeurism (active scopophilia). 2. a morbid desire to be seen; exhibitionism (passive scopophilia).

scopophobia (sko″po-fo′be-ah) morbid dread of being seen.

-scopy word element [Gr.], *examination of.*

scoracratia (sko″rah-kra′she-ah) fecal incontinence.

scorbutic (skor-bu′tik) pertaining to scurvy.

scorbutigenic (skor-bu″tĭ-jen′ik) causing scurvy.

scorbutus (skor-bu′tus) [L.] scurvy.

scordinemia (skor″dĭ-ne′me-ah) yawning and stretching with a feeling of lassitude.

score (skōr) a rating, usually expressed numerically, based on specific achievement or the degree to which certain qualities are manifest.

Apgar s., a numerical expression of an infant's condition at birth, based on heart rate, respiratory effort, muscle tone, reflex irritability, and color.

scoto- word element [Gr.], *darkness.*

scotochromogen (sko″to-kro′mo-jen) a microorganism whose pigmentation develops in the dark as well as in the light; specifically, a member of a group of the anonymous mycobacteria. adj., **scotochromogen′ic.**

scotodinia (sko″to-din′e-ah) dizziness with headache and dimness of vision.

scotogram, scotograph (sko′to-gram; sko′to-graf) 1. roentgenogram. 2. the effect produced on a photographic plate in the dark by certain substances.

scotoma (sko-to′mah) an area of depressed vision within the visual field, surrounded by an area of less depressed or of normal vision. adj., **scotom′atous.**

absolute s., an area within the visual field in which perception of light is entirely lost.

annular s., a circular area of depressed vision surrounding the point of fixation.

arcuate s., an arc-shaped defect of vision arising

in an area near the blind spot and extending toward it.

central s., an area of depressed vision corresponding with the fixation point and interfering with or abolishing central vision.

centrocecal s., a horizontal oval defect in the visual field situated between and embracing both the fixation point and the blind spot.

color s., an isolated area of depressed or defective vision for color in the visual field.

negative s., one which appears as a blank spot or hiatus in the visual field.

peripheral s., an area of depressed vision toward the periphery of the visual field.

physiologic s., that area of the visual field corresponding with the optic disk, in which the photosensitive receptors are absent.

positive s., one which appears as a dark spot in the visual field.

relative s., an area of the visual field in which perception of light is only diminished, or loss is restricted to light of certain wavelengths.

ring s., annular s.

scintillating s., blurring of vision with the sensation of a luminous appearance before the eyes, with a zigzag, wall-like outline; called also teichopsia.

scotomagraph (sko-to′mah-graf) an instrument for recording the size and shape of a scotoma.

scotometer (sko-tom′ĕ-ter) an instrument for diagnosing and measuring scotomas.

scotometry (sko-tom′ĕ-tre) the measurement of isolated areas of depressed vision (scotomas) within the visual field.

scotophilia (sko″to-fil′e-ah) love of darkness.

scotophobia (sko″to-fo′be-ah) morbid fear of darkness.

scotopia (sko-to′pe-ah) 1. night vision. 2. the adjustment of the eye for darkness; dark adaptation. adj., **scotop′ic.**

scotopsin (sko-top′sin) the protein moiety in the retinal rods that combines with 11-*cis*-retinal to form rhodopsin.

scr. scruple.

scratch test (skrach) a test for hypersensitivity in which a minute amount of the substance in question is inserted in small scratches made in the skin. A positive reaction is swelling and reddening at the site within 30 minutes. Used in allergy testing and in testing for tuberculosis (Pirquet's reaction). (See also SKIN TEST.)

screen (skrēn) 1. a framework or agent used as a shield or protector. 2. to examine.

Bjerrum s., tangent screen.

fluorescent s., a plate in the fluoroscope coated with crystals of a substance that fluoresces, permitting visualization of internal body structures by x-ray.

tangent s., a large square of black cloth with a central mark for fixation; used with a campimeter in mapping the field of vision.

screening (skrēn′ing) 1. examination of a large number of individuals to disclose certain characteristics, or a certain disease, as tuberculosis or diabetes mellitus. 2. fluoroscopy (Great Britain).

multiphasic s., multiple s., simultaneous examination of a population for several different diseases.

scrobiculate (skro-bik′u-lāt) marked with pits.

scrobiculus (skro-bik′u-lus) [L.] pit.

s. cor′dis, the pit of the stomach.

scrofula (skrof′u-lah) primary tuberculosis of the cervical lymph nodes; the inflamed structures being subject to a cheesy degeneration.

scrofuloderma (skrof″u-lo-der′mah) suppurating abscesses and fistulous passages opening on the skin, secondary to tuberculosis of the lymph nodes, especially those of the neck (scrofula).

scrofulous (skrof′u-lus) pertaining to or characterized by scrofuloderma or scrofula.

scrotectomy (skro-tek′to-me) excision of part of the scrotum.

scrotitis (skro-ti′tis) inflammation of the scrotum.

scrotocele (skro′to-sēl) scrotal hernia.

scrotoplasty (skro′to-plas″te) plastic reconstruction of the scrotum.

scrotum (skro′tum) the pouch that contains the testes and their accessory organs. It is composed of skin, the dartos, fascia, and the tunica vaginalis. adj., **scro′tal.** Each TESTIS is connected to a cremaster muscle descending from the abdominal wall. During cold weather these muscles draw the testes closer to the body to maintain their temperature. In hot weather the reverse occurs. The scrotum usually follows this movement.

The scrotum is subject to the same diseases as the rest of the skin, including cysts and cancer. Edema, whether caused by heart disease or the tropical disease ELEPHANTIASIS, can cause great enlargement of the scrotum by filling its loose tissues with fluid.

scruple (skroo′pl) a unit of weight of the apothecaries' system, equal to 20 grains; the equivalent of 1.296 gm.

scultetus bandage (binder) (skul-te′tus) a many-tailed bandage applied with the tails overlapping each other and held in position by safety pins.

scurvy (skur′ve) a condition due to deficiency of ASCORBIC ACID (vitamin C). Symptoms of infantile scurvy include poor appetite, digestive disturbances, failure to gain weight, and increasing irritability. Black and blue spots are scattered over the skin. Severe deficiency may cause changes in bone structure.

The only adults in the United States likely to develop scurvy are older people who live alone and neglect their diet. In adults, scurvy causes swollen and bleeding gums, looseness of the teeth, rupture of small blood vessels, and small black and blue spots on the skin. Later symptoms may include anemia, extreme weakness, soreness of the arms and legs, tachycardia, and dyspnea.

Treatment of scurvy consists of supplying the missing vitamin in prescribed doses, and supplying the proper diet, including fresh fruits and vegetables. When this is done, the symptoms quickly disappear.

Fruits and vegetables that are rich sources of vitamin C include the following: grapefruit, oranges, lemons, limes, cantaloupes, strawberries, raspberries, turnips, raw cabbage, potatoes (baked), and tomatoes.

scute (skūt) any squama or scalelike structure, especially the bony plate separating the upper part of the middle ear from the mastoid cells.

scutiform (sku′tĭ-form) shaped like a shield.

scutulum (sku′tu-lum), pl. *scu′tula* [L.] one of the disk- or saucer-like crusts characteristic of favus.

scutum (sku'tum) 1. scute. 2. a protective covering or shield, e.g., a chitin plate in the exoskeleton of hard-bodied ticks.

scybalous (sib'ah-lus) of the nature of a scybalum.

scybalum (sib'ah-lum), pl. *scyb'ala* [Gr.] a hard mass of fecal matter in the intestine.

scyphoid (si'foid) shaped like a cup or goblet.

SD streptodornase.

S.D. skin dose; standard deviation.

Se chemical symbol, *selenium.*

searcher (serch'er) an instrument (a sound) used in examining the bladder for calculi; called also stone searcher.

seasickness (se'sik-nes) discomfort caused by the motion of a boat under way, a form of MOTION SICKNESS. The unusual motion disturbs the organs of balance located in the inner ear. The symptoms are nausea and vomiting, dizziness, headache, pallor, and cold perspiration.

There are a number of ways to help ward off seasickness. It is best to stay in the fresh air instead of in a stuffy room, to eat lightly, and to avoid fatty, fried, or spicy foods. Antinausea medicines may be effective. If seasickness occurs, the sufferer should rest lying down with his head low, in a comfortable well ventilated place.

seatworm (sēt'werm) pinworm; an individual of the species *Enterobius vermicularis* (see also WORMS).

sebaceous (se-ba'shus) pertaining to or secreting sebum.

s. cyst, a benign retention cyst of a sebaceous gland containing the fatty secretion of the gland; called also wen. Sebaceous cysts may occur anywhere on the body except the palms of the hands and soles of the feet; they are most common on the scalp, back, and scrotum. A cyst may be a source of irritation or infection, and should be excised by a physician.

s. gland, one of the thousands of minute holocrine glands in the skin that secrete an oily, colorless, odorless fluid (sebum) through the hair follicles.

sebiferous, sebiparous (se-bif'er-us; se-bip'ah-rus) secreting or producing a fatty substance.

sebolith (seb'o-lith) a calculus in a sebaceous gland.

seborrhea (seb"o-re'ah) excessive discharge from the sebaceous glands, forming greasy scales or cheesy plugs on the body; it is generally attended with itching or burning.

s. sic'ca, dry, scaly seborrheic dermatitis.

seborrheic (seb"o-re'ik) affected with or of the nature of seborrhea.

s. dermatitis, an inflammatory condition of the skin of the scalp, with yellowish greasy scaling of the skin; commonly known as dandruff. It may spread to other areas about the face, neck, central part of the trunk and axillae.

The underlying cause is not known; the sebaceous glands become overactive and the hair and scalp are excessively oily. The scales are greasy, yellowish and crusty. Burning or itching and erythema of the involved areas may occur.

There is also a dry form of the condition, in which the scales are hard, dry and whitish gray in color and the hair is dry and brittle.

Although there is no specific cure for dandruff, various measures are used to control and relieve it. The most imperative point is cleanliness of the hair, scalp, combs and brushes. There are some helpful medical preparations which are prescribed for persistent cases. There usually contain sulfur, tar, salicylic acid, selenium sulfide, or steroids.

seborrheid (seb"o-re'id) a seborrheic eruption.

sebum (se'bum) the oily secretion of the sebaceous glands, whose ducts open into the hair follicles. It is composed of fat and epithelial debris from the cells of the malpighian layer, and it lubricates the skin.

secobarbital (sek"o-bar'bĭ-tal) a short- to intermediate-acting barbiturate.

sodium s., a hypnotic compound for oral or parenteral use.

Seconal (sek'ŏ-nal) trademark for preparations of secobarbital.

second-set phenomenon the accelerated and intensified rejection by the recipient of a second graft of tissue from the same donor as a consequence of the primary IMMUNE RESPONSE (i.e., antibody production and cell-mediated IMMUNITY) induced by the first graft.

secreta (se-kre'tah) [L., *pl.*] secretion products.

secretagogue (se-krēt'ah-gog) 1. causing a flow of secretion. 2. an agent that stimulates secretion.

secrete (se-krēt') to synthesize and release a substance.

secretin (se-kre'tin) a hormone secreted by the mucosa of the duodenum and jejunum when acid chyme enters the intestine; carried by the blood, it stimulates the secretion of pancreatic juice and, to a lesser extent, bile and intestinal secretion.

secretinase (se-kre'tin-ās) a substance in the serum that inactivates secretin.

secretion (se-kre'shun) 1. the cellular process of elaborating a specific product. This activity may range from separating a specific substance of the blood to the elaboration of a new chemical substance. 2. any substance produced by secretion. One example is the fatty substance produced by the sebaceous glands to lubricate the skin. Saliva, produced by the salivary glands, and gastric juice, secreted by specialized glands of the stomach, are both used in digestion. The secretions of the endocrine glands include various hormones and are important in the overall regulation of body processes.

internal s's, hormones.

secretoinhibitory (se-kre"to-in-hib'ĭ-tor"e) inhibiting secretion.

secretomotor (se-kre"to-mo'tor) stimulating secretion; said of nerves.

secretor (se-kre'tor) in genetics, one who secretes the ABH antigens of the ABO blood group in the saliva and other body fluids; also, the gene determining this trait.

secretory (se-kre'to-re) pertaining to secretion.

sectio (sek'she-o), pl. *sectio'nes* [L.] section.

section (sek'shun) 1. an act of cutting. 2. a cut surface. 3. a segment or subdivision of an organ.

abdominal s., laparotomy; incision of the abdominal wall.

cesarean s., delivery of a fetus by incision through the abdominal wall and uterus; see also CESAREAN SECTION.

frontal s., a section through the body passing at

right angles to the median plane, dividing the body into dorsal and ventral parts.

frozen s., a specimen cut by microtome from tissue that has been frozen; see also FROZEN SECTION.

perineal s., external urethrotomy.

sagittal s., a section through the body coinciding with the sagittal suture, thus dividing the body into right and left halves.

serial s's, histologic sections of a specimen made in consecutive order and so arranged for the purpose of microscopic examination.

sectorial (sek-to′re-al) cutting.

secundigravida (se-kun″dĭ-grav′ĭ-dah) a woman pregnant the second time; gravida II.

secundines (se-kun′dīnz) afterbirth; the placenta and the membranes expelled after childbirth.

secundipara (se″kun-dip′ah-rah) a woman who has had two pregnancies that resulted in viable offspring; para II.

Sedamyl (sed′ah-mil) trademark for a preparation of acetylcarbromal, a sedative.

sedation (se-da′shun) 1. the allaying of irritability or excitement, especially by administration of a sedative. 2. the state so induced.

sedative (sed′ah-tiv) 1. allaying irritabiliy and excitement. 2. an agent that calms nervousness, irritability, and excitement. In general, sedatives depress the central nervous system and tend to cause lassitude and reduced mental activity. They may be classified, according to the organ most affected, as cardiac, gastric, etc.

The degree of relaxation produced varies with the kind of sedative, the dose, the means of administration, and the mental state of the patient. By causing relaxation, a sedative may help a patient go to sleep, but it does not put him to sleep. Medicines that induce sleep are known as hypnotics. A drug may act as a sedative in small amounts and as a hypnotic in large amounts.

The BARBITURATES, such as phenobarbital, are the best-known sedatives. They are also widely used as hypnotics. Other effective sedatives are the bromides, paraldehyde, and chloral hydrate.

Sedatives are useful in the treatment of any condition in which rest and relaxation are important to recovery. Some sedatives are also useful in treatment of convulsive disorders or epilepsy and in counteracting the effect of convulsion-producing drugs. They are used to calm patients before childbirth or surgery. Restlessness in invalids, profound grief in adults, and overexcitement in children can be controlled by medically supervised sedation. Because many sedatives are habit-forming, they should be used only under the supervision of a physician.

Among drugs related to sedatives are the TRANQUILIZERS, which also have a calming effect but, unlike sedatives, usually do not suppress body reactions.

sedentary (sed′en-ter″e) of inactive habits; pertaining to a sitting posture.

sediment (sed′ĭ-ment) a precipitate, especially that formed spontaneously.

sedimentation (sed″ĭ-men-ta′shun) the settling out of sediment.

s. rate, the rate at which a sediment is deposited in a given volume of solution, especially when subjected to the action of a centrifuge. The *erythrocyte sedimentation rate* is the rate at which erythrocytes settle out of unclotted blood in an hour. Abbreviated sed. rate or E.S.R. The test is based on the fact that inflammatory processes cause an alteration in blood proteins, resulting in aggregation of the red cells, which makes them heavier and more likely to fall rapidly when placed in a special vertical test tube. Normal ranges vary according to the type of tube used, each type being of a different size. The most common methods and the normal range for each are: Wintrobe method—0 to 6.5 mm. per hour for men, 0 to 15 mm. per hour for women; Westergren method—0 to 15 mm. per hour for men, 0 to 20 mm. per hour for women.

The sedimentation rate is often inconclusive and is not considered specific for any particular disorder. It is most often used as gauge for determining the progress of an inflammatory disease such as rheumatic fever, rheumatoid arthritis, and respiratory infections. The information provided by this test must be used in conjunction with results from other tests and clinical evaluations.

seed (sēd) 1. the mature ovule of a flowering plant. 2. semen. 3. a small cylindrical shell of gold or other suitable material, used in application of radiation therapy. 4. to inoculate a culture medium with microorganisms.

plantago s., plantain s., psyllium s., cleaned, dried ripe seed of species of *Plantago;* used as a cathartic.

radon s., a small sealed container for radon, for insertion into the tissues of the body in radiotherapy.

Seessel's pouch (za′selz) an outpouching of the embryonic pharynx rostrad to the pharyngeal membrane and caudal to Rathke's pouch.

segment (seg′ment) a demarcated portion of a whole. adj., **segmen′tal.**

bronchopulmonary s., one of the smaller subdivisions of the lobe of a lung, separated from others by a connective tissue septum and supplied by its own branch of the bronchus leading to the particular lobe.

hepatic s's, subdivisions of the hepatic lobes based on arterial and biliary supply and venous drainage.

uterine s., either of the two portions into which the uterus becomes differentiated early in labor; the upper contractile portion (corpus uteri) becomes thicker as labor approaches, and the lower noncontractile portion (the isthmus) is thin walled and passive in character.

segmentation (seg″men-ta′shun) 1. division into similar parts. 2. cleavage.

segregation (seg″rĕ-ga′shun) 1. the separation of allelic genes during meiosis as homologous chromosomes begin to migrate toward opposite poles of the cell, so that eventually the members of each pair of allelic genes go to separate gametes.

segregator (seg′rĕ-ga′tor) an instrument for obtaining the urine from the ureter of each kidney separately.

Seidlitz powders (sĭd′litz) a mixture of sodium bicarbonate, potassium sodium tartrate, and tartaric acid; used as a cathartic.

seismotherapy (sīz″mo-ther′ah-pe) treatment of disease by mechanical vibration.

seizure (se′zhur) a sudden attack, as of a disease or EPILEPSY.

selenium (sĕ-le′ne-um) a chemical element, atomic number 34, atomic weight 78.96, symbol Se. (See table of ELEMENTS.)

s. sulfide, a bright orange, insoluble powder; used topically in solution in the treatment of seborrheic dermatitis.

self-antigen (self-an′tĭ-jen) any constituent of the body's own tissues capable of stimulating autoimmunity. (See also IMMUNITY.)

self-curing resin any resin which can be polymerized by addition of an activator and a catalyst without the use of external heat.

self-limited (self-lim′ĭ-ted) limited by its own peculiarities, and not by outside influence; said of a disease that runs a definite limited course.

self-suspension (self″sus-pen′shun) suspension of the body by the head and axillae for the purpose of stretching the vertebral column.

self-tolerance (self-tol′er-ans) immunological tolerance to self-antigens.

sella (sel′ah), pl. *sel′lae* [L.] a saddle-shaped depression. adj., **sel′lar.**

empty s., see EMPTY-SELLA SYNDROME.

s. tur′cica, a depression on the upper surface of the sphenoid bone, lodging the pituitary gland.

semantics (se-man′tiks) study of the meanings of words and the rules of their use; study of the relation between language and significance.

semeiography (se″mi-og′rah-fe) a description of the signs and symptoms of a disease.

semeiology (se″mi-ol′o-je) symptomatology.

semeiotic (se″mi-ot′ik) 1. pertaining to symptoms. 2. pathognomonic.

semelincident (sem″el-in′sĭ-dent) affecting a person only once.

semen (se′men) fluid discharged at ejaculation in the male, consisting of spermatozoa in their nutrient plasma, secretions from the prostate, seminal vesicles, and various other glands, epithelial cells and minor constituents. adj., **sem′inal.**

semi- word element [L.], *half.*

semicanal (sem″ĭ-kah-nal′) a trench or furrow open at one side.

semicircular (sem″ĭ-ser′ku-lar) shaped like a half-circle.

s. canals, the passages in the inner ear, in the bony labyrinth, which control the sense of balance. Each ear has three semicircular canals (anterior, lateral, and posterior) situated approximately at right angles to each other. The canals are filled with fluid and have enlarged portions at one end, called ampullae, which contain nerve endings.

The semicircular canals respond to movement of the head. When the head changes position in any direction, the fluid in the canal that lies in the plane of movement also moves but, because of its inertia, the fluid flow lags behind the head movement. Thus the fluid presses against the delicate hairs of the nerves in the ampulla, and these nerves then register the fact that the head is turning in such a direction. This helps the body maintain its equilibrium. (See also EAR and HEARING.)

It is the fluid movement in the semicircular canals that causes the feeling of dizziness or vertigo after spinning. When the spinning stops, the fluid in the horizontal canal continues to move for a moment in the direction of the spin, giving a temporary false reading that the head is turning in the other direction. Motion sickness is caused by the unusual and erratic motions of the head in an airplane, car, or ship, and the resulting stimulation of the semicircular canals.

semicoma (sem″ĭ-ko′mah) a stupor from which the patient may be aroused. adj., **semico′matose.**

semiflexion (sem″ĭ-flek′shun) the position of a limb midway between flexion and extension; the act of bringing to such a position.

Semikon (sem′ĭ-kon) trademark for preparations of methapyrilene, an antihistamine.

semilunar (sem″ĭ-lu′nar) shaped like a half-moon or crescent.

s. valves, valves guarding the entrances into the aorta and pulmonary trunk from the cardiac ventricles.

semination (sem″ĭ-na′shun) insemination.

seminiferous (sem″ĭ-nif′er-us) producing or carrying semen.

seminoma (sem″i-no′mah) a malignant tumor of the testis thought to arise from primitive gonadal cells.

seminormal (sem″ĭ-nor′mal) half of normal solution.

seminuria (se″mĭ-nu′re-ah) discharge of semen in the urine.

semipermeable (sem″ĭ-per′me-ah-bl) permitting passage only of certain molecules.

semis (se′mis) [L.] half; abbreviated *ss.*

semisulcus (sem″ĭ-sul′kus) a depression that, with an adjoining one, forms a sulcus.

semisupination (sem″ĭ-su″pĭ-na′shun) a position halfway toward supination.

semisynthetic (sem″ĭ-sin-thet′ik) produced by chemical manipulation of naturally occurring substances.

Semmelweiss (sem′el-vīs) Ignaz Philipp (1818–1965). Hungarian physician and pioneer of antisepsis in obstetrics. He was born at Buda and educated at the universities of Pest and Vienna. As assistant in an obstetrics ward of Allgemeines Krankenhaus in Vienna, where the mortality rate from puerperal fever was extremely high, Semmelweiss recognized that the infection was carried from patient to patient by the physicians, and he instituted preventive measures, such as cleansing of the physicians' hands with chlorinated lime. He met such fierce opposition from many of his colleagues that he left Vienna and returned to Pest, as physician in the maternity department.

Semoxydrine (sem-ok′sĭ-drin) trademark for a preparation of methamphetamine, a central nervous system stimulant.

senescence (sĕ-nes′ens) the process of growing old. adj., **senes′cent.**

Sengstaken-Blakemore tube (sengz′ta-ken blāk′mōr) a device used for the tamponade of bleeding esophageal varices, consisting of three tubes; one leading to a balloon that is inflated in the stomach, to retain the instrument in place and compress the vessels around the cardia; one leading to a long narrow balloon by which pressure is exerted against the wall of the esophagus; and the third attached to a suction apparatus for aspirating the contents of the stomach.

PATIENT CARE. Prior to insertion the tube is held under water to check for leaks. It is then chilled to make it more firm, and lubricated to facilitate passage. After the tube is in place, the physician may circulate ice water through the stomach balloon to help control hemorrhage.

Mild traction is applied to the tubing at the point at which it enters the nose. Because of the danger of tissue erosion and necrosis of the gastric and esophageal mucosa, it is recommended that the tube be deflated for 5 minutes at 8 to 12 hour intervals. The tubing is removed in 24 hours if bleeding is controlled.

The patient must be watched continuously for signs of either injury to or rupture of the esophagus, respiratory distress, and shock. It is possible that the tube may be pulled upward into the oropharyngeal area, causing acute respiratory distress and asphyxiation. A pair of scissors are kept readily at hand so that the tube may be cut in the event this occurs.

senile (se′nīl) pertaining to old age; manifesting senility.

senilism (se′nil-izm) premature old age.

senility (sĕ-nil′ĭ-te) old age; a pronounced loss of mental, physical, or emotional control in aged people, caused by physical or mental deterioration or a combination of the two. Certain types of psychosis are associated with senility.

By the age of 70, many people normally experience some degree of physical change, such as a slowing of the reflexes and a greater susceptibility to fatigue. In senility, however, these changes are often extreme in nature. Senility refers to psychologic changes; commonly the patient suffers lapses of memory and confuses the present with the past. Sudden uncontrolled outbursts of joy, rage, or despair may occur for no apparent reason. In severe cases, the patient may suffer from delusions of persecution or depression and apathy.

PSYCHOLOGIC CAUSES. Senility of psychologic origin is the most common type and is believed to be a reaction to loss of interests and stimulation and to the insecurities, frustrations, fears, and stresses of old age. There may be no physical damage to the brain. The patient may have reason to feel that he has become worthless or useless in his old age, and as a result he withdraws from everyday life. The period of old age makes necessary great adjustments to new physical conditions and living patterns, adjustments that many people are not able to make without professional help.

PHYSICAL CAUSES. The most common physical cause of senility is cerebral ARTERIOSCLEROSIS, which can cause slow, progressive brain damage. This may lead to a cerebral hemorrhage or thrombosis. The symptoms depend largely on the area of the brain that is damaged.

TREATMENT. The treatment for patients with psychologic changes of senility is primarily concerned with helping the patient adjust to his reduced capacities and limited physical activities. Psychotherapy is used to assist the patient in this adjustment. In addition, some effort should be made to reduce the demands and pressures of everyday living so that the patient will be better able to cope with his environment. Senility tends to become progressively worse, with irreversible changes in the patient's physical state and emotional makeup and personality.

PATIENT CARE. The patient with psychologic changes due to senility often is difficult to care for because he is irritable and uncooperative and often lacks good judgment. He must be supervised carefully so that he does not injure himself or wander away from his home or hospital room and become lost.

Unless his physical condition requires bed rest, a routine should be established for indoor exercise and walks out-of-doors when the weather permits. A schedule also should be established for taking the patient to the bathroom or offering him a bedpan if he is confined to bed. This will help avoid accidental soiling and wetting which can occur frequently because of forgetfulness and poor orientation. (See also BOWEL TRAINING and BLADDER TRAINING.)

Physical care includes special care of the skin, proper diet in small, frequent feedings and sufficient rest. (See also AGED.) A flexible plan for recreational and diversional activities must take into account the mental capacity and physical abilities of the patient, which may vary from day to day or even from one hour to the next. It is, however, harmful and degrading to the patient to make assumptions about his mental acuity. At all times he should be treated with dignity and every effort should be made to keep him alert and aware of his surroundings. Reality therapy, a technique that helps keep the patient in touch with reality and oriented as to time and place, can do much to prevent mental confusion in the senile patient.

senna (sen′ah) the dried leaflets of *Cassia acutiflora;* used in a syrup, fluidextract, or compound powder as a cathartic.

senopia (se-no′pe-ah) second sight; improvement of vision, especially near vision, in the aged, a sign of incipient cataract. Called also gerontopia.

sensation (sen-sa′shun) an impression produced by impulses conveyed by an afferent nerve to the sensorium.

girdle s., zonesthesia.

gnostic s's, sensations perceived by the more recently developed senses, such as those of light touch and the epicritic sensibility to muscle, joint, and tendon vibrations.

primary s., that resulting immediately and directly from application of a stimulus.

referred s., reflex s., one felt elsewhere than at the site of application of a stimulus.

subjective s., one originating with the organism and not occurring in response to an external stimulus.

sense (sens) a faculty by which the conditions or properties of things are perceived. Hunger, thirst, malaise, and pain are varieties of sense; a sense of equilibrium or of well-being (euphoria) and other senses are also distinguished. The five major senses comprise VISION, HEARING, SMELL, TASTE, and TOUCH.

The operation of all senses involves the reception of stimuli by sense organs. Each sense organ is sensitive to a particular kind of stimulus. The eyes are sensitive to light; the ears, to sound; the olfactory organs of the nose, to odor; and the taste buds of the tongue, to taste. Various sense organs of the skin and other tissues are sensitive to touch, pain, temperature, and other sensations.

On receiving stimuli, the sense organ translates them into nerve impulses that are transmitted along the sensory nerves to the brain. In the cerebral cortex, the impulses are interpreted, or perceived, as sensations. The brain associates them with other information, acts upon them, and stores them as memory. (See also NERVOUS SYSTEM and BRAIN.)

kinesthetic s., muscle sense.

light s., the faculty by which degrees of brilliancy are distinguished.

muscle s., muscular s., the faculty by which muscular movements are perceived.

posture s., a variety of muscular sense by which the position or attitude of the body or its parts is perceived.

pressure s., the faculty by which pressure upon the surface of the body is perceived.

sixth s., the general feeling of consciousness of the entire body; cenesthesia.

space s., the faculty by which relative positions and relations of objects in space are perceived.

special s., one of the five senses of seeing, feeling, hearing, taste, and smell.

stereognostic s., the sense by which form and solidity are perceived.

temperature s., the faculty by which differences of temperature are appreciated.

sensibility (sen″sĭ-bil′ĭ-te) susceptibility of feeling; ability to feel or perceive.

deep s., the sensibility of deep tissue (muscle, tendon, etc.) to pressure, pain, and movement.

epicritic s., the sensibility to gentle stimulations permitting fine discriminations of touch and temperature, localized in the skin.

proprioceptive s., the sensibility afforded by receptors in muscles, joints, and other parts, by which one is made aware of their position and state.

protopathic s., the sensibility to strong stimulations of pain and temperature; it is low in degree and poorly localized, existing in the skin and in the viscera, and acting as a defensive agency against pathologic changes in the tissues.

somesthetic s., proprioceptive sensibility.

splanchnesthetic s., the sensibility to stimuli received by splanchnic receptors.

sensible (sen′sĭ-bl) perceptible to the senses; capable of sensation.

sensitive (sen′sĭ-tiv) 1. able to receive or respond to stimuli. 2. unusually responsive to stimulation, or responding quickly and acutely.

sensitivity (sen″sĭ-tiv′ĭ-te) the state or quality of being sensitive.

sensitization (sen″sĭ-tĭ-za′shun) 1. the initial exposure of an individual to a specific antigen, resulting in an IMMUNE RESPONSE, subsequent exposure then inducing a much stronger immune response; said especially of such exposure resulting in a hypersensitivity reaction. 2. the coating of cells with antibody as a preparatory step in eliciting an immune reaction. 3. the preparation of a tissue or organ by one hormone so that it will respond functionally to the action of another.

active s., the sensitization that results from the injection of a dose of antigen into the animal.

autoerythrocyte s., see AUTOERYTHROCYTE SENSITIZATION SYNDROME.

passive s., that which results when blood serum of a sensitized animal is injected into a normal animal.

protein s., that bodily state in which the individual is sensitive or hypersusceptible to some foreign protein, so that when there is absorption of that protein a typical reaction is set up.

sensitized (sen′sĭ-tīzd) rendered sensitive.

sensomobile (sen″so-mo′bēl) moving in response to a stimulus.

sensomotor (sen″so-mo′tor) sensorimotor.

sensorial (sen-so′re-al) pertaining to the sensorium.

sensorimotor (sen″so-re-mo′tor) both sensory and motor.

sensorineural (sen″so-re-nu′ral) of or pertaining to a sensory nerve or sensory mechanism, as sensorineural deafness.

sensorium (sen-so′re-um) 1. the part of the cerebral cortex that receives and coordinates all the impulses sent to individual nerve centers. 2. the state of an individual as regards consciousness or mental awareness.

s. commu′ne, the part of the cerebral cortex that receives and coordinates all the impulses sent to individual nerve centers.

sensory (sen′so-re) pertaining to sensation.

s. nerve, a peripheral nerve that conducts impulses from a sense organ to the spinal cord or brain; called also afferent nerve.

sentient (sen′she-ent) able to feel; sensitive.

sepsis (sep′sis) the presence in the blood or other tissues of pathogenic microorganisms or their toxins; the condition associated with such presence.

puerperal s., sepsis occurring after childbirth, due to putrefactive matter absorbed from the birth canal (see also PUERPERAL FEVER).

septa (sep′tah) plural of *septum.*

septal (sep′tal) pertaining to a septum.

septan (sep′tan) recurring on the seventh day (every six days).

septate (sep′tāt) divided by a septum.

septectomy (sep-tek′to-me) excision of part of the nasal septum.

septic (sep′tik) pertaining to sepsis.

septicemia (sep″tĭ-se′me-ah) blood poisoning; systemic disease associated with the presence and persistence of pathogenic microorganisms or their toxins in the blood. adj., **septice′mic.**

cryptogenic s., septicemia in which the focus of infection is not evident during life.

puerperal s., that in which the focus of infection is a lesion of the mucous membrane received during childbirth.

septicophlebitis (sep″tĭ-ko-flĕ-bi′tis) septicemic inflammation of veins.

septicopyemia (sep″tĭ-ko-pi-e′me-ah) septicemia with pyemia.

septipara (sep-tip′ah-rah) a woman who has had seven pregnancies that resulted in living offspring; para VII.

septivalent (sep-tiv′ah-lent) having a valence of seven.

septomarginal (sep″to-mar′jin-al) pertaining to the margin of a septum.

septonasal (sep″to-na′zal) pertaining to the nasal septum.

septotomy (sep-tot′o-me) incision of the nasal septum.

septulum (sep′tu-lum), pl. *sep′tula* [L.] a small separating wall or partition.

septum (sep′tum), pl. *sep′ta* [L.] a wall or partition dividing a body space or cavity. adj., **sep′tal.** Some septa are membranous, some are composed of bone, and some of cartilage, and each is named according to its location. The wall separating the atria (upper chambers) of the heart, for instance, is called the septum atriorum, or interatrial septum.

Usually, however, the term septum is used to refer to the nasal septum, a plate of bone and cartilage covered with mucous membrane that divides the nasal cavity. An injury or malformation of this septum can produce a deviated septum, so that one part of the nasal cavity is smaller than the other. Occasionally the deviation may handicap breathing, block the normal flow of mucus from the sinuses during a cold, and prevent proper drainage of infected sinuses. Deviated septum is fairly common and seldom causes complications. In some cases surgery may be necessary to relieve the obstruction and reduce irritation and infection in the nose and sinuses. The surgical procedure is called a partial or complete submucous resection.

An opening, or defect, in the septum dividing the right and left sides of the heart sometimes is present at birth. The most common type is ventricular septal defect, an opening between the ventricles, often described by laymen as "a hole in the heart." (See also CONGENTITAL HEART DEFECT.)

atrioventricular s., the part of the membranous portion of the interventricular septum between the left ventricle and the right atrium.

interatrial s., the partition separating the right and left atria of the heart.

interventricular s., the partition separating the right and left ventricles of the heart.

s. lu′cidum, septum pellucidum.

pellucid s., s. pellu′cidum, the triangular double membrane separating the anterior horns of the lateral ventricles of the brain. Called also septum lucidum.

s. pri′mum, a septum in the embryonic heart, dividing the primitive atrium into right and left chambers. (See also CONGENTIAL HEART DEFECT.)

rectovaginal s., the membranous partition between the rectum and vagina.

rectovesical s., a membranous partition separating the rectum from the prostate and urinary bladder.

septuplet (sep-tup′let, sep-too′plet) one of seven offspring produced at one birth.

sequel (se′kwel) sequela.

sequela (se-kwel′lah), pl. *seque′lae* [L.] a morbid condition following or occurring as a consequence of another condition or event.

sequester (se-kwes′ter) to detach or separate abnormally a small portion from the whole.

sequestration (se″kwes-tra′shun) 1. abnormal separation of a part from a whole, as a portion of a bone by a pathologic process, or a portion of the circulating blood in a specific part occurring naturally or produced by application of a tourniquet. 2. isolation of a patient.

pulmonary s., loss of connection of lung tissue with the bronchial tree and the pulmonary veins.

sequestrectomy (se″kwes-trek′to-me) excision of a sequestrum.

sequestrum (se-kwes′trum), pl. *seques′tra* [L.] a piece of dead bone that has become separated during the process of necrosis from sound bone.

sera (se′rah) plural of *serum*.

Serenium (sĕ-re′ne-um) trademark for a preparation of ethoxazene, a urinary analgesic.

Serfin (ser′fin) trademark for a preparation of reserpine, an antihypertensive and tranquilizer.

sericeps (ser′ĭ-seps) a silken bag used in making traction on the fetal head.

series (se′rēz) a group or succession of events, objects, or substances arranged in regular order or forming a kind of chain; in electricity, parts of a circuit connected successively end to end to form a single path for the current. adj., **se′rial.**

aliphatic s., the open chain or fatty series of chemical compounds.

aromatic s., the compounds derived from benzene.

erythrocytic s., the succession of developing cells that ultimately culminates in the erythrocyte.

fatty s., methane and its derivatives and the homologous hydrocarbons.

granulocytic s., the succession of developing cells that ultimately culminates in mature granulocytes.

homologous s., a series of compounds each member of which differs from the one preceding it by the radical CH_2.

leukocytic s., the succession of developing cells that ultimately culminates in the leukocyte.

lymphocytic s., the succession of developing cells that ultimately culminates in mature lymphocytes.

monocytic s., the succession of developing cells that ultimately culminates in mature monocytes.

thrombocytic s., the succession of developing cells that ultimately culminates in mature blood platelets (thrombocytes).

serine (ser′ēn) a naturally occurring amino acid.

serocolitis (se″ro-ko-li′tis) inflammation of the serous coat of the colon.

seroconversion (se″ro-con-ver′zhun) the development of antibodies in response to administration of a vaccine.

seroculture (se″ro-kul′tūr) a bacterial culture on blood serum.

serodiagnosis (se″ro-di″ag-no′sis) diagnosis of disease based on serum reactions.

seroenteritis (se″ro-en″tĕ-ri′tis) inflammation of the serous coat of the intestine.

serofibrinous (se″ro-fi′brĭ-nus) marked by both a serous exudate and precipitation of fibrin.

seroflocculation (se″ro-flok″u-la′shun) flocculation produced in blood serum by an antigen.

seroimmunity (se″ro-ĭ-mu′nĭ-te) immunity produced by an antiserum; passive immunity.

serolipase (se″ro-li′pās) a lipase from blood serum.

serologist (se-rol′o-jist) a specialist in serology.

serology (se-rol′o-je) the study of antigen-antibody reactions *in vitro*. adj., **serolog′ic.**

serolysin (se-rol′ĭ-sin) a lysin of the blood serum.

seroma (se-ro′mah) a collection of serosanguineous fluid in the body, producing a tumor-like mass.

seromembranous (se″ro-mem′brah-nus) pertaining to or composed of serous membrane.

seromucous (se″ro-mu′kus) both serous and mucous.

seromuscular (se″ro-mus′ku-lar) pertaining to the serous and muscular coats of the intestine.

Seromycin (ser′o-mi″sin) trademark for preparations of cycloserine, an antibiotic.

seronegative (se″ro-neg′ah-tiv) showing a negative serum reaction.

seropositive (se″ro-poz′ĭ-tiv) showing positive results on serologic examination.

seroprognosis (se″ro-prog-no′sis) prognosis of disease based on serum reactions.

seroprophylaxis (se″ro-pro″fī-lak′sis) the injection of immune serum or convalescent serum for protective purposes.

seropurulent (se″ro-pu′roo-lent) both serous and purulent.

seropus (se″ro-pus′) serum mingled with pus.

seroreaction (se″ro-re-ak′shun) any reaction taking place in serum, or as a result of the action of a serum.

seroresistant (se″ro-re-zis′tant) showing a seropositive reaction to a pathogen after treatment.

serosa (se-ro′sah) any serous membrane. adj., **sero′sal.**

serosamucin (se-ro″sah-mu′sin) a protein from inflammatory serous exudates.

serosanguineous (se″ro-sang-gwin′e-us) composed of serum and blood.

seroserous (se″ro-se′rus) pertaining to two serous surfaces.

serositis (se″ro-si′tis) inflammation of a serous membrane.

serosity (se-ros′ĭ-te) the quality of serous fluids.

serosynovitis (se″ro-sin″o-vi′tis) synovitis with effusion of serum.

serotherapy (se″ro-ther′ah-pe) the treatment of infectious disease by the injection of serum from immune individuals.

serotonergic (se″ro-tŏn-er′jik) containing or activated by serotonin.

serotonin (se″ro-to′nin) a vasoconstrictor present in the blood, central nervous system, and other tissues. Produced enzymatically from tryptophan, it also stimulates smooth muscle and serves as a central neurotransmitter. Called also hydroxytryptamine.

serotype (se′ro-tīp) the type of a microorganism determined by its constituent antigens, or a taxonomic subdivision based thereon.

serous (se′rus) 1. pertaining to serum; thin and watery, like serum. 2. producing or containing serum.

serovaccination (se″ro-vak″sĭ-na′shun) injection of serum combined with bacterial vaccination to produce passive and active immunity.

Serpasil (ser′pah-sil) trademark for preparations of reserpine, an antihypertensive and tranquilizer.

serpiginous (ser-pij′ĭ-nus) creeping from part to part; having a wavy border.

serrated (ser′āt-ed) having a sawlike edge or border.

serration (sĕ-ra′shun) 1. the state of being serrated. 2. a serrated structure or formation.

Sertoli cell (ser-to′lē) any of the elongated cells in the tubules of the testes to which the spermatids become attached; they provide support, protection, and, apparently, nutrition until the spermatids are transformed into mature spermatozoa.

Sertoli-cell–only syndrome (ser-to′le) congenital absence of the germinal epithelium of the testes, the seminiferous tubules containing only Sertoli cells, marked by testes slightly smaller than normal, azoospermia, and elevated titers of follicle-stimulating hormone or of general gonadotropins.

serum (se′rum), pl. *se′ra* [L.], *serums.* the clear portion of any animal or plant fluid that remains after the solid elements have been separated out. The term usually refers to blood serum, the clear, straw-colored, liquid portion of the plasma that does not contain fibrinogen or blood cells, and remains fluid after clotting of blood.

Blood serum from persons or animals whose bodies have built up antibodies is called antiserum or immune serum. Inoculation with such an antiserum provides temporary, or passive, immunity against the disease, and is used when a person has already been exposed to or has contracted the disease. Diseases in which passive immunization is sometimes used include diphtheria, tetanus, botulism, and gas gangrene.

antilymphocyte s., ALS, serum from animals immunized with lymphocytes from a different species, used as an immunosuppressive agent, especially in organ transplantation. The gamma globulin fraction, antilymphocytic globulin (ALG), is now more commonly used.

foreign s., serum from an animal to be injected into one of another species.

s. glutamic oxaloacetic transaminase, SGOT, one of the enzymes that catalyze the transfer of an amino group (NH_2) from an alpha amino acid to an alpha keto acid. The enzyme is found normally in the serum and in various tissues, especially the heart and liver. An elevated SGOT level is seen in disease conditions in which dead or damaged cells leak the transaminase into the serum, as in myocardial infarction or in acute damage to hepatic cells. The SGOT test is not specific for any one disease condition. Its findings are compared with the results of other diagnostic tests and a physical examination. Normal range is 10 to 40 units.

Several drugs can cause elevated SGOT levels, and for this reason it is best to obtain the blood specimen before any drugs are given. About 5 ml. of venous blood is withdrawn, placed in a test tube and allowed to coagulate. It may be stored in a refrigerator until the testing is done.

s. glutamic pyruvic transaminase, SGPT, an enzyme similar to SGOT and found in several tissues of the body. Testing of SGPT levels is primarily a diagnostic test in liver disease. For example, SGPT levels can reach 4000 units in cases of hepatitis. The normal range is 5 to 40 units. A specimen for testing for SGPT is obtained in the same way as one for SGOT.

immune s., serum from an immunized individual, containing specific antibody or antibodies.

s. osmolality, a measure of the number of dissolved particles per unit of water in serum (see also serum OSMOLALITY).

pooled s., the mixed serum from a number of individuals.

s. sickness, a hypersensitivity reaction following a single, relatively large injection of foreign serum. It is marked by urticarial rashes, edema, adenitis, joint pains, high fever, and prostration.

Reactions to tetanus antitoxin derived from horse serum are especially common. When the serum-sensitive person is injected for the first time, the reaction usually occurs after a period of 8 to 12 days. Once a person has had a serum reaction, the serum responsible should be avoided, since a second reaction will be more severe.

It is customary to test a patient's sensitivity with

a small amount of serum before injecting the full dose. This precaution is especially important for patients who have other allergic susceptibilities.

serumal (se-roo′mal) pertaining to or formed from serum.

serum-fast (se′rum-fast) resistant to the effects of serum.

sesamoid (ses′ah-moid) 1. denoting a small nodular bone embedded in a tendon or joint capsule. 2. a sesamoid bone (see table of BONES).

sesqui- word element [L.], *one and one-half.*

sesquioxide (ses″kwe-ok′sīd) a compound of three parts of oxygen with two of another element.

sessile (ses′il) not pedunculated; attached by a broad base.

setaceous (se-ta′shus) bristle-like.

sex (seks) 1. a distinctive character of most animals and plants, based on the type of gametes produced by the gonads, ova being typical of the female, and sperm of the male, or the category in which the individual is placed on such basis. 2. to determine the sex of an individual.

s. character, primary, a trait directly concerned in reproductive function of the individual.

s. character, secondary, a trait typical of the sex but not directly concerned in reproductive function of the individual.

s. chromatin, the persistent mass of chromatin situated at the periphery of the nucleus in cells of normal females; it is the material of the inactivated sex chromosome. Called also Barr body.

chromosomal s., sex as determined by the presence of the XX (female) or the XY (male) genotype in somatic cells, without regard to phenotypic manifestations.

s. chromosomes, chromosomes that are associated with the determination of sex, in mammals constituting an unequal pair, called the X and the Y chromosome.

s. glands, the glands that regulate reproduction and manufacture the hormones that control the sex characters—the TESTES in the male, and the OVARIES in the female; called also GONADS.

gonadal s., the sex as determined on the basis of the gonadal tissue present (ovarian or testicular).

s. hormones, glandular secretions involved in the regulation of sexual functions. The principal sex hormone in the male is TESTOSTERONE, produced by the testes. In the female, the ovaries produce ESTROGEN and PROGESTERONE.

These hormones control the secondary sex characters, such as the shape and contour of the body, the distribution of body hair and the pitch of the voice. The male hormones stimulate production of sperm in men, and the female hormones control ovulation, pregnancy, and the menstrual cycle in women.

morphologic s., that determined on the morphology of the external genitalia.

psychologic s., that determined by the gender role assigned to and played by the growing individual.

sex-limited (seks-lim′ĭ-ted) affecting individuals of one sex only.

sex-linked (seks-linkt′) transmitted by a gene located on a sex (X or Y) chromosome.

sexology (sek-sol′o-je) the scientific study of sex and sexual relations.

sextan (seks′tan) recurring on the sixth day (every five days).

sextipara (seks-tip′ah-rah) a woman who has had six pregnancies that resulted in viable offspring; para VI.

sextuplet (seks-tup′let, seks-too′plet, seks′too-plet) any one of six offspring produced at the same birth.

sexual (seks′u-al) pertaining to sex.

s. deviation, sexual behavior that varies from that considered biologically or socially acceptable.

sexuality (seks″u-al′ĭ-te) 1. the characteristic quality of the male and female reproductive elements. 2. the constitution of an individual in relation to sexual attitudes and behavior.

Sézary syndrome an exfoliative erythroderma due to cutaneous infiltration of reticular lymphocytes, with alopecia, edema, hyperkeratosis, and pigment and nail changes.

S.G.O. Surgeon-General's Office.

SGOT serum glutamic oxaloacetic transaminase (see under SERUM).

SGPT serum glutamic pyruvic transaminase (see under SERUM).

shadow-casting (shad″o-kast′ing) application of a coating of gold, chromium, or other metal for the purpose of increasing the visibility of ultramicroscopic specimens under the microscope.

shaft (shaft) a long slender part, such as the portion of a long bone between the wider ends or extremities.

shank (shangk) the tibia or shin; a leglike part.

shaping (shāping) in BEHAVIOR THERAPY, the production of new behavior by providing reinforcement for progressively closer approximations of the final desired behavior.

Sharpey's fibers (shar′pēz) fibers that pass from the periosteum and embed in the periosteal lamellae.

sheath (shēth) a tubular case or envelope.

arachnoid s., the delicate membrane between the pial sheath and the dural sheath of the optic nerve.

carotid s., a portion of the cervical fascia enclosing the carotid artery, internal jugular vein, and vagus nerve.

connective tissue s. of Key and Retzius, Henle's sheath.

crural s., femoral sheath.

dural s., the external investment of the optic nerve.

femoral s., the fascial sheath of the femoral vessels.

Henle's s., the endoneurium, especially the delicate continuation around the terminal branches of nerve fibers; called also connective tissue sheath of Key and Retzius.

lamellar s., the perineurium.

medullary s., myelin s., the sheath surrounding the axon of some (myelinated) nerve fibers, consisting of myelin alternating with the spirally wrapped neurilemma.

pial s., the innermost of the three sheaths of the optic nerve.

root s., th epidermic layer of a hair follicle.

s. of Schwann, neurilemma.

synovial s., synovial membrane lining the cavity of a bone through which a tendon moves.

Sheehan's syndrome postpartum pituitary necrosis.

sheep cell agglutination test SCAT, a laboratory

test for infectious mononucleosis. When the antibody level of a person with this disease reaches a certain level, a sample of his blood will cause agglutination of sheep erythrocytes. If there is agglutination of these cells in concentrations up to 1:28, the findings are considered positive for infectious mononucleosis. The specimen for the test is 5 ml. of venous blood, placed in a test tube and allowed to coagulate. No special preparation of the patient is necessary.

Shenton's line (shen′tonz) a curved line seen in radiographs of the normal hip, formed by the top of the obturator foramen.

shield (shēld) any protecting structure.

shift (shift) a change or deviation.

chloride s., the exchange of chloride and carbonate between the plasma and the erythrocytes that takes place when the blood gives up oxygen and receives carbon dioxide. It serves to maintain ionic equilibrium between the cell and surrounding fluid.

s. to the left, a change in the blood picture, with a preponderance of young neutrophils.

s. to the right, a preponderance of older neutrophils in the blood picture.

Shigella (shĭ-gel′ah) a genus of bacteria that cause dysentery. They are gram-negative, rod-shaped bacteria.

S. boy′dii, the cause of an acute diarrheal disease in man, especially in the tropics.

S. dysente′riae, a species that produces a neurotropic exotoxin in addition to the endotoxin common to all members of the *Shigella* group; it is more common in tropical regions and produces severe dysentery. Called also Shiga bacillus.

S. flexner′i, a common agent of acute diarrheal disease of man.

S. son′nei, one of the commonest causes of bacillary dysentery in temperate climates.

shigella (shĭ-gel′ah), pl. *shigel′lae.* any individual organism of the genus *Shigella.*

shigellosis (shĭ-gel-o′sis) infection with *Shigella;* bacillary dysentery.

shin (shin) the prominent anterior edge of the tibia and leg.

s. bone, tibia.

saber s., marked anterior convexity of the tibia, seen in congenital syphilis.

s. splints, strain of the long flexor muscle of the toes occurring in athletes, marked by pain along the shin bone.

shingles (shing′gelz) herpes zoster.

shiver (shiv′er) 1. a slight tremor. 2. to tremble slightly, as from cold.

shivering (shiv′er-ing) involuntary shaking of the body, as with cold. It is caused by contraction or twitching of the muscles, and is a physiologic method of heat production in man and other mammals.

shock (shok) disruption of the circulation, which can upset all body functions; sometimes referred to as circulatory shock. It occurs when blood pressure is inadequate to force blood through the vital tissues. Shock is a dangerous condition which may be fatal.

MECHANISMS OF CIRCULATORY SHOCK. The essentials of circulatory shock are easier to understand if the circulatory system is thought of as a four-part mechanical device made up of a pump (the heart), a complex system of flexible tubes (the blood vessels), a circulating fluid (the blood), and a fine regulating system or "computer" (the nervous system) designed to control fluid flow and pressure. The diameter of the blood vessels is controlled by impulses from the nervous system which cause the muscular walls to contract. The nervous system also affects the rapidity and strength of the heartbeat, and thereby the blood pressure as well.

Shock, which is associated with a dangerously low blood pressure, can be produced by factors that attack the strength of the heart as a pump, decrease the volume of the blood in the system, or permit the blood vessels to increase in diameter.

TYPES OF CIRCULATORY SHOCK. There are five main types of circulatory shock. Low-volume shock occurs whenever there is insufficient blood to fill the circulatory system. Neurogenic shock is due to disorders of the nervous system. Two types of shock, allergic shock and septic shock, are due to reactions that impair the muscular functioning of the blood vessels. Cardiac shock is caused by impaired function of the heart.

Low-Volume Shock. This is a common form of shock that occurs when blood or plasma is lost in such quantities that the remaining blood cannot fill the circulatory system despite constriction of the blood vessels. The blood loss may be external, as when a vessel is severed by an injury, or the blood may be "lost" into spaces inside the body where it is no longer accessible to the circulatory system, as in severe gastrointestinal bleeding from ulcers, fractures of large bones with hemorrhage into surrounding tissues, or major burns that attract large quantities of blood fluids to the burn site outside blood vessels and capillaries. The treatment of low-volume shock requires replacement of the lost blood.

Neurogenic Shock. This form of shock, often called fainting, may be brought on by severe pain, fright, unpleasant sights, or other strong stimuli that overwhelm the usual regulatory capacity of the nervous system. The diameter of the blood vessels increases, the heart slows, and the blood pressure falls to the point where the supply of oxygen carried by the blood to the brain is insufficient. The patient then faints. Placing the head lower than the body is usually sufficient to relieve this form of shock.

Allergic Shock. Allergic shock, commonly called ANAPHYLACTIC SHOCK, is a rare phenomenon that occurs when a person receives an injection of a foreign protein to which he is highly sensitive. The blood vessels and other tissues are affected directly by the allergic reaction. Within a few minutes, the blood pressure falls and severe dyspnea develops. The sudden deaths that in rare cases follow bee stings or injection of certain medicines are due to anaphylactic reactions.

Septic Shock. Septic shock, resulting from bacterial infection, is being recognized with increasing frequency. Certain organisms contain a toxin that seems to act on the blood vessels when it is released into the bloodstream. The blood eventually pools within parts of the circulatory system that expand easily, causing the blood pressure to drop sharply. Gram-negative shock is a form of septic shock due to infection with gram-negative bacteria.

Cardiac Shock. Cardiac shock may be caused by conditions that interfere with the function of the heart as a pump, such as severe myocardial infarction, severe heart failure and certain disorders of rate and rhythm.

The Patient in Shock. The precise progression to a state of shock depends upon the cause of the disorder and the speed of onset. In hemorrhagic shock, for example, as blood is lost the patient with gradually progressing shock feels very restless at first. He becomes thirsty. His skin takes on a pallor and feels cold. Often he perspires profusely. The pulse speeds up but is weak and indistinct. He gradually feels lethargic and faint, and may show signs of air hunger (labored and difficult breathing). The nail beds and lips take on a bluish hue. As shock deepens and the blood pressure falls, the patient becomes comatose and eventually dies if untreated.

Treatment. Some relatively simple measures can be taken to reduce the effects of shock and slow its progress toward life-threatening proportions. In hypovolemic shock and endotoxic shock the patient is placed in supine position with the lower extremities elevated unless there is severe injury to the head, back, and neck. Patients in cardiogenic shock are placed in a sitting position. Measures are taken to minimize pain, but care must be taken not to administer a dosage of medication that may predispose the patient to arterial hypotension. Only small sips of water to relieve thirst are allowed in order to decrease the possibility of vomiting and aspiration.

More severe cases of shock require administration of oxygen to prevent tissue anoxia, and administration of intravenous fluids and possibly whole blood to restore blood volume and blood pressure.

ACIDOSIS frequently accompanies severe shock and thus requires administration of sodium bicarbonate intravenously. Other specific measures will depend on the type of shock that is manifested and the responsiveness of the patient to selected treatments. Fluid replacement, especially in hypovolemic shock, is most accurately guided by CENTRAL VENOUS PRESSURE measurements.

There is some controversy over the use of drugs that either constrict or dilate the blood vessels. It is generally the practice to administer vasoconstrictors first if the blood volume is normal or slightly expanded. These agents are used only briefly, however, and in as small doses as possible because, although they do increase blood flow to the brain and heart, they do so at the expense of other organs, particularly the kidneys. When blood volume expansion and efforts at peripheral vasoconstriction have not proved effective, vasodilators may be used. Serious renal injury that is a threat in unrelieved shock may be avoided by the use of diuretics.

Corticosteroids, such as hydrocortisone, are often administered in massive doses in the treatment of septic shock and other types that prove resistant to treatment.

allergic s., anaphylactic s., a violent attack of symptoms produced by a second injection of serum or protein and due to anaphylaxis.

colloidoclastic s., colloidoclasia.

electric s., shock caused by electric current passing through the body (see ELECTRIC SHOCK).

insulin s., a condition of circulatory insufficiency resulting from overdosage with insulin, which causes too sudden reduction of blood sugar. It is marked by tremor, sweating, vertigo, diplopia, convulsions, and collapse. Such a condition produced intentionally has been used in treatment of schizophrenia (See also INSULIN SHOCK and SHOCK THERAPY.)

respirator s., circulatory shock due to interference with the flow of blood through the great vessels and chambers of the heart, causing pooling of blood in the veins and the abdominal organs and a resultant vascular collapse. The condition sometimes occurs as a result of increased intrathoracic pressure in patients who are being maintained on a mechanical VENTILATOR.

shell s., condition of lost nervous control with numerous psychic symptoms, ranging from extreme fear to actual dementia, produced in soldiers under fire by the noise and concussion of bursting shells.

spinal s., the loss of spinal reflexes after injury of the spinal cord that appears in the muscles enervated by the cord segments situated below the site of the lesion.

s. therapy, a technique used in treating certain severe forms of mental illness. The patient is rendered temporarily unconscious, usually by means of an electric current. This form of psychiatric treatment is now frequently referred to as somatic therapy, rather than shock therapy, because it does not necessarily produce a state of shock in the medical sense. Shock therapy has been a method of treatment since the 1930's, but more recently the development of medicines such as tranquilizers and "mood elevators" has reduced its use.

Uses and Effects. The different types of shock have somewhat different effects. Electroshock is most useful in cases of severe depression and is sometimes used on patients with involutional reaction, a condition that appears in late middle age. It is also employed in patients who are in the depressive stage of affective psychosis.

Inhalant shock, which makes use of an ether compound, has much the same effect as electroshock. Alleviation of severe symptoms is rapid with these treatments.

Insulin shock, produced by administration of insulin, is a more prolonged form of treatment and is helpful primarily in treating cases of severe schizophrenia. It is rarely used, however.

Methods of Administration. In electroshock therapy, electrodes are placed on either side of the patient's forehead and a brief current is applied. The patient immediately becomes unconscious and retains no memory of a shock. Care is taken to prevent injury during the convulsions that follow treatment.

Inhalant therapy has the same effects, but is often accepted more readily by patients than electroshock therapy. Both treatments may be preceded by the administration of an anesthetic so that the patient is asleep during the entire procedure. Medication to relax the muscles so that the convulsion is very mild may also be employed.

In insulin therapy, a carefully measured quantity of insulin is injected into the patient, with coma and occasionally convulsions following. Sometimes insulin therapy is combined with electric shock for patients unresponsive to either treatment alone.

Objective. The objective of shock therapy is to enable patients who have withdrawn into phantasies or severe depression to reestablish contact with the world. It may then be possible to treat the causes of their mental illness with psychotherapy.

shoulder (shōl'der) the large joint where the humerus joins the scapula. The shoulder is a shallow ball-and-socket joint, similar to the hip joint.

At the shoulder, the smooth, rounded head of the humerus rests against the socket in the scapula. The joint is covered by a tough, flexible protective capsule and is heavily reinforced by ligaments that stretch across the joint. The ends of the bones where they meet at the joint are covered with a layer of cartilage that reduces friction and absorbs shock. A thin membrane, the synovial membrane, lines the socket and lubricates the joint with synovia. Further cushioning and lubrication are provided by fluid-filled sacs called bursae.

DISORDERS OF THE SHOULDER. One of the most common disorders of the shoulder is BURSITIS, or inflammation of the bursa, often caused by excessive use of the joint. The joint becomes painful and difficult to move.

The shoulder is one of the most common sites for a DISLOCATION, in which the ball of the humerus is disloged from its socket in the scapula. This injures the ligaments and the capsule, and may cause temporary paralysis of the arm as well as pain and swelling. A dislocated shoulder is usually caused by a blow or fall, but sometimes an unusual physical effort may pull the arm from the shoulder socket. A first dislocation often makes the joint more susceptible to future dislocations. Only a doctor should set a dislocated shoulder; inexpert efforts may do far more damage than the original injury.

Frozen shoulder is a disability of the shoulder joint due to chronic inflammation in and around the joint and characterized by pain and limitation of motion.

shoulder-hand syndrome a disorder of the upper extremity characterized by pain and stiffness in the shoulder, with puffy swelling and pain in the ipsilateral hand, sometimes occurring after myocardial infarction, but also produced by other causes.

show (sho) appearance of blood forerunning labor or menstruation.

shunt (shunt) 1. to turn to one side; to divert; to bypass. 2. a passage or anastomosis between two natural channels, especially between blood vessels. Such structures may be formed physiologically (e.g., to bypass a thrombosis), or they may be structural anomalies. 3. a surgical anastomosis.

arteriovenous (A-V) s., a U-shaped plastic tube inserted between an artery and a vein (usually between the radial artery and cephalic vein), bypassing the capillary network; commonly done to allow repeated access to the arterial system for the purpose of HEMODIALYSIS.

cardiovascular s., an abnormality of the blood flow between the sides of the heart or between the systemic and pulmonary circulation; see left-to-right SHUNT and right-to-left SHUNT.

jejunoileal s., an INTESTINAL BYPASS performed to control obesity.

left-to-right s., diversion of blood from the left side of the heart to the right side, or from the systemic to the pulmonary circulation through an anomalous opening such as a septal defect or patent ductus arteriosus.

portacaval s., postcaval s., surgical creation of an anastomosis between the portal vein and the vena cava.

reversed s., right-to-left shunt.

right-to-left s., diversion of blood from the right side of the heart to the left side or from the pulmonary to the systemic circulation through an anomalous opening such as septal defect or patent ductus arteriosus.

ventriculovenous s., surgical creation of a diversion of cerebrospinal fluid from the ventricles of the brain to the external jugular vein for the purpose of relieving HYDROCEPHALUS. The diversion is accomplished by insertion of a catheter. If the cardiac end of the catheter is threaded through the vena cava to

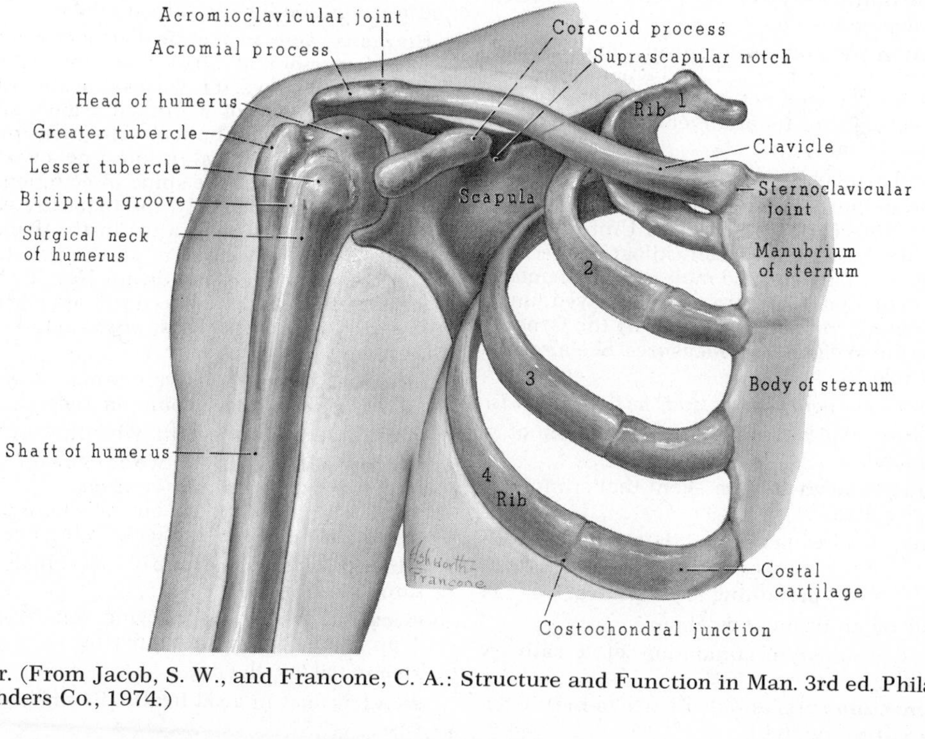

Shoulder. (From Jacob, S. W., and Francone, C. A.: Structure and Function in Man. 3rd ed. Philadelphia, W. B. Saunders Co., 1974.)

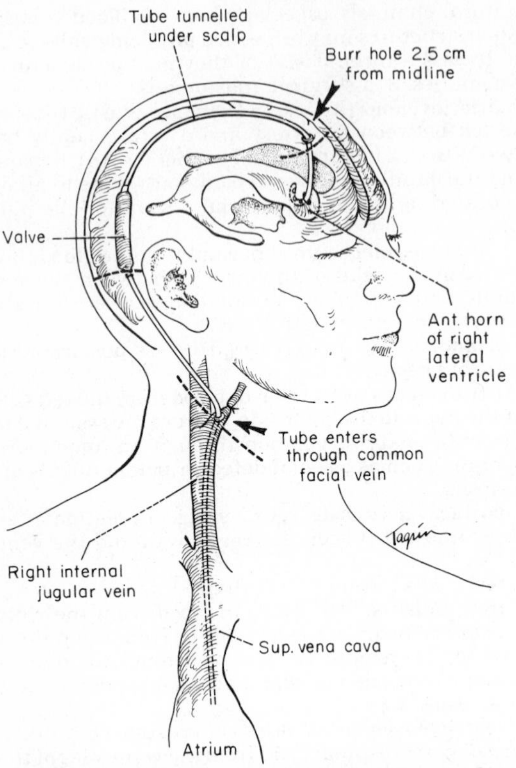

Schematic diagram to show placement of ventriculovenous shunt for hydrocephalus. (From Shillito and Ojemann, in Neurological Surgery. J. R. Youmans, Ed. Philadelphia, W. B. Saunders Co., 1973.)

the right atrium of the heart, the procedure is called a *ventriculoatrial* shunt.

Shwartzman phenomenon (shwarts′man) a local tissue reaction characterized by hemorrhagic necrosis due to an antigen-antibody reaction to certain bacterial substances. Its occurrence in humans is largely theoretical.

Si chemical symbol, *silicon.*

SI unit any of the units of the Systéme International d'Unites, or International System of Units. SI units comprise the base units (meter, kilogram, second, ampere, kelvin, candela, and mole), supplementary units (radian and steradian), and derived units (newton, pascal, and joule) adopted by the General Conference of Weights and Measures. See also Appendix, Table 10.

sial(o)- word element [Gr.], *saliva; salivary glands.*

sialadenitis (si″al-ad″ĭ-ni′tis) inflammation of a salivary gland.

sialagogue (si-al′ah-gog) an agent that stimulates the flow of saliva.

sialectasia (si″al-ek-ta′ze-ah) dilatation of a salivary duct.

sialine (si′ah-līn) pertaining to the saliva.

sialismus (si″ah-liz′mus) ptyalism.

sialitis (si″ah-li′tis) inflammation of a salivary gland or duct.

sialoadenectomy (si″ah-lo-ad″ĕ-nek′to-me) excision of a salivary gland.

sialoadenitis (si″ah-lo-ad″ĕ-ni′tis) inflammation of a salivary gland.

sialoadenotomy (si″ah-lo-ad′ĕ-not′o-me) incision of a salivary gland.

sialoaerophagia (si″ah-lo-a″er-o-fa′je-ah) the swallowing of saliva and air.

sialoangiectasis (si″ah-lo-an″je-ek′tah-sis) dilatation of a salivary duct.

sialoangiography (si″ah-lo-an″je-og′rah-fe) radiography of the ducts of the salivary glands after injection of radiopaque material.

sialocele (si′ah-lo-sēl) a salivary cyst.

sialodochitis (si″ah-lo-do-ki′tis) inflammation of a salivary duct.

sialodochoplasty (si″ah-lo-do′ko-plas″te) plastic repair of a salivary duct.

sialoductitis (si″ah-lo-duk-ti′tis) sialoangiitis.

sialogenous (si″ah-loj′ĕ-nus) producing saliva.

sialogogue (si-al′o-gog) sialagogue.

sialogram (si-al′o-gram) a film obtained by sialography.

sialography (si″ah-log′rah-fe) roentgen demonstration of the salivary ducts by means of the injection of substances opaque to x-rays.

sialolith (si-al′o-lith) a salivary calculus.

sialolithiasis (si″ah-lo-lĭ-thi′ah-sis) the formation of salivary calculi.

sialolithotomy (si″ah-lo-lĭ-thot′o-me) excision of a salivary calculus.

sialorrhea (si″ah-lo-re′ah) ptyalism.

sialoschesis (si″ah-los′kĕ-sis) suppression of secretion of saliva.

sialosis (si″ah-lo′sis) 1. the flow of saliva. 2. ptyalism. adj., **sialot′ic.**

sialostenosis (si″ah-lo-stĕ-no′sis) stenosis of a salivary duct.

sialosyrinx (si″ah-lo-sir′inks) 1. salivary fistula. 2. a syringe for washing out the salivary ducts, or a drainage tube for the salivary ducts.

Siamese twins identical (monozygotic) twins joined together at birth. The connection may be slight or extensive. It involves skin and usually muscles or cartilage of a limited region, such as the head, chest, hip, or buttock. The twins may share a single organ, such as an intestine, or occasionally may have parts of the spine in common.

If joined superficially, the twins are easily separated by surgery soon after birth. If more deeply united, they may have to go through life, if they survive, with their handicap. New techniques in surgery, however, are making it possible to separate some Siamese twins whose physical links are highly complex.

sib (sib) 1. a blood relative; one of a group of persons all descended from a common ancestor. 2. sibling.

sibilant (sib′ĭ-lant) shrill, whistling, or hissing.

sibling (sib′ling) any of two or more offspring of the same parents; a brother or sister.

half s., an individual one of whose parents was also a parent of the person of reference.

sibship (sib′ship) a group of individuals born of the same parents.

siccative (sik′ah-tiv) 1. drying; removing moisture. 2. an agent that produces drying.

siccus (sik′us) [L.] dry.

sick (sik) not in good health; ill; afflicted with disease.

s. sinus syndrome, a complex cardiac arrhythmia manifested as severe sinus bradycardia alone, sinus bradycardia alternating with tachycardia, or sinus bradycardia with atrioventricular block.

sickle cell (sik″l) a crescentic or sickle-shaped erythrocyte, the abnormal shape caused by the presence of varying proportions of hemoglobin S.

s. c. anemia, a genetically determined defect of hemoglobin synthesis, inherited as an autosomal recessive and confined for the most part to Negroes. In the homozygous state it is characterized by abnormal hemoglobin (hemoglobin S), anemia, reticulocytosis, and jaundice. Clinical findings include recurrent attacks of fever, and pain in the arms, legs, and abdomen from early childhood; a constant scleral icterus; and, in the crisis period, a tender, rigid abdomen resembling that seen in a surgical illness. Headache, paralysis, and convulsions may result from cerebral thrombosis due to increased viscosity of the blood. Treatment is symptomatic. There is a tendency to progressive renal damage in patients who survive the disease beyond the age of 50. (See also ANEMIA for patient care.)

s.c. trait, the condition, usually asymptomatic, of being heterozygous for hemoglobin S.

sicklemia (sik-le′me-ah) sickle cell anemia.

sickling (sik′ling) the development of sickle cells in the blood.

sickness (sik′nes) a condition of deviation from the normal healthy state.

S.I.D. Society for Investigative Dermatalogy.

side effect (sīd′ ĕ-fekt″) a consequence other than that for which an agent is used, especially an adverse effect on another organ system.

sidero- word element [Gr.], *iron.*

sideroblast (sid′er-o-blast″) a nucleated erythrocyte containing iron granules in its cytoplasm. adj., **sideroblas′tic.**

siderocyte (sid′er-o-sīt″) a red blood cell containing nonhemoglobin iron.

sideroderma (sid″er-o-der′mah) bronzed coloration of the skin due to disordered iron metabolism.

siderofibrosis (sid″er-o-fi-bro′sis) fibrosis associated with deposits of iron. adj., **siderofibrot′ic.**

sideropenia (sid″er-o-pe′ne-ah) deficiency of iron in the body or blood. adj., **siderope′nic.**

siderophil (sid′er-o-fil) 1. siderophilous. 2. a siderophilous cell or tissue.

siderophilin (sid″er-of′ĭ-lin) transferrin.

siderophilous (sid″er-of′ĭ-lus) tending to absorb iron.

siderophore (sid′er-o-fōr) a macrophage containing hemosiderin.

siderosis (sid″er-o′sis) 1. a form of PNEUMOCONIOSIS due to the inhalation of iron or other metallic particles. 2. excess of iron in the blood. 3. the deposit of iron in the tissues.

hepatic s., the deposit of an abnormal quantity of iron in the liver.

urinary s., the presence of hemosiderin granules in the urine.

SIDS sudden infant death syndrome.

sig. [L.] *sig′na* (mark).

sight (sīt) 1. the act or faculty of VISION, involving the EYE itself, the visual center in the brain, and the optic nerve and nerve fibers in the brain that connect the two. 2. a thing seen.

far s., hyperopia.

near s., myopia.

night s., hemeralopia; day blindness.

sigmatism (sig′mah-tizm) faulty enunciation or too frequent use of *s* sounds.

sigmoid (sig′moid) 1. shaped like the letter C or S. 2. the sigmoid colon, the distal part of the colon from the level of the iliac crest to the rectum.

sigmoidectomy (sig″moi-dek′to-me) excision of part of the sigmoid colon.

sigmoiditis (sig″moi-di′tis) inflammation of the sigmoid colon.

sigmoidopexy (sig-moi′do-pek″se) fixation of the sigmoid colon, as for rectal prolapse.

sigmoidoproctostomy, sigmoidorectostomy (sig-moi″do-prok-tos′to-me, sig-moi″do-rek-tos′-to-me) surgical anastomosis of the sigmoid colon to the rectum.

sigmoidoscope (sig-moi′do-skōp) an endoscope for use in sigmoidoscopy.

sigmoidoscopy (sig″moi-dos′ko-pe) direct examination of the interior of the sigmoid colon. (For preparation of the patient, see PROCTOSCOPY.)

sigmoidosigmoidostomy (sig-moi″do-sig″moi-dos′to-me) anastomosis of two previously remote portions of the sigmoid colon.

sigmoidostomy (sig″moi-dos′to-me) surgical creation of an opening from the surface of the body into the sigmoid colon.

sigmoidotomy (sig″moi-dot′o-me) incision of the sigmoid.

sigmoidovesical (sig-moi″do-ves′ĭ-kal) pertaining to or communicating with the sigmoid colon and the urinary bladder.

sign (sīn) 1. any objective evidence of disease or dysfunction. 2. an observable physical phenomenon so frequently associated with a given condition as to be considered indicative of its presence.

vital s′s, the signs of life, namely pulse, respiration, and temperature.

signa (sig′nah) [L.] mark, or write; abbreviated S. or sig. in prescriptions, followed by the signature.

signature (sig′nah-tūr) that part of a drug prescription that gives directions to be followed by the patient in its use.

Silastic (sĭ-las′tik) trademark for polymeric silicone substances having the properties of rubber; it is biologically inert and used in surgical prostheses.

silica (sil′ĭ-kah) silicon dioxide, a compound occurring naturally as quartz and in other forms, some of which are used in dental materials.

silicoanthracosis (sil″ĭ-ko-an″thrah-ko′sis) silicosis combined with pneumoconiosis of coal workers.

silicon (sil′ĭ-kon) a chemical element, atomic number 14, atomic weight 28.086, symbol Si. (See table of ELEMENTS.)

silicone (sil′ĭ-kōn) any organic compound in which all or part of the carbon has been replaced by silicon.

silicosis (sil″ĭ-ko′sis) a lung disease caused by the prolonged inhalation of silica dust. adj., **silicot′ic.** In the past it was called such colorful names as potter's asthma, stonecutter's cough, miner's mold, and grinder's rot, according to the occupation in which it was acquired. Besides silicosis, various other lung diseases result from inhaling industrial substances; together, these "dust diseases" are called the PNEUMOCONIOSES.

Today silicosis is most likely to be contracted in such industrial jobs as sandblasting in tunnels and hardrock mining, but it can occur in anyone who is habitually exposed to the dust of silica, one of the commonest minerals. All types of miners, for example, may be subject to it, from gold miners to coal miners.

Silicosis usually takes about 10 years of fairly constant exposure to develop. It may give few warning symptoms. As time goes on, an affected person experiences progressive shortness of breath, along with steady coughing which in the early stages is dry and unproductive of mucus. Later there may be mucus tinged with blood, loss of appetite, pain in the chest, and general weakness. The silica produces a nodular fibrotic reaction that scars the lungs and makes them receptive to the further complications of bronchitis and emphysema; persons with silicosis are also more susceptible to tuberculosis.

Since silicosis is a serious disease, those who must work near silica should take precautions to breathe as little of it as possible. This can usually be effected by the use of face masks, proper ventilation, and other safety devices. The cooperation of industry, labor, and government in developing various protective measures has made silicosis a much less common disease today than it used to be.

Regular chest x-rays are recommended for all workers exposed to silica as the quickest and easiest way to detect silicosis. If discovered in its early stages, the disease can usually be arrested by a change of occupation and appropriate therapy. Once fully developed, the disease rarely yields to treatment.

Silicote (sil′ĭ-kōt) trademark for preparations of dimethicone, a skin protective.

silicotuberculosis (sil″ĭ-ko-tu-ber″ku-lo′sis) tuberculous infection of the lung affected with silicosis.

silo-filler's disease pulmonary inflammation, often with acute pulmonary edema, due to inhalation of the irritant gases (especially oxides of nitrogen) which collect in recently filled silos.

silver (sil′ver) a chemical element, atomic number 47, atomic weight 107.870, symbol Ag. (See table of ELEMENTS.) It is used in medicine for its caustic, astringent and antiseptic effects.

colloidal s., a silver preparation in which the silver exists as free ions to only a small extent.

s. iodide, a yellowish, powdery compound; useful in syphilis and in nervous diseases, and also applied locally in conjunctivitis.

s. nitrate, colorless or white crystals, used as a caustic and local anti-infective, one important use being in prevention of ophthalmia neonatorum.

s. nitrate, toughened, a mixture of silver nitrate with hydrochloric acid, sodium chloride, or potassium nitrate, occurring as white crystalline masses molded into pencils or cones; a convenient means of applying silver nitrate locally.

s. protein, silver made colloidal by the presence of, or combination with, protein; an active germicide with a local irritant and astringent effect.

Silverman-Andersen score (sil′ver-man-an′dersen) a system for evaluation of breathing performance of premature infants. It consists of five items: (1) chest retraction as compared with abdominal retraction during inspiration; (2) retraction of the lower intercostal muscles; (3) xiphoid retraction; (4) flaring of the nares with inspiration; and (5) expiratory grunt. Each of the five factors is graded 0, 1, or 2. The sum of these factors yields the score. Adequate ventilation is indicated by a 0, severe respiratory distress is indicated by a score of 10.

simethicone (sĭ-meth′ĭ-kōn) an antiflatulent substance consisting of a mixture of dimethyl polysiloxanes and silica gel.

Simmonds' disease (sim′ondz) PANHYPOPITUITARISM in which cachexia is a prominent feature; called also pituitary cachexia. It follows the destruction of the pituitary gland by surgery, infection, injury, or tumor; it may also occur after difficult labor in childbirth.

Simmonds' disease was first described by Dr. Morris Simmonds of Hamburg, Germany, in 1914. Symptoms, which vary in intensity, are extreme weight loss, general debility, pallor, dry and yellowish skin, a slow pulse, hypotension, and atrophy of the genitalia and breasts, progressing to premature senility and apathy. Treatment is by regular administration of the various hormones whose release is normally dependent on pituitary function.

Sims (simz) James Marion (1813–1883). American surgeon and pioneer in gynecology. Born in South Carolina and graduated from Jefferson Medical College in Philadelphia, he is known chiefly for the semiprone position and the curved speculum that are named after him, and that contributed to his success in operating for vesicovaginal fistula. He established the State Hospital for Women in New York, and was president of the American Medical Association and honorary president of the International Medical Congress.

Sims' position (simz) the patient on his left side and chest, the right knee and thigh drawn up, the left arm along the back.

simulation (sim″u-la′shun) 1. the act of counterfeiting a disease; malingering. 2. the imitation of one disease by another.

Simulium (sĭ-mu′le-um) a genus of biting gnats, several species of which are the intermediate host of *Onchocerca volvulus*.

Sinaxar (sin′ak-sar) trademark for a preparation of styramate, a skeletal muscle relaxant.

sincalide (sin′kah-līd) a synthetic derivative of cholecystokinin, used intravenously to induce rapid contraction of the gallbladder.

sinciput (sin′sĭ-put) the upper and front part of the head. adj., **sincip′ital.**

Sinemet (sin′ĕ-met) trademark for a combination of carbidopa and levodopa, used in the treatment of Parkinson's disease.

sinew (sin′u) a tendon of a muscle.

weeping s., an encysted ganglion, chiefly on the back of the hand, containing synovial fluid.

Singoserp (sing′go-serp) trademark for preparations of syrosingopine, an antihypertensive.

singultus (sing-gul′tus) hiccup.

sinister (sin′is-ter) [L.] left; on the left side.

sinistr(o)- word element [L.], *left; left side.*

sinistrad (sin′is-trad) to or toward the left.

sinistral (sin′is-tral) pertaining to the left side.

sinistrality (sin″is-tral′ĭ-te) the preferential use, in voluntary motor acts, of the left member of the major paired organs of the body, as ear, eye, hand, and leg.

sinistraural (sin″is-traw′ral) hearing better with the left ear.

sinistrocardia (sin″is-tro-kar′de-ah) levocardia.

sinistrocerebral (sin″is-tro-ser′ĕ-bral) situated in the left hemisphere of the brain.

sinistrocular (sin″is-trok′u-lar) having the left eye dominant.

sinistrocularity (sin″is-trok″u-lar′ĭ-te) dominance of the left eye.

sinistrogyration (sin″is-tro-ji-ra′shun) a turning to the left.

sinistromanual (sin″is-tro-man′u-al) left-handed.

sinistropedal (sin″is-trop′ĕ-dal) using the left foot in preference to the right.

sinistrotorsion (sin″is-tro-tor′shun) a twisting toward the left, as of the eye.

sinoatrial (si″no-a′tre-al) pertaining to the sinus venosus and the atrium of the heart.

s. node, a collection of atypical muscle fibers (Purkinje fibers) in the wall of the right atrium where the rhythm of cardiac contraction is usually established; therefore also referred to as the pacemaker of the heart.

sinobronchitis (si″no-brong-ki′tis) chronic paranasal sinusitis with recurrent episodes of bronchitis.

Sintrom (sin′trom) trademark for a preparation of acenocoumarol, an anticoagulant.

sinuitis (sin″u-i′tis) sinusitis.

sinuotomy (si″nu-ot′o-me) sinusotomy.

sinuous (sin′u-us) bending in and out; winding.

sinus (si′nus) 1. a recess, cavity, or channel, as (a) one in bone or (b) a dilated channel for venous blood. 2. an abnormal channel or fistula, permitting escape of pus. In common usage, the word sinus refers to any of the eight cavities in the skull that are connected with the nasal cavity—the paranasal sinuses.

The paranasal sinuses are arranged in four pairs, with members of each pair on the left and right sides of the head. The pairs are the maxillary sinuses, located in the maxillae; the frontal sinuses, in the frontal bone; the sphenoid sinuses, in the sphenoid bone behind the nasal cavity; and the ethmoid sinuses, in the ethmoid bone, behind and below the frontal sinuses. (See also Plate 16.)

The functions of the sinuses are not certain. They are believed to help the nose in circulating, warming, and moistening the air as it is inhaled, thereby lessening the shock of cold, dry air to the lungs. They also are thought to have a minor role as resonating chambers for the voice.

anal s's, furrows, with pouchlike recesses at the distal end, separating the rectal columns; called also anal crypts.

aortic s's, pouchlike dilatations at the root of the aorta, one opposite each semilunar cusp of the aortic valve.

s. arrhythmia, the physiologic cyclic variation in heart rate related to vagal impulses to the sinoatrial node; it occurs commonly in children (juvenile arrhythmia) and in the aged, and requires no treatment.

carotid s., a dilatation of the proximal portion of the internal carotid or distal portion of the common carotid artery, containing in its wall pressoreceptors that are stimulated by changes in blood pressure. (See also CAROTID SINUS SYNDROME.)

cavernous s., an irregularly shaped venous channel between the layers of dura mater of the brain, one on either side of the body of the sphenoid bone and communicating across the midline. Several cranial nerves course through this sinus.

cerebral s., one of the ventricles of the brain.

cervical s., a temporary depression in the neck of the embryo containing the branchial arches.

circular s., the venous channel encircling the pituitary gland, formed by the two cavernous sinuses and the anterior and posterior intercavernous sinuses.

coccygeal s., a sinus or fistula just over or close to the tip of the coccyx.

coronary s., the dilated terminal portion of the great cardiac vein, receiving blood from other veins draining the heart muscle and emptying into the right atrium (see also CORONARY SINUS).

dermal s., a congenital sinus tract extending from the surface of the body, between the bodies of two adjacent lumbar vertebrae, to the spinal canal.

ethmoidal s., that paranasal sinus consisting of the ethmoidal cells collectively, and communicating with the nasal meatuses. (See Plate 16.)

frontal s., one of the paired paranasal sinuses in the frontal bone, each communicating with the middle meatus of the ipsilateral nasal cavity. (See Plate 16.)

intercavernous s's, channels connecting the two cavernous sinuses, one passing anterior and the other posterior to the stalk of the pituitary gland.

lymphatic s's, irregular, tortuous spaces within lymphoid tissues through which lymph flows.

marginal s., a venous channel near the edge of the placenta.

maxillary s., one of the paired paranasal sinuses in the body of the maxilla on either side, opening into the middle meatus of the ipsilateral nasal cavity. (See Plate 16.)

occipital s., a venous sinus between the layers of dura mater, passing upward along the midline of the cerebellum.

paranasal s's, mucosa-lined air cavities in bones of the skull, communicating with the nasal cavity and including ethmoidal, frontal, maxillary, and sphenoidal sinuses. (See Plate 16.)

petrosal s., inferior, a venous channel arising from the cavernous sinus and draining into the internal jugular vein.

petrosal s., superior, one arising from the cavernous sinus and draining into the transverse sinus of the dura mater.

pilonidal s., a suppurating sinus containing hair, occurring chiefly in the coccygeal region.

prostatic s., the posterolateral recess between the seminal colliculus and the wall of the urethra.

s's of pulmonary trunk, spaces between the wall of the pulmonary trunk and cusps of the pulmonary valve at its opening from the right ventricle.

renal s., a recess in the substance of the kidney, occupied by the renal pelvis, calices, vessels, nerves, and fat.

sagittal s., inferior, a small venous sinus of the dura mater, opening into the straight sinus.

sagittal s., superior, a venous sinus of the dura mater that ends in the confluence of sinuses.

sigmoid s., a venous sinus of the dura mater on

either side, continuous with the straight sinus and draining into the internal jugular vein of the same side.

sphenoidal s., one of the paired paranasal sinuses in the body of the sphenoid bone, opening into the highest meatus of the ipsilateral nasal cavity. (See Plate 16.)

sphenoparietal s., one of the venous sinuses of the dura mater, emptying into the cavernous sinus.

s's of spleen, dilated venous channels in the substance of the spleen.

straight s., a venous sinus of the dura mater formed by junction of the great cerebral vein and inferior sagittal sinus, and ending in the confluence of sinuses.

tarsal s., a space between the calcaneus and talus.

tentorial s., straight sinus.

transverse s. of dura mater, a large venous sinus on either side of the skull.

transverse s. of pericardium, a passage within the pericardial sac, behind the aorta and pulmonary trunk and in front of the left atrium and superior vena cava.

tympanic s., a deep recess on the medial wall of the middle ear.

urogenital s., an elongated sac formed by division of the cloaca in the early embryo which ultimately forms most of the vestibule of the vagina in the female, and of the urethra in the male.

uterine s's, venous channels in the wall of the uterus in pregnancy.

uteroplacental s's, blood spaces between the placenta and uterine sinuses.

s. of venae cavae, the posterior portion of the right atrium into which the inferior and the superior vena cava open.

venous s., s. veno'sus, 1. the common venous receptacle in the early embryo attached to the posterior wall of the primitive atrium. 2. sinus of venae cavae.

venous s's of dura mater, large channels for venous blood forming an anastomosing system between the layers of the dura mater of the brain, receiving blood from the brain and draining into the veins of the scalp or deep veins at the base of the skull.

venous s. of sclera, a circular channel at the junction of the sclera and cornea, into which aqueous humor filters from the anterior chamber of the eye.

sinusitis (si″nŭ-si′tis) inflammation of one or more of the paranasal SINUSES, often occurring during an upper respiratory infection, when infection in the nose spreads to the sinuses (sometimes encouraged by excessively strong blowing of the nose). Sinusitis also may be a complication of tooth infection, allergy, or certain infectious diseases, such as pneumonia and measles. There are many other causes of sinusitis, including air pollution, diving and underwater swimming, sudden extremes of temperature, and structural defects of the nose that interfere with breathing, such as deviated SEPTUM.

As the mucous membranes of the sinus become inflamed and swollen, the openings that lead from each sinus into the nasal passages become partially or wholly blocked. The mucus that accumulates in the sealed-off sinus causes pressure on the sinus walls, resulting in discomfort, fever, pain, and difficult breathing.

SYMPTOMS. The common symptoms of sinusitis are headache, usually located near the sinuses most involved, and nasal discharge. These may be accompanied by a slight rise in temperature, dizziness, and a general feeling of weakness and discomfort.

TREATMENT. Steam inhalations and antihistamine nose drops may help relieve the symptoms. An electric heating pad or a hot water bottle may ease pain if applied for 10 minutes every 2 hours over the painful area on the face or forehead. Aspirin will also give some relief.

Since sinusitis, either acute or chronic, can lead to complications of the middle ear or of adjacent bones, it is important to treat the condition early. Antibiotics may be necessary to combat infection.

Plenty of rest and sleep is recommended in acute attacks of sinusitis. Smoke, dust, and other irritants to the nasal passages should be avoided, and smoking should be stopped entirely.

When other methods fail to correct troublesome chronic sinusitis of long standing, surgery is sometimes required. The opening to the sinus may be made larger to ensure drainage and ventilation, but such measures cannot always guarantee complete cure.

Though a change of climate can sometimes help in cases of chronic sinusitis, it rarely is a necessity. Creating a better indoor climate with such devices as air conditioners and humidifiers often is equally beneficial in reducing the number and severity of sinus attacks.

Psychotherapy may be of help to some patients with disabling, chronic sinusitis because continual emotional strain is one of the factors that can intensify the symptoms.

sinusoid (si′nŭ-soid) 1. resembling a sinus. 2. a form of terminal blood channel consisting of a large, irregular, anastomosing vessel, having a lining of reticuloendothelium but little or no adventitia. Sinusoids are found in the liver, adrenal glands, heart, parathyroid glands, carotid bodies, spleen, hemolymph glands, and pancreas.

sinusotomy (si″nŭ-sot′o-me) incision of a sinus.

siphon (si′fon) 1. a bent tube with arms of unequal length, for drawing liquid from a higher to a lower level by force of atmospheric pressure. 2. to draw liquid by means of a siphon.

siphonage (si′fon-ij) the use of the siphon, as in gastric lavage or in draining the bladder.

Sippy diet (sip′e) a graduated diet for peptic ulcer and other conditions requiring a smooth diet, at first consisting of only milk and cream, with gradual addition of other foods, the amounts increasing until on day 28 the patient is placed on a regular ward diet.

sirenomelus (si″ren-om′ĕ-lus) a fetus with fused legs and no feet.

-sis word element [Gr.], *state; condition.*

sister (sis′ter) the nurse in charge of a hospital ward (Great Britain).

sitiology, sitology (sit″e-ol′o-je; si-tol′o-je) the science of food and nourishment.

sitomania (si″to-ma′ne-ah) excessive hunger, or morbid craving for food.

sitosterol (si″tos′ter-ol) one of a group of closely related plant sterols; a preparation of beta-sitosterol and certain saturated sterols is used as an antihypercholesterolemic agent.

sitotherapy (si″to-ther′ah-pe) treatment by food; dietotherapy.

sitotropism (si-tot′ro-pizm) tropism in response to the influence of food.

situs (si′tus), pl. *si′tus* [L.] site or position.

s. inver′sus, total or partial transposition of the body organs to the side opposite the normal.

sitz bath (sits) immersion in water of only the hips and buttocks, for relief of pain and discomfort following rectal surgery, cystoscopy, or vaginal surgery, or for cystitis or infections within the pelvic cavity (see also BATH).

Sjogren's syndrome (sho′grenz) keratoconjunctivitis sicca with pharyngitis sicca, enlargement of parotid glands, xerostomia, and chronic polyarthritis.

SK streptokinase.

skatole (skat′ōl) a compound formed in the putrefaction of proteins which contributes to the characteristic odor of the feces.

skatoxyl (skah-tok′sil) an oxidation product of skatole found in the urine in certain diseases of the large intestine.

skein (skān) spireme.

skelalgia (ske-lal′je-ah) pain in the leg.

skeletal (skel′ĕ-tal) pertaining to the skeleton.
s. system, the body's framework of bones; called also the skeleton. The skeleton of an average adult consists of 206 distinct bones (see also Plates 1 and 2).

FUNCTIONS OF THE SKELETAL SYSTEM. The bones of the skeleton give support and shape to the body and protect delicate internal organs. Muscles attached to the skeleton make motion possible. In addition to supporting the body, the bones store and help maintain the correct level of calcium (see also BONE). The bone marrow manufactures blood cells.

MAIN PARTS OF THE SKELETON. There are two main parts of the skeleton; the axial skeleton, including the bones of the head and trunk, and the appendicular skeleton, including the bones of the limbs. The axial skeleton has 80 bones; the appendicular skeleton, 126 bones.

Axial Skeleton. The axial skeleton includes the skull, the spine, and the ribs and sternum. The most important of these is the spine, called also the backbone and the vertebral column; it consists of 26 separate bones. Twenty-four vertebrae have holes through them, and the holes are lined up vertically, forming a hollow tube. The spinal cord runs through this bony tube and is protected by it.

The seven topmost spinal bones, the cervical vertebrae, are the neck bones. They support the skull, which encloses and protects the brain and provides protection for the eyes, the inner ears, and the nasal passages. The skull includes the cranium, the facial bones, and the auditory ossicles. Of the 28 bones of the skull, only one—the mandible—is movable.

Below the seven cervical vertebrae of the spine are 12 thoracic vertebrae; attached to them are 12 pairs of ribs, one pair to a vertebra. The ribs curve around to the front of the body, where most of them attach directly to the sternum or are indirectly attached to it by means of cartilage. The two bottom pairs of ribs remain unattached in front and so are called floating ribs. Together, the thoracic vertebrae, the ribs, and the sternum form a bony basket, called the thoracic (or rib) cage, that prevents the chest wall from collapsing and protects the heart and the lungs.

The remaining bones of the spine include five lumbar vertebrae, which support the small of the back, and the sacrum and coccyx.

The axial skeleton also includes a single bone in the neck, the hyoid bone, to which muscles of the mouth are attached. This is the only bone of the body that does not join with another bone.

Appendicular Skeleton. The appendicular skeleton includes the shoulder girdle, arm bones, pelvic girdle and leg bones. The shoulder (or pectoral) girdle, from which the arms hang, consists of the two clavicles (collarbones) and two scapulae (shoulder blades). The scapulae are joined to the sternum.

The arm has three long bones. One end of the upper arm bone, the humerus, fits into a socket in the shoulder girdle; the other end is connected at the elbow to the ulna and the radius, the two long bones of the lower arm. Eight small bones, the carpals, comprise the wrist. Five metacarpals form the palm of the hand, and the finger bones are made up of 14 phalanges in each hand.

At the lower end of the spine is the pelvic (or hip) girdle. This girdle and the last two bones of the spine, the sacrum and the coccyx, form the pelvis. This part of the skeleton encircles and protects the internal organs of the genitourinary system. In each side of the pelvis is a socket into which a femur fits.

Leg bones are similar in construction to arm bones, but are heavier and stronger. The thigh bone, or femur, which is the longest bone in the body, extends from the pelvis to the knee, and the tibia and fibula go from knee to ankle. The kneecap is a single bone, the patella. In each leg there are seven ankle bones, or tarsals; five foot bones, or metatarsals; and 14 toe bones, or phalanges.

JOINTS AND MOVEMENT. Any place in the skeleton where two or more bones come together is known as a JOINT. The way these bones are joined determines whether they can move and how they move. The elbow, for example, is a hinge joint, which allows bending in only one direction. In contrast, both bending and rotary movements are possible in the hip joint, a ball-and-socket joint. Many joints, such as most of those in the skull, are rigid and permit no movement whatsoever.

The force needed to move the bones is provided by MUSCLES, which are attached to the bones by tendons. A muscle typically spans a joint so that one end is attached by a tendon to one bone, and the other end to a second bone. Usually one bone serves as an anchor for the muscle, and the second bone is free to move. When the muscle contracts, it pulls the second bone. Actually, two sets of muscles that pull in opposite directions take part in any movement. When one set contracts, the opposing set relaxes.

skeletization (skel″ĕ-tĭ-za′shun) 1. extreme emaciation. 2. removal of soft parts from the skeleton.

skeletogenous (skel″ĕ-toj′ĕ-nus) producing skeletal structures or tissues.

skeleton (skel′ĕ-ton) the hardened tissues forming the supporting framework of an animal body (see SKELETAL SYSTEM).

Skene's glands (skēnz) the largest of the female urethral glands, which open within the urethral orifice; they are regarded as homologous with the prostate. Called also paraurethral ducts.

skenitis (ske-ni′tis) inflammation of Skene's glands.

skeocytosis (ske″o-si-to′sis) the presence of immature forms of leukocytes in the blood; shift to the left.

skeptophylaxis (skep″to-fi-lak′sis) 1. a condition in which a minute dose of a substance poisonous to animals will produce immediate temporary immunity to the action of the poison, although the blood of the animal may be highly toxic during that period of immunity. 2. the method of allergic desensitization by the preliminary injection of a small amount of the allergen, as is commonly done before the injection of an antiserum.

skia- word element [Gr.], *shadow* (especially as produced by x-rays).

skiameter (ski-am'ĕ-ter) an instrument for measuring the intensity of x-rays.

skiametry (ski-am'ĕ-tre) retinoscopy; observation of the pupil and retina under a beam of light projected into the eye, as a means of determining refractive errors of the eye.

skiascope (ski'ah-skōp) retinoscope; an instrument used in skiametry.

skiascopy (ski-as'ko-pe) 1. skiametry. 2. fluoroscopy.

skin (skin) the outer covering of the body. The skin is the largest organ of the body, and it performs a number of vital functions. It serves as a protective barrier against microorganisms. It helps shield the delicate, sensitive tissues underneath from mechanical and other injuries. It acts as an insulator against heat and cold, and helps eliminate body wastes in the form of perspiration. It guards against excessive exposure to the ultraviolet rays of the sun by producing a protective pigmentation, and it helps produce the body's supply of vitamin D. Its sense receptors enable the body to feel pain, cold, heat, touch, and pressure.

The skin consists of two main parts: an outer layer, the epidermis, and an inner layer, the corium (dermis, true skin).

EPIDERMIS. The epidermis is thinner than the corium, and is made up of several layers of different kinds of cells. The number of cells varies in different parts of the body; the greatest number is in the palms of the hands and soles of the feet, where the skin is thickest.

The cells in the outer or horny layer of the epidermis are constantly being shed and replaced by new cells from its bottom layers in the lower epidermis. The cells of the protective, horny layer are nonliving and require no supply of blood for nourishment. As long as the horny outer layer remains intact, microorganisms cannot enter.

CORIUM. Underneath the epidermis is the thicker part of the skin, the corium, or dermis, which is made up of connective tissue that contains blood vessels and nerves. The corium projects into the epidermis in ridges called papillae of the corium.

The nerves that extend through the corium end in the papillae. The various skin sensations, such as touch, pain, pressure, heat, and cold, are felt through these nerves. The reaction to heat and cold causes the expansion and contraction of the blood capillaries of the corium. This in turn causes more or less blood to flow through the skin, resulting in greater or smaller loss of body heat (see TEMPERATURE).

The sweat glands are situated deep in the corium. They collect fluid containing water, salt, and waste products from the blood and carry it away in canals that end in pores on the skin surface, where it is deposited as sweat. Perspiration helps regulate body temperature as well, because cooling of the skin occurs when sweat evaporates. The sebaceous glands are also in the corium. They secrete the oil that keeps the skin surface lubricated.

Beneath the corium is a layer of subcutaneous tissue. This tissue helps insulate the body against heat and cold, and cushions it against shock.

The hair and nails are outgrowths of the skin. The roots of the hair lie in follicles, or pockets of epidermal cells situated in the corium. Hair grows from the roots, but the hair cells die while still in the follicles, and the closely packed remains that are pushed upward form the hair shaft that is seen on the surface of the skin.

The nails grow in much the same way as the hair. The nail bed, like the hair root, is situated in the corium. The pink color of the nails is due to their translucent quality which allows the blood capillaries of the corium to show through.

DISORDERS OF THE SKIN. The skin reflects the general physical and emotional health. A skin disorder, for instance, may indicate disease within the body. For this reason, it is important that a particular skin condition be diagnosed and treated by a physician rather than by home treatments that may be unnecessary or actually harmful.

It is important to remember that the skin, given the opportunity, tends to heal itself. Overtreatment may be worse than no treatment at all. For common skin ailments, bland treatments, such as cool or warm compresses, lotions, and ointments, are usually recommended. Under no circumstances should one scratch, pick, or rub an incipient skin irritation or inflammation.

The medical name for an inflammation of the skin is DERMATITIS, and any itching of the skin is called PRURITUS. Dermatitis may occur without pruritus, and vice versa, but often they occur together.

Allergic reactions that may be manifested by skin disorders include URTICARIA (hives), ECZEMA, and various forms of contact dermatitis. Fungus infections of the skin include RINGWORM and ATHLETE'S FOOT.

BOILS and CARBUNCLES occur when bacteria gain entrance into the skin and cause the formation of pus. A related condition of the eyelid is a STY.

Streptococci or staphylococci cause IMPETIGO, which is marked by blisters and yellowish crusts and occurs most often in children.

A similar infection that affects the hair follicles at the pore openings of the skin is FOLLICULITIS. When such infection affects the follicles of the beard, it is called SYCOSIS BARBAE, or barber's itch.

ERYSIPELAS, or St. Anthony's fire, is a streptoccocal infection of the skin and underlying tissues that can be very serious if not treated. This condition is one of several forms of CELLULITIS that may affect the skin.

COLLAGEN DISEASES, which cause deterioration of the connective tissues, may affect the skin. They include the relatively uncommon LUPUS ERYTHEMATOSUS and scleroderma. PEMPHIGUS is a rare and serious disease that usually begins as a cluster of blisters on the nose or mouth and gradually involves the whole body.

Fever blisters, or coldsores, are caused by the virus of herpes simplex. Another virus disease affecting the skin is HERPES ZOSTER, or shingles, in which an infected nerve causes a skin eruption. WARTS are also caused by a virus.

The skin is subject to a number of pigmentary disorders. Some are congenital; others occur as the result of exposure to sunlight, heat, heavy metals, and other products, or as a result of local injury, or in association with various diseases.

Some persons lack pigmentation partially or completely. This condition, which is hereditary, is known as albinism. Vitiligo and leukoderma appear as white spots that occur because of decreased pigmentation. The cause of vitiligo is unknown. Leukoderma may accompany certain infections, or may result from injury or exposure to rubber products.

Excessive pigmentation includes the freckles that light-skinned persons tend to develop from overexposure to sunlight. LIVER SPOTS are brownish patches, somewhat larger and darker than freckles, that sometimes appear on the skin of an older person. Both conditions are harmless.

NEVI, or moles, are dark patches, varying in color from gray to brown to black. On the average, every person has at least 20. Some moles occasionally can become malignant and any change in their appearance should be brought to the attention of a physician.

A HEMANGIOMA is an area in which the blood vessels form an abnormally excessive network in the skin. They usually occur as birthmarks and some disappear with age; others can be treated surgically, with medications or with irradiation.

Bronzing of the skin sometimes is associated with ADDISON'S DISEASE and hemochromatosis ("bronze diabetes").

Various kinds of tumors or growths may be found on the skin. KELOIDS are benign tumors that usually originate in scar tissue. In many cases they can be removed with radium and x-ray therapy. XANTHOMAS are harmless yellow growths caused by deposits of fat in the skin. They may be associated with some underlying disorder of lipid metabolism. They can be eliminated by a physician if they are unsightly. Keratoses are wartlike growths, often brown in color, that appear most frequently in older persons. Because they can develop into cancers, they should receive medical attention. Generally a physician will recommend that they be removed.

CANCER of the skin is the most common of all cancers. Fortunately it is comparatively easy to treat successfully, especially if it is diagnosed early. As protection against skin cancer, sores that persist for more than 2 or 3 weeks and suspicious lumps or growths that suddenly begin to enlarge or change color should be brought to a physician's attention.

s. graft, a bit of skin implanted to replace a lost part of the integument (see also GRAFTING and PLASTIC SURGERY).

s. test, application of a substance to the skin, or intradermal injection of a substance, to permit observation of the body's reaction to it. Such a test detects a person's sensitivity to such allergens as dust and pollen, or to preparations of microorganisms believed to be the cause of a disorder.

There are several types of skin tests, including the patch test, the scratch test, and the intradermal test.

PATCH TEST. This is the simplest type of skin test. A small piece of gauze or filter paper is impregnated with a minute quantity of the substance to be tested and is applied to the skin, usually on the forearm. After a certain length of time the patch is removed and the reaction observed. If there is no reaction, the test result is said to be negative; if the skin is reddened or swollen, the result is positive.

The patch test is used most often in testing for skin allergies, especially contact DERMATITIS.

SCRATCH TEST. In this test, one or more small scratches or superficial cuts are made in the skin,

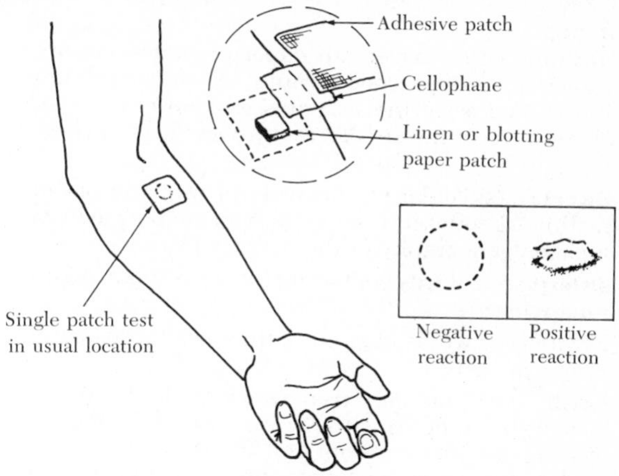

Patch test.

and a minute amount of the substance to be tested is inserted in the scratches and allowed to remain there for a short time. If no reaction has occurred after 30 minutes, the substance is removed and the test is considered negative. If there is redness or swelling at the scratch sites, the test is considered positive.

The scratch test is often used in testing for allergies. A complete screening for allergic sensitivity may require numerous skin tests. Only an extremely minute quantity of the substance can be used in each test since severe allergic reactions can occur.

The scratch test is also used in the diagnosis of tuberculosis. In Pirquet's reaction, for example, tuberculin is used, and the local inflammatory reaction that results is more marked in tuberculous persons than in normal ones.

INTRADERMAL TESTS. In these tests, the substance under study is injected between the layers of skin. Intradermal tests are used for diagnosis of infectious diseases and determination of susceptibiltiy to a disease or sensitivity to an allergen.

In the intradermal test for tuberculosis, the Mantoux test, a purified protein derivative (P.P.D.), prepared from tubercle bacilli, is injected. In a positive result, the area becomes reddened or inflamed within 72 hours. This indicates past or present infection. An infection that has been present for at least 2 to 8 weeks will usually be revealed by the test.

The Schick test, used to determine susceptibility to diphtheria, is one of the best-known intradermal skin tests. A very small dose of diphtheria antitoxin is injected into the forearm. In a positive reaction the area becomes red and remains so for about a week. If no reaction occurs, the person is immune to the disease.

The trichophytin test is sometimes used in diagnosing suspected cases of superficial fungus infection of the skin, such as ringworm. In the presence of infection by the fungus *Trichophyton,* an injection of trichophytin, which is prepared from cultures of the fungus, will produce a reaction similar to the tuberculin rection. Skin tests, of course, are always made in an area separate from the infected area.

In addition to their frequent use in testing for allergies, intradermal tests are employed in the diagnosis of parasitic infections, such as SCHISTOSOMIASIS, other fungus diseases besides trichophytosis, and mumps.

Skinner box (skin'er) an experimental enclosure for testing animal conditioning, in which the subject animal performs (e.g., presses a bar or lever) to obtain a reward (see also INSTRUMENTAL CONDITIONING).

Skiodan (ski'o-dan) trademark for preparations of methiodal sodium, used as a radiopaque medium for roentgenography of the urinary tract.

skler(o)- for words beginning thus, see those beginning *scler(o)-*.

skot(o)- for words beginning thus, see those beginning *scot(o)-*.

skull (skul) the bony framework of the head, enclosing and protecting the brain. The skull consists of two parts, the cranium and the facial section.

The cranium is the domed top, back, and sides of the skull. It is formed by comparatively large, smooth and gently curved bones connected to each other by dovetailed joints called sutures, which permit no movement and make the mature skull rigid. At birth, however, the skull joints are flexible, so that the infant's head can be compressed as it emerges from the birth canal. The joints remain flexible to allow expansion until the cranial bones are fully formed, around the second year of life. An infant's skull contains soft areas, or FONTANELS, where the bones of the cranium do not meet. (See illustration, page 928.)

The facial bones are smaller and more complex than the cranial bones. None of them are movable, except the mandible, which is hinged to the rest of the skull.

The skull protects the brain, the curve of the cranium serving to deflect blows, and it also protects the eyes, ears, and nose, which are surrounded by bone and recessed in the skull.

The skull is supported by the highest vertebra, called the atlas. This joint permits a back-and-forth, nodding motion. The atlas turns on the vertebra below it, the axis, which allows the skull to turn from side to side.

DISORDERS OF THE SKULL. The skull is rarely affected by disease. Uncommon ones like OSTEITIS DEFORMANS and ACROMEGALY cause the bones to increase in size. Like other bones, the skull may be fractured by blows, falls, or other accidents, but skull fracture can be far more dangerous because of its proximity to the brain. Concussion is almost always present with such fractures. If the fracture is simple, it will usually heal itself. There may be complications, however. If the fracture crosses an artery, surgery may be necessary. Another danger is that a bone or fragment of bone may be pushed in and exert pressure on the brain, possibly causing convulsions. Such a bone intrusion must be corrected by surgery. Open or compound fractures of the skull present the additional danger of infection to the brain. (See also HEAD INJURY.)

During infancy the bones of the skull may unite prematurely, causing the head to be misshapen and sometimes resulting in brain damage because of pressure effects on the growing brain.

sleep (slēp) a period of rest for the body and mind, during which volition and consciousness are in partial or complete abeyance and the bodily functions partially suspended. Sleep has also been described as a behavioral state marked by characteristic immobile posture and diminished but readily reversible sensitivity to external stimuli.

NREM AND REM SLEEP. Prior to the discovery and reporting of rapid eye movements (REM) during sleep, it was thought that sleep was a single state of passive recuperation in which the central nervous system was deactivated. Studies reported by Eugene Aserinsky and Nathaniel Kleitman in 1953, and subsequent studies by others concerned with the measurement of central and autonomic activities during sleep have led to the dividing of sleep into two categories: NREM, or non-rapid eye movement sleep, also called orthodox or synchronized (S) sleep; and REM, or rapid eye movement sleep, so called because of the rapid eye movements that are manifested during this stage of sleep. REM sleep is also called paradoxical or desynchronized (D) sleep.

On the basis of electroencephalographic (EEG) criteria, NREM sleep is subdivided into four stages. *Stage 1* is observed immediately after sleep begins

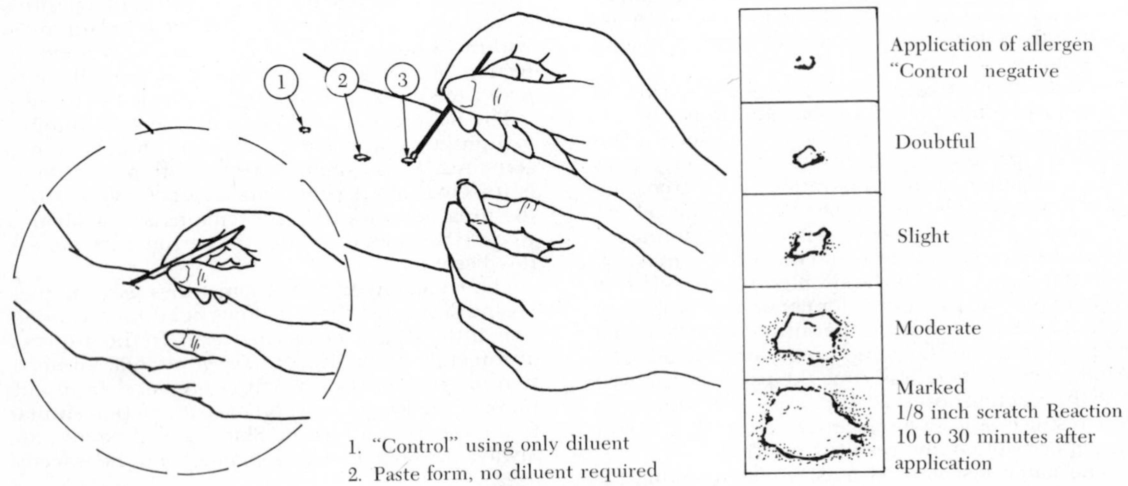

1. "Control" using only diluent
2. Paste form, no diluent required
3. Powder form, applied with a drop of diluent from end of toothpick

Scratch test.

or after momentary arousals and is characterized by low-voltage, mixed-frequency EEG tracing, with predominantly theta-wave activity (four to seven hertz, that is, cycles per second). *Stage 2* is characterized by intermittent waves of 12 to 16 hertz known as "sleep spindles." *Stages 3 and 4* consist of relatively high voltage EEG tracings with a predominance of delta wave activity (one to two hertz).

The EEG patterns of NREM sleep suggest that this kind of sleep is the kind of apparently restful state that supports the recuperative functions assigned to sleep. NREM sleep is increased after physical activity and has a relatively high priority among humans in the recovery sleep following extended periods of wakefulness.

Within 90 minutes after sleep begins, an adult progresses through all four stages of NREM sleep and then proceeds into the first of a series of REM periods of sleep. Brief cycles of about 10–30 minutes of REM sleep recur throughout the night, alternating with various stages of NREM sleep. During the latter part of the night there are decreasing periods of NREM sleep and longer periods of REM sleep.

Periods of REM sleep are usually accompanied by dreaming. There also are movement of the body and periodic twitching of the muscles of the face and extremities during REM sleep.

PATTERNS OF SLEEP. Although the average adult spends approximately 25 percent of total accumulated sleep in REM sleep and 75 percent in NREM sleep, the cyclic changes vary with individuals. The pattern of sleep, in addition to the REM and NREM states, also includes the periods of sleep and wakefulness within a 24-hour period.

Factors affecting the total sleep pattern include age, state of physical health, psychological state, and certain drugs. Newborn infants follow a pattern of several hours of sleep followed by a period of wakefulness. REM sleep occurs at the onset of sleep in infants; it rarely does in adults. As the child matures there is an increasing tendency toward longer periods of nocturnal sleep. Elderly persons sometimes return to the shorter periods of sleep that are typical of infants.

SLEEP REQUIREMENTS. There is a great variability in sleep requirements among individuals. Infants usually require 16 to 20 hours of total sleep during a 24-hour period with the number of hours decreasing as they mature. An adult usually requires 6 to 9 hours of total sleep.

The effects of *sleep deprivation* have been the subject of much research, including deprivation of total sleep, of REM sleep, and of NREM sleep. Total sleep deprivation usually leads to irritability and fatigue, difficulty in concentrating and remembering, poor muscle coordination, and visual or tactile hallucinations and illusions. There is no evidence that total sleep deprivation induces psychosis. Some bizarre behaviors may be manifested after an extended period of sleep loss, but these symptoms do not recur in most subjects once they have slept through a recovery period. It is suspected that when inappropriate behavior does persist after recovery sleep, the subject already had a tendency toward such behavior before sleep deprivation.

Selective sleep deprivation studies have shown that there is a need for both stage 4 NREM and REM sleep. REM sleep deprivation is not, however, psy-

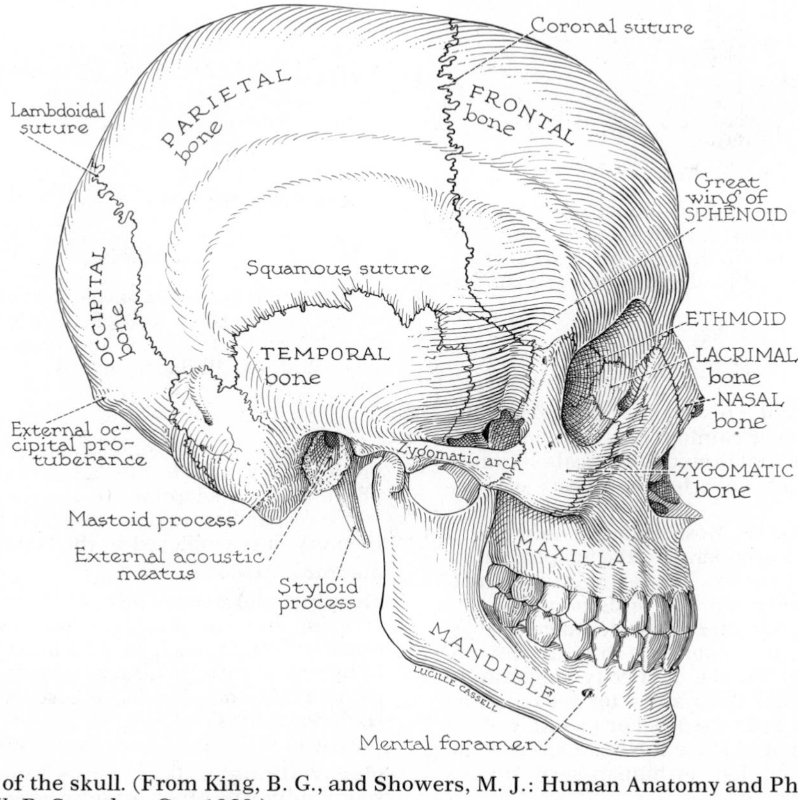

Lateral view of the skull. (From King, B. G., and Showers, M. J.: Human Anatomy and Physiology. 6th ed. Philadelphia, W. B. Saunders Co., 1969.)

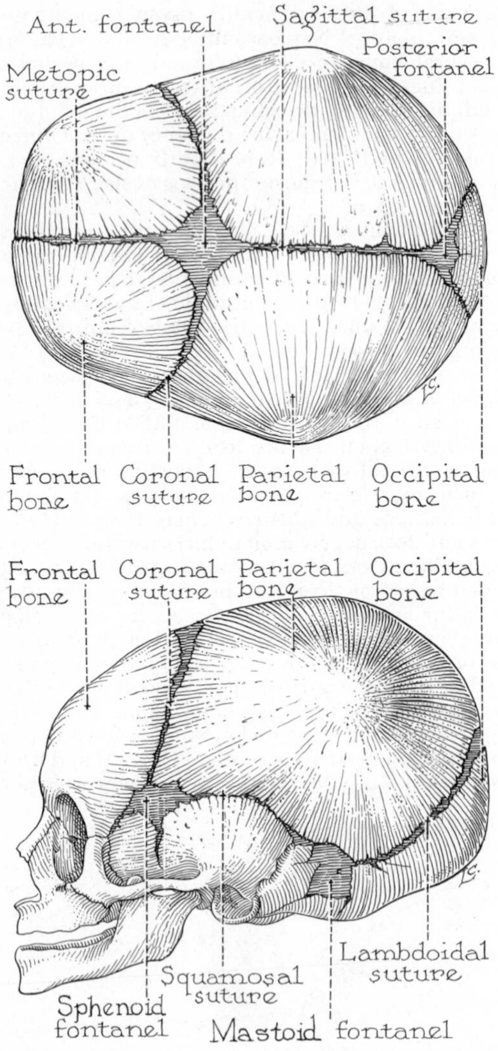

Skull at birth: Above, showing anterior and posterior fontanels; below, lateral view. (From King, B. G., and Showers, M. J.: Human Anatomy and Physiology. 6th ed. Philadelphia, W. B. Saunders Co., 1969.)

chologically harmful. This would seem to refute the freudian theory that dreaming (which accompanies REM sleep) is essential to emotional health because it serves as a safety valve for the release of emotional tensions.

BENEFITS OF SLEEP. Most theorists agree that sleep has value as a recuperative and adaptive function in the lives of humans. The relatively high metabolic needs of mammals and birds to maintain a constant body temperature in a wide range of environmental temperatures suggests that the periodic decreases in metabolic rate and body temperature that occur in NREM sleep allow for recuperation and restitution of body tissues. For example, even though the function of stage 2 NREM sleep is not clear, approximately half of human sleep time is spent in this stage.

It is also theorized that REM sleep provides a period of recuperation of mental activities and preparation for wakefulness. During REM sleep it is believed that there is increased metabolic activity in the brain so that during waking hours it is more receptive to new information and can assimilate it more easily.

SLEEP DISORDERS. Among the minor disorders of sleep are sleepwalking, sleep talking, ENURESIS, tooth-grinding (which is probably an orthodontic problem), and nightmares. Sleepwalking is not considered serious if it occasionally occurs in childhood. It should be considered pathological, however, if it persists into adulthood. Sleep talking is common to many persons and, while it may annoy others whose sleep it may disturb, it is not considered pathological.

A sleep disorder occurring in early childhood, and not to be confused with nightmares, is *night terrors* (pavor nocturnus). In this event, the child awakens with a scream, is in panic and cannot be consoled, and often is incoherent. There is poor recall of the event the following morning. Treatment usually involves reassurance of the parents. Adults who experience night terrors often have some psychological problem requiring treatment.

More serious disorders of sleep include persistent INSOMNIA, NARCOLEPSY, and chronic hypersomnia. Hypersomnia can occur with central nervous system damage and it may be secondary to some physical and mental illnesses, particularly depression.

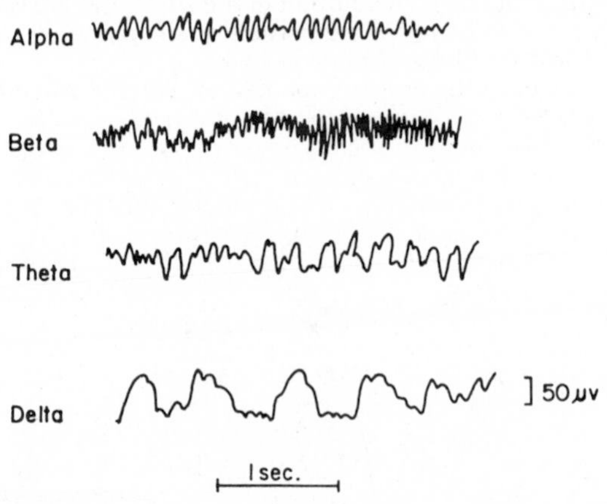

Different types of normal electroencephalographic waves. (From Guyton, A. C.: Basic Human Physiology: Normal Function and Mechanisms of Disease. 2nd ed. Philadelphia, W. B. Saunders Co., 1977.)

twilight s., a condition of analgesia and amnesia, produced by hypodermic administration of morphine and scopolamine. In this state the patient, while responding to pain, does not retain it in her memory. It is employed in the conduct of labor.

sleeping disease narcolepsy.

sleeping sickness a disease characterized by increasing drowsiness and lethargy, caused by a protozoal infection, such as African trypanosomiasis, or by a viral infection, such as lethargic encephalitis, St. Louis encephalitis, or eastern or western encephalomyelitis.

African s. s., African TRYPANOSOMIASIS.

sleepwalking walking while asleep; called also somnambulism. Much mystery has been attached to sleepwalking, although it is no more mysterious than dreaming. The principal difference between the two is that the sleepwalker, besides dreaming, is also using the part of his brain that stimulates walking.

Sleepwalking is most likely to happen during periods of emotional stress. Usually it ceases when the source of anxiety is removed. Often it occurs only once or twice and does not happen again. If sleepwalking recurs frequently, it may stem from serious emotional distress. (See also SLEEP.)

slide (slīd) a piece of glass or other transparent substance on which material is placed for examination under the microscope.

sling (sling) a bandage or suspensory for supporting a part.

slipped disk the popular name for a rupture of a disk, or pad of cartilage, between vertebrae (see slipped DISK).

slough (sluf) 1. a mass of dead tissue in, or cast out from, living tissue. 2. to shed or cast off.

slow-reacting substance a substance released in the anaphylactic reaction that induces slow, prolonged contraction of certain smooth muscles. Symbol SRS or SRS-A.

sludge (sluj) a suspension of solid or semisolid particles in a fluid.

sludging (sluj'ing) settling out of solid particles from solution.

s. of blood, intravascular agglutination of erythrocytes into irregular masses, interfering with circulation of blood.

Sm chemical symbol, *samarium*.

SMA Sequential Multiple Analysis, a sequence of tests performed on an automated instrument (AutoAnalyzer) used in the clinical laboratory for analysis of serum. The AUTOANALYZER is designed with multiple channels, with as many as 12 channels for a corresponding number of tests.

smallpox (smawl'poks) a highly contagious, often fatal viral disease; called also variola. Its most noticeable symptom is the appearance of blisters and pustules on the skin. Smallpox has become rare in most parts of the world because of widespread vaccination against the disease.

Smallpox is one of the most contagious diseases known. The virus that causes the disease is present in the nose and throat of the infected person, in the blisters on his skin, and in his excretions throughout the course of the disease.

The incubation period is generally 12 days, although it may vary from 7 to 21 days.

SYMPTOMS. The first symptoms of smallpox are severe headache, chills, and high fever. Children may suffer from vomiting and convulsions. Within 3 or 4 days, a rash of small, red pustules appears, first on the face, then on the arms, wrists, hands, and legs. A small number of spots appear on the trunk. In a day or two, the spots become blisters and fill with clear fluid. Over the next week, the fluid turns into a yellowish, puslike substance and begins to dry up, leaving a crust or scab on the skin. These scabs fall off after 3 or 4 weeks, leaving disfiguring pits in the skin, particularly on the face.

ISOLATION AND QUARANTINE. A smallpox patient must be rigorously isolated. All those known to have been in contact with the patient are quarantined for 16 days, unless they have just been revaccinated, in which case they may be released from quarantine as soon as the vaccination has "taken." Those in quarantine are kept under careful observation, so if the disease develops they can be isolated and treated immediately. All contaminated objects are destroyed by burning or sterilized with high-pressure steam or boiling water. The patient's home is thoroughly cleaned and disinfected.

TREATMENT. There is at present no cure for smallpox. One important consideration in treating the disease is the possibility of scarring caused by the blisters or pocks. To avoid this, medications may be given to prevent or soothe itching, and antibiotics are applied to the skin to counteract secondary infection. The patient's fingernails are cut short and his hands kept clean to further reduce the danger of infection.

Other than these measures, treatment consists largely of rest and proper nourishment. Medicines may be given to lower the patient's fever, along with sedatives.

PREVENTION. Regular revaccination induces a high degree of immunity and it is hoped that eventually a vigorous smallpox prevention program in the remaining areas of Asia and Africa will eradicate the disease throughout the world.

In countries in which smallpox is no longer a threat, vaccination is recommended only for persons at risk, that is, travelers to endemic areas and others likely to come in contact with such travelers.

Vaccination is no longer required of those persons leaving the United States and planning reentry at a later date.

smear (smēr) a specimen for microscopic study, the material being spread thinly and unevenly across the slide with a swab or loop, or with the edge of another slide.

Pap s., Papanicolaou s., see PAPANICOLAOU TEST.

smegma (smeg'mah) the secretion of sebaceous glands, especially the cheesy secretion, consisting principally of desquamated epithelial cells, found chiefly beneath the prepuce. adj., **smegmat'ic.**

smell (smel) the sense that enables one to perceive odors. The sense of smell depends on the stimulation of sense organs in the nose by small particles carried in inhaled air. It is important not only for the detection of odors, but also for the enjoyment of food. Flavor is a blend of taste and smell. Taste registers only four qualities: salt, sour, bitter, and sweet; other qualities of flavor depend on smell.

The organs of smell are small patches of special (olfactory) cells in the nasal mucosa. One patch is located in each of the two main compartments of the back of the nose. The olfactory cells are connected to the brain by the first cranial (olfactory) nerve. Air currents do not flow directly over the patches in breathing; this is why one must sniff to detect a faint odor or to enjoy a fragrance to the fullest.

When one sniffs, air currents carrying molecules of odorous chemicals enter special compartments, called olfactory chambers, where the chemicals are dissolved in mucus. There they can act on the organs of smell in much the same way that solutions act on the taste buds of the tongue. The endings of the sensory nerves that detect odors, the olfactory receptors, quickly adapt to an odor and cease to be stimulated by it after a few minutes of full exposure.

The sense of smell may be diminished or lost entirely, usually temporarily, as a result of an obstruction of the nose, a nasal infection, injury or deterioration of the nasal tissue, brain tumor, or mental illness. In rare instances, injury or disease causes such damage to the olfactory nerve that loss of the sense of smell is permanent. The complete absence of the sense of smell is known as anosmia.

Smith's fracture (smiths) reversed Colles' fracture.

Smith-Petersen nail (smith pe'ter-sen) a flanged nail for fixing the head of the femur in fracture of the femoral neck.

Smith-Strang disease (smith strănj) a hereditary defect in methionine absorption, in which the urine has a characteristic odor resembling that of the interior of an oasthouse due to alpha-hydroxybutyric acid formed by bacterial action on the unabsorbed methionine; it is marked by white hair, mental retardation, convulsions, and attacks of hyperpnea. Called also oasthouse urine disease.

smoking (smōk'ing) the act of drawing into the mouth and puffing out the smoke of tobacco contained in a cigarette, cigar, or pipe. For centuries, tobacco smoking has been suspected of being a health hazard. In recent years a close relationship between smoking and lung cancer and heart disease has definitely been established. While smoking is not the only cause of these diseases, its relationship to them and also to other diseases has been so strongly established that no smoker can afford to ignore the evidence. Parents especially owe it to their children to educate them in order that the cigarette habit will never begin.

In 1962 the Surgeon General of the United States organized a committee of experts to review some 8000 statistical studies on the effects of smoking. The report of this committee, issued in January 1964, stated:

> In view of the continuing and mounting evidence from many sources, it is the judgment of the Committee that cigarette smoking contributes substantially to mortality from certain specific diseases and to the overall death rate.
> Cigarette smoking is a health hazard of sufficient importance in the United States to warrant appropriate remedial action.

General Effects on Health. Tobacco smoke contains a number of harmful substances, including poisons such as nicotine, various irritants, and carcinogenic compounds. Because cigarette smokers usually inhale this smoke, they are much more subject to its harmful effects than pipe and cigar smokers, who generally do not inhale. In pipe and cigar smoking, however, there is some danger to the heart because of the nicotine that is absorbed by the mouth. There is also the possibility of cancer of the lips, tongue, and mouth. Statistically, there is no question that nonsmokers are far less subject to the diseases that affect smokers.

Among the respiratory diseases closely related to cigarette smoking are lung cancer, cancer of the larynx, chronic bronchitis, and emphysema. Coronary artery disease and hypertensive heart disease are also closely related to smoking, as are peptic ulcer, Buerger's disease (thromboangiitis obliterans), and cancer of the bladder. Other diseases have been linked with smoking. The risk of incurring any of these diseases increases with the number of cigarettes smoked daily, the length of each cigarette consumed, and the length of time the smoking habit has persisted. In general, heavy smokers as a group die younger than do nonsmokers.

S.M.P. Society of Medical Psychoanalysts.

Sn chemical symbol, *tin* (L. *stannum*).

snake (snāk) a limbless reptile, many species of which are poisonous.

snakebite (snāk'bīt) injury caused by the mouth parts of a snake. It is estimated that throughout the world the number of deaths resulting from venomous snakebites is between 20,000 and 25,000 per year. The greatest number of reported snakebite deaths is in the subcontinent of India. There are fewer than 20 snakebite deaths annually in the United States; far more persons die from hypersensitivity to insect stings.

Practices that increase the incidence of snakebites include failure to wear protective covering for the feet and legs, sleeping outdoors on the ground, and the ritual handling of venomous snakes in some religious ceremonies.

Recognition of Venomous Snakebite. The accurate diagnosis of venomous snakebite is greatly enhanced by capturing or killing the snake and correctly identifying it. Lacking this information, one must depend on clinical manifestations, which can be varied and confusing.

One should not depend on visual inspection of the pattern of marks left on the skin. Local swelling may blur the pattern of fang marks and it is possible that only one fang of the venomous snake entered the skin. Nonvenomous snakebites usually do not produce much local swelling and pain and they bleed freely. These symptoms may, however, occur in some types of venomous snakebites.

Symptoms of Venomous Snakebite. In general, venomous snakebites of the type found in the United States produce severe local pain, swelling that spreads from the site of puncture, and involvement of the lymph glands. The patient may experience nausea and vomiting, thirst, sweating, and a low grade fever. If no other symptoms develop, the prognosis is excellent.

More serious symptoms indicating neurotoxic poisoning include numbness and tingling of the face, hypotension, convulsions, and visual disturbances. If the snake is the type that produces hemorrhagic venom, there may be hemoptysis, hematuria, and increased prothrombin time.

Treatment. There are conflicting opinions among experts as to the value of incisions over the fang marks and suctioning of venom from the wound when done outside a medical facility and performed by someone other than a physician. Some continue to recommend emergency treatment consisting of immediate application of a tourniquet, deep incisions over the fang marks, and suctioning. Others feel that the application of a tourniquet to reduce peripheral circulation and packing the affected part in ice to reduce absorption of the venom is the best first aid treatment. The victim is kept calm and as physically inactive as possible and is quickly transported to a medical facility where adequate debridement of the wound and mechanical removal and neutralization of the venom can be done. This also minimizes the danger of introducing infectious agents into the wound.

In addition to local wound treatment, which may require skin grafting at a later date, treatment is concerned with administration of an immune serum (antisera or antivenin), counteraction of the specific pharmacologic effects of the venom, symptomatic relief, and prevention of complications.

PREVENTION OF SNAKEBITE. Most snakebites are inflicted on people who handle snakes or are senselessly incautious in localities where venomous snakes are prevalent. Certain common-sense precautions should be taken when visiting an area known to be inhabited by venomous snakes. Keep in mind that most of them are active in the early evening, that they often congregate on rocky south-facing or west-facing slopes to bask in the sunlight (especially in the spring and fall) and that they are not active at temperatures below 50° F.

snap (snap) a short, sharp sound.

opening s., a short, sharp, high-pitched click occurring in early diastole caused by opening of the mitral cusps, a characteristic sound in mitral stenosis.

snare (snār) a wire loop for removing polyps and other pedunculated growths by cutting them off at the base.

sneeze (snēz) 1. an involuntary, sudden, violent, and audible expulsion of air through the mouth and nose. 2. to expel air in such a manner. Sneezing is usually caused by the irritation of sensitive nerve endings in the mucous membrane that lines the nose. Allergies, drafts of cold air, and even bright light can produce sneezing.

Sneezing and coughing are similar in that both are reflex actions and are preceded by quick inhalations. (However, a cough may also be deliberate, to clear the throat or bronchi.) Sneezing and coughing both involve the glottis. The power for a cough is achieved by closing the glottis and holding the air under pressure for a moment, then suddenly forcing it out by action of the diaphragm and of the muscles of the chest wall and abdomen.

In a sneeze, the glottis is momentarily closed after air is inhaled and the tongue is pressed against the roof of the mouth. When the glottis is suddenly opened, part of the air goes through the nose and, when the tongue is released, part goes through the mouth; in this way mucus and other irritants are expelled from the nose.

Snellen chart (snel′en) a chart printed with block letters in gradually decreasing sizes, used in testing visual acuity.

snoring (snōr′ing) breathing during sleep accompanied by harsh sounds. It occurs when inhaled air causes the soft palate to vibrate. Snoring is common among persons who sleep with their mouths open.

Although snoring is a sign of sound sleep, it is sometimes desirable to eliminate or reduce it. If the mouth-breathing is stopped, the snoring will also stop. An obvious reason for mouth-breathing is lying on the back, in which position the mouth tends to hang open. Further, when a person is in deep sleep and lying on his back, his tongue may rest back in his throat, partly blocking the air passage and helping to make the snoring sounds. Gently rolling the snorer on his side can sometimes eliminate the snoring in these cases.

There may be some functional reason for mouth-breathing, such as a common cold or allergy, causing mucus to stop up the nose. Growths, called polyps, may obstruct the nasal passages. A deformity of the nasal SEPTUM, the bony portion that divides the nasal cavity into two compartments, may make nose-breathing difficult.

Correction of sleeping habits and of nose or throat troubles may lessen snoring or reduce it to a minimum. However, if an elderly person has been snoring regularly for many years, there is little that can be done to change his sleeping habits.

snow (sno) a freezing or frozen mixture consisting of discrete particles or crystals.

carbon dioxide s., the solid formed by rapid evaporation of liquid carbon dioxide, giving a temperature of about −110° F. (−79° C.); used locally in various skin conditions. (See also CARBON DIOXIDE SNOW.)

snowblindness (sno′blīnd-nes) temporary loss of sight due to injury to superficial cells of the cornea caused by ultraviolet rays of the sun reinforced by those reflected by snow.

S.N.S. Society of Neurological Surgeons.

snuffles (snuf′elz) catarrhal discharge from the nasal mucous membrane in congenital syphilis in infants.

SOAP subjective, objective assessment plan, a system utilized in PROBLEM-ORIENTED RECORD keeping.

soap (sōp) any compound of one or more fatty acids, or their equivalents, with an alkali. Soap is a detergent and is employed in liniments and enemas and in making pills. It is also a mild aperient, antacid, and antiseptic.

green s., a potassium soap made by saponification of vegetable oils, excluding coconut oil and palm kernel oil, without the removal of glycerin; it is the chief ingredient of green soap tincture.

soft s., medicinal, green soap.

sociobiology (so″se-o-bi-ol′o-je) the branch of theoretical biology which proposes that all animal (including human) behavior has a biological basis, which is controlled by the genes. adj., **sociobiolog′ical.**

sociologist (so″se-ol′o-jist) a specialist in sociology.

sociology (so″se-ol′o-je) the scientific study of social relationships and phenomena.

sociometry (so″se-om′ĕ-tre) the branch of sociology concerned with the measurement of human behavior.

sociopath (so′se-o-path″) a person with an antisocial personality; a psychopath. adj., **sociopath′ic.**

sociopathic personality (so″se-o-path′ik) psychopathic personality.

sociopathy (so″se-op′ah-the) the disorder of social behavior.

socket (sok′et) a hollow into which a corresponding part fits.

dry s., a condition sometimes occurring after tooth extraction, with exposure of bone, inflammation of an alveolar crypt, and severe pain.

soda (so′dah) sodium carbonate.

baking s., sodium bicarbonate.

caustic s., sodium hydroxide.

s. lime, calcium hydroxide with sodium or potassium hydroxide, or both; used as adsorbent of carbon dioxide in equipment for metabolism tests, inhalation anesthesia, or oxygen therapy.

sodium (so′de-um) a chemical element, atomic number 11, atomic weight 22.990, symbol Na. (See table of ELEMENTS.) Sodium is the chief cation of extracellular body fluids.

s. acetate, a systemic and urinary alkalizer.

s. acetrizoate, a substance used as contrast medium in angiocardiography and in x-ray visualization of the urinary and biliary tracts.

s. acid phosphate, sodium biphosphate.

s. alginate, a product derived from brown seaweeds, used in formulating various pharmaceutical preparations as an emulsifier, stabilizer, or thickening agent.

s. aminosalicylate, an antibacterial compound used in tuberculosis.

s. antimonyl-thioglycollate, an organic compound of antimony, used in leishmaniasis and schistosomiasis.

s. ascorbate, an antiscorbutic vitamin for parenteral administration.

s. benzoate, a white, odorless granular or crystalline powder, used chiefly as a test of liver function, and as a preservative for food and various pharmaceuticals.

s. bicarbonate, a white powder found in most households in the form of baking soda; called also bicarbonate of soda. Taken in water, it is a popular remedy for acid indigestion. It has a rapid and soothing effect on the stomach, but should not be used regularly since when taken in excess it tends to cause ALKALOSIS. It should never be taken by those who have a heart condition or who are on salt-restricted diet, because it is a source of sodium. A teaspoonful of milk of magnesia willl usually prove equally effective and is less harmful.

Sodium bicarbonate can also be mixed with water and applied as a paste for the relief of pain in the treatment of minor BURNS and insect stings. A cupful of bicarbonate of soda in the bath water will sometimes help to relieve itching caused by an allergic reaction. Applied in powder form, bicarbonate of soda is often a more effective deodorant than many commercial preparations.

s. biphosphate, a colorless or white crystalline compound, used as a urinary acidifier.

s. bisulfite, an antioxidant compound.

s. borate, a crystalline compound used in pharmaceutical preparations as an astringent for mucous membranes.

s. caprylate, a compound used in treatment of fungal infections of the skin.

s. carbonate, $Na_2CO_3 \cdot H_2O$, used as an alkalizing agent in pharmaceuticals, and has been used as a lotion or bath in the treatment of scaly skin, and as a detergent.

s. carboxymethyl cellulose, a compound used as a bulk-forming cathartic and gastric antacid.

s. chloride, a white, crystalline compound, a necessary constituent of the body and therefore of the diet; sometimes used parenterally in solution to replenish electrolytes in the body. Called also salt.

s. citrate, a crystalline compound, largely used as an anticoagulant in blood for transfusion.

s. cyclamate, a compound formerly used as a sweetening agent.

s. fluoride, a white, odorless powder used in fluoridation of drinking water or applied locally to teeth, in 1 to 2 per cent solution, to reduce the incidence of dental caries.

s. folate, a compound used in various anemias and in control of diarrhea in sprue.

s. glucosulfone, a compound used in treatment of leprosy and tuberculosis.

s. glutamate, the monosodium salt of L-glutamic acid; used in treatment of encephalopathies associated with liver diseases. Also used to enhance the flavor of foods.

s. hydrate, s. hydroxide, a compound used as an alkalizing agent in pharmaceuticals.

s. hypochlorite, a compound having germicidal, deodorizing, and bleaching properties; used in solution to disinfect utensils, and in diluted form (Dakin's solution) as a local antibacterial and to irrigate wounds.

s. indigotindisulfonate, a compound used in measurement of kidney function and as a stain in histology.

s. iodide, a compound used as a source of iodine and as an expectorant.

s. iodipamide, a water-soluble organic iodine compound used in roentgenography of the biliary tract.

s. iodohippurate, a compound used as a contrast medium in roentgenography of the urinary tract.

s. iodomethamate, a white, odorless powder used as a contrast medium in roentgenography of the urinary tract.

s. lactate, a compound used in solution to replenish body fluids and electrolytes.

s. lauryl sulfate, a surface-active agent used as a wetting agent; emulsifying aid and detergent in various cosmetic and dermatologic preparations and as an ingredient in toothpastes.

s. liothyronine, the sodium salt of L-3,3′,5-triiodothyronine; used in the treatment of hypothyroidism, metabolic insufficiency, and certain gynecologic disorders.

s. methicillin, a semisynthetic penicillin salt for parenteral administration.

s. morrhuate, sodium salts of the fatty acids of cod liver oil; used as a sclerosing agent in treatment of varicose veins.

s. nitrate, a compound used as a reagent and in certain industrial processes.

s. nitrite, a compound used as an antidote in cyanide poisoning and for relief of angina pectoris, Raynaud's disease, etc.

s. oxacillin, a semisynthetic penicillin salt for oral administration.

s. para-aminohippurate, a compound used in studies for measurement of effective renal plasma flow and determination of the functional capacity of the tubular excretory mechanism.

s. para-aminosalicylate, sodium aminosalicylate.

s. perborate, a compound used as an oxidant and local anti-infective.

s. peroxide, a white powder soluble in water; used as a dental bleach and in ointment form in acne and rosacea.

s. phosphate, a colorless or white granular salt, used as a cathartic.

s. polystyrene sulfonate, an ion-exchange resin used for removal of potassium ions in hyperpotassemia.

s. propionate, a compound used in fungal infections.

s. psylliate, the sodium salt of the liquid fatty acids obtained by hydrolysis of the fixed oil of the seeds of *Plantago ovata;* used as a sclerosing agent.

s. salicylate, an analgesic, antipyretic compound (see SALICYLIC ACID).

s. sulfate, a hydrogogue cathartic; also used as a diuretic and sometimes applied topically in solution to relieve edema and pain of infected wounds.

s. sulfocyanate, sodium thiocyanate.

s. sulfoxone, a compound used in treatment of leprosy.

s. tetradecyl sulfate, a white, waxy, odorless solid; used in solution as a sclerosing agent.

s. thiocyanate, white or colorless, odorless crystals

with a cooling, salty taste, used as a reagent and as a vasodilator.

s. thiosulfate, a compound used intravenously as an antidote for cyanide poisoning, in the prophylaxis of ringworm (added to foot baths), and as a topical application in tinea versicolor. Also used in measuring the volume of extracellular body fluid and the renal glomerular filtration rate.

sodoku (so'do-koo) a relapsing type of infection due to *Spirillum minus,* an organism transmitted by the bite of an infected rat; a form of RATBITE FEVER.

sodomy (sod'o-me) anal intercourse; also used to denote bestiality and fellatio.

soft palate the fleshy structure at the back of the mouth, which, together with the hard palate, forms the roof of the mouth. From the middle of the free border of the soft palate hangs the fleshy conical body called the uvula. In swallowing, the soft palate is drawn upward against the back of the pharynx and prevents food and fluids from straying into the nasal passage while they pass through the throat.

softening (sof'en-ing) a change of consistency, with loss of firmness or hardness.

red s., softening of a patch(es) of brain substance, with local redness due to congestion.

white s., the stage following yellow softening, in which the spot has become white from the presence of fatty deposit.

yellow s., the stage following red softening, in which the patch has become yellow due to degenerative changes in the brain substance.

sol (sol) a liquid colloid solution.

solid s., a colloid system in which both dispersed phase and disperse medium are solids.

sol. solution.

Solanum (so-la'num) a genus of herbs and shrubs, including the potato, several of the nightshades, and many poisonous and medicinal species.

solarization (so"lar-ĭ-za'shun) exposure to sunlight and the effects produced thereby.

solar plexus (so'lar) a netword of ganglia and nerves in the center of the abdomen; it is part of the autonomic nervous system. It is important in the control of the function of the liver, stomach, kidneys, and adrenal glands. A blow to it may knock a person out or cause great pain because the organs are momentarily thrown out of gear. Although the plexus recovers quickly, the effects on the body as a whole last longer.

solation (so-la'shun) the liquefaction of a gel.

sole (sōl) the bottom of the foot.

Solganal (sol'gah-nal) trademark for a preparation of aurothioglucose, an antirheumatic preparation of gold salts.

solid (sol'id) 1. not fluid or gaseous; not hollow. 2. a substance or tissue not fluid or gaseous.

solubility (sol"u-bil'ĭ-te) the quality of being soluble.

soluble (sol'u-b'l) susceptible of being dissolved.

Solu-Cortef (sol"u-kor'tef) trademark for a preparation of hydrocortisone, used as an anti-inflammatory agent.

solum (so'lum), pl. *so'la* [L.] the bottom or lowest part.

solute (sol'ūt) the substance that is dissolved in a liquid (solvent) to form a solution.

solution (so-loo'shun) 1. in pharmacology, a liquid preparation of one or more soluble chemical sub-

stances usually dissolved in water. 2. the process of dissolving or disrupting.

PREPARATION OF SOLUTIONS. Formula for preparing solutions from a pure drug:

pure drug : finished solution =
strength of solution
(expressed in percentage or ratio)

For example, to prepare 2000 ml. of a 2 per cent solution from boric acid crystals, the proportion would be

X gm. : 2000 ml. = 2 gm. : 100 ml.
X = 40 gm. pure drug

Formula for preparing solutions from stock solutions:

lesser amount of stock solution : greater amount of stock solution =
lesser strength : greater strength

For example, to prepare 1000 ml. of a 2 per cent solution from a 4 per cent stock solution, the proportion would be

X ml : 1000 ml. = 2 per cent : 4 per cent
X = 500 ml. stock solution

aqueous s., one in which water is used as the solvent.

buffer s., one that resists appreciable change in its hydrogen ion concentration (pH) when acid or alkali is added to it.

colloid s., colloidal s., a preparation consisting of minute particles of matter suspended in a solvent.

contrast s., a solution of a substance opaque to the x-ray, used to facilitate x-ray visualization of some organ or structure in the body.

hyperbaric s., one having a greater specific gravity than a standard of reference.

hypertonic s., one having an osmotic pressure greater than that of a standard of reference.

hypobaric s., one having a specific gravity less than that of a standard of reference.

hypotonic s., one having an osmotic pressure less than that of standard of reference.

iodine s., a transparent, reddish brown liquid, each 100 ml. of which contains 1.8 to 2.2 gm. of iodine and 2.1 to 2.6 gm. of sodium iodide; a local anti-infective.

iodine s., strong, Lugol's solution.

isobaric s., a solution having the same specific gravity as a standard of reference.

isotonic s., one having an osmotic pressure the same as that of a standard of reference.

molar s., a solution each liter of which contains 1 gram-molecule of the dissolved substance; designated M/1 or 1 M. The concentration of other solutions may be expressed in relation to that of molar solutions as tenth-molar (M/10 or 0.1 M), etc.

normal s., a solution each liter of which contains 1 gram equivalent weight of the dissolved substance; designated N/1 or 1 N.

ophthalmic s., a sterile solution, free from foreign particles, for instillation into the eye.

physiologic saline s., physiologic salt s., physiologic sodium chloride s., an aqueous solution of sodium chloride and other components, having an osmotic pressure identical to that of blood serum.

saline s., a solution of sodium chloride, or common salt, in purified water.

saturated s., a solution in which the solvent has taken up all of the dissolved substance that it can hold in solution.

sclerosing s., one containing an irritant substance that will cause obliteration of a space, as the lumen of a varicose vein or the cavity of a hernial sac.

standard s., one containing a fixed amount of solute.

supersaturated s., one containing a greater quantity of the solute than the solvent can hold in solution under ordinary conditions.

test s., a standard solution of a specified chemical substance used in performing a certain test procedure.

volumetric s., one that contains a specific quantity of solvent per stated unit of volume.

solvent (sol′vent) 1. capable of dissolving other material. 2. the liquid in which another substance (the solute) is dissolved to form a solution.

soma (so′mah) 1. the body as distinguished from the mind. 2. the body tissue as distinguished from the germ cells. 3. the cell body. adj., **so′mal, somat′ic.**

somasthenia (so″mas-the′ne-ah) bodily weakness with poor appetite and poor sleep.

somat(o)- word element [Gr.], *body.*

somatalgia (so″mah-tal′je-ah) bodily pain.

somatesthesia (so″mat-es-the′ze-ah) body consciousness or awareness.

somatic (so-mat′ik) pertaining to or characteristic of the body (soma).

somatization (so″mah-tĭ-za′shun) the conversion of mental experiences or states into bodily symptoms.

somatochrome (so-mat′o-krōm) any neuron which has a well marked cell body completely surrounding the nucleus, its colorable protoplasm having a distinct contour; used also adjectively.

somatogenic (so″mah-to-jen′ik) originating in the body.

somatology (so″mah-tol′o-je) the sum of what is known about the body.

somatome (so′mah-tōm) 1. an appliance for cutting the body of a fetus. 2. a somite.

somatomedin (so″mah-to-me′din) a peptide elaborated by the liver in response to stimulation by growth hormone; it stimulates skeletal growth by acting directly on cartilage cells.

somatometry (so″mah-tom′ĕ-tre) measurement of the dimensions of the entire body.

somatopagus (so″mah-top′ah-gus) a double fetus united at the trunks.

somatopathy (so″mah-top′ah-the) a bodily disorder rather than a mental one. adj., **somatopath′ic.**

somatoplasm (so-mat′o-plazm) the protoplasm of the body cells exclusive of the germ cells.

somatopsychic (so″mah-to-si′kik) pertaining to both mind and body.

somatopsychosis (so″mah-to-si-ko′sis) any mental disease symptomatic of bodily disease.

somatoschisis (so″mah-tos′kĭ-sis) splitting of the bodies of the vertebrae.

somatoscopy (so″mah-tos′ko-pe) examination of the body.

somatosexual (so″mah-to-seks′u-al) pertaining to both physical and sex characteristics or to physical manifestations of sexual development.

somatostatin (so″mah-to-stat′in) a polypeptide secreted by the hypothalamus that inhibits release of growth hormone from the pituitary, of insulin and glucagon from the pancreas, and of thyrotropin and gastrin; also produced synthetically.

somatotherapy (so″mah-to-ther′ah-pe) treatment aimed at relieving or curing ills of the body.

somatotonia (so″mah-to-to′ne-ah) a group of traits characterized by dominance of muscular activity and vigorous body assertiveness; considered typical of a mesomorph.

somatotopic (so″mah-to-top′ik) related to particular areas of the body; describing the organization of the motor area of the brain, specific regions of the cortex being responsible for the motor control of different areas of the body.

somatotrophin (so″mah-to-tro′fin) growth hormone (see also PITUITARY GLAND). adj., **somatotroph′ic.**

somatotropin (so″mah-to-tro′pin) growth hormone (see also PITUITARY GLAND). adj., **somatotro′pic.**

somatotype (so-mat′o-tīp) a particular type of body build.

somatotyping (so-mat″o-tīp′ing) objective classification of individuals according to type of body build.

Sombulex (som′bu-leks) trademark for a preparation of hexobarbital, an ultra–short-acting barbiturate.

somesthesia (so″mes-the′ze-ah) sensibility to bodily sensations. adj., **somesthet′ic.**

somite (so′mīt) one of the paired segments along the neural tube of a vertebrate embryo, formed by transverse subdivision of the thickened mesoderm next to the midplane, that develop into the vertebral column and muscles of the body.

somnambule (som-nam′būl) one who sleepwalks.

somnambulism (som-nam′bu-lizm) sleepwalking.

somnifacient (som″nĭ-fa′shent) causing sleep.

somniferous (som-nif′er-us) producing sleep.

somniloquism (som-nil′o-kwizm) habitual talking in one's sleep.

somnipathy (som-nip′ah-the) any disorder of sleep; a condition of hypnotic trance.

somnolence (som′no-lens) sleepiness; also, unnatural drowsiness.

somnolentia (som″no-len′she-ah) 1. incomplete sleep; drowsiness. 2. sleep drunkenness; a condition of incomplete sleep marked by loss of orientation and by excited or violent behavior.

Somnos (som′nos) trademark for preparations of chloral hydrate, a sedative and hypnotic.

sonitus (son′y-tus) tinnitus.

sonometer (so-nom′ĕ-ter) an apparatus for testing acuteness of hearing.

sonorous (so-nōr′us) resonant; sounding.

sopor (so′por) [L.] deep or profound sleep.

soporific (sop″ŏ-rif′ik, so″pŏ-rif′ik) 1. producing deep sleep. 2. an agent that induces sleep.

soporous (sop′or-us, so′por-us) associated with coma or deep sleep.

sorbefacient (sōr″bĕ-fa′shent) 1. promoting absorption. 2. an agent that promotes absorption.

sorbitan (sor′bĭ-tan) any of the anhydrides of sorbitol, the fatty acids of which are surfactants. (See also POLYSORBATE 80.)

sorbitol (sor'bĭ-tol) a crystalline, hexahydric alcohol, found in various berries and fruits; a pharmaceutical preparation is used as a flavoring agent and as an osmotic diuretic.

sordes (sōr'dēz) foul matter collected on the lips and teeth in low fevers, consisting of food, microorganisms, and epithelial elements.

s. gas'tricae, undigested food, mucus, etc., in the stomach.

sore (sōr) a popular term for any lesion of the skin or mucous membrane.

bed s., decubitus ulcer.

cold s., one around the mouth or lips due to herpes simplex virus. (See HERPES SIMPLEX.)

Delhi s., cutaneous leishmaniasis.

desert s., a form of tropical ulcer occurring in desert areas of Africa, Australia, and the Near East.

oriental s., cutaneous leishmaniasis.

pressure s., decubitus ulcer.

sorption (sorp'shun) 1. incorporation of water in a colloid. 2. processes involved in net movement of components of adjoining materials across the boundary separating them; applied to the bidirectional movements of substances across the mucosa of the gastrointestinal tract and the net result of such movements, including absorption, enterosorption, exsorption, and insorption.

S.O.S. [L.] *si o'pus sit* (if necessary).

sotalol (so'tah-lōl) an antiadrenergic (β-receptor) used as the hydrochloride salt.

soterenol (so-ter'ĕ-nol) an adrenergic with bronchodilator properties, used as the hydrochloride salt.

souffle (soo'f'l) a soft, blowing auscultatory sound.

cardiac s., any heart murmur of a blowing quality.

fetal s., a murmur sometimes heard over the pregnant uterus, supposed to be due to compression of the umbilical cord.

funic s., funicular s., a hissing souffle synchronous with fetal heart sounds, probably from the umbilical cord.

placental s., a souffle supposed to be produced by the blood current in the placenta; called also placental bruit.

uterine s., a sound made by the blood within the arteries of the gravid uterus.

sound (sownd) 1. percept resulting from stimulation of the ear by mechanical radiant energy of frequency between 20 and 20,000 cycles per second. 2. a slender instrument to be introduced into body passages or cavities, especially for the dilatation of strictures or detection of foreign bodies. 3. a noise, normal or abnormal, emanating from within the body.

ejection s's, high-pitched clicking sounds heard very shortly after the first heart sound, attributed to sudden distention of a dilated pulmonary artery or aorta or to forceful opening of the pulmonic or aortic cusps.

friction s., one produced by rubbing of two surfaces.

heart s's, the sounds produced by the functioning of the heart (see HEART SOUNDS).

Korotkoff s's, those heard during auscultatory blood pressure determination.

percussion s., any sound obtained by percussion.

physiologic s's, those heard when the external acoustic meatus are plugged, caused by the rush of blood through blood vessels in or near the inner ear and by adjacent muscles in continuous low-frequency vibration.

respiratory s., any sound heard on ausculation over the respiratory tract.

succussion s's, splashing sounds heard on succussion over a distended stomach or in hydropneumothorax.

to-and-fro s., a peculiar friction sound or murmur heard in pericarditis and pleurisy.

urethral s., a long, slender instrument for exploring and dilating the urethra.

white s., that produced by a mixture of all frequencies of mechanical vibration perceptible as sound.

space (spās) 1. a delimited area. 2. an actual or potential cavity of the body. 3. the areas of the universe beyond the earth and its atmosphere. adj., **spa'tial.**

dead s., 1. space remaining in tissues as a result of failure of proper closure of surgical or other wounds, permitting accumulation of blood or serum. 2. the portions of the respiratory tract (passages and space in the alveoli) occupied by gas not concurrently participating in oxygen-carbon dioxide exchange.

epidural s., the space between the dura mater and the lining of the spinal canal.

intercostal s., the space between two adjacent ribs.

interpleural s., mediastinum.

intervillous s., the cavernous space of the placenta into which the chorionic villi project and through which the maternal blood circulates.

lymph s's, open spaces filled with lymph in connective or other tissue, especially in the brain and meninges.

Meckel's s., a recess in the dura mater that lodges the trigeminal ganglion.

mediastinal s., mediastinum.

medullary s., the central cavity and the intervals between the trabeculae of bone that contain the marrow.

palmar s., a large fascial space in the hand, divided by a fibrous septum into a midpalmar and a thenar space.

parasinoidal s's, spaces in the dura mater along the superior sagittal sinus which receive the venous blood.

perivascular s., a lymph space within the walls of an artery.

plantar s., a fascial space on the sole of the foot, divided by septa into the lateral, middle, and median plantar spaces.

pneumatic s., a portion of bone occupied by air-containing cells, especially the spaces constituting the paranasal sinuses.

retroperitoneal s., the space between the peritoneum and the posterior abdominal wall.

retropharyngeal s., the space behind the pharynx, containing areolar tissue.

subarachnoid s., the space between the arachnoid and the pia mater, containing cerebrospinal fluid.

subdural s., the space between the dura mater and the arachnoid.

subphrenic s., the space between the diaphragm and subjacent organs.

subumbilical s., somewhat triangular space in the body cavity beneath the umbilicus.

Tenon's s., a lymph space between the sclera and Tenon's capsule.

sparganosis (spar″gah-no′sis) infection with spargana, which invade the subcutaneous tissues, causing inflammation and fibrosis. If the lymphatics are involved, elephantiasis results.

sparganum (spar-ga′num), pl. *sparga′na* [Gr.] a migrating larva of a tapeworm.

Sparine (spar′ēn) trademark for preparations of promazine, a tranquilizer.

spasm (spazm) 1. a sudden involuntary contraction of a muscle or group of muscles. 2. a sudden but transitory constriction of a passage, canal, or orifice. Spasms usually occur when the nerve supplying muscles are irritated, and are commonly accompanied by pain. Occasionally a spasm may occur in a blood vessel, and is then called vasospasm.

Spasms vary from mild twitches to severe CONVULSIONS and may be the symptoms of any number of disorders. Usually, spasms will cease when the cause is corrected, although sometimes the only treatment is to suppress the symptoms, as in EPILEPSY.

CLONIC SPASMS. Spasms in which contraction and relaxation of the muscle alternate are called clonic. This is the more common type of spasm and usually is not severe. A typical clonic spasm is the hiccup. Hiccups usually occur when the diaphragm is irritated, as by indigestion; very occasionally they may result from a serious condition, such as a brain tumor. Hiccups generally disappear by themselves or after a drink of water.

Spasms may be repetitive twitching motions, some of which are called tics. Tics often accompany other types of spasm, as in such diseases as cerebral palsy and Sydenham's chorea. They may also be seen in neuralgia. In tic douloureux (trigeminal neuralgia) the nerves of the face are involved.

Other types of repetitive twitching movements seem to be purposeless or without a cause and are called habit spasms. They include twitching of the face, blinking of the eyes, and grimacing. The movements are rapid and always repeated in the same way, unlike the spasms associated with chorea. The motions are carried out automatically in response to a stimulus that once may have existed but no longer does.

Spasms may also stem from emotional stress. Stuttering that continues after the age of 5 years is generally considered a habit spasm that is caused by emotional conflict or difficulty.

In a convulsive spasm the entire body is jerked by sudden violent movements that may involve almost all the muscles. These spasms may last from a fraction of a second to several seconds, or even minutes. Spasms accompanying epilepsy are usually convulsive. Treatment includes sedatives and any one of several anticonvulsants. In small children convulsions usually indicate a high fever and the onset of infection, or any general illness; at times they may be a symptom of severe disease.

TONIC SPASMS. If the contraction of a spasm is sustained or continuing, it is called tonic, or tetanic, spasm. Tonic spasms are generally severe because they are caused by diseases that affect the central nervous system or brain, as tetanus, rabies, and cerebral palsy. Severe tonic spasms can be fatal if not treated in time. Continued spasms can bring on exhaustion or asphyxiation. Treatment varies with the cause. If the disease is caused by a microorganism present in the system, as in tetanus, antiserum must be administered immediately. Antibiotics are also used to help curb infection. In many cases, tranquilizers, sedatives, and narcotics must be administered to help ease the spasms.

bronchial s., bronchospasm; spasmodic contraction of the muscular coat of the smaller divisions of the bronchi, as occurs in asthma.

nodding s., clonic spasm of the sternomastoid muscles, causing a nodding motion of the head.

spasmodic (spaz-mod′ik) of the nature of a spasm; occurring in spasms.

spasmolysis (spaz-mol′ĭ-sis) the arrest of spasm.

spasmolytic (spaz″mo-lit′ik) 1. arresting or checking spasms. 2. an agent that arrests spasms, especially of smooth muscle.

spasmophilia (spaz″mo-fil′e-ah) abnormal tendency to convulsions; abnormal sensitivity of motor nerves to stimulation with a resultant tendency to spasm.

spasmus (spaz′mus) [L.] spasm.

s. nu′tans, nodding spasm.

spastic (spas′tik) characterized by spasms, or tightening of the muscles, causing stiff and awkward movements and in some cases a scissors-like gait. The term is often used to describe a person suffering from CEREBRAL PALSY.

spasticity (spas-tis′ĭ-te) continuous resistance to stretching by a muscle due to abnormally increased tension, with heightened deep tendon reflexes.

spatial (spa′shal) pertaining to space.

spatium (spa′she-um), pl. *spa′tia* [L.] space.

spatula (spat′u-lah) a wide, flat, blunt, usually flexible instrument of little thickness, used for spreading material on a smooth surface or mixing.

spatulate (spach′ŭ-lāt) 1. having a flat blunt end. 2. to mix or manipulate with a spatula.

spatulation (spat″u-la′shun) the combining of materials into a homogeneous mixture by continuously heaping them together and smoothing the mass out on a smooth surface with a spatula.

spay (spa) to remove the ovaries.

SPCA serum prothrombin conversion accelerator (clotting factor VII). (See also CLOTTING.)

specialist (spesh′ah-list) a physician whose practice is limited to a particular branch of medicine or surgery, especially one who, by virtue of advanced training, is certified by a specialty board as being qualified to so limit his practice.

specialty (spesh′al-te) the field of practice of a specialist.

species (spe′shēz) a taxonomic category subordinate to a genus (or subgenus) and superior to a subspecies or variety; composed of individuals similar in certain morphologic and physiologic characteristics.

type s., the original species from which the description of the genus is formulated.

species-specific (spe′shēz-spĕ-sif′ik) characteristic of a particular species; having a characteristic effect on, or interaction with, cells or tissues of members of a particular species; said of an antigen, drug, or infective agent.

specific (spĕ-sif′ik) 1. pertaining to a species. 2. produced by a single kind of microorganism. 3. restricted in application, effect, etc., to a particular structure, function, etc. 4. a remedy specially indicated for any particular disease. 5. in immunology, pertaining to the special affinity of antigen for the corresponding antibody.

s. gravity, the weight of a substance compared with the weight of an equal amount of some other substance taken as a standard. For liquids the usual standard is water. The specific gravity of water is 1; if a sample of urine shows a specific gravity of 1.025, this means that the urine is 1.025 times heavier than water. Specific gravity is measured by means of a hydrometer.

specificity (spes″ĭ-fis′ĭ-te) the quality of having a certain action, as of affecting only certain organisms or tissues, or reacting only with certain substances, as antibodies with certain antigens (antigen specificity).

host s., the natural adaptability of a particular parasite to a certain species or group of hosts.

specimen (spes′ĭ-men) a small sample or part taken to show the nature of the whole, as a small quantity of urine for urinalysis, or a small fragment of tissue for microscopic study.

spectacles (spek′tĕ-kals) a pair of LENSES in a frame to assist vision (see also GLASSES).

spectinomycin (spek″tĭ-no-mi′sin) an antibiotic derived from *Streptomyces spectabilis,* used in treatment of gonorrhea.

spectra (spek′trah) plural of *spectrum.*

spectrocolorimeter (spek″tro-kul″er-im′ĕ-ter) an instrument for detecting color blindness.

spectrometry (spek-trom′ĕ-tre) determination of the place of lines in a spectrum.

spectrophotometer (spek″tro-fo-tom′ĕ-ter) 1. an apparatus for measuring light sense by means of a spectrum. 2. an apparatus for determining the quantity of coloring matter in a solution by measurement of transmitted light.

spectrophotometry (spek″tro-fo-tom′ĕ-tre) the use of the spectrophotometer.

spectroscope (spek′tro-skōp) an instrument for developing and analyzing the spectrum of a substance.

spectroscopy (spek-tros′ko-pe) examination by means of a spectroscope.

spectrum (spek′trum), pl. *spec′tra, spec′trums* [L.] 1. the series of images resulting from the refraction of electromagnetic radiation (e.g., light, x-rays) and their arrangement according to frequency or wavelength. 2. range of activity, as of an antibiotic, or of manifestations, as of a disease. adj., **spec′tral.**

absorption s., one obtained by passing radiation with a continuous spectrum through a selectively absorbing medium.

broad-s., effective against a wide range of microorganisms.

chromatic s., that portion of the electromagnetic spectrum including wavelengths of about 7700 to 3900 angstroms, giving rise to the perception of color by the normal eye.

electromagnetic s., the range of electromagnetic energy from cosmic rays to electric waves, including gamma, x- and ultraviolet rays, visible light and infrared rays and radio waves.

visible s., that portion of the range of wavelengths of electromagnetic vibrations (from 7700 to 3900 angstroms) which is capable of stimulating specialized sense organs and is perceptible as light.

speculum (spek′u-lum) an instrument for opening or distending a body orifice or cavity to permit visual inspection.

speech (spēch) the utterance of vocal sounds conveying ideas; the faculty of conveying thoughts and ideas by vocal sounds. The process is controlled through a speech center located in the frontal lobe of the human brain.

THE MECHANICS OF SPEECH. The voice originates in the larynx, which is in the upper end of the air passage to the lungs and is located behind the thyroid cartilage. The larynx, in cooperation with the mouth, throat, trachea, and lungs, works on the same principle as an organ or an oboe, in which air is forced over a thin reed to produce sound. The vocal cords, two reedlike bands, are attached at one end to the wall of the larynx behind the Adam's apple; the other ends are attached to movable cartilages. When the voice is not being used, muscles move these cartilages outward and hold the vocal cords against the sides of the larynx so that breathing is not obstructed. When one starts to speak, sing, grunt, or shout, the ends of the vocal cords connected to the cartilages are brought across the larynx, so that they partly obstruct it. As air is forced through, the cords vibrate, producing sound waves, the voice.

In speaking, the size and shape of the mouth and pharynx are varied as the sound goes through, by means of muscles of the mouth, throat, and tongue. Vowel sounds are initiated in the throat and are given their distinctive "shapes" by movements of the mouth and tongue. Consonants are formed by controlled interruptions of exhaled air.

VOLUME, PITCH, AND TIMBRE. The voice itself has three characteristics—volume, pitch, and timbre, or quality. Volume depends on the effort made in forcing air through the vocal cords.

Pitch of the voice depends on the amount of tension placed on the vocal cords, and on the length and thickness of the cords. Children's and women's vocal cords are short, giving them higher-pitched voices. A man's are longer and thicker and his voice is deeper.

Timbre is affected by the size and shape of the

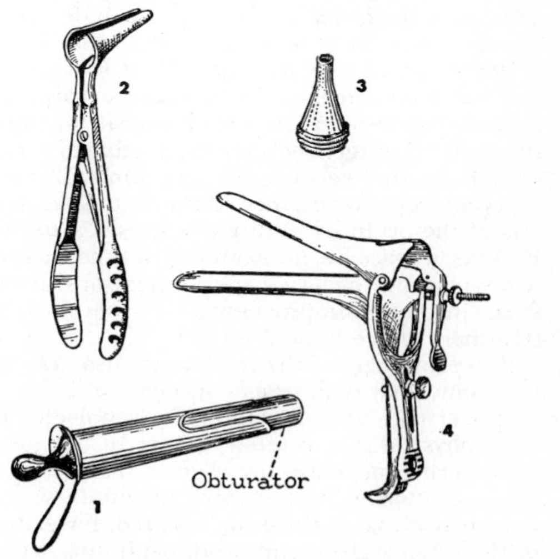

Speculums: 1, rectal (David); 2, nasal (Vienna model); 3, ear (Boucheron); 4, vaginal (Pederson). (From Dorland's Illustrated Medical Dictionary. 25th ed. Philadelphia, W. B. Saunders Co., 1974.)

individual's various resonating chambers—mouth, pharynx, chest, and others—and the way they are used. Bones in the head and chest also contribute to the quality of a voice. By long training in the use of the voice, singers are able to alter and control the mouth, throat, and chest cavities to produce a wide range of harmonics or overtones.

SPEECH DEFECTS. Over 100 muscles are involved in the utterance of a simple word, and the construction of a simple sentence is a feat so complicated that it is far beyond the capacity of any living thing except man. The process of learning to talk is obviously a difficult task for children, and it is not surprising that 5 to 7 per cent of them reach adulthood with a speech disorder serious enough to be a handicap.

The baby learns to make specific sounds with his voice by babbling and cooing. Gradually he becomes able, more or less unconsciously, to put these sounds together to form intelligible speech in imitation of his parents and other speakers around him. This complicated process is sometimes disturbed if the child is handicapped by congenital physical defects, illness, or psychologic difficulties. As a result, speech disorders may occur.

Congenital Causes. Prominent among the congenital defects that may cause speech problems are CLEFT LIP and CLEFT PALATE. These abnormalities are evident at birth and should be corrected by surgery at an early age.

Another congenital defect is tongue-tie, or abnormal shortness of the membrane connecting the base of the tongue to the floor of the mouth. This condition, which if uncorrected may cause lisping and other awkwardness, is easily corrected by surgical cutting of the membrane as soon as the difficulty becomes evident.

Congenital deafness will prevent a child from learning to speak in the usual way and may result in MUTISM. However, if the speech mechanisms are normal, the child can be taught to speak by a speech therapist.

Malformations of the nasal passages, larynx, or other parts of the voice-producing tract may cause oddities in the sound of the voice. Such defects also can be corrected in many cases by minor surgery.

Other Causes. By the age of 5 or 6 years, most children have mastered the basic art of talking. Serious difficulties that persist or appear for the first time after this age, and that are not due to congenital defects, are likely to arise from illness, injury, or a psychologic disturbance. Damage to speech centers of the brain by multiple sclerosis, syphilis, or Parkinson's disease, for example, may cause speech to be singsong, explosive, mechanical, or slurred. In such instances improvement of speech follows treatment of the basic disorder.

Poor alignment of the front teeth also may interfere somewhat with proper speech.

Stuttering. Speech defects of psychologic rather than physical origin often appear in the form of stammering, or stuttering. The terms are synonymous. Stuttering may involve involuntary hesitation in starting or finishing a sound, for example, difficulty in starting any word beginning with the letter *t*, or the inability to get beyond a first letter, such as *m* or *s*. There is often the spasmodic repetition of one sound with the apparent inability to pass on to the next one.

These difficulties can have many different specific causes, but generally they arise from feelings of insecurity and anxiety. Once the bad habits are formed, they may endure after the original cause no longer exists.

Various precautions by parents and other grownups in a household can help to encourage clear speech and to prevent the onset of stuttering. A child should be spoken to clearly so that he can learn how words should sound. Baby talk by grownups should be avoided, because it will only tend to prolong baby talk in the child. It is best to avoid criticism of the child's pronunciation and other speech habits—especially criticism in the form of nagging interruptions—that is likely to make him self-conscious, uncertain, and awkward.

Stuttering often occurs when a child is addressing an angry or impatient parent or someone else who represents authority. The child's speech may become disorganized by fear of punishment or disapproval, or by an accident or other upsetting event. He is often anxious to get his words out before his listener interrupts or turns away. This anxiety can be especially upsetting in children whose thoughts tend to outrace their ability to form their sentences. Patience and calm will alleviate a child's anxiety and encourage clear speech.

If speech defects persist when a child reaches school age, the help of a speech therapist may be required. Speech disorders resulting from mental illness are best dealt with by a psychiatrist.

esophageal s., speech produced by expelling swallowed air across one or more constrictions in the pharyngoesophageal segment; used after LARYNGECTOMY.

explosive s., loud, sudden enunciation, occurring in certain brain diseases.

mirror s., speech in which the order of syllables is reversed.

s. reading, understanding of speech through observation of the speaker's lip movements; called also lip reading.

scanning s., speech in which syllables are separated by pauses.

sperm (sperm) the male germ cell, which unites with an ovum in sexual reproduction to produce a new individual (see also SPERMATOZOON).

sperm(o)- word element [Gr.], *seed;* specifically used to refer to the male germinal element.

spermatic (sper-mat′ik) pertaining to the spermatozoa or to semen.

s. cord, the structure extending from the abdominal inguinal ring to the testis, comprising the pampiniform plexus, nerves, ductus deferens, testicular artery, and other vessels.

spermatid (sper′mah-tid) a cell produced by meiotic division of a secondary spermatocyte; it develops into the spermatozoon.

spermatitis (sper″mah-ti′tis) inflammation of a vas deferens; deferentitis.

spermato- word element [Gr.], *seed;* specifically used to refer to the male germinal element.

spermatoblast (sper-mat′o-blast) spermatid.

spermatocele (sper-mat′o-sēl) a cystic distention of the epididymis or rete testis, containing spermatozoa.

spermatocelectomy (sper″mah-to-se-lek′to-me) excision of a spermatocele.

spermatocidal (sper″mah-to-si′dal) destructive to spermatozoa.

spermatocyst (sper-mat′o-sist) 1. a seminal vesicle. 2. spermatocele.

spermatocystectomy (sper″mah-to-sis-tek′to-me) excision of a seminal vesicle.

spermatocystitis (sper″mah-to-sis-ti′tis) inflammation of a seminal vesicle.

spermatocystotomy (sper″mah-to-sis-tot′o-me) incision of a seminal vesicle, for the purpose of drainage.

spermatocyte (sper-mat′o-sīt) the mother cell of a spermatid.

primary s., the original large cell into which a spermatogonium develops before the first meiotic division.

secondary s., a cell produced by meiotic division of the primary spermatocyte, and which gives rise to the spermatid.

spermatocytogenesis (sper″mah-to-si″to-jen′ĕ-sis) the first stage of formation of spermatozoa, in which the spermatogonia develop into spermatocytes and then into spermatids.

spermatogenesis (sper″mah-to-jen′ĕ-sis) the development of mature spermatozoa from spermatogonia; it includes spermatocytogenesis and spermiogenesis.

spermatogenic (sper″mah-to-jen′ik) giving rise to sperm.

spermatogonium (sper″mah-to-go′ne-um), pl. *spermatogo′nia* [Gr.] an undifferentiated male germ cell, originating in a seminal tubule and dividing into two spermatocytes.

spermatoid (sper′mah-toid) resembling semen.

spermatolysin (sper″mah-tol′ĭ-sin) a lysin destructive to spermatozoa.

spermatolysis (sper″mah-tol′ĭ-sis) dissolution of spermatozoa. adj., **spermatolyt′ic.**

spermatopathia (sper″mah-to-path′e-ah) abnormality of the semen.

spermatorrhea (sper″mah-to-re′ah) involuntary escape of semen, without orgasm.

spermatoschesis (sper″mah-tos′kĕ-sis) suppression of the semen.

spermatoxin (sper″mah-tok′sin) a toxin that destroys spermatozoa.

spermatozoicide (sper″mah-to-zo′ĭ-sīd) an agent that destroys spermatozoa; spermicide.

spermatozoon (sper″mah-to-zo′on), pl. *spermatozo′a* [Gr.] a mature male germ cell, the specific output of the testes. It is the generative element of the semen that impregnates the ovum. adj., **spermatozo′al.**

The mature sperm cell is microscopic in size. It looks like a translucent tadpole, and has a flat, elliptical head containing a spherical center section, and a long tail by which it propels itself with a vigorous lashing movement.

Spermatozoa are produced in the testes. When mature, the sperm are carried in the semen. At the climax of coitus, the semen is discharged into the vagina of the female. A single discharge (about a teaspoonful of semen on the average) may contain more than 250 million spermatozoa. Only a few of these will travel as far as the uterine tubes; if an ovum is present there, and if the head of a single sperm penetrates the ovum, fertilization takes place. (See also REPRODUCTION.)

spermaturia (sper″mah-tu′re-ah) semen in the urine.

spermectomy (sper-mek′to-me) excision of part of the spermatic cord.

spermicide (sper′mĭ-sīd) an agent destructive to spermatozoa. adj., **spermici′dal.**

spermiduct (sper′mĭ-dukt) the ejaculatory duct and vas deferens together.

spermiogenesis (sper″me-o-jen′ĕ-sis) the second stage in the formation of spermatozoa, in which the spermatids transform into spermatozoa.

spermiogram (sper′me-o-gram″) a diagram or chart of various cells formed in development of the spermatozoon, or of the cells present in a specimen of semen.

spermioteleosis (sper″me-o-te″le-o′sis) progressive development of the spermatogonium through various stages to the mature spermatozoon.

spermolith (sper′mo-lith) a calculus in the vas deferens.

spermoneuralgia (sper″mo-nu-ral′je-ah) neuralgic pain in the spermatic cord.

spermophlebectasia (sper″mo-fle″bek-ta′ze-ah) varicose state of the spermatic veins.

spermotoxin (sper″mo-tok′sin) a toxin lethal to spermatozoa; especially an antibody produced by injection of an animal with spermatozoa.

sp. gr. specific gravity.

sphacelate (sfas′ĕ-lāt) to become gangrenous.

sphacelation (sfas″ĕ-la′shun) the formation of sphacelus; mortification.

sphacelism (sfas′ĕ-lizm) sphacelation or necrosis; sloughing.

sphaceloderma (sfas″ĕ-lo-der′mah) gangrene of the skin.

sphacelous (sfas′ĕ-lus) gangrenous; sloughing.

sphacelus (sfas′ĕ-lus) a slough; a mass of gangrenous tissue.

sphenion (sfe′ne-on) the point at the sphenoid angle of the parietal bone.

spheno- word element [Gr.], *wedge-shaped; sphenoid bone.*

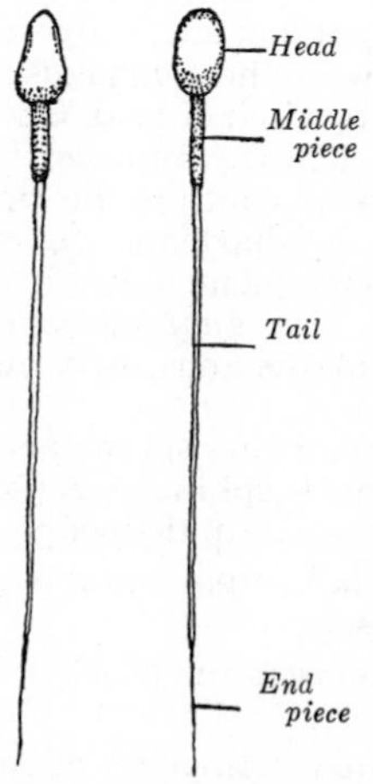

Human spermatozoon, side and flat views. (From Dorland's Illustrated Medical Dictionary. 25th ed. Philadelphia, W. B. Saunders Co., 1974.)

sphenoid (sfe'noid) wedge-shaped; designating especially a very irregular wedge-shaped bone at the base of the skull (sphenoid bone; see table of BONES).

sphenoidal (sfe-noi'dal) pertaining to the sphenoid bone.

sphenoiditis (sfe"noi-di'tis) inflammation of the sphenoid sinus.

sphenoidotomy (sfe"noi-dot'o-me) incision of a sphenoid sinus.

sphenomaxillary (sfe"no-mak'sĭ-ler"e) pertaining to the sphenoid bone and the maxilla.

sphenopalatine (sfe"no-pal'ah-tīn) pertaining to the sphenoid and palatine bones.

sphenotresia (sfe"no-tre'ze-ah) perforation of the base of the fetal skull in craniotomy.

sphenotribe (sfe'no-trīb) an instrument used for crushing the base of the fetal skull.

sphere (sfēr) a ball or globe. adj., **spher'ical.**
attraction s., centrosome.
segmentation s., 1. the morula. 2. a blastomere.

sphero- word element [Gr.], *round; a sphere.*

spherocyte (sfēr'o-sīt) a small, globular, completely hemoglobinated erythrocyte without the usual central pallor; characteristically found in hereditary spherocytosis but also in acquired hemolytic anemia. adj., **spherocyt'ic.**

spherocytosis (sfe"ro-si-to'sis) the presence of spherocytes in the blood.
hereditary s., a congenital hereditary form of hemolytic anemia characterized by spherocytosis, abnormal fragility of erythrocytes, jaundice, and splenomegaly.

spheroid (sfēr'oid) a spherelike body.

spheroidal (sfe-roi'dal) resembling a sphere.

spheroma (sfe-ro'mah) a globular tumor.

spherometer (sfe-rom'ĕ-ter) an apparatus for measuring the curvature of a surface.

sphincter (sfingk'ter) a circular muscle that constricts a passage or closes a natural orifice. When relaxed, a sphincter allows materials to pass through the opening. When contracted, it closes the opening.

There are four main sphincter muscles along the alimentary canal that aid in digestion: The *cardiac sphincter,* between the esophagus and the stomach, opens at the approach of food, which is then swept into the stomach by rhythmic peristaltic waves. The *pyloric sphincter* controls the opening from the stomach into the duodenum. It is usually closed, opening only for a moment when a peristaltic wave passes over it. Two *anal sphincters,* internal and external, control the anus, allowing the evacuation of feces.

In addition, there are sphincters in the iris of the eye, the bile duct (sphincter of Oddi), the urinary tract, and elsewhere in the body.

sphincteralgia (sfingk"ter-al'je-ah) pain in a sphincter muscle.

sphincterectomy (sfink"ter-ek'to-me) excision of a sphincter.

sphincterismus (sfingk"ter-iz'mus) spasm of a sphincter.

sphincteritis (sfingk"ter-i'tis) inflammation of a sphincter, particularly the sphincter of Oddi.

sphincterolysis (sfingk"ter-ol'ĭ-sis) surgical separation of the iris from the cornea in anterior synechia.

sphincteroplasty (sfingk'ter-o-plas"te) plastic reconstruction of a sphincter.

sphincterotomy (sfingk"ter-ot'o-me) incision of a sphincter.

sphingolipid (sfing"go-lip'id) a phospholipid containing sphingosine (e.g., ceramides, sphingomyelins, gangliosides, and cerebrosides), occurring in high concentrations in the brain and other nerve tissue.

sphingolipidosis (sfing"go-lip"ĭ-do'sis), pl. *sphingolipido'ses* [Gr.] a general designation applied to diseases characterized by abnormal storage of sphingolipids, such as Gaucher's disease, Niemann-Pick disease, Hurler's syndrome, and Tay-Sachs disease. All are associated with mental retardation and premature death.

sphingolipodystrophy (sfing"go-lip"o-dis'tro-fe) any of a group of disorders of sphingolipid metabolism. (See SPHINGOLIPIDOSIS.)

sphingomyelin (sfing"go-mi'ĕ-lin) a group of phospholipids that on hydrolysis yield phosphoric acid, choline, sphingosine, and a fatty acid.

sphingosine (sfing'go-sin) a basic amino alcohol present in sphingomyelin.

sphygmic (sfig'mik) pertaining to the pulse.
s. period, the second phase of ventricular systole (0.21–0.30 sec.), between the opening and closing of the semilunar valves, while the blood is discharged into the aorta and pulmonary artery.

sphymo- word element [Gr.], *the pulse.*

sphygmobolometer (sfig"mo-bo-lom'ĕ-ter) an instrument for recording the energy of the pulse wave, and so, indirectly, the strength of the systole.

sphygmochronograph (sfig"mo-kro'no-graf) a self-registering sphygmograph.

sphygmodynamometer (sfig"mo-di"nah-mom'ĕ-ter) an instrument for measuring the force of the pulse.

sphygmogram (sfig'mo-gram) the record or tracing made by a sphygmograph; called also pulse tracing.

sphygmograph (sfig'mo-graf) an apparatus for registering the movements of the arterial pulse. adj., **sphygmograph'ic.**

sphygmoid (sfig'moid) resembling the pulse.

sphygmomanometer (sfig"mo-mah-ncm'ĕ-ter) an instrument for measuring arterial blood pressure.

sphygmometer (sfig-mom'ĕ-ter) an instrument for measuring the force and frequency of the pulse.

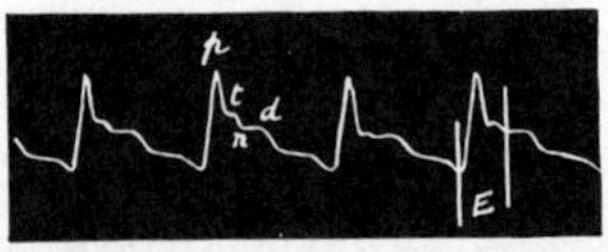

Radial sphygmogram from a healthy person. *p*, The percussion wave; *t*, tidal or predicrotic wave; *n*, dicrotic or aortic notch; *d*, dicrotic wave; *E*, the sphygmic period during which the semilunar valves are open. (From Dorland's Illustrated Medical Dictionary. 25th ed. Philadelphia, W. B. Saunders Co., 1974.)

sphygmoscope (sfig′mo-skōp) a device for rendering the pulse beat visible.

sphygmotonometer (sfig″mo-to-nom′ĕ-ter) an instrument for measuring the elasticity of arterial walls.

sphyrectomy (sfi-rek′to-me) excision of the malleus, or hammer, of the ear.

sphyrotomy (sfi-rot′o-me) division of the malleus.

spica (spi′kah) a figure-of-8 bandage, with turns crossing each other.

spicule (spik′ūl) a sharp, needle-like body or spike.

spider (spi′der) 1. an arthropod of the class Arachnida. 2. a spider-like nevus; a vascular spider.

black widow s., a poisonous spider, *Latrodectus mactans,* whose bite causes severe poisoning. (For first aid, see INSECT BITES AND STINGS.)

vascular s., a telangiectasis composed of small vessels radiating from a central arteriole, the whole resembling spider legs, occurring most often on the upper arms and chest, usually in children and pregnant women, but also in persons with liver disease. Called also nevus arachnoideus and spider nevus.

Spielmeyer-Vogt disease (spēl′mi-er-fogt) the juvenile form of AMAUROTIC FAMILIAL IDIOCY occurring between 5 and 10 years of age, and marked by "salt and pepper" pigmentation of the retinas. It differs from the infantile form (TAY-SACHS DISEASE) in that it shows no racial predilection.

spike (spīk) a sharp upward deflection in a curve or tracing, as on the encephalogram.

spina (spi′nah), pl. *spi′nae* [L.] spine; used in anatomic nomenclature to designate a slender, thornlike process such as occurs on many bones.

s. bif′ida, a defect of the vertebral column due to imperfect union of the paired vertebral arches at the midline; it may be so extensive (spi′na bif′ida cys′tica) as to allow herniation of the spinal cord and meninges, or it may be covered by intact skin (spi′na bif′ida occul′ta) and evident only on radiologic examination.

s. vento′sa, dactylitis of the bones of the hands or feet, occurring mostly in infants and children, with enlargement of digits, caseation, sequestration, and sinus formation.

spinal (spi′nal) pertaining to a spine or to the vertebral column.

s. canal, the canal formed by the series of vertebral foramina together, enclosing the spinal cord and meninges; called also vertebral canal.

s. column, the spine, or vertebral column.

s. cord, that part of the central nervous system lodged in the spinal canal, extending from the foramen magnum to the upper part of the lumbar region. (See Plates 12, 13, and 14.)

s. fusion, surgical creation of ankylosis of contiguous vertebrae; used in treatment of spondylosis and ruptured intervertebral (slipped) disk.

s. nerve, any of the 31 pairs of nerves arising from the spinal cord and passing out between the vertebrae, including eight cervical, twelve thoracic, five lumbar, five sacral, and one coccygeal. (See also Plate 13.)

s. puncture, introduction of a hollow needle into the subarachnoid space of the spinal canal, usually between the fourth and fifth lumbar vertebrae; called also LUMBAR PUNCTURE. In some cases the physician may choose to perform a CISTERNAL PUNCTURE, in which the needle is inserted immediately below the occipital bone into the cisterna cerebellomedullaris.

A spinal puncture may be done for diagnostic purposes to determine the pressure within the cerebrospinal cavities, to determine the presence of an obstruction to the flow of CEREBROSPINAL FLUID, to remove a specimen of cerebrospinal fluid for laboratory examination, or to inject air or other contrast medium into the spinal canal for the purpose of obtaining x-ray film of the cerebrospinal system.

PATIENT CARE. Before the procedure is begun the patient should be given a simple explanation of the nature and purpose of the test. He should be told that there is no danger of damage to the spinal cord during a lumbar puncture because the spinal cord does not extend below the second lumbar vertebra. For a cisternal puncture, the back of the neck may be shaved.

The patient is positioned so that his knees and head are flexed as much as possible, and he is assisted in maintaining this position during the entire procedure. A local anesthetic such as 1 per cent procaine is injected subcutaneously to anesthetize the skin and underlying tissues. The patient should be warned not to move suddenly and should be told that he will experience slight pressure when the puncture needle is inserted.

Strict adherence to the rules of aseptic technique is necessary to avoid the possibility of introducing microorganisms into the spinal canal. The attendant may be asked to assist in the Queckenstedt test during the spinal puncture. This test involves compression of the veins of the neck, first on one side, then on the other and finally on both sides at once. The cerebrospinal fluid pressure is measured each time the veins are compressed. This test determines whether there is an obstruction in the spinal canal. Care must be taken that the trachea is not constricted while the neck veins are being compressed.

After the procedure the patient is observed for signs of pulse changes, respiratory difficulty, or cyanosis. These rarely occur, but headache is common and may be partially relieved by keeping the patient flat in bed for 8 hours after the procedure. An ice cap and aspirin may help alleviate the discomfort.

spinalgia (spi-nal′je-ah) pain in the spinal region.

spinate (spi′nāt) thorn-shaped; having thorns.

spindle (spin′d′l) 1. the fusiform figure occurring during metaphase of cell division, composed of microtubules radiating from the centrioles and connecting the chromosomes at their centromeres. 2. muscle spindle.

muscle s., a mechanoreceptor found between the skeletal muscle fibers; the muscle spindles are arranged in parallel with muscle fibers, and respond to passive stretch of the muscle but cease to discharge if the muscle contracts isotonically, thus signaling muscle length. The muscle spindle is the receptor responsible for the stretch or myotatic reflex.

sleep s., a particular wave form in the electroencephalogram during sleep.

spine (spīn) 1. a thornlike process or projection; called also spina. 2. the backbone, or vertebral column. The spine is the axis of the skeleton; the skull and limbs are in a sense appendages. An intricate structure, the spine is composed of the vertebrae. These bones can move to a certain extent and so give flexibility to the spine, allowing it to bend forward, sideways and, to a lesser extent, backward. In the areas of the neck and lower back, the spine also can pivot, which permits the turning of the head and torso.

STRUCTURE OF THE SPINE. Each vertebra consists of two main parts: the body and, behind it, the vertebral arch. The body is a cylinder of bone, separated from the cylinders of neighboring vertebrae by intervertebral disks, layers of cartilage that act as cushions and allow some movement. Projecting backward from each body are two short, thick bony processes (projections) called pedicles. From the ends of these pedicles project two bony plates (laminae), which join together to form the hollow vertebral arch. Through this arch, and protected by it, passes the spinal cord, which is further protected by the meninges and bathed by the cerebrospinal fluid, which serves as a shock absorber.

There are usually 24 movable vertebrae and nine that are fused together. The topmost are the seven cervical vertebrae, which form the back of the neck, supporting the skull and allowing the head to turn from side to side by means of a pivotal motion between the two highest vertebrae. Below these are the 12 thoracic vertebrae, the supports on which the ribs are hinged, and then the five lumbar vertebrae, the largest movable vertebrae (the cervical are the smallest). Below the lumbar vertebrae, the spine terminates with two groups of vertebrae fused into single bones: the sacrum, composed of five vertebrae, and the coccyx, composed of four vertebrae.

Viewed from the side of the body, the spine as a whole has the shape of a gentle double S curve.

SPINAL INJURIES. Fracture, the most serious injury the spine can suffer, has become increasingly common as the number of automobile accidents has increased. When the spine is fractured, the greatest danger comes from the possibility that the spinal cord may be injured by movement of the fractured vertebrae. Injury to the cord can cause paralysis of

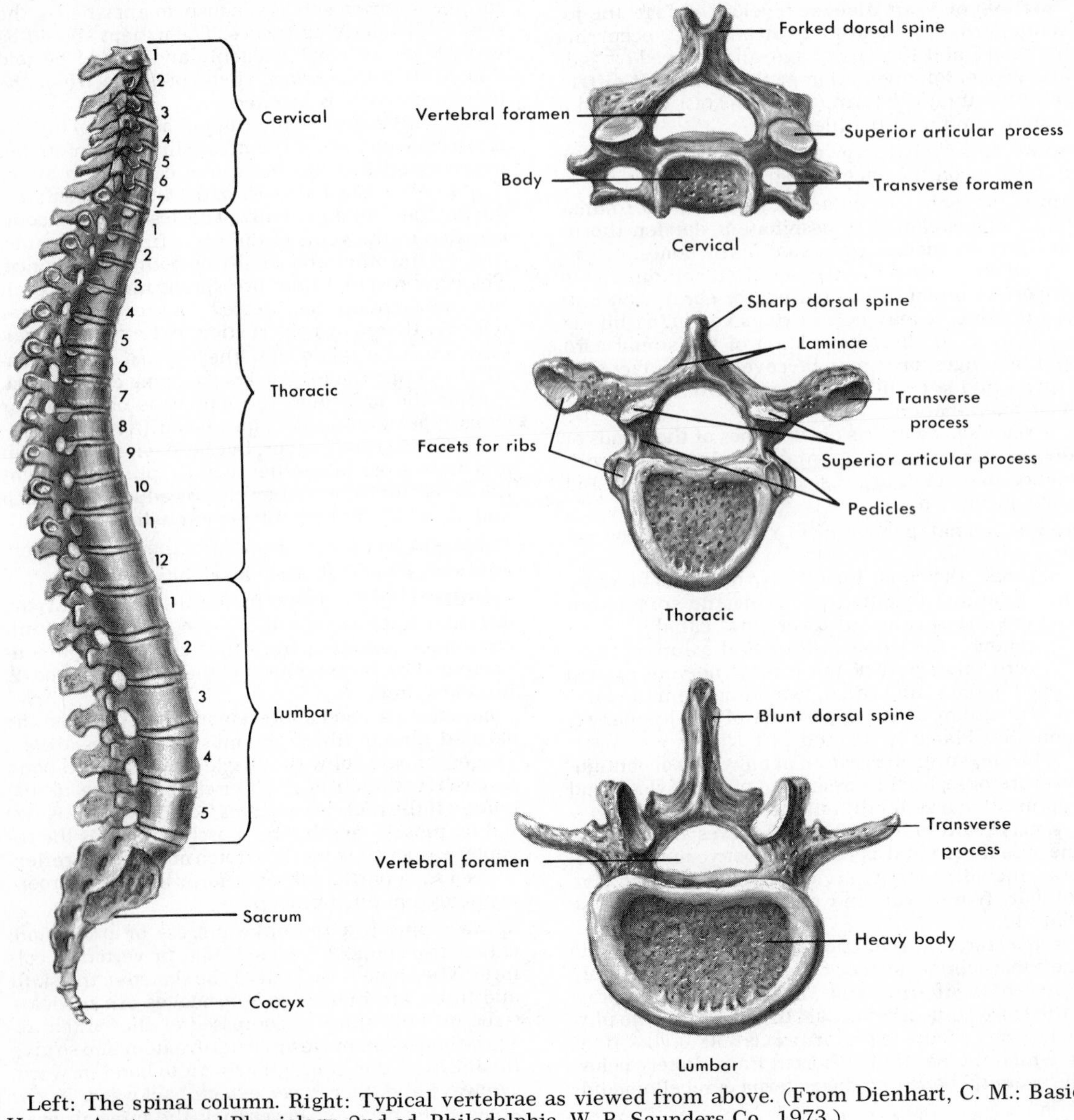

Left: The spinal column. Right: Typical vertebrae as viewed from above. (From Dienhart, C. M.: Basic Human Anatomy and Physiology. 2nd ed. Philadelphia, W. B. Saunders Co., 1973.)

all muscles lying below the point of injury. Therefore it is important not to lift or move a person who may have suffered fracture of the spine. If he must be moved before experienced first aid help arrives, he should be drawn carefully backwards or ahead, pulled by both legs or both armpits; any sideways motion must be avoided. (See also PARAPLEGIA and QUADRIPLEGIA.)

In a slipped DISK, one of the disks of cartilage between the vertebrae is moved partially out of place. The slipped disk may press on the spinal cord or one of the spinal nerves and cause pain, sometimes extremely severe. The disk may slip back into place after a period of bed rest, though sometimes the condition must be corrected surgically.

MALFORMATIONS OF THE SPINE. Of the various types of spinal malformations, some are congenital and others the result of postural defects or injuries. Spina bifida is congenital. KYPHOSIS (hunchback) may occasionally be congenital, but more often it is caused by one of the diseases that attack the structure of the bones. The most common of these is POTT'S DISEASE, or tuberculosis affecting the vertebrae and soft tissues of the spine. Another is osteitis deformans, a type of bone inflammation in which parts of the bone are replaced by softer tissue.

Less serious malformations include round shoulders, which may sometimes result from poor posture; the condition warrants corrective treatment for it may cause a strain on the heart. A curvature of the spine toward one side (scoliosis) sometimes is caused by a difference in the length of the legs and can be corrected with the use of a built-up shoe. Occasionally the spine is bent backward, perhaps in an effort to correct a heavy abdomen or for the sake of fashion.

Spinal curvature can also result from certain diseases; it can be the cause or symptoms of serious disorders.

OTHER SPINAL DISORDERS. Many of the various forms of arthritis may attack the spine. Among these is rheumatoid spondylitis, or Marie-Strümpell disease, which causes inflammation of cartilage between the vertebrae and eventually can cause the neighboring vertebrae to fuse together, preventing movement. Occasionally the whole spine becomes stiffened, a condition sometimes called poker spine. Loss of spinal flexibility may also be caused by osteoarthritis, the relatively mild arthritic condition that may develop in the later years. Spinal meningitis is an inflammation of the meninges, the membranes that cover the spinal cord.

spinifugal (spi-nif′u-gal) conducting or moving away from the spinal cord.

spinipetal (spi-nip′ĕ-tal) conducting or moving toward the spinal cord.

spinnbarkeit (spin′bahr-kīt) mucus of low viscosity from the cervix uteri, indicative of ovulation.

spinobulbar (spi″no-bul′bar) pertaining to the spinal cord and medulla oblongata.

spinocellular (spi″no-sel′u-lar) pertaining to prickle cells.

spinocerebellar (spi″no-ser″ĕ-bel′ar) pertaining to the spinal cord and cerebellum.

spinous (spi′nus) pertaining to or like a spine.

spiradenoma (spi″rad-ĕ-no′mah) adenoma of the sweat glands.

spiral (spi′ral) 1. winding like the thread of a screw. 2. a structure curving around a central point or axis.

Curschmann's s's, coiled fibrils of mucin sometimes found in the sputum of patients with asthma.

spireme (spi′rēm) the threadlike continuous or segmented figure formed by the chromosome material during prophase.

spirilla (spi-ril′ah) plural of *spirillum.*

spirillicidal (spi-ril″ĭ-si′dal) destroying spirilla.

spirillicide (spi-ril′ĭ-sīd) an agent that destroys spirilla.

spirillosis (spi″rĭ-lo′sis) a disease caused by presence of spirilla, such as rat-bite fever.

Spirillum (spi-ril′um) a genus of gram-negative bacteria, including one species, *S. mi′nus,* which is pathogenic for guinea pigs, rats, mice, and monkeys and is the cause of rat-bite fever (sodoku) in man.

spirillum (spi-ril′um), pl. *spiril′la* [L.] 1. a spiral-shaped bacterium. 2. a member of the genus *Spirillum.*

spirit (spir′it) 1. a volatile or distilled liquid. 2. a solution of a volatile material in alcohol.

ammonia s's, aromatic s's of ammonia, a mixture of ammonia, ammonium carbonate, and other agents for use as an inhalant to revive a person who has fainted.

rectified s., alcohol.

Spirochaeta (spi″ro-ke′tah) a genus of bacteria found in fresh-water or sea-water slime.

spirochete (spi′ro-kēt) 1. a highly coiled bacterium; a general term applied to any organism of the order Spirochaetales, which includes the causative organisms of syphilis (*Treponema pallidum*) and yaws (*Treponema pertenue*). 2. an organism of the genus Spirochaeta. adj., **spiroche′tal.**

spirocheticide (spi″ro-ke′tĭ-sīd) an agent that destroys spirochetes.

spirochetolysis (spi″ro-ke-tol′ĭ-sis) the destruction of spirochetes by lysis.

spirochetosis (spi″ro-ke-to′sis) infection with spirochetes.

spirogram (spi′ro-gram) a graph of respiratory movements made by the spirometer.

spirograph (spi′ro-graf) an apparatus for measuring and recording respiratory movements.

spiroid (spi′roid) resembling a spiral.

spirolactone (spi″ro-lak′tōn) a group of compounds capable of opposing the action of sodium-retaining steroids on renal transport of sodium and potassium.

spirometer (spi-rom′ĕ-ter) an instrument for measuring air taken into and expelled from the lungs. The spirometer provides a relatively simple method for determining most of the lung volumes and capacities that are measured in PULMONARY FUNCTION TESTS.

The device consists of a hollow drum floating over a chamber of water and counterbalanced by weights so that it can move freely up and down. Inside the drum is a mixture of gases, usually oxygen and air. Leading from the hollow space in the drum to the outside is a tube that has a mouthpiece through which the patient breathes. As he inhales and exhales through the tube the drum rises and falls, causing a needle to move on a nearby rotating chart. The tracing recorded on the chart is called a spirogram. (See illustration, page 944.)

spirometry (spi-rom′ĕ-tre) measurement of the

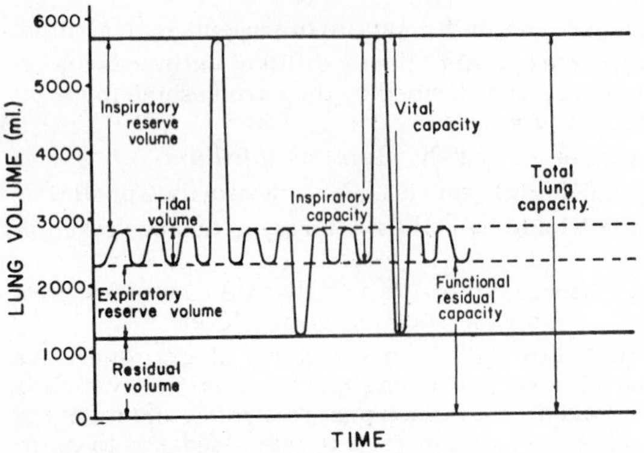

Diagram showing respiratory excursions during normal breathing and during maximal inspiration and normal expiration. (From Guyton, A. C.: Basic Human Physiology: Normal Function and Mechanisms of Disease. 2nd ed. Philadelphia, W. B. Saunders Co., 1977.)

breathing capacity by means of a spirometer.

spironolactone (spi-ro″no-lak′tōn) one of the spirolactones, an oral aldosterone antagonist which, when used with other diuretic drugs, is often successful in relieving edema or ascites in patients who have not responded to other diuretics.

splanchn(o)- word element [Gr.], *viscus (viscera); splanchnic nerve.*

splanchnapophysis (splangk″nah-pof′ĭ-sis) a skeletal element, such as the lower jaw, connected with the alimentary canal.

splanchnectopia (splangk″nek-to′pe-ah) displacement of a viscus or of the viscera.

splanchnesthesia (splangk″nes-the′ze-ah) visceral sensation. adj., **splanchnesthet′ic.**

splanchnic (splangk′nik) pertaining to the viscera.

s. nerves, a group of nerves serving the blood vessels and viscera. (See splanchnic NERVES and table of NERVES.)

splanchnicectomy (splangk″nĭ-sek′to-me) excision of part of the greater splanchnic nerve. The operation is combined with sympathectomy for relief of essential hypertension.

splanchnicotomy (splangk″nĭ-kot′o-me) transection of a splanchnic nerve.

splanchnocele (splangk′no-sēl) hernial protrusion of a viscus.

splanchnocoele (splangk′no-sēl) the portion of the embryonic body cavity from which the abdominal, pericardial, and pleural cavities are formed.

splanchnodiastasis (splangk″no-di-as′tah-sis) displacement of a viscus or viscera.

splanchnolith (splangk′no-lith) intestinal calculus.

splanchnology (splangk-nol′o-je) scientific study or description of the organs of the body, as of the digestive, respiratory, and genitourinary systems.

splanchnomegaly (splangk″no-meg′ah-le) enlargement of the viscera; visceromegaly.

splanchnopathy (splangk-nop′ah-the) any disease of the viscera.

splanchnopleure (splangk′no-plo͞or) the embryonic layer formed by union of the splanchnic meso-

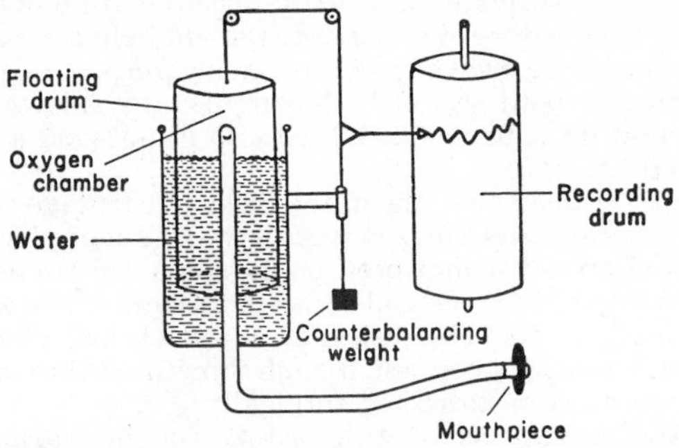

A spirometer. (From Guyton, A. C.: Basic Human Physiology: Normal Function and Mechanisms of Disease. 2nd ed. Philadelphia, W. B. Saunders Co., 1977.)

derm with entoderm; from it are developed the muscles and the connective tissue of the digestive tube.

splanchnoptosis (splangk″nop-to′sis) prolapse or downward displacement of the viscera.

splanchnosclerosis (splangk″no-sklĕ-ro′sis) hardening of the viscera.

splanchnoskeleton (splangk″no-skel′ĕ-ton) skeletal structures connected with viscera.

splanchnotomy (splangk-not′o-me) anatomy or dissection of the viscera.

splanchnotribe (splangk′no-trīb) an instrument for crushing the intestine to obliterate its lumen.

splayfoot (spla′foot) flatfoot; talipes valgus.

spleen (splēn) a large glandlike organ situated under the ribs in the upper left quadrant of the abdomen. Oblong and flattened in shape, it is dark red in color and weighs about 6 oz. adj., **splen′ic.**

In the unborn child the spleen, with the liver, produces erythrocytes. After birth, this function is taken over by the bone marrow. However, if there is bone marrow failure, the spleen may again produce red blood cells. In the normal adult the spleen is a reservoir for blood, and contains a high concentration of erythrocytes. In times of exertion, emotional stress, pregnancy, severe bleeding, carbon monoxide poisoning, or other occasions when the oxygen content of the blood must be increased, the spleen contracts rhythmically to release its store of red cells into the bloodstream.

The spleen also acts to help keep the blood free from unwanted substances, including wastes and infecting organisms. The blood is delivered to the spleen by the splenic artery, and passes through smaller branch arteries into a network of channels lined with leukocytes known as phagocytes (see RETICULOENDOTHELIAL SYSTEM). These clear the blood of old erythrocytes, damaged cells, parasites, and other toxic or foreign substances. Hemoglobin from the removed red cells is temporarily stored.

The spleen contains nodules of light-colored lymphoid tissue (white pulp) in which lymphocytes are manufactured. These cells also produce antibodies.

Although its functions are important, the spleen is not an indispensable organ. When ruptured or greatly enlarged because of disease, the spleen can be surgically removed (see SPLENECTOMY). Although this may leave the body less resistant to infection, the spleen's functions are generally taken over by other organs, particularly the liver.

accessory s., a small mass of tissue elsewhere in the body, histologically and functionally identical with that composing the normal spleen.

splen(o)- (sple′no) word element [Gr.], *spleen.*

splenadenoma (splēn″ad-ĕ-no′mah) hyperplasia of the spleen pulp.

splenalgia (sple-nal′je-ah) pain in the spleen.

splenectasis (sple-nek′tah-sis) splenomegaly.

splenectomy (sple-nek′to-me) excision of the SPLEEN. Indications for this procedure include severe trauma to or rupture of the spleen, enlargement (splenomegaly) when the destructive properties of the organ are greatly accelerated, and such blood disorders as idiopathic thrombocytopenic purpura and hereditary spherocytosis. The latter two conditions respond well to splenectomy. In blood dyscrasias in which parts of the reticuloendothelial system other than the spleen are involved, splenectomy may be of little value.

splenectopia, splenectopy (sple″nek-to′pe-ah; sple-nek′to-pe) displacement of the spleen.

splenic (splen′ik) pertaining to the spleen.

splenitis (sple-ni′tis) inflammation of the spleen, a condition that is attended by enlargement of the organ and severe local pain.

splenium (sple′ne-um) a compress or bandage; a bandlike structure.

s. cor′poris callo′si, the posterior, rounded end of the corpus callosum.

splenization (splen″ĭ-za′shun) the conversion of a tissue, as of the lung, into tissue resembling that of the spleen, due to engorgement and consolidation.

splenocele (sple′no-sēl) hernia of the spleen.

splenocolic (sple″no-kol′ik) pertaining to the spleen and colon.

splenocyte (splen′o-sīt) the monocyte characteristic of splenic tissue.

splenodynia (sple″no-din′e-ah) pain in the spleen.

splenography (sple-nog′rah-fe) 1. roentgenography of the spleen. 2. a description of the spleen.

splenohepatomegaly (sple″no-hep″ah-to-meg′ah-le) enlargement of the spleen and liver.

splenoid (sple′noid) resembling the spleen.

splenolysin (sple-nol′ĭ-sin) a lysin that destroys spleen tissue.

splenolysis (sple-nol′ĭ-sis) destruction of splenic tissue by a lysin.

splenoma (sple-no′mah) a splenic tumor.

splenomalacia (sple″no-mah-la′she-ah) abnormal softness of the spleen; lienomalacia.

splenomedullary (sple″no-med′u-ler″e) of or pertaining to the spleen and bone marrow; lienomedullary.

splenomegaly (sple″no-meg′ah-le) enlargement of the spleen.

congestive s., splenomegaly secondary to portal hypertension, with ascites, anemia, thrombocytopenia, leukopenia, and episodic hemorrhage from the intestinal tract.

hemolytic s., that associated with hemolytic anemia.

siderotic s., splenomegaly with deposit of iron and calcium.

splenometry (sple-nom′ĕ-tre) determination of the size of the spleen.

splenomyelogenous (sple″no-mi″ĕ-loj′ĕ-nus) formed in the spleen and bone marrow; lienomyelogenous.

splenomyelomalacia (sple″no-mi″ĕ-lo-mah-la′she-ah) softening of the spleen and bone marrow; lienomyelomalacia.

splenoncus (sple-nong′kus) splenoma.

splenopancreatic (sple″no-pan″kre-at′ik) pertaining to the spleen and pancreas.

splenopathy (sple-nop′ah-the) any disease of the spleen.

splenopexy (sple′no-pek″se) surgical fixation of the spleen.

splenopneumonia (splen″o-nu-mo′ne-ah) pneumonia attended with splenization of the lung.

splenoptosis (sple″nop-to′sis) downward displacement of the spleen.

splenorenal (sple″no-re′nal) pertaining to the spleen and kidney, or to splenic and renal veins.

splenorrhagia (sple″no-ra′je-ah) hemorrhage from the spleen.

splenorrhaphy (sple-nor′ah-fe) suture of the spleen.

splenotomy (sple-not′o-me) incision of the spleen.

splenotoxin (sple″no-tok′sin) a toxin produced by or acting on the spleen; lienotoxin.

splint (splint) a rigid or flexible appliance for fixation of displaced or movable parts.

USES. Splints are most commonly used to immobilize broken bones or dislocated joints. When a broken bone has been properly set, a splint permits complete rest at the site of the fracture and thus allows natural healing to take place with the bone in the proper position. Splints are also necessary to immobilize unset fractures when a patient is moved after an accident; they prevent motion of the fractured bone, which might cause greater damage.

In a pelvic or spinal fracture, the effect of splinting is achieved by placing the patient on a stretcher or board. Breaks of the ribs and of face and skull bones usually do not require the use of splints, since these parts are naturally splinted by adjacent bone and tissue.

MAKING AND APPLYING SPLINTS. A splint can be improvised from a variety of materials, but should usually be light, straight, and rigid. It should be long enough to extend beyond the joint above the injury and below the fracture site. A board used as a splint should be at least as wide as the injured part. Tightly rolled newspapers or magazines can be used to splint the arm or lower leg. Ice cream sticks have been used as splints for broken fingers.

Splints should be padded, at least on one side. Thick soft padding permits the injured part to swell and reduces interference with circulation. Bandages or strips of cloth or adhesive tape are used to hold splints in place.

After splinting, frequent examinations are necessary to determine whether the blood supply has been impaired. If the extremity becomes cold, pale, or blue, or if the affected part becomes too painful, the splint should be loosened. Splints should never be tight.

INTERNAL SPLINTS. Internal splints, as well as pins, wires, and other devices for the fixation of fractures, are among the more spectacular advances in orthopedics. They have worked wonders in the setting of hip fractures, especially in older people. Internal splints are available for almost every type of fracture. Stainless steel and Vitallium are the most commonly used materials. Splints and devices of this type require surgery for insertion, but are less cumbersome than external splints and permit earlier use of the fractured bone.

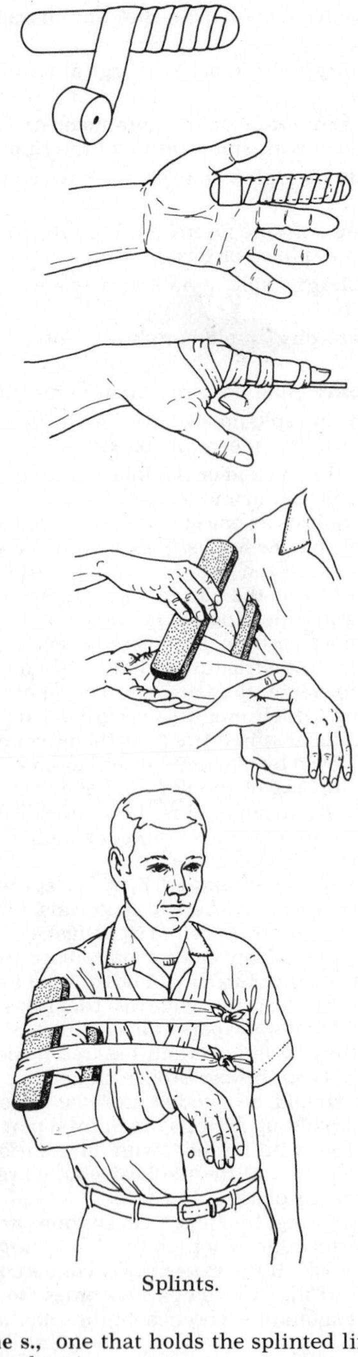

Splints.

airplane s., one that holds the splinted limb suspended in the air.

anchor s., one for fracture of the jaw, with metal loops fitting over the teeth and held together by a rod.

Balkan s., Balkan frame.

coaptation s's, small splints adjusted about a fractured limb for the purpose of producing coaptation of fragments.

dynamic s., functional s., a supportive or protective apparatus which aids in initiation and performance of motion by the supported or adjacent parts.

spodo- word element [Gr.], *waste material.*

spodogenous (spo-doj′ĕ-nus) caused by accumulation of waste material in an organ.

spondyl(o)- word element [Gr.], *vertebra; vertebral column.*

spondylalgia (spon″dĭ-lal′je-ah) pain in the vertebrae.

spondylarthritis (spon″dil-ar-thri′tis) arthritis of the spine.

spondylitic (spon″dĭ-lit′ik) pertaining to or marked by spondylitis.

spondylitis (spon″dĭ-li′tis) inflammation of the vertebrae. Almost always a serious chronic disorder, spondylitis may be associated with tuberculosis of the bones, in which case it is called POTT'S DISEASE. The vertebrae become eroded and collapse, causing KYPHOSIS (hunchback).

Spondylitis may also be associated with other infectious diseases, such as brucellosis, or undulant fever. The intervertebral disks and the vertebrae are affected and sometimes destroyed, and permanent stiffening, or ankylosis, of the back results.

A particularly serious ailment is rheumatoid spondylitis, called also Marie-Strümpell disease or ankylosing spondylitis. It is a form of rheumatoid arthritis that affects the spine, and is characterized by inflammation of the cartilage in the joints between vertebrae, and inflammation of the gliding joints between the vertebral arches. It affects males almost exclusively. There is stiffening of the spinal joints and ligaments, so that movement becomes increasingly painful and difficult. When it runs its full course, it results in bony ankylosis of the vertebral joints. The stiffening may extend to the ribs and limit the flexibility of the rib cage, so that breathing is impaired.

Kümmel's spondylitis or post-traumatic spondylitis, is compression fracture of a vertebra, with symptoms occurring a few weeks after injury (see also KÜMMEL'S DISEASE).

spondylizema (spon″dĭ-li-ze′mah) downward displacement of a vertebra because of destruction or softening of the one below it.

spondylocace (spon″dĭ-lok′ah-se) tuberculosis of the vertebrae.

spondylodymus (spon″dĭ-lod′ĭ-mus) twin fetuses united by the vertebrae.

spondylodynia (spon″dĭ-lo-din′e-ah) pain in a vertebra.

spondylolisthesis (spon″dĭ-lo-lis-the′sis) forward displacement of a vertebra over a lower segment, usually of the fifth lumbar over the sacrum, or of the fourth lumbar over the fifth. adj., **spondylolisthet′ic.**

spondylolysis (spon′dĭ-lol′ĭ-sis) the breaking down of a vertebra.

spondylopathy (spon″dĭ-lop′ah-the) any disease of the vertebrae.

spondylopyosis (spon″dĭ-lo-pi-o′sis) suppuration of a vertebra.

spondyloschisis (spon″dĭ-los′kĭ-sis) congenital fissure of a vertebral arch; spina bifida.

spondylosis (spon″dĭ-lo′sis) ankylosis of a vertebral joint; also, a general term for degenerative changes in the spine.

rhizomelic s., rheumatoid spondylitis.

spondylosyndesis (spon″dĭ-lo-sin′dĕ-sis) surgical creation of ankylosis between contiguous vertebrae; spinal fusion.

sponge (spunj) a porous, absorbent mass, as a pad of gauze or cotton surrounded by gauze, or the elastic fibrous skeleton of certain species of marine animals.

gelatin s., absorbable, a sterile, absorbable, water-insoluble, gelatin-base material used in the control of bleeding.

spongi(o)- word element [L., Gr.], *sponge; spongelike.*

spongiform (spun′jĭ-form) resembling a sponge.

spongioblast (spun′je-o-blast″) 1. any of the embryonic epithelial cells developed about the neural tube, which become transformed, some into neuroglial and some into ependymal cells. 2. amacrine (2).

spongioblastoma (spun″je-o-blas-to′mah) a tumor containing spongioblasts; gliosarcoma or glioblastoma.

spingiocyte (spun′je-o-sīt″) 1. a neuroglia cell. 2. one of the cells with spongy vacuolated protoplasm in the adrenal cortex.

spongioid (spun′je-oid) resembling a sponge.

spongioplasm (spun′je-o-plazm″) 1. a substance forming the network of fibrils pervading the cell substance and forming the reticulum of the fixed cell. 2. the granular material of an axon.

spongiosis (spun″je-o′sis) intercellular edema within the epidermis.

spongiositis (spun″je-o-si′tis) inflammation of the corpus spongiosum of the penis.

spongy (spun′je) of spongelike appearance or texture.

s. degeneration of central nervous system, s. degeneration of white matter, see spongy DEGENERATION of central nervous system.

sporadic (spo-rad′ik) occurring singly; widely scattered; not epidemic or endemic.

spore (spōr) the reproductive element of one of the lower organisms, such as a protozoon or certain plants.

sporicide (spōr′ĭ-sīd) an agent that kills spores. adj., **sporici′dal.**

sporocyst (spōr′o-sist) 1. any cyst or sac containing spores or reproductive cells; the oocyst of certain protozoa in which sporozoites develop. 2. the larval stages of flukes in snails.

sporogenic (spōr″o-jen′ik) producing spores.

sporogony (spo-rog′o-ne) the sexual stage in the life cycle of a sporozoan parasite, with development of the zygote into one or several haploid spores, each containing a distinctive number of sporozoites. adj., **sporogon′ic.**

sporont (spōr′ont) a mature protozoon in its sexual cycle.

sporoplasm (spōr′o-plazm) the protoplasm of reproductive cells.

Sporothrix (spo″ro-thriks) a genus of fungi, including *S. schenck′ii,* which causes sporotrichosis, and *S. car′nis,* which causes formation of white mold on meat in cold storage.

sporotrichosis (spo″ro-trĭ-ko′sis) a chronic fungal infection caused by *Sporothrix schenckii,* occurring in three forms. The *cutaneous lymphatic form* is characterized by a single pustule, papule, or nodule at the site of invasion, followed by lymphatic spread and the development of multiple, painless, subcutaneous granulomas, which tend to break down and form indolent ulcers or cold abscesses. The *disseminated form* is marked by multiple, painless, cutaneous or subcutaneous nodules, which may form cold abscesses, ulcers, or fistulas; this form may involve the muscles, joints, bones, eyes, gastrointestinal system, mucous membranes, and nervous system. The *pulmonary form* results from the inhalation of spores and causes acute disease or chronic granulomas similar to those seen in other mycoses.

Sporotrichum (spo-rot′rĭ-kum) a genus of fungi that once included *Sporothrix schenckii.*

Sporozoa (spo″ro-zo′ah) a subphylum of endoparasitic protozoa, marked by the lack of locomotor organs in adult stages and a complex life cycle usually involving an alternation of a sexual with an asexual cycle.

sporozoa (spo″ro-zo′ah) plural of *sporozoon.*

sporozoan (spo″ro-zo′an) 1. pertaining to the Sporozoa. 2. an individual of the Sporozoa.

sporozoite (spōr″o-zo′īt) a spore formed after fertilization; any one of the sickle-shaped nucleated germs formed by division of the protoplasm of a spore of a sporozoan organism. In malaria, the sporozoites are the forms of the plasmodium that are liberated from the oocysts in the mosquito, that accumulate in the salivary glands and that are transferred to man in the act of feeding.

sporozoon (spōr″o-zo′on), pl. *sporozo′a* [Gr.] an individual organism of the Sporozoa.

sporulation (spor″u-la′shun) formation of spores.

spotted fever a febrile disease characterized by a skin eruption, such as Rocky Mountain spotted fever, boutonneuse fever, and other infections due to tickborne rickettsiae.

sprain (sprān) wrenching or twisting of a joint, with partial rupture of its ligaments. There may also be damage to the associated blood vessels, muscles, tendons, and nerves.

A sprain is more serious than a strain, which is simply the overstretching of a muscle, without swelling. Severe sprains are so painful that the joint cannot be used. There is much swelling, with reddish to blue discoloration owing to hemorrhage from ruptured blood vessels.

First aid for a sprain involves immediate rest and the application of heat or cold by means of compresses. The sprained joint should be kept elevated if possible, and it should not be used.

sprue (sproo) a chronic form of malabsorption syndrome occurring in both tropical and nontropical forms.

nontropical s., a malabsorption syndrome affecting both children and adults, precipitated by ingestion of gluten-containing foods (see also CELIAC DISEASE).

tropical s., a chronic disease, affecting the digestive system, that is marked by imperfect absorption of food elements, especially fats but also certain vitamins, from the small intestine. The condition is closely related to CELIAC DISEASE and may be identical with it.

The name sprue derives from a Dutch word describing inflammation of the mouth, which is a frequent symptom. The disease has been recognized for more than 2000 years. It occurs mostly, but not exclusively, in the tropics.

SYMPTOMS AND TREATMENT. Symptoms are loss of appetite, flatulence, anemia, diarrhea, stomach cramps, and extreme loss of weight. Stools are usually pale, greasy, unformed, and foul-smelling, but at times become watery. If a deficiency of vitamin B complex is also present, cracks develop at the corners of the mouth and the tongue becomes smooth, glossy, and bright red.

Treatment consists of a special diet of foods that are low in fat, high in protein, and fairly bland. Diets free of gluten, a viscid grain protein, may be prescribed. Liver preparations, folic acid, calcium lactate tablets, vitamin B_{12}, and iron supplements to provide food elements that are not absorbed, as well as skimmed milk and ripe bananas, have produced favorable results. Antibiotics and cortisone have proved temporarily successful, but their prolonged use is not recommended. In critical cases, repeated small blood transfusions have been beneficial.

Cases of sprue that are recognized early respond better to treatment than do cases of long standing. Appetite and weight return rapidly. The time required for complete recovery is prolonged, however, especially in extreme cases.

spur (sper) a projecting body, as from a bone.

spurious (spūr′e-us) simulated; not genuine; false.

sputum (spu′tum) mucous secretion from the lungs, bronchi, and trachea which is ejected through the mouth, in contrast to saliva which is the secretion of the salivary glands.

s. specimen, a sample of mucous secretion from the bronchi and lungs. The specimen may be examined microscopically for the presence of malignant cells (*cytologic examination*) or tested to identify pathogenic bacteria (*bacteriologic examination*).

It is essential that the specimen obtained be mucus from the lungs and bronchi and not saliva. For those who are unable to produce sputum for examination, an AEROSOL may be used to increase the flow of secretions and stimulate coughing. The optimum time for collection of a sputum specimen is in the morning before breakfast. At this time secretions accumulated in the bronchi through the night are more readily available, and, should the coughing produce gagging, the patient is less likely to vomit if his stomach is empty. Specimens collected for bacteriologic culture must be placed in a sterile container and handled with care to avoid contamination from sources other than the sputum.

SQ subcutaneous.

squalene (skwa′lēn) an unsaturated terpin hydrocarbon from the liver oil of sharks and other elasmobranch fishes; it is an intermediate in cholesterol biosynthesis in all animals examined, and is found in small amounts in blood plasma and in increased amounts in viral influenza.

squama (skwa′mah), pl. *squa′mae* [L.] a scale, or thin, platelike structure.

squame (skwām) a scale or scalelike mass.

squamoparietal (skwa″mo-pah-ri′ĕ-tal) pertaining to the pars squamosa, or squamous portion of the temporal bone, and the parietal bone.

squamous (skwa′mus) scaly or platelike.

s. bone, the pars squamosa, or squamous portion of the temporal bone.

squatting (skwot′ing) a position with the hips and knees flexed, the buttocks resting on the heels; sometimes adopted by the parturient at delivery or by children with certain types of cardiac defects.

squill (skwil) the fleshy inner scales of the bulb of the white variety of *Urginea maritima;* it contains several cardioactive glycosides. The red variety is used as a rat poison.

squint (skwint) strabismus.

S.R. sedimentation rate.

Sr chemical symbol, *strontium.*

sRNA soluble RNA (ribonucleic acid).

SRS, SRS-A slow-reacting substance (of anaphylaxis).

ss. [L.] *se′mis* (one half).

S.T.37 (es″te thir″te-sev′en) trademark for a solution of hexylresorcinol, an anthelmintic.

stability (stah-bil′ĭ-te) the quality of maintaining a constant character despite forces that threaten to disturb it.

stabilization (sta″bĭ-lĭ-za′shun) the process of making firm and steady.

stable (sta′b′l) not readily subject to change.

stactometer (stak-tom′ĕ-ter) a device for measuring drops.

staff (staf) 1. a wooden rod or rodlike structure. 2. a grooved director used as a guide for the knife in lithotomy. 3. the professional personnel of a hospital.

s. of Æculapius, see ÆCULAPIUS.

attending s., the corps of attending physicians and surgeons of a hospital.

consulting s., specialists associated with a hospital and acting in an advisory capacity to the attending staff.

house s., the resident physicians and surgeons of a hospital.

stage (stāj) 1. a definite period or distinct phase, as of development of a disease or of an organism. 2. the platform of a microscope on which the slide containing the object to be studied is placed.

stain (stān) 1. a substance used to impart color to tissues or cells, to facilitate microscopic study and identification. 2. an area of discoloration of the skin.

acid s., one that is acid in reaction and more readily colors the cell protoplasm.

basic s., one in which the color is carried by a base and which has an affinity for cell nuclei.

contrast s., a second stain used in preparation of a specimen, which colors other elements than those colored by the first, increasing the contrast between them.

differential s., one which facilitates differentiation of various elements in a specimen.

Giemsa s., a solution containing azure II-eosin, azure II, glycerin, and methanol; used for staining protozoan parasites, such as trypanosomes, *Leishmania;* etc., and *Leptospira, Borrelia,* viral inclusion bodies, and *Rickettsia.*

Gram's s., a staining procedure in which bacteria are stained with crystal violet, treated with strong iodine solution, decolorized with ethanol or ethanol-acetone, and counterstained with a contrasting dye; those retaining the stain are gram-positive, and those losing the stain but staining with the counterstain are gram-negative.

hematoxylin and eosin s., a mixture of hematoxylin in distilled water and aqueous eosin solution, employed universally for routine examination of tissues.

metachromatic s., one that produces in certain elements color different from that of the stain itself.

neutral s., a combination of an acid and a basic stain for staining neutrophil tissues.

nuclear s., one that selectively stains cell nuclei, generally a basic stain.

port-wine s., nevus flammeus.

postvital s., a stain that appears after death of a tissue which has been previously stained by vital methods.

supravital s., a stain introduced in living tissue or cells that have been removed from the body.

tumor s., an area of increased density in a radiograph, due to collection of contrast material in distorted and abnormal vessels, prominent in the capillary and venous phases of arteriography, and presumed to indicate neoplasm.

vital s., a stain introduced into the living organism, and taken up selectively by various tissue or cellular elements.

Wright's s., a mixture of eosin and methylene blue, used for demonstrating blood cells and malarial parasites.

staining (stān′ing) artificial coloration of a substance to facilitate examination of tissues, microorganisms, or other cells under the microscope. For various techniques, see under STAIN.

stalagmometer (stal″ag-mom′ĕ-ter) an instrument for measuring surface tension by determining the exact number of drops in a given quantity of a liquid.

stammering (stam′er-ing) a speech problem characterized by involuntary pauses in speaking, often with repetition of sounds.

standard (stan′dard) something established as a measure or model to which other similar things should conform.

standstill (stand′stil) cessation of motion, as of the heart (cardiac standstill) or chest (respiratory standstill).

stannum (stan′um) [L.] tin (symbol Sn).

stanolone (stan′o-lōn) an androgen having the same actions and uses as testosterone.

stanozolol (stan′o-zo-lol″) an androgenic-anabolic steroid used to improve appetite and promote gain in weight by promoting nitrogen retention.

Stanton's disease (stan′tunz) melioidosis.

stapedectomy (sta″pe-dek′to-me) surgical removal of the stapes (stirrup of the middle ear), which is then replaced with a prosthetic device composed of stainless steel, Teflon, or a similar substance. The surgical procedure is performed for the relief of deafness produced by OTOSCLEROSIS, or fixation of the minute bones of the middle ear. Replacement of the fixed stapes with a device capable of vibrating permits the transmission of sound waves from the outer ear to the inner ear, and hearing is thus restored.

Because the stapes is one of the smallest bones in the body, this procedure is very delicate and must be performed under an operating microscope. Very fine instruments, designed specifically for this procedure, are used.

The procedure is done under local anesthesia and the patient is allowed out of bed within 48 hours after surgery and usually can go home on the third postoperative day. Vertigo (dizziness) is common following stapedectomy but it is only temporary. The patient must be protected from falls and self-injury until he regains his sense of balance. Care must also be taken to prevent infection and the patient must be cautioned against blowing his nose and getting water in his ear while bathing until the operative site is completely healed. (For additional information on patient care after stapedectomy, see surgery of the EAR.)

stapedial (stah-pe′de-al) pertaining to the stapes.

stapediotenotomy (stah-pe″de-o-tĕ-not′o-me) cutting of the tendon of the stapedius muscle.

stapediovestibular (stah-pe″de-o-ves-tib′u-lar) pertaining to the stapes and vestibule.

stapes (sta′pēz) the innermost of the three ossicles of the ear; called also stirrup. (See Plate 15.)

Staphcillin (staf-sil′in) trademark for a preparation of methicillin, an antibiotic of specific value in treatment of certain penicillin-resistant staphylococci.

staphyl(o)- word element [Gr.], *uvula; resembling a bunch of grapes; staphylococci.*

staphylectomy (staf″ĭ-lek′to-me) uvulectomy.

staphyledema (staf″il-ĕ-de′mah) edema of the uvula.

staphyline (staf′ĭ-līn) 1. pertaining to the uvula. 2. shaped like a bunch of grapes.

staphylitis (staf″ĭ-li′tis) inflammation of the uvula.

staphylococcemia (staf″ĭ-lo-kok-se′me-ah) staphylococci in the blood.

Staphylococcus (staf″ĭ-lo-kok′us) a genus of gram-positive bacteria made up of spherical microorganisms, tending to occur in grapelike clusters; they are constantly present on the skin and in the upper respiratory tract and are the most common cause of localized suppurating infections. There are several species, some of which are pathogenic, including *S. au′reus* and *S. pyog′enes* var. *S. al′bus.*

staphylococcus (staf″ĭ-lo-kok′us), pl. *staphylococ′ci* [Gr.] any organism of the genus *Staphylococcus.* adj., **staphylococ′cal, staphylococ′cic.**

staphyloderma (staf″ĭ-lo-der′mah) pyogenic skin infection by staphylococci.

staphylodialysis (staf″ĭ-lo-di-al′ĭ-sis) elongation of the uvula.

staphylokinase (staf″ĭ-lo-ki′nās) a bacterial kinase produced by certain strains of staphylococci; it induces fibrinolysis by converting plasminogen to plasmin.

staphylolysin (staf″ĭ-lol′ĭ-sin) a substance produced by staphylococci that causes hemolysis.

staphyloma (staf″ĭ-lo′mah) protrusion of the sclera or cornea, usually lined with uveal tissue, due to inflammation.

anterior s., staphyloma in the anterior part of the eye.

corneal s., 1. bulging of the cornea with adherent uveal tissue. 2. one formed by protrusion of the iris through a corneal wound.

posterior s., s. posti′cum, backward bulging of sclera at posterior pole of eye.

scleral s., protrusion of the contents of the eyeball where the sclera has become thinned.

staphyloncus (staf″ĭ-long′kus) a tumor or swelling of the uvula.

staphyloplasty (staf′ĭ-lo-plas″te) plastic repair of the soft palate and uvula.

staphyloptosis (staf″ĭ-lop-to′sis) elongation of the uvula.

staphylorrhaphy (staf″ĭ-lor′ah-fe) surgical correction of a midline cleft in the uvula and soft palate.

staphyloschisis (staf″ĭ-los′kĭ-sis) fissure of the uvula and soft palate.

staphylotomy (staf″ĭ-lot′o-me) 1. incision of the uvula. 2. excision of a staphyloma.

starch (starch) 1. any of a group of polysaccharides of the general formula, $(C_6H_{10}O_5)_n$; it is the chief storage form of CARBOHYDRATES in plants. 2. granular material separated from mature grain of *Zea mays* (Indian corn, or maize); used as a dusting powder and tablet disintegrant in pharmaceuticals.

animal s., glycogen.

s. glycerite, a preparation of starch, benzoic acid, purified water, and glycerin, used topically as an emollient.

starvation (star-va′shun) long-continued deprival of food and its morbid effects.

stasis (sta′sis) a stoppage or diminution of flow, as of blood or other body fluid, or of intestinal contents.

-stasis word element [Gr.], *maintenance of (or maintaining) a constant level; preventing increase or multiplication.* adj., **-stat′ic.**

stat. [L.] *sta′tim* (at once).

state (stāt) condition or situation.

dream s., a state of defective consciousness in which the environment is imperfectly perceived.

excited s., the condition of a nucleus, atom, or molecule produced by the addition of energy to the system as the result of absorption of photons or of inelastic collisions with other particles or systems.

ground s., the condition of lowest energy of a nucleus, atom or molecule.

refractory s., a condition of subnormal excitability of muscle and nerve following excitation.

resting s., the physiologic condition achieved by complete bed rest for at least 1 hour.

steady s., dynamic equilibrium.

State Health Planning and Development Agency (SHPDA) an agency designated by the governor of a state as the one responsible for performing the health planning and development functions prescribed by the National Health Planning and Resources Development Act of 1974 (Public Law 93-641). The Secretary of the Department of Health, Education and Welfare enters into and annually renews an agreement with each state governor for the selection of the SHPDA.

The SHPDA carries out its functions as prescribed by law and approved by the Secretary of HEW through a State Administration Program. The functions of the SHPDA, as stated by the law are: (1) Conduct the health planning activities of the State and implement those parts of the State Health Plan and the plans of the HEALTH SYSTEMS AGENCIES (HSAs) within each state which relate to the government of the state. (2) Prepare and review and revise as necessary (but at least annually) a preliminary statewide health plan which shall be made up of the health systems plans of the HSAs within the State. (3) Assist the Statewide Health Coordinating Council of the State in the review of the State medical facilities plan required under section 1603 of Public Law 93-641. (4) Make findings as to the need for institutional health services proposed by the HSAs. (5) Review all institutional health services being offered in the State and, after consideration of recommendations submitted by the HSAs respecting appropriateness of such services, make public its findings.

statim (sta′tim) [L.] at once; abbreviated stat.

statistics (stah-tis′tiks) 1. numerical facts pertaining to a particular subject or body of objects. 2. the science dealing with the collection, tabulation, and analysis of numerical facts.

vital s., that branch of biometry dealing with the data and laws of human mortality, morbidity, and natality.

statoconia (stat″o-ko′ne-ah), sing. *statoco′nium* [Gr.] minute calcareous particles in the gelatinous membrane surmounting the macula in the inner ear. Called also otoconia.

statolith (stat′o-lith) 1. a granule of the statoconia. 2. a solid or semisolid body occurring in the labyrinth of animals.

statolon (stat′o-lon) an antiviral agent derived from *Penicillium stoloniferum.*

statometer (stah-tom′ĕ-ter) an apparatus for measuring the degree of exophthalmos.

stature (stat′ūr) the height or tallness of a person standing.

status (sta′tus) [L.] condition or state.

s. asthmat′icus, asthmatic crisis; a sudden intense and continuous asthmatic attack, with dyspnea to the point of exhaustion and no response to the usual therapy.

s. epilep′ticus, rapid succession of epileptic spasms without intervals of consciousness; brain damage may result.

s. lymphat′icus, lymphatism.

s. thymicolymphat′icus, a condition resembling lymphatism, with enlargement of lymph-adenoid tissue and of the thymus as the special influencing factor; formerly thought to be the cause of sudden death in children.

s. verruco′sus, a wartlike appearance of the cerebral cortex, produced by disorderly arrangement of the neuroblasts, so that the formation of fissures and sulci is irregular and unpredictable.

steapsin (ste-ap′sin) the fat-splitting enzyme (lipase) of the pancreatic juice.

stear(o)- word element [Gr.], *fat.*

stearate (ste′ah-rāt) any compound of stearic acid.

stearic acid (ste-ar′ik) a saturated fatty acid from animal and vegetable fats; a pharmaceutical preparation of solid acids from fats, consisting chiefly of stearic acid and palmitic acid, is used in glycerin suppositories.

stearin (ste′ah-rin) a white, solid crystalline substance from fat.

stearopten (ste″ah-rop′ten) the solid constituent of a volatile oil.

steat(o)- word element [Gr.], *fat; oil.*

steatitis (ste″ah-ti′tis) inflammation of fatty tissue.

steatocystoma (ste″ah-to-sis-to′mah) a keratin cyst.

s. mul′tiplex, steatomatosis, a rare hereditary condition in which multiple sebaceous cysts occur on the trunk and limbs.

steatogenous (ste″ah-toj′ĕ-nus) producing fat; lipogenic.

steatolysis (ste″ah-tol′ĭ-sis) the emulsification of fats preparatory to absorption. adj., **steatolyt′ic.**

steatoma (ste″ah-to′mah) 1. lipoma. 2. a fatty mass retained within a sebaceous gland.

steatomatosis (ste″ah-to″mah-to′sis) the presence of numerous sebaceous cysts; steatocystoma multiplex.

steatonecrosis (ste″ah-to″nĕ-kro′sis) fat necrosis.

steatopathy (ste″ah-top′ah-the) disease of the sebaceous glands.

steatopygia (ste″ah-to-pij′e-ah) excessive fatness of the buttocks. adj., **steatop′ygous.**

steatorrhea (ste″ah-to-re′ah) excess fat in the feces due to a malabsorption syndrome caused by disease of the intestinal mucosa (e.g., sprue) or pancreatic enzyme deficiency.

steatosis (ste″ah-to′sis) fatty degeneration.

Steclin (stek′lin) trademark for preparations of tetracycline hydrochloride, an antibiotic.

stegnosis (steg-no′sis) constriction; stenosis.

Stein-Leventhal syndrome (stīn″lev′en-thal) secondary amenorrhea and absence of ovulation associated with bilateral polycystic ovaries, but normal excretion of follicle-stimulating hormone and 17-ketosteroids.

Steinert's disease (sti′nerts) myotonia dystrophica.

Steinmann extension (stīn′man) extension exerted on the distal fragment of a fractured bone by means of a nail or pin (Steinmann pin) driven into the fragment. Called also nail extension.

Steinmann pin (stīn′man) a metal rod for the internal fixation of fractures (see also STEINMANN EXTENSION).

Stelazine (stel′ah-zēn) trademark for preparations of trifluoperazine, a tranquilizer.

stella (stel′ah), pl. *stel′lae* [L.] star.

stellate (stel′āt) star-shaped; arranged in rosettes.
s. ganglion, cervicothoracic ganglion.

stellectomy (stel-ek′to-me) excision of a portion of the stellate (cervicothoracic) ganglion.

stem (stem) stalk; a stalklike supporting structure.
brain s., the stemlike portion of the brain connecting the cerebral hemispheres with the spinal cord, and comprising the pons, medulla oblongata, and midbrain; considered by some to include the diencephalon. (See also under BRAIN.)

Stenediol (sten′di-ol) trademark for preparations of methandriol, an anabolic stimulant.

steno- word element [Gr.], *narrow; contracted; constriction.*

stenocardia (sten″o-kar′de-ah) angina pectoris.

stenocephaly (sten″o-sef′ah-le) narrowness of the head or cranium. adj., **stenoceph′alous.**

stenochoria (sten″o-ko′re-ah) stenosis.

stenocoriasis (sten″o-ko-ri′ah-sis) contraction of the pupil.

stenopeic (sten″o-pe′ik) having a narrow opening or slit.

stenosed (stĕ-nōst′, stĕ-nōzd′) narrowed; constricted.

stenosis (stĕ-no′sis) narrowing or contraction of a body passage or opening.
aortic s., obstruction to the outflow of blood from the left ventricle into the aorta.
mitral s., a narrowing of the left atrioventricular orifice. (See also MITRAL COMMISSUROTOMY.)
pulmonary s., narrowing of the opening between the pulmonary artery and the right ventricle.
pyloric s., obstruction of the pyloric orifice of the stomach (see also PYLORIC STENOSIS).
tricuspid s., narrowing or stricture of the tricuspid orifice of the heart.

stenostomia (sten″o-sto′me-ah) narrowing of the mouth.

stenothermal, stenothermic (sten″o-ther′mal; sten″o-ther′mik) pertaining to or characterized by tolerance of only a narrow range of temperature.

stenothorax (sten″o-tho′raks) abnormal narrowness of the chest.

stenotic (stĕ-not′ik) marked by abnormal narrowing or constriction.

Sterane (ster′ān) trademark for preparations of prednisolone, a glucogenic corticosteroid.

sterco- word element [L.], *feces.*

stercobilin (ster″ko-bi′lin) a bile pigment derivative formed by air oxidation of stercobilinogen; it is a brown-orange-red pigmentation contributing to the color of feces and urine.

stercobilinogen (ster′ko-bi-lin′o-jen) a bilirubin metabolite and precursor of stercobilin, formed by reduction of urobilinogen.

stercorolith (ster′ko-ro-lith″) fecalith; an intestinal concretion formed around a center of fecal matter.

stercoroma (ster″ko-ro′mah) a tumor-like mass of fecal matter in the rectum; fecaloma.

Sterculia (ster-ku′le-ah) a genus of trees and shrubs, including many species, mostly tropical; some have edible seeds and others are medicinal, while still others afford a gum resembling tragacanth. The hairs of *S. apetala* of Panama may be very irritating. (See also KARAYA GUM.)

sterculia gum (ster-ku′le-ah) karaya gum.

stercus (ster′kus) [L.] dung or feces. adj., **ster′coral, ster′corous.**

stereo- word element [Gr.], *solid; firm; three dimensional.*

stereoarthrolysis (ster″e-o-ar-throl′ĭ-sis) surgical formation of a movable new joint in cases of bony ankylosis.

stereoauscultation (ster″e-o-aw″skul-ta′shun) auscultation with two stethoscopes, on different parts of the chest.

stereocampimeter (ster″e-o-kam-pim′ĕ-ter) an instrument for studying unilateral central scotomas and central retinal defects.

stereochemistry (ster″e-o-kem′is-tre) the branch of chemistry treating of the space relations of atoms in molecules. adj., **stereochem′ical.**

stereocinefluorography (ster″e-o-sin″ĕ-floo″or-og′rah-fe) recording by motion picture camera of images observed by steroscopic fluoroscopy, affording three-dimensional visualization.

stereoencephalotomy (ster″e-o-en-sef″ah-lot′o-me) stereotaxic surgery.

stereognosis (ster″e-og-no′sis) the sense by which the form of objects is perceived. adj., **stereognos′tic.**

stereoisomer (ster″e-o-i′so-mer) a compound showing stereoisomerism.

stereoisomerism (ster″e-o-i-som′ĕ-izm) isomerism in which the compounds have the same structural formulae, but the atoms are distributed differently in space. adj., **stereoisomer′ic.**

Stereo-orthopter (ster″e-o-or-thop′ter) trademark for a mirror-reflecting instrument for correcting strabismus.

stereoroentgenography (ster″e-o-rent″gen-og′-rah-fe) the making of a stereoscopic roentgenogram.

stereoscope (ster″e-o-skōp) an instrument for producing the appearance of solidity and relief by combining the images of two similar pictures of an object.

stereoscopic (ster″e-o-skop′ik) three-dimensional; having depth, as well as height and width.

stereospecific (ster″e-o-spĕ-sif′ik) pertaining to enzymes that interact only with substrates of very specific structure.

stereotactic (ster″e-o-tak′tik) stereotaxic.

stereotaxic (ster″e-o-tak′sik) 1. pertaining to or characterized by precise positioning in space; said especially of discrete areas of the brain that control specific functions. 2. pertaining to or exhibiting stereotaxis.

s. surgery, the production of sharply localized lesions in the brain after precise localization of the target tissue by use of three-dimensional coordinates.

stereotaxis, stereotropism (ster″e-o-tak′sis; ster″e-ot′ro-pizm) movement or growth in response to contact with a solid or rigid surface.

stereotypy (ster″e-o-ti″pe) persistent repetition of senseless acts or words. It may be a persistent maintaining of a bodily attitude (stereotypy of attitude), repetition of senseless movements (stereotypy of movement), or constant repetition of certain words or phrases (stereotypy of speech).

sterile (ster′il) 1. not fertile; barren; not producing young. (See also FERTILITY.) 2. aseptic; not producing microorganisms; free from living microorganisms.

sterility (stĕ-ril′ĭ-te) the state of being sterile.

sterilization (ster″il-ĭ-za′shun) 1. the process of rendering an individual incapable of reproduction, by castration, vasectomy, salpingectomy, or other procedure.

Endoscopic techniques for sterilization of the female involve *laparoscopy, culdoscopy,* and *hysteroscopy.* Each of these procedures may be performed under local or general anesthesia, do not involve major surgery, and usually do not require hospitalization. (See below.) 2. the process of destroying all microorganisms and their pathogenic products. It is accomplished by heat (wet steam under pressure at 120° C. for 15 minutes, or dry heat at 360° to 380° C. for 3 hours) or by bactericidal chemical compounds.

In sterilizing objects or substances, the high resistance of bacterial spore cells must be taken into account. Most dangerous bacteria are destroyed at a temperature of 50° to 60° C. (122° to 140° F.). Therefore, pasteurization of a fluid, which is the application of heat at about 60° C., destroys disease-causing bacteria. However, temperatures almost twice as high are usually required to destroy the spore cells.

The discovery that heat, in the form of flame, steam, or hot water, kills bacteria made possible the advances of modern surgery, which is based on freedom from microorganisms, or asepsis, and prevention of contamination. Sterilization of all equipment used during an operation, and of anything that in any way may touch the operative area, is carried out scrupulously in hospitals. Physicians and nurses wear sterile clothing. Instruments are sterilized by boiling, by chemical antiseptics, or by autoclaving.

In a physician's office needles for injections and any instruments used for treatment of wounds or other surgical procedures are also carefully sterilized, and other aseptic techniques are observed.

culdoscopic s., use of an endoscope to visualize the uterine tubes for the purpose of preventing conception. The endoscope is inserted through an incision in the vaginal wall behind the cervix. After the uterine tubes are located each tube is drawn out through the vaginal incision and severed. The major advantage of this procedure is that it can be done on an outpatient basis. A disadvantage is the complication of infection, a very real possibility owing to the unsterile nature of the vagina.

hysteroscopic s., use of an endoscopic instrument to visualize the interior of the uterus and uterine tubes for the purpose of preventing conception. The hysteroscope is inserted through the dilated cervix and on through the uterine cavity to the point at which each tube joins the uterus. A cautery is then used to electrocoagulate each tube. Occlusion of the tubes is accomplished by scar tissue that forms at the sites of cauterization.

laparoscopic s., that which employs an endoscope to visualize the uterine tubes and surrounding structures for the purpose of occluding the tubes. The instrument is guided into the abdominal cavity through a small puncture made by a trochar inserted immediately below the umbilicus. A second small puncture is made in the lower abdomen through which cautery forceps are inserted. The forceps are applied approximately 2 cm. from the point at which each of the tubes joins the uterus. In this way each tube is electrocoagulated and severed. An alternative to cauterization and severance of the tubes is the application of clips. However, there is the possibility that the clips may not completely occlude the tubes, allowing passage of the ovum and impregnation.

sterilize (ster′ĭ-līz) to subject to sterilization.

sterilizer (ster′ĭ-līz″er) an apparatus used in ridding instruments, dressings, etc., of all microorganisms and their pathogenic products. (See also AUTOCLAVE.)

Sterisol (ster′ĭ-sol) trademark for a preparation of hexetidine, a local antiseptic.

stern(o)- word element [L., Gr.], *sternum.*

sternal (ster′nal) pertaining to the sternum.

s. puncture, insertion of a hollow needle into the manubrium of the sternum for the purpose of obtaining a sample of bone marrow. The sternum is chosen because of its accessibility and because it is a thin, flat bone. The procedure must be done under surgical asepsis. The physician anesthetizes the skin and periosteum with 1 per cent procaine hydrochloride (Novocain) before introducing the sternal needle. The needle is designed with a special guard to prevent penetration beyond the desired depth. When the cells are being aspirated into the syringe the patient may experience a sharp pain; otherwise the procedure should not be painful.

The bone marrow samplings are examined for the presence of abnormal cells for the proportion of cells in their various stages of development and for the characteristics of the blood cells that predominate. This information is used in conjunction with clinical findings and other tests in the diagnosis of blood disorders such as the leukemias and anemia.

sternalgia (ster-nal′je-ah) pain in the sternum.

Sternberg's giant cells (stern′bergz) Sternberg-Reed cells.

Sternberg-Reed cells (stern′berg-rēd) enlarged, atypical histiocytes with multiple or hyperlobulated nucleoli; a characteristic feature of Hodgkin's disease.

Sterneedle (ster′ne-d′l) trademark for a controlled-depth, multiple-puncture apparatus used in diagnosing tuberculosis.

Sterneedle tuberculin test (ster′ne-d′l) an intracutaneous test for tuberculosis, 1 or 2 drops of tuberculin P.P.D. being forced to penetrate the outer layer of the skin by pressure of the six needle points of the Sterneedle.

sternoclavicular (ster″no-klah-vik′u-lar) pertaining to the sternum and clavicle.

sternocleidomastoid (ster″no-kli″do-mas′toid) pertaining to the sternum, clavicle, and mastoid process.

sternocostal (ster″no-kos′tal) pertaining to the sternum and ribs.

sternodymia (ster″no-dim′e-ah) union of two fetuses by the anterior chest wall.

sternodymus (ster-nod′ĭ-mus) conjoined twins united at the anterior chest wall.

sternohyoid (ster″no-hi′oid) pertaining to the sternum and hyoid bone.

sternoid (ster′noid) resembling the sternum.

sternomastoid (ster″no-mas′toid) pertaining to the sternum and the mastoid process of the temporal bone.

sternopericardial (ster″no-per″ĭ-kar′de-al) pertaining to the sternum and pericardium.

sternoschisis (ster-nos′kĭ-sis) congenital fissure of the sternum.

sternothyroid (ster″no-thy′roid) pertaining to the sternum and thyroid cartilage or gland.

sternotomy (ster-not′o-me) incision of the sternum.

sternum (ster′num) a plate of bone forming the middle of the anterior wall of the thorax and articulating with the clavicles and the cartilages of the first seven ribs. It consists of three parts, the manubrium, the body, and the xiphoid process.

sternutatory (ster-nu′tah-tor″e) 1. causing sneezing. 2. an agent that causes sneezing.

steroid (ste′roid) a complex molecule containing carbon atoms in four interlocking rings forming a hydrogenated cyclopentophenanthrene-ring system; three of the rings contain six carbon atoms each and the fourth contains five.

Steroids are important in body chemistry. Among them are the male and female sex hormones, such as testosterone and estrogen, and the hormones of the cortices of the adrenal glands, including cortisone. Vitamins of the D group are steroids involved in calcium metabolism. The cardiac glycosides, a group of compounds derived from certain plants, are partly steroids. Sterols, including cholesterol, are steroids. Cholesterol is the main building block of steroid hormones in the body; it is also converted into bile salts by the liver.

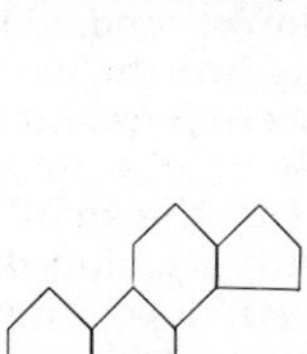

steroidogenesis (ste-roi″do-jen′ĕ-sis) production of steroids, as by the adrenal glands.

sterol (ste′rol) any steroid, e.g., cholesterol and ergosterol, having long (8–10 carbons) aliphatic side-chains at position 17 and at least one alcoholic hydroxyl group; the sterols have lipid-like solubility.

Sterosan (ster′o-san) trademark for preparations of chlorquinaldol, a bactericide and fungicide.

stertor (ster′tor) snoring; sonorous respiration, usually due to partial obstruction of the upper airway. adj., **ster′torous.**

steth(o)- word element [Gr.], *chest.*

stethalgia (steth-al′je-ah) pain in the chest or chest wall.

stethogoniometer (steth″o-go″ne-om′ĕ-ter) an apparatus for measuring the curvature of the chest.

stethoscope (steth′o-skōp) an instrument used to hear and amplify the sounds produced by the heart, lungs and other internal organs. adj., **stethoscop′ic.** As first introduced by the 19th century French physician, René Laënnec, the stethoscope was a simple wooden tube with a bell-shaped opening at one end. The modern stethoscope is binaural, with two earpieces and flexible rubber leading to them from the two-branched opening of the bell or cone. In this way, sound travels simultaneously through both of the branches to the earpieces.

stethospasm (steth′o-spazm) spasm of the chest muscles.

Stevens-Johnson syndrome (ste′venz-jon′son) a severe form of erythema multiforme in which the lesions may involve the oral and anogenital mucosa, associated with such constitutional symptoms as malaise, headache, fever, arthralgia, and conjunctivitis.

STH somatotropic (growth) hormone.

sthenic (sthen′ik) active; strong.

stibialism (stib′e-al-izm″) antimony poisoning.

stibium (stib′e-um) [L.] antimony (symbol Sb).

stibophen (stib′o-fen) an antimony-containing agent used as an antischistosomal and in the treatment of granuloma inguinale.

stichochrome (stik′o-krōm) any neuron having the stainable substance arranged in more or less regular layers.

Stieda's fracture (ste′dahz) fracture of the internal condyle of the femur.

stiff-man syndrome a condition of unknown etiology marked by progressive fluctuating rigidity of axial and limb muscles in the absence of signs of cerebral and spinal cord disease but with continuous electromyographic activity.

stigma (stig′mah), pl. *stig′mas, stig′mata* [Gr.] 1. any mental or physical mark or peculiarity that aids in identification or diagnosis of a condition. 2. [pl.] purpuric or hemorrhagic lesions of the hands and/or feet, resembling crucifixion wounds. adj., **stigmat'ic.**

stigmatization (stig″mah-tĭ-za'shun) the formation of stigmas.

stilbestrol (stil-bes'trol) diethylstilbestrol, a synthetic estrogen.

Stilbetin (stil-be'tin) trademark for a preparation of diethylstilbestrol, a synthetic estrogen.

stilet (sti'let) stylet.

Still's disease (stilz) juvenile rheumatoid arthritis.

Still's murmur (stilz) a functional cardiac murmur of childhood, heard in midsystole.

stillbirth (stil'berth) delivery of a dead child.

stillborn (stil'born) born dead.

stimulant (stim'u-lant) 1. producing stimulation. 2. an agent that stimulates.

stimulate (stim'u-lāt) to excite functional activity in a part.

stimulation (stim″u-la'shun) the act or process of stimulating; the condition of being stimulated.

stimulus (stim'u-lus), pl. *stim'uli* [L.] any agent, act, or influence that produces functional or trophic reaction in a receptor or an irritable tissue.

conditioned s., a neutral object or event that is psychologically related to a naturally stimulating object or event and which causes a CONDITIONED RESPONSE (see also CONDITIONING).

unconditioned s., any stimulus that is capable of eliciting an unconditioned response (see also CONDITIONING).

sting (sting) 1. injury caused by a poisonous substance produced by an animal or plant (biotoxin) introduced into an individual or with which he comes in contact, together with mechanical trauma incident to its introduction. (See also INSECT BITES AND STINGS.) 2. the organ used to inflict such injury.

stippling (stip'ling) a spotted condition or appearance, such as an appearance of the retina as if dotted with light and dark points, or the spotted appearance of the erythrocytes in basophilia.

stirrup (stir'up) the stapes, the innermost of the three ossicles of the ear.

stitch (stich) 1. a sudden transient cutting pain, generally in the flank. 2. a loop made in sewing or suturing.

stochastic (sto-kas'tik) arrived at by skillful conjecturing.

stoichiology (stoi″ke-ol'o-je) the science of elements, especially the physiology of the cellular elements of tissues. adj., **stoichiolog'ic.**

stoichiometry (stoi″ke-om'ĕ-tre) the science of the numerical relations of chemical elements and compounds and the mathematical laws of chemical changes. adj., **stoichiomet'ric.**

Stokes' disease (stōks) Graves' disease.

Stokes-Adams disease (stōks ad'amz) a condition caused by heart block and characterized by sudden attacks of unconsciousness, with or without convulsions; called also Adams-Stokes disease or syndrome.

stoma (sto'mah), pl. *sto'mas, sto'mata* [Gr.] 1. a mouthlike opening. 2. an incised opening that is kept open for drainage or other purposes, such as the opening in the abdominal wall for COLOSTOMY, URETEROSTOMY, and ILEAL CONDUIT. adj., **sto'mal.**

PATIENT CARE. Care of the patient with a stoma, for whatever reason it may have been created, is primarily concerned with developing in the patient an attitude of independence and freedom from restrictions on his physical, social, and recreational activities once he has been discharged from the hospital.

He will need instruction in obtaining and caring for the special appliance that is worn for the collection of body waste, fecal or urinary. Protection of the skin around the stoma is of particular concern, as is the control of odor and regulation of the flow of feces and urine. He must be aware of the complications that may develop and the signs and symptoms that should be reported to his physician.

In recent years there has been a new health care specialty developing to meet the particular needs of patients with stomas. Ostomy clubs composed of ostomates and conducted under the guidance of certified Enterostomal Therapists have been formed in many communities. At regularly held meetings the members find assistance in resolving their physical problems, and gain psychological support from one another in adjusting to their new body image. Those members of the club who have been able to adjust to their stomas are frequently available for visits to patients who are in the hospital or have just returned home after surgery.

Information about local resources available to the ostomate can be obtained from the American Cancer Society's Rehabilitation Program and from other agencies concerned with meeting the needs of patients with stomas. The United Ostomy Association, Inc., 1111 Wilshire Blvd., Los Angeles, California 90017, provides visiting services, printed material, and audio-visual teaching aids. Certified Enterostomal Therapists in a community can be located through the International Association for Enterostomal Therapy, Ravenswood Hospital and Medical Center, 4550 North Windchester, Chicago, Illinois 60640.

stomach (stum'ak) the curved, muscular, saclike structure that is an enlargement of the alimentary canal between the esophagus and the small intestine; called also gaster. (See also Plate 10.)

The wall of the stomach consists of four coats: an outer serous coat; a muscular coat, made up of longitudinal, circular, and oblique muscle fibers; a submucous coat; and a mucous coat or membrane forming the inner lining. The muscles account for the stomach's ability to expand when food enters it. The muscle fibers slide over one another, reducing the thickness of the stomach wall while increasing its area. When empty, the stomach has practically no cavity at all, since its walls are pressed tightly together. When full, the average stomach holds about $1\frac{1}{2}$ quarts.

The stomach muscles perform another function. When food enters the stomach, the muscles contract in rhythm. Their combined action sends a series of wavelike contractions from the upper end of the stomach to the lower end. These contractions, known as peristalsis, mix the partially digested food with the stomach secretions and ingested liquid until it has the consistency of a thick soup; the contractions then push it into the small intestine.

The stomach is emptied of its digested contents in 1 to 4 hours, or longer, depending upon the amount and type of food eaten. Foods rich in carbohydrates leave the stomach more rapidly than proteins, and proteins more rapidly than fats.

The stomach may continue to contract after it is empty. The contraction of the empty stomach stimulates nerves in its wall and may cause hunger pangs.

The mucous membrane lining the stomach contains innumerable gastric glands; their secretion, gastric juice, contains enzymes, mucin, and hydrochloric acid. Enzymes help to split the foot molecules into smaller parts during digestion. Mucin acts on certain sugars and also protects the mucous lining of the stomach from coarse particles and from the corrosive hydrochloric acid. Hydrochloric acid aids in dissolving the food before the enzymes begin working on it. (See also DIGESTIVE SYSTEM.)

DISORDERS OF THE STOMACH. Disturbances in the functioning of the stomach include indigestion and nausea; organic diseases include peptic ULCER and cancer.

Care given to establishing good eating habits will help to prevent stomach distress. Food should be wholesome, well prepared, and properly cooked. Heavy, fried and fatty foods, highly spiced food, too much roughage, and foods to which one has shown a sensitivity should be avoided. When nervous tension and anxiety are the underlying cause of a stomach disorder, an effort should be made to resolve the basic problems causing emotional distress.

Two common forms of gastric discomfort are belching (eructation) and heartburn. Usually belching results from swallowing air while eating, and heartburn, a burning sensation below the sternum, is thought to be caused by distention of the lower part of the esophagus, possibly from gulping food or other faulty eating habits. Both may be associated with peptic ulcer or hiatal hernia.

GASTRITIS, inflammation of the lining of the stomach, is a common disorder. It may be acute, chronic, or toxic.

SURGERY OF THE STOMACH. Surgical procedures of the stomach are most often done as treatment for malignant disease or for chronic ulcers that are complicated by hemorrhage or perforation. Surgical removal of the whole stomach is called total gastrectomy; excision of a portion of it is subtotal or partial gastrectomy. When partial gastrectomy is done, the remaining portion of the stomach is anastomosed to a loop of intestine (gastroenterostomy), usually of the jejunum (gastrojejunostomy). This is done to maintain continuity of the digestive tract. When total gastrectomy is performed, continuity is restored by an anastomosis between the end of the esophagus and the jejunum.

Another surgical procedure involving the stomach is GASTROSTOMY. This is a surgical incision into the stomach with the creation of a permanent opening to the surface of the body. Its purpose is the administration of feedings and fluids when strictures or obstruction of the esophagus makes swallowing impossible.

PATIENT CARE. Unless there is an emergency situation such as hemorrhage, the patient who is to undergo gastric surgery will have several diagnostic tests before the operation, including GASTRIC ANALYSIS, a gastrointestinal series of x-rays (see BARIUM TEST), and GASTROSCOPY.

Before the operation a Levin tube may be inserted and continuous suction used to remove gastric secretions and prevent distention. (For other routine preoperative procedures, see PREOPERATIVE CARE.)

Routine POSTOPERATIVE CARE, including observations of the patient and prevention of complications, is discussed under that heading. Immediately after surgery the patient who has undergone gastric surgery should be checked for tubes and drains that may have been inserted. In most instances the Levin tube will be left in place and suction resumed after surgery. Drainage from this tube will be dark brown at first and may be streaked with bright red blood. The color should gradually become lighter until it is a greenish yellow and the appearance of flecks or streaks of blood should diminish. If there is continued evidence of fresh bleeding the surgeon should be notified at once. The amount and character of drainage through the tube should be observed and recorded on the patient's chart every 8 hours.

Fluids by mouth are restricted until peristalsis resumes and the nasogastric tube is removed. Irrigation of the tube is done as ordered to assure proper drainage. The irrigations should be done gently and only as frequently as ordered because continuous washing can lead to excessive removal of electrolytes from the stomach. Mouth care and care of the nostrils are necessary as long as the tube is in place. Fluids are given intravenously until the patient is able to retain liquids and food by mouth.

After the tube is removed the surgeon will give written orders regarding liquids and foods permitted. Usually a very small amount of water is given at hourly intervals and the amount increased according to the patient's tolerance. Later, bland liquids and foods are added until the patient has progressed to a full diet. The hospital dietitian usually works closely with the patient in planning his diet so that when he returns home he will have well balanced meals that can be tolerated without difficulty.

Before the patient is discharged from the hospital he may be scheduled for another series of x-rays of the upper intestinal tract. This is done to observe the continuity of the digestive tract and to be sure it is functioning satisfactorily.

A group of symptoms known as the "dumping syndrome" sometimes develops after gastrectomy. They are the result of rapid emptying of gastric contents into the small intestine. These symptoms usually are mild and include palpitation, a feeling of weakness or fainting, and sweating; they may last for a few minutes or for as long as an hour. It is believed that meals high in carbohydrates and salt trigger the dumping syndrome because these substances must be diluted in the small intestine before they can be absorbed. To provide for this dilution, the jejunal loop becomes distended and fills with fluids that have shifted from the circulating blood. The symptoms produced by this condition can be relieved somewhat by limiting the intake of salt and carbohydrates and by restricting the amount of liquids taken with each meal.

When the stomach has been removed, the production of intrinsic factor, necessary for the absorption of vitamin B_{12} from the intestinal tract, is brought to a halt. This condition must be corrected by monthly injections of vitamin B_{12} for the rest of the patient's life.

cascade s., an atypical form of hourglass stomach, characterized roentgenologically by a drawing up of the posterior wall; an opaque medium first fills the upper sac and then cascades into the lower sac.

hourglass s., one shaped somewhat like an hourglass.

leather bottle s., linitis plastica.

s. pump, an apparatus used to remove material from the stomach. It consists of a rubber stomach tube to which a bulb syringe is attached. The tube is inserted into the mouth or nose and passed down the esophagus into the stomach. Suction from the syringe brings the contents of the stomach up through the tube.

A stomach pump can be used either to remove material from the stomach in case of emergency—for example, when a person has swallowed poison—or to obtain a specimen for chemical analysis, as in diagnosis of peptic ulcer or other stomach disorders.

s. tube, a flexible tube used for introducing food, medication, or other material directly into the stomach. It can be passed into the stomach by way of either the nose or the mouth. (See also TUBE FEEDING.)

A stomach tube may be employed in emergency feeding, during coma, or when patients refuse food. It is also used to dilute the contents of the stomach when a person has swallowed poison or to lavage the stomach before the contents are pumped out. Stomach tubes are also inserted to decompress the stomach when it becomes abnormally distended after certain abdominal operations.

water-trap s., a stomach with an extremely high pylorus, so that it does not readily empty itself.

stomachal (stum′ah-kal) pertaining to the stomach; stomachic.

stomachalgia (stum″ah-kal′je-ah) pain in the stomach.

stomachic (sto-mak′ik) 1. pertaining to the stomach. 2. a stimulant of gastric activity.

stomat(o)- word element [Gr.], *mouth.*

stomatalgia (sto″mah-tal′je-ah) pain in the mouth.

stomatitis (sto″mah-ti′tis) inflammation of the mucosa of the mouth. It may be caused by one of many diseases of the mouth or it may accompany another disease. Both gingivitis (inflammation of the gums) and glossitis (inflammation of the tongue) are forms of stomatitis.

CAUSES. The causes of stomatitis vary widely, from a mild local irritant to a vitamin deficiency or infection by a possibly dangerous disease-producing organism.

Inflammation may arise from actual injury to the inside of the mouth, as from cheek-biting, jagged teeth, tartar accumulations, and badly fitting dentures. Irritating substances, including alcohol, tobacco, and excessively hot or spicy food, may also cause stomatitis.

Other causes may be infectious bacteria, such as streptococci and gonococci or those causing TRENCH MOUTH, diphtheria, and tuberculosis; the fungus causing THRUSH; or the viruses causing herpes simplex and measles. Extreme vitamin deficiencies can result in mouth inflammation, as can certain blood disorders. Poisoning with heavy metals, such as lead or mercury, can cause stomatitis.

SYMPTOMS. There is generally swelling and redness of the tissues of the mouth, which may become quite sore, particularly during eating. The mouth may have an unpleasant odor. In some types of stomatitis the mouth becomes dry, but in others there is excessive salivation. Ulcerations may appear, and, in extreme cases, gangrene (gangrenous stomatitis).

Other forms of stomatitis may occasionally cause more severe symptoms, including chills, fever, and headache. Sometimes bleeding or white patches in the mouth can be seen. In thrush, the symptoms themselves may be slight (white spots in the mouth resembling milk clots) but the disease may give rise to serious infections elsewhere in the body. In some cases, stomatitis causes inflammation of the parotid glands.

Stomatitis resulting from certain diseases presents special identifying symptoms. Syphilitic stomatitis produces patches in the mouth; in scarlet fever the tongue first has a strawberry color, which then deepens to a raspberry hue; in measles, Koplik's spots appear.

TREATMENT AND PREVENTION. The treatment varies according to the cause. When the inflammation is caused by anemia, vitamin deficiency, or any infection of the body, both the underlying disease and the stomatitis are treated. Penicillin and various sulfonamide drugs often are effective against the inflammation and prevent its spreading to the parotid glands. Mouthwashes may be used under a physician's direction after he has determined the cause of the stomatitis. Gentian violet solution may be applied to the lesions of thrush; other forms of stomatitis may be swabbed with sodium bicarbonate, sodium perborate solution, or hydrogen peroxide.

With proper care, many cases of stomatitis can be prevented. Cleanliness is essential, especially of the mouth, teeth, dentures, and feeding utensils. Infants may acquire mouth infection from dirty bottles or from the mother's nipples. In the case of a prolonged fever or of any severe general illness, dryness of the mouth should be avoided by ingestion of increased amounts of fluids, particularly fruit juices.

angular s., superficial erosions and fissuring at the angles of the mouth; it may occur in riboflavin deficiency and in pellagra or result from overclosure of the jaws in denture wearers.

aphthous s., an acute infection of the oral mucosa caused by the virus of herpes simplex, with vesicle formation; called also canker sore.

gangrenous s., see NOMA.

herpetic s., an acute infection of the oral mucosa with vesicle formation, due to the herpes simplex virus.

necrotizing ulcerative s., necrotizing ulcerative gingivostomatitis.

stomatodynia (sto″mah-to-din′e-ah) pain in the mouth.

stomatogastric (sto″mah-to-gas′trik) pertaining to the stomach and mouth.

stomatology (sto″mah-tol′o-je) that branch of medicine which treats of the mouth and its diseases. adj., **stomatolog′ic.**

stomatomalacia (sto″mah-to-mah-la′she-ah) softening of the structures of the mouth.

stomatomenia (sto″mah-to-me′ne-ah) vicarious menstruation involving bleeding from the mouth.

stomatomycosis (sto″mah-to-mi-ko′sis) any fungal disease of the mouth.

stomatonecrosis (sto″mah-to-nĕ-kro′sis) gangrene of the mouth; see NOMA.

stomatopathy (sto″mah-top′ah-the) any disorder of the mouth.

stomatoplasty (sto′mah-to-plas″te) plastic reconstruction of the mouth. adj., **stomatoplas′tic.**

stomatorrhagia (sto″mah-to-ra′je-ah) hemorrhage from the mouth.

stomocephalus (sto″mo-sef′ah-lus) a fetus with rudimentary jaws and mouth.

stomodeum (sto″mo-de′um) the ectodermal depression at the head end of the embryo, which becomes the front part of the mouth.

-stomy word element [Gr.], *creation of an opening into* or *a communication between.*

stone (stōn) 1. a calculus. 2. a unit of weight, equivalent in the English system to 14 lb. avoirdupois.

stool (sto͞ol) the fecal discharge from the bowels (see also FECES).

lienteric s., feces containing much undigested food.

rice water s., the watery stool flecked with fragments of necrotic mucosal epithelium, characteristic of cholera.

stopcock (stop′kok) a valve that regulates the flow of fluid through a tube.

storage disease (stōr′ij) any metabolic disorder in which some substance (e.g., fats, proteins, or carbohydrates) accumulates in certain cells in abnormal amounts; called also thesaurismosis.

storax (sto′raks) a balsam obtained from the trunk of trees of the genus *Liquidambar;* used locally in scabies.

stosstherapy (stos′ther-ah-pe) treatment of a disease by a single massive dose of therapeutic agent or short-term administration of unphysiologically large doses.

strabismometer (strah-biz-mom′ĕ-ter) an apparatus for measuring the degree of strabismus.

strabismus (strah-biz′mus) deviation of the eye that the patient cannot overcome; the visual axes assume a position relative to each other different from that required by the physiological conditions. Called also squint. adj., **strabis′mic.** The various forms of strabismus are spoken of as tropias, their direction being indicated by the appropriate prefix, as *cyclo*tropia, *eso*tropia, *exo*tropia, *hyper*tropia, and *hypo*tropia.

During the first 3 to 6 months of life, the eyes of infants tend to waver and turn either inward or outward independently of one another; this usually corrects itself. If it persists, or if the eyes are continually crossed in the same way, even if the child is less than 6 months old, it may be a sign of strabismus. Children do not outgrow strabismus.

In an older child, a tendency to tilt the head when reading, or to close or rub one eye, may indicate crossed eyes.

Strabismus almost always appears at an early age. If not corrected, the condition may impair vision in the nonfocusing eye, as well as marring the child's appearance. In the great majority of cases the eyes can be straightened by proper medical treatment at any age, but vision of the malfunctioning eye may remain impaired. If treated early enough, preferably before 6 years, normal vision can usually be restored in the affected eye.

CAUSE. Strabismus may result from several factors, including a blow on the head, disease, or heredity. Many cases are caused by a malfunction of the muscles that move the eyes. This causes the eyes to focus differently, sending different images to the brain. As the child grows, he learns to ignore the image from one eye with the result that it fails to grow as strong as the eye on which he is depending.

TREATMENT. Treatment for strabismus varies with the individual case. A patch may be placed over the child's stronger eye for a period, forcing him to use the weaker eye and thus restoring its strength as far as possible, instead of letting it grow worse from lack of use. Eyeglasses or special eye exercises may correct the condition. In some cases, a relatively simple surgical operation on the eye muscles may be necessary. Since these muscles are outside the eye itself, there is no danger to the vision.

For further information on the functioning of the eyes, see EYE.

comitant s., concomitant s., that in which the angle of deviation of the visual axis of the squinting eye is always the same in relation to the other eye, no matter what the direction of the gaze; due to faulty insertion of the eye muscles.

convergent s., that in which the visual axes converge; esotropia, or cross-eye.

divergent s., that in which the visual axes diverge; called also exotropia and walleye.

horizontal s., that in which the visual axis of the squinting eye deviates in the horizontal plane (esotropia or exotropia).

nonconcomitant s., that in which the amount of deviation of the squinting eye varies according to the direction in which the eyes are turned.

vertical s., that in which the visual axis of the squinting eye deviates in the vertical plane (hypertropia or hypotropia).

strabotomy (strah-bot′o-me) cutting of an ocular tendon in treatment of strabismus.

strain (strān) 1. to overexercise. 2. to filter. 3. an overstretching or overexertion of some part of the musculature. 4. excessive effort. 5. a group of organisms within a species or variety, characterized by some particular quality, as rough or smooth strains of bacteria.

strait (strāt) a narrow passage.

s. jacket, straitjacket.

s's of the pelvis, the pelvic inlet (*superior pelvic strait*) and pelvic outlet (*inferior pelvic strait*).

straitjacket (strāt′jak″et) a contrivance for restraining the limbs, especially the arms, of a violently disturbed person.

stramonium (strah-mo′ne-um) dried leaves and flowering or fruiting tops of *Datura stramonium,* which contain the anticholinergic alkaloids atropine, hyoscamine, and scopolamine; used in treatment of asthma.

strangulated (strang′gu-lat″ed) congested by reason of constriction or hernial restriction, as strangulated HERNIA.

strangulation (strang″gu-la′shun) 1. arrest of respiration by occlusion of the air passages. 2. impairment of the blood supply to a part by mechanical constriction of the vessels.

strangury (strang′gu-re) slow and painful discharge of urine.

strap (strap) 1. a band or slip, as of adhesive plaster, used in attaching parts to each other. 2. to bind down tightly. (See illustration, page 958.)

Montgomery s's, straps made of lengths of adhesive tape, used to secure dressings that must be changed frequently.

stratification (strat″ĭ-fĭ-ka′shun) arrangement in layers.

stratiform (strat′ĭ-form) occurring in layers.

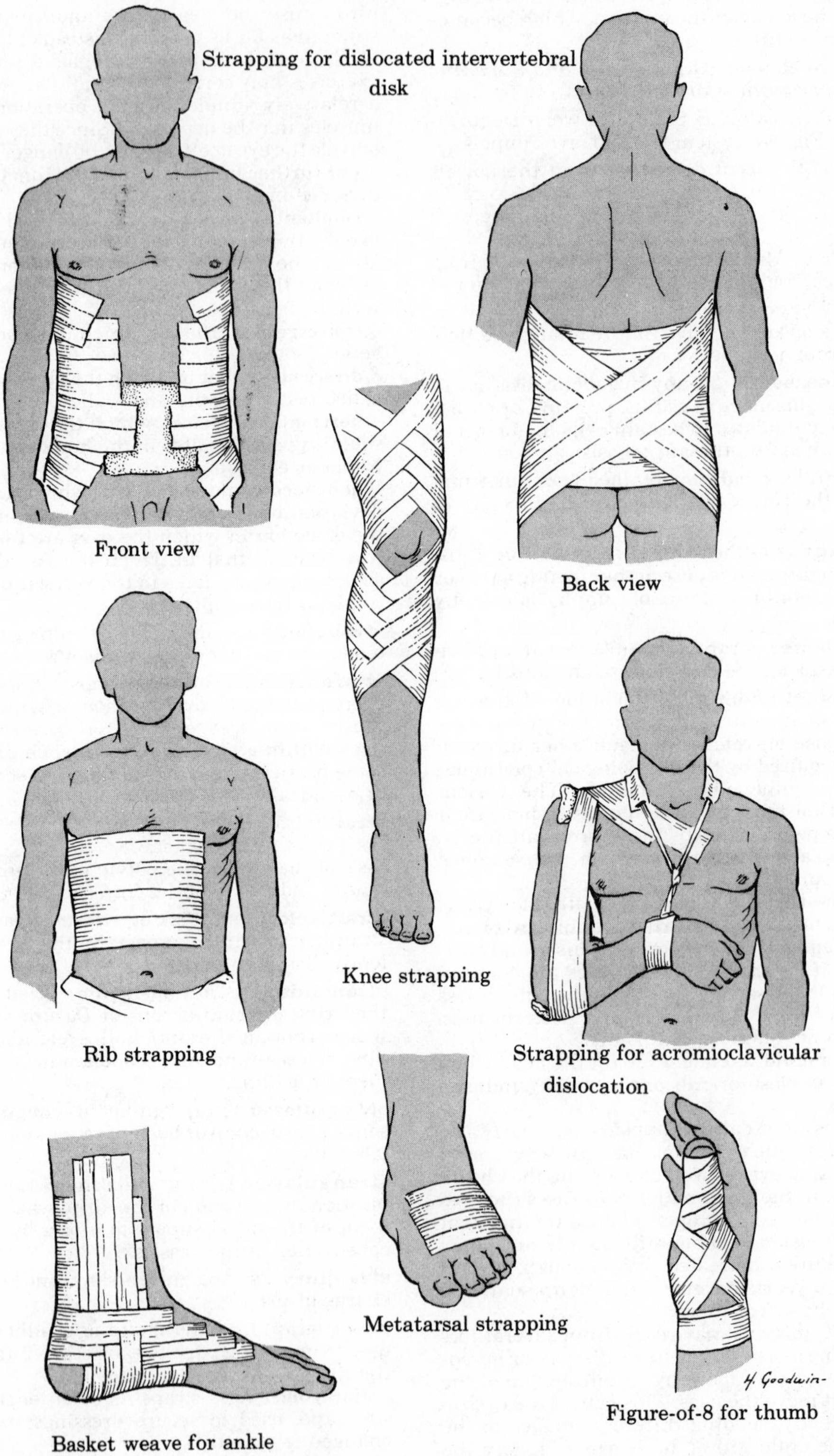

Types of strapping. (From Dorland's Illustrated Medical Dictionary. 25th ed. Philadelphia, W. B. Saunders Co., 1974.)

stratigraphy (strah-tig′rah-fe) a method of body-section roentgenography.

stratum (stra′tum), pl. *stra′ta* [L.] a sheetlike mass of tissue of fairly uniform thickness; used in anatomic nomenclature to designate distinct layers making up various tissues or organs, as of the skin, brain, retina.

s. cor′neum, the outer horny layer of the epidermis, consisting of cells that are dead and desquamating.

s. germinati′vum, 1. the basal layer and the prickle-cell layer of the skin considered together; called also malpighian layer. 2. the lower layer of the nail, from which the nail grows. Called also germinative layer.

s. granulo′sum, 1. the layer of cells between the stratum lucidum and the stratum spinosum of the skin. 2. the deep layer of the cortex of the cerebellum. 3. the layer of follicle cells lining the theca of the vesicular ovarian follicle. Called also granular layer.

s. lu′cidum, the clear translucent layer of the skin, just beneath the stratum corneum.

s. spino′sum, the layer of the epidermis between the stratum granulosum and the stratum basalis, marked by the presence of prickle cells; called also spinous layer and prickle-cell layer.

strawberry mark congenital hemangioma.

streak (strēk) a line or stripe.

angioid s's, red to black irregular bands in the ocular fundus running outward from the optic disk.

primitive s., a faint white trace at the caudal end of the embryonic disk, formed by movement of cells at the onset of mesoderm formation, providing the first evidence of the embryonic axis.

strephosymbolia (stref″o-sim-bo′le-ah) 1. a reading difficulty inconsistent with a child's general intelligence with confusion between similar but oppositely oriented letters (b-d, p-q), and a tendency to read backward. 2. a perceptual disorder in which objects are perceived as mirror images.

strepto- word element [Gr.], *twisted.*

Streptobacillus (strep″to-bah-sil′us) a genus of gram-negative bacteria.

s. monilifor′mis, an organism that causes Haverhill fever, a form of RATBITE FEVER.

streptobacillus (strep″to-bah-sil′lus), pl. *streptobacil′li.* 1. a group of rod-shaped bacteria that remain loosely attached end-to-end in long chains as a result of failure of daughter cells to separate after cell division. 2. an organism of the genus *Streptobacillus.*

streptococcal (strep″to-kok′al) pertaining to or due to a streptococcus.

s. sore throat, "strep throat," a sore throat caused by a streptococcus. The symptoms are more severe than in ordinary sore throat. There may be high fever, swelling of the glands of the neck, and a rash. Treatment is usually with penicillin or other antibiotics. (See also RHEUMATIC FEVER.)

streptococcemia (strep″to-kok-se′me-ah) the presence of streptococci in the blood.

Streptococcus (strep″to-kok′us) a genus of gram-positive bacteria. It is separable into the pyogenic group, the viridans group, the enterococcus group, and the lactic group. The first group includes the beta-hemolytic human and animal pathogens; the second and third include alpha-hemolytic parasitic forms occurring as normal flora in the upper respiratory tract and the intestinal tract, respectively; and the fourth is made up of saprophytic forms.

S. pneumo′niae, pneumococcus, the most common cause of lobar pneumonia, including some 80 serotypes distinguished by the polysaccharide hapten of the capsular substance. Called also *Diplococcus pneumoniae.*

S. pyog′enes, beta-hemolytic, toxigenic pyogenic streptococci causing septic sore throat, scarlet fever, rheumatic fever, puerperal fever, acute glomerulonephritis, and other conditions in man.

streptococcus (strep″to-kok′us), pl. *streptococ′ci* [Gr.] an organism of the genus *Streptococcus.* adj., **streptococ′cal, streptococ′cic.**

hemolytic s., any streptococcus capable of hemolyzing erythrocytes, classified as *α-hemolytic* or *viridans type,* producing a zone of greenish discoloration much smaller than the clear zone produced by the *β* type about the colony on blood agar; and the *β-hemolytic type,* producing a clear zone of hemolysis immediately around the colony on blood agar. The most virulent streptococci belong to the latter group.

streptodornase (strep″to-dor′nās) an enzyme produced by hemolytic streptococci that catalyzes the depolymerization of deoxyribonucleic acid (DNA).

streptokinase (strep″to-ki′nās) an enzyme produced by streptococci that catalyzes the conversion of plasminogen to plasmin. Streptokinase, when administered as a thrombolytic, requires detailed and skilled control to avoid hemorrhage. It also is capable of producing severe antigenic reactions upon readministration. (See also ANTICOAGULANT.)

s.-streptodornase, a mixture of enzymes elaborated by hemolytic streptococci; used as a proteolytic and fibrinolytic agent.

streptolysin (strep-tol′ĭ-sin) the hemolysin of hemolytic streptococci.

Streptomyces (strep″to-mi′sēz) a genus of bacteria, usually soil forms, but occasionally parasitic on plants and animals, and notable as the source of various antibiotics, e.g., the tetracyclines.

streptomycin (strep″to-mi′sin) an antibiotic substance produced by *Streptomyces griseus,* used chiefly in the treatment of tuberculosis.

streptonigrin (strep″to-ni′grin) an antineoplastic antibiotic produced by *Streptomyces flocculus.*

streptosepticemia (strep″to-sep″tĭ-se′me-ah) septicemia due to streptococci.

stress (stres) 1. forcibly exerted influence; pressure. 2. the sum of all the nonspecific biological phenomena elicited by adverse external influences, including damage and defense. Stress may be either physical or psychologic, or both. Just as a bridge is structurally capable of adjusting to certain physical stresses, the human body and mind are normally able to adapt to the stresses of new situations. However, this ability has definite limits beyond which continued stress may cause a breakdown, although this limit varies from person to person.

PHYSICAL STRESS. There are many kinds of physical stress, but they can be divided into two principal types, to which the body reacts in different ways. There is emergency stress, a situation that poses an immediate threat, such as a near accident in an automobile, a wound, or an injury. There is also continuing stress, such as that caused by changes in the body during puberty, pregnancy, menopause, acute and chronic diseases, and continuing exposure to excessive noise, vibration, fumes or chemicals.

The body's reaction to emergency stress is set off by the adrenal medulla. The medulla of each adrenal gland is directly connected to the nervous system. When an emergency arises, it pours the hormone epinephrine into the bloodstream. This has the effect of speeding up the heart and raising the blood pressure, emptying sugar supplies swiftly into the blood, and dilating the blood vessels in the muscles to give them immediate use of this energy. At the same time, the pupils of the eyes dilate. (See also ALARM REACTION.)

The reaction of the body to continuing stress is even more complex. Again the principal organs are the adrenal glands, but after the first phase of alarm, the glands continue to produce a steady supply of hormones that apparently increase the body's resistance. This is in addition to specific defenses such as the production of antibodies to fight infection. If the stress is overwhelming, as in the case of an extensive third-degree burn or an uncontrollable infectious disease, the third phase, exhaustion of the adrenal glands, sets in, sometimes with fatal results.

PSYCHOLOGIC STRESS. The emergency response of the body comes into play when a person merely foresees or imagines danger, as well as in real emergency situations. The thought of danger, or the vicarious experience of danger in a thrilling story, play, or film, may be enough to cause the muscles to tense and start the heart pounding. Psychologic situations can have the same effect. One of the best-known examples of this is "stage fright," often characterized by tensed muscles and an increased heart rate. At times the person may not even be aware of the unconscious thought that produces this dramatic reaction.

When stress is prolonged, the response may in fact damage the body. For example, peptic ULCER may result from prolonged nervous tension in response to real or imagined stresses in people who have a predisposition for ulcers. Such reactions to stress are discussed under PSYCHOSOMATIC ILLNESS.

The mind also responds to stress by adaptation. A healthy person can usually "get used" to situations that involve a certain amount of stress.

stress testing a technique for evaluating circulatory response to physical stress produced by exercise (see also EXERCISE TESTING).

stretcher (strech'er) a contrivance for carrying the sick or wounded.

stria (stri'ah), pl. *stri'ae* [L.] 1. a streak or line. 2. a narrow, bandlike structure; used in anatomic nomenclature to designate longitudinal collections of nerve fibers in the brain.

atrophic striae, stri'ae atroph'icae, atrophic, pinkish or purplish, scarlike lesions, later becoming white (lineae albicantes), on the breasts, thighs, abdomen, and buttocks, due to weakening of elastic tissues, associated with pregnancy (striae gravidarum), overweight, rapid growth during puberty and adolescence, Cushing's syndrome, and topical or prolonged treatment with corticosteroids.

stri'ae gravida'rum, striae atrophicae occurring in pregnancy.

stri'ae medulla'res, bundles of white fibers across the floor of the fourth ventricle.

striate, striated (stri'āt; stri'āt-ed) having streaks or striae.

striation (stri-a'shun) 1. the quality of being streaked. 2. a streak or scratch, or a series of streaks.

Striatran (stri'ah-tran) trademark for a preparation of emylcamate, a tranquilizer.

stricture (strik'tūr) an abnormal narrowing of a duct or passage.

stridor (stri'dor) a shrill, harsh sound, especially the respiratory sound heard during inspiration in laryngeal obstruction. adj., **strid'ulous.**

laryngeal s., that due to laryngeal obstruction. A *congenital* form, marked by stridor and dyspnea, is due to an infolding of a congenitally flabby epiglottis and aryepiglottic folds during inspiration; it is usually outgrown by two years of age.

striocerebellar (stri"o-ser"ĕ-bel'ar) pertaining to the corpus striatum and cerebellum.

strip (strip) 1. to press the contents from a canal, such as the urethra or a blood vessel, by running the finger along it. 2. to excise lengths of large veins and incompetent tributaries by subcutaneous dissection and the use of a stripper.

strobila (stro-bi'lah), pl. *strobi'lae* [L., Gr.] the chain of proglottids constituting the bulk of the body of adult tapeworms; considered by some to comprise the entire body, including the head, neck, and proglottids.

stroke (strōk) 1. a sudden and severe attack. 2. rupture or blockage of a blood vessel in the brain, depriving parts of the brain of blood supply, resulting in loss of consciousness, paralysis, or other symptoms depending on the site and extent of brain damage; see also CEREBRAL VASCULAR ACCIDENT.

heat s., a condition caused by exposure to excessive heat; see also SUNSTROKE.

s. syndrome, see CEREBRAL VASCULAR ACCIDENT.

stroma (stro'mah), pl. *stro'mata* [Gr.] the tissue forming the ground substance, framework, or matrix of an organ, as opposed to the functioning part or parenchyma. adj., **stro'mal, stromat'ic.**

stromuhr (strōm'oor) an instrument for measuring the velocity of the blood flow.

Strongyloides (stron"jĭ-loi'dēz) a genus of nematode parasites.

S. stercora'lis, a species found in the intestine of man and other mammals, primarily in the tropics and subtropics, usually causing diarrhea and intestinal ulceration.

strongyloidiasis, strongyloidosis (stron"jĭ-loi-di'ah-sis; stron"jĭ-loi-do'sis) infection with organisms of the genus *Strongyloides.*

strontium (stron'she-um) a chemical element, atomic number 38, atomic weight 87.62, symbol Sr. (See table of ELEMENTS.)

strophanthin (stro-fan'thin) a glycoside or a mixture of steroidal glycosides from the shrub *Strophanthus kombé;* used as a cardiotonic of rapid onset and short duration.

strophulus (strof'u-lus) a papular urticaria occurring in infants.

struma (stroo'mah) enlargement of the thyroid gland; goiter.

Hashimoto's s., s. lymphomato'sa, a progressive disease of the thyroid gland with degeneration of its epithelial elements and replacement by lymphoid and fibrous tissue.

s. **malig'na**, carcinoma of the thyroid gland.

s. **ova'rii**, a teratoid ovarian tumor composed of thyroid tissue.

Riedel's s., a chronic, proliferating, fibrosing, inflammatory process involving usually one but sometimes both lobes of the thyroid gland, as well as the trachea and other adjacent structures.

strumectomy (stroo-mek'to-me) excision of a goiter.

strumitis (stroo-mi'tis) thyroiditis.

Strümpell's disease (strim'pelz) 1. hereditary lateral sclerosis with the spasticity mainly limited to the legs. 2. polioencephalomyelitis.

Strümpell-Leichtenstern disease (strim'pel līk'ten-stern) hemorrhagic encephalitis.

Strümpell-Marie disease (strim'pel mah-re') rheumatoid spondylitis.

strychnine (strik'nīn) a very poisonous alkaloid from seeds of *Strychnos nux-vomica* and other species of *Strychnos.*

Stryker frame (strī'ker) an apparatus specially designed for care of patients with injuries of the spinal cord or paralysis. It is constructed of pipe and canvas and is designed so that one nurse can turn the patient without difficulty. The frame on which the patient lies while in the supine position is called the posterior frame; the anterior frame is used when the patient is turned on his abdomen. There are perineal openings in both frames for use of a bedpan. (See illustration.)

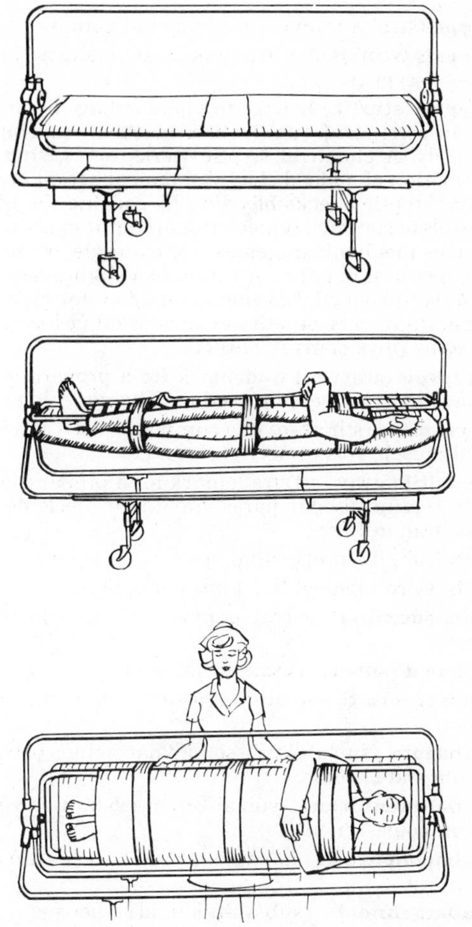

Stryker frame. (From Sutton, A. L.: Bedside Nursing Techniques. 2nd ed. Philadelphia, W. B. Saunders Co., 1969.)

S.T.S. serologic test for syphilis.

Stuart factor (stu'art) clotting factor X.

stump (stump) the distal end of a limb left after amputation.

stupe (stōōp) a hot, wet cloth or sponge, charged with a medication for external application.

stupefacient (stu″pĕ-fa'shent) 1. inducing stupor. 2. an agent that induces stupor.

stupefactive (stu″pĕ-fak'tiv) producing narcosis or stupor.

stupor (stu'por) partial or nearly complete unconsciousness; a state of lethargy and immobility with diminished responsiveness to stimulation. adj., **stu'porous.**

Sturge-Weber syndrome (disease) (sterj web'er) a congenital syndrome of nevus flammeus of the face, angiomas of the leptomeninges and choroid, and late glaucoma, frequently associated with intracranial calcification, mental retardation, contralateral hemiplegia, and epilepsy.

stuttering (stut'er-ing) a speech problem involving three definitive factors: (1) speech disfluency, most significantly the repetition of parts of words or whole words, prolongation of sounds or words and unduly prolonged pauses; (2) unfavorable reactions of listeners to the speaker's speech defect; and (3) the reactions of the speaker to the listeners' reactions, as well as to his own speech problems and to his conception of himself as a stutterer. (See also SPEECH.)

sty, stye (sti) inflammation of one or more of the sebaceous (meibomian or zeisian) glands of the eyelid; the lesion resembles a pimple. Called also hordeolum.

Hot compresses applied for 15 minutes every 2 hours may help localize the infection and promote drainage. In some cases a small surgical incision may be necessary. A mild antiseptic may be prescribed to prevent spread of the infection.

styl(o)- word element [L., Gr.], *stake; pole; styloid process of the temporal bone.*

stylet (sti'let) 1. a wire run through a catheter or cannula to render it stiff or to remove debris from its lumen. 2. a slender probe.

stylohyoid (sti″lo-hi'oid) pertaining to the styloid process and hyloid bone.

styloid (sti'loid) long and pointed, like a pen or stylus.

s. **process**, a bony projection, particularly a long spine projecting downward from the inferior surface of the temporal bone.

styloiditis (sti″loi-di'tis) inflammation of tissues around the styloid process.

stylomastoid (sti″lo-mas'toid) pertaining to the styloid and mastoid processes of the temporal bone.

stylomaxillary (sti″lo-mak'sĭ-ler″e) pertaining to the styloid process of the temporal bone and the maxilla.

stylus (sti'lus) 1. a stylet. 2. a pencil or stick, as of caustic.

stype (stīp) a tampon or pledget of cotton.

stypsis (stip′sis) 1. astringency; astringent action. 2. use of styptics.

styptic (stip′tik) 1. arresting hemorrhage by means of an astringent quality. 2. a markedly astringent remedy. A chemical styptic works by causing the formation of a blood clot by chemical action. A vascular styptic checks bleeding by causing the blood vessels to contract. A mechanical styptic causes clotting by mechanical means—for example, when one applies a bit of paper or cotton to a slight razor cut.

A styptic pencil is frequently used to stop bleeding from slight cuts. Styptics in various other forms are used by physicians in surgery.

Stypven (stip′ven) trademark for a preparation of Russell's viper venom; used as a hemostatic agent.

styramate (stir′ah-māt) a compound used as a skeletal muscle relaxant.

Suavitil (swav′ĭ-til) trademark for a preparation of benactyzine, used in parasympathetic blockade and as a tranquilizer.

sub (sub) [L.] preposition, *under.*

sub- word element [L.], *under; less than.*

subabdominal (sub″ab-dom′ĭ-nal) below the abdomen.

subacid (sub-as′id) somewhat acid.

subacromial (sub″ah-kro′me-al) below the acromion.

subacute (sub″ah-kūt′) somewhat acute; between acute and chronic.

subalimentation (sub″al-ĭ-men-ta′shun) insufficient nourishment.

subaponeurotic (sub″ap-o-nu-rot′ik) below an aponeurosis.

subarachnoid (sub″ah-rak′noid) between the arachnoid and the pia mater.

subareolar (sub″ah-re′o-lar) beneath the areola of the nipple.

subastragalar (sub″ah-strag′ah-lar) below the astragalus (talus).

subastringent (sub″ah-strin′jent) moderately astringent.

subaural (sub-aw′ral) below the ear.

subcapsular (sub-kap′su-lar) below a capsule, especially the capsule of the brain.

subcartilaginous (sub-kar″tĭ-laj′ĭ-nus) 1. below a cartilage. 2. partly cartilaginous.

subclavian, subclavicular (sub-kla′ve-an; sub″-klah-vik′u-lar) below the clavicle.

subclavian steal syndrome cerebral or brain stem ischemia resulting from diversion of blood flow from the basilar artery to the subclavian artery, in the presence of occlusive disease of the proximal portion of the subclavian artery.

subclinical (sub-klin′ĭ-kal) without clinical manifestations; said of the early stages or a very mild form of a disease.

subconjunctival (sub″kon-jungk-ti′val) beneath the conjunctiva.

subconscious (sub-kon′shus) 1. imperfectly or partially conscious, yet capable of being made conscious by an effort of memory or by association of ideas; called also preconscious. 2. the area of mental activity below the level of conscious perception.

subconsciousness (sub-kon′shus-nes) 1. partial unconsciousness. 2. the area of mental activity below the level of conscious perception.

subcoracoid (sub-kor′ah-koid) situated under the coracoid process.

subcortex (sub-kor′teks) the brain substance underlying the cortex. adj., **subcor′tical.**

subcostal (sub-kos′tal) below a rib or ribs.

subcranial (sub-kra′ne-al) below the cranium.

subcrepitant (sub-krep′ĭ-tant) somewhat crepitant in nature; said of a rale.

subculture (sub-kul′tūr) a culture of bacteria derived from another culture.

subcutaneous (sub″ku-ta′ne-us) beneath the layers of the skin.

s. **infusion**, infusion of fluids directly into the subcutaneous tissues (see also HYPODERMOCLYSIS).

s. **injection**, an injection made into the subcutaneous tissues (see also subcutaneous INJECTION).

subcuticular (sub″ku-tik′u-lar) below the epidermis.

subdiaphragmatic (sub-di″ah-frag-mat′ik) below the diaphragm.

subduct (sub-dukt′) to draw down.

subdural (sub-du′ral) between the dura mater and the arachnoid.

subendocardial (sub″en-do-kar′de-al) beneath the endocardium.

subendothelial (sub″en-do-the′le-al) beneath an endothelial layer.

subepidermal (sub″ep-ĭ-der′mal) beneath the epidermis.

subepithelial (sub″ep-ĭ-the′le-al) beneath the epithelium.

subfamily (sub-fam′ĭ-le) a taxonomic division sometimes established, subordinate to a family and superior to a tribe.

subfascial (sub-fash′al) beneath a fascia.

subfebrile (sub-feb′ril) somewhat febrile.

subgenus (sub-je′nus) a taxonomic category sometimes established, subordinate to a genus and superior to a species.

subglenoid (sub-gle′noid) beneath the glenoid (mandibular) fossa.

subglossal (sub-glos′al) below the tongue.

subgrondation (sub″gron-da′shun) depression of one fragment of bone beneath another.

subhepatic (sub″hĕ-pat′ik) below the liver.

subhyoid (sub-hi′oid) below the hyoid bone.

subiculum (su-bik′u-lum) an underlying or supporting structure.

subiliac (sub-il′e-ak) below the ilium.

subilium (sub-il′e-um) the lowest portion of the ilium.

subinvolution (sub″in-vo-lu′shun) incomplete involution; failure of a part to return to its normal size and condition after enlargement from functional activity.

subjacent (sub-ja′sent) located below.

subject (sub′jekt) a person or animal subjected to treatment, observation, or experiment.

subjective (sub-jek′tiv) perceived only by the affected individual and not by the examiner.

subjugal (sub-ju′gal) below the zygomatic bone.

sublatio retinae (sub-la′she-o ret′ĭ-ne) detachment

of the retina of the eye (see DETACHMENT OF RETINA).

sublesional (sub-le′zhun-al) performed or situated beneath a lesion.

sublethal (sub-le′thal) insufficient to cause death.

sublimate (sub′lĭ-māt) 1. a substance obtained by sublimation (1). 2. to accomplish sublimation.

sublimation (sub″lĭ-ma′shun) 1. the conversion of a solid directly into the gaseous state. 2. a defense mechanism in which an individual diverts his socially unacceptable instinctive drives into personally approved and socially acceptable channels. Mental conflicts may be resolved by this means although the person achieves only partial satisfaction of his impulses.

subliminal (sub-lim′ĭ-nal) below the threshold of sensation or conscious awareness.

sublingual (sub-ling′gwal) beneath the tongue.
s. gland, a salivary gland on either side under the tongue.

sublinguitis (sub″ling-gwi′tis) inflammation of the sublingual gland.

subluxation (sub″luk-sa′shun) incomplete or partial DISLOCATION.

submammary (sub-mam′ar-e) below the mammary gland.

submandibular (sub″man-dib′u-lar) below the mandible.

submaxilla (sub″mak-sil′ah) the mandible.

submaxillaritis (sub″mak-sĭ-ler-i′tis) inflammation of the submaxillary gland.

submaxillary (sub-mak′sĭ-ler″e) below the maxilla.
s. gland, a salivary gland on the inner side of each ramus of the lower jaw.

submental (sub-men′tal) below the chin.

submersion (sub-mer′zhun) the act of placing or the condition of being under the surface of a liquid.

submetacentric (sub-met″ah-sen′trik) having the centromere almost, but not quite, at the metacentric position.

submicron (sub-mi′kron) a colloidal particle invisible with the microscope, but visible with the ultramicroscope.

submicroscopic (sub-mi″kro-skop′ik) too small to be visible with the microscope.

submorphous (sub-mor′fus) neither amorphous nor perfectly crystalline.

submucosa (sub″mu-ko′sah) areolar tissue situated beneath a mucous membrane.

submucous (sub-mu′kus) beneath a mucous membrane.

subnarcotic (sub″nar-kot′ik) moderately narcotic.

subneural (sub-nu′ral) beneath a nerve.

subnormal (sub-nor′mal) below or less than normal.

subnormality (sub″nor-mal′ĭ-te) a state less than normal or that usually encountered, as mental subnormality, generally considered characterized by an intelligence quotient under 69.

suboccipital (sub″ok-sip′ĭ-tal) below the occiput.

suborbital (sub-or′bĭ-tal) beneath the orbit.

suborder (sub-or′der) a taxonomic category sometimes established, subordinate to an order and superior to a family.

suboxide (sub-ok′sīd) that oxide in any series which contains the least oxygen.

subpapular (sub-pap′u-lar) indistinctly papular.

subpatellar (sub″pah-tel′ar) below the patella.

subpericardial (sub″per-ĭ-kar′de-al) beneath the pericardium.

subperiosteal (sub″per-e-os′te-al) beneath the periosteum.

subperitoneal (sub″per-ĭ-to-ne′al) beneath the peritoneum.

subpharyngeal (sub″fah-rin′je-al) beneath the pharynx.

subphrenic (sub-fren′ik) beneath the diaphragm.

subphylum (sub-fi′lum), pl. *subphy′la* [L., Gr.] a taxonomic category sometimes established, subordinate to a phylum and superior to a class.

subplacenta (sub″plah-sen′tah) the decidua basalis.

subpleural (sub-ploo′ral) beneath the pleura.

subpreputial (sub″pre-pu′shal) beneath the prepuce.

subpubic (sub-pu′bik) beneath the pubic bone.

subpulmonary (sub-pul′mo-ner″e) beneath the lung.

subretinal (sub-ret′ĭ-nal) beneath the retina.

subscapular (sub-skap′u-lar) below the scapula.

subscription (sub-skrip′shun) the third chief part of a drug prescription, comprising directions to be followed by the pharmacist in its preparation.

subserous (sub-se′rus) beneath a serous membrane.

subspecies (sub-spe′shēz) a subdivision of a species; a variety or race.

substage (sub′stāj) the part of the microscope underneath the stage.

substance (sub′stans) the material constituting an organ or body.
black s., substantia nigra.
depressor s., a substance that tends to decrease activity or blood pressure.
gray s., nerve tissue composed of nerve cell bodies, unmyelinated nerve fibers, and supporting tissue; called also GRAY MATTER.
ground s., the gel-like material in which connective tissue cells and fibers are embedded.
medullary s., 1. the white matter of the central nervous system, consisting of axons and their myelin sheaths. 2. the soft, marrow-like substance of the interior of such structures as bone, kidney, and adrenal gland.
perforated s., 1. *anterior perforated substance,* an area anterolateral to each optic tract, pierced by branches of the anterior and middle cerebral arteries. 2. *posterior perforated substance,* an area between the cerebral peduncles, pierced by branches of the posterior cerebral arteries.
pressor s., a substance that raises blood pressure.
reticular s., the netlike mass of threads seen in erythrocytes after vital staining.
slow-reacting s., a substance released in the anaphylactic reaction that induces slow, prolonged contraction of certain smooth muscles. Symbol SRS or SRS-A.
threshold s's, those substances (e.g., glucose) excreted into the urine only when their concentration in plasma exceeds a certain value.
transmitter s., a chemical substance mediator that induces activity in an excitable tissue.

white s., tissue consisting mostly of myelinated nerve fibers and constituting the conducting portion of the brain and spinal cord; called also WHITE MATTER.

substantia (sub-stan′she-ah), pl. *substan′tiae* [L.] substance; used in anatomic nomenclature in naming various components of various tissues and structures of the body.

s. gelatino′sa, the substance sheathing the posterior horn of the spinal cord and lining its central canal.

s. ni′gra, the layer of gray substance separating the tegmentum of the midbrain from the crus cerebri.

substernal (sub-ster′nal) below the sternum.

substitution (sub″stĭ-tu′shun) 1. the act of putting one thing in the place of another, especially the chemical replacement of one substance by another. 2. a defense mechanism in which an individual replaces an unattainable or unacceptable goal, emotion, or motive with one that is attainable or acceptable.

substrate (sub′strāt) any substance upon which an enzyme acts.

substructure (sub′struk-tūr) the underlying or supporting portion of an organ or appliance.

subsylvian (sub-sil′ve-an) situated deep in the lateral sulcus (sylvian fissure).

subtarsal (sub-tar′sal) below the tarsus.

subtentorial (sub″ten-to′re-al) beneath the tentorium of the cerebellum.

subthalamus (sub-thal′ah-mus) a portion of the hypothalamus situated between the thalamus and the tegmentum of the midbrain. adj., **subthalam′ic.**

subtilin (sub′til-in) an antibiotic isolated from *Bacillus subtilis,* chiefly effective against gram-positive bacteria and certain acid-fast bacilli.

subtle (sut″l) 1. very fine, as a subtle powder. 2. very acute, as a subtle pain.

subtribe (sub′trīb) a taxonomic category sometimes established, subordinate to a tribe and superior to a genus.

subtrochanteric (sub″tro-kan-ter′ik) below the trochanter.

subtympanic (sub″tim-pan′ik) somewhat tympanic in quality.

subungual (sub-ung′gwal) beneath a nail.

suburethral (sub″u-re′thral) beneath the urethra.

subvaginal (sub-vaj′ĭ-nal) under a sheath, or below the vagina.

subvertebral (sub-ver′tĕ-bral) on the ventral side of the vertebrae.

subvirile (sub-vir′il) having deficient virility.

subvolution (sub″vo-lu′shun) the operation of turning over a flap to prevent adhesions.

Sucaryl (soo′kah-ril) trademark for preparations of calcium cyclamate and sodium cyclamate.

succenturiate (suk″sen-tu′re-āt) accessory; serving as a substitute.

succinate (suk′sĭ-nāt) any salt of succinic acid.

succinic acid (suk-sin′ik) an intermediate in the tricarboxylic acid cycle.

succinylcholine (suk″sĭ-nil-ko′lēn) a skeletal muscle relaxant used as the chloride salt.

succinylsulfathiazole (suk″sĭ-nil-sul″fah-thi′ah-zōl) an antibacterial agent used in infections of the intestinal tract.

succorrhea (suk″o-re′ah) excessive flow of a natural secretion.

succus (suk′us), pl. *suc′ci* [L.] any fluid derived from living tissue; bodily secretion; juice.

succussion (sŭ-kush′un) a splashing sound elicited when a patient is shaken, indicative of fluid and air in a body cavity.

Sucostrin (su-kos′trin) trademark for a preparation of succinylcholine, a skeletal muscle relaxant.

sucrase (soo′krās) β-fructofuranosidase.

sucrose (soo′krōs) a sugar obtained from sugar cane, sugar beet, or other sources; used as a food and sweetening agent.

suction (suk′shun) aspiration of gas or fluid by mechanical means.

post-tussive s., a sucking sound heard over a lung cavity just after a cough.

suctioning (suk′shun-ing) removal of material through the use of negative pressure, as in suctioning an operative wound during and after surgery to remove exudates, and in suctioning of the respiratory passages to remove secretions that the patient cannot remove by coughing.

Suctioning of the nose and mouth is a relatively simple procedure requiring only cleanliness and sensible care in the removal of liquids that are obstructing the nasal and oral passages. Suctioning of the deeper respiratory structures ("deep" and "endotracheal" suctioning) demand special skill and meticulous care to avoid traumatizing the delicate mucous membranes and introducing infection into the respiratory tree.

Another complication arising from improper tracheal suctioning is HYPOXIA, which occurs when prolonged suctioning removes the oxygen from the patient's airway and thus adds to his respiratory distress. The use of a catheter too large in diameter can cause obstruction of the bronchus and subsequent collapse of a lobe of the lung.

Because of the potential hazards inherent in the procedure, tracheal suctioning should be reserved only for those patients too weak and debilitated to cough up thick and tenacious sputum. When deep suctioning is necessary, it should be done only by those persons who are skillful in the technique and knowledgeable about the complications that can result from improper use of the suctioning equipment.

Suctoria (suk-to′re-ah) a class of protozoa (subphylum Ciliophora) whose members possess cilia only during the larval stage, the mature organism having suctorial tentacles that serve as locomotor and food-acquiring mechanisms; most are free-living, but some are parasites of other ciliates, of other protozoa, and of mammals.

suctorial (suk-to′re-al) adapted for sucking.

suctorian (suk-to′re-an) 1. any individual of the Suctoria. 2. of or pertaining to the Suctoria.

Sudafed (soo′dah-fed) trademark for preparations of pseudoephedrine, a nasal decongestant.

sudamen (soo-da′men), pl. *sudam′ina* [L.] a small whitish vesicle caused by retention of sweat in the layers of the epidermis.

Sudan (soo-dan′) a group of azo compounds used as biological stains for fats.

S. red III, a stain that colors fatty tissues red.

sudanophilia (soo-dan″o-fil′e-ah) 1. affinity for a Sudan stain. 2. a condition in which the leukocytes contain particles staining readily with Sudan red III.

sudation (soo-da′shun) the process of sweating.

sudatorium (soo″dah-to′re-um), pl. *sudato′ria* [L.] a hot air bath or sweat bath.

sudden infant death syndrome (SIDS) the sudden death, usually in its sleeping quarters, of an infant who is well or almost well prior to death and whose death remains unexplained after performance of an adequate autopsy. Called also cot, or crib, death. In the United States alone the disease accounts for around 10,000 infant deaths per year. The usual presenting picture is that of an apparently healthy baby, usually male and between the ages of two to four and a half months old, who is put to bed and is found the next morning to have died in its sleep. Disproportionate numbers of affected infants have been born prematurely, and most of them have had minor symptoms, such as a cold, shortly before death. The cause of crib death is not known. It is generally agreed that SIDS is a result of sudden interruption of a physiologic function. There is a possibility that it is caused by a malfunction in the central nervous system mechanism that controls cardiac and/or respiratory activities.

Through the efforts of the National Foundation for Sudden Infant Death, guilt and misunderstandings of the parents about the cause of their infant's death are being handled in a more sensitive and comforting way. Recent interest in research into causes of SIDS has resulted from pressure from parents and members of the national organizations concerned with child health and development. In 1974 Congress passed a bill to set up diagnostic centers throughout the country, and the National Institute of Child Health and Development now allocates more than half a million dollars annually for SIDS research. The address of the National Foundation for Sudden Infant Death, Inc., is 1501 Broadway, New York, New York 10036.

Sudeck's disease (soo′deks) post-traumatic osteoporosis.

sudomotor (soo″do-mo′tor) stimulating the sweat glands.

sudor (soo′dor) sweat; perspiration.

sudoral (soo′dor-al) characterized by profuse sweating.

sudoresis (soo″do-re′sis) profuse sweating.

sudoriferous (su″do-rif′er-us) 1. conveying sweat. 2. sudoriparous.

sudorific (su″do-rif′ik) 1. promoting sweating; diaphoretic. 2. an agent that causes sweating.

sudoriparous (soo″dŏ-rip′ah-rus) secreting or producing sweat.

suet (soo′et) the hard internal fat of the abdomen of ruminant animals.

mutton s., prepared s., the internal fat of the abdomen of sheep; used in formulating ointment bases and as an emollient.

suffocation (suf″ŏ-ka′shun) the stoppage of breathing, or the asphyxia that results from it. If suffocation is complete—that is, no air at all reaches the lungs—the lack of oxygen and excess of carbon dioxide in the blood will cause almost immediate loss of consciousness. Though the heart continues to beat briefly, death will follow in a matter of minutes unless emergency measures are taken to get breathing started again.

Suffocation can be caused by drowning, electric shock, gas or smoke poisoning, strangulation, or choking on a foreign body in the trachea. Once the cause of suffocation has been removed, the most important first-aid measure is ARTIFICIAL RESPIRATION, preferably the mouth-to-mouth technique.

FIRST AID IN CASES OF SUFFOCATION. In any emergency when breathing has stopped, have someone get help from the police, a fire department, a nearby hospital, or a physician. Meanwhile, give first aid as directed below. Artificial respiration, when called for, should be given preferably by the mouth-to-mouth method.

Drowning

1. Clear sand and other material from the mouth.
2. Give artificial respiration.

Gas Poisoning

1. Drag victim into open air.
2. Give artificial respiration.

Electric Shock

1. If victim is in contact with live wire or other electrical source, turn off electric current; if this is impossible, break contact by using a dry board or other nonconductor of electricity.
2. Give artificial respiration.

Strangulation

1. Remove whatever is causing strangulation if it is still present.
2. Give artificial respiration.

Choking on Foreign Body

1. Perform HEIMLICK MANEUVER.
2. Try to remove object with fingers or forceps.

suffusion (sŭ-fu′zhun) 1. the process of overspreading, or diffusion. 2. the condition of being moistened or permeated through.

sugar (shoog′ar) a sweet CARBOHYDRATE of both animal and vegetable origin, the two principal groups of which are the disaccharides and the monosaccharides.

beet s., sucrose from the sugar beet.

cane s., sucrose from sugar cane.

fruit s., fructose, or levulose.

grape s., dextrose.

invert s., a natural mixture of dextrose and levulose.

liver s., dextrose from the liver.

malt s., maltose.

milk s., lactose.

starch s., dextrin.

wood s., xylose.

suggestibility (sug-jes″tĭ-bil′ĭ-te) inclination to act on suggestions of others.

suggestible (sug-jes′tĭ-b′l) inclined to act on the suggestion of another.

suggestion (sug-jes′chun) 1. impartation of an idea to a subject from without. 2. an idea introduced from without.

hypnotic s., one imparted to a person in the hypnotic state.

posthypnotic s., implantation in the mind of a subject during hypnosis of a suggestion to be acted upon after recovery from the hypnotic state.

sugillation (sug″jĭ-la′shun) an ecchymosis.

suicide (soo′i-sīd) the taking of one's own life; also any person who voluntarily and intentionally takes his own life. Legally, a death suspected of being due to violence that is self-inflicted is not termed a suicide unless there is positive evidence of the victim's intent to destroy himself, or the method of death is such that a verdict of suicide is inevitable. This means that many deaths that would be termed suicide according to medicopsychological criteria are reported as accidental or from undetermined cause.

The difficulty of positively identifying a death as suicide is further complicated by the complexities of determining true intent and the psychological motivation a person may have had for ending his own life.

INCIDENCE. Statistical evidence of the actual suicide rate for a specific population is difficult to compile because of the ambiguity of the term, a lack of criteria by which a death may be judged suicidal, and a lack of agreement among those reporting deaths as to what does, indeed, constitute a suicide. In spite of these difficulties, some inferences can be drawn from the data at hand.

More males than females commit suicide, but more females than males *attempt* suicide. The actual suicide rate is higher among persons 55 to 64 years of age, whereas the suicide attempt rate is higher among those between 24 and 44 years of age. In recent years there has been an alarming increase in the incidence of suicide among university students throughout the world. In the U.S., suicide ranks third among the leading causes of death in adolescents.

Other high-risk groups include the elderly, the sick, and the mentally ill. There is a tendency of suicides to occur in families, but there is no evidence of a genetically determined suicidal behavior pattern. There are also seasonal fluctuations in the suicidal rates, with the highest number occurring in the spring.

Approximately one-third of all suicides have occurred in persons who have received psychiatric treatment. Depression is present in 95 percent of all suicidal cases, but these persons are most suicidal when they are just entering into or recovering from an attack of depression.

SUICIDAL TENDENCIES. All deeply depressed people are potential suicides. Their depression may be set off by illness or an external event, such as the death of a friend or relative, or there may be no apparent cause. However, depressed people do not always admit their suicidal thoughts; in fact, they often deny them. The suicidal impulse appears to arise in many cases from a combination of hate, rage, revenge, a sense of guilt, and a feeling of unbearable frustration. Suicide often appears to be an act of spite in which the person who takes his own life expresses toward himself the resentment he feels toward other people or the world in general. Simultaneously, he dramatically punishes himself for his own shortcomings.

Early signs of suicidal tendencies include low moods, with expressions of guilt, tension, and agitation; insomnia, early morning awakenings, requests for more sleeping pills; neglected personal appearance in one who is normally tidy; loss of weight and appetite; inability to concentrate; preoccupation with death; crumped copies of tentative suicide notes, left in wastebaskets or on desks; and heavier drinking, to give the person the courage to act.

TREATMENT AND PREVENTION. The suicidal person requires psychiatric care to relieve the depression, hostility, aggression, and other extremes of mood that cause him to contemplate taking his own life. Early recognition and treatment of mental illness, particularly depression, can do much to prevent many suicides.

The World Health Organization offers the following suggestions for prevention of suicide: (1) Availability of emergency medical services and poison control centers to prevent the fatal outcome of suicidal acts. (2) Recognition of the early signs of suicidal tendencies and prompt treatment. Any suicide threat must be taken seriously. The widespread belief that no one who talks about suicide is likely to attempt it is false. Of those who commit suicide, at least 80 percent have discussed it with someone else. (3) Special medical and social attention to high-risk groups. Measures should be taken against social isolation and neglect of those who are already suffering from a feeling of worthlessness and despair. These persons need satisfying social relations within the family and in the larger community so that they can receive continued support from others and experience a sense of self-worth and dignity.

The Save-A-Life League, founded about 1902 in New York City, and now also represented in numerous other cities throughout the United States, has helped to rescue more than 50,000 men and women from suicide. Many presuicidal people who are afraid to talk to doctors and clergymen will use this telephone service, maintained around the clock, to listen to the comforting voices of the professional "operators" until a member of the organization can visit the potential suicide and arrange for medical or psychiatric care. Other successful lay antisuicide organizations, relying primarily on telephone service, have been established throughout the world.

Sulamyd (sul'ah-mid) trademark for a preparation of sulfacetamide, a sulfonamide.

sulcate (sul'kāt) furrowed; marked with sulci.

sulcus (sul'kus), pl. *sul'ci* [L.] a groove or furrow; used in anatomic nomenclature to designate a linear depression, especially one separating the gyri of the brain.

calcarine s., a sulcus of the medial surface of the occipital lobe, separating the cuneus from the lingual gyrus.

central s., fissure of Rolando.

collateral s., collateral fissure.

sul'ci cu'tis, fine depressions of the skin between the ridges of the skin.

gingival s., the groove between the surface of the tooth and the epithelium lining the free gingiva.

hippocampal s., hippocampal fissure.

sulfa drugs (sul'fah) a group of chemical compounds used as antibacterial agents; called also sulfonamides.

sulfacetamide (sul"fah-set'ah-mīd) an antibacterial sulfonamide used in infections of the urinary tract.

sodium s., a form used topically in ointment or solution.

sulfacytine (sul"fah-si'tēn) a rapidly excreted, oral sulfonamide used in treatment of acute urinary tract infections.

sulfadiazine (sul"fah-di'ah-zēn) a rapidly absorbed and readily excreted antibacterial agent.

silver s., the silver derivative of sulfadiazine; used in the form of a cream in the treatment of burns.

sodium s., an antibacterial compound used intravenously.

sulfadimethoxine (sul″fah-di″meth-ok′sēn) a rapidly absorbed and slowly excreted antibacterial compound used in urinary tract and other infections.

sulfaethidole (sul″fah-eth′ĭ-dōl) a sulfonamide used as an antibacterial agent.

sulfaguanidine (sul″fah-gwan′ĭ-dēn) one of the sulfonamides used especially in intestinal tract infections.

sulfamerazine (sul″fah-mer′ah-zēn) a readily absorbed antibacterial sulfonamide.

sulfameter (sul′fah-me″ter) a long-acting sulfonamide, used in urinary tract infections.

sulfamethazine (sul″fah-meth′ah-zēn) an antibacterial substance.

sulfamethizole (sul″fah-meth′ĭ-zōl) an antibacterial compound used mainly in urinary tract infections.

sulfamethoxazole (sul″fah-meth-ok′sah-zōl) an antibacterial sulfonamide, especially useful in acute urinary tract infections and pyodermata and in infections of wounds and soft tissues.

sulfamethoxypyridazine (sul″fah-meth-ok″se-pi-rid′ah-zēn) an antibacterial sulfonamide used in urinary tract and other infections.

sulfamethyldiazine (sul″fah-meth″il-di′ah-zēn) sulfamerazine.

sulfamethylthiadiazole (sul″fah-meth″il-thi″ah-di′ah-zōl) sulfamethizole.

Sulfamezathine (sul″fah-mez′ah-thēn) trademark for a preparation of sulfamethazine.

Sulfamylon (sul″fah-mi′lon) trademark for preparations of mafenide.

sulfanilamide (sul″fah-nil′ah-mīd) a potent antibacterial compound, the first of the sulfonamides discovered.

sulfapyridine (sul″fah-pir′ĭ-dēn) a sulfonamide effective against pneumococci and staphylococci, but also used as a suppressant in dermatitis herpetiformis.

sulfasalazine (sul″fah-sal′ah-zēn) a combination of sulfapyridine and salicylic acid, used in the treatment and prophylaxis of ulcerative colitis.

Sulfasuxidine (sul″fah-suk′sĭ-dēn) trademark for preparations of succinylsulfathiazole.

sulfatase (sul′fah-tās) an enzyme that catalyzes the hydrolysis of sulfate esters.

sulfate (sul′fāt) a salt of sulfuric acid.

cupric s., a crystalline salt of copper used as an emetic, astringent, and fungicide. Called also copper sulfate.

ferrous s., an iron-containing compound used in treatment of iron deficiency anemia. (See also FERROUS SULFATE.)

Sulfathalidine (sul″fah-thal′ĭ-dēn) trademark for a preparation of phthalylsulfathiazole, an intestinal antibacterial.

sulfatide (sul′fah-tīd) any of a class of cerebroside sulfuric esters.

sulfhemoglobin (sulf″he-mo-glo′bin) sulfmethemoglobin.

sulfhemoglobinemia (sulf″he-mo-glo″bĭ-ne′me-ah) sulfmethemoglobin in the blood.

sulfhydryl (sulf-hi′dril) the univalent radical, —SH.

sulfide (sul′fīd) any binary compound of sulfur; a compound of sulfur with another element or base.

sulfinpyrazone (sul″fin-pi′rah-zōn) a uricosuric compound used in gout to promote excretion of uric acid.

sulfisomidine (sul″fĭ-som′ĭ-dēn) a compound closely related to sulfamethazine, used in urinary tract infections.

sulfisoxazole (sul″fĭ-sok′sah-zōl) an antibacterial compound used orally, topically, and parenterally, in infections of the urinary and respiratory tracts and of soft tissues.

sulfmethemoglobin (sulf″met-he″mo-glo′bin) a compound of hemoglobin and hydrogen sulfide.

sulfobromophthalein (sul″fo-bro″mo-thal′ēn) a sulfur- and bromine-containing compound used in liver function tests (see also BROMSULPHALEIN).

sulfonamide (sul-fon′ah-mīd) the chemical group SO_2NH_2; the sulfonamides are a group of compounds with one or more benzene rings, amino groups, and a sulfonamide group, including antibacterial drugs closely related to sulfanilamide.

sulfone (sul′fōn) 1. the radical SO_2. 2. any compound containing two hydrocarbon radicals attached to the radical SO_2.

sulfonethylmethane (sul″fōn-eth″il-meth′ān) a colorless crystalline substance, a hypnotic somnifacient.

sulfoxide (sul-fok′sīd) 1. the divalent radical =SO. 2. an organic compound intermediate between a sulfide and a sulfone.

sulfoxone (sul-fok′sōn) a dapsone derivative used in the form of the sodium salt as a leprostatic and a dermatitis herpetiformis suppressant.

sulfur (sul′fer) a chemical element, atomic number 16, atomic weight 32.064, symbol S. (See table of ELEMENTS.)

s. dioxide, a colorless, noninflammable gas, used as an antioxidant in pharmaceuticals; a dry form is used as an insecticide and rodenticide.

s. lo′tum, washed sulfur.

precipitated s., a fine, pale yellow powder; used in an ointment as a scabicide.

s. sublima′tum, sublimed s., a fine yellow crystalline powder; used as a parasiticide and scabicide.

washed s., sublimed sulfur purified by washing with water.

sulfurated (sul′fu-rāt″ed) combined with sulfur.

sulfuric acid (sul-fu′rik) an oily, highly caustic, poisonous compound, H_2SO_4.

sulph- for words beginning thus, see those beginning *sulf-*.

Sul-Spansion (sul-span′shun) trademark for a suspension of sulfaethidole, an antibacterial.

sumac (su′mak) name of various trees and shrubs of the genus *Rhus.*

poison s., a species, *Rhus vernix,* which causes an itching rash on contact with the skin (see also under POISON).

sunburn (sun′bern) inflammation—an actual burn—of the skin caused by exposure to ultraviolet rays of the sun. Depending on how severe the burn is, the skin may simply redden or it may become blistered and sore—a second-degree burn. In extreme cases there may be fever.

sunstroke (sun′strōk) a profound disturbance of the body's heat-regulating mechanism caused by prolonged exposure to excessive heat from the sun, particularly when there is little or no circulation of air. Persons over 40 and those in poor health are most susceptible to it.

The condition is called also heat stroke, a somewhat broader term that covers disorders caused by other forms of intense heat as well as those caused by the sun.

RECOGNITION. Sunstroke is not the same as HEAT EXHAUSTION, a less serious disorder in which the amount of salt and fluid in the body falls below normal. In sunstroke there is a disturbance in the mechanism that controls perspiration. Since sunstroke is much more dangerous than heat exhaustion and is treated differently, it is of the utmost importance to distinguish between the two. The first symptoms of both disorders may be similar: headache, dizziness, and weakness. But later symptoms differ sharply. In heat exhaustion, there is perspiration and a normal or below normal temperature, whereas in sunstroke there is extremely high fever and absence of sweating.

Sunstroke also may cause convulsions and sudden loss of consciousness. In extreme cases it may be fatal.

TREATMENT. In treatment of sunstroke, immediate steps must be taken to lower the body temperature, which may rise as high as 108° to 112° F. The patient should be placed in a shady, cool place and most of his clothing should be removed. Cold water is sprinkled on the patient or he is sprayed gently with a garden hose. The arms and legs should be massaged to maintain circulation.

Further treatment consists of measures to lower the body temperature, including ice packs, cold water enemas, and iced drinks by mouth. After the temperature has returned to normal, it is best for the patient to rest in bed for several days in a cool, well ventilated room.

super- word element [L.], *above; excessive.*

superalimentation (soo″per-al″ĭ-men-ta′shun) excessive feeding; sometimes used in the treatment of wasting diseases.

superalkalinity (soo″per-al″kah-lin′ĭ-te) excessive alkalinity.

supercilia (soo″per-sil′e-ah) (L., pl.) the hairs on the arching protrusion over either eye, the eyebrow.

supercilium (soo″per-sil′e-um) (L. sing.) eyebrow; the transverse elevation at the junction of the forehead and upper eyelid.

superclass (soo′per-klas) a taxonomic category sometimes established, subordinate to a phylum and superior to a class.

superego (soo″per-e′go) a part of the psyche derived from both the ID and the EGO, which acts, largely unconsciously, as a monitor over the ego. It is that part of the personality concerned with social standards, ethics, and conscience. Early in life the superego is formed by the infant's identification with his parents and other significant and esteemed persons in his life. The real or supposed expectations of these persons gradually are accepted as general rules of society and help form the "conscience." The superego tends to be self-critical and in psychotic and neurotic persons strong feelings of guilt and unworthiness can lead to self-punitive measures in an effort to resolve conflicts between the id, ego, and superego. (See also NEUROSIS and PSYCHOSIS.)

superexcitation (soo″per-ek″si-ta′shun) excessive excitation.

superfamily (soo″per-fam′ĭ-le) a taxonomic category sometimes established, subordinate to an order and superior to a family.

superfecundation (soo″per-fe″kun-da′shun) fertilization of two ova, liberated at the same time, by successive acts of coitus.

superfetation (soo″per-fe-ta′shun) fertilization of an ovum when there is already a developing embryo in the uterus; the presence in the uterus of two fetuses (but not twins) of different ages.

superficial (soo″per-fish′al) situated on or near the surface.

superficialis (soo″per-fish″e-a′lis) superficial.

superficies (soo″per-fish′e-ēz) an outer surface.

superinduce (soo″per-in-dūs′) to bring on in addition to an already existing condition.

superinfection (soo″per-in-fek′shun) a new infection complicating the course of antimicrobial therapy of an existing infection, due to invasion by bacteria or fungi resistant to the drug(s) in use.

superinvolution (soo″per-in″vo-lu′shun) prolonged involution of the uterus after delivery, to a size much smaller than the normal, occurring in nursing mothers.

superior (soo-pēr′e-or) situated above, or directed upward; in official anatomic nomenclature, used in reference to the upper surface of an organ or other structure, or to a structure occupying a higher position.

superjacent (soo″per-ja′sent) located just above.

superlactation (soo″per-lak-ta′shun) oversecretion of milk; hyperlactation.

superlethal (soo″per-le′thal) more than sufficient to cause death.

supermotility (soo″per-mo-til′ĭ-te) excessive motility.

supernatant (soo″per-na′tant) the liquid lying above a layer of precipitated insoluble material.

supernumerary (soo″per-nu′mer-ār″e) in excess of the regular number.

supernutrition (soo″per-nu-trish′un) excessive nutrition.

superolateral (soo″per-o-lat′er-al) above and to the side.

superphosphate (soo″per-fos′fāt) an acid phosphate.

supersaturate (soo″per-sat′u-rāt) to add more of an ingredient than can be held in solution permanently.

superscription (soo″per-skrip′shun) something written above; the first of four chief parts of a drug prescription, the ℞ or prescription sign ("Take thou").

supersoft (soo′per-soft) extremely soft; applied to x-rays of extremely long wavelength and low penetrating power.

supertension (soo″per-ten′shun) extreme tension.

supervoltage (soo′per-vol″tij) very high voltage; in x-ray therapy, generally considered to be in the range of 1 to 2 million volts.

supinate (soo′pĭ-nāt) the act of turning the palm foward or upward, or of raising the medial margin of the foot.

supination (soo″pĭ-na′shun) the act of assuming the

supine position; placing or lying on the back. Applied to the hand, the act of turning the palm upward.

supine (soo′pīn) lying with the face upward, or on the dorsal surface.

suppository (sŭ-poz′ĭ-to″re) an easily fusible medicated mass for introduction into the rectum, urethra, or vagina.

glycerin s., one made up of a mixture of glycerin and sodium stearate; used as a rectal evacuant.

suppressant (sŭ-pres′sant) 1. inducing suppression. 2. an agent that stops secretion, excretion, or normal discharge.

suppression (sŭ-presh′un) 1. sudden stoppage of a secretion, excretion, or normal discharge. 2. conscious inhibition as contrasted with repression, which is unconscious. 3. in genetics, restoration of a lost function by a second mutation either in a gene other than that involved in the primary mutation, or within the same gene.

suppurant (sup′u-rant) 1. promoting suppuration. 2. an agent causing suppuration.

suppuration (sup″u-ra′shun) formation or discharge of pus. adj., **sup′purative.**

supra- word element [L.], *above.*

supra-acromial (soo″prah-ah-kro′me-al) above the acromion.

supra-auricular (soo″prah-aw-rik′u-lar) above the auricle of the ear.

suprachoroid (soo″prah-ko′roid) above or upon the choroid.

suprachoroidea (soo″prah-ko-roi′de-ah) the outermost layer of the choroid.

supraclavicular (soo″prah-klah-vik′u-lar) above the clavicle.

supracondylar (soo″prah-kon′dĭ-lar) above a condyle.

supracostal (soo″prah-kos′tal) above or outside the ribs.

supracotyloid (soo″prah-kot′ĭ-loid) above the acetabulum.

supradiaphragmatic (soo″prah-di″ah-frag-mat′ik) above the diaphragm.

supraduction (soo″prah-duk′shun) sursumduction.

supraepicondylar (soo″prah-ep″ĭ-kon′dĭ-lar) above the epicondyle.

suprahyoid (soo″prah-hi′oid) above the hyoid bone.

supraliminal (soo″prah-lim′ĭ-nal) above the threshold of sensation.

supralumbar (soo″prah-lum′bar) above the loin.

supramaxillary (soo″prah-mak′sĭ-ler″e) pertaining to the upper jaw.

supraorbital (soo″prah-or′bĭ-tal) above the orbit.

suprapelvic (soo″prah-pel′vik) above the pelvis.

suprapontine (soo″prah-pon′tīn) above or in the upper part of the pons.

suprapubic (soo″prah-pu′bik) above the pubes.

suprarenal (soo″prah-re′nal) above a kidney; adrenal.

s. gland, adrenal gland.

suprarenalectomy (soo″prah-re″nal-ek′to-me) adrenalectomy; excision of one or both adrenal glands.

Suprarenin (soo″prah-ren′in) trademark for a preparation of epinephrine bitartrate, an adrenergic.

suprascapular (soo″prah-skap′u-lar) above the scapula.

suprascleral (soo″prah-skle′ral) on the outer surface of the sclera.

suprasellar (soo″prah-sel′ar) above the sella turcica.

supraspinal (soo″prah-spi′nal) above the spine.

suprasternal (soo″prah-ster′nal) above the sternum.

supratrochlear (soo″prah-trok′le-ar) above the trochlea.

supravaginal (soo″prah-vaj′ĭ-nal) outside or above a sheath, specifically, above the vagina.

supraversion (su″prah-ver′zhun) abnormal elongation of a tooth from its socket.

sura (soor′ah) [L.] calf of the leg. adj., **su′ral.**

suramin (soor′ah-min) an antitrypanosomal and antifilarial agent; used as the sodium salt.

surditas (ser′dĭ-tas) deafness.

Surfacaine (ser′fah-kān) trademark for preparations of cyclomethycaine, a surface anesthetic.

surface (ser′fas) the outer part or external aspect of a solid body.

s.-active agent, any substance capable of altering the physicochemical nature of surfaces and interfaces; an example is a detergent. Called also surfactant.

surfactant (ser-fak′tant) a surface-active agent, such as soap or a synthetic detergent. In pulmonary physiology, a mixture of lipoproteins (chiefly lecithin and sphingomyelin) secreted by the great alveolar (type II) cells into the alveoli and respiratory air passages, which reduces the surface tension of pulmonary fluids and thus contributes to the elastic properties of pulmonary tissue. (See also HYALINE MEMBRANE DISEASE.)

surgeon (ser′jun) 1. a physician who specializes in surgery. 2. the senior medical officer of a military unit.

surgery (ser′jer-e) 1. that branch of medicine which treats diseases, injuries, and deformities by manual or operative methods. 2. the place in a hospital, or doctor's or dentist's office where surgery is performed. 3. in Great Britain, a room or office where a doctor sees and treats patients. 4. the work performed by a surgeon. adj., **sur′gical.**

Surital (sur′ĭ-tal) trademark for preparations of thiamylal, an ultra–short-acting barbiturate.

surrogate (sur′o-gāt) a substitute; a thing or person that takes the place of something or someone else, as a drug used in place of another, or, in psychiatry, a person who takes the place of another in the subconscious or in dreams.

sursumduction (sur″sum-duk′shun) the turning upward of a part, especially the eyes.

sursumvergence (sur″sum-ver′jens) an upward movement, especially of an eye, the other eye not moving.

sursumversion (sur″sum-ver′zhun) an act of turning or directing upward, especially the simultaneous and equal upward turning of the eyes.

susceptibility (sŭ-sep″tĭ-bil′ĭ-te) the state of being susceptible.

susceptible (sŭ-sep′tĭ-b′l) readily affected or acted upon; lacking immunity or resistance.

suscitate (sus′ĭ-tāt) to arouse to great activity.

suscitation (sus″ĭ-ta′shun) arousal to greater activity.

suspension (sus-pen′shun) 1. temporary cessation, as of pain or a vital process. 2. a supporting from above, as in treatment of spinal disorders. 3. a preparation of a finely divided, undissolved substance dispersed in a liquid vehicle.

colloid s., one in which the suspended particles are very small.

suspensoid (sus-pen′soid) a colloid system in which the disperse phase consists of particles of any insoluble substance, as a metal, and the dispersion medium may be gaseous, liquid, or solid.

suspensory (sus-pen′so-re) 1. serving to hold up a part. 2. a ligament, bone, muscle, bandage, or sling for supporting a part.

sustentacular (sus″ten-tak′u-lar) supporting; sustaining.

sustentaculum (sus″ten-tak′u-lum), pl. *sustentac′uli* [L.] a support.

susurrus (sŭ-sur′us) [L.] murmur.

Sutton's disease (sut′onz) 1. halo nevus. 2. periadenitis mucosa necrotica recurrens.

Sutton's nevus (sut′onz) halo nevus.

sutura (soo-tu′rah), pl. *sutu′rae* [L.] suture; used in anatomic nomenclature to designate a type of joint in which the apposed bony surfaces are united by fibrous tissue, permitting no movement; found only between bones of the skull.

suturation (soo″tu-ra′shun) the process or act of suturing.

suture (soo′cher) 1. sutura, the line of union of adjoining bones of the skull. 2. a stitch or series of stitches made to secure apposition of the edges of a surgical or accidental wound; used also as a verb to indicate application of such stitches. 3. material used in closing a wound with stitches. adj., **su′tural.**

absorbable s., a strand of material used for closing wounds, which becomes dissolved in the body fluids and disappears, such as catgut and tendon.

apposition s., a superficial suture used for exact approximation of the cutaneous edges of a wound.

approximation s., a deep suture for securing apposition of the deep tissue of a wound.

buried s., one placed deep in the tissues and concealed by the skin.

catgut s., an absorbable suture, prepared from submucous connective tissue of the small intestine of healthy sheep.

cobbler's s., one made with suture material threaded through a needle at each end.

continuous s., one in which a continuous, uninterrupted length of material is used.

coronal s., the line of union between the frontal bone and the parietal bones.

cranial s., the lines of junction between the bones of the skull.

Czerny's s., 1. an intestinal suture in which the thread is passed through the mucous membrane only. 2. union of a ruptured tendon by splitting one of the ends and suturing the other end into the slit.

Czerny-Lembert s., a combination of the Czerny and the Lembert sutures.

false s., a line of junction between apposed surfaces without fibrous union of the bones.

Gély's s., a continuous stitch for wounds of the intestine, made with a thread having a needle at each end.

interrupted s., one in which each stitch is made with a separate piece of material.

lambdoid s., the line of union between the upper borders of the occipital and parietal bones, shaped like the Greek letter lambda; called also sutura lambdoidea.

Lembert s., an inverting suture used in gastrointestinal surgery.

lock-stitch s., a continuous hemostatic suture used in intestinal surgery, in which the needle is, after each stitch, passed through the loop of the preceding stitch.

mattress s., a method in which the stitches are parallel with (*horizontal mattress suture*) or at right angles to (*vertical mattress suture*) the wound edges.

purse-string s., a type of suture commonly used to bury the stump of the appendix, a continuous running suture being placed about the opening, and then drawn tight.

relaxation s., any suture so formed that it may be loosened to relieve tension as necessary.

sagittal s., the line of union of the two parietal bones, dividing the skull anteroposteriorly into two symmetrical halves; called also sutura sagittalis.

squamous s., the suture between the pars squamosa of the temporal bone and parietal bone.

subcuticular s., a method of skin closure involving placement of stitches in the subcuticular tissues parallel with the line of the wound.

Suvren (suv′ren) trademark for a preparation of captodiamine, a sedative and tranquilizer.

suxamethonium (suk″sah-mĕ-tho′ne-um) succinylcholine, a skeletal muscle relaxant.

swab (swahb) a small pledget of cotton or gauze wrapped around the end of a slender wooden stick or wire for applying medications or obtaining specimens of secretions, etc., from body surfaces or orifices.

swage (swāj) 1. to shape metal by hammering or by adapting it to a die. 2. to fuse, as suture material to the end of a suture needle.

swallowing (swahl′o-ing) the taking in of a substance through the mouth and pharynx and into the esophagus. It is a combination of a voluntary act and a series of reflex actions. Once begun, the process operates automatically. Called also deglutition.

THE THREE STAGES OF SWALLOWING. In the first, voluntary, stage of swallowing, the cheeks are sucked in slightly and the tongue is arched against the hard palate, so that the bolus, or ball of chewed food, is moved to the pharynx.

Normally, air is free to pass from the nose or mouth to the lungs and back again. But the moment the bolus approaches the fauces, the passage from the mouth to the pharynx, nerve centers are triggered that control a series of reflex actions. After one quick inhalation, breathing is halted for the brief instant of the next stage.

In this second, involuntary, stage of swallowing, the rear edge of the soft palate, which hangs down from the roof of the mouth, swings up against the back of the pharynx and blocks the passages to the nose. The back of the tongue fits tightly into the space between two muscular pillars at each side of the fauces, sealing the way back to the mouth. Simultaneously, the larynx moves upward against the epiglottis, effectively closing the entrance to the trachea.

Sometimes the larynx does not move up quickly enough and food gets into the air passage, stimulating a coughing reaction. With the one-way route to the stomach firmly established, however, the muscular coat of the pharynx contracts, squeezing the ball of food and forcing its passage into the esophagus.

In the third stage, the rhythmic contraction (peristalsis) of the muscles of the esophagus moves the food on to the stomach. The cardiac sphincter keeps the stomach entrance closed until food is swallowed. As the food approaches, moved by the wavelike contractions of the esophagus, the advancing portion of the wave causes the sphincter to relax and open, while the rear and contracting portion forces the ball of food through the entrance.

DISORDERS OF SWALLOWING. Difficulty in swallowing, dysphagia, is a symptom of most diseases of the esophagus. ACHALASIA is failure of the smooth muscles to relax sufficiently during swallowing. This disorder, found mostly in the elderly, may result in complete or partial esophageal obstruction. Acute and chronic esophagitis can produce difficulty in swallowing as can esophageal stricture. Although benign tumors of the esophagus may occur, most of them are malignant and are accompanied by progressive difficulty in swallowing.

The feeling that there is a lump in the throat or that food sticks there may also be caused by hysteria, in which case it is known as globus hystericus. It is rare and occurs most often in young girls.

The swallowing process can also be impeded by illnesses such as cerebral palsy, cerebral vascular accident, and paralysis.

In diagnosing disorders of swallowing, x-rays and ESOPHAGOSCOPY are used. Treatment may consist of a special diet, dilatation of the esophagus, or surgery. With proper care most cases can be cured; early treatment is important.

sweat (swet) the excretion of the sweat (sudoriparous) glands of the skin; PERSPIRATION. Sweating produces an evaporative cooling of the body and also serves an excretory function. Substances eliminated in sweat include water, sodium chloride, and small amounts of urea, lactic acid, and potassium ions. During maximal sweating, as in extremely hot weather, the amount of water eliminated can account for a loss of as much as 8 lb. of body weight per day.

Excessive sweating is called diaphoresis.

s. glands, the glands that secrete sweat, situated in the corium or subcutaneous tissue, and opening by a duct on the surface of the body. They are of two types: The ordinary or eccrine sweat glands are unbranched, coiled, tubular glands that are distributed over almost all of the body surface, and promote cooling by evaporation of their secretion. The apocrine sweat glands are large, branched, specialized glands that empty into the upper portion of a hair follicle instead of directly onto the skin surface, and are found only on certain areas of the body, such as around the anus and in the axilla. Called also sudoriferous, or sudoriparous, glands.

The sweat glands are innervated by cholinergic nerve fibers of the parasympathetic nervous system. They also can be stimulated by the hormones epinephrine and norepinephrine circulating in the blood.

swelling (swel'ing) 1. transient abnormal enlargement of a body part of area not due to cell proliferation. 2. an eminence, or elevation.

cloudy s., an early stage of toxic degenerative changes, especially in protein constituents of organs in infectious diseases, in which the tissues appear swollen, parboiled, and opaque but revert to normal when the cause is removed. Called also albuminoid, or albuminous, degeneration.

Swift's disease (swifts) acrodynia.

sycosiform (si-ko'sĭ-form) resembling sycosis.

sycosis (si-ko'sis) a papulopustular inflammation of the hair follicles, usually of the beard.

s. bar'bae, a staphylococcal infection and irritation of the hair follicles in the beard region. It may be associated with other superficial bacterial infections, such as impetigo or furunculosis.

The symptoms include burning, itching, and pain, with the formation of small papules and pustules that drain and form crusts. The pustules leave scars when they heal.

The condition is treated with bland hot compresses, antibiotics applied locally and administered parenterally, and manual epilation of the infected hairs. Scrupulous cleanliness and personal hygiene are necessary to prevent reinfection. Called also barber's itch, folliculitis barbae, and sycosis vulgaris.

lupoid s., a chronic, scarring form of deep sycosis barbae.

s. vulga'ris, sycosis barbae.

Sydenham's chorea (sid'en-hamz) a disorder of the central nervous system closely linked with rheumatic fever; called also Saint Vitus's dance.

The condition, usually self-limited, is characterized by purposeless, irregular movements of the voluntary muscles that cannot be controlled by the patient. The spasmodic jerking movements may be mild or severe and frequently begin as awkwardness and facial grimaces which can cause the child considerable embarassment since he has no control over them. Emotional instability and extreme nervousness usually accompany the physical symptoms.

Treatment and nursing care are based on relief of symptoms. Complete mental and physical rest are prescribed and mild sedatives such as phenobarbital or one of the tranquilizers may be given to promote relaxation. The prognosis for Sydenham's chorea is good and complete recovery is the rule.

sylvian fissure (sil'vĭ-an) a fissure extending laterally between the temporal and frontal lobes, and turning posteriorly between the temporal and parietal lobes. Called also fissure of Sylvius.

symballophone (sim-bal'o-fōn) a stethoscope with two chest pieces, making possible the comparison and localization of sounds.

symbiont (sim'bi-ont, sim'be-ont) an organism or species living in a state of symbiosis.

symbiosis (sim"bi-o'sis) 1. in parasitology, the biologic association of two individuals or populations of different species, classified as mutualism, commensalism, parasitism, amensalism, or synnecrosis, depending on the advantage or disadvantage derived from the relationship. 2. in pyschiatry, a mutually reinforcing relationship between persons who are dependent on each other. adj., **symbiot'ic.**

symbiote (sim'bi-ōt) symbiont.

symblepharon (sim-blef′ah-ron) adhesion of an eyelid(s) to the eyeball.

symblepharopterygium (sim-blef″ah-ro-tĕr-ij′e-um) symblepharon in which the adhesion is a cicatricial band resembling a pterygium.

symbolism (sim′bo-lizm) 1. an abnormal mental state in which every occurrence is conceived of as a symbol of the patient's own thoughts. 2. in psychoanalysis, a mechanism of unconscious thinking, usually of a sexual nature, whereby the real meaning becomes transformed so as not to be recognized as sexual by the superego.

symbolization (sim″bol-i-za′shun) a mental mechanism of the subconscious which consists in the representation of one object, idea, or quality by another.

symmelus (sim′ĕ-lus) a fetus with fused legs.

symmetry (sim′ĕ-tre) correspondence in size, form, and arrangement of parts on opposite sides of a plane, or around an axis. adj., **symmet′rical.**

bilateral s., the configuration of an irregularly shaped body (such as the human body or that of higher animals) that can be divided by a longitudinal plane into halves that are mirror images of each other.

radial s., that in which the body parts are arranged regularly around a central axis.

sympathectomize (sim″pah-thek′to-mīz) to deprive of sympathetic innervation.

sympathectomy (sim″pah-thek′to-me) excision or interruption of some portion of the sympathetic nervous pathway. The operation produces temporary vasodilation leading to improved nutrition of the part supplied by the vessel. It is done in cases of partial arterial obstruction with resultant trophic changes distally.

chemical s., the interruption of the transmission of impulses through a sympathetic nerve by chemical agents.

periarterial s., surgical removal of the sheath of an artery containing the sympathetic nerve fibers; it produces temporary vasodilation.

sympathetic (sim″pah-thet′ik) 1. pertaining to or caused by sympathy. 2. pertaining to the sympathetic nervous system.

s. blockade, block of nerve impulse transmission between a preganglionic sympathetic fiber and the ganglion cell.

s. nerves, 1. see SYMPATHETIC TRUNK. 2. any nerve of the sympathetic nervous system.

s. nervous system, the thoracolumbar part of the autonomic NERVOUS SYSTEM, the preganglionic fibers of which arise from cell bodies in the thoracic and first three lumbar segments of the spinal cord; postganglionic fibers are distributed to the heart, smooth muscle, and glands of the entire body. (See also Plate 14.)

s. trunk, two long ganglionated nerve strands, one on each side of the vertebral column, extending from the base of the skull to the coccyx.

sympathicoblast (sim-path′ĭ-ko-blast″) an embryonic cell that develops into sympathetic nerve cell.

sympathicoblastoma (sim-path″ĭ-ko-blas-to′mah) a malignant tumor containing sympathicoblasts.

sympathicolytic (sim-path″ĭ-ko-lit′ik) sympatholytic.

sympathicomimetic (sim-path″ĭ-ko-mi-met′ik) sympathomimetic.

sympathicotonia (sim-path″ĭ-ko-to′ne-ah) a stimulated condition of the sympathetic nervous system marked by vascular spasm, heightened blood pressure, and the dominance of other sympathetic functions. adj., **sympathicoton′ic.**

sympathicotripsy (sim-path″ĭ-ko-trip′se) surgical crushing of a nerve, ganglion, or plexus of the sympathetic nervous system.

sympathicotropic (sim-path″ĭ-ko-trop′ik) 1. having affinity for or exerting its principal effect on the sympathetic nervous system. 2. an agent with such properties.

sympathicus (sim-path′ĭ-kus) the sympathetic nervous system.

sympathin (sim′pah-thin) a neurohormonal mediator of nerve impulses at sympathetic nerve synapses; the term is used only when the nature of the mediator is unknown.

sympathism (sim′pah-thizm) suggestibility.

sympathoblast (sim-path′o-blast) sympathicoblast.

sympathoblastoma (sim″pah-tho-blast-to′mah) sympathicoblastoma.

sympathogonia (sim″pah-tho-go′ne-ah), sing. *sympathogo′nium* [Gr.] undifferentiated embryonic cells which develop into sympathetic cells.

sympathogonioma (sim″pah-tho-go″ne-o′ma) a tumor composed of sympathogonia.

sympathogonium (sim″pah-tho-go′ne-um), pl. *sympathogo′nia* [Gr.] an embryonic cell that develops into a sympathetic cell.

sympatholytic (sim″pah-tho-lit′ik) antiadrenergic: blocking transmission of impulses from the adrenergic (sympathetic) postganglionic fibers to effector organs or tissues, inhibiting such sympathetic functions as smooth muscle contraction and glandular secretion. Also, an agent that produces such an effect.

sympathomimetic (sim″pah-tho-mi-met′ik) adrenergic: producing effects resembling those of impulses transmitted by the postganglionic fibers of the sympathetic nervous system. Also, an agent that produces such an effect.

sympathy (sim′pah-the) 1. an influence produced in any organ by disease or disorder in another part. 2. compassion for another's grief or loss. 3. the influence exerted by one individual upon another, or received by one from another, and the effects thus produced, as in hypnotism or in yawning.

symphalangism (sim-fal′an-jizm) congenital ankylosis of the proximal phalangeal joints.

symphyseal, symphysial (sim-fiz′e-al) pertaining to a symphysis.

symphysiorrhaphy (sim-fiz″e-or′ah-fe) suture of a divided symphysis.

symphysiotomy (sim-fiz″e-ot′o-me) division of the symphysis pubis to facilitate delivery.

symphysis (sim′fĭ-sis), pl. *sym′physes* [Gr.] a site or line of union; a type of joint in which the apposed bony surfaces are firmly united by a plate of fibrocartilage.

pubic s., s. pu′bis, the line of union of the bodies of the pubic bones in the median plane.

sympodia (sim-po′de-ah) fusion of the lower extremities.

symptom (simp′tom) any indication of disease perceived by the patient.

cardinal s's, 1. symptoms of greatest significance to the physician, establishing the identity of the illness. 2. the symptoms shown in the temperature, pulse, and respiration.

dissociation s., anesthesia to pain and to heat and cold, without impairment of tactile sensibility.

objective s., one perceptible to others than the patient, as pallor, rapid pulse or respiration, restlessness, and the like.

presenting s., the symptom or group of symptoms about which the patient complains or from which he seeks relief.

signal s., a sensation, aura, or other subjective experience indicative of an impending epileptic or other seizure.

subjective s., one perceptible only to the patient, as pain, pruritus, vertigo, and the like.

withdrawal s's, symptoms which follow sudden abstinence from a drug on which a person is dependent (see also WITHDRAWAL SYMPTOMS).

symptomatic (simp″to-mat′ik) 1. pertaining to or of the nature of a symptom. 2. indicative (of a particular disease or disorder). 3. exhibiting the symptoms of a particular disease but having a different cause. 4. directed at the allaying of symptoms, as symptomatic treatment.

symptomatology (simp″to-mah-tol′o-je) 1. the branch of medicine dealing with symptoms. 2. the combined symptoms of a disease.

symptomatolytic (simp″to-mah″to-lit′ik) causing the disappearance of symptoms.

sympus (sim′pus) a fetus with feet and legs fused.

syn- word element [Gr.], *union; association.*

Synalar (sin′ah-lar) trademark for a preparation of fluocinolone acetonide, a steroid used as a topical anti-inflammatory agent.

synapse (sin′aps) the functional junction between two neurons, where a nerve impulse is transmitted from one neuron to another (see also NEURON).

axodendritic s., one between the axon of one neuron and the dendrites of another.

axodendrosomatic s., one between the axon of one neuron and the dendrites and body of another.

axosomatic s., one between the axon of one neuron and the body of another.

synapsis (sĭ-nap′sis) the pairing off and union of homologous chromosomes from male and female pronuclei at the start of meiosis.

synaptic (sĭ-nap′tik) pertaining to a synapse or to a synpasis.

synarthrodia (sin″ar-thro′de-ah) synarthrosis. adj., **synarthro′dial.**

synarthrophysis (sin″ar-thro-fi′sis) any ankylosing process.

synarthrosis (sin″ar-thro′sis), pl. *synarthro′ses* [Gr.] a form of joint in which the bony elements are united by continuous intervening fibrous tissue; called also fibrous joint.

syncanthus (sin-kan′thus) adhesion of the eyeball to the orbital structures.

syncephalus (sin-sef′ah-lus) a twin monster with heads fused into one, there being a single face, with four ears.

synchilia (sin-ki′le-ah) cogenital adhesion of the lips.

synchiria (sin-ki′re-ah) reference of sensation to the opposite side on application of a stimulus.

synchondrosis (sin″kon-dro′sis), pl. *synchondro′ses* [Gr.] a type of cartilaginous joint in which the cartilage is usually converted into bone before adult life.

synchondrotomy (sin″kon-drot′o-me) division of a synchondrosis.

synchronism (sin′kro-nizm) occurrence at the same time.

synchronous (sing′kro-nus) occurring at the same time.

synchysis (sin′kĭ-sis) a softening or fluid condition of the vitreous body of the eye.

s. scintil′lans, floating cholesterol crystals in the vitreous, developing as a secondary degenerative change.

synclitism (sin′klĭ-tizm) parallelism between the planes of the fetal head and those of the maternal pelvis. adj., **synclit′ic.**

synclonus (sin′klo-nus) muscular tremor or successive clonic contraction of various muscles together.

syncope (sing′ko-pe) a temporary suspension of consciousness due to cerebral anemia; fainting. adj. **syn′copal, syncop′ic.**

laryngeal s., tussive s., brief loss of consciousness associated with paroxysms of coughing.

vasovagal s., vasovagal attack.

Syncurine (sin′ku-rēn) trademark for a preparation of decamethonium, a muscle relaxant.

syncytioma (sin-sit″e-o′mah) syncytial endometritis.

s. malig′num, choriocarcinoma.

syncytiotrophoblast (sin-sit″e-o-trof′o-blast) the outer syncytial layer of the trophoblast.

syncytium (sin-sish′e-um) a multinucleate mass of protoplasm produced by the merging of cells. adj., **syncyt′ial.**

syndactyly (sin-dak′tĭ-le) the most common congenital anomaly of the hand, marked by the persistence of the webbing between adjacent digits, so they are more or less completely attached; generally considered an inherited condition, the anomaly may also occur in the foot.

syndectomy (sin-dek′to-me) peritectomy.

syndesis (sin′dĕ-sis) 1. arthrodesis. 2. synapsis.

syndesm(o)- word element [Gr.], *connective tissue; ligament.*

syndesmectomy (sin″des-mek′to-me) excision of a portion of ligament.

syndesmitis (sin″des-mi′tis) 1. inflammation of a ligament. 2. conjunctivitis.

syndesmography (sin″des-mog′rah-fe) a description of the ligaments.

syndesmology (sin″des-mol′o-je) scientific study of the ligaments and joints.

syndesmoma (sin″des-mo′mah) a tumor of connective tissue.

syndesmoplasty (sin-des′mo-plas″te) plastic repair of a ligament.

syndesmosis (sin″des-mo′sis), pl. *syndesmo′ses* [Gr.] a joint in which the bones are united by fibrous connective tissue forming an interosseous membrane or ligament.

syndesmotomy (sin″des-mot′o-me) incision of a ligament.

syndrome (sin′drōm) a combination of symptoms

resulting from a single cause or so commonly occurring together as to constitute a distinct clinical picture. For specific syndromes, see under the specific name, as ADRENOGENITAL SYNDROME.

syndromic (sin-drom′ik) occurring as a syndrome.

Syndrox (sin′droks) trademark for preparations of methamphetamine, a central nervous system stimulant.

synechia (sĭ-nek′e-ah), pl. *synech′iae* [Gr.] adhesion, as of the iris to the cornea or the lens.

annular s., adhesion of the whole rim of the iris to the lens.

anterior s., adhesion of the iris to the cornea.

posterior s., adhesion of the iris to the capsule of the lens or to the surface of the vitreous body.

total s., adhesion of the whole surface of the iris to the lens.

s. vul′vae, a congenital condition in which the labia minora are sealed in the midline, with only a small opening below the clitoris through which urination and menstruation may occur.

synechotomy (sin″ĕ-kot′o-me) incision of a synechia.

synencephalocele (sin″en-sef′ah-lo-sēl″) encephalocele with adhesions to adjoining parts.

syneresis (sĭ-ner′ĕ-sis) a drawing together of the particles of the disperse phase of a gel, with separation of some of the disperse medium and shrinkage of the gel, such as occurs in the clotting of blood.

synergism (sin′er-jizm) the joint action of agents so that their combined effect is greater than the algebraic sum of their individual parts. adj., **synergist′ic.**

synergist (sin′er-jist) an agent that acts with or enhances the action of another.

synergy (sin′er-je) correlated action or cooperation by two or more structures or drugs.

synesthesia (sin″es-the′ze-ah) a secondary sensation accompanying an actual perception; the experiencing of a sensation in one place, due to stimulation applied to another place; also, the condition in which a stimulus of one sense is perceived as sensation of a different sense, as when a sound produces a sensation of color.

synesthesialgia (sin″es-the″ze-al′je-ah) a condition in which a stimulus produces pain on the affected side but no sensation on the normal side of the body.

syngamy (sing′gah-me) a method of reproduction in which two individuals (gametes) unite permanently and their nuclei fuse; sexual reproduction.

syngeneic (sin″jen-e′ik) in transplantation biology, denoting individuals or tissues having identical genotypes, i.e., identical twins or animals of the same inbred strain, or their tissues. Called also isogeneic.

syngenesis (sin-jen′ĕ-sis) 1. the origin of an individual from a germ derived from both parents and not from either one alone. 2. the state of having descended from a common ancestor.

synkaryon (sin-kar′e-on) a nucleus formed by fusion of two pronuclei, the fertilization nucleus.

Synkayvite (sin′ka-vit) trademark for preparations of menadiol sodium diphosphate, a vitamin K preparation.

synkinesis (sin″ki-ne′sis) an associated movement; an unintentional movement accompanying a volitional movement. adj., **synkinet′ic.**

synnecrosis (sin″nĕ-kro′sis) symbiosis in which the relationship between populations (or individuals) is mutually detrimental.

synophthalmus (sin″of-thal′mus) cyclops.

Synophylate (sin″o-fi′lāt) trademark for preparations of theophylline sodium glycinate, a smooth muscle relaxant and diuretic.

synorchidism (sin-or′kĭ-dizm) synorchism.

synorchism (sin′or-kizm) congenital fusion of the testes into one mass.

synoscheos (sin-os′ke-os) adhesion between the penis and scrotum.

synosteotomy (sin″os-te-ot′o-me) dissection of the joints.

synostosis (sin″os-to′sis), pl. *synosto′ses* [Gr.] normal or abnormal union of two bones by osseous material. adj., **synostot′ic.**

synotia (sĭ-no′she-ah) a developmental anomaly with fusion of the ears, or their location near the midventral line in the upper part of the neck.

synotus (sĭ-no′tus) a fetus exhibiting synotia.

synovectomy (sin″o-vek′to-me) excision of a synovial membrane, as of that lining the capsule of the knee joint.

synovia (sĭ-no′ve-ah) synovial fluid; the transparent viscid fluid secreted by the synovial membrane and found in joint cavities, bursae, and tendon sheaths.

synovial (sĭ-no′ve-al) of, pertaining to, or secreting synovia.

s. fluid, synovia.

s. joint, a specialized form of articulation permitting more or less free movement, the union of the bony elements being surrounded by an articular capsule enclosing a cavity lined by synovial membrane; called also diarthrosis.

s. membrane, the inner of the two layers of the articular capsule of a synovial joint; composed of loose connective tissue and having a free smooth surface that lines the joint cavity; it secretes the synovia.

s. villi, slender projections from the surface of the synovial membrane into the cavity of a joint.

synovialis (sĭ-no″ve-a′lis) synovial.

synovialoma, synovioma (sĭ-no″ve-ah-lo′mah; sĭ-no″ve-o′mah) a tumor of synovial membrane origin.

synovitis (sin″o-vi′tis) inflammation of a synovial membrane, usually painful, particularly on motion, and characterized by fluctuating swelling, due to effusion in a synovial sac. It may be caused by rheumatic fever, rheumatoid arthritis, tuberculosis, trauma, gout, etc.

dry s., synovitis with little effusion.

purulent s., synovitis with effusion of pus in a synovial sac.

serous s., synovitis with copious nonpurulent effusion.

s. sic′ca, dry synovitis.

simple s., synovitis with clear or slightly turbid effusion.

tendinous s., inflammation of a tendon sheath.

synovium (sĭ-no′ve-um) a synovial membrane.

synthase (sin′thās) any enzyme, especially a lyase, which catalyzes a synthesis that does not involve the breakdown of a pyrophosphate bond, as opposed to *synthetase.*

synthesis (sin′thĕ-sis) 1. creation of a compound by

union of elements composing it, done artificially or as a result of natural processes. 2. the process of bringing back into consciousness activities or experiences that have become split off or disassociated. adj., synthet'ic.

synthesize (sin'thĕ-sīz") to produce by synthesis.

synthetase (sin'thĕ-tās) ligase; any of a class of enzymes that catalyze the joining together of two molecules coupled with the breakdown of a pyrophosphate bond in ATP or a similar triphosphate.

Synthroid (sin'throid) trademark for a preparation of sodium levothyroxine, used for replacement therapy in hypothyroidism.

Syntocinon (sin-to'sĭ-non) trademark for a solution of synthetic oxytocin, a uterine stimulant.

syntonic (sin-ton'ik) pertaining to a stable, integrated personality.

Syntropan (sin'tro-pan) trademark for a preparation of amprotropine phosphate, an anticholinergic.

syntrophoblast (sin-trof'o-blast) syncytiotrophoblast.

syntropic (sin-trop'ik) 1. turning or pointing in the same direction. 2. denoting correlation of several factors, as the relation of one disease to the development or incidence of another. 3. pertaining to a well-balanced personality.

syntropy (sin'tro-pe) the state of being syntropic.

syphilid (sif'ĭ-lid) any cutaneous lesion of syphilitic origin. It may be macular, papular, pustular, or, in tertiary syphilis, a gumma.

syphilis (sif'ĭ-lis) a contagious venereal disease leading to many structural and cutaneous lesions; called also lues.

Syphilis is caused by a spiral-shaped bacterium (spirochete), *Treponema pallidum.* It is transmitted primarily by coitus. The spirochetes enter the body through a break or abrasion of the skin or a mucous membrane. Since the bacteria can live only for a few minutes outside the body, the disease is seldom spread by contact with drinking or eating utensils previously used by a syphilitic person. It is never contracted from toilet seats.

Syphilis can be readily and completely cured, but if it is untreated or treated improperly, it can cause widespread damage. It is not hereditary but can be transmitted by an affected woman to her unborn child.

PRIMARY SYPHILIS. Within a few hours after the spirochetes penetrate the skin or a mucous membrane, they enter the bloodstream, and usually in about a week they spread throughout the body.

The first sign of primary syphilis is a painless sore, called a chancre, that appears 9 days to 3 months—usually 3 weeks—after infection. Usually firm or hard, the chancre may resemble a blister, pimple, or ulcerated open sore. In men, it appears usually on or near the head of the penis. In women, the chancre is commonly found on the labia, but it may be concealed inside the vagina, where it may not be felt or seen. Chancres sometimes develop elsewhere, such as on the lips of the mouth, a breast, or a finger. They also may appear in the anal region. The nearby lymph nodes become hard and swollen.

When the material from a chancre is examined under a microscope, the organism may be identified. Blood tests for syphilis, such as the Wassermann test and the Kahn test, may fail to detect the disease during this early stage.

Even though no treatment is given, the chancre will disapper in 10 to 40 days, often leading to the false conclusion that the disease is cured. Occasionally a chancre fails to develop or is too small to be noticed.

Primary syphilis can be cured with penicillin in adequate doses and other antibiotics, such as tetracycline.

SECONDARY SYPHILIS. Two to six months after the primary sore disappears, the secondary stage of syphilis begins; it may last up to 2 years.

A rash is usually one of the first symptoms. It may cover any part of the body and often spreads over the entire skin surface, including the palms and soles. It does not itch and may resemble the rash of measles as well as of many other diseases. It can be identified positively as a symptom of syphilis only by a blood test.

During secondary syphilis, thin white sores may appear on the mucosa of the mouth and throat and around the genitalia and rectum. Headache, fever, and a general feeling of illness are common. Hair may fall out in patches, bones and joints may be painful, and anemia may develop. Sometimes the eyes are affected.

Syphilis is highly contagious in this stage and of great danger to others. If mouth sores are present, the disease may be spread by kissing.

Like primary syphilis, the secondary stage disappears by itself, generally within 3 to 12 weeks, but may return later if the organisms are still present. As in the primary stage, the disease can be cured in the secondary stage by the use of penicillin or other antibiotics.

Together, the primary and secondary stages are known as "early syphilis."

TERTIARY SYPHILIS. The third, or tertiary, stage of the disease is known as "late syphilis." Its symptoms may develop soon after the secondary symptoms have vanished or they may lie hidden for 15 or more years. A person may be unaware that he has the disease. Even a blood test may be negative.

Late syphilis is less contagious to others but is extremely dangerous to the person who has it. It may be fatal, particularly if the central nervous system or heart is affected. The spirochete can invade any cell of the body and can damage any organ or structure of the body, including the internal organs, bones, joints, and skin. The characteristic lesion of tertiary syphilis is a soft gummy tumor called a gumma.

If late syphilis attacks the heart, aorta, or aortic valve, death may result from rupture of the weakened aorta or from heart failure. When it attacks the central nervous system, general paresis, a severe disease of the brain, may result; if not treated promptly, it will cause insanity and death. Another serious disorder of the nervous system caused by late syphilis is TABES DORSALIS, or locomotor ataxia, in which there is pain and loss of position sense.

Blindness may result if the infection involves the eyes. Other possible effects are deep ulcers on the legs or elsewhere, chronic inflammation of the bones, which is especially painful at night, and perforation of the soft palate.

Cure of late or tertiary syphilis takes longer and is more difficult than that of primary or secondary syphilis. Sometimes the disease cannot be completely cured. As with early syphilis, however, it may be successfully treated with penicillin and other antibiotics.

CONGENITAL SYPHILIS. Congenital syphilis is transmitted from a diseased mother to her unborn child through the placenta. Often this results in spontaneous abortion or stillbirth.

If the infant is born alive, he may have snuffles, caused by inflammation of the nose, and may be generally weak and sickly. Syphilitic rashes, especially in the genital area, may occur when the baby is 3 to 8 weeks old. Children with congenital syphilis are often born deformed, and may become blind, deaf, paralyzed, or insane.

To prevent congenital syphilis all pregnant women should have a blood test for syphilis during the early months of pregnancy. Treatment before the fifth month will always prevent infection of the unborn child. A syphilitic mother who is not treated early has only one chance in six of having a healthy child. If a child is born with syphilis, immediate treatment may be effective if the disease has not progressed too far.

BLOOD TESTS. Since a person infected with syphilis may not show all or even any of the symptoms of the first, second, or third stages of the disease, a routine blood test for syphilis becomes necessary for detection. The best known are the Wassermann test and the Kahn test.

There is no immunization against syphilis at present, but since the disease, if diagnosed and treated early, can be cured with penicillin and other antibiotics, it is advisable to have blood tests for syphilis during routine checkups. The genitalia and rectum should be examined periodically if exposure has occurred. Most states require a blood test for syphilis before marriage.

PREVENTION. The surest method of prevention is the avoidance of exposure to persons who may be infected with syphilis. Those who fail to heed such advice should at least follow recommended precautionary measures—use a rubber condom during the entire sexual act and the thorough cleansing of genitalia and surrounding parts with soap and water afterward.

In large measure, syphilis can be prevented and controlled through education. Educational campaigns have been effective in reducing the number of cases of syphilis, but the disease is still widespread.

nonvenereal s., a chronic treponemal infection mainly seen in children, occurring in many areas of the world, caused by an organism indistinguishable from *Treponema pallidum,* and transmitted by direct nonsexual contact and indirectly by common use of table and drinking utensils. The first lesions are usually oral mucous patches; subsequent lesions are concentrated in the axillae, inguinal region, and rectum. Then, after a latent period, there develop destructive lesions of the skin and bones.

syphilitic (sif″ĭ-lit′ik) affected with, caused by, or pertaining to syphilis.

syphiloderm (sif′ĭ-lo-derm″) syphilid.

syphilogenesis (sif″ĭ-lo-jen′ĕ-sis) the development of syphilis.

syphiloid (sif′ĭ-loid) 1. resembling syphilis. 2. a disease like syphilis.

syphilologist (sif″ĭ-lol′o-jist) a specialist in syphilology.

syphilology (sif″ĭ-lol′o-je) the sum of knowledge about syphilis, its pathology and treatment.

syphiloma (sif″ĭ-lo′mah) a tumor of syphilitic origin; a gumma.

syphilophyma (sif″ĭ-lo-fi′mah) any syphilitic growth or excrescence.

syring(o)- word element [Gr.], *tube; fistula.*

syringe (sir′inj) an instrument for introducing fluids into or withdrawing them from the body.

hypodermic s., one for introduction of liquids through a hollow needle into subcutaneous tissues.

syringectomy (sir″in-jek′to-me) excision of a fistula.

syringitis (sir″in-ji′tis) inflammation of the eustachian tube.

syringoadenoma (sĭ-ring″go-ad″ĕ-no′mah) syringocystadenoma.

syringobulbia (sĭ-ring″go-bul′be-ah) the presence of fluid-filled cavities in the medulla oblongata and pons.

syringocarcinoma (si-ring″go-kar″sĭ-no′mah) cancer of a sweat gland.

syringocele (sĭ-ring′go-sēl) a cavity-containing herniation of the spinal cord through the bony defect in spina bifida.

syringocoele (sĭ-ring′go-sēl) the central canal of the spinal cord.

syringocystadenoma (sĭ-ring″go-sist″ad-ĕ-no′mah) adenoma of the sweat glands; called also hidradenoma.

syringocystoma (sĭ-ring″go-sis-to′mah) a cystic tumor of a sweat gland.

syringoma (sir″ing-go′mah) syringocystadenoma.

syringomeningocele (sĭ-ring″go-mĕ-ning′go-sēl) meningocele resembling syringomyelocele.

syringomyelia (sĭ-ring″go-mi-e′le-ah) the presence of fluid-filled cavities in the substance of the spinal cord, with destruction of nerve tissue.

syringomyelitis (sĭ-ring″go-mi″ĕ-li′tis) inflammation of the spinal cord with the formation of cavities.

syringomyelocele (si-ring″go-mi′ĕ-lo-sēl″) hernial protrusion of the spinal cord through the bony defect in spina bifida, the mass containing a cavity connected with the central canal of the spinal cord.

syringotomy (sir″ing-got′o-me) incision of a fistula.

syrinx (sir′inks) a tube or pipe; a fistula.

syrosingopine (si″ro-sing′go-pēn) a white or slightly yellowish crystalline powder used as an antihypertensive.

syrup (sir′up) a viscous concentrated solution of a sugar, such as sucrose, in water or other aqueous liquid; combined with other ingredients, such a solution is used as a flavored vehicle for medications.

simple s., one compounded with purified water and sucrose.

systaltic (sis-tal′tik) alternately contracting and dilating; pulsating.

system (sis′tem) 1. a set or series of interconnected or interdependent parts or entities (objects, organs, or organisms) that act together in a common purpose or produce results impossible by action of one alone. 2. an organized set of principles or ideas. adj., **systemat′ic, system′ic.**

alimentary s., digestive system.

autonomic nervous s., the portion of the NERVOUS SYSTEM concerned with regulation of activity of cardiac muscle, smooth muscle, and glands. (See Plate 14.)

cardiovascular s., the heart and blood vessels, by which blood is pumped and circulated through the body (see also CIRCULATORY SYSTEM).

central nervous s., the portion of the NERVOUS SYSTEM consisting of the brain and spinal cord.

centrencephalic s., the neurons in the central core of the brain stem from the thalamus down to the medulla oblongata, connecting the two hemispheres of the brain.

circulatory s., the channels through which nutrient fluids of the body flow (see also CIRCULATORY SYSTEM).

conduction s., conductive s. (of heart), the system comprising the sinoatrial and atrioventricular nodes, atrioventricular bundle, and Purkinje fibers.

digestive s., the organs concerned with the ingestion and digestion of food (see also DIGESTIVE SYSTEM).

endocrine s., the system of glands and other structures that elaborate internal secretions (hormones) which are released directly into the circulatory system, influencing metabolism and other body processes; included are the pituitary, thyroid, parathyroid, and adrenal glands, gonads, pancreas, and paraganglia.

extrapyramidal s., a functional, rather than an anatomical, unit comprising the nuclei and fibers (excluding those of the pyramidal tract) involved in motor activities (see also EXTRAPYRAMIDAL SYSTEM).

genitourinary s., urogenital system; the organs concerned with production and excretion of urine, together with the REPRODUCTIVE ORGANS. (See Plate 11.)

haversian s., a haversian canal and its concentrically arranged lamellae, constituting the basic unit of structure in compact bone (osteon).

hematopoietic s., the tissues concerned in the production of blood, including bone marrow and lymph nodes.

heterogeneous s., a system or structure made up of mechanically separable parts, as an emulsion.

homogeneous s., a system or structure made up of parts that cannot be mechanicaly separated, as a solution.

hypophyseoportal s., the venules connecting the capillaries (gomitoli) in the median eminence of the hypothalamus with the sinusoidal capillaries of the anterior pituitary.

limbic s., a system of brain structures common to the brains of all mammals, comprising the phylogenetically old cortex (archipallium and paleopallium) and its primarily related nuclei. It is associated with olfaction, autonomic functions, and certain aspects of emotion and behavior.

lymphatic s., the lymphatic vessels and lymphoid tissue, considered collectively (see also CIRCULATORY SYSTEMS and LYMPHATIC SYSTEM).

metric s., a system of weights and measures based on the meter and having all units based on some power of 10 (see also Table of Weights and Measures in the Appendix).

nervous s., the organ system that along with the endocrine system, correlates the adjustments and reactions of an organism to internal and environmental conditions, comprising the central and peripheral nervous systems (see also NERVOUS SYSTEM).

parasympathetic nervous s., the craniosacral portion of the autonomic NERVOUS SYSTEM. Its preganglionic fibers leave the central nervous system with cranial nerves III, VII, IX and X and with the second to fourth sacral ventral roots; postganglionic fibers innervate the heart, smooth muscles, and glands of the head and neck, and thoracic, abdominal, and pelvic viscera. (See also Plate 14.)

peripheral nervous s., the portion of the NERVOUS SYSTEM consistng of the nerves and ganglia outside the brain and spinal cord.

portal s., an arrangement by which blood collected from one set of capillaries passes through a large vessel or vessels and another set of capillaries before returning to the systemic circulation, as in the pituitary gland and liver.

respiratory s., the tubular and cavernous organs that allow atmospheric air to reach the membranes across which gases are exchanged with the blood (see also RESPIRATORY SYSTEM and Plates 5 and 6).

reticuloendothelial s., a network of cells and tissues found throughout the body that is concerned in blood cell formation and destruction, storage of fatty materials and the metabolism of iron and pigment, and plays a defensive role in inflammation and immunity (see also RETICULOENDOTHELIAL SYSTEM.)

skeletal s., the body's framework of bones; the skeleton (see also SKELETAL SYSTEM).

sympathetic nervous s., the thoracolumbar part of the autonomic NERVOUS SYSTEM, the preganglionic fibers of which arise from cell bodies in the thoracic and first three lumbar segments of the spinal cord; postganglionic fibers are distributed to the heart, smooth muscle, and glands of the entire body. (See Plate 14.)

urinary s., the system formed in the body by the KIDNEYS, the urinary BLADDER, the URETERS, and the URETHRA, the organs concerned in the production and excretion of urine.

urogenital s., genitourinary system.

vascular s., the vessels of the body, especially the blood vessels.

vasomotor s., the part of the nervous system that controls the caliber of the blood vessels.

systema (sis-te'mah) [Gr.] system.

systemic (sis-tem'ik) pertaining to or affecting the body as a whole.

s. circulation, the flow of oxygenated blood from the left ventricle through the aorta, carrying oxygen and nutrient material to all the tissues of the body, and returning the venous blood through the superior and inferior venae cavae to the right atrium. (See also CIRCULATORY SYSTEM.)

systole (sis'to-le) the contraction, or period of contraction, of the heart, especially of the ventricles, during which blood is forced into the aorta and pulmonary artery. adj., **systol'ic.**

atrial s., contraction of the atria by which blood is forced into the ventricles; it precedes the true or ventricular systole.

extra s., an atrial or ventricular contraction occurring prematurely, while the basic rhythm of the heart is maintained.

ventricular s., contraction of the ventricles, forcing blood into the aorta and pulmonary artery.

systremma (sis-trem'ah) a cramp in the muscles of the calf of the leg.

Sytobex (si'to-beks) trademark for a parenteral preparation of crystalline vitamin B_{12}.

T

T. temperature; intraocular tension, normal intraocular tension being indicated by Tn, while T + 1, T + 2, etc., indicate increased tension, and T − 1, T − 2, etc., indicate decreased tension.

T_m tubular maximum (of the kidneys); used in reporting kidney function studies, with inferior letters representing the substance used in the test, as $T_{m_{PAH}}$ (tubular maximum for para-aminohippuric acid).

T.A. toxin-antitoxin.

Ta chemical symbol, *tantalum.*

T.A.B. a vaccine prepared from killed typhoid, paratyphoid A and paratyphoid B bacilli.

tabacosis (tab″ah-ko′sis) poisoning by tobacco, chiefly by inhaling tobacco dust; a form of PNEUMOCONIOSIS attributed to tobacco dust.

tabanid (tab′ah-nid) any gadfly of the family Tabanidae, including the horseflies and deerflies.

Tabanus (tah-ba′nus) a genus of bloodsucking biting flies (horseflies or gadflies) which transmit trypanosomes and anthrax to various animals.

tabardillo (tah″bar-dēl′yo) murine typhus, an infectious disease of Mexico resembling typhoid fever.

tabes (ta′bēz) 1. any wasting of the body; progressive atrophy of the body or a part of it. 2. tabes dorsalis. adj., **tabet′ic.**

t. dorsa′lis, a slowly progressive nervous disorder, from degeneration of the dorsal columns of the spinal cord and sensory nerve trunks, resulting in disturbances of sensation and interference with reflexes and consequently with movements; called also locomotor ataxia. It is caused by SYPHILIS and may appear 5 to 20 years after initial infection. The first symptoms are pain (frequently in the legs, although it may occur in the arms or trunk) and loss of position sense. The pupils are uneven and do not react to light (Argyll Robertson pupils). Unless the patient looks down at his legs he does not know where they are and he must depend on his vision for each step. The typical gait of a patient with this condition is jerky and wide-based. There is no cure for tabes dorsalis because there is destruction of nerve cells.

t. mesenter′ica, tuberculosis of the mesenteric glands in children.

tabescent (tah-bes′ent) growing emaciated; wasting away.

tabetiform (tah-bet′ĭ-form) resembling tabes.

tablature (tab′lah-tūr) separation of the chief cranial bones into inner and outer tables, separated by a diploë.

table (ta′b′l) a flat layer or surface.

inner t., the inner compact layer of the bones covering the brain.

outer t., the outer compact layer of the bones covering the brain.

vitreous t., inner table.

tablespoon (ta′b′l-spo͞on) a household unit of capacity, equivalent to about 15 ml. or 4 fluid drams.

tablet (tab′let) a solid dosage form containing a medicinal substance with or without a suitable diluent.

buccal t., one which dissolves when held between the cheek and gum, permitting direct absorption of the active ingredient through the oral mucosa.

enteric-coated t., one coated with material that delays release of the medication until after it leaves the stomach.

sublingual t., one that dissolves when held beneath the tongue, permitting direct absorption of the active ingredient by the oral mucosa.

taboo (tah-boo′) any of the negative traditions and behaviors generally regarded as harmful to social welfare.

taboparesis (ta″bo-pah-re′sis) tabes with general paresis.

tabular (tab′u-lar) resembling a table.

Tacaryl (tak′ah-ril) trademark for preparations of methdilazine, an antihistamine and antipruritic.

TACE (tās) trademark for preparations of chlorotrianisene, a synthetic estrogen.

tache (tahsh) [Fr.] a spot or blemish.

t. blanche ("white spot"), a white spot on the liver in certain infectious diseases.

t's bleuâtres ("bluish spots"), maculae caeruleae.

t. cérébrale ("cerebral spot"), a congested streak produced by drawing the nail across the skin; a concomitant of various nervous or cerebral diseases.

t. motrice ("motor spot"), a motor nerve ending in which the nerve fibril passes to a muscle cell, where it ends in a slight enlargement.

t. noire ("black spot"), an ulcer covered with a black crust, a characteristic local reaction at the presumed site of the infective bite in certain tick-borne rickettsioses.

tachogram (tak′o-gram) the graphic record produced by tachography.

tachography (tah-kog′rah-fe) the recording of the movement and speed of the blood current.

tachy- (tak′e) word element [Gr.], *rapid; swift.*

tachycardia (tak″e-kar′de-ah) abnormally rapid heart rate, usually taken to be over 100 beats per minute. adj., **tachycar′diac.**

atrial t., a rapid cardiac rate, usually 160–190 per minute, originating from an atrial locus.

ectopic t., rapid heart action in response to impulses arising outside the sinoatrial node.

paroxysmal t., rapid heart action that starts and stops abruptly.

ventricular t., an abnormally rapid ventricular rhythm with aberrant ventricular excitation, usually above 150 per minute, generated within the ventricle, and most often associated with atrioventricular dissociation.

tachylalia (tak″e-la′le-ah) rapidity of speech.

tachymeter (tah-kim′ĕ-ter) an instrument for measuring rapidity of motion.

tachyphagia (tak″e-fa′je-ah) rapid eating.

tachyphasia, tachyphrasia (tak″e-fa′ze-ah; tak″e-fra′ze-ah) extreme volubility of speech.

tachyphrenia (tak″e-fre′ne-ah) mental hyperactivity.

tachyphylaxis (tak″e-fi-lak′sis) 1. rapid immunization against the effect of toxic doses of an extract by previous injection of small doses of it. 2. the decreasing responses following consecutive injections made at short intervals. adj., **tachyphylac′tic.**

tachypnea (tak″ip-ne′ah) very rapid respiration; a respiratory neurosis marked by quick, shallow breathing.

tachyrhythmia (tak″e-rith′me-ah) tachycardia.

tachysterol (tah-kis′ter-ol) an isomer of ergosterol, an antirachitic substance, produced by irradiaton of ergosterol.

Tacosal (tak′o-sal) trademark for a preparation of phenytoin, an anticonvulsant.

tactile (tak′til) pertaining to touch.

tactometer (tak-tom′ĕ-ter) an instrument for measuring tactile sensibility; esthesiometer.

tactus (tak′tus) [L.] touch. adj., **tac′tual.**

t. erudi′tus, delicacy of touch acquired by practice.

Taenia (te′ne-ah) a genus of TAPEWORMS.

T. echinococ′cus, *Echinococcus granulosus.*

T. sagina′ta, a species 12–25 feet long, found in the adult form in the human intestine and in the larval state in muscles and other tissues of cattle and other ruminants; human infection usually results from eating inadequately cooked beef.

T. so′lium, a species 6–12 feet long, found in the adult intestine; the larval form most often is found in muscle and other tissues of the pig; human infection results from eating inadequately cooked pork.

taenia (te′ne-ah) 1. tenia (1). 2. a tapeworm of the genus *Taenia.*

taeniacide (te′ne-ah-sīd″) 1. lethal to tapeworms. 2. an agent lethal to tapeworms.

taeniafuge (te′ne-ah-fūj″) teniafuge.

taeniasis (te-ni′ah-sis) infection with tapeworms of the genus *Taenia.*

Tagathen (tag′ah-then) trademark for a preparation of chlorothen, an antihistamine.

Taka-diastase (tah′kah-di′as-tās) trademark for an amylolytic enzyme produced by the action of spores of the fungus *Aspergillus oryzae* on wheat bran; used as a digestant.

Takayasu's arteritis (disease) pulseless disease.

talbutal (tal′bu-tal) a hypnotic and sedative.

talc (talk) a native hydrous magnesium silicate, sometimes with a small amount of aluminum silicate; used as a dusting powder.

talcosis (tal-ko′sis) a condition due to inhalation or implantation in the body of talc.

talcum (tal′kum) talc.

talipes (tal′ĭ-pēz) CLUBFOOT; a congenital deformity of the foot, which is twisted out of shape or position; the foot may have an abnormally high longitudinal arch (talipes ca′vus) or it may be in dorsiflexion (talipes calca′neus) or plantar flexion (talipes equi′nus), abducted, everted (talipes val′gus), abducted, inverted (talipes va′rus), or various combinations of these (talipes calcaneoval′gus, talipes calcaneova′rus, talipes equinoval′gus or talipes equinova′rus).

talipomanus (tal″ĭ-pom′ah-nus) clubhand.

talocalcanean (ta″lo-kal-ka′ne-an) pertaining to the talus and calcaneus.

talocrural (ta″lo-kroo′ral) pertaining to the talus and the leg bones.

talofibular (ta″lo-fib′u-lar) pertaining to the talus and fibula.

talonavicular (ta″lo-nah-vik′u-lar) pertaining to the talus and navicular bone.

talus (ta′lus) ankle bone; the highest of the tarsal bones. (See also table of BONES.)

tampon (tam′pon) a pad or plug made of cotton, sponge, or other material, variously used in surgery to plug the nose, vagina, etc., for the control of hemorrhage or the absorption of secretions.

tamponade (tam″po-nād′) 1. surgical use of a tampon. 2. pathologic compression of a part.

cardiac t., compression of the heart due to collection of fluid or blood in the pericardium.

Tandearil (tan-de′ah-ril) trademark for a preparation of oxyphenbutazone, an anti-inflammatory agent.

Tangier disease (tan-jēr′) a familial disease characterized by a deficiency of high-density lipoproteins in the blood serum, with storage of cholesterol esters in the tonsils and other tissues.

tank (tank) an artificial receptacle for liquids.

Hubbard t., a tank in which exercises may be performed under water.

tannase (tan′ās) an enzyme that catalyzes the hydrolysis of ester linkages in gallic acid compounds.

tannate (tan′āt) any of the salts of tannic acid, all of which are astringent.

tannic acid (tan′ik) a substance obtained from bark and fruit of many plants, used as an astringent.

tannin (tan′in) tannic acid.

tantalum (tan′tah-lum) a chemical element, atomic number 73, atomic weight 180.948, symbol Ta. (See table of ELEMENTS.) It is a noncorrosive and malleable metal used for plates or disks to repair cranial defects, for wire sutures, and for making prosthetic appliances.

tantrum (tan′trum) a violent display of temper.

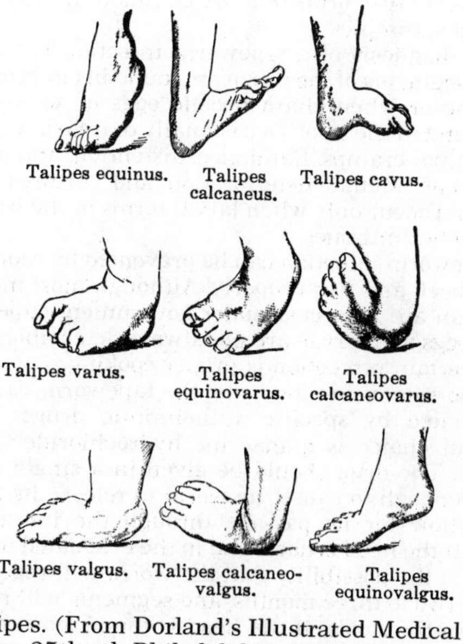

Talipes. (From Dorland's Illustrated Medical Dictionary. 25th ed. Philadelphia, W. B. Saunders Co., 1974.)

tap (tap) 1. a quick, light blow. 2. to drain off fluid by paracentesis.

spinal t., lumbar puncture.

Tapazole (tap′ah-zōl) trademark for a preparation of methimazole, used as a thyroid inhibitor.

tape (tāp) a long, narrow strip of fabric or other flexible material.

adhesive t., a strip of fabric or other material evenly coated on one side with a pressure-sensitive adhesive material.

tapeinocephaly (tah-pi″no-sef′ah-le) flattening or depression of the skull. adj., **tapeinocephal′ic.**

tapetum (tah-pe′tum), pl. *tape′ta* [L.] 1. a covering structure or layer of cells. 2. a stratum in the human brain composed of fibers from the body and splenium of the corpus callosum sweeping around the lateral ventricle.

t. lu′cidum, the iridescent epithelium of the choroid of animals that gives their eyes the property of shining in the dark.

tapeworm (tāp′werm) a parasitic cestode worm having a flattened bandlike form, which lodges in the intestines of animals and human beings. They are transmitted to man in larval form, embedded in cysts, in meat or fish that is not properly cooked. In the human they develop to maturity and attach themselves to the wall of the intestine, where they grow and release eggs.

Although a large number of adult tapeworms are considered human parasites, only a few infect man to any great degree. *Taenia saginata,* the beef tapeworm, and *T. solium,* the pork tapeworm, are widespread and quite common. Beef tapeworms grow to a length of 12 to 25 feet, and adult pork tapeworms average 6 to 12 feet in length. Both species release white, egg-containing proglottids, or segments of the body, which make their way to the anus and may be found in clothes or bedding. *Diphyllobothrium latum* is the fish tapeworm, and is found predominantly in the Great Lakes region of the United States, northern Europe, and Japan. It may grow as long as 60 feet. *Hymenolepis nana* and *H. diminuta* are dwarf tapeworms that are common in the tropics and subtropics.

The diagnosis of a tapeworm infection is made when segments of the worm are found in clothing or bedding or when characteristic eggs or segments are found in the stool. Occasionally diarrhea, vague abdominal cramps, flatulence, distention, and nausea occur. Mental deterioration and seizures are rare and occur only when larval forms of the worm invade brain tissue.

Tapeworm infection can be prevented by cooking pork, beef, and fish properly. Although most meats and fish are inspected under government supervision, eggs and larvae are not always detectable; the only certain protection is proper cooking.

Once it is inside the body, the tapeworm can be eliminated by specific anthelmintic drugs. The drug of choice is quinacrine hydrochloride (Atabrine). The drug should be given in a single dose large enough to cause the worm to release its hold and allow for its passage through the intestinal tract. If the head is not found in the evacuated feces, there is the possibility that the worm will regenerate in two to three months, and segments will reappear in the stools. If the head is found, no further treatment is necessary.

A newer drug said to be as effective and easy to administer is hydroxychlorobenzamide. It has the disadvantage of disintegrating the worm so that the head cannot be identified and thus there is no proof of cure. A follow-up within six months is recommended when this drug is used.

Echinococcus granulosis and *E. multilocularis* differ from other tapeworms in that the adults infect animal hosts and the larval forms are found in man. The larvae develop in the human intestine, penetrate its wall and are carried by the lymphatics to various organs of the body where they form slowly growing cysts (hydatid cysts). The liver is the organ most commonly involved. Treatment is by surgical removal of the cyst. Echinococcosis (HYDATID DISEASE) is uncommon in the United States.

armed t., *Taenia solium.*
beef t., *Taenia saginata.*
broad t., *Diphyllobothrium latum.*
dog t., *Dipylidium caninum.*
fish t., *Diphyllobothrium latum.*
hydatid t., *Echinococcus granulosus.*
pork t., *Taenia solium.*
unarmed t., *Taenia saginata.*

taphophilia (taf″o-fil′e-ah) morbid interest in graves and cemeteries.

tapotement (tah-pōt-maw′) [Fr.] a tapping manipulation in massage.

tar (tahr) a dark-brown or black, viscid liquid obtained from various species of pine or from bituminous coal.

coal t., a by-product obtained in destructive distillation of bituminous coal; used in ointment or solution in treatment of eczema.

juniper t., a volatile oil obtained from wood of *Juniperus oxycedrus;* used topically in the treatment of eczema.

pine t., a product of destructive distillation of the wood of various pine trees; used as a local antieczematic and rubefacient.

tarantula (tah-ran′tu-lah) a venomous spider (see also INSECT BITES AND STINGS).

tardive (tar′div) late; applied to a disease in which the characteristic lesion is late in appearing.

tare (tār) 1. the weight of the vessel in which a substance is weighed. 2. to weigh a vessel which is to contain a substance in order to allow for it when the vessel and substance are weighed together.

target (tar′get) an object or area toward which something is directed, such as the metal or plate of an x-ray tube on which the electrons impinge and from which the x-rays are sent out.

tarichatoxin (tar″ik-ah-tok′sin) a neurotoxin from the newt (*Taricha*), identical with TETRODOTOXIN.

tars(o)- (tar′so) word element [Gr.], *edge of eyelid; tarsus of the foot; instep.*

tarsadenitis (tahr″sad-ĕ-ni′tis) inflammation of the tarsus of the eyelid and the meibomian glands.

tarsal (tar′sal) pertaining to the tarsus of an eyelid or of the foot.

t. tunnel, the osseofibrous passage for the posterior tibial vessels, tibial nerve, and flexor tendons, formed by the flexor retinaculum and the tarsal bones.

t. tunnel syndrome, a complex of symptoms resulting from compression of the posterior tibial nerve or of the plantar nerves in the tarsal tunnel, with pain, numbness, and tingling paresthesia of the sole of the foot.

tarsalgia (tar-sal′je-ah) pain in a tarsus.

tarsalia (tar-sa′le-ah) the bones of the tarsus.

tarsalis (tar-sa′lis) [L.] tarsal.

tarsectomy (tar-sek′to-me) 1. excision of one or more bones of the tarsus. 2. excision of the cartilage of the eyelid.

tarsitis (tar-si′tis) inflammation of the cartilaginous portion of the eyelid; blepharitis.

tarsoclasis (tar-sok′lah-sis) surgical fracture of the tarsus of the foot.

tarsomalacia (tar″so-mah-la′she-ah) softening of the tarsal cartilage of an eyelid.

tarsometatarsal (tar″so-met″ah-tar′sal) pertaining to the tarsus and metatarsus.

tarsophyma (tar″so-fi′mah) any tumor of the tarsus.

tarsoplasty (tar′so-plas″te) plastic repair of the tarsus of the eyelid.

tarsoptosis (tar″sop-to′sis) falling of the tarsus; flatfoot.

tarsorrhaphy (tar-sor′ah-fe) suture of a portion of or the entire upper and lower eyelids for the purpose of shortening or closing the palpebral fissure.

tarsotomy (tar-sot′o-me) surgical incision of a tarsus, or an eyelid.

tarsus (tar′sus) 1. the seven bones—talus, calcaneus, navicular, medial, intermediate and lateral cuneiform, and cuboid—composing the articulation between the foot and leg; the ankle or instep. 2. the cartilaginous plate forming the framework of either (upper or lower) eyelid.

tartar (tar′tar) 1. the recrystallized sediment of wine casks; crude potassium bitartrate. 2. a yellowish film formed of calcium phosphate and carbonate, food particles, and other organic matter, deposited on the teeth by the saliva; called also dental calculus. Tartar should be removed regularly by a dentist. If neglected, it can cause bacteria to lodge between the gums and the teeth, causing gum infection, dental caries, loosening of the teeth, and other disorders.

tartaric acid (tar-tar′ik) a compound used in preparing refrigerant drinks and effervescent powders.

tartrate (tar′trāt) a salt of tartaric acid.

taste (tāst) the peculiar sensation caused by the contact of soluble substances with the tongue; the sense effected by the tongue, the gustatory and other nerves, and the gustatory center.

The organs of taste are the taste buds, bundles of slender cells with hairlike branches that are packed together in groups that form the projections called papillae at various places on the tongue. When a substance is introduced into the mouth, its molecules enter the pores of the papillae and stimulate the taste buds directly. In order to do this, the substance has to be dissolved in liquid. If it is not liquid when it enters the mouth, then it melts or is chewed and becomes mixed with saliva.

There are four basic tastes: sweet, salt, sour, and bitter. Sometimes alkaline and metallic are also included as basic tastes. All other tastes are combinations of these. The taste buds are specialized, and each responds only to the kind of basic taste that is its specialty. The sweet and salt taste buds are most numerous on the tip and front part of the tongue, sour taste buds are mainly along the edges, and bitterness is tasted at the back of the tongue. Bitter-sweet substances are tasted in two stages, first sweet, then bitter. The solid center of the tongue's surface has very few taste buds.

Other senses, including smell and touch, also play an important role in tasting.

taster (tās′ter) an individual capable of tasting a particular substance, such as phenylthiocarbamide, used in certain genetic studies.

tattooing (tah-too′ing) the introduction, by punctures, of permanent colors in the skin.

t. of cornea, permanent coloring of the cornea, chiefly to conceal leukomatous spots.

taurine (taw′rēn) a crystallized acid from the bile; found also in small quantities in lung and muscle tissues.

taurocholate (taw″ro-ko′lāt) a salt of taurocholic acid, one of the bile acids.

taurocholic acid (taw″ro-ko′lik) a bile acid; when hydrolyzed it splits into taurine and cholic acid.

Taussig-Bing syndrome (taw′sig-bing″) transposition of the great vessels of the heart and a ventricular septal defect straddled by a large pulmonary artery.

tautomer (taw′to-mer) a chemical compound exhibiting, or capable of exhibiting, tautomerism.

tautomeral (taw-tom′er-al) pertaining to the same part; said especially of neurons and neuroblasts sending processes to aid in formation of the white matter in the same side of the spinal cord.

tautomerase (taw-tom′er-ās) an enzyme that catalyzes tautomeric reactions.

tautomeric (taw″to-mer′ik) exhibiting, or capable of exhibiting, tautomerism.

tautomerism (taw-tom′er-izm) stereoisomerism in which the compounds are mutually interconvertible, under normal conditons, forming a mixture that is in dynamic equilibration.

taxis (tak′sis) 1. an orientation movement of a motile organism in response to a stimulus; it may be either toward (positive) or away from (negative) the source of the stimulus; used also as a word ending, affixed to a stem denoting the nature of the stimulus. 2. exertion of force in manual replacement of a displaced organ or part.

taxon (tak′son), pl. *tax′a* [Gr.] a particular group (category) into which living organisms are classified; the main categories (in ascending order) are species, genus, family, order, class, phylum, and kingdom.

taxonomy (tak-son′o-me) the orderly classification of organisms into appropriate categories (taxa), with application of suitable and correct names. adj., **taxonom′ic.**

Tay's spot (tāz) the choroid appearing as a red circular area surrounded by gray-white retina, as viewed through the fovea centralis in Tay-Sachs disease. Called also cherry-red spot.

Tay-Sach's disease (ta saks′) the infantile form of amaurotic familial idiocy, an inherited autosomal recessive condition belonging to a group of diseases classified as the sphingolipidoses. It affects chiefly Jewish infants and is distinguished by a cherry-red spot with a gray border on both retinas.

It is possible to test for this disease in the unborn fetus at 14 weeks of pregnancy. An absence of the enzyme hexoaminidase A indicates conclusively that the fetus has Tay-Sachs disease. Carriers of the trait have lowered levels of the enzyme in their blood, thus permitting screening of populations most susceptible to transmission of the trait to their offspring and genetic counseling of known carriers.

Taylor splint (ta'ler) a horizontal pelvic band and long lateral posterior bars; used to apply traction to the lower extremity.

Tb chemical symbol, *terbium.*

tb tuberculosis; tubercle bacillus.

Tc chemical symbol, *technetium.*

TCID tissue culture infective dose; that amount of a pathogenic agent that will produce pathologic change when inoculated on tissue cultures.

$TCID_{50}$ median tissue culture infective dose; that amount of a pathogenic agent that will produce pathologic change in 50 per cent of cell cultures inoculated.

Te chemical symbol, *tellurium.*

TEA tetraethylammonium, a ganglionic blocking agent, antihypertensive, and peripheral vasodilator.

tea (te) 1. the dried leaves of *Thea chinensis,* containing caffeine and tannic acid, or a decoction thereof. 2. any decoction or infusion.

pectoral t., an aqueous infusion of expectorant and demulcent herbs and aromatics.

TEAC tetraethylammonium chloride.

tears (tērz) the watery, slightly alkaline and saline secretion of the lacrimal glands that moistens the conjunctiva. (See also LACRIMAL APPARATUS and Plate 15.)

syndrome of crocodile t., spontaneous lacrimation occurring parallel with the normal salivation of eating. It follows facial paralysis and seems to be due to straying of the regenerating nerve fibers, some of those destined for the salivary glands going to the lacrimal glands.

tease (tēz) to pull apart gently with fine needles to permit microscopic examination.

teaspoon (te'spo͞on) a household unit of capacity containing about 4 ml. or 1 fluid dram.

teat (tēt) the nipple of the mammary gland.

technetium (tek-ne'she-um) a chemical element, atomic number 43, atomic weight 99, symbol Tc. (See table of ELEMENTS.)

technic (tek'nik) technique.

technician (tek'nish'an) a person skilled in the performance of technical procedures.

certified respiratory therapy t., one who has completed a one-year American Medical Association-approved program in respiratory therapy, has had one year of on-the-job training, and has passed the Technician Certification Board examination.

technique (tek-nēk') the method of procedure and details of a mechanical process or surgical operation.

tectorial (tek-to're-al) of the nature of a roof or covering.

tectorium (tek-to're-um) Corti's membrane.

tectospinal (tek"to-spi'nal) extending from the tectum of the midbrain to the spinal cord.

tectum (tek'tum) a rooflike structure.

t. of mesencephalon, t. of midbrain, the dorsal portion of the midbrain.

T.E.D. threshold erythema dose.

teeth (tēth) plural of *tooth.*

teething (tēth'ing) eruption of the teeth through the gums. The average infant cuts his first tooth between the sixth and ninth months. The full set of 20 baby teeth erupt gradually over a period up to about 30 months, the customary pattern being the arrival of two teeth, one on each side of the jaw, at a time.

Evidence of teething includes drooling, a compulsion to put objects into the mouth, and unusual crankiness. Some babies seem to be more bothered by teething than others, and different teeth affect the same baby in different ways.

It was long fashionable to ascribe any baby ailment to teething, despite the considerable harm such a hasty diagnosis often did by delaying recognition of the real trouble. Although teething sometimes may cause a slight fever, any such symptom should be watched carefully for further developments.

tegmen (teg'men), pl. *teg'mina* [L.] a covering structure or roof.

t. tym'pani, 1. the thin layer of bone separating the tympanic antrum from the cranial cavity. 2. the roof of the tympanic cavity, related to part of the petrous portion of the temporal bone.

tegmentum (teg-men'tum), pl. *tegmen'ta* [L.] 1. a covering. 2. the part of the cerebral peduncle dorsal to the substantia nigra. adj., **tegmen'tal.**

Tegretol (teg'rĕ-tol) trademark for a preparation of carbamazepine, and anticonvulsant.

teichopsia (ti-kop'se-ah) scintillating scotoma; the sensation of a luminous appearance before the eyes, with a zigzag, wall-like outline.

tela (te'lah), pl. *te'lae* [L.] a thin, weblike structure or tissue; used in naming various anatomic structures.

t. conjuncti'va, connective tissue.

t. elas'tica, elastic tissue.

t. subcuta'nea, the subcutaneous connective tissue or superficial fascia.

telalgia (tel-al'je-ah) referred pain; pain occurring in a part distant from the lesion.

telangiectasia (tel-an"je-ek-ta'ze-ah) a vascular lesion formed by dilation of a group of small blood vessels. adj., **telangiectat'ic.**

hereditary hemorrhagic t., a hereditary condition marked by multiple small angiomas of the skin and mucous membranes, often with nosebleed or gastrointestinal bleeding and sometimes with arteriovenous fistula of the lung or liver.

telangiectasis (tel-an"je-ek'tah-sis), pl. *telangiectases.* telangiectasia.

spider t., vascular spider.

telangiosis (tel-an"je-o'sis) any disease of the capillaries.

tele- (tel'e) word element [Gr.], *far away; operating at a distance; an end.*

telecardiography (tel"ĕ-kar"de-og'rah-fe) the recording of an electrocardiogram by transmission of impulses to a site at a distance from the patient.

telecardiophone (tel"ĕ-kar'de-o-fōn") an apparatus for making heart sounds audible at a distance from the patient.

teleceptor (tel'ĕ-sep"tor) a sensory nerve terminal that is sensitive to stimuli originating at a distance. Such nerve endings exist in the eyes and ears.

telecinesia (tel"ĕ-si-ne'ze-ah) telekinesis.

telefluoroscopy (tel"ĕ-floo"or-os'ko-pe) television transmission of fluoroscopic images for study at a distant location.

telekinesis (tel"ĕ-ki-ne'sis) 1. movement of an object produced without contact. 2. the ability to produce such movement. adj., **telekinet'ic.**

telemetry (tĕ-lem'ĕ-tre) the making of measurements at a distance from the subject, the measurable evidence of phenomena under investigation being transmitted by radio signals.

telencephalon (tel″en-sef'ah-lon) endbrain: 1. the paired brain vesicles, which are the anterolateral outpouchings of the forebrain, together with the median, unpaired portion, the terminal lamina of the hypothalamus; from it the cerebral hemispheres are derived. 2. the anterior of the two vesicles formed by specialization of the forebrain in embryonic development. adj., **telencephal'ic.**

teleneurite (tel″ĕ-nu'rīt) an end expansion of an axon.

teleneuron (tel″ĕ-nu'ron) a nerve ending.

teleological (te″le-o-loj'ĭ-kal) serving an ultimate purpose in development.

teleology (te″le-ol'o-je) the doctrine that the explanation of phenomena is to be found in terms of their purpose.

teleomitosis (tel″e-o-mi-to'sis) completed mitosis.

teleorganic (tel″e-or-gan'ik) necessary to life.

Telepaque (tel'ĕ-pāk) trademark for a preparation of iopanoic acid, a radiopaque medium used in cholecystography.

telepathy (tĕ-lep'ah-the) the communication of thought through extrasensory perception.

teleradiography (tel″ĕ-ra″de-og'rah-fe) teleroentgenography.

telergy (tel'er-je) 1. automatism. 2. a hypothetical action of one brain on another at a distance.

teleroentgenography (tel″ĕ-rent″gen-og'rah-fe) roentgenography with the x-ray tube 6½ to 7 feet away from the plate in order to more nearly secure parallelism of the rays.

telesthesia (tel″es-the'ze-ah) telepathy; perception at a distance.

teletherapy (tel″ĕ-ther'ah-pe) treatment in which the source of the therapeutic agent, e.g., radiation, is at a distance from the body.

telluric (tĕ-lu'rik) 1. pertaining to tellurium. 2. pertaining to or originating from the earth.

tellurium (tĕ-lu're-um) a chemical element, atomic number 52, atomic weight 127.60, symbol Te. (See table of ELEMENTS.)

telo- word element [Gr.], *end.*

telocentric (tel″o-sen'trik) having the centromere at one end of the replicating chromosome.

telodendron (tel″o-den'dron) any of the fine terminal branches of an axon.

telogen (tel'o-jen) the quiescent or resting phase of the hair cycle, following catagen, the hair having become a club hair and not growing further.

telognosis (tel″og-no'sis) diagnosis based on interpretation of roentgenograms transmitted by radio or telephonic communication.

telolecithal (tel″o-les'ĭ-thal) having a yolk concentrated at one of the poles.

telolemma (tel″o-lem'ah) the covering of a motor end-plate, made up of sarcolemma and an extension of Henle's sheath.

telomere (tel'o-mēr) an extremity of a chromosome, which has specific properties, one of which is a polarity that prevents reunion with any fragment after a chromosome has been broken.

telophase (tel'o-fāz) the last of the four stages of mitosis and of the two divisions of meiosis.

TEM triethylenemelamine, an antineoplastic agent.

Temaril (tem'ah-ril) trademark for preparations of trimeprazine, a systemic antipruritic.

temperament (tem'per-ah-ment) the peculiar physical character and mental cast of an individual.

lymphatic t., that characterized by a fair but not ruddy complexion, light hair, and a general softness or laxity of the tissues.

melancholic t., one characterized by melancholia and moroseness.

nervous t., that characterized by predominance of the nervous element and by great activity or susceptibility of the brain.

sanguine t., sanguineous t., that characterized by a fair and ruddy complexion, full, muscular development, large, full veins and an active pulse.

temperature (tem'per-ah-tūr) the degree of sensible heat or cold, expressed in terms of a specific scale.

Body temperature is measured by a clinical thermometer and represents a balance between the heat produced by the body and the heat it loses. Though heat production and heat loss vary with circumstances, the body regulates them, keeping a remarkably constant temperature. An abnormal rise in body temperature is called FEVER.

See also Table of Temperature Equivalents in the Appendix.

NORMAL BODY TEMPERATURE. Body temperature is usually measured by a thermometer placed in the mouth or in the rectum. The normal oral temperature is 98.6 degrees on the Fahrenheit scale; rectally, it is 99.2° F. On the Celsius (centigrade) scale, normal mouth temperature is 37° C.; rectally it is 37.3° C. These values are based on a statistical average. Normal temperature varies somewhat from person to person and at different times in each person.

Body temperature is usually slightly higher in the evening than in the morning. It is also somewhat higher during and immediately after eating, exercise, or emotional excitement. Temperature in infants and young children tends to vary somewhat more than in adults.

TEMPERATURE REGULATION. To maintain a constant temperature, the body must be able to respond to changes in the temperature of its surroundings. When the outside temperature drops, nerve endings near the skin surface sense the change and communicate it to the hypothalamus. Certain cells of the hypothalamus then signal for an increase in the body's heat production. This heat is conducted to the blood and distributed throughout the body. At the same time, the body acts to conserve its heat. The arterioles constrict so that less blood will flow near the body's surface. The skin becomes pale and cold. Sometimes it takes on a bluish color, the result of a color change in the blood, which occurs when the blood, flowing slowly, gives off more of its oxygen than usual.

Another signal from the brain stimulates muscular activity, which releases heat. Shivering is a form of this activity—a muscular reflex that produces heat.

When the outside temperature goes up, the body's cooling system is ordered into action. Sweat is released from sweat glands beneath the skin, and as it evaporates, the skin is cooled. Heat is also eliminated by the evaporation of moisture in the lungs. This process is accelerated by panting.

An important regulator of body heat is the peripheral capillary system. The vessels of this system form a network just under the skin. When these vessels dilate, they allow more warm blood from the interior of the body to flow through them, where it is cooled by the surrounding air.

ABNORMAL BODY TEMPERATURE. Abnormal temperatures occur when the body's temperature-regulating system is upset by disease or other physical disturbances. FEVER usually accompanies infection and many other disease processes. In most cases when the oral temperature is 37.8° C. (100° F.) or over, fever is present. Temperatures of 40° C. (104° F.) or over are common in serious illnesses, although occasionally very high fever accompanies an illness that causes little concern. Temperatures as high as 41.7° C. (107° F.) or higher sometimes accompany diseases in critical stages.

Subnormal temperatures, below 35.6° C. (96° F.) occur in cases of collapse (see also symptomatic HYPOTHERMIA).

absolute t., that reckoned from absolute zero (– 273.15° C. or – 459.67° F.).

critical t., that below which a gas may be converted to a liquid by pressure.

normal t., that usually registered by a healthy person (98.6° F. or 37° C.).

template (tem′plāt) a pattern or mold. In dentistry, a curved or flat plate used as an aid in setting teeth for a denture. In theoretical immunology, an antigen that determines the configuration of combining (antigen-binding) sites of antibody molecules. In genetics, a strand of DNA which specifies the synthesis of a complementary strand of RNA (mRNA), which in turn serves as a template for the synthesis of nucleic acids or proteins.

temple (tem′p'l) the lateral region on either side of the head, above the zygomatic arch.

tempolabile (tem″po-la′bil) subject to change with the passage of time.

tempora (tem′po-rah) [L.] the temples.

temporal (tem′po-ral) 1. pertaining to the temple. 2. pertaining to time; limited as to time; temporary.

t. bone, one of the two irregular bones forming part of the lateral surfaces and base of the skull, and containing the organs of hearing.

t. lobe, a long, tongue-shaped process constituting the lower lateral portion of the cerebral hemisphere.

temporomandibular (tem″po-ro-man″dib′u-lar) pertaining to the temporal bone and mandible.

temporomaxillary (tem″po-ro-mak′sĭ-ler″e) pertaining to the temporal bone and maxilla.

temporo-occipital (tem″po-ro-ok-sip′ĭ-tal) pertaining to the temporal and occipital bones.

temporosphenoid (tem″po-ro-sfe′noid) pertaining to the temporal and sphenoid bones.

tempostabile (tem″po-sta′bil) not subject to change with time.

Tempra (tem′prah) trademark for preparations of acetaminophen, an analgesic and antipyretic.

tenacious (tĕ-na′shus) viscid; adhesive.

tenaculum (tĕ-nak′u-lum) a hooklike surgical instrument for grasping and holding parts.

tenalgia (ten-al′je-ah) pain in a tendon.

tenderness (ten′der-nes) a state of unusual sensitivity to touch or pressure.

rebound t., a state in which pain is felt on the release of pressure over a part.

tendinitis (ten″dĭ-ni′tis) inflammation of tendons and of tendon-muscle attachments. It is one of the commonest causes of acute pain in the shoulder. Tendinitis is frequently associated with a calcium deposit (calcific tendinitis), which may also involve the bursa around the tendon or near the joint, causing bursitis.

Treatment may consist of the administration of steroids, given orally or by injection into the bursa, or it may take the form of injections of procaine or x-ray therapy. In severe cases, surgical removal of the calcium deposit may be required.

tendinoplasty (ten′dĭ-no-plas″te) tenoplasty.

tendinosuture (ten″dĭ-no-su′tūr) tenorrhaphy.

tendinous (ten′dĭ-nus) pertaining to, resembling, or of the nature of a tendon.

tendo (ten′do), pl. *ten′dines* [L.] tendon; used in anatomic nomenclature.

t. Achil′lis, t. calca′neus, Achilles tendon.

tendolysis (ten-dol′ĭ-sis) the freeing of a tendon from adhesions.

tendon (ten′don) a cord or band of strong white fibrous tissue that connects a muscle to a bone. When the muscle contracts, or shortens, it pulls on the tendon, which moves the bone. Tendons are so tough they are seldom torn, even when an injury is severe enough to break a bone or tear a muscle. One of the most prominent tendons is the Achilles tendon, which can be felt at the back of the ankle just above the heel; it attaches the triceps surae muscle to the calcaneus.

tendonitis (ten″do-ni′tis) tendinitis.

tendovaginal (ten″do-vaj′ĭ-nal) pertaining to a tendon and its sheath.

tenectomy (tĕ-nek′to-me) excision of a lesion of a tendon or of a tendon sheath.

tenesmus (tĕ-nez′mus) ineffectual and painful straining at stool or in urinating. adj., **tenes′mic.**

tenia (te′ne-ah), pl. *te′niae* [L.] 1. a flat band or strip of soft tissue; used in anatomic nomenclature to designate various structures. 2. a TAPEWORM of the genus *Taenia.*

te′niae co′li, the three thickened bands (te′nia li′bera, te′nia mesocol′ica, and te′nia omenta′lis) formed by longitudinal fibers in the tunica muscularis of the large intestine, extending from the root of the vermiform appendix to the rectum.

teniacide (te′ne-ah-sīd″) 1. lethal to tapeworms. 2. an agent lethal to tapeworms.

teniafuge (te′ne-ah-fūj″) a medicine for expelling tapeworms.

teniasis (te-ni′ah-sis) infection with tapeworms of the genus *Taenia.*

tennis elbow (ten′is) a painful condition localized to the outer aspect of the elbow, due to inflammation of the extensor tendon attachment to the lateral humeral condyle.

teno- word element [Gr.], *tendon.*

tenodesis (ten-od′ĕ-sis) suture of the end of a tendon to a bone.

tenodynia (ten″o-din′e-ah) tenalgia.

tenomyoplasty (ten″o-mi′o-plas″te) plastic repair of a tendon and muscle, applied especially to an operation for inguinal hernia.

tenomyotomy (ten″o-mi-ot′o-me) excision of a portion of a tendon and muscle.

Tenon's capsule (te′nonz) the connective tissue enveloping the posterior eyeball.

tenonectomy (ten″o-nek′to-me) excision of part of a tendon to shorten it.

tenonitis (ten″o-ni′tis) 1. tendinitis. 2. inflammation of Tenon's capsule, the connective tissue enclosing the eyeball.

tenonometer (ten″o-nom′ĕ-ter) an apparatus for measuring intraocular pressure.

tenontitis (ten″on-ti′tis) tendinitis.

tenonto- word element [Gr.], *tendon.*

tenontodynia (ten″on-to-din′e-ah) tenalgia.

tenontography (ten″on-tog′rah-fe) a written description or delineation of the tendons.

tenontology (ten″on-tol′o-je) the sum of what is known about the tendons.

tenontothecitis (ten-on″to-the-si′tis) tenosynovitis.

tenophyte (ten′o-fit) a growth or concretion in a tendon.

tenoplasty (ten′o-plas″te) plastic repair of a tendon. adj., **tenoplas′tic.**

tenoreceptor (ten″o-re-sep′tor) a nerve receptor in a tendon.

tenorrhaphy (ten-or′ah-fe) suture of a tendon.

tenositis (ten″o-si′tis) tendinitis.

tenostosis (ten″os-to′sis) conversion of a tendon into bone.

tenosuspension (ten″o-sus-pen′shun) attachment of the head of the humerus to the acromion by a strip of tendon; it is done for habitual dislocation of the shoulder.

tenosuture (ten″o-su′tūr) tenorrhaphy.

tenosynovectomy (ten″o-sin″o-vek′to-me) excision or resection of a tendon sheath.

tenosynovitis (ten″o-sin″o-vi′tis) inflammation of a tendon and its sheath, the lubricated layer of tissue in which the tendon is housed and through which it moves. Tenosynovitis occurs most frequently in the hands and wrists or feet and ankles, and is often the result of intense and continued use, as with pianists and typists. It is painful, and may temporarily disable the affected part.

Rheumatoid and other types of arthritis frequently involve tendon sheaths. A less common cause of tenosynovitis is injury to the tendon sheath and subsequent infection. It can also be the result of tuberculous or gonorrheal infection.

Treatment is by immobilization of the limb or, in severe cases, by surgery for the purpose of draining an infected sheath, or to release a tendon from a constricting sheath.

villonodular t., a condition marked by exaggerated proliferation of synovial membrane cells, producing a solid tumor-like mass, commonly occurring in periarticular soft tissues and less frequently in joints.

tenotomy (ten-ot′o-me) transection of a tendon.

graduated t., partial transection of a tendon.

tenovaginitis (ten″o-vaj″ĭ-ni′tis) tenosynovitis.

Tensilon (ten′sĭ-lon) trademark for a solution of edrophonium, a parasympathomimetic, muscle stimulant, curare antagonist, and diagnostic agent in myasthenia gravis.

tension (ten′shun) 1. the act of stretching or the condition of being stretched or strained. 2. the partial pressure of a component of a gas mixture.

arterial t., blood pressure within an artery.

intraocular t., intraocular pressure.

t. pneumothorax, accumulation of air or gas within the pleural cavity which, if not relieved, can lead to lung collapse and MEDIASTINAL SHIFT. (See also PNEUMOTHORAX.)

premenstrual t., a complex of symptoms, including emotional instability and irritability, sometimes occurring in the 10 days before menstruation; other symptoms include pain in the breasts, headache, nausea, anorexia, constipation, and pelvic discomfort (see also PREMENSTRUAL TENSION).

surface t., tension or resistance that acts to preserve the integrity of a surface.

tissue t., a state of equilibrium between tissues and cells that prevents overaction of any part.

tensometer (tens-om′ĕ-ter) an apparatus by which the tensile strength of materials can be determined.

tensor (ten′sor) any muscle that stretches or makes tense.

tent (tent) 1. a fabric covering designed to enclose an open space, especially such a covering over a patient's bed for administering oxygen or vaporized medication by inhalation. 2. a conical, expansible plug of soft material for dilating an orifice or for keeping a wound open, so as to prevent its healing except at the bottom.

sponge t., a conical plug made of compressed sponge used to dilate the os uteri.

tentacle (ten′tah-k′l) a slender, whiplike appendage in animals that may function in prehension and feeding or as a sense organ.

tentorium (ten-to′re-um), pl. *tento′ria* [L.] an anatomical part resembling a tent or covering. adj., **tento′rial.**

t. cerebel′li, the process of the dura mater supporting the occipital lobes and covering the cerebellum.

tephromyelitis (tef″ro-mi″ĕ-li′tis) inflammation of the gray matter of the spinal cord.

tephrosis (tĕ-fro′sis) incineration or cremation.

tepor (te′por) [L.] gentle heat.

ter- (ter) word element [L.], *three; three-fold.*

tera- (ter′ah) word element [Gr.], *monster;* used in naming units of measurement to designate an amount 10^{12} (a trillion, or million million) times the unit specified by the root to which it is joined, as teracurie; symbol T.

teracurie (ter″ah-ku′re) a unit of radioactivity, being one trillion (10^{12}) curies.

teras (ter′as), pl. *ter′ata* [L., Gr.] a monster. adj., **terat′ic.**

teratism (ter′ah-tizm) an anomaly of formation or development; the condition of a monster.

terato- (ter′ah-to) word element [Gr.], *monster; monstrosity.*

teratoblastoma (ter″ah-to-blas-to′mah) a neoplasm containing embryonic elements, differing from a teratoma in that its tissue does not represent all germinal layers.

teratogen (ter′ah-to-jen) an agent or influence that

causes physical defects in the developing embryo. adj., **teratogen'ic.**

teratogenesis (ter"ah-to-jen'ĕ-sis) the production of deformity in the developing embryo, or of a monster. adj., **teratogenet'ic.**

teratogenous (ter"ah-toj'ĕ-nus) developed from fetal remains.

teratogeny (ter"ah-toj'ĕ-ne) teratogenesis.

teratoid (ter'ah-toid) resembling a monster.

teratology (ter"ah-tol'o-je) that division of embryology and pathology dealing with abnormal development and congenital deformations. adj., **teratolog'ic.**

teratoma (ter"ah-to'mah) a true neoplasm made up of a number of different types of tissue, none of which is native to the area in which it occurs; usually found in the ovary or testis.

teratomatous (ter"ah-tom'ah-tus) pertaining to or of the nature of teratoma.

teratosis (ter"ah-to'sis) the condition of a monster.

terbium (ter'be-um) a chemical element, atomic number 65, atomic weight 158.924, symbol Tb. (See table of ELEMENTS.)

terchloride (ter-klo'rīd) trichloride.

terebene (ter'ĕ-bēn) a mixture of hydrocarbons from turpentine oil; antiseptic and expectorant.

terebration (ter"ĕ-bra'shun) an act of boring or trephining; also, a boring pain.

teres (te'rēz) [L.] long and round.

Terfonyl (ter'fo-nil) trademark for preparations of sulfamethazine, sulfadiazine, and sulfamerazine (trisulfapyrimidines).

ter in die (ter in de'a) [L.] three times a day.

term (term) a definite period, especially the period of gestation, or pregnancy.

terminal (ter'mĭ-nal) 1. forming or pertaining to an end. 2. a termination, end or extremity, especially a nerve ending.

terminatio (ter"mĭ-na'she-o), pl. *terminatio'nes* [L.] an ending; used in anatomic nomenclature to designate the site of discontinuation of a structure, as the free nerve endings (terminationes nervo'rum li'berae), in which the peripheral fiber divides into fine branches that terminate freely in connective tissue or epithelium.

terminology (ter"mĭ-nol'o-je) 1. the vocabulary of an art or science. 2. the science that deals with the investigation, arrangement, and construction of terms.

terminus (ter'mĭ-nus), pl. *ter'mini* [L.] an ending.

ternary (ter'nah-re) 1. third in order. 2. made up of three elements or radicals.

terpene (ter'pēn) any hydrocarbon of the formula $C_{10}H_{16}$.

terpin (ter'pin) a product obtained by the action of nitric acid on oil of turpentine and alcohol, used as an expectorant in the form of the hydrate salt.

Terramycin (ter'ah-mi"sin) trademark for preparations of oxytetracycline, an antibiotic.

terror (ter'or) an attack of extreme fear or dread.

night t., an extreme fear reaction in a child during sleep or at night.

tertian (ter'shan) recurring in 3-day cycles (every second day); applied to the type of fever caused by certain forms of malarial parasites (see also MALARIA).

tertiary (ter'she-a"re) third in order.

tertigravida (ter"she-grav'ĭ-dah) a woman pregnant for the third time; gravida III.

tertipara (ter-tip'ah-rah) tripara; a woman who has had three pregnancies that resulted in viable offspring; para III.

Tessalon (tes'ah-lon) trademark for a preparation of benzonatate, an antitussive.

tessellated (tes'ĕ-lāt"ed) divided into squares, like a checker board.

test (test) 1. an examination or trial. 2. a significant chemical reaction. 3. a reagent. See also specific names of tests, as ASCHHEIM-ZONDEK TEST.

acetic acid t., a test for albumin in the urine; acetic acid is added to boiled urine and a white precipitate forms.

agglutination t., one whose results depend on agglutination of bacteria or other cells; used in diagnosing certain infectious diseases and rheumatoid arthritis.

alkali-denaturation t., a spectrophotometric method for measuring the concentration of fetal (F) hemoglobin.

aptitude t., one designed to measure the capacity for developing general or specific skills.

association t., one based on associative reaction, usually by mentioning words to a patient and noting what other words the patient will give as the ones called up in his mind.

autohemolysis t., determination of spontaneous hemolysis in a blood specimen maintained under certain conditions, to detect the presence of certain hemolytic states.

barium t., roentgenographic examination using a barium sulfate mixture as the opaque contrast medium to locate digestive tract disorders.

biuret t., see BIURET.

chromatin t., determination of genetic sex of an individual by examination of body cells for the presence of sex chromatin, which is found in cells of the normal female.

cis-trans t., a test in microbial genetics to determine whether two mutations that have the phenotypic effect, in a haploid cell or a cell with single phage infection, are located in the same gene or in different genes; the test depends on the independent behavior of two alleles of a gene in a diploid cell or in a cell infected with two phages carrying different alleles.

coin t., a silver coin held flat on the anterior chest wall is struck with the edge of another silver coin; a clear, bell-like sound heard by stethoscope on the posterior chest wall indicates air in the pleural space.

complement-fixation t's, tests that utilize antigen-antibody reaction and result in hemolysis to determine the presence of various organisms in the blood (see also COMPLEMENT-FIXATION TESTS).

concentration t., a test of renal function based on the patient's ability to concentrate urine.

conjunctival t., itching and conjunctival congestion after instillation into the conjunctiva of a pollen or pollen extract to which the person is sensitive.

creatinine clearance t., a test for renal function based on the rate at which ingested creatinine is filtered through the renal glomeruli.

double-blind t., a study of the effects of a specific agent in which neither the administrator nor the recipient, at the time of administration, knows whether the active or an inert substance is being used.

finger-nose t., a test for coordinated movements of the extremities; the patient is directed to close his eyes, and, with arm extended to one side, slowly endeavor to touch the end of his nose with the tip of his index finger.

galactose tolerance t., a test of carbohydrate tolerance of the liver by measuring the amount of galactose eliminated in the urine after oral or intravenous administration of galactose.

guaiac t., one for determination of blood in a stain.

histamine t., 1. subcutaneous injection of 0.1 per cent solution of histamine to stimulate gastric secretion. 2. after rapid intravenous injection of histamine phosphate, normal persons experience a brief fall in blood pressure, but in those with pheochromocytoma, after the fall, there is a marked rise in blood pressure.

human erythrocyte agglutination t., one for rheumatoid arthritis, depending on agglutination by the patient's serum of human Rh-positive cells sensitized with incomplete anti-Rh antibody.

intracutaneous t., one that involves introduction of an antigen between the layers of the skin and evaluation of the reaction elicited by it.

latex-agglutination t., latex-fixation t., a serologic test for rheumatoid factor, helpful in the diagnosis of rheumatoid arthritis.

multiple-puncture t., an intracutaneous test in which the material used (e.g., tuberculin) is introduced into the skin by pressure of several needles or pointed tines or prongs.

neutralization t., one for the bacterial neutralization power of a substance by testing its action on the pathogenic properties of the organism concerned.

patch t., a test for hypersensitivity, performed by observing the reaction to application to the skin of filter paper or gauze saturated with the substance in question (see also SKIN TEST).

phlorhizin t., a test of kidney function based on injection of phlorhizin and sodium carbonate.

plasmacrit t., a rapid screening test for syphilis, using plasma from microhematocrit tubes.

precipitation t., precipitin t., any test in which the positive reaction consists in the formation and deposit of a precipitate in the fluid being tested.

pregnancy t's, laboratory procedures for early determination of pregnancy (see also PREGNANCY TESTS).

prothrombin consumption t., a test to measure the formation of intrinsic thromboplastin by determining the residual serum prothrombin after blood coagulation is complete.

pulmonary function t's, see under PULMONARY.

renal clearance t's, laboratory tests that determine the ability of the kidney to remove certain substances from the blood. The urea clearance test, which assesses the kidney's ability to extract urea from the blood and excrete it in the urine, has largely been replaced by the more precise CREATININE and PAH clearance tests.

scratch t., a test for hypersensitivity in which a minute amount of the substance in question is inserted in small scratches made in the skin. A positive reaction is swelling or redness at the site within 30 minutes. Used in ALLERGY testing and in testing for tuberculosis (Pirquet's reaction). (See also SKIN TEST.)

serologic t., one involving examination of blood serum.

sickling t., a method to demonstrate hemoglobin S and the sickling phenomenon in erythrocytes, performed by reducing the oxygen concentration to which the red cells are exposed.

single-blind t., a study of the effects of a specific agent in which the administrator, but not the recipient, knows whether the active or an inert substance is being used.

thematic apperception t., TAT, a psychologic test in which the patient constructs a story from a set of pictures. It is designed to reveal the patient's emotions, drives, sentiments, and conflicts.

three-glass t., a test to localize the site of urinary tract infection. The patient voids successively into three containers. In acute anterior urethritis the urine in only the first container will be turbid from pus or will contain blood. In posterior urethritis the urine in all three containers will be turbid or contain blood. Shreds in the third container point to chronic prostatitis.

tine t., a tuberculin skin test employing a multiple-puncture, disposable device (see also TINE TEST).

tolerance t., 1. an exercise test to determine the efficiency of the circulation. 2. a test to determine the body's ability to metabolize a substance or to endure administration of a drug.

tourniquet t., one involving the application of a tourniquet to an extremity, as in determination of capillary fragility (denoted by the appearance of petechiae) or of the status of the collateral circulation.

treponemal hemagglutination (TPHA) t., Treponema pallidum complement fixation (TPCF) t., Treponema pallidum cryolysis complement fixation (TPCP) t., Treponema pallidum immobilization (TPI) t., serologic tests related directly to the causative organism, used in the diagnosis of syphilis.

tuberculin t., a test for the presence of active or inactive TUBERCULOSIS, consisting in the subcutaneous injection of 5 mg. of tuberculin; a positive test is denoted by redness and induration at the injection site (see also MANTOUX TEST).

testalgia (tes-tal′je-ah) testicular pain.

Tes-Tape (tes′tāp) trademark for a reagent strip impregnated with glucose oxidase, peroxidase, and orthotolidine; used for determining the approximate concentration of glucose in the urine.

test meal a portion of food or foods given for the purpose of determining the functioning of the digestive tract.

barium t. m., a meal containing some preparation of barium as the opaque constituent (see also BARIUM TEST).

bismuth t. m., a meal containing some preparation of bismuth as the opaque constituent.

motor t. m., food or drink whose progress through the stomach, pylorus, and intestinal tract is observed fluoroscopically.

opaque t. m., a meal containing some substance opaque to x-rays, permitting visualization of the gastrointestinal tract.

test tube a tube of thin glass, closed at one end; used in chemical tests and other laboratory procedures.

test type printed letters of varying size, used in the testing of visual acuity.

testectomy (tes-tek′to-me) ORCHIECTOMY, the removal of a testis.

testes (tes′tēz) [L.] plural of *testis*.

testicle (tes'tĭ-k'l) testis.

testicular (tes-tik'u-lar) pertaining to the testis.

t. feminization syndrome, an extreme form of male pseudohermaphroditism, with external genitalia and secondary sex characters typical of the female, but with presence of testes and absence of uterus and uterine tubes.

testis (tes'tis), pl. *tes'tes* [L.] the male gonad; either of the paired, egg-shaped glands normally situated in the scrotum; called also testicle. The testes produce the spermatozoa, the male reproductive cells, which are ejaculated into the female vagina during coitus, and the male sex hormone, testosterone, which is responsible for the secondary sex characters of the male.

If the testes are removed (castration, bilateral ORCHIECTOMY) before puberty, the male is sterile and will never develop all the adult masculine characteristics. If the testes are removed after puberty, the male becomes sterile and his masculine characteristics will diminish unless he receives injections of male hormones. With aging, there is a gradual decrease in the production of testosterone.

In the unborn child, the testes lie close to the kidneys. During approximately the seventh month of fetal life, the testes begin to descend through the abdominal wall at the groin and enter the scrotum. As they descend they are accompanied by blood vessels, nerves, and ducts, all contained within the spermatic cord. The passageway through which the testes and spermatic cord descend is called the inguinal canal. Failure of a testis to descend into the scrotum is called CRYPTORCHIDISM.

The testis is divided internally into about 250 compartments or lobules, each of which contains one to three extremely small and convoluted tubules, within which spermatozoa are produced. When mature, the spermatozoa leave the tubules and enter the epididymis situated on top of and behind each testis. The spermatozoa are stored in the epididymis until such time as they are mixed in the semen and ejaculated during coitus. (See also REPRODUCTION and REPRODUCTIVE ORGANS, MALE.)

testitis (tes-ti'tis) inflammation of a testis; called also ORCHITIS.

testoid (tes'toid) a term applied to testicular hormones and other natural or synthetic compounds having a similar effect.

testolactone (tes"to-lak'tōn) an antineoplastic steroid prepared from testosterone or progesterone by microbial synthesis; used in the treatment of postmenopausal breast cancer.

testosterone (tes-tos'tĕ-rōn) one of the male sex hormones, or ANDROGENS, that are produced by the testes. Its chief function is to stimulate the development of the male reproductive organs, including the prostate, and the secondary sex characters, such as the beard. It encourages growth of bone and muscle, and helps maintain muscle strength.

Testosterone is obtained for therapeutic purposes by extraction from animal testes or by synthesis from cholesterol and certain other sterols in a laboratory. It is used generally in all cases of hypogonadism—that is, underfunctioning of the testes. It is also used to relieve some forms of breast cancer. Women normally secrete a certain amount of male hormones; however, if the hormone balance is disturbed and there is overproduction of male hormones in a woman, signs of masculinity may develop.

ethinyl t., ethisterone, a progestational steroid.

methyl t., an orally effective form of testosterone.

Testryl (tes'tril) trademark for a suspension of pure crystalline testosterone.

tetanic (tĕ-tan'ik) pertaining to tetanus.

tetaniform (tĕ-tan'ĭ-form) resembling tetanus.

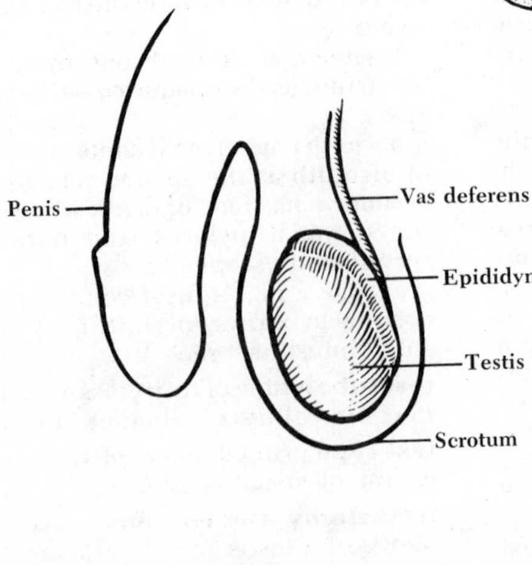

Testis.

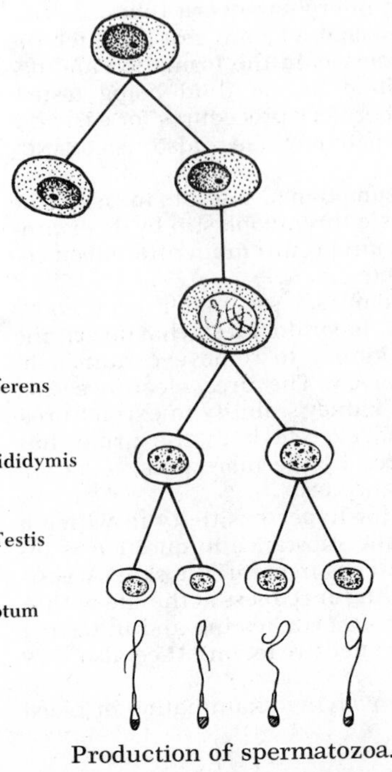
Production of spermatozoa.

tetanigenous (tet″an-nij′ĕ-nus) producing tetanic spasms.

tetanism (tet′ah-nizm) persistent muscular hypertonicity, as in the newborn.

tetanization (tet″ah-nĭ-za′shun) the induction of tetanic convulsions or symptoms.

tetanize (tet′ah-nīz) to induce tetanic convulsions or symptoms.

tetanode (tet′ah-nōd) the unexcited stage of tetany.

tetanoid (tet′ah-noid) resembling tetanus.

tetanolysin (tet″ah-nol′ĭ-sin) the hemolytic fraction of the exotoxin formed by *Clostridium tetani,* the causative organism of tetanus.

tetanospasmin (tet″ah-no-spaz′min) the neurotoxic component of the tetanus toxin, of primary importance in the pathogenesis of tetanus.

tetanus (tet′ah-nus) a highly fatal disease caused by the tetanus bacillus (*Clostridium tetani*) and characterized by muscle spasm and convulsions. Because stiffness of the jaw is often the first symptom, it is known also as lockjaw. adj., **tetan′ic.**

Tetanus is a serious illness, but because of widespread immunization, it now strikes only about 500 people in the United States each year.

Tetanus bacilli, which grow in the intestines of animals and man, are prevalent in rural areas. They are found in soil and dust, and are spread by animal and human feces. The organisms enter the body through a break in the skin, particularly in puncture wounds, including those caused by nails, splinters, insect bites, or gunshot. Occasionally, the original wound appears trivial and heals quickly; more often, there is obvious infection.

SYMPTOMS. Stiffness of the jaw is usually the first definite indication of tetanus. Difficulty in swallowing, stiffness of the neck, restlessness, irritability, headache, chills, fever, and convulsions are also among the early symptoms.

Muscles in the abdomen, back, neck, and face may go into spasm. If the infection is severe, convulsions are set off by slight disturbances, such as noises and drafts. During convulsions, there is difficulty in breathing and the possibility of asphyxiation.

TREATMENT. If there is any suspicion of contamination by tetanus bacilli, medical treatment should be obtained. This may include an adequate dose of antitoxin or a booster injection of tetanus toxoid (see below) to counteract any possible tetanus infection. Because of the possible danger of hypersensitivity to horse serum antitoxin, tetanus immune globulin —derived from human instead of horse serum—is preferred when available. In any case, the wound area must be carefully cleaned, and all dead tissue and foreign substances removed.

During a tetanus attack, sedatives are given to reduce the frequency of convulsions. Antibiotics are also used at times to help combat secondary infection. Most recently, hyperbaric oxygenation, providing oxygen under high pressure, has been used in treatment of tetanus.

PREVENTION. The most important weapon against tetanus is adequate IMMUNIZATION. Tetanus toxoid in combination with diphtheria toxoid and pertussis vaccine (DTP) is given at two months of age and repeated at four months, six months, 18 months, and four to six years of age.

At the time of an injury involving clean, minor wounds, no booster is needed for a fully immunized child unless it has been more than ten years since the last dose. For contaminated wounds a booster is recommended if more than five years have elapsed since the last dose. These recommendations for immunization against tetanus were approved by the American Academy of Pediatrics in 1971.

PATIENT CARE. Because the toxin from *Clostridium tetani* attacks the central nervous system it is extremely important to provide a nonstimulating environment for patients with tetanus. The room must be kept dark and quiet, and drafts of cold air, noises, and other external stimuli must be avoided because they may precipitate convulsive muscle spasms. As for any patient subject to convulsions, padded side rails are applied to the bed to prevent injury to the patient during a seizure. The head board is also padded with a cotton blanket or pillow, and a padded tongue depressor is kept at the bedside for insertion during seizures to prevent biting of the tongue. If the jaws are locked in a position that prevents proper insertion of the tongue blade, no attempt should be made to force the jaws open.

Fluids and nourishment usually are given intravenously during the acute stage of the disease. The patient's intake and output are carefully measured and recorded. Sedatives and antibiotic drugs are administered as ordered to reduce irritability and to combat secondary bacterial infections.

As long as the patient is acutely ill and likely to suffer from convulsive seizures, someone should be in constant attendance. Signs of respiratory difficulty, changes in pulse and blood pressure, and frequent and prolonged muscle spasms should be reported immediately to the physician in charge. A tracheostomy set should be readily available in the event severe dyspnea should develop.

infantile t., t. neonato′rum, tetanus of very young infants, usually due to infection of the umbilicus.

tetany (tet′ah-ne) 1. continuous tonic spasm of a muscle; steady contraction of a muscle without distinct twitching. 2. a syndrome manifested by sharp flexion of the wrist and ankle joints (carpopedal spasm), muscle twitchings, cramps, and convulsions, sometimes with attacks of stridor. It is caused by inadequate amounts of ionized calcium in the blood. This shortage of calcium causes irritability of the nerves and muscles, so that they respond to a stimulus with unnatural, violent contractions.

The drop in the calcium level can be caused by any one of several factors. It may occur in women during pregnancy or after childbirth if an excess amount of the mother's calcium is used. Tetany in a newborn baby is usually caused by temporarily underactive parathyroid glands. These glands normally keep the calcium and phosphate content of the blood at proper level. In children, tetany is more likely to occur because of an inadequate supply of calcium or vitamin D in the diet. Vitamin D is required for utilization of calcium in the body. Another cause of tetany in children is loss of calcium as a result of constant diarrhea.

An occasional cause of tetany in adults is the accidental removal or destruction of the parathyroid glands during thyroidectomy. This is sometimes unavoidable because the parathyroid glands are small and usually attached to the back of the thyroid gland or embedded in it.

Tetany often accompanies alkalosis, which may occur with prolonged vomiting, resulting in the loss of chlorides, or with excessive use of alkalis such as sodium bicarbonate. Alkalosis is also sometimes produced by hyperventilation.

TREATMENT. Treatment for tetany varies according to the cause and is usually successful. It may include the administration of vitamin D, calcium, parathyroid hormone, or other remedies. In chronic cases, as in the loss of the parathyroid glands, treatment may have to be continued indefinitely.

duration t., a continuous tetanic contraction in response to a strong continuous current, occurring especially in degenerated muscles.

gastric t., a severe form due to disease of the stomach, attended by difficult respiration and painful tonic spasms of the extremities.

hyperventilation t., tetany produced by forced inspiration and expiration continued for a considerable time.

latent t., tetany elicited by the application of electrical and mechanical stimulation.

parathyroid t., parathyroprival t., tetany due to removal or hypofunctioning of the parathyroid glands.

tetartanopia, tetartanopsia (tet″ar-tah-no′pe-ah, tet″ar-tah-nop′se-ah) 1. quadrantanopia; loss of vision in one-fourth of the visual field. 2. a type of defective color vision in which there is perception of red and green only, with blue and yellow perceived as an achromatic (gray) band.

tetra- (tĕ-trah) word element [Gr.], *four*.

tetrabasic (tĕ″trah-ba′sik) having four replaceable hydrogen atoms.

tetrabrachius (tĕ″trah-bra′ke-us) a double monster having four arms.

tetracaine (tet′rah-kān) a local and spinal anesthetic used in the form of the hydrochloride salt.

tetrachloride (tĕ″trah-klo′rīd) a compound of a radical with four atoms of chlorine.

tetrachloroethylene (tĕ″trah-klōr″o-eth′ĭ-lēn) a clear, colorless liquid used as an anthelmintic.

tetracrotic (tĕ″trah-krot′ik) having four sphygmographic waves or elevations to one beat of the pulse.

tetracycline (tĕ″trah-si′klēn) an antibiotic substance that is effective against many different microorganisms, including rickettsiae, certain viruses, and both gram-negative and gram-positive microorganisms. Preparations include chlortetracycline hydrochloride (Aureomycin), tetracycline hydrochloride (Achromycin), and demethylchlortetracycline (Declomycin).

Tetracyn (tĕ′trah-sin) trademark for preparations of tetracycline.

tetrad (tet′rad) a group of four similar or related entities, as (1) any element or radical having a valence, or combining power, of four; (2) a group of four chromosomal elements formed in meiosis; (3) a square of cells produced by division into two planes of certain cocci (Sarcina).

tetradactyly (tĕ″trah-dak′tĭ-le) the presence of four digits on the hand or foot.

tetraethylammonium (tĕ″trah-eth″il-ah-mo′ne-um) a radical used in the form of the bromide or chloride salt as a ganglionic blocking agent.

tetraethylthiuram disulfide (tĕ″trah-eth′il-thi′u-ram di-sul′fīd) a white or slightly yellow powder; used in treatment of alcoholism, because it produces a hypersensitivity reaction to alcohol (see also DISULFIRAM).

tetragonum (tĕ″trah-go′num) [L.] a four-sided figure.

t. lumba′le, the quadrangle bounded by the four lumbar muscles.

tetrahydrocannabinol (tet″rah-hi″dro-kah-nab′ĭ-nol) the active principle of cannabis, occurring in two isomeric forms, both considered psychomimetically active.

tetrahydrozoline (tĕ″trah-hi-dro′zo-lēn) an adrenergic used topically in the form of the hydrochloride salt to reduce nasal congestion.

tetraiodophthalein (tĕ″trah-i″o-do-thal′ēn) iodophthalein.

tetraiodothyronine (tĕ″trah-i″o-do-thi′ro-nēn) thyroxine.

tetralogy (tĕ-tral′o-je) a group or series of four.

t. of Fallot, a congenital defect of the heart that combines four structural anomalies: pulmonary stenosis (narrowing of the pulmonary artery); ventricular septal defect, or abnormal opening between the right and left ventricles; dextroposition of the aorta, in which the aortic opening overrides the septum and receives blood from both the right and left ventricles; and right ventricular hypertrophy, or increase of volume of the myocardium of the right ventricle.

Infants with this condition are sometimes referred to as blue babies because of the presence of cyanosis, an outstanding symptom of tetralogy of Fallot. The cyanosis is due to mixing of poorly oxygenated blood from the systemic circulation with oxygenated blood from the lungs, because of the position of the aorta. Other symptoms include clubbing of the ends of the fingers, hemoptysis, dyspnea on exertion, and a slight delay in growth and development.

Diagnosis is confirmed by electrocardiography, angiocardiography, and cardiac catheterization. These procedures demonstrate changes in the heart's electric impulses; defects in the ventricles, aorta, and pulmonary artery; and, from samplings of blood taken from the various chambers of the heart and great vessels, the oxygen content and pressure of the blood in these various areas.

Treatment of tetralogy of Fallot involves surgical correction whenever possible. Without corrective surgery the prognosis is extremely poor for children who are deeply cyanotic and have dyspnea on slight exertion.

Before surgery, medical treatment to avoid complications and to control dyspneic attacks is necessary. Since the hematocrit is high and polycythemia is common, efforts must be made to prevent dehydration and avoid the development of thrombi. Paroxysmal dyspnea, which often follows feeding or a spell of crying, usually can be relieved by placing the infant in knee-chest position, administering oxygen, or giving him a mild sedative or morphine.

Surgical procedures for correction of the defects in the heart and great vessels vary according to the severity of symptoms and the age of the patient. In some cases an anastomosis of the arteries may be done as a temporary measure until more extensive surgery is feasible. In most cases open heart surgery is most successful in relieving symptoms and produces the most lasting benefits. The risks of heart surgery have been reduced by the development of machines to provide extracorporeal circulation of the blood while the heart defects are being repaired (see also HEART SURGERY).

tetramastigote (tet″rah-mas′tĭ-gōt) 1. having four flagella. 2. an organism having four flagella.

tetrameric (tĕ″trah-mer′ik) having four parts.

tetranopsia (te″trah-nop′se-ah) obliteration of one quadrant of the visual field.

tetraparesis (tĕ″trah-pah-re′sis) muscular weakness affecting all four extremities.

tetrapeptide (tĕ″trah-pep′tīd) a peptide which, on hydrolysis, yields four amino acids.

tetraplegia (tĕ″trah-ple′je-ah) paralysis of all four extremities; QUADRIPLEGIA.

tetraploid (tet′rah-ploid) 1. characterized by tetraploidy. 2. an individual or cell having four sets of chromosomes.

tetraploidy (tĕ′trah-ploi″de) the state of having four sets of chromosomes (4n).

tetrapus (tĕ′trah-pus) a monster with four feet.

tetrasaccharide (tĕ″trah-sak′ah-rīd) a sugar, each molecule of which yields four molecules of monosaccharide on hydrolysis.

tetrascelus (tĕ-tras′ĕ-lus) a monster with four legs.

tetrasomy (tĕ′trah-so″me) the presence of two extra chromosomes of one type in an otherwise diploid cell. adj., **tetraso′mic.**

tetraster (tĕ-tras′ter) a figure in mitosis produced by quadruple division of the nucleus.

Tetrastoma (tĕ″trah-sto′mah) a genus of trematodes sometimes found in urine.

tetratomic (tĕ″trah-tom′ik) 1. containing four atoms in the molecule. 2. containing four replaceable hydrogen atoms. 3. containing four hydroxyl groups.

tetravalent (tĕ″trah-va′lent) having a valence of four.

tetrodotoxin (tet″ro-do-tok′sin) a highly lethal neurotoxin present in numerous species of puffer fish (suborder Tetraodontoidea) and in newts of the genus *Taricha* (tarichatoxin); ingestion results, within minutes, in malaise, dizziness, and tingling about the mouth, which may be followed by ataxia, convulsions, respiratory paralysis, and death.

tetroquinone (tet″ro-kwĭ-nōn) a systemic keratolytic.

tetroxide (tĕ-trok′sīd) a compound of an element or a radical with four oxygen atoms.

textiform (teks′tĭ-form) formed like a network.

textoblastic (teks″to-blas″tik) forming adult tissue; regenerative; said of cells.

texture (teks′chur) the structure or constitution of tissues. adj., **tex′tural.**

Th chemical symbol, *thorium.*

thalamencephalon (thal″ah-men-sef′ah-lon) that part of the diencephalon including the thalamus, metathalamus, and epithalamus.

thalamocoele (thal′ah-mo-sēl″) the third ventricle of the brain.

thalamocortical (thal″ah-mo-kor′tĭ-kal) pertaining to the thalamus and cerebral cortex.

thalamolenticular (thal″ah-mo-len-tik′u-lar) pertaining to the thalamus and lenticular nucleus.

thalamotomy (thal″ah-mot′o-me) the production of circumscribed lesions in the thalamus, formerly used in the treatment of certain psychotic states, and now sometimes used in the treatment of Parkinson's disease and certain other disorders of neuromuscular function.

thalamus (thal′ah-mus), pl. *thal′ami* [L.] either of two large ovoid structures composed of gray matter and situated at the base of the cerebrum. (See also BRAIN.) adj., **thalam′ic.** The thalamus functions as a relay station in which sensory pathways of the spinal cord and brain stem form synapses on their way to the cerebral cortex. Specific locations in the thalamus are related to specific areas on the body surface and in the cerebral cortex. A sensory impulse from the body surface travels upward to the thalamus, where it is received as a primitive sensation and then is sent on to the cerebral cortex for interpretation as to location, character, and duration.

The thalamus has numerous connections to other areas of the brain as well, and these are thought to be important in the integration of cerebral, cerebellar, and brain stem activity.

thalassemia (thal″ah-se′me-ah) a heterogeneous group of hereditary hemolytic anemias marked by a decreased rate of synthesis of one or more hemoglobin polypeptide chains, classified according to the chain involved (α, β, δ); the two major categories are α- and β-thalassemia.

α-t., alpha-t., that caused by diminished synthesis of alpha chains of hemoglobin. The *homozygous* form is incompatible with life, the stillborn infant displaying severe hydrops fetalis. The *heterozygous* form may be asymptomatic or marked by mild anemia.

β-t., beta-t., that caused by diminished synthesis of beta chains of hemoglobin. The *homozygous* form (Cooley's, Mediterranean, or erythroblastic anemia; thalassemia major), in which hemoglobin A is completely absent, appears in the newborn period and is marked by hemolytic, hypochromic, microcytic anemia, hepatosplenomegaly, skeletal deformation, mongoloid facies, and cardiac enlargement. The *heterozygous* form (thalassemia minor) is usually asymptomatic, but there is mild anemia.

t. major, see *beta-thalassemia.*

t. minor, see *beta-thalassemia.*

sickle cell-t., a hereditary anemia involving simultaneous heterozygosity for hemoglobin S and thalassemia.

thalassoposia (thah-las″o-po′ze-ah) the drinking of sea water.

thalassotherapy (thah-las″o-ther′ah-pe) treatment of disease by sea bathing, sea voyages, or sea air.

thalidomide (thah-lid′o-mīd) a sedative and hypnotic compound whose use during early pregnancy was frequently followed by the birth of infants showing serious developmental deformities, notably malformation of a limb or limbs.

thallium (thal′e-um) a chemical element, atomic number 81, atomic weight 204.37, symbol Tl. (See table of ELEMENTS.) Its salts are active poisons.

thallus (thal′us) 1. a simple plant body not differentiated into root, stem, and leaf, characteristic of mycelial fungi and some algae. 2. the actively growing vegetative organism as distinguished from reproductive or resting portions, as in fungi.

thanato- (than′ah-to) word element [Gr.], *death.*

thanatobiologic (than″ah-to-bi″o-loj′ik) pertaining to life and death.

thanatognomonic (than″ah-tog″no-mon′ik) indicating the approach of death.

thanatoid (than′ah-toid) resembling death.

thanatophobia (than″ah-to-fo′be-ah) unfounded apprehension of imminent death.

thebaine (the-ba′in) a crystalline, poisonous, and anodyne alkaloid from opium, having properties similar to those of strychnine.

thebesian foramina (the-be′ze-an) minute openings in the walls of the right atrium through which the smallest cardiac veins empty into the heart.

thebesian valve (the-be′ze-an) coronary vein.

thebesian veins (the-be′ze-an) smallest cardiac veins: numerous small veins arising in the muscular walls and draining independently into the cavities of the heart, and most readily seen in the atria.

theca (the′kah), pl. *the′cae* [L.] a case or sheath. adj., **the′cal.**

t. cor′dis, pericardium.

t. follic′uli, an envelope of condensed connective tissue surrounding a vesicular ovarian follicle, comprising an internal vascular layer (*theca interna*) and an external fibrous layer (*theca externa*).

thecitis (the-si′tis) tenosynovitis.

thecoma (the-ko′mah) theca cell tumor.

thecostegnosis (the″ko-steg-no′sis) contraction of a tendon sheath.

theine (the′in) the alkaloid of tea, isomeric with caffeine.

thelalgia (the-lal′je-ah) pain in the nipples.

thelarche (the-lar′ke) beginning of development of the breast at puberty.

theleplasty (the′le-plas″te) a plastic operation on the nipple.

thelerethism (thel-er′ĕ-thizm) erection of the nipple.

thelitis (the-li′tis) inflammation of a nipple.

thelium (the′le-um) 1. a papilla. 2. a nipple.

thelorrhagia (the″lo-ra′je-ah) hemorrhage from the nipple.

thelygenic (thel″ĭ-jen′ik) producing only female offspring.

thenad (the′nad) toward the thenar or toward the palm.

thenar (the′nar) 1. the fleshy part of the hand at the base of the thumb. 2. pertaining to the palm.

thenyldiamine (then″il-di′ah-mēn) a compound used as an antihistamine.

Thenylene (then′ĭ-lēn) trademark for a preparation of methapyrilene, an antihistamine.

thenylpyramine (then″il-pir′ah-mēn) methapyrilene, an antihistamine.

theobromine (the″o-bro′min) an alkaloid prepared from dried ripe seed of the tropical American tree *Theobroma cacao;* or made synthetically from xanthine; used as a diuretic, myocardial stimulant, vasodilator, and smooth muscle relaxant; available as theobromine calcium salicylate, theobromine sodium formate, theobromine sodium salicylate, and theobromine salicylate.

Theoglycinate (the″o-gli′sĭ-nāt) trademark for a preparation of theophylline sodium glycinate, used as a smooth muscle relaxant.

theophylline (the″o-fil′in) an alkaloid derived from tea or produced synthetically; used as a smooth muscle relaxant, myocardial stimulant, and diuretic; available as theophylline ethanolamine, theophylline methylglucamine, theophylline sodium acetate, and theophylline sodium glycinate.

t. cholinate, oxtriphylline, a smooth muscle relaxant, myocardial stimulant, and diuretic.

t. ethylenediamine, aminophylline, a smooth muscle relaxant, myocardial stimulant, and diuretic.

theory (the′o-re) 1. the doctrine or the principles underlying an art as distinguished from the practice of that particular art. 2. a formulated hypothesis or, loosely speaking, any hypothesis or opinion not based upon actual knowledge. See also names of specific theories, as LAMARCK'S THEORY.

cell t., all organic matter consists of cells, and cell activity is the essential process of life.

clonal-selection t. of immunity, immunologic specificity is preformed during embryonic life and mediated through cell clones.

germ t., 1. all organisms are developed from a cell. 2. infectious diseases are of microbial origin.

quantum t., radiation and absorption of energy occur in quantities (quanta) which vary in size with the frequency of the radiation.

recapitulation t., ontogeny recapitulates phylogeny (see also RECAPITULATION THEORY).

Thephorin (thef′o-rin) trademark for preparations of phenindamine, an antihistamine.

theque (tĕk) [Fr.] a round or oval collection, or nest, of melanin-containing nevus cells occurring at the dermoepidermal junction of the skin or in the dermis proper.

therapeutic (ther″ah-pu′tik) pertaining to therapeutics, or treatment of disease; curative.

therapeutics (ther″ah-pu′tiks) 1. the science and art of healing. 2. a scientific account of the treatment of disease.

therapeutist (ther″ah-pu′tist) therapist.

therapist (ther′-ah-pist) a person skilled in the treatment of disease or other disorder.

enterostomal t., one who is certified to assist in the specialized care of patients who have undergone enterostomy (see also STOMA).

physical t., a person skilled in the techniques of physical therapy and qualified to administer treatments prescribed by a physician (see also PHYSICAL THERAPIST).

registered respiratory t., one who holds at least an associate degree (AA or AD) in respiratory therapy from a college/hospital affiliation program, and has successfully completed the written and oral national examinations of the National Board of Respiratory Therapy (formerly of the American Registry of Inhalation Therapists).

speech t., a person specially trained and qualified to assist patients in overcoming speech and language disorders.

therapy (ther′ah-pe) the treatment of disease; therapeutics. (See also TREATMENT.)

anticoagulant t., the use of drugs to render the blood sufficiently incoagulable to discourage thrombosis.

aversion t., therapy directed at associating an undesirable behavior pattern with unpleasant stimulation.

collapse t., collapse and immobilization of the lung in treatment of pulmonary disease.

electroconvulsive t., electroshock t., the induction of convulsions by the passage of an electric current through the brain, as in the treatment of affective disorders (see also SHOCK THERAPY).

fever t., induction of high body temperature by

bacterial or physical means or by induction of fever-producing vaccines.

group t., psychotherapy carried out with a group of patients under the guidance of a single therapist.

immunosuppressive t., treatment with agents, such as x-rays, corticosteroids, and cytotoxic chemicals, which suppress the immune response to antigen(s); used in organ transplantation, autoimmune disease, allergy, multiple myeloma, etc.

inhalation t., treatment of pathophysiologic alterations of gas exchange in the cardiopulmonary system by the use of respirators, aerosols, oxygen, gas mixtures, etc.

insulin shock t., induction of hypoglycemic coma by the administration of insulin in the treatment of affective disorders (see also SHOCK THERAPY).

milieu t., daily participation in group psychiatric therapy at a hospital, providing for observation and utilization of the patients' interpersonal relationships in a social setting, as well as occupational, physical, and individual psychotherapy.

nonspecific t., treatment of disease by agents that produce a general effect on cellular activity.

occupational t., the teaching of useful skills or hobbies to sick or handicapped persons in order to promote their rehabilitation and recovery or to facilitate their ability to make a living (see also OCCUPATIONAL THERAPY).

oxygen t., the administration of supplemental oxygen to relieve hypoxemia and prevent damage to the tissue cells as a result of oxygen lack (hypoxia) (see also OXYGEN THERAPY).

physical t., use of physical agents and methods in rehabilitation and restoration of normal bodily function after illness or injury; it includes massage and manipulation, therapeutic exercises, hydrotherapy, and various forms of energy (electrotherapy, actinotherapy, and ultrasound) (see also PHYSICAL THERAPY).

radiation t., treatment of disease by means of ionizing radiation (see also RADIOTHERAPY).

replacement t., treatment to replace deficient formation or loss of body products by administration of the natural body products or synthetic substitutes.

serum t., serotherapy; treatment of disease by injection of serum from immune individuals.

shock t., treatment of affective disorders by induction of coma or convulsions by various means, including insulin injection, electroshock, etc. (see also SHOCK THERAPY).

specific t., treatment by measures that are effective against the organism causing the disease.

speech t., the use of special techniques for correction of speech and language disorders.

substitution t., the administration of a hormone to compensate for glandular deficiency.

vaccine t., injection of killed cultures of an organism to produce immunity to or modify the course of a disease.

therm (therm) a unit of heat. The word has been used as equivalent to (a) large calorie; (b) small calorie; (c) 1000 large calories; (d) 100,000 British thermal units.

therm(o)- (ther′mo) word element [Gr.], *heat.*

thermaerotherapy (therm-a″er-o-ther′ah-pe) treatment by application of hot air.

thermal (ther′mal) pertaining to heat.

thermalgesia (ther″mal-je′ze-ah) painful sensation produced by heat.

thermalgia (ther-mal′je-ah) causalgia.

thermanalgesia (therm″an-al-je′ze-ah) absence of sensibility to heat.

thermanesthesia (therm″an-es-the′ze-ah) inability to recognize heat and cold.

thermatology (ther″mah-tol′o-je) the study of heat as a therapeutic agent.

thermelometer (ther″mel-om′ĕ-ter) an electric thermometer for measuring small temperature changes.

thermesthesia (therm″es-the′ze-ah) perception of heat or cold.

thermesthesiometer (therm″es-the″ze-om′ĕ-ter) an instrument for measuring sensibility to heat.

thermhyperesthesia (therm″hi-per-es-the′ze-ah) increased sensibility to high temperatures.

thermhypesthesia (therm″hi-pes-the′ze-ah) decreased sensibility to high temperatures.

thermic (ther′mik) pertaining to heat.

thermistor (ther-mis′tor) a thermometer whose impedance varies with ambient temperature and so is able to measure extremely small temperature changes.

thermocautery (ther″mo-kaw′ter-e) cauterization by a heated wire or point.

thermochemistry (ther″mo-kem′is-tre) the aspect of physical chemistry dealing with temperature changes that accompany chemical reactions.

thermocoagulation (ther″mo-ko-ag″u-la′shun) coagulation of tissue with high-frequency currents.

thermocouple (ther′mo-kup″′l) a pair of dissimilar electric conductors so joined that with the application of heat an electromotive force is established; used for measuring small temperature differences.

thermodiffusion (ther″mo-dĭ-fu′zhun) diffusion influenced by a temperature gradient.

thermoduric (ther″mo-du′rik) able to endure high temperatures.

thermodynamics (ther″mo-di-nam′iks) the branch of science dealing with heat and energy, their interconversion, and problems related thereto.

thermoexcitory (ther″mo-ek-si′tor-e) stimulating production of bodily heat.

thermogenesis (ther″mo-jen′ĕ-sis) the production of heat, especially within the animal body. adj., **thermogenet′ic, thermogen′ic.**

thermogenics (ther″mo-jen′iks) the science of heat production.

thermogram (ther′mo-gram) 1. a graphic record of temperature variations. 2. the visual record obtained by thermography.

thermograph (ther′mo-graf) 1. an instrument for recording temperature variations. 2. thermogram (2). 3. the apparatus used in thermography.

thermography (ther-mog′rah-fe) a technique wherein an infrared camera photographically portrays the body's surface temperature, based on self-emanating infrared radiations; sometimes used as a means of diagnosing underlying pathologic conditions, such as breast tumors.

thermohyperalgesia (ther″mo-hi″per-al-je′ze-ah) extreme thermalgesia.

thermohyperesthesia (ther″mo-hi″per-es-the′ze-ah) extreme sensitiveness to heat.

thermoinhibitory (ther″mo-in-hib′ĭ-tor″e) retarding generation of bodily heat.

thermolabile (ther″mo-la′bil) easily affected by heat.

thermology (ther-mol′o-je) the science of heat.

thermolysis (ther-mol′ĭ-sis) 1. chemical dissociation by means of heat. 2. dissipation of bodily heat by radiation, evaporation, etc. adj., **thermolyt′ic.**

thermomassage (ther″mo-mah-sahzh′) massage with heat.

thermometer (ther-mom′ĕ-ter) an instrument for determining temperatures, in principle making use of a substance (such as alcohol or mercury) with a physical property that varies with temperature and is susceptible of measurement on some defined scale.

Celsius t., one employing the Celsius scale, that is, with the ice point at 0 and the normal boiling point of water at 100 degrees (100° C.). (For equivalents of Celsius and Fahrenheit temperatures, see Appendix.)

centigrade t., one having the interval between two established reference points divided into 100 equal units, as the Celsius thermometer.

clinical t., one used to determine the temperature of the human body.

electronic t., a clinical thermometer using a sensor based on thermistors, solid-state electronic devices whose electrical characteristics change with temperature. The reading is recorded within seconds, some having a red light or other device to indicate when maximum temperature is reached. Available models include hand-held, desk-top, and wall-mounted units, all having probes that are inserted orally or rectally. It is expected that in the future an electronic thermometer to be worn on the wrist will be available.

Fahrenheit t., one employing the Fahrenheit scale, that is, with the ice point at 32 and the normal boiling point of water at 212 degrees (212° F.). (For equivalents of Fahrenheit and Celsius temperatures, see Appendix.)

Kelvin t., one employing the KELVIN SCALE.

oral t., a clinical thermometer whose mercury containing bulb is placed under the tongue.

Rankine t., one employing the RANKINE SCALE.

Réaumur t., one employing the Réaumur scale, that is, having the ice point at 0 and the normal boiling point of water at 80 degrees (80° R.).

recording t., a temperature-sensitive instrument by which the temperature to which it is exposed is continuously recorded.

rectal t., a clinical thermometer that is inserted in the rectum for determining body temperature.

resistance t., one that uses the electric resistance of metals for determining temperature (thermocouple).

self-registering t., recording thermometer.

thermometry (ther-mom′ĕ-tre) measurement of temperature.

thermophile (ther′mo-fīl) a microorganism that grows best at elevated temperatures. adj., **thermophil′ic.**

thermophore (ther′mo-fōr) 1. a device or apparatus for retaining heat. 2. an instrument for estimating heat sensibility.

thermopile (ther′mo-pīl) a number of thermocouples in series, used to increase sensitivity to change in temperature or for direct conversion of heat into electric energy.

thermoplacentography (ther″mo-plas″en-tog′rah-fe) use of thermography for determination of the site of placental attachment.

thermoplegia (ther″mo-ple′je-ah) heat stroke or sunstroke.

thermopolypnea (ther″mo-pol″ip-ne′ah) quickened breathing due to great heat.

thermoreceptor (ther″mo-re-sep′tor) a nerve ending sensitive to stimulation by heat.

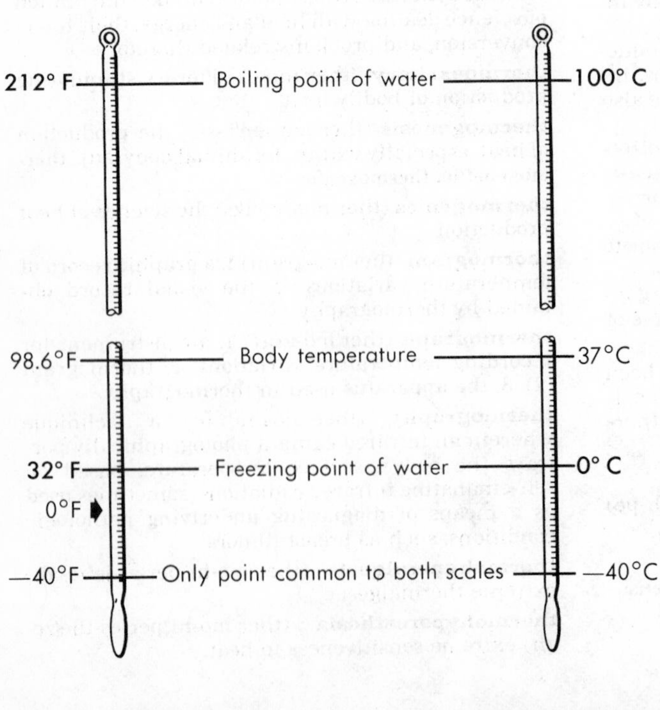

Comparison of the Fahrenheit and Celsius temperature scales. (From Lee, G. L., Van Orden, H. O., and Ragsdale, R. O.: General and Organic Chemistry. Philadelphia, W. B. Saunders Co., 1971.)

thermoregulation (ther″mo-reg″u-la′shun) heat regulation.

thermostabile (ther″mo-sta′b'l) not affected by heat.

thermostasis (ther″mo-sta′sis) maintenance of temperature, as in warm-blooded animals.

thermostat (ther′mo-stat) a device interposed in a heating system by which temperature is automatically maintained between certain levels.

thermosteresis (ther″mo-stē-re′sis) deprivation of heat.

thermosystaltic (ther″mo-sis-tal′tik) contracting under the stimulus of heat.

thermotaxis (ther″mo-tak′sis) 1. normal adjustment of bodily temperature. 2. movement of an organism in response to the stimulation of a temperature gradient. adj., **thermotac′tic, thermotax′ic.**

thermotherapy (ther″mo-ther′ah-pe) therapeutic use of heat.

thermotics (ther-mot′iks) the science of heat.

thermotonometer (ther″mo-to-nom′ĕ-ter) an instrument for measuring the amount of muscular contraction produced by heat.

thermotropism (ther″mot′ro-pizm) the orientation of a living cell in response to a heat stimulus. adj., **thermotrop′ic.**

thesaurismosis (the-saw″riz-mo′sis) a metabolic disorder in which some substance accumulates in certain cells in abnormal amounts. The stored substances may be fats, proteins, carbohydrates, or other substances.

thesaurosis (the″saw-ro′sis) a condition due to the storing up in the body of unusual amounts of normal or foreign substance.

thi(o)- (thi′o) word element [Gr.], *sulfur.*

thiabendazole (thi″ah-ben′dah-zol) a broad-spectrum anthelmintic found useful in ancylostomiasis and strongyloidiasis.

thiamazole (thi-am′ah-zōl) methimazole, a thyroid inhibitor.

thiamin (thi′ah-min) thiamine.

thiaminase (thi-am′ĭ-nās) an enzyme that catalyzes the splitting of thiamine into a pyrimidine and a thiazole derivative.

thiamine (thi′ah-min) vitamin B_1; a component of the B complex group of vitamins, found in various foodstuffs and present in the free state in blood plasma and cerebrospinal fluid. Deficiency results in neurological symptoms, cardiovascular dysfunction, edema, and reduced intestinal motility. (See also VITAMIN.)

t. hydrochloride, a vitamin supplement used in prophylaxis and treatment of thiamine deficiency.

t. mononitrate, a compound prepared by removing the chloride ions from thiamine hydrochloride and replacing them with nitric acid; used like thiamine hydrochloride.

phosphorylated t., t. pyrophosphate, the active form of thiamine, serving as a cofactor in certain reactions in carbohydrate metabolism. Called also cocarboxylase.

thiamylal (thi-am′ĭ-lal) an ultra-short-acting barbiturate; the sodium salt is used intravenously as a general anesthetic.

thiazide diuretics (thi′ah-zīd) a group of synthetic compounds that effect diuresis by enhancing the excretion of sodium and chloride.

thiemia (thi-e′me-ah) sulfur in the blood.

thiethylperazine (thi-eth″il-per′ah-zēn) a phenothiazine derivative useful as an antiemetic and antinauseant.

Thiersch graft (tērsh′) Ollier-Tiersch graft.

thigh (thi) the portion of the leg above the knee; the femur.

t. bone, femur.

thigmesthesia (thig″mes-the′ze-ah) tactile sensibility.

thigmotaxis (thig″mo-tak′sis) movement of an organism in response to contact. adj., **thigmotac′tic, thigmotax′ic.**

thigmotropism (thig-mot′ro-pizm) the orientation of an organism in response to the stimulus of contact. adj., **thigmotrop′ic.**

thihexinol (thi-hek′sĭ-nol) an anticholinergic used to inhibit intestinal hypermotility.

thimerosal (thi-mer′o-sal) a mercury-containing compound used as a local antibacterial agent.

thinking (thingk′ing) the formulation of images or concepts in one's mind.

thiobarbiturate (thi″o-bar-bit′u-rāt) a salt or derivative of thiobarbituric acid.

thiocyanate (thi″o-si′ah-nāt) a salt analogous in composition to a cyanate, but containing sulfur instead of oxygen.

thiodiphenylamine (thi″o-di-fen″il-am′ēn) phenothiazine, a compound whose derivatives are widely used as tranquilizers.

thioglucosidase (thi″glu-ko′sĭ-dās) an enzyme found in mustard seed that catalyzes the hydrolysis of thioglycosides to a thiol and a sugar.

thioguanine (thi″gwah′nēn) an antineoplastic (2-aminopurine-6-thiol) used in leukemia.

Thiomerin (thi″o-mer′in) trademark for a preparation of mercaptomerin, a mercurial diuretic.

thiomersalate (thi″o-mer′sah-lāt) thimerosal, a local antibacterial.

thionin (thi′o-nin) a dark-green powder, purple in solution, used as a metachromatic stain in microscopy.

thiopental (thi″o-pen′tal) an ultrashort-acting barbiturate, used in the form of the sodium salt, given intravenously or rectally to induce general ANESTHESIA. Psychiatrists use the drug as a sedative or sometimes in narcoanalysis.

thiopentone (thi″o-pen′tōn) thiopental.

thiopropazate (thi″o-pro′pah-zāt) a phenothiazine derivative used as a major tranquilizer in the form of the hydrochloride salt.

thioridazine (thi″o-rid′ah-zēn) a phenothiazine compound used in the form of the hydrochloride salt as a tranquilizer.

thiosulfate (thi″o-sul′fāt) any salt of thiosulfuric acid.

thiotepa (thi″o-te′pah) a compound used as an antineoplastic agent.

thiothixene (thi″o-thiks′ēn) a tranquilizer.

thiouracil (thi″o-u′rah-sil) a derivative of thiourea, used in treatment of hyperthyroidism because it suppresses thyroid hormone synthesis.

thiourea (th″o-u-re′ah) urea with its oxygen replaced by sulfur; an antithyroid substance that inhibits thyroid function.

thirst (therst) a sensation, often referred to the mouth and throat, associated with a craving for drink; ordinarily interpreted as a desire for water.

thixotropism, thixotropy (thik-sot′ro-pizm; thik-sot′ro-pe) the property of certain gels of becoming fluid when shaken and then becoming solid again.

thlipsencephalus (thlip″sen-sef′ah-lus) a monster with a defective skull.

Thomas splint (tom′as) two round iron rods joined at the upper end by an oval iron ring, or half-ring, and bent at the lower end to form the letter W; used to give support to the lower extremity and to remove the weight of the body from the knee joint by transferring it to the pelvis.

Thomsen's disease (tom′senz) myotonia congenita.

thonzylamine (thon-zil′ah-min) a compound used as an antihistamine.

thorac(o)- word element [Gr.], *chest.*

thoracalgia (tho″rah-kal′je-ah) pain in the chest wall.

thoracectomy (tho″rah-sek′to-me) thoracotomy with resection of part of a rib.

thoracentesis (tho″rah-sen-te′sis) surgical puncture and drainage of the thoracic cavity. The procedure may be done as an aid to the diagnosis of inflammatory or neoplastic diseases of the lung or pleura, or it may be used as a therapeutic measure to remove accumulations of fluid from the thoracic cavity.

The patient sits up for this procedure, his arms and head resting on the overbed table or over the back of a chair he is straddling. If the patient is unable to sit up he is turned onto his unaffected side. The skin at the site of insertion of the needle is cleansed with an antiseptic, and a local anesthetic is injected. The site most often used is the seventh intercostal space, just below the angle of the scapula.

Equipment needed includes a 50 ml. syringe and an aspirating needle, a stopcock and rubber tubing, a hemostat, sterile gauze dressings, sterile towels, and a sterile specimen tube.

After the procedure is completed the wound usually is sealed with collodion and covered with a sterile dressing. The site is checked frequently for signs of leakage, which should be reported to the physician.

The total amount and character of the fluid obtained is noted on the patient's chart. Samples of fluid are sent to the laboratory for evaluation if requested.

Immediately following the thoracentesis the patient is positioned on his unaffected side to rest the site of insertion of the trochar and allow it to seal itself. The patient is observed for signs of dizziness, changes in skin color, and respiratory and heart rate changes. Other signs of complications following thoracentesis include excessive coughing, blood-tinged sputum, and tightness of the chest.

Possible aftereffects of the procedure include PNEUMOTHORAX, subcutaneous emphysema (accumulation of air in the tissues of the skin), and bacterial infection. A MEDIASTINAL SHIFT resulting from removal of large amounts of fluid from the thoracic cavity may produce cardiac distress and pulmonary edema.

thoracic (tho-ras′ik) pertaining to the chest.

t. cage, the bony structure enclosing the thorax, consisting of the ribs, vertebral column, and sternum.

t. duct, a duct beginning in the receptaculum chyli and emptying into the venous system at the junction of the left subclavian and left internal jugular veins. It acts as a channel for the collection of the lymph from the portions of the body below the diaphragm and from the left side of the body above the diaphragm.

t. outlet syndrome, compression of the brachial plexus nerve trunks, with pain in the arms, paresthesia of fingers, vasomotor symptoms, and weakness and wasting of small muscles of the hand; it may be caused by drooping shoulder girdle, a cervical rib or fibrous band, an abnormal first rib, continual hyperabduction of the arm (as during sleep), or compression of the edge of scalenus anterior muscle.

t. surgery, surgical procedures involving entrance into the chest cavity. Until techniques for endotracheal anesthesia were perfected, this type of surgery was extremely dangerous because of the possibility of lung collapse. By administering anesthesia under pressure through an endotracheal tube it is now possible to keep one or both lungs expanded, even when they are subjected to atmospheric pressure.

Surgical procedures involving the lungs, heart, and great vessels are included under thoracic surgery. In order to give intelligent care to the patient before and after surgery, one must have adequate knowledge of the anatomy and physiology of the chest and thoracic cavity. It is especially important to know the difference in pressures within and outside the thoracic cavity. (See also LUNG, Mechanism of Inflation and Deflation.)

PATIENT CARE. Prior to surgery the care of the patient will depend on the specific operation to be done and the particular disorder requiring surgery. (See also surgery of the LUNG, and HEART surgery.) In general, the patient should be given an explanation of the operative procedure anticipated and the type of equipment that will be used in the postoperative period. He will be taught the proper method of coughing to remove secretions accumulated in the lungs. Although coughing may be painful in the immediate postoperative period and may require analgesic medication to relieve the discomfort, if the patient understands the need for coughing up the secretions he will be more cooperative. He may be given special exercises to preserve muscular action of the shoulder on the affected side and to maintain proper alignment of the upper portion of his body and arm. Usually the physical therapist supervises these exercises, but the nursing staff must cooperate in seeing that they are done.

Narcotics are rarely given before thoracic surgery because they can depress respiration. Usually the preoperative medication is atropine in combination with a barbiturate.

When the patient returns from the operating room the drainage catheters are usually protruding from above and below the area of surgery. The upper catheter allows for removal of air and the gradual expansion of the lung. The lower catheter provides for drainage of fluid. These catheters are attached to a closed drainage system. (See CHEST TUBE(S).)

When a patient cannot force out accumulated secretions by coughing, a chest suction machine may be used. These machines incorporate the principle of closed drainage and also provide negative pressure. Whatever the type of equipment used, the nurse should become familiar with its purpose and check frequently to be sure it is in good working order.

If the surgeon permits, the nursing staff may be responsible for measuring and recording the amount of drainage at regular intervals. This requires strict attention to proper clamping and reconnecting of the tubes before and after the bottles are removed.

As the operative site heals and the lung expands, the chest tubes can be safely removed. After their removal an airtight bandage is applied to the area. As a precaution against leakage of air into the chest cavity, the physician may apply petrolatum to the edges of the wound before applying the dressing.

t. vertebrae, the 12 vertebrae between the cervical and lumbar vertebrae, giving attachment to the ribs and forming part of the posterior wall of the thorax.

thoracoacromial (tho″rah-ko-ah-kro′me-al) pertaining to the chest and acromion.

thoracoceloschisis (tho″rah-ko-se-los′kĭ-sis) congenital fissure of the thorax and abdomen.

thoracocentesis (tho″rah-ko-sen-te′sis) thoracentesis.

thoracocyllosis (tho″rah-ko-sĭ-lo′sis) deformity of the thorax.

thoracocyrtosis (tho″rah-ko-sir-to′sis) abnormal curvature of the chest wall.

thoracodelphus (tho″rah-ko-del′fus) a double monster with one head, two arms, and four legs, the bodies being joined above the navel.

thoracodidymus (tho″rah-ko-did′ĭ-mus) thoracopagus.

thoracodynia (tho″rah-ko-din′e-ah) pain in the thorax.

thoracogastroschisis (tho″rah-ko-gas-tros′kĭ-sis) a developmental anomaly resulting from faulty closure of the body wall along the midventral line, involving both thorax and abdomen, i.e., fissure of the thorax and abdomen.

thoracolumbar (tho″rah-ko-lum′bar) pertaining to the thoracic and lumbar vertebrae.

thoracolysis (tho″rah-kol′ĭ-sis) the freeing of adhesions of the chest wall.

thoracomelus (tho″rah-kom′ĕ-lus) a monster with a supernumerary limb attached to the thorax.

thoracometer (tho″rah-kom′ĕ-ter) stethometer.

thoracomyodynia (tho″rah-ko-mi″o-din′e-ah) pain in the muscles of the chest.

thoracopagus (tho″rah-kop′ah-gus) conjoined twins united at the thorax.

thoracopathy (tho″rah-kop′ah-the) any disease of the thoracic organs or tissues.

thoracoplasty (tho′rah-ko-plas″te) surgical removal of ribs, allowing the chest wall to collapse a diseased lung.

thoracoschisis (tho″rah-kos′kĭ-sis) congenital fissure of the chest wall.

thoracoscope (tho-ra′ko-skōp) an endoscope for examining the pleural cavity through an intercostal space.

thoracoscopy (tho″rah-kos′ko-pe) examination of the pleural space with a thoracoscope.

thoracostenosis (tho″rah-ko-stĕn-o′sis) abnormal contraction of the thorax.

thoracostomy (tho″rah-kos′to-me) incision of the chest wall, with maintenance of the opening for drainage.

thoracotomy (tho″rah-kot′o-me) incision of the chest wall.

thorax (tho′raks) the part of the body between the neck and abdomen; the chest. It is separated from the abdomen by the diaphragm. The walls of the thorax are formed by the 12 pairs of ribs, attached to the sides of the spine and curving toward the front. The upper seven ribs are attached to the sternum, the next three connect with cartilage below and the last two (the floating ribs) are unattached in the front. The principal organs in the thoracic cavity are the heart with its major blood vessels, and the lungs with the bronchi, which bring in the body's air supply. The trachea enters the thorax to connect with the lungs, and the esophagus travels through it to connect with the stomach below the diaphragm. (See also THORACIC SURGERY.)

Thorazine (thor′ah-zēn) trademark for preparations of chlorpromazine, an antiemetic and tranquilizer.

Thorel's bundle (to′relz) a bundle of muscle fibers in the human heart connecting the sinoatrial and atrioventricular nodes.

thorium (tho′re-um) a chemical element, atomic number 90, atomic weight 232.038, symbol Th. (See table of ELEMENTS.) Formerly used as a roentgenographic contrast medium.

Thorn test (thorn) a test for adrenal cortical response after injection of ACTH or of epinephrine.

thoron (tho′ron) a radioactive isotope of radon.

thozalinone (tho-zal′ĭ-nōn) an antidepressant.

threadworm (thred′werm) any nematode worm, as *Enterobius vermicularis* (see also WORM).

threonine (thre′o-nin) a naturally occurring amino acid, one of those essential for human metabolism.

threpsology (threp-sol′o-je) the scientific study of nutrition.

threshold (thresh′old) the level that must be reached for an effect to be produced, as the degree of intensity of stimulus which just produces a sensation, or the concentration that must be present in the blood before certain substances are excreted by the kidney (renal threshold).

auditory t., the slightest perceptible sound.

t. of consciousness, the lowest limit of sensibility; the point of consciousness at which a stimulus is barely perceived.

thrill (thril) a vibration felt by the examiner on palpation.

diastolic t., one felt over the precordium during diastole in advanced aortic insufficiency.

hydatid t., one felt on percussing over a hydatid cyst.

presystolic t., one felt just before the systole over the apex of the heart.

systolic t., one felt over the precordium during systole in aortic stenosis, pulmonary stenosis, and ventricular septal defect.

thrix (thriks) hair.

t. annula′ta, a condition in which a hair appears

to be marked by alternating bands of white; called also ringed hair.

-thrix (thriks) word element [Gr.], *hair.*

throat (thrōt) 1. the area that includes the LARYNX and PHARYNX, passageways that link the nose and mouth with the respiratory and digestive systems of the body. 2. the fauces. 3. the anterior part of the neck.

DISORDERS OF THE THROAT. Sore throat is caused by inflammation or irritation of tissue in one or more areas of the pharynx or larynx. The disorder may be a disease in itself (see PHARYNGITIS and LARYNGITIS) or a symptom of a disease affecting other areas of the body. It also may be due to excess smoking or overuse of the voice.

Streptococcal sore throat, or "strep throat," is more severe than ordinary sore throat and may be accompanied by high fever, swelling of the cervical lymph nodes (swollen glands), and a rash. Penicillin or other antibiotics are usually used in treatment.

TONSILLITIS is often the cause of inflammation and discomfort in the throat.

Cancer of the throat, one of the least common forms of cancer, occurs most often in the larynx, and early diagnosis is essential to effective treatment. The first symptoms are persistent hoarseness and the feeling of a lump in the throat (although this feeling is usually caused by emotional stress, and is called globus hystericus).

CARE OF THE THROAT. Proper care of the throat does not require the use of sprays, gargles, or lozenges. On the contrary, nose drops and throat sprays, when inhaled, may irritate the trachea, bronchi, or lungs.

The people most concerned about their throats are usually those who depend on their voices in their occupations or professions. Proper training and use of the vocal muscles, not medications, are the best insurance against loss or change of voice. When muscular exhaustion from strain or overuse of the larynx does bring on laryngitis, rest for the voice muscles is the only real cure.

In serious cases the physician may recommend medication or the use of steam inhalants, but the essential aspect of treatment is silence, with any unavoidable talking done in a low voice. This "silent cure," if followed faithfully, is almost certain to result in the return of the normal voice.

throb (throb) a pulsating movement or sensation.

thromb(o)- (throm′bo) word element [Gr.], *clot; thrombus.*

thrombase (throm′bās) thrombin.

thrombasthenia (throm″bas-the′ne-ah) a platelet abnormality characterized by defective clot retraction and impaired ADP-induced platelet aggregation; it is manifested clinically as Glanzmann's disease, with epistaxis, inappropriate bruising, and excessive post-traumatic bleeding.

Glanzmann's t., thrombasthenia.

thrombectomy (throm-bek′to-me) surgical removal of a clot from a blood vessel.

medical t., enzymatic dissolution of a blood clot in situ.

thrombin (throm′bin) an enzyme resulting from activation of prothrombin, which catalyzes the conversion of fibrinogen to fibrin; a preparation from prothrombin of bovine origin is used as a topical hemostatic.

thromboangiitis (throm″bo-an″je-i′tis) inflammation of a blood vessel, with thrombosis.

t. oblit′erans, thromboangiitis with contraction of the vessel about the clot, leading to diminution of blood flow distal to the site; most frequently the lower extremities are affected. Called also BUERGER'S DISEASE.

thromboarteritis (throm″bo-ar″ter-i′tis) thrombosis associated with arteritis.

thromboclasis (throm-bok′lah-sis) the dissolution of a thrombus. adj., **thromboclas′tic.**

thrombocyst, thrombocystis (throm′bo-sist; throm″bo-sis′tis) a sac formed around a clot or thrombus.

thrombocyte (throm′bo-sīt) a blood platelet (see also PLATELET). adj., **thrombocyt′ic.**

thrombocythemia (throm″bo-si-the′me-ah) a fixed increase in the number of circulating blood platelets.

essential t., hemorrhagic t., a clinical syndrome with repeated spontaneous hemorrhages, either external or into the tissues, and greatly increased number of circulating platelets.

thrombocytocrit (throm″bo-si′to-krit) the volume of packed blood platelets in a given quantity of blood; also, the instrument used to measure platelet volume.

thrombocytolysis (throm″bo-si-tol′ĭ-sis) destruction of blood platelets (thrombocytes).

thrombocytopathy (throm″bo-si-top′ah-the) any qualitative disorder of blood platelets.

thrombocytopenia (throm″bo-si″to-pe′ne-ah) decrease in number of platelets in circulating blood. adj., **thrombocytope′nic.**

thrombocytopoiesis (throm″bo-si″to-poi-e′sis) the production of blood platelets (thrombocytes). adj., **thrombocytopoiet′ic.**

thrombocytosis (throm″bo-si-to′sis) increase in the number of platelets in the circulating blood.

thromboembolism (throm″bo-em′bo-lizm) obstruction of a blood vessel with thrombotic material carried by the blood from the site of origin to plug another vessel.

thromboendarterectomy (throm″bo-en″dar-ter-ek′to-me) excision of an obstructing thrombus together with a portion of the inner lining of the obstructed artery.

thromboendarteritis (throm″bo-en″dar-ter-i′tis) inflammation of the innermost coat of an artery, with thrombus formation.

thromboendocarditis (throm″bo-en″do-kar-di′tis) formation of a thrombus on a heart valve which has previously been eroded.

thrombogenesis (throm″bo-jen′ĕ-sis) clot formation. adj., **thrombogen′ic.**

thromboid (throm′boid) resembling a thrombus.

thrombokinase (throm″bo-ki′nās) activated clotting factor X.

thrombolymphangitis (throm″bo-lim″fan-ji′tis) inflammation of a lymph vessel due to a thrombus.

thrombolysis (throm-bol′ĭ-sis) dissolution of a thrombus.

thrombolytic (throm″bo-lit′ik) 1. dissolving or splitting up a thrombus. 2. an agent that dissolves or splits up a thrombus. The use of such thrombolytics as STREPTOKINASE and UROKINASE remains largely experimental in the United States (see also ANTICOAGULANT).

thrombon (throm′bon) the circulating blood platelets and their precursors.

thrombopathy (throm-bop′ah-the) thrombocytopathy.

thrombopenia (throm″bo-pe′ne-ah) thrombocytopenia.

thrombophilia (throm″bo-fil′e-ah) a tendency to the occurrence of thrombosis.

thrombophlebitis (throm″bo-flĕ-bi′tis) inflammation of a vein associated with thrombus formation. (See also venous THROMBOSIS.)

t. mi′grans, a recurrent condition involving different vessels simultaneously or at intervals.

postpartum iliofemoral t., thrombophlebitis of the iliofemoral vein following childbirth.

thromboplastic (throm″bo-plas′tik) causing or accelerating clot formation in the blood.

thromboplastid (throm″bo-plas′tid) a blood platelet.

thromboplastin (throm″bo-plas′tin) a substance in blood and tissues which, in the presence of ionized calcium, aids in the conversion of prothrombin to thrombin. Extrinsic and intrinsic thromboplastin are formed as the result of the interaction of different clotting factors; the factors that combine to form extrinsic thromboplastin are not all derived from intravascular sources, whereas those that form intrinsic thromboplastin are. Tissue thromboplastin, called also clotting factor III, is released by or derived from extravascular sources.

thrombopoiesis (throm″bo-poi-e′sis) 1. thrombogenesis. 2. thrombocytopoiesis. adj., **thrombopoiet′ic.**

thrombosis (throm-bo′sis) formation or presence of blood clots, or thrombi, inside a blood vessel or in one of the chambers of the heart. adj., **thrombot′ic.**

A thrombus may form whenever the flow of blood in the arteries or the veins is impeded. Many factors can interfere with the normal flow of the blood. Sometimes heart failure or physical inactivity retards circulation generally, or a change in the shape or inner surface of a vessel wall impedes the flow of blood, as in atherosclerosis. Any mass that has grown inside the body can exert pressure on a vessel, or the vessel wall can be injured and roughened by an accident, surgery, a burn, cold, inflammation, or infection. The blood may thicken in a reaction to the presence of a foreign serum or snake venom.

If the thrombus detaches itself from the wall and is carried along by the bloodstream, the clot is called an embolus. The condition is known as EMBOLISM.

A thrombus may form in the heart chambers. This sometimes occurs after coronary thrombosis (see below) at the place where the wall of the heart is weakened or in the dilated atria in some cases of mitral stenosis.

Because blood normally flows more slowly through the veins than through the arteries, thrombosis is more common in the veins than in the arteries.

VENOUS THROMBOSIS. Venous thrombosis occurs most often in the legs or pelvis. It may be a complication of phlebitis or may result from injury to a vein or from prolonged bed rest. The symptoms of venous thrombosis—a feeling of heaviness, pain, warmth, or swelling in the affected part, and possibly chills and fever—do not necessarily indicate its severity. Immediate medical attention is necessary in any case. Under *no* circumstances should the affected limb be massaged.

In a thrombosis of the superficial veins, bed rest with the legs elevated and application of heat to the affected area may be all that is necessary. In a thrombosis of the deep veins, the affected part must be immobilized to prevent the clot from spreading or turning into an embolus, and anticoagulant drugs may be given. With proper treatment, recovery occurs within a short time unless an embolism develops. Occasionally an operation is performed and the veins in which the clots have formed are tied off. Ordinarily, other veins take over their task and the circulation returns to normal.

PREVENTION. Immobility is a prime factor in the development of thrombosis; hence, all patients should be mobilized as soon as possible after surgery or an illness that requires bed rest or produces paralysis. Patients who cannot get out of bed should follow an exercise routine involving either active or passive motion of the extremities. For those who can perform active exercises, a footboard, rolled blanket, or pillow placed at the patient's feet can be used to encourage walking motions of the legs and stretching of the muscles. The bed clothes should be loose enough to permit free movement of the legs and feet.

The effectiveness of elastic stockings and elastic bandages is in dispute; however, the elastic stocking is becoming more acceptable. In either case, the bandages and the stocking must be applied so that they are smooth and free of wrinkles and fit snugly enough to provide firm support without restriction of circulation. Stockings applied to the lower legs should end two inches below the knee. Long stockings that extend above the knee should end two inches from the groin. Both stockings and bandages should be removed every eight hours to correct wrinkling and avoid skin breakdown.

ARTERIAL THROMBOSIS. The main types of arterial thrombosis are related to arteriosclerosis, although thrombosis can result from infection or from injury to an artery. Arteriosclerosis may be hereditary or may be brought on by diabetes mellitus.

Coronary thrombosis is a complication of coronary ATHEROSCLEROSIS. A blood clot in a coronary artery will block off part of the blood supply to the heart muscle and cause a severe heart attack. (See also MYOCARDIAL INFARCTION.) This constitutes a medical emergency.

In cerebral thrombosis, a clot obstructs the supply of blood to the brain and causes a CEREBRAL VASCULAR ACCIDENT (stroke). Besides hardening of the cerebral arteries, cerebral thrombosis can also be caused by hypertension, or may be a complication of syphilis or other infections, dehydration, diabetes mellitus, or a violent injury.

In advanced cases of arteriosclerosis, a clot may fill up whatever is left of a passageway, completely blocking off circulation to the area, and may eventually cause gangrene. This condition occurs most frequently in the arteries of the legs and is called peripheral thrombosis. The onset, which is often sudden, is characterized by either a tingling feeling or numbness and coldness in the limb. Pain is not always present. Immediate treatment with anticoagulants to discourage clotting is necessary. If this is not effective, surgery may be required. This condition is most common in the elderly and in diabetics. Modern methods of treatment can often save the limb.

In addition to the surgical removal of a thrombus or an embolus, surgery of the blood vessels also involves the removal of old, narrowed, or deteriorated vessels and their replacement with grafts.

thrombostasis (throm-bos′tah-sis) stasis of blood in a part with formation of thrombus.

thrombosthenin (throm″bo-sthe′nin) a substance liberated by blood platelets that is important for clot retraction and firmness of the clot.

thrombus (throm′bus) a solid mass formed in the living heart or vessels from constituents of the blood.

mural t., one attached to the wall of the endocardium in a diseased area.

occluding t., one that occupies the entire lumen of a vessel and obstructs blood flow.

parietal t., one attached to a vessel or heart wall.

thrush (thrush) infection of the oral mucous membrane by a fungus (*Candida albicans*). It is characterized by white patches on a red, moist inflamed surface, occurring anywhere in the mouth, including the tongue, but usually on the inner cheeks. These patches are occasionally accompanied by pain and fever.

Approximately 20 to 30 per cent of the population harbors *Candida albicans,* but the disease develops in only a very small number of this group. Those who are most susceptible are infants and adults who are in a weakened condition from infection, dietary deficiency (malnutrition), or uncontrolled diabetes mellitus, or who have been treated with antibiotics for a long time.

Any baby who has a sore throat and shows discomfort while nursing may have thrush. If the white patches that appear remain untreated, they will become larger and will tend to grow together; they may also spread to other parts of the body. If rubbed or irritated, they will become inflamed or bleed.

Thrush is sometimes regarded as a minor infection, yet it can persist for weeks or even months, especially in young babies. It is important that the cause of the infection be treated. Any dietary deficiency or diabetic condition that may exist must be corrected. Thrush itself is treated with antibiotics and fungicidal drugs. The best preventive measures are good general health, a well-balanced diet, and good mouth hygiene.

thrypsis (thrip′sis) a comminuted fracture.

thulium (thoo′le-um) a chemical element, atomic number 69, atomic weight 168.934, symbol Tm. (See table of ELEMENTS.)

thumb (thum) the radial or first digit of the hand; it has only two phalanges and is apposable to the four fingers of the hand.

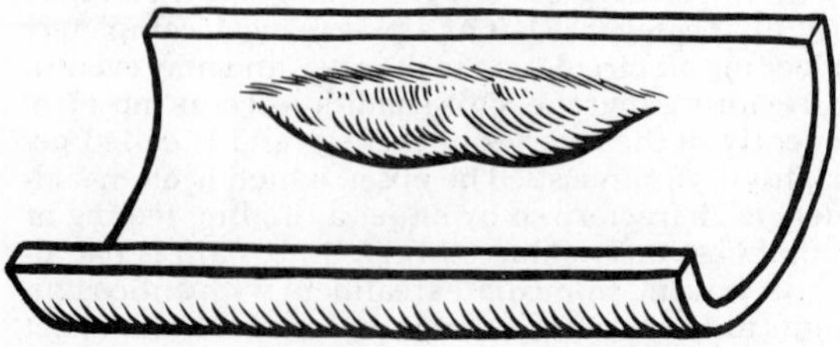

Thrombus on the inner wall of a blood vessel (shown here in section).

tennis t., tendinitis of the tendon of the long flexor muscle of the thumb, with calcification.

thym(o)- (thi′mo) word element [Gr.], *thymus; mind, soul,* or *emotions.*

thymectomize (thi-mek′to-mīz) to excise the thymus.

thymectomy (thi-mek′to-me) excision of the thymus.

thymelcosis (thi″mel-ko′sis) ulceration of the thymus.

thymergasia (thi″mer-ga′ze-ah) an affective or reaction-type psychosis, such as manic-depressive psychosis. adj., **thymergas′ic, thymergas′tic.**

-thymia (thi′me-ah) word element [Gr.], *condition of mind.* adj., **-thy′mic.**

thymic (thi′mik) pertaining to the thymus.

thymicolymphatic (thi″mĭ-ko-lim-fat′ik) pertaining to the thymus and lymphatic nodes.

thymidine (thi′mĭ-dēn) a nucleoside of DNA.

thymine (thi′min) a pyrimidine base in DNA.

thymitis (thi-mi′tis) inflammation of the thymus.

thymocyte (thi′mo-sīt) a lymphocyte arising in the thymus.

thymogenic (thi″mo-jen′ik) of affective or hysterical origin.

thymokinetic (thi″mo-ki-net′ik) tending to stimulate the thymus.

thymol (thi′mol) a phenol obtained from thyme oil and other volatile oils or produced synthetically; used as a topical antifungal and antibacterial, and as an antimicrobial agent in trichloroethylene.

t. iodide, a mixture of iodine derivatives of thymol, containing not less than 43 per cent of iodine; mild antiseptic.

thymoma (thi-mo′mah) a tumor derived from the epithelial or lymphoid elements of the thymus.

thymopathy (thi-mop′ah-the) any disease of the thymus.

thymoprivic, thymoprivous (thi″mo-priv′ik; thi-mop′rĭ-vus) pertaining to or resulting from removal or atrophy of the thymus.

thymosin (thi′mo-sin) a humoral factor secreted by the thymus, which promotes the growth of peripheral lymphoid tissue. Called also thymic hormone. (See also THYMUS.)

thymus (thi′mus) a ductless glandlike body lying in the upper mediastinum beneath the sternum, which reaches its maximum development during the early stages of life and continues to play an immunologic role throughout life, even though its function declines with age.

During the last stages of fetal life and the early neonatal period, the reticular structure of the thymus entraps immature "stem" cells arising from the bone marrow and circulating in the blood. The thymus preprocesses these cells, causing them to become sensitized and therefore capable of maturing into a type of lymphocyte that is essential to the development of cell-mediated IMMUNITY. After sensitization by the thymus, these lymphocytes reenter the blood and are transported to developing lymphoid tissue, where they seed the cells that eventually become thymus-dependent or T-lymphocytes. If the thymus is removed or becomes nonfunctional during fetal life, the lymphoid tissue fails to become seeded with the sensitized lymphocytes and the body's cell-mediated arm of immunity fails to develop. It is this arm of immunity that is mainly responsible for rejection of organ transplants and resistance to intracellular microbial infection, and perhaps plays a role in natural resistance to cancer.

In the 1960's Dr. Allan L. Goldstein and his associates at the University of Texas Medical Branch discovered and isolated a humoral factor, believed to be a hormone from the thymus, which they named thymosin. It is hoped that eventually this hormone will prove to be of value in restoring immunologic capability to immune-deficient patients. Another possibility is the development of an antithymosin serum, which could be effectively employed in the selective suppression of the immune systems of persons suffering from transplant rejection. It is proposed that the serum would suppress only the T-cell immune system, leaving the remaining humoral system intact and capable of producing antibodies against bacterial invasion.

DISORDERS OF THE THYMUS. A number of AUTOIMMUNE DISEASES have been related to defective immune responses in which the thymus plays or has played a role. Among these are agammaglobulinemia, certain leukemias, rheumatoid arthritis, and Hodgkin's disease.

Enlargement of the thymus has been associated with myasthenia gravis, decreased red blood cell formation, deficiency of gamma globulins with increase in infections, and deficiency of circulating small lymphocytes. There is also evidence that in thyroiditis and thyrotoxicosis the thymic parenchyma may be enlarged.

The factors and mechanisms involved in the effects of the thymus have yet to be verified by research. In animals, extracts of the thymus may increase or decrease carbohydrate metabolism, affect the rate of growth, regulate fertility, and suppress the proliferation of cancer cells. While there is no doubt that the thymus plays a major role in the complex immunologic system of man, the precise mechanisms by which this takes place and the ways in which these mechanisms can be manipulated to the benefit of man have yet to be determined.

thyro- (thi′ro) word element [Gr.], *thyroid.*

thyroadenitis (thi″ro-ad″ĕ-ni′tis) inflammation of the thyroid.

thyroaplasia (thi″ro-ah-pla′ze-ah) defective development of the thyroid with deficient activity of its secretion.

thyroarytenoid (thi″ro-ar″ĭ-te′noid) pertaining to the thyroid and arytenoid cartilages.

thyrocalcitonin (thi″ro-kal″sĭ-to′nin) calcitonin; a polypeptide hormone elaborated by the parafollicular cells of the thyroid gland in response to hypercalcemia, which lowers plasma calcium and phosphate levels, inhibits bone resorption, and serves as an antagonist to parathyroid hormone.

thyrocardiac (thi″ro-kar′de-ak) pertaining to the thyroid and heart.

t. disease, thyrotoxic heart disease.

thyrocele (thi′ro-sēl) tumor of the thyroid gland; goiter.

thyrochondrotomy (thi″ro-kon-drot′o-me) surgical incision of the thyroid cartilage.

thyrocricotomy (thi″ro-kri-kot′o-me) incision of the cricothyroid membrane, the lower part of the fibroelastic membrane of the larynx.

thyroepiglottic (thi″ro-ep″ĭ-glot′ik) pertaining to the thyroid and epiglottis.

thyrogenic, thyrogenous (thi″ro-jen′ik; thi-roj′ĕ-nus) originating in the thyroid.

thyroglobulin (thi″ro-glob′u-lin) an iodized glycoprotein characteristically present in the colloid of the thyroid follicles; thyroid hormone is bound to it in the gland.

thyroglossal (thi″ro-glos′al) pertaining to the thyroid and tongue.

thyrohyal (thi″ro-hi′al) pertaining to the thyroid cartilage and the hyoid bone.

thyrohyoid (thi″ro-hi′oid) pertaining to the thyroid gland or cartilage and the hyoid bone.

thyroid (thi′roid) 1. resembling a shield. 2. the thyroid gland. 3. a pharmaceutical preparation of cleaned, dried, powdered thyroid gland, obtained

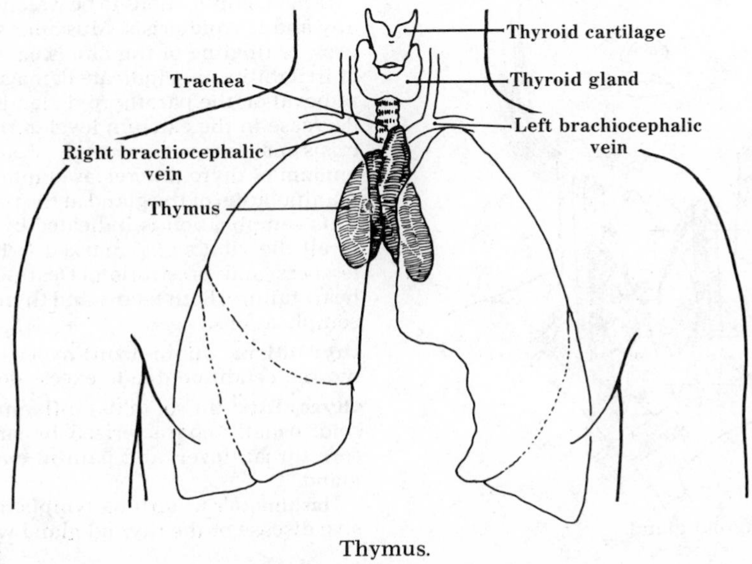

Thymus.

from those domesticated animals used for food by man.

t. cartilage, the shield-shaped cartilage of the larynx; the prominence it produces on the neck is the Adam's apple.

t. crisis, a sudden and dangerous increase of the symptoms of thyrotoxicosis; called also thyroid storm. The condition may occur in patients with severe HYPERTHYROIDISM and in the immediate postoperative period following THYROIDECTOMY. It is a serious event that can be fatal if not brought under control.

In thyroid crisis all of the body processes are accelerated to dangerously high levels. The pulse may rise to 200 beats per minute, and there is concurrent rise in the respiratory rate. The temperature control center loses control, bringing about a rapid and steady increase in body temperature.

Treatment is aimed at supplying the cells with oxygen and glucose and the reduction of body temperature. Oxygen is administered and glucose is given by mouth and intravenously. Measures to reduce hyperthermia include the application of ice packs or a hypothermia blanket.

t. extract, a pharmaceutical substance derived from thyroid glands from domesticated animals that are used for food by man, the glands having been deprived of connective tissue and fat and then cleaned, dried and powdered. It is used as a specific in hypothyroidism, in doses adjusted to the patient's needs.

t. gland, the largest of the ENDOCRINE GLANDS, situated in the front and sides of the neck just below the thyroid cartilage. It produces hormones that are vital in maintaining normal growth and metabolism. It also serves as a storehouse for iodine.

Excessive thyroid activity increases metabolism, causing nervousness, heart palpitations, restlessness, and insomnia (see also HYPERTHYROIDISM). Deficient thyroid activity produces drowsiness, fatigue, and lethargy (see also HYPOTHYROIDISM); marked deficiency can cause weight gain, coarsened features and thick, scaly skin (MYXEDEMA). Enlargement of the thyroid gland is called GOITER, and it often accompanies hyperthyroidism.

t. hormones, substances manufactured and secreted by the thyroid gland, including thyroxine and triiodothyronine. Together these substances act as a chemical agent or catalyst, stimulating specific organs, tissues, and cells. They are mainly responsible for an individual's energy or lack of it, and influence skeletal growth and sexual development, as well as the texture of the skin and luster of the hair. Calcitonin is also secreted by the thyroid gland.

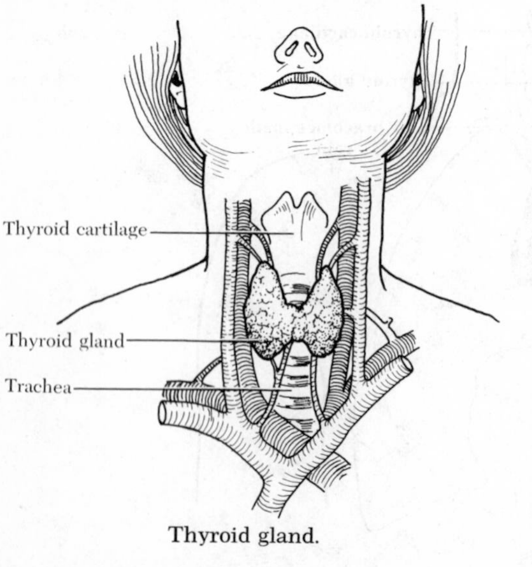

Thyroid gland.

thyroidectomize (thi″roi-dek′to-mīz) to subject to thyroidectomy.

thyroidectomy (thi″roi-dek′to-me) surgical excision of the thyroid gland. Total thyroidectomy, removal of the entire gland, may be performed in cases of cancer of the thyroid. Subtotal thyroidectomy, in which more than two-thirds of the gland is removed, is performed for certain patients suffering from HYPERTHYROIDISM. The remaining portion of the gland is left intact and continues to function and produce hormones.

PATIENT CARE. Prior to surgery the patient receives intensive therapy to maximize the possibility of a successful operation. This includes the administration of antithyroid drugs, iodine preparations, and supportive measures to promote rest and improve the nutritional status. Tests of thyroid function should indicate that the patient is eurythyroid; that is, the test results show no extremes of thyroid function and the patient presents mild or no symptoms of thyrotoxicosis.

When the patient is adequately prepared, the dangers of hemorrhage and THYROID CRISIS, the two major complications of thyroidectomy, are greatly diminished.

Immediately after surgery the patient is placed on his back in a low Fowler's or semi-Fowler's position. Motion of the head, unnecessary talking, and strenuous coughing should be discouraged. Temperature, pulse, and respirations are taken every 15 minutes until they remain within normal limits for several hours. The dressings are checked frequently for signs of hemorrhage or constriction of the throat. Special note should be made of the back of the neck, where blood may drain unnoticed. Hoarseness and slight difficulty in swallowing can be expected until the local edema subsides, but loss of the voice or severe dyspnea should be reported promptly to the surgeon. A tracheostomy set is kept at the bedside in case of respiratory obstruction.

Other complications to be watched for include tetany and thyroid crisis. Muscular twitching, numbness, or tingling of the hands or feet or other signs of irritability may indicate damage to, or accidental removal of, the parathyroid glands, and a resultant decrease in the calcium level of the blood. Thyroid crisis may occur as a result of an increase in the amount of thyroxine released into the blood during manipulation of the gland at the time of its removal. This complication is indicated by a rapid increase in all the vital signs, marked irritability and restlessness and prostration. Death may occur from heart failure. Both tetany and thyroid crisis are rare complications.

thyroidism (thi′roi-dizm) hyperthyroidism; also, a morbid condition due to excess doses of thyroid.

thyroiditis (thi″roi-di′tis) inflammation of the thyroid, usually characterized by such symptoms as sore throat, fever, and painful enlargement of the gland.

Hashimoto's t., struma lymphomatosa, a progressive disease of the thyroid gland with degeneration of its epithelial elements and replacement by lymphoid and fibrous tissue.

thyroidotomy (thi″roi-dot′o-me) incision of the thyroid.

thyroiodine (thi″ro-i′o-dīn) iodine as it exists in the hormones of the thyroid gland.

thyrolysin (thi-rol′ĭ-sin) a substance destructive to thyroid tissue. adj., **thyrolyt′ic.**

thyromegaly (thi″ro-meg′ah-le) goiter.

thyromimetic (thi″ro-mi-met′ik) producing effects similar to those of thyroid hormones or the thyroid gland.

thyroparathyroidectomy (thi″ro-par″ah-thi″roi-dek′to-me) excision of the thyroid and parathyroids.

thyroprival, thyroprivic (thi″ro-pri′val; thi″ro-priv′ik) pertaining to, marked by, or due to deprivation or loss of thyroid function.

thyroptosis (thi″rop-to′sis) downward displacement of a goitrous thyroid.

thyrosis (thi-ro′sis) any disease based on disordered thyroid action.

thyrotherapy (thi″ro-ther′ah-pe) treatment with preparations of thyroid.

thyrotomy (thi-rot′o-me) 1. surgical division of the thyroid cartilage. 2. the operation of cutting the thyroid gland.

thyrotoxic (thi″ro-tok′sik) marked by toxic activity of the thyroid.

t. crisis, a fulminating increase in all the symptoms of thyrotoxicosis.

t. heart disease, heart disease associated with hyperthyroidism, marked by atrial fibrillation, cardiac enlargement, and congestive heart failure. Called also thyrocardiac disease.

t. storm, thyrotoxic crisis.

thyrotoxicosis (thi″ro-tok″sĭ-ko′sis) a morbid condition due to overactivity of the thyroid gland.

thyrotoxin (thi″ro-tok′sin) a toxic substance produced in the thyroid gland.

thyrotrophic (thi″ro-trof′ik) thyrotropic.

thyrotrophin (thi″ro-trōf′in) thyrotropin.

thyrotropic (thi″ro-trop′ik) 1. pertaining to or marked by thyrotropism. 2. having an influence on the thyroid gland.

thyrotropin (thi″ro-trōp′in) a hormone secreted by the anterior lobe of the pituitary gland that has an affinity for and specifically stimulates the thyroid gland.

thyrotropism (thi-rot′ro-pizm) affinity for the thyroid gland.

thyroxine (thi-rok′sin) a hormone of the THYROID GLAND that contains iodine and is a derivative of the amino acid tyrosine. The chemical name for thyroxine is tetraiodothyronine; it is formed and stored in the thyroid follicles as thyroglobulin, the storage form. Thyroxine is released from the gland by the action of a proteolytic enzyme.

Thyroxine acts as a catalyst in the body and influences a great variety of effects, including metabolic rate (oxygen consumption); growth and development; metabolism of carbohydrates, fats, proteins, electrolytes, and water; vitamin requirements; reproduction; and resistance to infection.

Thyroxine can be extracted from animals or made synthetically; it is prescribed for hypothyroidism and for some types of goiter.

Ti chemical symbol, *titanium.*

TIA transient cerebral ischemic attacks (see CEREBROVASCULAR ACCIDENT).

tibia (tib′e-ah) the inner and larger bone of the leg below the knee; it articulates with the femur and head of the fibula above and with the talus below. (See Plate 1.) adj., **tib′ial.**

t. val′ga, a bowing of the leg in which the angulation is away from the midline of the body.

t. va′ra, a bowing of the leg in which the angulation is toward the midline of the body; bowleg.

tibialis (tib″e-a′lis) [L.] tibial.

tibiofemoral (tib″e-o-fem′o-ral) pertaining to the tibia and femur.

tibiofibular (tib″e-o-fib′u-lar) pertaining to the tibia and fibula.

tibiotarsal (tib″e-o-tar′sal) pertaining to the tibia and tarsus.

tic (tik) a spasmodic twitching movement made involuntarily by muscles that are ordinarily under voluntary control. Twitching of the eyelid, of muscles of the face, and of the diaphragm (hiccupping) are examples. In general, tics are of psychologic origin; they tend to develop in young persons of nervous temperament and occasionally persist into adulthood.

t. douloureux, trigeminal neuralgia, a painful disorder of the trigeminal nerve (the fifth cranial nerve). The disorder is characterized by severe pain in the face and forehead on the affected side. The pain extends to the midline of the face and head and may be triggered by cold drafts, chewing, drinking cold liquids, brushing the hair, or washing the face.

TREATMENT. Medical treatment is usually preferred, since surgical correction results in complete loss of sensation in the areas served by the nerve. The drugs employed include trichloroethylene administered by inhalation, niacin, potassium chloride, diethazine, and most recently carbamazepine (Tegretol).

When surgery is resorted to, the patient must be watched for signs of corneal infection, which frequently occurs. The infection usually develops as a result of loss of the corneal reflex, which normally provides a warning when foreign material or other injurious agents enter the eye. Postoperative instructions must be given the patient so that he can take necessary measures for the protection of his eye after discharge from the hospital.

facial t., spasm of the facial muscles.

tick (tik) a blood-sucking arachnid parasite. There are two types, hard and soft. Hard ticks have a smooth, hard cover that shields the entire back of the male but only the anterior portion of the back in the female. Soft ticks lack this shield.

Ticks are visible to the human eye. A hard tick can be seen on the skin, where it burrows into the outer layer with its knifelike tongue; it must be removed from the skin with care. Soft ticks do not bore into the skin. The two varieties carry different diseases but both thrive in the spring and early summer and inhabit wooded areas, brush, or grass.

Ticks serve as vectors for viruses causing Colorado tick fever and some forms of encephalitis and for rickettsiae that cause such diseases as ROCKY MOUNTAIN SPOTTED FEVER (also called tick fever and tick typhus) and boutonneuse fever. A progressive ascending flaccid paralysis (tick paralysis) may follow the bite of certain ticks, usually *Dermacentor andersoni.*

REMOVAL OF HARD TICKS. If hard ticks are extracted from the skin immediately, before they begin to suck blood, the chances of their transmitting disease are lessened; probably the only damage done will be an irritating itch at the site.

Ticks should be extracted whole; if they are carelessly pulled off the body, all or part of the mouth may be left in the skin. To loosen the tick's grasp, heavy oil, gasoline, or turpentine is applied to the area and left for half an hour. Once the tick has relinquished its hold, it should be carefully removed with tweezers. The tick should be destroyed, but not with the bare hands. The site should be washed with soap and water and an antiseptic should be applied to prevent infection.

t.i.d. [L.] *ter in di'e* (three times a day).

tidal volume (ti'dal) the amount of gas passing into and out of the lungs in each respiratory cycle.

tide (tīd) a physiologic variation or increase of a certain constituent in body fluids.

acid t., a temporary increase in the acidity of the urine that sometimes follows fasting.

alkaline t., a temporary increase in the alkalinity of the urine during gastric digestion.

fat t., the increase of a fat in the lymph and blood following a meal.

Tigan (ti'gan) trademark for preparations of trimethobenzamide, an antiemetic.

tigrolysis (ti-grol'ĭ-sis) chromatolysis (2).

timbre (tim'ber) the musical quality of a tone or sound.

time (tīm) a measure of duration. See under adjectives for specific times, e.g., BLEEDING TIME.

Timovan (tim'o-van) trademark for a preparation of prothipendyl, a tranquilizer.

tin (tin) a chemical element, atomic number 50, atomic weight 118.69, symbol Sn. (See table of ELEMENTS.)

tinct. tincture.

tinctorial (tingk-to're-al) pertaining to dyeing or staining.

tincture (tingk'tūr) an alcoholic or hydroalcoholic solution prepared from an animal or vegetable drug or a chemical substance.

belladonna t., a preparation of belladonna leaf in a menstruum of alcohol and water; used as an anticholinergic.

benzoin t., compound, a mixture of benzoin, aloes, storax, and tolu balsam in alcohol; used as a topical protectant.

digitalis t., finely powdered digitalis in a menstruum of alcohol and water; used as a cardiotonic.

green soap t., a mixture of green soap, lavender oil, and alcohol; a skin detergent.

iodine t., a mixture of iodine and sodium iodide in a menstruum of alcohol and water; used as an anti-infective for the skin.

nitromersol t., nitromersol, sodium hydroxide, and alcohol in hydroalcoholic solution; a local anti-infective.

opium t., an alcoholic solution of opium, each 100 ml. of which yields 0.95 to 1.05 gm. of anhydrous morphine; used as an intestinal sedative.

thimersol t., thimerosal, monoethanolamine, acetone, ethylenediamine solution, with alcohol and water; a local anti-infective.

Tindal (tin'dal) trademark for a preparation of acetophenazine, a tranquilizer.

tine test (tīn) a tuberculin skin test employing a multiple-puncture, disposable device. It is especially useful in mass screening of children, but is less accurate than the Mantoux test. Any doubtful reaction to the tine test should be rechecked by a Mantoux test before a follow-up chest x-ray is recommended. The test is read 48 to 72 hours after injection.

tinea (tin'e-ah) ringworm; a name applied to many different kinds of fungal infection of the skin, the specific type (depending on characteristic appearance, etiologic agent and site) usually being designated by a modifying term.

t. bar'bae, infection of the bearded parts of the face and neck caused by *Trichophyton;* called also ringworm of the beard.

t. cap'itis, fungal infection of the scalp caused by various species of *Microsporum* and *Trichophyton.* Generally it is characterized by one or more small, round, elevated patches, scaling of the scalp, and dry and brittle hair. Called also ringworm of the scalp.

t. cor'poris, fungal infection of the glabrous skin, usually due to species of *Tricophyton* or *Microsporum.*

t. cru'ris, a fungal infection common in males, starting in the perineal folds and extending onto the inner surface of the thighs, caused by *Epidermophyton floccosum* or species of *Trichophyton;* called also eczema marginatum, epidermophytosis cruris, and jock itch.

t. imbrica'ta, a distinctive type of tinea corporis occurring in tropical countries and caused by *Trichophyton concentricum;* the early lesion is annular, with a circle of scales at the periphery, characteristically attached along one edge. New and larger scaling rings form, sometimes reaching as many as 10 per lesion. Called also Malabar itch and Burmese ringworm.

t. ke'rion, a highly inflammatory and suppurative fungal infection of the scalp or beard region.

t. pe'dis, a chronic superficial fungal infection of the skin of the foot, especially of that between the toes and on the soles, characterized by maceration, scaling, and itching, and caused by species of *Trichophyton* or by *Epidermophyton floccosum* (see also ATHLETE'S FOOT).

t. profun'da, trichophytic granuloma.

t. syco'sis, an inflammatory, deep type of tinea barbae, due to *Trichophyton violaceum* or *T. rubrum.*

t. un'guium, onychomycosis; fungal infection of the nails.

t. versic'olor, a chronic, noninflammatory, usually asymptomatic disorder due to *Pityrosporon orbiculare,* marked only by multiple macular patches. Called also pityriasis versicolor.

Tinel's sign (tin-elz') a tingling sensation in the distal end of a limb when percussion is made over the site of a divided nerve; it indicates a partial lesion or the beginning regeneration of the nerve.

tingible (tin'jĭ-b'l) stainable.

tinnitus (tĭ-ni'tus) a noise in the ears, as ringing, buzzing, or roaring, which may at times be heard by others than the patient.

t. au'rium, a subjective sensation of noise in the ears.

tintometer (tin-tom′ĕ-ter) an instrument for determining the relative proportion of coloring matter in a liquid, as in blood.

tintometry (tin-tom′ĕ-tre) the use of the tintometer.

tirefond (tēr-faw′) [Fr.] an instrument like a corkscrew for raising depressed portions of bone.

tissue (tish′u) a group or layer of similarly specialized cells that together perform certain special functions.

adenoid t., lymphoid tissue.

adipose t., connective tissue made of fat cells in a meshwork of areolar tissue.

areolar t., connective tissue made up largely of interlacing fibers.

bony t., bone.

brown adipose t., brown fat t., a peculiar type of fat found in certain body regions in various mammals and in the human fetus.

cancellous t., the spongy tissue of bone.

cartilaginous t., the substance of cartilage.

chordal t., the tissue of the notochord.

chromaffin t., a tissue composed largely of chromaffin cells, well supplied with nerves and vessels; it occurs in the adrenal medulla and also forms the paraganglia of the body.

cicatricial t., the dense fibrous tissue forming a cicatrix, derived directly from granulation tissue.

connective t., the tissue that binds together and is the support of the various structures of the body; it consists mainly of fibroblasts and collagen and elastic fibrils. (See also CONNECTIVE TISSUE.)

elastic t., connective tissue made up of yellow elastic fibers, frequently massed into sheets.

endothelial t., peculiar connective tissue lining serous and lymph spaces.

epithelial t., a general name for tissues not derived from the mesoderm.

erectile t., spongy tissue that expands and becomes hard when filled with blood.

extracellular t., the total of tissues and body fluids outside the cells.

fatty t., connective tissue made of fat cells in a meshwork of areolar tissue.

fibrous t., the common connective tissue of the body, composed of yellow or white parallel elastic and collagen fibers.

t. fluid, the extracellular fluid that constitutes the environment of the body cells. It is low in protein, is formed by filtration through the capillaries, and drains away as lymph.

gelatinous t., mucous tissue.

glandular t., an aggregation of specialized form of epithelial tissue that elaborates secretions.

granulation t., material formed in repair of wounds of soft tissue, consisting of connective tissue cells and ingrowing young vessels; it ultimately forms cicatrix.

indifferent t., undifferentiated embryonic tissue.

interstitial t., connective tissue between the cellular elements of a structure.

lymphadenoid t., tissue resembling that of lymph nodes, spleen, bone marrow, tonsils, and lymph vessels.

lymphoid t., a lattice work of reticular tissue, the interspaces of which contain lymphocytes.

mesenchymal t., embryonic connective tissue composed of stellate cells and a ground substance of coagulable fluid.

mucous t., a jelly-like connective tissue, such as occurs in the umbilical cord.

muscular t., the substance of muscle.

myeloid t., red bone marrow.

nerve t., nervous t., the specialized tissue forming the elements of the nervous system.

osseous t., the specialized tissue forming the bones.

reticular t., reticulated t., connective tissue composed predominantly of reticulum cells and reticular fibers.

scar t., cicatricial tissue.

sclerous t's, the cartilaginous, fibrous, and osseous tissues.

skeletal t., the bony, ligamentous, fibrous, and cartilaginous tissue forming the skeleton and its attachments.

splenic t., red pulp.

subcutaneous t., the layer of loose connective tissue directly under the skin.

titanium (ti-ta′ne-um) a chemical element, atomic number 22, atomic weight 47.90, symbol Ti. (See table of ELEMENTS.)

t. dioxide, a white powder used in ointment or lotion to protect the skin from the rays of the sun.

titer (ti′ter) the quantity of a substance required to react with or to correspond to a given amount of another substance.

titrate (ti′trāt) to analyze by titration.

titration (ti-tra′shun) determination of a given component in solution by addition of a liquid reagent of known strength until a given reaction is produced.

titrimetry (ti-trim′ĕ-tre) analysis by titration. adj., **titrimet′ric.**

titubation (tit″u-ba′shun) the act of staggering or reeling; a staggering gait with shaking of the trunk and head, commonly seen in cerebellar disease.

Tl chemical symbol, *thallium.*

TLC tender loving care; thin layer chromatography; total lung capacity.

Tm 1. chemical symbol, *thulium.* 2. tubular maximum (in renal excretion).

TNT trinitrotoluene.

tobacco (to-bak′o) the dried prepared leaves of *Nicotiana tabacum,* an annual plant widely cultivated in the United States, the source of various alkaloids, the principal one being nicotine (see also SMOKING).

tobramycin (to″brah-mi′sin) an aminoglycoside antibiotic produced by *Streptomyces tenebrarius.*

Toclase (to′klās) trademark for preparations of carbetapentane, an antitussive.

toco- (to′ko) word element [Gr.], *childbirth; labor.* See also words beginning *toko-.*

tocology (to-kol′o-je) the science of reproduction and the art of obstetrics.

tocometer (to-kom′ĕ-ter) tokodynamometer.

tocopherol (to-kof′er-ol) an alcohol isolated from wheat germ oil or produced synthetically; it has the properties of vitamin E. In animals it is needed in the diet to insure reproduction, but its role in humans is unclear.

alpha t., vitamin E.

toe (to) a digit of the foot.

hammer t., deformity of a toe in which the proximal phalanx is extended and the second and distal phalanges are flexed, causing a clawlike appearance; it most often affects the second toe.

Morton's t., a painful condition of the third and

fourth toes due to thickening of the branch of the sensory nerve supplying them.

pigeon t., a permanent toeing-in position of the feet.

webbed t's, toes abnormally joined by strands of tissue at their base.

Tofranil (to-fra'nil) trademark for preparations of imipramine, an antidepressant.

togavirus (to"gah-vi'rus) a subgroup of arboviruses, including mosquito- and tickborne viruses that cause hemorrhagic fever; they are RNA viruses with envelopes (or "togas").

toilet (toi'let) the cleansing and dressing of a wound.

token economy a technique used in BEHAVIOR THERAPY in which the patient exchanges (pays) tokens, which he has earned through manifesting certain appropriate behavior, for something that he desires, such as food, privileges, or store items.

toko- (to'ko) word element [Gr.], *childbirth; labor.* See also words beginning *toco-*.

tokodynagraph (to"ko-di'nah-graf) a tracing obtained by the tokodynamometer.

tokodynamometer (to"ko-di"nah-mom'ĕ-ter) an instrument for measuring and recording the expulsive force of uterine contractions.

tolazamide (tol-az'ah-mīd) a hypoglycemic agent.

tolazoline (tol-az'o-lēn) a smooth muscle relaxant and peripheral vasodilator; used as the hydrochloride salt.

tolbutamide (tol-bu'tah-mīd) an oral hypoglycemic agent.

tolerance (tol'er-ans) the ability to endure without effect or injury. adj., **tol'erant.**

drug t., decrease of susceptibility to the effects of a drug due to its continued administration.

immunologic t., specific nonreactivity of lymphoid tissues to a particular antigen capable under other conditions of inducing immunity.

tolerogen (tol'er-o-jen) an antigen that induces a state of specific immunological unresponsiveness to subsequent challenging doses of the antigen.

Tolinase (tol'ĭ-nās) trademark for tolazamide, an oral hypoglycemic agent.

tolnaftate (tol-naf'tāt) a topical antifungal.

toluene (tol'u-ēn) the hydrocarbon C_7H_8.

toluidine (tol-u'ĭ-din) a compound made by reducing nitrotoluene.

tomatin (to-ma'tin) an antifungal antibiotic isolated from tomato plants affected with wilt.

-tome (-tōm) word element [Gr.], *an instrument for cutting; a segment.*

tomo- (to'mo) word element [Gr.], *a section; a cutting.*

tomogram (to'mo-gram) a radiograph produced by the tomograph.

tomograph (to'mo-graf) an apparatus for moving the x-ray tube through an arc during exposure, thus showing in detail a predetermined plane of tissue while blurring details of other planes.

tomography (tom-mog'rah-fe) a method of body-section roentgenography with the x-ray tube moved in only one direction, usually an arc.

computerized transverse axial t., a radiologic technique which utilizes a narrow beam (4 to 26 mm.) of x-rays, tomographic principles, and highly sensitive detectors to obtain a three-dimensional cross-sectional view of body parts. Also called computerized axial tomography (CAT).

The basic components of the CAT system are the scanner, computer, viewer, line printer, x-ray control, and teletype. The scanner is mounted on a gantry, which rotates one degree around the body part at the end of each traverse. The process is repeated through 180 degrees of rotation; that is, the machine moves in an arc or half-circle around the body part being examined.

The x-ray beam penetrates the body tissues and its action on the tissues of varying density is monitored by sodium iodide crystals positioned directly opposite the x-ray source and moving in conjunction with it. Information received by the crystals is relayed to a computer.

The computer processes the readings taken during the course of a scan and computes the absorption factors for each "slice" of tissue being viewed. Each cross-sectional slice represents an area that is 3 mm. square and 13 mm. thick. The image of each slice is projected on a matrix on the viewer, allowing the technologist to determine the density of a particular area. The areas of lesser density appear lighter on the viewer than do areas of greater density.

The line printer is a numerical printout of the computer which assigns a digit to each density gradient. The "picture" presented by the computer is based on its interpretation of varying densities of tissues, fluids, and bone.

Computerized axial tomography is a noninvasive radiologic technique that requires only one operator, presents no special risks to the patient, and can be done on an outpatient basis. It employs no opaque contrast material for revealing the size, shape, contour, density, and texture of an organ. It is not uncomfortable for the patient and therefore does not require sedation or anesthesia. Because it allows for three-dimensional visualization of body tissues without surgical intervention, it is believed that CAT will eventually revolutionize medical diagnosis.

-tomy (to'me) word element [Gr.], *incision; cutting.*

tone (tōn) 1. normal degree of vigor and tension; in muscle, the resistance to passive elongation or stretch. 2. a healthy state of a part; tonus. 3. a particular quality of sound or voice.

tongue (tung) a muscular organ on the floor of the mouth; it aids in chewing, swallowing, and speech, and is the location of organs of TASTE. The taste buds are located in the papillae, which are projections on the upper surface of the tongue.

The condition of the tongue can sometimes be a guide to the general condition of the body. Inflammation of the tongue, or glossitis, can accompany anemia, scarlet fever, nutritional deficiencies, and most general infections. Sometimes it is part of an adverse reaction to medication. One form of glossitis causes a smooth tongue, with a red, glazed appearance. A coated or furry tongue may be present in a variety of illnesses, but does not necessarily indicate illness. A dry tongue sometimes indicates insufficiency of fluids in the body, or it may result from fever. When the tongue is extremely dry and has a leathery appearance, the cause may be uremia.

bifid t., a tongue with a lengthwise cleft.

black t., blackening and elongation of the papillae of the tongue.

cleft t., bifid tongue.

coated t., one covered with a whitish or yellowish layer consisting of desquamated epithelium, debris, bacteria, fungi, etc.

fissured t., furrowed t., a tongue with numerous furrows or grooves on the dorsal surface, often radiating from a groove on the midline.

geographic t., a tongue with denuded patches, surrounded by thickened epithelium.

hairy t., one with the papillae elongated and hair-like.

raspberry t., a diffusely reddened and swollen, uncoated tongue, as seen several days after the onset of the rash in scarlet fever.

scrotal t., fissured tongue.

strawberry t., a coated tongue with enlarged red fungiform papillae, seen 24 hours after onset of the rash in scarlet fever.

trombone t., involuntary movement of the tongue, consisting of vigorous alternating protrusion and retraction.

tongue-tie (tung'ti) abnormal shortness of the frenulum of the tongue, resulting in limitation of its motion; called also ankyloglossia.

tonic (ton'ik) 1. producing and restoring normal tone. 2. characterized by continuous tension. 3. an agent that tends to restore normal tone.

tonicity (to-nis'ĭ-te) the state of tissue tone or tension; in body fluid physiology, the effective osmotic pressure equivalent.

tono- (to'no) word element [Gr.], *tone; tension.*

tonoclonic (ton″o-klon'ik) both tonic and clonic; said of muscular spasms.

tonofibril (ton'o-fi″bril) one of the fine fibrils in epithelial cells, thought to give a supporting framework to the cell.

tonogram (to'no-gram) the record produced by tonography.

tonograph (to'no-graf) a recording tonometer.

tonography (to-nog'rah-fe) the recording of changes in intraocular pressure due to sustained pressure on the eyeball.

tonometer (to-nom'ĕ-ter) an instrument for measuring tension or pressure, especially intraocular pressure.

tonometry (ton-nom'ĕ-tre) measurement of tension or pressure, e.g., intraocular pressure.

digital t., estimation of the degree of intraocular pressure by pressure exerted on the eyeball by the finger of the examiner.

tonoplast (ton'o-plast) the limiting membrane of an intracellular vacuole, the vacuole membrane.

tonoscope (ton'o-skōp) 1. an apparatus for rendering sound visible by registering the vibrations on a screen. 2. a device for examining the head or brain by means of sound. 3. tonometer.

tonsil (ton'sil) a small, rounded mass of tissue, especially of lymphoid tissue; generally used alone to designate the palatine tonsil. adj., **ton'sillar.**

There are three different kinds of tonsils. The structures usually referred to as the tonsils are the palatine tonsils, a pair of oval-shaped structures, about the size of almonds, partially embedded in the mucous membrane, one on each side of the back of the throat. Below them, at the base of the tongue, are the lingual tonsils. On the upper rear wall of the mouth cavity are the pharyngeal tonsils, or adenoids, which are of fair size in childhood but usually shrink after puberty.

These tissues are part of the lymphatic system and help to filter the circulating lymph of bacteria and any other foreign material that may enter the body, especially through the mouth and nose. In the process of fighting infection the palatine tonsils and the adenoids sometimes become enlarged and inflamed (see also TONSILLITIS).

t. of cerebellum, a rounded mass forming part of the cerebellum on its inferior surface.

tonsillectomy (ton″sĭ-lek'to-me) excision of tonsils. The procedure is performed in treatment of chronic infection of the tonsils.

PATIENT CARE. Since most patients undergoing tonsillectomy are children, it is important that the preoperative period include adequate emotional preparation of the patient and his family. The child should be told in advance of the admission to the hospital and given some idea of what he can expect. He should not be deceived about the possibility of discomfort, but it is best to stress the positive aspects of surgery, such as the fact that he will not suffer as many colds and attacks of sore throat once the surgery is performed and his throat has healed.

Although tonsillectomy may be considered minor surgery, there is always the possibility of serious hemorrhage after surgery. The child should be placed on his abdomen in bed immediately after surgery, to allow for adequate drainage of blood and mucus from the throat and mouth and avoid their aspiration into the respiratory passages. Signs of excessive bleeding from the operative site include bright red blood from the mouth or nose, frequent swallowing, and extreme restlessness. Efforts to keep the child quiet may include holding him, rocking him, or otherwise comforting him as he awakens from anesthesia. An ice collar is helpful in preventing edema, reducing blood loss, and eliminating nausea.

During the immediate postoperative period the diet is restricted to bland liquids. Citrus fruit juices are not allowed. As the throat heals and edema subsides, more solid foods are gradually added to the diet, but for at least a week after surgery all foods that are chemically, physically, or thermally irritating to the throat should be avoided.

tonsillitis (ton″sĭ-li'tis) inflammation and enlargement of a tonsil, especially the palatine tonsils.

Enlarged tonsils and adenoids need not be a cause for concern unless they become a source of chronic infection or interfere with swallowing or breathing. They may become enlarged in the process of filtering out frequent, mild infections. Also, the adenoids usually grow larger in children until about the age of 5 years, and then they may cease to be troublesome.

CAUSE. Tonsils are part of the lymphatic system, which aids the body in fighting off infections and "invasions" of foreign matter. Although the exact purpose of the tonsils is unknown, they are believed to act as filters and fighters of bacteria, guarding the entrances to the throat and nasal passages. Sometimes, however, they are overcome by the invading bacteria and become infected. One form of infection sometimes causing tonsillitis is streptococcal infection of the throat.

SYMPTOMS AND TREATMENT. A mild case of tonsillitis may appear to be only a slight sore throat. Symptoms of acute tonsillitis are inflamed, swollen tonsils and a very sore throat, with high fever, rapid pulse and general weakness. Swallowing is difficult and the lymph nodes in the neck may become swollen and painful.

Occasionally in an attack of severe tonsillitis an abscess may form around the tonsil, a condition called quinsy.

Treatment of tonsillitis usually consists of administration of antibiotics, gargles, and bed rest. When tonsillitis is recurrent and troublesome, however, it may be necessary to remove the tonsils surgically (see also TONSILLECTOMY).

follicular t., tonsillitis especially affecting the crypts.

parenchymatous t., acute, that affecting the whole substance of the tonsil.

pustular t., a variety characterized by formation of pustules.

tonsilloadenoidectomy (ton″sĭ-lo-ad″ĕ-noi-dek′to-me) excision of lymphoid tissue from the throat and nasopharynx (tonsils and adenoids).

tonsillolith (ton-sil′o-lith) a calculus in a tonsil.

tonsillotomy (ton″sĭ-lot′o-me) incision of a tonsil.

tonus (to′nus) tone or tonicity; the slight, continuous contraction of a muscle, which in skeletal muscles aids in the maintenance of posture and in the return of blood to the heart.

tooth (to͞oth), pl. *teeth.* one of the small, bonelike structures of the jaws for the biting and mastication of food; the teeth also assist in shaping sounds and forming words in speech.

STRUCTURE. The portion of a tooth that rises above the gum is the crown; the portion below is the root. The crown is covered by enamel, which is related to the epithelial tissue of the skin and is the hardest substance in the human body. The surface of the root is composed of a bonelike tissue called cementum. Underneath the surface enamel and cementum is a substance called dentin, which makes up the main body of the tooth. Within the dentin, in a space in the center of the tooth, is the dental pulp, a soft, sensitive tissue that contains nerves and blood and lymph vessels. The cementum, dentin, and pulp are formed from connective tissue. (See also Plate 9.)

Covering the root of the tooth and holding it in place in its socket, or alveolus, in the jaw is a fibrous connective tissue called the periodontium. Its many strong fibers are embedded in the cementum and also the wall of the tooth socket. The periodontium not only helps hold the tooth in place but also acts to cushion it against the pressure caused by biting and chewing.

There are 20 deciduous teeth, called also baby teeth or milk teeth, which are eventually replaced by 32 permanent teeth, evenly divided between upper and lower jaw.

Teeth have different shapes because they have different functions. The incisors, in the front of the mouth, are shaped like a cone with a sharp flattened end. They cut the food. There are eight deciduous and permanent incisors, four upper and four lower. The cuspids, at the corners of the mouth, shaped like simple cones, tear and shred food. There are four permanent cuspids; they are called also canines, and the two in the upper jaw are called eyeteeth. The premolars, or bicuspids, flanking the cuspids, consist of two cones, or cusps, fused together. They tear, crush, and grind the food. There are eight permanent premolars. The molars are in the back of the mouth. They have between three and five cusps each, and their function is to crush and grind food. There are 12 permanent molars in all, three on each side of both the upper and lower jaw. The hindmost molar in each of these groups, and the last one to emerge, is often called a wisdom tooth.

DEVELOPMENT AND ERUPTION. Both the deciduous teeth and the permanent teeth begin to develop before birth. Because of this, it is vitally important that expectant mothers receive foods that will supply the calcium, phosphorus, and vitamins necessary for healthy teeth.

The deciduous teeth begin to form about the sixth week of prenatal life, with calcification beginning about the sixteenth week. A considerable part of the crowns of these teeth is formed by the time the child is born.

Eruption, or cutting of teeth is slower in some children than others, but the deciduous teeth generally begin to appear when the infant is between 6 and 9 months of age, and the process is completed by the time a child is 2 to $2\frac{1}{2}$ years old.

When the child is about 6, the first permanent molar comes in just behind the second molar of the deciduous teeth. About the same time, shedding of the baby teeth begins. The permanent teeth form in the jaw even before the baby teeth have erupted, with the incisors and the cuspids beginning to calcify during the first 6 months of life. Calcification of the others takes place shortly after. As the adult teeth calcify, the roots of the baby teeth gradually disappear, or resorb, and are completely gone by the time the permanent teeth are ready to appear. Occasionally a baby tooth root does not resorb, and as a result the permanent tooth comes in outside its proper position. When resorption does not occur, it is necessary to remove the baby tooth and root.

The first teeth to be shed, about the sixth year, are the central incisors. The permanent incisors erupt shortly afterward. The lateral incisors are lost and replaced during the seventh to ninth years, and the cuspids in the ninth to twelfth years. The first premolars generally appear between the ages of 10 and 12, the second molars between 11 and 13 and the third molars, or wisdom teeth, between 17 and 22. It is not uncommon for the third molars to fail to erupt.

Occasionally there is a partial or total lack of either the deciduous or permanent teeth. In some cases this anodontia is hereditary, or it may be related to endocrine gland disturbances.

TOOTH DECAY AND ITS PREVENTION. Dental caries, the most common disease in the United States, begins on the outside of the teeth in the enamel. Bacteria and food adhere to the tooth surface to form a plaque. The action of the bacteria on starchy and sugary foods produces lactic acid, which is believed to dissolve the enamel. Once there is a breakthrough in the enamel, the decaying process moves on into the dentin and then to the pulp, attacking the nerves and causing toothache.

Flossing and Brushing the Teeth. Cleanliness is the best weapon against caries and PERIODONTITIS. Bacteria and food particles must be removed before the enamel is penetrated. This means thorough brushing regularly each day, preferably after every meal. If it is impossible to brush after every meal, it is helpful to rinse the mouth by swishing water vigorously back and forth between and around the teeth. When the teeth are brushed, food particles that lodge between the teeth should also be removed with dental floss.

The dental floss should be strung tightly between the two index fingers or between the bows of a floss holder. Flossing and brushing should be done in an orderly sequence so that no area is neglected. The usual pattern is beginning at the upper right, progressing to the upper left, and then from the lower left to the lower right. The floss is gently inserted between the teeth and pulled against the surface of one tooth to a point slightly under the tissue of the gum. It is then moved up and down for several strokes. The adjacent tooth is cleaned in the same manner.

The "sulcular" technique for brushing the teeth is so called because the bristles of the brush are worked beneath the free gingival margin and into the space between the tooth and the gum (the *sulcus*). To accomplish this the bristles are placed at a 45 degree angle to the gum line. Pressure is then used to move the brush back and forth horizontally. The brushing is continued around the mouth in the same pattern as the flossing.

A disclosing dye may be used to determine the presence of plaque on the teeth. Flavored mouthwash does not reduce plaque formation and is useful only to moisturize the tissues and improve mouth taste.

Proper Diet. In order to help maintain healthy teeth, the diet should include all the essential elements of good NUTRITION. Tooth decay can be reduced by limiting the intake of certain forms of sugar, especially the rich or highly concentrated ones such as candy or rich desserts.

Fluoridation. Another important means of preventing caries is through the use of fluoride. Many communities whose water is lacking in an adequate natural supply of fluoride add the chemical to their water supply. FLUORIDATION is effective for children and adolescents, and children raised on fluoridated water retain resistance to tooth decay when they become adults. In communities that do not have fluoridation, dentists may add a fluoride solution directly to the teeth or may suggest other means of obtaining fluoride protection.

Correction of Malocclusion. Another factor leading to tooth decay is poor position of the teeth, resulting in faulty closure of the jaws and uneven meeting of the teeth. This condition is called malocclusion. It should be corrected early because it also can lead to inadequate nutrition because of difficulty in chewing, and if it is severe enough to distort the face, it may have psychologic effects.

accessional teeth, the permanent molars, so called because they have no deciduous predecessors in the dental arch.

impacted t., one so placed in the jaw that it is unable to erupt or to attain its normal position in occlusion.

top(o)- word element [Gr.], *particular place or area.*

topagnosia (top″ag-no′ze-ah) 1. loss of touch localization. 2. loss of ability to recognize familiar surroundings.

topalgia (to-pal′je-ah) fixed or localized pain.

topectomy (to-pek′to-me) ablation of a small and specific area of the frontal cortex in the treatment of mental illness.

topesthesia (top″es-the′ze-ah) ability to recognize the location of a tactile stimulus.

tophaceous (to-fa′shus) gritty or sandy.

tophus (to′fus), pl. *to′phi* [L.] 1. a deposit of urates in the tissues about the joints in GOUT. 2. dental calculus.

t. syphilit′icus, a syphilitic node.

topical (top′ĭ-kal) pertaining to a particular area, as a topical anti-infective applied to a certain area of the skin and affecting only the area to which it is applied.

Topitracin (top″ĭ-tra′sin) trademark for a preparation of bacitracin, an antibiotic.

topoanesthesia (to″po-an″es-the′ze-ah) inability to recognize the location of a tactile stimulus.

topographic (top″o-graf′ik) describing or pertaining to special regions.

topography (to-pog′rah-fe) a special description of an anatomic region or a special part.

toponarcosis (top″o-nar-ko′sis) local anesthesia.

torcular Herophili (tor′ku-lar he-rof′ĭ-le) a depression in the occipital bone at the confluence of a number of cerebral venous sinuses.

torpid (tor′pid) not acting with normal vigor and facility.

torpor (tor′por) [L.] sluggishness.

t. ret′inae, sluggish response of the retina to the stimulus of light.

torque (tork) a rotatory force.

torsion (tor′shun) the act of twisting; the state of being twisted. adj., **tor′sive.**

torsiversion (tor″sĭ-ver′zhun) turning of a tooth on its long axis out of normal position.

torso (tor′so) the body, exclusive of the head and limbs.

torticollis (tor″tĭ-kol′is) wryneck, a contracted state of the cervical muscles, producing torsion of the neck. The deformity may be congenital, hysterical, or secondary to pressure on the accessory nerve, to inflammation of glands in the neck, or to muscle spasm.

tortipelvis (tor″tĭ-pel′vis) distortions of the spine and hip produced by a disorder marked by irregular muscular contractions of the trunk and extremities.

tortuous (tor′choo-us) twisted; full of turns and twists.

Torula (tor′u-lah) *Cryptococcus.*

T. hystolyt′ica, *Cryptococcus neoformans.*

toruloid (tor′u-loid) knotted or beaded, like a yeast cell.

torulus (tor′u-lus) [L.] a small elevation.

t. tac′tilis, a tactile elevation in the skin of the palms and soles.

torus (to′rus), pl. *to′ri* [L.] a swelling or bulging projection.

totipotential (to″tĭ-po-ten′shal) characterized by the ability to develop in any direction; said of cells that can give rise to cells of all orders, i.e., the complete individual.

touch (tuch) 1. the sense by which contact of an object with the skin is recognized. 2. palpation with the finger.

Touch is actually not a single sense, but several. There are separate nerves in the skin to register heat, cold, pressure, pain, and touch. These thousands of nerves are distributed unevenly over the body, so that some areas are more responsive to cold, others to pain, and others to heat or pressure.

Each of these types of nerves has a different structure at the receiving end. A touch nerve has an elongated bulb-shaped end, and a nerve responsive to cold a squat bulb; the nerve that registers warmth has what looks like twisted threads, and the nerve for deep pressure has an egg-shaped end. Pain receptors have no protective sheath.

If the sensory nerves were evenly distributed over the whole body, each square inch of skin would have about 50 heat receptors, 8 for cold, 100 for touch and 800 for pain. The sensitivity of a given spot depends in part on how thickly receptors of a particular kind are clustered in that spot, and localization of particular sensation depends on the concentration of the particular nerve endings in an area. Touch, pressure, and pain are sensations that can be localized quite accurately, but sensations of cold and heat are more diffuse.

The thickness of the skin in a given area and its supply of hairs also contribute to its touch sensitivity. A touch as light as one fifteen-thousandth of an ounce on the thin skin of the forehead can be felt, whereas a touch must be two and a half times as heavy to be felt on a fingertip. Hairs grow almost everywhere on the skin except the palms of the hands and the soles of the feet. They grow at a slant, and touch spots cluster in the skin near each of them. Even a light touch on the tip of a hair bends it back, and like a tiny lever it communicates the touch to the nerve endings.

The tactile sense develops with learning and experience. A simple test is to hold a pea between the first and second fingers. With the eyes closed, it is easy to tell that it is one object. However, if the fingers are crossed first, it will seem that there are two peas, because ordinarily it takes two objects to stimulate the touch receptors on the opposite sides of the fingers.

tourniquet (toor′nĭ-ket) a device for compression of an artery or vein. It is used to stop excessive bleeding, to prevent the spread of snake venom, and to facilitate obtaining blood samples or giving intravenous injections.

For hemorrhage, a tourniquet should be used only as a last resort, when the bleeding is so severe that it obviously threatens the life of the injured person and cannot be stopped by direct pressure.

In the case of snakebite, a moderately tight tourniquet that impedes the spread of venom but does not stop arterial blood flow may be applied.

A loosely applied tourniquet inhibits blood flow in the superficial veins, making them more prominent; this is helpful when a vein is being sought for an intravenous injection or for drawing blood.

APPLYING A TOURNIQUET. There are two places on the body where a tourniquet is effective in stopping profuse bleeding from an artery. If blood comes from a wound on the arm, the tourniquet is applied a hand's width below the armpit. If the bleeding is from a leg wound, the tourniquet should be placed a hand's width below the groin.

Any wide, flat piece of cloth long enough to circle the arm or leg twice may be used for a tourniquet. A necktie, scarf, or strip of heavy material is suitable. The cloth strip should be placed over a thick pad made of gauze or cloth, then wrapped around the limb and tied with a half knot. A small stick is placed over the half knot, and a square knot is tied over the stick. The tourniquet is tightened by slowly twisting the stick; bleeding will stop suddenly when the tourniquet is twisted tight enough.

Ten minutes after the tourniquet is applied, it should be loosened for exactly 1 minute to permit circulation of the blood in the arm or leg. During this period, a hand should be pressed against the wound. If severe bleeding does not recur during the time the tourniquet is loose, it need not be retightened but should be left in position in case bleeding becomes heavy again.

Tourniquets should never be covered by bandages, clothing, or blankets.

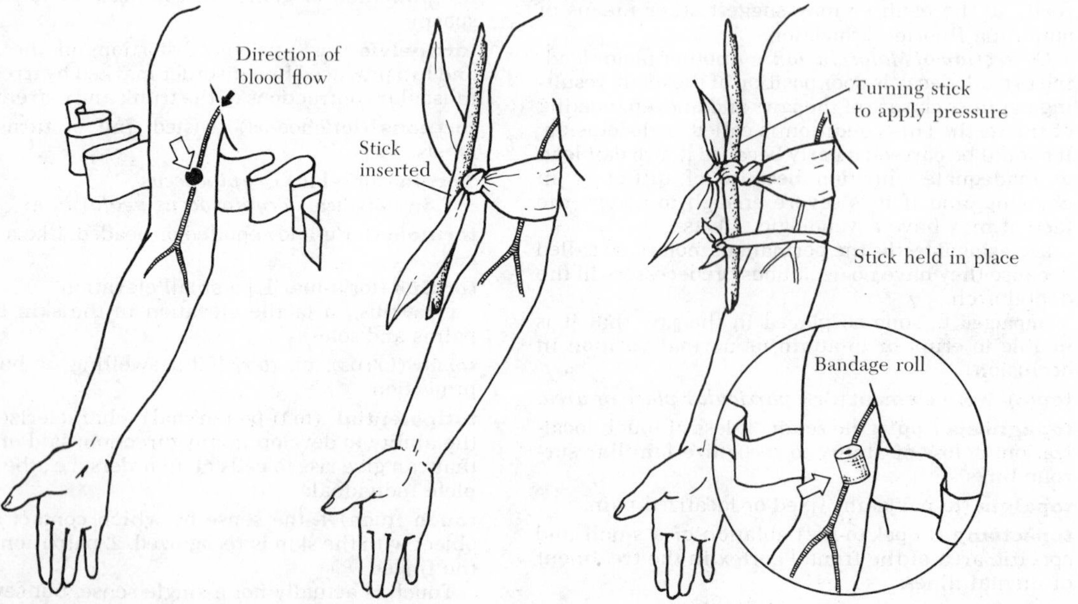

To apply a tourniquet for control of arterial bleeding from the arm: Wrap a gauze pad twice with a strip of cloth just below the armpit and tie with a half knot; tie a stick at the knot with a square knot. Slowly twist stick to tighten. Loosen tourniquet every 10 minutes.

A tourniquet applied after snakebite should not be tied with maximum pressure and should be loosened for 1 minute at 10-minute intervals. The tourniquet is always applied above the bite, to prevent flow of the venom toward the heart. If swelling increases, the tourniquet should be moved upward each time it is released (see also SNAKEBITE).

tox(o)- word element [Gr.; L.], *toxin; poison.*

toxemia (tok-se′me-ah) 1. a general intoxication sometimes due to absorption of bacterial products (toxins) formed at a local source of infection. 2. toxemia of pregnancy. adj., **toxe′mic.**

alimentary t., toxemia due to absorption from the alimentary canal of chemical poisons generated therein; a form of autointoxication.

t. of pregnancy, a group of pathologic conditions, essentially metabolic disturbances, occurring in pregnant women, manifested by preeclampsia and fully developed eclampsia.

toxic (tok′sik) poisonous; pertaining to poisoning.

toxic(o)- word element [Gr.], *poison; poisonous.*

toxicant (tok′sĭ-kant) 1. poisonous. 2. a poison.

toxicity (tok-sis′ĭ-te) the quality of being poisonous, especially the degree of virulence of a toxic microbe or of a poison.

toxicodendron (tok″sĭ-ko-den′dron) *Rhus toxicodendron.*

toxicogenic (tok″sĭ-ko-jen′ik) producing or elaborating toxins.

toxicoid (tok′sĭ-koid) resembling a poison.

toxicologist (tok″sĭ-kol′o-jist) a specialist in toxicology.

toxicology (tok″sĭ-kol′o-je) the science or study of poisons. adj., **toxicolog′ic.**

toxicomania (tok″sĭ-ko-ma′ne-ah) intense desire for poisons or intoxicants.

toxicopathy (tok″sĭ-kop′ah-the) toxicosis. adj., **toxicopath′ic.**

toxicopexy (tok′sĭ-ko-pek″se) the fixation or neutralization of a poison in the body. adj., **toxicopec′tic, toxicopex′ic.**

toxicophidia (tok″sĭ-ko-fid′e-ah) venomous serpents collectively.

toxicophobia (tok″sĭ-ko-fo′be-ah) morbid dread of poisons.

toxicophylaxin (tok″sĭ-ko-fi-lak′sin) a phylaxin that destroys the poisons produced by microorganisms.

toxicosis (tok″sĭ-ko′sis) any diseased condition due to poisoning.

toxiferous (tok-sif′er-us) conveying or producing a poison.

toxigenic (tok″sĭ-jen′ik) caused by or producing toxins.

toxigenicity (tok″sĭ-jĕ-nis′ĭ-te) the property of producing toxins.

toxin (tok′sin) a poison, especially a protein or conjugated protein produced by certain animals, some higher plants, and pathogenic bacteria.

It is characteristic of bacterial toxins that they do not cause symptoms until after a variable period of incubation while the microbes multiply, or, as is the case in botulism, the preformed toxin reaches and affects the tissue. Usually only a few toxin-producing agents are introduced into the body, and it is not until there are enough of them to overwhelm the leukocytes and other types of antibodies that symptoms occur. In some cases of food poisoning, symptoms are almost immediate because the toxin is taken directly with the food.

Toxins cause antitoxins to form in the body, thus providing a means for establishing IMMUNITY to certain diseases.

bacterial t′s, toxins produced by bacteria, including exotoxins, endotoxins, and toxic enzymes.

botulinus t., one of five type-specific, immunologically differentiable exotoxins (types A to E) produced by *Clostridium botulinum.*

dermonecrotic t., an exotoxin produced by certain bacteria that causes extensive local necrosis on intradermal inoculation.

Dick t., erythrogenic toxin.

diphtheria t., a protein exotoxin produced by *Corynebacterium diphtheriae* that is primarily responsible for the pathogenesis of diphtheritic infection; it is an enzyme that activates transferase II of the mammalian protein synthesizing system.

dysentery t., one produced by organisms of various species of *Shigella.*

erythrogenic t., a bacterial toxin from certain strains of *Streptococcus pyogenes* that produces an erythematous reaction when injected intradermally and is responsible for the rash in scarlet fever.

extracellular t., exotoxin.

fatigue t., kenotoxin.

intracellular t., endotoxin.

plant t., phytotoxin.

toxin-antitoxin (tok″sin-an′tĭ-tok″sin) a nearly neutral mixture of diphtheria toxin with its antitoxin; formerly used for vaccination against diphtheria, but now superseded by toxoid.

toxipathic (tok″sĭ-path′ik) pertaining to or caused by the pathogenic action of toxins, of whatever origin.

toxipathy (tok-sip′ah-the) toxicosis.

toxisterol (tok-sis′ter-ol) a poisonous isomer of ergosterol, produced by ultraviolet irradiation of the latter.

Toxocara (tok″so-ka′rah) a genus of nematode parasites found in the dog (*T. ca′nis*) and cat (*T. ca′ti*); both species are sometimes found in man.

toxocariasis (tok″so-ka-ri′ah-sis) infection by worms of the genus *Toxocara.*

toxoid (tok′soid) a toxin treated by heat or chemical agent to destroy its deleterious properties without destroying its ability to stimulate antibody production.

diphtheria t., a sterile preparation of formaldehyde-treated products of the growth of *Corynebacterium diphtheriae,* used as an active immunizing agent.

tetanus t., a sterile preparation of formaldehyde-treated products of the growth of *Clostridium tetani,* used as an active immunizing agent.

toxophilic (tok″so-fil′ik) easily susceptible to poison; having affinity for toxins.

toxophore (tok′so-fōr) the group of atoms in a toxin molecule that produces the toxic effect.

toxophorous (tok-sof′o-rus) bearing poison; producing the toxic effect.

Toxoplasma (tok″so-plaz′mah) a genus of sporozoan parasites in man, other mammals and some birds; it includes one species, *T. gon′dii,* which is frequently transmitted from an infected mother to an infant *in utero* or at birth. The infection may be asymptomatic or may produce encephalomyelitis with cerebral calcification and chorioretinitis (see TOXOPLASMOSIS).

toxoplasmin (tok″so-plaz′min) an antigen prepared from mouse peritoneal fluids rich with *Toxoplasma gondii;* injected intracutaneously as a test for toxoplasmosis.

toxoplasmosis (tok″so-plaz-mo′sis) a disease due to *Toxoplasma gondii.* The *congenital* form is marked by central nervous system lesions, which may lead to blindness, brain defects, and death. The *acquired* form is of two types: *lymphadenopathic toxoplasmosis,* closely resembling mononucleosis, and *disseminated toxoplasmosis,* with lesions involving the lungs, liver, heart, skin, muscle, brain, and meninges. Chorioretinitis invariably occurs in the congenital form, and often in the chronic form.

TPA total parenteral alimentation; see HYPERALIMENTATION.

TPN total parenteral nutrition; see HYPERALIMENTATION.

T.P.R. temperature, pulse, respiration.

tr. tincture.

trabecula (trah-bek′u-lah), pl. *trabec′ulae* [L.] a small beam or supporting structure; used in anatomic nomenclature to designate various fibromuscular bands or cords providing support in various organs, as heart, penis, and spleen, adj., **trabec′ular.**

trabeculate (trah-bek′u-lāt) marked with crossbars or trabeculae.

trabeculation (trah-bek″u-la′shun) the formation of trabeculae in a part.

tracer (trās′er) a means by which something may be followed, as (1) a mechanical device by which the outline or movements of an object can be graphically recorded, or (2) a material by which the progress of a compound through the body may be observed.

radioactive t., a radioactive isotope replacing a stable chemical element in a compound introduced into the body, enabling its metabolism, distribution and elimination to be followed.

trachea (tra′ke-ah) the air passage extending from the throat and larynx to the main bronchi; called also the windpipe. adj., **tra′cheal.** This tube, about three-fifths of an inch wide and 4 inches long, is reinforced at the front and sides by a series of C-shaped rings of cartilage that keep the passage uniformly open. The gaps between the rings are bridged by strong fibroelastic membranes.

The trachea is lined with mucous membrane covered with small hairlike processes called cilia. These continously sweep foreign material out of the breathing passages toward the mouth. The process is retarded by cold but speeded by heat.

Although the trachea is closed off during swallowing by the epiglottis, a sort of lid, a foreign body, such as a piece of meat, occasionally becomes lodged in it and causes choking. Surgical incision of the trachea, called tracheotomy, may be necessary for removal of the foreign body. (See also HEIMLICH MANEUVER).

TRACHEOSTOMY, incision of the trachea with insertion of a tube for passage of air, may be necessary if the trachea is obstructed by swelling due to infection or allergic reaction, by accumulation of tracheobronchial secretions or by a growth such as a polyp or tumor.

trachealgia (tra″ke-al′je-ah) pain in the trachea.

tracheitis (tra″ke-i′tis) inflammation of the trachea.

trachel(o)- word element [Gr.], *neck; necklike structure,* especially the cervix uteri.

trachelagra (tra″kĕ-lag′rah) gout in the neck.

trachelectomy (tra″kĕ-lek′to-me) excision of the uterine cervix.

trachelematoma (tra″kĕ-lem″ah-to′mah) a hematoma on the sternocleidomastoid muscle.

trachelism, trachelismus (tra′kĕ-lizm; tra″kĕ-liz′mus) spasm of the neck muscles; spasmodic reaction of the head in epilepsy.

trachelitis (tra″kĕ-li′tis) cervicitis; inflammation of the uterine cervix.

trachelocystitis (tra″kĕ-lo-sis-ti′tis) inflammation of the neck of the bladder.

trachelodynia (tra″kĕ-lo-din′e-ah) pain in the neck.

trachelomyitis (tra″kĕ-lo-mi-i′tis) inflammation of the muscles of the neck.

trachelopexy (tra′kĕ-lo-pek″se) fixation of the uterine cervix.

tracheloplasty (tra′kĕ-lo-plas″te) plastic repair of the uterine cervix.

trachelorrhaphy (tra″kĕ-lor′ah-fe) suture of the uterine cervix.

trachelotomy (tra″kĕ-lot′o-me) incision of the uterine cervix.

tracheo- (tra′ke-o) word element [Gr.], *trachea.*

tracheoaerocele (tra″ke-o-a′er-o-sēl″) tracheal hernia containing air.

tracheobronchial (tra″ke-o-brong′ke-al) pertaining to the trachea and bronchi.

tracheobronchitis (tra″ke-o-brong-ki′tis) inflammation of the trachea and bronchi.

tracheobronchoscopy (tra″ke-o-brong-kos′ko-pe) inspection of the interior of the trachea and bronchus.

tracheocele (tra″ke-o-sēl) hernial protrusion of the tracheal mucous membrane.

tracheoesophageal (tra″ke-o-e-sof″ah-je′al) pertaining to the trachea and esophagus.

tracheolaryngeal (tra″ke-o-lah-rin′je-al) pertaining to the trachea and larynx.

tracheolaryngotomy (tra″ke-o-lar″ing-got′o-me) incision of the larynx and trachea.

tracheomalacia (tra″ke-o-mah-la′she-ah) softening of the tracheal cartilages.

tracheopathy (tra″ke-op′ah-the) disease of the trachea.

tracheopharyngeal (tra″ke-o-fah-rin′je-al) pertaining to the trachea and pharynx.

tracheophony (tra″ke-of′o-ne) a sound heard in auscultation over the trachea.

tracheoplasty (tra′ke-o-plas′te) plastic repair of the trachea.

tracheopyosis (tra″ke-o-pi-o′sis) purulent tracheitis.

tracheorrhagia (tra″ke-o-ra′je-ah) hemorrhage from the trachea.

tracheoschisis (tra″ke-os′kĭ-sis) fissure of the trachea.

tracheoscopy (tra″ke-os′ko-pe) inspection of the interior of the trachea. adj., **tracheoscop′ic.**

tracheostenosis (tra″ke-o-stĕ-no′sis) constriction of the trachea.

tracheostomize (tra″ke-os′to-mīz) to perform tracheostomy upon.

tracheostomy (tra″ke-os′to-me) creation of an opening into the trachea through the neck, with insertion of an indwelling tube to facilitate passage of air or evacuation of secretions. The procedure may be an emergency measure or an elective one.

During the operation the patient is placed on his back with a pillow or roll of fabric under his shoulders so that the neck is extended and the trachea is prominent.

Tracheostomy Tray. The number and kinds of instruments available on a tracheostomy tray vary in different institutions, and although a tracheostomy may be done with very few instruments the following list includes those considered to be minimal: a scalpel, a curved blunt bistoury, dissecting scissors, a hemostat, forceps, two retractors, a tracheal dilator, gauze sponges, a pair of sterile gloves, and tracheostomy tubes.

Tracheostomy Tubes. There are many types of tracheostomy tubes available, but the basic structure is the same. All are curved to accommodate the anatomy of the trachea and most consist of an outer cannula to maintain the patency of the airway and an inner cannula that fits snugly inside the outer cannula and can be removed for cleaning and removal of accumulated secretions without disturbing the operative site. An accessory to the tracheostomy tubes is the obturator (pilot), which is an olive-tipped curved rod that is used to guide the outer cannula and prevent scraping of the tracheal walls while the tube is being inserted.

The earliest tracheostomy tubes were made of silver and consisted of only the three basic components. Later models came with an adaptor on the inner cannula to allow connection with a ventilator. The plastic tracheostomy tubes that are popular today may or may not have an inner cannula, but most have an inflatable cuff attached. The inflatable cuff may be built on the outer cannula, or it may be applied as needed. The cuff that is to be applied must be the proper size in order to be effective. The purpose of the cuff is to hold the tube in place and prevent the flow of air around the outside of the outer cannula. This allows for more effective ventilation of the patient and prevents the aspiration of liquids into the trachea.

There are two types of inflatable cuffs: single-lumen and double-lumen. In the single-lumen type, the cuff is inflated so that it distends evenly in all directions, exerting pressure against the walls of the trachea. The double-lumen cuff has two walls; the inflated inner wall presses against the tube to keep the tube in place and the inflated outer wall presses against the trachea to occlude the flow of air between the sides of the tube and the trachea. There are disadvantages to the use of these cuffs, especially that of displacement of the cuffs with motion of the patient and the danger of ischemic necrosis of the tracheal wall because of constant pressure.

There also is available a type of plastic tracheostomy tube that has no inner cannula and has two single-lumen cuffs attached to it. This allows for alternate inflation and deflation of the cuffs to prevent continuous pressure against any one area of the trachea mucosa.

Patient Care. The primary concern of tracheostomy care is maintenance of an adequate airway by keeping the tube free of secretions. During the first 24 hours after the operation the patient should have someone in constant attendance. Because he cannot call for help and will not be able to cough up and expectorate accumulations of secretions in the trachea, the patient may easily panic and feel that he is suffocating.

The patient is observed closely for signs of respiratory difficulty. If there is a change in the respiratory rate or a wheezing or crowing sound on inspiration the tube most likely is obstructed. If suctioning does not relieve the situation a physician should be called immediately. Restlessness, pallor, or the development of cyanosis is an indication of inadequate ventilation of the lungs resulting from obstruction of the airway.

Accidental expulsion of the outer cannula due to violent coughing or improperly tied tapes rarely occurs; should it happen, however, a dilator or hemostat must be used to hold open the incision while another tube is inserted.

The mucus will be slightly blood-tinged immediately after the tracheostomy is performed, but it should gradually assume a normal color. If there is evidence of persistent bleeding, this should be reported, as it may indicate internal hemorrhage. The mucus is suctioned as necessary with an electric or wall suction apparatus. The size of the catheter to be used for suctioning will depend on the size of the tracheostomy tube. The catheter should be small enough to move freely into and out of the tube and large enough to aspirate secretions effectively.

It is recommended by most authorities that aspiration of the tracheostomy tube be done under aseptic technique. Under no circumstances except dire emergency should the catheter used for suctioning the tracheostomy tube be the same as that used for oral and nasal suctioning, unless it is used first for the tracheostomy tube and then discarded after suctioning the nose and mouth. Suctioning should be done only as necessary. It is an irritating procedure that carries with it the hazards of infection and depletion of inhaled oxygen supply. (See also suction.)

Secretion buildup within the inner cannula can be minimized by (1) removing and cleaning the inner cannula every four hours or more frequently as needed, and (2) adequate humidification of inhaled air or gas (oxygen). There are many humidifier attachments available to compensate for the natural humidification mechanisms that have been bypassed by tracheostomy. In addition to maintaining the integrity of the respiratory mucosa and decreasing the buildup of dried secretions, the additional moisture helps reduce friction between the tracheostomy tube and the tracheal mucosa.

A sterile dressing, slit so that it fits around the tube, is applied at the time of the tracheostomy and is changed as often as necessary. If gauze squares are used, care must be taken that the edges are bound so that strings from the dressing will not be aspirated.

The outer cannula is not removed by the nurse unless the physician specifically writes an order to this effect. If the tracheostomy is permanent and the trachea has been sutured to the opening in the skin, there is less danger in removing the outer cannula because there are no loose flaps of skin to cover the opening while the tube is out of place.

The patient with a permanent tracheostomy must be taught self-care before he leaves the hospital. As he becomes accustomed to breathing through the tube, suctioning it as necessary and replacing the dressings, he will become less apprehensive. He must be cautioned against swimming, and should be warned to use care when taking a shower or bath that water is not aspirated through the tacheostomy.

tracheotome (tra′ke-o-tōm″) an instrument for incising the trachea.

tracheotomy (tra″ke-ot′o-me) incision of the trachea through the skin and muscles of the neck for exploration, for removal of a foreign body, or for obtaining a biopsy specimen or removing a local lesion.

trachoma (trah-ko′mah) a chronic infectious disease of the conjunctiva and cornea, producing photophobia, pain, and lacrimation, caused by an organism once thought to be a virus but now classified as a strain of the bacteria *Chlamydia trachomatis.*

Trachoma is more prevalent in Africa and Asia than in other parts of the world; in North Africa few persons reach adulthood without having contracted the infection. It is fairly common in parts of the United States, for example, in Indian reservations of the Southwest, where a hot dry climate and scarcity of water encourage its spread.

A condition closely related to trachoma in cause, manifestations, and epidemiologic pattern is inclusive conjunctivitis. This is fundamentally a disease of the adult genital tract, transmitted as a venereal disease. The agents of trachoma and inclusive conjunctivitis are called TRIC agents.

SYMPTOMS. Clinically, trachoma in children and adults begins with a conjunctivitis that is marked by tiny follicles on the upper eyelids and tarsal plate. The follicles become increasingly larger and there is granulation of the cornea and impairment of vision. Eventually there is severe scarring which results in blindness.

TREATMENT and PREVENTION. The drugs of choice in the treatment of trachoma are the tetracyclines and sulfonamides administered topically in the form of suspensions or ointments that adhere to the conjunctiva for prolonged effect.

Prevention of trachoma begins with an adequate water supply for washing the hands and bathing, control of flies, and education of the local population about the cause and spread of the disease. Early treatment of young children reduces the source of infection and avoids the complication of blindness. Repeated treatment programs for adults aid in controlling the spread of infection.

t. bodies, inclusion bodies found in clusters in the cytoplasm of the epithelial cells of the conjunctiva in trachoma.

trachomatous (trah-ko′mah-tus) pertaining to or of the nature of trachoma.

trachychromatic (tra″ke-kro-mat′ik) strongly or deeply staining.

trachyphonia (tra″ke-fo′ne-ah) roughness of the voice.

tracing (trās′ing) a graphic record produced by copying another, or scribed by an instrument capable of making a visual record of movements.

tract (trakt) a longitudinal assemblage of tissues or organs, especially a bundle of nerve fibers having a common origin, function, and termination, or a number of anatomic structures arranged in series and serving a common function.

alimentary t., alimentary canal.

biliary t., the organs, ducts, etc., participating in secretion (the liver), storage (the gallbladder), and delivery (hepatic and bile ducts) of bile into the duodenum.

digestive t., alimentary canal (see also DIGESTIVE SYSTEM).

dorsolateral t., a group of nerve fibers in the lateral funiculus of the spinal cord dorsal to the posterior column.

extrapyramidal t., see EXTRAPYRAMIDAL SYSTEM.

gastrointestinal t., the stomach and intestine in continuity (see also DIGESTIVE SYSTEM).

iliotibial t., a thickened longitudinal band of fascia lata extending from the tensor muscle downward to the lateral condyle of the tibia.

intestinal t., the small and large intestines in continuity (see also INTESTINAL TRACT).

optic t., the nerve tract proceeding backward from the optic chiasm, around the cerebral peduncle, and dividing into a lateral and medial root, which end in the superior colliculus and lateral geniculate body, respectively.

pyramidal t's, collections of motor nerve fibers arising in the brain and passing down through the spinal cord to motor cells in the anterior horns.

respiratory t., the organs that allow entrance of air into the lungs and exchange of gases with the blood, from the air passages in the nose to the pulmonary alveoli.

urinary t., the organs concerned in the production and excretion of urine: the KIDNEYS, the urinary BLADDER, the URETERS, and the URETHRA.

uveal t., the vascular tunic of the eye, comprising the choroid, ciliary body, and iris.

traction (trak′shun) the exertion of a pulling force, as that applied to a fractured bone or dislocated joint to maintain proper position and facilitate healing, or, in obstetrics, that along the axis of the pelvis to assist in delivery of a fetal part.

Traction also may be used to overcome muscle spasms in musculoskeletal disorders, such as "slipped disk," to lessen or prevent contractures and to correct or prevent a deformity.

Traction may be applied by means of a weight connected to a pulley mechanism over the patient's bed; this is known as weight traction. Elastic traction involves the use of an elastic appliance that exerts a pulling force upon the injured limb. In skeletal traction, force is applied directly upon a bone by means of surgically installed pins and wires or tongs. Splints and reinforced garments, such as surgical corsets and collars, also may be employed to provide forms of traction. In skin traction moleskin or some other type of adhesive bandage is used to cover the affected limb, and traction is applied to the bandage.

PATIENT CARE. The patient in constant traction must receive special skin care frequently to prevent breakdown of the skin. Since he often cannot move certain parts of his body without help, a regular schedule of changing and alternating positions should be instituted. Bony prominences are checked frequently for signs of pressure and irritation.

When allowed by the physician, the installation of a trapeze bar over the bed can give the patient greater freedom in moving himself about in bed and make him feel less dependent on the nursing staff. The patient should be instructed to lift himself

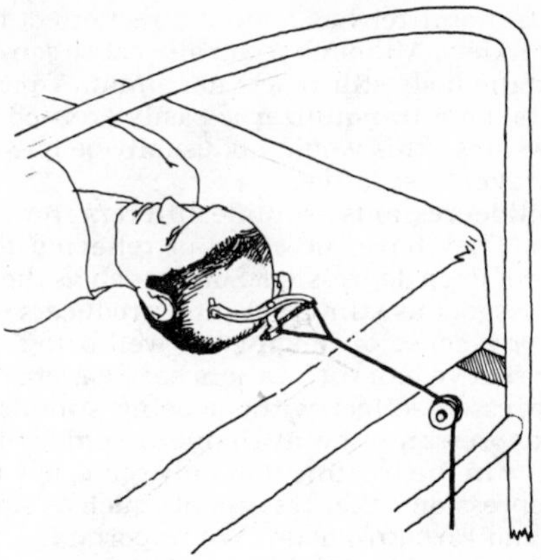

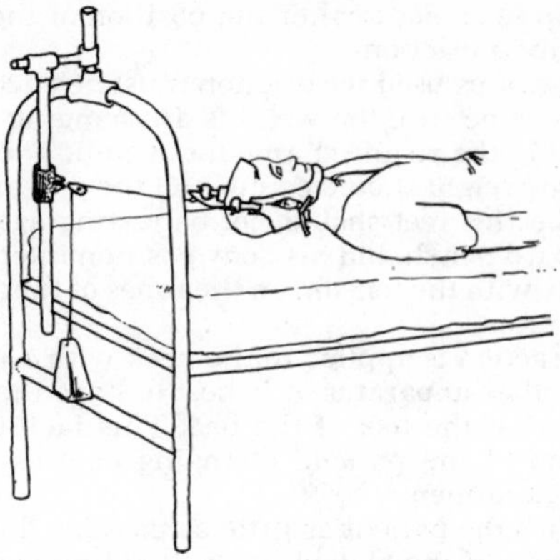

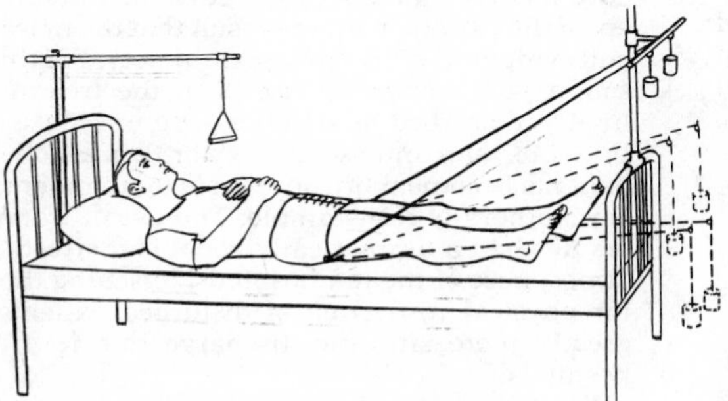

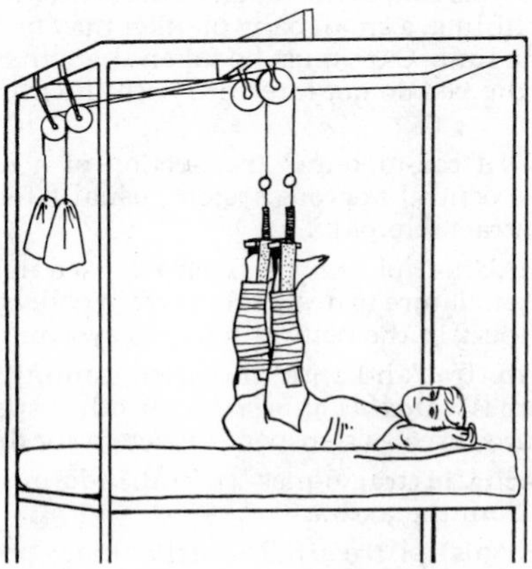

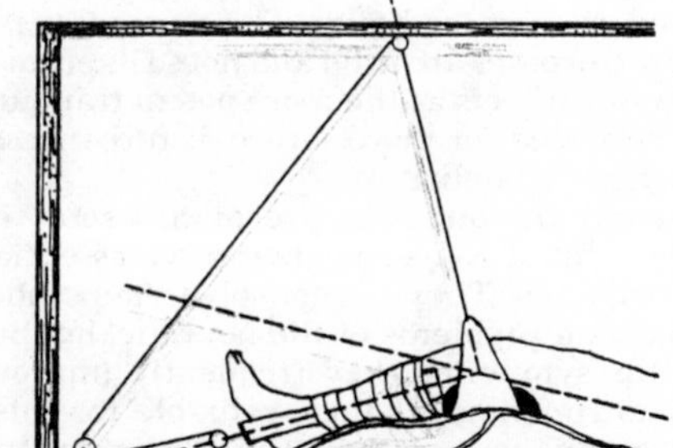

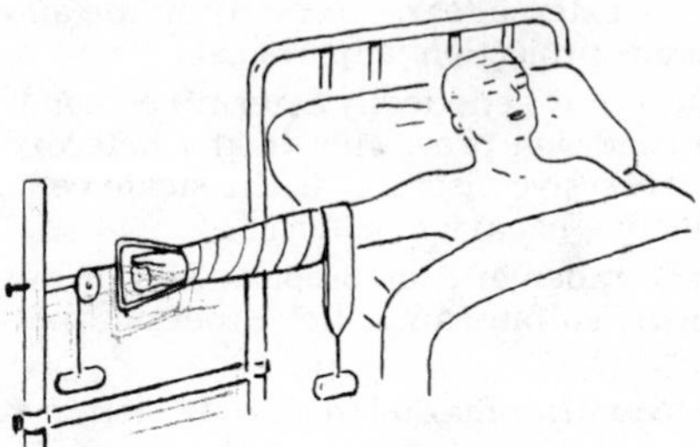

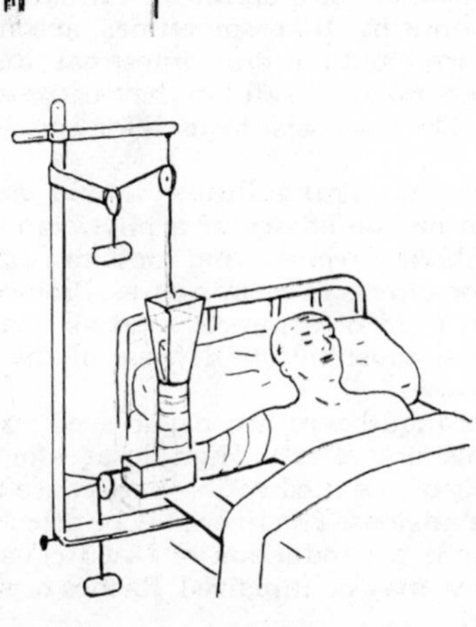

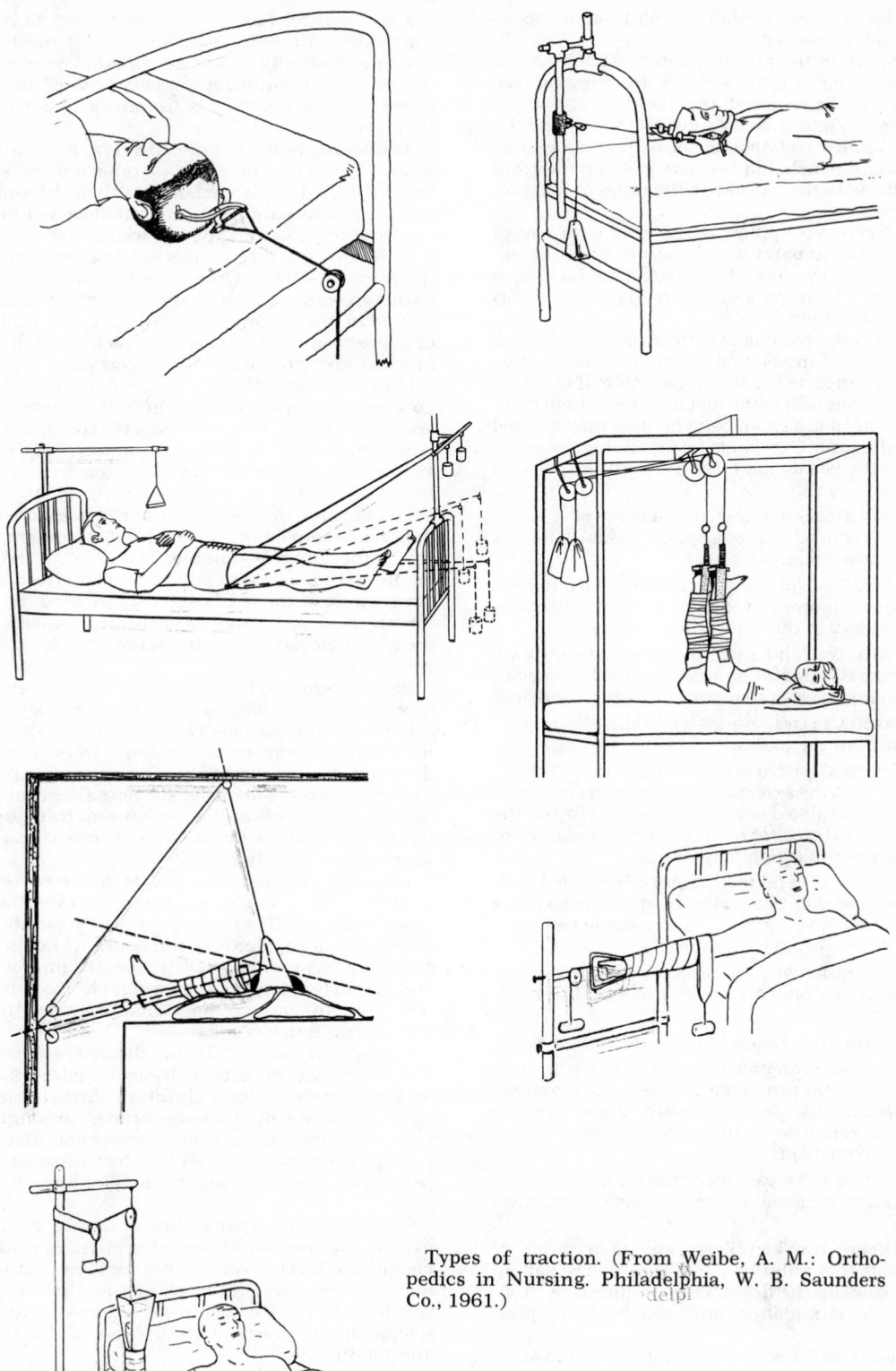

Types of traction. (From Weibe, A. M.: Orthopedics in Nursing. Philadelphia, W. B. Saunders Co., 1961.)

straight up so as not to alter the position of the affected limb in traction.

The apparatus used for traction must be checked frequently to be sure the weights are hanging free and exerting the required amount of pull. The patient's body weight should counteract the pull of the weights; i.e., his feet should not be resting against the footboard nor should his body position interfere in any way with the tension on the ropes of the traction apparatus.

When traction is applied to the neck with a head halter or other apparatus, it is best to have the patient's head at the foot of the bed. This facilitates observation of the patient, changing of dressings and other treatments.

To disturb the patient as little as possible during the changing of the bottom linen, it is best to start the linen change on the unaffected side. If the limb in traction feels cold to the touch or the patient complains of chilling, a small baby blanket may be used to cover the limb. Care must be taken that other top covers on the bed do not interfere with the traction apparatus.

tractotomy (trak-tot′o-me) transection of a nerve tract in the central nervous system, usually for the relief of intractable pain.

tractus (trak′tus), pl. *trac′tus* [L.] tract; used in anatomic nomenclature to designate certain collections of nerve fibers in the central nervous system.

tragacanth (trag′ah-kanth) the dried gummy exudation from *Astragalus gummifer* or other species of *Astragalus;* used as a suspending agent for drugs.

tragomaschalia (trag″o-mas-kal′e-ah) odorous perspiration from the axilla.

tragus (tra′gus), pl. *tra′gi* [L.] a cartilaginous projection anterior to the external opening of the ear; used also in the plural to designate hairs growing on the pinna of the external ear, especially on the anterior cartilaginous projection. adj., **tra′gal.**

trait (trāt) 1. any genetically determined condition; also, the condition prevailing in the heterozygous state of a recessive disorder, as the sickle cell trait. 2. a distinctive behavior pattern.

Tral (tral) trademark for preparations of hexocyclium methylsulfate, an anticholinergic and antispasmodic.

tramazoline (trah-maz′o-lēn) an adrenergic agent.

trance (trans) profound or abnormal sleep from which the patient cannot be aroused easily, and not due to organic disease. It is usually due to hysteria or other psychiatric disturbance and may be induced by hypnotism.

Trancopal (tran′ko-pal) trademark for a preparation of chlormezanone, a muscle relaxant and tranquilizer.

tranquilizer (tran′kwĭ-li″zer) any of a group of compounds that calm or quiet an anxious patient without causing the drowsiness produced by SEDATIVES or the stimulation produced by antidepressants.

Tranquilizers differ in important ways from other drugs used to reduce pain or relieve tension and anxiety. Sedatives, which include barbiturates and chloral hydrate, act as depressants of the nervous system and diminish the response to certain stimuli. They frequently bring about a lessening of anxiety. They may also cause the patient to become drowsy. Alcohol is well known for its effect in relieving emotional tension by a depressant action; it is essentially a sedative.

A tranquilizer has a more direct effect in lessening anxiety. Although it can also cause some drowsiness, the body still reacts to stimuli. A person who has taken a tranquilizer is easily aroused from his drowsiness; this would not usually be possible if he had taken a sedative.

Antidepressants are quite different from tranquilizers. They have the effect of relieving the symptoms of deep depression. Some, such as the amphetamines, act as stimulants and producers of euphoria, or a sense of heightened well-being, and may help relieve lethargy. Others have a more direct antidepressent effect without being stimulants. The antidepressants now available are unfortunately effective in the treatment of only some, not all, forms of depression; other treatments, such as SHOCK THERAPY and PSYCHOTHERAPY, are important.

USES. *In Mental Illness.* Tranquilizers do not cure mental illness. They relieve the intense anxiety of the patient, with the result that the more difficult symptoms of his disease disappear. For this reason, a very important use is in the treatment of highly disturbed psychotics (see PSYCHOSIS). Relieved of their intense anxiety or depression, these patients become more accessible to treatment, with psychotherapy for example. The use of tranquilizers has had a dramatically beneficial effect on the atmosphere of mental hospitals, lessening the need for physical restriction of disturbed patients, and greatly increasing the discharge rate from these hospitals.

In Anxiety and Neurosis. Tranquilizers are sometimes prescribed by physicians to relieve anxiety states from various causes. Chronic alcoholics may benefit from certain tranquilizers which reduce the craving for liquor. The tranquilizers used for these purposes are mild and not so likely to cause serious side effects as the more potent tranquilizers frequently used for more severe disturbances, such as psychosis or delirium.

Although tranquilizers are often useful in the management of NEUROSIS, they serve essentially to ease symptoms. They cannot solve the psychologic conflicts and problems of the neurotic, but by lessening his symptoms they frequently improve his ability to function. Though valuable for this purpose, tranquilizers are sometimes overused by people seeking quick results.

In Physical Illness. Tranquilizers are also effective in the relief of certain physical conditions. They may, for instance, be helpful as antinauseants to stop the vomiting that sometimes accompanies x-ray therapy and certain intestinal disorders. Tranquilizers may be useful in the treatment of hypertension. They may also be used for muscle relaxation.

SIDE EFFECTS. Tranquilizers should never be used except on the advice of a physician. All are potentially habit forming, and most can cause unpleasant side effects in certain cases. Prolonged use can lead to mild discomforts such as headaches, sleeplessness, constipation, dryness of the mouth, and nightmares.

Certain tranquilizers are capable of producing more serious side effects. High dosages or sudden withdrawals of the medication may cause tremors or even convulsions. The liver may be affected, producing jaundice. Production of blood cells by the bone marrow may be impaired. Rashes or sensitivity of the skin to sunlight may develop. There may be a possibility of damage to an unborn baby.

It is important to remember that each tranquilizer has its own range of effects and side effects. These are considered when a particular tranquilizer is selected by the physician; his advice should be followed carefully and any side effects should be reported to him.

Some persons take tranquilizers to relieve their tensions and then take stimulants such as amphetamine to give them "pep." These artificial efforts to make the body work both ways are likely to have unfortunate results for both body and mind. For these people, the answer usually is not medication but a return to normal life routines and rhythms—with the aid of a physician or a psychiatrist if necessary.

trans- (trans) word element [L.] *through; across; beyond;* in names of chemical compounds it indicates certain atoms or radicals on opposite sides of the molecule.

transabdominal (trans″ab-dom′ĭ-nal) across the abdominal wall or through the abdominal cavity.

transacetylation (trans-as″ĕ-til-a′shun) a chemical reaction involving the transfer of the acetyl radical.

transactional analysis (trans-ak′shun-al) a theory of personality structure and a psychotherapeutic method originated by Dr. Eric Berne. According to this theory the human personality is viewed as consisting of three ego states: the Parent, the Adult, and the Child. These ego states are described by Dr. Berne as being "coherent systems of thought and feeling manifested by corresponding patterns of behavior."

The word *transaction* in this term is in reference to the communication that takes place between two people. Or, more precisely, what occurs when a stimulus from the ego state of one person elicits a response from the ego state of another individual. *Analysis* refers to an investigation into the feelings and behavior patterns that are demonstrated during the transaction. In a successful or complementary transaction, the stimulus and response are between the same ego states; for example, Parent-Parent and Adult-Adult. In unsuccessful transactions one individual is speaking from one ego state, but gets a response from a different ego state. The interaction between the two is then either terminated or switched to another focus.

The therapeutic effect of transactional analysis is believed to be derived from an understanding of the origin of each of the three ego states, recognition of their influence on behavior, and an awareness of the options one has for dealing with reality in an effective and satisfying manner so that he can take care of his own needs and feel good about himself and other people.

transamidase (trans-am′ĭ-dās) an enzyme that catalyzes the transfer of an amide group from one molecule to another.

transaminase (trans-am′ĭ-nās) an enzyme that catalyzes the transfer of an amino group from one molecule to another.

glutamic oxaloacetic t., GOT, an enzyme normally present in serum (SGOT) and varius tissues, especially the heart and liver; it is released into serum as a result of tissue injury and is present in increased concentration in myocardial infarction or acute damage to liver cells.

glutamic pyruvic t., GPT, an enzyme normally present in the body, especially the liver, and observed in higher concentration in the serum of patients with acute damage to liver cells.

transamination (trans″am-ĭ-na′shun) the reversible exchange of amino groups between different amino acids.

transanimation (trans-an″ĭ-ma′shun) resuscitation of an asphyxiated person by mouth-to-mouth breathing (see also ARTIFICIAL RESPIRATION).

transaortic (trans″a-or′tik) performed through the aorta.

transatrial (trans-a′tre-al) performed through the atrium.

transaudient (trans-aw′de-ent) penetrable by sound waves.

transaxial (trans-ak′se-al) directed at right angles to the long axis of the body or a part.

transcalent (trans-ka′lent) penetrable by heat rays.

transcervical (trans-ser′vĭ-kal) 1. performed through the cervical opening of the uterus. 2. across or through the neck of a structure.

transcortical (trans-kor′tĭ-kal) connecting two parts of the cerebral cortex.

transcortin (trans″kor-tin) an α-globulin that binds and transports biologically active, unconjugated cortisol in plasma.

transcription (trans-krip′shun) the process by which genetic information contained in DNA produces a complementary series of bases in an RNA chain. (See also REVERSE TRANSCRIPTASE.)

transduction (trans-duk′shun) the transfer of a genetic fragment from one microorganism to another by bacteriophage.

transection (tran-sek′shun) a cross section; division by cutting transversely.

transfer factor TF, a factor occurring in sensitized lymphocytes that has the capacity to transfer delayed hypersensitivity to a normal (nonreactive) individual. It confers cell-mediated IMMUNITY and therefore has been found to be useful in treating conditions in which there is a disorder of IMMUNE RESPONSE. As an adjunct to antibiotic therapy it is useful in the treatment of such antibiotic-resistant diseases as candidiasis, coccidioidomycosis, and leprosy.

transferase (trans′fer-ās) an enzyme that catalyzes the transfer, from one molecule to another, of a chemical group that does not exist in free state during the transfer.

transference (trans-fer′ens) 1. the passage of a symptom or affection from one part to another. 2. in psychiatry, the shifting of an affect from one person to another or from one idea to another; especially the transfer by the patient to the analyst of emotional tones, of either affection or hostility, based on unconscious identification.

transferrin (trans-fer′in) a serum globulin that binds and transports iron.

transfix (trans-fiks′) to pierce through or impale.

transfixion (trans-fik′shun) a cutting through from within outward, as in amputation.

transforation (trans″fo-ra′shun) perforation of the fetal skull.

transformation (trans″for-ma′shun) change of form or structure; conversion from one form to another. In oncology, the change that a normal cell undergoes as it becomes malignant.

transformer (trans-for′mer) an induction apparatus for changing electrical energy at one voltage and current to electrical energy at another voltage and current, through the medium of magnetic energy, without mechanical motion.

closed-core t., one having a continuous core of magnetic material (usually iron) without any air gap.

step-down t., one for lowering the voltage of the original current.

step-up t., one for raising the voltage of the original current.

transfusion (trans-fu′zhun) introduction into the body circulation of blood or other fluid. Among the solutions employed are whole blood, plasma, serum, and various artificial blood substitutes.

Blood transfusions are used to replenish the depleted blood supply of the body in cases of hemorrhage, burns, injuries to blood vessels, shock during surgery, and certain blood dyscrasias such as anemia and leukemia.

TRANSFUSION METHODS. There are several different methods of transfusion. Direct transfusion, in which blood from one person is directly transferred to another person, is now rarely used. The usual method is indirect transfusion, in which blood is drawn from a donor, stored in a sterile container and later given to a recipient. Exchange transfusion, in which blood is removed from a person and simultaneously replaced by donor blood, is used mainly in treating ERYTHROBLASTOSIS FETALIS.

In reciprocal transfusion, blood from a person recovering from a contagious disease is transferred into the blood vessels of another person afflicted with the same disease in exchange for an equal amount of blood. This is designed to help the sick person by giving him antibodies developed by the person who is recovering.

Intrauterine Transfusion. Intrauterine transfusion involves direct transfusion of Rh-negative packed blood cells into the fetal peritoneal cavity. It is done to prevent death as a result of maternal-fetal blood incompatibility in which the fetal blood cells are destroyed (ERYTHROBLASTOSIS FETALIS).

The first step in a fetal transfusion is injection of a radiopaque dye into the amniotic fluid. After the fetus ingests the dye, his intestinal tract can be visualized by roentgenography and serves as a guidepost for location of the abdominal cavity. A long pudendal needle is then inserted through the mother's abdomen and guided through the uterine wall, through the fetal abdomen, and into the peritoneal cavity. Another x-ray is taken to confirm correct placement of the needle and then the erythrocytes are transfused.

This procedure is obviously not without hazard and is done only if the fetus cannot be expected to survive without it. The treatment may need to be repeated several times before birth.

BLOOD TYPING AND CROSSMATCHING. Transfusions were not practicable until the four main hereditary BLOOD GROUPS, A, B, AB, and O, were discovered at the beginning of this century. The different blood groups are caused by the presence of two substances, A and B, in the erythrocytes, and of their two antibodies, a and b, in the plasma. Various combinations of the substances and antibodies result in the four groups. Blood group is readily determined by a simple chemical test of two drops of blood.

A further precaution before transfusion is to mix small samples of the donor's and recipient's blood and to note the reaction; this is known as crossmatching.

Another matter to be considered is the RH FACTOR. Individuals lacking this factor are called Rh negative, and should always receive transfusions of Rh-negative blood.

ADVERSE REACTIONS. Among the most common transfusion reactions are those occurring as a result of blood group incompatibilities. They may range from mild reactions with rash, itching, and chills to severe and sometimes fatal shock and renal failure. When blood groups are incompatible there is agglutination (clumping) of the cells, hemolysis, and release of hemoglobin into the serum. Some symptoms may be manifested immediately, while others, such as jaundice, may not occur until several days after the transfusion.

Especially dangerous to patients with either cardiac or renal disease is HYPERKALEMIA, an excess of potassium in the blood. If the condition is not corrected, a flaccid paralysis develops, affecting the muscles of respiration and eventually the heart muscle, which can lead to cardiac arrest. High levels of potassium in donor blood are likely to occur when the bank blood is several days old. It is estimated that the breakdown of red cells in the stored blood increases the level of potassium at the rate of one milliequivalent per liter per day.

Another possible complication is hypocalcemia, which can occur when large amounts of blood containing the additive acid citrate dextrose (ACD) are given rapidly, as to a bleeding patient. The ACD anticoagulant binds with calcium ions in the recipient's blood, removing them from circulation and thereby reducing the calcium level below that essential for normal coagulation.

Circulatory overload is a possibility any time blood is administered rapidly in large amounts. Patients who are particularly susceptible to this eventuality are the very young, the very old, and those suffering from a pre-existing cardiopulmonary or renal problem. Another difficulty that may be encountered when blood is administered rapidly under pressure is that of air embolism.

PATIENT CARE. Every patient receiving a blood transfusion should be monitored closely for early signs of transfusion reactions and complications. Although transfusion of whole blood is a relatively common procedure, it is a highly complex one and not without danger to the patient. Should early signs of a reaction develop, the transfusion should be discontinued and the physician notified immediately.

Each unit of blood must be labeled carefully and accurately with the patient's name, room number, hospital number, and blood group. The label is read carefully immediately before administration to assure that the patient is receiving compatible blood. Although many complications and reactions cannot be anticipated and prevented, carelessness in the handling and administration of blood can result in unnecessary discomfort and danger to the patient.

transiliac (trans-il′e-ak) across the two ilia.

transillumination (trans″ĭ-lu″mĭ-na′shun) the passage of strong light through a body structure, to permit inspection by an observer on the opposite side.

translation (trans-la′shun) the formation of a polypeptide chain in the sequence directed by messenger RNA.

translocation (trans″lo-ka′shun) the attachment of a fragment of one chromosome to a nonhomologous chromosome.

reciprocal t., the mutual exchange of fragments between two broken chromosomes, one part of one uniting with part of the other.

translucent (trans-lu′sent) slightly penetrable by light rays.

transmethylase (trans-meth′ĭ-lās) an enzyme that catalyzes transmethylation.

transmethylation (trans″meth-ĭ-la′shun) the transfer of a methyl group (CH—) from the molecules of one compound to those of another.

transmigration (trans″mi-gra′shun) 1. diapedesis. 2. change of place from one side of the body to the other.

transmission (trans-mish′un) 1. transfer, as of a disease from one person to another. 2. heredity.

transmutation (trans″mu-ta′shun) 1. evolutionary change of one species into another. 2. the change of one chemical element into another.

transorbital (trans-or′bĭ-tal) performed through the bony socket of the eye.

transparent (trans-par′ent) permitting the passage of rays of light so that objects may be seen through the substance.

transpeptidase (trans-pep′tĭ-dās) an enzyme that catalyzes the transfer of an amino or peptide group from one molecule to another.

transphosphorylase (trans″fos-for′ĭ-lās) an enzyme that catalyzes the transfer of a phosphate group from one molecule to another.

transphosphorylation (trans″fos″for-ĭ-la′shun) the exchange of phosphate groups between organic phosphates, without their going through the stage of inorganic phosphates.

transpiration (trans″pĭ-ra′shun) discharge of air, vapor, or sweat through the skin.

transplacental (trans″plah-sen′tal) through the placenta.

transplant 1. (trans′plant) tissue used in grafting or transplanting. 2. (trans-plant′) to transfer tissue from one part to another.

transplantation (trans″plan-ta′shun) the transfer of living organs from one part of the body to another or from one individual to another. Transplantation and grafting mean the same thing, though the term grafting is more commonly used to refer to the transfer of skin (see GRAFTING).

In dentistry, transplantation refers to the insertion into a prepared dental alveolus of an autogenous or homologous tooth; it may be a developing tooth germ from the same mouth, or a frozen homologous transplant.

Occasionally an emergency requires an organ to be transplanted from one place to another within the body. Kidneys, for example, have been relocated to enable them to continue functioning after the ureters have been damaged. Organ transplants within the body, known as autotransplants, require delicate surgery, but otherwise pose no particular problem.

Kidney transplants have been performed since 1902, but the operation that advanced the procedure beyond the experimental stage was performed in 1954 in Boston. A kidney from one identical twin was successfully implanted in the other to replace his diseased kidneys. Since that time kidney transplantations have been the most successful of transplantations, primarily because there is an artificial kidney machine available, and also because the kidney is a paired organ. This means that the donor survives the removal of an organ for transplantation, and can be selected on the basis of tissue-type compatibility to avoid fatal rejection of the organ by the recipient.

In 1967 the South African surgeon Christiaan N. Barnard transplanted a human heart and set off a reaction from both medical and lay groups concerned about the ethical and legal implications of obtaining healthy organs for transplantation. These problems still have not been completely resolved to everyone's satisfaction.

Since the first human heart transplantation, attempts have been made to transplant the liver, pancreas, and lungs. A study co-sponsored by the American College of Surgeons and the National Institutes of Health reported that as of April 1, 1976, a worldwide total of 297 heart transplants had been done; of these recipients, 57 were still living. Since 1963, 252 recipients of liver transplants have been followed, and 31 were living in 1976. The longest period for a functioning liver transplant was 74 months at the time of the report. Only one pancreas recipient, out of the 47 pancreas transplantations reported, had survived 45 months. There had been no survivors of the 37 lung recipients reported.

REJECTION. The major problem to be overcome in transplantation therapy is the immune rejection phenomenon. Organs such as the cornea, skin, and bone can be transplanted successfully because, in the case of the cornea, the vascular supply is not involved, or, in skin and bone, the transplant serves as a structural foundation into which the new tissue grows. In the case of intact organs such as the kidney, heart, lung, liver, and pancreas, a generous blood supply is essential to their survival in the recipient's body. The blood of the recipient carries in it many of the tools used by the body in defense against foreign substances. As blood is drained from the transplanted organ into the host's general circulation, the body recognizes the transplanted tissue cells as foreign invaders (antigens) and immediately sets up an IMMUNE RESPONSE by producing antibodies. These antibodies are capable of inhibiting metabolism of the cells within the transplanted organ and eventually actively cause their destruction. They also play a role in delayed inflammatory response that can occur as late as weeks or months after implantation and adds to the destruction of the donor organ.

Control of the immune response in the recipient is attempted by the use of immunosuppressive agents such as antilymphocyte globulin (ALG), and antimetabolites, which tend to suppress the growth of rapidly dividing cells. Corticosteroids also are used because of their anti-inflammatory effect. All of the chemicals used in transplantation therapy interfere in some way with the body's normal defense mechanisms. For this reason a very delicate balance must be maintained in their administration so as to avoid tipping the scales in the direction of rejection of the organ on one side and a fatal infection on the other.

transport (trans′port) movement of materials in biologic systems, particularly into and out of cells and across epithelial layers.

active t., movement of materials across cell membranes and epithelial layers resulting directly from expenditure of metabolic energy.

transposition (trans″po-zish′un) displacement to the opposite side; in genetics, the nonreciprocal insertion of material deleted from one chromosome into another, nonhomologous chromosome.

t. of great vessels, a CONGENITAL HEART DEFECT, in which the position of the chief blood vessels of the heart is reversed.

transsegmental (trans″seg-men′tal) extending across segments.

transseptal (trans-sep′tal) extending or performed through or across a septum.

transsexual (trans-seks′u-al) 1. a person affected by transsexualism. 2. a person whose external anatomy has been changed to resemble that of the opposite sex.

transsexualism (trans-seks′u-al-izm″) a disturbance of gender identity in which the person has an overwhelming desire to be of the opposite sex, often seeking hormonal and surgical treatment to achieve this goal.

transthalamic (trans″thah-lam′ik) across the thalamus.

transthoracic (trans″tho-ras′ik) through the thoracic cavity or across the chest wall.

transtympanic (trans″tim-pan′ik) across the tympanic membrane or the cavity of the middle ear.

transudate (tran′su-dāt) a fluid substance that has passed through a membrane or has been extruded from a tissue; in contrast to an exudate, a transudate is characterized by high fluidity and a low content of protein, cells, or solid matter derived from cells.

transudation (tran″su-da′shun) 1. passage of serum or other body fluid through a membrane or tissue surface. 2. transudate.

transurethral (trans″u-re′thral) performed through the urethra.

transvaginal (trans-vaj′ĭ-nal) through the vagina.

transversalis (trans″ver-sa′lis) [L.] transverse.

transverse (trans-vers′) extending from side to side; situated at right angles to the long axis.

transversectomy (trans″ver-sek′to-me) excision of a transverse process of a vertebra.

transversus (trans-ver′sus) [L.] transverse.

transvesical (trans-ves′ĭ-kal) through the bladder.

transvestism (trans-ves′tizm) the condition of being a transvestite.

transvestite (trans-ves′tīt) a person who derives sexual pleasure from dressing in the attire of the opposite sex.

Trantas' dots (tran′tas) small, white calcareous-looking dots in the limbus of the conjunctiva in vernal conjunctivitis.

tranylcypromine (tran″il-si′pro-mēn) a compound used as an antidepressant.

trapezium (trah-pe′ze-um) an irregular, four-sided figure.

Trasentine (tras′en-tin) trademark for preparations of adiphenine, an anticholinergic and antispasmodic.

trauma (traw′mah) a wound or injury, especially damage produced by external force.

birth t., an injury to the infant during the process of being born. In some psychiatric theories, the psychic shock produced in an infant by the experience of being born.

psychic t., an emotional shock that makes a lasting impression.

traumat(o)- (traw′mah-to) word element [Gr.], *trauma.*

traumatic (traw-mat′ik) pertaining to, resulting from, or causing trauma.

traumatism (traw′mah-tizm) 1. the physical or psychic state resulting from an injury or wound. 2. a wound.

traumatology (traw″mah-tol′o-je) the branch of surgery dealing with wounds and disability from injuries.

traumatopnea (traw″mah-top-ne′ah) passage of air through a wound in the chest wall.

travail (trah-vāl′) labor; childbirth.

tray (tra) a flat-surfaced utensil for the conveyance of various objects or material.

Treacher Collins syndrome (tre′chur-kol′inz) see mandibulofacial DYSOSTOSIS.

treatment (trēt′ment) management and care of a patient or the combating of disease or disorder.

active t., treatment directed immediately to the cure of the disease or injury.

Banting t., treatment of obesity by a low carbohydrate diet rich in nitrogenous matter.

causal t., treatment directed against the cause of a disease.

conservative t., treatment designed to avoid radical medical therapeutic measures or operative procedures.

empiric t., treatment by means that experience has proved to be beneficial.

expectant t., treatment directed toward relief of untoward symptoms, leaving the cure of the disease to natural forces.

Karell T., treatment of heart and kidney disease by keeping the patient in bed and giving only 800 ml. of milk daily for 4 to 5 days, the diet then being gradually increased until, on the thirteenth day the regular diet is resumed.

Kenny's t., treatment of poliomyelitis by wrapping the patient in woolen cloths wrung out of hot water and re-educating muscles by passive exercise after pain has subsided.

palliative t., treatment that is designed to relieve pain and distress, but does not attempt a cure.

preventive t., prophylactic t., that in which the aim is to prevent the occurrence of the disease.

rational t., that based upon knowledge of disease and the action of the remedies given.

specific t., treatment particularly adapted to the special disease being treated.

supporting t., that which is mainly directed to sustaining the strength of the patient.

tree (tre) an anatomic structure with branches resembling a tree.

bronchial t., the bronchi and their branching structures. (See Plates 5 and 6.)

tracheobronchial t., the trachea, bronchi, and their branching structures. (See Plates 5 and 6.)

trehalose (tre-ha′lōs) a disaccharide from the cocoons of the beetle *Trehala manna* and yeast.

Trematoda (trem″ah-to′dah) a class of the phylum Platyhelminthes that includes the flukes. The trematodes or flukes are parasitic in man and animals, infections resulting from the ingestion or insufficiently cooked fish, crustaceans, or vegetation which contain their larvae. The important trematodes of man belong to the genera *Schistosoma, Echinostoma, Fasciolopsis, Gastrodiscoides, Heterophyes, Metagonimus, Clonorchis, Fasciola, Dicrocoelium, Opisthorchis,* and *Paragonimus.* (See also WORM.)

trematode (trem′ah-tōd) an individual of the class Trematoda.

tremor (trem′or, tre′mor) an involuntary trembling of the body or limbs. It may have either a physical or a psychologic cause.

Often tremors are associated with Parkinson's disease, in which nerve centers in the brain that control the muscles are affected. Early symptoms include trembling of the hands and nodding of the head. Tremors occur also in cerebral palsy and hyperthyroidism, and in narcotic addicts and alcoholics during withdrawal. They tend to develop as one of the results of aging.

Tremors are sometimes symptoms of temporary abnormal conditions, as, for example, insulin shock, or of poisoning, especially metallic poisoning. They sometimes appear with a high fever resulting from an infection.

Tremors of psychologic origin take many forms, some minor and some serious. If there is no physiologic cause, they may be a sign of general tension, as when a person holding a full cup of coffee seems compelled to shake and spill it. Violent, uncontrollable trembling is often seen in certain phases of severe mental disorder.

coarse t., that involving large groups of muscle fibers contracting slowly.

fibrillary t., rapidly alternating contraction of small bundles of muscle fibers.

fine t., one in which the vibrations are rapid.

flapping t., asterixis.

Hunt's t., tremor associated with every voluntary movement; characteristic of cerebellar lesions.

intention t., one occurring when the patient attempts voluntary movement.

senile t., tremor due to the infirmities of old age.

volitional t., trembling of the entire body during voluntary effort; seen in multiple sclerosis.

tremulous (trem′u-lus) shaking, trembling, or quivering.

trench fever a louseborne rickettsial disease due to *Rickettsia quintana,* with febrile paroxysms, leg pains, chills, sweating, rash, splenomegaly, and a tendency to relapse.

trench foot a condition of the feet resembling frostbite, due to the prolonged action of water on the skin combined with circulatory disturbance due to cold and inaction.

trench mouth an acute or chronic gingival infection; called also necrotizing ulcerative gingivitis. The name trench mouth was given to the disease during World War I, when it was common among soldiers in the trenches. It is relatively uncommon now and responds readily to antimicrobial therapy.

When the condition extends to other parts of the oral mucosa, with lesions involving the palate or pharynx, it is termed VINCENT'S ANGINA or necrotizing ulcerative gingivostomatitis.

Trendelenburg's position (tren-del′en-bergz) the patient is supine on a surface inclined 45 degrees, his head at the lower end and his legs flexed over the upper end.

trepan (trĕ-pan′) trephine.

trepanation, trephination (trep″ah-na′shun; tref″ĭ-na′shun) use of the trephine for creating an opening in the skull or in the sclera.

trephine (trĕ-fin′, trĕ-fēn′) 1. a crown saw for removing a circular disk of bone, chiefly from the skull. 2. an instrument for removing a circular area of cornea. 3. to remove with a trephine.

trepidation (trep″ĭ-da′shun) 1. a trembling or oscillatory movement. 2. nervous anxiety and fear. adj., **trep′idant.**

Treponema (trep″o-ne′mah) a genus of spirochetes (family Treponemataceae), some of them being pathogenic and parasitic for man and other animals, including the etiologic agents of pinta (*T. carate′um*), syphilis (*T. pal′lidum*), and yaws (*T. perten′ue*).

treponema (trep″o-ne′mah) an organism of the genus *Treponema.* adj., **trepone′mal.**

Treponemataceae (trep″o-ne″mah-ta′se-e) a family of bacteria that commonly occur as parasites in vertebrates, some of them causing disease. They are coarse or slender spiral forms, and are sometimes visible only with a darkfield microscope.

treponematosis (trep″o-ne″mah-to′sis) infection with organisms of the genus *Treponema.*

treponemicidal (trep″o-ne″mĭ-si′dal) destroying treponemas.

trepopnea (tre″pop-ne′ah) a condition in which respiration is more comfortable with the patient turned in a definite recumbent position.

treppe (trep′ĕ) [Ger.] the gradual increase in muscular contraction following rapidly repeated stimulation.

tresis (tre′sis) perforation.

tri- (tri) word element [Gr. L.], *three.*

triacetate (tri-as′ĕtāt) an acetate that contains three molecules of the acetic acid radical.

triacetin (tri-as′ĕ-tin) glyceryl triacetate; used as a topical antifungal.

triacetyloleandomycin (tri-as″ĕ-til-o″le-an″do-mi′sin) troleandomycin.

triad (tri′ad) 1. an element with a valence of three. 2. a group of three similar bodies, or a complex composed of three items or units.

triage (tre-ahzh′) [Fr.] the sorting out and classification of casualties of war or other disaster, to determine priority of need and proper place of treatment.

triambutosine (tri″am-bu′to-sīn) a drug used in the treatment of leprosy; not available in the United States.

triamcinolone (tri″am-sin′o-lōn) a prednisolone derivative used as an anti-inflammatory glucocorticoid in the form of the acetonide derivative and the diacetate ester.

triamterene (tri-am′ter-ēn) a diuretic which increases sodium and chloride excretion, but not potassium excretion.

triangle (tri′ang-g′l) a three-cornered object, figure, or area, as such an area on the surface of the body capable of fairly precise definition.

carotid t., inferior, that between the median line of the neck in front, the sternocleidomastoid muscle, and the anterior belly of the omohyoid muscle.

carotid t., superior, that between the anterior belly of the omohyoid muscle in front, the posterior belly of the digastric muscle above, and the sternocleidomastoid muscle behind.

cephalic t., one on the anteroposterior plane of the skull, between lines from the occiput to the forehead and to the chin, and from the chin to the forehead.

digastric t., submandibular triangle.

t. of elbow, a traingular area on the front of the elbow, bounded by the brachioradial muscle on the outside and the round pronator muscle inside, with the base toward the humerus.

t. of election, superior carotid triangle.

facial t., a triangular area whose points are the basion and the alveolar and nasal points.

femoral t., the area formed superiorly by the inguinal ligament, laterally by the sartorius muscle, and medially by the adductor longus muscle; called also Scarpa's triangle.

infraclavicular t., that formed by the clavicle above, the upper border of the greater pectoral muscle on the inside, and the anterior border of the deltoid muscle on the outside.

inguinal t., the triangular area bounded by the inner edge of the sartorius muscle, the inguinal ligament, and the outer edge of the long adductor muscle.

lumbocostoabdominal t., that lying between the external oblique muscle of the abdomen, the posterior inferior serratus muscle, the erector muscle of the spine, and the internal oblique muscle of the abdomen.

t. of necessity, inferior carotid triangle.

occipital t., the area bounded by the sternocleidomastoid muscle in front, the trapezius muscle behind, and the omohyoid muscle below.

Scarpa's t., femoral triangle.

subclavian t., a triangular area bounded by the clavicle, the sternocleidomastoid muscle, and the omohyoid muscle.

submaxillary t., that bounded by the lower jaw bone above, the posterior belly of the digastric muscle and the stylohyoid muscle below and the median line of the neck in front.

suboccipital t., that lying between the posterior greater rectus muscle of the head and the superior and inferior oblique muscles of the head.

triangular (tri-ang'gu-lar) having three angles or corners.

triangularis (tri-ang"gu-la'ris) [L.] triangular.

Triatoma (tri"ah-to'mah) a genus of bugs (order Hemiptera), the cone-nosed bugs, important in medicine as vectors of *Trypanosoma cruzi.*

triatomic (tri"ah-tom'ik) containing three atoms in the molecule.

tribe (trīb) a taxonomic category subordinate to a family (or subfamily) and superior to a genus (or subtribe).

triboluminescence (tri"bo-lu"mĭ-nes'ens) luminescence produced by mechanical energy, as by the grinding, rubbing, or breaking of certain crystals.

tribrachius (tri-bra'ke-us) a monster with three arms.

tribromoethanol (tri-bro"mo-eth'ah-nol) a white crystalline powder used in amylene hydrate solution as a basal anesthetic.

Triburon (trib'u-ron) trademark for preparations of triclobisonium, a topical and vaginal antiseptic.

TRIC agents those causing TRACHOMA and inclusive conjunctivitis.

tricarboxylic acid cycle (tri"car-bok-sil'ik) the cyclic metabolic mechanism by which the complete oxidation of the acetyl moiety of acetyl-coenzyme A is effected; the process is the chief source of mammalian energy, during which carbon chains of sugars, fatty acids, and amino acid are metabolized to yield carbon dioxide, water, and high-energy phosphate bonds. Called also Krebs cycle and citric acid cycle. See accompanying diagram.

tricephalus (tri-sef'ah-lus) a monster with three heads.

triceps (tri'seps) a muscle having three heads; the triceps muscle of the arm extends the forearm.

trich(o)- (trik'o) word element [Gr.], *hair.*

trichiasis (trĭ-ki'ah-sis) 1. a condition of ingrowing hairs about an orifice, or ingrowing eyelashes. 2. the appearance of hairlike filaments in the urine.

trichina (trĭ-ki'nah), pl. *trichi'nae* [Gr.] an individual organism of the genus *Trichinella.*

Trichinella (trik"ĭ-nel'ah) a genus of nematode parasites.

T. spira'lis, a species found in the striated muscle of various animals, a common cause of infection in man as a result of ingestion of poorly cooked pork.

trichinosis (trik"ĭ-no'sis) infection with the parasitic roundworm *Trichinella spiralis,* which enters the human body in infected pork eaten raw or insufficiently cooked.

The larvae, or early forms, of *T. spiralis* live embedded in tiny capsule-like cysts of muscle tissue of infected pork. When the meat is properly cooked, the larvae are killed by the high temperature. If, however, the pork is undercooked, they survive; when the meat is eaten, digestive juices dissolve the cyst capsules and free the larvae in the intestines, where they grow to maturity.

Trichinosis is found in most parts of the world with the exception of Australia and the Pacific islands. It is relatively common in Europe and the United States. In recent years there has been a decline in its incidence owing to enforcement of laws requiring the cooking of garbage fed to hogs. Other factors influencing the decline include storage of meat at low temperatures and education of the general public in the proper cooking of pork.

SYMPTOMS AND DEVELOPMENT. Trichinosis develops in stages that correspond to the worms' development in the intestine and, later, the movement of their larvae into other parts of the body. Symptoms and the severity vary according to the stage of the disease, the tissues invaded, and the total number of invading parasites.

During the initial stage of the disease, when larvae are developing into mature worms in the intestinal tract, there may be diarrhea, nausea, abdominal pain, and fever.

Symptoms that make identification of the disease more certain appear generally after an incubation period of 1 to 2 weeks. By this time, the mature worms have deposited their young in the intestinal wall and these new larvae are beginning to move through the body, causing a variety of reactions in one or several organs and areas. Edema may develop in the eyelids. This may be followed by hemorrhage of the retina, pain in the eyes, and extreme sensitivity to light.

As the larvae invade other parts of the body, there may be muscle soreness and pain, fever, thirst, chills, profuse sweating, and edema in the infected areas.

For most people there is more discomfort than

danger in this most serious phase of trichinosis—the time when the larvae are active in various parts of the body. Often the infection is mild enough for patients to be treated at home. The occasional fatal cases of the disease (fewer than 5 per cent of known cases) usually involve additional infections or disorders in organs weakened by the parasites.

In the usual course of the disease, there is a gradual decrease in symptoms as the larvae in muscle tissue become encysted and dormant and those in other types of tissue are destroyed. After about 3 months, most symptoms disappear, although vague muscular pain and fatigue may still continue for several months. Trichinosis almost never leaves any permanent disability.

TREATMENT AND PREVENTION. With its varying symptoms, trichinosis is sometimes difficult to diagnose, but a skin test has been developed that makes identification of the disease certain in most cases. Chest x-rays and microscopic examination of muscle tissue also can be useful in diagnosis.

There is no specific treatment for trichinosis; recovery is a matter of bed rest and time, which allow the body's natural defenses to overcome the parasites. Medications, including thiabendazol, cortisone, and ACTH, may be prescribed to relieve muscular pain and other symptoms.

The only certain safeguard against trichinosis is the thorough cooking of all pork products to ensure destruction of any encysted *Trichinella* larvae. Pork should be cooked at a temperature of 350° F., with a roasting time of 35 minutes per pound, until the meat is gray in color; if it is pink it is underdone. Cooking in this manner ensures that all parts of the

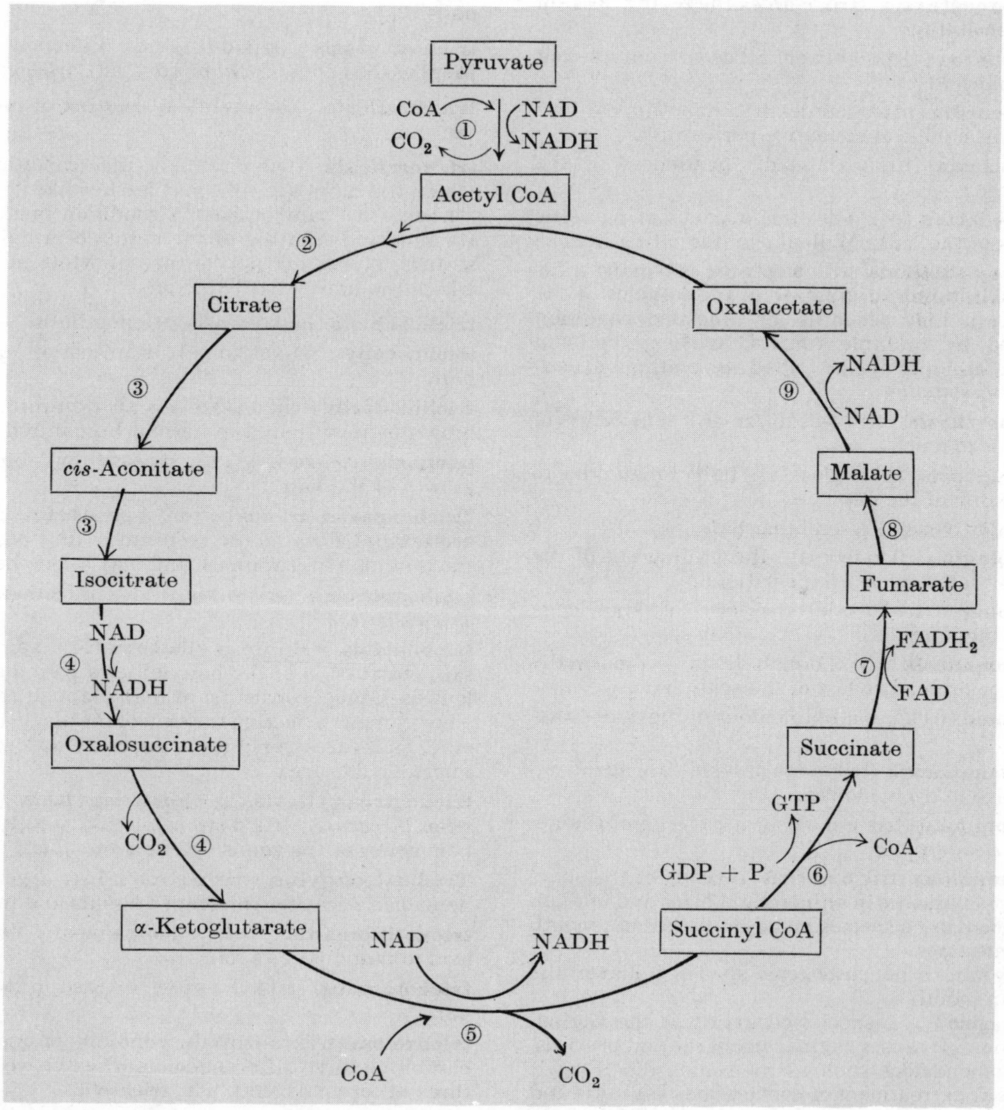

Diagrammatic representation of reactions by which carbon chains of sugars, fatty acids, and amino acids are metabolized to yield carbon dioxide, water, and high-energy phosphate bonds. Key to enzymes (circled numbers): 1 = pyruvate dehydrogenase. 2 = citrate synthase. 3 = aconitrate dehydrogenase. 4 = isocitric dehydrogenase. 5 = α-ketoglutarate dehydrogenase. 6 = succinyl-CoA synthetase. 7 = succinate dehydrogenase. 8 = fumarate hydratase (fumarase). 9 = malate dehydrogenase. (From Mazur, A., and Harrow, B.: Textbook of Biochemistry. 10th ed. Philadelphia, W. B. Saunders Co., 1971.)

roast will be heated to well above 140° F. (68 C.), the thermal death point of trichinae. Pork products such as frankfurters should never be eaten raw.

trichinous (trik'ĭ-nus) affected with or containing trichinae.

trichloride (tri-klo'rīd) any combination of three atoms of chloride with one of another element.

trichlormethiazide (tri-klōr"mĕ-thi'ah-zīd) a compound used as a diuretic and hypotensive and in the treatment of edema.

trichloroacetic acid (tri-klo"ro-ah-se'tic) colorless deliquescent crystals; germicidal, astringent, and caustic.

trichloroethylene (tri"klo-ro-eth'ĭ-lēn) a clear, mobile liquid used as an inhalation analgesic and anesthetic for short operative procedures.

trichoanesthesia (trik"o-an"es-the'ze-ah) loss of hair sensibility.

trichobezoar (trik"o-be'zōr) a bezoar composed of hair; hairball.

trichocardia (trik"o-kar'de-ah) a hairy appearance of the heart due to exudative pericarditis.

trichoclasia (trik"o-kla'se-ah) brittleness of the hair.

Trichodectes (trik"o-dek'tēz) a genus of parasitic insects of the order Mallophaga, the biting lice.

trichoepithelioma (trik"o-ep"ĭ-the"le-o'mah) a benign skin tumor originating in the follicles of the lanugo; it may occur as an inherited condition marked by multiple tumors (trichoepithelioma papillo'sum mul'tiplex). Called also epithelioma adenoides cysticum.

trichoesthesia (trik"o-es-the'ze-ah) sensibility of the hair to touch.

trichoglossia (trik"o-glos'e-ah) hairy tongue, due to thickening of the papillae.

trichoid (trik'oid) resembling hair.

trichologia (trik"o-lo'je-ah) the pulling out of the hair by delirious or insane patients.

trichology (trĭ-kol'o-je) the sum of knowledge about the hair.

trichomadesis (trik"o-mah-de'sis) abnormally rapid or premature loss of the scalp hair.

trichome (tri'kōm) a filamentous or hairlike structure.

trichomonacide (trik"o-mo'nah-sīd) an agent destructive to trichomonads.

trichomonad (trik"o-mo'nad) a parasite of the genus *Trichomonas.*

Trichomonas (trik"o-mo'nas) a genus of flagellate protozoa parasitic in animals and birds and in man.

T. homi'nis, a species found in the human mouth and intestines.

T. te'nax, a nonpathogenic species found in the human mouth.

T. vagina'lis, a species occurring in the vaginal secretions; it causes vaginal discharge and pruritus. Trichomonacides such as metronidazole (Flagyl) are used in treatment of trichomonas vaginitis and may be given also to the patient's husband, who may be an asymptomatic carrier of the infection.

trichomoniasis (trik"o-mo-ni'ah-sis) infection by organisms of the genus *Trichomonas.*

trichomycosis (trik"o-mi-ko'sis) any disease of the hair caused by fungi.

t. axilla'ris, infection of the axillary and sometimes of the pubic hair, due to *Corynebacterium tenuis* and not a fungus, with development of clumps of bacteria on the hairs, appearing as red, yellow, or black nodules. Called also leptothrix.

trichonodosis (trik"o-no-do'sis) a condition characterized by apparent or actual knotting of the hair.

trichopathy (trĭ-kop'ah-the) disease of the hair.

trichophytid (trĭ-kof'ĭ-tid) a secondary skin eruption that is the expression of an allergic reaction to a trichophyton infection and that occurs in an area remote from the site of infection.

trichophytin (trĭ-kof'ĭ-tin) a filtrate from cultures of *Trichophyton;* used in testing for trichophytosis.

trichophytobezoar (trik"o-fi"to-be'zōr) a bezoar composed of animal hair and vegetable fiber.

Trichophyton (trĭ-kof'ĭ-ton) a genus of fungi that may cause various infections of the skin, hair, and nails.

trichophytosis (trik"o-fi-to'sis) infection with fungi of the genus *Trichophyton.* adj., **trichophyt'ic.**

trichoptilosis (trik"o-tĭ-lo'sis) splitting of hairs at the end.

trichorrhexis (trik"o-rek'sis) the condition in which the hairs are split and feather-like.

t. nodo'sa, bamboo hair; a condition marked by fracture and splitting of the cortex of a hair into strands, giving the appearance of white nodes at which the hair is easily broken.

trichoschisis (trĭ-kos'kĭ-sis) trichoptilosis.

trichoscopy (trĭ-kos'ko-pe) examination of the hair.

trichosiderin (trik"o-sid'er-in) an iron-containing brown pigment found in normal human red hair.

trichosis (trĭ-ko'sis) any disease or abnormal growth of the hair.

Trichosporon (trĭ-kos'po-ron) a genus of fungi that are normal flora of the respiratory and digestive tracts of man and animals, and may infect the hair.

trichosporosis (trik"o-spo-ro'sis) infection with *Trichosporon.*

trichostasis spinulosa (trĭ-kos'tah-sis spin"u-lo'sah) obstruction of the hair follicles with a spinulous dark plug, consisting of many lanugo hairs in a horny mass, affecting the skin of the alae nasi and other facial areas, or of the arms, chest, abdomen, or interscapular area.

trichostrongyliasis, trichostrongylosis (trik"o-stron"jĭ-li'ah-sis; trik"o-stron"jĭ-lo'sis) infection by nematodes of the genus *Trichostrongylus.*

Trichostrongylus (trik"o-stron'jĭ-lus) a genus of nematode parasites infecting animals and man.

trichotillomania (trik"o-til"o-ma'ne-ah) compulsion to pull out one's hair.

trichotomous (trĭ-kot'o-mus) divided into three parts.

trichroism (tri'kro-izm) the condition or quality of exhibiting three different colors when viewed from three different aspects. adj., **trichro'ic.**

trichromatopsia (tri"kro-mah-top'se-ah) normal color vision for all three primary colors, red, green, and blue.

trichromic (tri-kro'mik) 1. pertaining to or exhibiting three colors. 2. able to distinguish only three of the seven colors of the spectrum.

trichuriasis (trik″u-ri′ah-sis) infection with *Trichuris.*

Trichuris (trik-u′ris) a genus of nematodes parasitic in the intestinal tract, including *T. trichiu′ra,* the whipworm, found in man, which may cause vomiting and diarrhea but often produces no symptoms.

tricipital (tri-sip′ĭ-tal) 1. three-headed. 2. relating to the triceps muscle.

triclobisonium (tri″klo-bi-so′ne-um) an anti-infective used topically as the chloride salt in superficial infections of the skin and vagina, and in vulvitis, vaginitis, and related infections due to *Trichomonas vaginalis, Candida albicans,* and *Hemophilus vaginalis.*

triclofos (tri′klo-fós) a hypnotic and sedative.

Tricofuron (tri″ko-fu′ron) trademark for preparations of furazolidone, used as an antibacterial and antiprotozoan agent.

Tricoloid (tri′ko-loid) trademark for preparations of tricyclamol, an anticholinergic.

tricornute (tri-kor′nūt) having three horns, cornua, or processes.

tricrotism (tri′krŏ-tizm) the quality of having three sphygmographic waves or elevations to one beat of the pulse. adj., **tricrot′ic.**

tricuspid (tri-kus′pid) having three points or cusps, as a valve of the heart.

t. valve, the valve that guards the opening between the right atrium and right ventricle.

tricyclamol (tri-si′klah-mol) an anticholinergic used in the form of the chloride salt to inhibit gastrointestinal hypermotility and to reduce gastric juice secretion.

tridactylism (tri-dak′tĭ-lizm) the presence of only three digits on the hand or foot.

tridentate (tri-den′tāt) having three prongs.

tridermic (tri-der′mik) derived from the ectoderm, entoderm, and mesoderm.

tridihexethyl (tri″di-heks-eth′il) an anticholinergic used as the chloride salt in the treatment of gastrointestinal disturbances.

Tridione (tri-di′ōn) trademark for preparations of trimethadione, an anticonvulsant.

triethanolamine (tri″eth-ah-nol′ah-mēn) a compound used as an alkalizing agent.

triethylamine (tri-eth″il-am′in) a ptomaine from putrefying fish.

triethylenemelamine (tri-eth″ĭ-lēn-mel′ah-mēn) a highly poisonous, white, crystalline powder used as an antineoplastic agent.

triethylenethiophosphoramide (tri-eth″ĭ-lēn-thi″o-fos-for′ah-mīd) thiotepa, an antineoplastic agent.

trifid (tri′fid) split into three parts.

trifluoperazine (tri″floo-o-per′ah-zēn) a phenothiazine derivative; its hydrochloride salt is used as a major tranquilizer.

triflupromazine (tri″floo-pro′mah-zēn) a phenothiazine derivative; its hydrochloride salt is used as a major tranquilizer.

trifluromethylthiazide (tri-flo͞or″o-meth″il-thi′-ah-zīd) flumethiazide.

trifurcation (tri″fur-ka′shun) division or the site of separation into three branches.

trigeminal (tri-jem′ĭ-nal) 1. triple. 2. pertaining to the fifth cranial (trigeminal) nerve.

t. nerve, the fifth cranial nerve; it arises in the pons, is composed of sensory and motor fibers, and has three divisions: ophthalmic, maxillary, and mandibular. The ophthalmic division supplies sensory fibers to the skin of the upper eyelid, side of the nose, forehead, and anterior half of the scalp. The maxillary division carries sensory impulses from the mucous membranes of the nose, the skin of the cheek and side of the forehead, and the upper lip and upper teeth. The mandibular division carries sensory impulses from the side of the head, chin, mucous membrane of the mouth, lower teeth, and anterior two-thirds of the tongue. (One can readily see why this nerve is sometimes called the great sensory nerve of the head.) The motor fibers are part of the mandibular branch and supply several of the muscles of chewing.

t. neuralgia, pain arising from irritation of the fifth cranial (trigeminal) nerve. The disorder is characterized by brief attacks of severe pain in the face and forehead of the affected side. The cause is unknown. Many patients describe sensitive areas about the nose and mouth which, when touched, excite an attack. Attacks also may be brought on by exposure to cold, eating and drinking, and washing the face. Treatment may be palliative or surgical. Called also TIC DOULOUREUX.

trigeminy (tri-jem′ĭ-ne) the condition of occurring in threes, especially the occurrence of three pulse beats in rapid succession.

triglyceride (tri-glis′er-īd) a compound consisting of three molecules of fatty acids bound with one molecule of glycerol; a neutral fat that is the usual storage form of lipids in animals.

Elevated serum triglycerides are now considered as important as high colesterol levels in the development of ischemic heart disease. The normal range for serum triglycerides is 0 to 160 mg./100 ml.

trigonal (tri′go-nal) 1. triangular. 2. pertaining to a trigone.

trigone (tri′gōn) a triangular area.

t. of bladder, vesical trigone.

carotid t., the triangular area bounded by the posterior belly of the digastric muscle, the sternocleidomastoid muscle, and the anterior midline of the neck.

olfactory t., the triangular area of gray matter between the roots of the olfactory tract.

vesical t., a triangular region of the wall of the urinary bladder, the three angles corresponding with the orifices of the ureters and urethra; it is an area in which the muscle fibers are closely adherent to the mucosa.

trigonectomy (tri″go-nek′to-me) excision of the vesical trigone.

trigonitis (tri″go-ni′tis) inflammation or localized hyperemia of the vesical trigone.

trigonocephalus (trig″o-no-sef′ah-lus) an individual exhibiting trigonocephaly.

trigonocephaly (tri″go-no-sef′ah-le) triangular shape of the head due to sharp forward angulation at the midline of the frontal bone. adj., **trigonocephal′ic.**

trigonum (tri-go′num), pl. *trigo′na* [L.] trigone, or triangle; used in anatomic nomenclature to designate various regions or structures.

trihexyphenidyl (tri-hek″se-fen′ĭ-dil) a compound

used as an anticholinergic and in treatment of Parkinson's disease.

trihybrid (tri-hi′brid) a hybrid offspring of parents differing in three mendelian characters.

triiodothyronine (tri″i-o″do-thi′ro-nēn) one of the thyroid hormones; an organic iodine-containing compound liberated from thyroglobulin by hydrolysis. It has several times the biologic activity of thyroxine.

trilabe (tri′lāb) a three-pronged lithotrite.

Trilafon (tri′lah-fon) trademark for preparations of perphenazine, a tranquilizer and antiemetic.

trilaminar (tri-lam′ĭ-nar) three-layered.

Trilene (tri′lēn) trademark for a preparation of trichloroethylene, an inhalation analgesic and anesthetic.

trilobate (tri-lo′bāt) having three lobes.

trilocular (tri-lok′u-lar) having three loculi or cells.

trilogy (tril′o-je) a group or series of three.

t. **of Fallot**, a term sometimes applied to concurrent pulmonic stenosis, atrial septal defect, and right ventricular hypertrophy.

trimanual (tri-man′u-al) accomplished by the use of three hands.

trimensual (tri-men′su-al) occurring every 3 months.

trimeprazine (tri-mep′rah-zēn) a drug with mild central nervous depressant, moderate antiemetic and anticonvulsant, and powerful antihistaminic action; used as an antipruritic in the form of the tartrate salt.

trimester (tri-mes′ter) a period of 3 months.

trimethadione (tri″meth-ah-di′ōn) a white, crystalline compound used as an anticonvulsant.

trimethaphan (tri-meth′ah-fan) a compound used in ganglionic blockade and as an antihypertensive.

trimethidinium (tri-meth″ĭ-din′e-um) a compound used in ganglionic blockade and as an antihypertensive.

trimethobenzamide (tri-meth″o-ben′zah-mīd) a compound used as an antiemetic.

trimethylene (tri-meth′ĭ-lēn) cyclopropane, a general anesthetic.

Trimeton (tri′mĕ-ton) trademark for preparations of pheniramine, an antihistamine.

trimorphous (tri-mor′fus) existing in three different forms.

trinitroglycerol (tri-ni″tro-glis′er-ol) nitroglycerin.

trinitrophenol (tri-ni″tro-fe′nol) a substance used as dye, tissue fixative, antiseptic, astringent, and stimulant of epithelialization; it can be detonated on percussion or by heating above 300° C. Called also picric acid.

trinitrotoluene (tri-ni″tro-tol′u-ēn) TNT: a high explosive derived from toluene; it sometimes causes poisoning in those who work with it, marked by dermatitis, gastritis, abdominal pain, vomiting, constipation, and flatulence.

triocephalus (tri″o-sef′ah-lus) a monster with no organs of sight, hearing, or smell, the head being a nearly shapeless mass.

triolism (tri′o-lizm) sexual interests or practices involving three persons of both sexes.

triorchidism (tri-or′kĭ-dizm) the presence of three testes.

triose (tri′ōs) a monosaccharide containing three carbon atoms in a molecule.

trioxsalen (tri-ok′sah-len) a psoralen used in conjunction with ultraviolet exposure in treatment of vitiligo and psoriasis.

tripara (trip′ah-rah) tertipara; a woman who has had three pregnancies that resulted in viable offspring; para III.

tripelennamine (tri″pĕ-len′ah-min) an antihistaminic used orally, parenterally, and topically in the symptomatic treatment of various allergic disorders.

tripeptide (tri-pep′tīd) a peptide formed from three amino acids.

triphalangism (tri-fal′an-jizm) three phalanges in a digit normally having only two.

triphasic (tri-fa′zik) having three phases.

triphenylmethane (tri-fen″il-meth′ān) a substance from coal tar, the basis of various dyes and stains, including aurin, rosaniline, basic fuchsin, and gentian violet.

triplegia (tri-ple′je-ah) paralysis of three extremities.

triplet (trip′let) 1. one of three offspring produced at one birth. 2. a combination of three objects or entities acting together, as three lenses or three nucleotides.

triplex (tri′pleks) triple or threefold.

triploid (trip′loid) having triple the haploid number of chromosomes (3n).

triplokoria (trip″lo-ko′re-ah) the presence of three pupils in an eye.

triplopia (trĭ-plo′pe-ah) defective vision, objects being seen as threefold; usually a hysterical symptom.

tripoding (tri′pod-ing) the use of three points of support, as adopted by paralyzed patients when changing from a sitting or standing position.

triprolidine (tri-pro′lĭ-dēn) a compound used as an antihistamine.

-tripsy (trip′se) word element [Gr.], *crushing;* used to designate a surgical procedure in which a structure is intentionally crushed.

tripus (tri′pus) a conjoined twin monster having three feet.

trisaccharide (tri-sak′ah-rīd) a sugar each molecule of which yields three molecules of monosaccharides on hydrolysis.

trismus (triz′mus) motor disturbance of the trigeminal nerve, especially spasm of the masticatory muscles, with difficulty in opening the mouth (lockjaw); a characteristic early symptom of tetanus.

trisomy (tri′som-e) the presence of an additional (third) CHROMOSOME of one type in an otherwise diploid cell (2n + 1). adj., **triso′mic.**

t. **D syndrome**, holoprosencephaly due to an aberration of the autosomes of the D group, in which central nervous system defects are associated with mental retardation, along with cleft lip and palate, polydactyly, and dermal pattern anomalies, and abnormalities of the heart, viscera, and genitalia.

t. **E syndrome**, neonatal hepatitis, mental retardation, scaphocephaly or other skull abnormality, micrognathia, blepharoptosis, low-set ears, corneal opacities, deafness, webbed neck, short digits, ventricular septal defects, Meckel's diverticulum, and other deformities; due to the presence of an extra E group chromosome.

t. **13–15 syndrome,** trisomy D syndrome.

t. **16–18 syndrome,** trisomy E syndrome.

t. **18 syndrome,** trisomy E syndrome.

t. **21 syndrome,** Down's syndrome.

trisplanchnic (tri-splangk′nik) pertaining to the three great visceral cavities, the skull, thorax, and abdomen.

tristichia (tri-stik′e-ah) the presence of three rows of eyelashes.

tristimania (tris″tĭ-ma′ne-ah) melancholia.

trisulcate (tri-sul′kāt) having three furrows.

trisulfate (tri-sul′fāt) a binary compound containing three sulfate groups in the molecule.

trisulfide (tri-sul′fīd) a sulfur compound containing three atoms of sulfur to one of the base.

tritanope (trit′ah-nōp) a person exhibiting tritanopia.

tritanopia (tri″tah-no′pe-ah) defective color vision, characterized by perception of only red and green and lacking blue and yellow. adj., **tritanop′ic.**

tritiate (trit′e-āt) to treat with tritium.

tritium (trit′e-um, trish′e-um) the mass 3 isotope of hydrogen, symbol ^3H, obtained by bombardment of beryllium in the cyclotron with deuterium ions. It has a half-life of about 31 years, and is used as an indicator or tracer in metabolic studies.

triturable (trit′u-rah-b′l) susceptible of being triturated.

triturate (trit′u-rāt) 1. to reduce to powder by rubbing. 2. a substance powdered fine by rubbing.

trituration (trit″u-ra′shun) 1. reduction to powder by friction or grinding. 2. a finely powdered substance.

triturator (trit″u-ra′tor) an apparatus in which substances can be continuously rubbed.

trivalent (tri-va′lent) having a valence of three.

tRNA transfer RNA (ribonucleic acid).

trocar (tro′kar) a sharp-pointed instrument used with a cannula for piercing a cavity wall.

Duchenne's t., a trocar for obtaining specimens of deep-seated tissues.

trochanter (tro-kan′ter) a broad, flat process on the femur, at the upper end of its lateral surface (greater trochanter), or a short conical process on the posterior border of the base of its neck (lesser trochanter). adj., **trochanter′ic, trochanter′ian.**

troche (tro′ke) a medicinal preparation for solution in the mouth, consisting of an active ingredient incorporated in a mass made of sugar and mucilage or fruit base.

trochlea (trok′le-ah), pl. *troch′leae* [L.] a pulley-shaped part or structure; used in anatomic nomenclature to designate various bony or fibrous structures through or over which tendons pass or with which other structures articulate.

trochlear (trok′le-ar) 1. pertaining to a trochlea. 2. pertaining to the fourth cranial (trochlear) nerve.

t. nerve, the fourth cranial nerve; it supplies muscle sense and the impulse for movement to the superior oblique muscle of the eyeball.

trochocephaly (tro″ko-sef′ah-le) a rounded appearance of the head due to synostosis of the frontal and parietal bones.

trochoid (tro′koid) pivot-like, or pulley-shaped.

trochoides (tro-koi′dēz) a pivot joint.

Troisier's node (trwah-ze-āz′) an enlarged supraclavicular lymph node, often the first sign of a malignant abdominal tumor. Called also sentinel, or signal, node.

troleandomycin (tro″le-an-do-mi″sin) an ester of oleandomycin, used as an antibacterial; called also triacetyloleandomycin.

trolnitrate (trol-ni′trāt) a compound used as a vasodilator, particularly in treatment of angina pectoris.

Trombicula (trom-bik′u-lah) a genus of acarine mites (family Trombiculidae), including *T. akamu′shi, T. delien′sis, T. fletch′eri, T. pal′lida,* and *T. scutella′ris,* whose larvae (CHIGGERS) are vectors of *Rickettsia tsutsugamushi,* the cause of scrub typhus.

T. alfreddugè′si, *Eutrombicula alfreddugèsi.*

trombiculiasis (trom-bik″u-li′ah-sis) infestation with mites of the genus *Trombicula.*

Trombiculidae (trom-bik′u-li″de) a family of mites cosmopolitan in distribution, whose parasitic larvae (CHIGGERS) infest vertebrates.

Tromexan (tro-mek′san) trademark for a preparation of ethyl biscoumacetate, an anticoagulant.

Tronothane (tron′o-thān) trademark for preparations of pramoxine, a topical anesthetic.

troph(o)- word element [Gr.], *food; nourishment.*

trophectoderm (trof-ek′to-derm) the earliest trophoblast.

trophedema (trof″ĕ-de′mah) a chronic disease with permanent edema of the feet or legs.

trophesy (trof′ĕ-se) defective nutrition due to disorder of the trophic nerves.

trophic (trof′ik) pertaining to nutrition.

-trophic, -trophin word element [Gr.], *nourishing; stimulating.*

trophoblast (trof′o-blast) the peripheral cells of the blastocyst, which attach the fertilized ovum to the uterine wall and become the placenta and the membranes that nourish and protect the developing organism. The inner cellular layer is the cytotrophoblast and the outer layer is the syntrophoblast.

trophoblastoma (trof″o-blas-to′mah) choriocarcinoma.

trophodermatoneurosis (trof″o-der″mah-to-nu-ro′sis) acrodynia.

trophology (tro-fol′o-je) the science of nutrition of the body.

trophoneurosis (trof″o-nu-ro′sis) 1. any functional nervous disease due to failure of nutrition from defective nerve influence. adj., **trophoneurot′ic.**

trophonosis (trof″o-no′sis) any disease due to nutritional causes.

trophonucleus (trof″o-nu′kle-us) macronucleus.

trophopathy (tro-fop′ah-the) any derangement of nutrition.

trophoplast (trof′o-plast) a granular protoplasmic body.

trophotaxis (trof″o-tak′sis) taxis in relation to nutritive materials.

trophotherapy (trof″o-ther′ah-pe) treatment of disease by dietary measures.

trophozoite (trof″o-zo′īt) the active, motile feeding stage of a sporozoan parasite.

tropia (tro′pe-ah) a manifest deviation of an eye

from the normal position when both eyes are open and uncovered. (See also STRABISMUS.)

-tropic (trop'ik) word element [Gr.], *turning toward; changing; tending to turn or change.*

tropical (trop'ĭ-kal) pertaining to the tropics, the regions of the earth lying between the tropic of Cancer above the Equator and the tropic of Capricorn below.

t. anhidrotic asthenia, a condition due to generalized absence of sweating in conditions of high temperature.

tropicamide (tro-pik'ah-mīd) an anticholinergic applied topically to the conjunctiva to produce mydriasis and cycloplegia.

tropine (tro'pēn) a crystalline alkaloid from atropine and various plants.

tropism (tro'pizm) a growth response in a nonmotile organism elicited by an external stimulus, and either toward (positive tropism) or away from (negative tropism) the stimulus; used as a word element combined with a stem indicating nature of the stimulus (e.g., phototropism) or material or entity for which an organism (or substance) shows a special affinity (e.g., neurotropism).

tropocollagen (tro"po-kol'ah-jen) the molecular unit of all forms of collagen; it is a helical structure of three polypeptides.

tropomyosin (tro"po-mi'o-sin) a muscle protein of the I band that inhibits contraction by blocking the interaction of actin and myosin, except when influenced by troponin.

troponin (tro'po-nin) a complex of muscle proteins which, when combined with Ca^{++}, influence tropomyosin to initiate contraction.

Trousseau's sign (troo-sōz') 1. spontaneous peripheral venous thrombosis, suggestive of visceral carcinoma, especially carcinoma of the pancreas. 2. a sign for tetany in which carpal spasm can be elicited by compressing the upper arm and causing ischemia to the nerves distally.

troxidone (trok'sĭ-dōn) trimethadione, an anticonvulsant.

T.R.U. turbidity reducing unit.

truncate (trung'kāt) 1. to amputate; to deprive of limbs. 2. having the end cut squarely off.

truncus (trung'kus), pl. *trun'ci* [L.] trunk; used in anatomic nomenclature.

t. arterio'sus, an artery connected with the fetal heart, developing into the aortic and pulmonary arches.

t. brachiocephal'icus, a vessel arising from the arch of the aorta and giving origin to the right common carotid and right subclavian arteries.

t. celi'acus, celiac trunk.

t. pulmona'lis, pulmonary trunk.

trunk (trungk) the main part, as the part of the body to which the head and limbs are attached, or a larger structure (e.g., vessel or nerve) from which smaller divisions or branches arise, or which is created by their union. adj., **trun'cal.**

celiac t., the arterial trunk arising from the abdominal aorta and giving origin to the left gastric, common hepatic, and splenic arteries.

lumbosacral t., a trunk formed by union of the lower part of ventral branch of the fourth lumbar nerve with the ventral branch of the fifth lumbar nerve.

pulmonary t., a vessel arising from the conus arteriosus of the right ventricle and bifurcating into the right and left pulmonary arteries.

sympathetic t., two long ganglionated nerve strands, one on each side of the vertebral column, extending from the base of the skull to the coccyx.

truss (trus) an elastic, canvas, or metallic device for retaining a reduced hernia within the abdominal cavity.

trypaflavine (trip"ah-fla'vin) acriflavine hydrochloride, an antiseptic dye.

trypanocidal (tri-pan"o-si'dal) destructive to trypanosomes.

trypanolysis (tri"pan-ol'ĭ-sis) the destruction of trypanosomes. adj., **trypanolyt'ic.**

Trypanosoma (tri"pan-o-so'mah) a multispecies genus of protozoa parasitic in the blood and lymph of invertebrates and vertebrates, including man; most species live part of their life cycle in the intestines of insects and other invertebrates, the typical adult stage being found only in the vertebrate host. Trypanosomal infections of man include Gambian and Rhodesian forms of African trypanosomiasis (caused by *T. gambien'se* and *T. rhodesien'se,* respectively) and South American trypanosomiasis (caused by *T. cru'zi*). Other species cause serious diseases of domestic animals, including *T. bru'cei, T. congolen'se, T. evan'si,* etc.

trypanosome (tri-pan'o-sōm) an individual of the genus *Trypanosoma.* adj., **trypanoso'mal, trypanoso'mic.**

trypanosomiasis (tri-pan"o-so-mi'ah-sis) infection with trypanosomes, parasitic protozoa found in the blood and lymph of infected animals and humans.

African t., a fatal disease of Africa caused by *Trypanosoma gambiense* or *T. rhodesiense* and involving the central nervous system. The parasites are transmitted to man from cattle or other animals by the bite of the tsetse fly. Usually the first symptom is inflammation at the site of the bite, appearing within 48 hours. Within several weeks the parasites invade the blood and lymph; eventually they attack the central nervous system. Characteristic symptoms include intermittent fever, rapid heartbeat, and enlargement of the lymph nodes and spleen. In the advanced stage of the disease there are personality changes, apathy, sleepiness, disturbances of speech and gait, and severe emaciation.

Suramin, pentamidine isethionate, and tryparsamide are used in the treatment of African trypanosomiasis. Prevention includes injections of pentamidine isethionate or suramin to remove the parasites from the blood or lymph nodes, but the most effective measure is eradication of the tsetse fly.

South American t., a form found in Mexico and Central and South America, caused by *Trypanosoma cruzi;* called also Chagas' disease. It is transmitted from wild animals by means of the feces of a blood-sucking bug. The parasites multiply around the points of entry before entering the blood and eventually attacking the heart, brain, and other tissues.

The acute form often attacks children. Early symptoms include swelling of the eyelids and the development of a hard, red, painful nodule on the skin. Enlargement of the lymph nodes, liver, and spleen occurs, along with inflammation of the heart muscle, psychic changes, and general debility. In adults the chronic form often resembles heart disease.

Preventive measures, such as the wearing of protective clothing and the use of insecticides, are of primary importance since there are no effective drugs for treatment.

trypanosomicide (tri-pan″o-so′mĭ-sīd) 1. lethal to trypanosomes. 2. an agent lethal to trypanosomes.

trypanosomid (tri-pan″o-so′mid) a skin eruption occurring in trypanosomiasis.

tryparsamide (trip-ar′sah-mīd) a white crystalline powder used in treatment of African trypanosomiasis.

trypsin (trip′sin) an enzyme that catalyzes the hydrolysis of practically all types of proteins, produced in the intestine by activation of trypsinogen. adj., **tryp′tic.**

crystallized t., a proteolytic enzyme crystallized from an extract of the pancreas of the ox; used in débridement of necrotic wounds and ulcers.

trypsinogen (trip-sin′o-jen) the inactive precursor of trypsin, secreted by the pancreas and activated to trypsin by contact with enterokinase.

tryptic (trip′tik) relating to or resulting from digestion by trypsin.

tryptophan (trip′to-fan) a naturally occurring amino acid, existing in proteins and essential for human metabolism.

tryptophanase (trip′to-fan″ās) an enzyme that catalyzes the cleavage of tryptophan into indole, pyruvic acid, and ammonia.

tryptophanuria (trip″to-fān-u′re-ah) excessive urinary excretion of trytophan.

T.S. test solution.

tsetse (tset′se) an African fly of the genus *Glossina*, which transmits trypanosomiasis.

TSH thyroid-stimulating hormone (thyrotropin, thyrotropic hormone).

tsutsugamushi fever (disease) (tsōōt″soo-gah-mōōsh′e) scrub typhus.

T.U. tuberculin unit.

Tuamine (too′ah-min) trademark for preparations of tuaminoheptane.

tuaminoheptane (tu-am″ĭ-no-hep′tān) an adrenergic used as a nasal decongestant in the form of the base (for inhalation) and sulfate salt (topical solution).

tuba (too′bah), pl. *tu′bae* [L.] tube.

Tubadil (too′bah-dil) trademark for a preparation of tubocurarine, a skeletal muscle relaxant.

Tubarine (too′bah-rin) trademark for a preparation of tubocurarine, a skeletal muscle relaxant.

tube (toob) a hollow cylindrical organ or instrument. adj., **tu′bal.**

auditory t., the narrow channel connecting the middle ear and nasopharynx (see also EUSTACHIAN TUBE).

chest t., one or more tubes inserted into the pleural space to provide relief from either PNEUMOTHORAX or accumulations of fluid within the thoracic cavity and to allow for re-expansion of the lung (see also CHEST TUBE).

Chaoul t., a tube used in x-ray therapy.

Coolidge t., a vacuum tube for the generation of x-rays (see also COOLIDGE TUBE).

Crookes′ t., an early form of vacuum tube by the use of which the roentgen rays were discovered.

drainage t., a tube used in surgery to facilitate escape of fluids.

Durham′s t., a jointed tracheotomy tube.

endobronchial t., a double-lumen tube inserted into the bronchus of one lung, permitting complete deflation of the other lung; used in anesthesia and thoracic surgery.

endotracheal t., an inflatable tube inserted into the mouth or nose and passed down into the trachea (see also ENDOTRACHEAL TUBE).

eustachian t., the narrow channel connecting the middle ear and the nasopharynx (see also EUSTACHIAN TUBE).

fallopian t., uterine tube.

feeding t., one for introducing high-caloric fluids into the stomach.

fermentation t., a U-shaped tube with one end closed, for determining gas production by bacteria.

Geissler′s t., an x-ray tube containing a highly rarefied gas.

intubation t., a breathing tube introduced into the air passage after tracheotomy.

Levin t., a gastroduodenal catheter of sufficiently small caliber to permit transnasal passage.

Miller-Abbott t., a double-channel intestinal tube with an inflatable balloon at its distal end, for use in treatment of obstruction of the small intestine, and occasionally as a diagnostic aid (see also MILLER-ABBOTT TUBE).

nasogastric t., a tube of soft rubber or plastic inserted through a nostril and into the stomach, for instilling liquid foods or other substances, or for withdrawing gastric contents. (See also TUBE FEEDING.)

neural t., the epithelial tube produced by folding of the neural plate in the early embryo.

otopharyngeal t., auditory tube.

Sengstaken-Blakemore t., an instrument used for tamponade of bleeding esophageal varices (see also SENGSTAKEN-BLAKEMORE TUBE).

stomach t., one that is passed through the esophagus to the stomach, for the introduction of nutrients or for gastric lavage (see also STOMACH TUBE).

test t., a tube of thin glass, closed at one end; used in chemical tests and other laboratory procedures.

thoracostomy t., one inserted through an opening in the chest wall for application of suction to the pleural cavity to facilitate reexpansion of the lung in spontaneous pneumothorax (see also CHEST TUBE).

tracheostomy t., a curved tube that is inserted into the trachea through the opening made in the neck at TRACHEOSTOMY.

uterine t., a slender tube extending laterally from the uterus toward the ovary on the same side, conveying ova to the cavity of the uterus and permitting passage of spermatozoa in the opposite direction; called also fallopian tube (see also UTERINE TUBE).

Wangensteen t., a small nasogastric tube connected with a special suction apparatus to maintain gastric and duodenal decompression.

tubectomy (too-bek′to-me) excision of a portion of the uterine tube.

tube feeding administration of liquid and semisolid foods through a nasogastric, gastrostomy, or enterostomy tube. Nasogastric tube feedings are administered to patients who are unable to take foods by mouth. These would include psychiatric patients who refuse to eat, debilitated and elderly patients who cannot swallow, and the newborn premature infant who has immature swallowing and gag reflexes. Gastrostomy tube feedings are administered directly into the stomach via a gastrostomy tube. Enterostomy tube feedings are administered into the small intestine to patients who are unable to take food into the stomach.

PATIENT CARE. The major goal of care of a patient being fed by tube is prevention of dehydration and subsequent fluid and electrolyte disturbances. This is particularly true in cases of prolonged tube feeding, in which there is always the possibility that fluid and electrolyte imbalances may become serious enough to present neurologic symptoms and even death. Early detection and correction of dehydration depend on careful monitoring of the patient and periodic evaluation of electrolyte status through laboratory tests. Many times patients receiving tube feedings are not aware of thirst or are unable to communicate their desire for water.

All tube-fed patients require good mouth care. If the feeding is through a nasogastric tube, the patient will be a mouth-breather, which contributes to dryness of the oral mucosa. Adequate mouth care can help in differentiating between thirst due to dryness of the mouth and thirst resulting from systemic dehydration.

tuber (too'ber) a swelling or protuberance.

t. cine'reum, an area of the undersurface of the forebrain to which the stalk of the pituitary gland is attached.

tubercle (too'ber-k'l) 1. a small, rounded nodule produced by the bacillus of tuberculosis (*Mycobacterium tuberculosis*). It is made up of small spherical cells that contain giant cells and are surrounded by spindle-shaped epithelioid cells. 2. a nodule or small eminence, especially one on a bone, for attachment of a tendon. adj., **tuber'cular.**

fibrous t., a tubercle of bacillary origin that contains connective tissue elements.

mental t., a prominence on the inner border of either side of the mental protuberance of the mandible.

miliary t., one of the many minute tubercles formed in many organs in acute miliary tuberculosis.

pubic t., a prominent tubercle at the lateral end of the pubic crest.

supraglenoid t., one on the scapula for attachment of the long head of the biceps muscle.

tuberculate, tuberculated (too-ber'ku-lāt"; too-ber'ku-lāt"ed) covered or affected with tubercles.

tuberculid (too-ber'ku-lid) a papular skin eruption usually attributed to allergy to tuberculosis.

papulonecrotic t., an eruption of crops of deep-seated papules or nodules, with central necrosis or ulceration.

tuberculigenous (too-ber"ku-lij'ĕ-nus) causing tuberculosis.

tuberculin (too-ber'ku-lin) a sterile liquid containing the growth products of, or specific substances extracted from, the tubercle bacillus; used in various forms in the diagnosis of tuberculosis.

New t., a suspension of the fragments of tubercle bacilli, freed from all soluble materials and with glycerin added.

Old t., a sterile solution of concentrated, soluble products of the growth of the tubercle bacillus, adjusted to standard potency by addition of glycerin and isotonic sodium chloride solution, final glycerin content being about 50 per cent.

purified protein derivative (P.P.D.) of t., a sterile, soluble, partially purified product of the growth of the tubercle bacillus in a special liquid medium free from protein.

tuberculitis (too-ber"ku-li'tis) inflammation of or near a tubercle.

tuberculocele (too-ber'ku-lo-sēl) tuberculous disease of a testis.

tuberculofibroid (too-ber"ku-lo-fi'broid) characterized by a tubercle that has undergone fibroid degeneration.

tuberculoid (too-ber'ku-loid) resembling a tubercle or tuberculosis.

tuberculoma (too-ber"ku-lo'mah) a tumor-like mass resulting from enlargement of a caseated tubercle.

tuberculosilicosis (too-ber"ku-lo-sil"ĭ-ko'sis) silicosis complicated by pulmonary tuberculosis.

tuberculosis (tu-ber'ku-lo'sis) an infectious, inflammatory, reportable disease that is chronic in nature and commonly affects the lungs (pulmonary tuberculosis), although it may occur in almost any part of the body.

The causative agent is the tubercle bacillus (*Mycobacterium tuberculosis*). Until recently, the only other mycobacteria thought to be pathogenic to humans were *M. bovis* and *M. avium*. It is now known that other "atypical" mycobacteria can produce diseases similar to true tuberculosis.

The most common mode of transmission of tuberculosis in the United States is inhalation of infected droplet nuclei. In some other parts of the world bovine tuberculosis, which is carried by milk and other dairy products from tuberculous cattle, is more prevalent. A rare mode of transmission is by infected urine, especially for young children using the same toilet facilities.

The tubercle bacillus is capable of surviving for months in dried sputum that is not exposed to sunlight. Within the body it can lie dormant for decades and then become reactivated years after an initial infection. This secondary tuberculosis infection (endogenous reinfection) can occur at any time the patient's resistance is lowered. For this reason, periodic evaluation for evidence of the disease is extremely important for anyone who has had a primary tuberculosis infection.

The tubercle bacillus is destroyed by boiling for 5 minutes, by autoclaving, by contact with coal tar preparations, e.g., phenol, and by ultraviolet radiation.

PRIMARY AND SECONDARY TUBERCULOSIS. The first or primary infection with tuberculosis bacilli usually presents no symptoms. In about 99 per cent of those who are infected, the disease remains quiescent after the development of a hypersensitivity to the tuberculin microorganism and is no longer clinically significant.

The primary infection usually involves the middle or lower lung area. The primary lesion consists of a small area of exudation in the lung parenchyma which quickly becomes caseous (cheeselike) and spreads to the bronchopulmonary lymph nodes, where it gains access to the blood stream. Thus the stage is set for the development of a chronic pulmonary and extrapulmonary tuberculosis at a later time. In most instances, however, a secondary reinfection from inside the body (endogenous) or outside the body (exogenous) does not occur because of the subsequent development of tuberculin hypersensitivity and cellular immunity. The presence of antigen concentrations at the initial site of infection brings about necrosis and eventually fibrosis and calcification of the tissues, which arrests the infection and renders the disease inactive. If, however, the infection is not controlled, the patient develops the symptoms of progressive primary tuberculosis.

Secondary tuberculosis develops as a result of either endogenous or exogenous reinfection by the tubercle bacillus. This is the most common form of clinical tuberculosis. In the United States development of secondary tuberculosis is almost always the result of an endogenous reinfection, which occurs when the primary lesion becomes active. This most frequently happens in debilitated persons who have lowered resistance to disease.

Resistance to tuberculosis depends on the general health and living conditions of the individual. Poor health, crowded and unsanitary housing, malnutrition, and other illnesses can lower the body's defenses. A second factor that can lead to activation of the disease is frequent exposure to the bacilli or exposure to such numbers that even a healthy person cannot escape infection.

TUBERCULIN TESTING. Within 3 to 10 days after the initial entry of the tubercle bacillus into the body, a sensitivity to the bacillus is present in all of the body cells. This sensitivity is the basis of tuberculin testing.

The most commonly used test is the MANTOUX TEST, which consists of an intradermal injection of a purified protein derivative of tuberculin. An indurated area (wheal) of 8 to 10 mm. in diameter 48 to 72 hours after injection is considered positive. Induration must be present; a reddened area is not indicative of a positive reaction. If the test is positive for tuberculin sensitivity, further studies, including x-rays, are indicated before a definite diagnosis of tuberculosis is established. False negative results can occur with acute viral infections and some neoplastic diseases, e.g., Hodgkin's disease. (See also IMMUNIZATION for the recommended tuberculin testing of children.)

SYMPTOMS. A child or young person with active tuberculosis usually suffers from one or more of the following symptoms: loss of energy, poor appetite, loss of weight, and fever. Even though these symptoms may have causes other than tuberculosis, they must be regarded as warning signals.

In adults, listlessness and vague pains in the chest may go unnoticed, since they are often not severe enough to attract attention. Unfortunately, the symptoms that most people associate with tuberculosis—cough, expectoration of purulent sputum, fever, night sweats, and hemorrhage from the lungs—do not appear in the early, most easily curable stage of the disease; often their appearance is delayed until a year or more after the initial exposure to the bacilli. Annual chest x-rays of all adults would permit discovery of almost all cases of tuberculosis at an early, easily curable stage.

Chronic pulmonary tuberculosis is often accompanied by pleurisy. Pleurisy with effusion often is the first symptom of tuberculosis. In certain cases, complications are possible and each has its characteristic symptoms. At a fairly late stage, the tuberculosis bacillus may cause ulcers or inflammation around the larynx (tuberculous laryngitis). Less often, tuberculous ulcers form on the tongue or tonsils. Sometimes intestinal infections develop; they are probably caused by swallowed bacteria-contaminated sputum. A most serious complication is the sudden collapse of a lung, the indication that a deep tuberculous cavity in the lung has perforated, or opened into the pleural cavity, allowing air and infected material to flow into it.

When a fairly large and previously walled-off lesion, or infected area, suddenly discharges its contents into the bronchial tree, the result is the infection of a large part of the lung, an acute and dangerous complication which causes tuberculous pneumonia.

Tuberculosis bacilli can spread to other parts of the body by way of the blood, producing the condition called miliary tuberculosis. When a large number of bacilli suddenly enter the circulatory system, they are carried to all areas of the body and may lodge in any organ. Minute tubercles form in the tissues of the organs affected; these lesions are about the size of a pinhead or millet seed (hence the name "miliary"). Unless promptly treated, and occasionally even then, the tiny lesions spread, join, and produce larger areas of infection.

Tuberculous pneumonia can begin in this way, as can tuberculosis of any other organ. Miliary infections involving the meninges produce a particularly serious disease; indeed, until the development of antibiotics and similar medicines, this condition nearly always proved fatal.

Practically all parts and organs of the body can be secondarily invaded by tubercle bacilli, a common type being involvement of the kidneys, which often spreads to the bladder and genitalia. Bone involvement, particularly of the spine (POTT'S DISEASE), was once common, especially among children.

Lupus, or lupus vulgaris, tuberculosis of the skin, is characterized by brown nodules on the corium; another form of tuberculosis of the skin is tuberculosis indurativa, a chronic disease in which indurated nodules form on the skin. When the adrenal glands are affected by tuberculosis, a rare occurrence, the condition can cause ADDISON'S DISEASE.

TREATMENT AND CARE. Most tuberculous patients are cared for at home under the supervision of a Public Health nurse who periodically visits the patient and his family. Hospitalization may be required for those patients who experience complications or who are beginning chemotherapy. The length of stay varies, but the advent of effective drug therapy has all but eradicated lengthy stays at special sanitoria and hospitals.

During hospitalization the patient should be taught how the disease is transmitted and how he can avoid spreading the infection to others. Patient education also should include information on the importance of a well-balanced diet and good health habits in the control of his disease.

It should be remembered that tuberculosis is an airborne infection. The patient's room should be adequately ventilated, but with the door to the hall kept closed. Ultraviolet radiation is most effective in decontamination. Masks may be necessary for those having intimate contact with a patient who is just beginning chemotherapy, and in caring for patients who cannot or will not take precautions against spreading the infection. Handwashing is essential to prevention of cross-infection. Fomites are not considered important in the transmission of tuberculosis and so no special precautions are required for eating utensils and other inanimate articles in the patient's room.

Drugs. Isoniazid (INH) remains the major antituberculous agent. It is usually administered in combination with ethambol (EMB) or another agent. The second major antituberculous drug is streptomycin, which often is used in the treatment of severe cases as the third medication in combination with INH and EMB. The three companion drugs may be administered for the first several months of therapy.

In INH-resistant cases, rifampin (RMP) is substituted as a companion drug for EMB. The advent of these drugs has revolutionized the treatment of tuberculosis and greatly improved its prognosis.

Surgical Procedures. In the past, the sanatorium rest cure frequently was augmented by one of the surgical procedures which aid healing by resting an infected lung for a period of time.

The best-known of these operations, artificial pneumothorax, involves collapsing the lung by injecting air into the pleural cavity. A lung also may be rested by inactivating the phrenic nerve, which carries impulses to the diaphragm from the brain and so helps to control breathing; if the left or right phrenic nerve is inactivated, the diaphragm and lung on the same side will not move.

With the successful treatment of tuberculosis by the new drugs, these operations have become relatively uncommon. In certain cases, however, when the disease is restricted to a lung and medication provides insufficient control, surgical removal of the diseased tissue is necessary.

PREVENTION. Tuberculosis is one of the most easily avoided of all the serious diseases. The best precautions are (1) maintenance of good health, (2) avoidance of unnecessary exposure to tuberculosis organisms, and (3) detection of the disease in its earliest stages.

BCG Vaccine. Some success in preventing tuberculosis has been attained by vaccination with BCG (bacille Calmette Guérin)—a vaccine evolved from strains of *Mycobacterium tuberculosis* taken from cattle. It provides at least partial immunity in most people, although it takes about 2 months to do so. BCG is now usually given to large groups under governmental auspices—for example, to school children living in slum areas in large cities. It has been widely used in many countries, but less widely in the United States. After vaccination with BCG, the patient will have a positive response to the tuberculin test. (See also BCG VACCINE.)

Isoniazid. This drug, one of the principal ones used in treating active cases, is given for a year to those, who convert from tuberculin negative to tuberculin positive, even though they may be asymptomatic.

avian t., a form affecting various birds, due to *Mycobacterium avium,* which may be communicated to man and other animals.

bovine t., an infection of cattle caused by *Mycobacterium bovis,* transmissible to man and other animals.

endogenous t., that arising from within the body and transmitted by blood to another organ.

exogenous t., that arising from a source outside the body.

hematogenous t., that carried through the blood stream to other organs from the primary site of infection.

open t., 1. that in which there are lesions from which tubercle bacilli are being discharged out of the body. 2. tuberculosis of the lungs with cavitation.

t. verruco'sa, warty t., a condition usually resulting from external inoculation of the tubercle bacilli into the skin, with wartlike papules coalescing to form distinctly verrucous patches with an inflammatory, erythematous border.

tuberculostatic (too-ber″ku-lo-stat′ik) 1. inhibiting the growth of *Mycobacterium tuberculosis.* 2. a tuberculostatic agent.

tuberculotic (too-ber″ku-lot′ik) pertaining to or affected with tuberculosis.

tuberculous (too-ber′ku-lus) pertaining to or affected with tuberculosis; caused by *Mycobacterium tuberculosis.*

tuberculum (too-ber′ku-lum), pl. *tuber′cula* [L.] a tubercle, nodule, or small eminence; used in anatomic nomenclature to designate principally a small eminence on a bone.

tuberosis (too″ber-o′sis) a condition characterized by the presence of nodules.

tuberositas (too″bĕ-ros′ĭ-tas), pl. *tuberosita′tes* [L.] tuberosity; used in anatomic nomenclature to designate elevations on bones to which muscles are attached.

tuberosity (too″bĕ-ros′ĭ-te) an elevation or protuberance.

tuberous (too′ber-us) covered with tubers; knobby.

t. sclerosis, a familial disease with tumors on the surfaces of the lateral ventricles of the brain and sclerotic patches on its surface, and marked by mental deterioration and epileptic attacks.

tubo- (too′bo) word element [L.], *tube.*

tubocurarine (too″bo-ku-rah′rēn) an alkaloid from the bark and stems of *Chondrodendron tomentosum,* used as a skeletal muscle relaxant.

tuboligamentous (too″bo-lig″ah-men′tus) pertaining to the uterine tube and broad ligament.

tubo-ovarian (too″bo-o-va′re-an) pertaining to the uterine tube and ovary.

tuboperitoneal (too″bo-per″ĭ-to-ne′al) pertaining to the uterine tube and the peritoneum.

tubouterine (too″bo-u′ter-in) pertaining to the uterine tube and uterus.

tubule (too′būl) a small tube. adj., **tu′bular.**

collecting t's, the terminal channels of the nephrons which open on the summits of the renal pyramids in the renal papillae.

convoluted t's, channels that follow a tortuous course; there are convoluted renal tubules and convoluted seminiferous tubules.

dentinal t's, the tubular structures of the teeth.

galactophorous t's, small channels for the passage of milk from the secreting cells in the mammary gland.

Henle's t's, the straight ascending and descending portions of a renal tubule forming Henle's loop.

lactiferous t's, galactophorous tubules.

mesonephric t's, the tubules comprising the mesonephros, or temporary kidney, of amniotes.

metanephric t's, the tubules comprising the permanent kidney of amniotes.

renal t's, the minute canals made up of basement membrane and lined with epithelium, composing the substance of the kidney and secreting, collecting and conducting the urine.

seminiferous t's, the tubules of the testis, in which spermatozoa develop and through which they leave the gland.

uriniferous t's, renal tubules; channels for the passage of urine.

tubulin (too'bu-lin) the constituent protein of microtubules; thought to be involved in phagocyte motility.

tubulorrhexis (too"bu-lo-rek'sis) rupture of the tubules of the kidney.

tubulus (too'bu-lus), pl. *tu'buli* [L.] tubule; a minute canal found in various structures or organs of the body.

tuft (tuft) a small clump or cluster; a coil.

malpighian t., renal glomerulus.

tugging (tug'ing) a pulling sensation, as a pulling sensation in the trachea (tracheal tugging), due to aneurysm of the arch of the aorta.

tularemia (too"lah-re'me-ah) a plaguelike disease of rodents, caused by *Francisella* (*Pasteurella*) *tularensis,* which is transmissible to man.

The illness can be contracted by handling diseased animals or their hides, eating infected wild game or being bitten by insects, such as horseflies and deer flies, that have fed on infected animals.

SYMPTOMS AND TREATMENT. Tularemia begins with a sudden onset of chills and fever, accompanied by headache, nausea, vomiting, and severe weakness. A day or so later, a small sore usually develops at the site of the infection, and it becomes ulcerated. There may also be enlargement and ulceration of the lymph nodes and a generalized red rash. In untreated cases, the fever may last for weeks or months.

Treatment is with antibiotics, such as tetracycline, streptomycin, and chloramphenicol.

PREVENTION. Tularemia is usually thought of as an occupational disease. Those who may be exposed to it, such as game wardens and hunters, should take certain precautions, such as wearing gloves when handling wild animals, particularly rabbits and squirrels, and wearing adequate clothing in the woods to prevent bites by insect vectors of the disease. Wild game must be especially well cooked, in order to kill the tularemia organism.

tumefacient (too"mĕ-fa'shent) producing tumefaction.

tumefaction (too"mĕ-fak'shun) a swelling; the state of being swollen, or the act of swelling; puffiness; edema.

tumescence (too-mes'ens) 1. the condition of being swollen. 2. a swelling.

tumid (too'mid) swollen; edematous.

tumor (too'mor) 1. swelling, one of the cardinal signs of inflammation; morbid enlargement. 2. neoplasm; a new growth of tissue in which cell multiplication is uncontrolled and progressive. adj., **tu'morous.** Tumors are called also neoplasms, which means that they are composed of new and actively growing tissue. Their growth is faster than that of normal tissue, continuing after cessation of the stimuli that evoked the growth, and serving no useful physiologic purpose.

Tumors are classified in a number of ways, one of the simplest being according to their origin and whether they are malignant or benign. Tumors of mesenchymal origin include fibroelastic tumors and those of bone, fat, blood vessels, and lymphoid tissue. They may be benign or malignant (sarcoma). Tumors of epithelial origin may be benign or malignant (carcinoma); they are found in glandular tissue or such organs as the breast, stomach, uterus, or skin. Mixed tumors contain different types of cells derived from the same primary germ layer, and teratomas contain cells derived from more than one germ layer; both kinds may be benign or malignant.

BENIGN TUMORS. Benign tumors do not endanger life unless they interfere with normal functions of other organs or affect a vital organ. They grow slowly, pushing aside normal tissue but not invading it. They are usually encapsulated, well demarcated growths. They are not metastatic; that is, they do not form secondary tumors in other organs. Benign tumors usually respond favorably to surgical treatment and some forms of RADIOTHERAPY.

MALIGNANT TUMORS. These tumors are composed of embryonic, primitive, or poorly differentiated cells. They grow in a disorganized manner and so rapidly that nutrition of the cells becomes a problem. For this reason necrosis and ulceration are characteristic of malignant tumors. They also invade surrounding tissues and are metastatic, initiating the growth of similar tumors in distant organs. (See also CANCER.)

carotid body t., a firm, round mass at the bifurcation of the common carotid artery.

connective tissue t., any tumor arising from a connective tissue structure, e.g., a fibroma or sarcoma.

desmoid t., a hard fibrous tumor.

erectile t., cavernous hemangioma.

Ewing's t., a malignant tumor of the bone which always arises in medullary tissue, occurring more often in cylindrical bones, with pain, fever, and leukocytosis as prominent symptoms; called also Ewing's sarcoma.

false t., structural enlargement due to extravasation, exudation, echinococcus, or retained sebaceous matter.

fibroid t., a common benign tumor of the uterus, properly designated as LEIOMYOMA, or myoma, of the UTERUS; a fibroma.

giant cell t., 1. a bone tumor, ranging from benign to frankly malignant, composed of cellular spindle cell stroma containing multinucleated giant cells resembling osteoclasts. 2. a benign, small, yellow, tumor-like nodule of tendon sheath origin, most often of the wrist and fingers or ankle and toes, laden with lipophages and containing multinucleated giant cells.

granulosa t., granulosa cell t., an ovarian tumor originating in the cells of the cumulus oophorus (see also GRANULOSA CELL TUMOR).

granulosa-theca cell t., an ovarian tumor composed of granulosa (follicular) cells and theca cells; either form may predominate (see also GRANULOSA-THECA CELL TUMOR).

heterologous t., one made up of tissue differing from that in which it grows.

homoiotypic t., homologous t., one made up of tissue resembling that in which it grows.

Hürthle cell t., a new growth of the thyroid gland composed wholly or predominantly of Hürthle cells (see also HÜRTHLE CELL TUMOR).

islet cell t., a tumor of the islands of Langerhans, which may result in hyperinsulinism.

Krukenberg's t., a type of carcinoma of the ovary, usually metastatic from gastrointestinal cancer, marked by areas of mucoid degeneration and by the presence of signet-ring–like cells (see also KRUKENBERG'S TUMOR).

lipoid cell t. of ovary, a usually benign ovarian

tumor composed of eosinophilic cells or cells with lipoid vacuoles; it causes masculinization.

mast cell t., a benign, local aggregation of mast cells forming a nodulous tumor.

melanotic neuroectodermal t., a benign, rapidly growing, dark tumor of the jaw and occasionally of other sites; almost always seen in infants.

mixed t., one composed of more than one type of neoplastic tissue.

organoid t., teratoma.

phantom t., abdominal or other swelling not due to structural change.

sand t., psammoma.

theca cell t., fibroid-like tumor of the ovary containing yellow areas of fatty material derived from theca cells.

true t., a neoplasm.

turban t's, multiple CYLINDROMAS of the scalp grouped together so as to cover the entire scalp.

Wilms' t., a rapidly developing malignant mixed tumor of the kidneys, made up of embryonal elements, and occurring chiefly in children before the fifth year; called also embryonal carcinosarcoma and nephroblastoma.

tumoricidal (too″mor-ĭ-si′dal) destructive to cancer cells.

tumorigenesis (too″mor-ĭ-jen′ĕ-sis) the production of tumors. adj., **tumorigen′ic.**

tumultus (too-mul′tus) excessive organic action or motility.

Tunga (tung′gah) a genus of fleas native to tropical and subtropical America and Africa.

T. pen′etrans, the chigoe flea, which attacks man, dogs, pigs, and other animals, as well as poultry, and causes intense skin irritation (see also CHIGOE).

tungsten (tung′sten) a chemical element, atomic number 74, atomic weight 183.85, symbol W. (See table of ELEMENTS.)

tunic (too′nik) a covering or coat.

Bichat's t., tunica intima.

tunica (too′nĭ-kah), pl. *tu′nicae* [L.] a covering or coat; used in anatomic nomenclature to designate a membranous covering of an organ or a distinct layer of the wall of a hollow structure, as a blood vessel.

t. adventi′tia, the outer coat of various tubular structures.

t. albugin′ea, a dense, white, fibrous sheath enclosing a part or organ.

t. conjuncti′va, the conjunctiva.

t. dar′tos, dartos.

t. ex′terna, an outer coat, especially the fibroelastic coat of a blood vessel.

t. in′tima, the innermost coat of blood vessels; called also Bichat's tunic.

t. me′dia, the middle coat of blood vessels.

t. muco′sa, the mucous membrane lining of various tubular structures.

t. muscula′ris, the muscular coat or layer surrounding the tela submucosa in most portions of the digestive, respiratory, urinary, and genital tracts.

t. pro′pria, the proper coat or layer of a part, as distinguished from an investing membrane.

t. sero′sa, the membrane lining the external walls of the body cavities and reflected over the surfaces of protruding organs; it secretes a watery exudate.

t. vagina′lis, the serous membrane covering the front and sides of the testis and epididymis.

t. vasculo′sa, a vascular coat, or a layer well supplied with blood vessels.

tunicin (too′nĭ-sin) a substance resembling cellulose, from the tissues of certain low forms of animal life.

tuning fork (to͞on′ing) a two-pronged forklike instrument of steel, the prongs of which give off a musical note when struck; used in detection of DEAFNESS.

tunnel (tun′el) a passageway of varying length through a solid body, completely enclosed except for the open ends, permitting entrance and exit.

carpal t., the osseofibrous passage for the median nerve and the flexor tendons, formed by the flexor retinaculum and the carpal bones (see also CARPAL TUNNEL SYNDROME).

flexor t., carpal tunnel.

tarsal t., the osseofibrous passage for the posterior tibial vessels, tibial nerve, and flexor tendons, formed by the flexor retinaculum and the tarsal bones.

t. vision, a condition of concentric reduction in the visual field, as though the subject were looking through a long tunnel or tube.

turbid (tur′bid) cloudy.

turbidimeter (tur″bĭ-dim′ĕ-ter) an apparatus for measuring turbidity of a solution.

turbidimetry (tur″bĭ-dim′ĕ-tre) the measurement of the turbidity of a liquid.

turbidity (tur-bid′ĭ-te) cloudiness; disturbance of solids (sediment) in a solution, so that it is not clear. adj., **tur′bid.**

turbinal, turbinate (tur′bĭ-nal; tur′bĭ-nāt) 1. shaped like a top. 2. turbinate bone (concha nasalis ossea).

turbinectomy (tur″bĭ-nek′to-me) excision of a turbinate bone (nasal concha).

turbinotomy (tur″bĭ-not′o-me) incision of a turbinate bone.

Turcot's syndrome familial polyposis of the colon associated with malignant tumors of the central nervous system.

turgescence (tur-jes′ens) distention or swelling of a part.

turgescent (tur-jes′ent) becoming swollen.

turgid (tur′jid) swollen and congested.

turgor (tur′gor) the condition of being turgid; normal or other fullness.

turista (tu-rēs′tah) Mexican name for traveler's diarrhea.

Turner's syndrome (tur′nerz) a syndrome characterized by retarded growth and sexual development, webbing of the neck, low posterior hair line margin, and other deformities; it is associated with absence or structural abnormality of the second sex chromosome. Called also gonadal dysgenesis.

turpentine (tur′pen-tīn) the concrete oleoresin from *Pinus palustris* and other species of pine trees; its volatile oil is used as a counterirritant and rubefacient.

turricephaly (tur″ĭ-sef′ah-le) oxycephaly.

tussis (tus′is) [L.] cough.

tussive (tus′iv) pertaining to or due to a cough.

tutamen (tu-ta′men), pl. *tutam′ina* [L.] a protective covering or structure.

tutam′ina oc′uli, the protecting appendages of the eye, as the eyelids, eyelashes, etc.

Tween 80, trademark for polysorbate 80, a surfactant.

twin (twin) one of two offspring produced in the same pregnancy. Twins occur approximately once in every 86 births.

Dizygotic, or fraternal, twins develop from two separate ova fertilized at the same time. They may be of the same sex or of opposite sexes, and are no more similar than any other two children of the same parents. Called also binovular, dichorial, dissimilar, and unlike twins.

Monozygotic, or identical, twins develop from a single ovum that divides after fertilization. Because they share the same set of chromosomes, they are always of the same sex, and are remarkably similar in hair color, finger and palm prints, teeth, and other respects. Monozygotic twins have exactly the same blood type and can accept tissue or organ transplants from each other. Called also enzygotic, monochorial, mono-ovular, similar, or true twins.

Approximately one-third of all twins are identical; the rest are fraternal. It is not clearly understood exactly what causes a single ovum to divide shortly after conception and thereby produce identical twins, although it seems to be a chance occurrence. The reasons for the production and fertilization of two separate ova that result in fraternal twins are not well understood either, but it is thought that a tendency toward fraternal twins runs in families and is transmitted through the genes of the mother. Women are more likely to have fraternal twins in their later childbearing years, between the ages of 30 and 38 years, than earlier. Older age in the father also seems to be a factor with fraternal twins.

conjoined t's, monozygotic twins whose bodies are joined (see also SIAMESE TWINS).

impacted t's, twins so situated during delivery that pressure of one against the other produces simultaneous engagement of both.

Siamese t's, conjoined twins.

unequal t's, twins of which one is incompletely developed.

twinning (twin'ing) 1. the production of symmetrical structures or parts by division. 2. the simultaneous intrauterine production of two or more embryos.

twitch (twich) a brief, contractile response of a skeletal muscle elicited by a single maximal volley of impulses in the neurons supplying it.

twitching (twich'ing) the occurrence of a single contraction or a series of contractions of a muscle.

tybamate (ti'bah-māt) a minor tranquilizer.

tychastics (ti-kas'tiks) the study of industrial accidents.

Tylenol (ti'lĕ-nol) trademark for preparations of acetaminophen, an analgesic and antipyretic.

tyloma (ti-lo'ma) a callus or callosity.

tylosis (ti-lo'sis) formation of callosities. adj., **tylot'ic.**

tympanal (tim'pah-nal) pertaining to the tympanum or to the tympanic membrane.

tympanectomy (tim"pah-nek'to-me) excision of the tympanic membrane.

tympanic (tim-pan'ik) 1. of or pertaining to the tympanum. 2. bell-like; resonant.

t. membrane, a thin, semitransparent membrane, nearly oval in shape, that stretches across the ear canal separating the tympanum (middle ear) from the external acoustic meatus (outer ear); called also the eardrum. It is composed of fibrous tissue, covered with skin on the outside and mucous membrane on the inside. It is constructed so that it can vibrate freely with audible sound waves that travel inward from outside. The handle of the malleus (hammer) of the middle ear is attached to the center of the tympanic membrane and receives the vibrations collected by the membrane, transmitting them to other bones of the middle ear (the incus and stapes) and eventually to the fluid of the inner ear.

Perforation of the tympanic membrane can cause some loss of hearing, the degree of loss depending on the size and location of the perforation. Since vibrations can still be transmitted to the inner ear by way of the bones of the skull, even nearly total destruction of the tympanic membrane does not produce total deafness. Surgical incision of the eardrum (myringotomy) may be done to relieve pressure and provide for drainage in an infection of the middle ear (see also OTITIS MEDIA).

t. membrane, secondary, the membrane enclosing the fenestra cochlearis; called also Scarpa's membrane.

t. notch, Rivinus' incisure.

t. plexus, a network of nerve fibers supplying the mucous lining of the tympanic tube.

tympanism, tympanites (tim'pah-nizm; tim"-pah-ni'tēz) drumlike distention of the abdomen due to air or gas in the intestine or peritoneal cavity. adj. **tympanit'ic.**

tympanitic (tim"pah-nit'ik) 1. pertaining to or affected with tympanites. 2. bell-like; tympanic.

tympanitis (tim"pah-ni'tis) otitis media.

tympanomastoiditis (tim"pah-no-mas"toi-di'tis) inflammation of the middle ear and the pneumatic cells of the mastoid process.

tympanoplasty (tim'pah-no-plas"te) plastic reconstruction of the bones of the middle ear, with establishment of ossicular continuity from the tympanic membrane to the oval window. This surgical procedure is performed when chronic infection or tumor has led to destruction of the ossicles, of the pars petrosa of the temporal bone, or both. Because the ossicles are so small, the surgery must be done under magnification with an operating microscope. Tympanoplasty requires great surgical skill and the use of specially designed instruments. It is often done in preference to radical MASTOIDECTOMY and offers the advantage of greater preservation of hearing. (For patient care after tympanoplasty, see surgery of the EAR.)

tympanosclerosis (tim"pah-no-sklĕ-ro'sis) a condition characterized by the presence of masses of hard, dense connective tissue around the auditory ossicles in the middle ear.

tympanotomy (tim"pah-not'o-me) myringotomy.

tympanous (tim'pah-nus) distended with gas.

tympanum (tim'pah-num) the part of the cavity of the middle ear, in the temporal bone, just medial to the tympanic membrane.

tympany (tim'pah-ne) 1. tympanitis. 2. a tympanic, or bell-like, percussion note.

type (tīp) the general or prevailing character of any particular case of disease, person, substance, etc.

asthenic t., a type of physical constitution, with long limbs, small trunk, flat chest, and weak muscles.

athletic t., a type of physical constitution with broad shoulders, deep chest, flat abdomen, thick neck, and good muscular development.

blood t's, see BLOOD GROUP.

phage t., an intraspecies type of bacterium demonstrated by phage TYPING. Called also lysotype and phagotype.

pyknic t., a type of physical constitution marked by rounded body, large chest, thick shoulders, broad head, and short neck.

sympatheticotonic t., a type of physical constitution characterized by sympathicotonia.

vagotonic t., a physical type characteristic of deficient adrenal activity; there are slow pulse, low blood pressure, localized sweating, high sugar tolerance, and oculocardiac reflex.

typhl(o)- word element [Gr.], *cecum; blindness.*

typhlectasis (tif-lek'tah-sis) distention of the cecum.

typhlitis (tif-li'tis) inflammation of the cecum.

typhlodicliditis (tif"lo-dik"lĭ-di'tis) inflammation of the ileocecal valve.

typhlolexia (tif"lo-lek'se-ah) visual aphasia; loss of ability to comprehend written language.

typhlolithiasis (tif"lo-lĭ-thi'ah-sis) the presence of calculi in the cecum.

typhlosis (tif-lo'sis) blindness.

typhlotomy (tif-lot'o-me) incision of the cecum.

typhoid (ti'foid) 1. resembling typhus. 2. typhoid fever.

t. fever, a bacterial infection transmitted by contaminated water, milk or other foods, especially shellfish. The causative organism is *Salmonella typhi,* harbored in human excreta.

Entering the body through the intestinal tract, the typhoid bacillus starts multiplying in the bloodstream, causing fever and diarrhea. The usual incubation period is 7 to 14 days. Later the bacilli localize in the intestinal tract or the gallbladder.

SYMPTOMS. The first symptoms of typhoid are headache, perhaps sore throat and a fever that may reach 40.5° C. (105° F.). The temperature rises daily, reaching a peak in 7 to 10 days, maintaining this level for about another week, and then subsiding by the end of the fourth week. Periods of chills and sweating may occur, with loss of appetite. A watery, grayish or greenish diarrhea is common, but constipation sometimes occurs instead. After 2 weeks, red spots begin to appear on the chest and abdomen. If the case is severe, the patient may lapse into states of delirious muttering and staring into space. About the third to fourth week an improvement is noticeable, and steady recovery follows. The disease is serious and sometimes fatal.

TRANSMISSION. A person who has had typhoid fever gains immunity from it but may become a carrier. Although perfectly well, he harbors the bacteria and passes them out in his feces and urine. The typhoid bacillus often lodges in the gallbladder of carriers, and when the gallbladder is removed the person may cease to be a carrier. In cities, food handled by carriers is the principal source of infection. In rural areas carriers may infect food—fruit and fresh vegetables, for example—that they raise. When sewage and sanitation systems are poor, the organisms may enter the water supply. They can also be spread to food and water by flies that have been in contact with body eliminations. Contamination is more likely if human feces are used to fertilize the crops, as they are in some areas.

PREVENTION AND TREATMENT. Once a widespread disease, typhoid fever has now been virtually eliminated in countries with advanced sanitation. Proper sanitation involves (1) good sewage systems to dispose of human wastes and (2) proper measures for keeping foods uncontaminated. Food should be carefully protected from flies. One should wash his hands carefully before eating and after going to the toilet.

Effective medicines, such as the antibiotic chloramphenicol, are available for the treatment of the disease.

A less serious disease whose symptoms resemble those of typhoid fever is paratyphoid, also transmitted by contaminated food or liquids.

PATIENT CARE. Patients with typhoid fever and paratyphoid are placed under enteric precautions until the urine and feces are free of bacilli. (See ISOLATION TECHNIQUE.) If sewage treatment for the community is adequate, the stools and urine need not be disinfected, but if there is danger of incomplete destruction of the bacilli by sewage treatment methods, the urine and feces should be disinfected by chlorinated lime or a 4 per cent Lysol solution before disposal. Other precautionary measures to prevent the spread of the disease include adequate screening of windows and doors so that flies may not come in contact with excreta.

Many patients with typhoid fever require measures to lower the body temperature when fever is extreme. These include cool sponge baths, application of ice bags, and administration of antipyretic drugs as ordered. Fluids should be forced, to prevent dehydration. The diet should consist of soft, bland, easily digested, and nourishing foods.

Observations of the patient include watching for sudden temperature changes, signs of intestinal bleeding, and symptoms of intestinal perforation.

Kaolin or a similar antidiarrheal may be needed to help control diarrhea. If constipation becomes a problem, a low saline enema should be given in preference to a cathartic because of the danger of intestinal perforation.

Good oral hygiene and care of the lips and mouth are essential, as for any patient with a prolonged febrile condition. In addition, the patient must be kept clean and dry and turned frequently to avoid the development of DECUBITUS ULCERS. During the convalescent period the patient will need adequate rest and a well-rounded diet to help him recover from this debilitating illness.

typhoidal (ti-foi'dal) resembling typhoid fever.

typhopneumonia (ti"fo-nu-mo'ne-ah) pneumonia with typhoid fever.

typhus (ti'fus) an acute infectious disease caused by species of the parasitic microorganism *Rickettsia.* The organisms are usually transmitted from infected rats and other rodents to man by lice, fleas, ticks and mites.

Rickettsiae enter the human body through cuts or breaks in the skin made by the bites of the lice or other pests.

TYPES AND TREATMENT. The principal types of the diseases are louse-borne typhus (epidemic or classic typhus) caused by *Rickettsia prowazekii,* murine (flea-borne) typhus caused by *R. typhi,* scrub typhus caused by *R. tsutsugamushi,* and recrudescent typhus.

Louse-Borne Typhus. Louse-borne typhus (epidemic or classic typhus) occurs after feces of an infected human body are rubbed into a break in the skin. After an incubation period of 6 to 15 days, the symptoms begin to appear—headache, running of the nose, cough, nausea, and chest pain. These are followed in a few days by high fever and chills, vomiting, constipation or diarrhea, muscular aching, and perhaps delirium or stupor. A red rash, which may bleed, appears on the trunk and spreads to the arms and legs.

After about 2 weeks the symptoms usually subside. Ordinarily louse typhus is not fatal, but it can be, particularly if pneumonia develops or if the afflicted person has heart disease.

Louse typhus is called epidemic typhus because of the devastation it has caused throughout history. It tends to appear where people are crowded together and are weakened by cold, disease, and starvation. It has many colloquial names, such as war fever, camp fever, or jail fever.

Murine Typhus. Murine typhus is a less common variety. It is called also endemic, rat, or flea typhus. As the name "murine" indicates, it is transmitted by the bites of rat or mouse fleas. The symptoms are like those of louse typhus but are less severe, and recovery occurs sooner. Antibiotics are used in treatment.

Scrub Typhus. Scrub typhus, called also Japanese river fever and tsutsugamushi fever, is prevalent in eastern Asia and has been carried to other areas by infected persons. It is transmitted by mites and hence is often called mite fever. The rodent responsible for this illness is the field mouse. The rickettsiae are transferred to humans by the bite of the larval form of the mite, usually in the groin or neck. The fever of scrub typhus and its other symptoms are very similar to those of other forms of typhus. It is treated with chloramphenicol and the tetracyclines.

Recrudescent Typhus. Recrudescent typhus, or Brill-Zinsser disease, is caused by *Rickettsia prowazekii,* the etiologic agent of louse-borne typhus. The rickettsiae, however, remain in the body after a first attack of typhus and can cause a recurrence (a recrudescence) as long as years after the first attack. The recrudescence is milder than the initial infection, however. Treatment is similar to that for epidemic typhus.

Closely related to these forms of typhus are tick-borne rickettsial diseases, such as ROCKY MOUNTAIN SPOTTED FEVER.

PREVENTION. Immunizing vaccines are available if an outbreak of typhus occurs or threatens. They greatly reduce the chance of infection, or modify the effects of the disease. Travelers should be vaccinated before visiting countries where the disease is prevalent. Some countries require proof of such protection before admitting a visitor.

Insect and rodent control are of great importance in the prevention and control of typhus. Adult lice can be destroyed by spraying garments with DDT. Frequent bathing and changes of underclothes are vital. Outer garments should be sterilized by steam to kill the louse eggs.

Fleas and mites are more difficult to control than lice. The best method is to destroy the rodents on which they live.

PATIENT CARE. The patient with typhus is initially isolated until he is free of body lice or mites. He is not capable of transmitting the disease without the aid of these vectors. To accomplish removal of lice or mites the patient should be washed with a 1 per cent solution of Lysol upon admission and his clothing must be disinfected or destroyed. Several shampoos may be necessary to eliminate parasites from the hair. Gentle, thorough cleaning is necessary and every effort must be made to avoid damage to the skin in one's enthusiasm for removing lice or mites.

The patient is given a soft diet and ample fluids, to prevent dehydration. Efforts are made to conserve the patient's strength and to protect him during periods of delirium, which are common.

Typhus is a very debilitating disease and requires a long period of convalescence in which the patient's general health must be improved. Nervous and mental symptoms may persist long after the acute phase of the disease subsides.

typing (tīp′ing) in transplantation immunology, a method of measuring the degree of organ, solid tissue, or blood compatibility between two individuals, in which specific histocompatibility antigens (e.g., those present on leukocytes or erythrocytes) are detected by means of suitable isoimmune antisera.

t. of blood, determining the character of the blood on the basis of agglutinogens in the erythrocytes. (See also BLOOD GROUP.)

phage t., characterization of bacteria, extending to strain differences, by demonstration of susceptibility to one or more (a spectrum) races of bacteriophage; widely applied to staphylococci, typhoid bacilli, etc., for epidemiological purposes.

tyramine (ti′rah-mēn) a decarboxylation product of tyrosine, which may be converted to cresol and phenol, found in decayed animal tissue, ripe cheese, and ergot. Closely related structurally to epinephrine and norepinephrine, it has a similar but weaker action.

tyrocidin, tyrocidine (ti″ro-si′din) a polypeptide antibiotic substance, the major component of tyrothricin.

tyrogenous (ti-roj′ĕ-nus) originating in cheese.

tyroid (ti′roid) of cheesy consistency; caseous.

tyroma (ti-ro′mah) a caseous tumor.

tyromatosis (ti″ro-mah-to′sis) a condition characterized by caseous degeneration.

tyrosine (ti′ro-sēn) a naturally occurring amino acid present in most proteins; it is a product of phenyalanine metabolism and a precursor of melanin, epinephrine, and thyroxine.

tyrosinosis (ti″ro-sĭ-no′sis) a condition characterized by a faulty metabolism of tyrosine in which an intermediate product, parahydroxyphenyl pyruvic acid, appears in the urine and gives it an abnormal reducing power.

tyrosinuria (ti″ro-sĭ-nu′re-ah) the presence of tyrosine in the urine.

tyrosis (ti-ro′sis) caseation (2).

tyrosyluria (ti″ro-sil-u′re-ah) increased urinary secretion of para-hydroxyphenyl compounds derived from tyrosine, as in tyrosinuria.

tyrothricin (ti″ro-thri′sin) an antibiotic substance produced by growth of a soil bacillus, *Bacillus brevis,* consisting principally of gramicidin and tyrocidin; used topically.

tyrotoxism (ti″ro-tok′sizm) poisoning from a toxin present in milk or cheese.

Tyson's glands (ti′sonz) sebaceous glands of the corona of the penis and inner surface of the prepuce, which secrete smegma; called also preputial glands.

tysonitis (ti″son-i′tis) inflammation of Tyson's glands (preputial glands).

tyvelose (ti″vel-ōs) an unusual sugar that is a polysaccharide somatic antigen of *Salmonella* species.

Tyvid (ti′vid) trademark for a preparation of isoniazid, used in treatment of tuberculosis.

Tzanck's test (tsankz) cytologic examination of scrapings from the base of herpetic lesions, useful in the diagnosis of HERPES SIMPLEX and herpes genitalis. The scrapings are fixed on a slide with absolute or methyl alcohol for 10 minutes and stained with Giesma stain. The findings of multinucleated giant cells or of typical eosinophilic intranuclear inclusions is diagnostic of herpesvirus infection.

tzetze (set′se) tsetse.

U

U chemical symbol, *uranium.*

U. unit.

ubiquinone (u-bik′kwĭ-nōn) coenzyme Q.

UDP uridine diphosphate.

UICC International Union Against Cancer (see CANCER).

ulcer (ul′ser) a local defect, or excavation of the surface of an organ or tissue, produced by sloughing of necrotic inflammatory tissue. As commonly used, the term often refers to a peptic ulcer of the inner wall, or lining, of the stomach (gastric ulcer) or of the duodenum (duodenal ulcer).

chronic leg u., ulceration of the lower leg caused by peripheral vascular disease involving either the arteries and arterioles or the veins and venules of the affected extremity. Arterial and venous ulcers are quite different and require different modes of treatment.

Arterial ulcer disease usually is caused by occlusion of small arteries or arterioles of the extremity. Ulceration is likely to occur in diabetics and in patients with atherosclerosis. The extremity is cold and pale with loss of hair and atrophy of the skin. If ulceration develops, it is treated by keeping the ulcer clean and dry and free from pressure. The patient must be taught to care for his feet and to avoid trauma from pressure and from physical injury.

Venous ulceration occurs as a result of one or more episodes of thrombophlebitis, which produce edema and stasis of the blood supply. The ulcers almost always occur in the lower third of the leg, where there is little subcutaneous tissue. Treatment consists of elevating the leg as much as possible to promote venous return and prevent engorgement of the blood vessels. Elastic bandages or support hose are worn to give support to the superficial veins and reduce edema. Local pressure may be applied directly over the granulating tissue of the ulcer by using 4 × 4 gauze squares cut to exact size. As the ulcer heals, the bandage is cut smaller. An elastic bandage is then wrapped around the leg up to the knee. The purpose of this treatment is to collapse perforating venules and prevent the transmission of hydrostatic pressure to the tissues under the ulcer.

Venous ulcers are treated very simply by daily washing, careful rinsing to remove all traces of soap, and thorough drying of the ulcerated area. The dry bandage is then applied so that local pressure is exerted against the ulcer and underlying venules. Medications in the form of topical antibiotics, steroids, and creams are not recommended. In most cases the simple cleansing, drying, and dressing of the ulcer and the application of pressure will promote rapid healing.

Curling's u., an ulcer of the duodenum seen after severe burns of the body.

decubitus u., bedsore; an ulceration caused by prolonged pressure on a body area in a patient confined to bed (see also DECUBITUS ULCER).

Hunner's u., one involving all layers of the bladder wall, occurring in chronic interstitial cystitis.

peptic u., a loss of tissues lining the lower esophagus, the stomach, and the duodenum. Acute lesions that do not extend through the muscularis mucosae are simply called lesions. Chronic lesions, which are almost always called ulcers, involve the muscular coat, destroying the musculature and replacing it with permanent scar tissue at the site of healing.

CAUSE. While it is known that gastric acid and pepsin are responsible for ulcer formation, it is not known why mucosal resistance to them should become impaired. Duodenal ulcers and some prepyloric gastric ulcers are associated with an increased amount or hyperacidity of the gastric juice. Gastric ulcers, on the other hand, are not associated with excessive acid levels.

Theories about genetic and environmental causes of peptic ulcer abound. Both gastric and duodenal ulcers tend to occur in families. Relatives of persons with gastric ulcers have three times the expected number of gastric ulcers. The same is true of duodenal ulcers. There is evidence that the increased familial incidence of both gastric and duodenal ulcers is not just due to a shared environment. There is as yet no direct evidence that either diets or particular elements of diets, such as hot spices, cause ulcers. However, gastric ulcer is more likely to occur in those who are poorly nourished and is primarily a disease of the lower socioeconomic levels of society. Despite the stereotype of the hard-driving executive who suffers from an ulcer, there is actually little difference in the incidence of ulcer in various occupations.

Psychosomatic factors do play some role in the development of peptic ulcers. Psychologic stress can and does alter gastric function. Prolonged psychologic or physiologic stress produces what is known as a *stress ulcer,* which is believed to be the result of persistent stimulation of the vagus nerves. A stress ulcer differs pathologically and clinically from a chronic peptic ulcer. It is more acute and more likely to produce hemorrhage; perforation occurs occasionally and pain is rare.

Conditions that are often associated with stress ulcers include severe trauma, surgery, advanced malignancy, extensive burns (Curling's ulcer), and brain injury.

Drug-induced ulcers are most commonly caused by the ingestion of aspirin, with alcohol running a close second. Other drugs that are strongly suspected of being ulcerogenic include the glucocorticoids, indomethacin, and phenylbutazone.

SYMPTOMS. The cardinal symptom of peptic ulcer is epigastric pain that may be described as burning, gnawing, cramping, or aching, and usually comes in waves that last several minutes. The daily pattern of pain is related to the secretion of acid and the presence of food in the stomach to act as a buffer. This pain is diminished in the morning when secretion is low and after meals when food is present. The pain is most severe before meals and at bedtime. It often appears for three or four days or weeks and then subsides only to reappear weeks or months later.

Other symptoms of uncomplicated peptic ulcer include nausea, loss of appetite, and sometimes weight loss. Spontaneous vomiting more often accompanies duodenal ulcers than gastric ulcers.

COMPLICATIONS. The three major complications of ulcer are hemorrhage, perforation, and obstruction. Bleeding may be manifested by emesis of bright red blood or of coffee-ground vomitus, and by tarry stools. The bleeding may vary from massive hemorrhage to occult (hidden) bleeding that occurs over a period of time.

Perforation frequently is a surgical emergency because of the possibility of a chemical peritonitis resulting from spilling of the gastric and intestinal contents into the peritoneal cavity.

Obstruction of the upper intestinal tract occurs as a result of scarring and loss of musculature at the pylorus. It is manifested by persistent vomiting that can quickly bring on ALKALOSIS because of the loss of gastric acids in the vomitus. The obstruction is treated by surgical removal of the scar tissue.

DIAGNOSIS. The most commonly used technique in the diagnosis of peptic ulcers is an upper gastrointestinal series utilizing a radiopaque material and radiography. GASTROSCOPY may be helpful in establishing the site of bleeding in a gastric ulcer, in differentiating between benign and malignant ulcerations, and between esophageal ulcer and diverticulum. Gastric analysis to determine level of acidity may be helpful in some cases but there is much individual variation in gastric acid secretions among patients with ulcer.

TREATMENT. The primary goals of medical treatment of peptic ulcers are: (1) relief of symptoms, (2) promotion of healing, (3) prevention of complications, and (4) prevention of recurrences. Because each patient responds differently to various modes of treatment, the medical regimen prescribed for him is planned according to his individual needs and responses.

In general the medical management of ulcers consists of antacid therapy, anticholinergic drugs and sedatives, dietary modification, and identifying and relieving sources of psychologic stress. Antacids, such as magnesium hydroxide and aluminum hydroxide, relieve the pain of ulcer by decreasing the levels of gastric acid and pepsin. The anticholinergic drugs usually are given before meals and at bedtime when gastric secretion is highest, because they decrease acid and pepsin secretion and decrease gastric and intestinal motility. Sedatives may be prescribed to reduce anxiety and tension.

Recently, Cimetidine (Tagamet), a histamine H_2-receptor antagonist that inhibits gastric acid secretion in response to all stimuli, has been shown to be effective in the treatment of peptic ulcer in a significant number of patients. It relieves pain, reduces the need for antacids, and promotes the rate of ulcer healing.

The dietary regimen prescribed for the ulcer patient will depend on his reaction to certain foods and the preference of his physician for certain dietary restrictions in the management of ulcers. Most authorities agree that caffeine and alcohol should be avoided and that smoking should be discouraged because it is known to slow down the healing of ulcers. Although there is no conclusive evidence that spices in moderate amounts cause ulcers or inhibit their healing, or that roughage has similar effects, some physicians restrict altogether or severely limit their intake by patients with peptic ulcers.

The practice of giving milk and cream hourly has been found to be ineffective, if not harmful. Studies have shown that this produces a lower intergastric pH than three regular meals, and in addition may accelerate the development of atherosclerosis.

Perhaps the most important aspect of dietary modification and of relief from stress, anxiety, and emotional unrest is the enlistment of the patient in a cooperative effort to determine what is most helpful for him and what he might do or refrain from doing in order to promote healing and prevent recurrences of his peptic ulcer.

Many ulcers can be treated without surgery when patients cooperate fully; however, surgery may be necessary in certain cases—when there is scarring of the ulcer (producing obstruction), recurrent bleeding, extreme pain and perforation. Gastric ulcers are more likely to require surgery than are duodenal ulcers. The operative procedure most frequently done in the treatment of gastric ulcer is subtotal gastrectomy in which the ulcerous portion of the stomach is removed (see also surgery of the

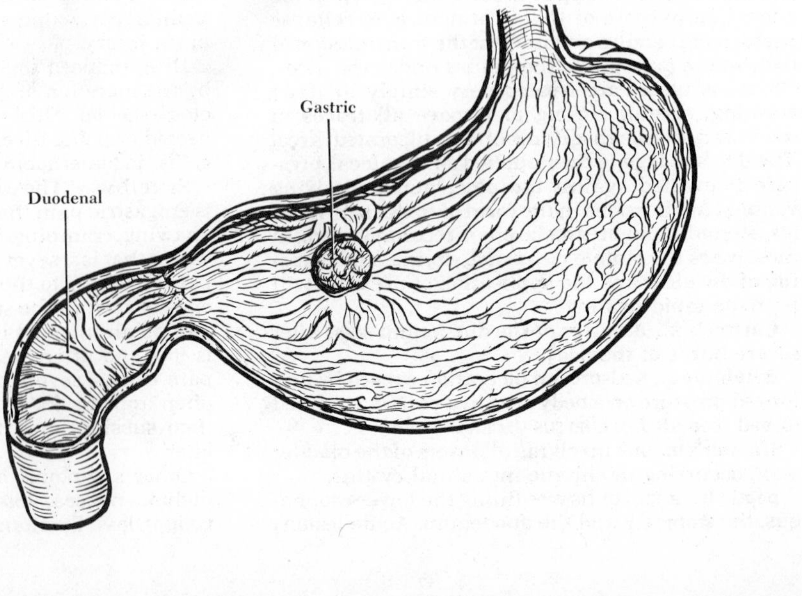

Ulcer.

STOMACH). This procedure is often done in conjunction with vagotomy, division of the vagus nerve, which eliminates cerebral stimuli of the stomach muscle and glands, thereby reducing gastric motility and secretion.

perforating u., one that involves the entire thickness of an organ, creating an opening on both surfaces.

phagedenic u., a necrotizing lesion in which tissue destruction is prominent.

rodent u., ulcerating basal cell carcinoma of the skin.

stress u., peptic ulcer, usually gastric, resulting from stress; possible predisposing factors include changes in the microcirculation of the gastric mucosa, increased permeability of the gastric mucosa barrier to H^+, and impaired cell proliferation.

trophic u., one due to imperfect nutrition of the part.

tropical u., a chronic, sloughing ulcer usually on the lower extremities, occurring in tropical regions.

varicose u., an ulcer due to varicose veins.

venereal u., a condition marked by formation of ulcers resembling chancre or chancroid about the vulvae of women not exposed to venereal disease.

ulcerate (ul′sĕ-rāt) to undergo ulceration.

ulceration (ul″sĕ-ra′shun) 1. formation or development of an ulcer. 2. an ulcer.

ulcerative (ul′sĕ-ra″tiv, ul′ser-ah-tiv) pertaining to or characterized by ulceration.

u. colitis, inflammation of the colon, with formation of ulcers in the intestinal mucosa. It is most likely to occur in young adults, but it can occur at any age. It is potentially serious and may be disabling or even fatal in rare instances.

The cause of ulcerative colitis is unknown. Emotional stress or acute infections frequently precipitate attacks.

SYMPTOMS. The chief symptom is severe diarrhea with as many as 15 or 20 watery stools a day, although none of the usual causes of diarrhea is present. There may be blood and mucus in the stool.

The patient feels weak, loses weight, and sometimes has anemia. He may suffer from pains in the joints or from skin disorders. As the disease progresses, it may spread to the covering of the colon, or it may cause intestinal perforation and peritonitis. Malignant degeneration may occur in these patients.

DIAGNOSIS. The lining of the colon can be examined and ulcerations visualized by PROCTOSCOPY. The existence of the disease can be determined also by barium enema (see BARIUM TEST).

TREATMENT. Rest is imperative. This includes not only physical rest in bed but complete freedom from emotional stress. A bland but nutritious diet that omits fruits and vegetables is also required. Antibiotics and cortisone may be prescribed, as well as sedatives and tranquilizers to relieve emotional distress. Counseling or PSYCHOTHERAPY may help the patient to deal with his anxieties and in this way reduce the causes of the disorder.

Treatment is difficult and the prognosis is poor. Advanced cases may respond to surgical procedures such as a colectomy or COLOSTOMY.

PATIENT CARE. The emotional aspects of ulcerative colitis are of primary importance in the care of these patients. Although these individuals may assume an outward appearance of calm and resignation to their illness, keeping their anxieties well hidden, they are almost always in need of help in coping with their anxieties and tensions.

The frequency and character of stools must be observed and recorded. Antidiarrheal drugs are administered as ordered and their effectiveness for the individual patient is noted on the chart. Special attention to cleanliness of the anal area will help prevent local irritation and discomfort produced by frequent elimination.

ulcerogangrenous (ul″ser-o-gang′grĕ-nus) characterized by both ulceration and gangrene.

ulcerogenic (ul″ser-o-jen′ik) causing ulceration; leading to the production of ulcers.

ulceromembranous (ul″ser-o-mem′brah-nus) characterized by ulceration and a membranous exudation.

ulcerous (ul′ser-us) 1. of the nature of an ulcer. 2. affected with ulceration.

ulcus (ul′kus), pl. *ul′cera* [L.] ulcer.

ulectomy (u-lek′to-me) 1. excision of scar tissue. 2. excision of the gingiva; gingivectomy.

ulerythema (u″ler-ĭ-the′mah) an erythematous disease of the skin with formation of cicatrices and atrophy.

u. ophryog′enes, a hereditary form in which keratosis pilaris involves the follicles of the eyebrow hairs.

ulitis (u-li′tis) inflammation of the gums.

ulna (ul′nah), pl. *ul′nae* [L.] the inner and larger bone of the forearm, on the side opposite the thumb. It articulates with the humerus and with the head of the radius at its proximal end; with the radius and bones of the carpus at the distal end. adj., **ul′nar.**

ulnad (ul′nad) toward the ulna.

ulnaris (ul-na′ris) [L.] ulnar.

ulnocarpal (ul″no-kar′pal) pertaining to the ulna and carpus.

ulnoradial (ul″no-ra′de-al) pertaining to the ulna and radius.

ulocace (u-lok′ah-se) ulceration of the gums.

ulocarcinoma (u″lo-kar″sĭ-no′mah) carcinoma of the gums.

uloglossitis (u″lo-glŏ-si′tis) inflammation of the gums and tongue; gingivoglossitis.

uloncus (u-long′kus) swelling of the gums.

olorrhagia (u″lo-ra′je-ah) a sudden discharge of blood from the gums.

ulotomy (u-lot′o-me) 1. incision of scar tissue. 2. incision of the gums.

Ultandren (ul-tan′dren) trademark for a preparation of fluoxymesterone, an androgen.

ultra- word element [L.], *beyond; excess.*

ultrabrachycephalic (ul″trah-brak″e-sĕ-fal′ik) having a cephalic index of more than 90.

ultracentrifugation (ul″trah-sen-trif″u-ga′shun) subjection of material to an exceedingly high centrifugal force, which will separate and sediment the molecules of a substance.

ultracentrifuge (ul″trah-sen′trĭ-fūj) the centrifuge used in ultracentrifugation.

ultrafilter (ul″trah-fil′ter) the filter used in ultrafiltration.

ultrafiltration (ul″trah-fil-tra′shun) filtration through a filter capable of removing very minute (ultramiscroscopic) particles.

ultramicroscope (ul″trah-mi′kro-skōp) a special darkfield microscope for examination of particles of colloidal size.

ultramicroscopic (ul″trah-mi″kro-skop′ik) 1. pertraining to the ultramicroscope. 2. too small to be seen with the ordinary light microscope.

ultramicroscopy (ul″trah-mi-kros′ko-pe) use of an ultramiscroscope.

Ultran (ul′tran) trademark for preparations of phenaglycodol, a sedative.

ultrasonic (ul″trah-son′ik) beyond the audible range; relating to sound waves having a frequency of more than 20,000 cycles per second.

ultrasonics (ul″trah-son′iks) that part of the science of acoustics dealing with the frequency range beyond the upper limit of perception by the human ear (above 20,000 cycles per second), but usually restricted to frequencies above 50,000 hertz. Ultrasonic radiation is injurious to tissues because of its thermal effects when absorbed by living matter, but in controlled doses it is used therapeutically to selectively break down pathologic tissues, as in treatment of arthritis and lesions of the nervous system, and also as a diagnostic aid by visually displaying echoes received from irradiated tissues, as in ECHOCARDIOGRAPHY and echoencephalography. (See also ULTRASONOGRAPHY.)

ultrasonogram (ul″trah-son′o-gram) the record obtained by ultrasonography.

ultrasonography (ul″trah-son-og′rah-fe) a radiologic technique in which deep structures of the body are visualized by recording the reflection of ultrasonic waves directed into the tissues. adj., **ultrasonograph′ic.** Frequencies in the range of 1 million to 10 million hertz are used in diagnostic ultrasonography. The lower frequencies provide a greater depth of penetration and are used to examine abdominal organs; those in the upper range provide less penetration and are used predominantly to examine more superficial structures such as the eye.

The basic principle of ultrasonography is the same as that of depth-sounding in oceanographic studies of the ocean floor. The ultrasonic waves are confined to a narrow beam that may be transmitted through, refracted, absorbed, or reflected by the medium toward which they are directed, depending on the nature of the surface they strike.

In diagnostic ultrasonography the ultrasonic waves are produced by electrically stimulating a crystal called a *transducer.* As the transducer moves across the body, the beam strikes an interface or boundary between tissues of varying density (e.g., muscle and blood), and some of the sound waves are reflected back to the transducer as echoes. The echoes are then converted into electrical impulses that are displayed on an oscilloscope, presenting a "picture" of the tissues under examination.

Ultrasonography can be utilized in examination of the heart (echocardiography), in location of aneurysms of the aorta and other abnormalities of the major blood vessels, and in identifying size and structural changes in organs in the abdominopelvic cavity. It is, therefore, of value in identifying and distinguishing cancers and benign cysts. The technique also may be used to evaluate tumors and foreign bodies of the eye, and to demonstrate retinal detachment. It is not, however, of much value in examination of the lungs because ultrasound waves do not pass through structures that contain air.

A particularly important use of ultrasonography is in the field of obstetrics and gynecology, where ionizing radiation is to be avoided whenever possible. The technique can evaluate fetal size and maturity and fetal and placental position. It is a fast, relatively safe, and reliable technique for diagnosing multiple pregnancies. Uterine tumors and other pelvic masses, including abscesses, can be identified by ultrasonography.

ultrasound (ul′trah-sownd) mechanical radiant energy of a frequency greater than 20,000 cycles per second; used in medicine in the technique of ULTRASONOGRAPHY.

ultrastructure (ul′trah-struk″chur) the structure visible only under the ultramicroscope and electron microscope.

ultraviolet (ul″trah-vi′o-let) denoting electromagnetic radiation of wavelength shorter than that of the violet end of the spectrum, having wavelengths of 4–400 nanometers.

u. rays, electromagnetic radiation beyond the violet end of the visible spectrum and therefore not visible to man. They are produced by the sun but are absorbed to a large extent by particles of dust and smoke in the earth's atmosphere. They are also produced by the so-called sun lamps.

Ultraviolet rays can produce sun-burning and affect the pigmentation of the skin, causing tanning. When they strike the skin surface, these rays transform provitamin D, secreted by the glands of the skin, into vitamin D, which is then absorbed into the body.

Because ultraviolet rays are capable of killing bacteria and other microorganisms, they are sometimes utilized in specially designed cabinets to sterilize objects, and may also be used to sterilize the air in operating rooms and other areas where destruction of bacteria is necessary.

u. therapy, the employment of ultraviolet radiation in the treatment of various diseases, particularly those affecting the skin. Among those diseases which respond to this form of therapy are ACNE VULGARIS, PSORIASIS, and ulcerations, as in DECUBITIS ULCERS.

DOSAGE. The dosage unit of ultraviolet radiation is expressed as minimal erythema dose (M.E.D.). Because of varying degrees of skin thickness and pigmentation, human skin varies widely in its sensitivity to ultraviolet radiation. The M.E.D. refers to the amount of radiation that will produce, within a few hours, minimal *erythema* (redness caused by engorgement of capillaries) in the average Caucasian skin. Dosage for individual patients is prescribed according to probable sensitivity as determined by that individual's skin type as compared to average sensitivity.

DEGREES OF ERYTHEMA. Minimal erythema is a *first degree* erythema. It usually is produced after about 15 seconds of exposure to a high-pressure mercury arc in a quartz burner that is placed at a distance of 30 inches from the skin. A *second degree* erythema results from a dose of about 2½ M.E.D. Its effects become apparent about four to six hours after application and is followed by slight peeling of the skin. A *third degree* erythema is produced by about 5 M.E.D. It may become apparent within two hours after application and is accompanied by edema followed by marked desquamation. A *fourth degree* erythema is produced by about 10 M.E.D. and is characterized by blistering.

PRECAUTIONS. It is apparent that ultraviolet therapy is safe only in the hands of a skilled and knowledgeable therapist. Areas of "thin skin" that may be burned more readily than that receiving treatment must be protected by wet towels or dressings. The eye is highly sensitive to ultraviolet radiation; therefore some form of protection, such as goggles, compresses, or cotton balls, should be provided the patient and the therapist to avoid damage to the conjunctiva and cornea.

Certain drugs, for example the sulfonamides, greatly increase sensitivity to ultraviolet radiation. All patients scheduled for this form of therapy should be questioned in regard to the medication they are taking so the dosage can be adjusted accordingly or the treatment deferred.

ululation (ul″u-la′shun) the loud crying or wailing of hysterical patients.

umbilical (um-bil′ĭ-kal) pertaining to the umbilicus.

u. cord, the structure that connects the fetus and placenta. This cord is the lifeline of the fetus in the uterus throughout pregnancy.

About 2 weeks after conception, the umbilical cord and the PLACENTA are sufficiently developed to begin their functions. Through two arteries and a vein in the cord, nourishment and oxygen pass from the blood vessels in the placenta to the fetus, and waste products pass from the fetus to the placenta.

Soon after birth, the umbilical cord is clamped or tied and then cut. The length of cord that is attached to the placenta, still in the uterus, is expelled with the placenta. The stump that remains attached to the baby's abdomen is about 2 inches long. After a few days it falls off naturally.

u. hernia, protrusion of abdominal contents through the abdominal wall at the umbilicus, the defect in the abdominal wall and protruding intestine being covered with skin and subcutaneous tissue.

During the growth of the fetus, the intestines grow more rapidly than the abdominal cavity. For a period, a portion of the intestines of the unborn child usually lies outside his abdomen in a sac within the umbilical cord. Normally, the intestines return to the abdomen, and the defect is closed by the time of birth. Occasionally the abdominal wall does not close solidly, and umbilical hernia results. This defect is more likely to be seen in premature infants and in girls rather than boys.

The defect in the abdominal wall usually closes by itself. Coughing, crying, and straining temporarily cause the sac to enlarge, but the hernia never bursts and digestion is not affected. The hernia may be strapped with adhesive or elastic tape or a truss may be used, but the effectiveness of these methods is doubtful. If the defect in the abdominal wall has not repaired itself by the time the child is 2 years old, surgery to correct the condition (HERNIORRAPHY) can then be performed.

Umbilical hernia should be distinguished from omphalocele, in which the intestines protrude directly into the umbilical cord and are covered only by a thin membrane. Omphalocele is a surgical emergency that must be treated immediately after birth.

umbilicated (um-bil′ĭ-kāt″ed) marked by depressed spots resembling the umbilicus.

umbilication (um-bil″ĭ-ka′shun) a depression resembling the umbilicus.

umbilicus (um-bil′ĭ-kus, um″bĭ-li′kus) the (usually) depressed scar marking the site of entry of the umbilical cord in the fetus; called also navel.

umbo (um′bo), pl. *umbo′nes* [L.] 1. a rounded elevation. 2. the slight projection at the center of the outer surface of the tympanic membrane.

unciform (un′sĭ-form) hooked or shaped like a hook.

uncinate (un′sĭ-nāt) 1. unciform. 2. relating to or affecting the uncinate gyrus.

uncipressure (un′sĭ-presh″ur) pressure with a hook to stop hemorrhage.

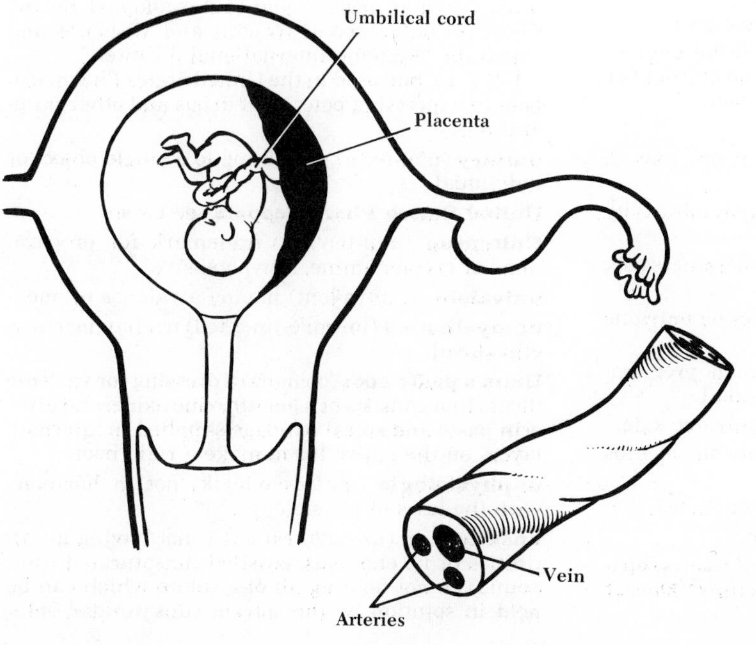

Umbilical cord. Left, in uterus; right, section.

unconscious (un-kon′shus) 1. insensible; incapable of responding to sensory stimuli and of having subjective experiences. 2. that part of the mental activity which includes primitive or repressed wishes, concealed from consciousness by the psychic censor.

collective u., the portion of the unconscious which is theoretically common to mankind.

unconsciousness (un-kon′shus-nes) an abnormal state of lack of response to sensory stimuli, resulting from injury, illness, shock or some other bodily disorder. A brief loss of unconsciousness from which the person recovers spontaneously or with slight aid is called fainting. Deep, prolonged unconsciousness is known as COMA. (See also levels of CONSCIOUSNESS.)

uncovertebral (un″ko-ver′tĕ-bral) pertaining to the uncinate processes of a vertebra.

unction (ungk′shun) 1. an ointment. 2. application of an ointment or salve; inunction.

unctuous (ungk′tu-us) greasy or oily.

uncus (ung′kus) the medially curved anterior part of the hippocampal gyrus. adj., **un′cal.**

undecylenic acid (un″des-ĭ-len′ik) an unsaturated fatty acid, used topically, in ointment or powder form, as an antifungal agent; toxic reactions are rare.

undifferentiated (un″dif-er-en′she-āt″ed) not differentiated; primitive.

undine (un′dēn) a small glass flask for irrigating the eye.

undulant fever (un′du-lant) brucellosis.

undulation (un″du-la′shun) a wavelike motion in any medium; a vibration.

ung. [L.] *unguen′tum* (ointment).

ungual (ung′gwal) pertaining to the nails.

unguent (ung′gwent) an ointment.

unguentum (ung-gwen′tum), pl. *unguen′ta* [L.] ointment.

unguiculate (ung-gwik′u-lāt) having claws; clawlike.

unguinal (ung′gwĭ-nal) pertaining to a nail.

unguis (ung′gwis), pl. *un′gues* [L.] the horny cutaneous plate on the surface of the distal end of finger or toe; a fingernail or toenail. (See also NAIL.)

uni- word element [L.], *one.*

uniaxial (u″ne-ak′se-al) 1. having only one axis. 2. developed in an axial direction only.

unicameral (u″nĭ-kam′er-al) having only one cavity or compartment.

unicellular (u″nĭ-sel′u-lar) made up of a single cell, as the bacteria.

uniglandular (u″nĭ-glan′du-lar) affecting only one gland.

unigravida (u″nĭ-grav′ĭ-dah) a woman pregnant for the first time; primigravida; gravida I.

unilateral (u″nĭ-lat′er-al) affecting only one side.

unilocular (u″nĭ-lok′u-lar) having only one loculus or compartment; monolocular.

uninucleated (u″nĭ-nu′kle-āt″ed) mononuclear.

uniocular (u″ne-ok′u-lar) monocular.

union (ūn′yun) the growing together of tissues separated by injury, as of the ends of a fractured bone, or of the edges of a wound.

uniovular (u″ne-ov′u-lar) arising from one ovum.

unipara (u-nip′ah-rah) a woman who has had one pregnancy that resulted in a viable infant; primipara; para I.

uniparous (u-nip′ah-rus) 1. producing only one ovum or offspring at a time. 2. primiparous.

unipolar (u″nĭ-po′lar) having a single pole or process, as a nerve cell.

unipotent, unipotential (u-nip′o-tent; u″nĭ-po-ten′shal) having only one power, as giving rise to cells of one order only.

unit (u′nit) 1. a single thing; one segment of a whole that is made up of identical or similar segments. 2. a specifically defined amount of anything subject to measurement, as of activity, dimension, velocity, volume, or the like.

Angström u., the unit of wavelength, equal to 10^{-10} meter; symbol A, Å, or A.U.

atomic mass u., the unit mass equal to $\frac{1}{12}$ the mass of the nuclide of carbon-12.

Bodansky u., the quantity of phosphatase in 100 ml. of serum that will liberate 1 mg. of phosphorus as phosphate ion from sodium β-glycerophosphate in 1 hour under standard conditions.

British thermal u., a unit of heat, being the amount necessary to raise the temperature of 1 pound of water from 39° to 40° F., generally considered the equivalent of 252 calories; abbreviated B.T.U.

electrostatic u's, that system of unit which is based on the fundamental definition of a unit charge as one that will repel a similar charge with a force of 1 dyne when the two charges are 1 cm. apart in a vacuum.

International u., a unit established by the International Conference for the Unification of Formulas; abbreviated I.U.

Kienböck's u., a unit of x-ray exposure equal to 0.1 erythema dose; symbol X.

motor u., the unit of motor activity formed by a motor nerve cell and its many innervated muscle fibers.

SI u., any of the base units (meter, kilogram, second, ampere, kelvin, candela, and mole), supplementary units (radian and steradian), and derived units (newton, pascal, and joule) adopted by the General Conference of Weights and Measures and called the "Système International d'Unités."

U.S.P. u., one used in the United States Pharmacopeia in expressing potency of drugs and other preparations.

unitary (u′nĭ-ter″e) pertaining to a single object or individual.

United States Pharmacopeia see U.S.P.

Unitensen (u″nĭ-ten′sen) trademark for preparations of cryptenamine, a hypotensive.

univalent (u″nĭ-va′lent) having a valence of one.

unmyelinated (un-mi′ĕ-lin-a″ted) not having a myelin sheath.

Unna's paste boot (oo′nahz) a dressing for varicose ulcers that consists of a gelatin, zinc oxide, and glycerin paste and spiral bandages applied in alternate layers on the entire leg to make a rigid boot.

unphysiologic (un″fiz-e-o-loj′ik) not in harmony with the laws of physiology.

unsaturated (un-sat′u-rāt″ed) 1. not having all affinities of its elements satisfied (unsaturated compound). 2. not holding all of a solute which can be held in solution by the solvent (unsaturated solution). 3. denoting compounds in which two or more atoms are united by double or triple bonds.

unsex (un-seks′) to deprive of the gonads.

unstriated (un-stri′āt-ed) having no striations, as smooth muscle.

Unverricht's disease (syndrome) (oon′fer-ikts) myoclonus epilepsy.

urachus (u′rah-kus) a fetal canal connecting the bladder with the allantois, persisting throughout life as a cord (median umbilical ligament). adj., **u′rachal.**

uracil (u′rah-sil) a pyrimidine base obtained from nucleic acid.

uracrasia (u″rah-kra′ze-ah) disordered state of the urine.

uragogue (u′rah-gog) diuretic.

uran(o)- word element [Gr.], *palate.*

uraniscus (u″rah-nis′kus) the palate.

uranium (u-ra′ne-um) a chemical element, atomic number 92, atomic weight 238.03, symbol U. (See table of ELEMENTS.)

uranoplasty (u-ran′o-plas″te) plastic repair of the palate; palatoplasty. adj., **uranoplas′tic.**

uranorrhaphy (u″rah-nor′ah-fe) suture of the palate; staphylorrhaphy.

uranoschisis (u″rah-nos′kĭ-sis) cleft palate.

uranostaphyloschisis (u″rah-no-staf″ĭ-los′kĭ-sis) fissure of the soft and hard palates.

uranyl (u′rah-nil) the UO^{++} ion, as in uranyl sulfate.

urarthritis (u″rar-thri′tis) gouty arthritis.

urate (u′rāt) a salt of uric acid.

uratemia (u″rah-te′me-ah) urates in the blood.

uratic (u-rat′ik) pertaining to urates or to gout.

uratoma (u″rah-to′mah) a concretion made up of urates; tophus.

uratosis (u″rah-to′sis) the deposit of urates in the tissues.

uraturia (u″rah-tu′re-ah) urates in the urine.

urceiform (ur-se′ĭ-form) pitcher-shaped.

ur-defense (ur″de-fens′) a belief essential to the psychologic integrity of the individual. Such beliefs include faith in personal survival, in religious, philosophic, or scientific systems, and in human succorance.

urea (u-re′ah) 1. the diamide of carbonic acid found in urine, blood, and lymph, the chief nitrogenous constituent of urine, and the chief nitrogenous end-product of protein metabolism; it is formed in the liver from amino acids and from ammonia compounds. 2. a pharmaceutical preparation of urea occasionally used to lower intracranial pressure. adj., **ure′al.**

The amount of urea in the urine increases with the quantity of protein in the diet. This is because urea is an endogenous and exogenous waste product: endogenous because some of it is derived from the breakdown of body protein as the tissues undergo disintegration and repair, and exogenous because some of it is derived from the deamination of amino acids absorbed from the intestinal tract but not utilized by the body.

In severe nephritis or other disorders leading to renal failure, the concentration of urea in the blood may be greatly increased, as revealed by measurement of the blood urea nitrogen (BUN).

u. cycle, a cyclic series of reactions that produce urea, a major route for removal of the ammonia produced in the metabolism of amino acids in the liver and kidney.

u. nitrogen, the nitrogen component of urea, a major excretory product of the kidneys. Elevation of urea nitrogen concentration in the blood (blood urea nitrogen, or BUN) indicates a disorder of kidney function. In determination of BUN the nitrogen fraction of the urea nitrogen compound is measured. No special preparation is necesary for the test. Venous blood is used and potassium oxalate is added to the specimen to prevent clotting. Normal range is 8 to 20 mg. per 100 ml. of blood.

ureametry (u″re-am′ĕ-tre) measurement of urea in urine.

ureapoiesis (u-re″ah-poi-e′sis) formation of urea. adj., **ureapoiet′ic.**

urease (u′re-ās) an enzyme that catalyzes the decomposition of urea to ammonia and carbon dioxide.

urecchysis (u-rek′ĭ-sis) an effusion of urine into cellular tissue.

Urecholine (u″re-ko′lin) trademark for preparations of bethanechol, a cholinergic agent.

uredema (u″rĕ-de′mah) swelling from extravasated urine.

ureide (u′re-īd) a compound of urea and an acid or aldehyde formed by the elimination of water.

urelcosis (u″rel-ko′sis) ulceration in the urinary tract.

uremia (u-re′me-ah) retention in the blood of substances ordinarily eliminated in the urine. adj., **ure′mic.** The condition develops when the kidneys lose most of their ability to filter out waste products from the blood, because of damage by disease or by severe trauma. It may be the result of a temporary poisoning or of obstruction of the kidneys, or it may occur in the final stage of a severe kidney disease.

Failure of the kidneys to excrete urine brings about potentially fatal consequences, as a result of an excess of potassium in the blood (hyperkalemia). Causes of the hyperkalemia are: (1) failure of the kidneys to excrete potassium in normal amounts, (2) diminished excretion of hydrogen ions, which in turn produces ACIDOSIS and a release of more potassium from the body tissues, and (3) increased rate of catabolism resulting from fever, trauma, infection, or other possible causes of the uremia.

Normally, the kidney excretes the end products of protein metabolism. In acute uremia these end products remain in the blood, causing an elevation in the BUN and creatinine levels.

SYMPTOMS. The first and most important symptom of acute uremia is always a sudden drop in the volume of urine (oliguria). In severe cases the production of urine may stop entirely (anuria).

Symptoms of hyperkalemia include severe muscle weakness and tingling around the mouth. If the condition is not corrected, cardiac arrest may occur very quickly and without warning unless the patient's ECG's are being monitored.

TREATMENT. Attempts are made to remove the excess potassium and other waste products that accumulate in the blood. DIALYSIS is employed and cationic exchange resins may be administered to promote excretion of potassium through the intestinal tract.

If anuria persists, fluid intake must be controlled so that the circulatory system is not overloaded. The intake of fluid in a 24-hour period is limited to 600 to 800 ml., the amount of insensible loss of fluid that normally occurs during that period of time.

Dietary sources of protein are restricted to prevent accumulations of the end products of protein metabolism and elevation of the BUN and creatinine levels.

As the patient's renal function returns and urinary flow increases, there may be a period of diuresis with excessive loss of electrolytes and fluids. During this phase of uremia it is imperative that accurate records of intake and output be kept as in other phases of the disease, and that the fluid and electrolyte status be carefully monitored.

PATIENT CARE. Disturbances in the normal fluid balance require strict measuring and recording of the patient's total intake and output. When severe edema is present, the fluid intake may be restricted and oral intake of fluids must then be spaced over a 24-hour period. Nausea and vomiting often present problems of adequate oral intake and should be recorded on the patient's chart so that fluids may be administered intravenously if necessary. The amount of fluid lost by emesis is carefully measured and recorded.

Mouth care is necessary at frequent intervals to prevent drying and cracking of the lips and oral mucosa and to reduce the foul breath which usually carries an odor of urine in uremic patients.

The skin is often dry, and deposits of urea salts cause severe itching. A sponge bath using a mild acid solution of vinegar and water (two tablespoons of vinegar to one pint of warm water) will relieve the irritation and discomfort. The bath should be followed by gentle application of a bland lotion. The presence of edema presents additional problems since edematous tissue breaks down more readily than normal tissue. To avoid rapidly developing DECUBITUS ULCERS the patient's position is changed and skin care is given at least every 2 hours. Extreme care must be used to keep the skin intact and to avoid friction against the bed linens when turning the patient.

Observations, in addition to intake and output and vital signs, include frequent checking for signs of developing convulsions. As intracranial pressure due to cerebral edema increases, the patient may exhibit extreme restlessness, irritability, and mental confusion. For this reason, and to avoid precipitation of a convulsive seizure, the patient's environment should be as quiet and nonstimulating as possible.

Uremia is often the final phase of severe renal damage. The process is frequently irreversible and death is the inevitable outcome. The patient and his family will need sympathetic understanding, warmth, and moral support during this time of emotional crisis.

uremigenic (u-re″mĭ-jen′ik) 1. caused by uremia. 2. causing uremia.

ureometry (u″re-om′ĕ-tre) ureametry.

ureotelic (u″re-o-tel′ik) having urea as the chief excretory product of nitrogen metabolism.

uresiesthesis (u-re″se-es-the′sis) the normal impulse to pass the urine.

uresis (u-re′sis) the passage of urine; urination.

-uresis word element [Gr.], *urinary excretion of.* adj., **-uret′ic.**

ureter (u-re′ter) the fibromuscular tube, 16 to 18 inches long, through which the urine passes from the kidney to the bladder. adj., **ure′teral, ureter′ic.** As urine is produced by each kidney, it passes into the ureter, which, contracting rhythmically, forces the urine along and empties it in spurts into the bladder. After being stored temporarily in the bladder, the urine passes out of the body by way of the urethra.

Rarely, a small calculus, or stone, formed in a kidney, passes into a ureter and obstructs it. The result is the sudden severe pain known as renal or ureteral colic. In such cases the aim of medical treatment is to relieve the pain and obstruction and to eliminate the condition that causes the stone.

ureter(o)- word element [Gr.], *ureter.*

ureteralgia (u-re″ter-al′je-ah) pain in the ureter.

ureterectasis (u-re″ter-ek′tah-sis) distention of the ureter.

ureterectomy (u-re″ter-ek′to-me) excision of a ureter.

ureteritis (u-re″ter-i′tis) inflammation of a ureter.

ureterocele (u-re′ter-o-sēl″) ballooning of the lower end of the ureter into the bladder.

ureterocelectomy (u-re″ter-o-se-lek′to-me) excision of a ureterocele.

ureterocolostomy (u-re″ter-o-ko-los′to-me) anastomosis of a ureter to the colon.

ureterocystoscope (u-re″ter-o-sis′to-skōp) a cystoscope with a catheter for insertion into the ureter.

ureterocystostomy (u-re″ter-o-sis-tos′to-me) ureteroneocystostomy.

ureterodialysis (u-re″ter-o-di-al′ĭ-sis) rupture of a ureter; ureterolysis.

ureteroenterostomy (u-re″ter-o-en″ter-os′to-me) anastomosis of one or both ureters to the wall of the intestine.

ureterography (u-re″ter-og′rah-fe) roentgenography of the ureter, after injection of a contrast medium.

ureteroheminephrectomy (u-re″ter-o-hem″ĭ-ne-frek′to-me) excision of the diseased portion of a reduplicated kidney and its ureter.

ureteroileostomy (u-re″ter-o-il″e-os′to-me) anastomosis of the ureters to an isolated loop of the ileum, drained through a stoma on the abdominal wall.

ureterolith (u-re′ter-o-lith″) a calculus in the ureter.

ureterolithiasis (u-re″ter-o-lĭ-thi′ah-sis) formation of a calculus in the ureter.

ureterolithotomy (u-re″ter-o-lĭ-thot′o-me) incision of a ureter for removal of calculus.

ureterolysis (u-re″ter-ol′ĭ-sis) 1. rupture of the ureter; ureterodialysis. 2. paralysis of the ureter. 3. the operation of freeing the ureter from adhesions.

ureteroneocystostomy (u-re″ter-o-ne″o-sis-tos′to-me) surgical transplantation of a ureter to a different site in the bladder; ureterocystostomy.

ureteroneopyelostomy (u-re″ter-o-ne″o-pi″ĕ-los′to-me) ureteropyeloneostomy.

ureteronephrectomy (u-re″ter-o-ne-frek′to-me) excision of a kidney and ureter.

ureteropathy (u-re″ter-op′ah-the) any disease of the ureter.

ureteropelvioplasty (u-re″ter-o-pel′ve-o-plas″te)

surgical reconstruction of the junction of the ureter and renal pelvis; ureteropyelostomy.

ureteroplasty (u-re′ter-o-plas″te) plastic repair of a ureter.

ureteropyelitis (u-re″ter-o-pi″ĕ-li′tis) inflammation of a ureter and renal pelvis.

ureteropyelography (u-re″ter-o-pi-ĕ-log′rah-fe) roentgenography of the ureter and renal pelvis.

ureteropyeloneostomy (u-re″ter-o-pi″ĕ-lo-ne-os′to-me) surgical creation of a new communication between a ureter and the renal pelvis; ureteroneopyelostomy; ureteropyelostomy.

ureteropyelonephritis (u-re″ter-o-pi″ĕ-lo-nĕ-fri′-tis) inflammation of the ureter, renal pelvis, and kidney.

ureteropyeloplasty (u-re″ter-o-pi′ĕ-lo-plas″te) plastic repair of the ureter and renal pelvis.

ureteropyelostomy (u-re″ter-o-pi″ĕ-los′to-me) ureteropelvioplasty.

ureteropyosis (u-re″ter-o-pi-o′sis) suppurative inflammation of the ureter.

ureterorrhagia (u-re″ter-o-ra′je-ah) discharge of blood from the ureter.

ureterorrhaphy (u-re″ter-or′ah-fe) suture of the ureter.

ureterosigmoidostomy (u-re″ter-o-sig″moi-dos′to-me) anastamosis of one or both ureters to the sigmoid colon. In this form of diversion of urinary flow there is no need for an appliance because the urine flows into the colon, which acts as a kind of reservoir. The urine liquefies the stool and creates difficulties in patients who are unable to regulate themselves successfully. A disadvantage of ureterosigmoidostomy is the constant danger of urinary infection by organisms from the bowel.

Indications for ureterosigmoidostomy are the same as for cutaneous URETEROSTOMY and ILEAL CONDUIT.

ureterostomy (u-re″ter-os′to-me) creation of a new outlet for a ureter.

cutaneous u., a type of urinary diversion in which one or both ureters are detached from the bladder and brought through the abdominal wall to form a STOMA. A collection pouch fitted with a belt is then worn snugly against the abdomen and over the "ureteral buds" or stomas to collect the urine as it passes through the ureters.

Indications for ureterostomy include malignancy or trauma which necessitates removal of the bladder, congenital defect or absence of portions of the urinary tract, and neurogenic bladder in which other devices for the collection of urine have proved unsatisfactory.

Patient care is similar to that for any patient with a diversion of urinary flow and is primarily concerned with teaching the patient how to care for his own appliance, and avoidance of complications arising from the creation of the stoma. (See also ILEAL CONDUIT.)

ureterotomy (u-re″ter-ot′o-me) incision of a ureter.

ureteroureterostomy (u-re″ter-o-u-re″ter-os′to-me) end-to-end anastomosis of the two portions of a transected ureter.

ureterovaginal (u-re″ter-o-vaj′ĭ-nal) pertaining to or communicating with a ureter and the vagina.

ureterovesical (u-re″ter-o-ves′ĭ-kal) pertaining to a ureter and the bladder.

urethan (u′rĕ-thăn) an antineoplastic, formed by esterification of carbamic acid.

urethr(o)- word element [Gr.], *urethra.*

urethra (u-re′thrah) the tubular passage through which urine is discharged from the bladder to the exterior of the body. adj., **ure′thral.** The external urinary opening is called the urinary meatus. In men the urethra conveys both urine and the secretions of the reproductive organs. In women its sole function is urination.

The female urethra is about 1½ inches long. The opening is situated between the clitoris and the opening of the vagina.

The male urethra is about 8 inches long and is narrower than that of the female. It has three sections—prostatic, membranous, and penile. It extends downward from the bladder through the prostate, which secretes into it a thin fluid. The membranous portion of the urethra receives the secretion of the bulbourethral glands. The urethra then extends down through the main body of the penis to the opening, or meatus, at the tip. Along the entire length of the passage are mucous glands.

DISORDERS OF THE URETHRA. Urethritis, inflammation of the urethra, occurs mainly in gonorrhea. Urethral strictures in men, caused by bands of fibrous tissue which obstruct the passage of urine, are also most often caused by neglected gonorrhea but may sometimes be caused by any infection, or by injury. They may be treated surgically or by dilatation. Kidney stones, or calculi, may rarely lodge in the urethra. They usually pass spontaneously but if not, may be removed with forceps or crushed.

In women, urethral caruncles, small, fleshy, red masses, sometimes form near the opening of the urethra, usually at the time of menopause. Caruncles are not dangerous unless they cause bleeding and painful urination; then surgical removal is required.

urethralgia (u″re-thral′je-ah) pain in a urethra; urethrodynia.

urethratresia (u-re″thrah-tre′ze-ah) imperforation of the urethra.

urethrectomy (u″re-threk′to-me) excision of the urethra.

urethremphraxis (u″re-threm-frak′sis) obstruction of the urethra.

urethrism (u-re′thrizm) irritability or chronic spasm of the urethra.

urethritis (u″re-thri′tis) inflammation of the urethra. The condition is frequently a symptom of gonorrhea but may be caused by other infectious organisms.

In urethritis the urethra swells and narrows, and the flow of urine is impeded. Both urination and the urgency to urinate increase. Urination is accompanied by burning pain. There may be a purulent discharge.

Urethritis usually responds to treatment with antibiotics or sulfonamides.

urethrobulbar (u-re″thro-bul′bar) pertaining to the urethra and the bulb of the penis.

urethrocele (u-re′thro-sēl) prolapse of the female urethra through the urinary meatus.

urethrocystitis (u-re″thro-sis-ti′tis) inflammation of the urethra and bladder.

urethrodynia (u-re″thro-din′e-ah) urethralgia.

urethrography (u″re-throg′rah-fe) roentgenography of the urethra.

urethrometry (u″re-throm′ĕ-tre) 1. determination of the resistance of various segments of the urethra to retrograde flow of fluid. 2. measurement of the urethra.

urethropenile (u-re″thro-pe′nīl) pertaining to the urethra and penis.

urethroperineal (u-re″thro-per″ĭ-ne′al) pertaining to the urethra and perineum.

urethroperineoscrotal (u-re″thro-per″ĭ-ne″o-skro′tal) pertaining to the urethra, perineum, and scrotum.

urethrophraxis (u-re″thro-frak′sis) obstruction of the urethra.

urethrophyma (u-re″thro-fi′mah) a tumor or growth in the urethra.

urethroplasty (u-re′thro-plas″te) plastic repair of the urethra.

urethroprostatic (u-re″thro-pros-tat′ik) pertaining to the urethra and prostate.

urethrorectal (u-re″thro-rek′tal) pertaining to the urethra and rectum.

urethrorrhagia (u-re″thro-ra′je-ah) a flow of blood from the urethra.

urethrorrhapy (u″re-thror′ah-fe) suture of a urethral fistula.

urethrorrhea (u-re″thro-re′ah) abnormal discharge from the urethra.

urethroscope (u-re′thro-skōp) an instrument for viewing the interior of the urethra.

urethroscopy (u″re-thros′ko-pe) visual inspection of the urethra. adj., **urethroscop′ic.**

urethrospasm (u-re′thro-spazm) spasm of the urethral muscular tissue.

urethrostaxis (u-re″thro-stak′sis) oozing of blood from the urethra.

urethrostenosis (u-re″thro-stĕ-no′sis) constriction of the urethra.

urethrostomy (u″re-thros′to-me) creation of a permanent opening for the urethra in the perineum.

urethrotome (u-re′thro-tōm) an instrument for cutting a urethral stricture.

urethrotomy (u″re-throt′o-me) incision of the urethra.

urethrotrigonitis (u-re″thro-tri″go-ni′tis) inflammation of the urethra and trigone of the bladder (vesical trigone).

urethrovaginal (u-re″thro-vaj′ĭ-nal) pertaining to the urethra and vagina.

urethrovesical (u-re″thro-ves′ĭ-kal) pertaining to the urethra and bladder.

urhidrosis (ur″hĭ-dro′sis) the presence in the sweat of urinous materials, chiefly uric acid and urea.

-uria word element [Gr.], *condition of the urine.* adj., **-u′ric.**

uric (u′rik) pertaining to the urine.

u. acid, the end product of purine metabolism or oxidation in the body. It is present in blood in a concentration of about 5 mg. per 100 ml. and is excreted in the urine in amounts of a little less than 1 gm. per day. In GOUT there is an excess of uric acid in the blood, and salts of uric acid—urates—form insoluble stones in the urinary tract, or they may crystallize and form deposits (tophi) in the joints and tissues.

The presence of high concentrations of uric acid in the urine is significant in the diagnosis of gout, but is of little significance in urinary disorders.

uricacidemia (u″rik-as″ĭ-de′me-ah) uric acid in the blood.

uricaciduria (u″rik-as″ĭ-du′re-ah) excess of uric acid in the urine.

uricase (u′rĭ-kās) an enzyme that catalyzes the conversion of uric acid to allantoin.

uricemia (u″rĭ-se′me-ah) uricacidemia.

uricolysis (u″rĭ-kol′ĭ-sis) the cleavage of uric acid or urates. adj., **uricolyt′ic.**

uricometer (u″rĭ-kom′ĕ-ter) an instrument for measuring uric acid in the urine.

uricosuria (u″rĭ-ko-su′re-ah) excretion of uric acid in the urine.

uricosuric (u″rĭ-ko-su′rik) 1. pertaining to, characterized by, or promoting uricosuria. 2. an agent that promotes uricosuria.

uricotelic (u″rĭ-ko-tel′ik) having uric acid as the chief excretory product of nitrogen metabolism.

uridine (u′rĭ-dēn) a ribonucleoside containing uracil.

u. diphosphate (UDP), a nucleotide that participates in glycogen metabolism and in some processes of nucleic acid synthesis.

uriesthesis (u″re-es-the′sis) uresiesthesis.

urin(o)- word element [Gr., L.], *urine.*

urina (u-ri′nah) [L.] urine.

urinal (u′rĭ-nal) a receptacle for urine.

urinalysis (u″rĭ-nal′ĭ-sis) analysis of the urine as an aid in the diagnosis of disease. Many types of tests are used in analyzing the urine to determine whether it contains abnormal substances indicative of disease. The most significant substances normally absent from urine and detected by urinalysis are protein, glucose, acetone, blood, pus, and casts.

urinary (u′rĭ-ner″e) pertaining to the urine; containing or secreting urine.

u. bladder, the musculomembranous sac in the anterior part of the pelvic cavity that serves as a reservoir for urine (see also BLADDER).

u. system, u. tract, the system formed in the body by the KIDNEYS, the urinary BLADDER, the URETERS, and the URETHRA, the organs concerned in the production and excretion of urine. (See also Plate 11.)

urinate (u′rĭ-nāt) to void urine.

urination (u″rĭ-na′shun) the discharge of urine from the bladder; called also voiding the urine and micturition. Urine from the kidneys is passed in spurts every few seconds along the ureters to the bladder, where it collects until voided. During the act of urination the urine passes from the bladder to the outside via the urethra.

THE URINARY PROCESS. Urination is a complex process controlled by several sets of muscles, including the internal and external sphincters, which are circular muscles surrounding the urethra; they have the power to contract and prevent flow through it. The internal sphincter is at the outlet of the bladder and works automatically. The external sphincter, situated along the urethra below the prostate in males and at an equivalent position in females, is controlled voluntarily.

As the bladder fills, the bladder muscle tends to contract automatically. The urge to urinate enters consciousness, but voiding may be controlled consciously to some extent. When the person decides to urinate, the bladder muscle contracts and both sphincters relax.

BED-WETTING AND INCONTINENCE. Control of the sphincters is late in developing. For the first year of life there is no control at all. Conscious control of the external sphincter develops in the second year, but complete control during sleep does not develop until the sphincters can deal automatically with the total amount of urine excreted during the night—about 10 oz. This is why bed-wetting can continue until comparatively late in young children.

Extreme fear in emergency situations may cause automatic relaxation of the sphincters with loss of control of urination, or INCONTINENCE. Incontinence also may occur in epileptic seizures, cerebral vascular accident (stroke), or other neurologic illness. In elderly men it may be due to hypertrophy of the prostate. Infection of the bladder or urethra in both men and women may impair control of urination.

Normally a quart or a quart and a half of urine is passed each day, but the amount is increased by a large intake of liquid or by cold weather. It is decreased in hot weather, when more fluid is eliminated through the skin by perspiration. Urination is usually necessary three or four times a day.

DISORDERS OF URINATION. Excessive secretion of urine (polyuria) may indicate diabetes mellitus, and diminution of urinary secretion (oliguria) may occur in nephritis. Frequent urination is a symptom of cystitis. Painful urination (dysuria) is characteristic of some bladder diseases, inflammation of the prostate, and certain infections, including gonorrhea. Nocturia, or excessive urination at night, is a symptom of some urinary system diseases. It often occurs in acute prostatitis.

Urinary suppression is failure of the kidneys to produce urine and results in uremia if not corrected. This condition is brought about by severe disease or injury to the renal cells. Urinary retention is the accumulation of urine within the bladder because of inability to urinate.

urine (u′rin) the fluid containing water and waste products that is secreted by the KIDNEYS, stored in the bladder and discharged by way of the urethra.

CONTENTS OF THE URINE. Several different types of waste products are eliminated in urine—for example, urea, uric acid, ammonia, and creatinine—none of which is useful in the blood. The largest component of urine by weight (apart from water) is urea, which is derived from the breakdown of proteins and amino acids in the diet and in the body itself. Its amount varies greatly from person to person, however, depending on the amount of protein in the diet. Besides waste materials, urine also contains surpluses of products that are necessary for bodily functioning. The kidneys remove not only excess water but also excess sodium chloride and other chemicals. Thus in a typical specimen of urine there will be sodium, potassium, calcium, magnesium, chloride, phosphate, and sulfate.

The color of urine is due to the presence of the yellow pigment urochrome. Individual ingredients of urine are not usually visible, but when the urine is alkaline some of the ingredients may form sediments of phosphates and urates. The urine may also become cloudy from the presence of mucus. Persistent cloudiness may indicate the presence of pus or blood.

URINE AS A SIGN OF ILLNESS. Changes in the urine can be an important warning of illness. The presence of glucose may signify the development of diabetes mellitus. If the urine is red or brown, this may indicate kidney disease, since the color may be due to blood in the urine (hematuria). A pink hue is not always caused by blood but may be due to certain foods such as beets and rhubarb, and cathartics containing senna, phenolphthalein, or cascara. A smoky color may indicate old blood in the urine. With jaundice the urine may become dark or brown-colored.

u. osmolality, a measure of the number of dissolved particles per unit of water in urine (see also urine OSMOLALITY).

residual u., urine remaining in the bladder after urination; seen in bladder outlet obstruction (as by prostatic hypertrophy) and disorders affecting nerves controlling bladder function.

urinemia (u″rĭ-ne′me-ah) uremia.

uriniferous (u″rĭ-nif′er-us) transporting or conveying urine.

uriniparous (u″rĭ-nip′ah-rus) excreting urine.

urinogenital (u″rĭ-no-jen′ĭ-tal) urogenital.

urinogenous (u″rĭ-noj′ĕ-nus) of urinary origin.

urinology (u″rĭ-nol′o-je) urology.

urinoma (u″rĭ-no′mah) a cyst containing urine.

urinometer (u″rĭ-nom′ĕ-ter) an instrument for determining the specific gravity of urine.

urinous (u′rĭ-nus) pertaining to or of the nature of urine.

uriposia (u″rĭ-po′ze-ah) the drinking of urine.

Uritone (u′rĭ-tōn) trademark for preparations of methenamine, an antibacterial used in urinary tract infections.

uro- word element [Gr.], *urine* (urinary tract, urination).

uroacidimeter (u″ro-as″ĭ-dim′ĕ-ter) an instrument for measuring the acidity of urine.

uroanthelone (u″ro-an′thĕ-lōn) urogastrone.

urobilin (u″ro-bi′lin) a brownish pigment formed by oxidation of urobilinogen; found in the feces and sometimes in the urine after standing in the air.

urobilinemia (u″ro-bi″lĭ-ne′me-ah) urobilin in the blood.

urobilinogen (u″ro-bi-lin′o-jen) a colorless compound formed in the intestines by the reduction of BILIRUBIN. Normally about 1 per cent of the bilirubin produced in the body by the breakdown of hemoglobin is excreted in the urine as urobilinogen. Increased amounts of urobilinogen in the urine indicate an excessive amount of bilirubin in the blood. Determination of the amount of urobilinogen excreted in a given period makes it possible to evaluate certain types of hemolytic anemia and also is of help in diagnosing liver dysfunction.

Laboratory tests for urobilinogen require collection of urine for a 24-hour period or for a 2-hour period. The 2-hour afternoon collection of urine is most commonly used because it is more convenient and also because it has been found that the excretion of urobilinogen reaches its maximum in the period from midafternoon to late evening. There is no special preparation of the patient for these tests. The exact time period in which the urine has been collected must be noted. The specimen should be taken to the laboratory immediately since bacteria which may be present in the urine can oxidize urobilinogen and change it to urobilin.

urocele (u′ro-sēl) distention of the scrotum with extravasated urine.

urochezia (u″ro-ke′ze-ah) discharge of urine in the feces.

urochrome (u′ro-krōm) a breakdown product of hemoglobin related to the bile pigments, found in the urine and responsible for its yellow color.

uroclepsia (u″ro-klep′se-ah) the involuntary escape of urine.

urocrisia (u″ro-kriz′e-ah) diagnosis by examining the urine.

urocyanogen (u″ro-si-an′o-jen) a blue pigment of urine, especially of cholera patients.

urocyanosis (u″ro-si″ah-no′sis) indicanuria.

urocyst (u′ro-sist) the urinary bladder. adj., **urocys′tic.**

urocystitis (u″ro-sis-ti′tis) inflammation of the urinary bladder.

urodynia (u″ro-din′e-ah) pain accompanying urination.

uroedema (u″ro-ĕ-de′mah) edema from infiltration of urine.

uroenterone (u″ro-en′ter-ōn) urogastrone.

uroerythrin (u″ro-er′ĭ-thrin) a reddish pigment of urine; purpurin.

uroflavin (u″ro-fla′vin) a fluorescent compound closely related to riboflavin, excreted in the urine.

urofuscohematin (u″ro-fus″ko-hem′ah-tin) a red-brown pigment from the urine in certain diseases.

urogastrone (u″ro-gas′trōn) a polypeptide derived from urine of man and other mammals that inhibits gastric secretion; called also anthelone U and uroanthelone.

urogenital (u″ro-jen′ĭ-tal) pertaining to the urinary system and genitalia; urinogenital; genitourinary.

u. system, genitourinary system.

urogenous (u-roj′ĕ-nus) 1. producing urine. 2. produced from or in the urine.

uroglaucin (u″ro-glaw′sin) indigo blue occurring in urine.

urogram (u′ro-gram) a film obtained by urography.

urography (u-rog′rah-fe) roentgenography of any part of the urinary tract.

ascending u., cystoscopic u., retrograde urography.

descending u., excretion u., excretory u., intravenous u., urography after intravenous injection of an opaque medium which is rapidly excreted in the urine.

retrograde u., urography after injection of contrast medium into the bladder through the urethra.

urogravimeter (u″ro-grah-vim′ĕ-ter) urinometer.

urohematin (u″ro-hem′ah-tin) the pigmentary substances of the urine.

urohematoporphyrin (u″ro-hem″ah-to-por′fĭ-rin) hematoporphyrin found in the urine.

urokinase (u″ro-ki′nās) an enzyme found in the urine of man and other mammals which converts plasminogen to plasmin and activates the fibrinolytic system.

urolith (u′ro-lith) a calculus in the urine or the urinary tract. adj., **urolith′ic.**

urolithiasis (u″ro-lĭ-thi′ah-sis) formation of urinary calculi, or the condition associated with urinary calculi.

urologist (u-rol′o-jist) a specialist in urology.

urology (u-rol′o-je) the branch of medicine dealing with the urinary system in the female and genitourinary system in the male. adj., **urolog′ic.**

urolutein (u″ro-lu′te-in) a yellow pigment of the urine.

uromelanin (u″ro-mel′ah-nin) a black pigment from urine.

uromelus (u-rom′ĕ-lus) a monster with fused legs and a single foot.

urometer (u-rom′ĕ-ter) urinometer.

uroncus (u-rong′kus) a swelling caused by retention or extravasation of urine.

uronephrosis (u″ro-nĕ-fro′sis) distention of the renal pelvis and tubules with urine.

uropathy (u-rop′ah-the) any disease in the urinary tract.

uropepsin (u″ro-pep′sin) a pepsin-like enzyme occurring in urine.

urophanic (u″ro-fan′ik) appearing in the urine.

urophein (u″ro-fe′in) an odoriferous gray pigment of urine.

uroplania (u″ro-pla′ne-ah) the presence of urine in, or its discharge from, organs not of the genitourinary system.

uropoiesis (u″ro-poi-e′sis) the formation of urine. adj., **uropoiet′ic.**

uroporphyria (u″ro-por-fir′e-ah) porphyria with excessive excretion of uroporphyrin.

uroporphyrin (u″ro-por′fĭ-rin) one of a group of porphyrins produced during biosynthesis of natural porphyrins and excreted in urine.

uroporphyrinogen (u″ro-por″fĭ-rin′o-jen) a precursor of uroporphyrin and coproporphyrinogen.

uropsammus (u″ro-sam′us) urinary gravel.

urorrhagia (u″ro-ra′je-ah) excessive secretion of urine.

urorrhea (u″ro-re′ah) involuntary flow of urine.

urorrhodin (u″ro-ro′din) a rose-colored pigment found in the urine in typhoid fever, tuberculosis, and other diseases.

urorrhodinogen (u″ro-ro-din′o-jen) a urinary chromogen that is decomposed into urorrhodin.

urorubin (u″ro-roo′bin) a red pigment from urine.

urorubrohematin (u″ro-roo″bro-hem′ah-tin) a red pigment rarely found in the urine in certain constitutional diseases, as in leprosy.

uroscheocele (u-ros′ke-o-sēl″) urocele.

uroschesis (u-ros′kĕ-sis) retention or suppression of the urine.

uroscopy (u-ros′ko-pe) diagnostic examination of the urine. adj., **uroscop′ic.**

urosemiology (u″ro-se″me-ol′o-je) uroscopy.

urosepsin (u″ro-sep′sin) a septic poison from urine in the tissues.

urosepsis (u″ro-sep′sis) septic poisoning from retained and absorbed urinary substances. adj., **urosep′tic.**

urostealith (u″ro-ste″ah-lith) a urinary calculus having fatty constituents.

urotoxia (u″ro-tok′se-ah) 1. the toxicity of the urine. 2. the toxic substances of the urine. 3. the unit of toxicity of the urine or a quantity sufficient to kill 1 kg. of living substance. adj., **urotox′ic.**

urotoxin (u″ro-tok′sin) the toxic constituents of urine.

Urotropin (u-rot′ro-pin) trademark for a preparation of methanamine, an antibacterial used in urinary tract infections.

uroureter (u″ro-u-re′ter) distention of the ureter with urine.

uroxanthin (u″ro-zan′thin) a yellow pigment of normal urine convertible into indigo blue.

ursone (ur′sōn) a crystallizable compound found in the waxlike coatings of various fruits and leaves.

Urtica (er-ti′kah) a genus of plants, the true nettles, which are covered with stinging hairs and secrete a poisonous fluid. *U. dio′ica,* of temperate regions, has stimulant, diuretic, and hemostatic properties.

urticant (er′tĭ-kant) producing urticaria.

urticaria (ur″tĭ-ka′re-ah) a vascular reaction of the skin marked by transient appearance of slightly elevated patches (wheals) which are redder or paler than the surrounding skin and often attended by severe itching; called also hives. The exciting cause may be certain foods, infection, or emotional stress. adj., **urtica′rial.**

giant u., u. gigan′tea, angioneurotic edema.

u. hemorrhag′ica, purpura with urticaria.

u. medicamento′sa, that due to use of a drug.

papular u., u. papulo′sa, an allergic reaction to the bite of various insects, with appearance of lesions that evolve into inflammatory, increasingly hard, red or brownish, persistent papules.

u. pigmento′sa, mastocytosis manifested as persistent pink to brown macules or soft plaques of various size; pruritus and urtication occur on stroking the lesions.

u. pigmento′sa, juvenile, urticaria pigmentosa present at birth or in the first few weeks of life, usually disappearing before puberty, taking the form of a single nodule or tumor or of a disseminated eruption of yellowish brown to yellowish red macules, plaques, or bullae.

solar u., a rare form produced by exposure to sunlight.

urtication (ur″tĭ-ka′shun) 1. the development or formation of urticaria. 2. a burning sensation, as of the sting of nettles.

urushiol (u-roo′she-ol) the toxic irritant principle of poison ivy and various related plants.

USAEC United States Atomic Energy Commission.

USAN United States Adopted Name, a nonproprietary designation for any compound used as a drug, established by negotiation between its manufacturer and a council sponsored jointly by the American Medical Association, American Pharmaceutical Association, United States Pharmacopeial Convention, Inc., and The National Formulary.

U.S.P. United States Pharmacopeia, a legally recognized compendium of standards for drugs, published by the United States Pharmacopeial Convention, Inc., and revised periodically; it also includes assays and tests for determination of strength, quality, and purity.

U.S.P.H.S. United States Public Health Service (see also PUBLIC HEALTH).

ustilaginism (us″tĭ-laj′ĭ-nizm) a condition resembling ergotism due to ingestion of maize containing *Ustilago maydis.*

Ustilago (us′tĭ-la′go) the smuts, a genus of fungi parasitic on plants. *U. may′dis* causes corn smut and ustilaginism.

uter(o)- word element [L.], *uterus.*

uteralgia (u″ter-al′je-ah) pain in the uterus.

uterine (u′ter-in, u′ter-īn) pertaining to the uterus.

u. tube, a slender tube extending laterally from the uterus to the ovary on the same side, conveying ova to the cavity of the uterus and permitting passage of spermatozoa in the opposite direction; called also fallopian tube and oviduct. When the mature ovum leaves the ovary it enters the fringed opening of the uterine tube, through which it travels slowly to the uterus. When conception takes place, the tube is usually the site of fertilization.

Infertility may be a result of obstruction or infection within the uterine tubes; the principal infections are gonorrhea and tuberculosis. A rare occurrence is the growth of a tumor in a tube. The removal of one tube by surgery, or the failure of a tube to function, ordinarily leaves the other tube intact and able to perform its function in reproduction. Occasionally the fertilized ovum implants in the wall of the uterine tube; this results in an ectopic, or tubal, PREGNANCY.

uteroabdominal (u″ter-o-ab-dom′ĭ-nal) pertaining to the uterus and abdomen.

uterocervical (u″ter-o-ser′vĭ-kal) pertaining to the uterus and cervix uteri.

uterofixation (u″ter-o-fik-sa′shun) hysteropexy; surgical fixation of the uterus.

uterogenic (u″ter-o-jen′ik) formed in the uterus.

uterogestation (u″ter-o-jes-ta′shun) uterine gestation; normal pregnancy.

uterography (u″ter-og′rah-fe) x-ray examination of the uterus; hysterography.

uterolith (u′ter-o-lith″) a uterine calculus; hysterolith.

uterometer (u″ter-om′ĕ-ter) an instrument for measuring the uterus; hysterometer.

utero-ovarian (u″ter-o-o-va′re-an) pertaining to the uterus and ovary.

uteropexy (u′ter-o-pek″se) hysteropexy.

uteroplacental (u″ter-o-plah-sen′tal) pertaining to the placenta and uterus.

uteroplasty (u′ter-o-plas″te) plastic repair of the uterus.

uterorectal (u″ter-o-rek′tal) pertaining to or communicating with the uterus and rectum.

uterosacral (u″ter-o-sa′kral) pertaining to the uterus and sacrum.

uterosalpingography (u″ter-o-sal″ping-gog′rah-fe) roentgenography of the uterus and uterine tubes; hysterosalpingography.

uteroscope (u′ter-o-skōp″) an instrument for viewing the interior of the uterus; hysteroscope.

uterotomy (u″ter-ot′o-me) hysterotomy; incision of the uterus.

uterotonic (u″ter-o-ton′ik) 1. increasing the tone of uterine muscle. 2. a uterotonic agent.

uterotubal (u″ter-o-tu′bal) pertaining to the uterus and uterine tubes.

uterovaginal (u″ter-o-vaj′ĭ-nal) pertaining to the uterus and vagina.

uterovesical (u″ter-o-ves′ĭ-kal) pertaining to the uterus and bladder.

uterus (u′ter-us) the hollow muscular organ in female mammals in which the fertilized ovum normally becomes embedded and in which the developing embryo and fetus is nourished. The uterus, or womb, is normally about the size and shape of a pear. The upper part, or fundus, is broad and flattened; the middle portion is the body, or corpus; the lower part, or cervix, is narrow and tubular. The cervix opens downward into the VAGINA. TWO UTERINE TUBES enter the uterus at the upper end, one on each side.

The walls of the uterus are composed of muscle; its lining is mucous membrane. The muscular substance of the uterus is called the myometrium; the inner lining is called endometrium. Between puberty and menopause, the lining goes through a monthly cycle of growth and discharge, known as the MENSTRUAL CYCLE. Menstruation occurs when the tissue prepared by the uterus for a possible embryo or fertilized egg, is unused and passes out through the vagina.

The menstrual cycle is interrupted by pregnancy when a mature ovum is fertilized by a spermatozoon. Fertilization usually takes place in the uterine tube; the fertilized ovum continues moving along the tube and comes to rest in the uterus, where it implants in the endometrium. The endometrium then serves to anchor the placenta, which filters nutrients from the mother's blood into the blood of the growing fetus. (See also REPRODUCTION and REPRODUCTIVE ORGANS, FEMALE.)

DISORDERS OF THE UTERUS. The main organs of the female reproductive system—uterus, uterine tubes, and ovaries—are connected to each other by ligaments that normally hold each in its proper place. Occasionally childbirth causes displacement of the uterus. The ligaments may stretch and weaken enough to permit the uterus to bulge into the vagina. This is called a prolapsed uterus. Uterine displacement may give rise to difficulties in urination and at times in conception. Internal supportive pessaries are sometimes prescribed for these conditions. Some can be corrected surgically.

The uterus is a frequent site of cancer, both of the cervix and of the corpus of the uterus. Regular medical examinations help to detect such growths promptly, and early diagnosis makes for successful treatment. Any irregular vaginal bleeding or discharge may be a symptom of such a growth and should have prompt attention.

Benign growths in the uterine walls, LEIOMYOMAS (called myomas, fibroid tumors, or, colloquially, fibroids) are common, and are not removed unless they produce symptoms or threaten to interfere with a desired pregnancy. They may occur in any part of the uterus, although they are most frequent in the myometrium. Occasionally, fibrous tissues are intertwined with the muscle fibers of the tumor, particularly in older women.

Leiomyomas are often numerous, although a single tumor may occur. They are usually small but sometimes grow quite large and may fill the whole uterus. After menopause, their growth usually ceases. Large tumors may cause pressure on neighboring organs, such as the bladder. Symptoms vary according to the location and size of the tumors. As they grow, they may cause painful menstruation, profuse and irregular menstrual bleeding, vaginal discharge, or frequent urination, as well as irregular enlargement of the uterus. If the tumor becomes twisted, there may be severe pelvic pain. They may also be the cause of infertility.

In pregnancy, the tumors may interfere with the natural enlargement of the uterus with the growing fetus. They may also cause spontaneous abortion and death of the fetus. Those in the lower part of the uterus may block the birth canal, in which case cesarean section may be necessary.

Medical examination is wise if one or more of the symptoms mentioned occur. Small leiomyomas are usually left undisturbed and are checked at frequent intervals. Larger tumors may be removed surgically. In some instances, hysterectomy is performed. It is reassuring that only a small percentage of such tumors ever become malignant, usually in later life.

Other frequent disorders associated with the uterus are menstrual problems, including painful menstruation (DYSMENORRHEA) and excess blood flow (menorrhagia). These disorders are among the most common causes of temporary female disability and are often difficult to correct, but they may also be symptoms of serious conditions. Excessive menstruation may cause anemia.

SURGERY OF THE UTERUS. Surgical procedures involving the uterus include various operations for shortening the ligaments supporting the uterus, for the purpose of correcting uterine displacement, and hysterectomy, or surgical removal of the uterus.

Subtotal (simple) hysterectomy involves removal

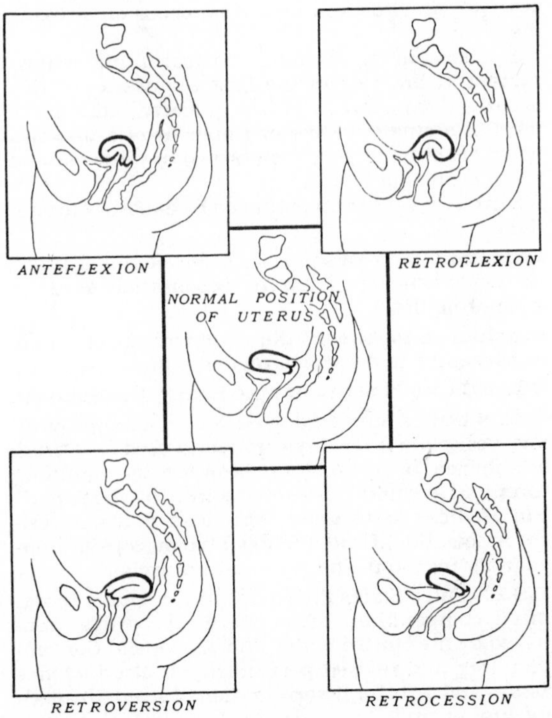

Types of forward and backward uterine displacements. (From Miller, N. F., and Avery, H.: Gynecology and Gynecologic Nursing. 5th ed. Philadelphia, W. B. Saunders Co., 1965.)

of all of the uterus except the cervix. This operation is most commonly performed in the case of a large leiomyoma. After the operation pregnancy is no longer possible and menstruation ceases, but glandular functions continue. MENOPAUSE does not occur prematurely, since the ovaries still produce estrogen and progesterone.

If the entire cervix as well as the corpus of the uterus is removed, the operation is called total (complete) hysterectomy. Sometimes one or both of the uterine tubes and the ovaries are removed as well. The operation is sometimes necessary in the case of benign conditions, such as cysts and large leiomyomas, and in malignant conditions.

As long as one ovary remains, menopause is not brought on by the operation. If both ovaries are removed, artificial menopause occurs; hormones or other medications may be given to facilitate this period of hormonal adjustment. Sexual activity is not affected.

Radical hysterectomy is one in which a portion of the vagina, the surrounding lymph nodes and the supporting ligaments of the pelvic organs are removed, in additon to the entire uterus. This operation may be performed in some cases of cancer of the cervix, although radiotherapy is usually preferred.

Usually in a hysterectomy the incision is made in the abdominal wall (abdominal hysterectomy), but in some instances the operation is performed by way of the vagina. A vaginal hysterectomy avoids the discomfort of an abdominal incision. This method may be used in certain benign conditions when other factors are favorable. When the cervix is not removed with the uterus, the procedure usually cannot be performed vaginally.

Patient Care. Preoperative procedures usually include complete shaving of the lower abdomen and perineum, administration of a cleansing enema and a vaginal douche the evening before surgery and restriction of food and fluids as for any other type of abdominal surgery.

Postoperatively, the patient is observed frequently for signs of hemorrhage. Although some serosanguineous discharge is to be expected, bleeding that exceeds a normal menstrual flow should be reported. The number of perineal pads soiled during a 8-hour period should be noted on the chart. Intra-abdominal bleeding may be recognized by such changes as restlessness, falling blood pressure, pallor, thirst, and excessive perspiration.

Complications to be avoided include thrombophlebitis, abdominal distention, and urinary retention. To avoid the development of a thrombus in the legs or pelvis the patient is encouraged to exercise her legs and to breathe deeply to improve pelvic circulation. Fowler's position and pillows beneath the knees are not allowed. Any complaint of pain, tenderness, or redness in the calf of the leg should be reported immediately. Early ambulation is the best preventive for most complications arising from a hysterectomy.

Abdominal distention is often avoided by insertion of a nasogastric tube prior to surgery. Urinary retention usually is prevented by insertion of a catheter while the patient is anesthetized; this is left in place until the third or fourth postoperative day.

Postoperative infection is relatively rare, but when it does occur the first symptoms develop about the third or fourth postoperative day. Elevation of temperature, malaise, and foul vaginal discharge are indicative of this complication.

utricle (u'trĭ-k'l) 1. any small sac. 2. the larger of the two divisions of the membranous labyrinth of the inner ear.

prostatic u., urethral u., a small blind pouch in the substance of the prostate.

utricular (u-trik'u-lar) 1. bladder-like. 2. pertaining to the utricle.

utriculitis (u-trik"u-li'tis) inflammation of the prostatic utricle or of the utricle of the ear.

utriculosaccular (u-trik"u-lo-sak'u-lar) pertaining to the utricle and saccule of the membranous labyrinth of the inner ear.

uve(o)- word element [L.], *uvea.*

uvea (u've-ah) [L.] the iris, ciliary body, and choroid together. adj., **u'veal.**

uveitis (u"ve-i'tis) inflammation of the uvea. adj., **uveit'ic.**

heterochromic u., heterochromic iridocyclitis.

sympathetic u., sympathetic opthalmia.

unveoparotid fever (u"ve-o-pah-rot'id) a manifestation of sarcoidosis, marked by chronic inflammation of the parotid gland and uvea, with chronic iridocyclitis, unilateral facial paralysis, lassitude, and a subfebrile temperature.

uveoparotitis (u"ve-o-par"o-ti'tis) unveoparotid fever.

uveoscleritis (u"ve-o-sklĕ-ri'tis) scleritis due to extension of uveitis.

uviform (u'vĭ-form) shaped like a grape.

uviofast (u've-o-fast") uvioresistant.

uviometer (u"ve-om'ĕ-ter) an instrument for measuring ultraviolet emanation.

uvioresistant (u"ve-o-re-zis'tant) resitant to or unaffected by ultraviolet rays; unviofast.

uviosensitive (u"ve-o-sen'sĭ-tiv) sensitive to ultraviolet rays.

uvula (u'vu-lah), pl. *u'vulae* [L.] a pendant, fleshy mass, specifically the palatine uvula. adj., **u'vular.**

u. of bladder, a rounded elevation at the neck of the bladder, formed by convergence of muscle fibers terminating in the urethra. Called also uvula vesicae.

u. cerebel'li, a lobule that is the posterior limit of the fourth ventricle of the brain. Called also uvula vermis.

u. palati'na, palatine u., the small, fleshy mass hanging from the soft palate above the root of the tongue.

u. ver'mis, the part of the vermis of the cerebellum between the pyramid and nodule.

u. vesi'cae, uvula of bladder.

uvulectomy (u"vu-lek'to-me) excision of the uvula.

uvulitis (u"vu-li'tis) inflammation of the uvula.

uvuloptosis (u"vu-lop-to'sis) a relaxed, pendulous state of the uvula.

uvulotomy (u"vu-lot'o-me) the cutting off of the uvula or a part of it.

V

V chemical symbol, *vanadium.*

V. vision; visual acuity.

v. vein, or [L.] *vena;* volt.

vaccigenous (vak-sij′ĕ-nus) producing vaccine.

vaccina (vak-si′nah) vaccinia.

vaccinable (vak-sin′ah-b′l) susceptible of being successfully vaccinated.

vaccinal (vak′sĭ-nal) 1. pertaining to vaccinia, to vaccine, or to vaccination. 2. having protective qualities when used by way of inoculation.

vaccinate (vak′sĭ-nāt) to inoculate with vaccine to produce immunity.

vaccination (vak″sĭ-na′shun) the introduction of vaccine into the body to produce immunity to a specific disease. The term vaccination comes from the Latin *vacca,* cow, and was coined when the first inoculations were given with organisms that caused the mild disease cowpox to produce immunity against smallpox. Today the word has the same meaning as inoculation and IMMUNIZATION.

vaccine (vak′sēn) a suspension of attenuated or killed microorganisms (viruses, bacteria, or rickettsiae), administered for prevention, amelioration, or treatment of infectious diseases.

autogenous v., a bacterial vaccine prepared from cultures of material derived from a lesion of the patient to be treated.

bacterial v., a preparation of attenuated or killed bacteria, used to increase immunity to the organisms injected, or sometimes for pyrogenetic effects in treatment of certain noninfectious diseases.

BCG v., a preparation used as an active immunizing agent against tuberculosis, consisting of a dried, living, avirulent culture of the Calmette-Guérin bacillus (see also BCG VACCINE).

v. lymph, material containing vaccinia virus collected from vaccinial vesicles of calves; used for active immunization against smallpox.

polyvalent v., one prepared from more than one strain or species of microorganisms.

vaccinia (vak-sin′e-ah) a viral disease of cattle; called also cowpox. When communicated to man, usually by vaccination, it confers immunity to SMALLPOX. Introduction of vaccinia virus for the purpose of immunization against smallpox results in a local reaction—a single lesion at the site of inoculation—or sometimes a general reaction.

In nonimmune patients a papule appears on the third or fourth day after inoculation. The lesion then changes to a vesicle (water-filled blister) and eventually to a pustule which lasts for about 12 days and then dries and forms a crust. During the following 7 days the crust detaches and leaves the characteristic vaccination scar.

Complications of vaccinia are rare. They include autoinoculation, in which other satellite lesions may appear over the body, secondary infection with streptococci or staphylococci, and postvaccinal encephalitis. Eczema vaccinatum can occur in persons in whom skin lesions of eczema are present at the time of vaccination. The eruption becomes generalized, particularly in the area where the primary dermatitis was located. To avoid this complication vaccination is contraindicated in patients who have eczema or other skin disorders.

No special treatment or dressing is required for the vaccinia. The lesion should be kept dry and open to the air.

v. gangreno′sa, generalized vaccinia marked by failure to develop antibodies against the virus (due to agammaglobulinemia), with spreading necrosis at the site and metastasis of lesions throughout the body.

generalized v., a condition of widespread vaccinal lesions resulting from sensitivity response to smallpox vaccination and delayed production of neutralizing antibodies.

progressive v., vaccinia gangrenosa.

vaccinial (vak-sin′e-al) pertaining to or characteristic of vaccinia (cowpox).

vacciniform (vak-sin′ĭ-form) resembling vaccinia.

vacciniola (vak″sĭ-ne-o′lah) generalized vaccinia.

vaccinotherapy (vak″sĭ-no-ther′ah-pe) therapeutic use of vaccines.

vacuolar (vak′u-o″lar) containing, or of the nature of, vacuoles.

vacuolated (vak′u-o-lāt″ed) containing vacuoles.

vacuolation (vak″u-o-la′shun) the process of forming vacuoles; the condition of being vacuolated.

vacuole (vak′u-ōl) a space or cavity in the protoplasm of a cell.

contractile v., a small fluid-filled cavity in the protoplasm of certain unicellular organisms; it gradually increases in size and then collapses, its function is thought to be respiratory and excretory.

vacuolization (vak″u-o-lĭ-za′shun) vacuolation.

vacuum (vak′u-um) a space devoid of air or other gas.

vagabond's disease discoloration of the skin in persons subjected to louse bites over long periods.

vagal (va′gal) pertaining to the vagus nerve.

v. attack, vasovagal attack.

vagina (vah-ji′nah) 1. any sheath or sheathlike structure. 2. the canal in the female, from the external genitalia (vulva) to the cervix uteri. The adult vagina is normally about 3 inches long and slopes upward and backward. Internally, the bladder is in front of the vagina and the rectum in back.

The vagina receives the erect penis in coitus. The spermatozoa are discharged into the vagina, swim through the cervical canal, and enter the uterus. The vagina is also the passage for menstrual discharge and functions as the birth canal.

The interior lining of the vagina is mucous membrane. Muscles and fibrous tissue form the vaginal walls. In pregnancy, changes occur in these tissues, enabling the vagina to stretch to many times its usual size during labor and childbirth.

In a virgin, the opening of the vagina is usually, but not necessarily, partially closed by a membrane, the hymen. Usually the hymen breaks at first intercourse; occasionally it ruptures during physical exercise.

In a normal state, the lining of the vagina secretes a fluid that is fermented to an acid by the bacteria that are usually present. This acidity probably helps to protect the vagina from invasion by other organisms. Douching as a regular practice should not be employed except when recommended by a physician.

Disorders of the Vagina. Symptoms of vaginal disorders include excessive discharge, soreness and burning, ulceration, pain on intercourse, itching, bleeding, swelling, and growths. A physician should be consulted for any of these complaints.

Infection is the most common cause of vaginal disease. A frequent chronic infection is caused by a protozoon called *Trichomonas vaginalis.* A yeast-like fungus, *Candida albicans,* causes another type of infectious vaginitis (candidiasis). The vagina may also be affected by gonorrhea, syphilis, and other venereal diseases. Diabetes mellitus may predispose a woman to vaginal infection.

Trauma during childbirth may damage the vagina. After menopause, the mucous lining tends to dry out and become irritated easily. Cysts and cancers may form in the vagina. Occasionally a fistula, or abnormal passage, may develop between the vagina and the bladder or rectum.

Vaginal Examination. Since cancer of the female reproductive organs is a relatively common occurrence and is curable if detected early, physicians recommend that women of reproductive age and beyond have a periodic vaginal or pelvis examination. Such an examination is also necessary during pregnancy and labor and in the postpartum examination 6 to 8 weeks after childbirth. This is a simple procedure that is rarely uncomfortable if the woman understands its purpose.

The patient lies on her back on a special table with her legs raised and spread by stirrups. The physician inserts a speculum to spread the vagina open. He is able to observe the cervix and the lining of the vagina directly, and may take smears for microscopic examination to detect infection or cancer. (See also PAPANICOLAOU TEST.)

After removing the speculum the examiner inserts rubber-gloved fingers into the vagina and places the other hand on the abdomen. In this way he is able to palpate the female reproductive organs, including the uterus and ovaries, between his hands. These organs are otherwise difficult or impossible to examine.

Patient Care. The patient should be prepared physically and emotionally for a vaginal examination. Since relaxation and cooperation of the patient are important to the success of the examination, she should be given a brief explanation of the procedure and encouraged to ask questions before the procedure is begun. The patient is draped with a top sheet so that the legs are covered and only the vulva is exposed. Privacy must be assured immediately before and during the examination. Equipment such as gloves, lubricant, vaginal speculum, and supplies needed for collecting specimens should be assembled before the examination is begun. After the examination is completed, the patient is assisted from the table.

Ideally, a vaginal examination should be done between menstrual periods; however, vaginal bleeding is not a contraindication to this procedure. Patients should be told this so that they will not postpone an appointment for examination when vaginal bleeding persists. They also should be instructed to avoid douching immediately before a vaginal examination as this may remove secretions that can be useful in diagnosis.

vaginal (vaj'ĭ-nal) pertaining to the vagina, the tunica vaginalis testis, or to any sheath.

vaginalectomy (vaj"ĭ-nal-ek'to-me) vaginectomy.

vaginalitis (vaj'ĭ-nal-i'tis) inflammation of the tunica vaginalis testis; periorchitis.

vaginate (vaj'ĭ-nāt) enclosed in a sheath.

vaginectomy (vaj"ĭ-nek'to-me) 1. resection of the tunica vaginalis testis. 2. excision of the vagina.

vaginismus (vaj"ĭ-niz'mus) painful spasms of the muscles of the vagina.

vaginitis (vaj"ĭ-ni'tis) 1. inflammation of the vagina; colpitis. 2. inflammation of a sheath.

adhesive v., that in which ulceration and exfoliation of the mucosa result in adhesions of the membranes.

atrophic v., that in postmenopausal women, with thinning and, often, ulceration of the vaginal epithelium; it may progress to adhesive vaginitis.

desquamative inflammatory v., a form resembling atrophic vaginitis but affecting women with normal estrogen levels.

emphysematous v., a variety marked by the formation of gas in the meshes of the connective tissue.

senile v., atrophic vaginitis.

vaginoabdominal (vaj"ĭ-no-ab-dom'ĭ-nal) pertaining to the vagina and abdomen.

vaginocele (vaj'ĭ-no-sēl") colpocele; vaginal hernia.

vaginodynia (vaj"ĭ-no-din'e-ah) pain in the vagina.

vaginofixation (vaj"ĭ-no-fik-sa'shun) vaginopexy; colpopexy.

vaginolabial (vaj"ĭ-no-la'be-al) pertaining to the vagina and labia.

vaginomycosis (vaj"ĭ-no-mi-ko'sis) any fungal disease of the vagina.

vaginopathy (vaj"ĭ-nop'ah-the) any disease of the vagina.

vaginoperineal (vaj"ĭ-no-per"ĭ-ne'al) pertaining to the vagina and perineum.

vaginoperineorrhaphy (vaj"ĭ-no-per"ĭ-ne-or'ah-fe) suture of the vagina and perineum; colpoperineorrhaphy.

vaginoperineotomy (vaj"ĭ-no-per"ĭ-ne-ot'o-me) incision of the vagina and perineum.

vaginoperitoneal (vaj"ĭ-no-per"ĭ-to-ne'al) pertaining to the vagina and peritoneum.

vaginopexy (vah-ji'no-pek"se) colpopexy; vaginofixation; suturing of the vagina to the abdominal wall in cases of vaginal relaxation.

vaginoplasty (vah-ji'no-plas"te) colpoplasty; plastic repair of the vagina.

vaginotomy (vaj"ĭ-not'o-me) colpotomy; incision of the vagina.

vaginovesical (vaj"ĭ-no-ves'ĭ-kal) pertaining to the vagina and bladder.

vagitus (vah-ji'tus) the cry of an infant.

v. uteri'nus, the cry of an infant in the uterus.

vagolysis (va-gol'ĭ-sis) surgical lysis of the vagus nerve.

vagolytic (va"go-lit'ik) having an effect resembling that produced by interruption of impulses transmitted by the vagus nerve; parasympatholytic.

vagomimetic (va″go-mi-met′ik) having an effect resembling that produced by stimulation of the vagus nerve.

vagotomy (va-got′o-me) interruption of the impulses carried by the vagus nerve or nerves; so called because it was first performed by surgical methods. The surgical procedure is done as part of the treatment of gastric or duodenal ULCER and often is performed in combination with gastroenterostomy or partial gastrectomy. The vagus nerve stimulates gastric secretion and affects gastric motility. Vagotomy thus reduces secretion of gastric juices and decreases physical activity of the stomach.

medical v., interruption of impulses carried by the vagus nerve by administration of suitable drugs.

vagotonia (va″go-to′ne-ah) irritability of the vagus nerve, characterized by vasomotor instability, sweating, disordered peristalsis, and muscle spasms. adj., **vagoton′ic.**

vagotonin (va-got′o-nin) a preparation of hormone from the pancreas that increases vagal tone, slows the heart, and increases the store of glycogen in the liver.

vagotropic (va″go-trop′ik) having an effect on the vagus nerve.

vagovagal (va″go-va′gal) arising as a result of afferent and efferent impulses mediated through the vagus nerve.

vagus nerve (va′gus) the tenth cranial nerve; it has the most extensive distribution of the cranial nerves, serving structures of the chest and abdomen as well as the head and neck.

Afferent fibers of the vagus nerve serve the mucous membrane of the larynx, trachea, and bronchi, lungs, arch of the aorta, esophagus, and stomach. Some of the functions affected by this nerve are coughing, sneezing, reflex inhibitions of the heart rate, and the sensation of hunger.

Motor fibers of the vagus nerve are concerned with swallowing, speech, peristalsis, and secretions from the glands of the stomach and the pancreas and contractions of the trachea, bronchi, and bronchioles.

vagusstoff (va′gus-stof) a substance liberated by the vagus nerve endings that inhibits cardiac activity; probably identical to acetylcholine.

valence (va′lens) the numerical measure of the capacity to combine; in chemistry, an expression of the number of atoms of hydrogen (or its equivalent) that one atom of a chemical element can hold in combination, if negative, or displace in a reaction, if positive; in immunology, an expression of the number of antigenic determinants with which one molecule of a given antibody can combine.

valethamate (val-eth′ah-māt) an anticholinergic used in the form of the bromide salt as an antispasmodic in hypermotility and spasm of the gastrointestinal, genitourinary, and biliary tracts.

valgus (val′gus) [L.] bent outward; twisted; denoting a deformity in which the angulation is away from the midline of the body, as in talipes valgus.

valine (va′lēn) a naturally occurring amino acid, one of those essential for human metabolism.

valinemia (val″ĭ-ne′me-ah) elevated levels of valine in the blood and urine.

Valium (val′e-um) trademark for a preparation of diazepam, a tranquilizer and skeletal muscle relaxant.

vallate (val′āt) having a wall or rim; rim-shaped.

vallecula (vah-lek′u-lah), pl. *vallec′ulae* [L.] a depression or furrow.

v. cerebel′li, a longitudinal fissure on the inferior cerebellum, in which the medulla oblongata rests.

v. syl′vii, a depression made by the fissure of Sylvius at the base of the brain.

v. un′guis, the sulcus of the matrix of the nail.

vallestril (val-les′tril) trademark for a preparation of methallenestril, an estrogenic compound.

Valleix's points (vahl-lāz′) tender points along the course of certain nerves in neuralgia; called also puncta dolorosa.

Valley fever coccidioidomycosis.

Valmid (val′mid) trademark for a preparation of ethinamate, sedative.

Valsalva's maneuver (val-sal′vahz) increase of intrathoracic pressure by forcible exhalation against the closed glottis. The maneuver causes a trapping of blood in the great veins, preventing it from entering the chest and right atrium. When the breath is released, the intrathoracic pressure drops and the trapped blood is quickly propelled through the heart, producing an increase in the heart rate (tachycardia) and the blood pressure. Immediately after this event a reflex bradycardia ensues.

Valsalva's maneuver occurs when one strains to defecate and urinate, uses his arm and upper trunk muscles to move up in bed, or strains during coughing, gagging, or vomiting. The increased pressure, immediate tachycardia, and reflex bradycardia can bring about cardiac arrest in vulnerable heart patients.

value (val′u) a measure of worth or efficiency; a quantitative measurement of the activity, concentration, etc., of specific substances.

normal v's, the range in concentration of specific substances found in normal healthy tissues, secretions, etc.

valva (val′vah,), pl. *val′vae* [L.] a valve.

valve (valv) a membranous fold in a canal or passage that prevents backward flow of material passing through it.

aortic v., that guarding the entrance to the aorta from the left ventricle.

atrioventricular v's, the valves between the right atrium and right ventricle (tricuspid valve) and the left atrium and left ventricle (mitral valve).

bicuspid v., mitral valve.

cardiac v's, valves that control flow of blood through and from the heart.

coronary v., a valve at entrance of the coronary sinus into right atrium.

ileocecal v., ileocolic v., that guarding the opening between the ileum and cecum.

mitral v., that between the left atrium and left ventricle, usually having two cusps (anterior and posterior).

pulmonary v., that at the entrance of the pulmonary trunk from the right ventricle.

pyloric v., a prominent fold of mucous membrane at the pyloric orifice of the stomach.

semilunar v's, valves made up of semilunar segments or cusps (valvulae semilunares), guarding the entrances into the aorta and pulmonary trunk from the cardiac ventricles.

thebesian v., coronary valve.

tricuspid v., that guarding the opening between the right atrium and right ventricle.

valvotomy (val-vot′o-me) incision of a valve.

valvula (val′vu-lah), pl. *val′vulae* [L.] a small valve.

valvular (val′vu-lar) pertaining to, affecting or of the nature of a valve.

valvulitis (val″vu-li′tis) inflammation of a valve, especially of a valve of the heart.

valvuloplasty (val′vu-lo-plas″te) plastic repair of a valve, especially a valve of the heart.

valvulotome (val′vu-lo-tōm″) an instrument for cutting a valve.

valvulotomy (val″vu-lot′o-me) valvotomy.

vanadium (vah-na′de-um) a chemical element, atomic number 23, atomic weight 50.942, symbol V. (See table of ELEMENTS.) Its salts have been used in treating various diseases. Absorption of its compounds, usually via the lungs, causes chronic intoxication, the symptoms of which include respiratory tract irritation, pneumonitis, conjunctivitis, and anemia.

vanadiumism (vah-na′de-um-izm″) poisoning by vanadium.

Vancocin (van′ko-sin) trademark for a preparation of vancomycin, an antibiotic.

vancomycin (van″ko-mi′sin) an antibiotic produced by *Streptomyces orientalis,* highly effective against gram-positive bacteria, especially against staphylococci; it is used as the hydrochloride salt. The toxic effects are quite severe and include damage to the eighth cranial (vestibulocochlear) nerve and renal disorders.

van den Bergh test (van den berg′) a laboratory test done to determine the concentration of BILIRUBIN in the blood. Blood is obtained by finger prick or venipuncture. Preparation of the patient requires only that he be in a fasting state. Normal range for this test is: direct bilirubin—0.0 to 0.1 mg. per 100 ml. of serum; total bilirubin—0.2 to 1.4 mg. per 100 ml. of serum.

van der Hoeve's syndrome (van der hōvz) see OSTEOGENESIS IMPERFECTA.

Van der Waals forces the relatively weak, short-range forces of attraction existing between atoms and molecules, which results in the attraction of nonpolar organic compounds to each other (hydrophobic bonding).

vanilla (vah-nil′ah) cured, full-grown, unripe fruit of species of *Vanilla;* used as a flavoring agent.

vanillin (vah-nil′in) a flavoring agent derived from vanilla and other plants or produced synthetically.

vanillism (vah-nil′izm) dermatitis, coryza, and malaise seen in handlers of raw vanilla, due to the mite *Acarus siro.*

vanillylmandelic acid (vah-nil″il-man-del′ik) an excretory product of the catecholamines, used as a test for epinephrine metabolism.

Vanogel (van′o-jel) trademark for an aqueous suspension of aluminum hydroxide gel, an antacid.

van't Hoff's rule (law) (vant-hofs′) the velocity of chemical reactions is increased twofold or more for each rise of 10° C. in temperature.

vapor (va′por) steam, gas, or exhalation.

vaporization (va″por-ĭ-za′shun) 1. the conversion of a solid or liquid into a vapor without chemical change; distillation. 2. treatment by vapors; vapotherapy.

vaporize (va′por-īz) to convert into vapor or to be transformed into vapor.

vapotherapy (va″po-ther′ah-pe) therapeutic use of steam, vapor, or spray.

Vaquez's disease (vah-kāz′) polycythemia vera.

varicella (var″ĭ-sel′ah) chickenpox.

varicelliform (var″ĭ-sel′ĭ-form) resembling chickenpox.

varices (var′ĭ-sēz) [L.] plural of *varix.*

variciform (vah-ris′ĭ-form) resembling a varix; varicose.

varicoblepharon (var″ĭ-ko-blef′ah-ron) a varicose swelling of the eyelid.

varicocele (var′ĭ-ko-sēl″) varicosity of the pampiniform plexus of the spermatic cord, forming a scrotal swelling that feels like a "bag of worms."

varicocelectomy (var″ĭ-ko-se-lek′to-me) excision of a varicocele.

varicography (var″ĭ-kog′rah-fe) x-ray visualization of varicose veins.

varicomphalos (var″ĭ-kom′fah-los) a varicose tumor of the umbilicus.

varicophlebitis (var″ĭ-ko-flĕ-bi′tis) varicose veins with inflammation.

varicose (var′ĭ-kōs) of the nature of or pertaining to a varix; unnaturally and permanently distended (said of a vein); variciform.

v. veins, swollen, distended, and knotted veins, usually in the subcutaneous tissues of the leg. They result from a stagnated or sluggish flow of the blood, in combination with defective valves and weakened walls of the veins.

Varicose veins occur most frequently in those who must stand or sit motionless for long periods of time. Pregnancy is sometimes responsible for the development of the condition. It also appears that a tendency to develop varicose veins may be inherited.

CAUSES. Blood returning to the heart from the legs must flow upward through the veins, against the pull of gravity. This blood is "milked" upward principally by the massaging action of the muscles against the veins. To prevent the blood from flowing backward, the veins contain flaplike valves, located at frequent intervals and operating in pairs. When the blood is flowing toward the heart, the venous valves are open and the blood can move freely. If the blood should attempt to flow backward, the valves close, effectively stopping the reverse movement of the blood.

Prolonged periods of standing or sitting without movement place a heavy strain on the veins. Without the massaging action of the muscles, the blood tends to back up. The weight of blood continually pressing downward against the closed venous valves causes the veins to distend; after a time, they lose their natural elasticity. When a number of valves no longer function efficiently, the blood collects in the veins, which gradually become swollen and more distended.

During pregnancy, more force often is necessary to push the blood through the veins because the pregnant uterus tends to press against the veins coming from the legs and thus prevents the free flow of blood. This increased back pressure can result in varicose veins.

SYMPTOMS. The development of varicose veins is

usually gradual. There may be feelings of fatigue in the legs and leg cramps at night; a continual dull ache may develop in the legs, and the ankles may swell.

If the condition is untreated and allowed to spread, as it often does, the veins become thick and hard to the touch, and dull or stabbing pains may be felt in time. Because of impaired circulation ulcers often develop on the lower legs.

TREATMENT. Treatment of mild cases of varicose veins includes rest periods at intervals during the day; the patient lies flat with his feet raised slightly above his body. Bathing the legs in warm water helps to stimulate the flow of blood, as does exercise. The daily routine should be changed to allow movement and changes in posture; even a brief walk will stimulate circulation grown stagnant during a time of standing or sitting in one position. Stockings lightly reinforced with elastic can be worn to help support the veins in the legs. Heavy elastic stockings, however, should be fitted and worn only under medical supervision, for if they do not fit correctly they may aggravate the condition by further restricting the flow of blood.

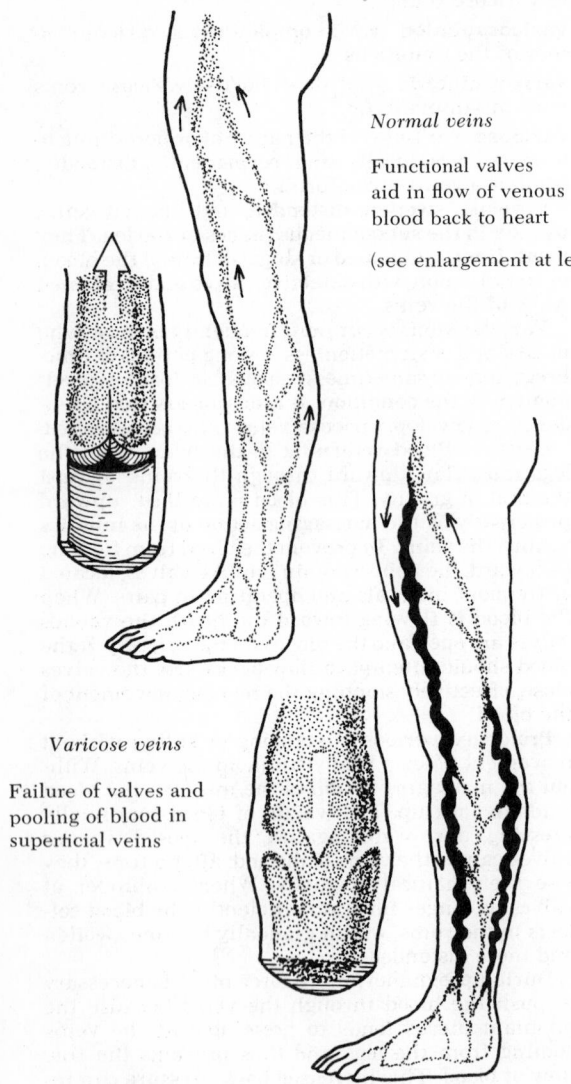

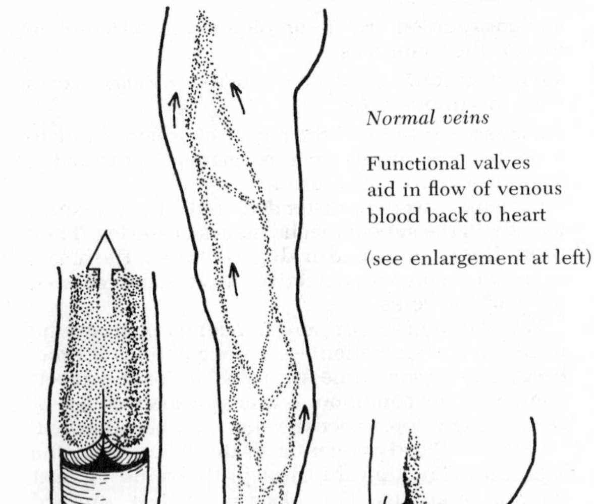

Comparison of normal veins and varicose veins in the leg.

Injections. Certain cases of varicose veins that have developed past the stage at which exercise and rest are helpful may be treated by injections of a hardening, or sclerosing, solution into the affected veins. A few hours after this treatment, which usually can be performed in the physician's office, the injected veins become hard, tender to the touch and painful. The pain subsides within a few days, however, and in about 2 months the varicose veins atrophy while the blood is channeled into other veins leading toward the heart.

The number of injections necessary depends upon the extent of the condition, and this form of treatment usually is not recommended for advanced cases because it has been found that in such cases recurrence is likely after a varying period of time following the injections.

Surgery. Varicose veins can cause much discomfort. The poor circulation involved means that any break in the skin of the leg is likely to develop into an ulcer that is painful and heals slowly and with difficulty. Therefore, chronic or well-advanced varicose conditions are best treated surgically. The operation consists of ligating (tying off) the affected vein and removing it.

PREVENTION. Regular leg exercises or long walks will stimulate the flow of blood through the legs. Those who have a predisposition to varicose veins should make such activities a part of their regular routine. If possible, they should avoid occupations that require them to stand or sit motionless for long periods of time, or should make it a point to walk about and exercise their leg muscles at frequent intervals during working hours. Tight stockings or garters should not be worn, nor should clothing that fits tightly or binds.

varicosity (var″ĭ-kos′ĭ-te) 1. a varicose condition; the quality or fact of being varicose. 2. a varix, or varicose vein.

varicotomy (var″ĭ-kot′o-me) excision of a varix or of a varicose vein.

varicula (vah-rik′u-lah) a varix of the conjunctiva.

Varidase (var′ĭ-dās) trademark for preparations of streptokinase-streptodornase, used as a proteolytic and fibrinolytic agent, for enzymatic débridement.

variety (vah-ri′ĕ-te) a taxonomic subcategory of a species.

variola (vah-ri′o-lah) smallpox. adj., **vari′olar, vari′olous.**

v. mi′nor, a mild form of smallpox having a low fatality rate.

variolate (va′re-o-lāt) 1. having the nature of appearance of smallpox. 2. to inoculate with smallpox virus.

variolation (va″re-o-la′shun) inoculation, application, or ingestion of crusts of dried variola pustules to produce immunity to natural infection by the virus of smallpox.

varioliform (va″re-o′lĭ-form) resembling smallpox.

varioloid (va′re-o-loid″) a modified and mild form of smallpox occurring in a person who has had a previous attack or has been vaccinated.

varix (vār′iks), pl. *var′ices* [L.] an enlarged, tortuous vein, artery, or lymphatic vessel.

aneurysmal v., a markedly dilated tortuous vessel;

sometimes used to denote a form of arteriovenous aneurysm in which the blood flows directly into a neighboring vein without the intervention of a connecting sac.

arterial v., a racemose aneurysm or varicose artery.

esophageal varices, varicosities of branches of the azygous vein which anastomose with tributaries of the portal vein in the lower esophagus, due to portal hypertension in cirrhosis of the liver.

lymph v., v. lymphat'icus, a soft, lobulated swelling of a lymph node, due to obstruction of lymphatic vessels.

varolian (vah-ro'le-an) pertaining to the pons varolii.

varus (va'rus) [L.] bent inward; denoting a deformity in which the angulation of the part is toward the midline of the body, as in talipes varus.

vas (vas), pl. *va'sa* [L.] a vessel. adj., **va'sal.**

v. aber'rans, 1. a blind tube sometimes connected with the epididymis; a vestigial mesonephric tube. 2. any anomalous or unusual vessel.

va'sa afferen'tia, vessels that convey fluid to a structure or part.

va'sa bre'via, short gastric arteries.

v. def'erens, the excretory duct of the testis, which unites with the excretory duct of the seminal vesicle to form the ejaculatory duct; called also ductus deferens.

va'sa efferen'tia, vessels that convey fluid away from a structure or part.

va'sa lymphat'ica, lymphatic vessels.

va'sa prae'via, the presentation, in front of the fetal head during labor, of the blood vessels of the umbilical cord where they enter the placenta.

va'sa rec'ta, long U-shaped vessels arising from the efferent glomerular arterioles of juxtamedullary nephrons and supplying the renal medulla.

va'sa vaso'rum, the small nutrient arteries and veins in the walls of the larger blood vessels.

vas(o)- word element [L.], *vessel; duct.*

vascular (vas'ku-lar) pertaining to blood vessels or indicative of a copious blood supply.

vascularity (vas″ku-lar'ĭ-te) the condition of being vascular.

vascularization (vas″ku-lar-ĭ-za'shun) the formation of new blood vessels in tissues.

vascularize (vas'ku-lar-īz″) to supply with vessels.

vasculature (vas'ku-lah-tūr″) 1. the vascular system of the body, or any part of it. 2. the supply of vessels to a specific region.

vasculitis (vas″ku-li'tis) inflammation of a vessel; angiitis.

vasculopathy (vas″ku-lop'ah-the) any disorder of blood vessels.

vasectomy (vah-sek'to-me) excision of the vas (ductus) deferens, or a portion of it; bilateral vasectomy results in sterility.

vasifactive (vas″ĭ-fak'tiv) vasoformative.

vasiform (vas'ĭ-form) resembling a vessel.

vasitis (vas-i'tis) inflammation of the vas (ductus) deferens.

vasoactive (vas″o-ak'tiv) exerting an effect on the caliber of blood vessels.

vasoconstriction (vas″o-kon-strik'shun) decrease in the caliber of blood vessels. adj., **vasoconstric'tive.**

vasoconstrictor (vas″o-kon-strik'tor) 1. causing constriction of the blood vessels. 2. a vasoconstrictive agent.

vasodentin (vas″o-den'tin) dentin provided with blood vessels, as in the teeth of some fishes.

vasodepression (vas″o-de-presh'un) decrease in vascular resistance with hypotension.

vasodepressor (vas″o-de-pres'sor) 1. having the effect of lowering the blood pressure through reduction in peripheral resistance. 2. an agent that causes vasodepression.

Vasodilan (vas″o-di'lan) trademark for preparations of isoxsuprine, a vasodilator.

vasodilatation (vas″o-dil″ah-ta'shun) a state of increased caliber of blood vessels. adj., **vasodi'lative.**

vasodilation (vas″o-di-la'shun) increase in the caliber of blood vessels.

vasodilator (vas″o-di-la'tor) 1. causing dilation of blood vessels. 2. a nerve or agent that causes dilation of blood vessels.

vasoepididymostomy (vas″o-ep″ĭ-did″ĭ-mos'to-me) anastomosis of the vas (ductus) deferens and the epididymis.

vasoformative (vas″o-for'mah-tive) pertaining to or promoting the formation of blood vessels.

vasoganglion (vas″o-gang'gle-on) a vascular ganglion or rete.

vasography (vas-og'rah-fe) roentgenography of the blood vessels.

vasohypertonic (vas″o-hi″per-ton'ik) vasoconstrictor.

vasohypotonic (vas″o-hi″po-ton'ik) vasodilator.

vasoinhibitor (vas″o-in-hib'ĭ-tor) an agent that inhibits vasomotor nerves. adj., **vasoinhib'itory.**

vasoligation (vas″o-li-ga'shun) ligation of the vas (ductus) deferens.

vasomotion (vas″o-mo'shun) change in caliber of blood vessels.

vasomotor (vas″o-mo'tor) 1. having an effect on the caliber of blood vessels. 2. a vasomotor agent or nerve.

vasoneuropathy (vas″o-nu-rop'ah-the) a condition caused by combined vascular and neurologic defect, resulting from simultaneous action or interaction of the vascular and nervous systems.

vasoneurosis (vas″o-nu-ro'sis) angioneurosis.

vaso-orchidostomy (vas″o-or″kĭ-dos'to-me) anastomosis of the epididymis to the severed end of the vas (ductus) deferens.

vasoparesis (vas″o-pah-re'sis) paralysis of vasomotor nerves.

vasopressin (vas″o-pres'in) a hormone secreted by cells of the hypothalamic nuclei and stored in the posterior pituitary for release as necessary; it constricts blood vessels, raising the blood pressure, and increases peristalsis, exerts some influence on the uterus, and influences resorption of water by the kidney tubules, resulting in concentration of urine. Also prepared synthetically or obtained from the posterior pituitary of domestic animals; used as an antidiuretic. Called also antidiuretic hormone.

vasopressor (vas″o-pres'or) 1. stimulating contraction of the muscular tissue of the capillaries and arteries. 2. a vasopressor agent.

vasopuncture (vas″o-pungk′tūr) surgical puncture of the vas (ductus) deferens.

vasoreflex (vas″o-re′fleks) a reflex of blood vessels.

vasorelaxation (vas″o-re″lak-sa′shun) decrease of vascular pressure.

vasorrhaphy (vas-or′ah-fe) suture of the vas (ductus) deferens.

vasosection (vas″o-sek′shun) the severing of a vessel or vessels, especially of the vasa deferentia (ductus deferentes).

vasosensory (vas″o-sen′so-re) supplying sensory filaments to the vessels.

vasospasm (vas′o-spazm) spasm of blood vessels, decreasing their caliber. adj., **vasospas′tic.**

vasostimulant (vas″o-stim′u-lant) stimulating vasomotor action.

vasostomy (vah-sos′to-me) surgical formation of an opening into the ductus (vas) deferens.

vasotomy (vah-sot′o-me) incision of the vas (ductus) deferens.

vasotonia (vas″o-to′ne-ah) tone or tension of the vessels.

vasotonic (vas″o-ton′ik) pertaining to, characterized by, or increasing vasotonia.

vasotrophic (vas″o-trof′ik) affecting nutrition through alterations of the caliber of the blood vessels.

vasotropic (vas″o-trop′ik) exerting an influence on the blood vessels, causing either constriction or dilatation.

vasovagal (vas″o-va′gal) vascular and vagal.

v. attack, v. syncope, a transient vascular and neurogenic reaction marked by pallor, nausea, sweating, bradycardia, and rapid fall in arterial blood pressure which, when below a critical level, results in loss of consciousness and characteristic electroencephalographic changes. It is most often evoked by emotional stress associated with fear or pain. Called also vagal attack.

vasovasostomy (vas″o-vah-sos′to-me) anastomosis of the ends of the severed vas (ductus) deferens.

vasovesiculectomy (vas″o-vě-sik″u-lek′to-me) excision of the vas (ductus) deferens and seminal vesicle.

Vasoxyl (vas-ok′sil) trademark for preparations of methoxamine, an adrenergic vasopressor.

vastus (vas′tus) [L.] great.

Vater's papilla (fah′terz) major duodenal papilla.

V.C. 1. vital capacity. 2. acuity of color vision.

V-Cillin (ve-sil′in) trademark for preparations of phenoxymethyl penicillin.

V.D. venereal disease.

V.D.G. venereal disease—gonorrhea.

V.D.H. valvular disease of the heart.

V.D.R.L. Venereal Disease Research Laboratory.

V.D.S. venereal disease—syphilis.

vection (vek′shun) the carrying of disease germs from an infected person to a well person.

vectis (vek′tis) a curved lever for making traction on the fetal head in labor.

vector (vek′tor) 1. a carrier, especially the animal (usually an arthropod) which transfers an infective agent from one host to another. The mosquito, which carries the malaria parasite, *Plasmodium,* from man to man, and the tsetse fly, which carries trypanosomes from beast to man, are vectors, as are dogs, bats, and other animals that transmit the rabies virus to man. 2. a quantity possessing magnitude, direction, and sense (positivity or negativity), and commonly represented by a straight line resembling an arrow: the length of the line denotes magnitude, the arrowhead denotes direction, and the position of the line with respect to an axis of reference denotes sense. adj., **vecto′rial.**

biologic v., an arthropod vector in whose body the infecting organism develops or multiplies before becoming infective to the recipient individual.

mechanical v., an arthropod vector that transmits the infective organisms from one host to another but is not essential to the life cycle of the parasite.

vectorcardiogram (vek″tor-kor′de-o-gram″) the record, usually a photograph, of the loop formed on the oscilloscope in vectorcardiography.

vectorcardiography (vek″tor-kar″de-og′rah-fe) the registration, usually by formation of a loop on an oscilloscope, of the direction and magnitude (vector) of the moment-to-moment electromotive forces of the heart during one complete cycle. adj., **vectorcardiograph′ic.**

vegan (vej′an) a vegetarian who excludes from his diet all protein of animal origin.

veganism (vej′ah-nizm) strict adherence to a vegetable diet, with exclusion of all protein of animal origin.

vegetable (vej′ĕ-tah-b′l) 1. pertaining to or derived from plants. 2. any plant or species of plant, especially one cultivated as a source of food.

vegetal (vej′ĕ-tal) 1. pertaining to plants or a plant. 2. vegetative.

vegetarian (vej″ĕ-ta′re-an) one who eats only foods of vegetable origin.

vegetarianism (vej″ĕ-ta′re-ah-nizm″) the restriction of one's food to substances of vegetable origin.

vegetation (vej″ĕ-ta′shun) any plantlike fungoid neoplasm or growth; a luxuriant fungus-like growth of pathologic tissue.

vegetative (vej′ĕ-ta″tiv) 1. concerned with growth and nutrition. 2. functioning involuntarily or unconsciously. 3. resting; denoting the portion of a cell cycle during which the cell is not replicating.

vegetoanimal (vej″ĕ-to-an′ĭ-mal) common to plants and animals.

vehicle (ve′ĭ-k′l) 1. a transporting agent, especially the component of a medication (prescription) serving as a solvent or to increase the bulk or decrease the concentration of the mixture. 2. any medium through which an impulse is propagated.

veil (vāl) 1. a covering structure. 2. a caul or piece of amniotic sac occasionally covering the face of a newborn child. 3. slight huskiness of the voice.

vein (vān) a vessel through which blood passes from various organs or parts back to the heart, in the systemic circulation carrying blood that has given up most of its oxygen. Veins, like arteries, have three coats, an inner, middle, and outer, but the coats are not so thick and they collapse when the vessel is cut. Many veins, especially the superficial, have valves formed of reduplication of their lining membrane. (For named veins of the body, see the table.) (See also Plate 7.)

afferent v's, veins that carry blood to an organ.

allantoic v's, paired vessels that accompany the

allantois, growing out from the primitive hindgut and entering the body stalk of the early embryo.

cardinal v's, embryonic vessels that include the pre- and postcardinal veins and the ducts of Cuvier (common cardinal veins).

emissary v., one passing through a foramen of the skull and draining blood from a cerebral sinus into a vessel outside the skull.

postcardinal v's, paired vessels in the early embryo that return blood from regions caudal to the heart.

precardinal v's, paired venous trunks in the embryo cranial to the heart.

pulp v's, vessels draining the venous sinuses of the spleen.

subcardinal v's, paired vessels in the embryo, replacing the postcardinal veins and persisting to some degree as definitve vessels.

sublobular v's, tributaries of the hepatic veins that receive the central veins of hepatic lobules.

supracardinal v's, paired vessels in the embryo developing later than the subcardinal veins and persisting chiefly as the lower segment of the inferior vena cava.

thebesian v., smallest cardiac veins: numerous small veins arising in the muscular walls and draining independently into the cavities of the heart, and most readily seen in the atria.

trabecular v's, vessels coursing in splenic trabeculae, formed by tributary pulp veins.

varicose v's, a permanently dilated, tortuous vein, usually in the subcutaneous tissues of the leg; incompetency of the venous valve is associated (see also VARICOSE VEINS).

vitelline v's, veins that return the blood from the yolk sac to the primitive heart of the early embryo.

Velacycline (val″ah-si′klēn) trademark for preparations of rolitetracycline, an antibiotic.

velamen (ve-la′men), pl. *velam′ina* [L.] a membrane, meninx, or velum.

velamentous (vel″ah-men′tus) membranous and pendent; like a veil.

Velban (vel′ban) trademark for a preparation of vinblastine sulfate, an antineoplastic agent.

vellus (vel′us) the coat of fine hairs that appears after the lanugo hairs are cast off and persists until puberty.

velopharyngeal (vel″o-fah-rin′je-al) pertaining to the velum palatinum (soft palate) and pharynx.

Velosef (vel′o-sef) trademark for preparations of cephradine, a cephalosporin antibiotic.

velum (ve′lum), pl. *ve′la* [L.] a covering structure or veil. adj., **ve′lar.**

v. interpos′itum, the membranous roof of the third ventricle of the brain.

medullary v., one of the two portions (superior medullary velum and inferior medullary velum) of the white matter of the hindbrain that form the roof of the fourth ventricle.

palatine v., v. palati′num, soft palate.

ven-, vene-, veni-, veno- word element [L.], *vein.*

vena (ve′nah), pl. *ve′nae* [L.] vein (see also table of VEINS).

venectasia (ve″nek-ta′ze-ah) phlebectasia.

venectomy (ve-nek′to-me) phlebectomy.

venenation (ven″ĕ-na′shun) poisoning; a poisoned condition.

venenous (ven′ĕ-nus) venomous.

venereal (vĕ-ne′re-al) due to or propagated by sexual intercourse.

v. disease, a contagious disease usually acquired in sexual intercourse or other genital contact, including SYPHILIS, GONORRHEA, CHANCROID, LYMPHOGRANULOMA VENEREUM, and GRANULOMA INGUINALE.

venereologist (vĕ-ne″re-ol′o-jist) a specialist in venereology.

venereology (vĕ-ne″re-ol′o-je) the study and treatment of venereal diseases.

venery (ven′er-e) coitus.

venesection (ven″ĕ-sek′shun) phlebotomy.

venipuncture (ven″ĭ-pungk′tūr) surgical puncture of a vein.

venisuture (ven″ĭ-su′tūr) phleborrhaphy.

venoclysis (ve-nok′lĭ-sis) injection of fluid into a vein; phleboclysis (see also INTRAVENOUS INFUSION).

venogram (ve′no-gram) phlebogram.

venography (ve-nog′rah-fe) phlebography.

venom (ven′om) poison, especially a toxic substance normally secreted by a serpent, insect, or other animal.

Russell's viper v., the venom of the Russell viper (*Vipera russelli*), which acts in vitro as an intrinsic thromboplastin and is useful in defining deficiencies of clotting factor X.

venomization (ven″om-ĭ-za′shun) treatment of a substance with snake venom.

venomotor (ve″no-mo′tor) controlling dilation or constriction of the veins.

venomous (ven′o-mus) secreting poison; poisonous.

veno-occlusive (ve″no-ŏ-kloo′siv) pertaining to or characterized by obstruction of the veins.

v. disease of liver, acute or chronic, partial or complete, occlusion of the branches of the hepatic veins by endophlebitis and thrombosis, leading to centrilobular necrosis, fibrosis, and ascites; most often seen in children.

venoperitoneostomy (ve″no-per″ĭ-to″ne-os′to-me) anastomosis of the saphenous vein with the peritoneum for drainage of ascites.

venosclerosis (ve″no-skle-ro′sis) sclerosis of veins; phlebosclerosis.

venosity (ve-nos′ĭ-te) 1. excess of venous blood in a part. 2. a plentiful supply of blood vessels or of venous blood.

venostasis (ve″no-sta′sis) retardation of the venous outflow in a part (see also PHLEBOSTASIS).

venotomy (ve-not′o-me) phlebotomy.

venous (ve′nus) pertaining to the veins.

v. return, the flow of blood into the heart from the peripheral vessels.

v. thrombosis, the presence of a thrombus in a vein (see also venous THROMBOSIS).

venovenostomy (ve″no-ve-nos′to-me) phlebophlebostomy.

vent (vent) an opening or outlet, such as an opening that discharges pus, or the anus.

venter (ven′ter), pl. *ven′tres* [L.] 1. any belly-shaped part; a fleshy contractible part of a muscle. 2. the abdomen or stomach. 3. a hollowed part or cavity.

ventilation (ven″tĭ-la′shun) 1. the process or act of supplying a house or room continuously with fresh air. 2. in respiratory physiology, the process of exchange of air between the lungs and the ambient

(*Text continued on page 1077.*)

Table of Veins

COMMON NAME*	NA TERM†	REGION*	RECEIVES BLOOD FROM*	DRAINS INTO*
accompanying v. of hypoglossal nerve	v. comitans nervi hypoglossi	accompanies hypoglossal nerve	formed by union of profunda linguae v. and sublingual v.	facial, lingual, or internal jugular
adrenal v's. *See* suprarenal v., left and right.				
anastomotic v., inferior	v. anastomotica inferior	interconnects superficial middle cerebral v. and transverse sinus		
anastomotic v., superior	v. anastomotica superior	interconnects superficial middle cerebral v. and superior sagittal sinus		
angular v.	v. angularis	between eye and root of nose	formed by union of supratrochlear v. and supraorbital v.	continues inferiorly as facial v.
antebrachial v., median	v. mediana antebrachii	forearm between cephalic v. and basilic v.	a palmar venous plexus	cephalic v. and/or basilic v., or median cubital v.
appendicular v.	v. appendicularis	accompanies appendicular artery		joins anterior and posterior cecal v's to form ileocolic v.
v. of aqueduct of vestibule	v. aqueductus vestibuli	passes through aqueduct of vestibule	internal ear	superior petrosal sinus
arcuate v's of kidney	vv. arcuatae renis	a series of complete arches across the bases of the renal pyramids, formed by union of interlobular v's and straight venules of kidney		interlobar v's
auditory v's, internal. *See* labyrinthine v's.				
auricular v's, anterior	vv. auriculares anteriores	anterior part of auricle		superficial temporal v.
auricular v., posterior	v. auricularis posterior	passes down behind auricle	a plexus on side of head	joins retromandibular v. to form external jugular v.
axillary v.	v. axillaris	the upper limb	formed at lower border of teres major muscle by junction of basilic v. and brachial v.	at lateral border of first rib is continuous with subclavian v.
azygos v.	v. azygos	intercepting trunk for right intercostal v's as well as connecting branch between superior and inferior venae cavae; it ascends in front of and on right side of vertebrae	ascending lumbar v.	superior vena cava
azygous v., left. *See* hemiazygos v.				

azygos v., lesser superior. *See* hemiazygos v., accessory.				
basal v.	v. basalis	passes from anterior perforated substance backward and around cerebral peduncle	anterior perforated substance	internal cerebral v.
basilic v.	v. basilica	forearm, superficially	ulnar side of dorsal rete of hand	joins brachial v's to form axillary v.
basilic v., median	v. mediana basilica	sometimes present as medial branch of a bifurcation of median antebrachial v.		basilic v.
basivertebral v's	vv. basivertebrales	venous sinuses in cancellous tissue of bodies of vertebrae, which communicate with venous plexus on anterior surface of vertebrae and with external and internal vertebral plexuses		
brachial v's	vv. brachiales	accompany brachial artery		joins basilic v. to form axillary v.
brachiocephalic v's	vv. brachiocephalicae (dextra et sinistra)	thorax	head, neck, and upper limbs; formed at root of neck by union of ipsilateral internal jugular and subclavian v's	unite to form superior vena cava
bronchial v's	vv. bronchiales		larger subdivisions of bronchi	azygos v. on left; hemiazygos or superior intercostal v. on right
v. of bulb of penis	v. bulbi penis		bulb of penis	internal pudendal v.
v. of bulb of vestibule	v. bulbi vestibuli		bulb of vestibule of vagina	internal pudendal v.
cardiac v's, anterior	vv. cordis anteriores		anterior wall of right ventricle	right atrium of heart, or lesser cardiac v.
cardiac v., great	v. cordis magna		anterior surface of ventricles	coronary sinus
cardiac v., middle	v. cordis media		diaphragmatic surface of ventricles	coronary sinus
cardiac v., small	v. cordis parva		right atrium and ventricle	coronary sinus
cardiac v's, smallest	vv. cordis minimae	numerous small veins arising in myocardium, draining independently into cavities of heart and most readily seen in the atria		
carotid v., external. *See* retromandibular v.				
cavernous v's of penis	vv. cavernosae penis		corpora cavernosa	deep v's and dorsal v. of penis
central v's of liver	vv. centrales hepatis	in middle of hepatic lobules	liver substance	hepatic v.

*v. = vein; v's = (pl.) veins. †v. = [L.] vena; vv. = [L.(pl.)] venae.

TABLE OF VEINS (*Continued*)

COMMON NAME*	NA TERM†	REGION*	RECEIVES BLOOD FROM*	DRAINS INTO*
central v. of retina	v. centralis retinae	eyeball	retinal v's	superior ophthalmic v.
central v. of suprarenal gland	v. centralis glandulae suprarenalis	the large single vein into which the various veins within the substance of the gland empty, and which continues at the hilus as the suprarenal v.		
cephalic v.	v. cephalica	winds anteriorly to pass along anterior border of brachioradial muscle; above elbow, ascends along lateral border of biceps of deltoid muscle	radial side of dorsal rete of hand	axillary v.
cephalic v., accessory	v. cephalica accessoria	forearm	dorsal rete of hand	joins cephalic v. just above elbow
cephalic v., median	v. mediana cephalica	sometimes present as lateral branch formed by bifurcation of median antebrachial v.		cephalic v.
cerebellar v's, inferior	vv. cerebelli inferiores		inferior surface of cerebellum	transverse, sigmoid, and inferior petrosal sinuses, or occipital sinus
cerebellar v's, superior	vv. cerebelli superiores		upper surface of cerebellum	straight sinus and great cerebral v., or transverse and superior petrosal sinuses
cerebral v., anterior	v. cerebri anterior	accompanies anterior cerebral artery		basal v.
cerebral v., great	v. cerebri magna	curves around splenium of corpus callosum	formed by union of the 2 internal cerebral veins	continues as or drains into straight sinus
cerebral v's, inferior	vv. cerebri inferiores	veins that ramify on base and inferolateral surface of brain, those on inferior surface of frontal lobe draining into inferior sagittal sinus and cavernous sinus; those on temporal lobe into superior petrosal sinus and transverse sinus; and those on occipital lobe into straight sinus		
cerebral v's, internal (2)	vv. cerebri internae	pass backward from interventricular foramen through tela choroidea	formed by union of thalamostriate v. and choroid v.; collect blood from basal ganglia	unite at splenium or corpus callosum to form great cerebral v.
cerebral v., middle, deep	v. cerebri media profunda	accompanies middle cerebral artery in floor of lateral sulcus		basal v.
cerebral v., middle, superficial	v. cerebri media superficialis	follows lateral cerebral fissure	lateral surface of cerebrum	cavernous sinus

cerebral v's, superior	vv. cerebri superiores	about 12 veins draining superolateral and medial surfaces of cerebrum toward longitudinal fissure		superior sagittal sinus
cervical v., deep	v. cervicalis profunda	accompanies deep cervical artery down neck	a plexus in suboccipital triangle	vertebral v. or brachiocephalic v.
cervical v's, transverse	vv. transversae colli	accompany transverse cervical artery		subclavian v.
choroid v.	v. choroidea	runs whole length of choroid plexus	choroid plexus, hippocampus, fornix, corpus callosum	joins thalamostriate v. to form internal cerebral v.
ciliary v's	vv. ciliares	anterior vessels follow anterior ciliary arteries; posterior follow posterior ciliary arteries	arise in eyeball by branches from ciliary muscle; anterior ciliary v's also receive branches from sinus venosus, sclerae, episcleral v's and conjunctiva of eyeball	superior ophthalmic v.; posterior ciliary v's empty also into inferior ophthalmic v.
circumflex femoral v's, lateral	vv. circumflexae femoris laterales	accompany lateral circumflex femoral artery		femoral v. or profunda femoris v.
circumflex femoral v's, medial	vv. circumflexae femoris mediales	accompany medial circumflex femoral artery		femoral v. or profunda femoris v.
circumflex iliac v., deep	v. circumflexa ilium profunda	a common trunk formed by veins accompanying deep circumflex iliac artery		external iliac v.
circumflex iliac v., superficial	v. circumflexa ilium superficialis	accompanies superficial circumflex iliac artery		great saphenous v.
v. of cochlear canal	v. canaliculi		cochlea	superior bulb of internal jugular v.
colic v., left	v. colica sinistra	accompanies left colic artery		inferior mesenteric v.
colic v., middle	v. colica media	accompanies middle colic artery		superior mesenteric v.
colic v., right	v. colica dextra	accompanies right colic artery		superior mesenteric v.
conjunctival v's	vv. conjunctivales		conjunctiva	superior ophthalmic v.
coronary v's. *See* entries under cardiac v's.				
cubital v., median	v. mediana cubiti	the large connecting branch passing obliquely upward across cubital fossa	cephalic v., below elbow	basilic v.
cutaneous v.	v. cutanea	one of the small veins that begin in papillae of skin, form subpapillary plexuses, and open into the subcutaneous veins		
cystic v.	v. cystica	within substance of liver	gallbladder	right branch of portal v.
deep v's of clitoris	vv. profundae clitoridis		clitoris	vesical venous plexus
deep v's of penis	vv. profundae penis	accompany deep artery of penis	penis	dorsal v. of penis

TABLE OF VEINS (*Continued*)

COMMON NAME*	NA TERM†	REGION*	RECEIVES BLOOD FROM*	DRAINS INTO*
digital v's of foot, dorsal	vv. digitales dorsales pedis	dorsal surfaces of toes		unite at clefts to form dorsal metatarsal v's
digital v's, palmar	vv. digitales palmares	accompany proper and common palmar digital arteries		superficial palmar venous arch
digital v's, plantar	vv. digitales plantares	plantar surfaces of toes		unite at clefts to form plantar metatarsal v's
diploic v., frontal	v. diploica frontalis		frontal bone	supraorbital v. externally, or superior sagittal sinus internally
diploic v., occipital	v. diploica occipitalis		occipital bone	occipital v. or transverse sinus
diploic v., temporal, anterior	v. diploica temporalis anterior		lateral portion of frontal bone, anterior part of parietal bone	sphenoparietal sinus internally, or a deep temporal v. externally
diploic v., temporal, posterior	v. diploica temporalis posterior		parietal bone	transverse sinus
dorsal v. of clitoris, deep	v. dorsalis clitoridis profunda	accompanies dorsal artery of clitoris		vesical plexus
dorsal v's of clitoris, superficial	vv. dorsales clitoridis superficiales		clitoris, subcutaneously	external pudendal v.
dorsal v. of penis, deep	v. dorsalis penis profunda	the single median vein lying subfascially in penis between the dorsal arteries; it begins in small veins around corona of glans, is joined by deep veins of penis as it passes proximally, and passes between arcuate pubic and transverse perineal ligaments, where it divides into a left and a right vein to join prostatic plexus		
dorsal v's of penis, superficial	vv. dorsales penis superficiales		penis, subcutaneously	external pudendal v.
dorsal v's of tongue. *See* lingual v's, dorsal.	vv. dorsales linguae			
emissary v., condylar	v. emissaria condylaris	a small vein running through condylar canal of skull, connecting sigmoid sinus with vertebral v. or internal jugular v.		
emissary v., mastoid	v. emissaria mastoidea	a small vein passing through mastoid foramen of skull, connecting sigmoid sinus with occipital v. or posterior auricular v.		
emissary v., occipital	v. emissaria occipitalis	an occasional small vein running through a minute foramen in occipital protuberance of skull, connecting confluence of sinuses with occipital v.		

emissary v., parietal	v. emissaria parietalis	a small vein passing through parietal foramen of skull, connecting superior sagittal sinus with superficial temporal v's		
epigastric v., inferior	v. epigastrica inferior	accompanies inferior epigastric artery		external iliac v.
epigastric v., superficial	v. epigastrica superficialis	accompanies superficial epigastric artery		great saphenous v. or femoral v.
epigastric v's, superior	vv. epigastricae superiores	accompany superior epigastric artery		internal thoracic v.
episcleral v's	vv. episclerales	around cornea		vorticose v's and ciliary v's
esophageal v's	vv. esophageae		esophagus	hemiazygos v. and azygos v., or left brachiocephalic v.
ethmoidal v's	vv. ethmoidales	accompany anterior and posterior ethmoidal arteries and emerge from ethmoidal foramina		superior ophthalmic v.
facial v.	v. facialis	the vein beginning at medial angle of eye as angular v., descending behind facial artery, and usually ending in internal jugular v.; sometimes joins retromandibular v. to form a common trunk		
facial v., deep	v. faciei profunda		pterygoid plexus	facial v.
facial v., posterior. *See* retromandibular v.				
facial v., transverse	v. transversa faciei	passes backward with transverse facial artery just below zygomatic arch		retromandibular v.
femoral v.	v. femoralis	follows course of femoral artery in proximal two thirds of thigh	continuation of popliteal v.	at inguinal ligament becomes external iliac v.
femoral v., deep	v. profunda femoris	accompanies deep femoral artery		femoral v.
fibular v's. *See* peroneal v's.	vv. fibulares (NA alternative for vv. peroneae)			
gastric v., left	v. gastrica sinistra	accompanies left gastric artery		portal v.
gastric v., right	v. gastrica dextra	accompanies right gastric artery		portal v.
gastric v's, short	vv. gastricae breves		left portion of greater curvature of stomach	splenic v.
gastroepiploic v., left	v. gastroepiploica sinistra	accompanies left gastroepiploic artery		splenic v.
gastroepiploic v., right	v. gastroepiploica dextra	accompanies right gastroepiploic artery		superior mesenteric v.
genicular v's	vv. genus	accompany genicular arteries		popliteal v.

TABLE OF VEINS (*Continued*)

COMMON NAME*	NA TERM†	REGION*	RECEIVES BLOOD FROM*	DRAINS INTO*
gluteal v's, inferior	vv. gluteae inferiores	accompany inferior gluteal artery; unite into a single vessel after passing through greater sciatic foramen	subcutaneous tissue of back of thigh, muscles of buttock	internal iliac v.
gluteal v's, superior	vv. gluteae superiores	accompany superior gluteal artery and pass through greater sciatic foramen	muscles of buttock	internal iliac v.
hemiazygos v.	v. hemiazygos	an intercepting trunk for lower left posterior intercostal v's; ascends on left side of vertebrae to eighth thoracic vertebra, where it may receive accessory branch, and crosses vertebral column	ascending lumbar v.	azygos v.
hemiazygos v., accessory	v. hemiazygos accessoria	the descending intercepting trunk for upper, often fourth through eighth, left posterior intercostal v's; it lies on left side and at eighth thoracic vertebra joins hemiazygos v. or crosses to right side to join azygos v. directly; above, it may communicate with left superior intercostal v.		
hemorrhoidal v's. *See* entries under rectal v's.				
hepatic v's	vv. hepaticae	2 or 3 large veins in an upper group and 6 to 20 small veins in a lower group, forming successively larger vessels	central v's of liver	inferior vena cava on posterior aspect of liver
hypogastric v. *See* iliac v., internal.				
ileal v's. *See* jejunal and ileal v's.				
ileocolic v.	v. ileocolica	accompanies ileocolic artery		superior mesenteric v.
iliac v., common	v. iliaca communis	ascends to right side of fifth lumbar vertebra	arises at sacroiliac joint by union of external and internal iliac v's	unites with fellow of opposite side to form inferior vena cava
iliac v., external	v. iliaca externa	extends from inguinal ligament to sacroiliac joint	continuation of femoral v.	joins internal iliac v. to form common iliac v.
iliac v., internal	v. iliaca interna	extends from greater sciatic notch to brim of pelvis	formed by union of parietal branches	joins external iliac v. to form common iliac v.
iliolumbar v.	v. iliolumbalis	accompanies iliolumbar artery		internal iliac v. and/or common iliac v.

innominate v's. *See* brachiocephalic v's.				
intercapital v's	vv. intercapitales	veins at clefts of fingers that pass between heads of metacarpal bones and establish communication between dorsal and palmar venous systems of hand		
intercostal v's, anterior (12 pairs)	vv. intercostales anteriores	accompany anterior thoracic arteries		internal thoracic v's
intercostal v., highest	v. intercostalis suprema	first posterior intercostal vein of either side, which passes over apex of lung		brachiocephalic, vertebral, or superior intercostal v.
intercostal v's, posterior, IV and XI	vv. intercostales posteriores (IV et XI)	accompany posterior intercostal arteries IV and XI		azygos v. on right; hemiazygos or accessory hemiazygos v. on left
intercostal v., superior, left	v. intercostalis superior sinistra	crosses arch of aorta	formed by union of second, third, and sometimes fourth posterior intercostal v's	left brachiocephalic v.
intercostal v., superior, right	v. intercostalis superior dextra		formed by union of second, third, and sometimes fourth posterior intercostal v's	azygos v.
interlobar v's of kidney	vv. interlobares renis	pass down between renal pyramids	venous arcades of kidney	unite to form renal v.
interlobular v's of kidney	vv. interlobulares renis		capillary network of renal cortex	venous arcades of kidney
interlobular v's of liver	vv. interlobulares hepatis	arise between hepatic lobules	liver	portal v.
interosseous v's of foot, dorsal. *See* metatarsal v's, dorsal.				
intervertebral v.	v. intervertebralis	vertebral column	vertebral venous plexuses	in neck, vertebral v.; in thorax, intercostal v's; in abdomen, lumbar v's; in pelvis, lateral sacral v's
jejunal v's. *See* jejunal and ileal v's.				
jejunal and ileal v's	vv. jejunales et ilei		jejunum and ileum	superior mesenteric v.
jugular v., anterior	v. jugularis anterior	arises under chin and passes down neck		external jugular v. or subclavian v., or jugular venous arch
jugular v., external	v. jugularis externa	begins in parotid gland behind angle of jaw and passes down neck	formed by union of retromandibular v. and posterior auricular v.	subclavian v., internal jugular v., or brachiocephalic v.
jugular v., internal	v. jugularis interna	from jugular fossa, descends in neck with internal carotid artery and then with common carotid artery	begins as superior bulb, draining much of head and neck	joins subclavian v. to form brachiocephalic v.
labial v's, anterior	vv. labiales anteriores		anterior aspect of labia in female	external pudendal v.

TABLE OF VEINS (*Continued*)

COMMON NAME*	NA TERM†	REGION*	RECEIVES BLOOD FROM*	DRAINS INTO*
labial v's, inferior	vv. labiales inferiores		region of lower lip	facial v.
labial v's, posterior	vv. labiales posteriores		labia in female	vesical venous plexus
labial v., superior	v. labiales superior		region of upper lip	facial v.
labyrinthine v's	vv. labyrinthi	pass through internal acoustic meatus	cochlea	inferior petrosal sinus or transverse sinus
lacrimal v.	v. lacrimalis		lacrimal gland	superior ophthalmic v.
laryngeal v., inferior	v. laryngea inferior		larynx	inferior thyroid v.
laryngeal v., superior	v. laryngea superior		larynx	superior thyroid v.
lingual v.	v. lingualis	a deep vein, following distribution of lingual artery		internal jugular v.
lingual v., deep	v. profunda linguae		deep aspect of tongue	joins sublingual v. to form accompanying v. of hypoglossal nerve
lingual v's, dorsal	vv. dorsales linguae	veins that unite with a small vein accompanying lingual artery and join main lingual trunk		
lumbar v's, I and II	vv. lumbales (I et II)	accompany first and second lumbar arteries		ascending lumbar v.
lumbar v's, III and IV	vv. lumbales (III et IV)	accompany third and fourth lumbar arteries		usually, inferior vena cava
lumbar v., ascending	v. lumbalis ascendens	an ascending intercepting vein for lumbar v's on either side; it begins in lateral sacral region and ascends to first lumbar vertebra, where by union with subcostal v. it becomes on right side the azygos v. and on left the hemiazygos v.		
maxillary v's	vv. maxillares	usually form a single short trunk with pterygoid plexus		joins superficial temporal v. in parotid gland to form retromandibular v.
mediastinal v's	vv. mediastinales		anterior mediastinum	brachiocephalic v., azygos v., or superior vena cava
meningeal v's	vv. meningeae	accompany meningeal arteries	dura mater (also communicate with lateral lacunae)	regional sinuses and veins
meningeal v's, middle	vv. meningeae mediae	accompany middle meningeal artery		pterygoid venous plexus
mesenteric v., inferior	v. mesenterica inferior	follows distribution of inferior mesenteric artery		splenic v.
mesenteric v., superior	v. mesenterica superior	follows distribution of superior mesenteric artery		joins splenic v. to form portal v.
metacarpal v's, dorsal	vv. metacarpeae dorsales	veins arising from union of dorsal veins of adjacent fingers and passing proximally to join in forming dorsal venous network of hand		

metacarpal v's, palmar	vv. metacarpeae palmares	accompany palmar metacarpal arteries		deep palmar venous arch
metatarsal v's, dorsal	vv. metatarseae dorsales		arise from dorsal digital v's of toes at clefts of toes	dorsal venous arch
metatarsal v's, plantar	vv. metatarseae plantares	deep veins of foot	arise from plantar digital v's at clefts of toes	plantar venous arch
musculophrenic v's	vv. musculophrenicae	accompany musculophrenic artery	parts of diaphragm and wall of thorax and abdomen	internal thoracic v's
nasal v's, external	vv. nasales externae	small ascending branches from nose		angular v., facial v.
nasofrontal v.	v. nasofrontalis		supraorbital v.	superior ophthalmic v.
oblique v. of left atrium	v. obliqua atrii sinistri	left atrium of heart		coronary sinus
obturator v's	vv. obturatoriae	enter pelvis through obturator canal	hip joint and regional muscles	internal iliac v. and/or inferior epigastric v.
occipital v.	v. occipitalis	scalp; follows distribution of occipital artery		opens under trapezius muscle into suboccipital venous plexus, or accompanies occipital artery to end in internal jugular v.
ophthalmic v., inferior	v. ophthalmica inferior	a vein formed by confluence of muscular and ciliary branches, and running backward either to join superior ophthalmic v. or to open directly into cavernous sinus; it sends a communicating branch through inferior orbital fissure to join pterygoid venous plexus		
ophthalmic v., superior	v. ophthalmica superior	a vein beginning at medial angle of eye, where it communicates with frontal, supraorbital, and angular v's; it follows distribution or ophthalmic artery, and may be joined by inferior ophthalmic v. at superior orbital fissure before opening into cavernous sinus		
ovarian v., left	v. ovarica sinistra		pampiniform plexus of broad ligament on left	left renal v.
ovarian v., right	v. ovarica dextra		pampiniform plexus of broad ligament on right	inferior vena cava
palatine v., external	v. palatina externa		tonsils and soft palate	facial v.
palpebral v's	vv. palpebrales	small branches from eyelids		superior ophthalmic v.
palpebral v's, inferior	vv. palpebrales inferiores		lower eyelid	facial v.
palpebral v's, superior	vv. palpebrales superiores		upper eyelid	angular v.
pancreatic v's	vv. pancreaticae		pancreas	splenic v., superior mesenteric v.

TABLE OF VEINS (*Continued*)

COMMON NAME*	NA TERM†	REGION*	RECEIVES BLOOD FROM*	DRAINS INTO*
pancreaticoduodenal v's	vv. pancreaticoduodenales	4 veins that drain blood from pancreas and duodenum, closely following pancreaticoduodenal arteries, a superior and an inferior vein originating from an anterior and a posterior venous arcade; anterior superior v. joins right gastroepiploic v., and posterior superior v. joins portal v.; anterior and posterior inferior v's join, sometimes as one trunk, uppermost jejunal v. or superior mesenteric v.		
paraumbilical v's	vv. paraumbilicales	veins that communicate with portal v. above and descend to anterior abdominal wall to anastomose with superior and inferior epigastric and superior vesical v's in region of umbilicus; they form a significant part of collateral circulation of portal v. in event of hepatic obstruction		
parotid v's	vv. parotideae		parotid gland	superficial temporal v.
perforating v's	vv. perforantes	accompany perforating arteries of thigh		profunda femoris v.
pericardiac v's	vv. pericardiaceae		pericardium	brachiocephalic, inferior thyroid, and azygos v's, superior vena cava
pericardiacophrenic v's	vv. pericardiacophrenicae		pericardium and diaphragm	left brachiocephalic v.
peroneal v's	vv. peroneae	accompany peroneal artery		posterior tibial v.
pharyngeal v's	vv. pharyngeae		pharyngeal plexus	internal jugular v.
phrenic v's, inferior	vv. phrenicae inferiores	accompany inferior phrenic arteries		on right, enters inferior vena cava; on left, enters left suprarenal or renal v., or inferior vena cava
phrenic v's, superior. *See* pericardiacophrenic v's.				
popliteal v.	v. poplitea	follows popliteal artery	formed by union of anterior and posterior tibial v's	at adductor hiatus becomes femoral v.
portal v.	v. portae	a short, thick trunk formed by union of superior mesenteric and splenic v's behind neck of pancreas; it ascends to right end of porta hepatis, where it divides into successively smaller branches, following branches of hepatic artery, until it forms a capillary-like system of sinusoids that permeates entire substance of liver		
posterior v. of left ventricle	v. posterior ventriculi sinistri cordis		posterior surface of left ventricle	coronary sinus

prepyloric v.	v. prepylorica	accompanies prepyloric artery, passing upward over anterior surface of junction between pylorus and duodenum		right gastric v.
profunda femoris v. *See* femoral v., deep.				
profunda linguae v. *See* lingual v., deep.				
v. of pterygoid canal	v. canalis pterygoidei	passes through pterygoid canal		pterygoid plexus
pudendal v's, external	vv. pudendae externae	follow distribution of external pudendal artery		great saphenous v.
pudendal v., internal	v. pudenda interna	follows course of internal pudendal artery		internal iliac v.
pulmonary v., inferior, left	v. pulmonalis inferior sinistra		lower lobe of left lung	left atrium of heart
pulmonary v., inferior, right	v. pulmonalis inferior dextra		lower lobe of right lung	left atrium of heart
pulmonary v., superior, left	v. pulmonalis superior sinistra		upper lobe of left lung	left atrium of heart
pulmonary v., superior, right	v. pulmonalis superior dextra		upper and middle lobes of right lung	left atrium of heart
pyloric v. *See* gastric v., right.				
radial v's	vv. radiales	accompany radial artery		brachial v's
ranine v. *See* sublingual v.				
rectal v's, inferior	vv. rectales inferiores		rectal plexus	internal pudendal v.
rectal v's, middle	vv. rectales mediae		rectal plexus	internal iliac and superior rectal v's
rectal v., superior	v. rectalis superior	establishes connection between portal and systemic systems	upper part of rectal plexus	inferior mesenteric v.
renal v's	vv. renales	short, thick trunks, one from either kidney, the one on the left being longer than that on the right	kidneys	inferior vena cava
retromandibular v.	v. retromandibularis	the vein formed in upper part of parotid gland behind neck of mandible by union of maxillary and superficial temporal v's; it passes downward through the gland, communicates with facial v. and, emerging from the gland, joins with posterior auricular v. to form external jugular v.		
sacral v's, lateral	vv. sacrales laterales	follow lateral sacral arteries		help form lateral sacral plexus; empty into internal iliac v. or superior gluteal v's
sacral v., median	v. sacralis mediana	follows median sacral artery		common iliac v.

TABLE OF VEINS (*Continued*)

COMMON NAME*	NA TERM†	REGION*	RECEIVES BLOOD FROM*	DRAINS INTO*
saphenous v., accessory	v. saphena accessoria		when present, medial and posterior superficial parts of thigh	great saphenous v.
saphenous v., great	v. saphena magna	extends from dorsum of foot to just below inguinal ligament		femoral v.
saphenous v., small	v. saphena parva	from behind ankle passes up back of leg to knee		popliteal v.
scrotal v's, anterior	vv. scrotales anteriores		anterior aspect of scrotum	external pudendal v.
scrotal v's, posterior	vv. scrotales posteriores	scrotum		vesical venous plexus
v. of septum pellucidum	v. septi pellucidi	septum pellucidum		thalamostriate v.
sigmoid v's	vv. sigmoideae		sigmoid colon	inferior mesenteric v.
spinal v's	vv. spinales	anastomosing networks of small veins that drain blood from spinal cord and its pia mater into internal vertebral venous plexuses		
spiral v. of modiolus	v. spiralis modioli	modiolus		labyrinthine v's
splenic v.	v. lienalis	passes from left to right of neck of pancreas	formed by union of several branches at hilus of spleen	joins superior mesenteric v. to form portal v.
stellate v's of kidney	venulae stellatae renis		superficial parts of renal cortex	interlobular v's of kidney
sternocleidomastoid v.	v. sternocleidomastidea	follows course of sternocleidomastoid artery		internal jugular v.
striate v.	v. striata		anterior perforated substance of brain	basal v.
stylomastoid v.	v. stylomastoidea	follows stylomastoid artery		retromandibular v.
subclavian v.	v. subclavia	follows subclavian artery	continues axillary v. as main venous channel of upper limb	joins internal jugular v. to form brachiocephalic v.
subcostal v.	v. subcostalis	accompanies subcostal artery		joins ascending lumbar v. to form azygos v. on right, hemiazygos v. on left
subcutaneous v's of abdomen	vv. subcutaneae abdominis	superficial layers of abdominal wall		
sublingual v.	v. sublingualis	follows sublingual artery		lingual v.
submental v.	v. submentalis	follows submental artery		facial v.
supraorbital v.	v. supraorbitalis	passes down forehead lateral to supratrochlear v.		joins supratrochlear v. at root of nose to form angular v.
suprarenal v., left	v. suprarenalis sinistra		left suprarenal gland	left renal v.
suprarenal v., right	v. suprarenalis dextra		right suprarenal gland	inferior vena cava

suprascapular v.	v. suprascapularis	accompanies suprascapular artery (sometimes as 2 veins that unite)		usually into external jugular v., occasionally into subclavian v.
supratrochlear v's (2)	vv. supratrochleares		venous plexuses high up on forehead	joins supraorbital v. at root of nose to form angular v.
temporal v's, deep	vv. temporales profundae		deep portions of temporal muscle	pterygoid plexus
temporal v., middle	v. temporalis media	descends deep to fascia to zygoma	arises in substance of temporal muscle	joins superficial temporal v.
temporal v's, superficial	vv. temporales superficiales	veins that drain lateral part of scalp in frontal and parietal regions, the branches forming a single superficial temporal v. in front of ear, just above zygoma; this descending vein receives middle temporal and transverse facial v's and, entering parotid gland, unites with maxillary v. deep to neck of mandible to form retromandibular v.		
testicular v., left	v. testicularis sinistra		left pampiniform plexus	left renal v.
testicular v., right	v. testicularis dextra		right pampiniform plexus	inferior vena cava
thalamostriate v.	v. thalamostriata		corpus striatum and thalamus	joins choroid v. to form internal cerebral v's
thoracic v's, internal	vv. thoracicae internae	2 veins formed by junction of the veins accompanying internal thoracic artery of either side; each continues along the artery to open into brachiocephalic v.		
thoracic v., lateral	v. thoracica lateralis	accompanies lateral thoracic artery		axillary v.
thoracoacromial v.	v. thoracoacromialis	follows thoracoacromial artery		subclavian v.
thoracoepigastric v's	vv. thoracoepigastricae	long, longitudinal, superficial veins in anterolateral subcutaneous tissue of trunk		superiorly into lateral thoracic v.; inferiorly into femoral v.
thymic v's	vv. thymicae		thymus	left brachiocephalic v.
thyroid v., inferior	v. thyroidea inferior	either of 2 veins, left and right, that drain thyroid plexus into left and right brachiocephalic v's; occasionally they may unite into a common trunk to empty, usually, into left brachiocephalic v.		
thyroid v's, middle	vv. thyroideae mediae		thyroid gland	internal jugular v.
thyroid v., superior	v. thyroidea superior	arises from side of upper part of thyroid gland	thyroid gland	internal jugular v., occasionally in common with facial v.
tibial v's, anterior	vv. tibiales anteriores	accompany anterior tibial artery		join posterior tibial v's to form popliteal v.
tibial v's, posterior	vv. tibiales posteriores	accompany posterior tibial artery		join anterior tibial v's to form popliteal v.

TABLE OF VEINS (*Concluded*)

COMMON NAME*	NA TERM†	REGION*	RECEIVES BLOOD FROM*	DRAINS INTO*
tracheal v's	vv. tracheales		trachea	brachiocephalic v.
tympanic v's	vv. tympanicae	small veins from middle ear that pass through petrotympanic fissure and open into the plexus around temporomandibular joint		retromandibular v.
ulnar v's	vv. ulnares	accompany ulnar artery		join radial v's at elbow to form brachial v's
umbilical v.	v. umbilicalis (formerly)	in the early embryo, either of the paired veins that carry blood from chorion to sinus venosus and heart; they later fuse and become left umbilical v. of fetus		
umbilical v. of fetus, left	v. umbilicalis sinistra	the vein formed by fusion of atrophied right umbilical v. with the left umbilical v., which carries all the blood from placenta to ductus venosus		
uterine v's	vv. uterinae		uterine plexus	internal iliac v's
vena cava, inferior	vena cava inferior	the venous trunk for the lower limbs and for pelvic and abdominal viscera; it begins at level of fifth lumbar vertebra by union of common iliac v's and ascends on right of aorta		right atrium of heart
vena cava, superior	vena cava superior	the venous trunk draining blood from head, neck, upper limbs, and thorax; it begins by union of 2 brachiocephalic v's and passes directly downward		right atrium of heart

air. *Pulmonary ventilation* (usually measured in liters per minute) refers to the total exchange, whereas *alveolar ventilation* refers to the effective ventilation of the alveoli, where gas exchange with the blood takes place. 3. in psychiatry, the free discussion of one's problems or grievances.

intermittent positive-pressure v. (IPPV), the provision of mechanical ventilation by a machine designed to deliver breathing gas until equilibrium is established between the patient's lungs and the VENTILATOR. IPPV machines are positive-pressure, pressure-cycled, assistor-controller (pneumatic) devices.

Because of their compact size and capability of operating independently of an electrical current, the IPPV machines have the most widespread applicability in the employment of a form of treatment called INTERMITTENT POSITIVE-PRESSURE BREATHING. Examples of the ventilators utilized in IPPV include the Bird respirator and the Bennett PR-2 model. Several newer machines employed specifically for IPPV and relatively simple in design are now available.

ventilator (ven″tĭ-la′tor) an apparatus designed to qualify the air that is breathed through it or to either intermittently or continuously assist or control pulmonary ventilation; called also respirator. Use of a mechanical ventilator is indicated as a supportive measure in patients suffering from respiratory paralysis and in those with ventilatory failure manifested by either alveolar hypoventilation or distributive HYPOXIA, or both.

In alveolar hypoventilation, gas exchange with the blood is inadequate for removal of carbon dioxide, oxygen delivery into the pulmonary system is thereby reduced, and tissue demands for oxygen cannot be met. As a result, the patient suffers from hypercapnia and ACIDOSIS. In distributive hypoxia, there may be normal functioning of ventilatory mechanics, but there is interference with the intrapulmonary distribution of the inspired air. As a result of this maldistribution, large amounts of carbon dioxide are removed from the blood, there is inadequate oxygenation of the blood, and the patient suffers from hypoxemia, hypocapnia, and ALKALOSIS.

In either case, the ventilator is used to improve alveolar ventilation, re-establish a normal ACID-BASE BALANCE, and correct the associated hypoxia. It is important, however, that the primary cause of a patient's ventilatory failure be known and that his blood gases be evaluated frequently during assisted or controlled ventilation so that the mechanical ventilator can be used to its best advantage and greatest benefit to the individual patient.

TYPES OF VENTILATORS. There are two major groups of ventilators: (1) those that generate negative pressure on the exterior surface of the chest, and (2) those that provide intrathoracic positive pressure.

Negative-Pressure Ventilators. Among the ventilators of this type are the body tank (IRON LUNG, or Drinker respirator) and the chest and chest-abdomen respirators such as the Emerson cuirass. These machines exert negative (subatmospheric) pressure on the exterior chest wall which is transmitted to the interior of the thorax, creating a suction effect and causing air to flow into the lungs. The lungs are allowed to exhale passively before the next inspiratory cycle. Full-body and chest ventilators are not effective in relief of ventilatory failure resulting from increased airway resistance due to intrapulmonary diseases, such as CHRONIC OBSTRUCTIVE PULMONARY DISEASE (COPD). They are, therefore, indicated in the treatment of patients whose ventilatory problems are caused by respiratory paralysis rather than obstructive lung disease and whose condition limits the employment of intubation.

Positive-Pressure Ventilators. These mechanical devices force air directly into the lungs under positive pressure, causing the lungs and chest to expand. Ventilators of this type are indicated in a wide variety of conditions that produce either acute respiratory distress or chronic respiratory insufficiency, or both.

Many positive-pressure ventilators are assistor-controller devices. This means that they can assist the respiratory efforts of a very weak patient, or they can be set to control the ventilation of a patient who cannot breathe normally on his own. In assisted ventilation the patient controls the ventilator through his inspiratory efforts. Each time he inhales, the machine is triggered to deliver a flow of air into his lungs and assist him in breathing more deeply and effectively. For patients who are very weak, a sensitivity control on the machine can be adjusted to respond to his efforts at inspiration.

The term controlled ventilation refers to the capability of the machine to ventilate automatically the lungs of the patient who cannot breathe on his own or whose breathing is erratic. Some ventilators combine the features of assisted and controlled ventilation while others are designed to provide either assisted or controlled ventilation only.

There is at the present time no mechanical ventilator that exactly duplicates all of the physiological mechanisms involved in the spontaneous breathing patterns of a healthy person during various stages of rest and activity. Each model is designed to utilize one or more physiologic and mechanical principles to assist the patient in respiratory failure; selection of the type of ventilator for the individual patient is based on that patient's particular needs.

Control Modes of Ventilation. Among the many models of positive-pressure ventilators are three general types that are classified according to the manner in which the cycling of the machine is controlled. These three control modes are *pressure cycling, volume cycling,* and *time cycling.*

Pressure-cycled ventilators are those in which cycling is primarily dependent upon a buildup of pressure within the patient's lungs. Each inspiratory phase of ventilation is triggered by the inspiratory effect of the patient's breathing and continues to deliver gas until an equilibrium is established between the patient's lungs and the ventilator. Controls that are basic components of all models of pressure-cycled ventilators include a pressure control, which governs the tidal volume delivered (usually between 10 and 30 mm. H_2O), and a sensitivity control, which determines the amount of inspiratory effort required of the patient to cycle the ventilator.

Volume-cycled ventilators rely upon volume as the cycling monitor. The volume-cycled machine is electrically powered and utilizes a motor-driven piston to deliver a predetermined volume of air from a cylinder. In order to avoid damage to the bronchi and lungs, both the volume-cycled and the time-cycled ventilators have devices that allow pressure to exert a limiting effect on the amount of air being forced into the lungs. Thus, when resistance to the flow of gas into the lungs reaches a certain level and pressure builds up, the inspiratory phase of ventilation is terminated.

The volume-cycled ventilator may be used when airway resistance is so great an adequate tidal volume cannot be maintained, for example, in patients suffering from severe COPD. Because of the danger of damaging the lungs from overinflation, these machines have a built in alarm system that is triggered by resistance to the flow of air, as in coughing or accumulations of secretions that increase the pressure beyond the pre-set level.

In *time-cycled ventilators* the cycling pattern is determined by controls which are manipulated to achieve the desired number of breaths per minute. These controls also can be adjusted for the inspiration phase and the expiration phase so that the ratio between the two phases can be set for maximum ventilation of the patient. In these ventilators the flow rate is adjusted so that the tidal volume prescribed by the physician can be delivered in the time allotted for inspiration. Although pressure plays no direct role in governing the cycling pattern, the variables of time and flow do, of course, affect the pressure.

Regardless of the mode of cycling and whether the machine provides assisted or controlled ventilation or both, all ventilators provide for the humidification of inspired air and the measurement of expired volumes. (See also INTERMITTENT POSITIVE-PRESSURE BREATHING.)

PATIENT CARE. Regardless of the model and capabilities of the mechanical ventilator being used in the treatment of a patient with inadequate ventilation, there are certain general principles that are basic to the competent care of that patient. It is essential that all those who accept responsibility for the care of the patient be fully aware of the physiologic effects of mechanical ventilation, particularly in regard to the relationship between the distribution of inspired air in the lung and the status of the BLOOD GASES and pH. A major contribution of mechanical ventilation should be the normalization of blood gases and avoidance of the extremes of ACIDOSIS and ALKALOSIS. Thus careful monitoring of the blood gases and the pH are an essential part of patient care during mechanical ventilation.

A second consideration in patient care and assessment of the effects of mechanical ventilation is that of its influence on circulation. It is apparent that increased intrathoracic pressure can interfere with the flow of blood through the great vessels and the chambers of the heart. The ultimate effect can be a pooling of blood in the veins and capillaries of the abdominal organs and a resultant vascular collapse that is sometimes called respirator shock. Frequent determinations of pulse rate and blood pressure are necessary to detect early development of this condition and correction of pressure levels to forestall shock. It should be noted that interference with the venous return to the right side of the heart can bring about a therapeutic effect in patients with pulmonary EDEMA. Thus a potentially hazardous side effect of an increase in intrathoracic pressure can be of benefit to the patient when used judiciously by a physician who is knowledgeable about all aspects of ventilatory therapy.

A third consideration is that of the effects of mechanical ventilation on the body fluid–antidiuretic hormone balance. It has long been recognized that pressure breathing, both positive and negative, influences the production of the antidiuretic hormone, causing an excess of this hormone and a resultant retention of water. If not corrected, the situation can lead to pulmonary edema and further interference with the patient's ventilation. The possibility of such an eventuality demands that accurate records be kept of the patient's intake and output and that a safe balance be maintained.

A thorough knowledge of the apparatus being used for mechanical ventilation is vital to competent care of the patient. No one should attempt to give patient care without prior instruction in the purpose of the machine and the physiologic and physical principles upon which it operates.

TRACHEOSTOMY care is of vital importance when the patient is being maintained on a respirator with controlled ventilation and positive pressure is being delivered via a tracheostomy tube. Suction is applied as necessary and some method for moisturizing the air is provided. In fact, whether the patient has a tracheostomy or not, the air passages must be kept moist whenever a respirator is used for a prolonged period.

If AEROSOL medications are administered by use of a respirator, it is important to know the type of medication being used, its desired effects and the signs and symptoms of overdosage or toxic side effects. When such symptoms appear the rate of nebulization requires adjustment.

The psychologic implications of the use of a respirator are manifold. If he is conscious or semiconscious, the patient is aware that the machine is concerned with maintaining his very "breath of life" and he is understandably apprehensive about its use and effects on his breathing. When a respirator is used for a brief period as a means of therapy, the patient can be told that he can control the cycle by the slightest effort on his part. Once he understands the way the machine works and his questions are answered to his satisfaction his fears can be allayed. The patient who is partially or totally dependent on a respirator will need more reassurance. He should be assured that someone will be near at all times in case the apparatus needs adjusting. Much of his panic and fear can be relieved if the nursing staff exercises patience and maintains a calm attitude when helping him adjust to the respirator.

Weaning from the Ventilator. Gradual withdrawal of the support of the ventilator ("weaning") begins as soon as the patient's blood gases, spontaneous breathing capabilities, and clinical status indicate that he may be able to start breathing on his own. Some patients view with alarm the prospect of trying to breathe without the aid of the ventilator while others may be overenthusiastic and wish to end their dependence on the machine before they are ready to do so. Difficulties are more likely to develop in those who have had prolonged controlled ventilation than in those who have had assisted ventilation for a short period of time.

Prior to the actual removal of ventilatory assistance the patient should be taught abdominal breathing and informed that a deep controlled breathing pattern will be more advantageous than rapid shallow breaths. He will need calm assurance that he will not be expected to endure any distress beyond his capability to cope with it, and that a person in whom he has confidence will remain with him while he is off the respirator.

It is recommended that weaning be initiated during the morning hours when the patient is most rested and relaxed. During the time the ventilator is first removed, the patient may be given humidified oxygen, or as in the case of the tracheotomized patient, warmed and humidified oxygenated air. Such measures will enhance the patient's tolerance to the weaning process. As his tolerance increases, the period of time he is off the ventilator is lengthened. Once he is able to breathe adequately independently of the ventilating machine, a simple ventilator may be kept close at hand in the event the patient should express or exhibit a need for it. During this time he is observed regularly to make certain he is able to breathe adequately on his own.

ventr(i)-, ventr(o)- word element [L.], *belly; front (anterior) aspect of the body; ventral aspect.*

ventrad (ven′trad) toward a belly, venter, or ventral aspect.

ventral (ven′tral) 1. pertaining to the abdomen or to any venter. 2. directed toward or situated on the belly surface; opposite of dorsal.

ventralis (ven-tra′lis) [L.] ventral.

ventricle (ven′trĭ-k'l) a small cavity or chamber, as in the brain or heart.

v. of Arantius, 1. the rhomboid fossa, especially its lower end. 2. fifth ventricle.

fifth v., the median cleft between the two laminae of the septum lucidum.

fourth v., a median cavity in the hindbrain, containing cerebrospinal fluid.

v. of larynx, the space between the true and false vocal cords.

lateral v., the cavity in each cerebral hemisphere, derived from the cavity of the embryonic tube, containing cerebrospinal fluid.

left v., the lower chamber of the left side of the heart, which pumps oxygenated blood out through the aorta to all the tissues of the body.

Morgagni's v., ventricle of larynx.

pineal v., an extension of the third ventricle into the stalk of the pineal body.

right v., the lower chamber of the right side of the heart, which pumps venous blood through the pulmonary trunk and arteries to the capillaries of the lung.

third v., a narrow cleft below the corpus callosum, within the diencephalon between the two thalami.

ventricornu (ven″trĭ-kor′nu) the anterior horn of gray matter in the spinal cord. adj., **ventricor′nual.**

ventricular (ven-trik′u-lar) pertaining to a ventricle.

v. septal defect, a CONGENITAL HEART DEFECT in which there is persistent patency of the ventricular septum in either the muscular or fibrous portion most often due to failure of the bulbar septum to completely close the interventricular foramen. The defect permits flow of blood directly from one ventricle to the other, resulting in bypassing of the pulmonary circulation and producing varying degrees of cyanosis because of oxygen deficiency.

ventriculitis (ven-trik″u-li′tis) inflammation of a ventricle, especially a cerebral ventricle.

ventriculoatriostomy (ven-trik″u-lo-a″tre-os′to-me) introduction of a catheter with a one-way valve to drain cerebrospinal fluid from a cerebral ventricle to the right atrium via the jugular vein, for relief of hydrocephalus.

ventriculocisternostomy (ven-trik″u-lo-sis″ter-nos′to-me) surgical creation of a communication between the third ventricle and the interpeduncular cistern, for drainage of cerebrospinal fluid.

ventriculocordectomy (ven-trik″u-lo-kor-dek′to-me) punch resection of the vocal cords.

ventriculogram (ven-trik′u-lo-gram″) a roentgenogram of the cerebral ventricles.

ventriculography (ven-trik″u-log′rah-fe) 1. roentgenography of the cerebral ventricles after introduction of air or other contrast medium. 2. roentgenography of a ventricle of the heart after injection of a contrast medium.

ventriculometry (ven-trik″u-lom′ĕ-tre) measurement of intracranial pressure.

ventriculonector (ven-trik″u-lo-nek′tor) the bundle of His.

ventriculopuncture (ven-trik″u-lo-pungk′tūr) surgical puncture of a lateral ventricle of the brain.

ventriculoscopy (ven-trik″u-los′ko-pe) endoscopic examination of the cerebral ventricles.

ventriculostomy (ven-trik″u-los′to-me) surgical creation of a free communication between the third ventricle and the interpeduncular cistern for relief of hydrocephalus.

ventriculosubarachnoid (ven-trik″u-lo-sub″ah-rak′noid) pertaining to the cerebral ventricles and subarachnoid space.

ventriculotomy (ven-trik″u-lot′o-me) incision of a ventricle of the heart.

ventriculus (ven-trik′u-lus), pl. *ventric′uli* [L.] 1. a ventricle. 2. the stomach.

ventricumbent (ven″trĭ-kum′bent) prone; lying on the belly.

ventriduct (ven″trĭ-dukt) to bring or carry ventrad.

ventrimeson (ven″trĭ-mes′on) the median line on the ventral surface. adj., **ventrime′sal.**

ventrofixation (ven″tro-fik-sa′shun) fixation of a viscus, e.g., the uterus, to the abdominal wall; ventrosuspension.

ventrohysteropexy (ven″tro-his′ter-o-pek″se) the uterus.

ventrolateral (ven″tro-lat′er-al) both ventral and lateral.

ventroscopy (ven-tros′ko-pe) illumination of the abdominal cavity for purposes of examination.

ventrose (ven′trōs) having a belly-like expansion.

ventrosuspension (ven″tro-sus-pen′shun) ventrofixation.

ventrotomy (ven-trot′o-me) celiotomy; opening of the abdominal cavity through an incision in its wall.

Venturi mask (ven-tu′re) any of three types of disposable masks used to administer controlled amounts of oxygen (see also OXYGEN THERAPY); each of these masks provides a constant oxygen concentration above that of the atmospheric concentration (21 per cent).

venturi meter (ven′tu-re) an instrumet for measuring the flow of liquids, as of the blood in vessels, by relating difference of pressures between a constricted and a nonconstricted portion of the tube through which fluid is flowing.

venula (ven′u-lah), pl. *ven′ulae* [L.] venule.

venule (ven′ūl) any of the small vessels that collect blood from the capillary plexuses and join to form veins. adj., **ven′ular.**

Veralba (ver-al′bah) trademark for preparations of

protoveratrines A and B, used as an antihypertensive.

Veratrum (ver-a'trum) a genus of poisonous liliaceous plants, including plants common *V. vi'ride* (American green hellbore) and *V. al'bum* (European white hellbore), both of which are the source of alkaloids used widely in treatment of hypertensive disorders.

verbigeration (ver-bij"er-a'shun) abnormal repetition of meaningless words and phrases.

verge (verj) a circumference or ring.

anal v., the opening of the anus on the surface of the body.

vergence (ver'jens) disjunctive movement of the eyes in opposite directions.

Veriloid (ver'ĭ-loid) trademark for a preparation of alkavervir, an antihypertensive.

vermicide (ver'mĭ-sīd) an agent lethal to worms or intestinal animal parasites.

vermicular (ver-mik'u-lar) wormlike in shape or appearance.

vermiculation (ver-mik"u-la'shun) peristaltic motion; peristalsis.

vermiculous (ver-mik'u-lus) 1. wormlike 2. infected with worms.

vermiform (ver'mĭ-form) worm-shaped.

v. appendix, a small appendage near the juncture of the small intestine and the large intestine (ileocecal valve); often called simply appendix. An apparently useless structure, it can be the source of a serious illness, APPENDICITIS.

vermifugal (ver-mif'u-gal) expelling worms or intestinal animal parasites.

vermifuge (ver'mĭ-fūj) an agent that expels worms or intestinal animal parasites; an anthelmintic.

vermilion border (ver-mil'yon) the exposed red portion of the upper or lower lip.

vermilionectomy (ver-mil"yon-ek'to-me) excision of the vermilion border of the lip.

vermin (ver'min) an external animal parasite; such parasites collectively.

vermination (ver"mĭ-na'shun) infestation with vermin or infection with worms.

verminous (ver'mĭ-nus) pertaining to, due to, or abounding in worms or in vermin.

vermis (ver'mis) [L.] 1. a worm, or wormlike structure. 2. vermis cerebelli.

v. cerebel'li, the median part of the cerebellum, between the two hemispheres.

nodule of v., the part of the vermis of the cerebellum, on the ventral surface, where the inferior medullary velum attaches.

Vernet's syndrome (ver-nāz') paralysis of the glossopharyngeal, vagus, and spinal accessory nerves due to a lesion in the region of the jugular foramen.

vernix (ver'niks) [L.] varnish.

v. caseo'sa, the unctuous substance composed of sebum and desquamated epithelial cells, covering the skin of the fetus.

verruca (vĕ-roo'kah), pl. *verru'cae* [L.] 1. a WART. 2. one of the wartlike elevations on the endocardium in various types of endocarditis. adj., **ver'rucose, verru'cous.**

v. pla'na, a small, smooth, usually skin-colored or light brown, slightly raised wart sometimes occurring in great numbers; seen most often in children.

v. planta'ris, a viral epidermal tumor on the sole of the foot (see also PLANTAR WART).

verruciform (vĕ-roo'sĭ-form) wartlike.

verruga (vĕ-roo'gah) wart.

v. perua'na, a hemangioma-like tumor or nodule occurring in Carrión's disease.

version (ver'zhun) the act of turning; especially the manual turning of the fetus in delivery.

bipolar v., turning effected by acting upon both poles of the fetus either by external or combined version.

cephalic v., turning of the fetus so that the head presents.

combined v., external and internal versions together.

external v., turning effected by outside manipulation.

internal v., turning effected by the hand or fingers inserted through the dilated cervix.

pelvic v., version by manipulation of the breech.

podalic v., conversion of a more unfavorable presentation into a footling presentation.

spontaneous v., one that occurs without aid from any extraneous force.

vertebr(o)- word element [L.], *vertebra; spine.*

vertebra (ver'tĕ-brah), pl. *ver'tebrae* [L.] any of the separate segments comprising the spine (vertebral column). (See also SPINE.)

The vertebrae support the body and provide the protective bony corridor through which the spinal cord passes. The 33 bones that make up the spine differ considerably in size and structure according to location. There are seven cervical (neck) vertebrae, 12 thoracic (high back), five lumbar (low back), five sacral (near the base of the spine), and four coccygeal (at the base). The five sacral vertebrae are fused to form the sacrum, and the four coccygeal vertebrae are fused to form the coccyx.

The weight-bearing portion of a typical vertebra is the vertebral body, the most forward portion. This is a cylindrical structure that is separated from the vertebral bodies above and below by disks of cartilage and fibrous tissue. These intervertebral disks act as cushions to absorb the mechanical shock of walking, running, and other activity. Rupture of an intervertebral disk is known popularly as slipped DISK.

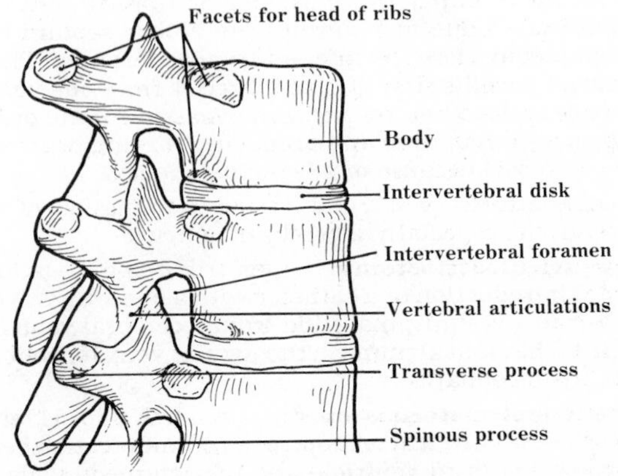

Structure of vertebrae.

A semicircular arch of bone protrudes from the back of each vertebral body, surrounding the spinal cord. Directly in its midline a bony projection, the spinous process, grows backward from the arch. The spinuous process can be felt on the back as a hard knob. Three pairs of outgrowths project from the arch. One of these protrudes horizontally on each side and in the thorax connects with the ribs. The remaining two form joints with the vertebrae above and below. The joints permit the spine to bend flexibly. The vertebrae are held firmly in place by a series of strong ligaments.

cranial v., the segments of the skull and facial bones, regarded by some as modified vertebrae.

v. denta'ta, the second cervical vertebra, or axis.

dorsal vertebrae, thoracic vertebrae.

false vertebrae, those vertebrae which normally fuse with adjoining segments: the sacral and coccygeal vertebrae.

v. mag'num, the sacrum.

odontoid v., the second cervical vertebra, or axis.

v. pla'na, a condition of spondylitis in which the body of the vertebra is reduced to a sclerotic disk.

true vertebrae, those segments of the vertebral column that normally remain unfused throughout life: the cervical, thoracic, and lumbar vertebrae.

vertebral (ver'tĕ-bral) of or pertaining to a vertebra.

v. canal, the canal formed by the series of vertebral foramina together, containing the spinal cord and meninges. Called also spinal canal.

v. column, the spine; the rigid structure in the midline of the back, composed of the vertebrae.

vertebrarium (ver"tĕ-bra're-um) the spine, or vertebral column.

Vertebrata (ver"tĕ-bra'tah) a subphylum of the Chordata, comprising all animals having a vertebral column, including mammals, birds, reptiles, amphibians, and fishes.

vertebrate (ver'tĕ-brāt) 1. having a vertebral column. 2. an animal with a vertebral column; any member of the Vertebrata.

vertebrectomy (ver"tĕ-brek'to-me) excision of a vertebra.

vertebrobasilar (ver"tĕ-bro-bas'ĭ-lar) pertaining to or affecting the vertebral and basilar arteries.

vertebrochondral (ver"tĕ-bro-kon'dral) pertaining to a vertebra and a costal cartilage.

vertebrocostal (ver"tĕ-bro-kos'tal) pertaining to a vertebra and a rib.

vertebrosternal (ver"tĕ-bro-ster'nal) pertaining to a vertebra and the sternum.

vertex (ver'teks) the summit or top, especially the top of the head (ver'tex cra'nii).

vertical (ver'tĭ-kal) 1. perpendicular to the plane of the horizon. 2. relating to the vertex.

verticalis (ver"tĭ-ka'lis) [L.] vertical.

verticillate (ver-tis'ĭ-lāt) arranged in whorls.

vertigo (ver'tĭ-go) a sensation of rotation or movement of one's self (subjective vertigo) or of one's surroundings (objective vertigo) in any plane. The term is sometimes used erroneously as a synonym for dizziness. Vertigo may result from diseases of the inner ear or may be due to disturbances of the vestibular centers or pathways in the central nervous system.

auditory v., aural v., Menière's disease.

central v., that due to disorder of the central nervous system.

labyrinthine v., a form associated with disease of the labyrinth of the ear.

organic v., that caused by vestibular brain disease or to tabes dorsalis.

peripheral v., vestibular vertigo.

positional p., postural p., that associated with a specific position of the head in space or with changes in position of the head in space.

vestibular v., vertigo due to disturbances of the vestibular centers or pathways in the central nervous system.

vertigraphy (ver-tig'rah-fe) body-section roentgenography.

verumontanitis (ver"oo-mon"tah-ni'tis) inflammation of the verumontanum.

verumontanum (ver"oo-mon-ta'num) a prominent portion of the male urethral crest, on which are the opening of the prostatic utricle and, on either side of it, the orifices of the ejaculatory ducts; called also seminal colliculus.

vesalianum (vĕ-sa"le-a'num) a sesamoid bone in the tendon of origin of the gastrocnemius muscle, or in the angle between the cuboid and fifth metatarsal bones.

Vesalius (ve-sa'le-us) Andreas (1514–1564). Flemish anatomist and physician, considered the most eminent anatomist of the 16th century. His *De humani corporis fabrica libri septum* (Seven Books on the Structure of the Human Body) was published in 1543. He was also a pioneer in ethnic craniology and experimental and comparative psychology.

vesic(o)- word element [L.], *blister; bladder.*

vesica (vĕ-si'kah), pl. *vesi'cae* [L.] bladder. adj., **ves'ical.**

vesicant (ves'ĭ-kant) 1. producing blisters. 2. an agent that produces blisters.

vesication (ves"ĭ-ka'shun) 1. the process of blistering. 2. a blistered spot or surface.

vesicle (ves'ĭ-k'l) 1. a small bladder or sac containng liquid. 2. a small circumscribed elevation of the epidermis containing a serous fluid; a small blister.

allantoic v., the internal hollow portion of the allantois.

auditory v., a detached ovoid sac formed by closure of the auditory pit in the early embryo, from which the percipient parts of the inner ear develop.

brain v's, the five divisions of the closed neural tube in the developing embryo, including the telencephalon, diencephalon, mesencephalon, metencephalon, and myelencephalon.

brain v's, primary, the three earlier subdivisions of the embryonic neural tube, including the forebrain, midbrain, and hindbrain.

brain v's, secondary, the four brain vesicles formed by specialization of the forebrain and of the hindbrain in later embryonic development.

chorionic v., the developing ovum at the time of its invasion of the endometrium of the uterus.

compound v., multilocular vesicle.

encephalic v's, brain vesicles.

germinal v., the fluid-filled nucleus of an oocyte toward the end of prophase of its meiotic division.

lens v., a vesicle formed from the lens pit of the embryo, developing into the crystalline lens.

multilocular v., one with multiple chambers or compartments.

optic v., an evagination on either side of the forebrain of the early embryo, from which the percipient parts of the eye develop.

otic v., auditory vesicle.

seminal v., paired sacculated pouches attached to the posterior urinary bladder; the duct of each joins the ipsilateral ductus deferens to form the ejaculatory duct.

umbilical v., the pear-shaped expansion of the yolk sac growing out into the cavity of the chorion, joined to the midgut by the yolk stalk.

vesicocele (ves′ĭ-ko-sēl″) hernia of the bladder.

vesicocervical (ves″ĭ-ko-ser′vĭ-kal) pertaining to the bladder and cervix uteri.

vesicoclysis (ves″ĭ-kok′lĭ-sis) introduction of fluid into the bladder.

vesicoenteric, vesicointestinal (ves″ĭ-ko-en-ter′ik; ves″ĭ-ko-in-tes′tĭ-nal) pertaining to or communicating with the urinary bladder and intestine.

vesicoprostatic (ves″ĭ-ko-pros-tat′ik) pertaining to the bladder and prostate.

vesicopubic (ves″ĭ-ko-pu′bik) pertaining to the bladder and pubes.

vesicosigmoidostomy (ves″ĭ-ko-sig″moi-dos′to-me) creation of a permanent communication between the urinary bladder and the sigmoid flexure.

vesicospinal (ves″ĭ-ko-spi′nal) pertaining to the bladder and spine.

vesicotomy (ves″ĭ-kot′o-me) incision into the bladder. In most cases the procedure is done to divert the flow of urine when the bladder can no longer function as a reservoir. After incising the bladder the surgeon moves it forward and sutures the bladder opening to the skin, forming a STOMA. Patient care is similar to that required for CUTANEOUS URETEROSTOMY and ILEAL CONDUIT. Called also cystotomy.

vesicoureteral (ves″ĭ-ko-u-re′ter-al) pertaining to the bladder and ureter.

vesicouterine (ves″ĭ-ko-u′ter-in) pertaining to the bladder and uterus.

vesicovaginal (ves″ĭ-ko-vaj′ĭ-nal) pertaining to the bladder and vagina.

vesicula (vĕ-sik′u-lah), pl. *vesic′ulae* [L.] vesicle.

vesicular (vĕ-sik′u-lar) 1. composed of or relating to small, saclike bodies. 2. pertaining to or made up of vesicles on the skin.

vesiculation (vĕ-sik″u-la′shun) formation of vesicles.

vesiculectomy (vĕ-sik″u-lek′to-me) excision of a vesicle, especially the seminal vesicle.

vesiculiform (vĕ-sik′u-lĭ-form) shaped like a vesicle.

vesiculitis (vĕ-sik″u-li′tis) inflammation of a vesicle, especially a seminal vesicle (seminal vesiculitis).

vesiculocavernous (vĕ-sik″u-lo-kav′er-nus) both vesicular and cavernous.

vesiculogram (vĕ-sik′u-lo-gram″) a roentgenogram of the seminal vesicles.

vesiculography (vĕ-sik″u-log′rah-fe) roentgenography of the seminal vesicles.

vesiculopapular (vĕ-sik″u-lo-pap′u-lar) marked by or having the characteristics of vesicles and papules.

vesiculopustular (vĕ-sik″u-lo-pus′tu-lar) marked by or having the characteristics of vesicles and pustules.

vesiculotomy (vĕ-sik″u-lot′o-me) incision into a vesicle, especially the seminal vesicles.

vesiculotympanic (vĕ-sik″u-lo-tim-pan′ik) having both a vesicular and tympanic quality; said of percussion sounds.

Vesprin (ves′prin) trademark for preparations of triflupromazine, a major tranquilizer.

vessel (ves′el) any channel for carrying a fluid, such as blood or lymph (see also VAS).

absorbent v's, lymphatic vessels.

blood v., any of the vessels conveying the blood; an artery, arteriole, vein, venule, or capillary.

collateral v's, 1. a vessel that parallels another vessel, a nerve, or other structure. 2. a vessel important in establishing and maintaining a collateral circulation.

great v's, the large vessels entering the heart, including the aorta, the pulmonary arteries and veins, and the venae cavae.

lacteal v's, those that take up chyle from the intestinal wall during digestion.

lymphatic v's, the capillaries, collecting vessels, and trunks that collect lymph from the tissues and carry it to the blood stream.

nutrient v's, vessels supplying nutritive elements to special tissues, as arteries entering the substance of bone or the walls of large blood vessels.

vestibule (ves′tĭ-būl) a space or cavity at the entrance to another structure. adj., **vestib′ular.**

v. of aorta, a small space at the root of the aorta.

v. of ear, an oval cavity in the middle of the bony labyrinth.

v. of mouth, the portion of the oral cavity bounded on the one side by teeth and gingivae, or the residual alveolar ridges, and on the other by the lips (labial vestibule) and cheeks (buccal vestibule).

v. of nose, the anterior part of the nasal cavity.

v. of pharynx, 1. the fauces. 2. oropharynx.

v. of vagina, the space between the labia minora into which the urethra and vagina open.

vestibulocochlear nerve (ves-tib″u-lo-kok′le-ar) the eighth cranial nerve, which emerges from the brain between the pons and medulla oblongata, behind the facial nerve. The vestibular division serves the vestibule of the ear and the semicircular canals, carrying impulses for equilibrium. The cochlear division serves the cochlea and carries impulses for the sense of hearing. Called also acoustic nerve and auditory nerve.

vestibuloplasty (ves-tib′u-lo-plas′te) surgical modification of gingiva–mucous membrane relationships in the vestibule of the mouth.

vestibulotomy (ves-tib″u-lot′o-me) incision into the vestibule of the ear.

vestibulourethral (ves-tib″u-lo-u-re′thral) pertaining to vestibule of the vagina and the urethra.

vestibulum (ves-tib′u-lum), pl. *vestib′ula* [L.] vestibule.

vestige (ves′tij) the remnant of a structure that functioned in a previous stage of species or individual development. adj., **vestig′ial.**

vestigium (ves-tij′e-um), pl. *vestig′ia* [L.] vestige.

veterinarian (vet″er-ĭ-na′re-an) a person trained and authorized to practice veterinary medicine and surgery; a doctor of veterinary medicine.

veterinary (vet′er-ĭ-ner″e) 1. pertaining to domestic animals and their diseases. 2. veterinarian.

V.F. vocal fremitus.

v.f. visual field.

via (vi'ah), pl. *vi'ae* [L.] way; channel.

viability (vi"ah-bil'ĭ-te) the state or quality of being viable.

viable (vi'ah-b'l) able to maintain an independent existence; able to live after birth.

Viadril (vi'ah-dril) trademark for a preparation of hydroxydione, a basal anesthetic.

vial (vi'al) a small bottle.

vibesate (vi'bĕ-sāt) a modified polyvinyl plastic applied topically as a spray to form an occlusive dressing for surgical wounds and other surface lesions.

vibex (vi'beks), pl. *vib'ices* [L.] a narrow linear mark or streak; a linear subcutaneous effusion of blood.

vibratile (vi'brah-tīl) swaying or moving to and fro; vibratory.

vibration (vi-bra'shun) 1. a rapid movement to and fro; oscillation. 2. the shaking of the body as a therapeutic measure. 3. a form of massage.

vibrator (vi'bra-tor) an apparatus used in vibratory treatment.

vibratory (vi'brah-tor"e) vibrating or causing vibration; vibritile.

Vibrio (vib're-o) a genus of gram-negative bacteria (family Spirillaceae).

V. chol'erae, the etiologic agent of classic (Asiatic) cholera in man; called also *Vibrio comma.*

V. com'ma, *Vibrio cholerae.*

vibrio (vib're-o) an organism of the genus *Vibrio,* or other spiral motile organism.

cholera v., *Vibrio cholerae.*

El Tor v., a biotype of *Vibrio cholerae.*

vibriocidal (vib"re-o-si'dal) destructive to organisms of the genus *Vibrio,* especially *V. cholerae.*

vibrion (ve"bre-on') a vibrio, or spiral motile organism.

v. septique, *Clostridium septicum.*

vibrissa (vi-bris'ah), pl. *vibris'sae* [L.] one of the hairs growing in the vestibule of the nose in man or about the nose (muzzle) of an animal.

vibrocardiogram (vi"bro-kar'de-o-gram") the record produced by vibrocardiography.

vibrocardiography (vi"bro-kar"de-og'rah-fe) graphic recording of vibrations of the chest wall of relatively high frequency that are produced by the action of the heart.

vibrotherapeutics (vi"bro-ther"ah-pu'tiks) the therapeutic use of vibrating appliances.

Vic d'Azyr's bundle (vĕk dah-zērz) a band of fibers extending from the mamillary body to the anterior nucleus of the thalamus.

Vicia (vish'e-ah) a genus of herbs.

V. fa'ba (V. fa'va), the fava or broad bean, whose beans or pollen contain a component capable of causing favism in susceptible persons.

vidarabine (vi-dār'ah-bēn) an antiviral ophthalmic agent used topically in the treatment of herpes simplex keratitis. Called also adenine arabinoside.

videognosis (vid"e-og-no'sis) diagnosis based on the interpretation of roentgenograms transmitted by television techniques to a radiologic center.

vigilambulism (vij"il-am'bu-lizm) a state resembling somnambulism, but not occurring in sleep; double or multiple personality.

Villaret's syndrome (ve-lah-rāz') unilateral paralysis of the glossopharyngeal, vagus, spinal accessory, and hypoglossal nerves and sometimes the facial nerve, due to a lesion in the retroparotid space.

villi (vil'i) [L.] plural of *villus.*

villikinin (vil"ĭ-ki'nin) a hypothetical hormone said to stimulate intestinal villus movement.

villoma (vĭ-lo'mah) a papilloma, chiefly of the rectum.

villose (vil'ōs) shaggy with soft hairs; covered with villi.

villositis (vil"o-si'tis) a bacterial disease with alterations in the villi of the placenta.

villosity (vĭ-los'ĭ-te) 1. condition of being covered with villi. 2. a villus.

villus (vil'us), pl. *vil'li* [L.] a small vascular process or protrusion, as from the free surface of a membrane.

arachnoid villi, microscopic projections of the arachnoid into some of the venous sinuses. (See also arachnoid GRANULATIONS.)

chorionic villi, threadlike projections originally occurring uniformly over the external surface of the chorion.

intestinal villi, multitudinous threadlike projections covering the surface of the mucous membrane lining the small intestine, serving as the sites of absorption of fluids and nutrients (see Plate 10).

synovial villi, slender projections from the surface of the synovial membrane into the cavity of a joint; called also haversian glands.

villusectomy (vil"ŭ-sek'to-me) synovectomy; excision of a synovial villus.

Vinactane (vin-ak'tān) trademark for a preparation of viomycin, a tuberculostatic antibiotic.

vinbarbital (vin-bar'bĭ-tal) an intermediate-acting barbiturate used orally as a sedative. Also used as the sodium salt and administered parenterally.

vinblastine (vin-blas'tēn) an antineoplastic alkaloid derived from *Vinca rosa;* used as the sulfate salt, especially for supplemental or alternative therapy in the treatment of Hodgkin's disease.

Vinca (vin'kah) a genus of apocynaceous woody herbs, including *V. ro'sea* (Madagascar periwinkle), which contains many alkaloids, such as vinblastine and vincristine.

Vincent's angina (vin'sents) gingivostomatitis caused by extension to the oral mucosa of necrotizing ulcerative gingivitis (TRENCH MOUTH), characterized by ulceration, pseudomembrane, and odor, with lesions involving the palate or pharynx as well as the oral mucosa. Called also necrotizing ulcerative gingivostomatitis.

Vincent's disease (gingivitis) (vin'sents) trench mouth.

vincristine (vin-kris'tēn) an antineoplastic alkaloid extracted from *Vinca rosea;* used as the sulfate salt.

vinculum (ving'ku-lum), pl. *vin'cula* [L.] a band or bandlike structure.

vin'cula ten'dinum, filaments that connect the phalanges with the flexor tendons.

vinegar (vin'ĕ-gar) 1. a weak and impure dilution of acetic acid. 2. a medicinal preparation of dilute acetic acid.

Vinethene (vin′ĕ-thēn) trademark for vinyl ether, an anesthetic.

Vinke tongs a type of tongs used to exert traction on the skull, as in surgery for fractures or cervical vertebrae.

vinleurosine (vin-lo͞or′o-sēn) an antineoplastic alkaloid from *Vinca rosea.*

vinyl (vi′nil) the univalent group, CH_2CH, from vinyl alcohol.

Viocin (vi′o-sin) trademark for a preparation of viomycin, a tuberculostatic antibiotic.

Vioform (vi′o-form) trademark for preparations of iodochlorhydroxyquin, a topical anti-infective.

violet (vi′o-let) 1. the reddish blue color produced by the shortest rays of the visible spectrum. 2. a dye that produces a reddish blue color.

crystal v., gentian v., methyl v., a dye derived from triphenylmethane, used as a topical anti-infective, stain, and internal anthelmintic; called also methylrosaniline chloride.

viomycin (vi″o-mi′sin) an antibiotic produced by *Streptomyces puniceus, S. floridae,* and *Actinomyces vinaceus,* or by other means; the sulfate salt is used as a tuberculostatic.

viosterol (vi-os′ter-ol) ergocalciferol.

viper (vi′per) any venomous snake of the Vipera, including the sand viper (*V. ammodytes*), the adder or European viper (*V. berus*), and Russell's viper (*V. russelli*).

viral (vi′ral) pertaining to or caused by a virus.

Virales (vi-ra′lēz) the taxonomic order comprising the viruses.

Virchow's node (vēr′kōz) an enlarged supraclavicular lymph node; often the first sign of a malignant abdominal tumor. Called also sentinel, or signal, node.

viremia (vi-re′me-ah) the presence of viruses in the blood.

virgin (vir′jin) a female who has not had coitus.

virile (vir′il) 1. peculiar to men or the male sex. 2. possessing masculine traits, especially copulative power.

virilescence (vir″ĭ-les′ens) the development of male secondary sex characters in the female.

virilism (vir′ĭ-lizm) the presence of male characteristics in the female. (See also VIRILIZATION.)

virility (vĭ-ril′ĭ-te) possession of normal primary sex characters in a male.

virilization (vir″ĭ-lĭ-za′shun) induction or development of male secondary sex characters, especially the appearance of such changes in the female. Called also masculinization.

virion (vi′re-on) the complete viral particle, found extracellullarly and capable of surviving in crystalline form and infecting a living cell; it comprises the nucleoid (genetic material) and the capsid.

virologist (vi-rol′o-jist) microbiologist specializing in virology.

virology (vi-rol′o-je) the study of viruses and viral diseases.

virucidal (vi″rŭ-si′dal) capable of neutralizing or destroying a virus.

virucide (vi′rŭ-sīd) an agent that neutralizes or destroys a virus.

virulence (vir′u-lens) the degree of pathogenicity of a microorganism as indicated by case fatality rates and/or its ability to invade the tissues of the host; the competence of any infectious agent to produce pathologic effects. adj., **vir′ulent.**

viruliferous (vir″u-lif′er-us) conveying or producing a virus or other noxious agent.

viruria (vi-roo′re-ah) the presence of viruses in the urine.

virus (vi′rus) a minute infectious agent, smaller than a bacterium, which is able to replicate only within a living host cell.

Viruses are so elusive that in most instances they cannot be identified and observed by the conventional methods of microbiology. The electron microscope makes it possible to "see" viruses, and they can be isolated by straining them through the minuscule pores of special filters. Viruses thrive only within the cells of living hosts, so that tissue cultures are used to grow viruses for use in vaccines.

CHARACTERISTICS OF VIRUSES. A virus has no metabolic activity of its own, but it has a very orderly structure, so uniform that some viruses can be crystallized much like common salt. The most important substance in viruses is nucleoprotein, a compound of protein and of nucleic acid, which is a substance common to all living matter. The nucleic acid, either deoxyribonucleic acid (DNA) or ribonucleic acid (RNA), contains the "instructions" and mechanisms that allow the virus to control the metabolic activity of the cells it infects. The nucleoprotein of the virus may be surrounded by one or more protein membranes.

Viruses are parasitic. They attach themselves to a living cell of a plant, animal, or human body, inject nucleoprotein into the cell and control the cell's normal metabolic mechanisms. The cell proceeds to make vital structures and assembles the units into complete viruses. The cell bursts, dies, and releases countless viruses, which can then invade other cells.

In some cases the virus may remain inactive for long periods before taking over control of cellular metabolism. In other cases, the virus may force the cell to make new cells as well as new viruses.

In addition to damaging the host by destroying cells, viruses may produce toxins. Viruses also act as antigens, substances the body recognizes as being foreign and combats by producing antibodies.

Viruses are causative organisms of a variety of infectious diseases, including the common cold, yellow fever, childhood diseases such as chickenpox, measles, mumps, and rubella, and certain types of pneumonia and encephalitis. Certain viruses have been shown to cause cancer in laboratory animals, but there is still no evidence that they can cause cancer in man. Viruses have the ability to change their individual characteristics so that they are able to continue to grow and propagate while adapting to new environments. This makes chemical treatment of viral diseases difficult since the viruses surviving an initial dose of a drug can change their characteristics so that they rapidly become resistant to the drug.

arbor (*ar*thropod-*borne*) **v.,** arbovirus.

attenuated v., one whose pathogenicity has been reduced by serial animal passage or other means.

bacterial v., one that is capable of producing transmissible lysis of bacteria (see also BACTERIOPHAGE).

Coxsackie v., coxsackievirus.

defective v., one that cannot be completely replicated or cannot form a protein coat; in some cases replication can proceed if missing gene functions are supplied by other viruses (see HELPER VIRUS).

ECHO (*e*nteric *c*ytopathogenic *h*uman *o*rphan) **v.**, echovirus.

EB v., Epstein-Barr virus.

encephalomyocarditis v., an enterovirus that causes mild aseptic meningitis and encephalomyocarditis.

enteric v., enterovirus.

enteric orphan v's, orphan viruses isolated from the intestinal tract of man and various other animals.

Epstein-Barr v., a herpesvirus that is the etiologic agent of infectious mononucleosis (see also EPSTEIN-BARR VIRUS).

filterable v., filtrable v., a pathogenic agent capable of passing through fine filters of diatomite or unglazed porcelain; ultravirus.

v. fixé, fixed v., rabies virus whose virulence and incubation period have been stabilized by serial passage and have remained fixed during further transmission; used for inoculating animals from which rabies vaccine is prepared.

helper v., one that aids in the development of a defective virus by supplying or restoring the activity of the viral gene or enabling it to form a protein coat.

herpes v., herpesvirus.

latent v., one that ordinarily occurs in a noninfective state and is demonstrable by indirect methods that activate it.

lytic v., one that is replicated in the host cell and causes death and lysis of the cell.

masked v., latent virus.

orphan v's, viruses isolated in tissue culture, but not found specifically associated with any disease.

parainfluenza v., one of a group of viruses isolated from patients with upper respiratory tract disease of varying severity.

plant v's, viruses that replicate in and may cause diseases of higher plants.

pox v., poxvirus.

respiratory syncytial v., a virus isolated from children with bronchopneumonia and bronchitis, characteristically causing syncytium formation in tissue culture.

street v., Pasteur's name for rabies virus derived from a dog with a naturally acquired case of the disease.

vis (vis), pl. *vi'res* [L.] force, energy.

viscer(o)- word element [L.], *viscera.*

viscera (vis'er-ah) [L.] plural of *viscus.*

viscerad (vis'er-ad) toward the viscera.

visceral (vis'er-al) pertaining to a viscus.

visceralgia (vis″er-al'je-ah) pain in any viscera.

visceroinhibitory (vis″er-o-in-hib'ĭ-tor″e) inhibiting the essential movements of any viscus.

visceromegaly (vis″er-o-meg'ah-le) splanchnomegaly.

visceromotor (vis″er-o-mo'tor) concerned in the essential movements of the viscera.

visceroparietal (vis″er-o-pah-ri'ĕ-tal) pertaining to the viscera and the abdominal wall.

visceroperitoneal (vis″er-o-per″ĭ-to-ne'al) pertaining to the viscera and peritoneum.

visceropleural (vis″er-o-ploo'ral) pertaining to the viscera and the pleura.

visceroptosis (vis″er-op-to'sis) splanchnoptosis; prolapse or downward displacement of the viscera.

viscerosensory (vis″er-o-sen'so-re) pertaining to sensation in the viscera.

visceroskeletal (vis″er-o-skel'ĕ-tal) pertaining to the visceral skeleton.

viscerosomatic (vis″er-o-so-mat'ik) pertaining to the viscera and the body.

viscerotonia (vis″er-o-to'ne-ah) a group of traits characterized by general relaxation, and love of comfort, sociability, and conviviality; considered typical of an endomorph.

viscerotropic (vis″er-o-trop'ik) acting primarily on the viscera; having a predilection for the abdominal or thoracic viscera.

viscid (vis'id) glutinous or sticky.

viscidity (vĭ-sid'ĭ-te) the property of being viscid.

viscosimeter (vis″ko-sim'ĕ-ter) an apparatus used in measuring viscosity of a substance.

viscosity (vis-kos'ĭ-te) resistance to flow; a physical property of a substance that is dependent on the friction of its component molecules as they slide by one another.

viscous (vis'kus) sticky or gummy; having a high degree of viscosity.

viscus (vis'kus), pl. *vis'cera* [L.] any large interior organ in any of the great body cavities, especially those in the abdomen.

vision (vizh'un) the faculty of seeing; sight. adj., **vis'ual.** The basic components of vision are the eye itself, the visual center in the brain, and the optic nerve, which connects the two. (See Plate 15.)

HOW THE EYE WORKS. The eye works like a camera. Light rays enter it through the adjustable iris and are focused by the lens onto the retina, a thin light-sensitive layer which corresponds to the film of the camera. The retina converts the light rays into nerve impulses, which are relayed to the visual center. There the brain interprets them as images.

Like a camera lens, the lens of the eye reverses images as it focuses them. The images on the retina are upside down and they are "flipped over" in the visual center. In a psychology experiment, a number of volunteers wore glasses that inverted everything. After 8 days, their visual centers adjusted to this new situation, and when they took off the glasses, the world looked upside down until their brain centers readjusted.

The retina is made up of millions of tiny nerve cells that contain specialized chemicals that are sensitive to light. There are two varieties of these nerve cells, rods and cones. Between them they cover the full range of the eye's adaptation to light. The cones are sensitive in bright light, and the rods in dim light. At twilight, as the light fades, the cones stop operating and the rods go into action. The momentary blindness experienced on going from bright to dim light, or from dim to bright, is the pause needed for the other set of nerve cells to take over.

The rods are spread toward the edges of the retina, so that vision in dim light is general but not very sharp or clear. The cones are clustered thickly in the center of the retina, in the fovea centralis. When the eyes are turned and focused on the object to be seen the image is brought to the central area of the retina. In very dim light, on the other hand, an object is seen more clearly if it is not looked at directly because then its image falls on an area where the rods are thicker.

COLOR VISION. Color vision is a function of the cones. The most widely accepted theory of color vision is that there are three types of cones, each type containing chemicals that respond to one of the three primary colors—red, green, and violet. White light stimulates all three sets of cones; any other color stimulates only one or two sets. The brain can then interpret the impulses from these cones as various colors. Man's color vision is amazingly delicate; a trained expert can distinguish among as many as 300,000 different hues.

COLOR BLINDNESS is the result of a disorder of one or more sets of cones. The great majority of people with some degree of color blindness lack either red or green cones, and cannot distinguish between the two colors. True color blindness, in which none of the sets of color cones works, is very rare. Most color blindness is inherited, and mostly by male children through their mothers from a color-blind grandfather.

STEREOSCOPIC VISION. Stereoscopic vision, or vision in depth, is caused by the way the eyes are placed. Each eye has a slightly different field of vision. The two images are superimposed on one another, but because of the distance between the eyes, the image from each eye goes slightly around its side of the object. From the differences between the images and from other indicators such as the position of the eye muscles when the eyes are focused on the object, the brain can determine the distance of the object.

Stereoscopic vision works best on nearby objects. As the distance increases, the difference between the left-eyed and the right-eyed views becomes less, and the brain must depend on other factors to determine distance. Among these are the relative size of the object, its color and clearness, and the receding lines of perspective. These factors may fool the eye; for example, in clear mountain air distant objects may seem to be very close. This is because their sharpness and color are not dulled by the atmosphere as much as they would be in more familiar settings.

DISORDERS OF VISION. Imperfect vision is most commonly caused by abnormal shape of the eyeball. In the normal eye, the lens focuses the image on the retina. This is 20/20 vision. The figures refer to the distance at which a standard object can be recognized. A person who is nearsighted, for example, may only be able to recognize at 20 feet an object that a person with perfect vision can recognize at 100 feet. In this case he is said to have 20/100 vision. For the sake of convenience, eye charts with letters of different sizes are used rather than objects placed at different distances.

Nearsightedness, or myopia, is the result of an eyeball that is longer than usual from front to back, so that the image falls in front of the retina. The lens can bring nearby objects into focus, but not those farther away. Farsightedness, or hyperopia, is caused by an eyeball that is shorter than normal, in which the image focuses behind the retina. ASTIGMATISM is impaired vision caused by irregularities in the curvature of the cornea or lens. All of these conditions can usually be corrected with prescription lenses.

achromatic v., vision characterized by lack of color vision.

binocular v., the use of both eyes together, without diplopia.

central v., that produced by stimulation of receptors in the fovea centralis.

day v., visual perception in the daylight or under conditions of bright illumination.

dichromatic v., that in which color perception is

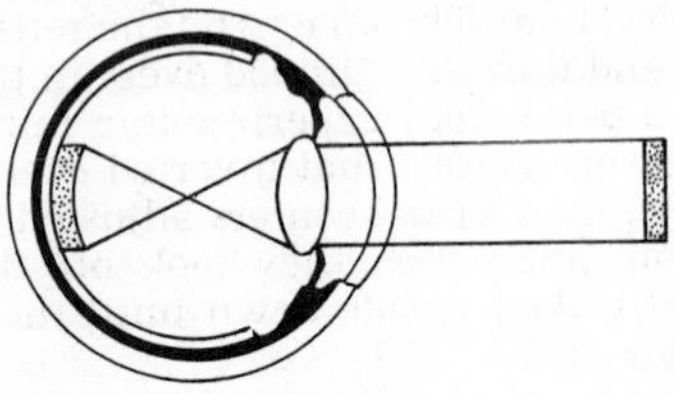

Normal vision

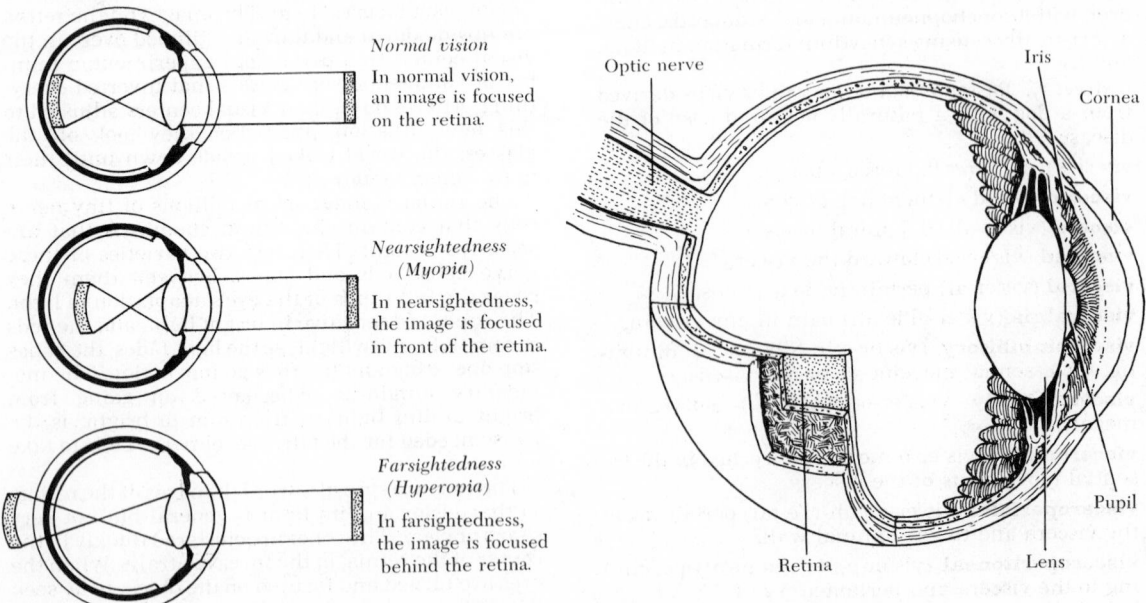

In normal vision, an image is focused on the retina.

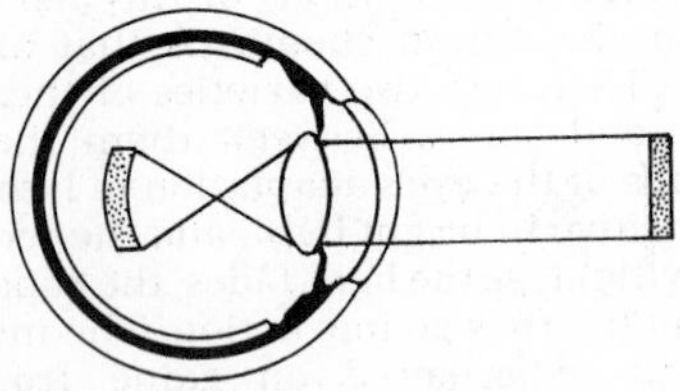

Nearsightedness (Myopia)

In nearsightedness, the image is focused in front of the retina.

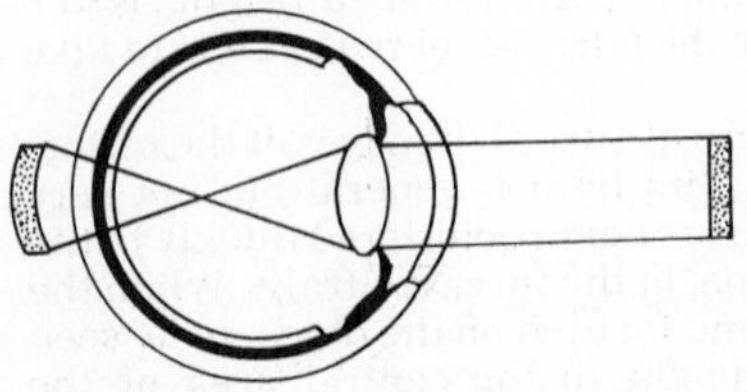

Farsightedness (Hyperopia)

In farsightedness, the image is focused behind the retina.

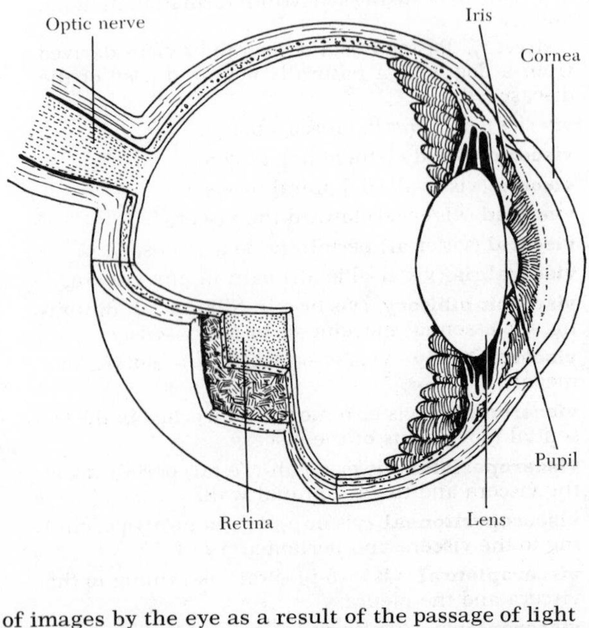

Right, anatomy of the eye. Vision is the reception of images by the eye as a result of the passage of light into the eye. Light is focused by the lens on the retina where it is converted into nerve impulses which are transmitted to the centers in the brain where images are interpreted.

restricted to a pair of primaries, either blue and yellow or (rarely) red and green.

double v., diplopia.

half v., hemianopia.

indirect v., peripheral vision.

monocular v., vision with one eye.

multiple v., polyopia.

night v., visual perception in the darkness of night or under conditions of reduced illumination.

oscillating v., oscillopsia.

peripheral v., that produced by stimulation of receptors in the retina outside the macula lutea.

tunnel v., a condition of concentric reduction in the visual field, as though the subject were looking through a long tunnel or tube.

visualization (vizh″u-al-ĭ-za′shun) the act of viewing or of achieving a complete visual impression of an object.

visuoauditory (vizh″u-o-aw′dĭ-to″re) pertaining to sight and hearing.

visuognosis (vizh″u-og-no′sis) recognition and interpretation of visual impressions.

visuopsychic (vizh″u-o-si′kik) visual and psychic; applied to the area of the cerebral cortex concerned in judgment of visual sensation.

visuosensory (vizh″u-o-sen′so-re) pertaining to perception of visual impressions.

vital (vi′tal) pertaining to life; necessary to life.

v. capacity, the volume of gas that can be expelled from the lungs from a position of full inspiration, with no limit to duration of expiration; equal to inspiratory capacity plus expiratory reserve volume.

v. signs, the signs of life, namely pulse, respiration, and temperature.

v. statistics, that branch of biometry dealing with the data and laws of human mortality, morbidity, natality, and demography.

vitalism (vi′tah-lizm) the theory that biological functions are produced by a distinct principal called vital force. adj., **vitalis′tic.**

vitalist (vi′tah-list) a believer in vitalism.

Vitallium (vi-tal′e-um) trademark for a cobalt-chromium alloy used for dentures and surgical appliances.

vitamer (vi′tah-mer) a substance or compound that has vitamin activity.

vitamin (vi′tah-min) an organic substance found in foods and essential in small quantities for growth, health, and the preservation of life itself. The body needs vitamins just as it requires other food constituents such as proteins, fats, carbohydrates, minerals, and water. Vitamins differ from these in chemical structure, however, and are required only in relatively minute quantities. The absence of one or more vitamins from the diet, or poor absorption of vitamins, can cause deficiency diseases such as rickets, scurvy, and beriberi.

Vitamins help transform other food substances into bones, skin, glands, nerves, brain, and blood.

The major vitamins are designated by the letters A, C, D, E, and K, and the term B complex. Some of these, the B vitamins and vitamin C, can be dissolved in water; the rest are soluble in fat. Vitamins do not resemble each other chemically except for their solubility. This quality of solubility is important in absorption of vitamins from the intestinal tract and in certain deficiency diseases.

VITAMIN A. Vitamin A helps to maintain epithelial tissues which cover the body and line certain internal organs. This vitamin also is essential for the proper growth of skeletal and soft tissues, and is necessary for light-sensitive pigments in the eye that make night vision possible. The particular manifestation of vitamin A deficiency depends upon the age of the patient. Among the commonest symptoms of vitamin A deficiency is night blindness. The skin may also be affected, becoming dry and pimply like a toad's skin.

Vitamin A occurs in nature in two forms: retinol (vitamin A_1) and dehydroretinol (vitamin A_2). It is manufactured by animals and man from carotenes found in green leafy and yellow vegetables, including kale, broccoli, spinach, carrots, squash, and sweet potatoes. It is obtained directly by eating animal products such as liver, eggs, whole milk, cream, and cheese.

THE B COMPLEX. The original "vitamin B" was found to be a group of vitamins, each differing chemically and each individually important in the body. For convenience, these vitamins are referred to as one group since they are often found together in foods. Deficiency in only one of these vitamins is rare, and the deficiency disease attributed to lack of one vitamin B usually is complicated by deficiencies of the others as well.

Vitamin B_1 (Thiamine). This vitamin is necessary to break down and release energy from carbohydrates. Lack of thiamine can cause loss of appetite, certain types of neuritis, and, in severe cases, BERIBERI, which affects the brain, heart, and nerves.

The best sources of thiamine are yeasts, ham, and certain pork cuts, liver, peanuts, whole and fortified cereals, and milk. The vitamin is easily destroyed by cooking and may also be lost by dissolving in the cooking water. Because the body does not store thiamine well, foods that are good sources of it should be included in each day's diet.

Vitamin B_2 (Riboflavin). This vitamin functions as a coenzyme concerned with oxidative processes. Riboflavin deficiency (ariboflavinosis) is believed to be one of the most common vitamin-deficiency diseases in the United States. The symptoms include open sores at the corners of the mouth and on the lips, a purple-red, inflamed tongue, seborrheic dermatitis, and corneal and other eye changes.

The main food sources of riboflavin are milk, liver, kidney, heart, green vegetables, dried yeasts, and enriched cereals. It is not usually affected by cooking, but is destroyed by light.

Niacin (Nicotinic Acid). This vitamin B appears to act in enzyme systems to utilize carbohydrates, fats, and amino acids. Niacin deficiency causes PELLAGRA, once a major deficiency disease in the United States. Symptoms of pellagra involve the skin and digestive and nervous systems. The vitamin also has vasodilating activity.

Food sources of niacin are various high-protein foods such as liver, yeast, bran, peanuts, lean meats, fish, and poultry.

Vitamin B_{12}. This vitamin contains a metal, cobalt. It is called also cyanocobalamin and extrinsic factor, and is needed for the efficient production of blood cells and for the health of the nervous system. Only small amounts of B_{12} are required by the body. The activity of this vitamin is associated with that of another B vitamin, folic acid.

Inability to absorb vitamin B_{12} occurs in PERNICIOUS ANEMIA, in which a substance normally secreted by the stomach, called intrinsic factor, is missing. Intrinsic factor is needed to absorb vitamin

B_{12} in the small intestine. Injections of vitamin B_{12} can control pernicious anemia. Poor absorption of vitamin B_{12} also occurs in sprue.

Vitamin B_{12} is not found in plant foods. The main source in the human diet are animal products such as milk, eggs, and liver. Probably the ultimate source of B_{12} is bacterial production in animal intestines. This production occurs in man, and in normal persons probably meets some or perhaps all of the body's requirements.

Other B Vitamins. These include vitamin B_6 (pyridoxine), biotin, folic acid, pantothenic acid, choline, inositol, and para-aminobenzoic acid. Vitamin B_6 deficiency can cause convulsions, lethargy, mental changes and retardation, inflammation of the skin, and anemia.

These vitamins, like most other members of the B complex, are widely found in fruits, vegetables, meat, and whole-grain cereals.

VITAMIN C (ASCORBIC ACID). This vitamin is necessary for the health of the supporting tissues of the body such as bone, cartilage, and connective tissue (see also ASCORBIC ACID). Vitamin C deficiency produces SCURVY.

Vitamin C is found in fresh fruits and vegetables, including citrus fruits, tomatoes, brussels sprouts, and to some extent whole potatoes. Cooking and storage destroys much of the vitamin C content of foods.

VITAMIN D. The action of sunlight on the skin changes certain substances in the body into vitamin D, a term for any of several active substances required for the utilization of calcium and phosphorus, essential for the growth and maintenance of bone, including cholecalciferol and ergocalciferol (know collectively as calciferol). Vitamin D deficiency causes RICKETS in children and OSTEOMALACIA and OSTEOPOROSIS in adults. Rickets is usually caused either by a diet deficient in vitamin D or by insufficient exposure to sunlight.

Few foods contain vitamin D. The only rich natural sources are fish liver oil and the livers of animals feeding on fish. For this reason vitamin D often is added to milk.

VITAMIN E. The role of this vitamin in human nutrition is uncertain. It is necessary in the diet of many species for normal reproduction, normal muscular development, normal resistance of erythrocytes to hemolysis, and various other biochemical functions; chemically, it is α-tocopherol, found in wheat germ oil, cereals, egg yolk, and beef liver, or produced synthetically.

VITAMIN K. Any of a group of vitamins found in alfalfa, spinach, cabbage, putrefied fish meal, and hempseed, which promote blood clotting by increasing the synthesis of prothrombin by the liver, therefore, deficiency of vitamin K delays clotting. Symptoms are excessive bleeding and bruises under the skin.

Generally, the bacteria of the intestine produce vitamin K in quantities that are adequate (provided it can be absorbed), except in newborn infants, in whom the deficiency is most frequently found.

VITAMIN SUPPLEMENTS. The exact vitamin requirements for good health often are not known with accuracy; they vary with age, weight, sex, and state of health. The need for certain vitamins increases with fever, some diseases, heavy exercise, pregnancy, and nursing.

If a person eats an adequate, varied diet of meats, fish, vegetables, and dairy products, he will receive enough vitamins to meet his usual requirements. Public health measures such as the addition of vitamin D to milk and the B vitamins to bread and other cereal products have helped to combat deficiency diseases.

The use of vitamin supplements is expensive and in general unnecessary. Specialists in nutrition advise against taking supplementary vitamins unless they are prescribed for a specific reason by a physician. Vitamins should not be used as "tonics." There is a distinct possibility that the indiscriminate use of vitamin preparations may sometimes lead to overdosage, a problem that has arisen in recent years. For example, overdoses of vitamins D, A, or K may result in serious disease, the excess vitamins acting like poisons. Also, tests suggest that large doses of vitamin D taken by a woman during pregnancy may have undesirable effects on her unborn child. Though these tests are not conclusive, they confirm the need for caution in the use of vitamins.

Vitamins are commonly prescribed in infancy and childhood, during pregnancy and nursing, for elderly patients whose dietary habits are poor, and in clearly diagnosed deficiency states. These include not only the more familiar deficiency diseases already described but also alcoholism and chronic wasting diseases.

vitellus (vi-tel′us) the yolk of egg.

vitellin (vi-tel′in) the phosphoprotein found in egg yolk.

vitelline (vi-tel′in) resembling or pertaining to the yolk of an egg or ovum.

vitellolutein (vi″tel-o-lu′te-in) yellow pigment obtainable from egg yolk.

vitellorubin (vi″tel-o-roo′bin) reddish pigment obtainable from egg yolk.

vitiligines (vit″ĭ-lij′ĭ-nēz) depigmented areas of the skin.

vitiligo (vit″ĭ-li′go) a condition in which destruction of melanocytes in small or large circumscribed areas results in patches of depigmentation often having a hyperpigmented border, and often enlarging slowly. adj., **vitilig′inous.**

vitrectomy (vĭ-trek′to-me) aspiration of the vitreous and replacement with a saline solution or vitreous; done to clear an opaque vitreous.

vitreodentin (vit″re-o-den′tin) an unusually hard and glasslike form of dentin.

vitreous (vit′re-us) 1. glasslike or hyaline. 2. the vitreous body.

v. body, the transparent gel filling the inner part of the eyeball between the lens and retina.

v. humor, 1. vitreous body. 2. the watery substance contained within the interstices of the stroma in the vitreous body.

persistent hyperplastic v., a congenital anomaly, usually unilateral, due to persistence of embryonic remnants of the fibromuscular tunic of the eye and part of the hyaloid vascular system. Clinically, there is a white pupil, elongated ciliary processes, and often microphthalmia; the lens, although clear initially, may become completely opaque.

vitriol (vit′re-ol) any crystalline sulfate.

blue v., copper sulfate.
green v., ferrous sulfate.
white v., zinc sulfate.

vitropression (vit′ro-presh′un) exertion of pressure

(*Text continued on page 1092.*)

The Principal Vitamins

Vitamin	Principal Sources	Properties	Physiologic Effects	Deficiency Symptoms	Daily Allowances	Usual Therapeutic Dosage
Vitamin A	Fish liver oils, liver, eggs, milk, butter, vitamin A-fortified margarine, green leafy or yellow vegetables	Oil-soluble; susceptible to oxidation, especially at high temperatures	Essential to normal function of epithelial cells and visual purple	Night blindness Xerophthalmia Hyperkeratosis of skin	Adults: 5,000–8,000 U.S.P. u.† Children: 1,500–5,000 U.S.P. u.‡	Up to 100,000 U.S.P. u./day
Vitamin B_1 (Thiamine)	Yeast, whole grains; meat, especially pork, liver; nuts, egg yolk, legumes, potatoes, most vegetables	Water-soluble; stable to heat, unstable to alkali, but heat-sensitive under neutral and alkaline conditions	Carbohydrate metabolism, nerve function; promotes growth	Beriberi Peripheral neuritis Cardiac disease	All ages: 0.4 mg./1,000 calories	5–30 mg./day
Vitamin B_2 (Riboflavin)	Milk, cheese, liver, organ meats, beef muscle, egg white	Slightly water-soluble; unstable to light and alkali	Promotes growth, general health; essential to cellular oxidation	Cheilosis Angular stomatitis Dermatitis Photophobia	All ages: 0.6 mg./1,000 calories	10–30 mg./day
Niacin (Nicotinic acid)	Yeast, liver, organ meats, peanuts, wheat germ	Water-soluble; stable; intolerance produces flushing, burning, itching (rare with niacinamide)	Essential for health, tissue respiration, tryptophan and carbohydrate metabolism, growth, gastrointestinal function and normal skin	Pellagra (Dermatitis, glossitis, gastrointestinal and nervous system dysfunction)	All ages: 6.6 mg. equivalent/1,000 calories	(Niacinamide) 100–1,000 mg./day
Vitamin B_6 Group (Pyridoxine, Pyridoxal, Pyridoxamine)	Yeast, liver, muscle meats, whole-grain cereals, fish, vegetables, molasses	Water-soluble; heat-, acid- and alkali-stable; sparingly soluble in alcohol; light-sensitive in neutral and alkaline solutions; nontoxic in recommended doses	Essential for cellular function and for metabolism of certain amino and fatty acids	Seborrhea-like skin lesions. Nerve inflammation Epileptiform convulsions in infants Anemias	Not established, but thought to be 1.5–2.0 mg./day	25–100 mg./day

THE PRINCIPAL VITAMINS (*Concluded*)

VITAMIN	PRINCIPAL SOURCES	PROPERTIES	PHYSIOLOGIC EFFECTS	DEFICIENCY SYMPTOMS	DAILY ALLOWANCES	USUAL THERAPEUTIC DOSAGE
Vitamin B_{12} (Cyanocobalamin)	Liver; meats, especially beef, pork, organ meats; eggs, milk and milk products	Water- and alcohol-soluble; nontoxic	Maturation of r.b.c.; neural function; may be a growth factor; may be implicated in carbohydrate and fat metabolism	Pernicious anemia; may have a beneficial effect in certain neuritides; tobacco-alcohol amblyopia	Not established, but thought to be about 3–5 (1.0–1.5 absorbed) mcg.	1–2 mcg./day I.M. to maintain remission in pernicious anemia
Vitamin C (Ascorbic acid)	Citrus fruits, tomatoes, potatoes, cabbage, green pepper	Water-soluble; stable in dry state but oxidized by heat and light; nontoxic in recommended doses	Essential to osteoid tissue, collagen formation, vascular function, tissue respiration and wound healing; relationship to adrenocortical hormones suggested	Scurvy (Hemorrhages, loose teeth, gingivitis)	Adults: 70 mg. Children: 30–80 mg.	100–1,000 mg. /day
Vitamin D Ergocalciferol (D_2) Cholecalciferol (D_3)	Fish liver oils, eggs, milk, butter, sunlight and irradiation	Oil-soluble; in large doses may cause hypercalcemia	Metabolism of Ca and K	Infantile rickets Infantile tetany Osteomalacia	Adults and Children: 400 U.S.P. u.	400–1,600 U.S.P. u./day
Folic acid (Pteroylglutamic acid)	Green leafy vegetables, liver and kidney, yeast	Soluble in boiling water or dilute aqueous alkali; nontoxic in recommended doses	Maturation of r.b.c.; may be concerned in synthesis of nucleoproteins	Nutritional macrocytic anemia; may be of value in the treatment of sprue; megaloblastic anemia of infancy	Not established, but 0.05 mg. (0.15 mg. total folic acid activity in foods)/day has been suggested	1–15 mg./day

Pantothenic acid (Calcium pantothenate)	Yeast, liver, kidneys, egg yolk, vegetables	Water-soluble viscous oil; unstable in hot acid or basic solutions	Involved in fat, protein and carbohydrate metabolism by its relation to acetylation processes	Exp'l def'cy in man charact'd by fatigue, malaise, headache, sleep disturbances, nausea, abdominal cramps, vomiting, paresthesias, muscle cramps and impaired coord'n. "Burning feet" syndrome may respond to pantothenate	Not yet established; thought to be about 10 mg. /day	Not known; not <50 mg./day should be used for therapeutic trial
Vitamin K (activity)	Intestinal bacterial synthesis and a normal diet		Prothrombin formation; normal blood coagulation	Hemorrhage from prolonged prothrombin time	Undetermined. In situations conducive to neonatal hemorrhage, 2–5 mg. may be given to mothers in labor, or 1–2 mg. to newborn infant	Varies with the needs of the patient and with the form selected
Menadione		Oil-soluble in water; unstable to light				
Menadione sodium bisulfite		Soluble in water; unstable with alkalis				
Phytonadione (Vitamin K_1)		Oily liquid; unstable to heat and light; insoluble in water				
Vitamin E Group (α, β, γ & δ tocopherol)	Vegetable oils, lettuce, eggs, cereal products	Slightly viscous oil; insoluble in water	Intracellular antioxidant	Abnormal fat deposits in muscles; creatinuria; macrocytic anemia when assoc. with protein def'cy	Not firmly established; may range from 10–30 mg. of d-α-tocopherol /day, depending on am't of polyunsaturated fats in diet	Not established. Perhaps between 50–300 mg.

Adapted from The Merck Manual. 11th ed. Copyright 1966, Merck & Co., Inc., Rahway, New Jersey.
†3,000–5,000 U.S.P. u., if all the activity is due to preformed vitamin A.
‡ 900–3,000 U.S.P. u., if all the activity is due to preformed vitamin A.

on the skin with a slip of glass, forcing blood from the area.

vitrum (vi′rum) [L.] glass.

vivi- word element [L.], *alive; life.*

vividialysis (viv″ĭ-di-al′ĭ-sis) dialysis through a living membrane (see also PERITONEAL DIALYSIS).

vividiffusion (viv″ĭ-dĭ-fu′zhun) circulation of the blood through a closed apparatus in which it is passed through a membrane for removal of substances ordinarily removed by the kidneys (see also artificial KIDNEY).

vivification (viv″ĭ-fĭ-ka′shun) conversion of lifeless into living protein matter by assimilation.

viviparous (vi-vip′ah-rus) giving birth to living young which develop within the maternal body.

vivisection (viv″ĭ-sek′shun) surgical procedures performed upon a living animal for purpose of physiologic or pathologic investigation.

vivisectionist (viv″ĭ-sek′shun-ist) one who practices or defends vivisection.

VLDL very low-density lipoproteins.

vocal (vo′kal) pertaining to the voice.

v. cords, the folds of mucous membrane in the LARYNX, the superior pair being called the false, and the inferior pair the true, vocal cords. These thin, reedlike bands vibrate to make vocal sounds during speaking, and are capable of producing a vast range of sounds.

One end of each cord is attached to the front wall of the larynx. These ends are close together. The opposite ends are connected to two tiny cartilages near the back wall of the larynx. The cartilages can be rotated so as to swing the cords far apart or bring them together. When the cords are apart, the breath passes through silently, unobstructed. When they are closer together, the cords partly obstruct the air passage, and as the air forced through them, the cords vibrate like the reeds of a pipe organ, producing sound waves. These waves are what we call the voice. (See also SPEECH.)

Various disorders may affect the larynx and vocal cords. LARYNGITIS may be acute or chronic and is usually caused by continual irritation of the vocal cords by overuse or by inhaled irritants such as tobacco smoke. The voice may be "lost" and then regained after a few days of rest and medication, if the cause has been removed. Prolonged or repeated impairment of the voice requires medical diagnosis.

LARYNGECTOMY, partial or total removal of the larynx, usually is performed as treatment for cancer of the larynx. Once the larynx is removed the patient must learn to speak without his vocal cords, by one of three methods: esophageal speech, pharyngeal speech, or use of an electronic voice box.

voice (vois) the sound produced by the SPEECH organs and uttered by the mouth.

void (void) to cast out as waste matter, especially the urine.

vol. volume.

vola (vo′lah) a concave or hollow surface.

v. ma′nus, the palm.

v. pe′dis, the sole.

volar (vo′lar) pertaining to the sole or palm; indicating the flexor surface of the forearm, wrist, or hand.

volaris (vo-la′ris) palmar.

volatile (vol′ah-til) evaporating rapidly.

volatilization (vol″ah-til-ĭ-za′shun) conversion into a vapor or gas without chemical change.

volition (vo-lish′un) the act or power of willing. adj., **voli′tional.**

Volkmann's canals (fōlk′mahnz) canals communicating with haversian canals, for passage of blood vessels through bone.

Volkmann's constracture (fōlk′mahnz) contraction of the fingers and sometimes of the wrist or of analogous parts of the foot, with loss of power, after severe injury or improper use of a tourniquet or cast.

Volkmann's disease (fōlk′mahnz) congenital deformity of the foot due to tibiotarsal dislocation.

Volkmann's paralysis (fōlk′mahnz) ischemic paralysis.

volley (vol′e) a rhythmical succession of muscular twitches artificially induced; the aggregate of nerve impulses set up by a single stimulus.

volsella (vol-sel′ah) vulsella.

volt (vōlt) the unit of electromotive force; 1 ampere of current against 1 ohm of resistance.

electron v., the energy acquired by an electron when accelerated by a potential of 1 volt, being equivalent to 3.82×10^{-20} calories, or 1.6×10^{-12} ergs; usually expressed in million electron volts or Mev.

voltage (vōl′tij) electromotive force measured in volts.

voltmeter (vōlt′me-ter) an instrument for measuring electromotive force in volts.

volume (vol′ūm) the space occupied by a substance or a three-dimensional region; the capacity of such a region or of a container.

expiratory reserve v., the maximal amount of gas that can be expired from the end-expiratory level.

inspiratory reserve v., the maximal amount of gas that can be inspired from the end-inspiratory position.

minute v., the volume of air expelled from the lungs per minute.

packed-cell v., the volume of packed red cells in milliliters per 100 ml. of centrifuged blood; abbreviated P.C.V.

residual v., the amount of gas remaining in the lung at the end of a maximal expiration.

stroke v., the quantity of blood ejected from a ventricle at each beat of the heart.

tidal v., the amount of gas passing into and out of the lungs in each respiratory cycle.

volumetric (vol″u-met′rik) pertaining to or accompanied by measurement in volumes.

volumometer (vol″u-mom′ĕ-ter) an instrument for measuring volume or changes in volume.

voluntary (vol′un-tār″e) accomplished in accordance with the will.

volute (vo-lūt) rolled up.

volvulosis (vol″vu-lo′sis) onchocerciasis due to *Onchocerca volvulus.*

volvulus (vol′vu-lus) [L.] torsion of a loop of intestine, causing obstruction with or without strangulation.

vomer (vo′mer) a bone forming part of the nasal septum (see also table of BONES). adj., **vo′merine.**

vomica (vom′ĭ-kah), pl. *vom′icae* [L.] 1. the profuse and sudden expectoration of pus and putrescent matter. 2. an abnormal cavity in an organ, especially in the lung, caused by suppuration and the breaking down of tissue.

vomit (vom′it) 1. matter expelled from the stomach by the mouth. 2. to eject stomach contents through the mouth.

black v., vomit consisting of blood which has been acted upon by the gastric juice, seen in yellow fever and other conditions in which blood collects in the stomach.

coffee-ground v., dark granular material ejected from the stomach, produced by mixture of blood with gastric contents; it is a sign of bleeding in the upper alimentary canal.

vomiting (vom′it-ing) forcible ejection of contents of stomach through the mouth.

cyclic v., recurring attacks of vomiting.

dry v., attempts at vomiting, with the ejection of nothing but gas.

pernicious v., vomiting in pregnancy so severe as to threaten life.

v. of pregnancy, vomiting occurring in pregnancy, especially early morning vomiting (see also MORNING SICKNESS).

projectile v., vomiting with the material ejected with great force; seen commonly in congenital pyloric obstruction.

stercoraceous v., vomiting of fecal matter.

vomitory (vom′ĭ-to″re) an emetic.

vomiturition (vom″ĭ-tu-rish′un) repeated ineffectual attempts to vomit; retching.

vomitus (vom′ĭ-tus) 1. vomiting. 2. matter vomited.

von Gierke's disease (von-gēr′kez) glycogenosis (type I) (see also GIERKE'S DISEASE).

von Hippel's disease (von hip′elz) angiomatosis confined chiefly to the retina.

von Hippel-Lindau disease (von-hip′el-lin′dow) Lindau-von Hippel disease.

von Jaksch's disease (von yaksh) anemia pseudoleukemia infantum.

von Recklinghausen's disease (von rek′ling-how″zenz) 1. neurofibromatosis. 2. see OSTEITIS FIBROSA CYSTICA.

von Willebrand's disease (von vil′ĕ-brandz) a congenital hemorrhagic diathesis with bleeding from the skin and mucosal surfaces, due to abnormal blood vessels, with or without platelet defects or deficiencies of blood CLOTTING factors VIII or IV. Called also angiohemophilia and pseudohemophilia.

vortex (vor′teks), pl. *vor′tices* [L.] a whorled or spiral arrangement or pattern, as of muscle fibers, or of the ridges or hairs of the skin.

vox (voks) [L.] voice.

v. choler′ica, the peculiar suppressed voice of true cholera.

voyeurism (voi′yer-izm) a form of sexual aberration in which gratification is derived from looking at sexual objects or acts.

V.R. vocal resonance.

V.S. volumetric solution.

v.s. vibration seconds (the unit of measurement of sound waves).

vuerometer (vu″er-om′ĕ-ter) an instrument for measuring the distance between the eyes.

vulgaris (vul-ga′ris) [L.] ordinary; common.

vulnerary (vul′ner-er″e) 1. pertaining to wounds or the healing of wounds. 2. an agent that promotes the healing of wounds.

vulnus (vul′nus), pl. *vul′nera* [L.] a wound.

vulsella, vulsellum (vul-sel′ah; vul-sel′um) a forceps with clawlike hooks at the end of each blade.

vulva (vul′vah) the external genital organs in the female. adj., **vul′val, vul′var.**

Two pairs of skin folds protect the vaginal opening, one on each side. The larger outer folds are the labia majora, and the more delicate inner folds are the labia minora. In a virgin, a thin membrane, the hymen, usually partially covers the opening of the vagina. Normally, the hymen is well perforated, to permit the menstrual flow. Occasionally it is not, and a minor surgical procedure may be necessary.

The upper or forward ends of the labia minora join around the clitoris, a small projection that is composed of erectile tissue like the male penis and has erotic functions. The opening of the urethra, which empties urine from the bladder, lies between the clitoris and the vagina. (See also REPRODUCTIVE ORGANS, FEMALE.)

vulvectomy (vul-vek′to-me) excision of the vulva.

vulvismus (vul-viz′mus) vaginismus.

vulvitis (vul-vi′tis) inflammation of the vulva.

vulvocrural (vol″vo-kroo′ral) pertaining to the vulva and thigh.

vulvouterine (vul″vo-u′ter-in) pertaining to the vulva and uterus.

vulvovaginal (vul″vo-vaj′ĭ-nal) pertaining to the vulva and vagina.

vulvovaginitis (vul″vo-vaj″ĭ-ni′tis) inflammation of the vulva and vagina.

vv. [L., pl.] *ve′nae* (veins).

v/v volume (of solute) per volume (of solvent).

W

W chemical symbol, *tungsten* (*wolfram*).

W. wehnelt (a unit of hardness of x-rays).

w. watt.

Waardenburg's syndrome a congenital hereditary syndrome of cochlear deafness, wide bridge of the nose, lateral displacement of medial canthi, confluent eyebrows, eyes of different color, white lashes and forelock, and leukoderma.

Wald (wawld) Lillian (1867–1940). American nurse; founder of the Henry Street Settlement in Manhattan's Lower East Side, one of the first nonsectarian visiting nurse services in the world.

Waldenström's disease (vahl'den-stremz) osteochondrosis of the capitular femoral epephysis.

Waldeyer's glands (vahl'di-erz) glands in the attached edge of the eyelid.

waist (wāst) the portion of the body between the thorax and the hips.

wall (wawl) a structure bounding or limiting a space or a definitive mass of material.

cell w., a structure outside of and protecting the cell membrane, present in all plant cells and in many bacteria and other types of cells.

wallerian degeneration (wahl-le're-an) fatty degeneration of a nerve fiber that has been severed from its nutritive source.

walleye (wawl'i) 1. leukoma, a white opacity of the cornea. A common cause is degeneration of the cornea from longstanding, untreated syphilis. Other possible causes include inflammation of the cornea, corneal ulcer, and trachoma. 2. STRABISMUS in which there is permanent deviation of the visual axis of one eye away from the other eye, resulting in diplopia; called also exotropia and divergent strabismus.

Walthard's islets microscopic inclusions of the ovarian germinal epithelium, which have been implicated in the development of Brenner tumors.

Walther's ganglion (vahl'terz) glomus coccygeum.

Wangensteen tube (wan'gen-stēn) a small nasogastric tube connected with a special suction apparatus to maintain gastric and duodenal decompression.

warfarin (wōr'fer-in) an anticoagulant, usually used as the sodium salt.

wart (wort) an epidermal tumor of viral origin; the term is also applied loosely to any of various benign, wartlike epidermal proliferations of nonviral origin. Called also verruca. Warts are generally more common among children and young adults than among older persons. Most warts are less than a quarter of an inch in diameter; they may be flat or raised, dry or moist. Usually they have a rough and pitted surface, either flesh-colored or darker than the surrounding skin.

Warts develop usually on the exposed parts of the fingers and hands, but also on the elbows, face, scalp, and other areas. When on especially vulnerable parts of the body, such as the knee or elbow, they are subject to irritation and may become quite tender. PLANTAR WARTS, which occur on the soles of the feet, become very sensitive because of pressure. Anal warts cause itching. Warts can also block a nostril or an external acoustic meatus.

A wart develops between 1 and 8 months after the virus becomes lodged in the skin. The virus is often spread by scratching, rubbing, and slight razor cuts. In more than half the cases, warts disappear without treatment, but some remain for years.

TREATMENT. Many popular "cures" for warts have been suggested, but are generally useless. Furthermore, self-treatment by cutting, scraping, or using acids or patent medicines, may cause bacterial infection, scarring, and other harm—without eliminating the warts.

A troublesome wart should be removed only by a physician, who may use acids, electrodesiccation, freezing with liquid nitrogen, or x-rays for the purpose. Warts are notoriously stubborn. Often the virus remains in the skin, and the wart grows again.

It is generally advised that warts on children be removed early. Otherwise they tend to be spread by the child's scratching and other activities. The tendency of warts to spread is less evident in adults.

wash (wosh) a solution used for cleansing or bathing a part, as an eye or the mouth.

Wassermann test (reaction) (wos'er-man) a complement-fixation test used in the diagnosis of syphilis.

Wassermann-fast (wos'er-man-fast") showing a positive reaction to the Wassermann test despite antisyphilitic treatment.

waste (wāst) 1. gradual loss, decay, or diminution of bulk. 2. useless and effete material, unfit for further use within the organism. 3. to pine away or dwindle.

water (wot'er) 1. a clear, colorless, odorless, tasteless liquid, H_2O. 2. an aqueous solution of a medicinal substance.

distilled w., water that has been purified by distillation.

heavy w., a compound analogous to water but containing the mass 2 isotope of hydrogen (deuterium), differing from ordinary water in having a higher freezing point (3.8° C.) and boiling point (101.4° C.), and in being incapable of supporting life. Called also deuterium oxide.

lime w., calcium hydroxide solution.

Waterhouse-Friderichsen syndrome (wot'er-hows frid"er-ik'sen) the malignant or fulminating form of meningococcal MENINGITIS, which is marked by sudden onset and short course, fever, coma, collapse, cyanosis, hemorrhages from the skin and mucous membranes, and bilateral adrenal hemorrhage.

waters (wot'erz) popular name for amniotic fluid.

Watson-Crick helix (wot'son krik) double helix; a representation of the structure of DEOXYRIBONUCLEIC ACID (DNA), consisting of two coiled chains, each of which contains information completely specifying the other chain.

Watson-Schwartz test (wot'son shwarts) a test for diagnosing acute porphyria, depending on the presence of porphobilinogen in the urine.

watt (wot) a unit of electric power, being the work done at the rate of 1 joule per second. It is equivalent to 1 ampere under pressure of 1 volt. Abbreviated w.

wattage (wot′ij) the output or consumption of an electric device expressed in watts.

wattmeter (wot′me-ter) an instrument for measuring wattage.

wave (wāv) a uniformly advancing disturbance in which the parts undergo a double oscillation, as a progressing disturbance on the surface of a liquid or the rhythmic variation occurring in the transmission of electromagnetic energy.

alpha w's, electroencephalographic waves having a frequency of 8 to 13 per second, typical of a normal person awake in a quiet resting state. (See also ELECTROENCEPHALOGRAPHY.)

beta w's, waves in the electroencephalogram having a frequency of 18 to 30 per second.

brain w's, changes in electric potential of different areas of the brain, as recorded by electroencephalography.

delta w's, 1. an early QRS vector in the electrocardiogram in Wolff-Parkinson-White syndrome. 2. electroencephalographic waves having a frequency below $3\frac{1}{2}$ per second, typical in deep sleep, in infancy, and in serious brain disorders. (See also ELECTROENCEPHALOGRAPHY.)

electromagnetic w's, the entire series of ethereal waves which are similar in character, and which move with the velocity of light, but which vary enormously in wavelength. The unbroken series is known from the hertzian waves used in radio transmission, which may be miles in length (one mile equals 1.6×10^5 cm.), through heat and light, the ultraviolet, roentgen rays, and gamma rays of radium to the cosmic rays, the wavelength of which may be as short as 0.0004 of an Angström unit (4×10^{-12} cm.).

hertzian w's, electromagnetic waves resembling light waves, but having greater wavelength; used in wireless telegraphy.

light w's, the electromagnetic waves that produce sensations on the retina. (See also VISION.)

P w., a deflection in the normal electrocardiogram produced by the wave of excitation passing over the atria.

pulse w., the elevation of the pulse felt by the finger or shown graphically in a recording of pulse pressure.

Q w., in the QRS complex, the initial electrocardiographic downward (negative) deflection, related to the initial phase of depolarization.

R w., the initial upward deflection of the QRS complex, following the Q wave in the normal electrocardiogram.

radio w's, electromagnetic radiation of wavelength between 10^{-1} and 10^6 cm. and frequency of about 10^{11} to 10^4 cycles per second.

S w., a downward deflection of the QRS complex following the R wave in the normal electrocardiogram.

T w., the second major deflection of the normal electrocardiogram, reflecting the potential variations occurring with repolarization of the ventricles.

theta w's, electroencephalographic waves having a frequency of 4 to 7 per second, occurring mainly in children but also in adults under emotional stress. (See also ELECTROENCEPHALOGRAPHY.)

ultrashort w's, electromagnetic waves of wavelength of less than 10 meters.

ultrasonic w's, waves similar to sound waves but of such high frequency that the human ear does not perceive them as sound.

wavelength (wāv′length) the distance between the top of one wave and the identical phase of the succeeding one in the advance of waves of radiant energy.

wax (waks) a plastic solid of plant or animal origin or produced synthetically. adj., **wax′y.**

ear w., cerumen.

W.B.C white blood cell (leukocyte); white blood (cell) count.

wean (wēn) to discontinue breast feeding and substitution of other feeding habits.

weanling (wēn′ling) an animal newly changed from breast feeding to other forms of nourishment.

webbed (webd) connected by a membrane or strand of tissue.

Weber's glands (va′berz) the tubular mucous glands of the tongue.

Weber test (va′ber) a hearing test made by placing a vibrating tuning fork at some point on the midline of the head and noting whether it is perceived as heard in the midline (normal) or referred to either ear (middle ear disease).

Weber-Christian disease (web′er kris′chan) nodular nonsuppurative panniculitis.

Wegener's granulomatosis (veg′ĕ-nerz) a progressive disease, with granulomatous lesions of the respiratory tract, focal necrotizing arteriolitis with mainly glomerular renal involvement and, finally, widespread inflammation of all organs of the body.

weight (wāt) heaviness; the degree to which a body is drawn toward the earth by gravity. (See also Tables of Weights and Measures in the Appendix.)

apothecaries' w., a system of weight used in compounding prescriptions based on the grain (equivalent 64.8 mg.). Its units are the scruple (20 grains), dram (3 scruples), ounce (8 drams), and pound (12 ounces).

atomic w., the weight of an atom of a chemical element, compared with the weight of an atom of carbon-12, which is taken as 12.00000.

avoirdupois w., the system of weight commonly used for ordinary commodities in English-speaking countries. Its units are the dram (27.344 grains), ounce (16 drams), and pound (16 ounces).

equivalent w., the weight in grams of a substance that is equivalent in a chemical reaction to 1.008 gm. of hydrogen.

molecular w., the weight of a molecule of a chemical compound as compared with the weight of an atom of carbon-12; it is equal to the sum of the weights of its constituent atoms. Abbreviated mol. wt.

Weil's disease (vīlz) leptospiral jaundice.

Weitbrecht's foramen (vīt′brekts) a foramen in the capsule of the shoulder joint.

Weitbrecht's ligament (vīt′brekts) a small ligamentous band extending from the ulnar tuberosity to the radius.

wen (wen) a sebaceous or epidermal inclusion cyst.

Wenckebach's period (ven′ke-bahks) a usually repetitive sequence seen in partial heart block, marked by progressive lengthening of the P–R interval until ventricular response occurs.

Wernicke's encephalopathy (ver'nĭ-kēz) an inflammatory hemorrhagic encephalopathy due to thiamine deficiency associated with chronic alcoholism, but also occurring as a complication of certain other diseases, with paralysis of the eye muscles, diplopia, nystagmus, ataxia, and mental changes ranging from deterioration and forgetfulness to delirium tremens and KORSAKOFF'S SYNDROME.

Wernicke's syndrome (ver'nĭ-kēz) presbyophrenia.

Westphal-Strümpell pseudosclerosis (disease) (vest'fahl strim'pel) hepatolenticular degeneration.

wet brain brain edema.

wet-nurse (wet'ners) a woman who suckles infants other than her own.

Wetzel grid (wet'zel) a direct-reading chart for evaluating physical fitness in terms of body build, development level, and basal metabolism.

Wharton's jelly (hwar'tunz) the soft, jelly-like intracellular substance of the umbilical cord.

wheal (hwēl) a localized area of edema on the body surface, often attended with severe itching and usually evanescent. It is the typical lesion of urticaria.

wheat germ (hwēt'jerm) the embryo of wheat, which contains tocopherol, thiamine, riboflavin, and other vitamins.

w. g. oil, oil derived from the germ of wheat kernels; it is rich in vitamin E.

wheeze (hwēz) a whistling respiratory sound.

wheezing (hwēz'ing) breathing with a rasp or whistling sound. It results from constriction or obstruction of the throat, pharynx, trachea, or bronchi.

Wheezing is commonly a symptom of ASTHMA. In an asthmatic attack, spasm of the bronchi occurs, and air can be forced only with difficulty into and from the lungs through the trachea.

Another cause of wheezing is congestive HEART FAILURE, in which there is difficulty in breathing, and frequently the lips have a bluish color and the veins in the neck are distended.

When wheezing is persistent and is not asthmatic, the cause may be an obstruction, such as a foreign body or tumor, somewhere in the breathing passages.

whiplash injury (hwip'lash) a nonspecific term applied to injury to the spinal cord and spine due to sudden extension of the neck, as in sudden stopping or propulsion of a vehicle.

Whipple's disease (hwip'elz) intestinal lipodystrophy.

whipworm (hwip'werm) *Trichuris trichiura.*

white cell, white blood cell leukocyte.

white matter, white substance the white nervous tissue, constituting the conducting portion of the brain and spinal cord, composed mostly of myelinated nerve fibers. Gray matter or substance is the term used to describe the tissues composed of unmyelinated fibers.

whitlow (hwit'lo) felon.

melanotic w., a malignant tumor of the nail bed characterized by formation of melanotic tissue.

Whitmore's disease (hwit'mōrz) melioidosis.

W.H.O. World Health Organization.

whoop (ho͞op) the sonorous and convulsive inspiration of whooping cough.

whooping cough (ho͞op'ing kof) an infectious disease characterized by catarrh of the respiratory tract and peculiar paroxysms of coughing, ending in a prolonged crowing or whooping respiration; called also pertussis. The causative organism is *Bordetella pertussis.* Whooping cough is a serious and widespread disease, with about 300,000 cases a year reported in the United States. Although it may attack at any age, most cases occur in children under 10, and half of these are in children under 5.

The organisms of whooping cough are spread by the victim's coughing and sneezing and by objects he has touched. The incubation period is usually about 7 days, although it may vary between 2 and 21 days. Unlike other respiratory diseases, whooping cough is more likely to occur in spring and summer than in winter. It affects females much more often than males.

SYMPTOMS. Whooping cough frequently starts with a running nose, a slight fever, and a persistent cough. This stage usually lasts about 2 weeks. After this, the child feels chilled and begins to vomit. His coughing increases. He begins to cough in spells of eight to ten times in one breath. This forces the air from the lungs, and the face may turn purple or blue from the effort and the shortage of air. Finally he catches his breath in long, noisy intake, or "whoop." In the very young (under 6 months) the true whoop is often not present, even when paroxysms are severe and frequent.

The coughing stage of the disease usually lasts 4 to 6 weeks, and the coughing may be very severe at night. Then the coughing spells become less frequent and less severe until the disease has run its course.

Stage three (convalescent stage) may last from 4 months to 2 years. The coughing spells diminish but the patient usually experiences them again each time he has an upper respiratory infection.

Complications of whooping cough include pneumonia, atelectasis, and emphysema; of these, pneumonia is the most serious, accounting for 90 per cent of the fatalities in young children. Brain damage, another complication, should be suspected if convulsive seizures occur in the pertussis patient.

IMMUNIZATION. An attack of whooping cough gives immunity, but second attacks are not unknown. The vaccine usually is given in combination with diphtheria and tetanus and is available as a depot preparation that should be given intramuscularly, preferably in the lateral thigh. Because of the possible neurologic effects of the pertussis component, it should not be given in the presence of nervous system illnesses. A history of severe reaction to the vaccine may require reduced amounts in divided dosages.

The American Academy of Pediatrics recommends that the DTP (diphtheria, tetanus, pertussis) immunizing agent be given at 2 months, 4 months, 6 months, 18 months, and at age 4 to 6 immediately before entering school.

TREATMENT AND PATIENT CARE. Precautions against the spread of the disease entail following the procedures of "respiratory isolation" during the entire hospitalization. Isolation is discontinued when the causative organisms are no longer present in the patient's throat, as determined by a bacterial culture of the sputum.

Treatment is primarily supportive, including bed rest as long as the fever persists, antibiotics to avoid secondary infections, and antipyretics to control fever.

In very serious cases, especially in infants, whooping cough may cause severe breathing difficulties. Suction may be necessary at frequent intervals to remove accumulations of mucus from the air passages. Fatalities, particularly in infants, are not uncommon.

A proper diet is essential during whooping cough. Because vomiting may be a problem, small frequent feedings of bland foods are considered best.

whorl (hwerl) a spiral arrangement, as in the ridges on the finger that make up a fingerprint.

Widal test (ve-dahl′) a test for the diagnosis of typhoid fever, based on agglutination of *Salmonella typhosa* by dilutions of the patient's serum.

Wilms' tumor (vilmz) a rapidly developing malignant mixed tumor of the kidneys, made up of embryonal elements, and occurring chiefly in children before the fifth year; called also embryonal carcinosarcoma and nephroblastoma.

Wilson's disease (wil′sunz) hepatolenticular degeneration.

Wilson-Mikity syndrome a rare form of pulmonary insufficiency in low-birth-weight infants, marked by hyperpnea and cyanosis of insidious onset during the first month of life and often resulting in death. Radiographically, there are multiple cyst-like foci of hyperaeration throughout the lung, with coarse thickening of the interstitial supporting structures. Called also pulmonary dysmaturity.

Winckel's disease (ving′kelz) a fatal disease of the newborn, with jaundice, hemoglobinuria, bloody urine, hemorrhage, cyanosis, collapse, and convulsions.

window (win′do) a circumscribed opening in a plane surface.

aortic w., a transparent region below the aortic arch, formed by the bifurcation of the trachea, visible in the left anterior oblique radiograph of the heart and great vessels.

oval w., an oval opening in the inner wall of the middle ear, which is closed by the stapes; called also fenestra vestibuli.

round w., a round opening in the middle ear covered by the secondary tympanic membrane; called also fenestra cochleae.

windpipe (wind′pīp) the trachea.

winking (wingk′ing) quick opening and closing of the eyelids.

jaw w., involuntary closing of the eyelids associated with jaw movements.

wintergreen oil (win′ter-grēn) methyl salicylate.

Wiskott-Aldrich syndrome (wis′kot awl′drich) a hereditary disorder characterized by thrombocytopenic purpura, eczema, and extreme susceptibility to infections (especially otitis media) due to immunodeficiency; it is transmitted as a sex-linked trait.

withdrawal (with-draw′al) 1. a pathological retreat from reality. 2. abstention from drugs to which one is habituated or addicted; also denoting the symptoms occasioned by such withdrawal (see also DRUG ADDICTION).

w. symptoms, a group of symptoms brought about by abrupt withdrawal of a narcotic or other drug to which a person has become addicted; called also abstinence syndrome. The usual reactions to alcohol withdrawal are anxiety, weakness, gastrointestinal symptoms, nausea and vomiting, tremor, fever, rapid heartbeat, convulsions, and delirium (see also DELIRIUM TREMENS). Similar effects are produced by withdrawal of barbiturates and in this case convulsions occur very frequently, often followed by psychosis with hallucinations.

Morphine withdrawal produces a standard pattern of reactions beginning with restlessness, which later becomes extreme. There may be slight fever, elevated blood pressure, and mild hyperglycemia, with lack of appetite and vomiting. The symptoms begin to decline by the third day and usually disappear by about the fourteenth day. The various morphine-like drugs produce similar symptoms, in some instances more acute and in others milder.

Treatment consists of providing a substitute drug such as a mild sedative, along with treatment of the symptoms as needed. Parenteral fluids are often required.

witzelsucht (vit′sel-zo͞okt) [Ger.] a mental condition marked by the making of poor jokes and puns and the telling of pointless stories at which the speaker is intensely amused; a condition characteristic of frontal lobe lesions.

Wohlfahrtia (vōl-fahr′te-ah) a genus of flies. The larvae of *W. magnif′ica* produce wound myiasis; those of *W. o′paca* and *W. vig′il* cause cutaneous myiasis.

Wolff-Parkinson-White syndrome (woolf-par′kin-sun-hwīt) the association of paroxysmal tachycardia (or atrial fibrillation) and preexcitation, in which the electrocardiogram displays a short P–R interval and a wide QRS complex which characteristically shows an early QRS vector (delta wave). Called also anomalous atrioventricular excitation.

wolffian body (woolf′e-an) mesonephros.

wolfram (wool′fram) tungsten (symbol W).

Wolman's disease primary familial xanthomatosis in infants; associated with involvement and calcification of the adrenal glands, failure to thrive, vomiting, diarrhea, hepatomegaly, splenomegaly, foam cells in the bone marrow and other tissues, and early death.

womb (wo͞om) uterus.

wood alcohol methyl alcohol.

Wood's filter (glass) (woodz) see WOOD'S LIGHT.

Wood's light (woodz) ultraviolet radiation from a mercury vapor source, transmitted through a nickel-oxide filter (Wood's filter, or glass), which holds back all but a few violet rays and passes ultraviolet wavelengths of about 365 nm.; used in diagnosis of fungal infections of the scalp and erythrasma, and to reveal the presence of porphyrins and fluorescent minerals.

woolsorter's disease pulmonary anthrax.

World Health Organization W.H.O.; the specialized agency of the United Nations that is concerned with health on an international level. The agency was founded in 1948 and in its constitution are listed the following objectives:

> Health is a state of complete physical and social well being, and not merely the absence of disease or infirmity. The enjoyment of the highest attainable standards of health is one of the fundamental rights of every human being without distinction of race, religion, political belief, economic or social condition. The health of all peoples is fundamental to the attainment of peace and security and is dependent upon the fullest cooperation of individuals and States. The achievement of any State in the promotion and protection of health is of value to all.

The major specific aims of the W.H.O. are:

1. To strengthen the health services of member nations, improving the teaching standards in medicine and allied professions, and advising and helping generally in the field of health.
2. To promote better standards for nutrition, housing, recreation, sanitation, economic and working conditions.
3. To improve maternal and child health and welfare.
4. To advance progress in the field of mental health.
5. To encourage and conduct research on problems of public health.

In carrying out these aims and objectives the W.H.O. functions as a directing and coordinating authority on international health. It serves as a center for all types of global and health information, promotes uniform quarantine standards and international sanitary regulations, provides advisory services through public health experts in control of disease and sets up international standards for the manufacture of all important drugs. Through its teams of physicians, nurses, and other health personnel it provides modern medical skills and knowledge to communities throughout the world.

worm (werm) any of the soft-bodies, elongated, naked invertebrates of the phyla Annelida, Acanthocephala, Aschelminthes, and Platyhelminthes. Worms are often found as parasites in man and other animals. The most common parasitic worms in North America are roundworms and tapeworms. (RINGWORM is not caused by a worm but is a form of fungal infection of the skin.)

Most worm infections are transmitted from person to person via feces that contaminate food and water. Serious worm infections may cause anemia, listlessness, fatigue, irritability, abdominal pain, diarrhea, and weight loss. Despite popular belief, worms do not cause convulsions in children.

Parasitic worms usually live in relative balance with their human hosts, taking enough nutrients to survive without destroying the health of the host. However, they reduce the strength and energy of the bodies they inhabit, often produce very uncomfortable symptoms and should never go untreated.

Suspected cases of worms should be brought to the attention of a physician, for self-treatment is likely to be ineffective and can be harmful. Effective medications against worms can be prescribed only by a physician.

ROUNDWORMS (NEMATODA). Roundworms, called also threadworms, somewhat resemble common earthworms in appearance. The varieties most frequently infecting man include *Ascaris lumbricoides,* pinworms, hookworms, filaria, and *Trichinella spiralis,* the cause of TRICHINOSIS, which is transmitted through inadequately cooked pork.

Ascaris lumbricoides. The largest of the roundworms that infect man, *Ascaris lumbricoides,* called also eelworm, is particularly common in the southern mountain regions of the United States. Often it is transmitted in human feces used as fertilizer. The *Ascaris* eggs develop into larvae in the soil and on growing plants on which the infected feces have been deposited. When vegetables from these areas are eaten without having been properly washed or thoroughly cooked, live larvae are carried into the digestive system along with the food. Migrating from the intestines into the blood, then to the lungs and the esophagus, the larvae finally return to the intestines, where they grow to maturity, reaching a length ranging from 6 to 14 inches.

Ascaris infection may go unsuspected until a worm is passed in the stool. But there may be colic or other abdominal symptoms, and occasionally the worms are vomited during their passage through the esophagus. In children, "wandering worms" may emerge through the skin near the navel, and in adults, near the groin. Infected children usually are thin because the worms consume vital nutrients and inhibit the digestion of proteins. Loss of appetite and angioneurotic edema are common, and the face may be swollen.

Accurate diagnosis of the presence and extent of *Ascaris* infection usually depends on the detection of eggs in a stool sample examined microscopically. Treatment involves the use of medications such as chenopodium oil and dithiazanine iodide to destroy and expel the parasites, and is completely successful in nearly every case.

Prevention of *Ascaris* infection depends primarily on the sanitary disposal of human feces and discontinuing their use as fertilizer. Also important are the thorough washing of hands before food is prepared, and the careful cleaning and cooking of possibly infected foods.

Enterobius vermicularis (Pinworm). Enterobius vermicularis, called also pinworm or seatworm, is a spindle-shaped roundworm less than half an inch long that inhabits the upper part of the large intestine, more commonly in children than adults. Pinworms do not produce the fatigue and loss of weight that characterize *Ascaris* infection, but instead the adult worms migrate to the anal region, usually at night, and deposit eggs, which cause irritation of the skin around the anus, leading to painful scratching and restless sleep.

This irritation is the usual sign of pinworm infection, although there may also be vague intestinal discomfort. Adult worms may appear in the feces, but the infection is transmitted by the eggs, which may be transferred to clothing, bedclothes, and toilet seats from the skin around the anus.

In scratching, the infected person is likely to collect the minute eggs on his hands and under his fingernails, and, until he washes thoroughly, he will shed the eggs on anything he touches.

The infection spreads to other persons when the eggs are carried to their mouths either by inhalation or on contaminated food, in beverages, or on hands. Widespread pinworm infection is explained by the fact that the eggs, which develop into mature worms only in a human body, can remain dormant but alive and infective for a considerable time in dust or air; they are not killed by most household disinfectants.

Enterobius vermicularis infection is treated by an anthelmintic such as pyrvinium pamoate, piperazine citrate, or gentian violet. The newer anthelmintic, mebendazole, is highly effective. Equally important, instructions for disinfecting bedclothes and other material that may harbor eggs must be followed carefully to avoid reinfection and spread of pinworms to other members of the family.

Prevention of pinworms is largely a matter of hygiene. Children should be taught to wash their hands well with soap and water before meals and after using the toilet. Care and cleanliness in the preparation of food is essential. If a case of pinworms develops in a family, extra precautions should be taken; toilet seats should be scrubbed daily with soap and water, and the bedding of the infected person should be disinfected by boiling at least twice a week.

Hookworm. Hookworms are small—about half an inch long—and are particularly widespread in the southeastern part of the United States. Their larvae develop in soil contaminated by feces from infected persons and they enter the body through the skin, usually through the sole of the foot. Children who go barefoot are especially susceptible. They travel by way of the blood to the lungs and then to the intestines, where the worms, by now full-grown, attach themselves to the intestinal wall and suck blood from it for nourishment. There may be no symptoms at all, or there may be severe blood loss and anemia, and eventually retardation of growth and mental development and even death. Diagnosis is made by detection of eggs in the feces. The infection is treated by administration of anthelmintic drugs such as mebendazole. It is prevented by improvement in sanitation facilities and wearing shoes out of doors. (See also HOOKWORM.)

Filaria. Another type of threadlike roundworm, often called filaria, causes a tropical disease known as FILARIASIS, which affects lymphoid tissues.

FLATWORMS (PLATYHELMINTHES). Flatworms infecting man include tapeworms, flukes, and *Echinococcus granulosus.*

Tapeworm. Several species of tapeworms infect man; all depend on two hosts, one human and one animal, for development through their full life cycle (egg to larva to adult). Usually larvae are found in animal hosts and adult worms in man.

The tapeworms commonly found in the United States enter human bodies in contaminated and insufficiently cooked pork (*Taenia solium*), beef (*T. saginata*), or fish (*Diphyllobothrium latum*). The larvae, embedded in cysts in the meat or fish, develop to maturity in the human intestine and attach themselves to the intestinal wall; from there they release eggs, or, in the case of *Taenia* species, egg-laden segments of the body called proglottids.

In mild or even moderate infections, tapeworms cause few or no symptoms. In heavy infections there may be diarrhea, abdominal cramps (resembling hunger pains), flatulence, distention, and nausea. In most cases, before these symtoms develop, the infected person discovers the tapeworm segments in his clothes or bedding.

Quinacrine hydrochloride (Atabrine) and aspidium oleoresin are used in treatment of tapeworm infection, quinacrine being the drug of choice because it is less toxic. After treatment the stool must be carefully examined for the parasite because if the head is retained in the intestine, the worm will grow again and treatment must be repeated. Prevention depends on thorough cooking of fish and meat. (See also TAPEWORM.)

Flukes (*Trematoda*). Flukes are not common in the United States but are a serious problem in many Asian, tropical, and subtropical countries. The Chinese liver fluke, *Clonorchis sinensis,* enters the body in raw or improperly cooked fish and may cause enlargement of the liver, jaundice, anemia, and weakness. Another liver fluke, *Fasciola hepatica,* is occasionally found in man; it causes obstruction of the bile ducts and enlargement of the liver. Blood flukes such as *Schistosoma* penetrate the skin, make

their way to the blood and travel to various parts of the body (see also SCHISTOSOMIASIS).

Treatment varies according to the type of fluke involved and requires careful medical supervision. Proper cooking of fish provides protection against liver fluke infection. Since snails are carriers of flukes, their destruction, usually by poison, is an effective preventive measure in areas where fluke infection is a problem.

Echinococcus granulosus. This tapeworm reverses the usual process of development in human and animal hosts. The adult *Echinococcus* is found in the intestine of dogs. The larva develops in the human intestine, penetrating the intestinal wall, and settling in various organs—most often the liver—where it forms a cyst (hydatid cyst) that grows slowly. Treatment is by surgical removal of the cyst. This type of worm infection is fortunately not common in the United States.

PATIENT CARE. The patient suffering from infection with worms is likely to be malnourished and suffering from anemia. Special attention should be given to the diet so that these conditions can be relieved. The patient also will need adequate rest and other general measures to improve his state of health.

The patient should have his own individual bedpan which is thoroughly washed and disinfected after each use. He is not allowed to use the bathroom if it is used by other persons. Some types of worms or eggs must be destroyed before they can be flushed into the sewage system. This will depend on the community's sewage treatment plant and the type of worm involved. If there is any doubt that the worms will be destroyed it is best to disinfect the stool with chlorinated lime before disposal in the sewage system.

wound (wo͞ond) a bodily injury caused by physical means, with disruption of the normal continuity of structures.

contused w., one in which the skin is unbroken.

incised w., one caused by a cutting instrument.

lacerated w., one in which the tissues are torn.

open w., one having a free outward opening.

penetrating w., puncture w., one caused by a sharp, usually slender object, which passes through the skin into the underlying tissues.

Wrisberg's ganglia (ris′bergs) cardiac ganglia.

wrist (rist) the region of the joint between the hand and the forearm; called also the carpus.

There are eight carpal bones in the wrist, arranged in two rows. The joint surfaces of these bones glide upon each other in four directions. The carpals join the bones of the forearm, the radius and ulna, and the bones of the hands, the metacarpals. The bones are bound together and protected by tough ligaments and capsules, the enveloping structures. The major arteries, nerves, veins, and tendons that serve the hand and fingers run across the wrist. Both tendons and the joint are lined with synovial membrane.

DISORDERS OF THE WRIST. The wrist is a strong but complicated joint and can suffer the same disorders as any other joint. The hands are constantly being used, and any sudden or strong movement or exertion may cause a structure to stretch, tear, or become dislocated.

A strained wrist, caused by overstretching or

Commonly Encountered Intestinal Parasitic Infections

Common Name	Scientific Name (Synonyms or Varieties)	Distribution	Portal of Entry (and Stage)	Diagnostic Stages(s) in Stool (or Other Medium)
ROUNDWORMS:				
Giant intestinal roundworm	*Ascaris lumbricoides*	Cosmopolitan, more common in warm moist climates	Mouth (embryonated eggs)	Immature eggs in stool. Worms evacuated in stool, occasionally vomited
Hookworm	a) *Ancylostoma duodenale* (Old World type) b) *Necator americanus* (Tropical type)	a) Temperate and warm moist climates b) Warm moist climates	Skin, usually feet, possibly mouth (filariform larvae)	Immature eggs in stool
Threadworm	*Strongyloides stercoralis*	Sou. U.S.A., moist tropics	Skin, usually feet (filariform larvae)	Larvae in stool
Whipworm	*Trichuris trichiura* (*Trichocephalus trichiurus*)	Gulf Coast, U.S.A.; warm moist climates	Mouth (embryonated eggs)	Immature eggs in stool
Pinworm or seatworm	*Enterobius vermicularis* (*Oxyuris vermicularis*)	Cosmopolitan, esp. in children	Mouth (embryonated eggs)	Eggs in perianal swabs; adult worms per anum
TAPEWORMS:				
Dwarf	*Hymenolepis nana*	Sou. U.S.A., in children	Mouth (eggs)	Eggs in stool
Beef	*Taenia saginata*	Cosmopolitan	Mouth (cysticercus larva in infected beef)	Eggs in stool; proglottids of adult worms per anum
Pork	*Taenia solium*	Rare in U.S.A.; common in Latin America	Mouth (cysticercus larva in infected pork)	Eggs in stool; proglottids of adult worms per anum
Fish	*Diphyllobothrium latum* (*Bothriocephalus latus*)	Northern Minn. and Mich.; Canada	Mouth (larva in infected fresh-water fish flesh)	Immature eggs in stool
Sparganum causing sparganosis	*Spirometra* spp. (*Sparganum mansoni* et al.)	Several areas, incl. Sou. U.S.A.	Usually mouth (larval stages)	Sparganum larva in subcutaneous tissues
PROTOZOA:				
Dysentery ameba	*Entamoeba histolytica* (*Ent. dysenteriae, Endamoeba histolytica*)	Cosmopolitan; common in warm moist climates	Mouth (cyst)	Vegetative stage or cyst in stool
Giardia	*Giardia lamblia* (*G. intestinalis, Lamblia intestinalis*)	In warm climates, prevalent, especially in children	Mouth (cyst)	Vegetative stage or cyst in stool
FLUKES:				
Intestinal	a) *Fasciolopsis buski* b) *Heterophyes, Metagonimus* c) *Echinostoma ilocanum* et al.	In U.S.A. only as rare infections imported from Orient or tropics	Mouth (encysted metacercarial larva)	Eggs in stool
Hepatic	*Fasciola hepatica* (sheep) liver fluke)	Cosmopolitan in sheep-raising countries	Mouth (encysted metacercarial larva)	Immature eggs in stool or biliary drainage
Pulmonary	*Paragonimus westermani* (Oriental lung fluke)	Orient, extensive foci	Mouth (encysted metacercarial larva)	Immature eggs in stool or sputum
Blood	a) *Schistosoma japonicum* b) *S. mansoni* c) *S. haematobium*	a) Orient b) Africa, Latin America c) Africa, Near East	Skin (active fork-tailed cercarial)	Embryonated eggs in stool (a, b), or urine (c)

*Note: Eosinophilia often accompanies intestinal helminthiasis.

Source of Infection	Most Common Symptoms	Therapeutic Agents	Remarks
Fecal contamination of soil (eggs)	Colicky pains, diarrhea "acute abdomen"	Piperazine Hexylresorcinol Dithiazanine iodide	May block intestine, biliary or pancreatic duct; bronchial symptoms (larval stage with eosinophilia*)
Fecal contamination of soil (larvae)	Melena, anemia, cardiac insufficiency, retarded growth	Tetrachloroethylene Hexylresorcinol Bephenium hydroxynaphthoate	Prophylaxis: Use sanitary latrines, wear shoes, treat infected persons
Fecal contamination of soil (larvae)	Radiating pain in pit of stomach, diarrhea	Dithiazanine iodide	Prophylaxis: Use sanitary latrines, wear shoes
Fecal contamination of soil (eggs)	Diarrhea, nausea, retarded growth	Dithiazanine iodide Hexylresorcinol enemas	May produce dysenteric syndrome, acute appendicitis, or prolapse of rectum in children
Eggs from contaminated fomites	Perianal and perineal pruritus	Piperazine	Often involves entire family
Eggs contaminating environment	Diarrhea, abdominal discomfort, dizziness, inanition in children	Quinacrine hydrochloride Hexylresorcinol	May be symptomless
Poorly cooked or raw infected beef	Systemic toxemia, abdominal distress, "acute appendix"	Quinacrine hydrochloride	Prophylaxis: Thoroughly cook all suspected beef
Poorly cooked infected pork	Similar to T. saginata	Quinacrine hydrochloride	Prophylaxis: Thoroughly cook all pork in infected areas. Ingested eggs may produce human cysticercosis
Infected fresh-water fish	Intestinal toxemia, bowel obstruction, may cause pernicious anemia	Aspidium oleoresin Quinacrine hydrochloride	
Drinking water containing infected Cyclops (primary host)	Inflamed subcutaneous tissue containing sparganum larva	Surgical excision	Adult worm in intestine of various nonhuman mammals
Feces-contaminated water, food, fomites	a) Diarrhea, dysentery, abdominal pain b) Amebic hepatitis	a) Oxytetracycline hydrochloride Diiodohydroxyquin Glycobiarsol b) Emetine hydrochloride Chloroquine phosphate	Amebiasis may be asyndromic in individuals or populations
Human feces	Mucous diarrhea, abdominal pain, loss of weight	Quinacrine hydrochloride	Infection acquired in childhood often spontaneously lost
a) Vegetation b) Fresh-water fish c) Snails	Intestinal toxemia, at times intestinal obstruction	a) Tetrachloroethylene b) Hexylresorcinol c) Aspidium oleoresin	Primary hosts are fresh-water snails
Watercress containing metacercarial cysts	Hepatic colic, cholecystiasis	Emetine hydrochloride	Sheep infected in U.S.A., but only 1 confirmed human infection
Crabs or crayfishes containing metacercarial cysts	Peribronchiolar distress, with hemoptysis	Emetine hydrochloride	Related species in wild mammals and hogs in U.S.A.
Infested water containing fork tailed larvae from snail hosts	Dysentery, intestinal and hepatic cirrhosis (a, b), hematuria, urinary fibrosis (c)	Antimony potassium tartrate Stibophen	Related flukes cause "swimmer's itch" in bathers in U.S.A. and elsewhere

overexertion, is usually treated by rest and the application of heat and light massage. Injury of the joint ligaments is called a SPRAIN and is a common disorder. DISLOCATION, or displacement of the bones of the wrist from their normal relationship, and FRACTURE, which causes swelling and pain on movement, may also occur. Often a fracture is difficult to distinguish from a bad sprain, and x-ray examination may be necessary for diagnosis.

Severe pain, swelling, and reddish blue discoloration may be a symptom of any of these cases of wrist injury. An ice pack is often recommended for swelling.

Other disorders of the wrist include ARTHRITIS, infection, ganglion (a form of cystic tumor), and TENOSYNOVITIS.

wristdrop (rist′drop) paralysis of the extensor muscles of the hand and fingers; it may be due to metallic poisoning.

wryneck (ri′neck) torticollis.

wt. weight.

Wuchereria (voo″ker-e′re-ah) a genus of filarial nematodes indigenous to the warmer regions of the world.

W. bancrof′ti, a species widely distributed in tropical and subtropical countries, causing ELEPHANTIASIS, lymphangitis, and chyluria by interfering with the lymphatic circulation (see also FILARIASIS).

wucheriasis (voo″ker-i′ah-sis) infection with worms of the genus *Wuchereria.*

w./v. weight (of solute) per volume (of solvent).

Wyamine (wi′ah-min) trademark for preparations of mephentermine, used as a sympathomimetic and a pressor substance.

Wycillin (wi-sil′in) trademark for a preparation of procaine penicillin G.

Wydase (wi′dās) trademark for preparations of hyaluronidase for injection, a spreading agent to promote diffusion and enhance absorption.

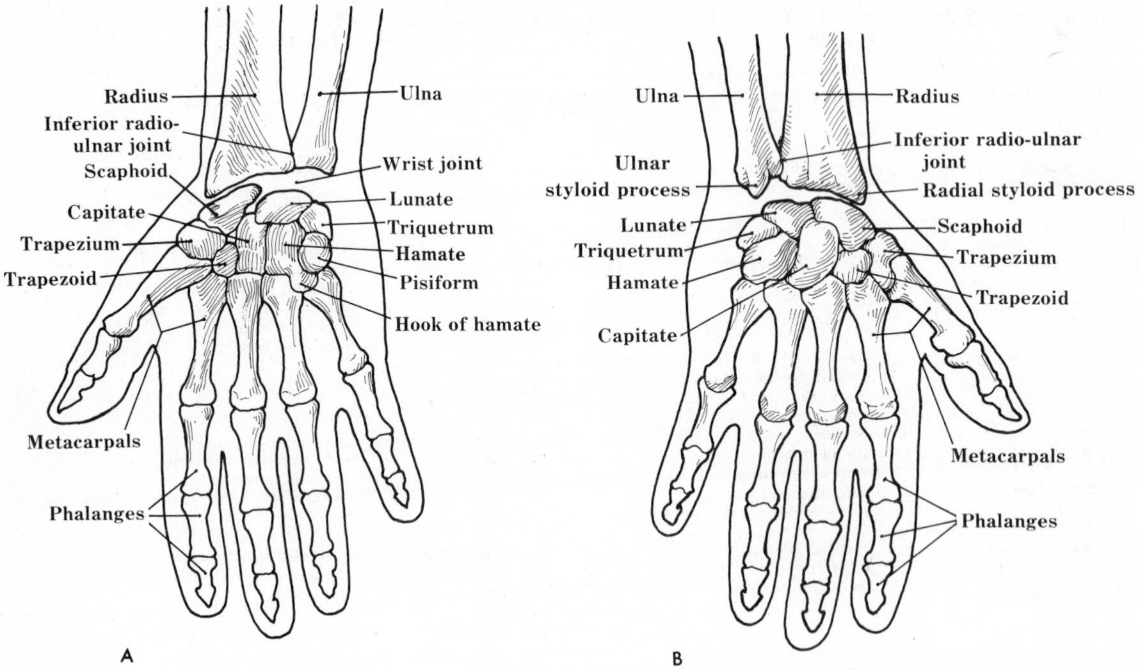

Bones of the wrist (carpal bones). *A,* Anterior view, right arm. *B,* Posterior view, right arm.

X

X symbol, *Kienböck's unit* (of x-ray exposure).

xanth(o)- word element [Gr.], *yellow.*

xanthelasma (zan″thel-az′mah) xanthoma affecting the eyelids and characterized by soft yellowish spots or plaques.

xanthematin (zan-them′ah-tin) a yellow substance derivable from heme (hematin).

xanthemia (zan-the′me-ah) the presence of yellow coloring matter in the blood; carotenemia.

xanthic (zan′thik) 1. yellow. 2. pertaining to xanthine.

xanthine (zan′thēn) a purine compound found in most bodily tissues and fluids; it is a precursor of uric acid.

dimethyl x., theobromine.

trimethyl x., caffeine.

xanthinuria (zan″thin-u′re-ah) excess of xanthine in the urine, due to a hereditary disorder of purine metabolism.

xanthochromatic (zan″tho-kro-mat′ik) yellow-colored.

xanthochromia (zan″tho-kro′me-ah) yellowish discoloration of the skin or spinal fluid. Xanthochromic spinal fluid usually indicates hemorrhage into the central nervous system and is due to the presence of xanthematin.

xanthochromic (zan″tho-kro-mat′ik) yellow-colored.

xanthocyanopsia (zan″tho-si″ah-nop′se-ah) inability to perceive red or green tints, vision being limited to yellow and blue.

xanthogranuloma (zan″tho-gran″u-lo′mah) a tumor having histologic characteristics of both granuloma and xanthoma.

juvenile x., a dermatosis in which groups of yellow, yellow-brown, reddish yellow, or brown papules occur on the extensor surfaces of the extremities, sometimes involving the eye, meninges, and testes, typically beginning in infancy or early childhood, usually with spontaneous remission in one to three years.

xanthoma (zan-tho′mah) a papule, nodule, or plaque in the skin due to lipid deposits; the color of a xanthoma is usually yellow, but may be brown, reddish, or cream. Microscopically, the lesions show light cells with foamy protoplasm (foam cells).

Xanthomas are usually harmless. They range in size from tiny pinheads to large nodules, and the shape may be round, flat, or irregular. They are often found around the eyes, the joints, the neck or the palms, or over tendons. Often these lipid deposits are not limited to the skin but are found throughout the body in bones, the heart, blood vessels, liver, and other organs.

The formation of xanthomas may indicate an underlying disease, usually related to abnormal metabolism of lipids, including cholesterol. Abnormally high levels of blood lipids may be found in diabetes mellitus (xanthoma diabeticorum), in diseases of the liver, kidney, and thyroid gland, and in several hereditary metabolic diseases. The excessive lipids carried in the blood may then be deposited as xanthomas.

Another group of diseases producing xanthomas affect the reticuloendothelial system, a widespread system of cells that have several functions, including an influence in the storage of fatty materials. These diseases are thought to have a similar basic mechanism but they have many different manifestations, which may include the formation of xanthomas. The xanthomas are usually found in the reticuloendothelial disorder called Hand-Schüller-Christian disease.

Treatment of xanthomas includes surgery, application of acids directly to the lipid deposits and management of the disease that causes them, as in diabetes mellitus.

xanthomatosis (zan″tho-mah-to′sis) an accumulation of excess lipids in the body due to disturbance of lipid metabolism and marked by the formation of foam cells in skin lesions.

x. bul′bi, fatty degeneration of the cornea due to disorder of lipid metabolism, marked by the presence of xanthomas.

xanthomatous (zan-tho′mah-tus) pertaining to xanthoma.

xanthophose (zan′tho-fōz) a yellow phose.

xanthophyll (zan′tho-fil) a yellow pigment of plants.

xanthoprotein (zan″tho-pro′te-in) an orange pigment produced by heating proteins with nitric acid.

xanthopsia (zan-thop′se-ah) chromatopsia in which objects are seen as yellow.

xanthopsin (zan-thop′sin) all-*trans* retinal (see RETINAL [2]).

xanthosine (zan′tho-sēn) a nucleoside composed of xanthine and ribose.

xanthosis (zan-tho′sis) yellowish discoloration; degeneration with yellowish pigmentation.

xanthurenic acid (zan″thu-ren′ik) a metabolite of L-tryptophan, present in normal urine and in increased amounts in vitamin B_6 deficiency.

Xe chemical symbol, *xenon.*

xenodiagnosis (zen″o-di″ag-no′sis) 1. diagnosis by means of finding, in the feces of clean laboratory-bred bugs fed on the patient, the infective forms of the organism causing the disease; used in the early stages of Chagas' disease. 2. diagnosis of trichinosis by means of feeding laboratory-bred rats or mice on meat suspected of being infected with *Trichinella,* and then examining the animals for the parasite.

xenogeneic (zen″o-jen-e′ik) in transplantation biology, denoting individuals or tissues from individuals of different species and hence of disparate cell type.

xenogenesis (zen″o-jen′ĕ-sis) 1. heterogenesis (1). 2. production of offspring unlike either parent.

xenogenous (zĕ-noj′ĕ-nus) caused by a foreign body, or originating outside the organism.

xenograft (zen′o-graft) a graft of tissue transplanted between animals of different species; a heterograft.

xenomenia (zen″o-me′ne-ah) vicarious menstruation.

xenon (ze′non) a chemical element, atomic number 54, atomic weight 131.30, symbol Xe. (See table of ELEMENTS.)

xenoparasite (zen″o-par′ah-sīt) an organism not usually parasitic on a particular species, but becomes so because of a weakened condition of the host.

xenophobia (zen″o-fo′be-ah) morbid dread of strangers.

xenophonia (zen″o-fo′ne-ah) alteration in the quality of the voice.

xenophthalmia (zen″of-thal′me-ah) inflammation caused by a foreign body in the eye; called also ophthalmoxerosis.

Xenopsylla (zen″op-sil′ah) a genus of fleas, including more than 30 species, many of which transmit disease-producing microorganisms.

X. cheo′pis, the rat flea, which transmits *Pasteurella pestis,* the causative organism of plague and *Rickettsia typhi,* the causative organism of murine typhus.

xer(o)- word element [Gr.], *dry; dryness.*

xerocheilia (ze″ro-ki′le-ah) dryness of the lips.

xeroderma (ze″ro-der′mah) a mild form of ichthyosis; excessive dryness of the skin.

x. pigmento′sum, a rare and often fatal hereditary pigmentary and atrophic disease in which the skin and eyes are extremely sensitive to light, beginning in childhood and progressing ' early development of freckles, telangiectases, keratoses, papillomas, and malignancy.

xerography (ze-rog′rah-fe) xeroradiography.

xeroma (ze-ro′mah) abnormal dryness of the conjunctiva; xerophthalmia.

xeromenia (ze″ro-me′ne-ah) the appearance of constitutional symptoms at the menstrual period without any flow of blood.

xerophagia (ze″ro-fa′je-ah) the eating of dry food.

xerophthalmia (ze″rof-thal′me-ah) abnormal dryness and thickening of the surface of the conjunctiva and cornea due to a deficiency of vitamin A or to local disease.

xeroradiography (ze″ro-ra″de-og′rah-fe) the making of radiographs by a dry, totally photoelectric process, using metal plates coated with a semiconductor, such as selenium.

The image produced by this process differs from conventional x-ray in that margins between tissues of varying densities are more clearly defined. Hence, xeroradiography is especially beneficial in the diagnosis of breast tumors. It does, however, require higher doses of radiation. Called also xerography.

xerosis (ze-ro′sis) abnormal dryness, as of the eye (xerophthalmia), skin (xeroderma), or mouth (xerostomia).

xerostomia (ze″ro-sto′me-ah) dryness of the mouth from lack of the normal secretion.

xiph(o)- word element [Gr.], *xiphoid process.*

xiphisternum (zif″ĭ-ster′num) xiphoid process. adj., **xiphister′nal.**

xiphocostal (zif″o-kos′tal) pertaining to the xiphoid process and ribs.

xiphoid (zif′oid, zi′foid) 1. sword-shaped; ensiform. 2. xiphoid process.

x. process, the pointed process of cartilage, supported by a core of bone, connected with the lower end of the body of the sternum.

xiphoiditis (zif″oi-di′tis) inflammation of the xiphoid process.

xiphopagus (zi-fop′ah-gus) symmetrical conjoined twins united in the region of the xiphoid process.

X-linked (eks′linkt) transmitted by genes on the X chromosome; sex-linked.

x-rays (ek′rāz) electromagnetic radiation of very short wavelength (5×10^{-6} to 5×10^{-4} μm.) used for diagnosis and treatment of various disorders; called also roentgen rays.

X-rays are commonly generated by passing a current of high voltage (from 10,000 volts up) through a Coolidge tube. They are able to penetrate most substances to some extent, some much more readily than others, and to affect photographic plate. These qualities make it possible to use them in taking roentgenograms of various parts of the body, thus revealing the presence and position of fractures or foreign bodies or of radiopaque substances that have been purposely introduced. They can also cause certain substances to fluoresce and thus make possible fluoroscopy, by which the size, shape, and movements of various organs such as the heart, stomach, and intestines can be observed. By reason of the high energy of their quanta, they strongly ionize tissue through which they pass by means of photoelectrons, both primary and secondary, which they liberate. Because of this effect they are used in treating various pathologic conditions. (See also RADIATION and RADIOTHERAPY.)

xylene (zi′lēn) a compound used as a cleaning solvent in microscopy.

xylenol (zi′lĕ-nol) any of a series of colorless crystalline substances resembling phenol.

Xylocaine (zi′lo-kān) trademark for preparations of lidocaine, a topical anesthetic.

xylol (zy′lol) xylene.

xylometazoline (zi″lo-met″ah-zo′lēn) an adrenergic used as a topical nasal decongestant in the form of the hydrochloride salt.

xylose (zi′lōs) a pentose occurring in mucopolysaccharides of connective tissue and sometimes in the urine; also obtained from vegetable gum.

xylulose (zi′lu-lōs) a pentose sugar occurring as D-xylulose and as L-xylulose, one of the few L sugars found in nature; it is sometimes excreted in the urine (see PENTOSURIA).

xylyl (zi′lil) the hydrocarbon radical $CH_3C_6H_4CH_2$.

xysma (zis′mah) material resembling bits of membrane in stools of diarrhea.

xyster (zis′ter) a filelike instrument used in surgery.

Y

Y chemical symbol, *yttrium.*

yaw (yaw) a lesion of YAWS.

mother y., the initial cutaneous lesion of YAWS; called also frambesioma.

yawning (yawn′ing) a deep, involuntary inspiration with the mouth open, often accompanied by the act of stretching.

yaws (yawz) a highly infectious disease caused by the spirochete *Treponema pertenue;* called also frambesia.

Athough almost nonexistent in the United States, yaws is common among people, especially children, who live under primitive conditions in equatorial Africa, South America, and the East and West Indies.

TRANSMISSION AND SYMPTOMS. Yaws is transmitted by direct contact. The first symptom, appearing usually about a month after exposure, is a single granulomatous lesion, an inflammatory but painless elevation of the skin. Called the "mother yaw," this soon ulcerates. Open, oozing sores appear a few weeks later on the hands, feet, face, scalp, and trunk. Eventually, after several years, the disease causes tissue destruction, bone changes, and shortening of the fingers or toes, in a cycle that has a resemblance to leprosy and is sometimes mistaken for it.

The causative organism of yaws is closely related to that of syphilis, and both diseases give a positive result in the Wassermann test. Yaws is classified as a nonvenereal disease and is not primarily communicated by coitus.

TREATMENT AND PREVENTION. Effective treatment is afforded by antibiotics, particularly penicillin.

Unsanitary living conditions unquestionably help spread the disease. Ideally, all clothing that has come in contact with yaws lesions should be sterilized and the sores cleaned with antiseptic and covered with clean dressings.

There is as yet no immunizing vaccine for yaws.

Yb chemical symbol, *ytterbium.*

yeast (yēst) a general term including unicellular, nucleated, usually rounded fungi that reproduce by budding; some are fermenters of carbohydrates, and a few are pathogenic for man.

brewer's y., *Saccharomyces cerevisiae,* used in brewing beer, making alcoholic liquors, and baking bread.

dried y., dried cells of any suitable strain of *Saccharomyces cerevisiae,* usually a by-product of the brewing industry; used as a natural source of protein and B-complex vitamins.

yellow (yel′o) 1. the color produced by stimulation by light waves of wavelength of 571.5 to 578.5 mμ. 2. a dye or stain that produces a yellow color.

y. fever, an acute infectious viral disease, transmitted by the female of certain types of mosquitoes, and characterized by fever, jaundice due to necrosis of the liver, and albuminuria.

Yellow fever is less rampant today largely because of vaccination and better control of the mosquitoes, but it is still a danger in most tropical countries. Among native inhabitants who contract the disease there is a mortality rate of about 5 per cent. In visitors from other climates, fatalities once ran as high as 40 per cent, but they are now much lower. With proper immunization precautions, a visitor from a temperate country today takes only a minimal risk.

The mosquito that transmits classic yellow fever is *Aedes aegypti.* In the jungles of Brazil and in parts of Africa, in the absence of *Aedes aegypti,* the disease may be carried by a different type of mosquito, which lives in treetops. These forest mosquitoes can communicate the disease to forest workers and also to certain animals, such as monkeys and marmosets, which then serve as virus reservoirs and as sources of reinfection for man. This form of the disease is called jungle or sylvan yellow fever, and is difficult to control because of the virtual impossibility of eradicating the tropical tree-inhabiting mosquitoes.

SYMPTOMS AND TREATMENT. Yellow fever has an incubation period of 3 to 6 days. It then manifests itself suddenly and intensely with fever, headache, muscular aches, and prostration. A few days later, the temperature suddenly falls, only to rise again. The pulse is originally very rapid, but then slows gradually to less than 50 beats per minute. In addition to the characteristic yellowing of the skin, the urine becomes darker. There may be frequent vomiting, and blood may become noticeable in the vomitus (so-called black vomit). There may also be bleeding from the mucous membranes.

The disease runs its course in a little more than a week. Those who survive (and the great majority do) suffer no permanent damage. The jaundice completely disappears. Furthermore, these persons are immune from a second attack. In fatal cases, death is usually due to liver or kidney failure.

There is no specific drug for the cure of yellow fever. The effects of the disease can be mitigated by analgesics, sedatives, bed rest, and a high-calorie, high-carbohydrate diet.

PATIENT CARE. The patient's fever is controlled with cold or tepid sponges and other measures to lower body temperature. (See also FEVER.) The diet consists of liquids and easily digested foods until the vomiting stops, and then is gradually increased. The patient's bed and room should be well screened to prevent transmission of the fever to others via mosquitoes.

visual y., all-*trans* retinal (see RETINAL [2]).

Yersinia (yer-sin′e-ah) a genus of gram-negative bacteria. *Y. pseudotuberculosis* causes pseudotuberculosis in rodents and mesenteric lymphadenitis in man.

yogurt (yo′gert) a form of curdled milk produced by fermentation with organisms of the genus *Lactobacillus.*

yoke (yōk) a connecting structure; a depression or ridge connecting two structures.

yolk (yōk) the stored nutrient of the ovum.

Young's rule (yungz) the dose of a drug for a child is obtained by multiplying the adult dose by the child's age in years and dividing the result by the sum of the child's age plus 12.

Young-Helmholtz theory (yung helm'hōlts) the theory that color vision depends on three sets of retinal receptors, corresponding to the colors red, green, and violet.

ytterbium (ī-ter'be-um) a chemical element, atomic number 70, atomic weight 173.04, symbol Yb. (See table of ELEMENTS.)

yttrium (ĭ'tre-um) a chemical element, atomic number 39, atomic weight 88.905, symbol Y. (See table of ELEMENTS.)

Z

Z symbol, *atomic number.*

Zactane (zak'tān) trademark for a preparation of ethoheptazine, an analgesic.

Zarontin (zah-ron'tin) trademark for a preparation of ethosuximide, an anticonvulsant.

zeatin (ze'ah-tin) a cytokinin or growth-stimulating factor of plants.

zeaxanthin (ze"ah-zan'thin) a carotenoid from yellow corn, egg yolk, and the seaweed *Fucus vesiculosis.*

zein (ze'in) a yellowish prolamine from corn.

Zenker's necrosis (degeneration) (zeng'kerz) hyaline degeneration and necrosis of striated muscle.

zeoscope (ze'o-skōp) an apparatus for determining the alcoholic strength of a liquid by means of its boiling point.

Zephiran (zef'i-ran) trademark for preparations of benzalkonium chloride, a topical antiseptic.

zero (ze'ro) the point on a thermometer scale from which the graduations begin. The zero of the Celsius (centigrade) scale is the ice point; on the Fahrenheit scale it is 32 degrees below the ice point.

absolute z., the lowest possible temperature, designated 0 on the Kelvin or Rankine scale, the equivalent of –273.15° C. or –459.67° F.

zinc (zingk) a chemical element, atomic number 30, atomic weight 65.37, symbol Zn. (See table of ELEMENTS.)

z. acetate, a salt used as an astringent and styptic.

z. bacitracin, the zinc salt of bacitracin, used as a topical antibacterial.

z. carbonate, a salt used as a dusting powder, or in the form of a cerate, and as an ingredient of medicinal zinc peroxide.

z. chloride, a salt used topically as an astringent desensitizer for dentin, caustic antiseptic, and deodorant.

z. gelatin, a mixture of zinc oxide, gelatin, glycerin and purified water; used topically as a protectant.

z. ointment, a preparation of zinc oxide and mineral oil in white ointment; used topically as an astringent and protectant.

z. oxide, a compound used as a topical astringent and protectant.

z. peroxide, medicinal, a mixture of zinc peroxide, zinc carbonate, and zinc hydroxide; used topically in 40 per cent solution as a local anti-infective and oxidant, and as an astringent and deodorant.

z. stearate, a compound of zinc with stearic and palmitic acids; used as a water-repellent protective powder in dermatoses.

z. sulfate, a compound used as an ophthalmic astringent.

z. undecylenate, a compound used topically in 20 per cent ointment as an antifungal agent.

white z., zinc oxide.

zirconium (zir-ko'ne-um) a chemical element, atomic number 40, atomic weight 91.22, symbol Zr. (See table of ELEMENTS.)

zn chemical symbol, *zinc.*

zo(o)- word element [Gr.], *animal.*

zoacanthosis (zo"ak-an-tho'sis) a dermatitis caused by penetration into the skin, of bristles, hairs, etc., of lower animals.

zoanthropy (zo-an'thro-pe) the delusion that one has become a beast adj., **zoanthrop'ic.**

zoetic (zo-et'ik) pertaining to life.

zoetrope (zo'ĕ-trōp) an apparatus affording pictures of objects apparently moving as in life.

Zollinger-Ellison syndrome (zol'in-jer-el'ĭ-sun) a triad comprising intractable, sometimes fulminating and in many ways atypical peptic ulcers; extreme gastric hyperacidity; and nonbeta-cell, gastrin-secreting islet cell tumors, which might be single or multiple, small or large, benign or malignant.

zona (zo'nah), pl. *zo'nae* [L.] 1. zone. 2. herpes zoster.

z. fascicula'ta, the thick middle layer of the adrenal gland.

z. glomerulo'sa, the outermost layer of the adrenal cortex.

z. ophthal'mica, herpetic infection of the cornea.

z. pellu'cida, the transparent, noncellular, secreted layer surrounding an ovum.

z. radia'ta, a zona pellucida exhibiting conspicuous radial striations.

z. reticula'ris, the innermost layer of the adrenal cortex.

z. stria'ta, a zona pellucida exhibiting conspicuous striations.

zone (zōn) an encircling region or area; by extension, any area with specific characteristics or boundary.

ciliary z., the outer of the two regions into which the anterior surface of the iris is divided by the angular line.

comfort z., an environmental temperature between 13 and 21° C. (55 and 70° F.) with a humidity of 30 to 55 per cent.

epileptogenic z., an area, stimulation of which may provoke an epileptic seizure.

erogenous z's, erotogenic z's, areas of the body whose stimulation produces erotic desire, e.g., the oral, anal, and genital orifices, and the nipples.

hypnogenic z., hypnogenous z., an area of the body pressure on which will characteristically induce sleep.

transitional z., the circle in the equator of the lens of the eye in which epithelial fibers are developed into lens fibers.

zonethesia (zo"nes-the'ze-ah) a sensation of constriction, as by a girdle.

zonifugal (zo-nif'u-gal) passing outward from a zone or region.

zoning (zōn'ing) the occurrence of a stronger fixation of complement in a lesser amount of suspected serum.

zonipetal (zo-nip'ĕ-tal) passing toward a zone or region.

zonula (zōn'u-lah), pl. *zon'ulae* [L.] zonule.

zonule (zōn'ūl) a small zone.

ciliary z., z. of Zinn, a series of fibers connecting

the ciliary body and lens of the eye, holding the lens in place.

zonulitis (zōn″u-li′tis) inflammation of the ciliary zonule.

zonulolysis (zon″u-lol′ĭ-sis) dissolution of the ciliary zonule by use of enzymes, to permit surgical removal of the lens.

zonulotomy (zon″u-lot′o-me) incision of the ciliary zonule.

zoo- word element [Gr.], *animal.*

zoobiology (zo″o-bi-ol′o-je) the biology of animals.

zoochemistry (zo″o-kem′is-tre) chemistry of animal tissues.

zoodermic (zo″o-der′mik) performed with the skin of an animal, especially in reference to skin grafts.

zoodynamics (zo″o-di-nam′iks) animal physiology.

zoogenous (zo-oj′ĕ-nus) 1. acquired from animals. 2. viviparous.

zoogeny (zo-oj′ĕ-ne) the development and evolution of animals.

zoogeography (zo″o-je-og′rah-fe) the scientific study of the distribution of animals.

zooglea (zo″o-gle′ah) a colony of bacteria embedded in a gelatinous matrix.

zoogony (zo-og′o-ne) the production of living young from within the body. adj., **zoog′onous.**

zoografting (zo′o-graft″ing) the grafting of animal tissue.

zooid (zo′oid) 1. animal-like. 2. an animal-like object or form. 3. an individual in a united colony of animals.

zoolagnia (zo″o-lag′ne-ah) sexual attraction toward animals.

zoology (zo-ol′o-je) the biology of animals.

Zoomastigophora (zo″o-mas″tĭ-gof′o-rah) a class of protozoa (subphylum Mastigophora), including all the flagellates that parasitize higher animals.

zoonosis (zo″o-no′sis), pl. *zoono′ses.* disease of animals transmissible to man adj., **zoonot′ic.**

zooparasite (zo″o-par′ah-sīt) any parasitic animal organism or species. adj., **zooparasit′ic.**

zoopathology (zo″o-pah-thol′o-je) the science of the diseases of animals.

zoophagous (zo-of′ah-gus) carnivorous.

zoophilia (zo″o-fil′e-ah) abnormal fondness for animals.

zoophobia (zo″o-fo′be-ah) abnormal fear of animals.

zooplankton (zo″o-plangk′ton) minute animal organisms floating free in practically all natural waters.

zooplasty (zo′o-plas″te) zoografting.

zoopsia (zo-op′se-ah) a hallucination with vision of animals.

zoospore (zo′o-spōr) a motile reproductive spore.

zoosterol (zo-os′ter-ol) a sterol of animal origin.

zootechnics (zo″o-tek′niks) the art of breeding, keeping, and handling of animals in domestication or captivity.

zootherapeutics (zo″o-ther″ah-pu′tiks) veterinary medicine.

zootomy (zo-ot′o-me) the dissection or anatomy of animals.

zootoxin (zo″o-tok′sin) a toxic substance of animal origin, e.g., venom of snakes, spiders, and scorpions.

zoster (zos″ter) herpes zoster.

zosteriform, zosteroid (zos-ter′ĭ-form; zos′ter-oid) resembling herpes zoster.

Z-plasty (ze′plas-te) repair of a skin defect by the transposition of two triangular flaps of adjacent skin, for relaxation of scar contractures.

Zr chemical symbol, *zirconium.*

zwitterion (tsvit′er-i″on) an ion that has both positive and negative regions of charge. Called also dipolar ion.

zyg(o)- word element [Gr.], *yoked; joined; a junction.*

zygal (zi′gal) shaped like a yoke.

zygapophysis (zi″gah-pof′ĭ-sis) the articular process of a vertebra.

zygion (zij′e-on) the most lateral point on the zygomatic arch.

zygodactyly (zi″go-dak′tĭ-le) union of digits by soft tissues (skin), without bony fusion of the phalanges involved.

zygoma (zi-go′mah) 1. the zygomatic process of the temporal bone. 2. zygomatic arch. 3. a term sometimes applied to the zygomatic bone.

zygomatic (zi″go-mat′ik) pertaining to zygomatic bone.

z. arch, the arch formed by the processes of the zygomatic and temporal bones.

z. bone, the bone forming the hard part of the cheek and the lower, lateral portion of the rim of the orbit (see also table of BONES).

z. process, a projection from the frontal or temporal bone, or from the maxilla, by which they articulate with the zygomatic bone.

zygomaticofacial (zi″go-mat″ĭ-ko-fa′shal) pertaining to the zygoma and face.

zygomaticotemporal (zi″go-mat″ĭ-ko-tem″por-al) pertaining to the zygoma and temporal bone.

zygon (zi′gon) the stem connecting the two branches of a zygal fissure.

zygosity (zi-gos′ĭ-te) the condition relating to conjugation, or to the zygote, as (*a*) the state of a cell or individual in regard to the alleles determining a specific character, whether identical (homozygosity) or different (heterozygosity); or (*b*) in the case of twins, whether developing from one zygote (monozygosity) or two (dizygosity).

zygote (zi′gōt) the cell resulting from union of a male and a female gamete; the fertilized ovum. More precisely, the cell after synapsis at the completion of fertilization until first cleavage. adj., **zygot′ic.** (See also REPRODUCTION.)

zygotene (zi′go-tēn) the synaptic stage of meiosis.

Zyloprim (zi′lo-prim) trademark for preparations of allopurinol, an inhibitor of uric acid production in the body; used in prevention of acute attacks of gout.

zym(o)- word element [Gr.], *enzyme; fermentation.*

zymase (zi′mās) enzyme.

zymic (zi′mik) pertaining to enzymes or fermentation.

zymogen (zi′mo-jen) an inactive precursor that is converted into an active enzyme by action of an acid or another enzyme or by other means; a proenzyme. adj., **zymogen′ic.**

zymogram (zi′mo-gram) a graphic representation of enzymatically active components of a material separated by electrophoresis.

zymohexase (zi″mo-hek′sās) an enzyme that catalyzes the splitting of fructose 1,6-diphosphate into dihydroxy acetone phosphate and phosphoglyceric aldehyde.

zymoid (zi′moid) resembling an enzyme.

zymolysis (zi-mol′ĭ-sis) fermentation or digestion by means of an enzyme. adj., **zymolyt′ic.**

zymophore (zi′mo-fōr) the group of atoms in a molecule of an enzyme that is responsible for its effect; the active site of an enzyme. adj., **zymoph′orous.**

zymoprotein (zi″mo-pro′te-in) any of a class of proteins having catalytic powers.

zymosan (zi′mo-san) a mixture of polysaccharides, proteins, and ash, derived from the cell walls or the entire cell of yeast. It is anticomplementary, and is used in assying properidin.

zymoscope (zi′mo-skōp) an apparatus for determining the fermenting power of yeast.

zymose (zi′mōs) β-fructofurosidase.

zymosis (zi-mo′sis) 1. fermentation. 2. the development of any infectious disease. 3. any infectious or contagious disease. adj., **zymot′ic.**

zymosterol (zi-mos′ter-ol) a sterol occurring in fungi and molds.

Appendix

1. Desirable Weights for Men and Women
2. Ideal Weights for Boys and Girls, According to Height and Age
3. Tables of Weights and Measures
4. Milliequivalent Conversion Factors
5. Approximate Household Equivalents
6. Table of Temperature Equivalents
7. Pulmonary Function (Normal Values)
8. Symbols Commonly Used in Pedigree Charts
9. Voluntary Health and Welfare Agencies
10. Food and Nutrition Board, National Academy of Sciences–National Research Council Recommended Daily Dietary Allowances (RDA), Revised 1974
11. Sources for Patient Education Materials
12. Laboratory Reference Values of Clinical Importance

1. Desirable Weights for Men and Women
Weight in Pounds According to Frame
(in Indoor Clothing)

Men of Ages 25 and Over

Height (with shoes on) 1-inch heels Feet	Inches	Small Frame	Medium Frame	Large Frame
5	2	112–120	118–129	126–141
5	3	115–123	121–133	129–144
5	4	118–126	124–136	132–148
5	5	121–129	127–139	135–152
5	6	124–133	130–143	138–156
5	7	128–137	134–147	142–161
5	8	132–141	138–152	147–166
5	9	136–145	142–156	151–170
5	10	140–150	146–160	155–174
5	11	144–154	150–165	159–179
6	0	148–158	154–170	164–184
6	1	152–162	158–175	168–189
6	2	156–167	162–180	173–194
6	3	160–171	167–185	178–199
6	4	164–175	172–190	182–204

Women of Ages 25 and Over

Height (with shoes on) 2-inch heels Feet	Inches	Small Frame	Medium Frame	Large Frame
4	10	92– 98	96–107	104–119
4	11	94–101	98–110	106–122
5	0	96–104	101–113	109–125
5	1	99–107	104–116	112–128
5	2	102–110	107–119	115–131
5	3	105–113	110–122	118–134
5	4	108–116	113–126	121–138
5	5	111–119	116–130	125–142
5	6	114–123	120–135	129–146
5	7	118–127	124–139	133–150
5	8	122–131	128–143	137–154
5	9	126–135	132–147	141–158
5	10	130–140	136–151	145–163
5	11	134–144	140–155	149–168
6	0	138–148	144–159	153–173

For girls between 18 and 25, subtract 1 pound for each year under 25.

Courtesy of Metropolitan Life Insurance Company.

2. Ideal Weights for Boys and Girls, According to Height and Age

Boys, Aged 14 to 19 Years

Height Feet	Inches	Age 14	15	16	17	18	19
4	6	72					
4	7	74					
4	8	78	80				
4	9	83	83				
4	10	86	87				
4	11	90	90	90			
5	0	94	95	96			
5	1	99	100	103	106		
5	2	103	104	107	111	116	
5	3	108	110	113	118	123	127
5	4	113	115	117	121	126	130
5	5	118	120	122	127	131	134
5	6	122	125	128	132	136	139
5	7	128	130	134	136	139	142
5	8	134	134	137	141	143	147
5	9	137	139	143	146	149	152
5	10	143	144	145	148	151	155
5	11	148	150	151	152	154	159
6	0		153	155	156	158	163
6	1		157	160	162	164	167
6	2		160	164	168	170	171

Girls, Aged 14 to 18 Years

Height Feet	Inches	Age 14	15	16	17	18
4	7	78				
4	8	83				
4	9	88	92			
4	10	93	96	101		
4	11	96	100	103	104	
5	0	101	105	108	109	111
5	1	105	108	112	113	116
5	2	109	113	115	117	118
5	3	112	116	117	119	120
5	4	117	119	120	122	123
5	5	121	122	123	125	126
5	6	124	124	125	128	130
5	7	130	131	133	133	135
5	8	133	135	136	138	138
5	9	135	137	138	140	142
5	10	136	138	140	142	144
5	11	138	140	142	144	145

From American Child Health Association.

3. Tables of Weights and Measures

Measures of Mass

Avoirdupois Weight

GRAINS	DRAMS	OUNCES	POUNDS	METRIC EQUIVALENTS, GRAMS
1	0.0366	0.0023	0.00014	0.0647989
27.34	1	0.0625	0.0039	1.772
437.5	16	1	0.0625	28.350
7000	256	16	1	453.5924277

Apothecaries' Weight

GRAINS	SCRUPLES (℈)	DRAMS (ʒ)	OUNCES (℥)	POUNDS(lb.)	METRIC EQUIVALENTS, GRAMS
1	0.05	0.0167	0.0021	0.00017	0.0647989
20	1	0.333	0.042	0.0035	1.296
60	3	1	0.125	0.0104	3.888
480	24	8	1	0.0833	31.103
5760	288	96	12	1	373.24177

Troy Weight

GRAINS	PENNYWEIGHTS	OUNCES	POUNDS	METRIC EQUIVALENTS, GRAMS
1	0.042	0.002	0.00017	0.0647989
24	1	0.05	0.0042	1.555
480	20	1	0.083	31.103
5760	240	12	1	373.24177

TABLES OF WEIGHTS AND MEASURES—*Continued*

MEASURES OF MASS

METRIC WEIGHT

MICROGRAM	MILLIGRAM	CENTIGRAM	DECIGRAM	GRAM	DECAGRAM	HECTOGRAM	KILOGRAM	EQUIVALENTS	
								AVOIRDUPOIS	APOTHECARIES'
1	...	...	...	...	...	...	...	0.000015 grains	
10^3	1	...	...	...	...	...	...	0.015432 grains	
10^4	10	1	...	...	...	...	...	0.154323 grains	
10^5	10^2	10	1	...	...	...	...	1.543235 grains	
10^6	10^3	10^2	10	1	...	...	...	15.432356 grains	
10^7	10^4	10^3	10^2	10	1	...	...	5.6438 dr.	7.7162 scr.
10^8	10^5	10^4	10^3	10^2	10	1	...	3.527 oz.	3.215 oz.
10^9	10^6	10^5	10^4	10^3	10^2	10	1	2.2046 lb.	2.6792 lb.
10^{12}	10^9	10^8	10^7	10^6	10^5	10^4	10^3	2204.6223 lb.	2679.2285 lb.

Measures of Capacity

Apothecaries' (Wine) Measure

MINIMS	FLUID DRAMS	FLUID OUNCES	GILLS	PINTS	QUARTS	GALLONS	EQUIVALENTS		
							CUBIC INCHES	MILLI-LITERS	CUBIC CENTIMETERS
1	0.0166	0.002	0.0005	0.00013	...	...	0.00376	0.06161	0.06161
60	1	0.125	0.0312	0.0078	0.0039	...	0.22558	3.6967	3.6967
480	8	1	0.25	0.0625	0.0312	0.0078	1.80468	29.5737	29.5737
1920	32	4	1	0.25	0.125	0.0312	7.21875	118.2948	118.2948
7680	128	16	4	1	0.5	0.125	28.875	473.179	473.179
15360	256	32	8	2	1	0.25	57.75	946.358	946.358
61440	1024	128	32	8	4	1	231	3785.434	3785.434

Tables of Weights and Measures—*Continued*

Measures of Capacity

Metric Measure

MICROLITER	MILLILITER	CENTILITER	DECILITER	LITER	DEKALITER	HECTOLITER	KILOLITER	MYRIALITER	EQUIVALENTS (APOTHECARIES' FLUID)	
1	...	...	...	...	...	...	...	...	0.01623108	min.
10^3	1	...	...	...	...	...	...	...	16.23	min.
10^4	10	1	...	...	...	...	...	...	2.7	fl. dr.
10^5	10^2	10	1	...	...	...	...	...	3.38	fl. oz.
10^6	10^3	10^2	10	1	...	...	...	...	2.11	pts.
10^7	10^4	10^3	10^2	10	1	...	...	...	2.64	gal.
10^8	10^5	10^4	10^3	10^2	10	1	...	...	26.418	gal.
10^9	10^6	10^5	10^4	10^3	10^2	10	1	...	264.18	gal.
10^{10}	10^7	10^6	10^5	10^4	10^3	10^2	10	1	2641.8	gal.

1 liter = 2.113363738 pints (Apothecaries').

Measures of Length

Metric Measure

Micron	Millimeter	Centimeter	Decimeter	Meter	Dekameter	Hectometer	Kilometer	Myriameter	Megameter	Equivalents
1	0.001	10^{-4}	...	...	...	...	...	...	...	0.000039 inch
10^3	1	10^{-1}	...	...	...	...	...	...	...	0.03937 inch
10^4	10	1	...	...	...	...	...	...	...	0.3937 inch
10^5	10^2	10	1	...	...	...	...	...	...	3.937 inch
10^6	10^3	10^2	10	1	...	...	...	...	...	39.37 inch
10^7	10^4	10^3	10^2	10	1	...	...	...	...	10.9361 yards
10^8	10^5	10^4	10^3	10^2	10	1	...	...	...	109.3612 yards
10^9	10^6	10^5	10^4	10^3	10^2	10	1	...	...	1093.6121 yards
10^{10}	10^7	10^6	10^5	10^4	10^3	10^2	10	1	...	6.2137 miles
10^{11}	10^8	10^7	10^6	10^5	10^4	10^3	10^2	10	1	62.1370 miles

Tables of Weights and Measures—*Continued*

Conversion Tables

AVOIRDUPOIS—METRIC WEIGHT

Ounces	Grams
1/16	1.772
1/8	3.544
1/4	7.088
1/2	14.175
1	28.350
2	56.699
3	85.049
4	113.398
5	141.748
6	170.097
7	198.447
8	226.796
9	255.146
10	283.495
11	311.845
12	340.194
13	368.544
14	396.893
15	425.243
16 (1 lb.)	453.59
Pounds	
1 (16 oz.)	453.59
2	907.18
3	1360.78 (1.36 kg.)
4	1814.37 (1.81 ")
5	2267.96 (2.27 ")
6	2721.55 (2.72 ")
7	3175.15 (3.18 ")
8	3628.74 (3.63 ")
9	4082.33 (4.08 ")
10	4535.92 (4.54 ")

APOTHECARIES'—METRIC LIQUID MEASURE

Minims	Milliliters
1	0.06
2	0.12
3	0.19
4	0.25
5	0.31
10	0.62
15	0.92
20	1.23
25	1.54
30	1.85
35	2.16
40	2.46
45	2.77
50	3.08
55	3.39
60 (1 fl.dr.)	3.70
Fluid drams	
1	3.70
2	7.39
3	11.09
4	14.79
5	18.48
6	22.18
7	25.88
8 (1 fl.oz.)	29.57
Fluid ounces	
1	29.57
2	59.15
3	88.72
4	118.29
5	147.87
6	177.44
7	207.01
8	236.58
9	266.16
10	295.73
11	325.30
12	354.88
13	384.45
14	414.02
15	443.59
16 (1 pt.)	473.18
32 (1 qt.)	946.36
128 (1 gal.)	3785.43

METRIC—AVOIRDUPOIS WEIGHT

GRAMS	OUNCES
0.001 (1 mg.)	0.000035274
1	0.035274
1000 (1 kg.)	35.274 (2.2046 lb.)

METRIC—APOTHECARIES' LIQUID MEASURE

MILLILITERS	MINIMS	MILLILITERS	FLUID DRAMS	MILLILITERS	FLUID OUNCES
1	16.231	5	1.35	30	1.01
2	32.5	10	2.71	40	1.35
3	48.7	15	4.06	50	1.69
4	64.9	20	5.4	500	16.91
5	81.1	25	6.76	1000 (1 L.)	33.815
		30	7.1		

TABLES OF WEIGHTS AND MEASURES—*Continued*

CONVERSION TABLES

APOTHECARIES'—METRIC WEIGHT

Grains	Grams
1/150	0.0004
1/120	0.0005
1/100	0.0006
1/80	0.0008
1/64	0.001
1/50	0.0013
1/48	0.0014
1/30	0.0022
1/25	0.0026
1/16	0.004
1/12	0.005
1/10	0.006
1/9	0.007
1/8	0.008
1/7	0.009
1/6	0.01
1/5	0.013
1/4	0.016
1/3	0.02
1/2	0.032
1	0.065
1 1/2	0.097 (0.1)
2	0.12
3	0.20
4	0.24
5	0.30
6	0.40
7	0.45
8	0.50
9	0.60
10	0.65
15	1.00
20 (1℈)	1.30
30	2.00
Scruples	
1	1.296 (1.3)
2	2.592 (2.6)
3 (1ʒ)	3.888 (3.9)
Drams	
1	3.888
2	7.776
3	11.664
4	15.552
5	19.440
6	23.328
7	27.216
8 (1℥)	31.103
Ounces	
1	31.103
2	62.207
3	93.310
4	124.414
5	155.517
6	186.621
7	217.724
8	248.828
9	279.931
10	311.035
11	342.138
12 (1 lb.)	373.242

METRIC—APOTHECARIES' WEIGHT

Milligrams	Grains
1	0.015432
2	0.030864
3	0.046296
4	0.061728
5	0.077160
6	0.092592
7	0.108024
8	0.123456
9	0.138888
10	0.154320
15	0.231480
20	0.308640
25	0.385800
30	0.462960
35	0.540120
40	0.617280
45	0.694440
50	0.771600
100	1.543240
Grams	
0.1	1.5432
0.2	3.0864
0.3	4.6296
0.4	6.1728
0.5	7.7160
0.6	9.2592
0.7	10.8024
0.8	12.3456
0.9	13.8888
1.0	15.4320
1.5	23.1480
2.0	30.8640
2.5	38.5800
3.0	46.2960
3.5	54.0120
4.0	61.728
4.5	69.444
5.0	77.162
10.0	154.324
	Equivalents
10	2.572 drams
15	3.858 "
20	5.144 "
25	6.430 "
30	7.716 "
40	1.286 oz.
45	1.447 "
50	1.607 "
100	3.215 "
200	6.430 "
300	9.644 "
400	12.859 "
500	1.34 lb.
600	1.61 "
700	1.88 "
800	2.14 "
900	2.41 "
1000	2.68 "

TABLES OF WEIGHTS AND MEASURES—*Concluded*

METRIC DOSES WITH APPROXIMATE APOTHECARY EQUIVALENTS*

These *approximate* dose equivalents represent the quantities usually prescribed, under identical conditions, by physicians trained, respectively, in the metric or in the apothecary system of weights and measures. In labeling dosage forms in both the metric and the apothecary systems, if one is the approximate equivalent of the other, the approximate figure shall be enclosed in parentheses.

When prepared dosage forms such as tablets, capsules, pills, etc., are prescribed in the metric system, the pharmacist may dispense the corresponding *approximate* equivalent in the apothecary system, and vice versa, as indicated in the following table.

Caution—For the conversion of specific quantities in a prescription which requires compounding, or in converting a pharmaceutical formula from one system of weights or measures to the other, *exact* equivalents must be used.

LIQUID MEASURE		LIQUID MEASURE	
METRIC	APPROX. APOTHECARY EQUIVALENTS	METRIC	APPROX. APOTHECARY EQUIVALENTS
1000 ml.	1 quart	3 ml.	45 minims
750 ml.	1 1/2 pints	2 ml.	30 minims
500 ml.	1 pint	1 ml.	15 minims
250 ml.	8 fluid ounces	0.75 ml.	12 minims
200 ml.	7 fluid ounces	0.6 ml.	10 minims
100 ml.	3 1/2 fluid ounces	0.5 ml.	8 minims
50 ml.	1 3/4 fluid ounces	0.3 ml.	5 minims
30 ml.	1 fluid ounce	0.25 ml.	4 minims
15 ml.	4 fluid drams	0.2 ml.	3 minims
10 ml.	2 1/2 fluid drams	0.1 ml.	1 1/2 minims
8 ml.	2 fluid drams	0.06 ml.	1 minim
5 ml.	1 1/4 fluid drams	0.05 ml.	3/4 minim
4 ml.	1 fluid dram	0.03 ml.	1/2 minim

WEIGHT		WEIGHT	
METRIC	APPROX. APOTHECARY EQUIVALENTS	METRIC	APPROX. APOTHECARY EQUIVALENTS
30 Gm.	1 ounce	30 mg.	1/2 grain
15 Gm.	4 drams	25 mg.	3/8 grain
10 Gm.	2 1/2 drams	20 mg.	1/3 grain
7.5 Gm.	2 drams	15 mg.	1/4 grain
6 Gm.	90 grains	12 mg.	1/5 grain
5 Gm.	75 grains	10 mg.	1/6 grain
4 Gm.	60 grains (1 dram)	8 mg.	1/8 grain
3 Gm.	45 grains	6 mg.	1/10 grain
2 Gm.	30 grains (1/2 dram)	5 mg.	1/12 grain
1.5 Gm.	22 grains	4 mg.	1/15 grain
1 Gm.	15 grains	3 mg.	1/20 grain
0.75 Gm.	12 grains	2 mg.	1/30 grain
0.6 Gm.	10 grains	1.5 mg.	1/40 grain
0.5 Gm.	7 1/2 grains	1.2 mg.	1/50 grain
0.4 Gm.	6 grains	1 mg.	1/60 grain
0.3 Gm.	5 grains	0.8 mg.	1/80 grain
0.25 Gm.	4 grains	0.6 mg.	1/100 grain
0.2 Gm.	3 grains	0.5 mg.	1/120 grain
0.15 Gm.	2 1/2 grains	0.4 mg.	1/150 grain
0.12 Gm.	2 grains	0.3 mg.	1/200 grain
0.1 Gm.	1 1/2 grains	0.25 mg.	1/250 grain
75 mg.	1 1/4 grains	0.2 mg.	1/300 grain
60 mg.	1 grain	0.15 mg.	1/400 grain
50 mg.	3/4 grain	0.12 mg.	1/500 grain
40 mg.	2/3 grain	0.1 mg.	1/600 grain

Note—A milliliter (ml.) is the approximate equivalent of a cubic centimeter (cc.).

*Adopted by the latest Pharmacopeia, National Formulary, and New and Nonofficial Remedies, and approved by the Federal Food and Drug Administration.

4. Milliequivalent Conversion Factors

mEq./L. of:	Divide mg./100 ml. or Vol. % by:	
Calcium	2.0	
Chlorides (from Cl)	3.5	
(from NaCl)	5.85	
CO_2 combining power	2.22	
Magnesium	1.2	
Phosphorus	3.1	(mM.)
Potassium	3.9	
Sodium	2.3	

From Brainerd, H., Margen, S., and Chatton, M. J.: Current Diagnosis and Treatment. Los Altos, Calif., Lange Medical Publications, 1967.

5. Approximate Household Equivalents

	Liquid	Weight
1 teaspoon	5 ml.	5 Gm.
1 tablespoon = 3 teaspoons	15 ml.	15 Gm.
1 cup = 16 tablespoons	237 ml.	240 Gm.
1 pint = 2 cups	473 ml.	480 Gm.
1 quart = 2 pints = 4 cups	946 ml.	960 Gm.

1	pound of butter	=	2 cups
8	average eggs	=	1 cup
4	cups sifted flour	=	1 pound
2	cups granulated sugar	=	1 pound
2⅔	cups confectioner's sugar	=	1 pound
2⅔	cups brown sugar	=	1 pound

6. Table of Temperature Equivalents

CELSIUS (CENTIGRADE): FAHRENHEIT SCALE

CELSIUS : FAHRENHEIT °F = (°C × 9/5) + 32				FAHRENHEIT : CELSIUS °C = (°F − 32) × 5/9					
C°	F°	C°	F°	F°	C°	F°	C°	F°	C°
−50	−58.0	49	120.2	−50	−46.7	99	37.2	157	69.4
−40	−40.0	50	122.0	−40	−40.0	100	37.7	158	70.0
−35	−31.0	51	123.8	−35	−37.2	101	38.3	159	70.5
−30	−22.0	52	125.6	−30	−34.4	102	38.8	160	71.1
−25	−13.0	53	127.4	−25	−31.7	103	39.4	161	71.6
−20	−4.0	54	129.2	−20	−28.9	104	40.0	162	72.2
−15	−5.0	55	131.0	−15	−26.6	105	40.5	163	72.7
−10	14.0	56	132.8	−10	−23.3	106	41.1	164	73.3
−5	23.0	57	134.6	−5	−20.6	107	41.6	165	73.8
0	32.0	58	136.4	0	−17.7	108	42.2	166	74.4
+1	33.8	59	138.2	+1	−17.2	109	42.7	167	75.0
2	35.6	60	140.0	5	−15.0	110	43.3	168	75.5
3	37.4	61	141.8	10	−12.2	111	43.8	169	76.1
4	39.2	62	143.6	15	−9.4	112	44.4	170	76.6
5	41.0	63	145.4	20	−6.6	113	45.0	171	77.2
6	42.8	64	147.2	25	−3.8	114	45.5	172	77.7
7	44.6	65	149.0	30	−1.1	115	46.1	173	78.3
8	46.4	66	150.8	31	−0.5	116	46.6	174	78.8
9	48.2	67	152.6	32	0	117	47.2	175	79.4
10	50.0	68	154.4	33	+0.5	118	47.7	176	80.0
11	51.8	69	156.2	34	1.1	119	48.3	177	80.5
12	53.6	70	158.0	35	1.6	120	48.8	178	81.1
13	55.4	71	159.8	36	2.2	121	49.4	179	81.6
14	57.2	72	161.6	37	2.7	122	50.0	180	82.2
15	59.0	73	163.4	38	3.3	123	50.5	181	82.7
16	60.8	74	165.2	39	3.8	124	51.1	182	83.3
17	62.6	75	167.0	40	4.4	125	51.6	183	83.8
18	64.4	76	168.8	41	5.0	126	52.2	184	84.4
19	66.2	77	170.6	42	5.5	127	52.7	185	85.0
20	68.0	78	172.4	43	6.1	128	53.3	186	85.5
21	69.8	79	174.2	44	6.6	129	53.8	187	86.1
22	71.6	80	176.0	45	7.2	130	54.4	188	86.6
23	73.4	81	177.8	46	7.7	131	55.0	189	87.2
24	75.2	82	179.6	47	8.3	132	55.5	190	87.7
25	77.0	83	181.4	48	8.8	133	56.1	191	88.3
26	78.8	84	183.2	49	9.4	134	56.6	192	88.8
27	80.6	85	185.0	50	10.0	135	57.2	193	89.4
28	82.4	86	186.8	55	12.7	136	57.7	194	90.0
29	84.2	87	188.6	60	15.5	137	58.3	195	90.5
30	86.0	88	190.4	65	18.3	138	58.8	196	91.1
31	87.8	89	192.2	70	21.1	139	59.4	197	91.6
32	89.6	90	194.0	75	23.8	140	60.0	198	92.2
33	91.4	91	195.8	80	26.6	141	60.5	199	92.7
34	93.2	92	197.6	85	29.4	142	61.1	200	93.3
35	95.0	93	199.4	86	30.0	143	61.6	201	93.8
36	96.8	94	201.2	87	30.5	144	62.2	202	94.4
37	98.6	95	203.0	88	31.0	145	62.7	203	95.0
38	100.4	96	204.8	89	31.6	146	63.3	204	95.5
39	102.2	97	206.6	90	32.2	147	63.8	205	96.1
40	104.0	98	208.4	91	32.7	148	64.4	206	96.6
41	105.8	99	210.2	92	33.3	149	65.0	207	97.2
42	107.6	100	212.0	93	33.8	150	65.5	208	97.7
43	109.4	101	213.8	94	34.4	151	66.1	209	98.3
44	111.2	102	215.6	95	35.0	152	66.6	210	98.8
45	113.0	103	217.4	96	35.5	153	67.2	211	99.4
46	114.8	104	219.2	97	36.1	154	67.7	212	100.0
47	116.6	105	221.0	98	36.6	155	68.3	213	100.5
48	118.4	106	222.8	98.6	37.0	156	68.8	214	101.1

7. PULMONARY FUNCTION (NORMAL VALUES)

Vital Capacity (liters)	Male: = [(27.63 − [0.112 × Age in yr.]) × Ht. in cm.] ÷ 1,000 Female: = [(21.78 − [0.101 × Age in yr.]) × Ht. in cm.] ÷ 1,000
Tidal Air	0.350–0.500 L.
Residual Volume*	1.0–1.5 L.
Total Lung Capacity	Vital Capacity + Residual Volume
Residual Volume: Total Lung Capacity	20–30%
Maximum Breathing Capacity	Male: 100–150 L./min. Female: 70–120 L./min. (approx. values) Male: L./min. = [86.5 − (0.522 × Age in yr.)] × sq.M. of B.S.A.** Female: L./min. = [71.3 − (0.474 × Age in yr.)] × sq.M. of B.S.A.**
Respiratory Rate (resting)	8–20/min.
Pulmonary Ventilation (resting)	3–4 L./min./sq.M. of B.S.A.
Pulmonary Compliance	0.200 L./cm. of H_2O intrapleural pressure change
O_2 Uptake (resting)	110–140 cc./min.sq.M. of B.S.A.
CO_2 Output (resting)	88–120 cc./min./sq.M. of B.S.A.
Respiratory Exchange Ratio (Resp. Quotient, R.Q.)	$\frac{CO_2}{O_2}$ = 0.77–0.90
Bronchospirometric Ratio (% total function)	Rt. lung: 52–58% Lt. lung: 48–42%
Timed Vital Capacity	First sec. = 83 + % of total vital capacity First 2 sec. = 94 + % of total vital capacity First 3 sec. = 97% of total vital capacity

From The Merck Manual. 11th ed. Copyright 1966, Merck & Co., Inc., Rahway, New Jersey.
*Air in lungs at maximal expiration.
**More accurate formulas.

8. Symbols Commonly Used in Pedigree Charts

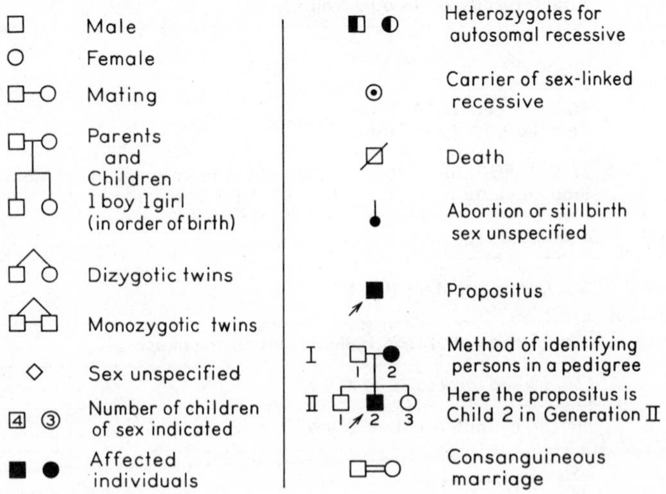

From Thompson, J. S., and Thompson, M. W.: Genetics in Medicine, 2nd ed. Philadelphia, W. B. Saunders Co., 1973.

9. Voluntary Health and Welfare Agencies

Addicts Anonymous
Box 2000, Lexington, KY 40501

Aging, National Council on the
315 Park Ave., South, New York, NY 10010

Alcoholics Anonymous, Inc.
P.O. Box 459, Grand Central Station, New York, NY 10017

Alcoholism, National Council on
2 East 103rd St., New York, NY 10029

Allergy, American Academy of
756 North Milwaukee St.,
Milwaukee, WS 53202

Allergy Foundation of America
801 Second Ave., New York, NY 10017

Arthritis Foundation, The
475 Riverside Drive, New York, NY 10027

Blind, American Foundation for the
15 West 16th St., New York, NY 10011

Blindness, National Society for the Prevention of
79 Madison Ave., New York, NY 10016

Cancer Research, The Institute for
7701 Burholme Ave., Philadelphia, PA 19111

Cancer Society, American
219 East 42nd St., New York, NY 10017

Cerebral Palsy Association, United
66 East 34th St., New York, NY 10016

Childbirth Education Association,
The International
Box 5852, Milwaukee, WS

Crippled Children and Adults,
National Easter Seal Society for
2023 West Ogden Ave., Chicago, IL 60612

Cystic Fibrosis Research Foundation, National
521 Fifth Ave., New York, NY 10017

Deaf, Alexander Graham Bell Association for the
1537 35th St., N.W., Washington, DC 20007

Deaf, The National Association of the
814 Thayer Ave., Silver Spring, MD 20910

Deafness Research Foundation
366 Madison Ave., New York, NY 10017

Diabetes Association, American
18 East 48th St., New York, NY 10017

Drug Abuse, The National Council on
8 South Michigan Ave., Suite 310,
Chicago, IL 60603

Epilepsy Foundation of America
733 15th St., Washington, DC 20005

Epilepsy League, National
203 North Wabash Ave., Chicago, IL 60601

Euthanasia Educational Council
250 West 57th St., New York, NY 10019

Family Service Association of America
44 East 23rd St., New York, NY 10010

Gerontological Society
One Dupont Circle, Suite 520,
Washington, DC 20036

Hearing and Speech Agencies,
National Association of
919 18th St., N.W., Washington, DC 20006

Heart Association, American
44 East 23rd St., New York, NY 10010

Kidney Foundation, National
342 Madison Ave., New York, NY 10017

LaLeche League International, Inc.
9616 Minneapolis Ave.,
Franklin Park, IL 60131

Leukemia Society
211 East 43rd St., New York, NY 10017

Lung Association, American
1740 Broadway, New York, NY 10019

Maternity Center Association
48 E. 92nd St., New York, NY 10028

Medic Alert Foundation
Box K-7, Turlock, CA 95380

Mental Health, National Association for
10 Columbus Circle, New York, NY 10019

Multiple Sclerosis Society, National
257 Park Ave. South, New York, NY 10010

Muscular Dystrophy Associations of America
1790 Broadway, New York, NY 10019

Narcotics Education
6830 Laurel Ave., Washington, DC 20012

Ostomy Association, Inc., United
1111 Wilshire Blvd., Los Angeles, CA 90017

Planned Parenthood Federation of America
515 Madison Ave., New York, NY 10022

Psychoprophylaxis in Obstetrics, Inc.,
American Society for
Suite 410, 1523 L St.,
N.W., Washington, DC 20005

9. Voluntary Health and Welfare Agencies—*Concluded*

Rehabilitation Association, National
1522 K St., N.W., Washington, DC 20005

Retarded Children, National Association for
420 Lexington Ave., New York, NY 10017

Retarded Citizens, National Association for
Publications Dept., P.O. Box 6109,
Arlington, TX 76011

Sex Information and Education of the U.S. (SIECUS)
1855 Broadway, New York, NY 10023

Social Health Association, American
1740 Broadway, New York, NY 10019

Speech and Hearing Association, American
1001 Connecticut Ave., N.W.,
Washington, DC 20006

Sudden Infant Death, Inc., National Foundation for
1501 Broadway, New York, NY 10036

Volta Bureau
1537 35th St., N.W., Washington, DC 20007

10. Food and Nutrition Board, National Academy of Sciences–National Research Council Recommended Daily Dietary Allowances (RDA),[a] Revised 1974

Designed for the maintenance of good nutrition of practically all healthy people in the U.S.A.

	Age (years)	Weight (kg)	Weight (lbs)	Height (cm)	Height (in)	Energy (kcal)[b]	Protein (g)	Fat-Soluble Vitamins: Vitamin A Activity (RE)[c]	Vitamin A Activity (IU)	Vitamin D (IU)	Vitamin E Activity[e] (IU)	Water-Soluble Vitamins: Ascorbic Acid (mg)	Folacin[f] (μg)	Niacin[g] (mg)	Riboflavin (mg)	Thiamin (mg)	Vitamin B_6 (mg)	Vitamin B_{12} (μg)	Minerals: Calcium (mg)	Phosphorus (mg)	Iodine (μg)	Iron (mg)	Magnesium (mg)	Zinc (mg)
Infants	0.0–0.5	6	14	60	24	kg × 117	kg × 2.2	420[d]	1,400	400	4	35	50	5	0.4	0.3	0.3	0.3	360	240	35	10	60	3
	0.5–1.0	9	20	71	28	kg × 108	kg × 2.0	400	2,000	400	5	35	50	8	0.6	0.5	0.4	0.3	540	400	45	15	70	5
Children	1–3	13	28	86	34	1,300	23	400	2,000	400	7	40	100	9	0.8	0.7	0.6	1.0	800	800	60	15	150	10
	4–6	20	44	110	44	1,800	30	500	2,500	400	9	40	200	12	1.1	0.9	0.9	1.5	800	800	80	10	200	10
	7–10	30	66	135	54	2,400	36	700	3,300	400	10	40	300	16	1.2	1.2	1.2	2.0	800	800	110	10	250	10
Males	11–14	44	97	158	63	2,800	44	1,000	5,000	400	12	45	400	18	1.5	1.4	1.6	3.0	1,200	1,200	130	18	350	15
	15–18	61	134	172	69	3,000	54	1,000	5,000	400	15	45	400	20	1.8	1.5	2.0	3.0	1,200	1,200	150	18	400	15
	19–22	67	147	172	69	3,000	54	1,000	5,000	400	15	45	400	20	1.8	1.5	2.0	3.0	800	800	140	10	350	15
	23–50	70	154	172	69	2,700	56	1,000	5,000		15	45	400	18	1.6	1.4	2.0	3.0	800	800	130	10	350	15
	51+	70	154	172	69	2,400	56	1,000	5,000		15	45	400	16	1.5	1.2	2.0	3.0	800	800	110	10	350	15
Females	11–14	44	97	155	62	2,400	44	800	4,000	400	12	45	400	16	1.3	1.2	1.6	3.0	1,200	1,200	115	18	300	15
	15–18	54	119	162	65	2,100	48	800	4,000	400	12	45	400	14	1.4	1.1	2.0	3.0	1,200	1,200	115	18	300	15
	19–22	58	128	162	65	2,100	46	800	4,000	400	12	45	400	14	1.4	1.1	2.0	3.0	800	800	100	18	300	15
	23–50	58	128	162	65	2,000	46	800	4,000		12	45	400	13	1.2	1.0	2.0	3.0	800	800	100	18	300	15
	51+	58	128	162	65	1,800	46	800	4,000		12	45	400	12	1.1	1.0	2.0	3.0	800	800	80	10	300	15
Pregnant						+300	+30	1,000	5,000	400	15	60	800	+2	+0.3	+0.3	2.5	4.0	1,200	1,200	125	18+[h]	450	20
Lactating						+500	+20	1,200	6,000	400	15	80	600	+4	+0.5	+0.3	2.5	4.0	1,200	1,200	150	18	450	25

[a] The allowances are intended to provide for individual variations among most normal persons as they live in the United States under usual environmental stresses. Diets should be based on a variety of common foods in order to provide other nutrients for which human requirements have been less well defined.

[b] Kilojoules (kJ) = 4.2 × kcal.

[c] Retinol equivalents.

[d] Assumed to be all as retinol in milk during the first six months of life. All subsequent intakes are assumed to be half as retinol and half as β-carotene when calculated from international units. As retinol equivalents, three fourths are as retinol and one fourth as β-carotene.

[e] Total vitamin E activity, estimated to be 80 percent as α-tocopherol and 20 percent other tocopherols. See text for variation in allowances.

[f] The folacin allowances refer to dietary sources as determined by *Lactobacillus casei* assay. Pure forms of folacin may be effective in doses less than one fourth of the recommended dietary allowance.

[g] Although allowances are expressed as niacin, it is recognized that on the average 1 mg of niacin is derived from each 60 mg of dietary tryptophan.

[h] This increased requirement cannot be met by ordinary diets; therefore, the use of supplemental iron is recommended.

11. Sources for Patient Education Materials

Abbott Film Services
Scientificom Distribution Center
708 No. Dearborn
Chicago, IL 60610

Abbott Laboratories
Professional Services – D383
Abbott Park
No. Chicago, IL 60064

*Alfred Higgins Prod., Inc.
9100 Sunset Blvd.
Los Angeles, CA 60069

*American Video Network
660 S. Bonnie Brae St.
Los Angeles, CA 90057

The Ames Co., Inc.
Division of Miles Laboratories
Elkart, IN 46514

Auburn University
Education Television Department
Auburn, AL 36830

Audience Planners
208 LaSalle St.
Chicago, IL 60604

Ayerst Laboratories
685 Third Ave.
New York, NY 10017

W. A. Baum Co., Inc.
Copiague, NY 11726

Becton Dickenson & Co.
Rutherford, NJ 07070
Re: "Getting Started" Program

Beecham-Massengill
Division of Beecham, Inc.
Bristol, TN 37620

Best Foods – Consumer Service Department
A Division of CPC International, Inc.
International Plaza
Englewood Cliffs, NJ 07632

Chaning L. Bete Co., Inc.
45 Federal St.
Greenfield, Mass 01301

Better Vision Institute
230 Park Ave.
New York, NY 10017

Blue Cross Association
Communications Division
840 N. Lake Shore Dr.
Chicago, IL 60611

Boehringer Ingleheim, Ltd.
23 West Tarrytown Rd.
Elmsford, NY 10523

*BNA Communications, Inc.
8371 Bernice Drive
Strongsville, OH 44136

Robert J. Brady Publishing Co.
Bowie, MD 20715

*Brookhaven Memorial Hospital
101 Brookhaven Hospital Road
Patchogue, NY 11772

Burroughs Wellcome Co.
Research Triangle Park, NC 27709

Campbell Soup Co.
Food Service Products Division
375 Memorial Ave.
Camden, NJ 08101

Carnation Co.
Medical Marketing Department
5045 Wilshire Blvd.
Los Angeles, CA 90036

Cereal Institute
135 S. LaSalle St.
Chicago, IL 60603

Children's Hospital Medical Center
Health Education Department
300 Longwood Ave.
Boston, Mass 02115

Churchill Films
622 N. Robertson Blvd.
Los Angeles, CA 90069

CIBA Pharmaceutical Co.
Division of CIBA–Geigy Corp.
556 Morris Ave.
Summit, NJ

CORE Communications in Health, Inc.
1290 Avenue of the Americas
New York, NY 10019

Davis and Geck
Director of Professional Relations
One Middletown Rd.
Pearl River, NY 10965

Davol, Inc.
69 Point St.
Providence, RI 02901

Diabetes Education Center
4959 Excelsior Blvd.
Minneapolis, MN 55416

Dorsey Laboratories
Division of Sandoy, Inc.
Lincoln, NB 68501

*Video Tape Programs

Sources for Patient Education Materials—*Continued*

Eaton Laboratories Division
Morton-Norwich Products, Inc.
Medical Film Library
Norwich, NY 13815

*EDCOA Productions, Inc.
520 S. Dean St.
Englewood, NJ 07631

Education for Health, Inc.
205 Deerwood Lane
Minneapolis, MN 55427

Ethicon
Modern Talking Picture Service, Inc.
Circulation Dept.
2323 New Hyde Park Rd.
New Hyde Park, NY 10040

*Fairview General Hospital
c/o the Greater Cleveland Hospital Association
1021 Euclid Ave.
Cleveland, OH 44115

*Family Communications, Inc.
4802 5th Ave.
Pittsburgh, PA 15213

Gerber Products Co.
445 State St. Box 33
Fremont, MI 49412

Graphics Co.
Nutritional Games
P.O. Box 331
Urbana, IL 61801

John F. Greer Co.
P.O. Box 2898
5335 College Ave.
Oakland, CA 94618

Health Films Library
P.O. Box 309
Madison, WI 53701

H. J. Heinz
Consumer Relations
P.O. Box 57
Pittsburgh, PA 15230

Hollister, Inc.
211 East Chicago, IL

*Holloran & Klein Video Prods.
4018 22nd St.
San Francisco, CA 94114

*Hospital Audiovisual Education
606 Halstead Ave.
Mamaroneck, NY 10543

*Indiana University School of Medicine
Medical Educational Resources Program
1100 W. Michigan St.
Indianapolis, IN 46202

*Video Tape Programs

Institute of Nutrition
Allied Health Services Bldg.
University of North Carolina, Chapel Hill
Chapel Hill, NC

Johnson & Johnson
New Brunswick, NJ 08903

Kaiser-Permanente Health Center
Audiovisual Workshop
3779 Piedmont Ave.
Oakland, CA 94611

Sister Kenny Institute
27th St. at Chicago Ave.
Minneapolis, MN 55504

Lawren Productions, Inc.
P.O. Box 1452
Burlingame, CA 94010

Learning Resources Facility
Institute of Rehabilitation Medicine
400 East 34th St.
New York, NY 10016

Lederle Laboratories
Film Library
1 Casoar St.
Danbury, CN 06810

Lee Creative Communications, Inc.
P.O. Box 1367
Rochester, NY 14603

Eli Lilly and Company
Educational Resources Program
P.O. Box 100B
Indianapolis, IN 46206

*Martland Hospital
Health Education Project
College of Medicine and Dentistry of New Jersey
65 Bergen Street
Newark, NJ 07107

Maternity Center Association
48 East 92nd St.
New York, NY 10028

McNeil Laboratories, Inc.
Camp Hill Road
Fort Washington, PA 19034

Mead Johnson & Co.
Public Relations Department
Evansville, IN 47721

*Medcom, Inc.
1633 Broadway
New York, NY

*Medfact, Inc.
420 Lake Ave., N.E.
Massilon, OH 44646

Media Medica, Inc.
555 5th Ave.
New York, NY 10017

Sources for Patient Education Materials—*Continued*

Medical Communications, Inc.
299 Park Ave.
New York, NY 10017

*Medi-Cine Corporation
3430-32 N. Illinois St.
Indianapolis, IN 46208

Merck, Sharpe & Dohme
Division of Merck & Co., Inc.
Audio Visual Services
West Point, PA 19486

Mercy Medical Center
Patient Education Division
Dubuque, IO 52001

Metropolitan Life Insurance Co.
P.O. Box 7750
San Francisco, CA 94120

Richard Milner
Milner, Fenwick
3800 Liberty Heights Ave.
Baltimore, MD 21215

National Academy of Sciences
National Resource Council
Food and Nutrition Board
2101 Constitution Ave.
Washington, DC 20418

National Dairy Council
6300 N. River Road
Rosemont, IL 60018

National Society for Medical Research
1330 Massachusetts Ave., N.W.
Washington, DC 20005

Nutrition Education Service
Montclair State College
Upper Montclair, NY 07043

Nutrition Foundation, Inc.
888 17th St., N.W.
Washington, DC 20006

Organon, Inc.
West Orange, NJ 07052

Ortho-Pharmaceutical Corp.
Professional Services
Route 202
Raritan, NJ 08869

Parke Davis & Co.
Joseph Campau at the River
Box 118—General Post Office
Detroit, MI 48232

Perennial Education, Inc.
1825 Willow Road
Northfield, IL 60083

Pfizer Laboratories
Pfizer, Inc.
235 East 42nd St.
New York, NY 10017

Pritchett & Hull Assoc., Inc.
2996 Grandview
Atlanta, GA 30305

*Professional Research, Inc.
660 S. Bonnie Brae Ave.
Los Angeles, CA 90057

Prudential Insurance Co. of America
Prudential Plaza
Chicago, IL 60601

*The Public Television Library
475 L'Enfant Plaza, S.W.
Washington, DC 20024

*Pyramid Films
Box 1048
Santa Monica, CA 90406

Research Media, Inc.
96 Mt. Suburn St.
Cambridge, Mass 02138

Riker Laboratories, Inc.
Subsidiary of 3M Co.
19901 Nordhoff St.
Northridge, CA 91324

Robins, Co.
1407 Cummins Drive
Richmond, VA 23220

Ross Laboratories
Creative Services and Information Department
625 Cleveland Ave.
Columbus, OH 43216

Sandoz Pharmaceuticals
East Hanover, NJ 07936

*W. B. Saunders Co.
West Washington Square
Philadelphia, PA 19105

Schering Corp.
Professional Film Library
c/o Association-Sterlings, Inc.
600 Grand Ave.
Ridgefield, NJ 07657

G. D. Searle & Co.
P.O. Box 5110
Chicago, IL 60680

Single Concept Films
Two Terrain Drive
Milwaukee, WI 53203

Smith, Kline & French Laboratories
Division of Smith, Kline Corp.
1500 Spring Garden St.
Philadelphia, PA 19101

E. R. Squibb & Sons, Inc.
P.O. Box 4000
Princeton, NJ 08540

---

*Video Tape Programs

Sources for Patient Education Materials—*Concluded*

Sunkist Growers, Inc.
Consumer Service
P.O. Box 7888
Valley Annex
Van Nuys, CA 91409

*Teach'em, Inc.
625 N. Michigan Ave.
Chicago, IL 60611

*University of Toronto
Division of Instructional Media Services
Toronto, Canada M5S 1A8

*Train-Aide
229 No. Central Ave.
Glendale, CA 91203

Train-Aide, Inc.
1015 Grandview
Glendale, CA 91201

Trainex Corp.
A Subsidiary of Medcom, Inc.
P.O. Box 116
Garden Grove, CA 92642

*Trainex Patient Video Corp.
10 Perimeter Place, N.W.
Atlanta, GA 30339

The Upjohn Co.
Professional Film Library
Attn: Ruth Watson
7000 Portage Rd.
Kalamazoo, MI 49001

*University of Illinois
Medical Center
Public Information Office
P.O. Box 6998
Chicago, IL 60680

*University of Kansas
College of Health Sciences and Hospital
39th and Rainbow Streets
Kansas City, KA 66102

*Video Tape Programs

University of Wisconsin
Bureau of Audiovisual Instruction
P.O. Box 2093
Madison, WI 53701

U.S. Department of Health, Education and Welfare
Diabetes and Arthritis Program
Washington, DC 20201

U.S. National Heart Institute
Heart Information Center
U.S. Government Printing Office
Washington, DC

Vidcom
2319 DeFoor Hills Road
P.O. Box 19978
Atlanta, GA

Video Communications, Inc.
Suite 904
Watergate Office Building
2600 Virginia Ave., N.W.
Washington, DC 21137

Vitamin Information Bureau, Inc.
383 Madison Ave.
New York, NY 10017

Warner/Chilicott
Division of Warner Lambert Co.
201 Taber Rd.
Morris Plains, NJ 07950

Washington State University
Cooperative Extension Service
Nutrition Games
Pullman, WA 99163

*Wells National Services Corporation
200 Park Ave.
New York, NY 10017

Winthrop Laboratories
90 Park Ave.
New York, NY 10016

Wyeth Laboratories
P.O. Box 8399
Philadelphia, PA 19101

12. LABORATORY REFERENCE VALUES OF CLINICAL IMPORTANCE*

prepared by
REX B. CONN, M.D.
The Johns Hopkins University School of Medicine, Baltimore, Maryland

THE INTERNATIONAL SYSTEM OF UNITS FOR LABORATORY MEASUREMENTS (LE SYSTÈME INTERNATIONAL D'UNITÉS)

Physicians are accustomed to receiving laboratory reports with measurements expressed in metric units such as the gram, liter, or milliliter; however, an extensive modification of the metric system has been adopted by clinical laboratories in many countries, and plans are being formulated to make a similar change in the United States. This adaptation is the International System of Units (Le Système International d'Unités), usually abbreviated S.I. Units. Whereas the metric system utilizes the centimeter, the gram, and the second as basic units, the International System uses the meter, the kilogram, and the second as well as four other basic units.

The overriding consideration for adopting the International System is that it will provide a common language among the various scientific disciplines throughout the world for unambiguous communication regarding all types of measurements. In the medical field, the advantages of conversion are that chemical relationships between various substances will become more readily apparent and there will be an international uniformity in laboratory reporting. The most serious disadvantage in making this conversion is that physicians will have to become accustomed to a new set of figures for almost all laboratory measurements. Because of this inconvenience, as well as a potential for serious misinterpretation of laboratory data, the conversion must be undertaken cautiously and only after a logical plan has been formulated and discussed. There appears to be little question, however, that the International System will be adopted in this country. Clinical laboratories in most western European countries, Canada, and Australia are already using S.I. Units, and American medical journals are adopting the practice of expressing measurements in both conventional and S.I. Units.

The International System

The International System is a coherent approach to all types of measurement which utilizes seven dimensionally independent basic quantities: mass, length, time, thermodynamic temperature, electric current, luminous intensity, and amount of substance. Each of these quantities is expressed in a clearly defined *basic unit* (Table 1).

Two or more basic units may be combined to provide *derived units* (Table 2) for expressing other measurements such as mass concentration (kilograms per cubic meter) and velocity (meters per second). Standardized prefixes (Table 3) for basic and derived units are used to express fractions or multiples of the basic units so that any measurement can be expressed in a value between 0.001 and 1000.

Medical Applications

The most profound change in laboratory reports will result from expressing concentration as amount per volume (moles per liter) rather than mass per volume (milligrams per 100 milliliters). The advantages in the former expression can be seen in the following:

Conventional Units

1.0 gram of hemoglobin
  Combines with 1.37 ml. of oxygen
  Contains 3.4 mg. of iron
  Forms 34.9 mg. of bilirubin

S.I. Units

1.0 mmol of hemoglobin
  Combines with 4.0 mmol of oxygen
  Contains 4.0 mmol of iron
  Forms 4.0 mmol of bilirubin

Chemical relationships between lactic acid and pyruvic acid and the glucose from which both are derived, as well as the relationship between bilirubin and the binding capacity of albumin, are other examples of chemical relationships that will be clarified by using the new system.

There are a number of laboratory and other medical measurements for which the S.I. Units appear to offer little advantage, and some which are disadvantageous because the change would require replacement or revision of instruments such as the sphygmomanometer. The cubic meter is the derived unit for volume; however, it is inappropriately large for medical measurements and the liter has been retained. Thermodynamic

TABLE 1. **Basic Units**

PROPERTY	BASIC UNIT	SYMBOL
Length	metre	m
Mass	kilogram	kg
Amount of substance	mole	mol
Time	second	s
Thermodynamic temperature	kelvin	K
Electric current	ampere	A
Luminous intensity	candela	cd

*From Howard F. Conn (Ed.): Current Therapy 1977. Philadelphia, W. B. Saunders Company, 1977.

LABORATORY REFERENCE VALUES OF CLINICAL IMPORTANCE—Continued

TABLE 2. **Derived Units**

DERIVED PROPERTY	DERIVED UNIT	SYMBOL
Area	square metre	m^2
Volume	cubic metre	m^3
	litre	l
Mass concentration	kilogram/cubic metre	kg/m^3
	gram/litre	g/l
Substance concentration	mole/cubic metre	mol/m^3
	mol/litre	mol/l
Temperature	degree Celsius	$C = K - 273.15$

temperature expressed in kelvins is not more informative for medical measurements. Since the Celsius degree is the same as the Kelvin degree, the Celsius scale will be used. Celsius rather than centigrade is the preferred term.

Selection of units for expressing enzyme activity presents certain difficulties. Literally dozens of different units have been used in expressing enzyme activity, and interlaboratory comparison of enzyme results is impossible unless the assay system is precisely defined. In 1964 the International Union of Biochemistry attempted to remedy the situation by proposing the International Unit for enzymes. This unit was defined as the amount of enzyme that will catalyze the conversion of 1 micromole of substrate per minute under standard conditions. Difficulties remain, however, as enzyme activity is affected by the temperature, pH, the type and amount of substrate, the presence of inhibitors, and other factors. Enzyme activity can be expressed in S.I. Units, and the katal has been proposed to express activities of all catalysts, including enzymes. The katal is that amount of enzyme which catalyzes a reaction rate of 1 mole per second. Thus adoption of the katal as the unit of enzyme activity would provide no more information than is obtained when results are expressed in International Units.

TABLE 3. **Standard Prefixes**

PREFIX	MULTIPLICATION FACTOR	SYMBOL
atto	10^{-18}	a
femto	10^{-15}	f
pico	10^{-12}	p
nano	10^{-9}	n
micro	10^{-6}	μ
milli	10^{-3}	m
centi	10^{-2}	c
deci	10^{-1}	d
deca	10^{1}	da
hecto	10^{2}	h
kilo	10^{3}	k
mega	10^{6}	M
giga	10^{9}	G
tera	10^{12}	T

Hydrogen ion concentration in blood is customarily expressed as pH, but in S.I. Units it would be expressed in nanomoles per liter. It appears unlikely that the very useful pH scale will be discarded.

Pressure measures, such as blood pressure and partial pressures of blood gases, would be expressed in S.I. Units, using the Pascal, a unit that can be derived from the basic units for mass, length, and time. This change probably will not be adopted in the early phases of the conversion to S.I. Units. Similarly, a proposed change in expressing osmolality in terms of the depression of freezing point is inappropriate, because osmolality may be calculated from vapor pressure as well as freezing point measurement.

Conventions

A number of conventions have been adopted to standardize usage of S.I. Units:

1. No periods are used after the symbol for a unit (kg not kg.), and it remains unchanged when used in the plural (70 kg not 70 kgs).
2. A half space rather than a comma is used to divide large numbers into groups of three (5 400 000 not 5,400,000).
3. Compound prefixes should be avoided (nanometer not millimicrometer).
4. Multiples and submultiples are used in steps of 10^3 or 10^{-3}.
5. The degree sign for the temperature scales is omitted (38 C not 38°C).
6. The preferred spelling is metre not meter, litre not liter.
7. Report of a measurement should include information on the system, the component, the kind of quantity, the numerical value, and the unit. For example: *System,* serum. *Component,* glucose. *Kind of quantity,* substance concentration. *Value,* 5.10. *Unit,* mmol/l.
8. The name of the component should be unambiguous; for example, "serum bilirubin" might refer to unconjugated bilirubin or to total bilirubin. For acids and bases, the maximally ionized form is used in naming the component; for example, lactate or urate rather than lactic acid or uric acid.

Tables of Reference Values

The following tables list "normal values" for most of the commonly performed laboratory tests. The term "normal values" has been changed to "reference values" to conform to current usage. The reference value is given in conventional units, the conversion factor is indicated when appropriate, and the value in S.I. Units is calculated from these figures. The letters in NOTES column refer to the additional information listed immediately following the tables.

REFERENCE VALUES IN HEMATOLOGY

	CONVENTIONAL UNITS	FACTOR	S.I. UNITS	NOTES
Acid hemolysis test (Ham)	No hemolysis	—	No hemolysis	
Alkaline phosphatase, leukocyte	Total score 14–100	—	Total score 14–100	
Carboxyhemoglobin	Up to 5% of total	0.01	0.05 of total	a
Cell counts				
Erythrocytes				
Males	4.6–6.2 million/cu. mm.	10^6	$4.6–6.2 \times 10^{12}/l$	
Females	4.2–5.4 million/cu. mm.		$4.2–5.4 \times 10^{12}/l$	
Children (varies with age)	4.5–5.1 million/cu. mm.		$4.5–5.1 \times 10^{12}/l$	
Leukocytes				
Total	4500–11,000/cu. mm.	10^6	$4.5–11.0 \times 10^9/l$	
Differential	*Percentage* / *Absolute*			
Myelocytes	0 / 0/cu. mm.	10^6	0/1	b
Band neutrophils	3–5 / 150–400/cu. mm.		$150–400 \times 10^6/l$	
Segmented neutrophils	54–62 / 3000–5800/cu. mm.		$3000–5800 \times 10^6/l$	
Lymphocytes	25–33 / 1500–3000/cu. mm.		$1500–3000 \times 10^6/l$	
Monocytes	3–7 / 300–500/cu. mm.		$300–500 \times 10^6/l$	
Eosinophils	1–3 / 50–250/cu. mm.		$50–250 \times 10^6/l$	
Basophils	0–0.75 / 15–50/cu. mm.		$15–50 \times 10^6/l$	
Platelets	150,000–350,000/cu. mm.	10^6	$150–350 \times 10^9/l$	
Reticulocytes	25,000–75,000/cu. mm. 0.5–1.5% of erythrocytes	10^6	$25–75 \times 10^9/l$	b
Coagulation tests				
Bleeding time (Duke)	1–5 min.	—	1–5 min	
Bleeding time (Ivy)	Less than 5 min.	—	Less than 5 min	
Clot retraction, qualitative	Begins in 30–60 min.	—	Begins in 30–60 min	
	Complete in 24 hrs.	—	Complete in 24 h	
Coagulation time (Lee-White)	5–15 min. (glass tubes)	—	5–15 min (glass tubes)	
	19–60 min. (siliconized tubes)	—	19–60 min (siliconized tubes)	
Fibrinogen	200–400 mg./100 ml.	0.0293	5.9–11.7 μmol/l	c
Fibrinolysins	0	—	0	
Partial thromboplastin time, activated (APTT)	35–45 sec.	—	35–45 s	
Prothrombin consumption	Over 80% consumed in 1 hr.	0.01	Over 0.80 consumed in 1 h	a
Prothrombin content	100% (calculated from prothrombin time)	0.01	1.0 (calculated from prothrombin time)	a
Prothrombin time (one stage)	12.0–14.0 sec.	—	12.0–14.0 s	
Thromboplastin generation test	Compared to normal control	—	Compared to normal control	
Tourniquet test	Ten or fewer petechiae in a 2.5 cm. circle after 5 min.	—	Ten or fewer petechiae in a 2.5 cm circle after 5 min	
Cold hemolysin test (Donath-Landsteiner)	No hemolysis	—	No hemolysis	

Corpuscular values of erythrocytes (values are for adults; in children, values vary with age)						
M.C.H. (mean corpuscular hemoglobin)	27–31 picogm.		0.0155	0.42–0.48 fmol		d
M.C.V. (mean corpuscular volume)	80–105 cu. micra		1.0	80–105 fl		
M.C.H.C. (mean corpuscular hemoglobin concentration)	32–36%		0.01	0.32–0.36		a
Haptoglobin (as hemoglobin binding capacity)	100–200 mg./100 ml.		0.155	16–31 μmol/l		d
Hematocrit						
Males	40–54 ml./100 ml.		0.01	0.40–0.54		a
Females	37–47 ml./100 ml.			0.37–0.47		
Newborn	49–54 ml./100 ml.			0.49–0.54		
Children (varies with age)	35–49 ml./100 ml.			0.35–0.49		
Hemoglobin						
Males	14.0–18.0 grams/100 ml.		0.155	2.17–2.79 mmol/l		d
Females	12.0–16.0 grams/100 ml.			1.86–2.48 mmol/l		
Newborn	16.5–19.5 grams/100 ml.			2.56–3.02 mmol/l		
Children (varies with age)	11.2–16.5 grams/100 ml.			1.74–2.56 mmol/l		
Hemoglobin, fetal	Less than 1% of total		0.01	Less than 0.01 of total		a
Hemoglobin A_2	1.5–3.0% of total		0.01	0.015–0.03 of total		a
Hemoglobin, plasma	0–5.0 mg./100 ml.		0.155	0–0.8 μmol/l		d
Methemoglobin	0–130 mg./100 ml.		0.155	4.7–20 μmol/l		e
Osmotic fragility of erythrocytes	Begins in 0.45–0.39% NaCl Complete in 0.33–0.30% NaCl		171	Begins in 77–67 mmol/l NaCl Complete in 56–51 mmol/l NaCl		
Sedimentation rate						
Wintrobe: Males	0–5 mm. in 1 hr.		—	0–5 mm/h		
Wintrobe: Females	0–15 mm. in 1 hr.		—	0–15 mm/h		
Westergren: Males	0–15 mm. in 1 hr.		—	0–15 mm/h		
Westergren: Females	0–20 mm. in 1 hr.		—	0–20 mm/h		
(May be slightly higher in children and during pregnancy)						
Bone marrow, differential cell count	*Range*	*Average*		*Range*	*Average*	
Myeloblasts	0.3–5.0%	2.0%	0.01	0.003–0.05	0.02	a
Promyelocytes	1.0–8.0%	5.0%		0.01–0.08	0.05	
Myelocytes: Neutrophilic	5.0–19.0%	12.0%		0.05–0.19	0.12	
Eosinophilic	0.5–3.0%	1.5%		0.005–0.03	0.015	
Basophilic	0.0–0.5%	0.3%		0.00–0.005	0.003	
Metamyelocytes	13.0–32.0%	22.0%		0.13–0.32	0.22	
Polymorphonuclear neutrophils	7.0–30.0%	20.0%		0.07–0.30	0.20	
Polymorphonuclear eosinophils	0.5–4.0%	2.0%		0.005–0.04	0.02	
Polymorphonuclear basophils	0.0–0.7%	0.2%		0.00–0.007	0.002	
Lymphocytes	3.0–17.0%	10.0%		0.03–0.17	0.10	
Plasma cells	0.0–2.0%	0.4%		0.00–0.02	0.004	
Monocytes	0.5–5.0%	2.0%		0.005–0.05	0.02	
Reticulum cells	0.1–2.0%	0.2%		0.001–0.02	0.002	
Megakaryocytes	0.3–3.0%	0.4%		0.003–0.03	0.004	
Pronormoblasts	1.0–8.0%	4.0%		0.01–0.08	0.04	
Normoblasts	7.0–32.0%	18.0%		0.07–0.32	0.18	

REFERENCE VALUES FOR BLOOD, PLASMA AND SERUM

(For some procedures the reference values may vary depending upon the method used)

	CONVENTIONAL UNITS	FACTOR	S.I UNITS	NOTES
Acetoacetate plus acetone, serum				
Qualitative	Negative	—	Negative	
Quantitative	0.3–2.0 mg./100 ml.	10	3–20 mg/l	
Aldolase, serum	0–11 milliunits/ml. (I.U.) (30°)	1.0	0–11 units/l (30 C)	f
Alpha amino nitrogen, serum	3.0–5.5 mg./100 ml.	0.714	2.1–3.9 mmol/l	
Ammonia, blood	80–110 mcg./100 ml.	0.587	47–65 μmol/l	
Amylase, serum	Less than 160 Caraway units/100 ml.	—	Less than 160 Caraway units/dl	f
Ascorbic acid, blood	0.4–1.5 mg./100 ml.	56.8	23–85 μmol/l	
Bilirubin, serum				
Direct	0.1–0.4 mg./100 ml.	17.1	1.7–6.8 μmol/l	
Indirect	0.2–0.7 mg./100 ml. (Total minus direct)	17.1	3.4–12 μmol/l (Total minus direct)	
Total	0.3–1.1 mg./100 ml.	17.1	5.1–19 μmol/l	
Bromsulphalein (BSP) (Inject 5 mg./kg. body weight, draw sample at 45 min.)	Less than 5%	0.01	Less than 0.05	a
Calcium, serum	4.5–5.5 mEq./liter	0.50	2.25–2.75 mmol/l	
	9.0–11.0 mg./100 ml.	0.25	2.25–2.75 mmol/l	
	(Slightly higher in children)		(Slightly higher in children)	
	(Varies with protein concentration)		(Varies with protein concentration)	
Calcium, ionized, serum	2.1–2.6 mEq./liter	0.50	1.05–1.30 mmol/l	
	4.25–5.25 mg./100 ml.	0.25	1.05–1.30 mmol/l	
Carbon dioxide content, serum				
Adults	24–30 mEq./liter	1.0	24–30 mmol/l	
Infants	20–28 mEq./liter	1.0	20–28 mmol/l	
Carbon dioxide tension (Pco_2), blood	35–45 mm. Hg	—	35–45 mm Hg	g
Carotene, serum	50–300 mcg./100 ml.	0.0186	0.93–5.58 μmol/l	
Ceruloplasmin, serum	23–44 mg./100 ml.	0.0662	1.5–2.9 μmol/l	h
Chloride, serum	96–106 mEq./liter	1.0	96–106 mmol/l	
Cholesterol, serum				
Total	150–250 mg./100 ml.	0.0259	3.9–6.5 mmol/l	
Esters	68–76% of total cholesterol	0.01	0.68–0.76 of total cholesterol	a
Cholinesterase				
Serum	0.5–1.3 pH units	—	0.5–1.3 pH units	f
Erythrocytes	0.5–1.0 pH unit	—	0.5–1.0 pH unit	f
Copper, serum				
Males	70–140 mcg./100 ml.	0.157	11–22 μmol/l	
Females	85–155 mcg./100 ml.	0.157	13–24 μmol/l	
Cortisol, plasma (8 A.M.)	6–16 mcg./100 ml.	27.6	170–440 nmol/l	
Creatine, serum	0.2–0.8 mg./100 ml.	76.3	15–61 μmol/l	

Males	0–50 milliunits/ml. (I.U.) (30°)	1.0	0–50 units/l (30 C)	f
Females	0–30 milliunits/ml. (I.U.) (30°) (Oliver-Rosalki)	1.0	0–30 units/l (30 C) (Oliver-Rosalki)	f
Creatine phosphokinase isoenzymes, serum				
CPK-MM	Present	—	Present	
CPK-MB	Absent	—	Absent	
CPK-BB	Absent	—	Absent	
Creatinine, serum	0.7–1.5 mg./100 ml.	88.4	62–133 μmol/l	
Cryoglobulins, serum	0	—	0	
Fatty acids, total, serum	190–420 mg./100 ml.	0.0352	7–15 mmol/l	i
Fibrinogen, plasma	200–400 mg./100 ml.	0.0293	5.9–11.7 μmol/l	c
Folate, serum	5–21 nanogm./ml.	2.27	11–48 nmol/l	
Gastrin, serum	0–200 picogm./ml.	1.0	0–200 ng/l	
Glucose (fasting)				
Blood	60–100 mg./100 ml.	0.0555	3.33–5.55 mmol/l	
Plasma or serum	70–115 mg./100 ml.	0.0555	3.89–6.38 mmol/l	
Haptoglobin, serum	100–200 mg./100 ml. (As hemoglobin binding capacity)	0.155	16–31 μmol/l (As hemoglobin binding capacity)	d
Hydroxybutyric dehydrogenase, serum	0–180 milliunits/ml. (I.U.) (30°) (Rosalki-Wilkinson)	1.0	0–180 units/l (30 C) (Rosalki-Wilkinson)	f
	114–290 units/ml. (Wroblewski)	—	114–290 units/ml (Wroblewski)	f
17-Hydroxycorticosteroids, plasma	8–18 mcg./100 ml.	0.0276	0.22–0.50 μmol/l	j
Immunoglobins, serum				
IgG	550–1900 mg./100 ml.	0.01	5.5–19.0 g/l	
IgA	60–333 mg./100 ml.	0.01	0.60–3.3 g/l	
IgM	45–145 mg./100 ml. (Varies with age in children)	0.01	0.45–1.5 g/l (Varies with age in children)	
Insulin, plasma (fasting)	5–25 microunits/ml.	1.0	5–25 milliunits/l	
Iodine, protein bound, serum	3.5–8.0 mcg./100 ml.	0.0788	0.28–0.63 μmol/l	k
Iron, serum	75–175 mcg./100 ml.	0.179	13–31 μmol/l	
Iron binding capacity, serum				
Total	250–410 mcg./100 ml.	0.179	45–73 μmol/l	
Saturation	20–55%	0.01	0.20–0.55	a
17-Ketosteroids, plasma	25–125 mcg./100 ml.	0.0347	0.87–4.34 μmol/l	l
Lactate, blood, venous	0.6–1.8 mEq./liter	1.0	0.6–1.8 mmol/l	
Lactate dehydrogenase, serum	0–300 milliunits/ml. (I.U.) (30°) (Wroblewski modified)	1.0	0–300 units/l (30 C) (Wroblewski modified)	f
	150–450 units/ml. (Wroblewski)	—	150–450 units/ml (Wroblewski)	
	80–120 units/ml. (Wacker)	—	80–120 units/ml (Wacker)	
Lactate dehydrogenase isoenzymes, serum				
LDH_1	22–37% of total	0.01	0.22–0.37 of total	a
LDH_2	30–46% of total		0.30–0.46 of total	
LDH_3	14–29% of total		0.14–0.29 of total	
LDH_4	5–11% of total		0.05–0.11 of total	
LDH_5	2–11% of total		0.02–0.11 of total	
Leucine aminopeptidase, serum	14–40 milliunits/ml. (I.U.) (30°)	1.0	14–40 units/l (30 C)	f
Lipase, serum	0–1.5 units (Cherry-Crandall)	—	0–1.5 units (Cherry-Crandall)	f
Lipids, total, serum	450–850 mg./100 ml.	0.01	4.5–8.5 g/l	m

Table continued on the following page

REFERENCE VALUES FOR BLOOD, PLASMA AND SERUM (*Continued*)

(For some procedures the reference values may vary depending upon the method used)

	CONVENTIONAL UNITS	FACTOR	S.I. UNITS	NOTES
Magnesium, serum	1.5–2.5 mEq./liter	0.50	0.75–1.25 mmol/l	
	1.8–3.0 mg./100 ml.	0.411		
5′-Nucleotidase, serum	Less than 1.6 milliunits/ml. (30°)	1.0	Less than 1.6 units/l (30 C)	f
Nitrogen, nonprotein, serum	15–35 mg./100 ml.	0.714	10.7–25.0 mmol/l	
Osmolality, serum	285–295 mOsm./kg. serum water	—	285–295 mmol/kg serum water	n
Oxygen, blood				
Capacity	16–24 vol.% (varies with hemoglobin)	0.446	7.14–10.7 mmol/l (varies with hemoglobin)	o
Content Arterial	15–23 vol.%	0.446	6.69–10.3 mmol/l	o
Venous	10–16 vol.%	0.446	4.46–7.14 mmol/l	o
Saturation Arterial	94–100% of capacity	0.01	0.94–1.00 of capacity	a
Venous	60–85% of capacity	0.01	0.60–0.85 of capacity	a
Tension, pO_2 Arterial	75–100 mm. Hg	—	75–100 mm Hg	g
pH, arterial, blood	7.35–7.45	—	7.35–7.45	p
Phenylalanine, serum	Less than 3 mg./100 ml.	0.0605	Less than 0.18 mmol/l	
Phosphatase, acid, serum	0–7.0 milliunits/ml. (I.U.) (30°)	1.0	0–7.0 units/l (30 C)	f
	1.0–5.0 units (King-Armstrong)	—	1.0–5.0 units (King-Armstrong)	
Phosphatase, alkaline, serum	10–32 milliunits/ml. (I.U.) (30°)	1.0	10–32 units/l (30 C)	f
	5.0–13.0 units (King-Armstrong)	—	5.0–13.0 units (King-Armstrong)	
	(Values are higher in children)		(Values are higher in children)	
Phosphate, inorganic, serum				
Adults	3.0–4.5 mg./100 ml.	0.323	1.0–1.5 mmol/l	
Children	4.0–7.0 mg./100 ml.		1.3–2.3 mmol/l	
Phospholipids, serum	6–12 mg./100 ml. (As lipid phosphorus)	0.323	1.9–3.9 mmol/l (As lipid phosphorus)	
Potassium, serum	3.5–5.0 mEq./liter	1.0	3.5–5.0 mmol/l	
Protein, serum				
Total	6.0–8.0 grams/100 ml.	10	60–80 g/l	m
Albumin	3.5–5.5 grams/100 ml.	10	35–55 g/l	q
		0.154	0.54–0.85 mmol/l	
Globulin	2.5–3.5 grams/100 ml.	10	25–35 g/l	
Electrophoresis				
Albumin	3.5–5.5 grams/100 ml.	10	35–55 g/l	q
	52–68% of total	0.01	0.52–0.68 of total	a
Globulin				
$Alpha_1$	0.2–0.4 gram/100 ml.	10	2–4 g/l	m
	2–5% of total	0.01	0.02–0.05 of total	a
$Alpha_2$	0.5–0.9 gram/100 ml.	10	5–9 g/l	m
	7–14% of total	0.01	0.07–0.14 of total	a
Beta	0.6–1.1 grams/100 ml.	10	6–11 g/l	m
	9–15% of total	0.01	0.09–0.15 of total	a
Gamma	0.7–1.7 grams/100 ml.	10	7–17 g/l	m
	11–21% of total	0.01	0.11–0.21 of total	a

Protoporphyrin, erythrocyte	27–61 mcg./100 ml. packed RBC	0.0178	0.48–1.09 μmol/l packed RBC	
Pyruvate, blood	0.01–0.11 mEq./liter	1.0	0.01–0.11 mmol/l	
Sodium, serum	136–145 mEq./liter	1.0	136–145 mmol/l	
Sulfates, inorganic, serum	0.8–1.2 mg./100 ml.	104	83–125 μmol/l	
Testosterone, plasma				
Males	275–875 nanogm./100 ml.	0.0347	9.5–30 nmol/l	
Females	23–75 nanogm./100 ml.	0.0347	0.8–2.6 nmol/l	
Pregnant	38–190 nanogm./100 ml.	0.0347	1.3–6.6 nmol/l	
Thyroid stimulating hormone (TSH), serum	0–7 microunits/ml.	1.0	0–7 milliunits/l	
Thyroxine, free, serum	1.0–2.1 nanogm./100 ml.	12.9	13–27 pmol/l	
Thyroxine (T_4), serum	4.4–9.9 mcg./100 ml.	12.9	57–128 nmol/l	
Thyroxine binding globulin (TBG), serum (as thyroxine)	10–26 mcg./100 ml.	12.9	129–335 nmol/l	
Tri-iodothyronine (T_3), serum	150–250 nanogm./100 ml.	0.0154	2.3–3.9 nmol/l	
Thyroxine iodine, serum	2.9–6.4 mcg./100 ml.	78.8	229–504 nmol/l	k
Transaminase, serum				
SGOT (aspartate aminotransferase)	0–19 milliunits/ml. (I.U.) (30°) (Karmen modified)	1.0	0–19 units/l (30 C) (Karmen modified)	f
	15–40 units/ml. (Karmen)		15–40 units/ml (Karmen)	
	18–40 units/ml. (Reitman-Frankel)		18–40 units/ml (Reitman-Frankel)	
SGPT (alanine aminotransferase)	0–17 milliunits/ml. (I.U.) (30°) (Karmen modified)	1.0	0–17 units/l (30 C) (Karmen modified)	f
	6–35 units/ml. (Karmen)		6–35 units/ml (Karmen)	
	5–35 units/ml. (Reitman-Frankel)		5–35 units/ml (Reitman-Frankel)	
Triglycerides, serum	40–150 mg./100 ml.	0.01	0.4–1.5 g/l	
		0.0114	0.45–1.71 mmol/l	r
Urate (serum)				
Males	2.5–8.0 mg./100 ml.	0.0595	0.15–0.48 mmol/l	
Females	1.5–7.0 mg./100 ml.	0.0595	0.09–0.42 mmol/l	
Urea				
Blood	21–43 mg./100 ml.	0.167	3.5–7.2 mmol/l	
Plasma or serum	24–49 mg./100 ml.	0.167	4.0–8.2 mmol/l	
Urea nitrogen				
Blood	10–20 mg./100 ml.	0.714	7.1–14.3 mmol/l	k
Plasma or serum	11–23 mg./100 ml.	0.714	7.9–16.4 mmol/l	
Vitamin A, serum	20–80 mcg./100 ml.	0.0349	0.70–2.8 μmol/l	
Vitamin B_{12}, serum	300–1000 picogm./ml.	0.738	220–740 pmol/l	

REFERENCE VALUES FOR URINE

(For some procedures the reference values may vary depending upon the method used)

	CONVENTIONAL UNITS	FACTOR	S.I. UNITS	NOTES
Acetone and acetoacetate, qualitative	Negative	—	Negative	
Addis count				
Erythrocytes	0–130,000/24 hrs.	—	0–130 000/24 h	
Leukocytes	0–650,000/24 hrs.	—	0–650 000/24 h	
Casts (hyaline)	0–2000/24 hrs.	—	0–2000/24 h	
Albumin				
Qualitative	Negative	—	Negative	
Quantitative	10–100 mg./24 hrs.	—	10–100 mg/24 h	q
		0.0154	0.15–1.5 μmol/24 h	
Aldosterone	3–20 mcg./24 hrs.	2.77	8.3–55 nmol/24 h	
Alpha amino nitrogen	50–200 mg./24 hrs.	0.0714	3.6–14.3 mmol/24 h	
Ammonia nitrogen	20–70 mEq./24 hrs.	1.0	20–70 mmol/24 h	
Amylase	35–260 Caraway units/hr.	—	35–260 Caraway units/h	f
Bilirubin, qualitative	Negative	—	Negative	
Calcium				
Low Ca diet	Less than 150 mg./24 hrs.	0.025	Less than 3.8 mmol/24 h	
Usual diet	Less than 250 mg./24 hrs.	0.025	Less than 6.3 mmol/24 h	
Catecholamines				
Epinephrine	Less than 10 mcg./24 hrs.	5.46	Less than 55 nmol/24 h	
Norepinephrine	Less than 100 mcg./24 hrs.	5.91	Less than 590 nmol/24 h	
Total free catecholamines	4–126 mcg./24 hrs.	5.91	24–745 nmol/24 h	s
Total metanephrines	0.1–1.6 mg./24 hrs.	5.07	0.5–8.1 μmol/24 h	t
Chloride	110–250 mEq./24 hrs. (Varies with intake)	1.0	110–250 mmol/24 h (Varies with intake)	
Chorionic gonadotropin	0	—	0	
Copper	0–50 mcg./24 hrs.	0.0157	0–0.80 μmol/24 h	
Creatine				
Males	0–40 mg./24 hrs.	0.00762	0–0.30 mmol/24 h	
Females	0–100 mg./24 hrs. (Higher in children and during pregnancy)	0.00762	0–0.76 mmol/24 h (Higher in children and during pregnancy)	
Creatinine	15–25 mg./kg. body weight/24 hrs.	0.00884	0.13–0.22 mmol·kg^{-1} body weight/24 h	
Creatinine clearance				
Males	110–150 ml./min.	—	110–150 ml/min	
Females	105–132 ml./min. (1.73 sq. meter surface area)	—	105–132 ml/min (1.73 m^2 surface area)	
Cystine or cysteine, qualitative	Negative	—	Negative	
Dehydroepiandrosterone	Less than 15% of total 17-ketosteroids	0.01	Less than 0.15 of total 17-ketosteroids	a
Delta aminolevulinic acid	1.3–7.0 mg./24 hrs.	7.63	10–53 μmol/24 h	

Estrogens				
Males				
Estrone	3–8 µg./24 hrs.	3.70	11–30 nmol/24 h	
Estradiol	0–6 µg./24 hrs.	3.67	0–22 nmol/24 h	
Estriol	1–11 µg./24 hrs.	3.47	3–38 nmol/24 h	
Total	4–25 µg./24 hrs.	3.60	14–90 nmol/24 h	u
Females				
Estrone	4–31 µg./24 hrs.	3.70	15–115 nmol/24 h	
Estradiol	0–14 µg./24 hrs.	3.67	0–51 nmol/24 h	
Estriol	0–72 µg./24 hrs.	3.47	0–250 nmol/24 h	
Total	5–100 µg./24 hrs. (Markedly increased during pregnancy)	3.60	18–360 nmol/24 h (Markedly increased during pregnancy)	u
Glucose (as reducing substance)	Less than 250 mg./24 hrs.	—	Less than 250 mg/24 h	
Gonadotropins, pituitary	10–50 mouse units/24 hrs.	—	10–50 mouse units/24 h	
Hemoglobin and myoglobin, qualitative	Negative	—	Negative	
Hemogentisic acid, qualitative	Negative	—	Negative	
17-Hydroxycorticosteroids				
Males	3–9 mg./24 hrs.	2.76	8.3–25 µmol/24 h	j
Females	2–8 mg./24 hrs.		5.5–22 µmol/24 h	
5-Hydroxyindoleacetic acid				
Qualitative	Negative	—	Negative	
Quantitative	Less than 9 mg./24 hrs.	5.23	Less than 47 µmol/24 h	
17-Ketosteroids				
Males	6–18 mg./24 hrs.	3.47	21–62 µmol/24 h	l
Females	4–13 mg./24 hrs. (Varies with age)		14–45 µmol/24 h (Varies with age)	
Magnesium	6.0–8.5 mEq./24 hrs.	0.5	3.0–4.3 mmol/24 h	
Metanephrines (see Catecholamines)				
Osmolality	38–1400 mOsm./kg. water	—	38–1400 mmol/kg water	n
pH	4.6–8.0, average 6.0 (Depends on diet)	—	4.6–8.0, average 6.0 (Depends on diet)	p
Phenosulfonphthalein excretion (PSP)	25% or more in 15 min. 40% or more in 30 min. 55% or more in 2 hrs. (After injection of 1 ml PSP intravenously)	0.01	0.25 or more in 15 min 0.40 or more in 30 min 0.55 or more in 2 h (After injection of 1 ml PSP intravenously)	a
Phenylpyruvic acid, qualitative	Negative	—	Negative	
Phosphorus	0.9–1.3 gm./24 hrs.	32.3	29–42 mmol/24 h	
Porphobilinogen				
Qualitative	Negative	—	Negative	
Quantitative	0–0.2 mg./100 ml.	4.42	0–0.9 µmol/l	
	Less than 2.0 mg./24 hrs.		Less than 9 µmol/24 h	
Porphyrins				
Coproporphyrin	50–250 mcg./24 hrs.	1.53	77–380 nmol/24 h	
Uroporphyrin	10–30 mcg./24 hrs.	1.20	12–36 nmol/24 h	
Potassium	25–100 mEq./24 hrs. (Varies with intake)	1.0	25–100 mmol/24 h (Varies with intake)	

Table continued on the following page

REFERENCE VALUES FOR URINE (*Continued*)

(For some procedures the reference values may vary depending upon the method used)

	CONVENTIONAL UNITS	FACTOR	S.I. UNITS	NOTES
Pregnanediol				
Males	0.4–1.4 mg./24 hrs.	3.12	1.2–4.4 μmol/24 h	
Females				
Proliferative phase	0.5–1.5 mg./24 hrs.		1.6–4.7 μmol/24 h	
Luteal phase	2.0–7.0 mg./24 hrs.		6.2–22 μmol/24 h	
Postmenopausal phase	0.2–1.0 mg./24 hrs.		0.6–3.1 μmol/24 h	
Pregnant 16 weeks	5–21 mg./24 hrs.		16–66 μmol/24 h	
Pregnant 20 weeks	6–26 mg./24 hrs.		19–81 μmol/24 h	
Pregnant 24 weeks	12–32 mg./24 hrs.		37–100 μmol/24 h	
Pregnant 28 weeks	19–51 mg./24 hrs.		59–159 μmol/24 h	
Pregnant 32 weeks	22–66 mg./24 hrs.		69–206 μmol/24 h	
Pregnant 36 weeks	23–77 mg./24 hrs.		72–240 μmol/24 h	
Pregnant 40 weeks	23–63 mg./24 hrs.		72–197 μmol/24 h	
Pregnanetriol	Less than 2.5 mg./24 hrs. in adults	2.97	Less than 7.4 μmol/24 h in adults	
Protein				
Qualitative	Negative	—	Negative	
Quantitative	10–150 mg./24 hrs.		10–150 mg/24 h	m
Sodium	130–260 mEq./24 hrs. (Varies with intake)	1.0	130–260 mmol/24 h (Varies with intake)	
Specific gravity	1.003–1.030	—	1.003–1.030	
Titratable acidity	20–40 mEq./24 hrs.	1.0	20–40 mmol/24 h	
Urate	200–500 mg./24 hrs. (With normal diet)	0.00595	1.2–3.0 mmol/24 h (With normal diet)	
Urobilinogen	Up to 1.0 Ehrlich unit/2 hrs. (1–3 P.M.)	—	Up to 1.0 Ehrlich unit/2 h (1–3 P.M.)	
	0–4.0 mg./24 hrs.	—	0–4.0 mg/24 h	
Vanillylmandelic acid (VMA) (4-hydroxy-3-methoxymandelic acid)	1–8 mg./24 hrs.	5.05	5–40 μmol/24 h	

REFERENCE VALUES FOR THERAPEUTIC DRUG MONITORING

	CONVENTIONAL UNITS	FACTOR	S.I. UNITS	NOTES
Carbamazepine, serum (Tegretol)	0 Therapeutic levels: 5.0–14.0 mg./liter	4.23	0 Therapeutic levels: 21–59 μmol/l	
Digoxin, serum With dose of 0.25 mg. per day	0 Therapeutic levels: 0.8–1.6 mcg./liter	1.28	0 Therapeutic levels: 1.0–2.3 nmol/l	

With dose of 0.5 mg. per day (Sample obtained 12 to 24 hrs. after last dose)	0.9–2.4 mcg./liter		1.2–3.1 nmol/l
Diphenylhydantoin, serum (Dilantin)	0 Therapeutic levels: 10–20 mg./liter Toxic levels: Above 20 mg./liter	3.65	0 Therapeutic levels: 37–73 μmol/l Toxic levels: Above 73 μmol/l
Ethosuximide, serum (Zarontin)	0 Therapeutic levels: 40–80 mg./liter	7.08	0 Therapeutic levels: 283–566 μmol/l
Lithium, serum	0 Therapeutic levels: 0.8–1.5 mEq./liter Toxic level: Above 2 mEq./liter	1.0	0 Therapeutic levels: 0.8–1.5 mmol/l Toxic level: Above 2 mmol/l
Phenobarbital, serum	0 Therapeutic levels: 10.0–25.0 mg./liter Toxic levels: Vary widely because of developed tolerance	4.31	0 Therapeutic levels: 43–108 μmol/l Toxic levels: Vary widely because of developed tolerance
Primidone, serum (Mysoline)	0 Therapeutic levels: 4.0–10.0 mg./liter	4.58	0 Therapeutic levels: 18–46 μmol/l
Procainamide, serum (Pronestyl)	0 Therapeutic levels: 4.0–8.0 mg./liter	4.24	0 Therapeutic levels: 17–34 μmol/l
Quinidine, serum	0 Therapeutic levels: 2.0–5.0 mg./liter Toxic levels: Over 10 mg./liter	3.08	0 Therapeutic levels: 6.2–15 μmol/l Toxic levels: Over 31 μmol/l
Salicylate, plasma	0 Therapeutic levels: 20–25 mg./100 ml. Toxic levels: Over 30 mg./100 ml. Death 45–75 mg./100 ml.	0.0555	0 Therapeutic levels: 1.0–1.4 mmol/l Toxic levels: Over 1.7 mmol/l Death 2.5–4.2 mmol/l
Theophylline, serum	0 Therapeutic levels: 5.0–20.0 mg./liter Toxic levels: Above 30.0 mg./liter	5.55	0 Therapeutic levels: 28–111 μmol/l Toxic levels: Above 167 μmol/l
Thiocyanate, serum (Metabolite of sodium nitroprusside)	0 Therapeutic levels: 80–120 mg./liter	0.0169	0 Therapeutic levels: 1.4–2.0 mmol/l

REFERENCE VALUES IN TOXICOLOGY

	CONVENTIONAL UNITS	FACTOR	S.I. UNITS	NOTES
Arsenic, blood	3.5–7.2 mcg./100 ml.	0.133	0.47–0.96 μmol/l	
Arsenic, urine	Less than 100 mcg./24 hrs.	0.0133	Less than 1.3 μmol/24 h	
Bromides, serum	0 Toxic levels: Above 17 mEq./liter	1.0	0 Toxic levels: Above 17 mmol/l	
Carbon monoxide, blood	Up to 5% saturation Symptoms occur with 20% saturation	—	Up to 0.05 saturation Symptoms occur with 0.20 saturation	a
Ethanol, blood	Less than 0.005%	217	Less than 1 mmol/l	
Marked intoxication	0.3–0.4%		65–87 mmol/l	
Alcoholic stupor	0.4–0.5%		87–109 mmol/l	
Coma	Above 0.5%		Above 109 mmol/l	
Lead, blood	0–40 mcg./100 ml.	0.0483	0–2 μmol/l	
Lead, urine	Less than 100 mcg./24 hrs.	0.00483	Less than 0.48 μmol/24 h	
Mercury, urine	Less than 10 mcg./24 hrs.	4.98	Less than 50 nmol/24 h	

REFERENCE VALUES FOR CEREBROSPINAL FLUID

	CONVENTIONAL UNITS	FACTOR	S.I. UNITS	NOTES
Cells	Fewer than 5/cu. mm.; all mononuclear	—	Fewer than 5/μl; all mononuclear	
Chloride	120–130 mEq./liter (20 mEq./liter higher than serum)	1.0	120–130 mmol/l (20 mmol/l higher than serum)	
Electrophoresis	Predominantly albumin	—	Predominantly albumin	
Glucose	50–75 mg./100 ml. (20 mg./100 ml. less than serum)	0.0555	2.8–4.2 mmol/l (1.1 mmol/l less than serum)	
IgG				
Children under 14	Less than 8% of total protein	—	Less than 0.08 of total protein	a,m
Adults	Less than 14% of total protein		Less than 0.14 of total protein	
Pressure	70–180 mm. water		70–180 mm water	g
Protein, total	15–45 mg./100 ml. (Higher, up to 70 mg./100 ml., in elderly adults and children)	0.01	0.150–0.450 g/l (Higher, up to 0.70 g/l, in elderly adults and children)	m

REFERENCE VALUES FOR GASTRIC ANALYSIS

	CONVENTIONAL UNITS	FACTOR	S.I. UNITS	NOTES
Basal gastric secretion (1 hour)				
Concentration	(Mean ± 1 S.D.)		(Mean ± 1 S.D.)	
Males	25.8 ± 1.8 mEq./liter	1.0	25.8 ± 1.8 mmol/l	
Females	20.3 ± 3.0 mEq./liter		20.3 ± 3.0 mmol/l	
Output	(Mean ± 1 S.D.)		(Mean ± 1 S.D.)	
Males	2.57 ± 0.16 mEq./hr.	1.0	2.57 ± 0.16 mmol/h	
Females	1.61 ± 0.18 mEq./hr.		1.61 ± 0.18 mmol/h	
After histamine stimulation				
Normal	Mean output 11.8 mEq./hr.	1.0	Mean output 11.8 mmol/h	
Duodenal ulcer	Mean output 15.2 mEq./hr.		Mean output 15.2 mmol/h	
After maximal histamine stimulation				
Normal	Mean output 22.6 mEq./hr.	1.0	Mean output 22.6 mmol/h	
Duodenal ulcer	Mean output 44.6 mEq./hr.		Mean output 44.6 mmol/h	
Diagnex blue (Squibb): Anacidity	0–0.3 mg. in 2 hrs.	1.0	0–0.3 mg in 2 h	
Doubtful	0.3–0.6 mg. in 2 hrs.		0.3–0.6 mg in 2 h	
Normal	Greater than 0.6 mg. in 2 hrs.		Greater than 0.6 mg in 2 h	
Volume, fasting stomach content	50–100 ml.	—	0.05–0.1 litre	
Emptying time	3–6 hrs.	—	3–6 h	
Color	Opalescent or colorless	—	Opalescent or colorless	
Specific gravity	1.006–1.009	—	1.006–1.009	
pH (adults)	0.9–1.5	—	0.9–1.5	p

GASTROINTESTINAL ABSORPTION TESTS

	CONVENTIONAL UNITS	FACTOR	S.I. UNITS	NOTES
d-Xylose absorption test	After an 8 hour fast, 10 ml./kg. body weight of a 0.05 solution of d-xylose is given by mouth. Nothing further by mouth is given until the test has been completed. All urine voided during the following 5 hours is pooled, and blood samples are taken at 0, 60, and 120 minutes. Normally 0.26 (range 0.16–0.33) of ingested xylose is excreted within 5 hours, and the serum xylose reaches a level between 25 and 40 mg./100 ml. after 1 hour and is maintained at this level for another 60 minutes.		No change	

Table continued on the following page

GASTROINTESTINAL ABSORPTION TESTS (*Continued*)

	CONVENTIONAL UNITS	FACTOR	S.I. UNITS	NOTES
Vitamin A absorption	A fasting blood specimen is obtained and 200,000 units of vitamin A in oil is given by mouth. Serum vitamin A level should rise to twice fasting level in 3 to 5 hours.		No change	

REFERENCE VALUES FOR FECES

	CONVENTIONAL UNITS	FACTOR	S.I. UNITS	NOTES
Bulk	100–200 grams/24 hrs.	—	100–200 g/24 h	
Dry matter	23–32 grams/24 hrs.	—	23–32 g/24 h	
Fat, total	Less than 6.0 grams/24 hrs.	—	Less than 6.0 g/24 h	
Nitrogen, total	Less than 2.0 grams/24 hrs.	—	Less than 2.0 g/24 h	
Urobilinogen	40–280 mg./24 hrs.	—	40–280 mg/24 h	
Water	Approximately 65%	0.01	Approximately 0.65	a

REFERENCE VALUES FOR SEMEN ANALYSIS

	CONVENTIONAL UNITS	FACTOR	S.I. UNITS	NOTES
Volume	2–5 ml.; usually 3–4 ml.	—	2–5 ml; usually 3–4 ml	
Liquefaction	Complete in 15 min.	—	Complete in 15 min	
pH	7.2–8.0; average 7.8	—	7.2–8.0; average 7.8	p
Leukocytes	Occasional or absent	—	Occasional or absent	
Count	60–150 million/ml.	—	60–150 million/ml	
	Below 60 million/ml. is abnormal	—	Below 60 million/ml is abnormal	
Motility	80% or more motile	—	0.80 or more motile	a
Morphology	80–90% normal forms	—	0.80–0.90 normal forms	a

REFERENCE VALUES FOR IMMUNOLOGIC PROCEDURES

	CONVENTIONAL UNITS	FACTOR	S.I. UNITS	NOTES
Syphilis serology (RPR and VDRL)	Negative		No change	
Mono screen	Negative		No change	
R.A. test (latex)	1:40 Negative 1:80–1:160 Doubtful 1:320 Positive		No change	
Rose test	1:10 Negative 1:20–1:40 Doubtful 1:80 Positive		No change	
Anti-streptolysin O titer	Normal up to 1:128. Single test usually has little significance. Rise in titer or persistently elevated titer is significant.		No change	
Anti-hyaluronidase titer	Less than 1:200. Significant if rising titer can be demonstrated at weekly intervals.		No change	
C-reactive protein	Negative		No change	
Anti-nuclear antibody	One specimen is sufficient, unless the result is inconsistent with the clinical impression. Most patients with active lupus have high ANA titers (160 or greater); some have lower titers (20–40). Patients with inactive lupus may have a negative test. Antinuclear antibodies are occasionally present in patients with no evidence of systemic lupus, usually in lower titers (20–40).		No change	
Febrile agglutinins	Titers of 1:80 or greater may be significant, particularly if subsequent samples show rise in titer.		No change	
Tularemia agglutinins	1:80 Negative 1:160 Doubtful 1:320 Positive		No change	
Proteus OX-19 agglutinins	Titers of 1:80 or greater may be significant, particularly if subsequent samples show rise in titer.		No change	
Complement fixation tests	Titers of 1:8 or less are usually not significant. Paired sera showing rise in titer of more than two tubes are usually considered significant.		No change	
C3 Test	80–140 mg./100 ml.	0.01	0.80–1.40 g/l	q
C4 Test	11–75 mg./100 ml.	0.01	0.11–0.75 g/l	

LABORATORY REFERENCE VALUES OF CLINICAL IMPORTANCE—Concluded

NOTES

a. Percentage is expressed as a decimal fraction.

b. Percentage may be expressed as a decimal fraction; however, when the result expressed is itself a variable fraction of another variable, the absolute value is more meaningful. There is no reason, other than custom, for expressing reticulocyte counts and differential leukocyte counts in percentages or decimal fractions rather than in absolute numbers.

c. Molecular weight of fibrinogen = 341,000.

d. Molecular weight of hemoglobin = 64,500. Because of disagreement as to whether the monomer or tetramer of hemoglobin should be used in the conversion, it has been recommended that the conventional grams per deciliter be retained. The tetramer is used in the table; values given should be multiplied by 4 to obtain concentration of the monomer.

e. Molecular weight of methemoglobin = 64,500. See note d above.

f. Enzyme units have not been changed in these tables because the proposed enzyme unit, the katal, has not been universally adopted (1 International Unit = 16.7 nkat).

g. It has been proposed that pressure be expressed in the Pascal (1 mm Hg = 0.133 kPa); however, this convention has not been universally accepted.

h. Molecular weight of ceruloplasmin = 151,000.

i. "Fatty acids" includes a mixture of different aliphatic acids of varying molecular weight. A mean molecular weight of 284 has been assumed in calculating the conversion factor.

j. Based upon molecular weight of cortisol 362.47.

k. The practice of expressing concentration of an organic molecule in terms of one of its constituent elements originated when measurements included a heterogeneous class of compounds (nonprotein nitrogenous compounds, iodine-containing compounds bound to serum proteins). It was carried over to expressing measurements of specific substances (urea, thyroxine), but the practice should be discarded. For iodine and nitrogen 1 mole is taken as the monoatomic form, although they occur as diatomic molecules.

l. Based upon molecular weight of dehydroepiandrosterone 288.41.

m. Weight per volume is retained as the unit because of the heterogeneous nature of the material measured.

n. The proposal that osmolality be reported as freezing point depression using the millikelvin as the unit has not been received with universal enthusiasm. The milliosmole is not an S.I. unit, and the unit used here is the millimole.

o. Volumes per cent might be converted to a decimal fraction; however, this would not permit direct correlation with hemoglobin content, which is possible when oxygen content and capacity are expressed in molar quantities. One millimole of hemoglobin combines with 4 millimoles of oxygen.

p. Hydrogen ion concentration in S.I. units would be expressed in nanomoles per liter; however, this change has not received general approval. Conversion can be calculated as antilog (−pH).

q. Albumin is expressed in grams per liter to be consistent with units used for other proteins. Concentration of albumin may be expressed in mmol/l also, an expression that permits assessment of binding capacity of albumin for substances such as bilirubin. Molecular weight of albumin is 65,000.

r. Most techniques for quantitating triglycerides measure the glycerol moiety, and the total mass is calculated using an average molecular weight. The factor given assumes a mean molecular weight of 875 for triglycerides.

s. Calculated as norepinephrine, molecular weight 169.18.

t. Calculated as metanephrine, molecular weight 197.23.

u. Conversion factor calculated from molecular weights of estrone, estradiol, and estriol in proportions of 2:1:2.